Goodman & Gilman's

Manual *of* Pharmacology and Therapeutics

Goodman & Gilman's

Manual *of* Pharmacology and Therapeutics

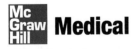 **Medical**

New York   Chicago   San Francisco   Lisbon   London   Madrid   Mexico City
Milan   New Delhi   San Juan   Seoul   Singapore   Sydney   Toronto

Goodman and Gilman's MANUAL OF PHARMACOLOGY AND THERAPEUTICS

Copyright © 2008 by The McGraw-Hill Companies, Inc. All rights reserved. Printed in the United States of America. Except as permitted under the United States Copyright Act of 1976, no part of this publication may be reproduced or distributed in any form or by any means, or stored in a data base or retrieval system, without the prior written permission of the publisher.

1 2 3 4 5 6 7 8 9 0   DOC/DOC   0 9 8 7

ISBN 978-0-07-144343-2
MHID 0-07-144343-6

This book was set in Times by International Typesetting and Composition.
The editors were James F. Shanahan and Christie Naglieri.
The production supervisor was Philip Galea.
Project management was provided by International Typesetting and Composition.
The cover designer was Janice Bielawa.
RR Donnelley was printer and binder.

This book is printed on acid-free paper.

Library of Congress Cataloging-in-Publication Data

Goodman and Gilman's manual of pharmacologyand therapeutics / [edited] by
    Laurence L. Brunton ... [et al.].
      p. ; cm.
    Companion v. to: Goodman & Gilman's the pharmacological basis of therapeutics. 11th ed. c2006.
    Includes index.
    ISBN-13: 978-0-07-144343-2 (pbk. : alk. paper)
    ISBN-10: 0-07-144343-6
    1. Pharmacology—Handbooks, manuals, etc. 2. Therapeutics—Handbooks, manuals, etc.
  I. Brunton, Laurence L. II. Goodman, Louis Sanford, 1906–2000
  III. Goodman & Gilman's the pharmacological basis of therapeutics.
  IV. Title: Manual of pharmacological therapeutics.
    [DNLM: 1. Pharmacology—Handbooks. 2. Drug Therapy—Handbooks.
  QV 39 G653   2007]
  RM301.12.G65   2007
  615′.1—dc22   2007014252

International Edition ISBN 978-0-07-110443-2
International MHID 0-07-110443-7

CONTENTS

v

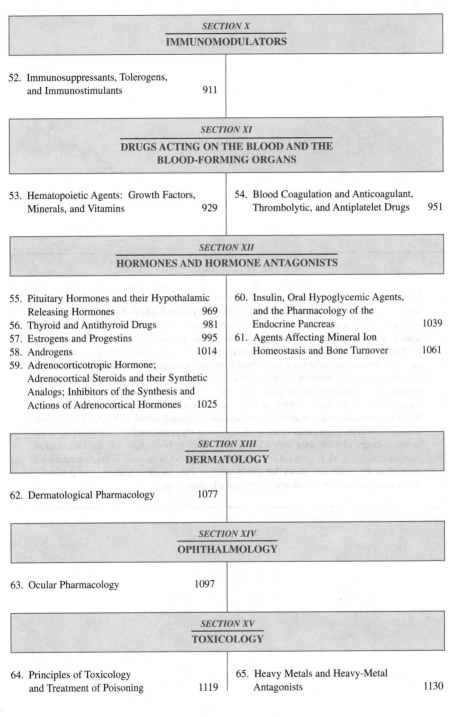

NOTICE

Medicine is an ever-changing science. As new research and clinical experience broaden our knowledge, changes in treatment and drug therapy are required. The authors and the publisher of this work have checked with sources believed to be reliable in their efforts to provide information that is complete and generally in accord with the standards accepted at the time of publication. However, in view of the possibility of human error or changes in medical sciences, neither the authors nor the publisher nor any other party who has been involved in the preparation or publication of this work warrants that the information contained herein is in every respect accurate or complete, and they disclaim all responsibility for any errors or omissions or for the results obtained from use of the information contained in this work. Readers are encouraged to confirm the information contained herein with other sources. For example and in particular, readers are advised to check the product information sheet included in the package of each drug they plan to administer to be certain that the information contained in this work is accurate and that changes have not been made in the recommended dose or in the contraindications for administration. This recommendation is of particular importance in connection with new or infrequently used drugs.

PREFACE

Perhaps there was once a time when most of pharmacological knowledge could fit into a relatively small volume, but that time has surely passed. Even as old knowledge has been pared, the addition of new knowledge has caused pharmacology textbooks to expand. Thanks to aggressive editing, the 11th edition of *Goodman & Gilman's The Pharmacological Basis of Therapeutics* is 5% shorter than its predecessor, yet the volume still weighs 4 kg. It's a wonderful book but clearly too heavy to carry around. Hence, this shorter, more portable version, *Goodman & Gilman's Manual of Pharmacology and Therapeutics*. The editors hope that this *Manual*, will affordably provide the essentials of medical pharmacology to a wide audience. The format of the parent text has been retained but the editors have tried to focus on core material, happy in the knowledge that the full text of the 11th edition, with its historical aspects, many chemical and clinical details, additional figures, and references, is available in print as well as online (at http://www.accessmedicine.com/), where updates are also published.

The editors of this volume thank the contributors and editors of the 11th edition of *Goodman & Gilman's*, which formed the basis of this manual. We are grateful to our editors at McGraw-Hill, James Shanahan and Christie Naglieri, to project manger Arushi Chawla, and to the long line of contributors and editors who have worked on *Goodman & Gilman's* since its original publication in 1941. It is a tribute to Alfred Gilman and Louis Goodman that their book is alive and vigorous after 66 years.

Laurence Brunton
San Diego, CA
July 1, 2007

1

PHARMACOKINETICS AND PHARMACODYNAMICS

The Dynamics of Drug Absorption, Distribution, Action, and Elimination

PHYSICOCHEMICAL FACTORS IN TRANSFER OF DRUGS ACROSS MEMBRANES

The absorption, distribution, metabolism, and excretion of a drug all involve its passage across cell membranes (Figure 1–1).

The plasma membrane consists of a bilayer of amphipathic lipids with their hydrocarbon chains oriented inward to the center of the bilayer to form a continuous hydrophobic phase and their hydrophilic heads oriented outward. Individual lipid molecules in the bilayer vary according to the particular membrane and can move laterally and organize themselves with cholesterol (e.g., sphingolipids), endowing the membrane with fluidity, flexibility, organization, electrical resistance, and relative impermeability to highly polar molecules. Membrane proteins embedded in the bilayer serve as receptors, ion channels, and transporters to transduce electrical or chemical signaling pathways; many of these proteins are targets for drugs. Cell membranes are relatively permeable to water and bulk flow of water can carry with it small drug molecules (<200 Da). Paracellular transport through intercellular gaps is sufficiently large that passage across most capillaries is limited by blood flow (e.g., glomerular filtration). Capillaries of the central nervous system (CNS) and a variety of epithelial tissues have tight intercellular junctions that limit paracellular transport.

PASSIVE MEMBRANE TRANSPORT

In passive transport, the drug molecule usually penetrates by diffusion along a concentration gradient by virtue of its solubility in the lipid bilayer. Such transfer is directly proportional to the magnitude of the concentration gradient across the membrane, to the lipid–water partition coefficient of the drug, and to the membrane surface area exposed to the drug. After a steady state is attained, the concentration of the unbound drug is the same on both sides of the membrane if the drug is a nonelectrolyte. For ionic compounds, the steady-state concentrations depend on the electrochemical gradient for the ion and on differences in pH across the membrane, which may influence the state of ionization of the molecule disparately on either side of the membrane.

WEAK ELECTROLYTES AND INFLUENCE OF pH Most drugs are weak acids or bases that are present in solution as both the lipid-soluble and diffusible nonionized form, and the relatively lipid-insoluble nondiffusible ionized species. Therefore, the transmembrane distribution of a weak electrolyte is determined by its pK_a (pH at which 50% is ionized) and the pH gradient across the membrane (*see* Figure 1–2). The ratio of nonionized to ionized drug at each pH is readily calculated from the Henderson–Hasselbalch equation:

$$\log \frac{[\text{Protonated form}]}{[\text{Unprotonated form}]} = pK_a - pH \qquad (1\text{–}1)$$

This equation relates the pH of the medium around the drug and the drug's acid dissociation constant (pK_a) to the ratio of the protonated (HA or BH^+) and unprotonated (A^- or B) forms, where $HA \rightarrow A^- + H^+$ ($K_a = [A^-][H^+]/[HA]$) describes the dissociation of an acid, and $BH^+ \rightarrow B + H^+$ ($K_a = [B][H^+]/[BH^+]$) describes the dissociation of the pronated form of a base. At steady state, an acidic drug will accumulate on the more basic side of the membrane and a basic drug on the more acidic side—a phenomenon termed *ion trapping*.

DRUG ABSORPTION, BIOAVAILABILITY, AND ROUTES OF ADMINISTRATION

Absorption is the movement of a drug from its site of administration into the central compartment (Figure 1–1) and the extent to which this occurs. For solid dosage forms, absorption first

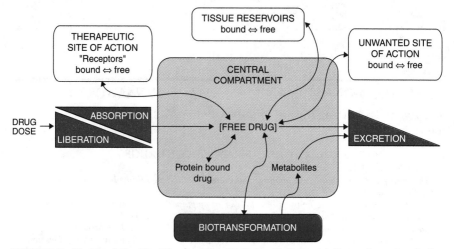

FIGURE 1–1 *The interrelationship of the absorption, distribution, binding, metabolism, and excretion of a drug and its concentration at its sites of action.* Possible distribution and binding of metabolites in relation to their potential actions at receptors are not depicted.

requires dissolution of the tablet or capsule, thus liberating the drug to be absorbed into the local circulation from which it will distribute to its sites of action. *Bioavailability* indicates the fractional extent to which a dose of drug reaches its site of action, taking into account, for example, the effects of hepatic metabolism and biliary excretion that may occur before a drug taken orally enters the systemic circulation. If hepatic elimination of the drug is large, bioavailability will be reduced substantially (the *first-pass effect*). This decrease in availability is a function of the anatomical site from which absorption takes place; other anatomical, physiological, and pathological factors can influence bioavailability (*see* below), and the choice of the route of drug administration must be based on an understanding of these conditions.

ORAL INGESTION

Absorption from the gastrointestinal (GI) tract is governed by factors such as surface area for absorption, blood flow to the site of absorption, the physical state of the drug (solution, suspension, or solid dosage form), its water solubility, and concentration at the site of absorption. For

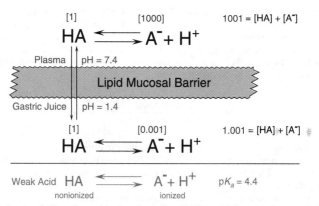

FIGURE 1–2 *Influence of pH on the partitioning of a weak acid (pK$_a$ = 4.4) between plasma (pH = 7.4) and gastric juice (pH = 1.4) separated by a lipid barrier.* The gastric mucosal membrane behaves as a lipid barrier permeable only to the lipid-soluble, nonionized form of the acid. The ratio of nonionized to ionized drug at each pH is readily calculated from the Henderson–Hasselbalch equation that relates the pH of the medium and the drug's dissociation constant (pK$_a$) to the ratio of the protonated (HA) and unprotonated (A$^-$) forms. The same principles apply to drugs that are weak bases (BH$^+$ ↔ B + H$^+$).

drugs given in solid form, the rate of dissolution may be the limiting factor in their absorption. Since most drug absorption from the GI tract occurs by passive diffusion, absorption is favored when the drug is in the nonionized and more lipophilic form. The epithelium of the stomach is lined with a thick mucous layer, and its surface area is small; by contrast, the villi of the upper intestine provide an extremely large surface area (~200 m²). *Accordingly, the rate of absorption of a drug from the intestine will be greater than that from the stomach even if the drug is predominantly ionized in the intestine and largely nonionized in the stomach. Thus, any factor that accelerates gastric emptying will be likely to increase the rate of drug absorption, whereas any factor that delays gastric emptying is expected to have the opposite effect. Gastric emptying is highly variable and influenced by numerous factors.*

Drugs that are destroyed by gastric secretions or that cause gastric irritation sometimes are administered in dosage forms with an enteric coating that prevents dissolution in the acidic gastric contents. The use of enteric coatings is helpful for drugs such as aspirin *that can cause significant gastric irritation.*

Controlled-Release Preparations

A slow rate of dissolution of a drug in GI fluids is the basis for controlled-release, extended-release, sustained-release, *and* prolonged-action *preparations that are designed to produce slow, uniform absorption of the drug for 8 hours or longer. Such preparations are offered for medications in all major drug categories. Potential advantages are reduction in the frequency of administration of the drug as compared with conventional dosage forms (possibly with improved compliance by the patient), maintenance of a therapeutic effect overnight, and decreased incidence and/or intensity of both undesired effects (by elimination of the peaks in drug concentration) and nontherapeutic blood levels of the drug (by elimination of troughs in concentration) that occur after administration of immediate-release dosage forms. Controlled-release dosage forms, while more expensive, are most appropriate for drugs with short $t_{1/2}$ (<4 hours) where patient non-compliance becomes a determinant of therapeutic failure.*

SUBLINGUAL ADMINISTRATION

Venous drainage from the mouth is to the superior vena cava, which protects highly soluble drugs like nitroglycerin *from rapid hepatic first-pass metabolism. If a tablet of nitroglycerin were swallowed, the accompanying hepatic metabolism would be sufficient to prevent the appearance of any active nitroglycerin in the systemic circulation.*

TRANSDERMAL ABSORPTION

Absorption of drugs able to penetrate the intact skin is dependent on the surface area over which they are applied and their lipid solubility (see Chapter 63*). The dermis is freely permeable to many solutes; consequently, systemic absorption of drugs occurs much more readily through inflamed, abraded, burned, or denuded skin. Unwanted effects can be produced by absorption through the skin of highly lipid-soluble substances (e.g., a lipid-soluble insecticide in an organic solvent). Transdermal absorption can be enhanced by suspending the drug in an oily vehicle and rubbing the resulting preparation into the skin. Hydration of the skin with an occlusive dressing may facilitate absorption.*

RECTAL ADMINISTRATION

The rectal route, though less predictable, can be used when oral ingestion is precluded because the patient is unconscious or when vomiting is present. Approximately 50% of the drug that is absorbed from the rectum will bypass the liver, thus reducing the hepatic first-pass effect.

PARENTERAL INJECTION

Intravenous

Factors relevant to absorption are circumvented by intravenous injection of drugs because bioavailability is rapid and complete. Also, drug delivery is controlled, can be adjusted to the response of the patient and is achieved with an accuracy and immediacy not possible by any other procedure. Irritating solutions can be given only in this manner because the drug, if injected slowly, is greatly diluted by the blood. Occasionally, a drug is injected directly into an artery to localize its effect. Diagnostic agents sometimes are administered by this route (e.g., technetium-labeled human serum albumin).

Unfavorable reactions can occur when transiently high concentrations of a drug or its vehicle are attained rapidly in plasma and tissues. There are therapeutic circumstances where it is advisable to administer a drug by bolus injection (e.g., tissue plasminogen activator) *and other circumstances where slower administration of drug is advisable (e.g.,* antibiotics).*

Subcutaneous

Injection of a drug into a subcutaneous site can be used only for drugs that are not irritating to tissue; otherwise, severe pain, necrosis, and tissue sloughing may occur. The rate of absorption following subcutaneous injection of a drug often is sufficiently constant and slow to provide a prolonged effect. Moreover, altering the period over which a drug is absorbed may be varied intentionally, as is accomplished with insulin for injection using particle size, protein complexation, and pH. Absorption of drugs implanted under the skin in a solid pellet form occurs slowly over a period of weeks or months; some hormones (e.g., contraceptives) are administered effectively in this manner.

Intramuscular

Drugs in aqueous solution are absorbed rapidly after intramuscular injection depending on the rate of blood flow to the injection site and the fat versus muscular composition of the site. This may be modulated to some extent by local heating, massage, or exercise. Generally, the rate of absorption following injection of an aqueous preparation into the deltoid or vastus lateralis is faster than when the injection is made into the gluteus maximus. The rate is particularly slower for females after injection into the gluteus maximus. Slow, constant absorption from the intramuscular site results if the drug is injected in solution, oil, or various other repository (depot) vehicles.

Intrathecal

The blood–brain barrier and the blood–cerebrospinal fluid (CSF) barrier often preclude or slow the entrance of drugs into the CNS. Therefore, when local and rapid effects on the meninges or cerebrospinal axis are desired, drugs sometimes are injected directly into the spinal subarachnoid space. Brain tumors may be treated by direct intraventricular drug administration.

PULMONARY ABSORPTION

Gaseous and volatile drugs may be inhaled and absorbed through the pulmonary epithelium and mucous membranes of the respiratory tract. Access to the circulation is rapid by this route because the lung's surface area is large (~140 m^2) and first-pass metabolism is avoided. The principles governing absorption and excretion of anesthetic and other therapeutic gases are discussed in Chapters 13 and 15.

TOPICAL APPLICATION
Mucous Membranes

Drugs are applied to the mucous membranes of the conjunctiva, nasopharynx, oropharynx, vagina, colon, urethra, and urinary bladder primarily for their local effects.

Eye

Topically applied ophthalmic drugs are used for their local effects (see Chapter 63) requiring absorption of the drug through the cornea; corneal infection or trauma thus may result in more rapid absorption. Ophthalmic delivery systems that provide prolonged duration of action (e.g., suspensions and ointments) are useful, as are ocular inserts providing continuous delivery of drug.

BIOEQUIVALENCE

Drug products are considered to be pharmaceutical equivalents if they contain the same active ingredients and are identical in strength or concentration, dosage form, and route of administration. Two pharmaceutically equivalent drug products are considered to be bioequivalent when the rates and extents of bioavailability of the active ingredient in the two products are not significantly different under suitable test conditions.

DISTRIBUTION OF DRUGS

Following absorption or systemic administration into the bloodstream, a drug distributes into interstitial and intracellular fluids depending on the particular physicochemical properties of the drug. Cardiac output, regional blood flow, capillary permeability, and tissue volume determine the rate of delivery and potential amount of drug distributed into tissues. Initially, liver, kidney, brain, and other well-perfused organs receive most of the drug, whereas delivery to muscle, most viscera, skin, and fat is slower. This second distribution phase may require minutes to several hours before the concentration of drug in tissue is in equilibrium with that in blood. The second phase also involves a far larger fraction of body mass than does the initial phase and generally accounts for most of the extravascularly distributed drug. With exceptions such as the brain, diffusion of drug into the interstitial fluid occurs rapidly. Thus, tissue distribution is determined by the partitioning of drug between blood and the particular tissue.

PLASMA PROTEINS   Many drugs circulate in the bloodstream reversibly bound to plasma proteins. Albumin is a major carrier for acidic drugs; α_1-acid glycoprotein binds basic drugs. Nonspecific binding to other plasma proteins generally occurs to a much smaller extent. In addition, certain drugs may bind to proteins that function as specific hormone carrier proteins, such as the binding of *thyroid hormone* to thyroxin-binding globulin.

The fraction of total drug in plasma that is bound is determined by the drug concentration, the affinity of binding sites for the drug, and the number of binding sites. For most drugs, the therapeutic range of plasma concentrations is limited; thus the extent of binding and the unbound fraction are relatively constant. The extent of plasma protein binding may be affected by disease-related factors (*e.g.*, hypoalbuminemia). Conditions resulting in the acute-phase reaction response (*e.g.*, cancer, arthritis, myocardial infarction, and Crohn's disease) lead to elevated levels of α_1-acid glycoprotein and enhanced binding of basic drugs.

Many drugs with similar physicochemical characteristics can compete with each other and with endogenous substances for protein binding. Drug toxicities based on competition between drugs for binding sites is not of clinical concern for most therapeutic agents. Steady-state unbound concentrations of drug will change significantly only when either input (dosing rate) or clearance of unbound drug is changed [see Equation (1–2)]. Thus, steady-state unbound concentrations are independent of the extent of protein binding. However, for narrow-therapeutic-index drugs, a transient change in unbound concentrations occurring immediately following the dose of a competing drug could be of concern, such as with the anticoagulant warfarin.

Importantly, binding of a drug to plasma proteins limits its concentration in tissues and at its site of action because only unbound drug is in equilibrium across membranes. Accordingly, after distribution equilibrium is achieved, the concentration of active, unbound drug in intracellular water is the same as that in plasma except when carrier-mediated transport is involved. Binding of a drug to plasma protein also limits the drug's glomerular filtration because this process does not immediately change the concentration of free drug in the plasma (water is also filtered). Drug transport and metabolism also are limited by binding to plasma proteins, except when these are especially efficient, and drug clearance, calculated on the basis of unbound drug, exceeds organ plasma flow.

TISSUE BINDING   Many drugs accumulate in tissues at higher concentrations than those in the extracellular fluids and blood. Tissue binding of drugs usually occurs with cellular constituents such as proteins, phospholipids, or nuclear proteins and generally is reversible. A large fraction of drug in the body may be bound in this fashion and serve as a reservoir that prolongs drug action in that same tissue or at a distant site reached through the circulation. Such tissue binding and accumulation also can produce local toxicity.

Fat as a Reservoir

Many lipid-soluble drugs are stored by physical solution in the neutral fat. In obese persons, the fat content of the body may be as high as 50%, and even in lean individuals it constitutes 10% of body weight; hence, fat may serve as a reservoir for lipid-soluble drugs. Fat is a rather stable reservoir because it has a relatively low blood flow.

REDISTRIBUTION   Termination of drug effect after withdrawal of a drug may result from redistribution of the drug from its site of action into other tissues or sites. Redistribution is a factor primarily when a highly lipid-soluble drug that acts on the brain or cardiovascular system is administered rapidly by intravenous injection or by inhalation. The highly lipid-soluble drug reaches its maximal concentration in brain within seconds of its intravenous injection; the plasma concentration then falls as the drug diffuses into other tissues, such as muscle. The concentration of the drug in brain follows that of the plasma because there is little binding of the drug to brain constituents. Thus, the onset of action is rapid, and its termination is rapid, related directly to the concentration of drug in the brain.

CENTRAL NERVOUS SYSTEM AND CEREBROSPINAL FLUID   Brain capillary endothelial cells have continuous tight junctions; therefore, drug penetration into the brain depends on transcellular rather than paracellular transport. The unique characteristics of brain capillary endothelial cells and pericapillary glial cells constitute the blood–brain barrier. At the choroid plexus, a similar blood–CSF barrier is present based on epithelial tight junctions. The lipid solubility of the nonionized and unbound species of a drug is therefore an important determinant of its uptake by the brain; the more lipophilic a drug is, the more likely it is to cross the blood–brain barrier. Drugs may penetrate into the CNS by specific uptake transporters (Chapter 2).

PLACENTAL TRANSFER OF DRUGS The transfer of drugs across the placenta is of critical importance because drugs may cause anomalies in the developing fetus. Lipid solubility, extent of plasma binding, and degree of ionization of weak acids and bases are important general determinants in drug transfer across the placenta. The fetal plasma is slightly more acidic than that of the mother (pH 7.0–7.2 vs. 7.4), so that ion trapping of basic drugs occurs. The view that the placenta is an absolute barrier to drugs is, however, completely inaccurate, in part because a number of influx transporters are also present. The fetus is to some extent exposed to all drugs taken by the mother.

EXCRETION OF DRUGS

Drugs are eliminated from the body either unchanged by the process of excretion or converted to metabolites (see Chapters 2 and 3). Excretory organs, the lung excluded, eliminate polar compounds more efficiently than substances with high lipid solubility. Lipid-soluble drugs thus are not readily eliminated until they are metabolized to more polar compounds.

The kidney is the most important organ for excreting drugs and their metabolites. Substances excreted in the feces are principally unabsorbed orally ingested drugs or drug metabolites excreted either in the bile or secreted directly into the intestinal tract and not reabsorbed. Excretion of drugs in breast milk is important not because of the amounts eliminated, but because the excreted drugs will have unwanted pharmacological effects in the nursing infant. Excretion from the lung is important mainly for the elimination of anesthetic gases (see Chapter 13).

RENAL EXCRETION Excretion of drugs and metabolites in the urine involves three distinct processes: glomerular filtration, active tubular secretion, and passive tubular reabsorption. Changes in overall renal function generally affect all three processes to a similar extent. In neonates, renal function is low compared with body mass but matures rapidly within the first few months after birth. During adulthood, there is a slow decline in renal function, ~1% per year, so that in elderly patients a substantial degree of functional impairment may be present.

The amount of drug entering the tubular lumen by filtration depends on the glomerular filtration rate and the extent of plasma binding of the drug; only unbound drug is filtered. In the proximal renal tubule, active, carrier-mediated tubular secretion also may add drug to the tubular fluid. Transporters such as P-glycoprotein and the multidrug-resistance–associated protein type 2 (MRP2), localized in the apical brush-border membrane, are responsible for the secretion of amphipathic anions and conjugated metabolites (e.g., glucuronides, sulfates, and glutathione adducts), respectively (see Chapters 2 and 3). Adenosine triphosphate (ATP)-binding cassette (ABC) transporters that are more selective for organic cationic drugs are involved in the secretion of organic bases. Membrane transporters, mainly located in the distal renal tubule, also are responsible for any active reabsorption of drug from the tubular lumen back into the systemic circulation.

In the proximal and distal tubules, the nonionized forms of weak acids and bases undergo net passive reabsorption. The concentration gradient for back-diffusion is created by the reabsorption of water with Na^+ and other inorganic ions. Since the tubular cells are less permeable to the ionized forms of weak electrolytes, passive reabsorption of these substances depends on the pH. When the tubular urine is made more alkaline, weak acids are largely ionized and thus are excreted more rapidly and to a greater extent. When the tubular urine is made more acidic, the fraction of drug ionized is reduced, and excretion is likewise reduced. Alkalinization and acidification of the urine have the opposite effects on the excretion of weak bases. In the treatment of drug poisoning, the excretion of some drugs can be hastened by appropriate alkalinization or acidification of the urine (see Chapter 64).

METABOLISM OF DRUGS

Renal excretion of unchanged drug plays only a modest role in the overall elimination of most therapeutic agents because lipophilic compounds filtered through the glomerulus are largely reabsorbed into the systemic circulation during passage through the renal tubules. The metabolism of drugs and other xenobiotics into more hydrophilic metabolites is essential for their elimination from the body, as well as for termination of their biological and pharmacological activity. In general, biotransformation reactions generate more polar, inactive metabolites that are readily excreted from the body. However, in some cases, metabolites with potent biological activity or toxic properties are generated.

Drug metabolism or biotransformation reactions are classified as either phase 1 functionalization reactions or phase 2 biosynthetic (conjugation) reactions. The enzyme systems involved in the biotransformation of drugs are localized primarily in the liver, although every tissue examined has some metabolic activity (see *Chapter 3 for details of drug metabolism*).

CLINICAL PHARMACOKINETICS

Clinical pharmacokinetics relies on a relationship between the pharmacological effects of a drug and a measurable concentration of the drug (*e.g.*, in blood or plasma). For some drugs, no clear or simple relationship has been found between pharmacological effect and concentration in plasma, whereas for other drugs, routine measurement of drug concentration is impractical as part of therapeutic monitoring. In most cases, the concentration of drug at its sites of action will be related to the concentration of drug in the systemic circulation. The pharmacological effect that results may be the clinical effect desired, or an adverse or toxic effect. Clinical pharmacokinetics provides a framework within which drug dose adjustments can be made.

The physiological and pathophysiological variables that dictate adjustment of dosage in individual patients often do so as a result of modification of pharmacokinetic parameters. The four most important parameters governing drug disposition are *clearance*, a measure of the body's efficiency in eliminating drug; *volume of distribution*, a measure of the apparent space in the body available to contain the drug; *elimination* $t_{1/2}$, a measure of the rate of removal of drug from the body; and *bioavailability*, the fraction of drug absorbed as such into the systemic circulation.

Clearance

Clearance is the most important concept to consider when designing a rational regimen for long-term drug administration. The clinician usually wants to maintain steady-state concentrations of a drug within a *therapeutic window* associated with therapeutic efficacy and a minimum of toxicity for a given agent. Assuming complete bioavailability, the steady-state concentration of drug in the body will be achieved when the rate of drug elimination equals the rate of drug administration. Thus:

$$\text{Dosing rate} = CL \cdot C_{ss} \qquad (1-2)$$

where CL is clearance of drug from the systemic circulation and C_{ss} is the steady-state concentration of drug.

Metabolizing enzymes and transporters (see *Chapters 2 and 3*) *usually are not saturated, and thus the* absolute *rate of elimination of the drug is essentially a linear function (first-order) of its concentration in plasma, where a constant* fraction *of drug in the body is eliminated per unit of time. If mechanisms for elimination of a given drug become saturated, the kinetics approach zero order, in which a constant* amount *of drug is eliminated per unit of time. Clearance of a drug is its rate of elimination by all routes normalized to the concentration of drug in some biological fluid where measurement can be made:*

$$CL = \text{rate of elimination}/C \qquad (1-3)$$

Thus, when clearance is constant, the rate of drug elimination is directly proportional to drug concentration. Clearance is the volume of biological fluid such as blood or plasma from which drug would have to be completely removed to account for the clearance (e.g., ml/min/kg). Clearance can be defined further as blood clearance (CL_b), plasma clearance (CL_p), depending on the measurement made (C_b, C_p).

Clearance of drug by several organs is additive. Elimination of drug may occur as a result of processes that occur in the GI tract, kidney, liver, and other organs. Division of the rate of elimination by each organ by a concentration of drug (e.g., plasma concentration) will yield the respective clearance by that organ. Added together, these separate clearances will equal systemic clearance:

$$CL_{renal} + CL_{hepatic} + CL_{other} = CL \qquad (1-4)$$

Systemic clearance may be determined at steady state by using Equation (1–2). For a single dose of a drug with complete bioavailability and first-order kinetics of elimination, systemic clearance may be determined from mass balance and the integration of Equation (1–3) over time:

$$CL = \text{Dose}/AUC \qquad (1-5)$$

where AUC is the total area under the curve that describes the measured concentration of drug in the systemic circulation as a function of time (from zero to infinity) as in Figure 1–5.

HEPATIC CLEARANCE

For a drug that is removed efficiently from the blood by hepatic processes (metabolism and/or excretion of drug into the bile), the concentration of drug in the blood leaving the liver will be low, the extraction ratio will approach unity, and the clearance of the drug from blood will become limited by hepatic blood flow (e.g., drugs with systemic clearances >6 mL/min/kg).

RENAL CLEARANCE

Renal clearance of a drug results in its appearance in the urine. The rate of filtration of a drug depends on the volume of fluid that is filtered in the glomerulus and the unbound concentration of drug in plasma because drug bound to protein is not filtered. The rate of secretion of drug by the kidney will depend on the drug's intrinsic clearance by the transporters involved in active secretion as affected by the drug's binding to plasma proteins, the degree of saturation of these transporters, and the rate of delivery of the drug to the secretory site. In addition, processes involved in drug reabsorption from the tubular fluid must be considered. These factors are altered in renal disease.

DISTRIBUTION

VOLUME OF DISTRIBUTION   The volume of distribution (V) relates the amount of drug in the body to the concentration of drug (C) in the blood. This volume does not necessarily refer to an identifiable physiological volume but rather to the fluid volume that would be required to contain all the drug in the body at the same concentration measured in the blood:

$$\text{Amount of drug in body} / V = C, \text{ or } V = \text{amount of drug in body} / C \qquad (1-6)$$

A drug's volume of distribution therefore reflects the extent to which it is present in extravascular tissues and not in the plasma. The plasma volume of a typical 70-kg man is 3 L, blood volume is about 5.5 L, extracellular fluid volume outside the plasma is 12 L, and the volume of total-body water is approximately 42 L.

Many drugs exhibit volumes of distribution far in excess of these values (see Appendix II in the 11th edition of the parent text). For drugs that are bound extensively to plasma proteins but that are not bound to tissue components, the volume of distribution will approach that of the plasma volume because drug bound to plasma protein is measurable. In contrast, certain drugs have high volumes of distribution even though the drug in the circulation is bound to albumin because these drugs are also sequestered elsewhere.

The volume of distribution may vary widely depending on the relative degrees of binding to high-affinity receptor sites, plasma and tissue proteins, the partition coefficient of the drug in fat, and accumulation in poorly perfused tissues. The volume of distribution for a given drug can differ according to patient's age, gender, body composition, and presence of disease. Total-body water of infants younger than 1 year of age, for example, is 75–80% of body weight, whereas that of adult males is 60% and that of adult females is 55%.

The volume of distribution defined in Equation 1–6 considers the body as a single homogeneous compartment. In this one-compartment model, all drug administration occurs directly into the central compartment, and distribution of drug is instantaneous throughout the volume (V). Clearance of drug from this compartment occurs in a first-order fashion; i.e., the amount of drug eliminated per unit of time depends on the amount (concentration) of drug in the body compartment. Figure 1–3A and Equation 1–7 describe the decline of plasma concentration with time for a drug introduced into this central compartment:

$$C = (\text{dose}/V) \cdot \exp(-kt) \qquad (1-7)$$

where k is the rate constant for elimination that reflects the fraction of drug removed from the compartment per unit of time. This rate constant is inversely related to the $t_{1/2}$ of the drug ($k = 0.693/t_{1/2}$).

The idealized one-compartment model does not describe the entire time course of the plasma concentration. That is, certain tissue reservoirs can be distinguished from the central compartment, and the drug concentration appears to decay in a manner that can be described by multiple exponential terms (Figure 1–3B). Nevertheless, the one-compartment model is sufficient to apply to most clinical situations for most drugs and the drug $t_{1/2}$ in the central compartment dictates the dosing interval for the drug.

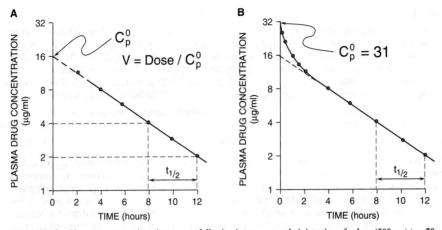

FIGURE 1–3 *Plasma concentration–time curves following intravenous administration of a drug (500 mg) to a 70-kg patient. A.* Drug concentrations are measured in plasma at 2-hour intervals following drug administration. The semilogarithmic plot of plasma concentration (C_p) *versus* time appears to indicate that the drug is eliminated from a single compartment by a first-order process (Equation 1–7) with a $t_{1/2}$ of 4 hours ($k = 0.693/t_{1/2} = 0.173$ hr^{-1}). The volume of distribution (V) may be determined from the value of C_p obtained by extrapolation to $t = 0$ ($C_p^0 = 16$ μg/mL). Volume of distribution (Equation 1–6) for the one-compartment model is 31.3 L, or 0.45 L/kg (V = dose/C_p^0). The clearance for this drug is 90 mL/min; for a one-compartment model, CL = kV. *B.* Sampling before 2 hours indicates that, in fact, the drug follows multiexponential kinetics. The terminal disposition half-life is 4 hours, clearance is 84 mL/min (Equation 1–5), V_{area} is 29 L (Equation 1–7), and V_{ss} is 26.8 L. The initial or "central" distribution volume for the drug ($V_1 = $ dose/C_p^0) is 16.1 L. The example chosen indicates that multicompartment kinetics may be overlooked when sampling at early times is neglected. In this particular case, there is only a 10% error in the estimate of clearance when the multicompartment characteristics are ignored. For many drugs, multicompartment kinetics may be observed for significant periods of time, and failure to consider the distribution phase can lead to significant errors in estimates of clearance and in predictions of the appropriate dosage. Also, the difference between the "central" distribution volume and other terms reflecting wider distribution is important in deciding a loading dose strategy. The multi-compartment model of drug disposition can be viewed as though the blood and highly perfused lean organs such as heart, brain, liver, lung, and kidneys cluster as a single central compartment, whereas more slowly perfused tissues such as muscle, skin, fat, and bone behave as the final compartment (*i.e.*, the tissue compartment). If the ratio of blood flow to various tissues changes within an individual or differs among individuals, rates of drug distribution to tissues will change. Changes in blood flow may cause some tissues that were originally in the "central" volume to equilibrate so slowly as to appear only in the "final" volume. This means that central volumes will appear to vary with disease states that cause altered regional blood flow (*e.g.*, liver cirrhosis). After an intravenous bolus dose, drug concentrations in plasma may be higher in individuals with poor perfusion (*e.g.*, shock). These higher systemic concentrations, in turn, may cause higher concentrations (and greater effects) in highly perfused tissues such as brain and heart. Thus, the effect of a drug at various sites of action can vary depending on perfusion of these sites.

Rate of Drug Distribution

In many cases, groups of tissues with similar perfusion–partition ratios all equilibrate at essentially the same rate such that only one apparent phase of distribution is seen (rapid initial fall of concentration of intravenously injected drug, as in Figure 1–3B). It is as though the drug starts in a "central" volume (Figure 1–1), which consists of plasma and tissue reservoirs that are in rapid equilibrium with it, and distributes to a "final" volume, at which point concentrations in plasma decrease in a log-linear fashion with a rate constant of k (Figure 1–3B).

The volume of distribution at steady state (V_{ss}) represents the volume in which a drug would appear to be distributed during steady state if the drug existed throughout that volume at the same concentration as that in the measured fluid (plasma or blood). V_{ss} also may be appreciated as shown in Equation (1–8), where V_C is the volume of distribution of drug in the central compartment and V_T is the volume term for drug in the tissue compartment:

$$V_{ss} = V_C + V_T \tag{1–8}$$

Half-Life

The $t_{1/2}$ is the time it takes for the plasma concentration or the amount of drug in the body to be reduced by 50%. For the simplest case, the one-compartment model (Figure 1–3A), $t_{1/2}$ may be determined readily by inspection and used to make decisions about drug dosage. However, drug concentrations in plasma often follow a multi-exponential pattern of decline (*see* Figure 1–3B); two or more $t_{1/2}$ terms thus may be calculated. Such prolonged half times can represent drug elimination from storage sites or poorly perfused tissue spaces and can be linked to drug toxicity.

A useful approximate relationship between the clinically relevant $t_{1/2}$, *clearance, and volume of distribution at steady state is given by*

$$t_{1/2} \cong 0.693 \cdot V_{ss}/CL \qquad (1-9)$$

As clearance of a drug decreases, owing to a disease process, for example, $t_{1/2}$ would be expected to increase as long as volume of distribution remains unchanged. However, increases in $t_{1/2}$ can result from changes in volume of distribution, *e.g.*, when changes in protein binding of a drug affect its clearance and lead to unpredictable changes in $t_{1/2}$. The $t_{1/2}$ provides a good indication of the time required to reach steady state after a dosage regimen is initiated or changed (*i.e.*, four half-lives to reach ~94% of a new steady state), the time for a drug to be removed from the body, and a means to estimate the appropriate dosing interval (*see* below).

STEADY STATE   Equation (1–2) indicates that a steady-state concentration eventually will be achieved when a drug is administered at a constant rate (Dosing rate = $CL \cdot C_{ss}$). At this point, drug elimination will equal the rate of drug availability. This concept also extends to regular intermittent dosage (*e.g.*, 250 mg of drug every 8 hours). During each interdose interval, the concentration of drug rises with absorption and falls by elimination. At steady state, the entire cycle is repeated identically in each interval (*see* Figure 1–4). Equation (1–2) still applies for intermittent dosing, but it now describes the average steady-state drug concentration (C_{ss}) during an interdose interval.

Extent and Rate of Bioavailability

BIOAVAILABILITY   It is important to distinguish between the rate and extent of drug absorption and the amount of drug that ultimately reaches the systemic circulation. This depends not only on the administered dose but also on the fraction of the dose (F) that is absorbed and escapes any first-pass elimination. This fraction is the drug's *bioavailability*.

If the hepatic blood clearance for the drug is large relative to hepatic blood flow, the extent of availability will be low when the drug is given orally (e.g., lidocaine or propranolol). *This reduction in availability is a function of the physiological site from which absorption takes place, and no modification of dosage form will improve the availability under conditions of linear kinetics. Incomplete absorption and/or intestinal metabolism following oral dosing will, in practice, reduce this predicted maximal value of F. When drugs are administered by a route that is subject to first-pass loss, the equations presented above that contain the terms* dose *or* dosing rate *also must include the bioavailability term F. For example, Equation (1–2) is modified to*

$$F \cdot \text{dosing rate} = CL \cdot C_{ss} \qquad (1-10)$$

where the value of F is between 0 and 1. The value of F varies widely for drugs administered by mouth and successful therapy can still be achieved for some drugs with F values as low as 0.03 (e.g., etidronate).

RATE OF ABSORPTION   Although the rate of drug absorption does not, in general, influence the average steady-state concentration of the drug in plasma, it may still influence drug therapy. If a drug is absorbed rapidly (*e.g.*, a dose given as an intravenous bolus) and has a small "central" volume, the concentration of drug initially will be high. It will then fall as the drug is distributed to its "final" (larger) volume (Figure 1–3B). If the same drug is absorbed more slowly (*e.g.*, by slow infusion), it will be distributed while it is being administered, and peak concentrations will be lower and will occur later. Controlled-release preparations are designed to provide a slow and sustained rate of absorption in order to produce smaller fluctuations in the plasma concentration–time profile during the dosage interval compared with more immediate-release formulations. Since the beneficial, nontoxic effects of drugs are based on knowledge of an ideal or desired plasma concentration range, maintaining that range while avoiding large swings between peak and trough concentrations can improve therapeutic outcome.

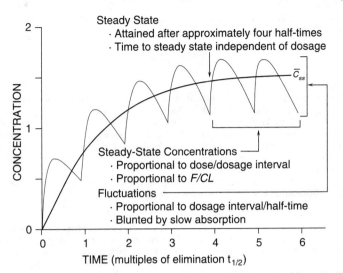

Steady State
· Attained after approximately four half-times
· Time to steady state independent of dosage

Steady-State Concentrations
· Proportional to dose/dosage interval
· Proportional to *F/CL*

Fluctuations
· Proportional to dosage interval/half-time
· Blunted by slow absorption

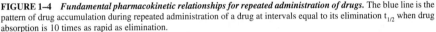

TIME (multiples of elimination $t_{1/2}$)

FIGURE 1–4 *Fundamental pharmacokinetic relationships for repeated administration of drugs.* The blue line is the pattern of drug accumulation during repeated administration of a drug at intervals equal to its elimination $t_{1/2}$ when drug absorption is 10 times as rapid as elimination.

As the rate of absorption increases, the concentration maxima approach 2 and the minima approach 1 during the steady state. The black line depicts the pattern during administration of equivalent dosage by continuous intravenous infusion. Curves are based on the one-compartment model. Average concentration ($\overline{C}_{ss}$) when the steady state is attained during intermittent drug administration is

$$\overline{C}_{ss} = \frac{F \cdot dose}{CL \cdot T}$$

where F is fractional bioavailability of the dose and T is dosage interval (time). By substitution of infusion rate for $F \cdot dose/T$, the formula is equivalent to Equation (1–2) and provides the concentration maintained at steady state during continuous intravenous infusion.

Nonlinear Pharmacokinetics

Nonlinearity in pharmacokinetics (i.e., changes in such parameters as clearance, volume of distribution, and $t_{1/2}$ as a function of dose or concentration of drug) usually is due to saturation of either protein binding, hepatic metabolism, or active renal transport of the drug.

SATURABLE PROTEIN BINDING

As the concentration of drug increases, the unbound fraction eventually also must increase (as all binding sites become saturated when drug concentrations in plasma are in the range of 10s to 100s of µg/mL). For a drug that is metabolized by the liver with a low intrinsic clearance–extraction ratio, saturation of plasma-protein binding will cause both V and CL to increase; $t_{1/2}$ thus may remain constant (Equation 1–9). For such a drug, C_{ss} will not increase linearly as the rate of drug administration is increased. For drugs that are cleared with high intrinsic clearance-extraction ratios, C_{ss} can remain linearly proportional to the rate of drug administration. In this case, hepatic clearance will not change, and the increase in V will increase the $t_{1/2}$ by reducing the fraction of the total drug in the body that is delivered to the liver per unit of time. Most drugs fall between these two extremes.

SATURABLE ELIMINATION

All active processes are undoubtedly saturable, but they will appear to be linear if values of drug concentrations encountered in practice are much less than K_m. When drug concentrations exceed K_m, nonlinear kinetics are observed. The major consequences of saturation of metabolism or transport are the opposite of those for saturation of protein binding. Saturation of metabolism or transport may decrease CL. Saturable metabolism causes oral first-pass metabolism to be less than *expected (higher F), and there is a greater fractional increase in C_{ss} than the corresponding fractional increase in the rate of drug administration.*

$$C_{ss} = \frac{\text{dosing rate} \cdot K_m}{v_m - \text{dosing rate}} \qquad (1\text{--}11)$$

As the dosing rate approaches the maximal elimination rate (v_m), the denominator approaches zero, and C_{ss} increases disproportionately. Because saturation of metabolism should have no effect on the volume of distribution, clearance and the relative rate of drug elimination decrease as the concentration increases; therefore, the log C_p time curve is concave-decreasing until metabolism becomes sufficiently desaturated and first-order elimination is present. Thus, the concept of a constant $t_{1/2}$ is not applicable to nonlinear metabolism occurring in the usual range of clinical concentrations. Consequently, changing the dosing rate for a drug with nonlinear metabolism is unpredictable because the resulting steady state is reached more slowly, and importantly, the effect is disproportionate to the alteration in the dosing rate.

Design and Optimization of Dosage Regimens

The intensity of a drug's effect is related to its concentration above a minimum effective concentration, whereas the duration of this effect reflects the length of time the drug level is above this value (Figure 1–5). These considerations, in general, apply to both desired and undesired

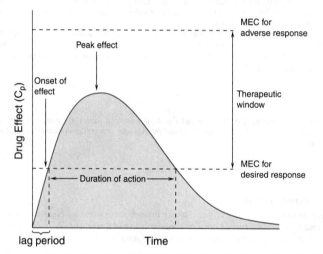

FIGURE 1–5 *Temporal characteristics of drug effect and relationship to the therapeutic window (e.g., single dose, oral administration).* A lag period is present before the plasma drug concentration (C_p) exceeds the minimum effective concentration (MEC) for the desired effect. Following onset of the response, the intensity of the effect increases as the drug continues to be absorbed and distributed. This reaches a peak, after which drug elimination results in a decline in C_p and in the effect's intensity. Effect disappears when the drug concentration falls below the MEC. Accordingly, the duration of a drug's action is determined by the time period over which concentrations exceed the MEC. An MEC exists for each adverse response, and if drug concentration exceeds this, toxicity will result. The therapeutic goal is to obtain and maintain concentrations within the therapeutic window for the desired response with a minimum of toxicity. Drug response below the MEC for the desired effect will be subtherapeutic; above the MEC for an adverse effect, the probability of toxicity will increase. Increasing or decreasing drug dosage shifts the response curve up or down the intensity scale and is used to modulate the drug's effect. Increasing the dose also prolongs a drug's duration of action but at the risk of increasing the likelihood of adverse effects. Unless the drug is nontoxic (e.g., penicillins), increasing the dose is not a useful strategy for extending the duration of action. Instead, another dose of drug should be given, timed to maintain concentrations within the therapeutic window. The area under the blood concentration-time curve (area under the curve, or AUC, shaded in gray) can be used to calculate the clearance (see Equation 1–5) for first-order elimination. The AUC is also used as a measure of bioavailability (defined as 100% for an intravenously administered drug). Bioavailability will be <100% for orally administered drugs, due mainly to incomplete absorption and first-pass metabolism and elimination. Thus, the therapeutic goal is to maintain steady-state drug levels within the therapeutic window. The application of pharmacokinetic monitoring to drug treatment in cases where the therapeutic index of a drug is narrow is beneficial since successful therapy is associated with a target blood level at steady-state.

(adverse) drug effects, and as a result, a therapeutic window *exists reflecting a concentration range that provides efficacy without unacceptable toxicity. Similar considerations apply after multiple dosing associated with long-term therapy, and they determine the amount and frequency of drug administration to achieve an optimal therapeutic effect. In general, the lower limit of the therapeutic range is approximately equal to the drug concentration that produces about half the greatest possible therapeutic effect, and the upper limit of the therapeutic range is such that no more than 5–10% of patients will experience a toxic effect. For some drugs, this may mean that the upper limit of the range is no more than twice the lower limit. Of course, these figures can be highly variable, and some patients may benefit greatly from drug concentrations that exceed the therapeutic range, whereas others may suffer significant toxicity at much lower values (e.g., digoxin).*

For a limited number of drugs, some effect of the drug is easily measured (e.g., blood pressure, blood glucose), and this can be used to optimize dosage using a trial-and-error approach. Even in an ideal case, certain quantitative issues arise, such as how often to change dosage and by how much. These usually can be settled with simple rules of thumb based on the principles discussed (e.g., change dosage by no more than 50% and no more often than every three to four half-lives). Alternatively, some drugs have very little dose-related toxicity, and maximum efficacy usually is desired. For these drugs, doses well in excess of the average required will ensure efficacy (if this is possible) and prolong drug action. Such a "maximal dose" strategy typically is used for penicillins.

For many drugs, however, the effects are difficult to measure (or the drug is given for prophylaxis), toxicity and lack of efficacy are potential dangers, or the therapeutic index is narrow. In these circumstances, doses must be titrated carefully, and drug dosage is limited by toxicity rather than efficacy.

MAINTENANCE DOSE

In most clinical situations, drugs are administered in a series of repetitive doses or as a continuous infusion to maintain a steady-state concentration of drug associated with the therapeutic window. Calculation of the appropriate maintenance dosage is a primary goal. To maintain the chosen steady-state or target concentration, the rate of drug administration is adjusted such that the rate of input equals the rate of loss. This relationship is expressed here in terms of the desired target concentration:

$$\text{Dosing rate} = \text{target } C_p \cdot CL/F \tag{1-12}$$

If the clinician chooses the desired concentration of drug in plasma and knows the clearance and bioavailability for that drug in a particular patient, the appropriate dose and dosing interval can be calculated.

Dosing Interval for Intermittent Dosage

In general, marked fluctuations in drug concentrations between doses are not desirable. If absorption and distribution were instantaneous, fluctuations in drug concentrations between doses would be governed entirely by the drug's elimination $t_{1/2}$. If the dosing interval T were chosen to be equal to the $t_{1/2}$, then the total fluctuation would be twofold; this is often a tolerable variation.

Pharmacodynamic considerations modify this. For drugs with a narrow therapeutic range, it may be important to estimate the maximal and minimal concentrations that will occur for a particular dosing interval. The minimal steady-state concentration $C_{ss,min}$ may be reasonably determined by the use of Equation (1–13):

$$C_{ss,\,min} = \frac{F \cdot \text{dose} / V_{ss}}{1 - \exp(-kT)} \cdot \exp(-kT) \tag{1-13}$$

where k equals 0.693 divided by the clinically relevant plasma $t_{1/2}$ and T is the dosing interval. The term exp(–kT) is, in fact, the fraction of the last dose (corrected for bioavailability) that remains in the body at the end of a dosing interval.

LOADING DOSE

A loading dose *is one dose or a series of doses given at the onset of therapy with the aim of achieving the target concentration rapidly. The appropriate magnitude for the loading dose is:*

$$\text{Loading dose} = \text{target } C_p \cdot V_{ss}/F \tag{1-14}$$

A loading dose may be desirable if the time required to attain steady state (and efficacy) by the administration of drug at a constant rate (four half-lives) is long relative to the demands of the condition being treated as is the case with the treatment of arrhythmias or cardiac failure.

The use of a loading dose also has significant disadvantages. The patient may be exposed abruptly to a toxic concentration of a drug that may take a long time to fall (i.e., long $t_{1/2}$). Loading doses tend to be large, and they are often given parenterally and rapidly; this can be particularly dangerous if toxic effects occur as a result of actions of the drug at sites that are in rapid equilibrium with the high concentration in plasma. It is therefore usually advisable to divide the loading dose into a number of smaller fractional doses administered over time, or to administer the loading dose as a continuous intravenous infusion over a period of time using computerized infusion pumps.

Therapeutic Drug Monitoring

The major use of measured concentrations of drugs (at steady state) is to refine the estimate of CL/F for the patient being treated [using Equation (1–10) as rearranged below]:

$$CL/F(\text{patient}) = \text{dosing rate}/C_{ss}(\text{measured}) \qquad (1\text{–}15)$$

The new estimate of CL/F can be used in Equation (1–12) to adjust the maintenance dose to achieve the desired target concentration.

PHARMACODYNAMICS

MECHANISMS OF DRUG ACTION AND THE RELATIONSHIP BETWEEN DRUG CONCENTRATION AND EFFECT

Pharmacodynamics—the study of the biochemical and physiological effects of drugs and their mechanisms of action—can provide the basis for the rational therapeutic use of a drug and the design of new and superior therapeutic agents.

Mechanisms of Drug Action

The effects of most drugs result from their interaction with macromolecular components of the organism. These interactions alter the function of the pertinent component and thereby initiate the biochemical and physiological changes that are characteristic of the response to the drug. The term *receptor* denotes the component of the organism with which the drug is presumed to interact.

Drug Receptors

Quantitatively proteins form the most important class of drug receptors. Examples include the receptors for hormones, growth factors, transcription factors, and neurotransmitters; the enzymes of crucial metabolic or regulatory pathways (*e.g.*, dihydrofolate reductase, acetylcholinesterase, and cyclic nucleotide phosphodiesterases); proteins involved in transport processes (*e.g.*, Na^+,K^+-ATPase); secreted glycoproteins (*e.g.*, Wnts); and structural proteins (*e.g.*, tubulin). Specific binding properties of other cellular constituents also can be exploited for therapeutic purpose. Thus, nucleic acids are important drug receptors, particularly for cancer chemotherapeutic agents.

A particularly important group of drug receptors consists of proteins that normally serve as receptors for endogenous regulatory ligands. Many drugs act on such physiological receptors and often are particularly selective because physiological receptors are specialized to recognize and respond to individual signaling molecules with great selectivity. Drugs that bind to physiological receptors and mimic the regulatory effects of the endogenous signaling compounds are termed *agonists*. Other drugs, termed *antagonists,* bind to receptors without regulatory effect, but their binding, blocks the binding of the endogenous agonist. Agents that are only partly as effective as agonists no matter the dose employed are termed *partial agonists*; those that stabilize the receptor in its inactive conformation are termed *inverse agonists* (Figure 1–6).

The strength of the reversible interaction between a drug and its receptor, as measured by their dissociation constant, is defined as the *affinity* of one for the other. Both the affinity of a drug for its receptor and its intrinsic activity are determined by its chemical structure.

CELLULAR SITES OF DRUG ACTION   Drugs act by altering the activities of their receptors. The sites at which drugs act and the extent of this action are determined by the location and functional capacity of receptors. Selective localization of drug action within an organism therefore

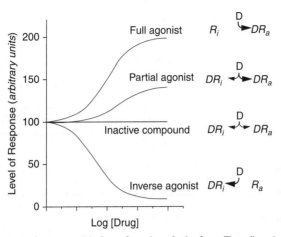

FIGURE 1-6 *Regulation of receptor activity by conformation-selective drugs.* The ordinate is some activity of the receptor produced by R_a, the active receptor conformation (*e.g.*, stimulation of adenylyl cyclase). If a drug D selectively binds to R_a, it will produce a maximal response. If D has equal affinity for R_i and R_a, it will not perturb the equilibrium between them and will have no effect on net activity; D would appear as an inactive compound. If the drug selectively binds to R_i, then the net amount of R_a will be diminished. If D can bind to receptor in an active conformation R_a but also bind to inactive receptor R_i with lower affinity, the drug will produce a partial response; D will be a partial agonist. If there is sufficient R_a to produce an elevated basal response in the absence of ligand (agonist-independent constitutive activity), then a drug binding to R_i will reduce activity; D will be an inverse agonist. Inverse agonists selectively bind to the inactive form of the receptor and shift the conformational equilibrium toward the inactive state. In systems that are without not constitutive activity, inverse agonists will behave like competitive antagonists. Receptors that have constitutive activity and are sensitive to inverse agonists include benzodiazepine, histamine, opioid, cannabinoid, dopamine, β adrenergic, calcitonin, bradykinin, and adenosine receptors.

does not necessarily depend on selective distribution of the drug. If a drug acts on a receptor that serves functions common to most cells, its effects will be widespread. If the function is a vital one, the drug may be particularly difficult or dangerous to use. Nevertheless, such a drug may be important clinically.

If a drug interacts with receptors that are unique to only a few types of differentiated cells, its effects are more specific. Hypothetically, the ideal drug would cause its therapeutic effect by such a discrete action. Side effects would be minimized, but toxicity might not be. If the differentiated function were a vital one, this type of drug also could be very dangerous. Even if the primary action of a drug is localized, the consequent physiological effects of the drug may be widespread.

Receptors for Physiological Regulatory Molecules

Postulating two functions of a receptor, ligand binding and message propagation (*i.e.*, signaling), suggests the existence of functional domains within the receptor: a *ligand-binding domain* and an *effector domain*. The structure and function of these domains often can be deduced from high-resolution structures of receptor proteins and by analysis of the behavior of intentionally mutated receptors.

The regulatory actions of a receptor may be exerted directly on its cellular target(s), *effector protein(s)*, or may be conveyed by intermediary cellular signaling molecules called *transducers*. The receptor, its cellular target, and any intermediary molecules are referred to as a *receptor–effector system* or *signal-transduction pathway*. Frequently, the proximal cellular effector protein is not the ultimate physiological target but rather is an enzyme or transport protein that creates, moves, or degrades a small metabolite (*e.g.*, a cyclic nucleotide or inositol trisphosphate) or ion (*e.g.*, Ca^{2+}) known as a *second messenger*. Second messengers can diffuse in the proximity of their binding sites and convey information to a variety of targets, which can respond simultaneously to the output of a single receptor binding a single agonist molecule. Even though these second messengers originally were thought of as freely diffusible molecules within the cell, their diffusion and their intracellular actions are constrained by compartmentation—selective localization of receptor–transducer–effector–signal termination complexes—established *via* protein–lipid and protein–protein interactions.

Receptors and their associated effector and transducer proteins also act as integrators of information as they coordinate signals from multiple ligands with each other and with the metabolic activities of the cell. An important property of physiological receptors that also makes them excellent targets for drugs is that they act catalytically. The catalytic nature of receptors is obvious when the receptor itself is an enzyme, but all known physiological receptors are formally catalysts. When, for example, a single agonist molecule binds to a receptor that is an ion channel, hundreds of thousands to millions of ions flow through the channel every second. Similarly, a single steroid hormone molecule binds to its receptor and initiates the transcription of many copies of specific mRNAs, which, in turn, can give rise to multiple copies of a single protein.

PHYSIOLOGICAL RECEPTORS: STRUCTURAL AND FUNCTIONAL FAMILIES

Receptors for physiological regulatory molecules can be assigned to a relatively few functional families whose members share both common mechanisms of action and similar molecular structures (Figure 1–7). For each receptor superfamily, there is now a context for understanding the structures of ligand-binding domains and effector domains and how agonist binding influences the regulatory activity of the receptor. The relatively small number of biochemical mechanisms and structural formats used for cellular signaling is fundamental to the ways in which target cells integrate signals from multiple receptors to produce additive, sequential, synergistic, or mutually inhibitory responses.

Receptors as Enzymes: Receptor Protein Kinases and Guanylyl Cyclases

A large group of receptors with intrinsic enzymatic activity consists of cell surface protein kinases, which exert their regulatory effects by phosphorylating diverse effector proteins at the inner face of the plasma membrane. Protein phosphorylation is a common mechanism for altering the biochemical activities of an effector or its interactions with other proteins. Most receptors that are protein kinases phosphorylate tyrosine residues in their substrates. A few receptor protein kinases phosphorylate serine or threonine residues. The most structurally simple receptor protein kinases are composed of an agonist-binding domain on the extracellular surface of the plasma membrane, a single membrane-spanning element, and a protein kinase domain on the inner membrane face. Many variations on this basic architecture exist, including assembly of multiple subunits in the mature receptor, obligate oligomerization of the liganded receptor, and the addition of multiple regulatory or protein-binding domains to the intracellular protein kinase domain that permit association of the liganded receptor with additional effector molecules and with substrates.

Another family of receptors, protein kinase–associated receptors, lack the intracellular enzymatic domains but, in response to agonists, bind or activate distinct protein kinases on the cytoplasmic face of the plasma membrane.

For the receptors that bind atrial natriuretic peptides and the peptides guanylin and uroguanylin, the intracellular domain is not a protein kinase but rather a guanylyl cyclase that synthesizes the second messenger cyclic guanosine monophosphate (cyclic GMP), which activates a cyclic GMP–dependent protein kinase (PKG) and can modulate the activities of several cyclic nucleotide phosphodiesterases, among other effectors.

Protease-Activated Receptor Signaling

Proteases that are anchored to the plasma membrane or that are soluble in the extracellular fluid (e.g., thrombin) can cleave ligands or receptors at the surface of cells to either initiate or terminate signal transduction. Peptide agonists often are processed by proteolysis to become active at their receptors. Targeting the proteolytic regulation of receptor mechanisms has produced successful therapeutic strategies, such as the use of angiotensin-converting enzyme (ACE) inhibitors in the treatment of hypertension (see Chapters 30 and 32) and the generation of new anticoagulants targeting the action of thrombin (see Chapter 54).

Ion Channels

Receptors for several neurotransmitters form agonist-regulated ion-selective channels in the plasma membrane, termed ligand-gated ion channels *or* receptor operated channels, *that convey their signals by altering the cell's membrane potential or ionic composition. This group includes the nicotinic cholinergic receptor, the γ-aminobutyric acid A (GABA$_A$) receptor, and receptors for glutamate, aspartate, and glycine (see Chapters 9, 12, and 16). They are all multisubunit proteins, with each subunit predicted to span the plasma membrane several times. Symmetrical association of the subunits allows each to form a segment of the channel wall, or pore, and to cooperatively*

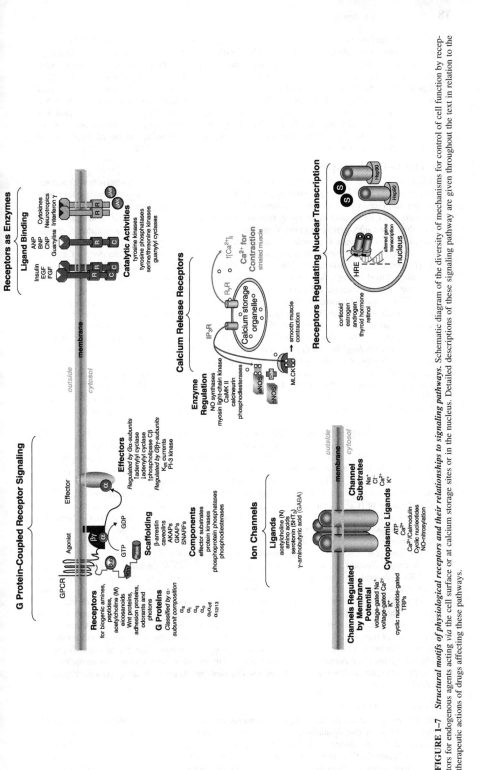

FIGURE 1–7 *Structural motifs of physiological receptors and their relationships to signaling pathways.* Schematic diagram of the diversity of mechanisms for control of cell function by receptors for endogenous agents acting *via* the cell surface or at calcium storage sites or in the nucleus. Detailed descriptions of these signaling pathway are given throughout the text in relation to the therapeutic actions of drugs affecting these pathways.

17

control channel opening and closing. Agonist binding may occur on a particular subunit that may be represented more than once in the assembled multimer (e.g., the nicotinic acetylcholine receptor) or may be conferred by a separate single subunit of the assembled channel, as is the case with the sulfonylurea receptor (SUR) that associates with a K^+ channel ($Kir_{6.2}$) to regulate the ATP-dependent K^+ channel (K_{ATP}) (see Chapter 60). Openers of the same channel (minoxidil) are used as vascular smooth muscle relaxants. Receptor-operated channels also are regulated by other receptor-mediated events, such as protein kinase activation following activation of G protein–coupled receptors (GPCRs) (see below). Phosphorylation of the channel protein on one or more of its subunits can confer both activation and inactivation depending on the channel and the nature of the phosphorylation.

G Protein–Coupled Receptors

A large superfamily of receptors that accounts for many known drug targets interacts with distinct heterotrimeric GTP-binding regulatory proteins known as G proteins. G proteins are signal transducers that convey information (i.e., agonist binding) from the receptor to one or more effector proteins. GPCRs include those for a number of biogenic amines, eicosanoids and other lipid-signaling molecules, peptide hormones, opioids, amino acids such as GABA, and many other peptide and protein ligands. G protein–regulated effectors include enzymes such as adenylyl cyclase, phospholipase C, phosphodiesterases, and plasma membrane ion channels selective for Ca^{2+} and K^+ (Figure 1–7). Because of their number and physiological importance, GPCRs are the targets for many drugs; perhaps half of all nonantibiotic prescription drugs are directed toward these receptors that make up the third largest family of genes in humans.

GPCRs span the plasma membrane as a bundle of seven α-helices. G proteins, composed of a GTP-binding α subunit, which confers specific recognition by receptor and effector, and an associated dimer of β and γ subunits that can confer both membrane localization of the G protein (e.g., via myristoylation) and direct signaling such as activation of inward rectifier K^+ (GIRK) channels and binding sites for G protein receptor kinases (GRKs), bind to the cytoplasmic face of the receptors promoting the binding of GTP to the G protein α subunit. GTP activates the G protein and allows it, in turn, to activate the effector protein. The G protein remains active until it hydrolyzes the bound GTP to GDP. Activation of the G_α subunit by GTP allows it to regulate an effector protein and to drive the release of $G_{\beta\gamma}$ subunits, which can also regulate effectors (e.g., K^+ channels), and which ultimately reassociate with GDP-liganded G_α, returning the system to the basal state.

Central to the effect of many GPCRs is release of Ca^{2+} from intracellular stores. For example, α receptors for norepinephrine activate G_q specific for the activation of phospholipase C_β. Phospholipase C_β (PLC_β) is a membrane-bound enzyme that hydrolyzes a membrane phospholipid, phosphatidylinositol-4,5-bisphosphate, to generate inositol-1,4,5-trisphosphate (IP_3) and the lipid, diacylglycerol. IP_3 binds to receptors on Ca^{2+} release channels in the IP_3-sensitive Ca^{2+} stores of the endoplasmic reticulum, triggering the release of Ca^{2+} and rapidly raising $[Ca^{2+}]_i$. The elevation of $[Ca^{2+}]_i$ is transient owing to its avid reuptake into stores. Ca^{2+} can bind to and directly regulate ion channels (e.g., large conductance Ca^{2+}-activated K^+ channels). Ca^{2+} can also bind to calmodulin; the resulting Ca^{2+}–calmodulin complex then can modulate a variety of effectors, including ion channels (e.g., the small conductance Ca^{2+}-activated K^+ channels), and cellular enzymes (e.g., Ca^{2+}–calmodulin–dependent protein kinases and PDEs).

Receptor–ligand interactions alone do not regulate all GPCR signaling. It is now clear that GPCRs undergo both homo- and heterodimerization and possibly oligomerization. Heterodimerization can result in receptor units with altered pharmacology compared with either individual receptor. Evidence is emerging that dimerization of receptors may regulate the affinity and specificity of the complex for G protein and regulate the sensitivity of the receptor to phosphorylation by receptor kinases and the binding of arrestin, events important in termination of the action of agonists and removal of receptors from the cell surface. Dimerization also may permit binding of receptors to other regulatory proteins such as transcription factors. Thus, the receptor–G protein effector systems are complex networks of convergent and divergent interactions involving both receptor–receptor and receptor–G protein coupling that permits extraordinarily versatile regulation of cell function.

Transcription Factors

Receptors for steroid hormones, thyroid hormone, vitamin D, and the retinoids are soluble DNA-binding proteins that regulate the transcription of specific genes. These receptors act as both hetero- and homo-dimers with homologous cellular proteins, but may be regulated by higher-order oligomerization with other modulators, often bound to these modulatory proteins in the cytoplasm, retaining them in an inactive state. Regulatory sites in DNA where agonists bind are receptor-specific: the sequence of a "glucocorticoid-response element," with only slight variation, is associated with each glucocorticoid-response gene, whereas a "thyroid-response element" confers specificity of the actions of the thyroid hormone nuclear receptor.

CYTOPLASMIC SECOND MESSENGERS

Binding of an agonist to a receptor provides the first message in receptor signal transduction to effector to affect cell physiology. The first messenger promotes the cellular production or mobilization of a second messenger, which initiates cellular signaling through a specific biochemical pathway. Physiological signals are integrated within the cell as a result of interactions between and among second-messenger pathways. Compared with the number of receptors and cytosolic signaling proteins, there are relatively few recognized cytoplasmic second messengers. However, their synthesis or release and degradation or excretion reflects the activities of many pathways. Well-studied second messengers include cyclic AMP, cyclic GMP, cyclic ADP–ribose, Ca^{2+}, inositol phosphates, diacylglycerol, and nitric oxide (NO). Second messengers influence each other both directly, by altering the other's metabolism, and indirectly, by sharing intracellular targets. This pattern of regulatory pathways allows the cell to respond to agonists, singly or in combination, with an integrated array of cytoplasmic second messengers and responses.

Cyclic AMP

Cyclic AMP, the prototypical second messenger, is synthesized by adenylyl cyclase under the control of many GPCRs; stimulation is mediated by G_s; inhibition, by G_i. There are nine membrane-bound isoforms of adenylyl cyclase (AC). The membrane-bound ACs are 120 kDa glycoproteins with six membrane-spanning helices; and two large cytoplasmic domains. Membrane-bound ACs exhibit basal enzymatic activity that is modulated by binding of GTP-liganded α subunits of stimulatory and inhibitory G proteins (G_s and G_i). ACs are catalogued based on their structural homology and their distinct regulation by G protein α and $\beta\gamma$ subunits, Ca^{2+}, protein kinases, and the actions of the diterpene forskolin. Because each AC isoform has its own tissue distribution and regulatory properties, different cell types respond differently to similar stimuli.

The role of drugs interacting at GPCRs as agonists is to accelerate the exchange of GDP for GTP on the α subunits of these G proteins. Once activated by α_s-GTP, AC remains activated until α_s hydrolyzes the bound GTP to GDP, which returns the system to its ground state. A single AC activation produces many molecules of cyclic AMP, which, in turn, can activate PKA. Cyclic AMP is eliminated by a combination of hydrolysis, catalyzed by cyclic nucleotide phosphodiesterases, and extrusion by several plasma membrane transport proteins.

Phosphodiesterase

Phosphodiesterases (PDEs) are regulated by controlled transcription as well as by second messengers (cyclic nucleotides and Ca^{2+}) and interactions with other signaling proteins such as β-arrestin and protein kinases. PDEs are responsible for the hydrolysis of the cyclic $3',5'$-phosphodiester bond found in cyclic AMP and cyclic GMP. PDEs comprise a superfamily with 11 subfamilies distinguished on the basis of amino acid sequence, substrate specificity, pharmacological properties, and allosteric regulation. The substrate specificities of the PDEs include enzymes that are specific for cyclic AMP, cyclic GMP, and both. PDEs play a highly regulated role that is important in controlling the intracellular levels of cyclic AMP and cyclic GMP. The importance of the PDEs as regulators of signaling is evident from their development as drug targets in diseases such as asthma and chronic obstructive pulmonary disease, cardiovascular diseases such as heart failure and atherosclerotic peripheral arterial disease, neurological disorders, and erectile dysfunction.

Cyclic GMP

Cyclic GMP is generated by two distinct forms of guanylyl cyclase (GC). NO stimulates soluble guanylyl cyclase (sGC), and the natriuretic peptides, guanylins, and heat-stable Escherichia coli *enterotoxin stimulate members of the membrane-spanning GCs (e.g., particulate GC).*

Actions of Cyclic Nucleotides

In most cases, cyclic AMP functions by activating the isoforms of cyclic AMP–dependent protein kinase (PKA), and cyclic GMP activates a PKG. Recently, a number of additional actions of cyclic nucleotides have been described, all with pharmacological relevance.

Cyclic Nucleotide–Dependent Protein Kinases

PKA holoenzyme consists of two catalytic (C) subunits reversibly bound to a regulatory (R) subunit dimer. The holoenzyme is inactive. Binding of four cyclic AMP molecules, two to each R subunit, dissociates the holoenzyme, liberating two catalytically active C subunits that phosphorylate serine and threonine residues on specific substrate proteins.

PKA diversity lies in both its R and C subunits. Molecular cloning has revealed α and β isoforms of both the classically described PKA regulatory subunits (RI and RII), as well as three C subunit isoforms Cα, Cβ, and Cγ. The R subunits exhibit different binding affinities for cyclic AMP, giving rise to PKA holoenzymes with different thresholds for activation. In addition to differential expression of R and C isoforms in various cells and tissues, PKA function is modulated by subcellular localization mediated by A-kinase-anchoring proteins (AKAPs).

PKA can phosphorylate both final physiological targets (metabolic enzymes or transport proteins) and numerous protein kinases and other regulatory proteins in multiple signaling pathways. This latter group includes transcription factors that allow cyclic AMP to regulate gene expression in addition to more acute cellular events.

Cyclic GMP activates a protein kinase, PKG, that phosphorylates some of the same substrates as PKA and some that are PKG-specific. Unlike PKA, PKG does not disassociate upon binding cyclic GMP. PKG is known to exist in two homologous forms. PKGI, with an acetylated N terminus, is associated with the cytoplasm and known to exist in two isoforms (Iα and Iβ) that arise from alternate splicing. PKGII, with a myristylated N terminus, is membrane-associated and may be compartmented by PKG-anchoring proteins in a manner similar to that known for PKA. Pharmacologically important effects of elevated cyclic GMP include modulation of platelet activation and regulation of smooth muscle contraction.

Cyclic Nucleotide–Gated Channels

In addition to activating protein kinases, cyclic AMP and cyclic GMP also bind to and directly regulate the activity of plasma membrane cation channels referred to as cyclic nucleotide–gated (CNG) channels. CNG ion channels have been found in kidney, testis, heart, and the CNS. These channels open in response to direct binding of intracellular cyclic nucleotides and contribute to cellular control of the membrane potential and intracellular Ca^{2+} levels. The CNG ion channels are multisubunit pore-forming channels that share structural similarity with the voltage-gated K^+ channels.

Calcium

The entry of Ca^{2+} into the cytoplasm is mediated by diverse channels: Plasma membrane channels regulated by G proteins, membrane potential, K^+ or Ca^{2+} itself, and channels in specialized regions of endoplasmic reticulum that respond to IP_3 or, in excitable cells, to membrane depolarization and the state of the Ca^{2+} release channel and its Ca^{2+} stores in the sarcoplasmic reticulum. Ca^{2+} is removed both by extrusion ($Na^+–Ca^{2+}$ exchanger and Ca^{2+} ATPase) and by reuptake into the endoplasmic reticulum (SERCA pumps). Ca^{2+} propagates its signals through a much wider range of proteins than does cyclic AMP, including metabolic enzymes, protein kinases, and Ca^{2+}-binding regulatory proteins (e.g., calmodulin) that regulate still other ultimate and intermediary effectors that regulate cellular processes as diverse as exocytosis of neurotransmitters and muscle contraction. Drugs such as chlorpromazine (an antipsychotic agent) are calmodulin inhibitors.

Regulation of Receptors

Receptors not only initiate regulation of biochemical events and physiological function but also are themselves subject to many regulatory and homeostatic controls. These controls include regulation of the synthesis and degradation of the receptor by multiple mechanisms, covalent modification, association with other regulatory proteins, and/or relocalization within the cell. Transducer and effector proteins are regulated similarly. Modulating inputs may come from other receptors, directly or indirectly, and receptors are almost always subject to feedback regulation by their own signaling outputs.

Continued stimulation of cells with agonists generally results in a state of *desensitization* (also referred to as *adaptation, refractoriness,* or *down-regulation*) such that the effect that follows continued or subsequent exposure to the same concentration of drug is diminished. This phenomenon, called *tachyphylaxis,* occurs rapidly and is important therapeutically; an example is attenuated response to the repeated use of β receptor agonists as bronchodilators for the treatment of asthma (*see* Chapters 10 and 27).

Desensitization can result from temporary inaccessibility of the receptor to agonist or from fewer receptors synthesized and available at the cell surface (e.g., down-regulation of receptor number). Phosphorylation of the receptor by specific GPCR kinases (GRKs) plays a key role in triggering rapid desensitization. Phosphorylation of agonist-occupied GPCRs by GRKs facilitates the binding of cytosolic proteins termed arrestins to the receptor, resulting in the uncoupling of

G protein from the receptor. The β-arrestins recruit proteins such as PDE4 (which limits cyclic AMP signaling), and others such as clathrin and β₂-adaptin, promoting sequestration of receptor from the membrane (internalization) and providing a scaffold that permits additional signaling steps.

Predictably, supersensitivity to agonists also frequently follows chronic reduction of receptor stimulation. Such situations can result, for example, following withdrawal from prolonged receptor blockade (e.g., the long-term administration of β receptor antagonists such as propranolol (see Chapter 10) or in the case where chronic denervation of a preganglionic fiber induces an increase in neurotransmitter release per pulse, indicating postganglionic neuronal supersensitivity. Supersensitivity can be the result of tissue response to pathological conditions, such as it happens in cardiac ischemia and is due to synthesis and recruitment of new receptors to the surface of the myocyte.

DISEASES RESULTING FROM RECEPTOR MALFUNCTION   Alteration in receptors and their immediate signaling effectors can be the cause of disease. The loss of a receptor in a highly specialized signaling system may cause a relatively limited, if dramatic, phenotypic disorder (*e.g.,* deficiency of the androgen receptor and androgen insensitivity syndrome; *see* Chapter 58). Deficiencies in widely employed signaling pathways have broad effects, as are seen in myasthenia gravis and some forms of insulin-resistant diabetes mellitus, which result from autoimmune depletion of nicotinic cholinergic receptors (*see* Chapter 9) or insulin receptors (*see* Chapter 60), respectively.

The expression of aberrant or ectopic receptors, effectors, or coupling proteins potentially can lead to supersensitivity, subsensitivity, or other untoward responses. Among the most significant events is the appearance of aberrant receptors as products of oncogenes that transform otherwise normal cells into malignant cells. Virtually any type of signaling system may have oncogenic potential (Chapter 51).

SIGNIFICANCE OF RECEPTOR SUBTYPES

Molecular cloning has accelerated discovery of novel receptor subtypes, and their expression as recombinant proteins has facilitated discovery of subtype-selective drugs. Distinct but related receptors may, but may not, display distinctive patterns of selectivity among agonist or antagonist ligands. When selective ligands are not known, the receptors are more commonly referred to as isoforms rather than as subtypes. The distinction between classes and subtypes of receptors, however, often is arbitrary or historical. The α₁, α₂, and β receptors differ from each other both in ligand selectivity among drugs and in coupling to G proteins (G_q, G_i, and G_s, respectively), yet α and β are considered receptor classes and α₁ and α₂ are considered subtypes. The α_{1A}, α_{1B}, and α_{1C} receptor isoforms differ little in their biochemical properties, although their tissue distributions are distinct. The β₁, β₂, and β₃ adrenergic receptor subtypes exhibit both differences in tissue distribution and phosphorylation by either GRKs or PKA.

Pharmacological differences among receptor subtypes are exploited therapeutically through the development and use of receptor-selective drugs. Such drugs may be used to elicit different responses from a single tissue when receptor subtypes initiate different intracellular signals, or they may serve to differentially modulate different cells or tissues that express one or another receptor subtype. Increasing the selectivity of a drug among tissues or among responses elicited from a single tissue may determine whether the drug's therapeutic benefits outweigh its unwanted effects.

Actions of Drugs Not Mediated by Receptors

Some drug effects do not occur *via* macromolecular receptors, such as therapeutic neutralization of gastric acid by a base (antacid). Drugs such as *mannitol* act according to colligative properties, increasing the osmolarity of various body fluids and causing changes in the distribution of water to promote diuresis, catharsis, expansion of circulating volume in the vascular compartment, or reduction of cerebral edema (*see* Chapter 28). The introduction of cholesterol-binding agents orally (*e.g., cholestyramine resin*) can be used to decrease dietary cholesterol absorption.

QUANTITATION OF DRUG–RECEPTOR INTERACTIONS AND EFFECTS
Receptor Pharmacology

Receptor occupancy theory, in which it is assumed that response emanates from a receptor occupied by a drug, has its basis in the law of mass action. The basic currency of receptor pharmacology is the dose–response curve, a depiction of the observed effect of a drug as a function of its

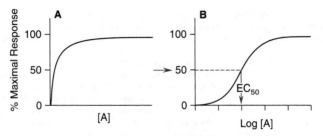

FIGURE 1-8   Graded respones expressed as a function of the concentration of drug A present at the receptor.
The hyperbolic shape of the curve in panel A becomes sigmoid when plotted semi-logarithmically, as in panel B. The concentration of drug that produces 50% of the maximal response quantifies drug activity and is referred to as the EC_{50} (effective concentration for 50% response). The range of concentrations needed to usefully depict the dose–response relationship (~3 $\log_{10}[10]$ units) is too wide to be useful in the linear format of Figure 1–8A; thus, most dose–response curves use log[D] on the abscissa (Figure 1–8B). Dose–response curves presented in this way are sigmoidal in shape and have three basic properties: threshold, slope, and maximal asymptote. These parameters characterize and quantitate the activity of the drug. The sigmoidal curve also depicts the law of mass action as expressed in Equation 1–16.

concentration in the receptor compartment. Figure 1–8A shows a typical dose–response curve; it reaches a maximal asymptotic value when the drug occupies all the receptor sites.

Some drugs cause low-dose stimulation and high-dose inhibition of response. These U-shaped relationships for some receptor systems are said to display hormesis. *Several drug–receptor systems can display this property (e.g., prostaglandins, endothelin, and purinergic and serotonergic agonists, among others), which is likely to be at the root of drug toxicity.*

Potency and Relative Efficacy

In general, the drug–receptor interaction is characterized first by binding of drug to receptor and second by generation of a response in a biological system. The first function is governed by the chemical property of *affinity,* ruled by the chemical forces that cause the drug to associate reversibly with the receptor.

$$D + R \overset{k_1}{\underset{k_2}{\rightleftarrows}} DR \rightarrow Response \tag{1-16}$$

This simple relationship, permits an appreciation of the reliance of the interaction of drug (D) with receptor (R) on both the forward or association rate (k_1) and the reverse or dissociation rate (k_2). At any given time, the concentration of agonist–receptor complex [DR] is equal to the product of k_1[D][R] minus the product k_2[DR]. At equilibrium (*i.e.*, when δ[DR]/$\delta\tau$ = 0), k_1[D][R] = k_2[DR]. The equilibrium dissociation constant (K_D) is then described by ratio of the off-rate and the on-rate (k_2/k_1).

$$\text{At equilibrium,} \quad K_D = \frac{[D][R]}{[DR]} = \frac{k_2}{k_1} \tag{1-17}$$

The affinity constant is the reciprocal of the equilibrium dissociation constant (affinity constant = $K_D = 1/K_A$). A high affinity means a small K_D. As a practical matter, the affinity of a drug is influenced most often by changes in its off-rate (k_2) rather than on its on-rate (k_1). Although a number of assumptions are made in this analysis, it is generally useful for considering the interactions of drugs with their receptors. Using this simple model of Equation 1–17 permits us to write an expression of the fractional occupancy (*f*) of receptors by agonist:

$$f = \frac{[\text{drug-receptor complexes}]}{[\text{total receptors}]} = \frac{[DR]}{[R] + [DR]} \tag{1-18}$$

This can be expressed in terms of K_A (or K_D) and [D]:

$$f = \frac{K_A[D]}{1+K_A[D]} = \frac{[D]}{[D]+K_D} \tag{1-19}$$

Thus, when $[D] = K_D$, a drug will occupy 50% of the receptors present. Potent drugs are those which elicit a response by binding to a critical number of a particular receptor type at low concentrations (high affinity) compared with other drugs acting on the same system and having lower affinity and thus requiring more drug to bind to the same number of receptors.

The generation of a response from the drug–receptor complex is governed by a property described as efficacy. Where agonism is the information encoded in a drug's chemical structure that causes the receptor to change conformation to produce a physiological or biochemical response when the drug is bound, efficacy *is that property* intrinsic *to a particular drug that determines how "good" an agonist the drug is. Historically, efficacy has been treated as a proportionality constant that quantifies the extent of functional change imparted to a receptor-mediated response system on binding a drug. Thus, a drug with high efficacy may be a full agonist eliciting, at some concentration, a full response, whereas a drug with a lower efficacy at the same receptor may not elicit a full response at any dose. When it is possible to describe the relative efficacy of drugs at a particular receptor, a drug with a low intrinsic efficacy will be a partial agonist.*

QUANTIFYING AGONISM   When the relative potency of two agonists of equal efficacy is measured in the same biological system, downstream signaling events are the same for both drugs, and the comparison yields a relative measure of the affinity and efficacy of the two agonists (Figure 1–9A). It is convenient to describe agonist response by determining the half-maximally effective concentration (EC_{50}) for producing a given effect. Thus, measuring agonist potency by comparison of EC_{50} values is one method of measuring the capability of different agonists to induce a response in a test system and for predicting comparable activity in another. Another method of estimating agonist activity is to compare maximal asymptotes in systems where the agonists do not produce maximal response (Figure 1–9B). The advantage of using maxima is that this property depends solely on efficacy, whereas potency is a mixed function of both affinity and efficacy.

QUANTIFYING ANTAGONISM   Characteristic patterns of antagonism are associated with certain mechanisms of blockade of receptors. One is straightforward *competitive antagonism*, whereby a drug that lacks intrinsic efficacy but retains affinity competes with the agonist for the binding site on the receptor. The characteristic pattern of such antagonism is the concentration-dependent production of a parallel shift to the right of the agonist dose–response curve with no change in the maximal response (Figure 1–10A). The magnitude of the rightward shift of the curve depends on the concentration of the antagonist and its affinity for the receptor.

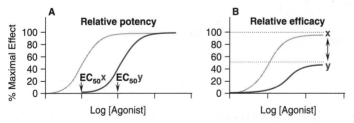

FIGURE 1–9 *Two ways of quantifying agonism. A.* The relative potency of two agonists (drug **x**, gray line; drug **y**, blue line) obtained in the same tissue is a function of their relative affinities and intrinsic efficacies. The half-maximal effect of drug **x** occurs at a concentration that is one-tenth the half-maximally effective concentration of drug **y**. Thus, drug **x** is more potent than drug **y**. *B.* In systems where the two drugs do not both produce the maximal response characteristic of the tissue, the observed maximal response is a nonlinear function of their relative intrinsic efficacies. Drug x is more efficacious than drug y; their asymptotic fractional responses are 100% (drug **x**) and 50% (drug **y**).

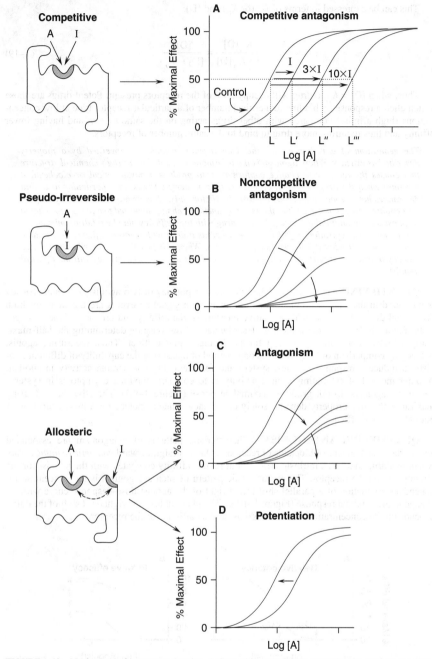

FIGURE 1–10 *Mechanisms of receptor antagonism.* **A.** Competitive antagonism occurs when the agonist A and antagonist I compete for the same binding site on the receptor. Response curves for the agonist are shifted to the right in a concentration-related manner by the antagonist such that the EC_{50} for the agonist increases (*e.g.,* L *versus* L′, L″, and L‴) with the concentration of the antagonist. **B.** If the antagonist binds to the same site as the agonist but does so irreversibly or pseudo-irreversibly (slow dissociation but no covalent bond), it causes a shift of the dose–response curve to the right, with further depression of the maximal response. Allosteric effects occur when the ligand I binds to a different site on the receptor to either inhibit response (*see* panel *C*) or potentiate response (*see* panel *D*). This effect is saturable; inhibition reaches a limiting value when the allosteric site is fully occupied.

A partial agonist similarly can compete with a "full" agonist for binding to the receptor. However, increasing concentrations of a partial agonist will inhibit response to a finite level characteristic of the drug's intrinsic efficacy; a competitive antagonist will reduce the response to zero. Partial agonists thus can be used therapeutically to buffer a response by inhibiting untoward stimulation without totally abolishing the stimulus from the receptor.

An antagonist may dissociate so slowly from the receptor as to be essentially irreversible in its action. Under these circumstances, the maximal response to the agonist will be depressed at some antagonist concentrations (Figure 1–10B). Operationally, this is referred to as *noncompetitive antagonism*, although the molecular mechanism of action really cannot be inferred unequivocally from the effect. An irreversible antagonist competing for the same binding site as the agonist also can produce the pattern of antagonism shown in Figure 1–10B.

Noncompetitive antagonism can be produced by another type of drug, referred to as an allosteric *antagonist. This type of drug produces its effect by binding a site on the receptor distinct from that of the primary agonist and thereby changing the affinity of the receptor for the agonist. In the case of an allosteric antagonist, the affinity of the receptor for the agonist is decreased by the antagonist (Figure 1–10C). In contrast, some allosteric effects could potentiate the effects of agonists (Figure 1–10D).*

For a complete Bibliographical listing see Goodman & Gilman's *The Pharmacological Basis of Therapeutics*, 11th ed., or Goodman & Gilman Online at www.accessmedicine.com.

2

MEMBRANE TRANSPORTERS AND DRUG RESPONSE

Transporters are membrane proteins that control the influx of essential nutrients and ions and the efflux of cellular waste, environmental toxins, and other xenobiotics. Approximately 6% of genes in the human genome encode transporters or transporter-related proteins. Drug-transporting proteins contribute to both therapeutic and adverse effects of drugs (Figure 2–1).

Two major superfamilies dominate the area of drug transporters: ATP-binding cassette (ABC) and solute carrier (SLC) transporters. Most ABC proteins are primary active transporters, which rely on adenosine triphosphate (ATP) hydrolysis to actively pump their substrates across membranes. The 49 known genes for ABC proteins are grouped into seven subclasses or families (ABCA to ABCG). Well known examples are P-glycoprotein (encoded by *ABCB1*) and the cystic fibrosis transmembrane regulator (CFTR, encoded by *ABCC7*). The SLC superfamily includes genes that encode facilitated transporters and ion-coupled secondary active transporters, 43 SLC families with ~300 transporters. Many mediate drug absorption and disposition. Prominent SLC transporters include the serotonin transporter (SERT, encoded by *SLC6A4*) and the dopamine transporter (DAT, encoded by *SLC6A3*).

MEMBRANE TRANSPORTERS IN THERAPEUTIC DRUG RESPONSES

PHARMACOKINETICS Important transporters located in intestinal, renal, and hepatic epithelia function in concert with metabolism of drugs in the selective absorption and elimination of endogenous substances and drugs (Figure 2–2). In addition, transporters mediate tissue-specific drug distribution (drug targeting); conversely, transporters also may serve as protective barriers to particular organs and cell types, controlling tissue distribution as well as the absorption and elimination of drugs.

PHARMACODYNAMICS: TRANSPORTERS AS DRUG TARGETS Membrane transporters are the targets of many drugs. For example, neurotransmitter transporters are the targets for drugs used in the treatment of neuropsychiatric disorders. SERT (*SLC6A4*) is a target for the selective serotonin reuptake inhibitors (SSRIs), a major class of antidepressant drugs. Other neurotransmitter reuptake transporters serve as drug targets for the tricyclic antidepressants, amphetamines (including amphetamine-like drugs used in the treatment of attention deficit disorder in children), and anticonvulsants. These transporters also may be involved in the pathogenesis of neuropsychiatric disorders, including Alzheimer's and Parkinson's diseases. Transporters that are nonneuronal also may be potential drug targets (*e.g.*, cholesterol transporters in cardiovascular disease, nucleoside transporters in cancers, glucose transporters in metabolic syndromes, and Na^+-H^+ antiporters in hypertension).

DRUG RESISTANCE Membrane transporters play critical roles in the development of resistance to anticancer drugs, antiviral agents, and anticonvulsants. P-glycoprotein, which exports many chemotherapeutics from cells, is overexpressed in tumor cells after exposure to cytotoxic anticancer agents. Other transporters (*e.g.*, breast cancer resistance protein [BCRP], organic anion transporters, and several nucleoside transporters) also have been implicated in resistance to anticancer drugs.

MEMBRANE TRANSPORTERS AND ADVERSE DRUG RESPONSES

Through import and export mechanisms, transporters ultimately control the exposure of cells to chemical carcinogens, environmental toxins, and drugs and thereby play critical roles in the cellular toxicities of these agents. Transporter-mediated adverse drug responses generally can be classified into three categories (Figure 2–3).

Transporters expressed in the liver and kidney—as well as metabolic enzymes—are key determinants of drug exposure (Figure 2–3, *top panel*) because they control the total clearance of drugs and thus influence the plasma concentration profiles and subsequent exposure to the toxicological target.

Transporters expressed in tissues that may be targets for drug toxicity (*e.g.*, brain) or in barriers to such tissues (*e.g.*, the blood–brain barrier [BBB]) can tightly control local drug concentrations and thus control the drug exposure of these tissues (Figure 2–3, *middle panel*). Drug-induced toxicity sometimes is caused by the concentrative tissue distribution mediated by influx transporters.

Transporters for endogenous ligands may be modulated by drugs and thereby exert adverse effects (Figure 2–3, *bottom panel*). If severe, these effects can lead to withdrawal of the drug

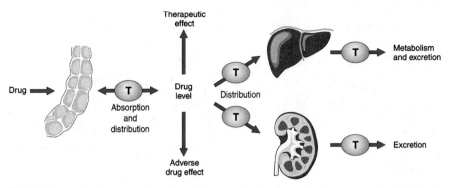

FIGURE 2–1 *Roles of membrane transporters in pharmacokinetic pathways.* Membrane transporters (T) play roles in pharmacokinetic pathways (drug absorption, distribution, metabolism, and excretion), thereby setting systemic drug levels. Drug levels often drive therapeutic and adverse drug effects.

(*e.g.*, the thiazolidinedione troglitazone). Thus, uptake and efflux transporters determine the plasma and tissue concentrations of endogenous compounds and xenobiotics, thereby influencing either systemic or site-specific drug toxicity.

BASIC MECHANISMS OF MEMBRANE TRANSPORT
TRANSPORTERS *VERSUS* CHANNELS

Both channels and transporters facilitate the membrane permeation of inorganic ions and organic compounds. Channels have two primary states, open *and* closed, *that are stochastic phenomena. Only in the open state do channels act as pores for their selected ions, allowing permeation across the plasma membrane. After opening, channels return to the closed state as a function of time.*

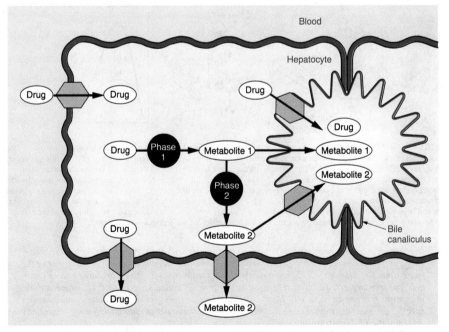

FIGURE 2–2 *Hepatic drug transporters.* Membrane transporters, shown as hexagons with arrows, work in concert with phase 1 and phase 2 drug-metabolizing enzymes in the hepatocyte to mediate the uptake and efflux of drugs and their metabolites.

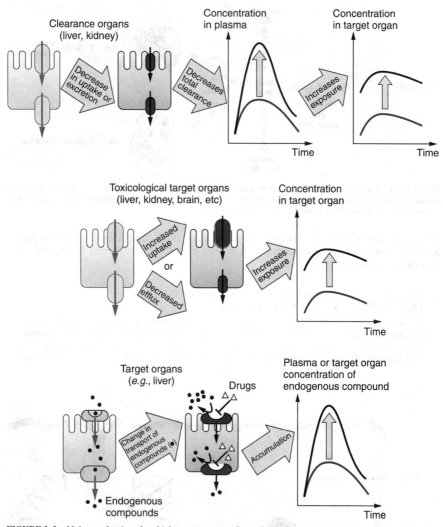

FIGURE 2–3 *Major mechanisms by which transporters mediate adverse drug responses.* Three cases are given. The left panel of each case provides a cartoon representation of the mechanism; the right panel shows the resulting effect on drug levels. (Top panel) Increase in the plasma concentrations of drug due to a decrease in the uptake and/or secretion in clearance organs such as the liver and kidney. (Middle panel) Increase in the concentration of drug in toxicological target organs due either to the enhanced uptake or to reduced efflux of the drug. (Bottom panel) Increase in the plasma concentration of an endogenous compound (*e.g.*, a bile acid) due to a drug's inhibiting the influx of the endogenous compound in its eliminating or target organ. The diagram also may represent an increase in the concentration of the endogenous compound in the target organ owing to drug-inhibited efflux of the endogenous compound.

In contrast, a transporter forms an intermediate complex with the substrate (solute); thereafter, a conformational change in the transporter induces substrate translocation to the other side of the membrane. Because of these different mechanisms, turnover rates differ markedly between channels and transporters. Turnover rate constants of typical channels are 10^6–10^8 s^{-1}, whereas those of transporters are, at most, 10^1–10^3 s^{-1}. Because transporters form intermediate complexes with specific compounds, transporter-mediated membrane transport is characterized by saturability and inhibition by substrate analogs.

    The basic mechanisms involved in solute transport across the plasma membrane include passive diffusion, facilitated diffusion, and active transport. Active transport can be further subdivided into primary and secondary active transport. These mechanisms are depicted in Figure 2–4.

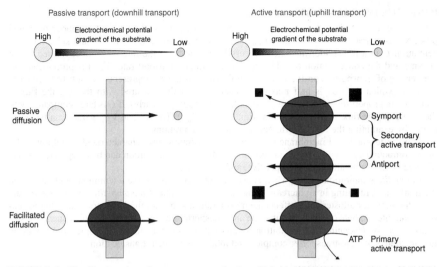

FIGURE 2–4 *Classification of membrane transport mechanisms. Light blue circles* depict the substrate. Size of the circles is proportional to the concentration of the substrate. *Arrows* show the direction of flux. *Black squares* represent the ion that supplies the driving force for transport (size is proportional to the concentration of the ion). *Dark blue ovals* depict transport proteins.

PASSIVE DIFFUSION Simple diffusion of a solute across the plasma membrane involves three processes: partition from the aqueous to the lipid phase, diffusion across the lipid bilayer, and repartition into the aqueous phase on the opposite side. Diffusion of any solute (including drugs) occurs down an electrochemical potential gradient of the solute and is dependent on both its chemical and electrical potential.

FACILITATED DIFFUSION Membrane transporters may facilitate diffusion of ions and organic compounds across the plasma membrane; this facilitated diffusion does not require energy input. Just as in passive diffusion, the transport of ionized and nonionized compounds across the plasma membrane occurs down their electrochemical potential gradient. Therefore, steady state will be achieved when the electrochemical potentials of the compound on both sides of the membrane become equal.

ACTIVE TRANSPORT Active transport requires energy input and transports solutes against their electrochemical gradients, leading to the concentration of solutes on one side of the plasma membrane and the creation of potential energy in the electrochemical gradient formed. Active transport plays an important role in the uptake and efflux of drugs and other solutes. Depending on the driving force, active transport can be subdivided into primary and secondary active transport (Figure 2–4).

Primary Active Transport Membrane transport that directly couples with ATP hydrolysis is called *primary active transport.* ABC transporters are examples of primary active transporters. They contain one or two highly conserved ATP binding cassettes that exhibit ATPase activity. ABC transporters mediate the unidirectional efflux of many solutes across biological membranes.

Secondary Active Transport In secondary active transport, the transport across the plasma membrane of one solute S_1 against its concentration gradient is driven energetically by the transport of another solute S_2 in accordance with its concentration gradient. The driving force for this type of transport therefore is stored in the electrochemical potential created by the concentration difference of S_2 across the plasma membrane. Depending on the transport direction of the solute, secondary active transporters are classified as either symporters or antiporters. *Symporters,* also termed *cotransporters,* transport S_2 and S_1 in the same direction, whereas *antiporters,* also termed *exchangers,* move their substrates in opposite directions (Figure 2–4).

KINETICS OF TRANSPORT

The flux of a substrate (rate of transport) across the plasma membrane *via* transporter-mediated processes is characterized by saturability. The relationship between the flux v and substrate concentration C in a transporter-mediated process is analogous to the rate of product formed by an enzyme and the concentration of substrate. The maximum transport rate (V_{max}) is proportional to the density of transporters on the plasma membrane, and the K_m represents the substrate concentration at which the flux is half maximal. When C is small compared with the K_m, the flux is increased in proportion to the substrate concentration (roughly linearly). If C is large compared with the K_m value, the flux approaches the maximal value (V_{max}). The K_m and V_{max} values can be determined by examining the flux at different substrate concentrations.

Transporter-mediated membrane transport of a substrate is also characterized by inhibition by other compounds. As with enzyme or receptor inhibition, this inhibition can be categorized as one of three types: competitive, noncompetitive, and uncompetitive.

Competitive inhibition occurs when substrates and inhibitors share a common binding site on the transporter, resulting in an increase in the apparent K_m value. *Noncompetitive* inhibition occurs when the inhibitor allosterically affects the transporter in a manner that does not inhibit the formation of an intermediate complex of substrate and transporter but does inhibit the subsequent translocation process. *Uncompetitive* inhibition assumes that inhibitors form a complex only with an intermediate substrate-transporter complex and inhibit subsequent translocation.

VECTORIAL TRANSPORT

The SLC transporters mediate either drug uptake or efflux, whereas ABC transporters mediate only unidirectional efflux. Asymmetrical transport across a monolayer of polarized cells, such as the epithelial and endothelial cells of brain capillaries, is called *vectorial transport* (Figure 2–5). Vectorial transport is important in the efficient transfer of solutes across epithelial or endothelial barriers; it plays a major role in hepatobiliary and urinary excretion of drugs from the blood to the lumen and in the intestinal absorption of drugs and nutrients. In addition, efflux of drugs from the brain *via* brain endothelial cells and brain choroid plexus epithelial cells involves vectorial transport.

For lipophilic compounds with sufficient membrane permeability, ABC transporters alone can achieve vectorial transport by extruding their substrates to the outside of cells without the help of influx transporters. For relatively hydrophilic organic anions and cations, coordinated uptake and efflux transporters in the polarized plasma membranes are necessary to achieve the vectorial movement of solutes across an epithelium. Common substrates of coordinated transporters are transferred efficiently across the epithelial barrier. In the liver, a number of transporters with different substrate specificities are localized on the sinusoidal membrane (facing blood). These transporters are involved in the uptake of bile acids, amphipathic organic anions, and hydrophilic organic cations into hepatocytes. Similarly, ABC transporters on the canalicular membrane (facing bile) export such compounds into the bile. Overlapping substrate specificities between the uptake

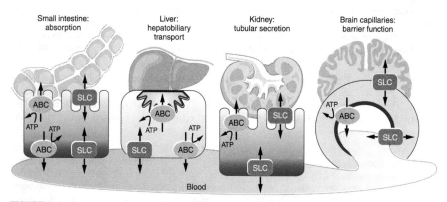

FIGURE 2–5 *Transepithelial or transendothelial flux.* Transepithelial or transendothelial flux of drugs requires distinct transporters at the two surfaces of the epithelial or endothelial barriers. These are depicted diagrammatically for transport across the small intestine (absorption), the kidney and liver (elimination), and the brain capillaries that comprise the blood–brain barrier.

transporters (Na⁺/taurocholate cotransporting polypeptide [NTCP] and organic anion transporting polypeptide [OATP] family) and efflux transporters (BSEP, MRP2, P-glycoprotein, and BCRP) make the vectorial transport of organic anions highly efficient. Similar transport systems also are present in the intestine, renal tubules, and endothelial cells of the brain capillaries (Figure 2–5).

REGULATION OF TRANSPORTER EXPRESSION

Transporter expression can be regulated transcriptionally in response to drug treatment and pathophysiological conditions, resulting in induction or down-regulation of transporter mRNAs. A number of nuclear receptors form heterodimers with the 9-cis-retinoic acid receptor (RXR) in regulating drug-metabolizing enzymes and transporters. Such receptors include pregnane X receptor (PXR/NR1I2), constitutive androstane receptor (CAR/NR1I3), farnesoid X receptor (FXR/NR1H4), peroxisome proliferator-activated receptor α (PPARα), and retinoic acid receptor (RAR). Except for CAR, these are ligand-activated nuclear receptors that, as heterodimers with RXR, bind specific elements in the enhancer regions of target genes. CAR has constitutive transcriptional activity that is antagonized by inverse agonists such as androstenol and androstanol and induced by barbiturates. PXR (SXR in humans) is activated by synthetic and endogenous steroids, bile acids, and drugs such as clotrimazole, phenobarbital, rifampin, sulfinpyrazone, ritonavir, carbamazepine, phenytoin, sulfadimidine, taxol, *and* hyperforin *(a constituent of St. John's wort). Table 2–1 summarizes the effects of drug activation of nuclear receptors on transporter expression. There is an overlap of substrates between CYP3A4 and P-glycoprotein, and PXR mediates coinduction of CYP3A4 and P-glycoprotein, supporting their cooperation in efficient detoxification.*

TRANSPORTER SUPERFAMILIES IN THE HUMAN GENOME

SLC TRANSPORTERS The SLC superfamily includes 43 families and contains ~300 human genes. Many of these genes are associated with genetic diseases (Table 2–2). SLC transporters transport diverse ionic and nonionic endogenous compounds and xenobiotics, acting either as facilitated transporters or as secondary active symporters or antiporters.

ABC SUPERFAMILY The ABC superfamily consists of 49 genes, each containing one or two conserved ABC regions. The ABC region—the core catalytic domain of ATP hydrolysis—contains Walker A and B sequences and an ABC transporter-specific signature C sequence. The ABC regions of these proteins bind and hydrolyze ATP, and the proteins use the energy for uphill transport of their substrates across the membrane. Although some ABC superfamily transporters contain only a single ABC motif, they form homodimers (BCRP/ABCG2) or heterodimers (ABCG5 and ABCG8) that exhibit a transport function. ABC transporters in prokaryotes are involved in the import of essential compounds that cannot be obtained by passive diffusion (*e.g.*, sugars, vitamins, and metals). Most ABC genes in eukaryotes transport compounds from the cytoplasm to the outside or into an intracellular compartment (*e.g.*, endoplasmic reticulum, mitochondria, and peroxisomes).

ABC transporters are divided into seven groups based on their sequence homology (Table 2–3). They are essential for many cellular processes, and mutations in at least 13 of the genes cause or contribute to human genetic disorders.

In addition to conferring multidrug resistance, an important pharmacological aspect of these transporters is xenobiotic export from healthy tissues. In particular, MDR1/ABCB1, MRP2/ABCC2, and BCRP/ABCG2 have been shown to be involved in overall drug disposition.

Properties of ABC Transporters Related to Drug Action

The tissue distribution of drug-related ABC transporters is summarized in Table 2–4, together with information about typical substrates.

TISSUE DISTRIBUTION OF DRUG-RELATED ABC TRANSPORTERS

MDR1 (ABCB1), MRP2 (ABCC2), and BCRP (ABCG2) are all expressed in the apical side of the intestinal epithelia, where they extrude xenobiotics, including many clinically relevant drugs. Key to the vectorial excretion of drugs into urine or bile, ABC transporters are expressed in polarized tissues, such as kidney and liver: MDR1, MRP2, and MRP4 (ABCC4) on the brush-border membrane of renal epithelia, and MDR1, MRP2, and BCRP on the bile canalicular membrane of hepatocytes. Some ABC transporters are expressed specifically on the blood side of the endothelial or epithelial cells that form barriers to the free entrance of toxic compounds into tissues: the BBB (MDR1 and MRP4 on the luminal side of brain capillary endothelial cells), the blood–cerebrospinal fluid (CSF) barrier (MRP1 and MRP4 on the basolateral blood side of choroid plexus epithelia), the blood–testis barrier (MRP1 on the basolateral membrane of mouse Sertoli

Table 2–1

Regulation of Transporter Expression by Nuclear Receptors

Transporter	Species	Transcription Factor	Ligand (Modulated by Drugs)	Effect of Ligand
MDR1 (P-gp)	Human	PXR	Rifampin (600 mg/day, 10 days)	↑ Transcription activity (promoter assay)
			Rifampin (600 mg/day, 10 days)	↑ Expression in duodenum in healthy subjects
				↓ Oral bioavailability of digoxin in healthy subjects
				↓ AUC of talinolol after IV and oral administration in healthy subjects
MRP2	Human	PXR	Rifampin (600 mg/day, 9 days)	↑ Expression in duodenum in healthy subjects
			Rifampin (600 mg/day, 9 days)	
			Rifampin/hyperforin	
	Mouse	FXR	GW4064/chenodeoxycholate	↑ Expression in human hepatocytes
		PXR	PCN/dexamethasone	↑ Expression in HepG2 cells
		CAR	Phenobarbital	↑ Expression in mouse hepatocyte
	Rat	PXR/FXR/CAR	PCN/GW4064/phenobarbital	↑ Expression in hepatocyte of PXR KO mice (promoter assay)
		PXR/FXR/CAR		↑ Expression in rat hepatocytes
BSEP	Human	FXR	Chenodeoxycholate, GW4064	↑ Transcription activity (promoter assay)
Ntcp	Rat	SHP1		↑ Transcription activity (promoter assay)
OATP1B1	Human	SHP1		↓ RAR mediated transcription
				Indirect effect on HNF1α expression
OATP1B3	Human	FXR	Chenodeoxycholate	↑ Expression in hepatoma cells
MDR2	Mouse	PPARα	Ciprofibrate (0.05% w/w in diet)	↑ Expression in the liver

Table 2–2

Families in the Human Solute Carrier Superfamily

Gene Name	Family Name	Number of Family Members	Selected Drug Substrates	Examples of Linked Human Diseases
SLC1	High-affinity glutamate and neutral amino acid transporter	7		Amyotrophic lateral sclerosis
SLC2	Facilitative GLUT transporter	14		
SLC3	Heavy subunits of the heteromeric amino acid transporters	2	Melphalin	Classic cystinuria type I
SLC4	Bicarbonate transporter	10		Hemolytic anemia, blindness–auditory impairment
SLC5	Na^+ glucose cotransporter	8	Glucosfamide	Glucose–galactose malabsorption syndrome
SLC6	Na^+- and Cl^--dependent neurotransmitter transporter	16	Paroxetine, fluoxetine	X-linked creatine deficiency syndrome
SLC7	Cationic amino acid transporter	14	Melphalan	Lysinuric protein intolerance
SLC8	Na^+/Ca^{2+} exchanger	3	Asymmetrical dimethylarginine	
SLC9	Na^+/H^+ exchanger	8	Thiazide diuretics	Congenital secretory diarrhea
SLC10	Na^+ bile salt cotransporter	6	Benzothiazepine	Primary bile salt malabsorption
SLC11	H^+ coupled metal ion transporter	2		Hereditary hemochromatosis
SLC12	Electroneutral cation–Cl^- cotransporter family	9		Gitelman's syndrome
SLC13	Na^+–sulfate/carboxylate cotransporter	5	Sulfate, cysteine conjugates	
SLC14	Urea transporter	2		Kidd antigen blood group
SLC15	H^+–oligopeptide cotransporter	4	Valacyclovir	
SLC16	Monocarboxylate transporter	14	Salicylate, atorvastatin	Muscle weakness
SLC17	Vesicular glutamate transporter	8		Sialic acid storage disease
SLC18	Vesicular amine transporter	3	Reserpine	Myasthenic syndromes
SLC19	Folate/thiamine transporter	3	Methotrexate	Thiamine-responsive megaloblastic anemia
SLC20	Type III Na^+–phosphate cotransporter	2		
SLC21/ SLC0	Organic anion transporter	11	Pravastatin	
SLC22	Organic cation/anion/zwitterion transporter	18	Pravastatin, metformin	Systemic carnitine deficiency syndrome
SLC23	Na^+-dependent ascorbate transporter	4	Vitamin C	
SLC24	$Na^+/(Ca^{2+}-K^+)$ exchanger	5		
SLC25	Mitochondrial carrier	27		Senger's syndrome
SLC26	Multifunctional anion exchanger	10	Salicylate, ciprofloxacin	Congenital Cl^--losing diarrhea

(Continued)

Table 2-2

Families in the Human Solute Carrier Superfamily (*Continued*)

Gene Name	Family Name	Number of Family Members	Selected Drug Substrates	Examples of Linked Human Diseases
SLC27	Fatty acid transporter protein	6		
SLC28	Na$^+$-coupled nucleoside transport	3	Gemcitabine, cladribine	
SLC29	Facilitative nucleoside transporter	4	Dipyridamole, gemcitabine	
SLC30	Zinc efflux	9		
SLC31	Copper transporter	2	Cisplatin	
SLC32	Vesicular inhibitory amino acid transporter	1	Vigabatrin	
SLC33	Acetyl-CoA transporter	1		
SLC34	Type II Na$^+$-phosphate cotransporter	3		Autosomal-dominant hypophosphatemic rickets
SLC35	Nucleoside-sugar transporter	17		Leukocyte adhesion deficiency type II
SLC36	H$^+$-coupled amino acid transporter	4	D-Serine, D-cycloserine	
SLC37	Sugar-phosphate/phosphate exchanger	4		Glycogen storage disease non-1a
SLC38	System A and N, Na$^+$-coupled neutral amino acid transporter	6		
SLC39	Metal ion transporter	14		Acrodermatitis enteropathica
SLC40	Basolateral iron transporter	1		Type IV hemochromatosis
SLC41	MgtE-like magnesium transporter	3		
SLC42	Rh ammonium transporter (pending)	3		Rh-null regulator
SLC43	Na$^+$-independent system-L–like amino acid transporter	2		

34

Table 2–3

The ATP Binding Cassette (ABC) Superfamily in the Human Genome and Linked Genetic Diseases

Gene Name	Family Name	Number of Family Members	Examples of Linked Human Diseases
ABCA	ABC A	12	Tangier disease (defect in cholesterol transport; ABCA1), Stargardt syndrome (defect in retinal metabolism; ABCA4)
ABCB	ABC B	11	Bare lymphocyte syndrome type I (defect in antigen-presenting; ABCB3 and ABCB4), progressive familial intrahepatic cholestasis type 3 (defect in biliary lipid secretion; MDR3/ABCB4), X-linked sideroblastic anemia with ataxia (a possible defect in iron homeostasis in mitochondria; ABCB7), progressive familial intrahepatic cholestasis type 2 (defect in biliary bile acid excretion; BSEP/ABCB11)
ABCC	ABC C	13	Dubin–Johnson syndrome (defect in biliary bilirubin glururonide excretion; MRP2/ABCC2), pseudoxanthoma (unknown mechanism; ABCC6), cystic fibrosis (defect in chloride channel regulation; ABCC7), persistent hyperinsulinemic hypoglycemia of infancy (defect in inwardly rectifying potassium conductance regulation in pancreatic B cells; SUR1)
ABCD	ABC D	4	Adrenoleukodystrophy (a possible defect in peroxisomal transport or catabolism of very long-chain fatty acids; ABCD1)
ABCE	ABC E	1	
ABCF	ABC F	3	
ABCG	ABC G	5	Sitosterolemia (defect in biliary and intestinal excretion of plant sterols; ABCG5 and ABCG8)

cells and MDR1 in several types of human testicular cells), and the blood–placenta barrier (MDR1, MRP2, and BCRP on the luminal maternal side and MRP1 on the antiluminal fetal side of placental trophoblasts).

MRP/ABCC Family

The substrates of transporters in the MRP/ABCC family are mostly organic anions. Both MRP1 and MRP2 accept glutathione and glucuronide conjugates, sulfated conjugates of bile salts, and nonconjugated organic anions of an amphipathic nature (at least one negative charge and some degree of hydrophobicity). They also transport neutral or cationic anticancer drugs, such as vinca alkaloids *and* anthracyclines, *possibly* via *a cotransport or symport mechanism with reduced glutathione. MRP3 also has a substrate specificity that is similar to that of MRP2 but with a lower transport affinity for glutathione conjugates compared with MRP1 and MRP2. MRP3 is expressed on the sinusoidal side of hepatocytes and is induced under cholestatic conditions. MRP3 functions to return toxic bile salts and bilirubin glucuronides into the blood circulation. MRP4 and MRP5 pump nucleotide analogs and clinically important anti–human immunodeficiency virus (HIV) drugs. No substrates for MRP6 have been identified that explain MRP6-associated pseudoxanthoma.*

ABC TRANSPORTERS IN DRUG ABSORPTION AND ELIMINATION

Systemic exposure to orally administered digoxin is increased by coadministration of MDR1 inducers and negatively correlated with MDR1 protein expression in the intestine. MDR1 is also expressed on the brush-border membrane of renal epithelia, and its function can be monitored using digoxin (>70% excreted in the urine). MDR1 inhibitors (e.g., quinidine, verapamil, vaspodar, spironolactone, clarithromycin, and ritonavir) all markedly reduce renal digoxin excretion. In view of this, drugs with narrow therapeutic windows (e.g., digoxin) should be used with great care if MDR1-based drug–drug interactions are likely.

Table 2-4

ABC Transporters Involved in Drug Absorption, Distribution, and Excretion

Transporter Name	Tissue Distribution	Physiological Function	Substrates
MDR1 (ABCB1)	Liver Kidney Intestine BBB BTB BPB	Detoxification of xenobiotics?	**Characteristics:** Neutral or cationic compounds with bulky structure **Anticancer drugs:** etoposide, doxorubicin, vincristine **Ca^{2+} channel blockers:** diltiazem, verapamil **HIV protease inhibitors:** indinavir, ritonavir **Antibiotics/antifungals:** erythromycin, ketoconazole **Hormones:** testosterone, progesterone **Immunosuppressants:** cyclosporine, FK506 (tacrolimus) **Others:** digoxin, quinidine
MRP1 (ABCC1)	Ubiquitous (kidney, BCSFB, BTB)	Leukotriene (LTC$_4$) secretion from leukocyte	**Characteristics:** Amphiphilic with at least one negative net charge **Anticancer drugs:** vincristine (with GSH), methotrexate **Glutathione conjugates:** LTC$_4$, glutathione conjugate of ethacrynic acid **Glucuronide conjugates:** estradiol-17-D-glucuronide, bilirubin mono(or bis) glucuronide **Sulfated conjugates:** estrone-3-sulfate (with GSH) **HIV protease inhibitors:** saquinavir **Antifungals:** grepafloxacin **Others:** folate, GSH, oxidized glutathione
MRP2 (ABCC2)	Liver Kidney Intestine BPB	Excretion of bilirubin glucuronide and GSH into bile	**Characteristics:** Amphiphilic with at least one negative net charge (similar to MRP1) **Anticancer drugs:** methotrexate, vincristine **Glutathione conjugates:** LTC$_4$, GSH conjugate of ethacrynic acid **Glucuronide conjugates:** estradiol-17-D-glucuronide, bilirubin mono(or bis) glucuronide **Sulfate conjugate of bile salts:** taurolithocholate sulfate **HIV protease inhibitors:** indinavir, ritonavir **Others:** pravastatin, GSH, oxidized glutathione
MRP3 (ABCC3)	Liver Kidney	?	**Characteristics:** Amphiphilic with at least one negative net charge (Glucuronide conjugates are better substrates than glutathione conjugates.)

Transporter	Tissue	Function	Substrates / Characteristics
	Intestine		**Anticancer drugs:** etoposide, methotrexate **Glutathione conjugates:** LTC_4, glutathione conjugate of 15-deoxy-delta prostaglandin J2 **Glucuronide conjugates:** estradiol-17-D-glucuronide, etoposide glucuronide **Sulfate conjugates of bile salts:** taurolithocholate sulfate **Bile salts:** glycocholate, taurocholate **Others:** folate, leucovorin
MRP4 (ABCC4)	Ubiquitous (kidney, prostate, lung, muscle, pancreas, testis, ovary, bladder, gallbladder, BBB, BCSFB)	?	**Characteristics:** Nucleotide analogues **Anticancer drugs:** 6-mercaptopurine, methotrexate **Glucuronide conjugates:** estradiol-17-D-glucuronide **Cyclic nucleotides:** cyclic AMP, cyclic GMP **HIV protease inhibitors:** adefovir **Others:** folate, leucovorin, taurocholate (with GSH)
MRP5 (ABCC5)	Ubiquitous	?	**Characteristics:** Nucleotide analogues **Anticancer drugs:** 6-mercaptopurine **Cyclic nucleotides:** cyclic AMP, cyclic GMP **HIV protease inhibitors:** adefovir
MRP6 (ABCC6)	Liver Kidney	?	**Anticancer drugs:** doxorubicin*, etoposide* **Glutathione conjugate of:** LTC_4 **Other:** BQ-123 (cyclic peptide ET-1 antagonist)
BCRP (MXR) (ABCG2)	Liver Intestine BBB	Normal heme transport during maturation of erythrocytes	**Anticancer drugs:** methotrexate, mitoxantrone, camptothecin analogs (SN-38, etc.), topotecan **Glucuronide conjugates:** 4-methylumbelliferone glucuronide, estradiol-17-D-glucuronide **Sulfate conjugates:** dehydroepiandrosterone sulfate, estrone-3-sulfate **Others:** cholesterol, estradiol
MDR3 (ABCB4)	Liver	Excretion of phospholipids into bile	**Characteristics:** Phospholipids
BSEP (ABCB11)	Liver	Excretion of bile salts into bile	**Characteristics:** Bile salts
ABCG5 and ABCG8	Liver Intestine	Excretion of plant sterols into bile and intestinal lumen	**Characteristics:** Plant sterols

NOTE: Representative substrates and cytotoxic drugs with increased resistance (*) are included in this table (cytotoxicity with increased resistance is usually caused by the decreased accumulation of the drugs). Although MDR3 (ABCB4), BSEP (ABCB11), ABCG5, and ABCG8 are not directly involved in drug disposition, inhibition of these physiologically important ABC transporters will lead to unfavorable side effects.

Little clinically applicable information regarding MRP2 and BCRP drug-handling is available. Most MRP2 or BCRP substrates also can be transported by the OATP family transporters on the sinusoidal membrane.

GENETIC VARIATION IN MEMBRANE TRANSPORTERS: IMPLICATIONS FOR CLINICAL DRUG RESPONSE

Inherited disorders of membrane transport have been identified (Tables 2–2 and 2–3), and polymorphisms in membrane transporters that play a role in drug response are yielding new insights in pharmacogenetics (*see* Chapter 4). The most widely studied drug transporter is P-glycoprotein (MDR1, *ABCB1*); the *ABCB1* genotype is associated with responses to anticancer drugs, antiviral agents, immunosuppressants, antihistamines, cardiac glycosides, and anticonvulsants. *ABCB1* SNPs also have been associated with tacrolimus and *nortriptyline* neurotoxicity and susceptibility for developing ulcerative colitis, renal cell carcinoma, and Parkinson's disease.

TRANSPORTERS INVOLVED IN PHARMACOKINETICS
Hepatic Transporters
HMG-CoA REDUCTASE INHIBITORS

Statins are cholesterol-lowering agents that reversibly inhibit HMG-CoA reductase, which catalyzes a rate-limiting step in cholesterol biosynthesis (see Chapter 35). Most of the statins in the acid form are substrates of uptake transporters that mediate hepatic uptake and enterohepatic circulation (Figures 2–5 and 2–6). In this process, hepatic uptake transporters such as OATP1B1 and efflux transporters such as MRP2 cooperate to produce vectorial transcellular transport of bisubstrates in the liver. The efficient first-pass hepatic uptake of statins by OATP1B1 helps them to exert their pharmacological effect and also minimizes the systemic drug distribution, thereby minimizing adverse effects in smooth muscle. Recently, two common SNPs in SLCO1B1 (OATP1B1) have been associated with elevated plasma levels of pravastatin.

DRUG–DRUG INTERACTIONS INVOLVING TRANSPORTER-MEDIATED HEPATIC UPTAKE   Transporter-mediated hepatic uptake can cause drug–drug interactions among drugs that are actively taken up into the liver and metabolized and/or excreted in the bile. When an inhibitor of drug-metabolizing enzymes is highly concentrated in hepatocytes by active transport,

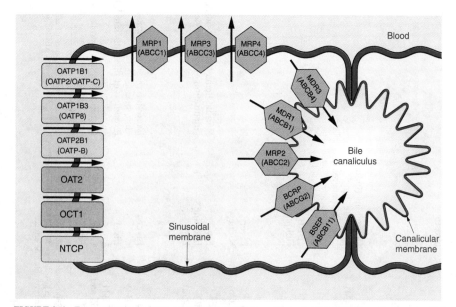

FIGURE 2–6 *Transporters in the hepatocyte that function in the uptake and efflux of drugs across the sinusoidal membrane and efflux of drugs into the bile across the canalicular membrane.* See *text for details of the transporters pictured.*

extensive inhibition of the drug-metabolizing enzymes may be observed because of the high concentration of the inhibitor in the vicinity of the drug-metabolizing enzymes.

Renal Transporters

ORGANIC CATION TRANSPORT   Structurally diverse organic cations are secreted in the proximal tubule. Many secreted organic cations are endogenous compounds (*e.g.,* choline, *N*-methylnicotinamide, and dopamine), and renal secretion appears to be important in eliminating excess concentrations of these substances. However, a primary function of organic cation secretion is to rid the body of xenobiotics, including many positively charged drugs and their metabolites (*e.g., cimetidine, ranitidine,* metformin, *procainamide,* and *N-acetylprocainamide*), and toxins from the environment (*e.g., nicotine*). Organic cations that are secreted by the kidney may be either hydrophobic or hydrophilic. Hydrophilic organic drug cations generally have molecular weights of <400; a current model for their secretion in the proximal tubule of the nephron is shown in Figure 2–7.

For the transepithelial flux of a compound (e.g., secretion), it is essential for the compound to traverse two membranes sequentially, the basolateral membrane facing the blood side and the apical membrane facing the tubular lumen. Distinct transporters on each membrane mediate the sequential steps of transport. Organic cations cross the basolateral membrane by three distinct transporters in the SLC family 22 (SLC22): OCT1 (SLC22A1), OCT2 (SLC22A2), and OCT3 (SLC22A3). Organic cations are transported across this membrane down their electrochemical gradient (–70 mV). The SLC22 members have 12 putative transmembrane domains with N-linked glycosylation sites.

Transport of organic cations from cell to tubular lumen across the apical membrane occurs via an electroneutral proton–organic cation exchange mechanism. Transporters on the apical

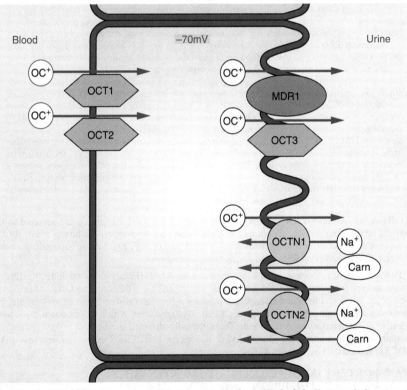

FIGURE 2–7   *Model of organic cation secretory transporters in the proximal tubule. Hexagons* depict transporters in the SLC22 family, SLC22A1 (OCT1), SLC22A2 (OCT2), and SLC22A3 (OCT3). *Circles* show transporters in the same family, SLC22A4 (OCTN1) and SLC22A5 (OCTN2). MDR1 (ABCB1) is depicted as a *dark blue oval.* Carn, carnitine; OC$^+$, organic cation.

membrane are in the SLC22 family and termed novel organic cation transporters *(Octns) OCTN1 (SLC22A4) and OCTN2 (SLC22A5). These bifunctional transporters mediate both organic cation secretion and carnitine reabsorption. In the reuptake mode, the transporters function as* Na^+ *cotransporters, relying on the inwardly driven* Na^+ *gradient created by* Na^+,K^+*-ATPase to move carnitine from tubular lumen into the cell. In the secretory mode, the transporters function as proton–organic cation exchangers: protons move from tubular lumen to cell interior in exchange for organic cations, which move from cytosol to tubular lumen.*

OCT1 has four splice variants, one of which is functionally active, OCT1G/L554. OCT1 is expressed primarily in the liver, with some expression in heart, intestine, and skeletal muscle. In humans, very modest levels of OCT1 transcripts are detected in the kidney. The transport mechanism of OCT1 is electrogenic and saturable for transport of small-molecular-weight organic cations including tetraethylammonium (TEA) and dopamine. OCT1 also can mediate organic cation–organic cation exchange. Organic cations can trans-inhibit OCT1. When present on the cytosolic side of a membrane, the hydrophobic organic cations quinine and quinidine, which are poor substrates of OCT1, can trans-inhibit influx of organic cations via OCT1.

Human OCT1 (SLC22A1) *accepts a wide array of monovalent organic cations with molecular weights of <400, including many drugs (e.g., procainamide, metformin, and* pindolol*). Inhibitors of OCT1 are generally more hydrophobic. Since OCT1 mammalian orthologs have >80% amino acid identity, evolutionarily nonconserved residues among mammalian species clearly are involved in specificity differences.*

OCT2 is located adjacent to OCT1 on chromosome 6 (6q26). A single splice variant of human OCT2, termed OCT2-A, in the kidney is a truncated form of OCT2 that appears to have a lower K_m *for substrates than OCT2. In the kidney, OCT2 is localized to the proximal tubule, distal tubules, and collecting ducts. In the proximal tubule, OCT2 is restricted to the basolateral membrane. The transport mechanism of OCT2 is similar to that of OCT1.*

Like OCT1, OCT2 generally accepts a wide array of monovalent organic cations with molecular weights of <400. OCT2 is also present in neuronal tissues and may play a housekeeping role in neurons, taking up excess concentrations of neurotransmitters and recycling neurotransmitters by taking up breakdown products that then reenter monoamine synthetic pathways.

Human OCT3 is expressed in the liver, kidney (weakly), intestine, and placenta. Like OCT1 and OCT2, OCT3 appears to support electrogenic potential-sensitive organic cation transport. Some studies have suggested that OCT3 is the extraneuronal monoamine transporter based on its substrate specificity and potency of interaction with monoamine neurotransmitters. Because of its relatively low abundance in the kidney, OCT3 may play only a limited role in renal drug elimination.

OCTN1 (SLC22A4) is expressed in the kidney, trachea, and bone marrow and operates as an organic cation–proton exchanger. OCTN1 likely functions as a bidirectional pH- and ATP-dependent transporter at the apical membrane in renal tubular epithelial cells.

OCTN2 (SLC22A5) is expressed predominantly in the renal cortex, with very little expression in the medulla, and is localized to the apical membrane of the proximal tubule. OCTN2 transports L*-carnitine with high affinity in a* Na^+*-dependent manner, whereas,* Na^+ *does not influence OCTN2-mediated transport of organic cations. Thus, OCTN2 is thought to function as both a* Na^+*-dependent carnitine transporter and a* Na^+*-independent organic cation transporter. Mutations in OCTN2 cause primary systemic carnitine deficiency.*

ORGANIC ANION TRANSPORT   Structurally diverse organic anions are secreted in the proximal tubule. The primary function of organic anion secretion appears to be the removal from the body of xenobiotics, including many weakly acidic drugs (*e.g.*, pravastatin, captopril, p-amino-hippurate [PAH], and penicillins) and toxins (*e.g.*, ochratoxin).

Two primary transporters on the basolateral membrane (Figure 2–8) mediate the flux of organic anions from interstitial fluid to tubule cells: OAT1 (*SLC22A6*) and OAT3 (*SLC22A8*). Hydrophilic organic anions are transported across the basolateral membrane against an electrochemical gradient in exchange with intracellular α-ketoglutarate, which moves down its concentration gradient from cytosol to blood. The outwardly directed gradient of α-ketoglutarate is maintained by a basolateral Na^+-dicarboxylate transporter (NaDC3). The Na^+ gradient that drives NaDC3 is maintained by Na^+,K^+-ATPase.

TRANSPORTERS INVOLVED IN PHARMACODYNAMICS: DRUG ACTION IN THE BRAIN

Neurotransmitters are packaged in vesicles in presynaptic neurons, released in the synapse by vesicle fusion with the plasma membrane, and—except for acetylcholine—are then taken back into the presynaptic neurons or postsynaptic cells (*see* Chapter 6). Transporters involved in the neuronal

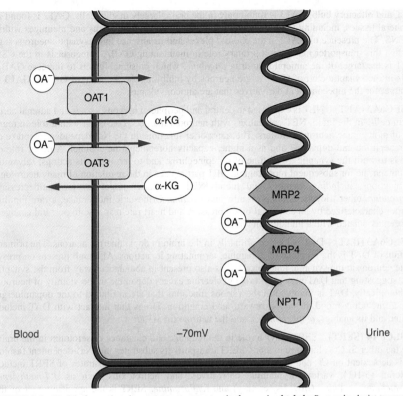

FIGURE 2–8 *Model of organic anion secretory transporters in the proximal tubule.* *Rectangles* depict transporters in the SLC22 family, OAT1 (SLC22A6) and OAT3 (SLC22A8), and *hexagons* depict transporters in the ABC superfamily, MRP2 (ABCC2) and MRP4 (ABCC4). NPT1 (SLC17A1) is depicted as a *circle.* OA⁻, organic anion; α-KG, α-ketoglutarate.

reuptake of neurotransmitters and the regulation of their levels in the synaptic cleft belong to two major superfamilies, SLC1 and SLC6. Transporters in both families play roles in reuptake of γ-aminobutyric acid (GABA), glutamate, and the monoamine neurotransmitters norepinephrine, serotonin, and dopamine. These transporters may serve as pharmacologic targets for neuropsychiatric drugs.

SLC6 family members localized in the brain and involved in neurotransmitter reuptake into presynaptic neurons include the norepinephrine transporter (NET, *SLC6A2*), the dopamine transporter (DAT, *SLC6A3*), the serotonin transporter (SERT, *SLC6A4*), and several GABA reuptake transporters (GAT1, GAT2, and GAT3). Each of these transporters appears to have 12 transmembrane domains and a large extracellular loop with glycosylation sites between transmembrane domains 3 and 4. Typically, these proteins are ~600 amino acids in length. SLC6 family members depend on the Na⁺ gradient to actively transport their substrates into cells. Cl⁻ is also required, although to a variable extent depending on the family member.

Through reuptake mechanisms, the neurotransmitter transporters in the SLC6A family regulate the concentrations and persistence of neurotransmitters in the synaptic cleft; the extent of transmitter uptake also influences subsequent vesicular storage of transmitters. Further, the transporters can function in the reverse direction by exporting neurotransmitters in a Na⁺-independent fashion. Many of these transporters also are present in other tissues (*e.g.,* kidney and platelets), where they may serve other roles.

SLC6A1 (GAT1), SLC6A11 (GAT3), AND SLC6A13 (GAT2) GAT1 is the most important GABA transporter in the brain; it predominantly is expressed in presynaptic GABAergic neurons. GAT1 is found in abundance in the neocortex, cerebellum, basal ganglia, brainstem, spinal cord, retina, and olfactory bulb. GAT3 is found only in the brain, largely in glial cells. GAT2 is found in peripheral tissues, including the kidney and liver, and in the choroid plexus and meninges within the CNS. The presence of GAT2 in the choroid plexus and its absence in presynaptic neurons suggest that this transporter may play a primary role in maintaining GABA homeostasis in the CSF. GAT1 is the target of the antiepileptic drug *tiagabine*, which presumably acts to increase GABA levels in the synaptic cleft of GABAergic neurons by inhibiting the reuptake of GABA. GAT3 is the target for the nipecotic acid derivatives that are anticonvulsants.

SLC6A2 (NET)   NET is expressed in central and peripheral nervous tissues and adrenal chromaffin cells. In the brain, NET colocalizes with neuronal markers, consistent with a role in reuptake of monoamine neurotransmitters. The transporter functions in the Na^+-dependent reuptake of norepinephrine and dopamine and as a higher-capacity norepinephrine channel. A major role of NET is to limit the synaptic dwell time of norepinephrine and to terminate its actions, salvaging norepinephrine for subsequent repackaging. NET participates in the regulation of many neurological functions, including memory and mood. NET is a drug target for the antidepressant *desipramine*, other tricyclic antidepressants, and *cocaine*. Orthostatic intolerance, a rare familial disorder characterized by an abnormal blood pressure and heart rate response to postural changes, has been associated with a mutation in NET.

SLC6A3 (DAT)   DAT is located primarily in the brain in dopaminergic neurons. The primary function of DAT is the reuptake of dopamine, terminating its actions. Although present on presynaptic neurons at the synaptic junction, DAT is also present in abundance away from the synaptic cleft, suggesting that DAT may play a role in clearing excess dopamine in the vicinity of neurons. Physiologically, DAT is involved in the various functions that are attributed to the dopaminergic system, including mood, behavior, reward, and cognition. Drugs that interact with DAT include cocaine and its analogs, *amphetamines,* and the neurotoxin *MPTP*.

SLC6A4 (SERT)   SERT plays a role in the reuptake and clearance of serotonin in the brain. Like the other SLC6A family members, SERT transports its substrates in a Na^+-dependent fashion and is dependent on Cl^- and possibly on the countertransport of K^+. Substrates of SERT include serotonin (5-HT), various tryptamine derivatives, and neurotoxins such as *3,4-methylenedioxymethamphetamine* (MDMA; ecstasy) and *fenfluramine*. SERT is the specific target of the selective serotonin reuptake inhibitors (*e.g., fluoxetine* and *paroxetine*) and one of several targets of tricyclic antidepressants (*e.g., amitriptyline*). Genetic variants of SERT have been associated with an array of behavioral and neurological disorders. The precise mechanism by which a reduced activity of SERT, caused by either a genetic variant or an antidepressant, ultimately affects mood and behavior is not known.

BLOOD–BRAIN AND BLOOD–CSF BARRIERS

Drugs acting in the CNS must either cross the BBB or the blood–CSF barrier, which are formed by brain capillary endothelial cells or epithelial cells of the choroid plexus, respectively. Efflux transporters play a role in these dynamic barriers. P-glycoprotein extrudes its substrate drugs on the luminal membrane of the brain capillary endothelial cells into the blood, complicating CNS therapy for some drugs (*see* Chapter 1). Other transporters in the BBB and the blood–CSF barrier include members of organic anion transporting polypeptide (OATP1A4 and OATP1A5) and organic anion transporter (OAT3) families, which facilitate the uptake of organic compounds such as β-lactam antibiotics, statins, PAH, H_2-receptor antagonists, and bile acids on the plasma membrane facing the brain–CSF. Further understanding of influx and efflux transporters in these barriers should translate into more effective delivery of drugs to the CNS while avoiding undesirable CNS side effects and may help to define the mechanisms of drug–drug interactions and interindividual differences in the therapeutic CNS effects.

For a complete Bibliographical listing see Goodman & Gilman's *The Pharmacological Basis of Therapeutics*, 11th ed., or Goodman & Gilman Online at www.accessmedicine.com.

3

DRUG METABOLISM

Substances foreign to the body, or xenobiotics, are metabolized by the same enzymatic pathways and transport systems that are utilized for dietary constituents. Xenobiotics to which humans are exposed include environmental pollutants, food additives, cosmetic products, agrochemicals, processed foods, and drugs. Many xenobiotics are lipophilic chemicals that, in the absence of metabolism, would not be efficiently eliminated and would accumulate in the body, possibly causing toxicity. Most xenobiotics are subjected to metabolic pathways that convert these hydrophobic chemicals into more hydrophilic derivatives that are readily eliminated in urine or bile.

The processes of drug metabolism that lead to elimination also play a major role in diminishing the biological activity of drugs. For example, *phenytoin*, an anticonvulsant used in the treatment of epilepsy, is virtually insoluble in water. Metabolism by phase 1 cytochrome P450 enzymes (CYPs) makes 4-OH-phenytoin, which is a substrate for phase 2 uridine diphosphate-glucuronosyltransferases (UGTs) that produce a water soluble 4-glucuronate adduct that is readily eliminated. Metabolism also terminates the biological activity of the drug.

Paradoxically, these same enzymes can also convert certain chemicals to highly reactive toxic and carcinogenic metabolites. Depending on the structure of the chemical substrate, xenobiotic-metabolizing enzymes produce electrophilic metabolites that can react with nucleophilic cellular macromolecules such as DNA, RNA, and protein. Reaction of these electrophiles with DNA can sometimes result in cancer through the mutation of genes such as oncogenes or tumor suppressor genes. This potential for carcinogenic activity makes testing the safety of drug candidates of vital importance, particularly for drugs that will be used chronically.

THE PHASES OF DRUG METABOLISM Xenobiotic metabolism consists of phase 1 reactions (oxidation, reduction, or hydrolytic reactions) and phase 2 reactions, in which enzymes form a conjugate of the phase 1 product (Table 3–1). Phase 1 enzymes introduce functional groups (*e.g.*, -OH, -COOH, -SH, -O-, or NH_2) into the compound; these moieties do little to increase the water solubility of the drug but usually lead to drug inactivation. Metabolism, usually the hydrolysis of an ester or amide linkage, sometimes results in bioactivation of a drug. Inactive drugs that undergo metabolism to an active drug are called *prodrugs*. The antitumor drug *cyclophosphamide* is bioactivated to a cell-killing electrophilic derivative (*see* Chapter 51). Phase 2 enzymes facilitate the elimination of drugs and the inactivation of electrophilic and potentially toxic metabolites produced by oxidation. While many phase 1 reactions result in drug inactivation, phase 2 reactions produce a metabolite with improved water solubility and increased molecular weight, thereby facilitating drug elimination.

Phase 1 oxidation reactions are catalyzed by the superfamilies of CYPs, flavin-containing monooxygenases (FMOs), and epoxide hydrolases (EHs). The CYPs and FMOs comprise superfamilies containing multiple genes. The phase 2 enzymes include several superfamilies of conjugating enzymes, such as the glutathione-S-transferases (GSTs), UDP-glucuronosyltransferases (UGTs), sulfotransferases (SULTs), *N*-acetyltransferases (NATs), and methyltransferases (MTs). These conjugation reactions usually require the substrate to have oxygen (hydroxyl or epoxide groups), nitrogen, or sulfur atoms that serve as acceptor sites for a hydrophilic moiety (*e.g.*, glutathione, glucuronic acid, sulfate, or an acetyl group) that is covalently conjugated to an acceptor site on the molecule, as in the example of phenytoin. In general, oxidation by phase 1 enzymes either adds or exposes a functional group, permitting the products to then serve as substrates for phase 2 conjugating or synthetic enzymes.

SITES OF DRUG METABOLISM Xenobiotic-metabolizing enzymes are expressed in most tissues in the body; the highest levels are found in the gastrointestinal (GI) tract (*e.g.*, liver, small intestine, and colon). The high concentration of xenobiotic-metabolizing enzymes in GI epithelium mediates the initial metabolic processing of most oral drugs and is the initial site for first-pass metabolism of drugs. Absorbed drug then enters the portal circulation and transits to the liver, which is the major "metabolic clearing house" for both endogenous chemicals (*e.g.*, cholesterol, steroid hormones, fatty acids, and proteins) and xenobiotics. While some active drug may escape first-pass metabolism in the GI tract and liver, subsequent passes through the liver result in further metabolism of the parent drug until it is eliminated. Other organs that contain significant xenobiotic-metabolizing enzymes include the nasal mucosa and lung, which play important roles in the first-pass metabolism of airborne pollutants and of drugs that are administered as aerosols.

Table 3–1

Xenobiotic Metabolizing Enzymes

Enzymes	Reactions
Phase 1 "oxygenases"	
Cytochrome P450s (P450 or CYP)	C and O oxidation, dealkylation, others
Flavin-containing monooxygenases (FMO)	N, S, and P oxidation
Epoxide hydrolases (mEH, sEH)	Hydrolysis of epoxides
Phase 2 "transferases"	
Sulfotransferases (SULT)	Addition of sulfate
UDP-glucuronosyltransferases (UGT)	Addition of glucuronic acid
Glutathione-S-transferases (GST)	Addition of glutathione
N-acetyltransferases (NAT)	Addition of acetyl group
Methyltransferases (MT)	Addition of methyl group
Other enzymes	
Alcohol dehydrogenases	Reduction of alcohols
Aldehyde dehydrogenases	Reduction of aldehydes
NADPH-quinone oxidoreductase (NQO)	Reduction of quinones

mEH and sEH are microsomal and soluble epoxide hydrolase. UDP, uridine diphosphate; NADPH, reduced nicotinamide adenine dinucleotide phosphate.

    The phase 1 CYPs, FMOs, and EHs, and some phase 2 conjugating enzymes, notably the UGTs, are located in the endoplasmic reticulum (ER) of the cell (Figure 3–1). The ER lumen is physically distinct from the rest of the cytosolic components and is ideally suited for the metabolic function of these enzymes: hydrophobic molecules enter the cell and embed in the lipid bilayer, where they encounter the phase 1 enzymes. Once oxidized, drugs are conjugated in the membrane by the UGTs

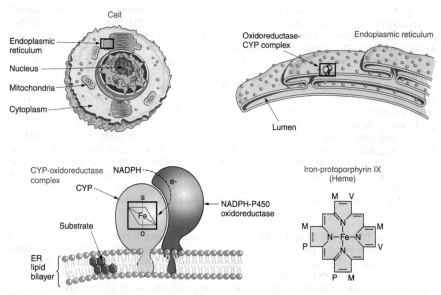

FIGURE 3–1 *Location of CYPs in the cell.* The figure shows increasingly microscopic levels of detail, sequentially expanding the areas within the black boxes. CYPs are embedded in the phospholipid bilayer of the endoplasmic reticulum (ER). Most of the enzyme is located on the cytoplasmic surface of the ER. A second enzyme, NADPH-cytochrome P450 oxidoreductase, transfers electrons to the CYP where it can, in the presence of O_2, oxidize xenobiotic substrates, many of which are hydrophobic and dissolved in the ER. A single NADPH-CYP oxidoreductase species transfers electrons to all CYP isoforms in the ER. Each CYP contains a molecule of iron-protoporphyrin IX that functions to bind and activate O2. Substituents on the porphyrin ring are methyl (M), propionyl (P), and vinyl (V) groups.

or by the cytosolic transferases such as GST and SULT. The metabolites are then transported out of the cell and into the bloodstream. Hepatocytes, which constitute >90% of the cells in the liver, carry out most drug metabolism and produce conjugated substrates that can also be transported though the bile canalicular membrane into the bile for elimination in the gut (*see* Chapter 2).

THE CYPs CYPs are heme proteins (Figure 3–1). The heme iron binds oxygen in the CYP active site, where oxidation of substrates occurs. Electrons are supplied by the enzyme NADPH-cytochrome P450 oxidoreductase and its cofactor, NADPH. Metabolism of a substrate by a CYP consumes one molecule of O_2 and produces an oxidized substrate and a molecule of water. Depending on the nature of the substrate, the reaction for some CYPs is partially "uncoupled," consuming more O_2 than substrate metabolized and producing "activated oxygen" or O_2^-. The O_2^- is usually converted to water by the enzyme superoxide dismutase.

Among the diverse reactions carried out by mammalian CYPs are *N*-dealkylation, *O*-dealkylation, aromatic hydroxylation, *N*-oxidation, *S*-oxidation, deamination, and dehalogenation (Table 3–2). CYPs are involved in the metabolism of dietary and xenobiotic agents, as well as the synthesis of endogenous compounds that are derived from cholesterol (*e.g.,* steroid hormones and bile acids).

The CYPs that carry out xenobiotic metabolism have the capacity to metabolize a large number of structurally diverse chemicals. This is due both to multiple forms of CYPs and to the capacity of a single CYP to metabolize structurally dissimilar chemicals. A single compound can be metabolized by multiple CYPs and CYPs can metabolize a single compound at multiple positions. This promiscuity of CYPs (Table 3–2), due to their large and fluid substrate binding sites, occurs at the cost of relatively slow catalytic rates. Eukaryotic CYPs metabolize substrates at a fraction of the rate of more typical enzymes involved in intermediary metabolism and mitochondrial electron transfer. As a result, drugs generally have half-lives in the range of 3–30 hours, while endogenous compounds have half-lives of seconds to minutes.

The broad substrate specificity of CYPs is one of the underlying reasons for the high frequency of drug interactions. When two coadministered drugs are both metabolized by a single CYP, they compete for binding to the enzyme's active site. This can result in the inhibition of metabolism of one or both of the drugs, leading to elevated plasma levels. For drugs with a narrow therapeutic index, the elevated serum levels may elicit unwanted toxicities. Drug-drug interactions are among the leading causes of adverse drug reactions.

THE NAMING OF CYPs

There are 57 functional CYP genes and 58 pseudogenes in humans. These genes are grouped into families and subfamilies. CYPs are named with the root "CYP" followed by a number designating the family, a letter denoting the subfamily, and a second number designating the CYP isoform. Thus, CYP3A4 is family 3, subfamily A, and gene number 4. In humans, 12 CYPs in families 1–3 (CYP1A1, 1A2, 1B1, 2A6, 2B6, 2C8, 2C9, 2C19, 2D6, 2E1, 3A4, and 3A5) are primarily responsible for xenobiotic metabolism. The liver contains the greatest abundance of xenobiotic-metabolizing CYPs; CYPs also are expressed throughout the GI tract, and, in lower amounts, in lung, kidney, and the central nervous system (CNS). The most important CYPs for drug metabolism are those in the CYP2C, CYP2D, and CYP3A subfamilies. CYP3A4—the most abundantly expressed—is involved in the metabolism of ~50% of clinically used drugs (Figure 3–2A). The CYP1A, CYP1B, CYP2A, CYP2B, and CYP2E subfamilies are rarely involved in the metabolism of therapeutic drugs, but they catalyze the metabolic activation of many protoxins and procarcinogens.

There are large interindividual variations in CYP activity due to genetic polymorphisms and differences in gene regulation (see below). Several human CYP genes exhibit polymorphisms, including CYP2A6, CYP2C9, CYP2C19, and CYP2D6.

DRUG-DRUG INTERACTIONS Interactions at the level of drug metabolism form the basis of many drug interactions. Most commonly, an interaction occurs when two drugs (*e.g.,* a statin and a macrolide antibiotic or antifungal) are metabolized by the same enzyme and affect each other's metabolism. Thus, it is important to determine the identity of the CYP that metabolizes a particular drug and to avoid coadministering drugs that are metabolized by the same CYP. Some drugs can also inhibit CYPs independently of being substrates. For example, the common antifungal agent, *ketoconazole* (NIZORAL) is a potent inhibitor of CYP3A4 and other CYPs. Coadministration of ketoconazole with the anti-HIV viral protease inhibitors reduces the clearance of the protease inhibitor and increases its plasma concentration and the risk of toxicity. For most drugs, the package insert lists the CYP that carries out its metabolism and notes the potential for drug interactions. Some drugs are CYP inducers that can induce not only their own metabolism but also the metabolism of coadministered

Table 3–2

Major Reactions Involved in Drug Metabolism

	Reaction	Examples
I. Oxidative reactions		
N-Dealkylation	$RNHCH_3 \longrightarrow RNH_2 + CH_2O$	Imipramine, diazepam, codeine, erythromycin, morphine, tamoxifen, theophylline, caffeine
O-Dealkylation	$ROCH_3 \longrightarrow ROH + CH_2O$	Codeine, indomethacin, dextromethorphan
Aliphatic hydroxylation	$RCH_2CH_3 \longrightarrow RCHOHCH_3$	Tolbutamide, ibuprofen, phenobarbital, meprobamate, cyclosporine, midazolam
Aromatic hydroxylation	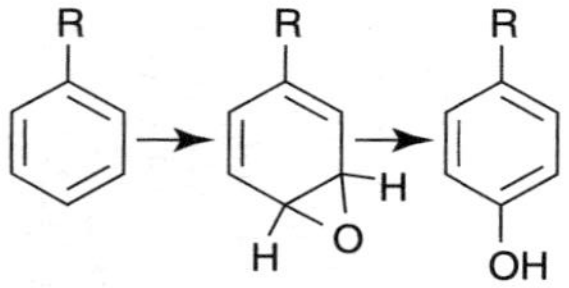 (aromatic ring R) $\longrightarrow$ arene oxide $\longrightarrow$ (phenol R—OH)	Phenytoin, phenobarbital, propanolol, ethinyl estradiol, amphetamine, warfarin
N-Oxidation	$RNH_2 \longrightarrow RNHOH$; $\begin{array}{c} R_1 \\ \quad \diagdown NH \\ R_2 \diagup \end{array} \longrightarrow \begin{array}{c} R_1 \\ \quad \diagdown N—OH \\ R_2 \diagup \end{array}$	Chlorpheniramine, dapsone, meperidine
S-Oxidation	$\begin{array}{c} R_1 \\ \quad \diagdown S \\ R_2 \diagup \end{array} \longrightarrow \begin{array}{c} R_1 \\ \quad \diagdown S{=}O \\ R_2 \diagup \end{array}$	Cimetidine, chlorpromazine, thioridazine, omeprazole
Deamination	$R\underset{\underset{NH_2}{\mid}}{CH}CH_3 \longrightarrow R\underset{\underset{NH_2}{\mid}}{\overset{\overset{OH}{\mid}}{C}}CH_3 \longrightarrow R\overset{\overset{O}{\|}}{C}-CH_3 + NH_3$	Diazepam, amphetamine

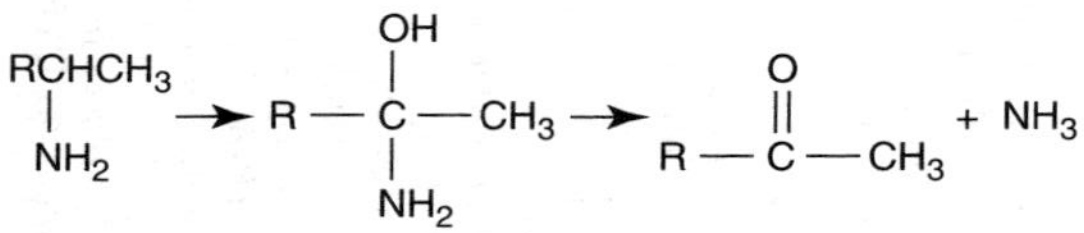

46

II. Hydrolysis reactions

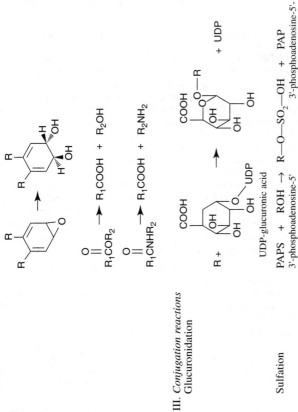

R_1COR_2 ⟶ $R_1COOH + R_2OH$

R_1CNHR_2 ⟶ $R_1COOH + R_2NH_2$

Carbamazepine

Procaine, aspirin, clofibrate, meperidine, enalapril, cocaine
Lidocaine, procainamide, indomethacin

III. Conjugation reactions
Glucuronidation

$R +$ UDP-glucuronic acid ⟶ + UDP

Acetaminophen, morphine, oxazepam, lorazepam

Sulfation

PAPS + ROH → R—O—SO$_2$—OH + PAP
3'-phosphoadenosine-5'-phosphosulfate   3'-phosphoadenosine-5'-phosphate

Acetaminophen, steroids, methyldopa

Acetylation

CoAS—CO—CH$_3$ + RNH$_2$ → RNH—CO—CH$_3$ + CoA-SH

Sulfonamides, isoniazid, dapsone, clonazepam (*see* Table 3–3)

Methylation

RO, RS-, RN- + AdoMet → RO-CH$_3$ + AdoHomCys

L-Dopa, methyldopa, mercaptopurine, captopril

Glutathione conjugation

GSH + R → GS-R

Adriamycin, fosfomycin, busulfan

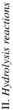

drugs (*see* below and Figure 3–5). Steroid hormones and herbal products such as St. John's wort can increase hepatic levels of CYP3A4, thereby increasing the metabolism of many drugs. Drug metabolism can also be influenced by diet. CYP inhibitors and inducers are commonly found in foods and in some cases these can influence drug toxicity and efficacy. Components of grapefruit juice are potent inhibitors of CYP3A4; thus, drug inserts may warn that taking a medication with grapefruit juice could increase the drug's bioavailability. The antihistamine *terfenadine* was withdrawn from the market because its metabolism was blocked by CYP3A4 substrates such as *erythromycin* and grapefruit juice. Terfenadine is a prodrug that requires oxidation by CYP3A4 to its active metabolite, and at high doses the parent compound causes arrhythmias. Thus, elevated levels of parent drug in the plasma as a result of CYP3A4 inhibition caused ventricular tachycardia in some individuals. Interindividual differences in drug metabolism are significantly influenced by polymorphisms in CYPs. The CYP2D6 polymorphism has led to the withdrawal of several drugs (*e.g., debrisoquine* and *perhexiline*) and the cautious use of others that are CYP2D6 substrates (*e.g., encainide* and *flecainide* [antiarrhythmics], *desipramine* and *nortriptyline* [antidepressants], and *codeine*).

FLAVIN-CONTAINING MONOOXYGENASES (FMOs) FMOs are another superfamily of phase 1 enzymes that are expressed at high levels in the liver and localized to the ER. There are six families of FMOs, with FMO3 being most abundant in liver. FMOs are minor contributors to drug metabolism and generally produce benign metabolites. FMOs are not induced by any of the xenobiotic receptors (*see* below) or easily inhibited; thus, in distinction to CYPs, FMOs are less involved in drug interactions. This distinction has practical consequences, as illustrated by two drugs used in the control of gastric motility, *itopride* and *cisapride*. Itopride is metabolized by FMO3; cisapride is metabolized by CYP3A4. Thus, itopride is less likely to be involved in drug interactions than is cisapride. CYP3A4 participates in drug interactions through induction and inhibition of metabolism, whereas FMO3 is not induced or inhibited by any clinically used drugs (although FMOs may become important as new drugs are developed). FMO3 metabolizes nicotine as well as H_2-receptor antagonists (*cimetidine* and *ranitidine*), antipsychotics (*clozapine*), and antiemetics (*itopride*).

HYDROLYTIC ENZYMES Epoxides are highly reactive electrophiles that can bind to cellular nucleophiles found in protein, RNA, and DNA, resulting in cell toxicity and transformation. Two forms of *epoxide hydrolase* (EH) hydrolyze epoxides produced by CYPs: a soluble form (sEH) is expressed in the cytosol and a microsomal form (mEH) is localized to the ER membrane. These EHs participate in the deactivation of potentially toxic derivatives generated by CYPs. The antiepileptic drug *carbamazepine* (Chapter 19) is a prodrug that is converted to its pharmacologically active derivative, carbamazepine-10,11-epoxide by CYP3A4. This metabolite is efficiently hydrolyzed by mEH to a dihydrodiol, resulting in drug inactivation. The tranquilizer *valnoctamide* and anticonvulsant *valproic acid* inhibit mEH, resulting in clinically significant drug interactions with carbamazepine by causing elevations of the active derivative. This has led to the development of new antiepileptic drugs (*e.g., gabapentin* and *levetiracetal*) that are metabolized by CYPs but not by EHs.

The *carboxylesterase* superfamily catalyzes the hydrolysis of ester- and amide-containing compounds. These enzymes are found in both the ER and cytosol of many cell types and are involved in detoxification or metabolic activation of drugs, environmental toxins, and carcinogens. Carboxylesterases also catalyze the activation of prodrugs to their respective free acids. For example, the prodrug and cancer chemotherapeutic agent *irinotecan* is bioactivated by plasma and intracellular carboxylesterases to the potent topoisomerase inhibitor SN-38.

PHASE 2 METABOLISM: CONJUGATING ENZYMES The phase 2 conjugation reactions are synthetic in nature. The contributions of different phase 2 reactions to drug metabolism are shown in Figure 3–2B. Two of the reactions, glucuronidation and sulfation, result in the formation of metabolites with significantly increased hydrophilicity. Glucuronidation also markedly increases the molecular weight of the compound, which favors biliary excretion. Characteristic of the phase 2 reactions is the participation of cofactors such as UDP-glucuronic acid (UDP-GA) for UGTs and 3′-phosphoadenosine-5′-phosphosulfate (PAPS) for SULTs; these cofactors react with functional groups on the substrates that often are generated by the phase 1 CYPs. With the exception of glucuronidation, which is localized to the luminal side of the ER, all phase 2 reactions are carried out in the cytosol. The catalytic rates of phase 2 reactions are significantly faster than the rates of the CYPs. Thus, if a drug is targeted for phase 1 oxidation through the CYPs followed by a phase 2 conjugation reaction, the rate of elimination usually will depend on the phase 1 reaction.

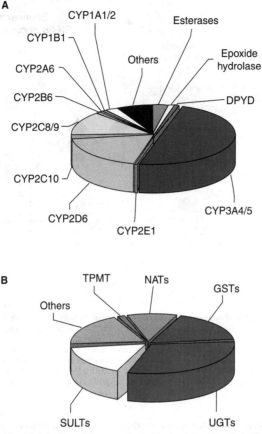

A

CYP1A1/2

CYP1B1

CYP2A6

CYP2B6

CYP2C8/9

CYP2C10

CYP2D6

Others

Esterases

Epoxide hydrolase

DPYD

CYP3A4/5

CYP2E1

B

TPMT   NATs

Others

GSTs

SULTs   UGTs

FIGURE 3–2 *The fraction of clinically used drugs metabolized by the major phase 1 and phase 2 enzymes.* The relative size of each pie section represents the estimated percentage of drugs metabolized by the major phase 1 (panel *A*) and phase 2 (panel *B*) enzymes. In some cases, more than a single enzyme is responsible for metabolism of a single drug. CYP, cytochrome P450; DPYD, dihydropyrimidine dehydrogenase; GST, glutathione-S-transferase; NAT, N-acetyltransferase; SULT, sulfotransferase; TPMT, thiopurine methyltransferase; UGT, UDP-glucuronosyltransferase.

GLUCURONIDATION   UGTs catalyze the transfer of glucuronic acid from the cofactor UDP-GA to a substrate to form β-D-glucopyranosiduronic acids (glucuronides), metabolites that are sensitive to cleavage by β-glucuronidase. The generation of glucuronides can be formed through alcoholic and phenolic hydroxyl groups, carboxyl, sulfuryl, and carbonyl moieties, as well as through primary, secondary, and tertiary amine linkages. Examples of glucuronidation reactions are shown in Table 3–2. The broad specificity of UGTs assures that most clinically used drugs are excreted as glucuronides. There are 19 human genes that encode the UGT proteins; nine are encoded by the *UGT1* locus on chromosome 2; ten are encoded by the *UGT2* gene cluster on chromosome 4. Both families of proteins are involved in the metabolism of drugs and xenobiotics, while the UGT2 family appears to have greater specificity for the glucuronidation of endogenous substances such as steroids.

UGTs are expressed in a tissue-specific and often inducible fashion, with the highest concentration in the GI tract and liver. Based upon their physicochemical properties, glucuronides are excreted by the kidneys into the urine or through active transport processes through the apical surface of the liver hepatocytes into the bile ducts and thence to the duodenum with bile. Many drugs that are glucuronidated and excreted in the bile reenter the circulation by "enterohepatic recirculation": β-D-glucopyranosiduronic acids are targets for β-glucuronidase activity found in strains of

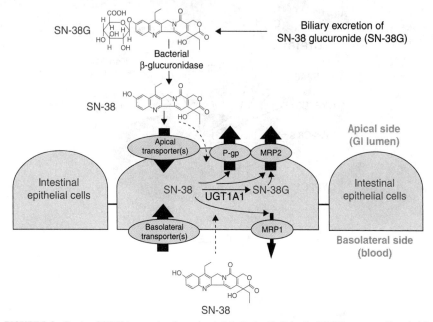

SN-38G ← **Biliary excretion of SN-38 glucuronide (SN-38G)**

Bacterial β-glucuronidase

SN-38

Apical transporter(s) · P-gp · MRP2

Apical side (GI lumen)

Intestinal epithelial cells

SN-38 $\xrightarrow{\text{UGT1A1}}$ SN-38G

Intestinal epithelial cells

Basolateral transporter(s) · MRP1

Basolateral side (blood)

SN-38

FIGURE 3–3 Routes of SN-38 transport and exposure to intestinal epithelial cells. SN-38 is transported into the bile following glucuronidation by liver UGT1A1 and extrahepatic UGT1A7. Following cleavage of luminal SN-38 glucuronide (SN-38G) by bacterial β-glucuronidase, reabsorption into epithelial cells can occur by passive diffusion (indicated by the dashed arrows entering the cell) as well as by apical transporters. Movement into epithelial cells may also occur from the blood by basolateral transporters. Intestinal SN-38 can efflux into the lumen through P-glycoprotein (P-gp) and multidrug resistance protein 2 (MRP2) and into the blood *via* MRP1. Excessive accumulation of the SN-38 in intestinal epithelial cells, resulting from reduced glucuronidation, can lead to cellular damage and toxicity.

bacteria that are common in the lower GI tract; the result is the liberation of free drug into the intestinal lumen; free drug is transported by passive diffusion or through apical transporters back into the intestinal epithelial cells, and enters the portal circulation (Figure 3–3).

UGT1A1 is of great importance in drug metabolism. For instance, the glucuronidation of bilirubin by UGT1A1 is the rate-limiting step in assuring efficient bilirubin clearance; this rate can be affected by both genetic variation and competing substrates (drugs). Bilirubin is the breakdown product of heme, 80% of which originates from circulating hemoglobin and 20% from other heme-containing proteins such as the CYPs. Bilirubin must be metabolized further by glucuronidation to assure its elimination. The failure to efficiently metabolize bilirubin by glucuronidation leads to elevated serum levels (hyperbilirubinemia). There are more than 50 genetic lesions in the UGT1A1 gene that can lead to inherited unconjugated hyperbilirubinemia. Two UGT1A1 deficiencies are Crigler-Najjar syndrome type I, diagnosed as a complete lack of bilirubin glucuronidation, and Crigler-Najjar syndrome type II, differentiated by the detection of low amounts of bilirubin glucuronides in duodenal secretions. These rare syndromes result from mutations in the UGT1A1 gene and the consequent production of little or no functional UGT1A1 protein.

Gilbert's syndrome is a generally benign condition, present in up to 10% of the population, that is diagnosed clinically because circulating bilirubin levels are 60–70% higher than those in normal subjects. The most common genetic polymorphism associated with Gilbert's syndrome is a mutation in the UGT1A1 gene promoter, which leads to reduced expression of UGT1A1. Subjects with Gilbert's syndrome may be predisposed to adverse drug reactions resulting from a reduced capacity to metabolize drugs by UGT1A1. In these patients, there is competition for drug metabolism with bilirubin glucuronidation, resulting in pronounced hyperbilirubinemia as well as reduced formation of the glucuronide metabolites of drugs. Gilbert's syndrome alters patient responses to irinotecan. Irinotecan, a prodrug used in chemotherapy of solid tumors (see Chapter 51), is metabolized to its active form SN-38 by serum carboxylesterases. SN-38, a potent topoisomerase inhibitor, is inactivated by UGT1A1 and excreted in the bile (Figure 3–3). Once in the lumen of the intestine, the SN-38 glucuronide undergoes cleavage by bacterial β-glucuronidase and reenters the circulation through intestinal absorption. Elevated levels of SN-38 in the blood lead to hematological toxicities characterized by leukopenia and neutropenia, and damage to the intestinal epithelial cells, resulting in severe diarrhea. Patients with Gilbert's syndrome who are receiving irinotecan therapy are predisposed to hematological and GI toxicities resulting from elevated serum levels of SN-38, the net result of insufficient UGT1A activity and consequent accumulation of a toxic drug in the GI epithelium.

SULFATION The sulfotransferases (SULTs) are located in the cytosol and conjugate sulfate derived from 3'-phosphoadenosine-5'-phosphosulfate (PAPS) to the hydroxyl groups of aromatic and aliphatic compounds. In humans, 11 SULT isoforms have been identified. SULTs metabolize a wide variety of endogenous and exogenous substrates and play important roles in normal human homeostasis. For example, SULT1B1 is the predominant form expressed in skin and brain, carrying out sulfation of cholesterol and thyroid hormones; cholesterol sulfate is an essential regulator of keratinocyte differentiation and skin development. SULT1A3 is highly selective for catecholamines, while estrogens are sulfated by SULT1E1 and dehydroepiandrosterone (DHEA) is sulfated by SULT2A1; as a consequence, significant fractions of circulating catecholamines, estrogens, iodothyronines, and DHEA exist in the sulfated form.

The SULT1 family isoforms are the major SULT forms involved in drug metabolism, with SULT1A1 being the most important. SULT1C2 and SULT1C4 are expressed abundantly in fetal tissues and decline in abundance in adults; little is known about their substrate specificities. SULT1E catalyzes the sulfation of endogenous and exogenous steroids, and has been found localized in liver as well as in hormone-responsive or producing tissues such as the testis, breast, adrenal gland, and placenta.

Metabolism of drugs through sulfation often leads to the generation of chemically reactive metabolites, where the sulfate is electron withdrawing and may be heterolytically cleaved, leading to the formation of an electrophilic cation. Examples of the generation by sulfation of a carcinogenic or toxic response in mutagenicity assays occur with chemicals derived from the environment or from food mutagens generated from well-cooked meat. Thus, it is important to understand whether human SULT polymorphisms are associated with cancers related to environmental exposure. Since SULT1A1 is the most abundant form in human tissues and displays broad substrate specificity, the polymorphic profiles associated with this gene and the onset of various human cancers are of considerable interest.

GLUTATHIONE CONJUGATION The glutathione-S-transferases (GSTs) catalyze the transfer of glutathione to reactive electrophiles, a function that serves to protect cellular macromolecules from interacting with electrophilic heteroatoms (-O, -N, and -S). The cosubstrate in the reaction is the tripeptide glutathione(γ-glutamic acid, cysteine, and glycine (*see* Figure 3–4). Cellular glutathione may be oxidized (GSSG) or reduced (GSH), and the ratio of GSH:GSSG is critical in maintaining a cellular environment in the reduced state. In addition to affecting xenobiotic

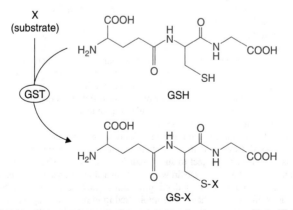

FIGURE 3–4 *Glutathione as a cosubstrate in the conjugation of a drug or xenobiotic (X) by glutathione-S-transferase (GST).*

conjugation with GSH, a severe reduction in GSH content can predispose cells to oxidative damage, a state linked to a number of disease states.

The formation of glutathione conjugate generates a thioether linkage of drug or xenobiotic to the cysteine moiety of the tripeptide. Since the concentration of glutathione in hepatic cells is high, typically in the 10 mM range, many drugs and xenobiotics can react nonenzymatically with glutathione. However, the GSTs have been found to comprise up to 10% of the total cellular protein, assuring efficient enzymatic conjugation of glutathione to reactive electrophiles. The high concentration of GSTs also provides a reservoir of intracellular binding sites that facilitates noncovalent and sometimes covalent interactions with compounds that are not substrates for glutathione conjugation. The cytosolic pool of GSTs has been shown to bind steroids, bile acids, bilirubin, cellular hormones, and environmental toxicants, in addition to complexing with other cellular proteins.

The 20+ human GSTs are divided into two subfamilies that differ in their substrate specificities. The cytosolic forms predominate in the metabolism of drugs and xenobiotics, whereas the microsomal GSTs metabolize endogenous compounds such as leukotrienes and prostaglandins. Despite the apparent overcapacity of GSTs and GSH, there is always concern that some reactive intermediates will escape detoxification, bind to cellular components, and cause toxicity. The potential for such an occurrence is heightened if GSH is depleted or if a specific polymorphism of GST is less active. While it is difficult to deplete cellular GSH levels, drugs that require large doses to be clinically efficacious have the greatest potential to lower cellular GSH levels. Acetaminophen, which normally is metabolized by glucuronidation and sulfation, is also a substrate for oxidative metabolism by CYP2E1 to generate the toxic metabolite N-acetyl-p-benzoquinone imine (NAPQI). An overdose of acetaminophen can deplete cellular GSH levels, increase NAPQI levels, and enhance the potential for NAPQI to interact with other cellular components.

The GSTs are all polymorphic, and several of the polymorphic forms express a null phenotype. Individuals who carry these polymorphisms are predisposed to toxicities by agents that are selective substrates for the GSTs. The allele GSTM1*0 is observed in 50% of the Caucasian population and has been associated with human malignancies of the lung, colon, and bladder. Null activity in the GSTT1 gene has been associated with adverse side effects and toxicity in cancer chemotherapy with cytostatic drugs; the toxicities result from insufficient drug clearance via GSH conjugation. Expression of the null genotype can reach 60% in Chinese and Korean populations. Activities of GSTs in cancerous tissues also have been linked to the development of drug resistance toward chemotherapeutic agents.

N-ACETYLATION The cytosolic N-acetyltransferases (NATs) are responsible for the metabolism of drugs and environmental agents containing an aromatic amine or hydrazine group. The addition of the acetyl group from the cofactor acetyl-coenzyme A often leads to a metabolite that is less water soluble because the ionizable amine is neutralized by covalent addition of an acetyl group. NATs are among the most polymorphic of all human xenobiotic drug-metabolizing enzymes. There are two functional NAT genes in humans, *NAT1* and *NAT2*. Over 25 allelic variants of *NAT1* and *NAT2* have been characterized, and homozygous genotypes for at least two variant alleles are required to predispose to lowered drug metabolism. *Slow* acetylation patterns are attributed mostly to *NAT2* polymorphisms.

Following the introduction of *isoniazid* for the treatment of tuberculosis, toxicities were noted in 5–15% of the patients (*see* Chapter 47) Individuals suffering from the toxic effects of isoniazid excreted large amounts of unchanged drug and low amounts of acetylated isoniazid. Pharmacogenetic studies led to the classification of "rapid" and "slow" acetylators, with the "slow" phenotype being predisposed to toxicity. Molecular analysis of the *NAT2* gene revealed polymorphisms that correspond to the "slow" and "fast" acetylator phenotypes. Polymorphisms in the *NAT2* gene and their association with the slow acetylation of isoniazid provided the first link between pharmacogenetic phenotype and a genetic polymorphism.

Drugs that are subject to acetylation and their known toxicities are listed in Table 3–3. Many classes of clinically used drugs contain an aromatic amine or a hydrazine group that can be acetylated. If a drug is known to be subject to such modification, the acetylation phenotype of an individual patient can be important. Adverse drug reactions in a slow acetylator resemble drug overdose; thus, a "slow acetylator" requires dose reduction or an increased dosing interval. Several drugs that are acetylated (*e.g.*, sulfonamides) have been implicated in idiosyncratic hypersensitivity reactions. Sulfonamides are transformed into hydroxylamines that interact with cellular proteins, generating haptens that can elicit autoimmune responses. Individuals who are slow acetylators are predisposed

Table 3–3

Indications and Unwanted Side Effects of Drugs Metabolized by N-Acetyltransferases

Drug	Indication	Major Side Effects
Acebutolol	Arrhythmias, hypertension	Drowsiness, weakness, insomnia
Amantadine	Influenza A, parkinsonism	Appetite loss, dizziness, headache, nightmares
Aminobenzoic acid	Skin disorders, sunscreens	Stomach upset, contact sensitization
Aminoglutethimide	Adrenal cortex carcinoma, breast cancer	Clumsiness, nausea, dizziness, agranulocytosis
Aminosalicylic acid	Ulcerative colitis	Allergic fever, itching, leukopenia
Amonafide	Prostate cancer	Myelosuppression
Amrinone	Advanced heart failure	Thrombocytopenia, arrhythmias
Benzocaine	Local anesthesia	Dermatitis, itching, rash, methemoglobinemia
Caffeine	Neonatal respiratory distress syndrome	Dizziness, insomnia, tachycardia
Clonazepam	Epilepsy	Ataxia, dizziness, slurred speech
Dapsone	Dermatitis, leprosy, AIDS-related complex	Nausea, vomiting, hyperexcitability, methemoglobinemia, dermatitis
Dipyrone (metamizole)	Analgesic	Agranulocytosis
Hydralazine	Hypertension	Hypotension, tachycardia, flushing, headache
Isoniazid	Tuberculosis	Peripheral neuritis, hepatotoxicity
Nitrazepam	Insomnia	Dizziness, somnolence
Phenelzine	Depression	CNS excitation, insomnia, orthostatic hypotension, hepatotoxicity
Procainamide	Ventricular tachyarrhythmia	Hypotension, systemic lupus erythematosus
Sulfonamides	Antibacterial agents	Hypersensitivity, hemolytic anemia, fever, lupus-like syndromes

to such drug-induced reactions. Thus, knowledge of a patient's acetylating phenotype can be important in avoiding drug toxicity.

Tissue-specific NAT expression can affect toxicity of environmental pollutants. NAT1 is ubiquitously expressed in human tissues, whereas NAT2 is found in liver and the GI tract. Both enzymes have a capacity to form N-hydroxy–acetylated metabolites from bicyclic aromatic hydrocarbons, a reaction that leads to the nonenzymatic release of the acetyl group and the generation of highly reactive nitrenium ions. Thus, N-hydroxy acetylation is thought to activate certain environmental toxicants. In contrast, direct N-acetylation of the environmentally generated bicyclic aromatic amines is stable and leads to detoxification. NAT2 fast acetylators efficiently metabolize and detoxify bicyclic aromatic amine through liver-dependent acetylation. Slow acetylators (NAT2 deficient) accumulate bicyclic aromatic amines, which are metabolized by CYPs to N-OH metabolites that are eliminated in the urine. In bladder epithelium, NAT1 efficiently catalyzes the N-hydroxy acetylation of bicyclic aromatic amines, a process that leads to deacetylation and the formation of the mutagenic nitrenium ion. Slow acetylators due to NAT2 deficiency are predisposed to bladder cancer if exposed to environmental bicyclic aromatic amines.

METHYLATION In humans, xenobiotics can undergo O-, N-, and S-methylation. Methyltransferases (MTs) are identified by substrate and methyl conjugate. Humans express three N-methyltransferases, one catechol-O-methyltransferase (COMT), a phenol-O-methyltransferase (POMT), a thiopurine S-methyltransferase (TPMT), and a thiol methyltransferase (TMT). All MTs use S-adenosyl-methionine as the methyl donor. Except for a conserved signature sequence, there is limited overall sequence conservation among the MTs, indicating that each MT has evolved to display a unique catalytic function. Although all MTs generate methylated products, the substrate specificity of each is high.

Nicotinamide N-methyltransferase (NNMT) methylates serotonin, tryptophan, and pyridine-containing compounds such as nicotinamide and nicotine. Phenylethanolamine N-methyltransferase (PNMT) is responsible for the methylation of norepinephrine to form epinephrine; the histamine N-methyltransferase (HNMT) metabolizes substances containing an imidazole ring (e.g., histamine). *COMT methylates neurotransmitters containing a catechol moiety* (e.g., dopamine and norepinephrine, methyldopa, *and drugs of abuse such as ecstasy). The most important MT clinically may be TPMT, which catalyzes the S-methylation of aromatic and heterocyclic sulfhydryl compounds, including the thiopurine drugs* azathioprine *(AZA),* 6-mercaptopurine *(6-MP), and* thioguanine. *AZA and 6-MP are used for inflammatory bowel disease (see Chapter 38) and autoimmune disorders such as systemic lupus erythematosus and rheumatoid arthritis. Thioguanine is used in acute myeloid leukemia, and 6-MP is used to treat childhood acute lymphoblastic leukemia (see Chapter 51). Because TPMT is responsible for the detoxification of 6-MP, a genetic deficiency in TPMT can result in severe toxicities in patients taking these drugs. The toxic side effects arise when a lack of 6-MP methylation by TPMT causes accumulation of 6-MP, resulting in the generation of toxic levels of 6-thioguanine nucleotides. Tests for TPMT activity have made it possible to identify individuals who are predisposed to the toxic side effects of 6-MP therapy, who therefore should receive a decreased dose.*

INDUCTION OF DRUG METABOLISM Xenobiotics can influence the extent of drug metabolism by activating transcription and inducing the expression of genes encoding drug-metabolizing enzymes. Thus, a drug may induce its own metabolism. One potential consequence of this is a decrease in plasma drug concentration as the autoinduced metabolism of the drug exceeds the rate at which new drug enters the body, resulting in loss of efficacy. Ligands and the receptors through which they induce drug metabolism are shown in Table 3–4. Figure 3–5 shows the scheme by which a drug may interact with nuclear receptors to induce its own metabolism. A particular receptor, when activated by a ligand, can induce the transcription of a battery of target genes, including CYPs and drug transporters. Any drug that is a ligand for a receptor that induces CYPs and transporters could cause altered drug metabolism and drug interactions.

The aryl hydrocarbon receptor (AHR) is a basic helix-loop-helix transcription factor that induces expression of genes encoding CYP1A1 and CYP1A2, which metabolically activate chemical carcinogens, including environmental contaminants and carcinogens derived from food. Many of these substances are inert unless metabolized by CYPs. Induction of CYPs by AHR could result in an increase in the toxicity and carcinogenicity of these procarcinogens. For example, *omeprazole*, a proton pump inhibitor used to treat ulcers (*see* Chapter 36), is an AHR ligand and can induce CYP1A1 and CYP1A2, possibly activating toxins/carcinogens.

Another induction mechanism involves members of the nuclear receptor superfamily. Many of these receptors were originally termed "orphan receptors" because they had no known endogenous ligands. The nuclear receptors relevant to drug metabolism and drug therapy include the pregnane X receptor (PXR), constitutive androstane receptor (CAR), and the peroxisome proliferator activated receptor (PPAR). PXR is activated by a number of drugs, including antibiotics (*rifampin* and *troleandomycin*), Ca^{2+} channel blockers (*nifedipine*), statins (*mevastatin*), antidiabetic drugs (*rosiglitazone*), HIV protease inhibitors (*ritonavir*), and anticancer drugs (*paclitaxel*). Hyperforin, a component of St. John's wort, also activates PXR. This activation is thought to be the basis for the decreased efficacy of oral contraceptives in individuals taking St. John's wort: activated PXR induces CYP3A4, which can metabolize steroids found in oral contraceptives. PXR also induces the expression of genes encoding certain drug

Table 3–4

Nuclear Receptors that Induce Drug Metabolism

Receptor	Ligands
Aryl hydrocarbon receptor (AHR)	Omeprazole
Constitutive androstane receptor (CAR)	Phenobarbital
Pregnane X receptor (PXR)	Rifampin
Farnesoid X receptor (FXR)	Bile acids
Vitamin D receptor	Vitamin D
Peroxisome proliferator activated receptor (PPAR)	Fibrates
Retinoic acid receptor (RAR)	*all-trans*-Retinoic acid
Retinoid X receptor (RXR)	*9-cis*-Retinoic acid

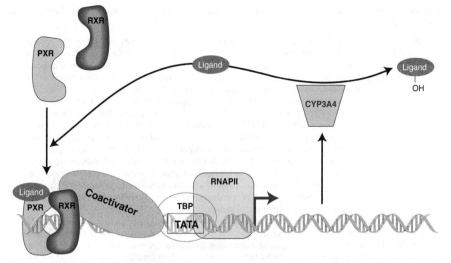

FIGURE 3–5 *Induction of drug metabolism by nuclear receptor–mediated signal transduction.* When a drug such as atorvastatin (Ligand) enters the cell, it can bind to a nuclear receptor such as the pregnane X receptor (PXR). PXR then forms a complex with the retinoid X receptor (RXR), binds to DNA upstream of target genes, recruits coactivator (which binds to the TATA box binding protein, TBP), and activates transcription. Among PXR target genes are CYP3A4, which can metabolize the atorvastatin and decrease its cellular concentration. Thus, atorvastatin induces its own metabolism, undergoing both ortho- and para-hydroxylation.

transporters and phase 2 enzymes including SULTs and UGTs. Thus, PXR facilitates the metabolism and elimination of xenobiotics, including drugs, with notable consequences (*see* legend to Figure 3–5).

The nuclear receptor CAR was discovered based on its capacity to activate genes in the absence of ligand. Steroids such as *androstanol*, the antifungal agent *clotrimazole*, and the antiemetic *meclizine* are inverse agonists that inhibit gene activation by CAR, while the pesticide 1,4-bis (2-[3,5-dichloropyridyloxy]) benzene, the steroid 5β-pregnane-3,20-dione, and probably other endogenous compounds are agonists that activate gene expression when bound to CAR. Genes induced by CAR include those encoding CYP2B6, CYP2C9, and CYP3A4, various phase 2 enzymes (including GSTs, UGTs, and SULTs), and drug and endobiotic transporters. CYP3A4 is induced by both PXR and CAR; thus, its level is highly influenced by a number of drugs and other xenobiotics. In addition to a potential role in inducing drug degradation, CAR may function in the control of bilirubin degradation, the process by which the liver decomposes heme. As with the xenobiotic-metabolizing enzymes, species differences also exist in the ligand specificities of these nuclear receptors. For example, rifampin activates human PXR but not mouse or rat PXR, while meclizine preferentially activates mouse CAR but inhibits gene induction by human CAR.

The PPAR family has three members, α, β, and γ. PPARα is the target for the fibrate hyperlipidemic drugs (*e.g., gemfibrozil* and *fenofibrate*). While PPARα activation induces target genes encoding fatty acid metabolizing enzymes that lower serum triglycerides, it also induces CYP4 enzymes that carry out the oxidation of fatty acids and drugs with fatty acid–containing side chains, such as *leukotrienes* and *arachidonic acid* analogs.

DRUG METABOLISM, DRUG DEVELOPMENT, AND THE SAFE AND EFFECTIVE USE OF DRUGS Drug metabolism influences drug efficacy and safety. A substantial percentage (~50%) of drugs associated with adverse responses are metabolized by xenobiotic-metabolizing enzymes, notably the CYPs. Many of these CYPs are subject to induction and inhibition by drugs, dietary factors, and other environmental agents. This can result in decreases in drug efficacy and half life; conversely, changes in CYP activity can result in drug accumulation to toxic levels. Thus, before a new drug application is filed with the FDA, the routes of metabolism and the enzymes involved in this metabolism must be established, so that relevant polymorphisms of metabolic enzymes are identified and potential drug interactions can be predicted and avoided.

Historically, drug candidates have been administered to rodents at doses well above the human target dose in order to predict acute toxicity. For drug candidates that will be used chronically in humans, long-term carcinogenicity studies are carried out in rodent models. For determination of metabolism, the compound is subjected to interaction with human liver cells or extracts from these cells that contain the drug-metabolizing enzymes. Such studies determine how humans will metabolize a particular drug, and to a limited extent, predict its rate of metabolism. If a CYP is involved, a panel of recombinant CYPs can be used to determine which CYP predominates in the metabolism of the drug. If a single CYP, such as CYP3A4, is found to be the sole CYP that metabolizes a drug candidate, then a decision can be made about the likelihood of drug interactions. Interactions arise when multiple drugs are simultaneously administered, for example in elderly patients, who on a daily basis may take prescribed anti-inflammatory drugs, cholesterol-lowering drugs, blood pressure medications, a gastric-acid suppressant, an anticoagulant, and a number of over-the-counter medications. Ideally, a candidate drug would be metabolized by several CYPs, so that variability in expression levels of one CYP or drug-drug interactions would not significantly impact its overall metabolism and pharmacokinetics.

Similar studies can be carried out with phase 2 enzymes and drug transporters in order to predict the metabolic fate of a drug. In addition to the use of recombinant human xenobiotic-metabolizing enzymes in predicting drug metabolism, human receptor–based (PXR and CAR) systems should also be used to determine whether a particular drug candidate could be a ligand for PXR, CAR, or PPARα.

For a complete Bibliographical listing see Goodman & Gilman's *The Pharmacological Basis of Therapeutics*, 11th ed., or Goodman & Gilman Online at www.accessmedicine.com.

4

PHARMACOGENETICS

Pharmacogenetics is the study of the genetic basis for variation in drug response; it also encompasses pharmacogenomics, which employs tools for surveying the entire genome to assess multigenic determinants of drug response. Technical advances in genomics permit genotype-to-phenotype analyses in which genomic polymorphisms are exploited to assess whether a particular genomic variability translates into phenotypic variability of drug response.

Importance of Pharmacogenetics to Variability in Drug Response

An individual's response to a given drug depends on a complex interplay among many environmental and genetic factors (Figure 4–1). Genetic factors account for most of the variation in metabolic rates for many drugs. Heritability can account for 75–85% of the variability in pharmacokinetic half-lives for drugs that are eliminated by metabolism. Cytotoxicity of drugs also appears to be heritable.

Several genetic polymorphisms of drug-metabolizing enzymes result in monogenic traits in which genotype predicts phenotype. In retrospective analyses, half of adverse drug reactions were associated with drugs that are substrates for polymorphic drug-metabolizing enzymes. Thus, drugs metabolized by enzymes that exhibit polymorphic activity, which make up only 22% of all drugs, disproportionately account for adverse drug reactions. Prospective genotype determinations of these enzymes may allow us to avoid many adverse drug reactions.

GENOMIC BASIS OF PHARMACOGENETICS
Types of Genetic Variants

A *polymorphism* is a variation in the DNA sequence that is present at an allele frequency of 1% or greater in a population. Two major types of sequence variation have been associated with variation in human phenotype: *single nucleotide polymorphisms* (SNPs) and *insertions/deletions* (indels) (Figure 4–2). SNPs are present in the human genome at approximately one SNP every few hundred to a thousand base pairs, depending on the gene region. Indels are much less frequent, particularly in coding regions of genes.

SNPs in the coding region are termed *cSNPs* and are further classified as nonsynonymous (or *missense*) if the base pair change results in an amino acid substitution, synonymous (or *sense*) if the base pair substitution within a codon does not alter the encoded amino acid, and *nonsense* if they introduce a stop codon. Typically, substitutions of the third base pair in a codon, the *wobble position*, do not alter the encoded amino acid. In addition, about 10% of SNPs can have more than two possible alleles (*e.g.*, a C can be replaced by either an A or G), so that the same polymorphic site can be associated with amino acid substitutions in some alleles but not others.

Polymorphisms in noncoding regions of genes may occur in the 5′ and 3′ untranslated regions, in promoter or enhancer regions, in intronic regions, or in large intergenic regions between genes. Intronic polymorphisms found near exon-intron boundaries are often treated as a distinct category from other intronic polymorphisms, since they may affect splicing and thereby affect function. Noncoding SNPs in promoters/enhancers or in 5′ and 3′ untranslated regions may affect gene transcription or transcript stability. Noncoding SNPs in introns or exons may create alternative splicing sites, and the altered transcript may have fewer or more exons, or shorter or larger exons, than the wild-type transcript. Introduction or deletion of exonic sequence can cause a frame shift in the translated protein and thereby change protein structure or function, or can result in an early stop codon, producing an unstable or nonfunctional protein. Because 95% of the genome is intergenic, most polymorphisms are unlikely to directly affect the encoded transcript or protein. However, intergenic polymorphisms may have biological consequences by affecting DNA tertiary structure, interaction with chromatin and topoisomerases, or DNA replication. Thus, intergenic polymorphisms cannot be assumed to be pharmacogenetically insignificant.

A remarkable degree of diversity is evident in the types of insertions/deletions that are tolerated as germline polymorphisms. One common polymorphism in glutathione-S-transferase M1 (*GSTM1*) is caused by a 50-kilobase (kb) germline deletion; the null allele has a population frequency of 0.3–0.5, depending on race/ethnicity. In biochemical studies, homozygous null individuals have only ~50% of the liver glutathione conjugating capacity of those with at least one copy of the *GSTM1* gene. In the *UGT1A1* promoter, the number of TA repeats affects the quantitative

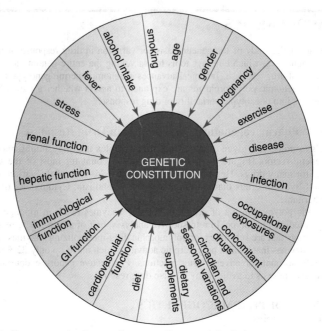

FIGURE 4–1 *Exogenous and endogenous factors contribute to variation in drug response.*

expression of this crucial glucuronosyl transferase in liver. Finally, a common 68 base pair indel polymorphism in cystathionine β-synthase has been linked to folate levels.

A *haplotype*, defined as a series of linked polymorphisms on a chromosome, specifies the DNA sequence variation on one chromosome. For example, consider two SNPs in *ABCB1* encoding the P-glycoprotein multidrug resistance protein: a T to A base pair substitution at position 3421 and a C to T change at position 3435. Possible haplotypes are $T_{3421}C_{3435}$, $T_{3421}T_{3435}$, $A_{3421}C_{3435}$, and $A_{3421}T_{3435}$. For any gene, individuals will have two haplotypes, one maternal and one paternal in origin, which may or may not be identical. Haplotypes are important because they are the functional unit of the gene. That is, a haplotype represents the constellation of variants that occur together for the gene on each chromosome. In some cases, this constellation of variants, rather than the individual variant or allele, may be functionally important. In others, however, a single mutation may be functionally important regardless of other variants within the haplotype(s).

Ethnic Diversity

Polymorphisms differ in their frequencies within human populations. Among coding region SNPs, synonymous SNPs are present, on average, at higher frequencies than nonsynonymous SNPs. For most genes, the nucleotide diversity, which reflects the number and the frequency of the SNPs, is greater for synonymous than for nonsynonymous SNPs. This reflects selective pressures (termed *negative* or *purifying selection*) that act to preserve the functional activity, and hence the amino acid sequence, of proteins. In human population studies using whole genome scanning, polymorphisms have been classified as either cosmopolitan (*i.e.*, present in all ethnic groups) or population (or race and ethnic) specific. Cosmopolitan polymorphisms are present in all ethnic groups, although frequencies may differ among ethnic groups; they usually are found at higher allele frequencies in comparison to population-specific polymorphisms and are evolutionarily older.

African Americans have the highest number of population-specific polymorphisms in comparison to European Americans, Mexican Americans, and Asian Americans. Africans are believed to be the oldest population and therefore carry both recently derived, population-specific polymorphisms, and older cosmopolitan polymorphisms that occurred before migrations out of Africa.

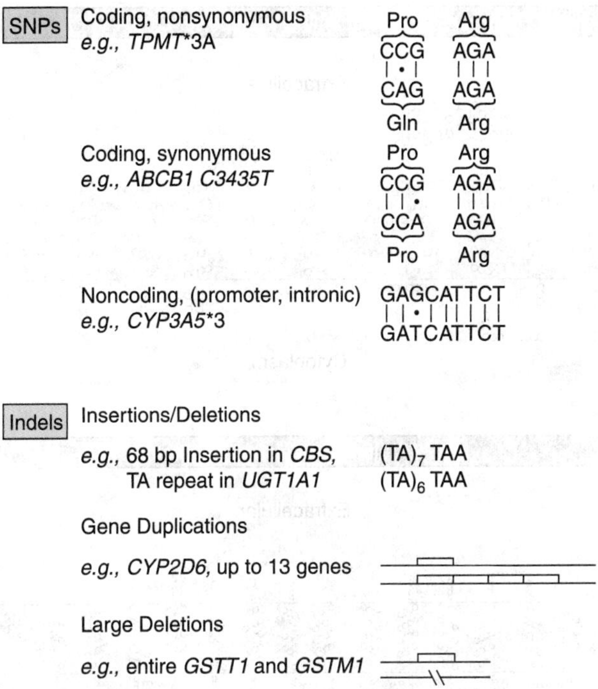

SNps	Coding, nonsynonymous e.g., TPMT*3A	Pro CCG | • | CAG Gln	Arg AGA | | | AGA Arg

Coding, synonymous
e.g., ABCB1 C3435T

Pro Arg
CCG AGA
\| \| • \| \| \|
CCA AGA
Pro Arg

Noncoding, (promoter, intronic)
e.g., CYP3A5*3

GAGCATTCT
\| \| • \| \| \| \| \| \|
GATCATTCT

Indels	Insertions/Deletions

e.g., 68 bp Insertion in CBS,   (TA)$_7$ TAA
        TA repeat in UGT1A1   (TA)$_6$ TAA

Gene Duplications

e.g., CYP2D6, up to 13 genes

Large Deletions

e.g., entire GSTT1 and GSTM1

FIGURE 4–2 *Molecular mechanisms of genetic polymorphisms.* The most common genetic variants are single nucleotide polymorphism substitutions (SNPs). *Coding nonsynonymous* SNPs result in a nucleotide substitution that changes the amino acid codon (here proline to glutamine), which could change protein structure, stability, substrate affinities, or introduce a stop codon. *Coding synonymous* SNPs do not change the amino acid codon, but may have functional consequences (transcript stability, splicing). Noncoding SNPs may be in promoters, introns, or other regulatory regions that may affect transcription factor binding, enhancers, transcript stability, or splicing. The second major types of polymorphism are *indels* (*insertion/deletions*). Indels can have any of the same effects as SNP substitutions: short repeats in the promoter (which can affect transcript amount), or larger insertions/deletions that add or subtract amino acids. Indels can also involve gene duplications, stably transmitted inherited germline gene replication that causes increased protein expression and activity, or gene deletions that result in the complete lack of protein production. All of these mechanisms have been implicated in common germline pharmacogenetic polymorphisms. TPMT, thiopurine methyltransferase; ABCB1, the multidrug resistance transporter (P-glycoprotein); CYP, cytochrome P450; CBS, cystathionine β-synthase; UGT, UDP-glucuronyl transferase; GST, glutathione-S-transferase.

Consider the coding region variants of two membrane transporters (Figure 4–3). Shown are nonsynonymous and synonymous SNPs; population-specific nonsynonymous cSNPs are indicated in the figure. The multidrug resistance associated protein, MRP2, has a large number of nonsynonymous cSNPs. There are fewer synonymous variants than nonsynonymous variants, but the allele frequencies of the synonymous variants are greater than those of the nonsynonymous variants. By comparison, the dopamine transporter DAT has a number of synonymous variants but no nonsynonymous variants, suggesting that selective pressures have acted against substitutions that led to changes in amino acids.

In a survey of coding region haplotypes in ~300 different genes in 80 ethnically diverse DNA samples, most genes were found to have between 2 and 53 haplotypes, with the average number of haplotypes in a gene being 14. Like SNPs, haplotypes may be cosmopolitan or population specific and ~20% of the over 4000 identified haplotypes were cosmopolitan. Considering the frequencies of the haplotypes, cosmopolitan haplotypes actually accounted for over 80% of all haplotypes, whereas population-specific haplotypes accounted for only 8%.

Polymorphism Selection

Genetic variations sometimes cause a "disease" phenotype. Due to the disease, some evolutionary selection against these single-gene polymorphisms is present. Cystic fibrosis, sickle-cell anemia,

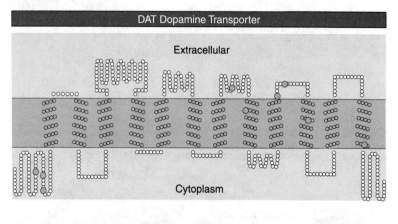

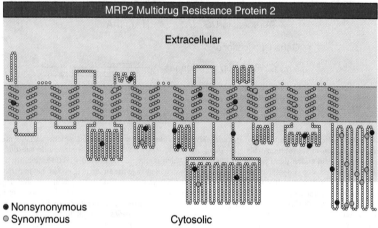

● Nonsynonymous
◎ Synonymous

FIGURE 4–3 *Coding region polymorphisms in two membrane transporters.* Shown are the dopamine transporter, DAT (encoded by SLCGA3) and multidrug resistance associated protein, MRP2 (encoded by ABCC2). Coding region variants were identified in 247 ethnically diverse DNA samples (100 African Americans, 100 European Americans, 30 Asians, 10 Mexicans, and 7 Pacific Islanders). Shown in light gray are synonymous variants, and in black, nonsynonymous variants.

and Crigler-Najjar syndrome are examples of inherited diseases caused by single gene defects. Crigler-Najjar syndrome is a severe genetic disorder caused by rare inactivating mutations in *UGT1A1*. More common and less deleterious polymorphisms in *UGT1A1* are associated with modest hyperbilirubinemia and altered drug clearance. Polymorphisms in other genes are highly penetrant in subjects challenged with certain drugs; these polymorphisms thus are the causes of monogenic pharmacogenetic traits. Because they are not deleterious in the constitutive state, there is unlikely to be any selective pressure for or against these polymorphisms. Most genetic polymorphisms have a modest impact on the affected genes, are part of a large array of multigenic factors that impact drug effect, or affect genes whose products play a minor role in drug action relative to large nongenetic effects. For example, phenobarbital induction of metabolism may be such an overwhelming "environmental" effect that polymorphisms in the affected transcription factors and drug-metabolizing enzymes have relatively modest effects.

PHARMACOGENETIC STUDY DESIGN CONSIDERATIONS
Pharmacogenetic Measures

A *pharmacogenetic trait* is any measurable or discernible trait associated with a drug, including enzyme activity, drug or metabolite levels in plasma or urine, effects on blood pressure or lipid levels, and drug-induced gene expression patterns. Directly measuring a trait (*e.g.*, enzyme activity) has the advantage that the net effect of the contributions of all genes that influence the trait is reflected in the phenotypic measure but the disadvantage is that it also reflects nongenetic influences (*e.g.*, diet, drug interactions, diurnal, or hormonal fluctuation) and thus, may be "unstable." For example, if a patient is given an oral dose of *dextromethorphan*, and the urinary ratio of parent drug to metabolite is assessed, the phenotype reflects the CYP2D6 genotype. If dextromethorphan instead is given with *quinidine*, a potent CYP2D6 inhibitor, the ratio may indicate a poor metabolizer genotype even though the subject carries wild-type CYP2D6 alleles. In other words, quinidine coadministration may result in a drug-induced enzymatic deficiency, and the false assignment to a CYP2D6 poor metabolizer phenotype. Lack of consistency for a given subject in a phenotypic measure, such as the erythromycin breath test for CYP3A, indicates that the phenotype is influenced by nongenetic factors and may indicate a multigenic or weakly penetrant effect of a monogenic trait. Because most pharmacogenetic traits are multigenic rather than monogenic (Figure 4–4), considerable effort is being made to identify the important genes and their polymorphisms that influence variability in drug response.

Most genotyping methods use genomic DNA that is extracted from somatic, diploid cells, usually white blood cells or buccal cells due to their ready accessibility. DNA is extremely stable if appropriately extracted and stored; unlike many laboratory tests, genotyping need be performed only once because DNA sequence is generally constant throughout an individual's lifetime. Although tremendous progress has been made in molecular biological techniques to determine genotypes, relatively few pharmacogenetic tests are used routinely in patient care. Genotyping tests are directed at each specific known polymorphic site using a variety of strategies that generally depend at some level on the specific and avid annealing of at least one oligonucleotide to a region of DNA flanking or overlapping the polymorphic site. Because genomic variability is so common (with polymorphic sites every few hundred nucleotides), "cryptic" or unrecognized polymorphisms may interfere with oligonucleotide annealing, thereby resulting in false-positive or false-negative genotype assignments. Full integration of genotyping into therapeutics will require high standards for genotyping technology, perhaps with more than one method required for each polymorphic site.

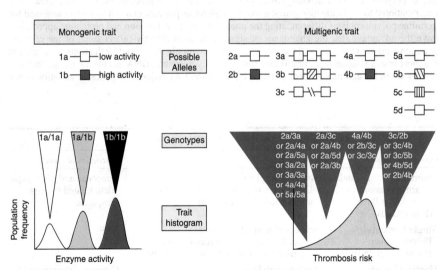

FIGURE 4–4 *Monogenic versus multigenic pharmacogenetic traits.* Possible alleles for a monogenic trait (*upper left*), in which a single gene has a low-activity (1a) and a high-activity (1b) allele. The population frequency distribution of a monogenic trait (*bottom left*), here depicted as enzyme activity, may exhibit a trimodal frequency distribution with relatively distinct separation among low activity (homozygous for 1a), intermediate activity (heterozygous for 1a and 1b), and high activity (homozygous for 1b). This is contrasted with multigenic traits (*e.g.*, an activity influenced by up to four different genes, genes 2 through 5), each of which has 2, 3, or 4 possible alleles (a through d). The population histogram for activity is unimodal-skewed, with no distinct differences among the genotypic groups. Multiple combinations of alleles coding for low activity and high activity at several of the genes can translate into low-, medium-, and high-activity phenotypes.

Because polymorphisms are so common, the allelic structure that indicates whether polymorphisms within a gene are on the same or different alleles (their haplotype) may also be important. Experimental methods to unambiguously confirm whether polymorphisms are allelic are technically challenging so statistical probability is often used to assign putative or inferred haplotypes.

Candidate Gene *versus* Genome-Wide Approaches

After genes in drug response pathways are identified, the next step in the design of a candidate gene association pharmacogenetic study is to identify genetic polymorphisms that are most likely to contribute to the therapeutic and/or adverse responses. There are several databases that contain information on polymorphisms and mutations in human genes (Table 4–1) that allow the investigator to search by gene for reported polymorphisms. Some databases, such as the Pharmacogenetics and Pharmacogenomics Knowledge Base, include phenotypic and genotypic data.

Because it is currently impractical to analyze all polymorphisms in a candidate gene association study, it is important to select polymorphisms that most likely are associated with the drug-response phenotype. For this purpose, there are two categories of polymorphisms. Some polymorphisms do not directly alter function of the expressed protein (*e.g.*, they don't affect the enzyme that metabolizes the drug or the drug receptor). Rather, these polymorphisms are linked to the variant allele that alters function. If they are very tightly linked with the causative polymorphism, these polymorphisms nonetheless may serve as surrogates for drug-response phenotype.

The second type of polymorphism is the *causative polymorphism,* which directly produces the phenotype. Whenever possible, it is desirable to select polymorphisms for pharmacogenetic studies that are likely to be causative. If biological information indicates that a particular polymorphism alters function, this polymorphism is an excellent candidate to use in an association study.

A potential drawback of the candidate gene approach is that the wrong genes may be studied. Genome-wide approaches, using gene expression arrays, genome-wide scans, or proteomics, can complement the candidate gene approach by providing a relatively unbiased survey of the genome to identify previously unrecognized candidate genes. For example, RNA, DNA, or protein from patients who have unacceptable toxicity from a drug can be compared with corresponding material from identically treated patients who did not exhibit such toxicity. Patterns of gene expression, clusters of polymorphisms or heterozygosity, or relative amounts of proteins can be ascertained using computational tools, to identify genes, genomic regions, or proteins that can be further assessed for germline polymorphisms differentiating the phenotype. Gene expression and proteomic approaches have the advantage that the abundance of signal may itself directly reflect some of the relevant genetic variation; however, both types of expression are highly influenced by the tissue studied, and the most relevant tissue (*e.g.*, brain) may not be readily available. DNA has the advantage that it is readily available and independent of tissue type, but the vast majority of genomic variation is not

Table 4–1

Databases Containing Information on Human Genetic Variation

Database Name	URL (Agency)	Description of Contents
Pharmacogenetics and Pharmacogenomics Knowledge Base (PharmGKB)	www.pharmgkb.org (NIH Sponsored Research Network and Knowledge Database)	Genotype and phenotype data related to drug response
Single Nucleotide Polymorphism Database (dbSNP)	www.ncbi.nlm.nih.gov/entrez query.fcgi?db=snp (National Center for Biotechnology Information, NCBI)	SNP
Human Genome Variation Database (HGVbase)	hgvbase.cgb.ki.se	Genotype/phenotype associations
Human Gene Mutation Database (HGMD)	www.hgmd.org	Mutations/SNPs in human genes
Online Mendelian Inheritance in Man	www.ncbi.nlm.nih.gov/entrez/ query.fcgi?db=OMIM (NCBI)	Human genes and genetic disorders

in genes, and the large number of SNPs raises the danger of type I error (finding differences that are false-positives).

Functional Studies of Polymorphisms

For most polymorphisms, functional information is not available. Therefore, it is important to predict whether a given polymorphism may result in a change in protein function, stability, or subcellular localization. One approach to understanding the functional effects of various types of genomic variations is to survey the mutations that have been associated with human Mendelian disease. DNA variations associated with diseases or traits most frequently are missense and nonsense mutations, followed by deletions. Of amino acid replacements associated with human disease, there is a high representation at residues that are most conserved evolutionarily. More radical changes in amino acids also are more likely to be associated with disease than more conservative changes; substitution of a charged amino acid (Arg) for a nonpolar, uncharged amino acid (Cys) is more likely to affect function than substitution of residues that are more chemically similar (*e.g.*, Arg to Lys).

With an increasing number of SNPs being identified by large-scale SNP discovery projects, computational methods are needed to predict the functional consequences. To this end, predictive algorithms have been developed to identify potentially deleterious amino acid substitutions. These methods can be classified into two groups. The first group relies on sequence comparisons alone to identify and score substitutions according to their degree of conservation across multiple species. The second group of methods relies on mapping of SNPs onto protein structures, in addition to sequence comparisons.

For many proteins—including enzymes, transporters, and receptors—the mechanisms by which amino acid substitutions alter function have been characterized in kinetic studies. Figure 4–5 shows simulated curves depicting the rate of metabolism of a substrate by two amino acid variants of an enzyme and the most common genetic form of the enzyme. The metabolism of substrate by one variant enzyme, Variant A, is characterized by an increased K_m. Such an effect can occur if the amino acid substitution alters the binding site of the enzyme leading to a decreased affinity for the substrate. An amino acid variant may also alter the maximum rate of substrate metabolism (V_{max}) by the enzyme, as exemplified by Variant B. Such reductions in V_{max} generally reflect reduced expression of the enzyme, which may occur because of decreased protein stability or changes in protein trafficking or recycling.

In contrast to studies with coding region SNPs, predicting the function of SNPs in noncoding regions of genes represents a major challenge in human genetics and pharmacogenetics. The principles of evolutionary conservation that have been validated in predicting the function of

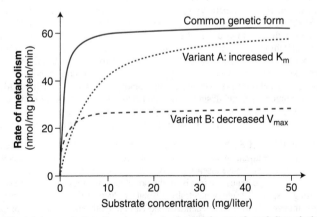

FIGURE 4–5 *Simulated concentration–dependence curves showing the rate of metabolism of a hypothetical substrate by the common genetic form of an enzyme and two nonsynonymous variants.* Variant A exhibits an increased K_m and likely reflects a change in the substrate binding site of the protein by the substituted amino acid. Variant B exhibits a change in the maximum rate of metabolism (V_{max}) of the substrate. This may be due to reduced expression level of the enzyme or to a decrease in its catalytic efficiency. Altered K_m and V_{max} may also be coexpressed in a single variant (not shown).

nonsynonymous variants in the coding region need to be refined and tested as predictors of function of SNPs in noncoding regions.

Pharmacogenetic Phenotypes

Candidate genes for therapeutic and adverse response can be divided into three categories: pharmacokinetic, receptor/target, and disease-modifying.

PHARMACOKINETICS Germline variability in genes that encode factors that determine the pharmacokinetics of a drug, in particular enzymes and transporters, affect drug concentrations and are therefore major determinants of therapeutic and adverse drug response (Table 4–2). Multiple enzymes and transporters may affect the pharmacokinetics of a given drug. Several polymorphisms in drug metabolizing enzymes are monogenic phenotypic trait variations and thus are referenced using their phenotypic designations (*e.g.*, slow *vs.* fast acetylation, extensive *vs.* poor metabolizers of debrisoquine or *sparteine*) rather than using genotypic designations that reference the gene that is the target of polymorphisms in each case (*e.g.*, NAT2 and CYP2D6, respectively). A large number of medications (~15–25% of all medicines in use) are known substrates for CYP2D6 (Table 4–2). The molecular and phenotypic characterization of multiple racial and ethnic groups has shown that seven variant alleles account for >90% of the "poor metabolizer" low-activity CYP2D6 alleles in most racial groups, that the frequency of variant alleles varies with geographic origin, and that a small percentage of individuals carry stable duplications of CYP2D6, with "ultrarapid" metabolizers having up to 13 copies of the active gene. Phenotypic consequences of the deficient CYP2D6 phenotype include increased risk of toxicity of antidepressants or antipsychotics (catabolized by the enzyme), and lack of analgesic effect of codeine (anabolized by the enzyme); conversely, the ultra-rapid phenotype is associated with extremely rapid clearance and thus decreased efficacy of antidepressants.

CYP2C19, historically termed mephenytoin hydroxylase, displays pharmacogenetic variability, with just a few SNPs accounting for the majority of the deficient, poor metabolizer phenotype. The deficient phenotype is much more common in Chinese and Japanese populations. Several proton pump inhibitors (*e.g.*, omeprazole and *lansoprazole*) are inactivated by CYP2C19. Thus, the deficient patients have higher exposure to active parent drug, a greater pharmacodynamic effect (higher gastric pH), and a higher probability of ulcer cure than heterozygotes or homozygous wild-type individuals.

The anticoagulant *warfarin* is catabolized by CYP2C9. Inactivating polymorphisms in *CYP2C9* are common—with 2–10% of most populations being homozygous for low-activity variants—and are associated with lower warfarin clearance, lower dose requirements, and a higher risk of bleeding complications.

Thiopurine methyltransferase (TPMT) methylates thiopurines such as *mercaptopurine* (an antileukemic drug that is also the product of *azathioprine* metabolism). One in 300 individuals is homozygous deficient, 10% are heterozygotes, and about 90% are homozygous for wild-type *TPMT* alleles. Three SNPs account for over 90% of the inactivating alleles. Because methylation of mercaptopurine competes with activation of the drug to thioguanine nucleotides, the concentration of the active (but also toxic) thioguanine metabolites is inversely related to TPMT activity and directly related to the probability of pharmacologic effects. Dose reductions (from that appropriate for the "average" population) may be required to avoid myelosuppression in 100% of homozygous deficient patients, 35% of heterozygotes, and only 7–8% of those with homozygous wild-type activity. Mercaptopurine has a narrow therapeutic range, and dosing by trial and error can place patients at higher risk of toxicity; thus, prospective adjustment of thiopurine doses based on *TPMT* genotype has been proposed, both for leukemia and for nonmalignant diseases such as Crohn's disease and transplant rejection.

PHARMACOGENETICS AND DRUG TARGETS Gene products that are direct drug targets have important roles in pharmacogenetics. Whereas highly penetrant genetic variants with profound functional consequences may cause disease phenotypes that confer negative selective pressure, more subtle variations in the same genes can persist in the population without causing disease but nonetheless affecting drug response. Methylenetetrahydrofolate reductase (MTHFR), the target of several antifolate drugs, interacts with folate-dependent one-carbon synthesis reactions. Complete inactivation *via* rare point mutations in MTHFR causes severe mental retardation and premature cardiovascular disease. Whereas rare variants in *MTHFR* may result in the severe phenotype, the C677T SNP causes an amino acid substitution that is maintained in the population at a high frequency. The T variant is associated with modestly lower MTHFR activity (~30% less than the 677C allele) and modest, but significantly elevated, plasma homocysteine concentrations This polymorphism does not alter

Table 4–2

Examples of Genetic Polymorphisms Influencing Drug Response

Gene Product (Gene)	Drugs	Responses Affected
Drug metabolizing enzymes		
CYP2C9	Tolbutamide, warfarin, phenytoin, nonsteroidal anti-inflammatories	Anticoagulant effect of warfarin
CYP2C19	Mephenytoin, omeprazole, hexobarbital, mephobarbital, propranolol, proguanil, phenytoin	Peptic ulcer response to omeprazole
CYP2D6	β blockers, antidepressants, antipsychotics, codeine, debrisoquine, dextromethorphan, encainide, flecainide, fluoxetine, guanoxan, N-propylajmaline, perhexiline, phenacetin, phenformin, propafenone, sparteine	Tardive dyskinesia from antipsychotics, narcotic side effects, codeine efficacy, imipramine dose requirement, β blocker effect
CYP3A4/3A5/3A7	Macrolides, cyclosporine, tacrolimus, Ca²⁺ channel blockers, midazolam, terfenadine, lidocaine, dapsone, quinidine, triazolam, etoposide, teniposide, lovastatin, alfentanil, tamoxifen, steroids	Efficacy of immunosuppressive effects of tacrolimus
Dihydropyrimidine dehydrogenase	Fluorouracil	5-Fluorouracil neurotoxicity
N-acetyltransferase (*NAT2*)	Isoniazid, hydralazine, sulfonamides, amonafide, procainamide, dapsone, caffeine	Hypersensitivity to sulfonamides, amonafide toxicity, hydralazine-induced lupus, isoniazid neurotoxicity
Glutathione transferases (*GSTM1, GSTT1, GSTP1*)	Several anticancer agents	Decreased response in breast cancer, more toxicity and worse response in acute myelogenous leukemia
Thiopurine methyl-transferase (*TPMT*)	Mercaptopurine, thioguanine, azathioprine	Thiopurine toxicity and efficacy, risk of second cancers
UDP-glucuronosyl-transferase (*UGT1A1*)	Irinotecan, bilirubin	Irinotecan toxicity
P-glycoprotein (*ABCB1*)	Natural product anticancer drugs, HIV protease inhibitors, digoxin	Decreased CD4 response in HIV-infected patients, decreased digoxin AUC, drug resistance in epilepsy
UGT2B7	Morphine	Morphine plasma levels
COMT	Levodopa	Enhanced drug effect
CYP2B6	Cyclophosphamide	Ovarian failure

(Continued)

65

Table 4-2

Examples of Genetic Polymorphisms Influencing Drug Response (Continued)

Gene Product (Gene)	Drugs	Responses Affected
Targets and receptors		
Angiotensin-converting enzyme (ACE)	ACE inhibitors (e.g., enalapril)	Renoprotective effects, hypotension, left ventricular mass reduction, cough
Thymidylate synthase	Methotrexate	Leukemia response, colorectal cancer response
β_2-Adrenergic receptor (*ADBR2*)	β_2 Antagonists (e.g., albuterol, terbutaline)	Bronchodilation, susceptibility to agonist-induced desensitization, cardiovascular effects (e.g., increased heart rate, cardiac index, peripheral vasodilation)
β_1-Adrenergic receptor (*ADBR1*)	β_1 Antagonists	Response to β_1 antagonists
5-Lipoxygenase (*ALOX5*)	Leukotriene receptor antagonists	Asthma response
Dopamine receptors (D_2, D_3, D_4)	Antipsychotics (e.g., haloperidol, clozapine, thioridazine, nemonapride)	Antipsychotic response (D_2, D_3, D_4), antipsychotic-induced tardive dyskinesia (D_3) and acute akathisia (D_3), hyperprolactinemia in females (D_2)
Estrogen receptor α	Estrogen hormone replacement therapy	High-density lipoprotein cholesterol
Serotonin transporter (SERT)	Antidepressants (e.g., clomipramine, fluoxetine, paroxetine, fluvoxamine)	Clozapine effects, 5-HT neurotransmission, antidepressant response
Serotonin receptor (5-HT_{2A})	Antipsychotics	Clozapine antipsychotic response, tardive dyskinesia, paroxetine antidepression response, drug discrimination
HMG-CoA reductase	Pravastatin	Reduction in serum cholesterol
Modifiers		
Adducin	Diuretics	Myocardial infarction or strokes
Apolipoprotein E	Statins (e.g., simvastatin), tacrine	Lipid-lowering; clinical improvement in Alzheimer's
Modifiers, continued		
Human leukocyte antigen	Abacavir	Hypersensitivity reactions
Cholesteryl ester transfer protein	Statins (e.g., pravastatin)	Slowing atherosclerosis progression
Ion channels (*HERG*, *KvLQT1*, *Mink*, *MiRP1*)	Erythromycin, cisapride, clarithromycin, quinidine	Increased risk of drug-induced *torsades de pointes*, increased QT interval
Methylguanine-deoxyribonucleic acid methyltransferase	Carmustine	Response of glioma to carmustine
Parkin	Levodopa	Parkinson's disease response
MTHFR	Methotrexate	Gastrointestinal toxicity
Prothrombin, factor V	Oral contraceptives	Venous thrombosis risk
Stromelysin-1	Statins (e.g., pravastatin)	Reduction in cardiovascular events and in repeat angioplasty
Vitamin D receptor	Estrogen	Bone mineral density

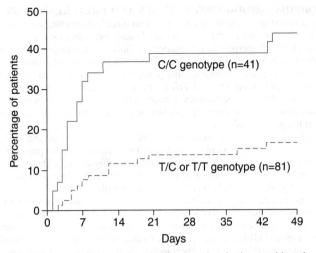

FIGURE 4-6 *Pharmacodynamics and pharmacogenetics.* The proportion of patients requiring a dosage decrease for the antidepressant drug paroxetine was greater ($p = 0.001$) in the approximately one-third of patients who have the C/C genotype for the serotonin 2A receptor ($5HT_{2A}$) compared to the two-thirds of patients who have either the T/C or T/T genotype at position 102. The major reason for dosage decreases in paroxetine was the occurrence of adverse drug effects.

drug pharmacokinetics but apparently modulates pharmacodynamics by predisposing to GI toxicity of the antifolate drug *methotrexate* in transplant recipients. Following prophylactic treatment with methotrexate for graft-*versus*-host disease, mucositis was three times more common in patients homozygous for the 677T allele than in those homozygous for the 677C allele.

Many polymorphisms in drug targets predict responsiveness to drugs (Table 4–2). Serotonin receptor polymorphisms predict not only the responsiveness to antidepressants (Figure 4–6), but also the overall risk of depression. β adrenergic receptor polymorphisms have been linked to asthma responsiveness after β agonist therapy, renal function following angiotensin-converting enzyme (ACE) inhibitors, and heart rate following β-blockers. Polymorphisms in 3-hydroxy-3-methylglutaryl coenzyme A reductase have been linked to the degree of lipid lowering following statins, which are inhibitors of this enzyme (*see* Chapter 35), and to the degree of elevation of high-density lipoproteins among women on estrogen replacement therapy (Figure 4–7).

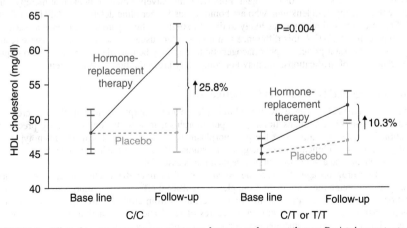

FIGURE 4-7 *Effect of genotype on response to estrogen hormone replacement therapy.* Depicted are pretreatment (base line) and posttreatment (follow-up) high-density lipoprotein (HDL) cholesterol levels in women of the C/C *vs.* C/T or T/T HMG-CoA reductase genotype.

POLYMORPHISM-MODIFYING DISEASES AND DRUG RESPONSES   Some genes may affect the underlying disease being treated without directly interacting with the drug. Modifier polymorphisms are important for the *de novo* risk of some events and for the risk of drug-induced events. The *MTHFR* polymorphism, for example, is linked to homocysteinemia, which in turn affects thrombosis risk. The risk of a drug-induced thrombosis is dependent not only on the use of prothrombotic drugs, but on environmental and genetic predisposition to thrombosis, which may be affected by germline polymorphisms in *MTHFR*, factor V, and prothrombin. These polymorphisms do not directly affect the pharmacokinetics or pharmacodynamics of prothrombotic drugs, such as glucocorticoids, estrogens, and asparaginase, but may modify the risk of the phenotypic event (thrombosis) in the presence of the drug.

Likewise, polymorphisms in ion channels (*e.g., HERG*, KvLQT1, Mink, and *MiRP1*) may affect the overall risk of cardiac dysrhythmias, which may be accentuated in the presence of a drug that can prolong the QT interval (*e.g.,* macrolide antibiotics, antihistamines). These modifier polymorphisms may impact on the risk of "disease" phenotypes even in the absence of drug challenges; in the presence of drug, the "disease" phenotype may be elicited.

In addition to the underlying germline variation of the host, tumors also harbor somatically-acquired mutations, and the efficacy of some anticancer drugs depends on the genetics of both the host and the tumor. For example, non-small-cell lung cancer is treated with epidermal growth factor receptor (EGFR), such as *gefitinib*. Patients whose tumors have activating mutations in the tyrosine kinase domain of *EGFR* appear to respond better to gefitinib than those without such mutations. Thus, the receptor is altered, and at the same time, individuals with the activating mutations may be considered to have a distinct category of non-small-cell lung cancer.

Pharmacogenetics and Drug Development

Pharmacogenetics will likely impact drug development in several ways. Genome-wide approaches hold promise for identification of new drug targets and new drugs. In addition, accounting for genetic/genomic interindividual variability may lead to genotype-specific development of new drugs and to genotype-specific dosing regimens.

Pharmacogenetics may identify subsets of patients who will have a very high or a very low likelihood of responding to an agent. This will permit testing of the drug in a selected population that is more likely to respond, minimizing the possibility of adverse events in patients who derive no benefit, and more tightly defining the parameters of response in the subset more likely to benefit.

A related role for pharmacogenomics in drug development is to identify genetic subsets of patients who are at highest risk for a serious adverse drug effect and to avoid testing the drug in that subset of patients. For example, the identification of HLA subtypes associated with hypersensitivity to the HIV-1 reverse transcriptase inhibitor *abacavir* could theoretically identify a subset of patients who should receive alternative therapy, and thereby minimize or even abrogate hypersensitivity as an adverse effect of this agent. Following intensively timed antileukemic therapy, children with acute myeloid leukemia who are homozygous for germline deletions in GSH transferase (*GSTT1*) are almost three times as likely to die of toxicity as those patients who have at least one wild-type copy of *GSTT1*; this difference is not seen after "usual" doses of therapy. These results suggest an important principle: pharmacogenetic testing may help to identify patients who require altered dosages of medications, but may not completely preclude the use of the agents.

Pharmacogenetics in Clinical Practice

Three major types of evidence are needed to implicate a polymorphism in clinical care: screens of tissues from multiple humans linking the polymorphism to a trait; complementary preclinical functional studies indicating that the polymorphism is plausibly linked with the phenotype; and multiple supportive clinical phenotype/genotype studies. Because of the high probability of error in genotype/phenotype association studies, replication is essential.

Adjusting drug dosages for variables such as renal or liver dysfunction is accepted in drug dosing. Even though there are many examples of significant effects of polymorphisms on drug disposition (*e.g.,* Table 4–2), there is much more hesitation from clinicians to adjust doses based on genetic testing than on indirect clinical measures of renal and liver function. Existing resources permit clinicians to access information on pharmacogenetics (*see* Table 4–1).

The high frequency of functionally important polymorphisms ensures that dosing complexity will increase. Even if only one polymorphism were considered when dosing a drug, the scale of

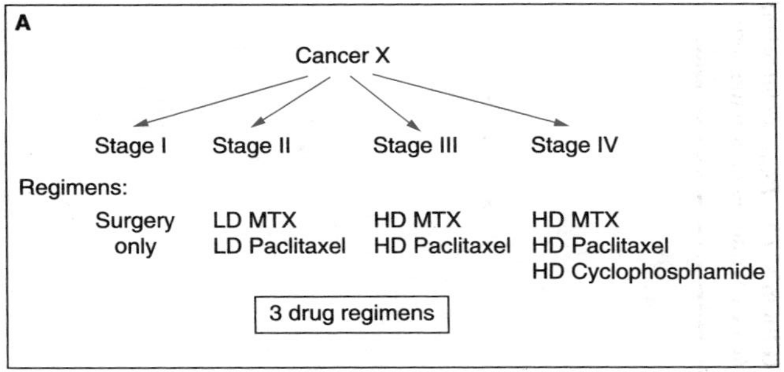

A

Cancer X → Stage I, Stage II, Stage III, Stage IV

Regimens:

Stage I	Stage II	Stage III	Stage IV
Surgery only	LD MTX, LD Paclitaxel	HD MTX, HD Paclitaxel	HD MTX, HD Paclitaxel, HD Cyclophosphamide

3 drug regimens

B Each Gene Has 2 Major Alleles / Each Drug Affected by 1 Polymorphism

Multilocus Genotype	TYMS Low	TYMS High	MDR1 Low	MDR1 High	GSTM1 Low	GSTM1 High
A	X		X		X	
B	X		X			X
C	X			X	X	
D	X			X		X
E		X	X		X	
F		X	X			X
G		X		X	X	
H		X		X		X

C Use Genotypes to Individualize Drug Regimens for Cancer X

Multilocus Genotype	Stage II MTX	Stage II Paclitaxel	Stage II Cyclo	Stage III MTX	Stage III Paclitaxel	Stage III Cyclo	Stage IV MTX	Stage IV Paclitaxel	Stage IV Cyclo
A	Low	Low	0	Low	Low	0	Low	Low	Low
B	Low	High	0	Low	High	0	Low	High	Low
C	Low	Low	0	Low	Low	0	Low	Low	High
D	Low	High	0	Low	High	0	Low	High	High
E	High	Low	0	High	Low	Low	High	High	Low
F	High	High	0	High	High	Low	High	High	High
G	High	Low	0	High	Low	Low	High	Low	Low
H	High	High	0	High	High	High	High	High	High

3 drug regimens expand to 11 regimens

FIGURE 4-8 *Potential impact of incorporation of pharmacogenetics into dosing of drugs for a relatively simple therapeutic regimen.* The traditional approach to treatment for a disease (A), in this case a cancer, is based purely on stage of the cancer. With this strategy, some with stage II disease are not receiving as much drug as they could tolerate; some patients with stage III or IV disease are undertreated and some are overtreated. Panel **B** illustrates a hypothetical patient population with eight different multilocus genotypes. It is assumed that each of the three drugs is affected by just one genetic polymorphism (*TYMS* for methotrexate [MTX], *MDR1* for paclitaxel, and *GSTM1* for cyclophosphamide), and each polymorphism has just two important genotypes (one coding for low and one for high activity). The possible multilocus genotypes are designated by the letters A to H, and the combinations of *TYMS*, *MDR1* and *GSTM1* genotypes giving rise to those multilocus genotypes are indicated in the table. If these three genotypes, along with stage of cancer, are used to individualize dosages (C), so that those with low activity receive lower doses and those with higher activity receive higher doses of the relevant drug, what began as a total of three drug regimens in the absence of pharmacogenetics becomes 11 regimens (distinguished by different backgrounds and font colors) by using pharmacogenetics for dosage individualization.

complexity could be large. Many individuals take multiple drugs simultaneously for different diseases, while many therapeutic regimens for a single disease include multiple agents. All of this translates into a plethora of possible drug-dose combinations. The promise of human genomics has emphasized the potential to discover individualized "magic bullets", while ignoring the reality of the added complexity of additional testing and need for interpretation of results to capitalize on individualized dosing. This is illustrated in Figure 4–8. In this case, a traditional anticancer treatment regimen is replaced with one that incorporates pharmacogenetic information with the stage of the cancer determined by a variety of standardized pathological criteria. Assuming just one important genetic polymorphism for each of the three different anticancer drugs, 11 individual drug regimens are generated.

The potential utility of pharmacogenetics in drug therapy is great. Once adequate genotype/phenotype studies have been conducted, molecular diagnostic tests will be developed that detect >95% of the important genetic variants for the most polymorphisms; such genetic tests have the advantage that they need only be conducted once in a given individual. Continued incorporation of pharmacogenetics into clinical trials will identify important genes and polymorphisms demonstrate whether dosage individualization can improve outcomes and decrease adverse effects. Significant covariates will be identified to refine dosing in the context of drug interactions and disease influences. Although the challenges are substantial, accounting for the genetic basis of variability in response to medications is likely to be a fundamental component of disease diagnosis and pharmacotherapy.

For a complete Bibliographical listing see Goodman & Gilman's *The Pharmacological Basis of Therapeutics*, 11th ed., or Goodman & Gilman Online at www.accessmedicine.com.

5

THE SCIENCE OF DRUG THERAPY

Optimal therapeutic decisions are based on an evaluation of the patient and assessment of the evidence for efficacy and safety of treatment. Therapy must be guided by an understanding of drug pharmacokinetics and pharmacodynamics that is integrated with patient-focused information. Well-designed and executed clinical trials provide the scientific evidence that informs most therapeutic decisions; they may be supplemented by *observational studies*, particularly in assessing adverse effects that elude detection in clinical trials.

Clinical Trials

In clinical trials, random assignment of patients or volunteers to the control group or the group receiving the experimental therapy is the optimal method for distributing the known and unknown variables that affect outcome between the treatment and control groups. Randomized clinical trials may be impossible to use studying all experimental therapies; for patients who cannot—by regulation, ethics, or both—be studied with this design (*e.g.*, children or fetuses) or for disorders with a typically fatal outcome (*e.g.*, rabies), it may be necessary to use historical controls.

Concealing participant assignment is referred to as *blinding* or *masking*. Participants in the control group will receive an inactive replica of the drug, a *placebo*. In a *single-blind study*, participants are blinded to treatment assignment, but investigators are not. In a *double-blind study*, neither the participants nor the investigators know whether the active agent is being given. Blinding the investigators not only removes bias in patient management and outcome interpretation but also eliminates selectivity in the enthusiasm for therapy typically conveyed by clinicians. By eliminating participant and observer bias, the randomized, double-blind, placebo-controlled trial has the highest likelihood of revealing the truth about the effects of a drug. This design permits evaluation of subjective end points, such as pain, that are powerfully influenced by the administration of placebo. Striking examples include pain in labor, where a placebo produces ~40% of the relief provided by the opioid analgesic *meperidine* with a remarkably similar time course, angina pectoris, where as much as a 60% improvement in symptoms is achieved with placebo, and depression, where the response to placebo is often 60–70% as great as that of an active antidepressant drug.

The existence of a therapy known to improve disease outcome provides an ethical basis for comparing a new drug with the established treatment rather than placebo. If the aim is to show that the new drug is as effective as the comparator, then the size of the trial must be sufficiently large to have the statistical power needed to demonstrate a meaningful difference. Trials conducted against comparators as controls can be misleading if they claim equal efficacy based on the lack of a statistical difference between the drugs in a trial that was too small to demonstrate such a difference. When trials against comparator drugs examine the relative incidence of side effects, it also is important that equally effective doses of the drugs are used.

A clear hypothesis should guide the selection of a *primary endpoint*, which should be specified before the trial is initiated. Ideally, this primary endpoint will measure a clinical outcome, either a disease-related outcome, such as improvement of survival or reduction of myocardial infarction, or a symptomatic outcome, such as pain relief or quality of life. Examination of a single, prospectively selected endpoint will most likely yield a valid result. A few additional (secondary) endpoints also may be designated in advance; the greater the number of such endpoints examined, the greater the likelihood that apparently significant changes in one of them will occur by chance. The least rigorous examination of trial results comes from retrospective selection of endpoints after viewing the data. This introduces a selection bias and increases the probability of a chance result; retrospective selection therefore should be used only as the basis to generate hypotheses that then can be tested prospectively.

Therapeutic decisions sometimes must be based on trials evaluating surrogate endpoints—measures such as clinical signs or laboratory findings that are correlated with but do not directly measure clinical outcome. Such surrogate endpoints include measurements of blood pressure (for antihypertensive drugs), plasma glucose (drugs for diabetes), and level of viral RNA in plasma (for antiretroviral drugs). The extent to which surrogate endpoints predict clinical outcome varies, and two drugs with the same effect on a surrogate endpoint may have different effects on clinical outcome. The effect of a drug on a surrogate endpoint may lead to erroneous conclusions about the clinical consequences of drug administration. In one compelling example, the CAST study showed that—despite the ability of certain antiarrhythmics to suppress ventricular ectopy after myocardial infarction—the drugs actually increased the frequency of sudden cardiac death. Thus, the ultimate test of a drug's efficacy must arise from actual clinical outcomes rather than surrogate markers.

The *sample* of patients selected for a clinical trial may not be representative of the entire *population* of patients with that disease. Patients entered into a trial usually are selected according to the severity of their disease and other characteristics (*inclusion criteria*) or are excluded because of coexisting disease, concurrent therapy, or specific features of the disease itself (*exclusion criteria*). It always is important to ascertain that the clinical characteristics of an individual patient correspond with those of patients in the trial. For example, the Randomized Aldactone Evaluation Study (RALES) showed that treatment with the mineralocorticoid-receptor antagonist *spironolactone* was associated with a 30% reduction in death in patients with severe congestive heart failure. Hyperkalemia, a potential adverse effect, was seen only rarely in this study, which excluded patients with serum creatinine levels >2.5 mg/dL. With the expanded use of spironolactone after RALES was published, numerous patients, many of whom did not meet the RALES inclusion criteria, developed severe hyperkalemia. Therefore, knowledge of the criteria for selecting the patients in a trial must inform the application of study results to a given patient.

Determination of efficacy and safety is an ongoing process usually based on results from multiple randomized, double-blind, controlled trials. A *meta-analysis* of similarly designed studies that measured the same endpoint can be used to better assess possible significance of drug treatment; by narrowing confidence limits; they can strengthen the likelihood that an apparent effect is (or is not) due to the drug rather than chance.

Observational Studies

Important but infrequent adverse drug effects may escape detection in the randomized, controlled trials that demonstrate efficacy and form the basis for approval of drugs for marketing (*e.g.*, COX-2 inhibitors, *see* Chapter 26). The number of patient-years of drug exposure during a clinical trial is small relative to exposure after the drug is marketed. Furthermore, some adverse effects may have a long latency or may affect patients not included in the controlled trials. Observational studies therefore are used to examine those adverse effects that only become apparent with widespread, prolonged use.

The quality of information derived from observational studies varies with the design and depends highly on the selection of controls and the accuracy of the information on medication use. *Cohort studies* compare the occurrence of events in users and nonusers of a drug; this is the more powerful of the observational study designs. *Case-control studies* compare drug exposure among patients with an adverse outcome *versus* that in control patients. Because the control and treatment groups in an observational study are not selected randomly, they may be different in unknown ways that determine outcome independent of drug use. Because of the limitations of observational studies, their validity cannot be equated with that of randomized, controlled trials (Table 5–1). Observational studies raise questions and pose hypotheses about adverse reactions; if it is not feasible to test these hypotheses in controlled trials, then clinical decisions may be made from replicated findings from observational studies.

PATIENT-CENTERED THERAPEUTICS

Interindividual differences in drug delivery to its site(s) of action can profoundly influence therapeutic effectiveness and adverse effects. Some of the determinants of interindividual variation are

Table 5–1

A Ranking of the Quality of Comparative Studies

Randomized, controlled trials
  Double blinded
  Single blinded
  Unblinded

Observational studies
  Prospective cohort study
  Prospective case-control study
  Retrospective cohort study
  Retrospective case control study

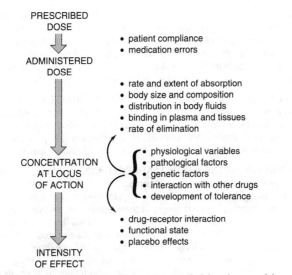

PRESCRIBED
DOSE

- patient compliance
- medication errors

ADMINISTERED
DOSE

- rate and extent of absorption
- body size and composition
- distribution in body fluids
- binding in plasma and tissues
- rate of elimination

CONCENTRATION
AT LOCUS
OF ACTION

- physiological variables
- pathological factors
- genetic factors
- interaction with other drugs
- development of tolerance

- drug-receptor interaction
- functional state
- placebo effects

INTENSITY
OF EFFECT

FIGURE 5–1 *Factors that determine the relationship between prescribed drug dosage and drug effect.*

indicated in Figure 5–1. Therapeutic success and safety result from integrating evidence of efficacy and safety with knowledge of the individual factors that determine response in a given patient.

Drug History

The starting point in the drug history is the documentation of current prescription drug use. It often is very helpful for patients to bring all current medications with them to the clinical encounter. Specific prompting is required to elicit the use of over-the-counter drugs and herbal supplements. Similarly, information about medications that are used only sporadically (*e.g., sildenafil* for erectile dysfunction) may not be volunteered. With cognitively impaired patients, it may be necessary to include caregivers and pharmacy records in the drug history process. Adverse reactions to drugs should be documented with specifics regarding severity. It is revealing to ask whether patients or their physicians have discontinued any medications in the past. A review of current drug profile and list of adverse effects are required for each patient encounter, both during hospital rounds and during outpatient visits, to maximize effectiveness and safety of treatment.

DETERMINANTS OF INTERINDIVIDUAL VARIATION IN RESPONSE TO DRUGS
Disease-Induced Alterations in Pharmacokinetics

IMPAIRED RENAL CLEARANCE OF DRUGS If a drug is cleared primarily by the kidney, dose modification should be considered in patients with renal dysfunction. When renal clearance is diminished, the desired effect can be maintained either by decreasing the dose or lengthening the dose interval. Estimation of the glomerular filtration rate (GFR) based on serum creatinine, ideal body weight, and age provides an approximation of the renal clearance of many drugs.

With knowledge of the GFR, initial dosing reductions can be estimated. The accuracy of initial dosing should be monitored by clinical assessment and plasma drug concentration where feasible.

Drug metabolites that may accumulate with impaired renal function may be pharmacologically active or toxic. Although *meperidine* is not dependent on renal function for elimination, its metabolite *normeperidine* is cleared by the kidney and accumulates when renal function is impaired. Because normeperidine has greater convulsant activity than meperidine, its high levels in renal failure probably account for the central nervous system (CNS) excitation, with irritability, twitching, and seizures, that can occur when multiple doses of meperidine are given to patients with impaired renal function (*see* Chapter 21).

IMPAIRED HEPATIC CLEARANCE OF DRUGS   The effect of liver disease on the hepatic biotransformation of drugs cannot be predicted from any measure of hepatic function. Thus, even though the metabolism of some drugs is decreased with impaired hepatic function, there is no quantitative basis for dose adjustment other than assessment of the clinical response and plasma concentration. The oral bioavailability of drugs with extensive first-pass hepatic clearance (*e.g., morphine,* meperidine, *midazolam,* and *nifedipine*) may be increased in liver disease.

CIRCULATORY INSUFFICIENCY OWING TO CARDIAC FAILURE OR SHOCK   In circulatory failure, neuroendocrine compensation can substantially reduce renal and hepatic blood flow, thereby reducing elimination of many drugs. Particularly affected are drugs with high hepatic extraction ratios, such as *lidocaine,* whose clearance is a function of hepatic blood flow; in this setting, only half the usual infusion rate of lidocaine is required to achieve therapeutic plasma levels.

ALTERED DRUG BINDING TO PLASMA PROTEINS   When a drug is highly bound to plasma proteins, its egress from the vascular compartment is limited to the unbound (free) drug. Hypoalbuminemia owing to renal insufficiency, hepatic disease, or other causes can reduce the extent of binding of acidic and neutral drugs; in these conditions, measurement of free drug provides a more accurate guide to therapy than does analysis of total drug. Changes in protein binding are particularly important for drugs that are >90% bound to plasma protein, where a small change in the extent of binding produces a large change in the level of free drug. Metabolic clearance of such highly bound drugs also is a function of the unbound fraction of drug. Thus, clearance is increased in those conditions that reduce protein binding; shorter dosing intervals therefore must be employed to maintain therapeutic plasma levels.

INTERACTIONS BETWEEN DRUGS

Marked alterations in the effects of some drugs can result from coadministration with another agent. Such interactions can cause toxicity or inhibit the drug effect and the therapeutic benefit.

Drug interactions always should be considered when unexpected responses to drugs occur. Understanding the mechanisms of drug interaction provides a framework for preventing them. Drug interactions may be *pharmacokinetic* (*i.e.,* the delivery of a drug to its site of action is altered by a second drug) or *pharmacodynamic* (*i.e.,* the response of the drug target is modified by a second drug).

Pharmacokinetic Interactions Caused by Diminished Drug Delivery to the Site of Action

For drugs administered orally, impaired gastrointestinal (GI) absorption is an important consideration. For example, aluminum ions in certain antacids or ferrous ions in oral iron supplements form insoluble chelates of *tetracycline antibiotics,* thereby preventing their absorption. The antifungal *ketoconazole* is a weak base that is only soluble at acid pH. Drugs that inhibit gastric acidity, such as the proton pump inhibitors and histamine H_2 receptor antagonists, impair the dissolution and absorption of ketoconazole.

Many drug interactions involve the CYPs that perform phase 1 metabolism of a large number of drugs (*see* Chapter 3). Their expression can be induced by a plethora of drugs, including antibiotics (*e.g., rifampin*), anticonvulsants (*e.g., phenobarbital,* phenytoin, and *carbamazepine*), nonnucleoside reverse transcriptase inhibitors (*e.g., efavirenz* and *nevirapine*), and herbal supplements (*e.g., St. John's wort*). Although these drugs most potently induce CYP3A4, the expression of CYPs in the 1A, 2B, and 2C families also can be induced. Induction of these enzymes accelerates the metabolism of drugs that are their substrates, including *cyclosporine, tacrolimus, warfarin, verapamil, methadone, dexamethasone, methylprednisolone, estrogen,* and the *HIV protease inhibitors.* The decrease in oral bioavailability from increased first-pass metabolism in the liver results in loss of efficacy.

Pharmacokinetic Interactions that Increase Drug Delivery to the Site of Action

INHIBITION OF DRUG-METABOLIZING ENZYMES   For drugs whose clearance depends on biotransformation, inhibition of a metabolizing enzyme leads to reduced clearance, prolonged $t_{1/2}$, and drug accumulation during maintenance therapy, sometimes with severe adverse effects. Knowledge of the CYP isoforms that catalyze the principal pathways of drug metabolism provides a basis for understanding and even predicting drug interactions (*see* Chapter 3).

Hepatic CYP3A isozymes catalyze the metabolism of many drugs that are subject to significant drug interactions owing to inhibition of metabolism. Drugs metabolized predominantly by CYP3A isozymes include immunosuppressants (*e.g.*, cyclosporine and tacrolimus); HMG-CoA reductase inhibitors (*e.g.*, *lovastatin, simvastatin*, and *atorvastatin*); HIV protease inhibitors (*e.g.*, *indinavir, nelfinavir, saquinavir, amprinavir,* and *ritonavir*); Ca^{2+} channel antagonists (*e.g.*, *felodipine, nifedipine, nisoldipine*, and *diltiazem*); glucocorticoids (*e.g.*, dexamethasone and *methylprednisolone*); benzodiazepines (*e.g.*, *alprazolam*, midazolam, and *triazolam*); and lidocaine.

The inhibition of CYP3A isoforms may vary even among structurally related members of a given drug class. For example, the antifungal azoles ketoconazole and *itraconazole* potently inhibit CYP3A enzymes, whereas the related *fluconazole* inhibits minimally except at high doses or in the setting of renal insufficiency. Similarly, certain macrolide antibiotics (*e.g.*, *erythromycin* and *clarithromycin*) potently inhibit CYP3A isoforms, but *azithromycin* does not. In one instance, the inhibition of CYP3A4 activity is turned to therapeutic advantage: the HIV protease inhibitor ritonavir inhibits CYP3A4 activity; when coadministered with other protease inhibitors metabolized by this pathway, ritonavir increases their half-lives and permits less frequent dosing.

Drug interactions mediated by CYP3A inhibition can be severe (*e.g.*, nephrotoxicity induced by cyclosporine and tacrolimus and rhabdomyolysis resulting from increased levels of statins). Whenever an inhibitor of the CYP3A isoforms is administered, the clinician must be cognizant of the potential for serious interactions with drugs metabolized by CYP3A.

Drug interactions also can result from inhibition of other CYPs. *Amiodarone* and its active metabolite *desethylamiodarone* promiscuously inhibit several CYPs, including CYP2C9, the principal enzyme that eliminates the active *S*-enantiomer of warfarin. Because many patients treated with amiodarone (*e.g.*, subjects with atrial fibrillation) are also receiving warfarin, the potential exists for major bleeding complications.

Knowledge of the specific pathways of metabolism of a drug and the molecular mechanisms of enzyme induction can help to identify potential interactions; thus, the pathways of drug metabolism often are determined during preclinical drug development. For example, if *in vitro* studies indicate that a compound is metabolized by CYP3A4, studies can focus on commonly used drugs that either inhibit (*e.g.*, ketoconazole) or induce (*e.g.*, rifampin) this enzyme. Other probes for the evaluation of potential drug interactions targeted at human CYPs include midazolam or erythromycin for CYP3A4 and *dextromethorphan* for CYP2D6.

INHIBITION OF DRUG TRANSPORT Drug transporters are key determinants of the availability of certain drugs to their site(s) of action, and clinically significant drug interactions can result from inhibition of drug transporters (*see* Chapter 2). P-glycoprotein, which actively transports multiple chemotherapeutic drugs out of cancer cells and renders them resistant to drug action, is expressed on the luminal aspect of intestinal epithelial cells (where it functions to inhibit xenobiotic absorption), on the luminal surface of renal tubular cells, and on the canalicular aspect of hepatocytes. Since this transporter is responsible for the elimination of certain drugs (*e.g.*, digoxin), inhibition of P-glycoprotein-mediated transport results in increased plasma levels of drug at steady state. Inhibitors of P-glycoprotein include verapamil, diltiazem, amiodarone, *quinidine,* ketoconazole, itraconazole, and erythromycin. P-glycoprotein on the capillary endothelium that forms the blood–brain barrier exports drugs from the brain, and inhibition of P-glycoprotein enhances CNS distribution of some drugs (*e.g.*, HIV protease inhibitors).

Pharmacodynamic Interactions

Combinations of drugs often are employed to therapeutic advantage when their beneficial effects are additive or synergistic or because therapeutic effects can be achieved with fewer drug-specific adverse effects by using submaximal doses of drugs in concert. Combination therapy often constitutes optimal treatment for many conditions, including heart failure (*see* Chapter 33), hypertension (*see* Chapter 32), and cancer (*see* Chapter 51). This section addresses pharmacodynamic interactions that produce adverse effects.

Nitrovasodilators (*see* Chapter 31) produce vasodilation by NO–dependent elevation of cyclic GMP in vascular smooth muscle. The pharmacologic effects of sildenafil, *tadalafil*, and *vardenafil* result from inhibition of the type 5 cyclic nucleotide phosphodiesterase (PDE5) that hydrolyzes cyclic GMP to 5′GMP in the vasculature. Thus, coadministration of an NO donor (*e.g.*, nitroglycerin) with a PDE5 inhibitor can cause potentially catastrophic hypotension.

The oral anticoagulant warfarin has a narrow margin between therapeutic inhibition of clot formation and bleeding complications and is subject to several important drug interactions (*see* Chapter 54). Nonsteroidal anti-inflammatory drugs cause gastric and duodenal ulcers (*see* Chapter 36), and their concurrent administration with warfarin increases the risk of GI bleeding almost fourfold compared with warfarin alone. By inhibiting platelet aggregation, *aspirin* increases the incidence of bleeding in warfarin-treated patients. Finally, antibiotics that alter the intestinal flora reduce the bacterial synthesis of vitamin K, thereby enhancing the effect of warfarin.

A subset of nonsteroidal anti-inflammatory drugs, including *indomethacin, ibuprofen, piroxicam,* and the *cyclooxygenase (COX)-2 inhibitors,* can antagonize antihypertensive therapy, especially with regimens employing angiotensin-converting enzyme inhibitors, angiotensin receptor antagonists, and β adrenergic receptor antagonists. The effect on arterial pressure ranges from trivial to severe. In contrast, aspirin and *sulindac* produce little, if any, elevation of blood pressure when used concurrently with these antihypertensive drugs.

Antiarrhythmic drugs that block potassium channels, such as *sotalol* and quinidine, can cause the polymorphic ventricular tachycardia known as *torsades de pointes* (*see* Chapter 34). The abnormal repolarization that leads to polymorphic ventricular tachycardia is potentiated by hypokalemia, and diuretics that produce potassium loss increase the risk of this drug-induced arrhythmia.

AGE AS A DETERMINANT OF RESPONSE TO DRUGS Most drugs are evaluated in young and middle-aged adults, and data on their use in children and the elderly are sparse. At the extremes of age, drug pharmacokinetics and pharmacodynamics can be altered, possibly requiring substantial alteration in the dose or dosing regimen to safely produce the desired clinical effect.

Children Drug disposition in childhood does not vary linearly with either body weight or body surface area, and there are no reliable, broadly applicable formulas for converting drug doses used in adults to those that are safe and effective in children. An important generality is that pharmacokinetic variability is likely to be greatest at times of physiological change (*e.g.,* the newborn or premature baby or at puberty) such that dosing adjustment, often aided by drug monitoring for drugs with narrow therapeutic indices, becomes critical for safe, effective therapeutics.

Most drug-metabolizing enzymes are expressed at low levels at birth, followed by an isozyme-specific postnatal induction. CYP2E1 and CYP2D6 appear in the first day, followed within 1 week by CYP3A4 and the CYP2C subfamily. CYP2A1 is not expressed until 1–3 months after birth. Some glucuronidation pathways are decreased in the newborn, and an inability of newborns to glucuronidate *chloramphenicol* was responsible for the "gray baby syndrome" (*see* Chapter 46). When adjusted for body weight or surface area, hepatic drug metabolism in children after the neonatal period often exceeds that of adults. Studies using *caffeine* as a model substrate illustrate the developmental changes in CYP1A2 that occur during childhood (Figure 5–2). The mechanisms regulating such developmental changes are uncertain, and other pathways of drug metabolism probably mature with different patterns.

Renal elimination of drugs also is reduced in the neonatal period. Neonates at term have markedly reduced GFR (2–4 mL/min/1.73 m^2), and prematurity reduces renal function even further. As a result, neonatal dosing regimens for a number of drugs (*e.g.,* aminoglycosides) must be

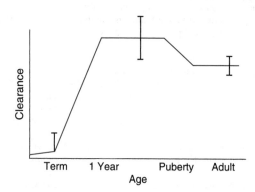

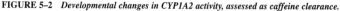

FIGURE 5–2 *Developmental changes in CYP1A2 activity, assessed as caffeine clearance.*

reduced to avoid toxic drug accumulation. GFR (corrected for body surface area) increases progressively to adult levels by 8–12 months of age. Dosing guidelines for children—where they exist—are drug- and age-specific.

Drug pharmacodynamics in children also may differ from those in adults. *Antihistamines* and *barbiturates* that generally sedate adults may be excitatory in children. The enhanced sensitivity to the sedating effects of *propofol* in children has led to the administration of excessive doses that produced myocardial failure, metabolic acidosis, and multiorgan failure. Unique features of childhood development also may provide special vulnerabilities to drug toxicity; for example, tetracyclines can permanently stain developing teeth, and glucocorticoids can attenuate linear growth of bones.

The Elderly   As adults age, gradual changes in pharmacokinetics and pharmacodynamics increase the interindividual variability of doses required for a given effect. Pharmacokinetic changes result from changes in body composition and the function of drug-eliminating organs. The reduction in lean body mass, serum albumin, and total-body water, coupled with the increase in percentage of body fat, alters drug distribution in a manner dependent on lipid solubility and protein binding. The clearance of many drugs is reduced in the elderly. Renal function variably declines to ~50% of that in young adults. Hepatic blood flow and drug metabolism also are reduced in the elderly but vary considerably. In general, the activities of hepatic CYPs are reduced, but conjugation mechanisms are relatively preserved. Frequently, the elimination half-lives of drugs are increased as a consequence of larger apparent volumes of distribution of lipid-soluble drugs and/or reductions in the renal or metabolic clearance.

Changes in pharmacodynamics are important factors in treating the elderly. Drugs that depress the CNS produce increased effects at any given plasma concentration due to age-related pharmacokinetic changes, physiological changes, and loss of homeostatic resilience, resulting in increased sensitivity to unwanted effects of drugs (*e.g.,* hypotension from psychotropic medications and hemorrhage from anticoagulants).

The number of elderly in developed nations is increasing rapidly. These individuals have more illnesses than younger people and consume a disproportionate share of prescription and over-the-counter drugs; they also are a population in whom drug use is especially likely to be marred by serious adverse effects and drug interactions. They therefore should receive drugs only when absolutely necessary for well-defined indications and at the lowest effective doses. Appropriate monitoring of drug levels and frequent reviews of the patient's drug history, with discontinuation of those drugs that did not achieve the desired end point or are no longer required, would greatly improve the health of the elderly.

THE PHARMACODYNAMIC CHARACTERISTICS OF A DRUG THAT DETERMINE ITS USE IN THERAPY

When drugs are administered to patients, there is no single characteristic relationship between the drug concentration in plasma and the measured effect; the concentration–effect curve may be concave upward, concave downward, linear, sigmoid, or an inverted-U shape. Moreover, the concentration–effect relationship may be distorted if the response being measured is a composite of several effects, such as the change in blood pressure produced by a combination of cardiac, vascular, and reflex effects. However, such a composite concentration–effect curve often can be resolved into simpler curves for each of its components. These simplified concentration–effect relationships, regardless of their exact shape, can be viewed as having four characteristic variables: *potency, maximal efficacy, slope,* and *individual variation.* These concepts are discussed in more detail in Chapter 1.

Potency can be viewed as the location of the concentration–effect curve along the concentration axis. Potency can be useful in the design of dosage forms, but more potent drugs are not always superior therapeutic agents. Maximal efficacy is the maximal effect that can be produced by a drug, as determined principally by the properties of the drug and its receptor–effector system and is reflected in the plateau of the concentration–effect curve. In clinical use, undesired effects may limit a drug's dosage such that its true maximal efficacy may not be achievable and clinical efficacy is then seen at a lower concentration. The slope of the concentration–effect curve reflects the mechanism of action of a drug, including the shape of the curve that describes drug binding to its receptor. The steepness of the curve dictates the range of doses that are useful for achieving a clinical effect (Figure 5–3).

Pharmacodynamic Variability

Individuals vary in the magnitude of their response to the same concentration of a single drug or to similar drugs, and a given individual may not always respond in the same way to the same drug

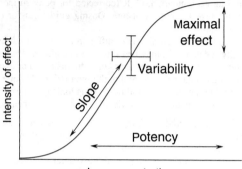

FIGURE 5–3 *The Log concentration–effect relationship.* Representative log concentration-effect curve illustrating its four characterizing variables. Here, the effect is measured as a function of increasing drug concentration in the plasma. Similar relationships also can be plotted as a function of the dose of drug administered. These plots are referred to as dose–effect curves. (*See* text for further discussion.)

concentration. A concentration–effect curve applies only to a single individual at one time or to an average individual. The intersecting brackets in Figure 5–3 indicate that an effect of varying intensity will occur in different individuals at a specified drug concentration or that a range of concentrations is required to produce an effect of specified intensity in all patients.

Attempts have been made to define and measure individual "sensitivity" to drugs in the clinical setting, and progress has been made in understanding some of the determinants of sensitivity to drugs that act at specific receptors. Drug responsiveness may change because of disease or because of previous drug administration. Receptors are dynamic, and their concentration and function may be up- or down-regulated by endogenous and exogenous factors.

Data on the association of drug levels with efficacy and toxicity must be interpreted in the context of the pharmacodynamic variability in the population (*e.g.*, genetics, age, disease, and other drugs). The variability in pharmacodynamic response in the population may be analyzed by constructing a quantal concentration–effect curve (Figure 5–4A).

The Therapeutic Index

The dose of a drug required to produce a specified effect in 50% of the population is the *median effective dose* (ED_{50}, Figure 5–4B). In preclinical studies of drugs, the *median lethal dose* (LD_{50}) is determined in experimental animals. The LD_{50}/ED_{50} ratio is an indication of the *therapeutic index*, which is a statement of how selective the drug is in producing its desired *versus* its adverse effects. In clinical studies, the dose, or preferably the concentration, of a drug required to produce toxic effects can be compared with the concentration required for therapeutic effects in the population to evaluate the *clinical therapeutic index*. Since pharmacodynamic variation in the population may be marked, the concentration or dose of drug required to produce a therapeutic effect in most of the population usually will overlap the concentration required to produce toxicity in some of the population, even though the drug's therapeutic index in an individual patient may be large. Also, the concentration–percent curves for efficacy and toxicity need not be parallel, adding yet another complexity to determination of the therapeutic index in patients. Finally, no drug produces a single effect, and the therapeutic index for a drug will vary depending on the effect being measured.

ADVERSE DRUG REACTIONS AND DRUG TOXICITY

Any drug, no matter how trivial its therapeutic actions, has the potential to do harm. Adverse reactions are a cost of modern medical therapy. Although the mandate of the Food and Drug Administration (FDA) is to ensure that drugs are safe and effective, these terms are relative. The anticipated benefit from any therapeutic decision must be balanced by the potential risks.

It has been estimated that 3–5% of all hospitalizations can be attributed to adverse drug reactions, resulting in 300,000 hospitalizations annually in the U.S. Once hospitalized, patients have about a 30% chance of an untoward event related to drug therapy, and the risk attributable to each course of drug therapy is about 5%. The chance of a life-threatening drug reaction is about 3% per

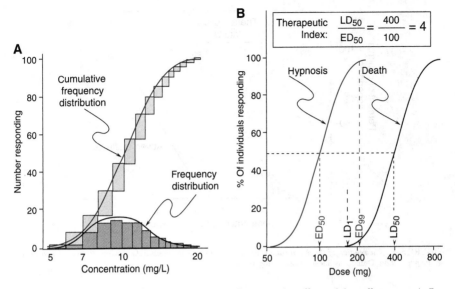

FIGURE 5–4 *Frequency distribution curves and quantal concentration–effect and dose–effect curves. A. Frequency distribution curves.* An experiment was performed on 100 subjects, and the effective plasma concentration that produced a quantal response was determined for each individual. The number of subjects who required each dose is plotted, giving a log-normal frequency distribution (*colored bars*). The gray bars demonstrate that the normal frequency distribution, when summated, yields the cumulative frequency distribution—a sigmoidal curve that is a quantal concentration–effect curve. *B. Quantal dose–effect curves.* Animals were injected with varying doses of sedative-hypnotic, and the responses were determined and plotted. The calculation of the therapeutic index, the ratio of the LD_{50} to the ED_{50}, is an indication of how selective a drug is in producing its desired effects relative to its toxicity. (*See* text for additional explanation.)

patient in the hospital and about 0.4% per each course of therapy. *Adverse reactions to drugs are the most common cause of iatrogenic disease.*

Mechanism-based adverse drug reactions are extensions of the principal pharmacological action of the drug. These would be expected to occur with all members of a class of drugs having the same mechanism of action.

When an adverse effect is encountered infrequently, it may be referred to as *idiosyncratic (i.e.,* it does not occur in the population at large). Idiosyncratic adverse effects may be mechanism-based (*e.g.,* angioedema on angiotensin-converting enzyme inhibitors) or off-target reactions (*e.g.,* anaphylaxis to *penicillin*). Investigations of idiosyncratic reactions often have identified a genetic or environmental basis for the unique host factors leading to the unusual effects.

THERAPEUTIC DRUG MONITORING

Given the multiple factors that alter drug disposition, measurement of the concentration in body fluids can assist in individualizing therapy with selected drugs. Determination of the concentration of a drug is particularly useful when well-defined criteria are met:

1. A demonstrated relationship exists between the concentration of drug in plasma and the desired therapeutic effect or the toxic effect to be avoided. The range of plasma levels between that required for efficacy and that at which toxicity occurs for a given individual is designated the *therapeutic window.*
2. There is sufficient variability in plasma level that the level cannot be predicted from the dose alone.
3. The drug produces effects, intended or unwanted, that are difficult to monitor.
4. The concentration required to produce the therapeutic effect is close to the level that causes toxicity (*i.e.,* there is a low therapeutic index).

A clear demonstration of the relation of drug concentration to efficacy or toxicity is not achievable for many drugs; even when such a relationship can be determined, it usually predicts only

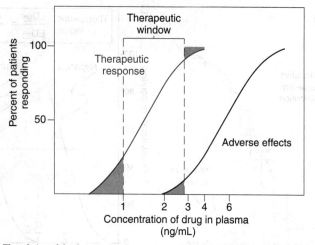

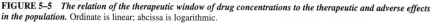

FIGURE 5–5   *The relation of the therapeutic window of drug concentrations to the therapeutic and adverse effects in the population.* Ordinate is linear; abcissa is logarithmic.

a probability of efficacy or toxicity. In trials of antidepressant drugs, such a high proportion of patients respond to placebo that it is difficult to determine the plasma level associated with efficacy. There is a quantal concentration–response curve for efficacy and adverse effects (Figure 5–5); for many drugs, the concentration that achieves efficacy in all the population may produce adverse effects in some individuals. Thus, a *population therapeutic window* expresses a range of concentrations at which the likelihood of efficacy is high and the probability of adverse effects is low. It does not guarantee either efficacy or safety. *Therefore, use of the population therapeutic window to adjust dosage of a drug should be complemented by monitoring appropriate clinical and surrogate markers for drug effect.*

THE DYNAMIC INFORMATION BASE

The information available to guide drug therapy is continually evolving. Among the available sources are textbooks of pharmacology and therapeutics, medical journals, published treatment guidelines, analytical evaluations of drugs, drug compendia, professional seminars and meetings, and advertising. A strategy to extract objective and unbiased data is required for the practice of rational, evidence-based therapeutics. Patient-centered acquisition of relevant information is a centerpiece of such a strategy. This requires access to the information in the practice setting and increasingly is facilitated by electronic availability of information resources including the primary medical literature (available *via* PubMed, *www.ncbi.nlm.nih.gov/entrez/query.fcgi*).

Depending on their aim and scope, textbooks of pharmacology may provide, in varying proportions, basic pharmacological principles, critical appraisal of useful categories of therapeutic agents, and detailed descriptions of individual drugs or prototypes that serve as standards of reference for assessing new drugs. In addition, pharmacodynamics and pathophysiology are correlated. Therapeutics is considered in virtually all textbooks of medicine but often superficially. The PDR offers industry-collated data and can be used for indication and dosing information. Industry promotion—in the form of direct-mail brochures, journal advertising, displays, professional courtesies, or the detail person or pharmaceutical representative—is intended to be persuasive rather than educational. The pharmaceutical industry cannot, should not, and indeed does not purport to be responsible for the education of physicians in the use of drugs.

DRUG NOMENCLATURE

The existence of many names for each drug, even when the names are reduced to a minimum, has led to a lamentable and confusing situation in drug nomenclature (*see* Appendix I in the 11th edition of the parent text). In addition to its formal *chemical* name, a new drug is usually assigned a *code* name by the pharmaceutical manufacturer. If the drug appears promising and the manufacturer wishes to place it on the market, a *U.S. adopted name* (USAN) is selected by the USAN Council, which is jointly sponsored by the American Medical Association, the American Pharmaceutical Association, and the United States Pharmacopeial Convention, Inc. This *nonproprietary* name often is referred to as the *generic name*. If the drug is eventually admitted to the *United States Pharmacopeia* (*see* below), the USAN becomes the *official name*. However, the nonproprietary and official names of an older drug may differ. Subsequently, the drug also will be assigned a *proprietary name*, or *trademark*, by the manufacturer. If more than one company markets the drug, then it may have several proprietary names. If mixtures of the drug with other agents are marketed, each such mixture also may have a separate proprietary name.

There is increasing worldwide adoption of the same *nonproprietary name* for each therapeutic substance. For newer drugs, the USAN is usually adopted for the nonproprietary name in other countries, but this is not true for older drugs. International agreement on drug names is mediated through the World Health Organization and the pertinent health agencies of the cooperating countries.

Except for a few drugs such as *levodopa* and *dextroamphetamine*, nonproprietary names usually give no indication of the drug's stereochemistry. This issue becomes important when a drug's different diastereomers produce different pharmacologic effects, as is the case with *labetalol* (*see* Chapters 10 and 32).

The nonproprietary or official name of a drug should be used whenever possible, and such a practice has been adopted in this book. The use of the nonproprietary name is clearly less confusing when the drug is available under multiple proprietary names and when the nonproprietary name more readily identifies the drug with its pharmacological class. The facile argument for the proprietary name is that it is frequently more easily pronounced and remembered as a result of advertising. *For purposes of identification, representative proprietary names, designated by* SMALLCAP TYPE, *appear throughout the text and in the index.* Not all proprietary names for drugs are included because the number of proprietary names for a single drug may be large and because proprietary names differ from country to country.

DRUG DEVELOPMENT AND ITS REGULATION
Drug Regulation

The history of drug regulation in the U.S. reflects the growing involvement of governments in most countries to ensure some degree of efficacy and safety in marketed medicinal agents. The first legislation, the Federal Food and Drug Act of 1906, was concerned with the interstate transport of adulterated or misbranded foods and drugs. There were no obligations to establish drug efficacy and safety. This act was amended in 1938, after the deaths of 105 children that resulted from the marketing of a solution of *sulfanilamide* in diethylene glycol, an excellent but highly toxic solvent. The amended act, the enforcement of which was entrusted to the FDA, was concerned primarily with the truthful labeling and safety of drugs. Toxicity studies, as well as approval of a new drug application (NDA), were required before a drug could be promoted and distributed. However, no proof of efficacy was required, and extravagant claims for therapeutic indications were made commonly.

In this relatively relaxed atmosphere, research in basic and clinical pharmacology burgeoned in industrial and academic laboratories. The result was a flow of new drugs, called "wonder drugs" by the lay press. Because efficacy was not rigorously defined, a number of therapeutic claims could not be supported by data. The risk-to-benefit ratio was seldom mentioned but emerged dramatically early in the 1960s. At that time, *thalidomide*, a hypnotic with no obvious advantage over other drugs in its class, was introduced in Europe. After a short period, it became apparent that the incidence of a relatively rare birth defect, phocomelia, was increasing. It soon reached epidemic proportions, and retrospective epidemiological research firmly established the causative agent to be thalidomide taken early in the course of pregnancy. The reaction to the dramatic demonstration of the teratogenicity of a needless drug was worldwide. In the U.S., it resulted in the Harris-Kefauver Amendments to the Food, Drug, and Cosmetic Act in 1962, which require sufficient pharmacological and toxicological research in animals before a drug can be tested in human beings. The data from such studies must be submitted to the FDA in the form of an application for an investigational new drug (IND) before clinical studies can begin. Three phases of clinical testing have evolved to provide the data that are used to support an NDA. Proof of efficacy is required, as is documentation of relative safety in terms of the risk-to-benefit ratio for the disease entity to be treated.

Drug Development

By the time an IND application has been initiated and a drug reaches the stage of testing in humans, its pharmacokinetic, pharmacodynamic, and toxic properties have been evaluated in vivo *in several species of animals in accordance with regulations and guidelines published by the FDA. Although the value of many requirements for preclinical testing is self-evident, such as those that screen for direct toxicity to organs and characterize dose-related effects, the value of others is controversial, particularly because of the well-known interspecies variation in the effects of drugs.*

Trials of drugs in human beings in the U.S. generally are conducted in three phases, which must be completed before an NDA can be submitted to the FDA for review; these are outlined in Figure 5–6. Although assessment of risk is a major objective of such testing, this is far more difficult than is the determination of whether a drug is efficacious for a selected clinical condition. Usually about 2000–3000 carefully selected patients receive a new drug during phase 3 clinical trials. At most, only a few hundred are treated for more than 3–6 months regardless of the likely

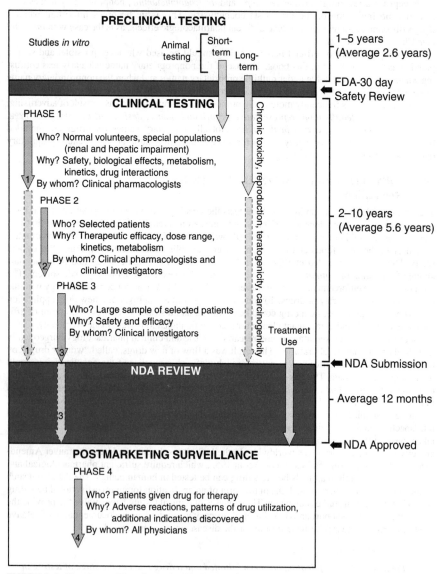

FIGURE 5–6   *The phases of drug development in the United States.*

duration of therapy that will be required in practice. Thus, the most profound and overt risks that occur almost immediately after the drug is given can be detected in a phase 3 study if they occur more often than once per 100 administrations. Risks that are medically important but delayed or less frequent than 1 in 1000 administrations may not be revealed prior to marketing (e.g., COX-2 inhibitors). Consequently, a number of unanticipated adverse and beneficial effects of drugs are detectable only after the drug is used broadly. Many countries, including the U.S., have established systematic methods for the surveillance of the effects of drugs after they have been approved for distribution (see below).

Postmarketing Surveillance for Adverse Reactions

For idiosyncratic adverse reactions, current approaches to "safety assessment" in clinical trials are problematic. The relative rarity of severe idiosyncratic reactions (e.g., severe dermatological, hematological, or hepatological toxicities) poses an epidemiological challenge. It is clear that a risk of 1 in 1000 is not distributed evenly across the population; some patients, due to unique genetic or environmental factors, are at an extremely high risk, whereas the remainder of the population may be at low or no risk. In contrast to the human heterogeneity underlying idiosyncratic risk, the standard process of drug development, particularly preclinical safety assessment using inbred healthy animals maintained in a defined environment on a defined diet and manifesting predictable habits, limits the identification of risk for idiosyncratic adverse drug reactions in the human population. Understanding the genetic and environmental bases of idiosyncratic adverse events holds the promise of assessing individual rather than population risk, thereby improving the overall safety of pharmacotherapy.

Formal approaches for estimating the magnitude of an adverse drug effect are the follow-up *or* cohort *study of patients who are receiving a particular drug, the case-control study, where the frequency of drug use in cases of adverse reactions is compared with controls, and meta-analyses of pre- and postmarketing studies. Cohort studies can estimate the incidence of an adverse reaction but cannot, for practical reasons, discover rare events. To have any significant advantage over the premarketing studies, a cohort study must follow at least 10,000 patients who are receiving the drug to detect with 95% confidence one event that occurs at a rate of 1 in 3300, and the event can be attributed to the drug only if it does not occur spontaneously in the control population. Meta-analyses combine the data from several studies in an attempt to discern benefits or risks that are sufficiently uncommon that an individual study lacks the power to discover them.*

The Key Role of the Clinician in Surveillance for Adverse Reactions

Because of the shortcomings of cohort and case-control studies and meta-analyses, additional approaches are needed. Spontaneous reporting of adverse reactions has proven to be an effective way to generate an early signal that a drug may cause an adverse event. In the past few years, considerable effort has gone into improving the reporting system in the U.S., which is now called MEDWATCH. Still, the voluntary reporting system in the U.S. is deficient compared with the legally mandated systems of many other nations.

For a complete Bibliographical listing see Goodman & Gilman's *The Pharmacological Basis of Therapeutics*, 11th ed., or Goodman & Gilman Online at www.accessmedicine.com.

6

NEUROTRANSMISSION: THE AUTONOMIC AND SOMATIC MOTOR NERVOUS SYSTEMS

The autonomic nervous system (ANS) is the primary moment-to-moment regulator of the internal environment of the organism, regulating specific functions that occur without conscious control, for example, respiration, circulation, digestion, body temperature, metabolism, sweating, and the secretions of certain endocrine glands. The endocrine system, in contrast, provides slower, more generalized regulation by secreting hormones into the systemic circulation to act at distant, widespread sites over periods of minutes to hours to days.

In the periphery, the ANS consists of nerves, ganglia, and plexuses that innervate the heart, blood vessels, glands, other visceral organs, and smooth muscle in various tissues. Based on considerations of anatomy and neurotransmitters, we divide the ANS into sympathetic and parasympathetic branches. The sympathetic branch, including the adrenal medulla, is not essential to life in a controlled environment, but the lack of sympathoadrenal functions becomes evident with stress (*e.g.*, compensatory cardiovascular responses to altered posture and exercise do not occur; fainting ensues). The sympathetic system normally is continuously active, adjusting moment-to-moment to a changing environment. The sympathoadrenal system also can discharge as a unit, particularly during rage and fright, and affect sympathetically-innervated structures over the entire body simultaneously, increasing heart rate and blood pressure, shifting blood flow from skin and splanchnic regions to the skeletal muscles, elevating blood glucose, dilating the bronchioles and pupils, and generally preparing the organism for "fight or flight."

The parasympathetic system, organized mainly for discrete and localized discharge, slows the heart rate, lowers the blood pressure, stimulates GI movements and secretions, aids absorption of nutrients, protects the retina from excessive light, and empties the urinary bladder and rectum. Many parasympathetic responses are rapid and reflexive. Although the parasympathetic branch of the ANS is concerned primarily with conservation of energy and maintenance of organ function during periods of satiety and minimal activity, its elimination is incompatible with life.

VISCERAL AFFERENT FIBERS

Afferent fibers from visceral structures are the first link in the reflex arcs of the autonomic system. With certain exceptions, such as local axon reflexes, most visceral reflexes are mediated through the central nervous system (CNS). Information on the status of the visceral organs is transmitted to the CNS through the cranial nerve (parasympathetic) visceral sensory system and the spinal (sympathetic) visceral afferent system. The cranial visceral sensory system carries mainly mechanoreceptor and chemosensory information; the afferents of the spinal visceral system principally convey sensations related to temperature and tissue injury of mechanical, chemical, or thermal origin. Cranial visceral sensory information enters the CNS via four cranial nerves: the trigeminal (V), facial (VII), glossopharyngeal (IX), and vagus (X). These four cranial nerves transmit visceral sensory information from the internal face and head (V), tongue (taste, VII), hard palate, upper part of the oropharynx, and carotid body (IX), and lower part of the oropharynx, larynx, trachea, esophagus, and thoracic and abdominal organs (X), with the exception of the pelvic viscera, which are innervated by nerves from the second through fourth sacral spinal segments. The visceral afferents from these four cranial nerves terminate topographically in the solitary tract nucleus (STN).

Sensory afferents from visceral organs also enter the CNS via the spinal nerves. Those concerned with muscle chemosensation may arise at all spinal levels; sympathetic visceral sensory afferents generally arise at the thoracic levels where sympathetic preganglionic neurons are found. Pelvic sensory afferents from spinal segments S2–S4 enter at that level and are important for the regulation of sacral parasympathetic outflow. In general, visceral afferents that enter the spinal nerves convey information concerned with temperature as well as nociceptive visceral inputs.

Neurotransmitters that mediate transmission from sensory fibers have not been characterized unequivocally. Substance P and calcitonin gene–related peptide are leading candidates for communicating nociceptive stimuli from the periphery to the CNS. Somatostatin, vasoactive intestinal polypeptide (VIP), and cholecystokinin may play a role in the transmission of afferent impulses from autonomic structures. ATP appears to be a neurotransmitter in certain sensory neurons, including those that innervate the urinary bladder. Enkephalins, present in interneurons in the dorsal spinal cord (within an area termed the substantia gelatinosa), *have antinociceptive effects that appear to arise from presynaptic and postsynaptic actions to inhibit the release of substance P and diminish the activity of cells that project from the spinal cord to higher centers in the CNS. The excitatory amino acids glutamate and aspartate also play major roles in transmission of sensory responses to the spinal cord.*

CENTRAL AUTONOMIC CONNECTIONS

There probably are no purely autonomic or somatic centers of integration; extensive overlap occurs; somatic responses always are accompanied by visceral responses, and vice versa. *Autonomic reflexes can be elicited at the level of the spinal cord and are manifested by sweating, blood pressure alterations, vasomotor responses to temperature changes, and reflex emptying of the urinary bladder, rectum, and seminal vesicles. The hypothalamus and the STN are principal loci of integration of ANS functions, including regulation of body temperature, water balance, carbohydrate and fat metabolism, blood pressure, emotions, sleep, respiration, and reproduction. Signals are received through ascending spinobulbar pathways, the limbic system, neostriatum, cortex, and to a lesser extent other higher brain centers.*

The CNS can produce a wide range of patterned autonomic and somatic responses. Highly integrated patterns of response generally are organized at the hypothalamic level and involve autonomic, endocrine, and behavioral components. More limited patterned responses are organized at other levels of basal forebrain, brainstem, and spinal cord.

DIVISIONS OF THE PERIPHERAL AUTONOMIC SYSTEM: EFFERENT NERVES

On the efferent side, the ANS consists of two large divisions: (1) the sympathetic or thoracolumbar, and, (2) the parasympathetic or craniosacral (*see* Figure 6–1).

The neurotransmitter of all preganglionic autonomic fibers, all postganglionic parasympathetic fibers, and a few postganglionic sympathetic fibers is *acetylcholine* (ACh). Adrenergic fibers comprise the majority of the postganglionic sympathetic fibers; here, the transmitter is *norepinephrine* (NE, *noradrenaline*). The terms *cholinergic* and *adrenergic* are used to describe neurons that release ACh or NE, respectively.

SYMPATHETIC BRANCH OF THE ANS

The cells that give rise to the preganglionic fibers of this division lie mainly in the intermediolateral columns of the spinal cord and extend from the first thoracic to the second or third lumbar segment. The axons from these cells are carried in the anterior (ventral) nerve roots and synapse with neurons lying in sympathetic ganglia outside the cerebrospinal axis. Sympathetic ganglia are found in three locations: paravertebral, prevertebral, and terminal.

The 22 pairs of paravertebral sympathetic ganglia form the lateral chains on either side of the vertebral column. The ganglia are connected to each other by nerve trunks and to the spinal nerves by rami communicantes. *The white rami are restricted to the segments of the thoracolumbar outflow; they carry the preganglionic myelinated fibers that exit the spinal cord via the anterior spinal roots. The gray rami arise from the ganglia and carry postganglionic fibers back to the spinal nerves for distribution to sweat glands and pilomotor muscles and to blood vessels of skeletal muscle and skin. The prevertebral ganglia lie in the abdomen and the pelvis near the ventral surface of the bony vertebral column and consist mainly of the celiac (solar), superior mesenteric, aorticorenal, and inferior mesenteric ganglia. The terminal ganglia are few in number, lie near the organs they innervate, and include ganglia connected with the urinary bladder and rectum and the cervical ganglia in the region of the neck. Small intermediate ganglia lie outside the conventional vertebral chain, especially in the thoracolumbar region, usually proximally to the communicating rami and the anterior spinal nerve roots.*

Preganglionic fibers issuing from the spinal cord may synapse with the neurons of more than one sympathetic ganglion. Their principal ganglia of termination need not correspond to the original level from which the preganglionic fiber exits the spinal cord. Many of the preganglionic fibers from the fifth to the last thoracic segment pass through the paravertebral ganglia to form the splanchnic nerves. Most of the splanchnic nerve fibers do not synapse until they reach the celiac ganglion; others directly innervate the adrenal medulla (see below).

Postganglionic fibers arising from sympathetic ganglia innervate visceral structures of the thorax, abdomen, head, and neck. The trunk and the limbs are supplied by the sympathetic fibers in spinal nerves, as described earlier. The prevertebral ganglia contain cell bodies whose axons

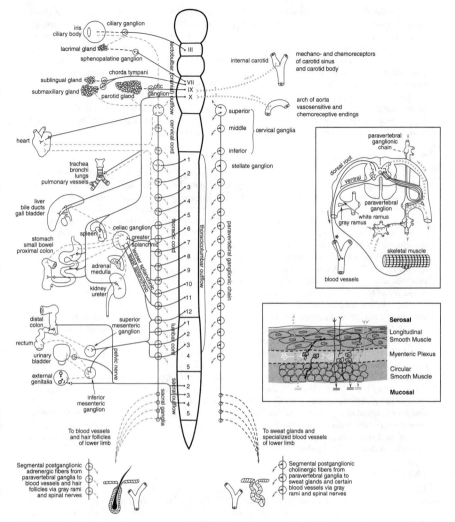

FIGURE 6–1   *The autonomic nervous system (ANS).* Schematic representation of the autonomic nerves and effector organs based on chemical mediation of nerve impulses. Blue, cholinergic; gray, adrenergic; dotted blue, visceral afferent; solid lines, preganglionic; broken lines, postganglionic. In the upper rectangle at the right are shown the finer details of the ramifications of adrenergic fibers at any one segment of the spinal cord, the path of the visceral afferent nerves, the cholinergic nature of somatic motor nerves to skeletal muscle, and the presumed cholinergic nature of the vasodilator fibers in the dorsal roots of the spinal nerves. The asterisk (*) indicates that it is not known whether these vasodilator fibers are motor or sensory or where their cell bodies are situated. In the lower rectangle on the right, vagal preganglionic (*solid blue*) nerves from the brainstem synapse on both excitatory and inhibitory neurons found in the myenteric plexus. A synapse with a postganglionic cholinergic neuron (*blue with varicosities*) gives rise to excitation, whereas synapses with purinergic, peptide (VIP), or an NO-generating neuron (*black with varicosities*) lead to relaxation. Sensory nerves (*dotted blue lines*) originating primarily in the mucosal layer send afferent signals to the CNS but often branch and synapse with ganglia in the plexus. Their transmitter is substance P or other tachykinins. Other interneurons (*white*) contain serotonin and will modulate intrinsic activity through synapses with other neurons eliciting excitation or relaxation (*black*). Cholinergic, adrenergic, and some peptidergic neurons pass through the circular smooth muscle to synapse in the submucosal plexus or terminate in the mucosal layer, where their transmitter may stimulate or inhibit GI secretion.

innervate the glands and smooth muscles of the abdominal and the pelvic viscera. Many of the upper thoracic sympathetic fibers from the vertebral ganglia form terminal plexuses, such as the cardiac, esophageal, and pulmonary plexuses. The sympathetic distribution to the head and the neck (vasomotor, pupillodilator, secretory, and pilomotor) is via the cervical sympathetic chain and its three ganglia. All postganglionic fibers in this chain arise from cell bodies located in these three ganglia; all preganglionic fibers arise from the upper thoracic segments of the spinal cord, there being no sympathetic fibers that leave the CNS above the first thoracic level.

The adrenal medulla and other chromaffin tissue are embryologically and anatomically similar to sympathetic ganglia. The adrenal medulla differs from sympathetic ganglia in that its principal catecholamine is epinephrine *(Epi,* adrenaline*), not NE. The chromaffin cells in the adrenal medulla are innervated by typical preganglionic fibers that release ACh.*

PARASYMPATHETIC BRANCH OF THE ANS

The parasympathetic branch of the ANS consists of preganglionic fibers that originate in the CNS and their postganglionic connections. The regions of central origin are the midbrain, the medulla oblongata, and the sacral part of the spinal cord. The midbrain, or tectal, outflow consists of fibers arising from the Edinger–Westphal nucleus of the third cranial nerve and going to the ciliary ganglion in the orbit. The medullary outflow consists of the parasympathetic components of the seventh, ninth, and tenth cranial nerves. The fibers in the seventh (facial) cranial nerve form the chorda tympani, which innervates the ganglia lying on the submaxillary and sublingual glands. They also form the greater superficial petrosal nerve, which innervates the sphenopalatine ganglion. The autonomic components of the ninth (glossopharyngeal) cranial nerve innervate the otic ganglia. Postganglionic parasympathetic fibers from these ganglia supply the sphincter of the iris (pupillary constrictor muscle), the ciliary muscle, the salivary and lacrimal glands, and the mucous glands of the nose, mouth, and pharynx. These fibers also include vasodilator nerves to these same organs. The tenth (vagus) cranial nerve arises in the medulla and contains preganglionic fibers, most of which do not synapse until they reach the many small ganglia lying directly on or in the viscera of the thorax and abdomen. In the intestinal wall, the vagal fibers terminate around ganglion cells in the myenteric and submucosal plexuses. Thus, preganglionic fibers are very long, whereas postganglionic fibers are very short. The vagus nerve also carries a far greater number of afferent fibers (but apparently no pain fibers) from the viscera into the medulla; the cell bodies of these fibers lie mainly in the nodose ganglion.

The parasympathetic sacral outflow consists of axons that arise from cells in the second, third, and fourth segments of the sacral cord and proceed as preganglionic fibers to form the pelvic nerves (nervi erigentes). They synapse in terminal ganglia lying near or within the bladder, rectum, and sexual organs. The vagal and sacral outflows provide motor and secretory fibers to thoracic, abdominal, and pelvic organs (Figure 6–1).

ENTERIC NERVOUS SYSTEM

The activities of the GI tract are controlled locally through a restricted part of the peripheral nervous system called the enteric nervous system *(ENS). The ENS is involved in sensorimotor control and consists of both afferent sensory neurons and a number of motor nerves and interneurons that are organized principally into two nerve plexuses: the myenteric (Auerbach's) plexus and the submucosal (Meissner's) plexus. The myenteric plexus, located between the longitudinal and circular muscle layers, plays an important role in the contraction and relaxation of GI smooth muscle. The submucosal plexus is involved with secretory and absorptive functions of the GI epithelium, local blood flow, and neuroimmune activities. The ENS consists of components of the sympathetic and parasympathetic branches of the ANS and has sensory nerve connections through the spinal and nodose ganglia (see Chapter 37).*

Parasympathetic input to the GI tract is excitatory; preganglionic neurons in the vagus innervate the parasympathetic ganglia of the enteric plexuses. Postganglionic sympathetic nerves also synapse with the intramural enteric parasympathetic ganglia. Sympathetic nerve activity induces relaxation primarily by inhibiting the release of ACh from the preganglionic fibers.

The intrinsic primary afferent neurons are present in both the myenteric and submucosal plexuses. They respond to luminal chemical stimuli, to mechanical deformation of the mucosa, and to stretch. The nerve endings of the primary afferent neurons can be activated by endogenous substances (e.g., serotonin) arising from local enterochromaffin cells or possibly from serotonergic nerves.

The muscle layers of the GI tract are dually innervated by excitatory and inhibitory motor neurons whose cell bodies are in the gut wall. ACh, in addition to being the transmitter of parasympathetic nerves to the ENS, is the primary excitatory transmitter acting on nicotinic acetylcholine receptors (nAChRs) in ascending intramural pathways. Pharmacological blockade of cholinergic neurotransmission, however, does not completely abolish this excitatory transmission because cotransmitters, such as substance P and neurokinin A, are coreleased with ACh and contribute to the excitatory response; similarly, ATP acts as an excitatory neurotransmitter via P2X receptors.

Inhibitory neurons of the ENS release a variety of transmitters and cotransmitters, including nitric oxide (NO), ATP (acting on P2Y receptors), VIP, and pituitary adenylyl cyclase–activating peptide (PACAP); NO is a primary inhibitory transmitter. Interstitial cells of Cajal (ICC) relay signals from the nerves to the smooth muscle cells to which they are electrically coupled. The ICC have receptors for both the inhibitory transmitter NO and the excitatory tachykinins. Disruption of the ICC impairs excitatory and inhibitory neurotransmission.

DIFFERENCES AMONGST SYMPATHETIC, PARASYMPATHETIC, AND MOTOR NERVES

A preganglionic sympathetic fiber may traverse a considerable distance of the sympathetic chain and pass through several ganglia before it finally synapses with a postganglionic neuron; also, its terminals contact a large number of postganglionic neurons, and one ganglion cell may be supplied by several preganglionic fibers, such that the ratio of preganglionic axons to ganglion cells may be >1:20. This organization permits a diffuse discharge of the sympathetic system.

The parasympathetic system, in contrast, has terminal ganglia very near or within the organs innervated and thus is more circumscribed in its influences. In some organs, there is a 1:1 relationship between the number of preganglionic and postganglionic fibers (this distinction does not apply to all sites; in the myenteric plexus, this ratio is ~1:8000).

The cell bodies of somatic motor neurons reside in the ventral horn of the spinal cord (*see* Figure 6–1); the axon divides into many branches, each of which innervates a single muscle fiber, so more than 100 muscle fibers may be supplied by one motor neuron to form a motor unit. At each neuromuscular junction, the axonal terminal loses its myelin sheath and forms a terminal arborization that lies in apposition to a specialized surface of the muscle membrane, the *motor end plate* (*see* Figure 9–2).

RESPONSES OF EFFECTOR ORGANS TO AUTONOMIC NERVE IMPULSES

From the responses of the various effector organs to autonomic nerve impulses and the knowledge of the intrinsic autonomic tone, one can predict the actions of drugs that mimic or inhibit the actions of these nerves. In some instances, the sympathetic and parasympathetic neurotransmitters can be viewed as physiological or functional antagonists. Most viscera are innervated by both divisions of the ANS, and the level of activity at any moment represents the sum of influences of the two components. Effects of sympathetic and parasympathetic stimulation of the heart and the iris show a pattern of functional antagonism in controlling heart rate and pupillary aperture, respectively, whereas their actions on male sexual organs are complementary and are integrated to promote sexual function. The control of peripheral vascular resistance is due primarily, but not exclusively, to sympathetic control of the contraction of arteriolar smooth muscle. The effects of stimulating the sympathetic and parasympathetic nerves to various organs, visceral structures, and effector cells are summarized in Table 6–1.

NEUROTRANSMISSION

Nerve impulses elicit responses by liberating specific chemical neurotransmitters. Understanding the chemical mediation of nerve impulses provides the framework for our knowledge of the mechanism of action of drugs at these sites. The sequence of events involved in neurotransmission is of particular importance because pharmacologically active agents modulate the individual steps.

AXONAL CONDUCTION

Conduction *refers to the passage of an impulse along an axon or muscle fiber;* transmission *refers to the passage of an impulse across a synaptic or neuroeffector junction. Axonal conduction has its basis in transmembrane ionic gradients and in selectively permeable membrane channels. At rest, the interior of the typical mammalian axon is ~70 mV negative to the exterior. The resting potential is essentially a K^+ Nernst potential based on the higher concentration of K^+ [~40x] in the axoplasm* versus *the extracellular fluid and the relatively high permeability of the resting axonal membrane to K^+. Na^+, and Cl^- are present in higher concentrations in the extracellular fluid than in the axoplasm, but the axonal membrane at rest is considerably less permeable to these ions; hence, their contribution to the resting potential is small. These ionic gradients are maintained by the Na^+, K^+-ATPase.*

In response to depolarization to a threshold level, an action potential (AP) is initiated locally in the membrane. The AP consists of two phases. Following a small gating current resulting from

Table 6-1

Responses of Effector Organs to Autonomic Nerve Impulses

Organ System	Sympathetic Effect[a]	Adrenergic Receptor Type[b]	Parasympathetic Effect[a]	Cholinergic Receptor Type[b]
Eye				
Radial muscle, iris	Contraction (mydriasis)++	α_1		
Sphincter muscle, iris			Contraction (miosis)+++	M_3, M_2
Ciliary muscle	Relaxation for far vision+	β_2	Contraction for near vision+++	M_3, M_2
Lacrimal glands	Secretion+	α	Secretion+++	M_3, M_2
Heart[c]				
Sinoatrial node	Increase in heart rate++	$\beta_1 > \beta_2$	Decrease in heart rate+++	$M_2 >> M_3$
Atria	Increase in contractility and conduction velocity++	$\beta_1 > \beta_2$	Decrease in contractility++ and shortened AP duration	$M_2 >> M_3$
Atrioventricular node	Increase in automaticity and conduction velocity++	$\beta_1 > \beta_2$	Decrease in conduction velocity; AV block+++	$M_2 >> M_3$
His–Purkinje system	Increase in automaticity and conduction velocity	$\beta_1 > \beta_2$	Little effect	$M_2 >> M_3$
Ventricle	Increase in contractility, conduction velocity, automaticity and rate of idioventricular pacemakers+++	$\beta_1 > \beta_2$	Slight decrease in contractility	$M_2 >> M_3$
Blood vessels (Arteries and arterioles)[d]				
Coronary	Constriction+; dilation[e,d]++	$\alpha_1, \alpha_2, \beta_2$	No innervation[h]	—
Skin and mucosa	Constriction+++	α_1, α_2	No innervation[h]	—
Skeletal muscle	Constriction; dilation[e,d]++	α_1, β_2	Dilation[h] (?)	—
Cerebral	Constriction (slight)	α_1	No innervation[h]	—
Pulmonary	Constriction+; dilation	α_1, β_2	No innervation[h]	—
Abdominal viscera	Constriction +++; dilation +	α_1, β_2	No innervation[h]	—
Salivary glands	Constriction+++	α_1, α_2	Dilation[h]++	—
Renal	Constriction++; dilation++	$\alpha_1, \alpha_2, \beta_1, \beta_2$	No innervation[h]	M_3
(Veins)[d]	Constriction; dilation	$\alpha_1, \alpha_2, \beta_2$		

	Adrenergic response	Receptor type[b]	Cholinergic response	Receptor type[b]
Endothelium			Activation of NO synthase[h]	M_3
Lung				
Tracheal and bronchial smooth muscle	Relaxation	β_2	Contraction	$M_2 = M_3$
Bronchial glands	Decreased secretion, increased secretion	α_1 β_2	Stimulation	M_3, M_2
Stomach				
Motility and tone	Decrease (usually)[i]+	$\alpha_1, \alpha_2, \beta_1, \beta_2$	Increase[i]+++	$M_2 = M_3$
Sphincters	Contraction (usually)+	α_1	Relaxation (usually)+	M_3, M_2
Secretion	Inhibition	α_2	Stimulation++	M_3, M_2
Intestine				
Motility and tone	Decrease[h]+	$\alpha_1, \alpha_2, \beta_1, \beta_2$	Increase[i]+++	M_3, M_2
Sphincters	Contraction+	α_1	Relaxation (usually)+	M_3, M_2
Secretion	Inhibition	α_2	Stimulation++	M_3, M_2
Gallbladder and ducts	Relaxation+	β_2	Contraction+	M
Kidney				
Renin secretion	Decrease+; increase++	α_1, β_1	No innervation	—

[a] Responses are designated + to +++ to provide an approximate indication of the importance of sympathetic and parasympathetic nerve activity in the control of the various organs and functions listed.

[b] Adrenergic receptors: α_1, α_2, and subtypes thereof; β_1, β_2, β_3. Cholinergic receptors: nicotinic (N); muscarinic (M), with subtypes 1–4. The receptor subtypes are described more fully in Chapters 7 and 10 and in Tables 6–2, 6–3 and 6–6. When a designation of subtype is not provided, the nature of the subtype has not been determined unequivocally. Only the principal receptor subtypes are shown. Transmitters other than acetylcholine and norepinephrine contribute to many of the responses.

[c] In the human heart, the ratio of β_1 to β_2 is about 3:2 in atria and 4:1 in ventricles. While M_2 receptors predominate, M_3 receptors are also present.

[d] The predominant α_1 receptor subtype in most blood vessels (both arteries and veins) is α_{1A} (see Table 6–8), although other α_1 subtypes are present in specific vessels. The α_{1D} is the predominant subtype in the aorta.

[e] Dilation predominates in situ owing to metabolic autoregulatory mechanisms.

[f] Over the usual concentration range of physiologically released circulating epinephrine, the β-receptor response (vasodilation) predominates in blood vessels of skeletal muscle and liver; the α-receptor response (vasoconstriction) in other abdominal viscera. The renal and mesenteric vessels also contain specific dopaminergic receptors whose activation causes dilation.

[g] Sympathetic cholinergic neurons cause vasodilation in skeletal muscle beds, but this is not involved in most physiological responses.

[h] The endothelium of most blood vessels releases NO, which causes vasodilation in response to muscarinic stimuli. However, unlike the receptors innervated by sympathetic cholinergic fibers in skeletal muscle blood vessels, these muscarinic receptors are not innervated and respond only to exogenously added muscarinic agonists in the circulation.

[i] While adrenergic fibers terminate at inhibitory β receptors and at inhibitory α receptors on parasympathetic (cholinergic) excitatory ganglion cells of the myenteric plexus, the primary inhibitory response is mediated via enteric neurons through NO, P2Y receptors, and peptide receptors.

(Continued)

Table 6-1

Responses of Effector Organs to Autonomic Nerve Impulses (*Continued*)

Organ System	Sympathetic Effect[a]	Adrenergic Receptor Type[b]	Parasympathetic Effect[a]	Cholinergic Receptor Type[b]
Urinary bladder				
Detrusor	Relaxation+	β_2	Contraction+++	$M_3 > M_2$
Trigone and sphincter	Contraction++	α_1	Relaxation++	$M_3 > M_2$
Ureter				
Motility and tone	Increase	α_1	Increase (?)	M
Uterus	Pregnant contraction;	α_1	Variable[j]	M
	Relaxation	β_2		
	Nonpregnant relaxation	β_2		
Sex organs, male	Ejaculation+++	α_1	Erection+++	M_3
Skin				
Pilomotor muscles	Contraction++	α_1		
Sweat glands	Localized secretion[k]++	α_1		M_3, M_2
	Generalized secretion+++			
Spleen capsule	Contraction+++	α_1	—	—
	Relaxation+	β_2	—	
Adrenal medulla	— Secretion of Epi and NE			$N (\alpha_3)_2(\beta_4)_3$; M (secondarily)
Skeletal muscle	Increased contractility; glycogenolysis; K^+ uptake	β_2	—	—
Liver	Glycogenolysis and gluconeogenesis+++	α_1, β_2	—	—
Pancreas				
Acini	Decreased secretion+	α	Secretion++	M_3, M_2
Islets (β cells)	Decreased secretion+++	α_2	—	—
	Increased secretion+	β_2		

Tissue	Adrenergic response	Adrenergic receptor	Cholinergic response	Cholinergic receptor
Fat cells[l]	Lipolysis+++; (thermogenesis)	$\alpha_1, \beta_1, \beta_2, \beta_3$		—
	Inhibition of lipolysis	α_2		
Salivary glands	K$^+$ and water secretion+	α_1	K$^+$ and water secretion+++	M$_3$, M$_2$
Nasopharyngeal glands			Secretion++	M$_3$, M$_2$
Pineal	Melatonin synthesis	β	—	
Posterior pituitary	Vasopressin secretion	β_1	—	
Autonomic nerve endings				
Sympathetic terminals				
Autoreceptor	Inhibition of NE release	$\alpha_{2A} > \alpha_{2C}\ (\alpha_{2B})$		
Heteroreceptor			Inhibition of NE release	M$_2$, M$_4$
Parasympathetic terminal				
Autoreceptor			Inhibition of ACh release	M$_2$, M$_4$
Heteroreceptor	Inhibition of ACh release	$\alpha_{2A} > \alpha_{2C}$		

[l] Uterine responses depend on stages of menstrual cycle, amount of circulating estrogen and progesterone, and other factors.

[k] Palms of hands and some other sites ("adrenergic sweating").

[m] There is significant variation among species in the receptor types that mediate certain metabolic responses. All three β adrenergic receptors have been found in human fat cells. Activation of β₃ adrenergic receptors produces a vigorous thermogenic response as well as lipolysis. The significance is unclear. Activation of β adrenergic receptors also inhibits leptin release from adipose tissue.

ADH, antidiuretic hormone, arginine vasopressin; AV, atrioventricular; AP, action potential.

depolarization inducing an open conformation of the channel, the initial phase is caused by a rapid increase in the permeability of Na^+ through voltage-sensitive Na^+ channels. The result is inward movement of Na^+ and a rapid depolarization from the resting potential, which continues to a positive overshoot. The second phase results from the rapid inactivation of the Na^+ channel and the delayed opening of a K^+ channel, which permits outward movement of K^+ to terminate the depolarization.

The transmembrane ionic currents produce local circuit currents around the axon. As a result, adjacent resting channels in the axon are activated, exciting an adjacent portion of the axonal membrane and causing propagation of the AP without decrement along the axon. The region that has undergone depolarization remains momentarily in a refractory state. In myelinated fibers, permeability changes occur only at the nodes of Ranvier, thus causing a rapidly progressing type of jumping, or saltatory, conduction. The puffer fish poison tetrodotoxin and a congener found in shellfish, saxitoxin, selectively block axonal conduction by blocking the voltage-sensitive Na^+ channel and preventing the increase in Na^+ permeability associated with the rising phase of the AP. In contrast, batrachotoxin, a potent steroidal alkaloid secreted by a South American frog, produces paralysis through a selective increase in permeability of the Na^+ channel, which induces a persistent depolarization. Scorpion toxins are peptides that cause persistent depolarization by inhibiting the inactivation process. For more details on Na^+ and Ca^{2+} channels, see Chapters 14, 31, and 34.

JUNCTIONAL TRANSMISSION   The arrival of the AP at the axonal terminals initiates a series of events that trigger transmission of an excitatory or inhibitory impulse across the synapse or neuroeffector junction (*see* Figure 6–2):

1. *Release of stored neurotransmitter; prejunctional regulation.* Nonpeptide (small molecule) neurotransmitters are largely synthesized in the axonal terminals and stored there in synaptic

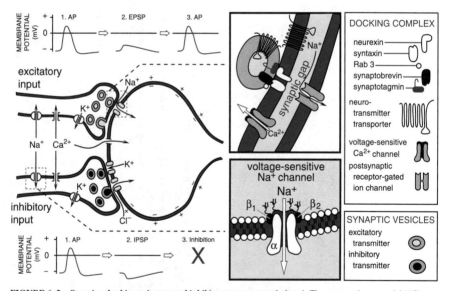

FIGURE 6–2   *Steps involved in excitatory and inhibitory neurotransmission.* 1. The nerve action potential (AP) consists of a transient self-propagated reversal of charge on the axonal membrane. (The internal potential E_i goes from a negative value, through zero potential, to a slightly positive value primarily through increases in Na^+ permeability and then returns to resting values by an increase in K^+ permeability.) When the AP arrives at the presynaptic terminal, it initiates release of the excitatory or inhibitory transmitter. Depolarization at the nerve ending and entry of Ca^{2+} initiate docking and then fusion of the synaptic vesicle with the membrane of the nerve ending. Docked and fused vesicles are shown. 2. Combination of the excitatory transmitter with postsynaptic receptors produces a localized depolarization, the excitatory postsynaptic potential (EPSP), through an increase in permeability to cations, most notably Na^+. The inhibitory transmitter causes a selective increase in permeability to K^+ or Cl^-, resulting in a localized hyperpolarization, the inhibitory postsynaptic potential (IPSP). 3. The EPSP initiates a conducted AP in the postsynaptic neuron; this can be prevented, however, by the hyperpolarization induced by a concurrent IPSP. Transmitter action is terminated by enzymatic destruction, by reuptake into the presynaptic terminal or adjacent glial cells, or by diffusion.

vesicles. Peptide neurotransmitters (or precursor peptides) are found in large dense-core vesicles that are transported down the axon from their site of synthesis in the cell body. The arrival of an AP and depolarization of the axonal terminal membrane causes the synchronous release of several hundred quanta of neurotransmitter; a critical step in most but not all nerve endings is the influx of Ca^{2+}, which enters the axonal cytoplasm and promotes fusion between the axoplasmic membrane and those vesicles in close proximity to it. The contents of the vesicles, including enzymes, other proteins, and cotransmitters (*e.g.*, ATP, NPY) then are discharged to the exterior by *exocytosis* (*see* Figure 6-2).

Receptors on soma, dendrites, and axons of neurons respond to neurotransmitters or modulators released from the same neuron or from adjacent neurons or cells. Soma–dendritic receptors are located on or near the cell body and dendrites; when activated, they primarily modify functions of the soma–dendritic region such as protein synthesis and generation of action potentials. Presynaptic receptors are located on axon terminals or varicosities; when activated, they modify functions such as synthesis and release of transmitters. Two main classes of presynaptic receptors have been identified on most neurons, including sympathetic and parasympathetic terminals. Heteroreceptors are presynaptic receptors that respond to neurotransmitters, neuromodulators, or neurohormones released from adjacent neurons or cells. For example, NE can influence the release of ACh from parasympathetic neurons by acting on α_{2A}, α_{2B}, and α_{2C} receptors, whereas ACh can influence the release of NE from sympathetic neurons by acting on M_2 and M_4 receptors (see below). The other class of presynaptic receptors are autoreceptors, *located on axon terminals of a neuron and activated by the neuron's own transmitter to modify subsequent transmitter synthesis and release. For example, NE may interact with α_{2A} and α_{2C} receptors to inhibit neurally-released NE. Similarly, ACh may interact with M_2 and M_4 receptors to inhibit neurally-released ACh. Adenosine,* dopamine (DA), *glutamate, γ-aminobutyric acid* (GABA), *prostaglandins, and enkephalins influence neurally-mediated release of neurotransmitters, in part by altering the function of prejunctional ion channels.*

2. *Combination of the transmitter with postjunctional receptors and production of the postjunctional potential.* The released transmitter diffuses across the synaptic or junctional cleft and combines with specialized receptors on the postjunctional membrane; this often results in a localized increase in the ionic permeability, or conductance, of the membrane. With certain exceptions (noted below), one of three types of permeability change can occur: (a) a generalized increase in the permeability to cations (notably Na^+ but occasionally Ca^{2+}), resulting in a localized depolarization of the membrane, i.e., an excitatory postsynaptic potential (EPSP); (b) a selective increase in permeability to anions, usually Cl^-, resulting in stabilization or hyperpolarization of the membrane (an inhibitory postsynaptic potential or IPSP); or (c) an increased permeability to K^+ (the K^+ gradient is directed outward; thus, hyperpolarization results, *i.e.*, an IPSP).

Electrical potential changes associated with the EPSP and IPSP generally result from passive fluxes of ions down concentration gradients. The changes in channel permeability that cause these potential changes are specifically regulated by the specialized postjunctional neurotransmitter receptors (see Chapter 12 and below). In the presence of an appropriate neurotransmitter, the channel opens rapidly to a high-conductance state, remains open for about a millisecond, and then closes. A short pulse of current is observed as a result of the channel's opening and closing. The summation of these microscopic events gives rise to the EPSP. High-conductance ligand-gated ion channels usually permit passage of Na^+ or Cl^-; K^+ and Ca^{2+} are involved less frequently. The preceding ligand-gated channels belong to a large superfamily of ionotropic receptor proteins that includes the nicotinic, glutamate, serotonin ($5-HT_3$) and P2X receptors, which conduct primarily Na^+, cause depolarization, and are excitatory, and GABA and glycine receptors, which conduct Cl^-, cause hyperpolarization, and are inhibitory. Neurotransmitters also can modulate the permeability of K^+ and Ca^{2+} channels indirectly, often via receptor-G protein interactions (see Chapter 1). Other receptors for neurotransmitters act by influencing the synthesis of intracellular second messengers (e.g., cyclic AMP, cyclic GMP, IP_3) and do not necessarily cause a change in membrane potential.

3. *Initiation of postjunctional activity.* If an EPSP exceeds a certain threshold value, it initiates an action potential in the postsynaptic membrane by activating voltage-sensitive channels in the immediate vicinity. In certain smooth muscle types in which propagated impulses are minimal, an EPSP may increase the rate of spontaneous depolarization, cause Ca^{2+} release, and enhance muscle tone; in gland cells, the EPSP initiates secretion through Ca^{2+} mobilization. An IPSP, which occurs in neurons and smooth muscle but not in skeletal muscle, will tend to oppose excitatory potentials simultaneously initiated by other neuronal sources. The ultimate response depends on the summation of all the potentials.

4. *Destruction or dissipation of the transmitter and termination of action.* To sustain high frequency transmission and regulation of function, the synaptic dwell-time of the primary neurotransmitter must be relatively short. At cholinergic synapses involved in rapid neurotransmission, high and localized concentrations of *acetylcholinesterase* (AChE) are localized to hydrolyze ACh. When AChE is inhibited, removal of the transmitter occurs principally by diffusion, and the effects of ACh are potentiated and prolonged (*see* Chapter 8).

Termination of the actions of catecholamines occurs by a combination of simple diffusion and reuptake by the axonal terminals of the released transmitter by the SLC6 family of transporters using energy stored in the transmembrane Na^+ gradient (*see* Tables 2–2 and 6–5). Termination of the actions of 5-HT and GABA and other amino acid transmitters also results from their transport into neurons and surrounding glia by SLC1 and SLC6 family members. Peptide neurotransmitters are hydrolyzed by various peptidases and dissipated by diffusion; specific uptake mechanisms have not been demonstrated for these substances.

5. *Nonelectrogenic functions.* During the resting state, there is a continual slow release of isolated quanta of the transmitter that produces electrical responses at the postjunctional membrane [miniature end-plate potentials (*mepps*)] that are associated with the maintenance of physiological responsiveness of the effector organ. A low level of spontaneous activity within the motor units of skeletal muscle is particularly important because skeletal muscle lacks inherent tone. The activity and turnover of enzymes involved in the synthesis and inactivation of neurotransmitters, the density of presynaptic and postsynaptic receptors, and other characteristics of synapses probably are controlled by trophic actions of neurotransmitters or other trophic factors released by the neuron or the target cells.

Cholinergic Transmission

The synthesis, storage, and release of ACh (Figure 6–3) follow a similar life cycle in all cholinergic synapses, including those at skeletal neuromuscular junctions, preganglionic sympathetic and parasympathetic terminals, postganglionic parasympathetic varicosities, postganglionic sympathetic varicosities innervating sweat glands in the skin, and in the CNS.

CHOLINE ACETYLTRANSFERASE

Choline acetyltransferase catalyzes the synthesis of ACh—the acetylation of choline with acetyl coenzyme A (CoA). Choline acetyltransferase, like other protein constituents of the neuron, is synthesized within the perikaryon and then is transported along the length of the axon to its terminal. Axonal terminals contain a large number of mitochondria, where acetyl CoA is synthesized. Choline is taken up from the extracellular fluid into the axoplasm by active transport. The synthetic step occurs in the cytosol; most of the ACh is then sequestered within synaptic vesicles. Inhibitors of choline acetyltransferase have no therapeutic utility, in part because the uptake of choline, not the activity of the acetyltransferease, is rate-limiting in ACh biosynthesis.

CHOLINE TRANSPORT Transport of choline from the plasma into neurons is rate-limiting in ACh synthesis and is accomplished by distinct high- and low-affinity transport systems. The high-affinity system ($K_m = 1–5\ \mu M$) is unique to cholinergic neurons, dependent on extracellular Na^+, and inhibited by *hemicholinium*. Plasma concentrations of choline approximate 10 μM. Much of the choline formed from AChE-catalyzed hydrolysis of ACh is recycled into the nerve terminal.

STORAGE OF ACh

After its synthesis, ACh is taken up by storage vesicles principally at the nerve terminals. The vesicles contain both ACh and ATP, at an estimated ratio of 10:1, in the fluid phase with Ca^{2+} and Mg^{2+}, and vesiculin, a negatively charged proteoglycan thought to sequester Ca^{2+} or ACh. In some cholinergic vesicles there are peptides (e.g., VIP) that act as cotransmitters. The vesicular ACh transporter, has considerable concentrating power, is saturable, and is ATP-dependent. The process is inhibited by vesamicol (Figure 6–3). Inhibition by vesamicol is noncompetitive and reversible and does not affect the vesicular ATPase. Estimates of the ACh content of synaptic vesicles range from 1000 to over 50,000 molecules per vesicle; a single motor nerve terminal contains 300,000 or more vesicles.

RELEASE OF ACETYLCHOLINE AND ITS MODULATION BY TOXINS

The release of ACh and other neurotransmitters by exocytosis is inhibited by botulinum and tetanus toxins from Clostridium. Botulinum toxin acts in the nerve ending to reduce ACh vesicular release (see Chapters 9 and 63 for therapeutic uses of botulinum toxin).

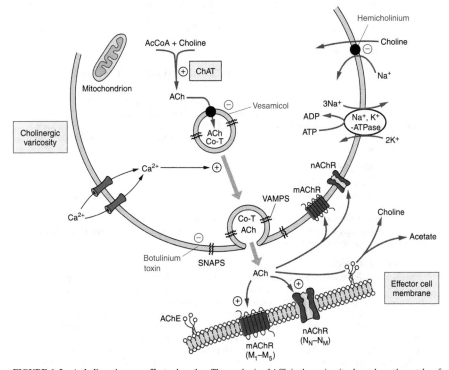

FIGURE 6–3 *A cholinergic neuroeffector junction.* The synthesis of ACh in the varicosity depends on the uptake of choline *via* a sodium-dependent carrier. This uptake can be blocked by *hemicholinium*. Choline and the acetyl moiety of acetyl coenzyme A, derived from mitochondria, form ACh, a process catalyzed by the enzyme choline acetyltransferase (ChAT). ACh is transported into the storage vesicle by a carrier that can be inhibited by *vesamicol*. ACh is stored in vesicles along with other potential cotransmitters (Co-T) such as ATP and VIP. Release of ACh and the Co-T occurs following depolarization of the membrane, which allows the entry of Ca^{2+} through voltage-dependent Ca^{2+} channels. Elevated $[Ca^{2+}]_{in}$ promotes fusion of the vesicular membrane with the cell membrane and exocytosis of vesicular contents. This fusion process involves the interaction of specialized proteins of the vesicular membrane (VAMPs, vesicle-associated membrane proteins) and the membrane of the varicosity (SNAPs, synaptosome-associated proteins). The exocytotic release of ACh can be blocked by *botulinum toxin*. Once released, ACh can interact with the muscarinic receptors (mAChR), which are GPCRs, or nicotinic receptors (nAChR), which are ligand-gated ion channels, to produce the characteristic response of the effector. ACh also can act on presynaptic mAChRs or nAChRs to modify its own release. The action of ACh is terminated by hydrolysis to choline and acetate by acetylcholinesterase (AChE) associated with the effector cell membrane.

By contrast, tetanus toxin primarily has a central action: it is transported in retrograde fashion up the motor neuron to its soma in the spinal cord. From there the toxin migrates to inhibitory neurons that synapse with the motor neuron and blocks exocytosis in the inhibitory neuron. The block of release of inhibitory transmitter gives rise to tetanus or spastic paralysis. The toxin from the venom of black widow spiders (α-latrotoxin) binds to neurexins, transmembrane proteins that reside on the nerve terminal membrane, resulting in massive synaptic vesicle exocytosis.

ACETYLCHOLINESTERASE (AChE)

ACh must be removed or inactivated within the time limits imposed by the response characteristics of the synapse. At the neuromuscular junction, immediate removal is required to prevent lateral diffusion and sequential activation of adjacent receptors. This removal is accomplished in <1 ms by hydrolysis of ACh by AChE. The K_m of AChE for ACh is ~50–100 µM. The resulting choline has only $10^{-3}–10^{-5}$ the potency of ACh at the neuromuscular junction. AChE is found in cholinergic neurons (dendrites, perikarya, and axons) and is highly concentrated at the postsynaptic end plate of the neuromuscular junction. A similar esterase, butyrylcholinesterase (BuChE; also known as pseudocholinesterase*), is present in low abundance in glial or satellite cells but is virtually absent in neuronal elements of the central and peripheral nervous systems.*

BuChE is synthesized primarily in the liver and is found in liver and plasma. AChE and BuChE typically are distinguished by the relative rates of ACh and butyrylcholine hydrolysis and by effects of selective inhibitors (see Chapter 8). Almost all pharmacological effects of the anti-ChE agents are due to the inhibition of AChE, with the consequent accumulation of endogenous ACh in the vicinity of the nerve terminal.

CHARACTERISTICS OF CHOLINERGIC TRANSMISSION AT VARIOUS SITES

Skeletal Muscle

At the neuromuscular junction (Figure 9–2), ACh interacts with nicotinic ACh receptors and induces an immediate, marked increase in cation permeability. Upon activation by ACh, the nicotinic receptor's intrinsic channel opens for about 1 ms, admitting ~50,000 Na^+ ions. The channel-opening process is the basis for the localized depolarizing EPP within the end plate, which triggers the muscle AP and leads to contraction.

Autonomic Ganglia

The primary pathway of cholinergic transmission in autonomic ganglia is similar to that at the neuromuscular junction of skeletal muscle. The initial depolarization is the result of activation of nicotinic ACh receptors, which are ligand-gated cation channels with properties similar to those found at the neuromuscular junction. Several secondary transmitters or modulators either enhance or diminish the sensitivity of the postganglionic cell to ACh. Ganglionic transmission is discussed in more detail in Chapter 9.

Autonomic Effectors

Stimulation or inhibition of autonomic effector cells by ACh results from interaction of ACh with muscarinic ACh receptors. In this case, the effector is coupled to the receptor by a G protein (see Chapter 1). In contrast to skeletal muscle and neurons, smooth muscle and the cardiac conduction system (sinoatrial [SA] node, atrium, atrioventricular [AV] node, and the His–Purkinje system) normally exhibit intrinsic activity, both electrical and mechanical, that is modulated but not initiated by nerve impulses. At some smooth muscle, ACh causes a decrease in the resting potential (i.e., the membrane potential becomes less negative) and an increase in the frequency of spike production, accompanied by a rise in tension. A primary action of ACh in initiating these effects through muscarinic receptors is probably partial depolarization of the cell membrane brought about by an increase in Na^+ and, in some instances, Ca^{2+} conductance; activation of muscarinic receptors can also activate the G_q-PLC-IP_3 pathway leading to the mobilization of stored Ca^{2+}. Hence, ACh stimulates ion fluxes across membranes and/or mobilizes intracellular Ca^{2+} to cause contraction.

In the heart, spontaneous depolarizations normally arise from the SA node. In the cardiac conduction system, particularly in the SA and AV nodes, stimulation of the cholinergic innervation or the direct application of ACh causes inhibition, associated with hyperpolarization of the membrane and a marked decrease in the rate of depolarization. These effects are due, at least partly, to a selective increase in permeability to K^+ and are mediated by muscarinic cholinergic receptors.

PREJUNCTIONAL SITES

Both cholinergic and adrenergic nerve terminal varicosities contain autoreceptors and heteroreceptors. ACh release therefore is subject to complex regulation by mediators, including ACh itself acting on M_2 and M_4 autoreceptors, and other transmitters (e.g., NE acting on α_{2A} and α_{2C} adrenergic receptors) or locally-produced substances (e.g., NO). ACh-mediated inhibition of ACh release following activation of M_2 and M_4 autoreceptors is thought to represent a physiological negative-feedback control mechanism. At some neuroeffector junctions (e.g., the myenteric plexus in the GI tract or the SA node in the heart), sympathetic and parasympathetic nerve terminals often are juxtaposed. The opposing effects of NE and ACh, therefore, result not only from the opposite effects of the two transmitters on the smooth muscle or cardiac cells but also from their mutual inhibition of each other's release via actions on heteroreceptors. Muscarinic autoreceptors and heteroreceptors are targets for both agonists and antagonists. Muscarinic agonists can inhibit the electrically-induced release of ACh; antagonists will enhance the evoked release of transmitter. In addition to α_{2A} and α_{2C} adrenergic receptors, other inhibitory heteroreceptors on parasympathetic terminals include A_1, H_3, and opioid receptors. Evidence also exists for β_2 adrenergic facilitatory receptors.

EXTRANEURONAL CHOLINERGIC SYSTEMS   ACh is present in the vast majority of human cells and organs, including epithelial cells (airways, alimentary tract, epidermis, glandular tissue), mesothelial and endothelial cells, circulating cells (platelets), and immune cells (mononuclear cells, macrophages). The exact function of nonneuronal ACh is not known; proposed roles include regulation of mitosis, locomotion, automaticity, ciliary activity, cell–cell contact, barrier function, respiration and secretion, and the regulation of lymphocyte function.

CLASSIFICATION OF CHOLINERGIC RECEPTORS

ACh elicits responses similar to those of either nicotine or muscarine, depending on the physiological preparation. Thus, the receptors for ACh are classified as nicotinic or muscarinic. Tubocurarine and atropine block nicotinic and muscarinic effects of ACh, respectively, providing pharmacological evidence of two receptor types for ACh.

Subtypes of Nicotinic Acetylcholine Receptors

The nicotinic ACh receptors (nAChRs) are members of a superfamily of ligand-gated ion channels. The receptors exist at the skeletal neuromuscular junction, autonomic ganglia, adrenal medulla and in the CNS. They are the natural targets for ACh as well as pharmacologically administered drugs, including nicotine. The receptor forms a pentameric structure consisting of homomeric α and β subunits. In humans, 8 α subunits (α_2 through α_7, α_9, and α_{10}) and three β subunits (β_2 through β_4) have been cloned. Both the muscle and neuronal nAChRs share structural and functional properties with other ligand-gated channels such as the $GABA_A$, 5-HT_3, and glycine receptors. The muscle nAChR is the best-characterized form. The muscle nicotinic receptor contains four distinct subunits in a pentameric complex ($\alpha_2\beta\delta\gamma$ or $\alpha_2\beta\delta\varepsilon$; *see* Table 6–2). The muscle and neuronal subunits share the basic topography of a large extracellular N-terminal domain that contributes to agonist binding, four hydrophobic transmembrane domains (TM_1 through TM_4), a large cytoplasmic loop between TM_3 and TM_4, and a short extracellular C terminus. The M_2 transmembrane region is thought to form the ion pore of the nAChR (*see* Chapter 9). Autonomic ganglia form homomeric α_7 and heteromeric α_3/β_4, with $(\alpha_3)_2(\beta_4)_3$ being the most prevalent.

The pentameric structure of the neuronal nAChR and the considerable molecular diversity of its subunits offer the possibility of a large number of nAChRs with different physiological properties. These receptors may subserve a variety of discrete functions and thus represent novel drug targets for a wide variety of therapeutic agents. The stoichiometry of most nAChRs in brain is still uncertain. Distinctions amongst nAChRs are listed in Table 6–2. The structure, function, distribution, and subtypes of nicotinic receptors are described in more detail in Chapter 9.

SUBTYPES OF MUSCARINIC RECEPTORS

In mammals, five distinct subtypes of muscarinic ACh receptors (mAChRs) have been identified, each produced by a different gene. Like the different forms of nicotinic receptors, these variants have distinct anatomical locations in the periphery and CNS and differing chemical specificities. The mAChRs are GPCRs (see **Table 6–3***). Muscarinic AChRs are present in virtually all organs, tissues, and cell types, although certain subtypes often predominate at specific sites. For example, the M_2 receptor is the predominant subtype in the heart, whereas the M_3 receptor is the predominant subtype in the bladder. In the periphery, mAChRs mediate the classical muscarinic actions of ACh in organs and tissues innervated by parasympathetic nerves; mAChRs are also present at sites that lack parasympathetic innervation (e.g., on endothelial and smooth muscle cells of most blood vessels). In the CNS, mAChRs are involved in regulating a large number of cognitive, behavior, sensory, motor, and autonomic functions. The basic functions of muscarinic cholinergic receptors (Table 6–3) are mediated by interactions with G proteins and thus by G protein–induced changes in the function of distinct member-bound effector molecules. The M_1, M_3, and M_5 subtypes couple through the pertussis toxin–insensitive G_q, G_{11}, and $G_{12/13}$ to stimulate the PLC-IP$_3$-Ca^{2+} pathway, with activation of Ca^{2+}-dependent phenomena such as contraction of smooth muscle and secretion (see Chapter 1). Another product of PLC activation, diacylglycerol, in conjunction with Ca^{2+}, activates PKC, resulting in the phosphorylation of numerous proteins and leading to various physiological responses. Activation of M_1, M_3, and M_5 receptors can also cause the activation of phospholipase A_2, leading to the release of arachidonic acid and consequent eicosanoid synthesis, resulting in autocrine/paracrine stimulation of adenylyl cyclase.*

Stimulation of M_2 and M_4 cholinergic receptors leads to interaction with other G proteins, (e.g., G_i and G_o) with a resulting inhibition of adenylyl cyclase, a decrease in cyclic AMP, activation of inwardly rectifying K^+ channels, and inhibition of voltage-gated Ca^{2+} channels, with the functional consequences of hyperpolarization and inhibition of excitability. These are most clear in myocardium, where inhibition of adenylyl cyclase and activation of K^+ conductances account for the negative chronotropic and inotropic effects of ACh.

Table 6–2

Characteristics of Subtypes of Nicotinic Acetylcholine Receptors (nAChRs)

Receptor (Primary Receptor Subtype)*	Main Synaptic Location	Membrane Response	Molecular Mechanism	Agonists	Antagonists
Skeletal muscle (N_M) $(\alpha_1)_2\beta_1\varepsilon\delta$ adult $(\alpha_1)_2\beta_1\gamma\delta$ fetal	Skeletal neuromuscular junction (postjunctional)	Excitatory; end-plate depolarization; skeletal muscle contraction	Increased cation permeability ($Na^+; K^+$)	ACh Nicotine Succinylcholine	Atracurium Vecuronium d-Tubocurarine Pancuronium α-Conotoxin α-Bungarotoxin
Peripheral neuronal (N_N) $(\alpha_3)_2(\beta_4)_3$	Autonomic ganglia; adrenal medulla	Excitatory; depolarization; firing of postganglion neuron; depolarization and secretion of catecholamines	Increased cation permeability ($Na^+; K^+$)	ACh Nicotine Epibatidine Dimethylphenyl-piperazinium	Trimethaphan Mecamylamine
Central neuronal (CNS) $(\alpha_4)_2(\beta_4)_3$ (α-btox-insensitive)	CNS; pre- and postjunctional	Pre- and postsynaptic excitation Prejunctional control of transmitter release	Increased cation permeability ($Na^+; K^+$)	Cytisine, epibatidine Anatoxin A	Mecamylamine Dihydro-β-erythrodine Erysodine Lophotoxin
$(\alpha_7)_5$ (α-btox-sensitive)	CNS; Pre- and postsynaptic	Pre- and postsynaptic excitation Prejunctional control of transmitter release	Increased cation permeability (Ca^{2+})	Anatoxin A	Methyllycaconitine α-Bungarotoxin α-Conotoxin IMI

*Nine individual subunits have been identified and cloned in human brain, which combine in various conformations to form individual receptor subtypes. The structure of individual receptors and the subtype composition are incompletely understood. Only a finite number of naturally occurring functional nAChR constructs have been identified. α-btox, α-bungarotoxin.

Table 6-3

Characteristics of Muscarinic Acetylcholine Receptor Subtypes (mAChRs)

Receptor	Size; Chromosome Location	Cellular and Tissue Location[*]	Cellular Response[†]	Functional Response[‡]
M_1	460 aa 11q 12–13	CNS; Most abundant in cerebral cortex, hippocampus and striatum Autonomic ganglia Glands (gastric and salivary) Enteric nerves	Activation of PLC; ↑IP_3 and ↑DAG → ↑Ca^{2+} and PKC Depolarization and excitation (↑sEPSP) Activation of PLD₂, PLA₂; ↑AA Couples via $G_{q/11}$	Increased cognitive function (learning and memory) Increased seizure activity Decrease in dopamine release and locomotion Increase in depolarization of autonomic ganglia Increase in secretions
M_2	466 aa 7q 35–36	Widely expressed in CNS, heart, smooth muscle, autonomic nerve terminals	Inhibition of adenylyl cyclase, ↓cAMP Activation of inwardly rectifying K^+ channels Inhibition of voltage-gated Ca^{2+} channels Hyperpolarization and inhibition Couples via G_i/G_o (PTX-sensitive)	*Heart:* SA node: slowed spontaneous depolarization; hyperpolarization, ↓HR AV node: decrease in conduction velocity Atrium: ↓ refractory period, ↓ contraction Ventricle: slight ↓ contraction *Smooth muscle:* ↑ Contraction *Peripheral nerves:* Neural inhibition via autoreceptors and heteroreceptor ↓ Ganglionic transmission *CNS:* Neural inhibition ↑ Tremors; hypothermia; analgesia
M_3	590 aa 1q 43–44	Widely expressed in CNS (< than other mAChRs) Abundant in smooth muscle and glands	Activation of PLC; ↑IP3 and ↑DAG → ↑Ca^{2+} and PKC Depolarization and excitation (↑sEPSP) Activation of PLD₂, PLA₂; ↑AA Couples via $G_{q/11}$	*Smooth muscle* ↑ Contraction (predominant in some, e.g. bladder) *Glands:* ↑ Secretion (predominant in salivary gland)

(Continued)

Table 6–3

Characteristics of Muscarinic Acetylcholine Receptor Subtypes (mAChRs) (Continued)

Receptor	Size; Chromosome Location	Cellular and Tissue Location*	Cellular Response†	Functional Response‡
		Heart		Increases food intake, body weight, fat deposits Inhibition of dopamine release Synthesis of NO
M_4	479 aa 11p 12–11.2	Preferentially expressed in CNS, particularly forebrain	Inhibition of adenylyl cyclase, $\downarrow$cAMP Activation of inwardly rectifying K^+ channels Inhibition of voltage-gated Ca^{2+} channels Hyperpolarization and inhibition Couples via G_i/G_o (PTX-sensitive)	Autoreceptor- and heteroreceptor-mediated inhibition of transmitter release in CNS and periphery Analgesia; cataleptic activity Facilitation of dopamine release
M_5	532 aa 15q 26	Expressed in low levels in CNS and periphery Predominant mAChR in dopamine neurons in VTA and substantia nigra	Activation of PLC; $\uparrow$IP$_3$ and $\uparrow$DAG $\rightarrow$ $\uparrow$Ca^{2+} and PKC Depolarization and excitation ($\uparrow$sEPSP) Activation of PLD$_2$, PLA$_2$; $\uparrow$AA Couples via $G_{q/11}$	Mediator of dilation in cerebral arteries and arterioles (?) Facilitates dopamine release Augmentation of drug-seeking behavior and reward (e.g., opiates, cocaine)

*Most organs, tissues, and cells express multiple mAChRs.

†M_1, M_3, and M_5 mAChRs appear to couple to the same G proteins and signal through similar pathways. Likewise, M_2 and M_4 mAChRs couple through similar G proteins and signal through similar pathways.

‡Despite the fact that in many tissues, organs, and cells multiple subtypes of mAChRs coexist, one subtype may predominate in producing a particular function; in others, there may be equal predominance.

ABBREVIATIONS: PLC, phospholipase C; IP$_3$, inositol-1,4,5-trisphosphate; DAG, diacylglycerol; PLD, phospholipase D; AA, arachidonic acid; PLA, phospholipase A; cAMP, cyclic AMP; SA node, sinoatrial node; AV node, atrioventricular node; HR, heart rate; PTX, pertussis toxin; VTA, ventral tegmentum area.

Following activation by agonists, mAChRs can be phosphorylated by a variety of receptor kinases and second-messenger regulated kinases; the phosphorylated mAChR subtypes then can interact with β-arrestin and presumably other adaptor proteins. As a result, the various mAChR signaling pathways may be differentially altered, leading to short- or long-term desensitization of a particular signaling pathway, receptor-mediated activation of the MAP kinase pathway downstream of mAChR phosphorylation, and long-term potentiation of mAChR-mediated PLC stimulation. Agonist activation of mAChRs also may induce receptor internalization and down-regulation.

Adrenergic Transmission

Norepinephrine (NE), dopamine (DA), and epinephrine (Epi) are catecholamines. NE is the principal transmitter of most sympathetic postganglionic fibers and of certain tracts in the CNS. DA is the predominant transmitter of the mammalian extrapyramidal system and of several mesocortical and mesolimbic neuronal pathways. Epi is the major hormone of the adrenal medulla. There are important interactions between the endogenous catecholamines and many of the drugs used in the treatment of hypertension, mental disorders, and a variety of other conditions described in subsequent chapters. The basic physiological, biochemical, and pharmacological features are presented here. Almost every step in the synthesis, storage, release, reuptake/metabolism, and action of catecholamine can be usefully modulated by pharmacological agents.

SYNTHESIS, STORAGE, AND RELEASE OF CATECHOLAMINES *Synthesis*—The steps in the synthesis of DA, NE (known outside the U.S. as noradrenaline), and Epi (known as adrenaline) are shown in Figure 6–4. Tyrosine is sequentially 3-hydroxylated and decarboxylated to form DA. DA is β-hydroxylated to yield NE (the transmitter in postganglionic nerves of the sympathetic branch of the ANS), which is N-methylated in chromaffin tissue to give Epi. The enzymes involved are not completely specific; consequently, other endogenous substances and some drugs are also substrates. 5-hydroxytryptamine (5-HT, serotonin) can be produced from 5-hydroxy-L-tryptophan by aromatic L-amino acid decarboxylase (AAD or dopa decarboxylase). AAD also converts dopa into DA, and methyldopa into α-methyl-DA, which is converted to α-methyl-NE by dopamine β-hydroxylase (DβH; Table 6–4).

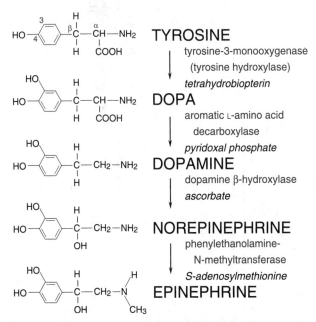

FIGURE 6–4 *The biosynthesis of dopamine, norepinephrine, and epinephrine.* The enzymes involved are shown in blue; essential cofactors in italics. The final step occurs only in the adrenal medulla and in a few epinephrine-containing neuronal pathways in the brainstem.

Table 6-4

Enzymes for Synthesis of Catecholamines

Enzyme	Occurrence	Subcellular Distribution	Cofactor Requirement	Substrate Specificity	Comments
Tyrosine hydroxylase	Widespread; sympathetic nerves	Cytoplasmic	Tetrahydrobiopterin, O_2, Fe^{2+}	Specific for L-tyrosine	Rate-limiting step Inhibition can lead to depletion of NE
Aromatic L-amino acid decarboxylase	Widespread; sympathetic nerves	Cytoplasmic	Pyridoxal phosphate	Nonspecific	Inhibition does not alter tissue NE and Epi appreciably
Dopamine β-hydroxylase	Widespread; sympathetic nerves	Synaptic vesicles	Ascorbic acid, O_2 (contains copper)	Nonspecific	Inhibition can decrease NE and Epi levels
Phenylethanolamine N-methyltransferase	Largely in adrenal gland	Cytoplasmic	S-Adenosyl methionine (CH_3 donor)	Nonspecific	Inhibition leads to decrease in adrenal catecholamines; under control of glucocorticoids

Tyrosine hydroxylase, the rate-limiting enzyme, is a substrate for PKA, PKC, and CaM kinase; phosphorylation may increase hydroxylase activity, an important acute mechanism whereby NE and Epi, acting at autoreceptors, enhance catecholamine synthesis in response to elevated nerve stimulation. In addition, there is a delayed increase in tyrosine hydroxylase gene expression after nerve stimulation, occurring at the levels of transcription, RNA processing, regulation of RNA stability, translation, and enzyme stability. Thus, multiple mechanisms maintain the content of catecholamines in response to increased transmitter release. In addition, tyrosine hydroxylase is subject to allosteric feedback inhibition by catecholamines.

The main features of the mechanisms of synthesis, storage, and release of catecholamines and their modifications by drugs are summarized in Figure 6–5. NE or Epi is stored in vesicles with ATP and other cotransmitters (e.g., neuropeptide Y [NPY]), depending on the site. The adrenal medulla has two distinct catecholamine-containing cell types: those with NE and those that express the enzyme phenylethanolamine-N-methyltransferase (PNMT) and contain primarily Epi (in these cells, the NE formed in the granules leaves these structures, is methylated in the cytoplasm to Epi, then reenters the chromaffin granules, where it is stored until released. In adults, Epi accounts for ~80% of the catecholamines of the adrenal medulla. A major factor that controls the rate of synthesis of Epi, and hence the size of the store available for release from the adrenal medulla, is the level of glucocorticoids secreted by the adrenal cortex. The intraadrenal portal vascular system carries the corticosteroids directly to the adrenal medullary chromaffin cells, where they induce the synthesis of PNMT (Figure 6–4). The activities of both tyrosine hydroxylase and DβH also are increased in the adrenal medulla when the secretion of glucocorticoids is stimulated. Thus, any stress that persists sufficiently to evoke an enhanced secretion of corticotropin mobilizes the appropriate hormones of both the adrenal cortex (predominantly cortisol in humans) and medulla (Epi). This relationship occurs only in certain mammals, including humans, in which adrenal chromaffin cells are enveloped by steroid-secreting cortical cells. There is evidence for PMNT expression and extra-adrenal chromaffin tissue in mammalian tissues such as brain, heart, and lung, leading to extra-adrenal Epi synthesis.

In addition to synthesis of new transmitter, NE stores are also replenished by transport of NE previously released to the extracellular fluid by the combined actions of a NE transporter (NET, or uptake 1) that terminates the synaptic actions of released NE and returns NE to the neuronal cytosol, and VMAT-2, the vesicular monoamine transporter, that refills the storage vesicles from the cytosolic pool of NE (see below). In the removal of NE from the synaptic cleft, uptake by the NET is more important than extraneuronal uptake (ENT, uptake 2). The sympathetic nerves as a whole remove ~87% of released NE via NET compared with 5% by extraneuronal ENT and 8% via diffusion to the circulation. By contrast, clearance of circulating catecholamines is primarily by nonneuronal mechanisms, with liver and kidney accounting for >60% of the clearance. Because VMAT-2 has a much higher affinity for NE than does the metabolic enzyme, monoamine oxidase, over 70% of recaptured NE is sequestered into storage vesicles.

STORAGE OF CATECHOLAMINES   Vesicular storage of catecholamines ensures their regulated release and protects them from intraneuronal metabolism by oxidative deamination by monoamine oxidase (MAO) (*see* below and Figure 6–6). The vesicular monoamine transporter (VMAT-2) is driven by a pH gradient established by an ATP-dependent proton pump. Monoamine transporters are relatively promiscuous and transport DA, NE, Epi, and 5-HT. *Reserpine* inhibits VMAT-2, making the catecholamine susceptible to degradation and leading to depletion of catecholamine from sympathetic nerve endings and in the brain.

There are two neuronal membrane transporters for catecholamines, the NE transporter (NET) and the DA transporter (DAT) (*see* Table 6–5). NET is Na^+-dependent and is blocked selectively by a number of drugs, including *cocaine* and tricyclic antidepressants such as *imipramine*. This transporter has a high affinity for NE and a somewhat lower affinity for Epi; the synthetic β adrenergic receptor agonist *isoproterenol* is not a substrate for this system. A number of other highly specific, high affinity neurotransmitter transporters have been identified, including those for 5-HT and a variety of amino acid transmitters. These plasma membrane transporters appear to have greater substrate specificity than do vesicular transporters and may be viewed as targets ("receptors") for specific drugs such as cocaine (NET, DAT) or *fluoxetine* (SERT, the serotonin transporter).

Certain sympathomimetic drugs (e.g., ephedrine and tyramine) produce some of their effects indirectly by displacing NE from the nerve terminals to the extracellular fluid by a nonexocytotic mechanism, and then the released NE acts at receptor sites of the effector cells. The mechanisms by which these drugs release NE from nerve endings are complex. All such drugs are substrates for NET. As a result of their transport across the neuronal membrane into the axoplasm, they make carrier

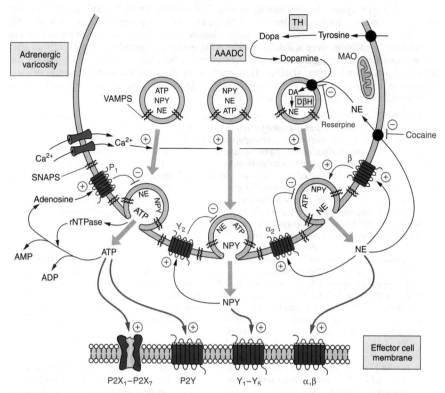

FIGURE 6–5 *An adrenergic neuroeffector junction.* Tyrosine is transported into the varicosity and converted to DOPA by tyrosine hydroxylase (TH) and DOPA to dopamine *via* the action of aromatic L-amino acid decarboxylase (AAADC). Dopamine is taken up into storage vesicles by a transporter that can be blocked by reserpine; cytoplasmic NE also can be taken up by this transporter. Dopamine is converted to NE within the vesicle *via* the action of dopamine-β-hydroxylase (DβH). NE is stored in vesicles along with cotransmitters (e.g., NPY and ATP), depending on the particular neuroeffector junction; different populations of vesicles may preferentially store different proportions of the cotransmitters. Release of the transmitters occurs upon depolarization of the varicosity, which allows entry of Ca^{2+} through voltage-dependent Ca^{2+} channels. Elevated $[Ca^{2+}]_{in}$ promotes fusion of the vesicular membrane with the membrane of the varicosity, with subsequent exocytosis of transmitters. This fusion process involves the interaction of specialized proteins associated with the vesicular membrane (VAMPs, vesicle-associated membrane proteins) and the membrane of the varicosity (SNAPs, synaptosome-associated proteins). Once in the synapse, NE can interact with α- and β-adrenergic receptors to produce the characteristic response of the effector. The adrenergic receptors are GPCRs. α and β receptors also can be located presynaptically where NE can either diminish (α_2), or facilitate (β) its own release and that of the cotransmitters. The principal mechanism by which NE is cleared from the synapse is *via* a cocaine-sensitive neuronal uptake transporter. Once transported into the cytosol, NE can be restored in the vesicle or metabolized by monoamine oxidase (MAO). NPY produces its effects by activating NPY receptors, of which there are at least five types (Y_1 through Y_5). NPY receptors are GPCRs. NPY can modify its own release and that of the other transmitters *via* presynaptic receptors of the Y_2 type. NPY is removed from the synapse by the action of peptidases. ATP produces its effects by activating P2X receptors (ligand-gated ion channels) and P2Y receptors (GPCRs). There are multiple subtypes of both P2X and P2Y receptors. As with the other cotransmitters, ATP can act prejunctionally to modify its own release *via* receptors for ATP or *via* its metabolic breakdown to adenosine that acts on P1 (adenosine) receptors. ATP is cleared from the synapse primarily by releasable nucleotidases (rNTPase) and by cell-fixed ectonucleotidases.

available at the inner surface of the membrane for the outward transport of NE ("facilitated exchange diffusion"). In addition, these indirect-acting sympathomimetic drugs mobilize NE stored in the vesicles by competing for the vesicular uptake process. By contrast, reserpine, which depletes vesicular stores of NE, inhibits VMAT-2, but enters the adrenergic nerve ending by passive diffusion.

Three extraneuronal transporters handle a range of endogenous and exogenous substrates (*see* Table 6–4). ENT, the extraneuronal amine transporter (*uptake 2 or OCT3*), is an organic cation transporter. Relative to NET, ENT exhibits lower affinity for catecholamines, favors Epi over NE or DA, and shows a higher maximal rate of catecholamine uptake. ENT is not Na^+-dependent and

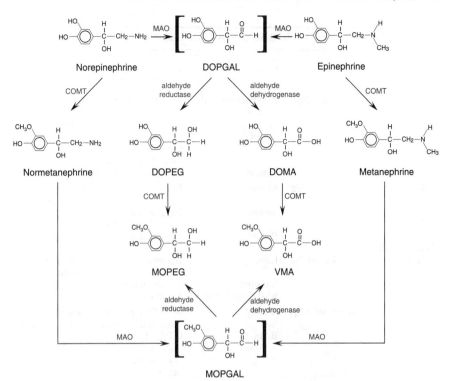

FIGURE 6–6 *Metabolism of catecholamines.* Norepinephrine and epinephrine are first oxidatively deaminated by monoamine oxidase (MAO) to 3,4-dihydroxyphenylglycoaldehyde (DOPGAL) and then either reduced to 3,4-dihydroxyphenylethylene glycol (DOPEG) or oxidized to 3,4-dihydroxymandelic acid (DOMA). Alternatively, they can be methylated initially by catechol-*O*- methyltransferase (COMT) to normetanephrine and metanephrine, respectively. Most of the products of either enzyme then are metabolized by the other enzyme to form the major excretory products in blood and urine, 3-methoxy-4-hydroxyphenylethylene glycol (MOPEG or MHPG) and 3-methoxy-4-hydroxymandelic acid (vanillylmandelic acid, VMA). Free MOPEG is largely converted to VMA. The glycol and, to some extent, the *O*-methylated amines and the catecholamines may be conjugated to the corresponding sulfates or glucuronides.

displays a completely different profile of pharmacological inhibition. Other members of this family are OCT1 and OCT2 (*see* Chapter 2). In addition to catecholamines, OCT1-3 can transport other organic cations, including 5-HT, histamine, choline, spermine, guanidine, and creatinine.

RELEASE OF CATECHOLAMINES Details of excitation-secretion coupling in sympathetic neurons and the adrenal medulla are not completely known. The triggering event is the entry of Ca^{2+}, which results in the exocytosis of the granular contents, including NE or Epi, ATP, some neuroactive peptides or their precursors, chromogranins, and DβH. Ca^{2+}-triggered secretion involves interaction of molecular scaffolding proteins and fusion proteins, leading to docking of granules at the plasma membrane and thence to secretion (*see* Figure 6–5).

Prejunctional Regulation of Norepinephrine Release

The release of the three sympathetic cotransmitters (catecholamine, ATP, NPY; *see* Figure 6–5) can be modulated by prejunctional autoreceptors and heteroreceptors. Following their release from sympathetic terminals, all three cotransmitters—NE, NPY, and ATP—can feedback on prejunctional receptors to inhibit the subsequent exocytosis. The α_{2A} and α_{2C} adrenergic receptors are the principal prejunctional receptors that inhibit sympathetic neurotransmitter release; the α_{2B} adrenergic receptors also may inhibit transmitter release at selected sites. Antagonists of this receptor, in turn, can enhance the electrically-evoked release of sympathetic neurotransmitter. NPY, acting on Y$_2$ receptors, and ATP-derived adenosine, acting on P1 receptors, also can inhibit sympathetic

Table 6–5

Characteristics of Transporters for Endogenous Catecholamines

Type of Transporter	Substrate Specificity	Tissue	Region/Cell Type	Inhibitors
Neuronal				
NET	DA > NE > Epi	All sympathetically innervated tissue	Sympathetic nerves	Desipramine, cocaine, nisoxetine
		Adrenal medulla	Chromaffin cells	
		Liver	Capillary endothelial cells	
		Placenta	Syncytiotrophoblast	
DAT	DA >> NE > Epi	Kidney	Endothelium	Cocaine, imazindol
		Stomach	Parietal and endothelial cells	
		Pancreas	Pancreatic duct	
Nonneuronal:				
OCT 1	DA ≈ Epi >> NE	Liver	Hepatocytes	Isocyanines, corticosterone
		Intestine	Epithelial cells	
		Kidney (not human)	Distal tubule	
OCT 2	DA >> NE > Epi	Kidney	Medullary proximal and distal tubules	Isocyanines, corticosterone
		Brain	Glial cells of DA-rich regions, some nonadrenergic neurons	
ENT (OCT 3)	Epi >> NE >DA	Liver	Hepatocytes	Isocyanines, corticosterone, O-methyl-isoproterenol
		Brain	Glial cells, others	
		Heart	Myocytes	
		Blood vessels	Endothelial cells	
		Kidney	Cortex, proximal and distal tubules	
		Placenta	Syncytiotrophoblast (basal membrane)	
		Retina	Photoreceptors, ganglion amacrine cells	

ABBREVIATIONS: NET, norepinephrine transporter, originally known as uptake 1; DAT, dopamine transporter; ENT (OCT3), extraneuronal transporter, originally known as uptake 2; OCT1, OCT2, organic cation transporters; Epi, epinephrine; NE, norepinephrine; DA, dopamine.

neurotransmitter release. Numerous heteroreceptors on sympathetic nerve varicosities also inhibit the release of sympathetic neurotransmitters; these include: M_2 and M_4 muscarinic, 5-HT, PGE_2, histamine, enkephalin, and DA receptors. Enhancement of sympathetic neurotransmitter release can be produced by activation of β_2 adrenergic receptors, angiotensin II receptors, and nACh receptors. All these receptors are targets for agonists and antagonists.

TERMINATION OF THE ACTIONS OF CATECHOLAMINES The actions of NE and Epi are terminated by (1) reuptake into nerve terminals by NET; (2) dilution by diffusion out of the junctional cleft and uptake at end organs and extraneuronal sites by ENT, OCT1, and OCT2. Subsequent to uptake, the catecholamines are subject to metabolic transformation by MAO and catechol-O-methyltransferase (COMT). In addition, catecholamines are metabolized by sulfotransferases (*see* Chapter 3). Termination of action by a powerful degradative enzymatic pathway, such as that provided by AChE in cholinergic transmission, is absent from the adrenergic system. Inhibitors of neuronal reuptake of catecholamines (*e.g.*, cocaine, imipramine) potentiate the effects of the neurotransmitter, whereas inhibitors of MAO and COMT have relatively little effect, demonstrating the predominant role of uptake in termination of effect. However, MAO metabolizes transmitter that is released within the nerve terminal cytosol. COMT, particularly in the liver, plays a major role in the metabolism of endogenous circulating and administered catecholamines.

Both MAO and COMT are distributed widely throughout the body, including the brain; the highest concentrations of each are in the liver and the kidney. However, little or no COMT is found in sympathetic neurons. In the brain, there is also no significant COMT in presynaptic terminals, but it is found in some postsynaptic neurons and glial cells. In the kidney, COMT is localized in proximal tubular epithelial cells, where DA is synthesized, and is thought to exert local diuretic and natriuretic effects. The physiological substrates for COMT include L-dopa, all three endogenous catecholamines (DA, NE, and Epi), their hydroxylated metabolites, catecholestrogens, ascorbate, and dihydroxyindolic intermediates of melanin. MAO and COMT are differentially localized: MAO associated chiefly with the outer surface of mitochondria, COMT largely cytosolic. These factors help to determine the primary metabolic pathways followed by catecholamines in various circumstances and to explain effects of certain drugs. Two different isozymes of MAO (MAO-A and MAO-B) are found in widely varying proportions in different cells in the CNS and in peripheral tissues. In the periphery, MAO-A is located in the syncytiotrophoblast layer of term placenta and liver, whereas MAO-B is located in platelets, lymphocytes, and liver. In the brain, MAO-A is located in all regions containing catecholamines, with the highest abundance in the locus ceruleus. MAO-B, on the other hand, is found primarily in regions that are known to synthesize and store serotonin. MAO-B is most prominent in the nucleus raphe dorsalis but also in the posterior hypothalamus and in glial cells in regions known to contain nerve terminals. MAO-B is also present in osteocytes around blood vessels.

Selective inhibitors of these two isozymes are available (see Chapter 17). Irreversible antagonists of MAO (e.g., phenelzine, tranylcypromine, and isocarboxazid) enhance the bioavailability of tyramine contained in many foods by inhibiting MAO-A; tyramine-induced NE release from sympathetic neurons may lead to markedly increased blood pressure (hypertensive crisis); selective MAO-B inhibitors (e.g., selegiline) or reversible MAO-A–selective inhibitors (e.g., moclobemide) are less likely to cause this potential interaction. MAO inhibitors are useful in the treatment of Parkinson's disease and mental depression (see Chapters 17 and 20).

Most of the Epi and NE that enters the circulation—from the adrenal medulla, sympathetic discharge or exogenous administration—is methylated by COMT to metanephrine or normetanephrine, respectively (Figure 6–6). NE that is released intraneuronally by drugs such as reserpine is deaminated initially by MAO and the aldehyde is reduced by aldehyde reductase or oxidized by aldehyde dehydrogenase. 3-Methoxy-4-hydroxymandelic acid [generally but incorrectly called vanillylmandelic acid (VMA)] is the major metabolite of catecholamines excreted in the urine. The corresponding product of the metabolic degradation of DA, which contains no hydroxyl group in the side chain, is homovanillic acid (HVA). Other metabolic reactions are described in Figure 6–6. Measurement of the concentrations of catecholamines and their metabolites in blood and urine is useful in the diagnosis of pheochromocytoma, a catecholamine-secreting tumor of the adrenal medulla/chromaffin tissue.

Inhibitors of MAO (e.g., pargyline and nialamide) can cause an increase in the concentration of NE, DA, and 5-HT in the brain and other tissues accompanied by a variety of pharmacological effects. No striking pharmacological action in the periphery can be attributed to the inhibition of COMT. However, the COMT inhibitors entacapone and tocapone are efficacious in the therapy of Parkinson's disease (see Chapter 20).

CLASSIFICATION OF ADRENERGIC RECEPTORS Understanding the diverse effects of the catecholamines and sympathomimetic agents requires understanding the properties of the different types of adrenergic receptors and their distribution on various tissues and organs (Tables 6–1, 6–5, 6–6, 6–7, and 10–6).

MOLECULAR BASIS OF ADRENERGIC RECEPTOR FUNCTION Adrenergic receptors are divided into two main classes, α and β, and thence into subclasses. All of the adrenergic receptors are GPCRs that link to heterotrimeric G proteins, each receptor showing a preference for a particular class of G proteins, that is, α_1 to G_q, α_2 to G_i, and all β to G_s (Table 6–6). The responses that follow activation of adrenergic receptors result from G protein–mediated effects on the generation of second messengers and on the activity of ion channels.

β ADRENERGIC RECEPTORS

β Receptors regulate numerous functional responses, including heart rate and contractility, smooth muscle relaxation, and multiple metabolic events (Table 6–1). All three of the β receptor

Table 6-6

Characteristics of Subtypes of Adrenergic Receptors*

Receptor	Agonists	Antagonists	Tissue	Responses
α_1[†]	Epi ≥ NE >> Iso Phenylephrine	Prazosin	Vascular smooth muscle	Contraction
			GU smooth muscle	Contraction
			Liver[‡]	Glycogenolysis; gluconeogenesis
			Intestinal smooth muscle	Hyperpolarization and relaxation
			Heart	Increased contractile force; arrhythmias
α_2[†]	Epi ≥ NE >> Iso Clonidine	Yohimbine	Pancreatic islets (β cells)	Decreased insulin secretion
			Platelets	Aggregation
			Nerve terminals	Decreased release of NE
			Vascular smooth muscle	Contraction
β_1	Iso > Epi = NE Dobutamine	Metoprolol CGP 20712A	Juxtaglomerular cells	Increased renin secretion
			Heart	Increased force and rate of contraction and AV nodal conduction velocity
β_2	Iso > Epi >> NE Terbutaline	ICI 118551	Smooth muscle (vascular, bronchial, GI, and GU)	Relaxation
			Skeletal muscle	Glycogenolysis; uptake of K^+
			Liver[‡]	Glycogenolysis; gluconeogenesis
β_3[§]	Iso = NE > Epi BRL 37344	ICI 118551 CGP 20712A	Adipose tissue	Lipolysis

ABBREVIATIONS: Epi, epinephrine; NE, norepinephrine; Iso, isoproterenol; GI, gastrointestinal; GU, genitourinary.

*This table provides examples of drugs that act on adrenergic receptors and of the location of subtypes of adrenergic receptors.

[†]At least three subtypes each of α_1 and α_2 adrenergic receptors are known, but distinctions in their mechanisms of action have not been clearly defined.

[‡]In some species (e.g., rat), metabolic responses in the liver are mediated by α_1 adrenergic receptors, whereas in others (e.g., dog) β_2 adrenergic receptors are predominantly involved. Both types of receptors appear to contribute to responses in human beings.

[§]Metabolic responses in adipocytes and certain other tissues with atypical pharmacological characteristics may be mediated by this subtype of receptor. Most β adrenergic receptor antagonists (including propranolol) do not block these responses.

Table 6-7

Adrenergic Receptors and Their Effector Systems

Adrenergic Receptor	G Protein	Examples of Some Biochemical Effectors
β_1	G_s	↑ adenylyl cyclase, ↑ L-type Ca^{2+} channels
β_2	G_s	↑ adenylyl cyclase
β_3	G_s	↑ adenylyl cyclase
α_1 Subtypes	G_q	↑ phospholipase C
	G_q	↑ phospholipase D
	G_q, G_i/G_o	↑ phospholipase A_2
	G_q	? ↑ Ca^{2+} channels
α_2 Subtypes	$G_{i\,1,2,\,or\,3}$	↓ adenylyl cyclase
	G_i ($\beta\gamma$ subunits)	↑ K^+ channels
	G_o	↓ Ca^{2+} channels (L- and N-type)
	?	↑ PLC, PLA_2

subtypes (β_1, β_2, and β_3) couple to G_s and activate adenylyl cyclase (Table 6–6). Thus, stimulation of β adrenergic receptors leads to the accumulation of cyclic AMP, activation of PKA, and altered function of numerous cellular proteins as a result of their phosphorylation (see Chapter 1). In addition, G_s can enhance directly the activation of voltage-sensitive Ca^{2+} channels in the plasma membrane of skeletal and cardiac muscle. Catecholamines promote β receptor feedback regulation, i.e., desensitization and receptor down-regulation, and β receptors differ in the extent to which they undergo such regulation, with the β_2 receptor being the most susceptible. β_1, β_2, and β_3 receptors may differ in their signaling pathways and subcellular location in experimental systems, and coupling to G_i is possible, probably due to subtype-selective association with intracellular scaffolding and signaling proteins. The activation of PKA by cyclic AMP and the importance of compartmentation of components of the cyclic AMP pathway are discussed in Chapter 1.

α ADRENERGIC RECEPTORS

The α_1 receptors (α_{1A}, α_{1B}, and α_{1D}) and α_2 receptors (α_{2A}, α_{2B}, and α_{2C}) are GPCRs. α_2 receptors couple to a variety of effectors (Table 6–6), generally inhibiting adenylyl cyclase and activating G protein–gated K^+ channels, resulting in membrane hyperpolarization (possibly via Ca^{2+}-dependent processes or from direct interaction of liberated $\beta\gamma$ subunits with K^+ channels). α_2 receptors also can inhibit voltage-gated Ca^{2+} channels, an effect mediated by G_o. Other second-messenger systems linked to α_2-receptor activation include acceleration of Na^+/H^+ exchange, stimulation of phospholipase $C_{\beta2}$ activity and arachidonic acid mobilization, increased phosphoinositide hydrolysis, and increased intracellular availability of Ca^{2+}. The latter is involved in the smooth muscle–contracting effect of α_2 adrenergic receptor agonists. The α_{2A} receptor plays a major role in inhibiting NE release from sympathetic nerve endings and suppressing sympathetic outflow from the brain, leading to hypotension. In the CNS, α_{2A} receptors, the most dominant adrenergic receptor, probably produce the antinociceptive effects, sedation, hypothermia, hypotension, and behavioral actions of α_2 agonists. The α_{2B} receptor is the main receptor mediating α_2-induced vasoconstriction, whereas the α_{2C} receptor is the predominant receptor inhibiting the release of catecholamines from the adrenal medulla and modulating DA neurotransmission in the brain.

Stimulation of α_1 receptors results in the regulation of multiple effector systems, primarily activation of the G_q-PLC_β-IP_3-Ca^{2+} pathway and the activation of other Ca^{2+}- and calmodulin-sensitive pathways and the activation of PKC. PKC phosphorylates many substrates, including membrane proteins such as channels, pumps, and ion-exchange proteins (e.g., Ca^{2+}-transport ATPase). These effects presumably lead to regulation of various ion conductances α_1-receptor stimulation of phospholipase A_2 leads to the release of free arachidonate, which is then metabolized via the cyclooxygenase and lipoxygenase pathways to the bioactive prostaglandins and leukotrienes, respectively (see Chapter 25). Stimulation of phospholipase A_2 activity by various agonists (including Epi acting at α_1 receptors) is found in many tissues, suggesting that this effector is physiologically important. Phospholipase D hydrolyzes phosphatidylcholine to yield phosphatidic acid (PA). Although PA itself may act as a second messenger by releasing Ca^{2+} from intracellular stores, it also is metabolized to the second messenger DAG. Phospholipase D is an effector for ADP-ribosylating factor (ARF), suggesting that phospholipase D may play a role in membrane trafficking. Finally, some evidence in vascular smooth muscle suggests that α_1 receptors are capable of regulating a Ca^{2+} channel via a G protein.

In most smooth muscles, the increased concentration of intracellular Ca^{2+} ultimately causes contraction as a result of activation of Ca^{2+}-sensitive protein kinases such as the calmodulin-dependent myosin light-chain kinase; phosphorylation of the light chain of myosin is associated with the development of tension. In contrast, the increased concentration of intracellular Ca^{2+} that results from stimulation of α_1 receptors in GI smooth muscle causes hyperpolarization and relaxation by activation of Ca^{2+}-dependent K^+ channels. The α_{1A} receptor is the predominant receptor causing vasoconstriction in many vascular beds, including the mammary, mesenteric, splenic, hepatic, omental, renal, pulmonary, and epicardial coronary arteries. It is also the predominant subtype in the vena cava and the saphenous and pulmonary veins. Together with the α_{1B} receptor subtype, its activation promotes cardiac growth. The α_{1B} receptor subtype is the most abundant subtype in the heart, whereas the α_{1D} receptor subtype is the predominant receptor causing vasoconstriction in the aorta. Some evidence suggests that α_{1B} receptors mediate behaviors such as reaction to novelty and exploration and are involved in behavioral sensitizations and in the vulnerability to addiction (see Chapter 23).

Localization of Adrenergic Receptors—Presynaptically located α_2 and β_2 receptors fulfill important roles in the regulation of neurotransmitter release from sympathetic nerve endings (see above). Presynaptic α_2 receptors also may mediate inhibition of release of neurotransmitters other than NE in the central and peripheral nervous systems. Both α_2 and β_2 receptors are located *on many types of neurons in the brain. In peripheral tissues, postsynaptic α_2 receptors are found in vascular and other smooth muscle cells (where they mediate contraction), adipocytes, and many types of secretory epithelial cells (intestinal, renal, endocrine). Postsynaptic β_2 receptors are found in the myocardium (where they mediate contraction) as well as on vascular and other smooth muscle cells (where they mediate relaxation). Both α_2 and β_2 receptors may be situated at sites that are relatively remote from nerve terminals releasing NE. Such extrajunctional receptors typically are found on vascular smooth muscle cells and blood elements (platelets and leukocytes) and may be activated preferentially by circulating catecholamines, particularly Epi. In contrast, α_1 and β_1 receptors appear to be located mainly in the immediate vicinity of sympathetic adrenergic nerve terminals in peripheral target organs, strategically placed to be activated during stimulation of these nerves. These receptors also are distributed widely in the mammalian brain.*

The cellular distributions of the three α_1 and three α_2 receptor subtypes still are incompletely understood. Recent findings indicate that α_{2A} subtype functions as a presynaptic autoreceptor in central noradrenergic neurons.

REFRACTORINESS TO CATECHOLAMINES Exposure of catecholamine-sensitive cells and tissues to adrenergic agonists causes a progressive diminution in their capacity to respond to such agents. This phenomenon, variously termed *refractoriness, desensitization,* downregulation, or *tachyphylaxis,* can limit the therapeutic efficacy and duration of action of catecholamines and other agents (*see* Chapter 1).

PHARMACOLOGICAL CONSIDERATIONS

Each step in neurotransmission (Figures 6–2, 6–3, and 6–5) represents a potential point of therapeutic intervention. This is depicted in the diagrams of the cholinergic and adrenergic terminals and their postjunctional sites (Figures 6–3 and 6–5). Drugs that affect processes involved in each step of transmission at both cholinergic and adrenergic junctions are summarized in Table 6–7.

OTHER AUTONOMIC NEUROTRANSMITTERS

Both central and peripheral neurons generally contain more than one transmitter substance (see Chapter 12). The anatomical separation of the parasympathetic and sympathetic components of the ANS and the actions of ACh and NE provide the essential framework for studying autonomic function, but a host of other chemical messengers (e.g., purines, eicosanoids, NO, peptides) also modulate or mediate responses in the ANS. ATP and ACh can coexist in cholinergic vesicles; ATP, NPY, and catecholamines are found within storage granules of sympathetic nerves and the adrenal medulla. Many peptides are found in the adrenal medulla, nerve fibers, or ganglia of the ANS or in the structures that are innervated by the ANS, including the enkephalins, substance P and other tachykinins, somatostatin, gonadotropin-releasing hormone, cholecystokinin, calcitonin gene–related peptide, galanin, pituitary adenylyl cyclase–activating peptide, VIP, chromogranins, and NPY. Some of the orphan GPCRs discovered in the course of genome-sequencing projects may represent receptors for undiscovered peptides or other cotransmitters. The evidence for widespread transmitter function in the ANS is substantial for VIP and NPY. ATP and its metabolites may act postsynaptically and exert presynaptic modulatory effects on transmitter release via P2 receptors and receptors for adenosine. In addition to acting as a cotransmitter with NE, ATP may be a cotransmitter with ACh in certain postganglionic parasympathetic nerves, for example, in the urinary bladder. NPY is colocalized and coreleased with NE and ATP in most peripheral sympathetic nerves, especially those innervating blood vessels. Thus, NPY, together with NE and ATP, may be the third sympathetic cotransmitter. The functions of NPY include (1) direct postjunctional contractile effects; (2) potentiation of the contractile effects of the other sympathetic cotransmitters; and (3) inhibitory modulation of the nerve stimulation–induced release of all three sympathetic cotransmitters.

VIP and ACh coexist in peripheral autonomic neurons, and it seems likely that VIP is a parasympathetic cotransmitter in certain locations, such as the nerves regulating GI sphincters.

NANC TRANSMISSION BY PURINES Autonomic neurotransmission may be nonadrenergic and noncholinergic (NANC). The existence of purinergic neurotransmission in the GI tract, genitourinary tract, and certain blood vessels is compelling; ATP fulfills the criteria for a neurotransmitter. Adenosine, generated from the released ATP by ectoenzymes and releasable nucleotidases, acts as a modulator, causing feedback inhibition of release of the transmitter. Purinergic receptors may be divided into the adenosine (P1) receptors and ATP receptors (P2X and P2Y receptors); both P1 and P2 receptors have various subtypes. Methylxanthines such as caffeine and theophylline preferentially block adenosine receptors (see Chapter 27). The P1 and P2Y receptors mediate their responses *via* G proteins; P2X receptors are a subfamily of ligand-gated ion channels.

ENDOTHELIUM-DERIVED FACTORS AND NITRIC OXIDE   Intact endothelium is necessary to achieve vascular relaxation in response to ACh. This inner cellular layer of the blood vessel now is known to modulate autonomic and hormonal effects on the contractility of blood vessels. In response to a variety of vasoactive agents and even physical stimuli, the endothelial cells release a short-lived vasodilator called *endothelium-derived relaxing factor* (EDRF), now known to be NO. Products of inflammation and platelet aggregation (*e.g.,* 5-HT, histamine, bradykinin, purines, thrombin) exert all or part of their actions by stimulating NO production. Endothelium–dependent relaxation is important in a variety of vascular beds, including the coronary circulation. Activation of receptors linked to the G_q-PLC-IP_3 pathway on endothelial cells mobilizes stored Ca^{2+}, activates endothelial NO synthase, and promotes NO production. NO diffuses to the underlying smooth muscle and induces relaxation of vascular smooth muscle by activating the soluble guanylyl cyclase, which increases cyclic GMP concentrations. Nitrate vasodilators used to lower blood pressure or to treat ischemic heart disease act as NO donors (*see* Chapter 31). NO also is released from certain nerves (*nitrergic*) innervating blood vessels and smooth muscles of the GI tract. NO has a negative inotropic action on the heart. Alterations in the production or action of NO may affect a number of conditions such as atherosclerosis and septic shock.

NO is synthesized from L-arginine and molecular oxygen by Ca^{2+}-calmodulin-sensitive *nitric oxide synthase* (NOS). There are three known forms of this enzyme. One form (eNOS) is constitutive, residing in the endothelial cell and synthesizing NO over short periods in response to receptor-mediated increases in cellular Ca^{2+}. A second form (nNOS) is responsible for the Ca^{2+}-dependent NO synthesis in neurons. The third form of NOS (iNOS) is induced after activation of cells by cytokines and bacterial endotoxins. Once expressed, iNOS binds Ca^{2+} tightly, is independent of fluctuations in $[Ca^{2+}]_i$, and synthesizes NO for long periods of time. This inducible, high-output form is responsible for the toxic manifestations of NO. Glucocorticoids inhibit the expression of inducible, but not constitutive, forms of NOS in vascular endothelial cells. However, other endothelium-derived factors also may be involved in vasodilation and hyperpolarization of the smooth muscle cell. NOS inhibitors might have therapeutic benefit in septic shock and neurodegenerative diseases. Conversely, diminished production of NO by the endothelial cell layer in atherosclerotic coronary arteries may contribute to the risk of myocardial infarction.

For a complete Bibliographical listing see Goodman & Gilman's *The Pharmacological Basis of Therapeutics*, 11th ed., or Goodman & Gilman Online at www.accessmedicine.com.

7

MUSCARINIC RECEPTOR AGONISTS AND ANTAGONISTS

MUSCARINIC RECEPTORS AND MUSCARINIC AGONISTS

Actions of acetylcholine (ACh) are referred to as *muscarinic* based on the observation that muscarine acts selectively at certain sites and, qualitatively, produces the same effects as ACh. Peripheral muscarinic acetylcholine receptors are found primarily on autonomic effector cells innervated by postganglionic parasympathetic nerves and on some cells that receive little or no cholinergic innervation but express muscarinic receptors (*e.g.*, vascular endothelial cells). There are also muscarinic receptors in ganglia and the adrenal medulla, where muscarinic stimulation seems to modulate the effects of nicotinic stimulation. Within the central nervous system (CNS), the hippocampus, cortex, and thalamus have high densities of muscarinic receptors.

Muscarinic agonists mimic the muscarinic effects of ACh and typically are longer-acting congeners of ACh or natural alkaloids that display little selectivity for the various subtypes of muscarinic receptors. The muscarinic, or parasympathomimetic, actions of the drugs considered in this chapter are practically equivalent to the effects of postganglionic parasympathetic nerve impulses listed in Table 6–1. All of the actions of ACh and its congeners at muscarinic receptors can be blocked by *atropine*.

Subtypes of Muscarinic Receptors

The cloning of complementary DNAs (cDNAs) encoding muscarinic receptors has identified five distinct gene products, designated as M_1 through M_5 (see Table 6–3). All of the muscarinic receptor subtypes are G protein–coupled receptors (GPCRs). Although selectivity is not absolute, stimulation of M_1 and M_3 receptors generally activates the G_q-PLC-IP$_3$ pathway and mobilizes intracellular Ca^{2+}, resulting in a variety of Ca^{2+}-mediated events, either directly or as a consequence of the phosphorylation of target proteins. In contrast, M_2 and M_4 muscarinic receptors couple to G_i to inhibit adenylyl cyclase and to G_i and G_0 to regulate specific ion channels (e.g., enhancement of K^+ conductance in cardiac sinoatrial [SA] nodal cells) through βγ subunits of the G proteins.

Pharmacological Effects of Muscarinic Stimulation

CARDIOVASCULAR SYSTEM ACh has four primary effects on the cardiovascular system: vasodilation, a decrease in cardiac rate (the negative chronotropic effect), a decrease in the rate of conduction in the specialized tissues of the SA and atrioventricular (AV) nodes (the negative dromotropic effect), and a decrease in the force of cardiac contraction (the negative inotropic effect). The last effect is of lesser significance in ventricular than in atrial muscle. Certain of the above responses can be obscured by baroreceptor and other reflexes that dampen or counteract the direct responses to ACh.

Although ACh rarely is given systemically, its cardiac actions are important because of the involvement of cholinergic vagal impulses in the baroreceptor reflex and in the actions of the cardiac glycosides, antiarrhythmic agents, and many other drugs; afferent stimulation of the viscera during surgical interventions also stimulates vagal release of ACh.

The intravenous injection of a small dose of ACh produces a transient fall in blood pressure owing to generalized vasodilation, usually accompanied by reflex tachycardia. A considerably larger dose is required to elicit bradycardia or block of AV nodal conduction from a direct action of ACh on the heart. If large doses of ACh are injected after the administration of atropine, an increase in blood pressure is observed due to stimulation of nicotinic receptors on the adrenal medulla and sympathetic ganglia resulting in the release of catecholamines into the circulation and at postganglionic sympathetic nerve endings.

ACh produces dilation of essentially all vascular beds, including those of the pulmonary and coronary vasculature; the effect is mediated by stimulation of endothelial NO production. Vasodilation of coronary beds may be elicited by baroreceptor or chemoreceptor reflexes or by direct electrical stimulation of the vagus; however, neither parasympathetic vasodilator nor sympathetic vasoconstrictor tone plays a major role in the regulation of coronary blood flow relative to the effects of local oxygen tension and autoregulatory metabolic factors such as adenosine.

Dilation of vascular beds by exogenous ACh is due primarily to M_3 receptors on endothelial cells. Most vessels lack cholinergic innervation, but their endothelial and smooth muscle cells express muscarinic receptors. In each cell type, stimulation of the muscarinic receptors activates the G_q-PLC-IP$_3$ pathway and mobilizes cell Ca^{2+}. In endothelial cells, this leads to Ca^{2+}-calmodulin–dependent activation of endothelial NO synthase (eNOS, NOS-3) and production of NO which diffuses to adjacent smooth muscle cells, where it stimulates the soluble guanylyl cyclase and causes relaxation (*see* Chapters 1 and 6). Vasodilation also may arise indirectly due to inhibition of norepinephrine (NE) release from adrenergic nerve endings by ACh. If the endothelium is damaged, as occurs under various pathophysiological conditions, the direct effect of ACh on the muscarinic receptors on vascular smooth muscle cells predominates, and the resultant mobilization of cell Ca^{2+} causes vasoconstriction. There is also evidence of NO-based (nitrergic) neurotransmission in peripheral blood vessels.

Cholinergic stimulation affects cardiac function both directly and by inhibiting the effects of adrenergic activation. The latter depends on the level of sympathetic drive to the heart and results in part from inhibition of cyclic AMP formation and reduction in L-type Ca^{2+} channel activity, mediated through M_2 receptors. Inhibition of adrenergic stimulation of the heart also results from the capacity of M_2 receptors to inhibit the release of NE from sympathetic nerve endings. Cholinergic innervation of the ventricular myocardium is less dense, and the parasympathetic fibers terminate largely on specialized conduction tissue such as the Purkinje fibers but also on some ventricular myocytes, which express M_2 receptors.

In the SA node, each normal cardiac impulse is initiated by the spontaneous depolarization of the pacemaker cells (*see* Chapter 34). When a threshold is reached, an action potential is initiated and conducted through the atrial muscle fibers to the AV node and thence through the Purkinje system to the ventricular muscle. ACh slows the heart rate by decreasing the rate of spontaneous diastolic depolarization (the pacemaker current) and by increasing the repolarizing K^+ current at the SA node (a direct effect of $\beta\gamma$ subunits of G_i/G_o); in sum, the membrane potential is more negative and attainment of the threshold potential and the succeeding events in the cardiac cycle are delayed.

In atrial muscle, ACh decreases the strength of contraction. This occurs largely indirectly, as a result of decreasing cyclic AMP and Ca^{2+} channel activity. Direct inhibitory effects are seen at higher ACh concentrations and result from M_2 receptor–mediated activation of G protein–regulated K^+ channels. The rate of impulse conduction in the normal atrium is either unaffected or may increase in response to ACh, due to the activation of additional Na^+ channels, possibly in response to the ACh-induced hyperpolarization. The combination of these factors is the basis for the perpetuation or exacerbation by vagal impulses of atrial flutter or fibrillation arising at an ectopic focus. In contrast, primarily in the AV node and to a much lesser extent in the Purkinje conducting system, ACh slows conduction and increases the refractory period. The decrease in AV nodal conduction usually is responsible for the complete heart block that may be observed when large quantities of cholinergic agonists are administered systemically. With an increase in vagal tone, such as is produced by *digoxin*, the increased refractory period can contribute to the reduction in the frequency with which aberrant atrial impulses are transmitted to the ventricle, and thus protect the ventricle during atrial flutter or fibrillation.

Although the effect is smaller than that observed in the atrium, ACh produces a negative inotropic effect in the ventricle. This inhibition is most apparent when there is concomitant adrenergic stimulation or underlying sympathetic tone. ACh suppresses automaticity of Purkinje fibers and increases the threshold for ventricular fibrillation. To the extent that the ventricle receives cholinergic innervation, sympathetic and vagal nerve terminals lie in close proximity, and muscarinic receptors are believed to exist at presynaptic as well as postsynaptic sites.

GASTROINTESTINAL AND URINARY TRACTS   Although stimulation of vagal input to the gastrointestinal (GI) tract increases tone, amplitude of contraction, and secretory activity of the stomach and intestine, such responses are inconsistently seen with administered ACh. Poor perfusion of visceral organs and rapid hydrolysis by plasma butyrylcholinesterase limit access of systemically administered ACh to visceral muscarinic receptors. Parasympathetic sacral innervation causes detrusor muscle contraction, increased voiding pressure, and ureter peristalsis, but for similar reasons these responses are not evident with administered ACh.

MISCELLANEOUS EFFECTS

The influence of ACh and parasympathetic innervation on various organs and tissues is discussed in detail in Chapter 6. ACh and its analogs stimulate secretion by all glands that receive parasympathetic innervation, including the lacrimal, tracheobronchial, salivary, and digestive glands. The effects on the respiratory system, in addition to increased tracheobronchial secretion, include bronchoconstriction and stimulation of the chemoreceptors of the carotid and aortic bodies. When instilled into the eye, muscarinic agonists produce miosis (see Chapter 63).

Table 7–1

Some Pharmacological Properties of Choline Esters and Natural Alkaloids

Muscarinic Agonist	Susceptibility to Cholinesterases	Muscarinic Activity					Nicotinic Activity
		Cardiovascular	Gastrointestinal	Urinary Bladder	Eye (Topical)	Antagonism by Atropine	
Acetylcholine	+++	++	++	++	+	+++	++
Methacholine	+	+++	++	++	+	+++	+
Carbachol	–	+	+++	+++	++	+	+++
Bethanechol	–	±	+++	+++	++	+++	–
Muscarine	–	++	+++	+++	++	+++	–
Pilocarpine	–	+	+++	+++	++	+++	–

CHOLINOMIMETIC CHOLINE ESTERS AND NATURAL ALKALOIDS

Muscarinic cholinergic receptor agonists can be divided into two groups: (1) ACh and several synthetic choline esters, and (2) the naturally occurring cholinomimetic alkaloids (particularly pilocarpine, *muscarine*, and *arecoline*) and their synthetic congeners. The structures and pharmacologic properties of a congeneric series are summarized by Table 7–1 and Figure 7–1.

Methacholine (acetyl-β-methylcholine) differs from ACh chiefly in its greater duration and selectivity of action. Its action is more prolonged because the added methyl group increases its resistance to hydrolysis by cholinesterases. Carbachol and bethanechol, unsubstituted carbamoyl esters, are completely resistant to hydrolysis by cholinesterases and thus survive long enough to be distributed to areas of low blood flow. Carbachol retains substantial nicotinic activity, particularly on autonomic ganglia; both its peripheral and its ganglionic actions are probably due, in part, to the release of endogenous ACh from the terminals of cholinergic fibers.

Of the three major natural plant alkaloids, muscarine acts almost exclusively at muscarinic receptor sites, arecoline also acts at nicotinic receptors, and pilocarpine has a dominant muscarinic action but causes anomalous cardiovascular responses (the sweat glands are particularly sensitive to this drug). Although these naturally occurring alkaloids are valuable as pharmacological tools, present clinical use is restricted largely to pilocarpine as a sialagogue and miotic agent (*see* Chapter 63).

Pharmacological Properties

GASTROINTESTINAL TRACT

All muscarinic agonists can stimulate GI smooth muscle, increasing tone and motility; large doses will cause spasm and tenesmus. Unlike methacholine, carbachol, bethanechol, and pilocarpine stimulate the GI tract without significant cardiovascular effects.

URINARY TRACT

Choline esters and pilocarpine contract the detrusor muscle of the bladder, increase voiding pressure, decrease bladder capacity, and increase ureteral peristalsis. In addition, the trigone and external sphincter muscles relax. Bethanechol shows some selectivity for bladder stimulation relative to cardiovascular activity (see Table 7–1).

EXOCRINE GLANDS

Choline esters and muscarinic alkaloids stimulate secretion of glands that receive parasympathetic or sympathetic cholinergic innervation, including the lacrimal, salivary, digestive, tracheobronchial, and sweat glands. Pilocarpine in particular causes marked diaphoresis (2–3 L of sweat may be secreted) and markedly increases salivation. Muscarine and arecoline also are potent diaphoretic agents. Accompanying side effects may include hiccough, salivation, nausea, vomiting, weakness, and occasionally collapse. These alkaloids also stimulate the lacrimal, gastric, pancreatic, and intestinal glands, and the mucous cells of the respiratory tract.

RESPIRATORY SYSTEM

In addition to tracheobronchial secretions, bronchial smooth muscle is stimulated by the muscarinic agonists. Asthmatic patients respond with intense bronchoconstriction, secretions, and a reduction in vital capacity. These actions form the basis of the methacholine challenge test used to diagnose airway hyperreactivity.

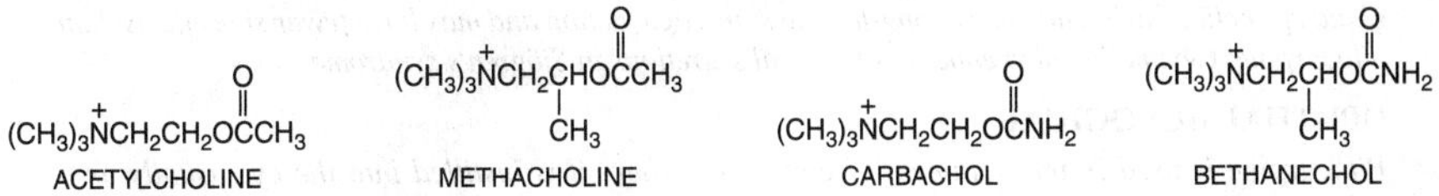

$$
\underset{\substack{+ \\ \text{(CH}_3)_3\text{NCH}_2\text{CH}_2\text{OCCH}_3 \\ \text{ACETYLCHOLINE}}}{\overset{\text{O}}{\parallel}} \qquad
\underset{\substack{+ \\ \text{(CH}_3)_3\text{NCH}_2\text{CHOCCH}_3 \\ | \\ \text{CH}_3 \\ \text{METHACHOLINE}}}{\overset{\text{O}}{\parallel}} \qquad
\underset{\substack{+ \\ \text{(CH}_3)_3\text{NCH}_2\text{CH}_2\text{OCNH}_2 \\ \text{CARBACHOL}}}{\overset{\text{O}}{\parallel}} \qquad
\underset{\substack{+ \\ \text{(CH}_3)_3\text{NCH}_2\text{CHOCNH}_2 \\ | \\ \text{CH}_3 \\ \text{BETHANECHOL}}}{\overset{\text{O}}{\parallel}}
$$

FIGURE 7–1   *Acetylcholine and choline esters.*

CARDIOVASCULAR SYSTEM

Continuous intravenous infusion of methacholine elicits hypotension and bradycardia, just as ACh does but at 1/200 the dose. Muscarine, at small doses, leads to a marked fall in blood pressure and a slowing or temporary cessation of the heartbeat. In contrast, carbachol and bethanechol generally cause only a transient fall in blood pressure at doses that affect the GI and urinary tracts.

EYE

Muscarinic agonists stimulate the pupillary constrictor and ciliary muscles when applied locally to the eye, causing pupil constriction and a loss of ability to accommodate to far vision.

CENTRAL NERVOUS SYSTEM

Quaternary choline esters do not cross the blood–brain barrier.

Therapeutic Uses

Acetylcholine (MIOCHOL-E) is available as an ophthalmic surgical aid for rapid production of miosis. Bethanechol chloride (URECHOLINE, others) is available in tablets and as an injection for use as a stimulant of GI smooth muscle, especially the urinary bladder. Pilocarpine hydrochloride (SALAGEN) is available as 5- or 7.5-mg oral doses for treatment of xerostomia or as ophthalmic solutions (PILOCAR, others) of varying strength. Methacholine chloride (PROVOCHOLINE) may be administered for diagnosis of bronchial hyperreactivity. The unpredictability of absorption and intensity of response has precluded its use as a vasodilator or cardiac vagomimetic agent. Cevimeline (EVOXAC) is a newer muscarinic agonist available orally for use in treatment of xerostomia.

GASTROINTESTINAL DISORDERS

Bethanechol can be of value in certain cases of postoperative abdominal distention and in gastric atony or gastroparesis. Oral administration is preferred; the usual dosage is 10–20 mg, three or four times daily. Bethanechol is given by mouth before each main meal in cases without complete retention; when gastric retention is complete and nothing passes into the duodenum, the subcutaneous route is necessary because of poor stomach absorption. Bethanechol has been used to advantage in certain patients with congenital megacolon and with adynamic ileus secondary to toxic states. Prokinetic agents with combined cholinergic-agonist and dopamine-antagonist activity (e.g., metoclopramide) or serotonin-antagonist activity (see Chapter 37) have largely replaced bethanechol in gastroparesis and esophageal reflux disorders.

URINARY BLADDER DISORDERS

Bethanechol may be useful in treating urinary retention and inadequate emptying of the bladder when organic obstruction is absent, as in postoperative and postpartum urinary retention and in certain cases of chronic hypotonic, myogenic, or neurogenic bladder. α Adrenergic antagonists are useful adjuncts in reducing outlet resistance of the internal sphincter (see Chapter 10). Bethanechol may enhance contractions of the detrusor muscle after spinal injury if the vesical reflex is intact, and some benefit has been noted in partial sensory or motor paralysis of the bladder. Catheterization thus can be avoided. For acute retention, multiple subcutaneous doses of 2.5 mg of bethanechol may be administered. The stomach should be empty when the drug is injected. In chronic cases, 10–50 mg of the drug may be given orally two to four times daily with meals to avoid nausea and vomiting. When voluntary or spontaneous voiding begins, bethanechol is then slowly withdrawn.

XEROSTOMIA

Pilocarpine is administered orally in 5–10-mg doses given three times daily for the treatment of xerostomia that follows head and neck radiation treatments or that is associated with Sjögren's syndrome, an autoimmune disorder occurring primarily in women in whom secretions, particularly salivary and lacrimal, are compromised. Side effects typify cholinergic stimulation, with sweating being the most common complaint. Bethanechol is an oral alternative that produces less diaphoresis. Cevimeline (EVOXAC) has activity at M_3 muscarinic receptors, such as those on lacrimal and salivary *gland epithelia. Cevimeline has a long-lasting sialogogic action and may have fewer side effects than pilocarpine. Cevimeline also enhances lacrimal secretions in Sjögren's syndrome.*

OPHTHALMOLOGICAL

Pilocarpine is used in the treatment of glaucoma, where it is instilled into the eye usually as a 0.5–4% solution. An ocular insert (OCUSERT PILO-20) that releases 20 µg of pilocarpine per hour over 7 days also is marketed for the control of elevated intraocular pressure. Pilocarpine usually is better tolerated than are the anticholinesterases and is the standard cholinergic agent for the treatment of open-angle glaucoma. Reduction of intraocular pressure occurs within a few minutes and lasts 4–8 hours. The ophthalmic use of pilocarpine alone and in combination with other agents is discussed in Chapter 63. The miotic action of pilocarpine is useful in reversing a narrow-angle glaucoma attack and overcoming the mydriasis produced by atropine; alternated with mydriatics, pilocarpine is employed to break adhesions between the iris and the lens.

CENTRAL NERVOUS SYSTEM

Agonists that selectively stimulate postsynaptic M_1 receptors in the CNS without concomitantly stimulating the presynaptic M_2 receptors (that inhibit release of endogenous ACh) have been in clinical trial for treating the cognitive impairment associated with Alzheimer's disease. However, lack of efficacy in improvement of cognitive function has diminished enthusiasm for this approach.

Precautions, Toxicity, and Contraindications

Muscarinic agonists are administered subcutaneously to achieve an acute response and orally to treat more chronic conditions. Should serious toxic reactions to these drugs arise, atropine sulfate *(0.5–1 mg in adults) should be given subcutaneously or intravenously.* Epinephrine *(0.3–1 mg, subcutaneously or intramuscularly) also is of value in overcoming severe cardiovascular or bronchoconstrictor responses.*

Major contraindications to the use of the muscarinic agonists are asthma, hyperthyroidism, coronary insufficiency, and acid-peptic disease. Their bronchoconstrictor action is liable to precipitate an asthma attack; hyperthyroid patients may develop atrial fibrillation. Hypotension induced by these agents can severely reduce coronary blood flow, especially if it is already compromised. Other possible undesirable effects of the cholinergic agents are flushing, sweating, abdominal cramps, belching, a sensation of tightness in the urinary bladder, difficulty in visual accommodation, headache, and salivation.

Toxicology

Poisoning from pilocarpine, muscarine, or arecoline is characterized chiefly by exaggeration of their parasympathomimetic effects. Treatment consists of the parenteral administration of atropine in doses sufficient to cross the blood–brain barrier and measures to support the respiratory and cardiovascular systems and to counteract pulmonary edema.

MUSHROOM POISONING (MYCETISM)

Mushrooms are a rich source of toxins; mushroom poisoning has increased as the result of the popularity of hunting wild mushrooms. High concentrations of muscarine are present in various species of Inocybe *and* Clitocybe. *The symptoms of muscarine intoxication (salivation, lacrimation, nausea, vomiting, headache, visual disturbances, abdominal colic, diarrhea, bronchospasm, bradycardia, hypotension, shock) develop within 30–60 minutes of ingestion. Treatment with atropine (1–2 mg intramuscularly every 30 minutes) effectively blocks these effects.*

Intoxication produced by Amanita muscaria *and related* Amanita *species arises from the neurologic and hallucinogenic properties of muscimol, ibotenic acid, and other isoxazole derivatives that stimulate excitatory and inhibitory amino acid receptors. Symptoms range from irritability, restlessness, ataxia, hallucinations, and delirium to drowsiness and sedation. Treatment is mainly supportive; benzodiazepines are indicated when excitation predominates; atropine often exacerbates the delirium.*

Mushrooms from Psilocybe *and* Panaeolus *species contain psilocybin and related derivatives of tryptamine that cause short-lasting hallucinations.* Gyromitra *species (false morels) produce GI disorders and a delayed hepatotoxicity. The toxic substance, acetaldehyde methylformylhydrazone, is converted in the body to reactive hydrazines. Although fatalities from liver and kidney failure have been reported, they are far less frequent than with amatoxin-containing mushrooms.*

The most serious form of mycetism is produced by Amanita phalloides, *other* Amanita *species,* Lepiota, *and* Galerina *species. These species account for >90% of fatal cases. Ingestion of as little as 50 g of* A. phalloides *(deadly nightcap) can be fatal. The principal toxins are the amatoxins (α- and β-amanitin), a group of cyclic octapeptides that inhibit RNA polymerase II and hence block messenger RNA (mRNA) synthesis. This causes cell death, particularly in the GI mucosa, liver, and kidneys. Initial symptoms include diarrhea and abdominal cramps. A symptom-free period lasting up to 24 hours is followed by hepatic and renal malfunction. Death occurs in 4–7 days from renal and hepatic failure. Treatment is largely supportive;* penicillin, thioctic acid, and silibinin *may be effective antidotes, but the evidence is anecdotal.*

Because the toxicity and treatment strategies for mushroom poisoning depend on the species ingested, their identification is key. Regional poison control centers in the U.S. maintain up-to-date information on the incidence of poisoning in the region and treatment procedures.

MUSCARINIC RECEPTOR ANTAGONISTS

General comments—Muscarinic receptor antagonists reduce the effects of ACh by competitively inhibiting its binding to muscarinic cholinergic receptors. In general, muscarinic antagonists cause little blockade at nicotinic receptors; however, the quaternary ammonium derivatives of atropine are generally more potent at muscarinic receptors and exhibit a greater degree of nicotinic blocking activity, and consequently are more likely to interfere with ganglionic or neuromuscular transmission. At high or toxic doses, central effects of atropine and related drugs are observed, generally CNS stimulation followed by depression; since quaternary compounds penetrate the blood–brain barrier poorly, they have little or no effect on the CNS.

Parasympathetic neuroeffector junctions in different organs vary in their sensitivity to muscarinic receptor antagonists (Table 7–2). Effects such as reduction of gastric secretions occur only at doses that produce severe undesirable effects. This hierarchy of relative sensitivities is not a consequence of differences in the affinity of atropine for the muscarinic receptors at these sites; atropine lacks receptor subtype selectivity. More likely determinants include the degree to which the functions of various end organs are regulated by parasympathetic tone and the involvement of intramural neurons and reflexes. Actions of most clinically available muscarinic receptor antagonists differ only quantitatively from those of atropine. No antagonist in the receptor-selective category, including pirenzepine, is completely selective; in fact, clinical efficacy may arise from a balance of antagonistic actions on two or more receptor subtypes.

Pharmacological Properties: The Prototypical Alkaloids Atropine and Scopolamine

Atropine and scopolamine differ quantitatively in antimuscarinic actions, particularly in their ability to affect the CNS. Atropine has almost no detectable effect on the CNS at doses that are used clinically. In contrast, scopolamine has prominent central effects at low therapeutic doses. The basis for this difference is probably the greater permeation of scopolamine across the blood–brain barrier. Because atropine has limited CNS effects, it is preferred to scopolamine for most purposes.

CENTRAL NERVOUS SYSTEM Atropine in therapeutic doses (0.5–1 mg) causes only mild vagal excitation as a result of stimulation of the medulla and higher cerebral centers. With toxic doses of atropine, central excitation becomes more prominent, leading to restlessness, irritability,

Table 7–2

Effects of Atropine in Relation to Dose

Dose	Effects
0.5 mg	Slight cardiac slowing; some dryness of mouth; inhibition of sweating
1 mg	Definite dryness of mouth; thirst; acceleration of heart, sometimes preceded by slowing; mild dilation of pupils
2 mg	Rapid heart rate; palpitation; marked dryness of mouth; dilated pupils; some blurring of near vision
5 mg	All the above symptoms marked; difficulty in speaking and swallowing; restlessness and fatigue; headache; dry, hot skin; difficulty in micturition; reduced intestinal peristalsis
10 mg and more	Above symptoms more marked; pulse rapid and weak; iris practically obliterated; vision very blurred; skin flushed, hot, dry, and scarlet; ataxia, restlessness, and excitement; hallucinations and delirium; coma

disorientation, hallucinations, or delirium (*see* discussion of atropine poisoning, below). With still larger doses, stimulation is followed by depression, leading to circulatory collapse and respiratory failure after a period of paralysis and coma.

Scopolamine in therapeutic doses normally causes CNS depression manifested as drowsiness, amnesia, fatigue, and dreamless sleep, with a reduction in rapid eye movement (REM) sleep. Scopolamine also causes euphoria and is therefore subject to some abuse. Scopolamine is effective in preventing motion sickness.

The belladonna alkaloids and related muscarinic receptor antagonists have long been used in parkinsonism. These agents can be effective adjuncts to treatment with *levodopa* (*see* Chapter 20). Muscarinic receptor antagonists also are used to treat the extrapyramidal symptoms that commonly occur as side effects of conventional antipsychotic drug therapy (*see* Chapter 18). Certain antipsychotic drugs are relatively potent muscarinic receptor antagonists, and these cause fewer extrapyramidal side effects.

GANGLIA AND AUTONOMIC NERVES Cholinergic neurotransmission in autonomic ganglia is mediated primarily by activation of nicotinic ACh receptors (*see* Chapters 6 and 9). ACh and other cholinergic agonists also cause the generation of slow excitatory postsynaptic potentials (EPSPs) that are mediated by ganglionic M_1 receptors. This response is particularly sensitive to blockade by pirenzepine. The extent to which the slow EPSPs can alter impulse transmission through the different sympathetic and parasympathetic ganglia is difficult to assess, but the effects of pirenzepine on responses of end organs suggest a physiological modulatory function for the ganglionic M_1 receptor.

Pirenzepine inhibits gastric acid secretion at doses that have little effect on salivation or heart rate. Since the muscarinic receptors on the parietal cells do not appear to have a high affinity for pirenzepine, the M_1 receptor responsible for alterations in gastric acid secretion may be localized in intramural ganglia. Blockade of ganglionic muscarinic receptors (rather than those at the neuroeffector junction) apparently underlies the capacity of pirenzepine to inhibit relaxation of the lower esophageal sphincter. Likewise, blockade of parasympathetic ganglia may contribute to the response to muscarinic antagonists in lung and heart.

Presynaptic muscarinic receptors on terminals of sympathetic and parasympathetic neurons generally inhibit transmitter release; thus, blockade of these presynaptic receptors will augment transmitter release. Nonselective muscarinic blocking agents may thus augment ACh release, partially counteracting their effective postsynaptic receptor blockade. Since muscarinic receptor antagonists can alter autonomic activity at the ganglion and postganglionic neuron, the ultimate response of end organs to blockade of muscarinic receptors is difficult to predict. Thus, while direct blockade at neuroeffector sites predictably reverses the usual effects of the parasympathetic nervous system, concomitant inhibition of ganglionic or presynaptic receptors may produce paradoxical responses.

EYE

Muscarinic receptor antagonists block the cholinergic responses of the pupillary sphincter muscle of the iris and the ciliary muscle controlling lens curvature (see Chapter 63). Thus, they dilate the pupil (mydriasis) and paralyze accommodation (cycloplegia). Locally applied atropine and scopolamine produce ocular effects of considerable duration; accommodation and pupillary reflexes may not fully recover for 7–12 days; thus, other muscarinic antagonists with shorter durations of action are preferred as mydriatics (see Chapter 63). Muscarinic receptor antagonists administered systemically have little effect on intraocular pressure except in patients predisposed to narrow-angle glaucoma, in whom the pressure may occasionally rise dangerously.

CARDIOVASCULAR SYSTEM

Heart Although the dominant response to atropine is tachycardia, the heart rate often decreases slightly (4–8 beats/min) transiently with average clinical doses (0.4–0.6 mg). The slowing is usually absent after rapid intravenous injection. Larger doses of atropine cause progressively increasing tachycardia by blocking vagal effects on M_2 receptors on the SA node. Resting heart rate increased by 35–40 beats/min in young men given 2 mg of atropine intramuscularly. The maximal heart rate (*e.g.*, in response to exercise) is not altered by atropine. The influence of atropine is most noticeable in healthy young adults, in whom vagal tone is considerable. In infancy and old age, even large doses of atropine may fail to accelerate the heart. Atropine often produces cardiac arrhythmias, but without significant cardiovascular symptoms.

With low doses of scopolamine (0.1–0.2 mg), the cardiac slowing is greater than with atropine. With higher doses, a transient cardioacceleration may be observed.

Adequate doses of atropine can abolish many types of reflex vagal cardiac slowing or asystole— for example, from inhalation of irritant vapors, stimulation of the carotid sinus, pressure on the eyeballs, peritoneal stimulation, or injection of contrast dye during cardiac catheterization. Atropine also prevents or abruptly abolishes bradycardia or asystole caused by choline esters, acetylcholinesterase inhibitors, or other parasympathomimetic drugs, as well as cardiac arrest from electrical stimulation of the vagus. The removal of vagal influence on the heart by atropine also may facilitate AV conduction.

Circulation Atropine, alone, has little effect on blood pressure, an expected result since most vessels lack cholinergic innervation. However, in clinical doses, atropine completely counteracts the peripheral vasodilation and sharp fall in blood pressure caused by choline esters. Atropine in toxic, and occasionally therapeutic, doses can dilate cutaneous blood vessels, especially those in the blush area (atropine flush).

RESPIRATORY TRACT Belladonna alkaloids inhibit secretions of the nose, mouth, pharynx, and bronchi, and thus dry the mucous membranes of the respiratory tract. Reduction of mucous secretion and mucociliary clearance resulting in mucus plugs are undesirable side effects of atropine in patients with airway disease. Inhibition by atropine of bronchoconstriction caused by histamine, bradykinin, and the eicosanoids presumably reflects the participation of parasympathetic efferents in the bronchial reflexes elicited by these agents. The ability to block the indirect bronchoconstrictive effects of these mediators that are released during attacks of asthma forms the basis for the use of anticholinergic agents, along with β-adrenergic receptor agonists, in the treatment of asthma (*see* Chapter 27).

GASTROINTESTINAL TRACT Atropine can completely abolish the effects of ACh (and other parasympathomimetic drugs) on the motility and secretions of the GI tract, but can only incompletely inhibit the effects of vagal impulses. This difference is particularly striking in the effects of atropine on gut motility. Preganglionic vagal fibers that innervate the GI tract synapse not only with postganglionic cholinergic fibers, but also with a network of noncholinergic intramural neurons. These neurons of the enteric plexus release numerous neurotransmitters and neuromodulators (*e.g.*, 5-HT, DA, myriad peptides) whose actions atropine does not block and which can effect changes in motility. Similarly, while vagal activity modulates gastrin-elicited histamine release and gastric acid secretion, the actions of gastrin can occur independently of vagal tone. Histamine H_2 receptor antagonists and proton pump inhibitors have replaced nonselective muscarinic antagonists as inhibitors of acid secretion (*see* Chapter 36).

Secretions

Salivary secretion, *mediated through M_3 receptors, is particularly sensitive to inhibition by muscarinic receptor antagonists, which can completely abolish the copious, watery, parasympathetically induced secretion. The mouth becomes dry, and swallowing and talking may become difficult. Gastric secretions during the cephalic and fasting phases are reduced markedly by muscarinic antagonists; the intestinal phase of gastric secretion is only partially inhibited. Atropine also reduces the cytoprotective secretions (HCO_3^-, mucus) of the superficial epithelial cells* (see *Figure 36–1*).

Motility

The parasympathetic nerves enhance both tone and motility and relax sphincters, thereby favoring intestinal transit. Muscarinic antagonists produce prolonged inhibitory effects on the motor activity of the GI tract; relatively large doses are needed to produce such inhibition. The complex myenteric nervous system can regulate motility independently of parasympathetic control, however (see *Chapter 6*).

OTHER SMOOTH MUSCLES

Urinary Tract

Muscarinic antagonists decrease the normal tone and amplitude of contractions of the ureter and bladder, and often eliminate drug-induced enhancement of ureteral tone, but at doses of atropine that inhibit salivation and lacrimation and cause blurring of vision (Table 7–2). Control of bladder contraction is complex, involving mainly M_2 receptors at multiple sites and also M_3 receptors that can mediate detrusor muscle contraction.

Biliary Tract

Atropine exerts a mild antispasmodic action on the gallbladder and bile ducts, an effect that usually is insufficient to overcome or prevent the marked spasm and increase in biliary duct pressure induced by opioids, for which nitrites (see *Chapter 31*) *are more effective.*

SWEAT GLANDS AND TEMPERATURE

Small doses of atropine or scopolamine inhibit the activity of sweat glands innervated by sympathetic cholinergic fibers, making the skin hot and dry. After large doses or at high environmental temperatures, sweating may be sufficiently depressed to raise the body temperature.

Pharmacologic Properties: The Quaternary Derivatives Ipratropium and Tiotropium

Ipratropium bromide (ATROVENT, others) is a quaternary ammonium derivative of atropine. O*xitropium bromide* is a quaternary derivative of scopolamine. Ipratropium blocks all subtypes of muscarinic receptors and thus blocks presynaptic muscarinic inhibition of ACh release. The most recently developed and bronchoselective member of this family, tiotropium bromide (SPIRIVA), has a longer duration of action and shows some selectivity for M_1 and M_3 receptors, with lower affinity for M_2 receptors, and thus less presynaptic effect on ACh release.

Ipratropium and tiotropium can produce bronchodilation, tachycardia, and inhibition of secretion similar to that of atropine but with less inhibitory effect on mucociliary clearance relative to atropine. Hence, inhaled ipratropium and tiotropium provide useful anticholinergic therapy of chronic obstructive pulmonary disease and asthma while minimizing the increased accumulation of lower airway secretions encountered with atropine.

Actions of inhaled ipratropium or tiotropium are confined almost exclusively to the mouth and airways. Dry mouth is the only side effect reported frequently. Selectivity results from the very inefficient absorption of the quaternary drug from the lungs or the GI tract. These drugs cause a marked reduction in sensitivity to methacholine in asthmatic subjects, but only modest inhibition of responses to histamine, bradykinin, or $PGF_{2\alpha}$, and little protection against bronchoconstriction induced by 5-HT or leukotrienes. The therapeutic uses of ipratropium and tiotropium are discussed further in Chapter 27.

ABSORPTION, FATE, AND EXCRETION OF MUSCARINIC ANTAGONISTS The belladonna alkaloids and the tertiary synthetic and semisynthetic derivatives are absorbed rapidly from the GI tract and mucosal surfaces; absorption from intact skin is limited, although efficient absorption does occur in the postauricular region for some agents, allowing delivery *via* transdermal patch. Systemic absorption of inhaled or orally ingested quaternary muscarinic antagonists is minimal, even from the conjunctiva of the eye; the quaternary agents do not cross the blood–brain barrier.

Atropine has a $t_{1/2}$ of ~4 hours; hepatic metabolism accounts for the elimination of about half of a dose; the remainder is excreted unchanged in the urine. Ipratropium is administered as an aerosol or solution for inhalation; tiotropium is administered as a dry powder. As with most drugs administered by inhalation, ~90% of the dose is swallowed and appears in the feces. After inhalation, maximal responses usually develop over 30–90 minutes, with tiotropium having the slower onset. The effects of ipratropium last for 4–6 hours; tiotropium's effects persist for 24 hours, and the drug is amenable to once-daily dosing.

THERAPEUTIC USES OF MUSCARINIC RECEPTOR ANTAGONISTS

The major limitation in the use of the nonselective muscarinic antagonists is the failure to obtain desired therapeutic responses without concomitant side effects. Some selectivity and reduction in side effects have been achieved by local administration and by the use of minimally absorbed quaternary compounds. Subtype-selective muscarinic receptor antagonists hold the most promise for treating specific clinical symptoms, but few show absolute selectivity.

RESPIRATORY TRACT These drugs reduce secretion in both the upper and lower respiratory tracts. This effect in the nasopharynx may provide symptomatic relief of acute rhinitis associated with coryza or hay fever. The contribution of antihistamines employed in "cold" mixtures is likely due to their antimuscarinic properties, except in conditions with an allergic basis.

Systemic administration of belladonna alkaloids or their derivatives for bronchial asthma or COPD carries the disadvantage of reducing bronchial secretions and inspissation of the residual secretions. This viscid material is difficult to remove from the respiratory tree, and its presence can dangerously obstruct airflow and predispose to infection. By contrast, ipratropium and tiotropium, administered by inhalation, do not produce adverse effects on mucociliary clearance, and can be used safely in the treatment of airway disease (*see* Chapter 27).

GENITOURINARY TRACT

Overactive urinary bladder disease can be successfully treated with muscarinic antagonists, primarily tolterodine and trospium chloride, which lower intravesicular pressure, increase capacity, and reduce the frequency of contractions by antagonizing parasympathetic control of the bladder. Oxybutynin is used as a transdermal system (OXYTROL) that delivers 3.9 mg/day and is associated with a lower incidence of side effects than the oral immediate- or extended-release formulations. Tolterodine is metabolized by CYP2D6 to a 5-hydroxymethyl metabolite; since this metabolite possesses similar activity to the parent drug, variations in CYP2D6 levels do not affect the duration of drug action. Trospium is as effective as oxybutynin, with better tolerability. Solifenacin is newly approved for overactive bladder with a favorable efficacy: side effect ratio. Stress urinary incontinence has been treated with some success with duloxetine *(YENTREVE), which acts centrally to influence 5-HT and NE levels.*

GASTROINTESTINAL TRACT   In the management of acid-peptic disease, antisecretory doses of muscarinic antagonists produce limiting side effects (Table 7–2) and, consequently, poor patient compliance. Pirenzepine has selectivity for M_1 over M_2 and M_3 receptors. However, pirenzepine's affinities for M_1 and M_4 receptors are comparable, so it does not possess total M_1 selectivity. *Telenzepine* is an analog of pirenzepine that has higher potency and similar selectivity for M_1 muscarinic receptors. Both drugs are used in the treatment of acid-peptic disease in Europe, Japan, and Canada, but not currently in the U.S. At therapeutic doses of pirenzepine, the incidence of dry mouth, blurred vision, and central muscarinic disturbances are relatively low. Central effects are not seen because of the drug's limited penetration into the CNS. Pirenzepine's relative selectivity for M_1 receptors is a marked improvement over atropine. Pirenzepine (100–150 mg/day) produces about the same rate of healing of duodenal and gastric ulcers as the H_2 antagonists *cimetidine* or *ranitidine*. Side effects necessitate drug withdrawal in <1% of patients. H_2-receptor antagonists and proton pump inhibitors generally are drugs of choice to reduce gastric acid secretion (*see* Chapter 36). The belladonna alkaloids and synthetic substitutes are very effective in reducing excessive salivation, such as drug-induced salivation and that associated with heavy-metal poisoning and parkinsonism.

The belladonna alkaloids (atropine, *belladonna tincture*, l-hyoscyamine sulfate [ANASPAZ, LEVSIN, others], and scopolamine), and combinations with sedatives (*e.g., phenobarbital* [DONNATAL, others] or *butabarbital* [BUTIBEL]), antianxiety agents (*e.g., chlordiazepoxide* [LIBRAX, others], or *ergotamine* [BELLAMINE]) also have been used in a wide variety of conditions of irritable bowel and increased tone (spasticity) or motility of the GI tract. Pharmacotherapy of inflammatory bowel disease is discussed in Chapter 38. Therapy of disorders of bowel motility and water flux are discussed in Chapter 37.

USES IN OPHTHALMOLOGY

Effects limited to the eye are obtained by local administration of muscarinic receptor antagonists to produce mydriasis and cycloplegia. Cycloplegia is not attainable without mydriasis and requires higher concentrations or more prolonged application of a given agent. In instances in which complete cycloplegia is required, more effective agents such as atropine or scopolamine are preferred to drugs such as cyclopentolate *and* tropicamide. Homatropine hydrobromide *(ISOPTO HOMATROPINE, others), a semisynthetic derivative of atropine (Figure 7–2)* cyclopentolate hydrochloride *(CYCLOGYL, others), and* tropicamide *(MYDRIACYL, others) are preferred to topical atropine or scopolamine because of their shorter duration of action (see Chapter 63).*

CARDIOVASCULAR SYSTEM

The cardiovascular effects of muscarinic receptor antagonists are of limited clinical application. Atropine may be considered in the initial treatment of patients with acute myocardial infarction in whom excessive vagal tone causes sinus or nodal bradycardia. Dosing must be judicious; doses that are too low can cause a paradoxical bradycardia; excessive doses will cause tachycardia that may extend the infarct by increasing O_2 demand. Atropine occasionally is useful in reducing the severe bradycardia and syncope associated with a hyperactive carotid sinus reflex. Atropine will protect the SA and AV nodes from the effects of excessive ACh in instances of poisoning with anticholinesterase pesticides.

CENTRAL NERVOUS SYSTEM

Certain muscarinic antagonists are effective against motion sickness. They should be given prophylactically; they are much less effective after severe nausea or vomiting has developed. Scopolamine is the most effective prophylactic agent for short (4–6 hours) exposures to severe motion, and probably for exposures of up to several days. A transdermal preparation of scopolamine (TRANSDERM SCOP) is highly effective when used prophylactically. Scopolamine, incorporated into a multilayered adhesive unit, is applied to the postauricular mastoid region, where transdermal

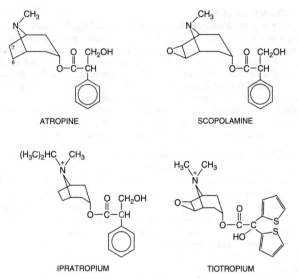

FIGURE 7–2 *Muscarinic Antagonists: belladonna alkaloids and quaternary analogs.* The blue **C** identifies an asymmetric carbon atom.

absorption is especially efficient, and over a period of about 72 hours, ~0.5 mg of scopolamine is delivered. Dry mouth is common, drowsiness is not infrequent, and blurred vision occurs in some individuals. Mydriasis and cycloplegia can occur by inadvertent transfer of the drug to the eye from the fingers after handling the patch. Rare but severe psychotic episodes have been reported.

Benztropine mesylate *(COGENTIN, others),* biperiden *(AKINETON),* procyclidine *(KEMADRIN), and* trihexyphenidyl hydrochloride *(ARTANE, others) are tertiary-amine muscarinic receptor antagonists (together with the ethanolamine antihistamine* diphenhydramine *[BENADRYL, others]) that gain access to the CNS and can therefore be used when anticholinergics are indicated to treat parkinsonism and the extrapyramidal side effects of antipsychotic drugs* (see *Chapter 20).*

USES IN ANESTHESIA

Atropine commonly is given to block responses to vagal reflexes induced by surgical manipulation of visceral organs. Atropine or glycopyrrolate is used with neostigmine *to block its parasympathomimetic effects when the latter agent is used to reverse skeletal muscle relaxation after surgery* (see *Chapter 9).*

ANTICHOLINESTERASE POISONING

The use of atropine in large doses for the treatment of poisoning by anticholinesterase organophosphorus insecticides is discussed in Chapter 8. Atropine also may be used to antagonize the parasympathomimetic effects of pyridostigmine *or other anticholinesterase agents administered in the treatment of myasthenia gravis.*

OTHER MUSCARINIC ANTAGONISTS
METHSCOPOLAMINE

Methscopolamine bromide (PAMINE), a quaternary ammonium derivative of scopolamine, lacks the central actions of scopolamine and is used chiefly in GI diseases. It is less potent than atropine and is poorly absorbed; however, its action is more prolonged, the usual oral dose (2.5 mg) acting for 6–8 hours.

HOMATROPINE METHYLBROMIDE

Homatropine methylbromide is the quaternary derivative of homatropine. It is less potent than atropine in antimuscarinic activity, but it is four times more potent as a ganglionic blocking agent. It is available in combination with hydrocodone *as an antitussive combination (HYCODAN) and has been used for relief of GI spasms and as an adjunct in peptic ulcer disease.*

GLYCOPYRROLATE

Glycopyrrolate *(ROBINUL, others) is employed orally to inhibit GI motility and is used parenterally to block the effects of vagal stimulation during anesthesia and surgery.*

MISCELLANEOUS ANTISPASMODICS

Dicyclomine hydrochloride *(BENTYL, others)*, flavoxate hydrochloride *(URISPAS, others)*, oxybutynin chloride *(DITROPAN, others)*, *and* tolterodine tartrate *(DETROL) are tertiary amines;* trospium chloride *(SANCTURA) is a quaternary amine; in therapeutic doses they decrease spasm of the GI tract, biliary tract, ureter, and uterus.*

MEPENZOLATE BROMIDE

Mepenzolate bromide *(CENTIL), a quaternary amine, has peripheral actions similar to those of atropine. It is indicated for adjunctive therapy of peptic ulcer disease and has been used as a GI antispasmodic.*

PROPANTHELINE

Propantheline bromide *(PRO-BANTHINE) is a widely used synthetic nonselective muscarinic receptor antagonist. High doses produce the symptoms of ganglionic blockade; toxic doses block the skeletal neuromuscular junction. Its duration of action is comparable to that of atropine.*

POISONING BY MUSCARINIC RECEPTOR ANTAGONISTS AND OTHER DRUGS WITH ANTICHOLINERGIC PROPERTIES

The deliberate or accidental ingestion of natural belladonna alkaloids is a major cause of poisonings. Many histamine H_1-receptor antagonists, phenothiazines, and tricyclic antidepressants also block muscarinic receptors, and in sufficient dosage, produce syndromes that include features of atropine intoxication.

Among the tricyclic antidepressants, *protriptyline* and *amitriptyline* are potent muscarinic receptor antagonists, with an affinity for the receptor that is approximately one-tenth that reported for atropine. Since these drugs are administered in therapeutic doses considerably higher than the effective dose of atropine, antimuscarinic effects often are observed clinically (*see* Chapter 17), and overdose with suicidal intent is a danger in the population using antidepressants. Fortunately, most of the newer antidepressants and SSRIs are far less anticholinergic. In contrast, the newer antipsychotic drugs ("atypical", characterized by their low propensity for inducing extrapyramidal side effects) include agents that are potent muscarinic receptor antagonists (*e.g., clozapine, olanzapine*). Accordingly, dry mouth is a prominent side effect of these drugs (a paradoxical side effect of clozapine is increased salivation and drooling, possibly the result of its partial agonist properties).

Infants and young children are especially susceptible to the toxic effects of muscarinic antagonists. Indeed, cases of intoxication in children have resulted from conjunctival instillation for ophthalmic purposes. Systemic absorption occurs either from the nasal mucosa after the drug has traversed the nasolacrimal duct or from the GI tract if the drug is swallowed. Poisoning with *diphenoxylate*-atropine (LOMOTIL, others), used to treat diarrhea, has been extensively reported in the pediatric literature. Transdermal preparations of scopolamine used for motion sickness may cause toxic psychoses, especially in children and in the elderly. Serious intoxication may occur in children who ingest berries or seeds containing belladonna alkaloids. Poisoning from ingestion and smoking of jimson weed, or thorn apple, is seen with some frequency.

Table 7–2 shows the oral doses of atropine causing undesirable responses or symptoms of overdosage. Measures to limit intestinal absorption should be initiated without delay if the poison has been taken orally (see Chapter 64). For symptomatic treatment, intravenous physostigmine rapidly abolishes the delirium and coma caused by large doses of atropine, but carries some risk of overdose in mild atropine intoxication. Since physostigmine is metabolized rapidly, the patient may again lapse into coma within 1–2 hours, and repeated doses may be needed (see Chapter 8). If marked excitement is present and more specific treatment is not available, a benzodiazepine is the most suitable agent for sedation and for control of convulsions. Phenothiazines or agents with antimuscarinic activity should not be used, because their antimuscarinic action is likely to intensify toxicity. Support of respiration and control of hyperthermia may be necessary.

For a complete Bibliographical listing see Goodman & Gilman's *The Pharmacological Basis of Therapeutics,* 11th ed., or Goodman & Gilman Online at www.accessmedicine.com.

8

ACETYLCHOLINESTERASE INHIBITORS

Acetylcholinesterase (AChE) terminates the action of acetylcholine (ACh) at the junctions of the various cholinergic nerve endings with their effector organs or postsynaptic sites. Inhibitors of AChE, or *anticholinesterase* (anti-ChE) *agents*, cause ACh to accumulate in the vicinity of cholinergic nerve terminals and thus can produce effects equivalent to excessive stimulation of cholinergic receptors throughout the central and peripheral nervous systems; such is the basis of their clinical use and their adverse effects. Since cholinergic neurotransmission is widely distributed across animal species, anti-ChE agents are also effective toxins (*e.g.*, agricultural insecticides, pesticides, and, regrettably, chemical warfare "nerve gases").

MECHANISM OF ACTION OF AChE INHIBITORS

AChE inhibitors may be divided into three groups: noncovalent or "reversible" inhibitors, carbamoylating inhibitors, and organophosphorus compounds. The mechanisms of the action of compounds that typify these three classes of anti-ChE agents are shown in Figure 8–1. Three distinct domains on AChE constitute binding sites for inhibitory ligands and form the basis for specificity differences between AChE and butyrylcholinesterase: the acyl pocket of the active center, the choline subsite of the active center, and the peripheral anionic site. Reversible inhibitors (e.g., edrophonium, tacrine) bind to the choline subsite. Edrophonium has a brief duration of action because it binds reversibly and its quaternary structure facilitates renal elimination. Additional reversible inhibitors, such as donepezil, bind with higher affinity to the active center. Other reversible inhibitors (e.g., propidium and the snake peptidic toxin fasciculin) bind to the peripheral anionic site on AChE.

Drugs that have a carbamoyl ester linkage (e.g., physostigmine and neostigmine) are hydrolyzed by AChE (much more slowly than is ACh), generating a carbamoylated enzyme (Figure 8–1C). In contrast to the acetyl enzyme, methylcarbamoyl AChE and dimethylcarbamoyl AChE are far more stable (the $t_{1/2}$ for hydrolysis of the dimethylcarbamoyl enzyme is 15–30 minutes), precluding enzyme-catalyzed hydrolysis of ACh for extended periods of time. In vivo, the duration of inhibition by the carbamoylating agents is 3–4 hours.

The organophosphorus inhibitors (e.g., DFP), form stable conjugates with AChE, with the active center serine phosphorylated or phosphonylated (Figure 8–1D). If the alkyl groups in the phosphorylated enzyme are ethyl or methyl, spontaneous regeneration of active enzyme requires several hours. Secondary (as in DFP) or tertiary alkyl groups further enhance the stability of the phosphorylated enzyme, and significant regeneration of active enzyme usually does not occur. Hence, the return of AChE activity depends on synthesis of a new enzyme. The stability of the phosphorylated enzyme is enhanced through "aging," which results from the loss of one of the alkyl groups.

Thus, the terms *reversible* and *irreversible* as applied to the carbamoyl ester and organophosphorate anti-ChE agents, respectively, reflect only quantitative differences in rates of decarbamoylation or dephosphorylation of the conjugated enzyme. Both chemical classes react covalently with the enzyme serine in essentially the same manner as does ACh.

Action at Effector Organs The characteristic pharmacological effects of the anti-ChE agents are due primarily to the accumulation of ACh at sites of cholinergic transmission. Virtually all acute effects of moderate doses of organophosphates are attributable to this action. The consequences of enhanced concentrations of ACh at motor endplates are unique to these sites and are discussed below. The tertiary amine and particularly the quaternary ammonium anti-ChE compounds may have additional direct actions at certain cholinergic receptor sites (*e.g.*, effects of neostigmine on the spinal cord and neuromuscular junction reflect anti-ChE activity and direct cholinergic stimulation).

CHEMISTRY AND STRUCTURE–ACTIVITY RELATIONSHIPS

Noncovalent Inhibitors

These agents share mechanism (above and Figure 8–1) but differ in their disposition in the body and their affinity for the enzyme. Edrophonium, a quaternary drug whose activity is limited to peripheral nervous system synapses, has a moderate affinity for AChE. Its volume of distribution is limited and renal elimination is rapid, accounting for its short duration of action. By contrast, tacrine and donepezil (Figure 8–2) have higher affinities for AChE and are more hydrophobic, contributing to their longer durations of action; they readily cross the blood–brain barrier to inhibit AChE in the central nervous system (CNS).

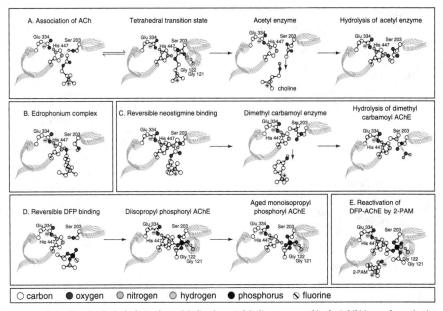

FIGURE 8–1 *Steps in the hydrolysis of acetylcholine by acetylcholinesterase and in the inhibition and reactivation of AChE.* Only the three residues of the catalytic triad are depicted. The associations and reactions shown are: *A.* Acetylcholine (ACh) catalysis: binding of ACh, formation of a tetrahedral transition state, formation of the acetyl enzyme with liberation of choline, rapid hydrolysis of the acetyl enzyme with return to the original state. *B.* Reversible binding and inhibition by edrophonium. *C.* Neostigmine reaction with and inhibition of acetylcholinesterase (AChE): reversible binding of neostigmine, formation of the dimethyl carbamoyl enzyme, slow hydrolysis of the dimethyl carbamoyl enzyme. *D.* Diisopropyl fluorophosphate (DFP) reaction and inhibition of AChE: reversible binding of DFP, formation of the diisopropyl phosphoryl enzyme, formation of the aged monoisopropyl phosphoryl enzyme. Hydrolysis of the diisopropyl enzyme is very slow and is not shown. The aged monoisopropyl phosphoryl enzyme is virtually resistant to hydrolysis and reactivation. The tetrahedral transition state of ACh hydrolysis resembles the conjugates formed by the tetrahedral phosphate inhibitors and accounts for their potency. Amide bond hydrogens from Gly 121 and 122 stabilize the carbonyl and phorphoryl oxygens. *E.* Reactivation of the diisopropyl phosphoryl enzyme by pralidoxime (2-PAM). 2-PAM attack of the phosphorus on the phosphorylated enzyme will form a phospho-oxime with regeneration of active enzyme.

"Reversible" Carbamate Inhibitors

Therapeutically useful drugs of this class of interest are shown in Figure 8–2; the essential moiety of physostigmine is a methylcarbamate of an amine-substituted phenol. An increase in anti-ChE potency and duration of action results from the linking of two quaternary ammonium moieties. One such example is the miotic agent demecarium *(2 neostigmine molecules connected by a series of 10 methylene groups). The second quaternary group confers additional stability to the drug–AChE interaction. Carbamoylating inhibitors with high lipid solubilities (e.g., rivastigmine), which readily cross the blood–brain barrier and have longer durations of action, are approved or in clinical trial for the treatment of Alzheimer's disease (see Chapter 20).*

The carbamate insecticides carbaryl *(SEVIN),* propoxur *(BAYGON), and* aldicarb *(TEMIK), which are used extensively as garden insecticides, inhibit ChE in a fashion identical with other carbamoylating inhibitors.*

Organophosphorus Compounds

The prototypic compound is DFP, which produces virtually irreversible inactivation of AChE and other esterases by alkylphosphorylation. Its high lipid solubility, low molecular weight, and volatility facilitate inhalation, transdermal absorption, and penetration into the CNS. After desulfuration, the insecticides in current use form the dimethoxy or diethoxyphosphoryl enzyme.

Malathion, parathion, and methylparathion *have become popular insecticides. Acute and chronic toxicity has limited the use of parathion and methylparathion, and potentially less hazardous compounds have replaced them. The parent compounds are inactive in inhibiting AChE in* vitro; *they must be activated* in vivo *via a phosphoryl oxygen for sulfur substitution (phosphothioate to*

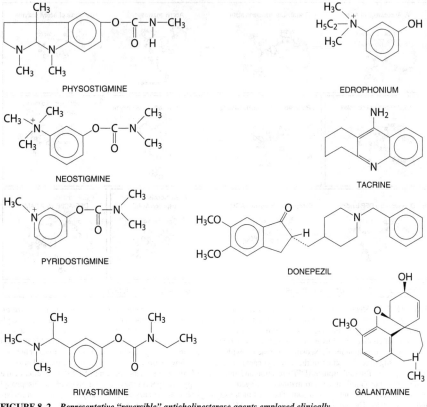

PHYSOSTIGMINE

EDROPHONIUM

NEOSTIGMINE

TACRINE

PYRIDOSTIGMINE

DONEPEZIL

RIVASTIGMINE

GALANTAMINE

FIGURE 8–2 *Representative "reversible" anticholinesterase agents employed clinically.*

phosphate), a conversion carried out predominantly by hepatic CYPs. This reaction also occurs in the insect, typically with more efficiency. Other insecticides possessing the phosphorothioate structure have been widely employed, including diazinon *(SPECTRACIDE, others) and* chlorpyrifos *(DURSBAN, LORSBAN). Chlorpyrifos recently has been placed under restricted use because of evidence of chronic toxicity in the newborn animal. For the same reason, diazinon has been banned in the U.S.*

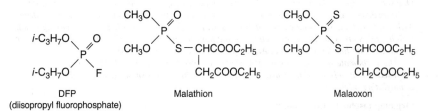

DFP
(diisopropyl fluorophosphate)

Malathion

Malaoxon

Malathion (CHEMATHION, MALA-SPRAY) requires conversion to malaoxon (replacement of a sulfur atom with oxygen in vivo, conferring resistance to mammalian species). Malathion can be detoxified by hydrolysis of the carboxyl ester linkage by plasma carboxylesterases, and plasma carboxylesterase activity dictates species resistance to malathion. The detoxification reaction is much more rapid in mammals and birds than in insects. Malathion has been employed in aerial spraying of relatively populous areas for control of Mediterranean fruit flies and mosquitoes that harbor and transmit viruses harmful to human beings (e.g., West Nile encephalitis virus). Evidence of acute toxicity from malathion arises only with suicide attempts or deliberate poisoning.

The lethal dose in mammals is ~1 g/kg. Exposure to the skin results in a small fraction (<10%) of systemic absorption. Malathion is used topically in the treatment of pediculosis (lice) infestations. Among the quaternary ammonium organophosphorus compounds, only echothiophate *is useful clinically (limited to ophthalmic administration). It is not volatile and does not readily penetrate the skin.*

PHARMACOLOGICAL PROPERTIES

The pharmacological properties of anti-ChE agents can be predicted by knowing where ACh is released physiologically by nerve impulses, the degree of nerve impulse activity, and the responses of the corresponding effector organs to ACh (*see* Chapter 6). The anti-ChE agents potentially can produce all the following effects: (1) stimulation of muscarinic receptor responses at autonomic effector organs; (2) stimulation, followed by depression or paralysis, of all autonomic ganglia and skeletal muscle (nicotinic actions); and (3) stimulation, with occasional subsequent depression, of cholinergic receptor sites in the CNS.

In general, compounds containing a quaternary ammonium group do not penetrate cell membranes readily; hence, anti-ChE agents in this category are absorbed poorly from the gastrointestinal (GI) tract or across the skin and are excluded from the CNS by the blood–brain barrier after moderate doses. On the other hand, such compounds act preferentially at the neuromuscular junctions of skeletal muscle, exerting their action both as anti-ChE agents and as direct agonists. They have comparatively less effect at autonomic effector sites and ganglia.

The more lipid-soluble agents are well absorbed after oral administration, have ubiquitous effects at both peripheral and central cholinergic sites, and may be sequestered in lipids for long periods of time. Lipid-soluble organophosphorus agents also are well absorbed through the skin, and the volatile agents are transferred readily across the alveolar membrane.

The therapeutically important sites of action of anti-ChE agents are the CNS, eye, intestine, and the neuromuscular junction of skeletal muscle; other actions are of toxicological consequence.

EYE   When applied locally to the conjunctiva, anti-ChE agents cause conjunctival hyperemia and constriction of the pupillary sphincter muscle around the pupillary margin of the iris (miosis) and the ciliary muscle (block of accommodation reflex with resultant focusing to near vision). Miosis is apparent in a few minutes and can last several hours to days. The block of accommodation generally disappears before termination of miosis. Intraocular pressure, when elevated, usually falls as the result of facilitation of outflow of the aqueous humor (*see* Chapter 63).

GASTROINTESTINAL TRACT   Neostigmine enhances gastric contractions, increases the secretion of gastric acid, and stimulates the lower potion of the esophagus. In patients with marked achalasia and dilation of the esophagus, the drug can cause a salutary increase in tone and peristalsis.

Neostigmine augments GI motor activity; the colon is particularly stimulated. Propulsive waves are increased in amplitude and frequency, and movement of intestinal contents is thus promoted. The effect of anti-ChE agents on intestinal motility probably represents a combination of actions at the ganglion cells of Auerbach's plexus and at the smooth muscle fibers (*see* Chapter 37).

NEUROMUSCULAR JUNCTION   Most of the effects of potent anti-ChE drugs on skeletal muscle can be explained by their inhibition of AChE at neuromuscular junctions. However, there is good evidence for an accessory direct action of neostigmine and other quaternary ammonium anti-ChE agents on skeletal muscle.

The lifetime of free ACh in the nerve-muscle synapse (~200 μsec) is normally shorter than the decay of the end-plate potential or the refractory period of the muscle. After inhibition of AChE, the residence time of ACh in the synapse increases, allowing for lateral diffusion and rebinding of the transmitter to multiple receptors and a prolongation of the decay time of the endplate potential. Asynchronous excitation and fasciculations of muscle fibers occur. With sufficient inhibition of AChE, depolarization of the endplate predominates, and blockade owing to depolarization ensues (*see* Chapter 9). The anti-ChE agents will reverse the antagonism caused by competitive neuromuscular blocking agents but not that caused by depolarizing agents (*e.g.*, *succinylcholine*), whose depolarization will be further enhanced by AChE inhibition (*see* Chapter 9).

ACTIONS AT OTHER SITES   Secretory glands that are innervated by postganglionic cholinergic fibers include the bronchial, lacrimal, sweat, salivary, gastric (antral G cells and parietal cells), intestinal, and pancreatic acinar glands. Low doses of anti-ChE agents augment secretory responses to nerve stimulation; higher doses actually produce an increase in the resting rate of secretion.

Anti-ChE agents increase contraction of smooth muscle fibers of the bronchioles and ureters. The cardiovascular actions of anti-ChE agents are complex, since they reflect both ganglionic and postganglionic effects of accumulated ACh on the heart and blood vessels and actions in the CNS. The predominant effect on the heart from the peripheral action of accumulated ACh is bradycardia, resulting in a fall in cardiac output. Higher doses usually cause a fall in blood pressure, often due to effects of anti-ChE agents on medullary vasomotor centers of the CNS. Anti-ChE agents augment vagal influences on the heart. At the ganglia, accumulating ACh initially is excitatory on nicotinic receptors, but at higher concentrations, ganglionic blockade ensues as a result of persistent depolarization. Excitation of parasympathetic ganglion cells reinforces diminished cardiac function, whereas enhanced function results from the action of ACh on sympathetic ganglion cells. Excitation followed by inhibition also is elicited by ACh at the central medullary vasomotor and cardiac centers. These effects are complicated further by the hypoxemia resulting from the bronchoconstrictor and secretory actions of increased ACh on the respiratory system; hypoxemia, in turn, can reinforce both sympathetic tone and ACh-induced discharge of epinephrine from the adrenal medulla. Hence, it is not surprising that an increase in heart rate is seen with severe ChE inhibitor poisoning. Hypoxemia probably is a major factor in the CNS depression that appears after large doses of anti-ChE agents. Atropine antagonizes CNS-stimulant effects, although not as completely as muscarinic effects at peripheral autonomic effector sites.

ABSORPTION, FATE, AND EXCRETION Physostigmine is absorbed readily from the GI tract, subcutaneous tissues, and mucous membranes. The conjunctival instillation of solutions of the drug may result in systemic effects if measures (*e.g.*, pressure on the inner canthus) are not taken to prevent absorption from the nasal mucosa. Parenterally administered physostigmine is largely destroyed within 2 hours, mainly by hydrolytic cleavage by plasma esterases; renal excretion plays only a minor role in its elimination.

Neostigmine and pyridostigmine are absorbed poorly after oral administration, such that much larger doses are needed than by the parenteral route (effective parenteral dose of neostigmine, 0.5–2 mg; equivalent oral dose, 15–30 mg or more). Neostigmine and pyridostigmine are destroyed by plasma esterases, with half-lives of 1–2 hours.

Organophosphorus anti-ChE agents with the highest risk of toxicity are highly lipid-soluble liquids; many have high vapor pressures. Agents used as agricultural insecticides (e.g., diazinon, malathion) generally are dispersed as aerosols or dusts that are absorbed rapidly through the skin and mucous membranes following contact with moisture, by the lungs after inhalation, and by the GI tract after ingestion. Absorbed organophosphorus compounds are hydrolyzed by plasma and liver esterases to the corresponding phosphoric and phosphonic acids, which are excreted in the urine. Young animals are deficient in these esterases (carboxylesterases and paraoxonases), which could contribute to toxicity in neonates and children.

TOXICOLOGY
ACUTE INTOXICATION

Acute intoxication by anti-ChE agents causes muscarinic and nicotinic signs and symptoms, and, except for compounds of extremely low lipid solubility, affects the CNS. Systemic effects appear within minutes after inhalation of vapors or aerosols. The onset of symptoms is delayed after GI and percutaneous absorption. Duration of effects is determined largely by the properties of the compound: lipid solubility, whether it must be activated to the oxon, stability of the organophosphorus-AChE bond, and whether "aging" of phosphorylated enzyme has occurred.

After local exposure to vapors or aerosols or after their inhalation, ocular and respiratory effects generally appear first. Ocular manifestations include marked miosis, ocular pain, conjunctival congestion, diminished vision, ciliary spasm, and brow ache. With acute systemic absorption, miosis may not be evident due to sympathetic discharge in response to hypotension. In addition to rhinorrhea and hyperemia of the upper respiratory tract, respiratory effects include tightness in the chest and wheezing due to bronchoconstriction and increased bronchial secretion. GI symptoms occur earliest after ingestion and include anorexia, nausea and vomiting, abdominal cramps, and diarrhea. With percutaneous absorption of liquid, localized sweating and muscle fasciculations in the immediate vicinity are generally the earliest symptoms. Severe intoxication is manifested by extreme salivation, involuntary defecation and urination, sweating, lacrimation, penile erection, bradycardia, and hypotension.

Nicotinic actions at the neuromuscular junctions of skeletal muscle usually consist of fatigability and generalized weakness, involuntary twitchings, scattered fasciculations, and eventually severe weakness and paralysis. The most serious consequence is paralysis of the respiratory muscles.

The broad spectrum of effects of acute AChE inhibition on the CNS includes confusion, ataxia, slurred speech, loss of reflexes, Cheyne-Stokes respiration, generalized convulsions, coma, and central respiratory paralysis. Actions on the vasomotor and other cardiovascular centers in the medulla oblongata lead to hypotension.

The time of death after a single acute exposure may range from <5 minutes to nearly 24 hours, depending on the dose, route, agent, and other factors. The cause of death primarily is respiratory failure, usually accompanied by a secondary cardiovascular component. Peripheral muscarinic and nicotinic as well as central actions all contribute to respiratory compromise; effects include laryngospasm, bronchoconstriction, increased tracheobronchial and salivary secretions, compromised voluntary control of the diaphragm and intercostal muscles, and central respiratory depression. Blood pressure may fall to alarmingly low levels and cardiac arrhythmias intervene. These effects usually result from hypoxemia and often are reversed by assisted pulmonary ventilation.

Delayed symptoms appearing after 1–4 days and marked by persistent low blood ChE and severe muscle weakness are termed the intermediate syndrome. *A delayed neurotoxicity also may be evident after severe intoxication (see below).*

Diagnosis and Treatment

The diagnosis of severe, acute anti-ChE intoxication is made readily from the history of exposure and the characteristic signs and symptoms. In suspected cases of milder, acute, or chronic intoxication, determination of the ChE activities in erythrocytes and plasma generally will establish the diagnosis. Although these values vary considerably in the normal population, they usually are depressed well below the normal range before symptoms are evident.

Atropine in sufficient dosage effectively antagonizes the actions at muscarinic receptor sites, and to a moderate extent, at peripheral ganglionic and central sites. Atropine should be given in doses sufficient to cross the blood–brain barrier. Following an initial injection of 2–4 mg (intravenously if possible, otherwise intramuscularly), 2 mg should be given every 5–10 minutes until muscarinic symptoms disappear, if they reappear, or until signs of atropine toxicity appear. More than 200 mg may be required on the first day. A mild degree of atropine block should then be maintained for as long as symptoms are evident. Atropine is virtually without effect against the peripheral neuromuscular compromise, which may be reversed by pralidoxime (2-PAM), *a cholinesterase reactivator. AChE reactivators are beneficial in the therapy of organophosphorus anti-ChE intoxication, but their use is supplemental to the administration of atropine.*

In moderate or severe intoxication with an organophosphorus anti-ChE agent, the recommended adult dose of pralidoxime is 1–2 g, infused intravenously over not less than 5 minutes. If weakness is not relieved or if it recurs after 20–60 minutes, the dose should be repeated. Early treatment is very important to assure that the oxime reaches the phosphorylated AChE while the latter still can be reactivated. Many of the alkylphosphates are extremely lipid soluble, and if extensive partitioning into body fat has occurred and desulfuration is required for inhibition of AChE, toxicity will persist and symptoms may recur after initial treatment. With severe toxicities from the lipid-soluble agents, it is necessary to continue treatment with atropine and pralidoxime for a week or longer.

General supportive measures are important, including: (1) termination of exposure, by removal of the patient or application of a gas mask if the atmosphere remains contaminated, removal and destruction of contaminated clothing, copious washing of contaminated skin or mucous membranes with water, or gastric lavage; (2) maintenance of a patent airway; (3) artificial respiration, if required; (4) administration of oxygen; (5) alleviation of persistent convulsions with diazepam (5–10 mg, intravenously); and (6) treatment of shock.

CHOLINESTERASE REACTIVATORS Although the phosphorylated esteratic site of AChE undergoes hydrolytic regeneration at a slow or negligible rate, nucleophilic agents, such as hydroxylamine (NH_2OH), hydroxamic acids ($RCONH–OH$), and oximes ($RCH=NOH$), reactivate the enzyme more rapidly than does spontaneous hydrolysis. Reactivation with pralidoxime (Figure 8–1E) occurs at a million times the rate of that with hydroxylamine. Several *bis*-quaternary oximes are even more potent as reactivators for insecticide and nerve gas poisoning (*e.g.*, HI-6, used in Europe as an antidote).

PHARMACOLOGY, TOXICOLOGY, AND DISPOSITION The reactivating action of oximes *in vivo* is most marked at the skeletal neuromuscular junction. Following a dose of an organophosphorus compound that produces total blockade of transmission, the intravenous injection of an oxime restores responsiveness of the motor nerve to stimulation within minutes. Antidotal effects are less striking at autonomic effector sites, and the quaternary ammonium group restricts entry into the CNS.

Although high doses or accumulation of oximes can inhibit AChE and cause neuromuscular blockade, they should be given until one can be assured of clearance of the offending organophosphate. Many organophosphates partition into lipid and are released slowly as the active entity. Current antidotal therapy for organophosphate exposure resulting from warfare or terrorism includes parenteral atropine, an oxime (2-PAM or HI-6), and a benzodiazepine as an anticonvulsant. Oximes and their metabolites are readily eliminated by the kidney.

THERAPEUTIC USES

AVAILABLE THERAPEUTIC AGENTS

The compounds described here are those commonly used as anti-ChE drugs and ChE reactivators in the U.S. Ophthalmic preparations are described in Chapter 63. Conventional dosages and routes of administration are given in the discussion of therapeutic applications.

Physostigmine salicylate *(ANTILIRIUM), for injection.* Physostigmine sulfate ophthalmic ointment; physostigmine salicylate ophthalmic solution. Pyridostigmine bromide, *for oral (MESTINON) or parenteral (REGONOL, MESTINON) use.* Neostigmine bromide *(PROSTIGMIN), for oral use.* Neostigmine methylsulfate *(PROSTIGMIN), for parenteral use.* Ambenonium chloride *(MYTELASE), for oral use.* Tacrine *(COGNEX),* donepezil *(ARICEPT),* rivastigmine *(EXELON),* and galantamine *(REMINYL), approved for the treatment of Alzheimer's disease.*

Pralidoxime chloride *(PROTOPAM CHLORIDE), the only AChE reactivator currently available in the U.S., available in a parenteral formulation. The AChE reactivator HI-6 is available in several European and Near Eastern countries.*

PARALYTIC ILEUS AND ATONY OF THE URINARY BLADDER

In the treatment of both these conditions, neostigmine generally is preferred among the anti-ChE agents. The direct parasympathomimetic agents (Chapter 7) are employed for the same purposes. The usual subcutaneous dose of neostigmine methylsulfate for postoperative paralytic ileus is 0.5 mg, given as needed. Peristaltic activity commences 10–30 minutes after parenteral administration, whereas 2–4 hours are required after oral administration of neostigmine bromide (15–30 mg). It may be necessary to assist evacuation with a small low enema or gas with a rectal tube.

A similar dose of neostigmine is used for the treatment of atony of the detrusor muscle of the urinary bladder.

Neostigmine should not be used when the intestine or urinary bladder is obstructed, when peritonitis is present, when the viability of the bowel is doubtful, or when bowel dysfunction results from inflammatory bowel disease.

GLAUCOMA AND OTHER OPHTHALMOLOGIC INDICATIONS

For a complete account of the pharmacotherapy of glaucoma and the roles of anti-ChE agents in ocular therapy, see *Chapter 63.*

MYASTHENIA GRAVIS

Myasthenia gravis is a neuromuscular disease characterized by weakness and marked fatigability of skeletal muscle; exacerbations and partial remissions occur frequently. The defect in myasthenia gravis is in synaptic transmission at the neuromuscular junction, such that mechanical responses to nerve stimulation are not well sustained. Myasthenia gravis is caused by an autoimmune response primarily to the ACh receptor at the postjunctional endplate. These antibodies reduce the number of receptors detectable by receptor-binding assays and electrophysiological measurements of ACh sensitivity. The similarity of the symptoms of myasthenia gravis and curare poisoning suggested that physostigmine might be of therapeutic value; 40 years elapsed before this suggestion was tried, successfully.

In a subset of ~10% of patients with myasthenic syndrome, muscle weakness has a congenital rather than an autoimmune basis, with mutations in the ACh receptor that affect ligand-binding and channel-opening kinetics, or in a form of AChE tethered by a collagen-like tail. Administration of anti-ChE agents does not result in subjective improvement in most congenital myasthenic patients.

Diagnosis

Although the diagnosis of autoimmune myasthenia gravis usually can be made from the history, signs, and symptoms, its differentiation from certain neurasthenic, infectious, endocrine, congenital, neoplastic, and degenerative neuromuscular diseases can be challenging. Myasthenia gravis is the only condition in which the muscular weakness can be improved dramatically by anti-ChE medication. The edrophonium test *for evaluation of possible myasthenia gravis is performed by rapid intravenous injection of 2 mg of* edrophonium chloride, *followed 45 seconds later by an additional 8 mg if the first dose is without effect; a positive response consists of brief improvement in strength, unaccompanied by lingual fasciculation (which generally occurs in nonmyasthenic patients). An excessive dose of an anti-ChE drug results in a* cholinergic crisis, *characterized by skeletal muscle weakness (due to depolarization blockade of nicotinic receptors at the neuromuscular junction) and other features (see above) from excess ACh at muscarinic receptors. The distinction between the weakness of cholinergic crisis/anti-AChE overdose and myasthenic weakness is of practical importance: the former is treated by withholding, and the latter by administering, the anti-ChE agent. When the edrophonium test is performed cautiously (limiting the dose to 2 mg and with facilities for respiratory resuscitation available) a further decrease in strength indicates cholinergic crisis, while improvement signifies myasthenic weakness.* Atropine sulfate, 0.4–0.6 mg *or more intravenously, should be given immediately if a severe muscarinic reaction ensues. Detection of antireceptor antibodies in muscle biopsies or plasma is now widely employed to establish the diagnosis.*

Treatment

Pyridostigmine, neostigmine, and ambenonium are the standard anti-ChE drugs used in the symptomatic treatment of myasthenia gravis. All can increase the response of myasthenic muscle to repetitive nerve impulses, primarily by the preservation of endogenous ACh. The optimal single oral dose of an anti-ChE agent is determined empirically. Baseline recordings are made for grip strength, vital capacity, and a number of signs and symptoms that reflect the strength of various muscle groups. The patient then is given an oral dose of pyridostigmine (30–60 mg), neostigmine (7.5–15 mg), or ambenonium (2.5–5 mg). The improvement in muscle strength and changes in other signs and symptoms are noted at frequent intervals until there is a return to the basal state. After an hour or longer in the basal state, the drug is readministered at 1.5 times the initial amount, and the functional observations are repeated. This sequence is continued, with increasing increments of one-half the initial dose, until an optimal response is obtained.

The interval between oral doses required to maintain a reasonably even level of strength usually is 2–4 hours for neostigmine, 3–6 hours for pyridostigmine, and 3–8 hours for ambenonium. However, the required dose may vary from day to day; physical and emotional stress, infections, and menstruation usually necessitate an increase in the frequency or size of the dose. In addition, unpredictable exacerbations and remissions of the myasthenic state may require adjustment of dosage. Patients can be taught to modify their dosage regimens according to their changing requirements.

Pyridostigmine is available in sustained-release tablets containing a total of 180 mg, of which 60 mg is released immediately and 120 mg over several hours; this preparation is of value in maintaining patients for 6–8-hour periods but should be limited to use at bedtime. Muscarinic cardiovascular and GI side effects of anti-ChE agents generally can be controlled by atropine or other anticholinergic drugs (see Chapter 7), remembering that anticholinergic drugs mask many side effects of an excessive dose of an anti-ChE agent. In most patients, tolerance develops eventually to the muscarinic effects, so that anticholinergic medication is not necessary.

A number of drugs, including curariform agents and certain antibiotics and general anesthetics, interfere with neuromuscular transmission (see Chapter 9); their administration to patients with myasthenia gravis is hazardous without proper adjustment of anti-ChE dosage and other appropriate precautions. Glucocorticoids and immunosuppressant therapies are also used in the treatment of myasthenia gravis.

INTOXICATION BY ANTICHOLINERGIC DRUGS

In addition to atropine and other muscarinic agents, phenothiazines, antihistamines, and tricyclic antidepressants have central and peripheral anticholinergic activity. The effectiveness of physostigmine in reversing the anticholinergic effects of these agents has been documented. However, other toxic effects of the tricyclic antidepressants and phenothiazines (see Chapters 17 and 18), such as intraventricular conduction deficits and ventricular arrhythmias, are not reversed by physostigmine. In addition, physostigmine may precipitate seizures; hence, its usually small potential benefit must be weighed against this risk. The initial intravenous or intramuscular dose of physostigmine is 2 mg, with additional doses given as necessary. Physostigmine, a tertiary amine, crosses the blood–brain barrier, in contrast to the quaternary anti-AChE drugs.

ALZHEIMER'S DISEASE

A deficiency of intact cholinergic neurons, particularly those extending from subcortical areas such as the nucleus basalis of Meynert, has been observed in patients with progressive dementia of the Alzheimer type. Using a rationale similar to that in other CNS degenerative diseases, therapy for enhancing concentrations of cholinergic neurotransmitters in the CNS has been used in mild-to-moderate Alzheimer's disease. Therapeutic strategies are directed at maximizing the ratio of central to peripheral ChE inhibition and using ChE inhibitors in conjunction with selective cholinergic agonists and antagonists.

Donepezil, 5 and 10 mg/day oral doses, may improve cognition and global clinical function and delay symptomatic progression of the disease. The drug is well tolerated in single daily doses; side effects are largely attributable to excessive cholinergic stimulation (nausea, diarrhea, and vomiting). Usually, 5 mg doses are administered at night for 4–6 weeks; if this dose is well tolerated, the dose can be increased to 10 mg daily. Rivastigmine, a long-acting carbamoylating inhibitor, has efficacy, tolerability, and side effects similar to those of donepezil. Galantamine, a recently approved AChE inhibitor, has a side-effect profile similar to those of donepezil and rivastigmine. Tacrine is approved for mild-to-moderate Alzheimer's disease, but a high incidence of hepatotoxicity limits this drug's utility. See Chapter 20 for further discussion of therapies for this disease.

For a complete Bibliographical listing see Goodman & Gilman's *The Pharmacological Basis of Therapeutics*, 11th ed., or Goodman & Gilman Online at www.accessmedicine.com.

9

AGENTS ACTING AT THE NEUROMUSCULAR JUNCTION AND AUTONOMIC GANGLIA

The nicotinic acetylcholine (ACh) receptor mediates neurotransmission postsynaptically at the neuromuscular junction and peripheral autonomic ganglia; in the central nervous system (CNS), it largely controls release of neurotransmitters from presynaptic sites. The receptor is called the *nicotinic acetylcholine* receptor because it is stimulated by both the neurotransmitter ACh and the alkaloid *nicotine.*

THE NICOTINIC ACETYLCHOLINE RECEPTOR
ACh interacts with the nicotinic ACh receptor to initiate an end-plate potential (EPP) in muscle or an excitatory postsynaptic potential (EPSP) in peripheral ganglia (Chapter 6). The nicotinic receptor of vertebrate skeletal muscle is a pentamer composed of 4 distinct subunits (α, β, γ, and δ) in the stoichiometric ratio of 2:1:1:1, respectively. In mature, innervated muscle end plates, the γ subunit is replaced by the closely related ε subunit. The nicotinic receptor is prototypical of other pentameric ligand-gated ion channels, which include the receptors for the inhibitory amino acids (γ-aminobutyric acid [GABA] and glycine) and 5-HT_3 serotonin receptors (Figure 9–1).

NEUROMUSCULAR BLOCKING AGENTS
Classification and Overview of Chemical Properties of Neuromuscular Blocking Agents
A single depolarizing agent, succinylcholine, is in general clinical use; multiple competitive or nondepolarizing agents are available (Figure 9–2). Therapeutic selection should be based on achieving a pharmacokinetic profile consistent with the duration of the interventional procedure and minimizing cardiovascular compromise or other adverse effects (Table 9–1). Two general classifications are useful in distinguishing side effects and pharmacokinetic behavior. The first relates to the duration of drug action; these agents are categorized as long-, intermediate-, and short-acting. The persistent blockade and difficulty in complete reversal after surgery with D-tubocurarine, metocurine, *pancuronium*, and *doxacurium* led to the development of *vecuronium* and *atracurium*, agents of intermediate duration, followed by development of a short-acting agent, *mivacurium*. Often, the long-acting agents are the more potent, requiring the use of low concentrations. The necessity of administering potent agents in low concentrations delays their onset. Rocuronium is an agent of intermediate duration but of rapid onset and lower potency. Its rapid onset allows it to be used as an alternative to succinylcholine in rapid-induction anesthesia and in relaxing the laryngeal and jaw muscles to facilitate tracheal intubation.

The second useful designation is the chemical class of the agents (Table 9–1). The natural alkaloid D-tubocurarine and the semisynthetic alkaloid alcuronium seldom are used. Apart from a shorter duration of action, the newer agents exhibit greatly diminished frequency of side effects, chief of which are ganglionic blockade, block of vagal responses, and histamine release. The prototype ammonio steroid, pancuronium, induces virtually no histamine release; however, it blocks muscarinic receptors, and this antagonism is manifested primarily in vagal blockade and tachycardia. Tachycardia is eliminated in the newer ammonio steroids, vecuronium and rocuronium. The benzylisoquinolines lack vagolytic and ganglionic blocking actions but show a slight propensity for histamine release. Mivacurium is extremely sensitive to catalysis by cholinesterase or other plasma hydrolases, therein accounting for its short duration of action.

Pharmacological Properties
Table 9–1 summarizes the pharmacological properties of various neuromuscular blocking agents. The anatomy, physiology, and pharmacology of the motor end plate are shown in Figure 9–3.

SKELETAL MUSCLE Competitive antagonists competitively block the binding of ACh to the nicotinic ACh receptor at the end plate. The depolarizing agents, such as succinylcholine, act by a different mechanism: initially, they depolarize the membrane by opening channels in the same manner as ACh. However, they persist for longer durations at the neuromuscular junction because of their resistance to AChE. The depolarization is thus longer-lasting, resulting in a brief period of repetitive excitation (fasciculations), followed by block of neuromuscular transmission (and flaccid paralysis). Paralysis occurs because released ACh binds to receptors on an already depolarized end

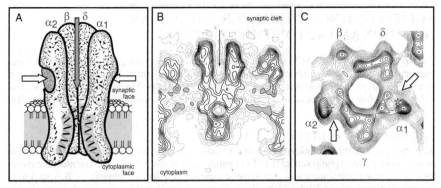

FIGURE 9–1 *Subunit organization of the nicotinic ACh receptor and related pentameric ligand-gated ion channels.* For each subunit (MW ~40–60 kDa), the amino terminal region (~210 amino acids) is at the extracellular surface, followed by 4 transmembrane domains (TM_1–TM_4), with a small carboxyl terminus at the extracellular surface. Five subunits aggregate to form the receptor/pore/ion channel; the α-helical TM_2 regions from each subunit of the pentameric receptor line the internal pore of the receptor. One disulfide motif is conserved throughout the family of receptors.

plate (an end plate depolarized from –80 to –55 mV by a depolarizing blocking agent is resistant to further depolarization by ACh). The exact sequence from fasciculations to paralysis is influenced by such factors as the anesthetic agent used concurrently, the type of muscle, and the rate of drug adminis- tra-tion. The characteristics of depolarization and competitive blockade are contrasted in Table 9–2.

SEQUENCE AND CHARACTERISTICS OF PARALYSIS Following intravenous administration of an appropriate dose of a competitive antagonist, motor weakness progresses to a total flaccid paralysis. Small, rapidly moving muscles (*e.g.,* those of the eyes, jaw, and larynx) relax before those of the limbs and trunk. Ultimately, intercostal muscles and finally the diaphragm are paralyzed, and respiration then ceases. Recovery of muscles usually occurs in the reverse order to that of their paralysis, and thus the diaphragm ordinarily is the first muscle to regain function.

After a single intravenous dose of 10–30 mg of a depolarizing agent such as succinylcholine, muscle fasciculations, particularly over the chest and abdomen, occur briefly; relaxation occurs within 1 minute, becomes maximal within 2 minutes, and generally disappears within 5 minutes. Transient apnea usually occurs at the time of maximal effect. Muscle relaxation of longer duration is achieved by continuous intravenous infusion. After infusion is discontinued, the effects of the drug usually disappear rapidly because of its rapid hydrolysis by plasma and hepatic butyryl-cholinesterase. Muscle soreness may follow the administration of succinylcholine. Small prior doses of competitive blocking agents have been employed to minimize fasciculations and muscle pain caused by succinylcholine, but this procedure is controversial because it increases the requirement for the depolarizing drug.

During prolonged depolarization, muscle cells may lose significant quantities of K^+ and gain Na^+, Cl^-, and Ca^{2+}. In patients in whom there has been extensive injury to soft tissues, the efflux of K^+ following continued administration of succinylcholine can be life-threatening. Thus, there are many conditions for which succinylcholine administration is contraindicated or should be undertaken with great caution. Under clinical conditions, with increasing concentrations of succinylcholine and over time, the block may convert slowly from a depolarizing to a nondepolarizing type (termed *phase I* and *phase II* blocks). This change in the nature of the blockade produced by succinylcholine (from phase I to phase II) presents an additional complication with long-term infusions (*see* Table 9–3).

Central Nervous System

Tubocurarine and other quaternary neuromuscular blocking agents are virtually devoid of central effects following ordinary clinical doses because of their inability to penetrate the blood–brain barrier.

AUTONOMIC GANGLIA AND MUSCARINIC SITES Neuromuscular blocking agents show variable potencies in producing ganglionic blockade. Clinical doses of tubocurarine produce partial blockade both at autonomic ganglia and at the adrenal medulla, resulting in a fall in blood pressure and tachycardia. Pancuronium shows less ganglionic blockade at standard clinical doses.

Competitive Agents

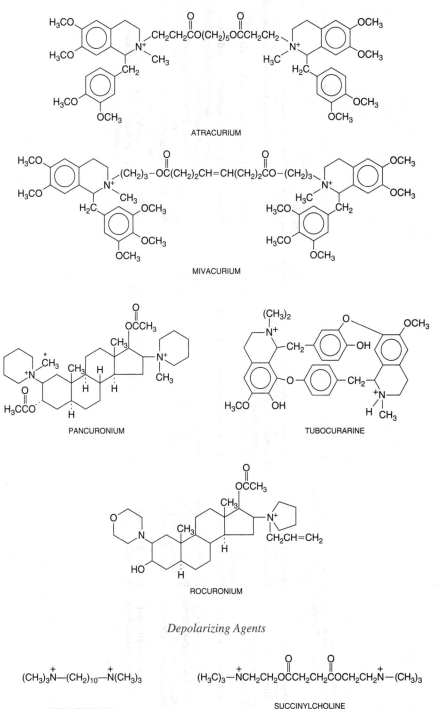

FIGURE 9–2 *Neuromuscular blocking agents.* (* *This methyl group is absent in vecuronium.*)

Table 9-1

Classification of Neuromuscular Blocking Agents

Agent (TRADE NAME)	Chemical Class	Pharmacological Properties	Time of Onset, min	Clinical Duration, min	Mode of Elimination
Succinylcholine (ANECTINE, others)	Dicholine ester	Ultrashort duration; depolarizing	1–1.5	5–8	Hydrolysis by plasma cholinesterases
D-Tubocurarine	Natural alkaloid (cyclic benzylisoquinoline)	Long duration; competitive	4–6	80–120	Renal elimination; liver clearance
Atracurium (TRACRIUM)	Benzylisoquinoline	Intermediate duration; competitive	2–4	30–60	Hofmann degradation; hydrolysis by plasma esterases; renal elimination
Doxacurium (NUROMAX)	Benzylisoquinoline	Long duration; competitive	4–6	90–120	Renal elimination
Mivacurium (MIVACRON)	Benzylisoquinoline	Short duration; competitive	2–4	12–18	Hydrolysis by plasma cholinesterases
Pancuronium (PAVULON)	Ammonio steroid	Long duration; competitive	4–6	120–180	Renal elimination
Pipecuronium (ARDUAN)	Ammonio steroid	Long duration; competitive	2–4	80–100	Renal elimination; liver metabolism and clearance
Rocuronium (ZEMURON)	Ammonio steroid	Intermediate duration; competitive	1–2	30–60	Liver metabolism
Vecuronium (NORCURON)	Ammonio steroid	Intermediate duration; competitive	2–4	60–90	Liver metabolism and clearance; renal elimination

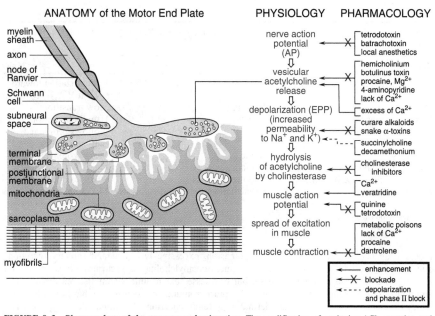

ANATOMY of the Motor End Plate   PHYSIOLOGY   PHARMACOLOGY

FIGURE 9–3 *Pharmacology of the neuromuscular junction.* The modification of excitation-ACh secretion and nicotinic receptor activation-contraction coupling by various agents is shown on the *right; an arrow marked with an X indicates inhibition or block; a plain arrow indicates enhancement or activation.*

Atracurium, vecuronium, doxacurium, *pipecuronium* (no longer marketed in the U.S.), mivacurium, and rocuronium are even more selective. The maintenance of cardiovascular reflex responses usually is desired during anesthesia.

Pancuronium has a vagolytic action, presumably from blockade of muscarinic receptors, that leads to tachycardia. Of the depolarizing agents, succinylcholine, at doses producing skeletal muscle relaxation, rarely causes effects attributable to ganglionic blockade. However, cardiovascular effects are sometimes observed, probably owing to the successive stimulation of vagal ganglia (manifested by bradycardia) and sympathetic ganglia (resulting in hypertension and tachycardia).

HISTAMINE RELEASE   Tubocurarine produces typical histamine-like wheals when injected intracutaneously or intra-arterially in humans; some clinical responses to neuromuscular

Table 9–2

Comparison of Competitive (D-Tubocurarine) and Depolarizing (Decamethonium) Blocking Agents

	D-Tubocurarine	Decamethonium
Effect of D-tubocurarine administered previously	Additive	Antagonistic
Effect of decamethonium administered previously	No effect, or antagonistic	Some tachyphylaxis, but may be additive
Effect of anticholinesterase agents on block	Reversal of block	No reversal
Effect on motor end plate	Elevated threshold to acetylcholine; no depolarization	Partial, persisting depolarization
Initial excitatory effect on striated muscle	None	Transient fasciculations
Character of muscle response to indirect tetanic stimulation during *partial* block	Poorly sustained contraction	Well-sustained contraction

Table 9-3

Clinical Responses and Monitoring of Phase I and Phase II Neuromuscular Blockade by Succinylcholine Infusion

Response	Phase I	Phase II
End-plate membrane potential	Depolarized to −55 mV	Repolarization toward −80 mV
Onset	Immediate	Slow transition
Dose-dependence	Lower	Usually higher or follows prolonged infusion
Recovery	Rapid	More prolonged
Train of four and tetanic stimulation	No fade	Fade*
Acetylcholinesterase inhibition	Augments	Reverses or antagonizes
Muscle response	Fasciculations → flaccid paralysis	Flaccid paralysis

*Post-tetanic potentiation follows fade.

blocking agents (*e.g.,* bronchospasm, hypotension, excessive bronchial and salivary secretion) appear to be caused by the release of histamine. Succinylcholine, mivacurium, doxacurium, and atracurium also cause histamine release, but to a lesser extent unless administered rapidly. The ammonio steroids, pancuronium, vecuronium, pipecuronium, and rocuronium, have even less tendency to release histamine after intradermal or systemic injection. Histamine release typically is a direct action of the muscle relaxant on the mast cell rather than IgE-mediated anaphylaxis.

ACTIONS OF NEUROMUSCULAR BLOCKING AGENTS WITH LIFE-THREATEN-ING IMPLICATIONS   Depolarizing agents can release K^+ rapidly from intracellular sites; this may be a causative factor in production of the prolonged apnea in patients who receive these drugs while in electrolyte imbalance.

Succinylcholine-induced hyperkalemia is a life-threatening complication of that drug (*e.g.,* in patients with congestive heart failure who are receiving digoxin or diuretics). Likewise, caution should be used or depolarizing blocking agents should be avoided in patients with extensive soft tissue trauma or burns. A higher dose of a competitive blocking agent often is indicated in these patients. In addition, succinylcholine administration is contraindicated or should be given with great caution in patients with nontraumatic rhabdomyolysis, ocular lacerations, spinal cord injuries with paraplegia or quadriplegia, or muscular dystrophies. Succinylcholine no longer is indicated for children ≤8 years of age unless emergency intubation or securing an airway is necessary. Hyperkalemia, rhabdomyolysis, and cardiac arrest have been reported; a subclinical dystrophy frequently is associated with these adverse responses. Neonates also may have an enhanced sensitivity to competitive neuromuscular blocking agents.

DRUG INTERACTIONS   From a clinical viewpoint, important pharmacological interactions of these drugs occur with certain general anesthetics, certain antibiotics, Ca^{2+} channel blockers, and anti-ChE compounds. Since the anti-ChE agents *neostigmine, pyridostigmine,* and *edrophonium* preserve endogenous ACh and also act directly on the neuromuscular junction, they can be used in the treatment of overdosage with competitive blocking agents. Similarly, on completion of the surgical procedure, many anesthesiologists employ neostigmine or edrophonium to reverse and decrease the duration of competitive neuromuscular blockade. Succinylcholine should never be administered after reversal of competitive blockade with neostigmine; in this circumstance, a prolonged and intense blockade often results (*see* Table 9-2). A muscarinic antagonist (atropine or glycopyrrolate) is used concomitantly to prevent stimulation of muscarinic receptors and thereby to avoid slowing of the heart rate. Many inhalational anesthetics (*e.g.,* halothane, isoflurane, enflurane) "stabilize" the postjunctional membrane and act synergistically with the competitive blocking agents; this requires a reduction in the dose of the nicotinic receptor blocking drugs.

Aminoglycoside antibiotics produce neuromuscular blockade by inhibiting ACh release from the preganglionic terminal (through competition with Ca^{2+}) and to a lesser extent by noncompetitively blocking the receptor. Tetracyclines also can produce neuromuscular blockade, possibly by chelation of Ca^{2+}. Additional antibiotics that have neuromuscular blocking action, through both presynaptic *and postsynaptic actions, include* polymyxin B, colistin, clindamycin, and lincomycin. Ca^{2+} channel blockers *enhance neuromuscular blockade produced by both competitive and depolarizing antagonists. When neuromuscular blocking agents are administered to patients receiving these agents, dose adjustments should be considered; if recovery of spontaneous respiration is delayed, Ca^{2+} salts may facilitate recovery.*

Miscellaneous drugs that may have significant interactions with either competitive or depolarizing neuromuscular blocking agents include trimethaphan *(no longer marketed in the U.S.),* opioid analgesics, procaine, lidocaine, quinidine, phenelzine, phenytoin, propranolol, magnesium salts, corticosteroids, digitalis glycosides, chloroquine, catecholamines, *and* diuretics.

TOXICOLOGY The important untoward responses of the neuromuscular blocking agents include prolonged apnea, cardiovascular collapse, those resulting from histamine release, and, rarely, anaphylaxis. Related factors may include alterations in body temperature; electrolyte imbalance, particularly of K^+ (discussed earlier); low plasma butyrylcholinesterase levels, resulting in a reduction in the rate of destruction of succinylcholine; the presence of latent myasthenia gravis or of malignant disease such as small cell carcinoma of the lung (Eaton-Lambert myasthenic syndrome); reduced blood flow to skeletal muscles, causing delayed removal of the blocking drugs; and decreased elimination of the muscle relaxants secondary to reduced renal function. Great care should be taken when administering these agents to dehydrated or severely ill patients.

MALIGNANT HYPERTHERMIA Malignant hyperthermia is a potentially life-threatening event triggered by certain anesthetics and neuromuscular blocking agents. Clinical features include contracture, rigidity, and heat production from skeletal muscle resulting in severe hyperthermia, accelerated muscle metabolism, metabolic acidosis, and tachycardia. Uncontrolled release of Ca^{2+} from the sarcoplasmic reticulum of skeletal muscle is the initiating event. Although the halogenated hydrocarbon anesthetics (*e.g.,* halothane, isoflurane, and *sevoflurane*) and succinylcholine alone reportedly precipitate the response, most incidents arise from the combination of depolarizing blocking agent and anesthetic.

Susceptibility to malignant hyperthermia, an autosomal dominant trait, is associated with certain congenital myopathies such as central core disease. In the majority of cases, however, no clinical signs are visible in the absence of anesthetic intervention.

Susceptibility relates to a mutation in RyR-1, the gene encoding the skeletal muscle ryanodine receptor (RYR-1); other loci have been identified on the L-type Ca^{2+} channel and on associated proteins.

Treatment entails intravenous administration of *dantrolene* (DANTRIUM), which blocks Ca^{2+} release and its sequelae in skeletal muscle. Rapid cooling, inhalation of 100% oxygen, and control of acidosis should be considered adjunct therapy in malignant hyperthermia.

Central core disease has five allelic variants of RyR-1; patients with central core disease are highly susceptible to malignant hyperthermia with the combination of an anesthetic and a depolarizing neuromuscular blocker. Patients with other muscle syndromes or dystonias also have an increased frequency of contracture and hyperthermia in the anesthesia setting.

RESPIRATORY PARALYSIS Treatment of respiratory paralysis arising from an adverse reaction or overdose of a neuromuscular blocking agent includes positive-pressure artificial respiration with oxygen and maintenance of a patent airway until recovery of normal respiration is ensured. With the competitive blocking agents, this may be hastened by the administration of neostigmine methylsulfate (0.5–2 mg intravenously) or edrophonium (10 mg intravenously, repeated as required).

INTERVENTIONAL STRATEGIES FOR OTHER TOXIC EFFECTS Neostigmine effectively antagonizes only the skeletal muscular blocking action of the competitive blocking agents *and may aggravate side effects (e.g., hypotension) or induce bronchospasm. In such circumstances,* sympathomimetic amines may be given to support the blood pressure. Atropine or glycopyrrolate is administered to counteract muscarinic stimulation. *Antihistamines* will counteract the responses that follow the release of histamine, particularly when administered before the neuromuscular blocking agent.

ABSORPTION, FATE, AND EXCRETION Quaternary ammonium neuromuscular blocking agents are poorly and irregularly absorbed from the gastrointestinal (GI) tract. Absorption is adequate from intramuscular sites. Rapid onset is achieved with intravenous administration. The more potent agents must be given in lower concentrations, and diffusional requirements slow their rate of onset.

With long-acting competitive blocking agents (*e.g.,* D-tubocurarine, pancuronium), blockade may diminish after 30 minutes owing to redistribution of the drug, yet residual blockade and plasma levels of the drug persist. Subsequent doses show diminished redistribution. Long-acting agents may accumulate with multiple doses.

The ammonio steroids contain ester groups that are hydrolyzed in the liver. Typically, the metabolites have about half the activity of the parent compound and contribute to the total relaxation profile. Ammonio steroids of intermediate duration of action (*e.g.,* vecuronium, rocuronium; *see* Table 9–1) are cleared more rapidly by the liver than is pancuronium. The more rapid decay of neuromuscular blockade with compounds of intermediate duration argues for sequential dosing of these agents rather than administering a single dose of a long duration neuromuscular blocking agent.

Atracurium is converted to less active metabolites by plasma esterases and spontaneous degradation. Because of these alternative routes of metabolism, atracurium does not exhibit an increased $t_{1/2}$ in patients with impaired renal function and therefore is the agent of choice in this setting. Mivacurium shows an even greater susceptibility to butyrylcholinesterases, and thus has the shortest duration among nondepolarizing blockers. The extremely brief duration of action of succinylcholine also is due largely to its rapid hydrolysis by the butyrylcholinesterase of liver and plasma. Among the occasional patients who exhibit prolonged apnea following the administration of succinylcholine or mivacurium, most (but not all) have atypical or deficient plasma cholinesterase, hepatic or renal disease, or a nutritional disturbance.

Therapeutic Uses

Neuromuscular blocking agents are used mainly as adjuvants in surgical anesthesia to relax skeletal muscle, particularly of the abdominal wall, to facilitate operative manipulations; with muscle relaxation not dependent on the depth of general anesthesia, a much lighter level of anesthesia suffices, minimizing risk of respiratory and cardiovascular depression and shortening postanesthetic recovery. Neuromuscular blocking agents will not substitute for inadequate depth of anesthesia.

Muscle relaxation is useful in orthopedic procedures (*e.g.,* correction of dislocations, alignment of fractures). Neuromuscular blocking agents of short duration often are used to facilitate endotracheal intubation and have been used to facilitate laryngoscopy, bronchoscopy, and esophagoscopy in combination with a general anesthetic agent.

Neuromuscular blocking agents are administered parenterally, generally intravenously. These drugs are hazardous and should be administered to patients only by clinicians who have had extensive training in their use and in a setting where facilities for respiratory and cardiovascular resuscitation are immediately at hand.

MEASUREMENT OF NEUROMUSCULAR BLOCKADE IN HUMANS

Assessment of neuromuscular block usually is performed by stimulation of the ulnar nerve. Responses are monitored from compound action potentials or muscle tension developed in the adductor pollicis (thumb) muscle. Responses to repetitive or tetanic stimuli are most useful for evaluation of blockade of transmission. Thus, stimulus schedules such as the "train of four" and the "double burst" or responses to tetanic stimulation are preferred procedures. Rates of onset of blockade and recovery are more rapid in the airway musculature (jaw, larynx, and diaphragm) than in the thumb. Hence, tracheal intubation can be performed before onset of complete block at the adductor pollicis, whereas partial recovery of function of this muscle allows sufficient recovery of respiration for extubation.

PREVENTING TRAUMA DURING ELECTROSHOCK THERAPY

Electroconvulsive therapy (ECT) of psychiatric disorders occasionally is complicated by trauma to the patient; the seizures induced may cause dislocations or fractures. Inasmuch as the muscular component of the convulsion is not essential for benefit from the procedure, neuromuscular blocking agents and thiopental are employed. Succinylcholine or mivacurium is used most often because of the brevity of relaxation.

CONTROL OF MUSCLE SPASMS Agents that act in the CNS to block spasms are considered in Chapter 20. Two peripherally-acting agents are used, *botulinum toxin* (*see* Chapter 6) and dantrolene. Botulinum toxin A (BOTOX), by blocking ACh release, produces flaccid paralysis of skeletal muscle and diminished activity of parasympathetic and sympathetic cholinergic synapses. Inhibition lasts from several weeks to 3–4 months, and restoration of function requires nerve sprouting. Uses of BOTOX in dermatology and ophthalmology are described in Chapters 62 and 63.

In addition to its use in managing an acute attack of malignant hyperthermia (*see* above), dantrolene has been used in the treatment of spasticity and hyperreflexia. Dantrolene causes a generalized weakness; thus, its use should be restricted to nonambulatory patients with severe spasticity. Hepatotoxicity has been reported with continued use, requiring liver function tests.

GANGLIONIC NEUROTRANSMISSION

Neurotransmission in autonomic ganglia is a more complex process than that described by a single neurotransmitter–receptor system, with at least 4 distinct changes in membrane potential elicited by stimulation of the preganglionic nerve. The primary event involves a rapid depolarization of postsynaptic sites by ACh. An action potential is generated in the postganglionic neuron when the initial EPSP attains sufficient amplitude; in mammalian sympathetic ganglia *in vivo*, effective transmission likely requires activation at multiple synapses. The EPSP is followed by a slow inhibitory postsynaptic potential (IPSP), a slow EPSP, and a late, slow EPSP; slow IPSP and slow EPSP are not seen in all ganglia. The initial EPSP is mediated through nicotinic (N) receptors, the slow IPSP and EPSP through M_2 and M_1 muscarinic receptors, and the late, slow EPSP through various peptidergic receptors in response to peptides released from presynaptic nerve endings or interneurons in specific ganglia (*see* Chapter 7). The slow EPSPs result from decreased K^+ conductance (the M current, which regulates the sensitivity of the cell to repetitive fast-depolarizing events). The IPSP is unaffected by nicotinic receptor antagonists but is generally sensitive to blockade by both atropine and α adrenergic receptor antagonists; apparently, ACh released at the preganglionic terminal acts on catecholamine-containing interneurons to stimulate the release of dopamine (DA) or norepinephrine (NE); the catecholamine, in turn, produces hyperpolarization (an IPSP) of ganglion cells. Small, intensely fluorescent (SIF) cells containing DA and NE and adrenergic nerve terminals are present in ganglia and presumably participate in IPSP generation (*see* Figure 9–5 in the 11th edition of the parent text).

The relative importance of secondary pathways and the identity of modulating transmitters differ amongst individual ganglia and between parasympathetic and sympathetic ganglia. Myriad peptides (gonadotropin-releasing hormone, substance P, angiotensin, calcitonin gene-related peptide [CGRP], vasoactive intestinal polypeptide, neuropeptide Y, and enkephalins), are present in ganglia and are presumed to mediate the late slow EPSP. Other neurotransmitters, such as 5-HT and GABA, are known to modify ganglionic transmission. Precise details of their modulatory actions are not understood; they are most closely associated with the late slow EPSP and inhibition of the M current. Secondary transmitters (and their antagonists) only modulate the initial EPSP. By contrast, conventional ganglionic blocking agents can inhibit ganglionic transmission completely.

Drugs that stimulate cholinergic receptor sites on autonomic ganglia can be grouped into two categories. The first group consists of drugs with nicotinic specificity, including nicotine itself. Their excitatory effects on ganglia are rapid in onset, are blocked by ganglionic nicotinic receptor antagonists, and mimic the initial EPSP. The second group is composed of agents such as *muscarine, McN-A-343,* and *methacholine.* Their excitatory effects on ganglia are delayed in onset, blocked by atropine-like drugs, and mimic the slow EPSP.

Ganglionic blocking agents acting on the nicotinic receptor may be classified into two groups. The first group includes drugs that initially stimulate the ganglia by an ACh-like action and then block them because of a persistent depolarization (*e.g.*, nicotine); prolonged application of nicotine results in desensitization of the cholinergic receptor site and continued blockade. Drugs in the second group of blockers, of which hexamethonium and trimethaphan are prototypes, impair transmission either by competing with ACh for ganglionic nicotinic receptor sites (trimethaphan) or by blocking the channel after it opens (hexamethonium). Regardless of the mechanism, the initial EPSP is blocked, and ganglionic transmission is inhibited.

GANGLIONIC STIMULATING DRUGS

Nicotine and several other compounds stimulate ganglionic nicotinic receptors (Figure 9–4).

Nicotine

Nicotine is medically and socially significant because of its presence in tobacco, its toxicity, and its propensity to cause dependence in its users. The chronic effects of nicotine and the untoward effects of the chronic use of tobacco are considered in Chapter 23. Nicotine is one of the few natural liquid alkaloids. It is a colorless, volatile base ($pK_a = 8.5$) that turns brown and acquires the odor of tobacco on exposure to air.

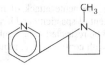

NICOTINE

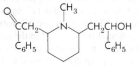

LOBELINE

$$CH_3 \underset{\underset{CH_3}{|}}{\overset{\overset{CH_3}{|}}{\overset{+}{N}}} CH_3$$

TETRAMETHYLAMMONIUM (TMA)

1,1-DIMETHYL-4-PHENYLPIPERAZINIUM (DMPP)

FIGURE 9–4 *Ganglionic stimulants.*

PHARMACOLOGICAL ACTIONS

The complex and often unpredictable changes that occur in the body after administration of nicotine are due not only to its actions on a variety of neuroeffector and chemosensitive sites but also to the fact that the alkaloid can stimulate and desensitize receptors. The ultimate response of any one system represents the summation of stimulatory and inhibitory effects of nicotine. For example, the drug can increase heart rate by excitation of sympathetic or paralysis of parasympathetic cardiac ganglia, or it can slow heart rate by paralysis of sympathetic or stimulation of parasympathetic cardiac ganglia. In addition, the effects of the drug on the chemoreceptors of the carotid and aortic bodies and on brain centers influence heart rate, as do the cardiovascular compensatory reflexes resulting from changes in blood pressure caused by nicotine. Finally, nicotine elicits a discharge of epinephrine from the adrenal medulla, which accelerates heart rate and raises blood pressure.

Peripheral Nervous System

The major action of nicotine consists initially of transient stimulation followed by a more persistent depression of all autonomic ganglia. Small doses of nicotine stimulate the ganglion cells directly and may facilitate impulse transmission. When larger doses of the drug are applied, the initial stimulation is followed very quickly by a blockade of transmission. Nicotine also possesses a biphasic action on the adrenal medulla; small doses evoke the discharge of catecholamines, and larger doses prevent their release in response to splanchnic nerve stimulation.

The effects of nicotine on the neuromuscular junction are similar to those on ganglia. However, the stimulant phase is obscured largely by the rapidly developing paralysis. In the latter stage, nicotine also produces neuromuscular blockade by receptor desensitization.

Nicotine, like ACh, will stimulate a number of sensory receptors. These include mechanoreceptors that respond to stretch or pressure of the skin, mesentery, tongue, lung, and stomach; chemoreceptors of the carotid body; thermal receptors of the skin and tongue; and pain receptors. Prior administration of hexamethonium prevents stimulation of the sensory receptors by nicotine but has little, if any, effect on the activation of sensory receptors by physiological stimuli.

Central Nervous System

Nicotine markedly stimulates the CNS. Low doses produce weak analgesia; with higher doses, tremors leading to convulsions at toxic doses are evident. The excitation of respiration is a prominent action of nicotine; although large doses act directly on the medulla oblongata, smaller doses augment respiration reflexly by excitation of the chemoreceptors of the carotid and aortic bodies.

Stimulation of the CNS with large doses is followed by depression, and death results from failure of respiration owing to both central paralysis and peripheral blockade of muscles of respiration. Nicotine induces vomiting by both central and peripheral actions. The primary sites of action of nicotine in the CNS are prejunctional, causing the release of other transmitters. Accordingly, the stimulatory and pleasure–reward actions of nicotine appear to result from release of excitatory amino acids, DA, and other biogenic amines from various CNS centers. Release of excitatory amino acids may account for much of nicotine's stimulatory action. Chronic exposure to nicotine increases the density or number of nicotinic receptors.

Cardiovascular System

In general, the cardiovascular responses to nicotine are due to stimulation of sympathetic ganglia and the adrenal medulla, together with the discharge of catecholamines from sympathetic nerve endings. Also contributing to the sympathomimetic response to nicotine is the activation of chemoreceptors of the aortic and carotid bodies, which reflexly results in vasoconstriction, tachycardia, and elevated blood pressure.

Gastrointestinal Tract

The combined activation of parasympathetic ganglia and cholinergic nerve endings by nicotine results in increased tone and motor activity of the bowel. Nausea, vomiting, and occasionally diarrhea are observed following systemic absorption of nicotine in an individual who has not been exposed to nicotine previously.

Exocrine Glands

Nicotine causes an initial stimulation of salivary and bronchial secretions that is followed by inhibition.

ABSORPTION, FATE, AND EXCRETION

Nicotine is readily absorbed from the respiratory tract, buccal membranes, and skin. Severe poisoning has resulted from percutaneous absorption. Being a relatively strong base, its absorption from the stomach is limited. Intestinal absorption is far more efficient. Nicotine in chewing tobacco, because it is absorbed more slowly than inhaled nicotine, has a longer duration of effect. The average cigarette contains 6–11 mg nicotine and delivers about 1–3 mg nicotine systemically to the smoker; bioavailability can increase as much as threefold with intensity of puffing and technique of the smoker.

Nicotine is available in several dosage forms to help achieve abstinence from tobacco use. Efficacy results primarily from preventing a withdrawal or abstinence syndrome. Nicotine may be administered orally as a gum (nicotine polacrilex, NICORETTE), transdermal patch (NICODERM, HABITROL, others), a nasal spray (NICOTROL NS), and a vapor inhaler (NICOTROL INHALER). The first two are used most widely, and the objective is to obtain a sustained plasma nicotine concentration lower than venous blood concentrations after smoking (arterial blood concentrations immediately following inhalation can be as much as tenfold higher than venous concentrations). The efficacy of these dosage forms in producing abstinence from smoking is enhanced when linked to counseling and motivational therapy (see Chapter 23).

Approximately 80–90% of nicotine is altered in the body, mainly in the liver but also in the kidney and lung; cotinine is the major metabolite. The profile of metabolites and the rate of metabolism appear to be similar in smokers and nonsmokers. The $t_{1/2}$ of nicotine following inhalation or parenteral administration is ~2 hours. Nicotine and its metabolites are eliminated rapidly by the kidney. The rate of urinary excretion of nicotine diminishes when the urine is alkaline. Nicotine also is excreted in the milk of lactating women who smoke; the milk of heavy smokers may contain 0.5 mg/L.

ACUTE NICOTINE POISONING

Poisoning from nicotine may occur from accidental ingestion of nicotine-containing insecticide sprays or in children from ingestion of tobacco products. The acutely fatal dose of nicotine for an adult is probably ~60 mg of the base. Smoking tobacco usually contains 1–2% nicotine. Apparently, the gastric absorption of nicotine from tobacco taken by mouth is delayed because of slowed gastric emptying, so vomiting caused by the central effect of the initially absorbed fraction may remove much of the tobacco remaining in the GI tract.

The onset of symptoms of acute, severe nicotine poisoning is rapid: nausea, salivation, abdominal pain, vomiting, diarrhea, cold sweat, headache, dizziness, disturbed hearing and vision, mental confusion, and marked weakness. Faintness and prostration ensue; the blood pressure falls; breathing is difficult; the pulse is weak, rapid, and irregular; and collapse may be followed by terminal convulsions. Death may result within a few minutes from respiratory failure.

Therapy

Vomiting may be induced, or gastric lavage should be performed. Alkaline solutions should be avoided. A slurry of activated charcoal is then passed through the tube and left in the stomach. Respiratory assistance and treatment of shock may be necessary.

Other Ganglionic Stimulants

Stimulation of ganglia by tetramethylammonium (TMA) or 1,1-dimethyl-4-phenylpiperazinium iodide (DMPP) differs from that produced by nicotine in that the initial stimulation is not followed by a dominant blocking action. DMPP is about three times more potent and slightly more ganglion-selective than nicotine. Although parasympathomimetic drugs stimulate ganglia, their effects usually are obscured by stimulation of other neuroeffector sites. McN-A-343 is an exception; it can stimulate muscarinic M_1 receptors in ganglia.

GANGLIONIC BLOCKING DRUGS

A chemically diverse group of compounds blocks autonomic ganglia without causing prior stimulation (Figure 9–5).

PHARMACOLOGICAL PROPERTIES

Most of the physiological alterations observed after the administration of ganglionic blocking agents can be anticipated by a careful inspection of Figure 6–1 and by knowing which division of the autonomic nervous system exercises dominant control of various organs (Table 9–4). For example, blockade of sympathetic ganglia interrupts adrenergic control of arterioles and results in vasodilation, improved peripheral blood flow in some vascular beds, and a fall in blood pressure.

Generalized ganglionic blockade also may result in atony of the bladder and GI tract, cycloplegia, xerostomia, diminished perspiration, and postural hypotension (via abolition of circulatory reflex pathways); these changes are the generally undesirable effects that limit the therapeutic efficacy of ganglionic blocking agents.

Cardiovascular System

Existing sympathetic tone is critical in determining the degree to which blood pressure is lowered by ganglionic blockade; thus, blood pressure may be decreased only minimally in recumbent normotensive subjects but may fall markedly in sitting or standing subjects. Postural hypotension limits use of ganglionic blockers in ambulatory patients.

Changes in heart rate following ganglionic blockade depend largely on existing vagal tone. Mild tachycardia usually accompanies the hypotension, a sign that indicates fairly complete

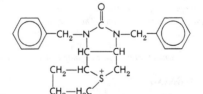

HEXAMETHONIUM (C6)

TRIMETHAPHAN

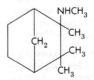

MECAMYLAMINE

FIGURE 9–5 *Ganglionic blocking agents.*

Table 9–4

Usual Predominance of Sympathetic or Parasympathetic Tone at Various Effector Sites, and Consequences of Autonomic Ganglionic Blockade

Site	Predominant Tone	Effect of Ganglionic Blockade
Arterioles	Sympathetic (adrenergic)	Vasodilation; increased peripheral blood flow; hypotension
Veins	Sympathetic (adrenergic)	Dilation: peripheral pooling of blood; decreased venous return; decreased cardiac output
Heart	Parasympathetic (cholinergic)	Tachycardia
Iris	Parasympathetic (cholinergic)	Mydriasis
Ciliary muscle	Parasympathetic (cholinergic)	Loss of visual accommodation
Gastrointestinal tract	Parasympathetic (cholinergic)	Reduced tone and motility; constipation; decreased gastric and pancreatic secretions
Urinary bladder	Parasympathetic (cholinergic)	Urinary retention
Salivary glands	Parasympathetic (cholinergic)	Xerostomia
Sweat glands	Sympathetic (cholinergic)	Anhidrosis
Genital tract	Sympathetic and parasympathetic	Decreased stimulation

ganglionic blockade. However, a decrease may occur if the heart rate is high initially. In patients with normal cardiac function, these drugs may reduce cardiac output as a consequence of diminished venous return resulting from venous dilation and peripheral pooling of blood. In patients with cardiac failure, ganglionic blockade frequently results in increased cardiac output owing to a reduction in peripheral resistance. In hypertensive subjects, cardiac output, stroke volume, and left ventricular work are diminished.

Although ganglionic blockade decreases total systemic vascular resistance, changes in blood flow and vascular resistance of individual vascular beds vary: reduction of cerebral blood flow is small unless mean systemic blood pressure falls below 50–60 mm Hg; skeletal muscle blood flow is unaltered; splanchnic and renal blood flow decrease.

ABSORPTION, FATE, AND EXCRETION
Absorption of quaternary ammonium and sulfonium compounds from the GI tract is incomplete and unpredictable, due to the limited ability of these ionized substances to penetrate cell membranes and depression of propulsive movements of the small intestine and gastric emptying.

Absorption of mecamylamine is less erratic, but reduced bowel activity and paralytic ileus are a danger. After absorption, the quaternary ammonium- and sulfonium-blocking agents are confined primarily to the extracellular space and are excreted mostly unchanged by the kidney. Mecamylamine concentrates in the liver and kidney and is excreted slowly in an unchanged form.

UNTOWARD RESPONSES AND SEVERE REACTIONS
Milder untoward responses are: visual disturbances, dry mouth, conjunctival suffusion, urinary hesitancy, decreased potency, subjective chilliness, moderate constipation, occasional diarrhea, abdominal discomfort, anorexia, heartburn, nausea, eructation, and bitter taste and the signs and symptoms of syncope caused by postural hypotension. More severe reactions include marked hypotension, constipation, syncope, paralytic ileus, urinary retention, and cycloplegia.

FORMULATIONS AND THERAPEUTIC USES
Only mecamylamine (INVERSINE) is currently available in the U.S. Ganglionic blocking agents have been supplanted by superior agents for the treatment of chronic hypertension (see Chapter 32), acute hypertensive crises and the production of controlled hypotension (e.g., reduction in blood pressure during surgery to minimize hemorrhage in the operative field).

For a complete Bibliographical listing see Goodman & Gilman's *The Pharmacological Basis of Therapeutics*, 11th ed., or Goodman & Gilman Online at www.accessmedicine.com.

10

ADRENERGIC AGONISTS AND ANTAGONISTS

I. CATECHOLAMINES AND SYMPATHOMIMETIC DRUGS

Actions of catecholamines and sympathomimetic agents can be classified into seven broad types: (1) peripheral excitatory actions on smooth muscles (*e.g.*, in blood vessels supplying skin, kidney, and mucous membranes) and on gland cells (*e.g.*, in salivary and sweat glands); (2) peripheral inhibitory action on certain other types of smooth muscle (*e.g.*, in the wall of the gut, bronchial tree, and blood vessels supplying skeletal muscle); (3) cardiac excitatory action (increased rate and force of contraction); (4) metabolic actions (*e.g.*, enhanced glycogenolysis in liver and muscle, accelerated liberation of free fatty acids from adipose tissue); (5) endocrine actions (*e.g.*, modulation of secretion of insulin, renin, and pituitary hormones); (6) actions in the central nervous system (CNS) (*e.g.*, respiratory stimulation, increased wakefulness and psychomotor activity, reduced appetite); and (7) prejunctional actions (inhibition or facilitation of neurotransmitter release, inhibition being physiologically more important). Not all sympathomimetic drugs show each of the above types of action to the same degree; however, many of their differences are only quantitative.

Understanding the pharmacological properties of sympathomimetics and their antagonists depends on knowledge of the classification, distribution, and mechanism of action of α and β adrenergic receptors (*see* Tables 6–1, 6–6, 6–7, Figure 10–1, and Table 10–6).

CLASSIFICATION OF SYMPATHOMIMETIC DRUGS

Catecholamines and sympathomimetic drugs are classified as direct, indirect, or mixed acting. Direct-acting agents act directly on one or more of the adrenergic receptors. Indirect-acting drugs increase the availability of norepinephrine (NE) or epinephrine (Epi) to stimulate adrenergic receptors (by releasing or displacing NE from sympathetic nerve varicosities [*e.g.*, amphetamine]; by blocking the transport of NE into sympathetic neurons [*e.g.*, cocaine]; or by blocking the metabolizing enzymes, MAO [*e.g., pargyline*] or COMT [*e.g., entacapone*]). Drugs that indirectly release NE and also directly activate receptors are referred to as mixed-acting sympathomimetic drugs (*e.g., ephedrine*). The classification is not absolute and activities may overlap; prototypical drugs are listed in Figure 10–1.

β-phenylethylamine, a benzene ring with an ethylamine side chain, may be viewed as a parent structure for sympathomimetic amines (Table 10–1). NE, Epi, dopamine (DA), isoproterenol, and a few other agents have hydroxyl groups substituted at positions 3 and 4 of the benzene ring. Since o-dihydroxybenzene is also known as catechol, sympathomimetic amines with these hydroxyl substitutions in the aromatic ring are termed catecholamines. *Many directly acting sympathomimetic drugs influence both α and β receptors, but the ratio of activities varies among drugs in a continuous spectrum from predominantly α activity (phenylephrine) to predominantly β activity (isoproterenol). Maximal α and β activity depends on the presence of hydroxyl groups on positions 3 and 4. The response to noncatecholamines is partly determined by their capacity to release NE from storage sites. Phenylethylamines that lack hydroxyl groups on the ring and the β-hydroxyl group on the side chain act almost exclusively by causing the release of NE from sympathetic nerve terminals. Unsubstituted or alkyl-substituted compounds cross the blood–brain barrier more readily and have more central activity. Thus, ephedrine, amphetamine, and* methamphetamine *exhibit considerable CNS activity, and the absence of polar hydroxyl groups results in a loss of direct sympathomimetic activity.*

Catecholamines have only a brief duration of action and are ineffective when administered orally because they are rapidly inactivated in the intestinal mucosa and the liver (see Chapter 6). Compounds without one or both hydroxyl substituents are not substrates for COMT, and their oral effectiveness and duration of action are enhanced. Substitution on the α-carbon *blocks oxidative deamination by MAO, prolonging the duration of action of noncatecholamines. Thus, the duration of action of ephedrine and amphetamine is measured in hours rather than minutes. Substitution of an –OH on the β carbon generally decreases actions within the CNS (largely by reducing lipid solubility) but greatly enhances agonist activity at both α and β adrenergic receptors.*

PHYSIOLOGICAL EFFECTS OF ADRENERGIC RECEPTOR STIMULATION   In the response of any cell or organ to sympathomimetic amines, the density and proportion of α and β adrenergic receptors are key. For example, the receptors in bronchial smooth muscle are largely of the β_2 subtype; thus, NE (stimulating predominantly $\beta_1 + \alpha$ receptors) has relatively little capacity to increase bronchial airflow. In contrast, isoproterenol (a β agonist) and Epi (an $\alpha + \beta$ agonist)

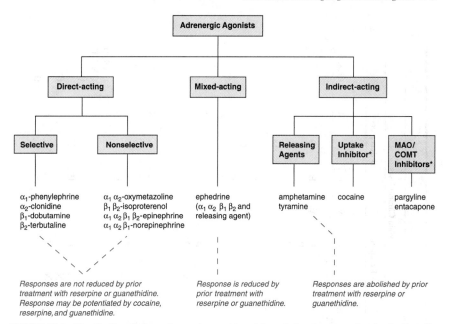

FIGURE 10–1 *Classification of adrenergic receptor agonists and drugs that produce sympathomimetic effects.* For each category, a prototypical drug is shown. *Not actually sympathetic drugs but produce sympathomimetic effects.

are potent bronchodilators. Cutaneous blood vessels physiologically express almost exclusively α receptors; thus, NE and Epi cause constriction of such vessels, whereas isoproterenol has little effect. The smooth muscle of blood vessels that supply skeletal muscles has both β_2 and α receptors; activation of β_2 receptors causes vasodilation, and stimulation of α receptors constricts these vessels. In such vessels, the threshold concentration for activation of β_2 receptors by Epi is lower than that for α receptors, but when both types of receptors are activated at high concentrations of Epi, the response to α receptors predominates; physiological concentrations of Epi primarily cause vasodilation.

The integrated response of an organ to sympathomimetic amines results not only from their direct effects, but also from reflex homeostatic adjustments. A striking effect of many sympathomimetic amines is a rise in arterial blood pressure caused by stimulation of vascular α adrenergic receptors. This stimulation elicits compensatory reflexes (mediated by the carotid–aortic baroreceptor system) that adjust CNS outflow to the cardiovascular system. As a result, sympathetic tone is diminished and vagal tone is enhanced; each of these responses leads to slowing of the heart rate. Conversely, when a drug (e.g., a β_2 agonist) lowers mean blood pressure at the mechanoreceptors of the carotid sinus and aortic arch, the baroreceptor reflex works to restore pressure by reducing parasympathetic (vagal) outflow from the CNS to the heart, and increasing sympathetic outflow to the heart and vessels. The baroreceptor reflex effect is of special importance for drugs that have little capacity to activate β receptors directly. With diseases (e.g., atherosclerosis) that may impair baroreceptor mechanisms, effects of sympathomimetic drugs may be magnified.

ENDOGENOUS CATECHOLAMINES
Epinephrine (Epi)

Epinephrine (adrenaline) is a potent stimulant of both α and β adrenergic receptors, and its effects on target organs are thus complex. Most of the responses listed in Table 6–1 are seen after injection of Epi (although sweating, piloerection, and mydriasis depend on the physiological state of the subject). Particularly prominent are the actions on the heart and on vascular and other smooth muscle. Effects of Epi reproduce those of adrenal medullary stimulation and are often described by the paradigm of "fight or flight."

Table 10-1

Chemical Structures and Main Clinical Uses of Important Sympathomimetic Drugs[†]

Structure: benzene ring (positions 5, 6, 1, 2, 3, 4) — βCH — αCH — NH

Drug	Substitution	β	α	N	A	N	P	V	B	C	U	CNS
					α Receptor				β Receptor			Main Clinical Uses
Phenylethylamine		H	H	H								
Epinephrine	3-OH,4-OH	OH	H	CH$_3$	A		P	V	B	C		
Norepinephrine	3-OH,4-OH	OH	H	H			P					
Dopamine	3-OH,4-OH	H	H	H			P					
Dobutamine	3-OH,4-OH	H	H	1*						C		
Colterol	3-OH,4-OH	OH	H	C(CH$_3$)$_3$					B			
Ethylnorepinephrine	3-OH,4-OH	OH	CH$_2$CH$_3$	H					B			
Isoproterenol	3-OH,4-OH	OH	H	CH(CH$_3$)$_2$					B	C		
Isoetharine	3-OH,4-OH	OH	CH$_2$CH$_3$	CH(CH$_3$)$_2$					B			
Metaproterenol	3-OH,5-OH	OH	H	CH(CH$_3$)$_2$					B			
Terbutaline	3-OH,5-OH	OH	H	C(CH$_3$)$_3$					B		U	
Metaraminol	3-OH	OH	CH$_3$	H		N	P					
Phenylephrine	3-OH	OH	H	CH$_3$			P					
Tyramine	4-OH	H	H	H								
Hydroxyamphetamine	4-OH	OH	CH$_3$	H								
Ritodrine	4-OH	OH	CH$_3$	2*						C	U	
Prenalterol	4-OH	OH‡	H	CH(CH$_3$)$_2$								
Methoxamine	2-OCH$_3$,5-OCH$_3$	OH	CH$_3$	H			P					
Albuterol	3-CH$_2$OH,4-OH	OH	H	C(CH$_3$)$_3$					B	C	U	
Amphetamine		H	CH$_3$	H		N	P					CNS, 0
Methamphetamine		H	CH$_3$	CH$_3$		N	P					CNS, 0
Benzphetamine		H	CH$_3$	3*		N			B			0
Ephedrine		OH	CH$_3$	CH$_3$			P		B	C		
Phenylpropanolamine		OH	CH$_3$	H			P					0
Mephentermine		H	4*³	CH$_3$								
Phentermine		H	4*	H								0

150

Propylhexedrine	5*	H	CH_3	CH_3	N	
Diethylpropion			6*			0
Phenmetrazine			7*			0
Phendimetrazine			8*			0

1
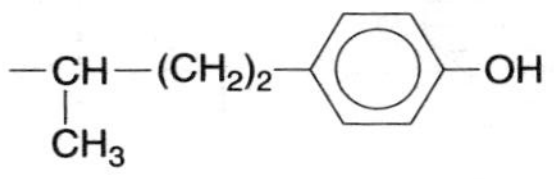

2
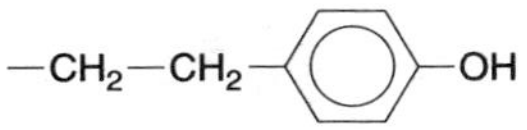

3
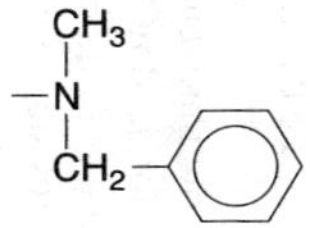

4
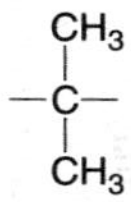

5
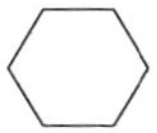

6
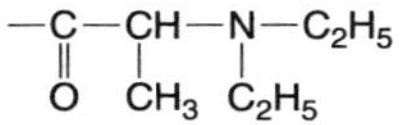

7
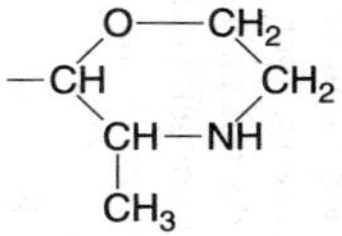

8
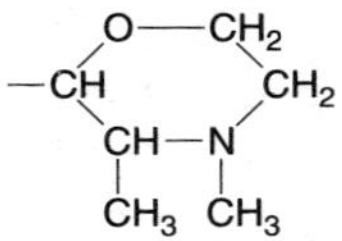

α Activity	*β Activity*	
A = Allergic reactions (includes β action)	B = Bronchodilator	CNS = Central nervous system
N = Nasal decongestion	C = Cardiac	0 = Anorectic
P = Pressor (may include β action)	U = Uterus	
V = Other local vasoconstriction (*e.g.*, in local anesthesia)		

*Numbers bearing an asterisk refer to the substituents numbered in the bottom rows of the table; substituent 3 replaces the N atom, substituent 5 replaces the phenyl ring, and 6, 7, and 8 are attached directly to the phenyl ring, replacing the ethylamine side chain.

†The α and β in the prototypical formula refer to positions of the C atoms in the ethylamine side chain.

‡Prenalterol has —OCH_2— between the aromatic ring and the carbon atom designated as β in the prototypical formula.

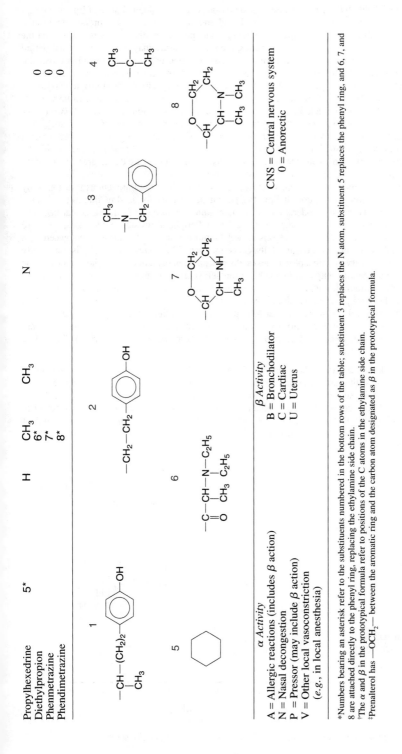

BLOOD PRESSURE   Epi is a potent vasopressor. A pharmacological dose of Epi, given rapidly by an intravenous route, rapidly increases blood pressure to a peak that is proportional to the dose. The increase in systolic pressure is greater than the increase in diastolic pressure, so that the pulse pressure increases. As the response wanes, the mean pressure may fall below normal before returning to control levels. The mechanism of the rise in blood pressure due to Epi is threefold: (1) a direct myocardial stimulation that increases the strength of ventricular contraction (positive inotropic action, via β_1 receptors); (2) an increased heart rate (positive chronotropic action, via β_1 receptors); and (3) vasoconstriction in many vascular beds (especially in the precapillary resistance vessels of skin, mucosa, and kidney) along with marked constriction of the veins (*via* α receptors). The pulse rate, at first accelerated by the direct positive chrontropic effect of Epi, may slow down markedly as blood pressure rises, due to the compensatory baroreceptor reflex (bradycardia due to vagal discharge). Small doses of Epi (0.1 μg/kg) may cause the blood pressure to fall; the depressor effect of small doses and the biphasic response to larger doses are due to greater sensitivity to Epi of vasodilator β_2 receptors than of constrictor α receptors.

The effects are somewhat different when the drug is given by slow intravenous infusion or by subcutaneous injection. Absorption of Epi after subcutaneous injection is slow due to local vasoconstrictor action. There is a moderate increase in systolic pressure due to increased cardiac contractile force and a rise in cardiac output (Figure 10–2). Peripheral resistance decreases, owing to a dominant action on β_2 receptors of vessels in skeletal muscle, where blood flow is enhanced; as a consequence, diastolic pressure usually falls. Since the mean blood pressure usually is not greatly elevated, compensatory baroreceptor reflexes do not appreciably antagonize the direct cardiac actions. Heart rate, cardiac output, stroke volume, and left ventricular stroke work increase as a result of direct cardiac stimulation and increased venous returns to the heart, which is reflected by an increase in right atrial pressure. At slightly higher rates of infusion, there may be no change or a slight rise in peripheral resistance and diastolic pressure, depending on the dose and the resultant ratio of α to β responses in the various vascular beds; compensatory reflexes also may come into play. The effects of intravenous infusion of Epi, NE, and isoproterenol are compared in Table 10–2 and Figure 10–2.

VASCULAR EFFECTS   The chief vascular action of Epi is on the smaller arterioles and precapillary sphincters, although veins and large arteries also respond. Various vascular beds react differently, resulting in substantial redistribution of blood flow. Injected Epi markedly decreases cutaneous blood flow, constricting precapillary vessels and small venules. Cutaneous vasoconstriction accounts for a marked decrease in blood flow in the hands and feet. The "after congestion" of mucosa following the vasoconstriction from locally applied Epi probably is due to changes in

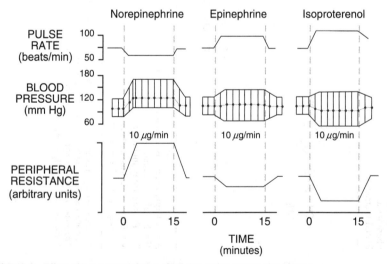

FIGURE 10–2   *Effects of intravenous infusion of NE, Epi, and isoproterenol in humans.*

Table 10-2

Comparison of the Effects of Intravenous Infusion of Epinephrine and Norepinephrine in Human Beings[*]

Effect	EPI	NE
Cardiac		
Heart rate	+	$-$[†]
Stroke volume	++	++
Cardiac output	+++	0, –
Arrhythmias	++++	++++
Coronary blood flow	++	++
Blood pressure		
Systolic arterial	+++	+++
Mean arterial	+	++
Diastolic arterial	+, 0, –	++
Mean pulmonary	++	++
Peripheral circulation		
Total peripheral resistance	–	++
Cerebral blood flow	+	0, –
Muscle blood flow	+++	0, –
Cutaneous blood flow	– –	– –
Renal blood flow	–	–
Splanchnic blood flow	+++	0, +
Metabolic effects		
Oxygen consumption	++	0, +
Blood glucose	+++	0, +
Blood lactic acid	+++	0, +
Eosinopenic response	+	0
Central nervous system		
Respiration	+	+
Subjective sensations	+	+

[*]0.1–0.4 μg/kg/min.

ABBREVIATIONS: Epi, epinephrine; NE, norepinephrine; +, increase; 0, no change; –, decrease; [†], after atropine, +.

vascular reactivity as a result of tissue hypoxia rather than to β agonist activity of the drug on mucosal vessels.

Blood flow to skeletal muscles is increased by therapeutic doses, due in part to powerful β_2-mediated vasodilation that is only partially counterbalanced by vasoconstrictor via the α receptors that also are present. If an α receptor antagonist is given, vasodilation in muscle is more pronounced, total peripheral resistance is decreased, and mean blood pressure falls (*Epi reversal*). After the administration of a nonselective β receptor antagonist, Epi produces only vasoconstriction and a considerable pressor effect.

In usual therapeutic doses, Epi has little constrictor action on cerebral arterioles. The cerebral circulation does not constrict in response to activation of the sympathetic nervous system by stressful stimuli; indeed, autoregulatory mechanisms tend to limit the increase in cerebral blood flow caused by increased blood pressure.

Doses of Epi that have little effect on mean arterial pressure consistently increase renal vascular resistance and reduce renal blood flow. All segments of the renal vascular bed contribute to the increased resistance. Since the glomerular filtration rate is only slightly and variably altered, the filtration fraction is consistently increased. Excretion of Na^+, K^+, and Cl^- is decreased. Maximal tubular reabsorptive and excretory capacities are unchanged. The secretion of renin is increased as a consequence of the stimulation of β_1 receptors on the juxtaglomerular cells (see Figure 30–2).

Epi increases arterial and venous pulmonary pressures. Although direct pulmonary vasoconstriction occurs, redistribution of blood from the systemic to the pulmonary circulation, due to constriction of the more powerful musculature in the systemic great veins, contributes to an increase in pulmonary pressure. Very high concentrations of Epi may cause pulmonary edema precipitated by elevated pulmonary capillary filtration pressure and possibly by "leaky" capillaries.

Coronary blood flow is enhanced by Epi or by cardiac sympathetic stimulation under physiological conditions. The increased flow, which occurs even with doses that do not increase the aortic blood pressure, is the result of two factors. The first is the increased relative duration of diastole at higher heart rates (see below); this is partially offset by decreased blood flow during systole because of more forceful contraction of the surrounding myocardium and an increase in mechanical compression of the coronary vessels. The increased flow during diastole is further enhanced if aortic blood pressure is elevated by Epi; as a consequence, total coronary flow may be increased. The second factor is a metabolic dilator effect that results from the increased strength of contraction and myocardial O_2 consumption due to direct effects of Epi on cardiac myocytes. This vasodilation is mediated in part by adenosine released from cardiac myocytes, which tends to override a direct vasoconstrictor effect of Epi that results from activation of α receptors in coronary vessels.

CARDIAC EFFECTS   Epi is a powerful cardiac stimulant. Direct responses to Epi include increase in the rate of tension development, peak contractile force, and rate of relaxation; decreased time to peak tension; increased excitability, acceleration of the rate of spontaneous beating, and induction of automaticity in specialized regions of the heart. Epi acts directly on the predominant β_1 receptors of the myocytes and of the cells of the pacemaker and conducting tissues. The heart rate increases, and the rhythm often is altered. Cardiac systole is shorter and more powerful, cardiac output is enhanced, and the work of the heart and its O_2 consumption are markedly increased. Cardiac efficiency (work done relative to O_2 consumption) is lessened.

By increasing the rates of ventricular contraction and relaxation, Epi preferentially shortens systole and usually does not reduce the duration of diastole. Epi speeds the heart by accelerating the slow depolarization of sinoatrial (SA) nodal cells that takes place during phase 4 of the action potential (see Chapter 34). The amplitude of the AP and the maximal rate of depolarization (phase 0) also are increased. A shift in the location of the pacemaker within the SA node often occurs, owing to activation of latent pacemaker cells. In Purkinje fibers, Epi accelerates diastolic depolarization and may activate latent pacemakers. If large doses of Epi are given, premature ventricular contractions occur and may herald more serious ventricular arrhythmias. Conduction through the Purkinje system depends on the level of membrane potential at the time of excitation. Epi often increases the membrane potential and improves conduction in Purkinje fibers that have been excessively depolarized.

Epi normally shortens the refractory period of the atrioventricular (AV) node by direct effects on the heart, although doses of Epi that elicit a vagal reflex may indirectly slow the heart and prolong the AV node's refractory period. Epi decreases the grade of AV block that occurs as a result of disease, drugs, or vagal stimulation. Supraventricular arrhythmias may occur from the combination of Epi and cholinergic stimulation. Depression of sinus rate and AV conduction by vagal discharge probably plays a part in Epi-induced ventricular arrhythmias, since various drugs that block the vagal effect confer some protection. The actions of Epi in enhancing cardiac automaticity and in causing arrhythmias are effectively antagonized by β receptor antagonists. However, activation of cardiac α_1 receptors prolongs the refractory period and strengthens myocardial contractions. Cardiac arrhythmias have been seen in patients after inadvertent intravenous administration of conventional subcutaneous doses of Epi.

Epi and other catecholamines may cause myocardial cell death, particularly after intravenous infusions. Acute toxicity is associated with contraction band necrosis and other pathological changes; prolonged sympathetic stimulation of the heart, such as in congestive cardiomyopathy, may promote apoptosis of cardiomyocytes.

NONVASCULAR SMOOTH MUSCLES   The effects of Epi on smooth muscle depend on the types and densities of adrenergic receptors expressed by the muscle (*see* Table 6–1). In general, Epi relaxes GI smooth muscle, due to activation of both α and β receptors. Intestinal tone and the frequency and amplitude of spontaneous contractions are reduced. The stomach usually is relaxed. By contrast, the pyloric and ileocecal sphincters are contracted (but these effects depend on the pre-existing tone of the muscle; if tone already is high, Epi causes relaxation; if low, contraction).

The responses of uterine muscle to Epi vary with phase of the sexual cycle, state of gestation, and dose. During the last month of pregnancy and at parturition, Epi inhibits uterine tone and contractions. β_2-Selective agonists (e.g., ritodrine or terbutaline) can delay premature labor, although *their efficacy is limited (see below). Epi relaxes the detrusor muscle of the bladder (via activation of β receptors) and contracts the trigone and sphincter muscles (via α agonist activity). This can result in hesitancy in urination and may contribute to retention of urine in the bladder. Activation of smooth muscle contraction in the prostate promotes urinary retention.*

RESPIRATORY EFFECTS

Acting at β_2 receptors on bronchial smooth muscle, Epi is a powerful bronchodilator, especially when bronchial muscle is contracted because of disease or in response to drugs or various autacoids. Beneficial effects of Epi in asthma also may arise from β_2-mediated inhibition of antigen-induced release of inflammatory mediators from mast cells, and to a lesser extent from an α adrenergic effect to diminish bronchial secretions and congestion within the mucosa. Other drugs, such as glucocorticoids and leukotriene-receptor antagonists, have more profound anti-inflammatory effects in asthma (see Chapter 27).

EFFECTS ON THE CNS

Epi, a polar compound, penetrates poorly into the CNS and, at conventional therapeutic doses, is not a powerful CNS stimulant. While Epi may cause restlessness, apprehension, headache, and tremor, these effects in part may be secondary to the effects of Epi on the cardiovascular system, skeletal muscles, and intermediary metabolism (i.e., the result of somatic manifestations of anxiety).

METABOLIC EFFECTS   Epi elevates the concentrations of glucose and lactate in blood (*see* Chapter 6), and can inhibit (α_2 effect) or stimulate (β_2 effect) insulin secretion; inhibition is the predominant effect. Glucagon secretion is enhanced via activation of β receptors of the α cells of pancreatic islets. Epi also decreases the uptake of glucose by peripheral tissues, in part because of its effects on the secretion of insulin, but also possibly due to direct effects on skeletal muscle. Glycosuria rarely occurs. The effect of Epi to stimulate glycogenolysis in most tissues and in most species involves β receptors.

Epi raises the plasma concentration of free fatty acids by stimulating β receptors in adipocytes, activating triglyceride lipase and accelerating triglyceride breakdown to free fatty acids and glycerol. The calorigenic action of Epi (increase in metabolism) is reflected by an increase of 20–30% in O_2 consumption, mainly due to enhanced breakdown of triglycerides in brown adipose tissue, providing an increase in oxidizable substrate.

MISCELLANEOUS EFFECTS

Epi rapidly increases the number of circulating polymorphonuclear leukocytes, likely due to β receptor–mediated demargination of these cells. Epi accelerates blood coagulation and promotes fibrinolysis. The effects of Epi on secretory glands are not marked; in most glands, secretion is inhibited, partly owing to the reduced blood flow caused by vasoconstriction. Epi stimulates lacrimation and a scanty mucus secretion from salivary glands. Sweating and pilomotor activity are minimal after systemic administration of Epi, but occur after intradermal injection of dilute solutions of either Epi or NE; such effects are inhibited by α receptor antagonists.

Mydriasis is readily seen during physiological sympathetic stimulation but not when Epi is instilled into the conjunctival sac of normal eyes. Epi usually lowers intraocular pressure (see Chapter 63).

Epi facilitates neuromuscular transmission, particularly that following prolonged rapid stimulation of motor nerves; stimulation of α receptors promotes transmitter release from the somatic motor neuron, perhaps as a result of enhanced influx of Ca^{2+}. These responses likely are mediated by α_1 receptors and may explain in part the ability of intra-arterial Epi to briefly increase strength in patients with myasthenia gravis. Epi also acts directly on white, fast-twitch muscle fibers to prolong the active state, thereby increasing peak tension. Of greater physiological and clinical importance is the capacity of Epi and selective β_2 agonists to increase physiological tremor, at least in part due to β receptor–mediated enhancement of discharge of muscle spindles.

Via activation of β_2 receptors, Epi promotes a fall in plasma K^+, largely due to stimulation of K^+ uptake into cells, particularly skeletal muscle. This is associated with decreased renal K^+ excretion.

ABSORPTION, FATE, AND EXCRETION   Epi is ineffective after oral administration because it is rapidly metabolized in the GI mucosa and liver. Absorption from subcutaneous tissues occurs relatively slowly because of local vasoconstriction, and the rate may be further decreased by systemic hypotension (*e.g.*, in shock). Absorption is more rapid after intramuscular injection. In emergencies, it may be necessary to administer Epi intravenously. When relatively concentrated solutions (1%) are nebulized and inhaled, the actions of the drug largely are restricted to the respiratory tract; however, systemic reactions such as arrhythmias may occur, particularly if larger amounts are used.

Epi is rapidly inactivated, especially by the liver, which is rich in COMT and MAO (*see* Figure 6–6 and Table 6–5).

FORMULATIONS

Epi injection is available in 1 mg/mL (1:1000), 0.1 mg/mL (1:10,000), and 0.5 mg/mL (1:2000) solutions. The usual adult dose given subcutaneously ranges from 0.3 to 0.5 mg. The intravenous route is used cautiously if an immediate and reliable effect is mandatory. If the solution is given by vein, it must be adequately diluted and injected very slowly. The dose is seldom as much as 0.25 mg, except for cardiac arrest, when larger doses may be required. Epi suspensions are used to slow subcutaneous absorption and must never be injected intravenously. Also, a 1% (10 mg/mL; 1:100) formulation is available for administration via inhalation; every precaution must be taken not to confuse this 1:100 solution with the 1:1000 solution designed for parenteral administration; inadvertent injection of the 1:100 solution can be fatal. Epi is unstable in alkaline solution; when exposed to air or light, it turns pink from oxidation to adrenochrome and then brown from polymer formation; thus, an antioxidant or acid must be included.

TOXICITY, ADVERSE EFFECTS, AND CONTRAINDICATIONS

Epi may cause restlessness, throbbing headache, tremor, and palpitations; these effects rapidly subside with rest, quiet, recumbency, and reassurance. More serious reactions include cerebral hemorrhage and cardiac arrhythmias. The use of large doses or the accidental, rapid intravenous injection of Epi may result in cerebral hemorrhage from the sharp rise in blood pressure. Ventricular arrhythmias may follow the drug's administration. Epi may induce angina in patients with coronary artery disease. Use of Epi generally is contraindicated in patients receiving nonselective β receptor–blocking drugs, since its unopposed actions on vascular α_1 receptors may lead to severe hypertension and cerebral hemorrhage.

THERAPEUTIC USES

Clinical uses of Epi are based on its actions on blood vessels, heart, and bronchial muscle. A major use is to provide rapid relief of hypersensitivity reactions, including anaphylaxis, to drugs and other allergens. Epi is used to prolong the action of local anesthetics, presumably by vasoconstriction and a consequent reduction in absorption (see Chapter 14). It may restore cardiac rhythm in patients with cardiac arrest. Epi also is used as a topical hemostatic agent on bleeding surfaces such as in the mouth or in bleeding peptic ulcers during endoscopy of the stomach and duodenum. Systemic absorption of the drug can occur with dental application. In addition, inhalation of Epi may be useful in the treatment of postintubation and infectious croup. The therapeutic uses of Epi, in relation to other sympathomimetic drugs, are discussed later in this chapter.

Norepinephrine

NE (LEVARTERENOL, *l*-noradrenaline) is released by mammalian postganglionic sympathetic nerves (Table 10–1). NE constitutes 10–20% of the catecholamine content of human adrenal medulla and as much as 97% in some pheochromocytomas, which may not express phenylethanolamine-*N*-methyltransferase.

PHARMACOLOGICAL PROPERTIES   The pharmacological actions of NE and Epi have been extensively compared *in vivo* and *in vitro* (Table 10–2). They are approximately equipotent in stimulating β_1 receptors; they differ mainly in their effectiveness in stimulating α and β_2 receptors. NE is a potent α agonist and has relatively little action on β_2 receptors; however, it is somewhat less potent than Epi on the α receptors of most organs. Isoproterenol stimulates all β receptors but not α receptors. Figure 10–2 compares the cardiovascular effects of infusions of NE, Epi, and isoproterenol.

Cardiovascular Effects   In response to infused NE, systolic and diastolic pressures, and usually pulse pressure, increase (*see* Figure 10–2). Cardiac output is unchanged or decreased, and total peripheral resistance is raised. Compensatory vagal reflex activity slows the heart, overcoming direct cardioaccelerator action; stroke volume increases. Peripheral vascular resistance increases in most vascular beds, and renal blood flow is reduced. NE constricts mesenteric vessels and reduces splanchnic and hepatic blood flow. Coronary flow usually is increased, probably owing both to indirectly induced coronary dilation, as with Epi, and to elevated blood pressure. Although generally a poor β_2 agonist, NE may increase coronary blood flow directly by stimulating β_2 receptors on coronary vessels. Patients with Prinzmetal's variant angina may be supersensitive to the α constrictor effects of NE.

ABSORPTION, FATE, AND EXCRETION

NE, like Epi, is ineffective when given orally and is absorbed poorly from sites of subcutaneous injection. It is rapidly inactivated in the body by uptake and the actions of COMT and MAO. Small amounts normally are found in the urine. The excretion rate may be greatly increased in patients with pheochromocytoma.

ADVERSE EFFECTS; PRECAUTIONS

The untoward effects of NE resemble those of Epi, although there typically is greater elevation of blood pressure with NE. Excessive doses cause severe hypertension. Care must be taken that necrosis and sloughing do not occur at the site of intravenous injection owing to extravasation of the drug. The infusion should be made high in the limb, preferably through a long plastic cannula extending centrally. Impaired circulation at injection sites, with or without extravasation of NE, may be relieved by infiltrating the area with phentolamine, *an α receptor antagonist. Blood pressure must be determined frequently. Reduced blood flow to organs such as kidney and intestines is a constant danger with the use of NE.*

THERAPEUTIC USES

NE (LEVOPHED, others) has limited therapeutic value. Its use in shock is discussed below. In the treatment of low blood pressure, the dose is titrated to the desired pressor response.

Dopamine

DA (3,4-dihydroxyphenylethylamine; Table 10–1) is the metabolic precursor of NE and Epi; it is a central neurotransmitter particularly important in the regulation of movement (*see* Chapters 12, 18, and 20). In the periphery, DA is synthesized in epithelial cells of the proximal tubule and is thought to exert local diuretic and natriuretic effects. DA is a substrate for both MAO and COMT and thus is ineffective when administered orally. Classification of DA receptors is described in Chapters 12 and 20.

PHARMACOLOGICAL PROPERTIES

Cardiovascular Effects The cardiovascular effects of DA are mediated by several distinct types of receptors that vary in their affinity for DA. At low concentrations, the primary interaction of DA is with vascular D_1 receptors, especially in the renal, mesenteric, and coronary beds; this interaction leads to smooth muscle vasodilation (via the G_s-adenylyl cyclase-cAMP pathway). Infusion of low doses of DA causes an increase in glomerular filtration rate, renal blood flow, and Na^+ excretion. Activation of D_1 receptors on renal tubular cells decreases sodium transport by cAMP-dependent and cAMP-independent mechanisms. Increasing cAMP production in the proximal tubular cells and the medullary part of the thick ascending limb of the loop of Henle inhibits the Na^+-H^+ exchanger and the Na^+,K^+-ATPase. Renal tubular actions of DA that cause natriuresis may be augmented by the increase in renal blood flow and in glomerular filtration rate that follow its administration. The resulting increase in hydrostatic pressure in the peritubular capillaries and reduction in oncotic pressure may contribute to diminished Na^+ reabsorption by the proximal tubular cells. Thus, DA has pharmacologically appropriate effects in the management of states of low cardiac output associated with compromised renal function, such as severe congestive heart failure.

At higher concentrations, DA acts on cardiac β_1 receptors to produce a positive inotropic effect. DA also causes the release of NE from nerve terminals, which contributes to its effects on the heart. DA usually increases systolic blood pressure and pulse pressure and either has no effect on diastolic blood pressure or increases it slightly. Total peripheral resistance usually is unchanged when low or intermediate doses of DA are given, probably because of reduced regional arterial resistance in some vascular beds (e.g., mesenteric and renal) with minor increases in others. At high concentrations, DA activates vascular α_1 receptors, leading to more general vasoconstriction.

CNS

Although there are specific DA receptors in the CNS, injected DA usually has no central effects because it does not readily cross the blood–brain barrier.

THERAPEUTIC USES Dopamine (INTROPIN, others) is used in the treatment of severe congestive failure, particularly in patients with oliguria and low or normal peripheral vascular resistance. The drug also may improve physiological parameters in the treatment of cardiogenic and septic shock. While DA may acutely improve cardiac and renal function in severely ill patients with chronic heart disease or renal failure, there is little evidence supporting long-term benefit in clinical outcome. The management of shock is discussed below.

Dopamine hydrochloride is used only intravenously, initially at a rate of 2–5 μg/kg/min, increasing gradually to 20–50 μg/kg/min if necessary. During the infusion, patients require clinical assessment of myocardial function, perfusion of vital organs such as the brain, and the production of urine. Reduction in urine flow, tachycardia, or the development of arrhythmias may be indications to slow or terminate the infusion. The duration of action of DA is brief; thus, the rate of administration can be used to control the intensity of effect.

Related drugs include fenoldopam and dopexamine. Fenoldopam (CORLOPAM), a benzazepine derivative, is a rapidly acting vasodilator used for control of severe hypertension (e.g., malignant hypertension with end-organ damage) in hospitalized patients for not more than 48 hours. Fenoldopam is an agonist for peripheral D_1 receptors and binds with moderate affinity to α_2 adrenergic receptors; it has no significant affinity for D_2 receptors or α_1 or β adrenergic receptors. Fenoldopam is a racemate; the R-isomer is the active component. It dilates a variety of blood vessels, including coronary arteries, afferent and efferent arterioles in the kidney, and mesenteric arteries. Of an orally administered dose, <6% is absorbed because of extensive first-pass metabolism. The elimination $t_{1/2}$ of intravenously infused fenoldopam is ~10 minutes. Adverse effects are related to vasodilation and include headache, flushing, dizziness, and tachycardia or bradycardia.

Dopexamine (DOPACARD) is a synthetic analog with intrinsic activity at D_1, D_2, and β_2 receptors; it may also inhibit catecholamine uptake. Dopexamine has favorable hemodynamic actions in patients with severe congestive heart failure, sepsis, and shock. In patients with low cardiac output, dopexamine infusion significantly increases stroke volume and decreases systemic vascular resistance. Tachycardia and hypotension can occur, but usually only at high infusion rates. Dopexamine is not available in the U.S.

PRECAUTIONS, ADVERSE REACTIONS, AND CONTRAINDICATIONS Before DA is administered to patients in shock, hypovolemia should be corrected. Untoward effects due to overdosage generally are attributable to excessive sympathomimetic activity (although this also may be the response to worsening shock). Nausea, vomiting, tachycardia, anginal pain, arrhythmias, headache, hypertension, and peripheral vasoconstriction may be encountered during DA infusion. Extravasation of large amounts of DA during infusion may cause ischemic necrosis and sloughing. Rarely, gangrene of the fingers or toes has followed prolonged infusion of the drug. DA should be avoided or used at reduced dosage (one-tenth or less) if the patient has received an MAO inhibitor. Careful adjustment of dosage also is necessary in patients who are taking tricyclic antidepressants.

β ADRENERGIC RECEPTOR AGONISTS

β Adrenergic receptor agonists play a major role only in the treatment of bronchoconstriction in patients with asthma (reversible airway obstruction) or chronic obstructive pulmonary disease (COPD). Minor uses include management of preterm labor, treatment of complete heart block in shock, and short-term treatment of cardiac decompensation after surgery or in patients with congestive heart failure or myocardial infarction. The chronotropic effect of β agonists is useful in the emergency treatment of arrhythmias such as torsades de pointes, bradycardia, or heart block (see Chapter 34).

Isoproterenol

Isoproterenol (isopropylarterenol, isopropyl NE, isoprenaline; *see* Table 10–1) is a potent, nonselective β receptor agonist with very low affinity for α receptors. Consequently, isoproterenol has powerful effects on all β receptors and almost no action at α receptors.

PHARMACOLOGICAL ACTIONS The major cardiovascular effects of isoproterenol (compared with Epi and NE) are illustrated in Figure 10–2. Intravenous infusion of isoproterenol lowers peripheral vascular resistance, primarily in skeletal muscle but also in renal and mesenteric vascular beds. Diastolic pressure falls. Systolic blood pressure may remain unchanged or rise; mean arterial pressure typically falls. Cardiac output increases due to the positive inotropic and chronotropic effects of the drug in the face of diminished peripheral vascular resistance. The cardiac effects of isoproterenol may lead to palpitations, sinus tachycardia, and more serious arrhythmias.

Isoproterenol relaxes almost all varieties of smooth muscle when the tone is high, an action that is most pronounced on bronchial and GI smooth muscle. Isoproterenol's effect in asthma may be due in part to inhibition of antigen-induced release of histamine and other mediators of inflammation, an action shared by β_2-selective agonists.

ABSORPTION, FATE, AND EXCRETION

Isoproterenol is readily absorbed when given parenterally or as an aerosol. It is metabolized in the liver and other tissues by COMT. Isoproterenol is a relatively poor substrate for MAO and is not taken up by sympathetic neurons via NET to the same extent as Epi and NE. Isoproterenol's duration of action exceeds that of Epi but still is brief.

TOXICITY AND ADVERSE EFFECTS

Palpitations, tachycardia, headache, and flushing are common. Cardiac ischemia and arrhythmias may occur, particularly in patients with underlying coronary artery disease.

THERAPEUTIC USES

Isoproterenol (ISUPREL, others) may be used in emergencies to stimulate heart rate in patients with bradycardia or heart block, particularly in anticipation of inserting an artificial cardiac pacemaker or in patients with the ventricular arrhythmia torsades de pointes. In asthma and shock, isoproterenol largely has been replaced by other sympathomimetic drugs (see below and Chapter 27).

Dobutamine

The pharmacological effects of *dobutamine* (*see* Table 10–1 for structure) result from direct interactions with α and β receptors and are complex. The preparation of dobutamine used clinically is a racemate. The (–) isomer of dobutamine is a potent α_1 agonist and pressor; (+) dobutamine is a potent α_1 antagonist that can block the effects of (–) dobutamine. Both isomers are full agonists at β receptors, but the (+) isomer is more potent than the (–) isomer by ~tenfold.

CARDIOVASCULAR EFFECTS

The cardiovascular effects of racemic dobutamine are a composite of the pharmacological properties of the (–) and (+) stereoisomers. Dobutamine has relatively more prominent inotropic than chronotropic effects, compared to isoproterenol. This useful selectivity may arise because peripheral resistance is relatively unchanged due to a counterbalancing of α_1 receptor–mediated vasoconstriction and β_2 receptor–mediated vasodilation. Alternatively, cardiac α_1 receptors may contribute to the inotropic effect. At equivalent inotropic doses, dobutamine enhances automaticity of the sinus node to a lesser extent than does isoproterenol; however, enhancement of AV and intraventricular conduction is similar for both drugs.

ADVERSE EFFECTS

Blood pressure and heart rate may increase significantly during dobutamine administration, requiring reduction of infusion rate; hypertensive patients may exhibit such an exaggerated pressor response more frequently. Since dobutamine facilitates AV conduction, patients with atrial fibrillation are at risk of marked increases in ventricular response rates; digoxin or other measures may be required to prevent this from occurring. Some patients may develop ventricular ectopic activity. As with any inotropic agent, dobutamine may increase the size of an infarct by increasing myocardial O_2 demand. The efficacy of dobutamine for more than a few days is uncertain; there is evidence of the development of tolerance.

THERAPEUTIC USES; PHARMACOKINETICS

Dobutamine (DOBUTREX, others) is indicated for the short-term treatment of cardiac decompensation post cardiac surgery or in patients with congestive heart failure or acute myocardial infarction. An infusion of dobutamine in combination with echocardiography is useful in the noninvasive assessment of patients with coronary artery disease; stressing the heart with dobutamine may reveal cardiac abnormalities in selected patients.

A loading dose is not required, and steady-state concentrations generally are achieved within 10 minutes of initiation of the infusion. The rate of infusion required to increase cardiac output typically is 2.5–10 μg/kg/min; higher infusion rates occasionally are required. The rate and duration of the infusion are determined by the clinical and hemodynamic responses of the patient. The onset of effect is rapid. Dobutamine has a t$_{1/2}$ of ~2 minutes; the major metabolites are conjugates of dobutamine and 3-O-methyldobutamine.

β_2-Selective Adrenergic Receptor Agonists

In treating asthma, preferential activation of β_2 receptors without stimulation of β_1 receptors in the heart is desirable. Drugs with preferential affinity for β_2 receptors over β_1 receptors have been *developed, but selectivity is not absolute and is lost at high concentrations. Administration by inhalation of small doses of a β_2 agonist in aerosol form leads to effective activation of β_2 receptors in the bronchi but very low systemic drug concentrations. Consequently, there is less potential to activate cardiac β_1 receptors or to stimulate β_2 receptors in skeletal muscle (which can cause tremor). The use of β agonists for the treatment of asthma is discussed in Chapter 27.*

METAPROTERENOL *Metaproterenol* (called *orciprenaline* in Europe), *terbutaline*, and *fenoterol* belong to the structural class of resorcinol bronchodilators that have hydroxyl groups at positions 3 and 5 of the phenyl ring (rather than at positions 3 and 4 as in catechols; *see* Table 10–1). Consequently, these agents are resistant to methylation by COMT, and a substantial fraction (40%) is absorbed in active form after oral administration. Metaproterenol is excreted primarily as glucuronic acid conjugates. Metaproterenol is β_2 selective, although probably less selective than albuterol or terbutaline; thus, metaproterenol is more prone to cause cardiac stimulation.

Effects occur within minutes of inhalation and persist for several hours. After oral administration, onset of action is slower, but effects last 3 to 4 hours. Metaproterenol (ALUPENT, others) is used for the long-term treatment of obstructive airway diseases, asthma, and for treatment of acute bronchospasm (see Chapter 27). Side effects are similar to the short- and intermediate-acting sympathomimetic bronchodilators.

TERBUTALINE
Terbutaline is a β_2-selective bronchodilator that contains a resorcinol ring and thus is not a substrate for COMT. It is effective when taken orally, subcutaneously, or by inhalation. Effects are observed rapidly after inhalation or parenteral administration; after inhalation, its action may persist for 3–6 hours. With oral administration, the onset of effect may be delayed for 1–2 hours. Terbutaline (BRETHINE, others) is used for the long-term treatment of obstructive airway diseases and acute bronchospasm; a parenteral formulation is used for the emergency treatment of status asthmaticus (see Chapter 27).

ALBUTEROL
Albuterol (VENTOLIN, PROVENTIL, others) is a selective β_2 agonist with pharmacological properties and therapeutic indications similar to those of terbutaline. It is administered by inhalation or orally for the symptomatic relief of bronchospasm. When administered by inhalation, terbutaline produces significant bronchodilation within 15 minutes; effects persist for 3–4 hours. Cardiovascular effects of albuterol are considerably weaker than those of isoproterenol that produce comparable bronchodilation when administered by inhalation. Oral albuterol may delay preterm labor. Rare CNS and respiratory side effects are sometimes observed.

ISOETHARINE
The selectivity of isoetharine for β_2 receptors may not approach that of other agents. Although resistant to metabolism by MAO, it is a catecholamine and thus is a good substrate for COMT (Table 10–1). It is used only by inhalation for acute episodes of bronchoconstriction.

PIRBUTEROL
Pirbuterol is a relatively selective β_2 agonist structurally related to albuterol. Pirbuterol acetate (MAXAIR) is available for inhalation therapy; dosing is typically every 4–6 hours.

BITOLTEROL
Bitolterol (TORNALATE) is a novel β_2 agonist prodrug in which the OH groups in the catechol moiety are protected by esterification. Esterase activities thought to be higher in lung than heart hydrolyze the prodrug to the active form, colterol, or terbutylne (Table 10–1). The duration of bitolterol's effect after inhalation is 3–6 hours.

FENOTEROL
Fenoterol (BEROTEC) is a β_2-selective agonist administered by inhalation. Fenoterol has a prompt onset of action, and a sustained effect (4–6 hours). Possible association of fenoterol use with increased deaths from asthma in New Zealand is controversial. Fenoterol is under investigation for use in the U.S.

FORMOTEROL
Formoterol (FORADIL) is a long-acting, lipophilic, high-affinity β_2-selective agonist. Significant bronchodilation occurs within minutes of inhalation and may persist for up to 12 hours, an advantage over many β_2-selective agonists in settings such as nocturnal asthma. Formoterol is

FDA-approved for treatment of asthma, bronchospasm, prophylaxis of exercise-induced bronchospasm, and COPD.

PROCATEROL

Procaterol (MASCACIN, *others; not available in U.S.), a β_2-selective agonist, is administered by inhalation and has a prompt onset of action that is sustained for ~5 hours.*

SALMETEROL

Salmeterol (SEREVENT) is a lipophilic β_2-selective receptor agonist with prolonged action (>12 hours) and relatively high selectivity (50× that of albuterol) for β_2 receptors. Since the onset of action of inhaled salmeterol is relatively slow, it is not suitable monotherapy for acute breakthrough attacks of bronchospasm. Salmeterol or formoterol are the agents of choice for nocturnal asthma in patients who remain symptomatic despite anti-inflammatory agents and other standard management. Salmeterol provides symptomatic relief and improved lung function in patients with COPD. Salmeterol should not be used more than twice daily (morning and evening) and should not be used to treat acute asthma symptoms, which should be treated with a short-acting β_2 agonist when breakthrough symptoms occur. Salmeterol is metabolized by CYP3A4 to α-hydroxy-salmeterol, which is eliminated primarily in the feces.

RITODRINE

Ritodrine is a selective β_2 agonist originally developed as a uterine relaxant. Ritodrine is rapidly but incompletely (30%) absorbed following oral administration; 90% of the drug is excreted in the urine as inactive conjugates; ~50% of ritodrine is excreted unchanged after intravenous administration. The pharmacokinetic properties of ritodrine are complex and incompletely defined, especially in pregnant women. Administered intravenously to selected patients, ritodrine can arrest premature labor and prolong pregnancy; however, β_2-selective agonists may not have clinically significant benefits on perinatal mortality and may actually increase maternal morbidity. In one trial comparing nifedipine with ritodrine in managing preterm labor, nifedipine was associated with a longer postponement of delivery, fewer maternal side effects, and fewer admissions to the neonatal intensive care unit.

ADVERSE EFFECTS OF β_2-SELECTIVE AGONISTS

The major adverse effects of β-receptor agonists occur as a result of excessive activation of β receptors: tremor, to which tolerance develops and which can be minimized by starting oral therapy with a low dose of drug and progressively increasing the dose as tolerance to the tremor develops; feelings of restlessness, apprehension, and anxiety, which may limit therapy; and tachycardia, primarily via β_1 receptors but also possibly via cardiac β_2 receptors, or to reflex effects that stem from β_2 receptor–mediated peripheral vasodilation. During a severe asthma attack, heart rate actually may decrease during therapy with a β agonist, presumably because of improvement in pulmonary function with consequent reduction in endogenous cardiac sympathetic stimulation. In patients without cardiac disease, β agonists rarely cause significant arrhythmias or myocardial ischemia; however, patients with underlying coronary artery disease or preexisting arrhythmias are at greater risk. The risk of adverse cardiovascular effects is increased in patients receiving MAO inhibitors; 2 weeks should elapse between use of MAO inhibitors and administration of β_2 agonists or other sympathomimetics. Severe pulmonary edema has been reported in women receiving ritodrine or terbutaline for premature labor.

Epidemiologic studies suggest a connection between prolonged use of β receptor agonists and death or near-death from asthma, raising questions about the role of β agonists in the treatment of chronic asthma. Tolerance to the pulmonary effects of these drugs is not a major clinical problem for the majority of asthmatics. Regular use of β_2-selective agonists may cause increased bronchial hyperreactivity and deterioration in disease control; whether this potential adverse association may be more unfavorable for long-acting β agonists or excess doses is not yet known. For patients requiring regular use of β agonists over prolonged periods, strong consideration should be given to additional or alternative therapy (e.g., inhaled glucocorticoids). In some diabetic patients, β agonists may worsen hyperglycemia, and higher doses of insulin may be required. All these adverse effects are far less likely with inhalation therapy than with parenteral or oral therapy.

α_1-SELECTIVE ADRENERGIC RECEPTOR AGONISTS

Activation of α adrenergic receptors in vascular smooth muscle results in contraction, causing increases in peripheral vascular resistance and blood pressure. Although the clinical utility of α agonists is limited, they may be useful in the treatment of hypotension and shock. Some of the properties of the drugs listed below may be inferred from their structures (Table 10–1).

Phenylephrine

Phenylephrine (NEO-SYNEPHRINE, others) is a selective α_1 receptor agonist; it activates β receptors only at much higher concentrations. The drug causes marked arterial vasoconstriction during intravenous infusion. Phenylephrine also is used as a nasal decongestant and as a mydriatic in various nasal and ophthalmic formulations (*see* Chapter 63 for ophthalmic uses).

Mephentermine

Mephentermine (WYAMINE SULFATE) acts both directly and indirectly. After an intramuscular injection, the onset of action is prompt (within 5–15 minutes), and effects may last for several hours. Since the drug releases NE, cardiac contraction is enhanced, and cardiac output and systolic and diastolic pressures usually are increased. The change in heart rate is variable, depending on the degree of vagal tone. Adverse effects are related to CNS stimulation, excessive rises in blood pressure, and arrhythmias. Mephentermine is used to prevent hypotension, which frequently accompanies spinal anesthesia.

Metaraminol

Metaraminol (ARAMINE) is a mixed-acting agent: an agonist at vascular α adrenergic receptors and an indirectly acting agent that stimulates the release of NE. The drug has been used in the treatment of hypotensive states or off-label to relieve attacks of paroxysmal atrial tachycardia, particularly those associated with hypotension (see Chapter 34 for preferable treatments of this arrhythmia).

Midodrine

Midodrine (PROAMATINE) is an orally effective α_1 receptor agonist. It is a prodrug; its activity is due to its conversion to an active metabolite, desglymidodrine, which achieves peak concentrations ~1 hour after a dose of midodrine. The $t_{1/2}$ of desglymidodrine is ~3 hours; its duration of action is 4–6 hours. Midodrine stimulates contraction of both arterial and venous smooth muscle, and has useful effects in treating autonomic insufficiency and postural hypotension. A frequent complication in these patients is supine hypertension, which can be minimized by avoiding dosing prior to bedtime and by elevating the head of the bed. Typical dosing, achieved by careful titration of blood pressure responses, is 2.5–10 mg 3 times daily.

α_2-SELECTIVE ADRENERGIC RECEPTOR AGONISTS

α_2-selective adrenergic agonists are used primarily for the treatment of systemic hypertension, a surprising use since many blood vessels contain postsynaptic α_2 adrenergic receptors that promote vasoconstriction; indeed, increased blood pressure is a transient immediate response to these agents. Thus, all α_2 agonists must be used with caution in patients with cardiovascular disease. Some α_2 agonists usefully decrease intraocular pressure.

Clonidine

Intravenous infusion of clonidine causes an acute rise in blood pressure due to activation of postsynaptic α_2 receptors in vascular smooth muscle. The affinity of clonidine for these receptors is high, although the drug is a partial agonist with relatively low efficacy at these sites. The hypertensive response that follows parenteral administration of clonidine generally is not seen when the drug is given orally. After either oral or parenteral administration, the transient vasoconstriction is followed by a more prolonged hypotensive response that results from decreased sympathetic outflow from the CNS, apparently from activation of α_2 receptors in the lower brainstem region. Clonidine also stimulates parasympathetic outflow, which may contribute to the slowing of heart rate. In addition, some of the antihypertensive effects of clonidine may be mediated by activation of presynaptic α_2 receptors that suppress the release of NE, ATP, and NPY from postganglionic sympathetic nerves. Clonidine decreases the plasma concentration of NE and reduces its excretion in the urine.

ABSORPTION, FATE, AND EXCRETION

Clonidine is well absorbed after oral administration, with bioavailability ~100%. The peak concentration in plasma and the maximal hypotensive effect are observed 1–3 hours after an oral dose; plasma concentrations of clonidine and its pharmacological effects correlate well. The elimination $t_{1/2}$ of the drug ranges from 6–24 hours (mean ~12 hours). About half of an administered dose appears unchanged in the urine; the $t_{1/2}$ of the drug may increase with renal failure. A transdermal delivery patch permits continuous administration of clonidine at a relatively constant rate for a week; 3–4 days are required to reach steady-state concentrations in plasma. When the patch *is removed, plasma concentrations remain stable for ~8 hours and then decline gradually over a period of several days; this decrease is associated with a rise in blood pressure.*

ADVERSE EFFECTS

The major adverse effects of clonidine are dry mouth and sedation, which may diminish in intensity after several weeks of therapy. Sexual dysfunction and marked bradycardia may occur. These effects of clonidine frequently are dose-related; their incidence may be lower with transdermal administration of clonidine, which avoids the relatively high peak concentrations that occur after oral administration. About 15–20% of patients develop contact dermatitis when using clonidine in the transdermal system. Withdrawal reactions follow abrupt discontinuation of long-term therapy with clonidine in some hypertensive patients.

THERAPEUTIC USES

The major therapeutic use of clonidine (CATAPRES, others) is in the treatment of hypertension (see Chapter 32). Clonidine also has apparent efficacy in the off-label treatment of a range of other disorders: reducing diarrhea in some diabetic patients with autonomic neuropathy; treating and preparing addicted subjects for withdrawal (see Chapter 23); ameliorating some of the adverse sympathetic nervous activity associated with withdrawal, and decreasing craving for the drug. Transdermal administration of clonidine (CATAPRES-TTS) may be useful in reducing the incidence of menopausal hot flashes.

The capacity of clonidine to activate postsynaptic α_2 receptors in vascular smooth muscle has been exploited in a limited number of patients whose autonomic failure is so severe that reflex sympathetic responses on standing are absent; postural hypotension is thus marked. Since the central effect of clonidine on blood pressure is unimportant in these patients, the drug can elevate blood pressure and improve the symptoms of postural hypotension. Among the other off-label uses of clonidine are atrial fibrillation, attention-deficit/hyperactivity disorder (ADHD), constitutional growth delay in children, cyclosporine-associated nephrotoxicity, Tourette's syndrome, hyperhidrosis, mania, posthepatic neuralgia, psychosis, restless leg syndrome, ulcerative colitis, and allergy-induced inflammatory reactions in patients with extrinsic asthma.

Apraclonidine

Apraclonidine (IOPIDINE) is a relatively selective α_2 agonist that is used topically to reduce intraocular pressure with minimal systemic effects; apraclonidine seems not to cross the blood–brain barrier and is more useful than clonidine for ophthalmic therapy. The drug is useful as short-term adjunctive therapy in glaucoma patients whose intraocular pressure is not well controlled by other pharmacological agents and to control or prevent elevations in intraocular pressure that occur in patients after laser trabeculoplasty or iridotomy (see Chapter 63).

Brimonidine

Brimonidine (ALPHAGAN), a clonidine derivative and α_2 agonist, is administered topically to lower intraocular pressure in patients with ocular hypertension or open-angle glaucoma; brimonidine both decreases aqueous humor production and increases outflow (see Chapter 63). Unlike apraclonidine, brimonidine crosses the blood–brain barrier and can produce hypotension and sedation, although these effects are slight compared to those of clonidine.

Dexmedetomidine (PRECEDEX), a relatively selective α_2 agonist with sedative properties, produces preoperative sedation and anxiolysis, drying of secretions, and analgesia; the drug is used as an anesthetic adjunct.

Guanfacine

Guanfacine (TENEX), an α_2 agonist, is more selective for α_2 receptors than is clonidine. Guanfacine lowers blood pressure by activation of brainstem receptors with resultant suppression of sympathetic activity. The drug is well absorbed after oral administration. About 50% of guanfacine appears unchanged in the urine; the rest is metabolized. The $t_{1/2}$ for elimination ranges from 12–24 hours. Guanfacine and clonidine appear to have similar efficacy for the treatment of hypertension and a similar pattern of adverse effects. A withdrawal syndrome may occur after abrupt discontinuation, but it is less frequent and milder than the syndrome that follows clonidine withdrawal, perhaps reflecting the longer $t_{1/2}$ of guanfacine.

Guanabenz

Guanabenz *(WYTENSIN, others) and guanfacine are closely related chemically and pharmacologically. Guanabenz is a centrally acting α_2 agonist that decreases blood pressure. Guanabenz has a $t_{1/2}$ of 4–6 hours and is extensively metabolized by the liver. Dosage adjustment may be necessary* *in patients with hepatic cirrhosis. The adverse effects of guanabenz (e.g., dry mouth and sedation) are similar to those of clonidine.*

Methyldopa

In the brain, methyldopa *(α-methyl-3,4-dihydroxyphenylalanine) is metabolized to α-methylNE, and this compound is thought to activate central α_2 receptors and lower blood pressure in a manner similar to that of clonidine (see Chapter 32).*

Tizanidine

Tizanidine *(ZANAFLEX, others) is an α_2 agonist with some properties similar to those of clonidine. The drug is also a muscle relaxant used for the treatment of spasticity associated with cerebral and spinal disorders.*

MISCELLANEOUS SYMPATHOMIMETIC AGONISTS
Amphetamine

Amphetamine (racemic β-phenylisopropylamine; see Table 10–1) acts indirectly to produce powerful stimulant actions in the CNS and α and β receptor stimulation in the periphery. Unlike Epi, amphetamine is effective after oral administration, and its effects last for several hours.

CARDIOVASCULAR RESPONSES
Amphetamine given orally raises systolic and diastolic blood pressure. Heart rate often is reflexly slowed; with large doses, cardiac arrhythmias may occur.

OTHER SMOOTH MUSCLES
In general, smooth muscles respond to amphetamine as they do to other sympathomimetic amines. The contractile effect on the sphincter of the urinary bladder is particularly marked, and for this reason amphetamine has been used in treating enuresis and incontinence. Pain and difficulty in micturition occasionally occur. GI effects are unpredictable: relaxation if enteric activity is pronounced, stimulation if the gut already is relaxed. The response of the human uterus varies, but there usually is an increase in tone.

CNS
Amphetamine is one of the most potent sympathomimetic amines in stimulating the CNS. It stimulates the medullary respiratory center, lessens the degree of central depression caused by various drugs, and produces other signs of CNS stimulation; the d-isomer (dextroamphetamine) *is three to four times more potent than the l-isomer. Psychic effects depend on the dose and the mental state and personality of the individual. The main results of an oral dose of 10–30 mg include wakefulness, alertness, and a decreased sense of fatigue; elevation of mood, with increased initiative, self-confidence, and ability to concentrate; often, elation and euphoria; and increase in motor and speech activities. Performance of simple mental tasks is improved; although more work may be accomplished, the number of errors may increase. Physical performance—in athletes, for example—is often improved, and the drug often is abused for this purpose. Prolonged use or large doses are nearly always followed by depression and fatigue. Many individuals given amphetamine experience headache, palpitation, dizziness, vasomotor disturbances, agitation, confusion, dysphoria, apprehension, delirium, or fatigue (see Chapter 23).*

FATIGUE AND SLEEP
In general, amphetamine prolongs the duration of adequate performance before fatigue appears, and partly reverses the effects of fatigue, most noticeably when performance has been reduced by fatigue and lack of sleep. The need for sleep may be postponed, but it cannot be avoided indefinitely. When the drug is discontinued after long use, the pattern of sleep may take as long as 2 months to return to normal.

Analgesia
Amphetamine and some other sympathomimetic amines have a small analgesic effect that is not sufficiently pronounced to be therapeutically useful. Amphetamine can enhance the analgesia produced by opiates.

Respiration
Amphetamine stimulates the respiratory center, increasing the rate and depth of respiration. In normal individuals, usual doses of the drug do not appreciably increase respiratory rate or minute volume. Nevertheless, when respiration is depressed by centrally acting drugs, amphetamine may stimulate respiration.

Appetite

Weight loss in obese humans treated with amphetamine is almost entirely due to reduced food intake and only in small measure to increased metabolism. In humans, tolerance to the appetite suppression develops rapidly.

Mechanisms of Action in the CNS

Amphetamine appears to exert most or all of its CNS effects indirectly by releasing biogenic amines from storage sites in nerve terminals. The alerting effect of amphetamine, its anorectic effect, and at least a component of its locomotor-stimulating action presumably are mediated by release of NE from central noradrenergic neurons. Some aspects of locomotor activity and the stereotyped behavior induced by amphetamine probably result from the release of DA from dopaminergic nerve terminals in the neostriatum. Higher doses are required to produce these behavioral effects. With still higher doses of amphetamine, disturbances of perception and overt psychosis occur, possibly due to release of 5-HT from serotonergic neurons and of DA in the mesolimbic system.

TOXICITY AND ADVERSE EFFECTS   The acute toxic effects of amphetamine usually are extensions of its therapeutic actions and as a rule result from overdosage. CNS effects commonly include restlessness, dizziness, tremor, hyperactive reflexes, talkativeness, tenseness, irritability, weakness, insomnia, fever, and sometimes euphoria. Confusion, aggressiveness, changes in libido, anxiety, delirium, paranoid hallucinations, panic states, and suicidal or homicidal tendencies occur, especially in mentally ill patients. However, these psychotic effects can be elicited in any individual if sufficient quantities of amphetamine are ingested for a prolonged period. Fatigue and depression usually follow central stimulation. Cardiovascular effects are common and include headache, chilliness, pallor or flushing, palpitation, cardiac arrhythmias, anginal pain, hypertension or hypotension, and circulatory collapse. Excessive sweating occurs. GI symptoms include dry mouth, metallic taste, anorexia, nausea, vomiting, diarrhea, and abdominal cramps. Fatal poisoning usually terminates in convulsions and coma; cerebral hemorrhages are the main pathological findings.

Toxicity shows great biological variability, occasionally occurring after as little as 2 mg, but rare with <15 mg. Severe reactions have occurred with 30 mg, yet doses of 400–500 mg are not uniformly fatal. Larger doses can be tolerated after chronic use of the drug. Treatment of acute amphetamine intoxication may include acidification of the urine with ammonium chloride to enhance the rate of elimination. Sedatives may be required for the CNS symptoms. Severe hypertension may require administration of sodium nitroprusside *or an α adrenergic receptor antagonist. Chronic amphetamine intoxication causes symptoms similar to those of acute overdosage, but abnormal mental conditions are more common. Weight loss may be marked. A psychotic reaction with vivid hallucinations and paranoid delusions, often mistaken for schizophrenia, is the most common serious effect. Recovery usually is rapid after withdrawal of the drug, but the condition can become chronic, with amphetamine hastening the onset of incipient schizophrenia.*

Amphetamines are schedule II drugs and should be used only under medical supervision. Amphetamine use is inadvisable in patients with anorexia, insomnia, asthenia, psychopathic personality, or a history of homicidal or suicidal tendencies.

DEPENDENCE AND TOLERANCE

Psychological dependence often occurs when amphetamine or dextroamphetamine is used chronically, as discussed in Chapter 23. Tolerance almost invariably develops to the anorexigenic effect of amphetamines, and often is seen also in the need for increasing doses to maintain improvement of mood in psychiatric patients, yet cases of narcolepsy have been treated for years without requiring an increase in the initially effective dose.

THERAPEUTIC USES

*Dextroamphetamine (*DEXEDRINE, *others), with greater CNS action and less peripheral action, is FDA approved for the treatment of narcolepsy and attention-deficit/hyperactivity disorder (see below).*

Methamphetamine

*Methamphetamine (*DESOXYN*) acts centrally to release DA and other biogenic amines and to inhibit neuronal and vesicular monoamine transporters and MAO. Small doses have prominent central stimulant effects without significant peripheral actions; somewhat larger doses produce a sustained rise in systolic and diastolic blood pressures, due mainly to cardiac stimulation and an increase in cardiac output secondary to venoconstriction. Methamphetamine is a schedule II drug and is widely abused (see Chapter 23).*

Methylphenidate

Methylphenidate *(RITALIN, others), structurally related to amphetamine, is a mild CNS stimulant with more prominent effects on mental than on motor activities. However, large doses produce signs of generalized CNS stimulation and convulsions. Its pharmacological properties are essentially the same as those of the amphetamines, including the potential for abuse. Methylphenidate is a schedule II-controlled substance in the U.S. Methylphenidate is effective in the treatment of narcolepsy and attention-deficit/hyperactivity disorder (see below). Racemic methylphenidate is readily absorbed after oral administration and reaches peak concentrations in plasma in ~2 hours. The more potent (+) enantiomer has a $t_{1/2}$ of ~6 hours. Concentrations in the brain exceed those in plasma. The main urinary metabolite is a deesterified product, ritalinic acid, which accounts for 80% of the dose. Methylphenidate is contraindicated in patients with glaucoma.*

Dexmethylphenidate

Dexmethylphenidate *(FOCALIN) is the d-threo enantiomer of racemic methylphenidate. It is FDA approved for the treatment of attention-deficit/hyperactivity disorder and is a schedule II-controlled substance in the U.S.*

Pemoline

Pemoline *(CYLERT, others), structurally dissimilar to methylphenidate, elicits similar changes in CNS function with minimal effects on the cardiovascular system. It is a schedule IV-controlled substance in the U.S. and is used in treating attention-deficit/hyperactivity disorder. It can be given once daily because of its long $t_{1/2}$. Clinical improvement may require treatment for 3–4 weeks. Pemoline has been associated with severe hepatic failure.*

Ephedrine

Ephedrine *is an agonist at both α and β receptors and also enhances release of NE from sympathetic neurons; thus, it is a* mixed-acting *sympathomimetic. Ephedrine does not contain a catechol moiety and is effective after oral administration. The drug stimulates heart rate and cardiac output and variably increases peripheral resistance; as a result, it usually increases blood pressure. Activation of β receptors in the lungs promotes bronchodilation. Ephedrine is a potent CNS stimulant. After oral administration, effects of the drug may persist for several hours. Ephedrine is eliminated in the urine largely as unchanged drug, with a $t_{1/2}$ of ~3–6 hours. A steroisomer of ephedrine,* pseudoephedrine, *is used as a nasal mucosal vasoconstrictor and decongestant (see below)*

TOXICITY

Untoward effects of ephedrine include hypertension and insomnia. Tachyphylaxis may occur with repetitive dosing. Usual or higher-than-recommended doses may cause adverse cardiovascular effects in individuals with underlying cardiovascular disease. Herbal preparations containing ephedrine (ma huang, ephedra) are widely utilized; these preparations vary in their content of ephedrine; thus, their use may lead to inadvertent consumption of dangerously high doses of ephedrine and its isomers. Because of this, the FDA has banned the sale of dietary supplements containing ephedra in the U.S.

Other Sympathomimetics

Several sympathomimetic drugs are used primarily as vasoconstrictors for local application to the nasal mucous membrane or the eye: propylhexedrine *(BENZEDREX, others)*, naphazoline *(PRIVINE, NAPHCON, others)*, oxymetazoline *(AFRIN, OCUCLEAR, others)*, and xylometazoline *(OTRIVIN, others) [see Table 10–1]. Ethylnorepinephrine (BRONKEPHRINE) is a β agonist that is used as a bronchodilator; the drug also has α agonist activity, which may cause local vasoconstriction and thereby reduce bronchial congestion.* Phenylephrine *(see above)*, pseudoephedrine *(SUDAFED, others) (a stereoisomer of ephedrine), and phenylpropanolamine are sympathomimetics used most commonly in oral preparations for the relief of nasal congestion. Pseudoephedrine is available without a prescription in a variety of solid and liquid dosage forms. Phenylpropanolamine shares the pharmacological properties of ephedrine and is approximately equal in potency except that it causes less CNS stimulation. The drug has been available over-the-counter (OTC), and numerous proprietary mixtures marketed for the oral treatment of nasal and sinus congestion contain one of these sympathomimetic amines, usually in combination with an H_1 histamine antagonist. Because phenylpropanolamine increases the risk of hemorrhagic stroke, most manufacturers have voluntarily stopped marketing products containing phenylpropanolamine in the U.S. and the FDA is withdrawing approval for the drug.*

THERAPEUTIC USES OF SYMPATHOMIMETIC DRUGS

SHOCK

Shock is a life-threatening condition characterized by inadequate perfusion of tissues, hypotension, and, ultimately, failure of organ systems. Treatment of shock consists of specific efforts to reverse the underlying pathogenesis as well as nonspecific measures aimed at correcting hemodynamic abnormalities. Regardless of etiology, the accompanying fall in blood pressure generally leads to marked activation of the sympathetic nervous system. This, in turn, causes peripheral vasoconstriction and an increase in the rate and force of cardiac contraction. In the initial stages of shock, these mechanisms may maintain blood pressure and cerebral blood flow, although blood flow to the kidneys, skin, and other organs may be decreased, leading to impaired production of urine and metabolic acidosis.

The initial therapy of shock involves basic life-support measures (maintenance of blood volume, etc.). Specific therapy (e.g., antibiotics for patients in septic shock) should be initiated immediately. If these measures do not lead to an adequate therapeutic response, it may be necessary to use vasoactive drugs in an effort to improve abnormalities in blood pressure and flow. This therapy generally is empirically based on response to hemodynamic measurements. Many of these pharmacological approaches, while reasonable, are of uncertain efficacy. Adrenergic receptor agonists may be used in an attempt to increase myocardial contractility or to modify peripheral vascular resistance. In general terms, β receptor agonists increase heart rate and force of contraction, α receptor agonists increase peripheral vascular resistance, and DA promotes dilation of renal and splanchnic vascular beds, in addition to activating β and α receptors.

Cardiogenic shock due to myocardial infarction has a poor prognosis; therapy is aimed at improving peripheral blood flow. Medical intervention is designed to optimize cardiac filling pressure (preload), myocardial contractility, and peripheral resistance (afterload). Preload may be increased by administration of intravenous fluids or reduced with drugs such as diuretics and nitrates. Sympathomimetic amines have been used to increase the force of contraction of the heart. Some of these drugs have disadvantages: isoproterenol is a powerful chronotropic agent and can greatly increase myocardial O_2 demand; NE intensifies peripheral vasoconstriction; Epi increases heart rate and may predispose the heart to dangerous arrhythmias. DA is an effective inotropic agent that causes less increase in heart rate than does isoproterenol and also promotes renal arterial dilation (possibly useful in preserving renal function). When given in high doses (>10–20 μg/kg/min), DA activates α receptors, causing peripheral and renal vasoconstriction. Dobutamine has complex pharmacological actions that are mediated by its stereoisomers; it increases myocardial contractility with little increase in heart rate or peripheral resistance.

In some patients, hypotension is so severe that vasoconstrictors are required to maintain a blood pressure sufficient for CNS perfusion. Alpha agonists (e.g., NE, phenylephrine, metaraminol, mephentermine, midodrine, ephedrine, Epi, DA, and methoxamine) have been used. This approach may be advantageous in patients with hypotension due to failure of the sympathetic nervous system (e.g., after spinal anesthesia or injury). In patients with other forms of shock, such as cardiogenic shock, reflex vasoconstriction generally is intense, and α receptor agonists may further compromise blood flow to organs such as the kidneys and gut and adversely increase the work of the heart. Indeed, vasodilating drugs such as nitroprusside are more likely to improve blood flow and decrease cardiac work in such patients by decreasing afterload if a minimally adequate blood pressure can be maintained.

The hemodynamic abnormalities in septic shock are complex and poorly understood. Most patients with septic shock initially have low or marginal peripheral vascular resistance, possibly reflecting excessive nitric oxide (NO) production. If the syndrome progresses, myocardial depression, increased peripheral resistance, and impaired tissue oxygenation occur. The primary treatment of septic shock is antibiotics. Therapy with vasoactive drugs must be individualized according to hemodynamic monitoring.

HYPOTENSION

Drugs with predominantly α agonist activity can be used to raise blood pressure in patients with decreased peripheral resistance in conditions such as spinal anesthesia or intoxication with antihypertensive medications. However, hypotension per se is not an indication for treatment with these agents unless there is inadequate perfusion of organs such as the brain, heart, or kidneys. Furthermore, adequate replacement of fluid or blood may be more appropriate than drug therapy for many patients with hypotension.

Patients with orthostatic hypotension (excessive fall in blood pressure with standing) often represent a pharmacological challenge. There are diverse causes for this disorder, including the Shy-Drager syndrome and idiopathic autonomic failure. Therapeutic approaches include physical maneuvers and a variety of drugs (fludrocortisone, *prostaglandin synthesis inhibitors, somato-statin analogs,* caffeine, *vasopressin analogs, and DA antagonists). The ideal agent would enhance venous constriction prominently and produce relatively little arterial constriction so as to avoid supine hypertension. No such agent currently is available. Drugs used include* α_1 *agonists and indirect-acting agents. Midodrine shows promise in treating orthostatic hypotension.*

HYPERTENSION

Centrally acting α_2 *receptor agonists such as clonidine are useful in the treatment of hypertension. Drug therapy of hypertension is discussed in Chapter 32.*

CARDIAC ARRHYTHMIAS

During cardiopulmonary resuscitation, Epi and other α *agonists increase diastolic pressure and improve coronary blood flow.* α *agonists also help to preserve cerebral blood flow. Thus, during external cardiac massage, Epi facilitates distribution of the limited cardiac output to the cerebral and coronary circulations. The optimal dose of epinephrine in patients with cardiac arrest is unclear. Once a cardiac rhythm has been restored, it may be necessary to treat arrhythmias, hypotension, or shock. Treatment of cardiac arrhythmias is detailed in Chapter 34.*

HEART FAILURE

Use of β *agonists and* β *antagonists in the treatment of heart failure is described in Chapter 33.*

LOCAL VASCULAR EFFECTS OF α ADRENERGIC RECEPTOR AGONISTS

Epi is used in many surgical procedures in the nose, throat, and larynx to shrink the mucosa and improve visualization by limiting hemorrhage. Simultaneous injection of Epi with local anesthetics retards the absorption of the anesthetic and increases the duration of anesthesia (see *Chapter 14). Injection of* α *agonists into the penis may be useful in reversing priapism, a complication of the use of* α *receptor antagonists or PDE5 inhibitors* (e.g., *sildenafil) in the treatment of erectile dysfunction. Both phenylephrine and oxymetazoline are efficacious vasoconstrictors when applied locally during sinus surgery.*

NASAL DECONGESTION

α *Receptor agonists are used extensively as nasal decongestants, as discussed above. Sympathomimetic decongestants should be used with great caution in patients with hypertension and in men with prostatic enlargement and not used by patients who are taking MAO inhibitors. Oral decongestants are much less likely to cause rebound congestion but carry a greater risk of inducing adverse systemic effects. Indeed, patients with uncontrolled hypertension or ischemic heart disease generally should avoid the oral consumption of OTC products or herbal preparations containing sympathomimetics.*

ASTHMA

Use of β *adrenergic agonists in the treatment of asthma is discussed in Chapter 27.*

ALLERGIC REACTIONS

Epi is the drug of choice to reverse the manifestations of serious acute hypersensitivity reactions (e.g., *from food, bee sting, or drug allergy). A subcutaneous injection of Epi rapidly relieves itching, hives, and swelling of lips, eyelids, and tongue. In some patients, careful intravenous infusion of Epi may be required to ensure prompt pharmacological effects. This treatment may be life saving when edema of the glottis threatens airway patency or when there is hypotension or shock in patients with anaphylaxis. In addition to its cardiovascular effects, Epi activates* β *receptors that suppress the release from mast cells of mediators such as histamine and leukotrienes. Although glucocorticoids and antihistamines frequently are administered to patients with severe hypersensitivity reactions, Epi remains the mainstay.*

OPHTHALMIC USES

Ophthalmic uses are discussed in Chapter 63.

NARCOLEPSY

Narcolepsy is characterized by hypersomnia. Some patients respond to treatment with tricyclic antidepressants or MAO inhibitors. Alternatively, CNS stimulants such as amphetamines may be useful. Therapy with amphetamines is complicated by the risk of abuse and the likelihood of the development of tolerance and a variety of behavioral changes (see *above). Amphetamines may disturb nocturnal sleep, which increases the difficulty of avoiding daytime attacks of sleep in these patients. Modafinil (PROVIGIL), a CNS stimulant, may be beneficial via an unknown mechanism. In the U.S., modafinil is a schedule IV-controlled substance.*

Occasionally, narcolepsy results from mutations in orexin neuropeptides (also called hypocretins), which are expressed in the lateral hypothalamus, or in their G protein–coupled receptors. Although such mutations are not present in most subjects with narcolepsy, the levels of orexins in the CSF are diminished, suggesting that deficient orexin signaling may play a pathogenic role. The association of these neuropeptides and their cognate GPCRs with narcolepsy provides an attractive target for the development of novel pharmacotherapies for this disorder.

WEIGHT REDUCTION

Optimally, weight loss is achieved by a gradual increase in energy expenditure from exercise combined with dieting to decrease the caloric intake. Amphetamine promotes weight loss by suppressing appetite rather than by increasing energy expenditure. Other anorexic drugs include methamphetamine, dextroamphetamine, phentermine, benzphetamine, phendimetrazine, phenmetrazine, diethylpropion, mazindol, phenylpropanolamine, and sibutramine (a mixed adrenergic/serotonergic drug). These agents may be effective adjuncts in the treatment of obesity but they all present significant risk of adverse effects (see above). Available evidence does not support the isolated use of these drugs in the absence of a more comprehensive program that stresses exercise and diet modification.

ATTENTION-DEFICIT/HYPERACTIVITY DISORDER

ADHD, usually first evident in childhood, is characterized by excessive motor activity, difficulty in sustaining attention, and impulsiveness. A variety of stimulant drugs have been utilized in the treatment of ADHD, and they are particularly indicated in moderate-to-severe cases. Methylphenidate is effective in children with ADHD and is the most common intervention; treatment may start with a dose of 5 mg in the morning and at lunch, increasing gradually over a period of weeks depending on the response as judged by parents, teachers, and the clinician. The total daily dose generally should not exceed 60 mg. Methylphenidate has a short duration of action; thus, most children require 2–3 doses/day, with the timing individualized for effect. Methylphenidate, dextroamphetamine, and amphetamine probably have similar efficacy in ADHD. Pemoline appears to be less effective, although like sustained release preparations of methylphenidate (RITALIN SR, CONCERTA, METADATE) and amphetamine (ADDERAL XR), pemoline may be used once daily in children and adults. Potential adverse effects of these medications include insomnia, abdominal pain, anorexia, and weight loss that may be associated with suppression of growth in children. Minor symptoms may be transient or may respond to adjustment of dosage or administration of the drug with meals.

II. ADRENERGIC RECEPTOR ANTAGONISTS

Adrenergic receptor *antagonists* inhibit the interaction of NE, Epi, and other sympathomimetic drugs with α and β receptors (*see* Figure 10–3). Detailed knowledge of the localization of adrenergic receptors and of effector-response coupling is essential for understanding the pharmacological properties and therapeutic uses of this important class of drugs (see Tables 6–1, 6–6, 6–7, 6–8, 10–2 and 10–6).

α ADRENERGIC RECEPTOR ANTAGONISTS

Effects of α adrenergic antagonists may be predicted from the consequences of α receptor stimulation. The α_1 adrenergic receptors mediate contraction of arterial and venous smooth muscle. The α_2 receptors are involved in suppressing sympathetic outflow from the CNS, increasing vagal tone, facilitating platelet aggregation, inhibiting the release of NE and ACh from nerve endings, and regulating metabolic effects (*e.g.*, suppression of insulin secretion and inhibition of lipolysis) and contraction of some arteries and veins.

α receptor antagonists are chemically heterogeneous and have a wide spectrum of pharmacological specificities (Figure 10–3, Table 10–3). Prazosin is much more potent in blocking α_1 than α_2 receptors (i.e., α_1 selective), whereas yohimbine is α_2 selective; phentolamine has similar affinities for both of these receptor subtypes. Newer agents discriminate amongst the subtypes of a particular receptor (e.g., tamsulosin has higher potency at α_{1A} than at α_{1B} receptors). Table 10–3 summarizes the properties of three chemically distinct groups of α blockers.

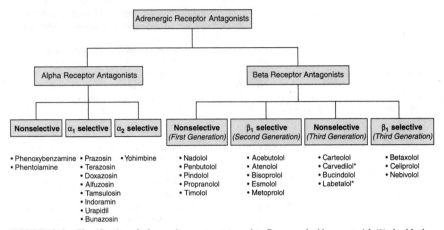

FIGURE 10–3 *Classification of adrenergic receptor antagonists.* Drugs marked by an asterisk (*) also block α_1 receptors.

Pharmacological Properties

CARDIOVASCULAR SYSTEM

α_1 Receptor Antagonists Blockade of α_1 adrenergic receptors inhibits vasoconstriction induced by endogenous catecholamines; vasodilation may occur in both arteriolar resistance vessels and veins. The result is a fall in blood pressure due to decreased peripheral resistance; the magnitude of such effects depends on the activity of the sympathetic nervous system, is less in supine than in upright subjects, and is enhanced by hypovolemia. For most α receptor antagonists, the fall in blood pressure is opposed by baroreceptor reflexes that cause increases in heart rate and cardiac output, as well as fluid retention. These compensatory reflexes are exaggerated if the antagonist also blocks α_2 receptors on peripheral sympathetic nerve endings, leading to enhanced release of NE and increased stimulation of postsynaptic β_1 receptors in the heart and on juxtaglomerular cells. Since blockade of α_1 receptors inhibits vasoconstriction, pressor responses to Epi may be transformed to vasodepressor effects ("epinephrine reversal") due to unopposed stimulation of β_2 receptors in the vasculature with resultant vasodilation.

α_2 Adrenergic Receptor Antagonists Activation of α_2 receptors in the pontomedullary region of the CNS inhibits sympathetic nervous system activity and leads to a fall in blood pressure; these receptors are a site of action for drugs such as clonidine. Activation of presynaptic α_2 receptors inhibits the release of NE and cotransmitters from peripheral sympathetic nerve endings. Thus, blockade of peripheral α_2 receptors with selective antagonists such as yohimbine increases sympathetic outflow and potentiates the NE release, leading to activation of α_1 and β_1 receptors in the heart and peripheral vasculature with a consequent rise in blood pressure. Antagonists that simultaneously block α_1 and α_2 receptors cause similar effects on sympathetic outflow and NE release, but the net increase in blood pressure is prevented by inhibition of vasoconstriction (α_1 blockade).

The physiological role of vascular α_2 receptors in the regulation of blood flow within various vascular beds is uncertain. Vacular α_2 receptors probably are preferentially stimulated by circulating catecholamines, whereas α_1 receptors are activated by NE released from sympathetic nerves.

OTHER ACTIONS

Catecholamines increase the output of glucose from the liver, predominantly via β receptors, although α receptors may contribute, and thus, α receptor antagonists may reduce glucose release. α_{2A} Receptors facilitate platelet aggregation; the effect of blockade of platelet α_2 receptors in vivo is not clear. Activation of α_2 receptors in the pancreatic islets suppresses insulin secretion; conversely, their blockade may facilitate insulin release (see Chapter 60). Alpha receptor antagonists reduce smooth muscle tone in the prostate and neck of the bladder, thereby decreasing resistance to urine outflow in benign prostatic hypertrophy (see below).

Table 10–3

Comparative Information About α Adrenergic Receptor Antagonists

	Haloalkylamines	Imidazolines	Quinazolines
Prototype	Phenoxybenzamine (PBZ)	Phentolamine	Prazosin
Others		Tolazoline	Terazosin Doxazosin Trimazosin Alfuzosin
Antagonism Selectivity	Irreversible α_1 with some α_2	Competitive Nonselective between α_1 and α_2	Competitive Selective for α_1; does not distinguish among α_1 subtypes
Hemodynamic effects	Decreased PVR and blood pressure Venodilation is prominent Cardiac stimulation (cardiovascular reflexes and enhanced NE release due to α_2 antagonism)	Similar to PBZ	Decreased PVR and blood pressure Veins less susceptible than arteries; thus, postural hypotension less of a problem Cardiac stimulation is less (NE release is not enhanced due to α_1 selectivity)
Actions other than α blockade	Some antagonism of ACh, 5-HT, and histamine Blockade of neuronal and extraneuronal uptake	Cholinomimetic; adrenomimetic; histamine-like actions Antagonism of 5-HT	At high doses some direct vasodilator action, probably due to PDE inhibition
Routes of administration	Intravenous and oral; oral absorption incomplete and erratic	Similar to PBZ	Oral
Adverse reactions	Postural hypotension, tachycardia, miosis, nasal stuffiness, failure of ejaculation	Same as PBZ, plus GI disturbances due to cholinomimetic and histamine-like actions	Some postural hypotension, especially with the first dose; less of a problem overall than with PBZ or phentolamine
Therapeutic uses	Conditions of catecholamine excess (*e.g.*, pheochromocytoma) Peripheral vascular disease	Same as PBZ	Primary hypertension Benign prostatic hypertrophy

ABBREVIATIONS: ACh, acetylcholine; 5-HT, 5-hydroxytryptamine; PBZ, phenoxybenzamine; NE, norepinephrine; PVR, peripheral vascular resistance.

Phenoxybenzamine

Phenoxybenzamine (PBZ), a haloalkylamine that blocks α_1 and α_2 receptors, is covalently conjugated with α receptors. Consequently, receptor blockade is irreversible and restoration of cellular responsiveness to α receptor agonists probably requires the synthesis of new receptors. Table 10–3 summarizes salient properties of PBZ, the major physiological effects of which result from blockade of α receptors in smooth muscle.

PBZ causes a progressive decrease in peripheral resistance, an increase in cardiac output (due, in part, to reflex sympathetic nerve stimulation), tachycardia accentuated by enhanced release of NE (due to α_2 blockade), and decreased clearance of NE (due to inhibition of NET and ENT by the drug). PBZ impairs pressor responses to exogenously administered catecholamines and causes "epinephrine reversal" (β_2 predominance in the vasculature). PBZ has little effect on supine blood pressure in normotensive subjects but causes a marked fall in blood pressure on standing (antagonism of compensatory vasoconstriction). The drug impairs the ability to respond to hypovolemia and anesthetic-induced vasodilation. At higher doses, PBZ also irreversibly inhibits responses to 5-HT, histamine, and ACh.

THERAPEUTIC USES

A major use of PBZ (DIBENZYLINE) is in the treatment of pheochromocytoma, tumors of the adrenal medulla and sympathetic neurons that secrete enormous quantities of catecholamines. The usual result is hypertension, which may be episodic and severe. PBZ is almost always used to treat the patient in preparation for surgical removal of the tumor. The standard therapy is to initiate PBZ (at a dosage of 10 mg twice daily) 1–3 weeks before the operation, increasing the dose every other day until the desired effect on blood pressure is achieved. Therapy may be limited by postural hypotension; nasal stuffiness is another frequent adverse effect. Prolonged treatment with PBZ may be necessary in patients with inoperable or malignant pheochromocytoma; the usual daily dose is 40–120 mg given in 2–3 divided portions. Metyrosine, a competitive inhibitor of tyrosine hydroxylase, may be a useful adjuvant. Beta receptor antagonists also are used to treat pheochromocytoma, but only after the administration of an α receptor antagonist (see below).

PBZ has been used off-label to control the manifestations of autonomic hyperreflexia in patients with spinal cord transection.

TOXICITY AND ADVERSE EFFECTS

The major adverse effect of PBZ is postural hypotension, often accompanied by reflex tachycardia and other arrhythmias. Hypotension can be particularly severe in hypovolemic patients or under conditions that promote vasodilation (administration of vasodilator drugs, exercise, ingestion of alcohol or large quantities of food). Reversible inhibition of ejaculation may occur because of impaired smooth muscle contraction in the vas deferens and ejaculatory ducts. PBZ is mutagenic in the Ames test; the clinical significance of this finding is unknown.

Phentolamine and Tolazoline

Phentolamine, an imidazoline, is a competitive α receptor antagonist that has similar affinities for α_1 and α_2 receptors. Its effects on the cardiovascular system are very similar to those of PBZ (see Table 10–3).

THERAPEUTIC USES

Phentolamine (REGITINE) can be used in short-term control of hypertension in patients with pheochromocytoma. Rapid infusions of phentolamine may cause severe hypotension, so the drug should be administered cautiously. Phentolamine also may be useful to relieve pseudo-obstruction of the bowel in patients with pheochromocytoma; this condition may result from the inhibitory effects of catecholamines on intestinal smooth muscle. Phentolamine has been used locally to prevent dermal necrosis after the inadvertent extravasation of an α receptor agonist. The drug also may be useful for the treatment of hypertensive crises that follow the abrupt withdrawal of clonidine or that may result from the ingestion of tyramine-containing foods during the use of nonselective MAO inhibitors. Phentolamine administered buccally, orally, or by intracavernous injection into the penis may have efficacy in some men with sexual dysfunction.

TOXICITY AND ADVERSE EFFECTS

Hypotension is the major adverse effect of phentolamine; reflex cardiac stimulation may cause tachycardia, arrhythmias, and ischemic cardiac events. GI stimulation may result in abdominal pain, nausea, and exacerbation of peptic ulcer. Phentolamine should be used with particular caution in patients with coronary artery disease or a history of peptic ulcer.

Quinazoline α Antagonists

Prazosin

Prazosin, the prototypic quinazoline α blocker, is a potent and selective α_1 receptor antagonist. The quinazoline class of α receptor antagonists has largely replaced the nonselective haloalkylamine (e.g., PBZ) and imidazoline (e.g., phentolamine) α receptor antagonists. The affinity of prazosin for α_1 adrenergic receptors is ~1000× that for α_2 adrenergic receptors; prazosin has similar potencies at α_{1A}, α_{1B}, and α_{1D} subtypes. Interestingly, the drug also is a relatively potent inhibitor of cyclic nucleotide PDEs. Prazosin frequently is used for the treatment of hypertension (see Chapter 32). The major effects of prazosin result from its blockade of α_1 receptors in arterioles and veins, leading to a fall in peripheral vascular resistance and in venous return to the heart. With little or no α_2 receptor–blocking effect at concentrations achieved clinically, prazosin probably does not promote the release of NE from sympathetic nerve endings in the heart. In addition, prazosin decreases cardiac preload and thus has little tendency to increase cardiac output and rate, in contrast to vasodilators such as hydralazine that have minimal dilatory effects on veins. Prazosin also may act in the CNS to suppress sympathetic outflow. Prazosin appears to depress baroreflex function in hypertensive patients. Prazosin and related drugs in this class tend to have favorable effects on serum lipids in humans, decreasing low-density lipoproteins (LDL) and triglycerides while increasing concentrations of high-density lipoproteins (HDL).

Prazosin (MINIPRESS, others) is well absorbed after oral administration, with a bioavailability of 50–70% and peak plasma concentrations 1–3 hours after an oral dose. Because prazosin binds avidly α_1-acid glycoprotein (only 5% of the drug is free), diseases that modify the concentration of this protein (e.g., inflammatory processes) may change the free fraction. Prazosin is extensively metabolized in the liver; the plasma $t_{1/2}$, 2–3 hours, may be prolonged to 6–8 hours in congestive heart failure). In the treatment of hypertension, the duration of action of the drug is 7–10 hours. Therapy is begun with 1 mg given 2–3 times daily, and the dose is increased to achieve target blood pressure. The initial dose should be 1 mg, usually given at bedtime (recumbency reduces the risk of syncopal reactions that may follow the first dose of prazosin). A maximal antihypertensive effect generally is observed with a total daily dose of 20 mg. In treating benign prostatic hyperplasia (BPH), doses from 1 to 5 mg twice daily typically are used. The twice-daily dosing requirement for prazosin is a disadvantage compared with newer α_1 receptor antagonists.

Terazosin

Terazosin (HYTRIN, others), a prazosin congener, is less potent than prazosin but retains high specificity for α_1 receptors; terazosin does not discriminate among α_{1A}, α_{1B}, and α_{1D} receptors. The major distinction between the two drugs is in their pharmacokinetic properties: terazosin is more water soluble, has a higher bioavailability (>90%), a longer $t_{1/2}$ (~12 hours), and a longer duration of action at typical doses (>18 hours). Consequently, the drug may be taken once daily to treat hypertension and BPH in most patients. Terazosin and doxazosin induce apoptosis in prostate smooth muscle cells, an action that may lessen the symptoms associated with chronic BPH. This apoptotic effect apparently relates to the quinazoline moiety rather than α_1 receptor antagonism. An initial dose of 1 mg is recommended. Doses are titrated upward depending on the therapeutic response; 10 mg/day may be required for maximal effect in BPH.

Doxazosin

Doxazosin (CARDURA, others), a structural analog of prazosin, is a highly selective α_1 antagonist, although nonselective among α_1 receptor subtypes. Doxasin has effects similar to those of prazosin but differs pharmacokinetically: long $t_{1/2}$ (~20 hours) and long duration of action (36 hours). Bioavailability and extent of metabolism of doxazosin and prazosin are similar; most doxazosin metabolites are eliminated in the feces. Doxazosin is given initially as a 1-mg dose in the treatment of hypertension or BPH. Similarly to terazosin, doxazosin may have beneficial actions related to apoptosis in the long-term management of BPH.

ALFUZOSIN

Alfuzosin (UROXATRAL), a quinazoline-based, non-subtype-selectiveα_1 antagonist, has been used extensively in treating BPH (recommended dosage, one 10-mg extended-release tablet daily, after the same meal each day).

TAMSULOSIN

Tamsulosin (FLOMAX), a benzenesulfonamide, is an α_1 receptor antagonist with some selectivity for α_{1A} and α_{1D} subtypes, favoring α_{1A} blockade in prostate. Tamsulosin is efficacious in the treatment of BPH with little effect on blood pressure. The drug is well absorbed, has a $t_{1/2}$ of 5–10 hours, and is extensively metabolized by CYPs. Tamsulosin may be administered at a 0.4-mg starting dose. Abnormal ejaculation is an adverse effect of tamsulosin.

ADVERSE EFFECTS

An adverse effect of prazosin and its congeners is the first-dose effect; marked postural hypotension and syncope may occur 30–90 minutes after the initial dose. The mechanisms responsible for exaggerated hypotensive response and the subsequent development of tolerance to the effect are not clear; an action in the CNS to reduce sympathetic outflow may contribute. Risk of the first-dose phenomenon is minimized by limiting the initial dose (e.g., 1 mg at bedtime), by increasing the dosage slowly, and by introducing additional antihypertensive drugs cautiously. Since orthostatic hypotension may be a problem during long-term use, standing and recumbent blood pressures should be checked. Nonspecific adverse effects (e.g., headache, dizziness, and asthenia) rarely limit treatment with prazosin. The adverse effects of structural analogs of prazosin are similar to those of prazosin.

THERAPEUTIC USES *Hypertension* Prazosin and its congeners are used in the treatment of hypertension (*see* Chapter 32).

Congestive Heart Failure

Prazosin provides short-term symptomatic relief in heart failure but is not a drug of choice (see Chapter 33).

Benign Prostatic Hyperplasia (BPH)

The symptoms of BPH (e.g., urethral obstruction leading to weak stream, urinary frequency, and nocturia) result from mechanical pressure on the urethra (due to an increase in smooth muscle mass) and an α_1-mediated increase in smooth muscle tone in the prostate and neck of the bladder. α_1 receptors in the trigone muscle of the bladder and urethra contribute to the resistance to outflow of urine; prazosin reduces this. The efficacy and importance of α receptor antagonists in the medical treatment of BPH have been demonstrated in multiple controlled clinical trials. Finasteride (PROPECIA) and dutasteride (AVODART), which inhibit conversion of testosterone to dihydrotestosterone (See Chapter 58), can reduce prostate volume in some patients; however, their overall efficacy appears less than that of α_1 receptor antagonists. Selective α_1 receptor antagonists have efficacy in BPH owing to relaxation of smooth muscle in the bladder neck, prostate capsule, and prostatic urethra. Recent studies show that combination therapy with doxazosin and finasteride reduces the risk of overall clinical progression of BPH significantly more than treatment with either drug alone. Prazosin, terazosin, doxazosin, tamsulosin, and alfuzosin have been studied extensively and used widely in patients with BPH. With the exception of tamsulosin, the comparative efficacies of each of these drugs appear similar. Tamsulosin at the recommended dose of 0.4 mg daily is less likely to cause orthostatic hypotension than are the other drugs. The predominant α_1 receptor subtype in the human prostate appears to be α_{1A}.

Other Disorders

Prazosin can decrease the incidence of digital vasospasm in patients with Raynaud's disease; however, its efficacy relative to Ca^{2+} channel blockers is not known. Prazosin may be useful in treating vasospastic disorders, and in patients with mitral or aortic valvular insufficiency (presumably because of afterload reduction).

Additional a Adrenergic Receptor Antagonists
ERGOT ALKALOIDS

For information on ergot alkaloids, see *Chapter 11.*

INDORAMIN

Indoramin *is a competitive α_1 antagonist that also antagonizes agonist effects at H_1 and 5-HT receptors. Via α_1 antagonism, indoramin lowers blood pressure with minimal tachycardia and decreases the incidence of attacks of Raynaud's phenomenon. Indoramin has modest bioavailability (<30%, with considerable variability), with extensive first-pass metabolism and an elimination $t_{1/2}$ ~5 hours; some metabolites may be biologically active. Adverse effects include sedation, dry mouth, and failure of ejaculation. Indoramin is an effective antihypertensive, but has complex pharmacokinetics and lacks a well-defined therapeutic niche. Indoramin is not available in the U.S.*

KETANSERIN

Ketanserin, a 5-HT receptor/α_1 receptor antagonist, is discussed in Chapter 11.

URAPIDIL

Urapidil *is a selective α_1 receptor antagonist whose role in the treatment of hypertension remains to be determined. Urapidil is not available in the U.S.*

BUNAZOSIN

Bunazosin, *a quinazoline α_1-selective antagonist, lowers blood pressure in patients with hypertension. Bunazosin is not available in the U.S.*

YOHIMBINE

Yohimbine (YOCON), *a competitive α_2 antagonist, is an indolealkylamine alkaloid found in the bark of the tree* Pausinystalia yohimbe *and in* Rauwolfia *root; structurally, yohimbine resembles reserpine.*

Yohimbine readily enters the CNS, where it acts to increase blood pressure and heart rate; it also enhances motor activity and produces tremors. Yohimbine also is an antagonist of 5-HT. In the past, yohimbine was used to treat male sexual dysfunction, although efficacy never was clearly demonstrated; yohimbine also may be useful for diabetic neuropathy and in the treatment of postural hypotension.

NEUROLEPTIC AGENTS

Chlorpromazine, haloperidol, *and other phenothiazine and butyrophenone neuroleptics produce significant blockade of both α and D_2 receptors (see Chapter 18).*

β ADRENERGIC RECEPTOR ANTAGONISTS

β Adrenergic receptor *antagonists* inhibit the interaction of NE, Epi, and sympathomimetic drugs with *β* receptors. Detailed knowledge of autonomic tone, localization of *β* receptor subtypes, effector-response coupling, and the multiplicity of possible actions of these drugs is essential for understanding their pharmacological effects and therapeutic uses (*see* Tables 6–1, 6–6, 6–7, 6–8, 10–2, 10–6, and Figure 10–3). Effects of *β* adrenergic antagonists may be predicted from the consequences of *β* receptor stimulation (generally equivalent to the effects of elevated cyclic AMP). Effects of *β* antagonists at a particular site depend on the level of receptor stimulation, or tone, at that site. Effects of antagonists are more prominent when receptor stimulation by agonist is high.

β antagonists can be distinguished by: relative specificity for $β_1$ over $β_2$ receptors, intrinsic sympathomimetic activity, capacity to block β receptors, differences in lipid solubility, capacity to induce vasodilation, and pharmacokinetic properties. β Adrenergic antagonists may be classified as Non-Subtype Selective *(First Generation),* $β_1$-Selective *(Second Generation), and* Antagonists with Additional Cardiovascular Actions *(Third Generation). Table 10–4 summarizes pharmacological and pharmacokinetic properties of β receptor antagonists.*

Table 10–4

Pharmacological/Pharmacokinetic Properties of β Receptor Blocking Agents

Drug	Membrane-Stabilizing Activity	Intrinsic Agonist Activity	Lipid Solubility	Extent of Absorption (%)	Oral Bioavailability (%)	Plasma $t_{\frac{1}{2}}$ (hours)	Protein Binding (%)
Classical nonselective β blockers: First generation							
Nadolol	0	0	Low	30	30–50	20–24	30
Penbutolol	0	+	High	~100	~100	~5	80–98
Pindolol	+	+++	Low	>95	~100	3–4	40
Propranolol	++	0	High	<90	30	3–5	90
Timolol	0	0	Low to Moderate	90	75	4	<10
$β_1$-Selective β blockers: Second generation							
Acebutolol	+	+	Low	90	20–60	3–4	26
Atenolol	0	0	Low	90	50–60	6–7	6–16
Bisoprolol	0	0	Low	≤90	80	9–12	~30
Esmolol	0	0	Low	NA	NA	0.15	55
Metoprolol	+*	0	Moderate	~100	40–50	3–7	12
Nonselective β blockers with additional actions: Third generation							
Carteolol	0	++	Low	85	85	6	23–30
Carvedilol	++	0	Moderate	>90	~30	7–10	98
Labetalol	+	+	Low	>90	~33	3–4	~50
$β_1$-selective β blockers with additional actions: Third generation							
Betaxolol	+	0	Moderate	>90	~80	15	50
Celiprolol	0	+	Low	~74	30–70	5	4–5

*Detectable only at doses much greater than required for β blockade.

CARDIOVASCULAR SYSTEM The major therapeutic effects of β receptor antagonists are on the cardiovascular system. It is important to distinguish these effects in normal subjects from those in subjects with cardiovascular disease such as hypertension or myocardial ischemia.

Since catecholamines have positive chronotropic and inotropic actions, β antagonists slow the heart rate and decrease myocardial contractility. When tonic stimulation of β receptors is low, this effect is correspondingly modest. However, when the sympathetic nervous system is activated, as during exercise or stress, β receptor antagonists attenuate the expected rise in heart rate. Short-term administration of β receptor antagonists decreases cardiac output; peripheral resistance increases in proportion to maintain blood pressure as a result of blockade of vascular β_2 receptors and compensatory reflexes, such as increased sympathetic nervous system activity, leading to activation of vascular β receptors. With long-term use of β receptor antagonists, total peripheral resistance returns to initial values or decreases in patients with hypertension. With β antagonists that also are β_1 receptor antagonists (*e.g.*, labetalol, carvedilol, bucindolol) or direct vasodilators (celiprolol, nebivolol, nipradilol, carteolol, betaxolol, bopindolol, bevantolol), cardiac output is maintained with a greater fall in peripheral resistance.

β Receptor antagonists have significant effects on cardiac rhythm and automaticity, to which blockade of both β_1 and β_2 receptors likely contributes. β_3 receptors occur in normal myocardial tissue, where they can couple to G_i and inhibit cardiac contraction and relaxation. The physiological role of cardiac β_3 receptors remains to be established. β antagonists reduce sinus rate, decrease the spontaneous rate of depolarization of ectopic pacemakers, slow conduction in the atria and in the AV node, and increase the functional refractory period of the AV node.

ACTIVITY AS ANTIHYPERTENSIVE AGENTS β Receptor antagonists generally do not reduce blood pressure in patients with normal blood pressure but will lower blood pressure in patients with hypertension. Reduction of β_1-stimulated renin release from the juxtaglomerular cells is a putative contributing mechanism (*see* Chapter 30).

Since presynaptic β receptors enhance the release of NE from sympathetic neurons, diminished release of NE resulting from β blockade is a possible response, but its relationship to the antihypertensive effects of β antagonists is unclear. Although β blockade would not be expected to decrease the contractility of vascular smooth muscle, long-term administration of these drugs to hypertensive patients ultimately decreases peripheral vascular resistance. The mechanism of this effect is unknown, but the delayed fall in peripheral vascular resistance in the face of a persistently reduced cardiac output appears to account for much of the antihypertensive effect of these drugs. There is relatively little evidence to support a postulated CNS effect of β blockers that contributes to their antihypertensive effects. Indeed, drugs that poorly penetrate the blood–brain barrier are effective antihypertensive agents.

Some β receptor antagonists produce peripheral vasodilation; at least six properties may contribute to this effect, including production of nitric oxide, activation of β_2 receptors, blockade of α_1 receptors, blockade of Ca^{2+} entry, opening of K^+ channels, and antioxidant activity (*see* Table 10–5 and Figure 10–4). These mechanisms appear to contribute to the antihypertensive effects by enhancing hypotension, increasing peripheral blood flow, and decreasing afterload. Two of these agents (*e.g.*, celiprolol and nebivolol) may produce vasodilation and thereby reduce preload. Nebivolol reportedly activates endothelial β_3 receptors, leading to NO production and dilation of human coronary microvessels.

Table 10–5

Third-Generation β Receptor Antagonists with Additional Cardiovascular Actions: Proposed Mechanisms Contributing to Vasodilation

Nitric Oxide Production	β_2 Receptor Agonism	α_1 Receptor Antagonism	Ca^{2+} Entry Blockade	K^+ Channel Opening	Antioxidant Activity
Celiprolol*	Celiprolol*	Carvedilol	Carvedilol	Tilisolol*	Carvedilol
Nebivolol*	Carteolol	Bucindolol*	Betaxolol		
Carteolol	Bopindolol*	Bevantolol*	Bevantolol*		
Bopindolol*		Nipradilol*			
Nipradilol*		Labetalol			

*Not currently available in the United States, where most are under investigation for use.

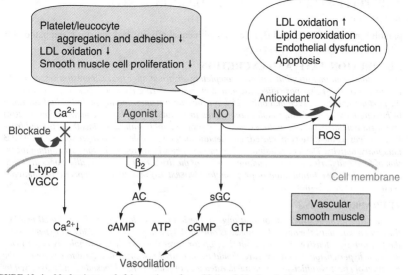

FIGURE 10–4 *Mechanisms underlying actions of vasodilating β blockers in blood vessels.* ROS, reactive oxygen species; sGC, soluble guanylyl cyclase; AC, adenylyl cyclase; L-type VGCC, L-type voltage-gated Ca^{2+} channel.

Propranolol and other nonselective β receptor antagonists inhibit the vasodilation caused by isoproterenol and augment the pressor response to Epi. This action is significant in patients with pheochromocytoma, in whom β receptor antagonists should be used only after adequate α receptor blockade has been established. This sequence avoids uncompensated α receptor–mediated vasoconstriction caused by catecholamines secreted by the tumor.

PULMONARY SYSTEM   Nonselective β receptor antagonists such as propranolol block β_2 receptors in bronchial smooth muscle, with little effect on pulmonary function in normal individuals. In patients with COPD, such blockade can lead to life-threatening bronchoconstriction. Although β_1-selective antagonists or antagonists with intrinsic sympathomimetic activity are less likely than propranolol to increase airway resistance, these drugs should be used only with great caution, if at all, in patients with bronchospastic diseases. Drugs with β_1 selectivity and β_2 receptor partial agonism (*e.g.*, celiprolol) have potential here, although clinical experience is limited.

METABOLIC EFFECTS   Catecholamines promote glycogenolysis and mobilize glucose in response to hypoglycemia. Nonselective β blockers blunt these responses and may delay recovery from hypoglycemia in type 1 (insulin-dependent) diabetes mellitus, but infrequently in type 2 diabetes mellitus. β receptor antagonists can interfere with the counterregulatory effects of catecholamines secreted during hypoglycemia by blunting the perception of symptoms such as tremor, tachycardia, and nervousness. Thus, β adrenergic receptor antagonists should be used with great caution in patients with labile diabetes and frequent hypoglycemic reactions; if a β antagonist must be used, a β_1-selective antagonist is preferred. In contrast to classical β blockers, which decrease insulin sensitivity, the vasodilating β receptor antagonists increase insulin sensitivity in patients with insulin resistance.

> β Receptor antagonists can reduce activation of hormone-sensitive lipase and attenuate the release of free fatty acids from adipose tissue. Nonselective β receptor antagonists consistently reduce HDL cholesterol, increase LDL cholesterol, and increase triglycerides. In contrast, β_1-selective antagonists improve the serum lipid profile of dyslipidemic patients. Propranolol and atenolol increase triglycerides, whereas chronic celiprolol, carvedilol, and carteolol reduce plasma triglycerides.

OTHER EFFECTS

> β Receptor antagonists block catecholamine-induced tremor and inhibit mast-cell degranulation by catecholamines.

NON-SUBTYPE-SELECTIVE β RECEPTOR ANTAGONISTS
Propranolol

Propranolol interacts with β_1 and β_2 receptors with equal affinity, lacks intrinsic sympathomimetic activity, and does not block α receptors.

ABSORPTION, FATE, AND EXCRETION
Propranolol is highly lipophilic, almost completely absorbed after oral administration, and subject to a prominent first-pass effect (hepatic metabolism during the drug's first passage through the portal circulation), such that only ~25% reaches the systemic circulation. Individual variation in hepatic clearance of propranolol contributes to variability in plasma concentrations (~20×) after oral administration. Hepatic extraction of propranolol is saturable, thus the extracted fraction declines as the dose is increased; one hepatic metabolite, 4-hydroxypropranolol, has some β antagonist activity. The bioavailability of propranolol may be increased by the concomitant ingestion of food and during long-term administration of the drug. Propranolol readily enters the CNS. A sustained-release formulation of propranolol (INDERAL LA) maintains therapeutic plasma concentrations over a 24-hour period.

THERAPEUTIC USES
For the treatment of hypertension and angina, the initial oral dose generally is 40–80 mg/day, titrated upward until the desired response is obtained, typically at <320 mg/day. In hypertension, the full antihypertensive effect may not develop for several weeks. If propranolol is taken twice daily for hypertension, blood pressure should be measured just prior to a dose to ensure that the duration of effect is sufficiently prolonged. Adequacy of β adrenergic blockade can be assessed by measuring suppression of exercise-induced tachycardia.

Propranolol also is used to treat various arrhythmias (Chapter 34), myocardial infarction (Chapter 31), congestive heart failure (Chapter 33), pheochromocytoma, and migraine (prophylactically). Propranolol also has been used for several off-label indications including parkinsonian tremors (sustained-release only), akathisia induced by antipsychotic drugs, variceal bleeding in portal hypertension, and generalized anxiety disorder.

Nadolol

Nadolol (CORGARD, others) is a long-acting antagonist with equal affinity for β_1 and β_2 receptors. Its pharmacological and pharmacokinetic properties are summarized in Table 10–4. Nadolol is used in hypertension and angina pectoris. Unlabeled uses have included migraine prophylaxis, parkinsonian tremors, and variceal bleeding in portal hypertension. Nadolol is water soluble and incompletely absorbed from the gut. The drug is largely excreted intact in the urine; thus, nadolol may accumulate in patients with renal failure, in whom dosage should be reduced. With its long $t_{1/2}$, nadolol may be administered once daily.

Timolol

Timolol (BLOCADREN, others) is a potent, non-subtype-selective β receptor antagonist, with properties summarized in Table 10–4. It is used for hypertension, congestive heart failure, migraine prophylaxis, open-angle glaucoma, and intraocular hypertension. Timolol is well absorbed from the GI tract. The drug is subject to first-pass metabolism and is metabolized extensively by hepatic CYP2D6 in the liver. The ophthalmic formulation of timolol (TIMOPTIC, others), used for the treatment of glaucoma, may be extensively absorbed systemically (see Chapter 63), causing adverse effects in susceptible patients (e.g., those with asthma or congestive heart failure).

Pindolol

Pindolol (VISKEN, others) is a non-subtype-selective β receptor antagonist, as described in Table 10–4. Notably, pindolol is a weak partial β agonist; such drugs may be preferred as antihypertensive agents in individuals with diminished cardiac reserve or a propensity for bradycardia.

β_1-SELECTIVE ADRENERGIC ANTAGONISTS
Metoprolol

Metoprolol (LOPRESSOR, others) is a β_1-selective antagonist lacking intrinsic sympathomimetic activity and membrane-stabilizing activity (see Table 10–4). Despite almost complete GI absorption, metoprolol's bioavailability is relatively low because of first-pass metabolism. Plasma concentrations vary widely, which may relate to genetically determined differences in hepatic CYP2D6 activity. The $t_{1/2}$ of metoprolol (3–4 hours) can double in CYP2D6 poor metabolizers, who have a 5× higher risk for developing adverse effects compared to normal metabolizers. An extended-release formulation (TOPROL XL) is available for once-daily administration.

For hypertension, the usual initial dose is 100 mg/day, increasing at weekly intervals until optimal reduction of blood pressure is achieved. If the drug is taken only once daily, confirm that blood pressure is controlled for the entire 24-hour period. Metoprolol generally is used in two divided doses for the treatment of stable angina. For the initial treatment of patients with acute myocardial infarction, an intravenous formulation of metoprolol tartrate is available; initiate oral dosing as soon as the clinical situation permits. Metoprolol generally is contraindicated for the treatment of acute MI in patients with heart rates <45 beats/min, heart block greater than first-degree (PR interval ≥0.24 second), systolic blood pressure <100 mm Hg, or moderate-to-severe heart failure. Metoprolol is also effective in chronic heart failure (see Chapter 33).

Atenolol

Atenolol (TENORMIN, others) is a β_1-selective antagonist (see Table 10–4). The drug is excreted largely unchanged in the urine; thus, atenolol accumulates in patients with renal failure, and dosage should be reduced when creatinine clearance is <35 ml/min. The initial dose of atenolol for the treatment of hypertension usually is 50 mg/day, given once daily. The daily dose may be increased to 100 mg; higher doses are unlikely to provide any greater antihypertensive effect. Atenolol has been shown to be efficacious, in combination with a diuretic, in elderly patients with isolated systolic hypertension.

Esmolol

Esmolol (BREVIBLOC, others) is a β_1-selective antagonist that is administered intravenously when β blockade of short duration is desired or in critically ill patients in whom adverse effects of brady-cardia, heart failure, or hypotension may necessitate rapid withdrawal of the drug. The duration of action of esmolol is brief because esterases in erythrocytes rapidly degrade the drug. Onset and cessation of esmolol's β blockade are rapid; peak effects occur within 6–10 minutes of administration of a loading dose, and there is substantial attenuation of β blockade within 20 minutes of stopping an infusion. Because esmolol is used in urgent settings where immediate onset of β blockade is warranted, a partial loading dose typically is administered, followed by a continuous infusion of the drug. If an adequate therapeutic effect is not observed within 5 minutes, the same loading dose is repeated, followed by a maintenance infusion at a higher rate. This process may be repeated until the desired endpoint (e.g., lowered heart rate or blood pressure) is reached.

Acebutolol

Acebutolol (SECTRAL, others) is a selective β_1 adrenergic receptor antagonist. The drug undergoes significant first-pass metabolism to an active metabolite, diacetolol, which accounts for most of the drug's activity. The elimination $t_{1/2}$ of acebutolol is ~3 hours, that of diacetolol, 8–12 hours. The initial dose of acebutolol in hypertension usually is 400 mg/day, given as a single dose or as two divided doses, as required to control blood pressure. Optimal responses usually occur with doses of 400–800 mg/day. For treatment of ventricular arrhythmias, acebutolol should be given twice daily.

Bisoprolol

Bisoprolol (ZEBETA) is a highly selective β_1 receptor antagonist that is approved for the treatment of hypertension. Bisoprolol can be considered a standard treatment option when selecting a β blocker for use in combination with ACE inhibitors and diuretics in patients with stable, moderate-to-severe chronic heart failure (in whom it lowers all-case mortality; see Chapter 33) and in treating hypertension. Bisoprolol generally is well-tolerated; side effects include dizziness, bradycardia, hypotension, and fatigue.

β Antagonists with Additional Cardiovascular Effects (Third Generation β Blockers)

Some β adrenergic antagonists have additional vasodilating actions that are produced through a variety of mechanisms summarized in Table 10–5 and Figure 10–4.

Labetalol

Labetalol (NORMODYNE, TRANDATE, others) is a competitive antagonist at both α_1 and β receptors. The pharmacological properties of labetolol are complex, because each of four isomers displays

Table 10–6

Summary of Adrenergic Agonists and Antagonists

Class	Drugs	Prominent Pharmacological Actions	Principal Therapeutic Applications	Untoward Effects	Comments
Direct-acting nonselective agonists	Epinephrine (α_1, α_2, β_1, β_2, β_3)	Increase in heart rate Increase in blood pressure Increased contractility Slight decrease in PVR Increase in cardiac output Vasoconstriction (viscera) Vasodilation (skeletal muscle) Increase in blood glucose and lactic acid	Open-angle glaucoma With local anesthetics to prolong action Anaphylactic shock Complete heart block or cardiac arrest Bronchodilator in asthma	Palpitation Cardiac arrhythmias Cerebral hemorrhage Headache Tremor Restlessness	Not given orally Life saving in anaphylaxis or cardiac arrest
	Norepinephrine (α_1, α_2, β_1, $>> \beta_2$)	Increase in systolic and diastolic blood pressure Vasoconstriction Increase in PVR Direct increase in heart rate and contraction Reflex decrease in heart rate	Hypotension	Similar to Epi Hypertension	Not absorbed orally
β receptor agonists					
Nonselective ($\beta_1 + \beta_2$)	Isoproterenol	IV administration Decrease in PVR Increase in cardiac output Tachyarrhythmias Bronchodilation	Bronchodilator in asthma Complete heart block or cardiac arrest Shock	Palpitations Tachycardia Headache Flushed skin Cardiac ischemia in patients with CAD Increase in blood pressure and heart rate	Administered by inhalation in asthma
β_1-selective	Dobutamine	Increase in contractility Some increase in heart rate Increase in AV conduction	Short-term treatment of cardiac decompensation after surgery, or patients with CHF or MI	Use with caution in patients with hypertension or cardiac arrhythmias Used only IV	

β_2-selective (intermediate-acting)	Albuterol Bitolterol Fenoterol Isoetharine Metaproterenol Procaterol Terbutaline Ritodrine	Relaxation of bronchial smooth muscle Relaxation of uterine smooth muscle Activation of other β_2 receptors after systemic administration	Bronchodilators for treatment of asthma and COPD Short/intermediate-acting drugs for acute bronchospasm	Skeletal muscle tremor Tachycardia and other cardiac effects seen after systemic administration (much less with inhalational use)	Use with caution in patients with CV disease (reduced by inhalational administration) Minimal side effects
(Long-acting)	Formoterol Salmeterol		Best choice for prophylaxis due to long action		Long action favored for prophylaxis
α Receptor agonists					
α_1-selective	Methoxamine Phenylephrine Mephentermine Metaraminol Midodrine	Vasoconstriction	Nasal congestion (used topically) Postural hypotension	Hypertension Reflex bradycardia Dry mouth, sedation, rebound hypertension upon abrupt withdrawal	Mephentermine and metaraminol also act indirectly to release NE Midodrine is a prodrug converted *in vivo* to an active compound
α_2-selective	Clonidine Apraclonidine Guanfacine Guanabenz Brimonidine α-methyldopa	Decrease sympathetic outflow from brain to periphery resulting in decreased PVR and blood pressure Decrease nerve-evoked release of sympathetic transmitters Decrease production of aqueous humor	Adjunctive therapy in shock Hypertension To reduce sympathetic response to withdrawal from narcotics, alcohol, and tobacco Glaucoma		Apraclonidine and brimonidine used topically for glaucoma and ocular hypertension Methyldopa is converted in CNS to α-methyl NE, an effective α_2 agonist
Indirect-acting	Amphetamine Methamphetamine Methyphenidate (releases NE peripherally; NE, DA, 5-HT centrally)	CNS stimulation Increase in blood pressure Myocardial stimulation	Treatment of ADHD Narcolepsy Obesity (rarely)	Restlessness Tremor Insomnia Anxiety Tachycardia Hypertension Cardiac arrhythmias	Schedule II drugs Marked tolerance occurs Chronic use leads to dependence Can result in hemorrhagic stroke in patients with underlying disease Long-term use can cause paranoid schizophrenia

(Continued)

Table 10–6

Summary of Adrenergic Agonists and Antagonists (*Continued*)

Class	Drugs	Prominent Pharmacological Actions	Principal Therapeutic Applications	Untoward Effects	Comments
Mixed-acting	Dopamine (α_1, α_2, β_1, D_1; releases NE)	Vasodilation (coronary, renal mesenteric beds) Increase in glomerular filtration rate and natriuresis Increase in heart rate and contractility Increase in systolic blood pressure	Cardiogenic shock Congestive heart failure Treatment of acute renal failure	High doses lead to vasoconstriction	Important for its ability to maintain renal blood flow Administered IV
	Ephedrine (α_1, α_2, β_1, β_2; releases NE)	Similar to epinephrine but longer lasting CNS stimulations	Bronchodilator for treatment of asthma Nasal congestion Treatment of hypotension and shock	Restlessness Tremor Insomnia Anxiety Tachycardia Hypertension	Administered by all routes Not commonly used
α blockers					
Nonselective (classical α blockers)	Phenoxybenzamine Phentolamine Tolazoline	Decrease in PVR and blood pressure Venodilation	Treatment of catecholamine excess (*e.g.*, pheochromocytoma)	Postural hypotension Failure of ejaculation	Cardiac stimulation due to initiation of reflexes and to enhanced release of NE via α_2 receptor blockade
α_1-selective	Prazosin Terazosin Doxazosin Trimazosin Alfuzosin Tamsulosin	Decrease in PVR and blood pressur Relax smooth muscles in neck of urinary bladder and in prostate	Primary hypertension Increase urine flow in BPH	Postural hypotension when therapy instituted	Phenoxybenzamine produces long-lasting α-receptor blockade and at high doses can block neuronal and extraneuronal uptake of amines

182

α₁-selective (Continued)				Prazosin and related quinazolines are selective for α_1 receptors but not among α_1 subtypes Tamsulosin exhibits some selectivity for α_{1A} receptors
β blockers Non-selective (1st generation)	Nadolol Penbutolol Pindolol Propranolol Timolol	Decrease in heart rate Decrease in contractility Decrease in cardiac output Slow conduction in atria and AV node Increase refractory period, AV node Bronchoconstriction Prolonged hypoglycemia Decrease in plasma FFA Reduction in HDL cholesterol Increase in LDL cholesterol and triglycerides Hypokalemia	Angina pectoris Hypertension Cardiac arrhythmias CHF Pheochromocytoma Glaucoma Hypertropic obstructive cardiomyopathy Hyperthyroidism Migraine prophylaxis Acute panic symptoms Substance abuse withdrawal Variceal bleeding in portal hypertension	Bradycardia Negative inotropic effect Decrease in cardiac output Bradyarrhythmias Reduction in AV conduction Bronchoconstriction Fatigue Sleep disturbances (insomnia, nightmares) Prolongation of hypoglycemia Sexual dysfunction in men Drug interactions	Pharmacological effects depend largely on degree of sympathoadrenal tone Bronchoconstriction (of concern in asthmatics and COPD) Hypoglycemia (concern in hypoglycemics and diabetics) Membrane stabilizing effect (propranolol, acebutolol, carvedilol, and betaxolol only) ISA (strong for pindolol; weak for penbutolol, carteolol, labetalol, and betaxolol)
β_1-selective (2nd generation)	Acebutolol Atenolol Bisoprolol Esmolol Metoprolol				

(Continued)

Table 10-6

Summary of Adrenergic Agonists and Antagonists (*Continued*)

Class	Drugs	Prominent Pharmacological Actions	Principal Therapeutic Applications	Untoward Effects	Comments
Nonselective (3rd generation) vasodilators	Carteolol Carvedilol Bucindolol Labetalol	Membrane stabilizing effect ISA Vasodilation			Vasodilation seen in 3rd generation drugs; multiple mechanisms (α_1 antagonism; β_2 agonism; release of NO; Ca^{2+} channel blockade; opening of K^+ channels; others)
β_1-selective (3rd generation) vasodilators	Betaxolol Celiprolol Nebivolol				

ADHD, attention-deficit/hyperactivity disorder; AV, atrioventricular; BPH, benign prostatic hypertrophy; CAD, coronary artery disease; CHF, congestive heart failure; COPD, chronic obstructive pulmonary disease; CV, cardiovascular; DA, dopamine; D1, subtype 1 dopamine receptor; Epi, epinephrine; FFA, free fatty acids; 5-HT, serotonin; ISA, intrinsic sympathomimetic activity; MI, myocardial infarction; NE, norepinephrine; NO, nitric oxide; PVR, peripheral vascular resistance.

different relative activities. The properties of the racemic mixture include selective blockade of α_1 receptors (as compared with the α_2 subtype), blockade of β_1 and β_2 receptors, partial agonist activity at β_2 receptors, and inhibition of neuronal uptake of NE (cocaine-like effect). The potency of the mixture for β receptor blockade is 5–10× that for α_1 receptor blockade. Actions of labetalol on both α_1 and β-receptors contribute to the fall in blood pressure observed in patients with hypertension. β_1 receptor blockade leads to relaxation of arterial smooth muscle and vasodilation, particularly in the upright position. β_1 Blockade contributes to a fall in blood pressure, in part by blocking reflex sympathetic stimulation of the heart. In addition, intrinsic sympathomimetic activity of labetalol at β_2 receptors may contribute to vasodilation.

Although labetalol is completely absorbed from the gut, there is extensive first-pass clearance; bioavailability may be increased by food intake. The rate of hepatic metabolism of labetalol is sensitive to changes in hepatic blood flow. The various isomers have different elimination kinetics.

Two forms are available, an oral form for therapy of chronic hypertension, and an intravenous formulation for hypertensive emergencies. Labetalol has been associated with hepatic injury in a limited number of patients.

Carvedilol

Carvedilol (COREG) blocks β_1, β_2, and α_1 receptors and also has myriad additional cardiovascular effects (see Tables 10–4 and 10–5). Carvedilol produces vasodilation; its antioxidant and antiproliferative effects may be beneficial in treating congestive heart failure. Carvedilol improves ventricular function and reduces mortality and morbidity in patients with mild-to-severe congestive heart failure. Combined with conventional therapy, carvedilol reduces mortality in myocardial infarction. There are no significant changes in the pharmacokinetics of carvedilol in elderly hypertensives. Since the drug is metabolized by hepatic CYPs, no change in dosage is needed in patients with moderate-to-severe renal insufficiency.

Bucindolol

Bucindolol (SANDONORM) is a third-generation non-selective β antagonist with some α_1 receptor blocking as well as β_2 and β_3 agonistic properties. Bucindolol reduces afterload and increases plasma HDL cholesterol, but does not affect plasma triglycerides. In contrast to other β receptor antagonists studied in multicenter trials, bucindolol was not associated with improved survival. Bucindolol is not available in the U.S.

Celiprolol

Celiprolol (SELECTOR) is a third-generation cardioselective, β receptor antagonist with weak vasodilating and bronchodilating effects attributed to partial β_2 agonist activity. It may block peripheral α_2-adrenergic receptors and promote NO production (see Tables 10–4 and 10–5). Celiprolol is safe and effective for hypertension and angina.

Nebivolol

Nebivolol is a racemate: the d-isomer is a highly selective β_1 antagonist; the l-isomer enhances NO production, possibly via activation of endothelial β_3 receptors. Nebivolol has a distinct hemodynamic profile: it acutely lowers arterial blood pressure without depressing left ventricular function, and reduces systemic vascular resistance. Nebivolol is devoid of intrinsic sympathomimetic activity, inverse agonistic activity, and α_1 receptor–blocking properties. It is effective in treating hypertension and diastolic heart failure. A New Drug Application has been submitted to the FDA for nebivolol's use in hypertension.

Other β Receptor Antagonists

Other β antagonists have been evaluated to varying extents. Oxprenolol (no longer marketed in the U.S.) and penbutolol (LEVATOL) are non-subtype-selective β blockers with intrinsic sympathomimetic activity. Medroxalol is a nonselective β blocker with α_1 receptor–blocking activity. Levobunolol (BETAGAN LIQUIFILM, others) is a non-subtype-selective β antagonist used topically in the treatment of glaucoma. Betaxolol (BETOPTIC), a β_1-selective antagonist, is available as an ophthalmic preparation for glaucoma and an oral formulation for systemic hypertension. Betaxolol may be less likely to induce bronchospasm than are the ophthalmic preparations of the nonselective β blockers timolol and levobunolol. Similarly, ocular administration of carteolol (OCUPRESS) may be less likely than timolol to have systemic effects. Sotalol (BETAPACE, BETAPACE AF, others) is a nonselective β antagonist that has antiarrhythmic actions independent of its ability to block β adrenergic receptors (see Chapter 34).

Propafenone (RYTHMOL), a Na^+-channel blocking drug, is also a β receptor antagonist (see Chapter 34).

ADVERSE EFFECTS AND PRECAUTIONS

The most common adverse effects of β receptor antagonists arise as pharmacological consequences of blockade of β receptors; serious adverse effects unrelated to β receptor blockade are rare.

CARDIOVASCULAR SYSTEM β receptor blockade may cause or exacerbate heart failure in patients with compensated heart failure, acute myocardial infarction, or cardiomegaly. Nonetheless, chronic administration of β receptor antagonists is efficacious in prolonging life in the therapy of heart failure in selected patients (*see* below and Chapter 33). The bradycardia caused by β antagonists may cause life-threatening bradyarrhythmias in patients with partial or complete AV conduction defects. Particular caution is indicated in patients who are taking other drugs, such as *verapamil* or various antiarrhythmic agents, which may impair sinus-node function or AV conduction.

Some patients complain of cold extremities while taking β blockers. Symptoms of peripheral vascular disease may worsen (this is uncommon), or Raynaud's phenomenon may develop.

After prolonged β blockade, there is enhanced sensitivity to β adrenergic stimulation when the β blocker is withdrawn abruptly, possibly related to upregulation of β *receptors during* β blockade. Thus, abrupt discontinuation of β receptor antagonists after long-term treatment can exacerbate angina and may increase the risk of sudden death. Optimal strategies for discontinuation of β blockers are not known, but it is prudent to decrease the dose gradually (over several weeks) and to restrict exercise during this period.

PULMONARY FUNCTION A major adverse effect of β receptor antagonists is the bronchconstriction resulting from blockade of β_2 receptors in bronchial smooth muscle. β Blockers may cause a life-threatening increase in airway resistance in patients with bronchospastic disease. β_1-selective antagonists or those with intrinsic sympathomimetic activity at β_2 adrenergic receptors may be somewhat less likely to induce bronchospasm; however, the selectivity of current β_1 blockers is modest, and these drugs should be avoided if possible in patients with asthma.

CNS CNS-related adverse effects may include fatigue, sleep disturbances (including insomnia and nightmares), and depression. There is no clear correlation between the incidence of the adverse effects of β receptor antagonists and their lipophilicity.

METABOLISM β adrenergic blockade may blunt recognition of hypoglycemia and may delay recovery from insulin-induced hypoglycemia. β receptor antagonists should be used with caution in diabetic patients who are prone to hypoglycemic reactions; β_1-selective agents may be preferable.

MISCELLANEOUS

Despite anecdotal evidence, the incidence of sexual dysfunction in hypertensive males treated with β receptor antagonists is not clearly defined. Information about the safety of β antagonists during pregnancy still is limited.

OVERDOSAGE

Manifestations of poisoning with β receptor antagonists depend on the pharmacological properties of the ingested drug. Hypotension, bradycardia, prolonged AV conduction times, and widened QRS complexes are common manifestations. Seizures and depression may occur. Hypoglycemia is rare, and bronchospasm is uncommon in the absence of pulmonary disease. Significant bradycardia should be treated with atropine, but a cardiac pacemaker often is required. Large doses of isoproterenol or an α receptor agonist may be necessary to treat hypotension.

DRUG INTERACTIONS

Aluminum salts, cholestyramine, and colestipol may decrease absorption of β blockers. Phenytoin, rifampin, and phenobarbital, as well as smoking, induce hepatic biotransformation enzymes and may decrease plasma concentrations of β receptor antagonists that are metabolized extensively (e.g., propranolol). Cimetidine and hydralazine may increase bioavailability of propranolol and metoprolol by affecting hepatic blood flow. β Receptor antagonists can impair the clearance of lidocaine.

Other drug interactions have pharmacodynamic explanations. For example, β antagonists and Ca^{2+} channel blockers have additive effects on the cardiac conducting system. Additive effects on blood pressure between β blockers and other antihypertensive agents often are employed to *clinical advantage. The antihypertensive effects of β receptor antagonists can be opposed by* indomethacin *and other NSAIDs (see Chapter 26).*

THERAPEUTIC USES
Cardiovascular Diseases

β Receptor antagonists are used extensively in the treatment of hypertension (*see* Chapter 32), angina and acute coronary syndromes (*see* Chapter 31), and congestive heart failure (*see* Chapter 33). These drugs also are used frequently in the treatment of supraventricular and ventricular arrhythmias (*see* Chapter 34).

MYOCARDIAL INFARCTION
β Receptor antagonists lacking intrinsic sympathomimetic activity, administered during the early phases of acute myocardial infarction and continued long-term, may decrease mortality by ~25%.

CONGESTIVE HEART FAILURE
The reflex sympathetic responses to heart failure may stress the failing heart and exacerbate the progression of the disease, and blocking those responses is beneficial (*see* Chapter 33). β Receptor antagonists are highly effective treatment for all grades of heart failure secondary to left ventricular systolic dysfunction. The drugs improve myocardial function and the quality of life, and prolong life. Thus, β blockers have moved from being contraindicated to being the standard of care in many settings of heart failure.

USE OF β ANTAGONISTS IN OTHER CARDIOVASCULAR DISEASES
β Receptor antagonists, particularly propranolol, are used in the treatment of hypertrophic obstructive cardiomyopathy, for relieving angina, palpitations, and syncope. β Blockers also may attenuate catecholamine-induced cardiomyopathy in pheochromocytoma.

β Blockers are used frequently in the medical management of acute dissecting aortic aneurysm; their usefulness comes from reduction in the force of myocardial contraction and in $\delta P/\delta t$. Patients with Marfan's syndrome may develop progressive dilation of the aorta, which may lead to aortic dissection and regurgitation, a major cause of death in these patients; chronic treatment with propranolol may slow the progression of aortic dilation and its complications.

Glaucoma

β Receptor antagonists are very useful in the treatment of chronic open-angle glaucoma. Six drugs currently are available: carteolol (OCUPRESS, others), betaxolol (BETAOPTIC, others), levobunolol (BETAGAN, others), *metipranolol* (OPTIPRANOLOL, others), timolol (TIMOPTIC, others), and *levobetaxolol* (BETAXON). Timolol, levobunolol, carteolol, and metipranolol are nonselective; betaxolol and levobetaxolol are β_1 selective; none has significant membrane-stabilizing or intrinsic sympathomimetic activity. Topically administered β blockers have little or no effect on pupil size or accommodation and are devoid of blurred vision and night blindness often seen with miotics. These agents decrease the production of aqueous humor, which appears to be the mechanism for their clinical effectiveness. For details of the treatment of glaucoma, *see* Chapter 63.

Other Uses

β Receptor antagonists control many of the cardiovascular signs and symptoms of hyperthyroidism and are useful adjuvants to more definitive therapy. Propranolol, timolol, and metoprolol are effective for the prophylaxis of migraine; the mechanism of this effect is not known; these drugs are not useful for treating acute migraine attacks. By reducing signs of increased sympathetic activity (tachycardia, muscle tremors, etc.), propranolol and other β blockers are effective in controlling acute panic symptoms in individuals who are required to perform in public or in other anxiety-provoking situations. Propranolol also may be useful in the treatment of essential tremor.

β Blockers may be of some value in the treatment of patients undergoing withdrawal from alcohol or those with akathisia. Propranolol and nadolol are efficacious in the primary prevention of variceal bleeding in patients with portal hypertension caused by hepatic cirrhosis.

For a complete Bibliographical listing see Goodman & Gilman's *The Pharmacological Basis of Therapeutics,* **11th ed., or Goodman & Gilman Online at www.accessmedicine.com.**

11

5-HYDROXYTRYPTAMINE (SEROTONIN)

5-Hydroxytryptamine (5-HT, serotonin, 3-[β-aminoethyl]-5-hydroxyindole) is widely distributed, occurring in vertebrates, tunicates, mollusks, arthropods, coelenterates, fruits, and nuts. In humans, 5-HT is found in enterochromaffin cells throughout the gastrointestinal (GI) tract, in storage granules in platelets, and broadly throughout the central nervous system (CNS). 5-HT is also present in venoms (e.g., those of the common stinging nettle, wasps, and scorpions).

SYNTHESIS AND METABOLISM

5-HT is synthesized by a two-step pathway from tryptophan *(Figure 11–1), which is actively transported into the brain by a carrier protein that also transports other large neutral and branched-chain amino acids.* Tryptophan hydroxylase, *a mixed-function oxidase that requires O_2 and a reduced pteridine cofactor, is the rate-limiting enzyme in the synthetic pathway. Unlike tyrosine hydroxylase, tryptophan hydroxylase is not regulated by end-product inhibition, although regulation by phosphorylation is common to both enzymes. Brain tryptophan hydroxylase is not generally saturated with substrate; consequently the concentration of tryptophan in the brain influences the synthesis of 5-HT.*

The enzyme that converts L-5-hydroxytryptophan to 5-HT, aromatic L-amino acid decarboxylase, *is the same enzyme that decarboxylates L-dopa in catecholamine synthesis (see Chapter 6). 5-HT is stored in secretory granules by a vesicular transporter and released by exocytosis. The action of released 5-HT is terminated by neuronal uptake mediated by a specific 5-HT transporter localized in the membrane of serotonergic axon terminals (where it terminates the action of 5-HT in the synapse) and in the membrane of platelets (where it takes up 5-HT from the blood). This uptake system is the only way that platelets acquire 5-HT (they lack the enzymes required to synthesize 5-HT). The 5-HT transporter, SERT, has been cloned (see Chapters 2 and 12).*

The principal route of metabolism of 5-HT involves oxidative deamination by MAO, with subsequent conversion of the aldehyde to 5-hydroxyindole acetic acid (5-HIAA) by an aldehyde dehydrogenase (Figure 11–1). Reduction of the acetaldehyde to an alcohol, 5-hydroxytryptophol, is normally insignificant. 5-HIAA is actively transported out of the brain by a process that is sensitive to probenecid. Since 5-HIAA formation accounts for nearly 100% of the metabolism of 5-HT in brain, the turnover rate of brain 5-HT is estimated by measuring the rate of rise of 5-HIAA after administration of probenecid. 5-HIAA from brain and peripheral sites of 5-HT storage and metabolism is excreted in the urine (range of urinary excretion of 5-HIAA by a normal adult, 2–10 mg/day). Larger amounts are excreted by patients with carcinoid syndrome, providing a reliable diagnostic test for the disease. Ingestion of ethyl alcohol results in elevated amounts of nicotinamide adenine dinucleotide (NADH), which diverts 5-hydroxyindole acetaldehyde from the oxidative route to the reductive pathway, increasing excretion of 5-hydroxytryptophol and reducing excretion of 5-HIAA. MAO-A preferentially metabolizes 5-HT and NE. Neurons contain both isoforms of monoamine oxidase (MAO-A and MAO-B); MAO-B is the principal isoform in platelets.

A close relative of 5-HT, melatonin *(5-methoxy-N-acetyltryptamine), is formed by sequential N-acetylation and O-methylation (Figure 11–1). Melatonin is the principal indoleamine in the pineal gland, where it may be said to constitute a pigment of the imagination. External factors including environmental light control melatonin synthesis. Melatonin induces pigment lightening in skin cells and suppresses ovarian functions; it also serves a role in regulating biological rhythms and shows promise in the treatment of jet lag and other sleep disturbances.*

PHYSIOLOGICAL FUNCTIONS OF SEROTONIN
Multiple 5-HT Receptors

The multiple 5-HT receptor subtypes comprise the largest known neurotransmitter-receptor family. 5-HT receptor subtypes are expressed in distinct but often overlapping patterns and couple to different transmembrane-signaling mechanisms (Table 11–1). Four 5-HT receptor families are recognized: $5\text{-}HT_1$ through $5\text{-}HT_4$. The $5\text{-}HT_1$, $5\text{-}HT_2$, and $5\text{-}HT_{4-7}$ receptor families are members of the superfamily of GPCRs (*see* Chapter 1). The $5\text{-}HT_3$ receptor, on the other hand, is a ligand-gated ion channel that gates Na^+ and K^+ and has a predicted membrane topology akin to that of the nicotinic cholinergic receptor (*see* Chapter 9).

$5\text{-}HT_1$ RECEPTORS All 5 members of the $5\text{-}HT_1$ receptor subfamily inhibit adenylyl cyclase. At least one $5\text{-}HT_1$ receptor subtype, the $5\text{-}HT_{1A}$ receptor, also activates a receptor-operated K^+ channel and inhibits a voltage-gated Ca^{2+} channel, a common property of receptors coupled to

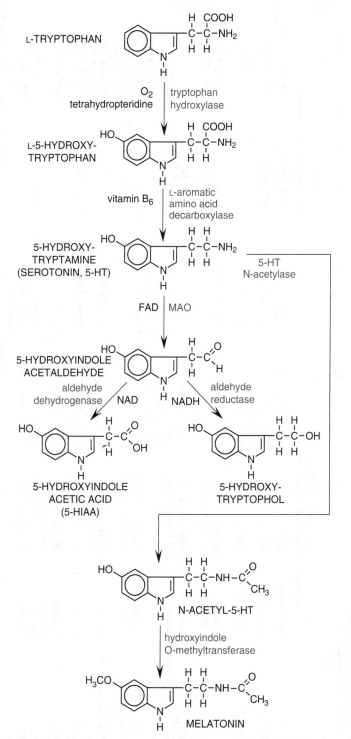

FIGURE 11–1 *Synthesis and inactivation of serotonin.* Synthetic enzymes are identified in blue lettering, and cofactors are shown in black lowercase letters.

Table 11-1

Serotonin Receptor Subtypes

Structural Families

Subtype	Gene Structure**	Signal Transduction	Localization	Function	Selective Agonist	Selective Antagonist
	5-HT₁, 5-HT₂, 5-HT₄₋₇ G protein–coupled receptor (heptaspan)				5-HT₃ 5-HT–gated ion channel (quadrispan)	
5-HT$_{1A}$	Intronless	Inhibition of AC	Raphe nuclei Hippocampus	Autoreceptor	8-OH-DPAT	WAY 100135 WAY 405
5-HT$_{1B}$*	Intronless	Inhibition of AC	Subiculum Substantia nigra	Autoreceptor	—	SB 216641
5-HT$_{1D}$	Intronless	Inhibition of AC	Cranial blood vessels Cortex	Vasoconstriction	Sumatriptan	GR 127935
5-HT$_{1E}$	Intronless	Inhibition of AC	Striatum	—	5-fluorolryptamine	Fluspirilene
5-HT$_{1F}$†	Intronless	Inhibition of AC	Brain and periphery	—	Ly 334370	—
5-HT$_{2A}$ (D receptor)	Introns	Activation of PLC	Platelets Smooth muscle Cerebral cortex	Platelet aggregation Contraction Neuronal excitation	α-Methyl-5-HT, DOI	Ketanserin LY53857 MDL 100,907
5-HT$_{2B}$	Introns	Activation of PLC	Stomach fundus	Contraction	α-Methyl-5-HT, DOI	LY53857
5-HT$_{2C}$	Introns	Activation of PLC	Choroid plexus	—	α-Methyl-5-HT, DOI	LY53857 Mesulergine
5-HT$_3$ (M receptor)	Introns	Ligand-operated ion channel	Peripheral nerves Area postrema	Neuronal excitation	2-Methyl-5-HT	Ondansetron Tropisetron
5-HT$_4$	Introns	Activation of AC	Hippocampus GI tract	Neuronal excitation	Renzapride	GR 113808
5-HT$_{5A}$	Introns	Inhibition of AC	Hippocampus	Unknown	—	SB 699551
5-HT$_{5B}$	Introns	Unknown				
5-HT$_6$	Introns	Activation of AC	Striatum	Synaptic modulation?	CGS 12066	SB 271046
5-HT$_7$	Introns	Activation of AC	Hypothalamus; GI	Nociception/ thermo reg.	Lisuride	Pirenperone

*Also referred to as 5-HT$_{1D\beta}$. †Also referred to as 5-HT$_{1E\beta}$. **Presence of introns may result in splice variants of the receptor.
ABBREVIATIONS: AC, adenylyl cyclase; PLC, phospholipase C; 8-OH-DPAT, 8-hydroxy-(2-N,N-dipropylamino)-tetraline; DOI, 1-(2,5-dimethoxy-4-iodophenyl) isopropylamine.

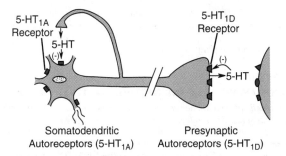

FIGURE 11–2 *Two classes of 5-HT autoreceptors with differential localizations.* Somatodendritic 5-HT$_{1A}$ autoreceptors decrease raphe cell firing when activated by 5-HT released from axon collaterals of the same or adjacent neurons. The receptor subtype of the presynaptic autoreceptor on axon terminals in the human forebrain has different pharmacological properties and has been classified as 5-HT$_{1D}$; this receptor modulates the release of 5-HT. Postsynaptic 5-HT$_1$ receptors are also indicated.

the pertussis toxin–sensitive G$_i$/G$_o$ family of G proteins. The 5-HT$_{1A}$ receptor is found in the raphe nuclei of the brainstem, where it functions as an inhibitory, somatodendritic autoreceptor on cell bodies of serotonergic neurons (Figure 11–2). Another subtype, the 5-HT$_{1D}$ receptor, functions as an autoreceptor on axon terminals, inhibiting 5-HT release. 5-HT$_{1D}$ receptors, abundantly expressed in the substantia nigra and basal ganglia, may regulate the firing rate of dopamine (DA)-containing cells and the release of DA at axonal terminals.

5-HT$_2$ RECEPTORS The three subtypes of 5-HT$_2$ receptors couple to pertussis toxin–insensitive G proteins (*e.g.*, G$_q$ and G$_{11}$) and thence to PLC to generate *diacylglycerol* (a cofactor in the activation of PKC) and *inositol trisphosphate* (which mobilizes intracellular stores of Ca^{2+}). 5-HT$_{2A}$ receptors are broadly distributed in the CNS, primarily in serotonergic terminal areas. High densities of 5-HT$_{2A}$ receptors are found in prefrontal, parietal, and somatosensory cortex, claustrum, and in platelets. 5-HT$_{2A}$ receptors in the GI tract are thought to correspond to the D subtype of 5-HT receptor. 5-HT$_{2B}$ receptors originally were described in stomach fundus. The expression of 5-HT$_{2B}$ receptor messenger RNA (mRNA) is highly restricted in the CNS. 5-HT$_{2C}$ receptors have a very high density in the choroid plexus, an epithelial tissue that is the primary site of cerebrospinal fluid production. The 5-HT$_{2C}$ receptor has been implicated in feeding behavior and susceptibility to seizure.

5-HT$_3$ RECEPTORS The 5-HT$_3$ receptor is the only monoamine neurotransmitter receptor that is known to function as a ligand-operated ion channel. The 5-HT$_3$ receptor corresponds to the originally described M receptor. Activation of 5-HT$_3$ receptors elicits a rapidly desensitizing depolarization, mediated by the gating of cations. These receptors are located on parasympathetic terminals in the GI tract, including vagal and splanchnic afferents. In the CNS, a high density of 5-HT$_3$ receptors is found in the solitary tract nucleus and the area postrema. 5-HT$_3$ receptors in both the GI tract and the CNS participate in the emetic response, providing an anatomical basis for the antiemetic property of 5-HT$_3$ receptor antagonists.

5-HT$_4$ RECEPTORS 5-HT$_4$ receptors are widely distributed throughout the body. In the CNS, the receptors are found on neurons of the superior and inferior colliculi and in the hippocampus. In the GI tract, 5-HT$_4$ receptors are located on neurons of the myenteric plexus and on smooth muscle and secretory cells. The 5-HT$_4$ receptor is thought to evoke secretion in the alimentary tract and to facilitate the peristaltic reflex. 5-HT$_4$ receptors couple to G$_s$ to activate adenylyl cyclase, leading to a rise in intracellular levels of cyclic AMP, possibly accounting for the utility of prokinetic benzamides in GI disorders (*see* Chapter 37).

ADDITIONAL CLONED 5-HT RECEPTORS

Two other cloned receptors, 5-HT$_6$ and 5-HT$_7$, are linked to activation of adenylyl cyclase. Multiple splice variants of the 5-HT$_7$ receptor have been found, although functional distinctions are not clear. Circumstantial evidence suggests that 5-HT$_7$ receptors play a role in smooth-muscle relaxation in the GI tract and the vasculature. The atypical antipsychotic drug clozapine has a high *affinity for 5-HT$_6$ and 5-HT$_7$ receptors, but whether this relates to the broader effectiveness of clozapine as an antipsychotic is not known (see Chapter 18). Two subtypes of the 5-HT$_5$ receptor have been cloned; the 5-HT$_{5A}$ receptor couples to inhibit adenylyl cyclase; functional coupling of the cloned 5-HT$_{5B}$ receptor has not been described.*

Sites of 5-HT Action

ENTEROCHROMAFFIN CELLS AND GASTROINTESTINAL TRACT

Enterochromaffin cells of the GI mucosa (highest density in the duodenum) synthesize and store 5-HT and other autacoids. Basal release of enteric 5-HT is augmented by mechanical stretching and efferent vagal stimulation. 5-HT probably has an additional role in stimulating motility via the myenteric network of neurons (see Chapters 6 and 37). 5-HT released from enterochromaffin cells enters the portal vein and is subsequently metabolized by MAO-A in the liver. 5-HT that survives hepatic oxidation is rapidly removed by the endothelium of lung capillaries and then inactivated by MAO. 5-HT released by mechanical or vagal stimulation also acts locally to regulate GI function. Motility of gastric and intestinal smooth muscle may be either enhanced or inhibited via at least six subtypes of 5-HT receptors (Table 11–2). Abundant 5-HT$_3$ receptors on vagal and other afferent neurons and on enterochromaffin cells play a pivotal role in emesis (see Chapter 37). Enteric 5-HT is released in response to ACh, sympathetic nerve stimulation, increases in intraluminal pressure, and lowered pH, triggering peristaltic contraction.

PLATELETS

Platelets differ from other formed elements of blood in expressing mechanisms for uptake, storage, and endocytotic release of 5-HT. 5-HT is not synthesized in platelets, but is taken up from the circulation and stored in secretory granules by active transport, similar to the uptake and storage of NE by sympathetic nerve terminals (see Chapters 6 and 12). Measuring the rate of Na$^+$-dependent 5-HT uptake by platelets provides a sensitive assay for 5-HT-uptake inhibitors.

A complex local interplay of multiple factors, including 5-HT, regulates thrombosis and hemostasis (see Chapters 25 and 54). When platelets contact injured endothelium, they release substances that promote platelet aggregation, and secondarily, they release 5-HT (Figure 11–3). 5-HT binds to platelet 5-HT$_{2A}$ receptors and elicits a weak aggregation response that is markedly augmented by the presence of collagen. If the damaged blood vessel is injured to a depth where vascular smooth muscle is exposed, 5-HT exerts a direct vasoconstrictor effect, thereby contributing to hemostasis, which is enhanced by locally released autacoids (thromboxane A$_2$, kinins, and vasoactive peptides). Conversely, 5-HT may stimulate production of NO and antagonize its own vasoconstrictor action, as well as the vasoconstriction produced by other locally released agents.

CARDIOVASCULAR SYSTEM

The classical response of blood vessels to 5-HT is contraction, particularly in the splanchnic, renal, pulmonary, and cerebral vasculatures. This response also occurs in bronchial smooth muscle. 5-HT induces a variety of cardiac responses that result from activation of multiple 5-HT receptor subtypes, stimulation or inhibition of autonomic nerve activity, and reflex responses to 5-HT. Thus, 5-HT has positive inotropic and chronotropic actions on the heart that may be blunted by simultaneous stimulation of afferent nerves from baroreceptors and chemoreceptors. An effect

Table 11–2

Some Actions of 5-HT in the Gastrointestinal Tract

Site	Response	Receptor
Enterochromaffin cells	Release of 5-HT	5-HT$_3$
	Inhibition of 5-HT release	5-HT$_4$
Enteric ganglion cells (presynaptic)	Release of ACh	5-HT$_4$
	Inhibition of ACh release	5-HT$_{1P}$, 5-HT$_{1A}$
Enteric ganglion cells (postsynaptic)	Fast depolarization	5-HT$_3$
	Slow depolarization	5-HT$_{1P}$
Smooth muscle, intestinal	Contraction	5-HT$_{2A}$
Smooth muscle, stomach fundus	Contraction	5-HT$_{2B}$
Smooth muscle, esophagus	Contraction	5-HT$_4$

ABBREVIATION: ACh, acetylcholine

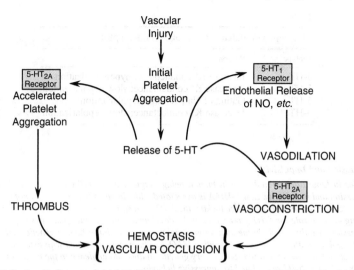

FIGURE 11–3 *Local influences of platelet 5-HT.* Aggregation triggers the release of 5-HT stored in platelets. Local actions of 5-HT include feedback actions on platelets (shape change and accelerated aggregation) mediated by 5-HT_{2A} receptors, stimulation of NO production mediated by 5-HT_1-like receptors on vascular endothelium, and contraction of vascular smooth muscle mediated by 5-HT_{2A} receptors. These influences act in concert with many other mediators (not shown) to promote thrombus formation and hemostasis. See Chapter 54 for details of adhesion and aggregation of platelets and factors contributing to thrombus formation and blood clotting.

on vagus nerve endings elicits the Bezold-Jarisch reflex, causing bradycardia and hypotension. The local response of arterial blood vessels to 5-HT also may be inhibitory, the result of stimulated NO and prostaglandin synthesis and blockade of NE release from sympathetic nerves. On the other hand, 5-HT amplifies the local constrictor actions of NE, AngII, and histamine, which reinforce the hemostatic response to 5-HT.

CENTRAL NERVOUS SYSTEM

A multitude of brain functions are influenced by 5-HT, including sleep, cognition, sensory perception, motor activity, temperature regulation, nociception, mood, appetite, sexual behavior, and hormone secretion. All of the cloned 5-HT receptors are expressed in the brain, often in overlapping domains. The principal cell bodies of 5-HT neurons are located in raphe nuclei of the brainstem and project throughout the brain and spinal cord. In addition to being released at discrete synapses, release of serotonin also seems to occur at sites of axonal swelling, termed varicosities, *which do not form distinct synaptic contacts. 5-HT released at nonsynaptic varicosities is thought to diffuse to outlying targets, rather than acting on discrete synaptic targets, perhaps acting as a neuromodulator as well as a neurotransmitter (see Chapter 12). Serotonergic nerve terminals contain all of the proteins needed to synthesize 5-HT from L-tryptophan (Figure 11–1). Newly formed 5-HT is rapidly accumulated in synaptic vesicles, where it is protected from MAO. 5-HT released by nerve-impulse flow is reaccumulated into the presynaptic terminal by the 5-HT transporter, SERT (see Chapter 2); thus, reuptake terminates the neurotransmitter action of 5-HT. 5-HT taken up by nonneuronal cells is destroyed by MAO. 5-HT has direct excitatory and inhibitory actions (Table 11–3), which may occur in the same preparation, but with distinct temporal patterns.*

Behavior

Sleep-Wake Cycle

5-HT plays a role in control of the sleep-wake cycle. Depletion of 5-HT elicits insomnia that is reversed by the 5-HT precursor, 5-hydroxytryptophan; treatment with L-tryptophan or nonselective 5-HT agonists accelerates sleep onset and prolongs total sleep time. 5-HT antagonists reportedly can increase and decrease slow-wave sleep, probably reflecting interacting or opposing roles for subtypes of 5-HT receptors. One relatively consistent finding in humans and in laboratory animals is an increase in slow-wave sleep following administration of a selective $5\text{-HT}_{2A/2C}$ receptor antagonist such as ritanserin.

Table 11–3

Electrophysiological Effects of 5-HT Receptors

Subtype	Response
$5\text{-}HT_{1A,B}$	Increase K^+ conductance; hyperpolarization
$5\text{-}HT_{2A}$	Decrease K^+ conductance; slow depolarization
$5\text{-}HT_3$	Gating of Na^+, K^+; fast depolarization
$5\text{-}HT_4$	Decrease K^+ conductance; slow depolarization

Aggression and Impulsivity

Studies in laboratory animals and in human beings suggest that 5-HT serves a critical role in aggression and impulsivity. Low 5-HIAA is associated with violent suicidal acts, but not with suicidal ideation per se. Knockout mice lacking the 5-HT$_{1B}$ receptor exhibit extreme aggression, suggesting either a role for 5-HT$_{1B}$ receptors in the development of neuronal pathways important in aggression or a direct role in the mediation of aggressive behavior. A human genetic study identified a point mutation in the gene encoding MAO-A, which was associated with extreme aggressiveness and mental retardation. Laboratory genetic studies add credence to the proposition that abnormalities in 5-HT are related to aggressive behaviors.

Anxiety and Depression

A mechanism for altering synaptic availability of 5-HT is inhibition of presynaptic reaccumulation of neuronally released 5-HT. Selective serotonin reuptake inhibitors (SSRIs; e.g., fluoxetine [PROZAC]) potentiate and prolong the action of 5-HT released by neuronal activity. Effects of 5-HT-active drugs, like the SSRIs, in anxiety and depressive disorders strongly suggest an effect of 5-HT in the neurochemical mediation of these disorders. SSRIs are the most widely used treatment for endogenous depression (see Chapter 17).

Appetite

Two halogenated amphetamines, fenfluramine and dexfenfluramine, have been used to reduce appetite; these drugs were withdrawn from the U.S. market after reports of cardiac toxicity associated with their use. The mechanism of action of this class of drugs is controversial. A profound reduction in levels of 5-HT in the brain lasts for weeks and is accompanied by a loss of proteins (5-HT transporter and tryptophan hydroxylase) selectively localized in 5-HT neurons, suggesting that the halogenated amphetamines have a neurotoxic action, although neuroanatomical signs of neuronal death are not readily apparent.

Sibutramine (MERIDIA), an inhibitor of the reuptake of 5-HT, NE, and DA, is used as an appetite suppressant in the management of obesity; two active metabolites probably account for sibutramine's therapeutic effects. Whether effects on a single neurotransmitter system are primarily responsible for sibutramine's effects in obese patients is unclear.

5-HT RECEPTOR AGONISTS AND ANTAGONISTS

5-HT Receptor Agonists

Direct-acting 5-HT receptor agonists have diverse chemical structures and diverse pharmacological properties (Table 11–4), not surprising considering the plethora of 5-HT receptor subtypes. 5-HT$_{1A}$ receptor–selective agonists have helped elucidate the functions of this receptor in the brain and have resulted in a new class of antianxiety drugs including buspirone, *gepirone,* and *ipsapirone* (*see* Chapter 17). 5-HT$_{1D}$ receptor–selective agonists (*e.g., sumatriptan)* cause constriction of intracranial blood vessels and are used for treatment of acute migraine attacks (*see* below). A number of 5-HT$_4$ receptor–selective agonists have been developed or are being developed for the treatment of disorders of the GI tract (*see* Chapter 37).

5-HT RECEPTOR AGONISTS AND MIGRAINE Migraine headaches afflict 10–20% of the population in the U.S., producing a morbidity estimated at 64 million missed workdays/year. Although migraine is a specific neurological syndrome, manifestations vary widely: migraine without aura (common migraine); migraine with aura (classic migraine), which includes subclasses of migraine with typical aura, migraine with prolonged aura, migraine without headache, and migraine

Table 11–4

Serotonergic Drugs: Primary Actions and Clinical Uses

Receptor	Action	Drug Examples	Clinical Disorder
5-HT$_{1A}$	Partial agonist	Buspirone, ipsapirone	Anxiety, depression
5-HT$_{1D}$	Agonist	Sumatriptan	Migraine
5-HT$_{2A/2C}$	Antagonist	Methysergide, trazodone, risperidone, ketanserin	Migraine, depression, schizophrenia
5-HT$_3$	Antagonist	Ondansetron	Chemotherapy-induced emesis
5-HT$_4$	Agonist	Cisapride mosapride, renzapride	GI disorders
5-HT transporter	Inhibitor	Fluoxetine, sertraline	Depression; panic, obsessive-compulsive, and posttraumatic stress disorders; social phobia

with acute-onset aura; and several other rarer types. Auras also may appear without a subsequent headache. Premonitory aura may begin as long as 24 hours before the onset of pain and often is accompanied by photophobia, hyperacusis, polyuria, and diarrhea, and by disturbances of mood and appetite. A migraine attack may last for hours or days and be followed by prolonged pain-free intervals. The frequency of migraine attacks is extremely variable, but usually ranges from 1–2/year to 1–4/month.

Therapy of migraine headaches is complicated by the variable responses among and within individual patients and by the lack of a firm understanding of the pathophysiology of the syndrome. The efficacy of antimigraine drugs varies with the absence or presence of aura, duration of the headache, its severity and intensity, and as yet undefined environmental and genetic factors. A rather vague and inconsistent pathophysiological characteristic of migraine is the spreading depression of neural impulses from a focal point of vasoconstriction followed by vasodilation. However, it is unlikely that vasoconstriction followed by vasodilation (spreading depression) or vasodilation alone accounts for the local edema and focal tenderness often observed in migraine patients.

Consistent with the hypothesis that 5-HT is a key mediator in the pathogenesis of migraine, 5-HT receptor agonists have become the mainstay for acute treatment of migraine headaches. New treatments for the prevention of migraines, such as botulinum toxin and newer antiepileptic drugs, have unique mechanisms of action, presumably unrelated to 5-HT.

5-HT$_1$ Receptor Agonists: The Triptans

The triptans are indole derivatives, with substituents on the 3 and 5 positions (Figure 11–4). The selective pharmacological effects of the triptans *(sumatriptan [IMITREX], zolmitriptan [ZOMIG], naratriptan [AMERGE], and rizatriptan [MAXALT and MAXALT-MLT]) at 5-HT$_1$ receptors have provided*

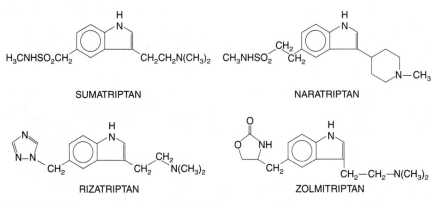

FIGURE 11–4 *Structures of the triptans (selective 5-HT$_1$ receptor agonists).*

insights into the pathophysiology of migraine. Clinically, the drugs are effective, acute antimigraine agents. Their capacity to decrease the nausea and vomiting of migraine is an important advance in the treatment of the condition.

Pharmacological Properties In contrast to ergot alkaloids (*see* below), the pharmacological effects of the triptans appear to be limited to the 5-HT_1 family of receptors, providing evidence that this receptor subclass plays an important role in the acute relief of a migraine attack. The triptans are much more selective agents than are ergot alkaloids, interacting potently with 5-HT_{1D} and 5-HT_{1B} receptors, with low or no affinity for other subtypes of 5-HT receptors or for α_1 and α_2 adrenergic, β adrenergic, dopaminergic, muscarinic cholinergic, and $GABA_A$ receptors. Clinically effective doses of the triptans correlate well with their affinities for 5-HT_{1B} and 5-HT_{1D} receptors. Current data are thus consistent with the hypothesis that 5-HT_{1B} and/or 5-HT_{1D} receptors are the most likely 5-HT receptors involved in the mechanism of action of acute antimigraine drugs.

Mechanism of Action

Two hypotheses have been proposed to explain the efficacy of $5\text{-HT}_{1B/1D}$ receptor agonists in migraine. According to one pathophysiological model of migraine, unknown events lead to the abnormal dilation of carotid arteriovenous anastomoses in the head, diverting blood from the capillary beds and thereby producing cerebral ischemia and hypoxia. In this model, an effective antimigraine agent constricts intracranial blood vessels, including arteriovenous anastomoses, and restores blood flow to the brain. Indeed, ergotamine, dihydroergotamine, and sumatriptan share the capacity to produce this vascular effect with a pharmacological specificity that mirrors the effects of these agents on 5-HT_{1B} and 5-HT_{1D} receptor subtypes.

An alternative hypothesis relates to the observation that both 5-HT_{1B} and 5-HT_{1D} receptors serve as presynaptic autoreceptors, modulating neurotransmitter release from neuronal terminals (Figure 11–2). 5-HT_1 agonists may block the release of proinflammatory neuropeptides at the level of the nerve terminal in the perivascular space. Ergotamine, dihydroergotamine, and sumatriptan can block the development of neurogenic plasma extravasation in dura mater associated with depolarization of perivascular axons following capsaicin injection or unilateral electrical stimulation of the trigeminal nerve. The capacity of potent 5-HT_1 receptor agonists to inhibit endogenous neurotransmitter release in the perivascular space could account for their efficacy in the acute treatment of migraine.

Absorption, Fate, and Excretion When given subcutaneously, sumatriptan reaches its peak plasma concentration in ~12 minutes. Following oral administration, peak plasma concentrations occur within 1–2 hours. Bioavailability following subcutaneous administration is ~97%; after oral administration or nasal spray, bioavailability is 14–17%. The elimination $t_{1/2}$ is ~1–2 hours. Sumatriptan is metabolized predominantly by MAO-A, and its metabolites are excreted in the urine.

Zolmitriptan reaches its peak plasma concentration 1.5–2 hours after oral administration. Its bioavailability is ~40% following oral ingestion. Zolmitriptan is converted to an active N-desmethyl metabolite, which has severalfold higher affinity for 5-HT_{1B} and 5-HT_{1D} receptors than does the parent drug. Both the metabolite and the parent drug have half-lives of 2–3 hours.

Naratriptan, administered orally, reaches its peak plasma concentration in 2–3 hours and has an absolute bioavailability of ~70%. It is the longest acting of the triptans, having a $t_{1/2}$ of ~6 hours. Fifty percent of a dose of naratriptan is excreted unchanged in the urine; ~30% is excreted as products of oxidation by CYPs.

Rizatriptan has an oral bioavailability of ~45% and reaches peak plasma levels within 1–1.5 hours after oral ingestion of tablets of the drug. An orally disintegrating dosage form has a somewhat slower rate of absorption, yielding peak plasma levels of the drug 1.6–2.5 hours after administration. Rizatriptan is principally metabolized *via* oxidative deamination by MAO-A.

Adverse Effects and Contraindications Rare but serious cardiac events have been associated with the administration of 5-HT_1 agonists, including coronary artery vasospasm, transient myocardial ischemia, atrial and ventricular arrhythmias, and myocardial infarction, predominantly in patients with risk factors for coronary artery disease. Generally, only minor side effects are seen with the triptans in the acute treatment of migraine. Up to 83% of patients experience at least one side effect after subcutaneous injection of sumatriptan; most report transient mild pain, stinging, or burning sensations at the site of injection. The most common side effect of sumatriptan nasal spray is a bitter taste. Orally administered triptans can cause paresthesias; asthenia and fatigue; flushing; feelings of pressure, tightness, or pain in the chest, neck, and jaw; drowsiness; dizziness; nausea; and sweating. Triptans are contraindicated in patients with a history of significant cardiovascular disease. Because triptans may cause an acute, usually small, increase in blood pressure, they also are contraindicated in patients with uncontrolled hypertension. Naratriptan is contraindicated in patients with severe renal or hepatic impairment. Rizatriptan should be used with caution in patients with renal or hepatic disease but is not contraindicated in such patients. Sumatriptan, rizatriptan, and zolmitriptan are contraindicated in patients who are taking MAO inhibitors.

Use in Treatment of Migraine   Triptans are effective in the acute treatment of migraine (with or without aura), but are not intended for use in prophylaxis of migraine. Treatment should begin as soon as possible after onset of a migraine attack. Oral dosage forms of the triptans are the most convenient but may not be practical in patients experiencing migraine-associated nausea and vomiting. Approximately 70% of individuals report significant headache relief from a 6-mg subcutaneous dose of sumatriptan. This dose may be repeated once within a 24-hour period if the first dose does not relieve the headache. An oral formulation and a nasal spray of sumatriptan also are available. The onset of action is as early as 15 minutes with the nasal spray. The recommended oral dose of sumatriptan is 25–100 mg, repeatable after 2 hours up to a total dose of 200 mg over a 24-hour period. When administered by nasal spray, from 5–20 mg of sumatriptan is recommended. The dose can be repeated after 2 hours up to a maximum dose of 40 mg over a 24-hour period. Zolmitriptan is given orally in a 1.25–2.5-mg dose, repeatble after 2 hours, up to a maximum dose of 10 mg over 24 hours, if the migraine attack persists. Naratriptan is given orally in a 1–2.5-mg dose, which should not be repeated until 4 hours after the previous dose; the maximum dose over a 24-hour period should not exceed 5 mg. The recommended oral dose of rizatriptan is 5–10 mg, repeatable after 2 hours up to a maximum dose of 30 mg over a 24-hour period. The safety of treating more than 3–4 headaches over a 30-day period with triptans has not been established. Triptans should not be used concurrently with (or within 24 hours of) an ergot derivative (*see* below), nor should one triptan be used concurrently or within 24 hours of another.

Ergot and the Ergot Alkaloids   Ergot is the product of a fungus (*Claviceps purpurea*) that grows on rye and other grains. The contamination of an edible grain by a poisonous, parasitic fungus spread death (called "holy fire" or "St. Anthony's fire") for centuries, causing gangrene of the extremities and limbs, and abortion when ingested during pregnancy. Pharmacological effects of the ergot alkaloids are varied and complex; the complexity of their actions limits their therapeutic uses. In general, the effects result from their actions as partial agonists or antagonists at adrenergic, dopaminergic, and serotonergic receptors (*see also* Chapter 10). The spectrum of effects depends on the agent, dosage, species, tissue, physiological and endocrinological state, and experimental conditions.

For chemical structures of ergot alkaloids, see Table 11–6 in the 11th edition of the parent text. A synthetic ergot derivative, bromocriptine (2-bromo-α-ergocriptine), is used to control the secretion of prolactin (see Chapter 55), a property derived from its DA agonist effect. Other agents of this series include lysergic acid diethylamide (LSD), a potent hallucinogenic drug, and methysergide, a 5-HT antagonist.

Absorption, Fate, and Excretion

Oral administration of ergotamine generally results in low or undetectable systemic drug concentrations, because of extensive first-pass metabolism. Bioavailability after sublingual administration probably is <1% and is inadequate for therapeutic purposes. The bioavailability after administration of rectal suppositories is greater. Ergotamine is metabolized in the liver by largely undefined pathways; 90% of the metabolites are excreted in the bile; traces of unmetabolized drug are found in urine and feces. Despite a plasma $t_{1/2}$ of ~2 hours, ergotamine produces vasoconstriction that lasts for 24 hours or longer. Dihydroergotamine is eliminated more rapidly than ergotamine, presumably due to its rapid hepatic clearance.

Ergonovine and methylergonovine are rapidly absorbed after oral administration and reach peak concentrations in plasma within 60–90 minutes that are >10 times those achieved with an equivalent dose of ergotamine. A uterotonic effect in postpartum women can be observed within 10 minutes after oral administration of 0.2 mg of ergonovine. Judging from the relative durations of action, ergonovine is metabolized and/or eliminated more rapidly than is ergotamine. The $t_{1/2}$ of methylergonovine in plasma is 0.5–2 hours.

Use in the Treatment of Migraine

The multiple pharmacological effects of ergot alkaloids complicate determination of their precise mechanism of action in the acute treatment of migraine. Actions of ergot alkaloids at $5\text{-}HT_{1B/1D}$ receptors likely mediate their acute antimigraine effects. The ergot derivative methysergide, a 5-HT receptor antagonist, has been used for the prophylactic treatment of migraine headaches and is discussed below (see 5-HT Receptor Antagonists).

The use of ergot alkaloids for migraine should be restricted to patients having frequent, moderate migraine or infrequent, severe migraine attacks. The patient should take ergot preparations as soon as possible after the onset of a headache. GI absorption of ergot alkaloids is erratic, perhaps contributing to the large variation in patient response. Available preparations in the U.S. include sublingual tablets of ergotamine tartrate (ERGOMAR) and a nasal spray and solution for injection of dihydroergotamine mesylate (MIGRANAL and D.H.E. 45, respectively). The recommended dose for ergotamine tartrate is 2 mg sublingually, which can be repeated at 30-minute intervals if necessary up to a total dose of 6 mg in a 24-hour period or 10 mg/week. Dihydroergotamine mesylate injections can be given intravenously, subcutaneously, or intramuscularly. The recommended dose is 1 mg, which can be repeated after 1 hour if necessary up to a total dose of 2 mg (intravenously) or 3 mg (subcutaneously or intramuscularly) in a 24-hour period or 6 mg in a week. The dose of dihydroergotamine mesylate administered as a nasal spray is 0.5 mg (one spray) in each nostril, repeated after 15 minutes for a total dose of 2 mg (4 sprays). The safety of more than 3 mg over 24 hours or 4 mg over 7 days has not been established.

Adverse Effects and Contraindications

Nausea and vomiting, due to a direct effect on CNS emetic centers, occur in ~10% of patients after oral administration of ergotamine, and in about twice that number after parenteral administration. Noticing this side effect may be difficult, since nausea and sometimes vomiting are part of the symptomatology of migraine. Leg weakness is common; muscle pains, occasionally severe, may occur in the extremities, as well as numbness and tingling of extremities. Precordial distress, angina-like pain, and transient tachycardia or bradycardia, also have been noted, presumably as a result of coronary vasospasm induced by ergotamine. Localized edema and itching may occur in an occasional hypersensitive patient, but usually do not necessitate interruption of ergotamine therapy. In the event of acute or chronic poisoning (ergotism), treatment consists of complete withdrawal of the offending drug and maintenance of adequate circulation. Dihydroergotamine has lower potency than does ergotamine as an emetic, vasoconstrictor, and oxytocic.

Ergot alkaloids are contraindicated in women who are or may become pregnant; the drugs may cause fetal distress and miscarriage. Ergot alkaloids also are contraindicated in patients with peripheral vascular disease, coronary artery disease, hypertension, impaired hepatic or renal function, and sepsis. Ergot alkaloids should not be taken within 24 hours of the use of the triptans, and should not be used concurrently with other drugs that can cause vasoconstriction.

Use of Ergot Alkaloids in Postpartum Hemorrhage

All natural ergot alkaloids markedly increase the motor activity of the uterus. As the dose is increased, contractions become more forceful and prolonged, resting tone is dramatically increased, and sustained contracture can result. Although this precludes their use for induction or facilitation of labor, it is compatible with their use postpartum or after abortion to control bleeding and maintain uterine contraction. The gravid uterus is very sensitive, and small doses of ergot alkaloids can be given immediately postpartum to obtain a marked uterine response, usually without significant side effects. Ergot alkaloids are used primarily to prevent postpartum hemorrhage. Although all natural ergot alkaloids have qualitatively the same effect on the uterus, ergonovine is the most active and also is less toxic than ergotamine. Thus, ergonovine and its semisynthetic derivative methylergonovine have replaced other ergot preparations as uterine-stimulating agents in obstetrics.

D-Lysergic Acid Diethylamide (LSD)

LSD (see Table 11–6 in the 11th edition of the parent text) is a nonselective 5-HT agonist. This ergot derivative profoundly alters human behavior, eliciting perception disturbances such as sensory distortion (especially visual and auditory) and hallucinations at doses as low as 1 μg/kg. The potent, mind-altering effects of LSD explain its abuse by human beings (see Chapter 23) and the fascination of scientists with the mechanism of action of LSD. LSD interacts with brain 5-HT receptors as an agonist/partial agonist. LSD mimics 5-HT at $5-HT_{1A}$ autoreceptors on raphe cell bodies, producing a marked slowing of the firing rate of serotonergic neurons. Current theories focus on the ability of hallucinogens such as LSD to promote glutamate release in thalamocortical terminals, thus causing a dissociation between sensory relay centers and cortical output. LSD and other hallucinogenic drugs act as partial or full agonists at $5-HT_{2A}$ and $5-HT_{2C}$ receptors. Whether the agonist property of hallucinogenic drugs at $5-HT_{2C}$ receptors contributes to the behavioral alterations is not known. The hallucinogenic phenethylamine derivatives such as 1-(4-bromo-2,5-dimethoxyphenyl)-2-aminopropane are selective $5-HT_{2A/2C}$ receptor agonists.

m-Chlorophenylpiperazine (mCPP)   The actions of mCPP *in vivo* primarily reflect activation of
5-HT$_{1B}$ and/or 5-HT$_{2A/2C}$ receptors, although this agent is not subtype-selective in radioligand-binding studies *in vitro*. mCPP is an active metabolite of the antidepressant drug *trazodone* (DESYREL).

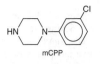

mCPP

mCPP has been employed to probe brain 5-HT function in human beings. The drug alters a
number of neuroendocrine parameters and elicits profound behavioral effects, with anxiety as a
prominent symptom. mCPP elevates corticotropin and prolactin secretion (probably *via* a combination of 5-HT$_1$ and 5-HT$_{2A/2C}$ receptor activation) and increases growth hormone secretion (apparently by a 5-HT-independent mechanism). 5-HT$_{2A/2C}$ receptors appear to mediate at least part of the
anxiogenic effects of mCPP, since 5-HT$_{2A/2C}$ receptor antagonists attenuate mCPP-induced anxiety.

5-HT Receptor Antagonists

Clinical effects of 5-HT-related drugs often exhibit a significant delay in onset, notable in drugs
used to treat affective disorders such as anxiety and depression (*see* Chapter 17). This delayed onset
may relate to adaptive changes in 5-HT receptor density and sensitivity after chronic drug treatments. Laboratory studies have documented agonist-promoted receptor subsensitivity and down-
regulation of 5-HT receptor subtypes. However, an unusual adaptive process, *antagonist*-induced
down-regulation of 5-HT$_{2C}$ receptors, occurs in laboratory animals after chronic treatment with
receptor antagonists. Many clinically effective drugs, including clozapine, ketanserin, and
amitriptyline, exhibit this unusual property. These drugs, as well as several other 5-HT$_{2A/2C}$ receptor antagonists, possess negative intrinsic activity or inverse agonism, reducing constitutive
(spontaneous) receptor activity as well as blocking agonist occupancy (competitive antagonism).
Other 5-HT$_{2A/2C}$ receptor antagonists act in the classical manner, simply blocking receptor occupancy by agonists. Even though there is modest evidence for constitutive activity *in vivo*, drug
development has been further refined by focusing on reduction of preexisting constitutive neuronal
activity as opposed to blockade of excess neurotransmitter action.

Ketanserin

Ketanserin *(SUFREXAL) potently blocks 5-HT$_{2A}$ receptors, less potently blocks 5-HT$_{2C}$ receptors,
and has no significant effect on 5-HT$_3$ or 5-HT$_4$ receptors or any members of the 5-HT$_1$ receptor
family. Ketanserin also has high affinity for α adrenergic and histamine H$_1$ receptors.*
   *Ketanserin lowers blood pressure in patients with hypertension, causing a reduction compa-
rable to that seen with β adrenergic-receptor antagonists or diuretics. The drug appears to reduce
the tone of both capacitance and resistance vessels. This effect likely relates to its blockade of
α$_1$ adrenergic receptors, not its blockade of 5-HT$_{2A}$ receptors. Ketanserin inhibits 5-HT-induced
platelet aggregation but does not greatly reduce the capacity of other agents to cause aggregation. Severe side effects after treatment with ketanserin have not been reported. Its oral bioavailability is ~50%; its plasma t$_{1/2}$ is 12–25 hours. The primary mechanism of inactivation is hepatic
metabolism. Ketanserin is available in Europe but not in the U.S.*
   *Chemical relatives of ketanserin such as ritanserin are more selective 5-HT$_{2A}$ receptor antago-
nists with low affinity for α$_1$ adrenergic receptors. However, ritanserin, as well as most other 5-HT$_{2A}$
receptor antagonists, also potently antagonize 5-HT$_{2C}$ receptors. The physiological significance of
5-HT$_{2C}$-receptor blockade is unknown. MDL 100,907 is the prototype of a new series of potent
5-HT$_{2A}$ receptor antagonists, with high selectivity for 5-HT$_{2A}$ versus 5-HT$_{2C}$ receptors.*

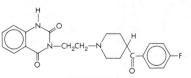

KETANSERIN

Atypical Antipsychotic Drugs   Clozapine (CLOZARIL), a 5-HT$_{2A/2C}$ receptor antagonist, represents a class of atypical antipsychotic drugs with reduced incidence of extrapyramidal side effects compared to the classical neuroleptics, and possibly a greater efficacy for reducing negative symptoms of schizophrenia (*see* Chapter 18). Clozapine also has a high affinity for subtypes of DA receptors.

One of the newest strategies for the design of additional atypical antipsychotic drugs is to combine 5-HT$_{2A/2C}$ and DA D$_2$-receptor blocking actions in the same molecule. *Risperidone* (RISPERDAL), for example, is a potent 5-HT$_{2A}$ and D$_2$ receptor antagonist. Low doses of risperidone have been reported to attenuate negative symptoms of schizophrenia with a low incidence of extrapyramidal side effects. Extrapyramidal effects are commonly seen, however, with doses of risperidone in excess of 6 mg/day. Other atypical antipsychotic agents—*quetiapine* (SEROQUEL) and *olanzapine* (ZYPREXA)—act on multiple receptors, but their antipsychotic properties are thought to be due to antagonism of DA and 5-HT.

Methysergide   Methysergide (SANSERT; 1-methyl-*d*-lysergic acid butanolamide) is a congener of methylergonovine (*see* Table 11–6 in the 11th edition of the parent text). Methysergide blocks 5-HT$_{2A}$ and 5-HT$_{2C}$ receptors but has partial agonist activity in some preparations. Methysergide inhibits the vasoconstrictor and pressor effects of 5-HT, as well as the actions of 5-HT on various types of extravascular smooth muscle. It can both block and mimic the central effects of 5-HT. Methysergide is not selective: it also interacts with 5-HT$_1$ receptors, but its therapeutic effects appear primarily to reflect blockade of 5-HT$_2$ receptors. Although methysergide is an ergot derivative, it has only weak vasoconstrictor and oxytocic activity.

Methysergide has been used for the prophylactic treatment of migraine and other vascular headaches, including Horton's syndrome. It is without benefit when given during an acute migraine attack. The protective effect takes 1–2 days to develop and disappears slowly when treatment is terminated, possibly due to the accumulation of an active metabolite of methysergide, methylergometrine, which is more potent than the parent drug. Methysergide also has been used to combat diarrhea and malabsorption in patients with carcinoid tumors, and in the postgastrectomy dumping syndrome; these conditions have a 5-HT–mediated component. However, methysergide is ineffective against other substances (*e.g.,* kinins) released by carcinoid tumors. The preferred agent to treat malabsorption in carcinoid patients is a somatostatin analog, *octreotide acetate* (SANDOSTATIN), which inhibits the secretion of all mediators released by carcinoid tumors (*see* Chapter 55).

Side effects of methysergide are usually mild and transient, although drug withdrawal is infrequently required to reverse more severe reactions. Common side effects include GI disturbances (heartburn, diarrhea, cramps, nausea, and vomiting), and symptoms related to vasospasm-induced ischemia (numbness and tingling of extremities, pain in the extremities, and low back and abdominal pain). Effects attributable to central actions include unsteadiness, drowsiness, weakness, lightheadedness, nervousness, insomnia, confusion, excitement, hallucinations, and even frank psychotic episodes. Reactions suggestive of vascular insufficiency and exacerbation of angina pectoris have been observed in a few patients. A potentially serious complication of prolonged treatment is inflammatory fibrosis, giving rise to various syndromes that include retroperitoneal fibrosis, pleuropulmonary fibrosis, and coronary and endocardial fibrosis. Usually the fibrosis regresses after drug withdrawal, although persistent cardiac valvular damage has been reported. Because of this danger, other drugs are preferred for the prophylactic treatment of migraine (*see* earlier discussion of migraine therapy). If methysergide is used chronically, treatment should be interrupted for 3 weeks or more every 6 months.

Cyproheptadine   The structure of *cyproheptadine* (PERIACTIN; *see* below) resembles that of the phenothiazine histamine H$_1$ receptor antagonists; indeed, cyproheptadine is an effective H$_1$ receptor antagonist. The drug also has prominent 5-HT blocking activity on smooth muscle via its binding to 5-HT$_{2A}$ receptors. In addition, it has weak anticholinergic activity and mild CNS depressant properties. Cyproheptadine shares the properties and uses of other H$_1$ receptor antagonists (*see* Chapter 24). It is effective in controlling skin allergies, particularly the accompanying pruritus. In allergic conditions, the action of cyproheptadine as a 5-HT receptor antagonist is irrelevant, since 5-HT$_{2A}$ receptors are not involved in human allergic responses. Some physicians recommend cyproheptadine to counteract the sexual side effects of selective 5-HT reuptake inhibitors such as fluoxetine and sertraline (*see* Chapter 17). The 5-HT blocking actions of cyproheptadine explain its value in the postgastrectomy dumping syn-

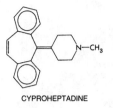

CYPROHEPTADINE

drome, GI hypermotility of carcinoid syndrome, and migraine prophylaxis. Cyproheptadine is not, however, a preferred treatment for these conditions. Side effects of cyproheptadine include those common to other H_1 receptor antagonists, such as drowsiness. Weight gain and increased growth observed in children have been attributed to impaired regulation of growth hormone secretion.

For a complete Bibliographical listing see Goodman & Gilman's *The Pharmacological Basis of Therapeutics,* **11th ed., or Goodman & Gilman Online at www.accessmedicine.com.**

12

NEUROTRANSMISSION AND THE CENTRAL NERVOUS SYSTEM

CELLULAR ORGANIZATION OF THE BRAIN: A PHARMACOLOGICAL VIEW OF NEURONS

Neurons are classified according to function (sensory, motor, or interneuron), location, and identity of the transmitter(s) that they synthesize and release. They exhibit the cytological characteristics of highly active secretory cells with large nuclei: large amounts of smooth and rough endoplasmic reticulum; and frequent clusters of specialized smooth endoplasmic reticulum (Golgi complex), in which secretory products of the cell are packaged into membrane-bound organelles for transport from the cell body proper to the axon or dendrites (Figure 12–1). Neurons are rich in microtubules, which support the complex cellular structure and assist in the reciprocal transport of essential macromolecules and organelles between the cell body and the distant axon or dendrites. The sites of interneuronal communication in the CNS are termed synapses. *Although synapses are functionally analogous to "junctions" in the somatic motor and autonomic nervous systems, the central junctions contain an array of specific proteins presumed to be the active zone for transmitter release and response. Like peripheral "junctions," central synapses also are denoted by accumulations of tiny (500–1500 Å) organelles, termed* synaptic vesicles. *The proteins of these vesicles have been shown to have specific roles in transmitter storage, vesicle docking onto presynaptic membranes, voltage- and Ca^{2+}-dependent secretion (see Chapter 6), and recycling and restorage of released transmitter.*

SUPPORTIVE CELLS

According to most estimates, neurons are outnumbered, perhaps by an order of magnitude, by various supportive cells: the macroglia, the microglia, the cells of the vascular elements comprising the intracerebral vasculature and cerebrospinal fluid (CSF)–forming cells of the choroid plexus found within the intracerebral ventricular system, and the meninges, which cover the brain surface and comprise the CSF–containing envelope. Macroglia are the most abundant supportive cells; some are categorized as astrocytes *(cells interposed between the vasculature and the neurons, often surrounding individual compartments of synaptic complexes), which play a variety of metabolic support roles including furnishing energy intermediates and supplementary removal of extracellular neurotransmitter secretions. The* oligodendroglia, *a second category of macroglia, are the myelin-producing cells. Myelin, made up of multiple layers of their compacted membranes, insulates segments of long axons bioelectrically and accelerates action potential conduction velocity.* Microglia *are derived from mesoderm and are related to the macrophage/monocyte lineage. Some microglia reside within the brain, while additional microglial cells may be recruited to the brain by inflammation following microbial infection or other brain injury (see Chapter 52).*

BLOOD–BRAIN BARRIER

Apart from instances in which drugs are introduced directly into the CNS, the concentration of the agent in the blood after oral or parenteral administration differs substantially from its concentration in the brain. The blood–brain barrier *(BBB) is a boundary between the periphery and the CNS that forms a permeability barrier to the passive diffusion of substances from the bloodstream into various regions of the CNS. Evidence of the barrier is provided by the greatly diminished rate of access of chemicals from plasma to the brain (see Chapters 1 and 2). This barrier is nonexistent in the peripheral nervous system, and is much less prominent in the hypothalamus and in several small, specialized organs (the circumventricular organs) lining the third and fourth ventricles of the brain: the median eminence, area postrema, pineal gland, subfornical organ, and subcommissural organ. Selective barriers to permeation into and out of the brain also exist for small, charged molecules such as neurotransmitters, their precursors and metabolites, and some drugs. These diffusional barriers are viewed as a combination of the partition of solute across the vasculature (which governs passage by definable properties such as molecular weight, charge, and lipophilicity) and the presence or absence of energy-dependent transport systems (see Chapter 2).*

DENDRODENDRITIC

AXOAXODENDRITIC
("SERIAL")

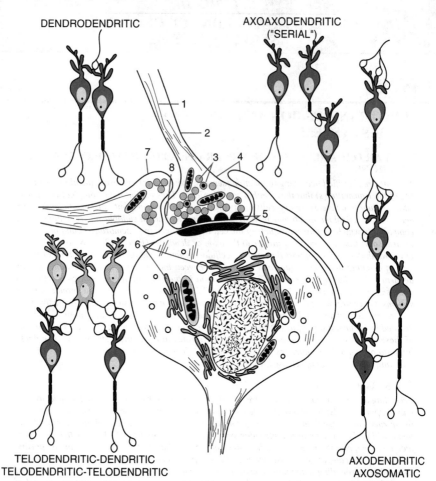

TELODENDRITIC-DENDRITIC
TELODENDRITIC-TELODENDRITIC

AXODENDRITIC
AXOSOMATIC

FIGURE 12–1 *Schematic view of the drug-sensitive sites in prototypical synaptic complexes.* In the center, a post-synaptic neuron receives a somatic synapse (shown greatly oversized) from an axonic terminal; an axoaxonic terminal is shown in contact with this presynaptic nerve terminal. Drug-sensitive sites include: (1) microtubules and molecular motors responsible for bidirectional transport of macromolecules between the neuronal cell body and distal processes; (2) electrically conductive membranes; (3) sites for the synthesis and storage of transmitters; (4) sites for the active uptake of transmitters by nerve terminals or glia; (5) sites for the release of transmitter; (6) postsynaptic receptors, cytoplasmic organelles, and postsynaptic proteins for expression of synaptic activity and for long-term mediation of altered physiological states; (7) presynaptic receptors on adjacent presynaptic processes; and (8) on nerve terminals (autoreceptors). Around the central neuron are schematic illustrations of the more common synaptic relationships in the CNS.

The brain clears metabolites of transmitters into the CSF by excretion via the acid transport system of the choroid plexus. Substances that rarely gain access to the brain from the bloodstream often can reach the brain when injected directly into the CSF. Under certain conditions, it may be possible to open the BBB, at least transiently, to permit the entry of chemotherapeutic agents. Cerebral ischemia and inflammation also modify the BBB, increasing access to substances that ordinarily would not affect the brain.

INTEGRATIVE CHEMICAL COMMUNICATION IN THE CNS AND NEUROPHARMACOLOGY

A central underlying concept of neuropsychopharmacology is that drugs that influence behavior and improve the functional status of patients with neurological or psychiatric diseases act by enhancing or blunting the effectiveness of specific combinations of synaptic transmitter actions.

Four research strategies provide the neuroscientific substrates of neuropsychological phenomena: molecular (or biochemical), cellular, multicellular (or systems), and behavioral. Molecular mechanisms include: (1) ion channels, which provide for changes in excitability induced by neurotransmitters; (2) neurotransmitter receptors; (3) auxiliary intramembranous and cytoplasmic transductive molecules that couple these receptors to intracellular effectors for short-term changes in excitability and for longer-term regulation through alterations in gene expression; and (4) transporters for the conservation of released transmitter molecules by reaccumulation into nerve terminals, and then into synaptic vesicles (see Chapter 6). Vesicular transporters are distinct from the plasma membrane proteins involved in transmitter uptake into nerve terminals. Electrical excitability of neurons occurs through modifications of the transmembrane ion channels that all neurons express in abundance. Discriminative ion channels (Figures 12–2 and Chapter 9) regulate the flow of the three major cations, Na^+, K^+ and Ca^{2+}, and Cl^- anions. Two other families of channels regulate ion fluxes: cyclic nucleotide–modulated channels, and transient receptor potential (TRP) channels.

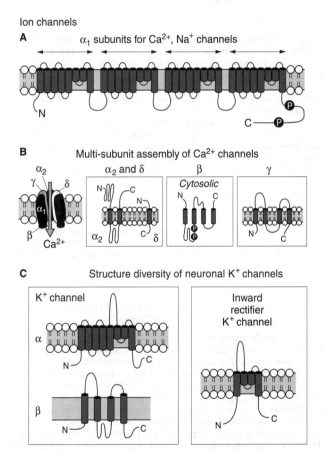

FIGURE 12–2 *The major molecular motifs of ion channels that establish and regulate neuronal excitability in the central nervous system. A.* The α subunits of the Ca^{2+} and Na^+ channels share a similar presumptive six-transmembrane structure, repeated four times, in which an intramembranous segment separates transmembrane segments 5 and 6. *B.* The Ca^{2+} channel also requires several auxiliary small proteins (α_2, β, γ, and δ). The α_2 and δ subunits are linked by a disulfide bond (*not shown*). Regulatory subunits also exist for Na^+ channels. *C.* Voltage-sensitive K^+ channels (K_v) and the rapidly activating K^+ channel (K_a) share a similar presumptive six-transmembrane domain similar in overall configuration to one repeat unit within the Na^+ and Ca^{2+} channel structure, while the inwardly rectifying K^+ channel protein (K_{ir}) retains the general configuration of just loops 5 and 6. Regulatory β subunits (cystosolic) can alter K_v channel functions. Channels of these two overall motifs can form heteromultimers.

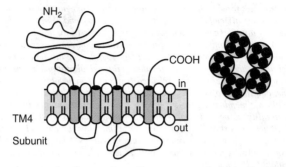

FIGURE 12–3 *Ionophore receptors for neurotransmitters are composed of subunits with four transmembrane domains and are assembled as tetramers or pentamers (at right).* The predicted motif shown likely describes nicotinic cholinergic receptors for ACh, GABA_A receptors for gamma-aminobutyric acid, and receptors for glycine.

Voltage-dependent ion channels (Figure 12–2) provide for rapid changes in ion permeability along axons and within dendrites and for the excitation-secretion coupling that releases neurotransmitters from presynaptic sites. Ligand-gated ion channels, regulated by the binding of neurotransmitters, form a distinct group of ion channels (Figure 12–3). Within the CNS, variants of the K^+ channels (the delayed rectifier, the Ca^{2+}-activated K^+ channel, and the after-hyperpolarizing K^+ channel) regulated by intracellular second messengers repeatedly have been shown to underlie complex forms of synaptic modulation.

Cyclic nucleotide–modulated channels consist of two groups: the cyclic nucleotide–gated (CNG) channels, which play key roles in sensory transduction for olfactory and photoreceptors, and the hyperpolarization-activated, cyclic nucleotide–gated (HCN) channels. HCN channels are cation channels that open with hyperpolarization and close with depolarization; upon direct binding of cyclic AMP or cyclic GMP, the activation curves for the channels are shifted to more hyperpolarized potentials. These channels play essential roles in cardiac pacemaker cells and presumably in rhythmically discharging neurons.

TRP channels, named for their role in Drosophila phototransduction, are a family of hexaspanning receptors with a pore domain between the fifth and sixth transmembrane segments and a common 25-amino acid TRP "box" C-terminal of the sixth transmembrane domain; these channels are found across the phylogenetic scale from bacteria to mammals. Members of the TRPV subfamily serve as the receptors for endogenous cannabinoids, such as anandamide, and the hot pepper toxin, capsaicin.

Identification of Central Transmitters

The criteria for the identification of central transmitters require the same data used to establish the transmitters of the autonomic nervous system (*see* Chapter 6).

1. *The transmitter must be shown to be present in the presynaptic terminals of the synapse and in the neurons from which those presynaptic terminals arise.* Extensions of this criterion involve the demonstration that the presynaptic neuron synthesizes the transmitter substance, rather than simply storing it after accumulation from a nonneural source.
2. *The transmitter must be released from the presynaptic nerve concomitantly with presynaptic nerve activity.* This criterion is best satisfied by electrical stimulation of the nerve pathway *in vivo* and collection of the transmitter in an enriched extracellular fluid within the synaptic target area. The release of all known transmitter substances, including presumptive transmitter release from dendrites, is voltage-dependent and requires Ca^{2+} influx into the presynaptic terminal. However, transmitter release is relatively insensitive to extracellular Na^+ or to tetrodotoxin, which blocks transmembrane movement of Na^+.
3. *When applied experimentally to the target cells, the effects of the putative transmitter must be identical to the effects of stimulating the presynaptic pathway.* This criterion can be met loosely by qualitative comparisons (*e.g.*, both the substance and the pathway inhibit or excite the target cell). More convincing is the demonstration that the ionic conductances activated by the pathway are the same as those activated by the candidate transmitter. The criterion can be satisfied less rigorously by demonstration of the pharmacological identity of receptors (order of potency of agonists and antagonists). Generally, pharmacological antagonism of the actions of the pathway

and those of the candidate transmitter should be achieved by similar concentrations of antagonist. To be convincing, the antagonistic drug should not affect responses of the target neurons to other unrelated pathways or to chemically distinct transmitter candidates. Actions that are qualitatively identical to those that follow stimulation of the pathway also should be observed with synthetic agonists that mimic the actions of the transmitter.

Many brain and spinal cord synapses, especially those involving peptide neurotransmitters, apparently contain more than one transmitter substance. Substances that coexist in a given synapse are presumed to be released together, but in a frequency-dependent fashion, with higher frequency bursts mediating peptide release. Coexisting substances may either act jointly on the postsynaptic membrane, or affect release of transmitter from the presynaptic terminal. Clearly, if more than one substance transmits information, no single agonist or antagonist would faithfully mimic or fully antagonize activation of a given presynaptic element. Costorage and corelease of ATP and NE are an example.

RECEPTOR PROPERTIES
Biochemical techniques and molecular cloning studies have revealed two major motifs and one minor motif of transmitter receptors. The first, oligomeric ion channel receptors, are composed of multiple subunits, usually with four transmembrane domains (Figure 12–3). The ion channel receptors (ionotropic receptors or IRs) for neurotransmitters contain sites for reversible phosphorylation by protein kinases and phosphoprotein phosphatases and for voltage gating. Receptors with this structure include nicotinic cholinergic receptors; the receptors for the amino acids GABA, glycine, glutamate, and aspartate; and the $5\text{-}HT_3$ receptor.

The second major motif comprises the G protein–coupled receptors (GPCRs), a large family of heptahelical receptors (see Figures 1–7 and 10–1). Activated receptors (themselves subject to reversible phosphorylation at one or more functionally distinct sites) can interact with the heterotrimeric GTP-binding protein complex. Such protein–protein interactions can activate, inhibit, or otherwise regulate effector systems such as adenylyl cyclase or phospholipase C, and ion channels, such as voltage-gated Ca^{2+} channels or receptor-operated K^+ channels (see Chapter 1). GPCRs are employed by muscarinic cholinergic receptors, one subtype each of GABA and glutamate receptors, and all other aminergic and peptidergic receptors.

A third receptor motif is the growth factor receptor (GFR), a monospanning membrane protein that has an extracellular binding domain that regulates an intracellular catalytic activity, such as the atrial natriuretic peptide–binding domain that regulates the activity of the membrane-bound guanylyl cyclase (see Figure 1–7). Dimerization of GPCRs and GFRs apparently contributes to their activities, as does localization within or outside of caveolae in the membrane.

Postsynaptic receptivity of CNS neurons is regulated continuously in terms of the number of receptor sites and the threshold required to generate a response. Receptor number often depends on the concentration of agonist to which the target cell is exposed. Thus, chronic excess of agonist can lead to a reduced number of receptors (desensitization or down-regulation) and consequently to subsensitivity or tolerance to the transmitter. For many GPCRs, short-term down-regulation is achieved by the actions of G protein–linked receptor kinases (GRKs) and internalization of the receptors (see Chapter 1). *Conversely, deficit of agonist or prolonged pharmacologic blockade of receptors can lead to increased numbers of receptors and supersensitivity of the system. These adaptive processes become especially important when drugs are used to treat chronic illness of the CNS. After prolonged exposure to drug, the actual mechanisms underlying the therapeutic effect may differ strikingly from those that operate when the agent is first introduced. Similar adaptive modifications of neuronal systems also can occur at presynaptic sites, such as those concerned with transmitter synthesis, storage, and release.*

TRANSMITTERS, HORMONES, AND MODULATORS: CONTRASTING PRINCIPLES OF NEURONAL REGULATION
NEUROTRANSMITTERS   Transmitters may produce minimal effects on bioelectric properties, yet activate or inactivate biochemical mechanisms necessary for responses to other circuits. Alternatively, the action of a transmitter may vary with the context of ongoing synaptic events—enhancing excitation or inhibition, rather than operating to impose direct excitation or inhibition. Each chemical substance that fits within the broad definition of a transmitter may therefore require operational definition within the spatial and temporal domains of a specific cell–cell circuit. Those same properties may not necessarily be generalized to other cells contacted by the same presynaptic neurons; differences in operation may relate to differences in postsynaptic receptors and the mechanisms by which an activated receptor produces its effects.

Classically, electrophysiological signs of the action of a *bona fide* transmitter fall into two major categories: (1) *excitation*, in which ion channels are opened to permit net influx of positively charged ions, leading to depolarization with a reduction in the electrical resistance of the membrane; and (2) *inhibition*, in which selective ion movements lead to hyperpolarization, also with decreased membrane resistance. There also may be many "nonclassical" transmitter mechanisms operating in the CNS. In some cases, either depolarization or hyperpolarization is accompanied by a *decreased* ionic conductance (increased membrane resistance) as actions of the transmitter lead to the closure of ion channels (so-called leak channels) that normally are open in some resting neurons. For transmitters such as monoamines and certain peptides, a "conditional" action may be involved, *i.e.*, a transmitter substance may enhance or suppress the response of the target neuron to classical excitatory or inhibitory transmitters while producing little or no change in membrane potential or ionic conductance when applied alone. Such conditional responses are termed *modulatory*. Regardless of the mechanisms that underlie such synaptic operations, their temporal and biophysical characteristics differ substantially from the rapid onset-offset effects previously thought to describe all synaptic events. These differences raise the issue of whether substances that produce slow synaptic effects should be described as neurotransmitters. Some of the alternative terms and the relevant molecules are described below.

NEUROHORMONES

Peptide-secreting cells of the hypothalamic-hypophyseal circuits originally were described as neurosecretory cells, receiving synaptic information from other central neurons, yet secreting transmitters in a hormone-like fashion into the circulation. The transmitter released from such neurons was termed a neurohormone, *i.e., a substance secreted into the blood by a neuron. These hypothalamic neurons also may form traditional synapses with central neurons, and cytochemical evidence indicates that the same substances that are secreted as hormones from the posterior pituitary (oxytocin, arginine-vasopressin; see Chapters 29 and 55) mediate transmission at these sites. Thus, the designation* hormone *relates to the release at the posterior pituitary and does not necessarily describe all actions of the peptide.*

NEUROMODULATORS

The distinctive feature of a modulator is that it originates from nonsynaptic sites, yet influences the excitability of nerve cells. Substances such as CO_2 and ammonia, arising from active neurons or glia, are potential modulators through nonsynaptic actions. Similarly, circulating steroid hormones, steroids produced in the nervous system (i.e., neurosteroids), locally released adenosine, other purines, eicosanoids, and NO are regarded as modulators (see below).

NEUROMEDIATORS

Substances that participate in eliciting the postsynaptic response to a transmitter fall under this heading. The clearest examples of such effects are provided by the involvement of cyclic AMP, cyclic GMP, and inositol phosphates as second messengers at specific sites of synaptic transmission (see Chapters 1, 6, 7, 10, and 11). Changes in the concentration of second messengers may enhance the generation of synaptic potentials, and second messenger–dependent protein phosphorylation can initiate a complex cascade of molecular events that regulate the properties of membrane and cytoplasmic proteins central to neuronal excitability. These possibilities are particularly pertinent to the action of drugs that augment or reduce transmitter effects (see below).

NEUROTROPHIC FACTORS

Neurotrophic factors are substances produced within the CNS by neurons, astrocytes, microglia, or transiently invading peripheral inflammatory or immune cells that assist neurons in their attempts to repair damage. Seven categories of neurotrophic peptides are recognized: (1) the classic neurotrophins (NGF, brain-derived neurotrophic factor, and the related neurotrophins); (2) the neuropoietic factors, which have effects both in brain and in myeloid cells (e.g., cholinergic differentiation factor [also called leukemia inhibitory factor], ciliary neurotrophic factor, and some interleukins); (3) growth factor peptides, such as EGF, TGF α and β, glial cell–derived neurotrophic factor, and activin A; (4) the fibroblast growth factors; (5) insulin-like growth factors; (6) platelet-derived growth factors; and (7) axon guidance molecules.

CENTRAL NEUROTRANSMITTERS

Table 12–1 summarizes the pharmacological properties of the transmitters in the CNS that have been studied extensively. Neurotransmitters are discussed below as groups of substances within given chemical categories: amino acids, amines, and neuropeptides.

Table 12–1

Overview of Transmitter Pharmacology in the Central Nervous System

Transmitter	Transporter Blocker[a]	Receptor	Agonists	Receptor-Effector Coupling	Selective Antagonists
		Subtype		Motif (IR/GPCR)	
GABA	Guvacine, nipecotic acid	$GABA_A$; $\alpha, \beta, \gamma, \delta, \sigma$ isoforms	Muscimol Isoguvacine THIP	IR: classical fast inhibitory transmission via Cl^- channels	Bicuculline Picrotoxin SR 95531
	(β-Alanine for glia)	$GABA_B$	Baclofen 3-Aminopropylphosphinic acid	IR: pre- and postsynaptic effects	2-hydroxy-s-Saclofen CGP35348 CGP55845
		$GABA_C$	β-Alanine; taurine	IR: slow, sustained responses via Cl^- channels	
Glycine	? Sarcosine	α and β subunits		IR: classical fast inhibitory transmission via Cl^- channels (insensitive to bicuculline and picrotoxin)	Strychnine
Glutamate	TFB-TBOA	AMPA	Quisqualate	IR: classical fast excitatory transmission via cation channels	NBQX
Aspartate	—	GLU 1–4	Kainate AMPA		CNQX GYK153655
		KA GLU 5–7; KA 1,2	Domoic acid Kainate		CNQX LY294486
		NMDA NMDA $1,2_{A-D}$	NMDA GLU, ASP	IR: depolarization Mg^{2+}-gated slow excitatory transmission	MK801 AP5 Ketamine, PCP
		mGLU 1,5 (Group I mGluRs)	3,5-DHPG	GPCRs: modulatory; regulate ion channels, second messenger production, and protein phosphorylation	
		mGLU 2,3 (Group II mGluRs)	APDC		
		mGLU 4,6,7,8 (Group III mGluRs)	LY354740 L-AP4	*In vitro* coupling: Group I, G_q; Groups II and III, G_i	

(Continued)

209

Table 12-1

Overview of Transmitter Pharmacology in the Central Nervous System (Continued)

Transmitter	Transporter Blocker*	Receptor / Subtype	Agonists	Receptor-Effector Coupling Motif (IR/GPCR)	Selective Antagonists
Acetylcholine	—	Nicotinic		IR: classical fast excitatory transmission *via* cation channels	α-Bungarotoxin
		α_{2-4} and β_{2-4} isoforms $\alpha7$			Me-Lycaconitine
		Muscarinic M_{1-4}		GPCR: modulatory M_1, M_3: G_q, $\uparrow IP_3/Ca^{2+}$ M_2, M_4: G_i, $\downarrow$cAMP	M_1: Pirenzepine; M_2: Methoctramine; M_3: Hexahydrosiladifenidol; M_4: Tropicamide
Dopamine	Cocaine; mazindol; GBR12-395; nomifensine	D_{1-5}	D_1: SKF38393; D_2: Bromocriptine; D_3: 7-OH-DPAT	GPCR: D_1 D_5: G_s coupled; $D_{2,3,4}$: G_i coupled	D_1: SCH23390; D_2: Sulpiride, domperidone
Norepinephrine	Desmethylimipramine; mazindol, cocaine	α_{1A-D}	α_{1A}: NE > EPI	GCPR: $G_{q/11}$ coupled	WB4101
		α_{2A-C}	α_{2A}: Oxymetazoline	GCPR: $G_{i/o}$ coupled	α_{2A-C}: Yohimbine α_{2B}, α_{2C}: Prazosin
		β_{1-3}	β_1: EPI = NE; β_2: EPI >> NE; β_3: NE > EPI	GPCR: G_s coupled GPCR: $G_s/G_{i/o}$ coupled GPCR: $G_{i/o}$ coupled	β_1: Atenolol; β_2: Butoxamine; β_3: BRL 37344
Serotonin	Clomipramine; sertraline; fluoxetine	5-HT_{1A-F}	5-HT_{1A}: 8-OH-DPAT; 5-HT_{1B}: CP93129; 5-HT_{1D}: LY694247	GPCR: $G_{q/11}$ coupled	5-HT_{1A}: WAY101135 5-HT_{1D} GR127935
		5-HT_{2A-C}	α-Me-5-HT, DOB		LY53857; ritanserin; mesulergine; ketanserin
		5-HT_3	2-Me-5-HT; m-CPG	IR: classical fast excitatory transmission *via* cation channels	Tropisteron: ondansetron; granisetron
		5-HT_{4-7}	5-HT_4: BIMU8; RS67506; renzapride	GPCR: $5\text{-HT}_{4,6,7}$: G_s coupled 5-HT_5: G_s coupled?	5-HT4: GR113808; SB204070

Transmitter		Receptor	Agonist	Structural information	Antagonist
Histamine	—	H_1	2-Pyridylethylamine	GPCR: $G_{q/11}$ coupled	Mepyramine
		H_2	2-Me-histamine; Methylhistamine; dimaprit, impromadine	GPCR: G_s coupled	Ranitidine, famotidine, cimetidine
		H_3	H_3: R-α-Me-histamine	GPCR: $G_{i/o}$ coupled? Autoreceptor function: inhibits transmitter release	H_3; Thioperamide
		H_4	Imetit, clobenpropit	GPCR: G_i, G_i coupled?	JNJ777120
Vasopressin	—	$V_{1A,B}$	—	GPCR: G_q, $G_{q/11}$ coupled; modulatory; regulates ion channels, second messenger production, and protein phosphorylation	V_{1A}: SR49059
		V_2	DDAVP	GPCR: G_s coupled	d(CH$_2$)$_5$ [dIle^{2}Ile^4]AVP
Oxytocin	—		[Thr^4,Gly^7]OT	GPCR: $G_{q/11}$ coupled	d(CH$_2$)$_5$ [Tyr(Me)^2, Thr^4, Orn^8]OT$_{1-8}$, atosiban
Tachykinins	—	NK_1 (SP > NKA > NKB)	Substance P Me ester	GPCR: $G_{q/11}$ coupled; modulatory; regulates ion channels, second messenger production, and protein phosphorylation	SR140333, LY303870, CP99994
		NK_2 (NKA > NKB > SP)	β-[Ala^8]NKA$_{4-10}$		GR94800, GR159897
		NK3 (NKB > NKA > SP)	GR138676		SR142802, SR223412, [Pro^7]NKB
CCK	—	CCK_A	CCK8 >> gastrin, 5 = CCK4	GPCR: $G_{q/11}$ and G_s coupled	Devazepide; lorglumide
		CCK_B	CCK8 > gastrin, 5 = CCK4	GPCR: $G_{q/11}$ coupled	CI988; L365260; YM022
NPY	—	Y_1	[Pro^{34}]NPY	GPCR: $G_{i/o}$ coupled	—
		Y_2	NPY$_{13-36}$; NPY$_{18-36}$		
		Y_{4-6}	NPY$_{13-36}$; NPY$_{18-36}$		
Neurotensin	—	NTS1	—	GPCR: $G_{q/11}$ coupled	SR48692
		NTS2	—		

(Continued)

211

Table 12-1

Overview of Transmitter Pharmacology in the Central Nervous System (Continued)

Transmitter	Transporter Blocker[*]	Receptor	Agonists	Receptor-Effector Coupling	Selective Antagonists
		Subtype		Motif (IR/GPCR)	
Opioid peptides	—	μ (β-endorphin)	DAMGO, sufentanil; DALDA	GPCR: $G_{i/o}$ coupled	CTAP; CTOP; β-FNA
		δ (Met^5-Enk)	DPDPE; DSBULET; SNC-80		Naltrindole; DALCE; ICI174864; SB205588
		κ (Dyn A)	U69593; CI977; ICI74864		Nor-binaltorphimine; 7-[3-(1-piperidinyl) propanamido] morphan
Somatostatin	—	sst$_{1A-C}$	SRIF1A; seglitide	GPCR: $G_{i/o}$ coupled	—
		sst$_{2A,B}$	Octreotide; seglitide, BIM23027		Cyanamid 154806
		sst$_{3,4}$	BIM23052, NNC269100		
		sst$_5$	L362855		BIM23056
Purines	—	P1 (A$_{1,2a,2b,3}$)	A$_1$: N6-cyclopentyladenosine A$_{2a}$: CGS21680; APEC; HENECA	GPCR: $G_{i/o}$ coupled GPCR: G_s coupled	8-Cyclopentyltheophylline; DPCPX CO66713; SCH58261; ZM241385
		P2X$_{3,4,6}$	α,β-methylene ATP, ATPXS	IR: transductive effects not yet determined	Suramin (nonselective)
		P2Y	ADPβF, ATPXS 2 methylthio ATP	GPCR: $G_{i/o}$ and $G_{q/11}$ coupled	Suramin, PPADS

[*]In some instances (e.g., acetylcholine, purines), agents that inhibit metabolism of the transmitter(s) have effects that are analogous to those of inhibitors of transport of other transmitters.

Receptor-effector coupling consists of ion channel mechanisms for ionotropic receptors (IR) or coupling to G proteins for GPCRs. All GPCRs modulate neuronal activity by affecting second messenger production, protein phosphorylation, and ion channel function by mechanisms described in Chapter 1. In general, G_s couples to adenylyl cyclase to activate cyclic AMP production, while coupling to G_i inhibits adenylyl cyclase; coupling to G_q activates the PLC-IP$_3$-Ca^{2+} pathway; $\beta\gamma$ subunits of G proteins may modulate ion channels directly.

ABBREVIATIONS: 7-OH-DPAT, 7-hydroxy-2 (di-n-propylamino) tetralin; 5-HT, 5-hydroxytryptamine (serotonin); L-AP4, L-amino-4-phosphonobutyrate; APDC, 1S, 4R-4-aminopyrrolidine2-4-dicarboxylate; AVP, arginine vasopressin; CCK, cholecystokinin; CTAP, DPhe-Cys-Tyr-DTrp-Arg-Thr-Pen-Thr-NH$_2$; CTOP, DPhe-Cys-Tyr-DTrp-Orn-Thr-Pen-Thr-NH$_2$; DALCE, [DAla^2, Leu^5, Cys^6]enkephalin; DAMGO, [D-Ala^2,N-Me-Phe^4,Gly^5-ol]– enkephalin; DDAVP, 1-desamino-8-D-arginine vasopressin; DHPG, dihydroxyphenylglycine; DPDPE, [d-Pen^2, d-Pen^5] enkephalin; DSBULET, Tyr-d-Ser-o-rbutyl-Gly-Phe-Leu-Thr; EPI, epinephrine; NE, norepinephrine; NK, neurokinin; NPY, neuropeptide Y; OT, oxytocin; PCP, phencyclidine; SP, substance P; SRIF, somatotropin release-inhibiting factor; THIP, 4,5,6,7-tetrahydroisoxazolo [5,4-c]-pyridone; VP, vasopressin. All other abbreviations represent experimental drugs coded by their manufacturers.

AMINO ACIDS The CNS contains high concentrations of certain amino acids, notably glutamate and gamma-aminobutyric acid (GABA). The dicarboxylic amino acids (*e.g.*, glutamate and aspartate) produce near universal excitation, while the monocarboxylic ω-amino acids (*e.g.*, GABA, glycine, β-alanine, and taurine) produce qualitatively similar, consistent inhibitions. The availability of selective antagonists has permitted identification of selective amino acid receptors and receptor subtypes. These data, together with the development of methods for mapping the ligands and their receptors, demonstrate that the amino acids GABA, glycine, and glutamate are central transmitters. The structures of glycine, glutamate, GABA, and some related compounds are shown in Figure 12–4.

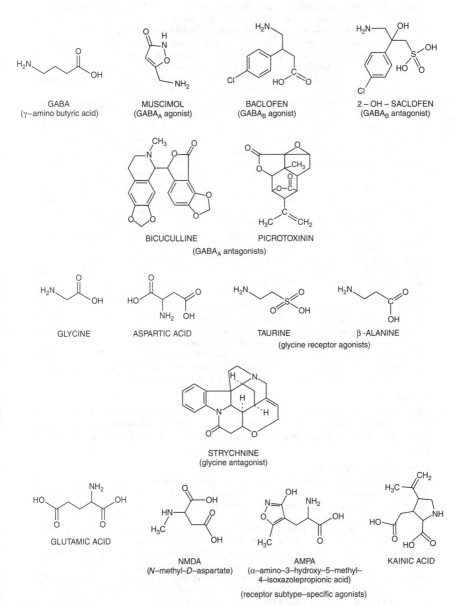

FIGURE 12–4 *Amino acid transmitters and congeners.* Endogenous compounds are shown in blue.

GABA

GABA is the major inhibitory neurotransmitter in the mammalian CNS; it mediates the inhibitory actions of local interneurons in the brain and may also mediate presynaptic inhibition within the spinal cord. Presumptive GABA-containing inhibitory synapses have been demonstrated most clearly between cerebellar Purkinje neurons and their targets in Deiter's nucleus; between small interneurons and the major output cells of the cerebellar cortex, olfactory bulb, cuneate nucleus, hippocampus, and lateral septal nucleus; and between the vestibular nucleus and the trochlear motoneurons. GABA also mediates inhibition within the cerebral cortex and between the caudate nucleus and the substantia nigra. GABA-containing neurons and nerve terminals can be localized with immunocytochemical methods that visualize glutamic acid decarboxylase, the enzyme that catalyzes the synthesis of GABA from glutamic acid, or by in situ hybridization of the mRNA for this protein. GABA-containing neurons frequently coexpress one or more neuropeptides (see below). The most useful compounds for confirmation of GABA-mediated effects have been bicuculline and picrotoxin (Figure 12–4); however, many convulsants whose actions previously were unexplained (including penicillin and pentylenetetrazol) also may act as relatively selective antagonists of GABA action. Useful therapeutic effects have not yet been obtained through the use of agents that mimic GABA (e.g., muscimol), inhibit its active reuptake (e.g., 2,4-diaminobutyrate, nipecotic acid, and guvacine), or alter its turnover (e.g., aminooxyacetic acid).

GABA receptors have been divided into three main types: A, B, and C. The most prominent subtype, the $GABA_A$ receptor, is a ligand-gated Cl^- ion channel, an "ionotropic receptor" that is opened after release of GABA from presynaptic neurons. The $GABA_B$ receptor is a GPCR. The $GABA_C$ receptor is a transmitter-gated Cl^- channel. The $GABA_A$ receptor subunit proteins have been well characterized due to their abundance. The receptor also has been extensively characterized as the site of action of many neuroactive drugs (see Chapters 16 and 22), notably benzodiazepines, barbiturates, ethanol, anesthetic steroids, and volatile anesthetics. Based on sequence homology, more than 15 other subunits have been cloned and appear to be expressed in multiple multimeric, pharmacologically distinctive combinations. In addition to these subunits, which are products of separate genes, splice variants for several subunits have been described. The $GABA_A$ receptor, by analogy with the nicotinic cholinergic receptor, may be either a pentameric or tetrameric protein in which the subunits assemble together around a central ion pore typical for all ionotropic receptors (see below). The major form of the $GABA_A$ receptor contains at least three different subunits—α, β, and γ—but their stoichiometry is not known. All three subunits are required to interact with benzodiazepines with the profile expected of the native $GABA_A$ receptor, and inclusion of variant α, β, or γ subunits alters the pharmacological profiles. The $GABA_B$ or metabotropic GABA receptor interacts with G_i to inhibit adenylyl cyclase, activate K^+ channels, and reduce Ca^{2+} conductance. Presynaptic $GABA_B$ receptors function as autoreceptors, inhibiting GABA release, and may play the same role on neurons releasing other transmitters. There are two subtypes of $GABA_B$ receptors, 1a and 1b. The $GABA_C$ receptor is less widely distributed than the A and B subtypes and is pharmacologically distinct: GABA is more potent by an order of magnitude at $GABA_C$ than at $GABA_A$ receptors, and a number of $GABA_A$ agonists (e.g., baclofen) and modulators (e.g., benzodiazepines and barbiturates) seem not to interact with $GABA_C$ receptors. $GABA_C$ receptors are found in the retina, spinal cord, superior colliculus, and pituitary.

Glycine

Many of the features described for the $GABA_A$ receptor family apply to the inhibitory glycine receptor that is prominent in the brainstem and spinal cord. Multiple subunits assemble into a variety of glycine receptor subtypes, the complete functional significance of which is not known.

Glutamate and Aspartate

Glutamate and aspartate have powerful excitatory effects on neurons in virtually every region of the CNS. Glutamate and possibly aspartate are the principal fast ("classical") excitatory transmitters throughout the CNS. Glutamate receptors are classed functionally either as ligand-gated ion channel ("ionotropic") receptors or as "metabotropic" GPCRs. Neither the precise number of subunits that form a functional glutamate ionotropic receptor ion channel in vivo nor the intramembranous topography of the subunits has been established unequivocally. The ligand-gated ion channels are further classified according to the identity of agonists that selectively activate each receptor subtype and are broadly divided into N-methyl-D-aspartate (NMDA) receptors and "non-NMDA" receptors. The non-NMDA receptors include the α-amino-3-hydroxy-5-methyl-4-isoxazole propionic acid (AMPA), and kainate receptors (Figure 12–4). Selective agonists and antagonists for NMDA receptors are available; the latter include open-channel blockers such as phencyclidine (PCP or "angel dust"), antagonists such as 5,7-dichlorokynurenic acid, which act *at an allosteric glycine-binding site, and the novel antagonist ifenprodil, which may act as a closed channel blocker. In addition, the activity of NMDA receptors can be modulated by pH and a variety of endogenous modulators including Zn^{2+}, some neurosteroids, arachidonic acid, redox reagents, and polyamines (e.g., spermine). Diversity of glutamate receptors arises by alternative splicing or by single-base editing of mRNAs encoding the receptors or receptor subunits. Alternative splicing has been described for metabotropic receptors and for subunits of NMDA, AMPA, and kainate receptors. AMPA and kainate receptors mediate fast depolarization at most glutamatergic synapses in the brain and spinal cord. NMDA receptors also are involved in normal synaptic transmission, but activation of NMDA receptors is associated more closely with the induction of various forms of synaptic plasticity rather than with fast point-to-point signaling in the brain. AMPA or kainate receptors and NMDA receptors may be co-localized at many glutamatergic synapses. A well-characterized phenomenon involving NMDA receptors is the induction of long-term potentiation (LTP). LTP refers to a prolonged (hours to days) increase in the size of a postsynaptic response to a presynaptic stimulus of given strength. Activation of NMDA receptors is obligatory for the induction of one type of LTP that occurs in the hippocampus. NMDA receptors normally are blocked by Mg^{2+} at resting membrane potentials. Thus, activation of NMDA receptors requires not only binding of synaptically released glutamate but also simultaneous depolarization of the postsynaptic membrane. This is achieved by activation of AMPA/kainate receptors at nearby synapses by inputs from different neurons. AMPA receptors also are dynamically regulated to affect their sensitivity to the synergism with NMDA. Thus, NMDA receptors may function as coincidence detectors, being activated only when there is simultaneous firing of two or more neurons. NMDA receptors also can induce long-term depression (LTD; the converse of LTP) at CNS synapses.*

Glutamate Excitotoxicity

High concentrations of glutamate produce neuronal cell death. The cascade of events leading to neuronal death is thought to be triggered by excessive activation of NMDA or AMPA/kainate receptors, allowing significant influx of Ca^{2+} into the neurons. Following a period of ischemia or hypoglycemia in the brain, NMDA receptor antagonists can attenuate neuronal cell death induced by activation of these receptors but cannot prevent all such damage. Glutamate-induced depletion of Na^+ and K^+ and small elevations of extracellular Zn^{2+} can activate necrotic and proapoptotic cascades, leading to neuronal death. Glutamate receptors are targets for therapeutic interventions (e.g., in chronic neurodegenerative diseases and schizophrenia; see Chapters 18 and 20).

ACETYLCHOLINE   In most regions of the CNS, the effects of ACh, assessed either by iontophoresis or by radioligand-binding assays, appear to be generated by interaction with a mixture of nicotinic and muscarinic receptors. Several presumptive cholinergic pathways have been proposed in addition to that of the motoneuron-Renshaw cell. Eight major clusters of ACh neurons and their pathways have been characterized.

CATECHOLAMINES   The brain contains separate neuronal systems that utilize three different catecholamines—dopamine (DA), norepinephrine (NE), and epinephrine (Epi). Each system is anatomically distinct and serves separate, but similar, functional roles within its field of innervation.

Dopamine

The CNS distributions of DA and NE differ markedly. More than half the CNS content of catecholamine is DA, with large amounts in the basal ganglia (especially the caudate nucleus), the nucleus accumbens, the olfactory tubercle, the central nucleus of the amygdala, the median eminence, and restricted fields of the frontal cortex. Most attention has been directed to the long projections between the major DA-containing nuclei in the substantia nigra and ventral tegmentum and their targets in the striatum, in the limbic zones of the cerebral cortex, and in other major limbic regions (but generally not in the hippocampus).

Initial pharmacological studies distinguished two subtypes of DA receptors: D_1 (which couples to G_s and adenylyl cyclase) and D_2 (which couples to G_i to inhibit adenylyl cyclase). Subsequent cloning studies identified three additional genes encoding subtypes of DA receptors: one resembling the D_1 receptor, D_5; and two resembling the D_2 receptor, D_3 and D_4, as well as two isoforms of the D_2 receptor that differ in the predicted length of their third intracellular loops, D_2 short and D_2 long. The D_1 and D_5 receptors activate adenylyl cyclase. The D_2 receptors couple to multiple effector systems, including the inhibition of adenylyl cyclase activity, suppression of Ca^{2+} currents, and activation of K^+ currents. The effector systems to which the D_3 and D_4 receptors *couple are not well defined. DA receptors have been implicated in the pathophysiology of schizophrenia and Parkinson's disease (see Chapters 18 and 20).*

Norepinephrine

There are relatively large amounts of NE within the hypothalamus and in certain zones of the limbic system (e.g., the central nucleus of the amygdala, the dentate gyrus of the hippocampus). NE also is present in lower amounts in most brain regions. Mapping studies indicate that noradrenergic neurons of the locus ceruleus innervate specific target cells in a large number of cortical, subcortical, and spinomedullary fields.

Three types of adrenergic receptors (α_1, α_2, and β) and their subtypes occur in the CNS; all are GPCRs and can be distinguished in terms of their pharmacological properties and their distribution (see Chapter 10). The β adrenergic receptors are coupled to stimulation of adenylyl cyclase activity. The α_1 adrenergic receptors are associated predominantly with neurons, while α_2 adrenergic receptors are more characteristic of glial and vascular elements. The α_1 receptors couple to G_q to stimulate phospholipase C. The α_1 receptors on noradrenergic target neurons of the neocortex and thalamus respond to NE with prazosin-sensitive, depolarizing responses due to decreases in K^+ conductances (both voltage sensitive and voltage insensitive). Stimulation of α_1 receptors also can augment cyclic AMP accumulation in neocortical slices in response to vasoactive intestinal polypeptide, possibly an example of G_q-G_S cross-talk involving Ca^{2+}/calmodulin and/or PKC. α_2 Adrenergic receptors are prominent on noradrenergic neurons, where they presumably couple to G_i, inhibit adenylyl cyclase, and mediate a hyperpolarizing response due to enhancement of an inwardly rectifying K^+ channel.

Epinephrine

Epinephrine-containing neurons are found in the medullary reticular formation and make restricted connections to a few pontine and diencephalic nuclei, coursing as far rostrally as the paraventricular nucleus of the dorsal midline thalamus. Their physiological properties have not been identified.

5-HYDROXYTRYPTAMINE

In the mammalian CNS, neurons containing 5-hydroxytryptamine (5-HT) are found in nine nuclei lying in or adjacent to the midline (raphe) regions of the pons and upper brainstem. Cells receiving 5-HT input, such as the suprachiasmatic nucleus, ventrolateral geniculate body, amygdala, and hippocampus, exhibit a uniform and dense investment of reactive terminals.

There are 14 distinct mammalian 5-HT receptor subtypes (see Chapter 11) that exhibit characteristic ligand-binding profiles, couple to different intracellular signaling systems, exhibit subtype-specific distributions within the CNS, and mediate distinct behavioral effects of 5-HT. The 5-HT receptors fall into four broad classes: the $5-HT_1$ and $5-HT_2$ classes both are GPCRs and include multiple isoforms within each class; the $5-HT_3$ receptor is a ligand-gated ion channel with structural similarity to the α subunit of the nicotinic ACh receptor. Members of the $5-HT_4$, $5-HT_5$, $5-HT_6$, and $5-HT_7$ classes all are GPCRs but have not been fully characterized in the CNS.

The $5-HT_1$ receptor subset contains at least five receptor subtypes ($5-HT_{1A}$, $5-HT_{1B}$, $5-HT_{1D}$, $5-HT_{1E}$, and $5-HT_{1F}$) that are linked to inhibition of adenylyl cyclase activity or to regulation of K^+ or Ca^{2+} channels. The $5-HT_{1A}$ receptors are abundantly expressed on 5-HT neurons of the dorsal raphe nucleus, where they are thought to be involved in temperature regulation. They also are found in regions of the CNS associated with mood and anxiety such as the hippocampus and amygdala. Activation of $5-HT_{1A}$ receptors opens an inwardly rectifying K^+ conductance, which leads to hyperpolarization and neuronal inhibition. These receptors can be activated by the drugs buspirone and ipsapirone, which are used to treat anxiety and panic disorders (see Chapter 17). In contrast, $5-HT_{1D}$ receptors are activated by the drug sumatriptan (used for acute management of migraine headaches; see Chapters 11 and 21).

The $5-HT_2$ receptor class has three subtypes: $5-HT_{2A}$, $5-HT_{2B}$, and $5-HT_{2C}$; all couple to pertussis toxin–insensitive G proteins (e.g., G_q and G_{11}) and link to activation of phospholipase C. $5-HT_{2A}$ receptors are enriched in forebrain regions such as the neocortex and olfactory tubercle, as well as in several nuclei arising from the brainstem. The $5-HT_{2C}$ receptor, similar in sequence and pharmacology to the $5-HT_{2A}$ receptor, is expressed abundantly in the choroid plexus, where it may modulate CSF production (see Chapter 11).

The $5-HT_3$ receptors function as ligand-gated ion channels and are expressed in the area postrema and solitary tract nucleus, where they couple to potent depolarizing responses that show rapid desensitization to continued 5-HT exposure. Actions of 5-HT at central $5-HT_3$ receptors can lead to emesis and antinociceptive actions, and $5-HT_3$ antagonists are beneficial in the management of chemotherapy-induced emesis (see Chapter 37).

5-HT$_4$ receptors occur on neurons within the inferior and superior colliculi and in the hippocampus. Activation of 5-HT$_4$ receptors stimulates the G$_s$-adenylyl cyclase–cyclic AMP pathway. The 5-HT$_6$ and 5-HT$_7$ receptors also couple to G$_s$-adenylyl cyclase; their affinity for clozapine may relate to its antipsychotic efficacy (see Chapters 11 and 18). Of the two subtypes of 5-HT$_5$ receptors, the 5-HT$_{5A}$ receptor seems to inhibit cyclic AMP synthesis, while 5-HT$_{5B}$ receptor-effector coupling has not been described.

The hallucinogen lysergic acid diethylamide (LSD) interacts with 5-HT, primarily through 5-HT$_2$ receptors. When applied iontophoretically, LSD and 5-HT both potently inhibit the firing of raphe (5-HT) neurons, whereas LSD and other hallucinogens are far more potent excitants on facial motoneurons that receive innervation from the raphe. The inhibitory effect of LSD on raphe neurons offers a plausible explanation for its hallucinogenic effects, namely that these effects result from depression of activity in a system that tonically inhibits visual and other sensory inputs. However, typical LSD-induced behavior is still seen in animals with destroyed raphe nuclei or after blockade of the synthesis of 5-HT by p-chlorophenylalanine.

HISTAMINE   Histaminergic neurons are located in the ventral posterior hypothalamus; they give rise to long ascending and descending tracts to the entire CNS. Based on the central effects of histamine antagonists, the histaminergic system is thought to regulate arousal, body temperature, and vascular dynamics.

There are four subtypes of histamine receptors; all are GPCRs. H$_1$ receptors, the most prominent, are located on glia, vessels, and neurons and act to mobilize Ca^{2+} in receptive cells through the G$_q$-PLC pathway. H$_2$ receptors couple via G$_S$ to the activation of adenylyl cyclase, perhaps in concert with H$_1$ receptors in certain circumstances. H$_3$ receptors, which have the greatest sensitivity to histamine, are localized in basal ganglia and olfactory regions; consequences of H$_3$ receptor activation remain unresolved but may include reduced Ca^{2+} influx and feedback inhibition of transmitter synthesis and release (see Chapter 24). The expression of H$_4$ receptors is confined to cells of hematopoietic origin: eosinophils, T cells, mast cells, basophils, and dendritic cells. H$_4$ receptors appear to couple to G$_{i/o}$ and G$_q$, and are postulated to play a role in inflammation and chemotaxis.

PEPTIDES   There are novel peptides in the CNS, each capable of regulating neural function, and peptides thought to be restricted to the gut or endocrine glands. While some CNS peptides may function individually, most appear to act in concert with coexisting transmitters (amines and amino acids). Some neurons may contain two or more transmitters, and their release can be independently regulated.

Since almost all peptides were identified initially on the basis of bioassays, their names reflect these biologically assayed functions (e.g., thyrotropin-releasing hormone and vasoactive intestinal polypeptide). A parsimonious view is that each peptide has unique messenger roles at the cellular level that are used repeatedly in functionally similar pathways within functionally distinct systems.

Peptides differ in several important respects from monoamine and amino acid transmitters. Peptide synthesis is performed in the rough endoplasmic reticulum. The propeptide is cleaved to the secreted form as secretory vesicles are transported from the perinuclear cytoplasm to the nerve terminals. Furthermore, no active recycling mechanisms for peptides have been described. This increases the dependency of peptidergic nerve terminals on distant sites of synthesis.

Since linear chains of amino acids can assume many conformations at their receptors, it is difficult to define the sequences and their steric relationships that are critical for activity. Thus, development of nonpeptidic synthetic agonists or antagonists that interact with specific peptide receptors has been difficult; similarly, morphine is only natural product that acts selectively at peptidergic synapses.

OTHER REGULATORY SUBSTANCES
Purines

Adenosine *and* uridine di- *and* triphosphates *have roles as extracellular signaling molecules. ATP is a component of the adrenergic storage vesicle and is released with catecholamines. Intracellular nucleotides may also reach the cell surface by other means and extracellular adenosine can result from cellular release or extracellular production from adenine nucleotides. Extracellular nucleotides and adenosine act on a family of purinergic receptors that is divided into two classes, P1 and P2. The P1 receptors are GPCRs that interact with adenosine; two of these receptors (A$_1$ and A$_3$) couple to G$_i$ and two (A$_{2a}$ and A$_{2b}$) couple to G$_s$; methylxanthines antagonize A$_1$ and A$_3$ receptors (see Chapter 27). Activation of A$_1$ receptors is associated with inhibition of adenylyl* *cyclase, activation of K^+ currents, and in some instances, with activation of PLC; stimulation of A_2 receptors activates adenylyl cyclase. The P2 class consists of a large number of P2X receptors that are ligand-gated ion channels, and of the P2Y receptors, a large subclass of GPCRs that couple to G_q or G_s and their associated effectors. $P2Y_{14}$ receptors are expressed in the CNS, interact with UDP-glucose, and may couple to G_q. The costorage of ATP and catecholamines in adrenergic storage vesicles and their co-release from adrenergic nerves suggests that P2Y receptors in the synaptic region will be stimulated whenever a nerve releases catecholamine. There is in vitro evidence for synergistic $G_q{\rightarrow}G_s$ cross talk (enhanced β adrenergic response) when β_2 receptors and G_q-linked P2Y receptors are activated simultaneously.*

Much current interest stems from pharmacological rather than physiological observations. Adenosine can act presynaptically throughout the cortex and hippocampal formation to inhibit the release of amine and amino acid transmitters. ATP-regulated responses have been linked pharmacologically to a variety of supracellular functions, including anxiety, stroke, and epilepsy.

Diffusible Mediators

Arachidonic acid can be liberated during phospholipid hydrolysis (by pathways involving phospholipases A_2, C, and D; see Chapter 1) and converted to local regulatory molecules by cyclooxygenases (leading to prostaglandins *and* thromboxanes), *lipoxygenases (leading to the* leukotrienes *and other transient catabolites of eicosatetraenoic acid), and CYPs (which are expressed at low levels in brain and are inducible)* (see *Chapter 25). Arachidonic acid metabolites have been implicated as diffusible modulators in the CNS, particularly for LTP and other forms of plasticity.*

In addition to its importance in the periphery as a regulator of vascular tone and inflammation, nitric oxide (NO) has roles in the CNS. Both constitutive and inducible forms of nitric oxide synthase (NOS) are expressed in the brain. Studies with potent inhibitors of NOS (e.g., *methyl arginine and nitroarginine) and NO donors* (e.g., *nitroprusside) have implicated NO in a host of CNS phenomena, including LTP, activation of the soluble guanylyl cyclase, neurotransmitter release, and enhancement of glutamate (NMDA)-mediated neurotoxicity. Carbon monoxide (CO) may be a second gaseous, labile, diffusible intercellular regulator.*

Cytokines

Cytokines are a family of polypeptide regulators produced throughout the body by cells of diverse embryological origin. Effects of cytokines are regulated by the conditions imposed by other cytokines, interacting as a network with variable effects leading to synergistic, additive, or opposing actions. Tissue-produced peptidic factors termed chemokines *serve to attract cells of the immune and inflammatory lines into interstitial spaces. These special cytokines have received much attention as potential regulators in nervous system inflammation (as in early stages of dementia, following infection with human immunodeficiency virus, and during recovery from traumatic injury). Neurons and astrocytes may be induced under some pathophysiological conditions to express cytokines or other growth factors.*

ACTIONS OF DRUGS IN THE CNS

SPECIFICITY AND NONSPECIFICITY OF CNS DRUG ACTIONS   Specificity of CNS-active drugs often is a property of the dose–response relationship of the drug and the cell or mechanisms under scrutiny (*see* Chapters 1 and 5). Even a drug that is highly specific when tested at a low concentration may exhibit nonspecific actions at higher doses. Conversely, even generally acting drugs may not act equally on all levels of the CNS. For example, sedatives, hypnotics, and general anesthetics would have very limited utility if central neurons that control the respiratory and cardiovascular systems were especially sensitive to their actions. Drugs with specific actions may produce nonspecific effects if the dose and route of administration produce high tissue concentrations.

Drugs whose mechanisms currently appear to be primarily general or nonspecific are classed according to whether they produce behavioral depression or stimulation. Specifically acting CNS drugs can be classed more definitively according to their locus of action or specific therapeutic usefulness. The absence of overt behavioral effects does not rule out the existence of important central actions for a given drug. For example, the impact of muscarinic cholinergic antagonists on the behavior of normal animals may be subtle, but these agents are used extensively in the treatment of movement disorders and motion sickness (*see* Chapter 7).

The specificity of a drug's action frequently is overestimated, partly because the drug is identified with the effect that is implied by the class name. Although selectivity of action may be remarkable, a drug usually affects several CNS functions to varying degrees.

General (Nonspecific) CNS Depressants

This category includes the anesthetic gases and vapors, the aliphatic alcohols, and some hypnotic-sedative drugs. These agents can depress excitable tissue at all levels of the CNS, leading to a decrease in the amount of transmitter released by the nerve impulse, as well as to general depression of postsynaptic responsiveness and ion movement. At sub-anesthetic concentrations, these agents (e.g., ethanol) can exert relatively specific effects on certain groups of neurons, which may account for differences in their behavioral effects, especially the propensity to produce dependence (see Chapters 13, 16, and 22).

General (Nonspecific) CNS Stimulants

In this category are pentylenetetrazol and related agents that are capable of powerful excitation of the CNS, and the methylxanthines, which have a much weaker stimulant action. Stimulation may be accomplished by one of two general mechanisms: (1) by blockade of inhibition or (2) by direct neuronal excitation (which may involve increased transmitter release, more prolonged transmitter action, labilization of the postsynaptic membrane, or decreased synaptic recovery time).

Drugs That Selectively Modify CNS Function

Modifiers may cause either depression or excitation, in some instances producing both effects simultaneously on different systems. Some modifiers have little effect on excitability in therapeutic doses. The principal classes of CNS modifiers are: anticonvulsants, drugs used in treating Parkinson's disease, opioid and nonopioid analgesics, appetite suppressants, antiemetics, analgesic-antipyretics, certain stimulants, neuroleptics (antidepressants and antimanic and antipsychotic agents), tranquilizers, sedatives, and hypnotics. Medications employed in the treatment of Alzheimer's disease (cholinesterase inhibitors and antiglutamate neuroprotectants) and compounds promising in the symptomatic treatment of Huntington's disease (tetrabenazine for the depletion of monoamines and reduction in tremor) may be included.

GENERAL CHARACTERISTICS OF CNS DRUGS Combinations of centrally acting drugs frequently are administered to therapeutic advantage (*e.g.*, an anticholinergic drug and levodopa for Parkinson's disease). However, other combinations of drugs may be detrimental because of potentially dangerous additive or mutually antagonistic effects.

The effect of a CNS drug is additive with the physiological state and with the effects of other depressant and stimulant drugs. For example, anesthetics are less effective in a hyperexcitable subject than in a normal patient; the converse is true for stimulants. In general, the depressant effects of drugs from all categories are additive (*e.g.*, the fatal combination of barbiturates or benzodiazepines with ethanol), as are the effects of stimulants. Therefore, respiration depressed by morphine is further impaired by depressant drugs, while stimulant drugs can augment the excitatory effects of morphine to produce vomiting and convulsions.

Antagonism between depressants and stimulants is variable. Some instances of true pharmacological antagonism among CNS drugs are known; for example, opioid antagonists selectively block the effects of opioid analgesics. However, the antagonism exhibited between two CNS drugs is usually physiological in nature. Thus, an individual whose CNS is depressed by an opiate cannot be returned entirely to normal by stimulation by caffeine.

The selective effects of drugs on specific neurotransmitter systems may be additive or competitive. This potential for drug interaction must be considered whenever such drugs are administered concurrently. To minimize such interactions, a drug-free period may be required when modifying therapy, and development of desensitized and supersensitive states with prolonged therapy may limit the speed with which one drug may be halted and another started. An excitatory effect is commonly observed with low concentrations of certain depressant drugs due either to depression of inhibitory systems or to a transient increase in the release of excitatory transmitters. Examples are the stage of excitement during induction of general anesthesia and the effects of alcohol to relieve inhibitions. The excitatory phase occurs only with low concentrations of the depressant; uniform depression ensues with increasing drug concentration. The excitatory effects can be minimized, when appropriate, by pretreatment with a depressant drug that is devoid of such effects (*e.g.*, benzodiazepines in preanesthetic medication). Acute, excessive stimulation of the cerebrospinal axis normally is followed by depression, which is in part a consequence of neuronal fatigue and exhaustion of stores of transmitters. Postictal depression is additive with the effects of depressant drugs. Acute, drug-induced depression generally is not followed by stimulation. However, chronic drug-induced sedation or depression may be followed by prolonged hyperexcitability upon abrupt withdrawal of the medication (barbiturates or alcohol). This type of hyperexcitability can be controlled effectively by the same or another depressant drug (*see* Chapters 16, 17, and 18).

Attempts to predict the behavioral or therapeutic consequences of drugs designed to elicit precise and restricted receptor actions in simple model systems may fail as a consequence of the complexity of the interactions possible, including differences between normal and diseased tissue.

For a complete Bibliographical listing see Goodman & Gilman's *The Pharmacological Basis of Therapeutics,* 11th ed., or Goodman & Gilman Online at www.accessmedicine.com.

GENERAL ANESTHETICS

General anesthetics depress the central nervous system (CNS) sufficiently to permit the performance of surgery and other noxious or unpleasant procedures. General anesthetics have low therapeutic indices and require great care in administration. While all general anesthetics produce a relatively similar anesthetic state, they differ in their secondary actions (side effects) on other organ systems. The selection of specific drugs and routes of administration to produce general anesthesia is based on their pharmacokinetic properties and on the secondary effects of the various drugs, in the context of the proposed diagnostic or surgical procedure and with the consideration of the individual patient's age, associated medical condition, and medication use. Anesthesiologists also employ sedatives (*see* Chapter 16), neuromuscular blocking agents (*see* Chapter 9), and local anesthetics (*see* Chapter 14)

GENERAL PRINCIPLES OF SURGICAL ANESTHESIA

The practice of anesthesia is usually neither therapeutic nor diagnostic, and the exceptions to this (*e.g.,* treatment of status asthmaticus with halothane and intractable angina with epidural local anesthetics) should not obscure this critical point. Hence, administration of general anesthesia and developments of new anesthetic agents and physiologic monitoring technology have been driven by three general objectives:

1. *Minimizing the potentially deleterious effects of anesthetic agents and techniques.*
2. *Sustaining physiologic homeostasis during surgical procedures* that may involve major blood loss, tissue ischemia, reperfusion of ischemic tissue, fluid shifts, exposure to a cold environment, and impaired coagulation.
3. *Improving postoperative outcomes* by choosing techniques that block or treat components of the *surgical stress response,* which may lead to short- or long-term sequelae.

Hemodynamic Effects of General Anesthesia The most prominent physiological effect of anesthesia induction is a decrease in systemic arterial blood pressure. The causes include direct vasodilation, myocardial depression, a blunting of baroreceptor control, and a generalized decrease in central sympathetic tone. The hypotensive response is enhanced by underlying volume depletion or preexisting myocardial dysfunction. Even anesthetics that show minimal hypotensive tendencies under normal conditions (*e.g., etomidate* and *ketamine*) must be used with caution in trauma victims, in whom intravascular volume depletion is being compensated by intense sympathetic discharge. Smaller-than-normal anesthetic dosages are employed in patients presumed to be sensitive to hemodynamic effects of anesthetics.

Respiratory Effects of General Anesthesia Airway maintenance is essential following induction of anesthesia, as nearly all general anesthetics reduce or eliminate both ventilatory drive and the reflexes that maintain airway patency. Therefore, ventilation generally must be assisted or controlled for at least some period during surgery. The gag reflex is lost, and the stimulus to cough is blunted. Lower esophageal sphincter tone also is reduced, so both passive and active regurgitation may occur. Endotracheal intubation is a major reason for a decline in the number of aspiration deaths during general anesthesia. Muscle relaxation is valuable during the induction of general anesthesia where it facilitates management of the airway, including endotracheal intubation. Neuromuscular blocking agents commonly are used to effect such relaxation (*see* Chapter 9), reducing the risk of coughing or gagging during laryngoscopic-assisted instrumentation of the airway and of aspiration prior to secure placement of an endotracheal tube. Alternatives to an endotracheal tube include a facemask and a laryngeal mask, an inflatable mask placed in the oropharynx forming a seal around the glottis.

Hypothermia Prevention of hypothermia has emerged as a major goal of anesthetic care. Patients commonly develop hypothermia (body temperature <36°C) during surgery. The reasons for hypothermia include low ambient temperature, exposed body cavities, cold intravenous fluids, altered thermoregulatory control, reduced metabolic rate, and peripheral vasodilation produced by anesthetics that permits heat transfer from the core to peripheral body compartments. General anesthetics lower the core temperature set point at which thermoregulatory vasoconstriction is activated to defend against heat loss. Metabolic rate and total body oxygen consumption decrease with general anesthesia by ~30%, reducing heat generation. Even small drops in body temperatures may increase perioperative morbidity, including cardiac complications, wound infections, and impaired coagulation.

Modalities to maintain normothermia include using warm intravenous fluids, heat exchangers in the anesthesia circuit, forced-warm-air covers, and new technology involving water-filled garments with microprocessor feedback control to a core temperature set point.

Nausea and Vomiting   Nausea and vomiting in the postoperative period continue to be significant problems following general anesthesia and are caused by an action of anesthetics on the chemoreceptor trigger zone and the brainstem vomiting center, which are modulated by serotonin (5-HT), histamine, acetylcholine, and dopamine. The 5-HT$_3$ receptor antagonist *ondansetron* (*see* Chapter 37) is very effective in suppressing nausea and vomiting. Common treatments also include *droperidol, metoclopramide, dexamethasone,* and avoidance of N$_2$O. The use of *propofol* as an induction agent and the nonsteroidal anti-inflammatory drug *ketorolac* as a substitute for opioids may decrease the incidence and severity of postoperative nausea and vomiting.

Other Emergence and Postoperative Phenomena   Physiological changes accompanying emergence from general anesthesia can be profound. Hypertension and tachycardia are common as the sympathetic nervous system regains its tone, which is enhanced by pain. Myocardial ischemia can appear or markedly worsen during emergence in patients with coronary artery disease. Emergence excitement occurs in 5–30% of patients and is characterized by tachycardia, restlessness, crying, moaning and thrashing, and various neurological signs. Postanesthesia shivering occurs frequently because of core hypothermia. A small dose of *meperidine* (12.5 mg) lowers the shivering trigger temperature and effectively stops the activity. The incidence of these emergence phenomena is greatly reduced when opioids are employed as part of the intraoperative regimen.

Airway obstruction may occur during the postoperative period because residual anesthetic effects continue to partially obtund consciousness and reflexes (especially in patients who normally snore or who have sleep apnea). Strong inspiratory efforts against a closed glottis can lead to negative-pressure pulmonary edema. Pulmonary function is reduced postoperatively following all types of anesthesia and surgery, and hypoxemia may occur. Hypertension can be prodigious, often requiring aggressive treatment.

Pain control can be complicated in the immediate postoperative period. Respiratory suppression associated with opioids can be problematic among postoperative patients with a substantial residual anesthetic effect. Patients can alternate between screaming in apparent agony and being deeply somnolent with airway obstruction, all in a matter of moments. The nonsteroidal antiinflammatory agent ketorolac (30–60 mg intravenously) frequently is effective, and the development of injectable cyclooxygenase-2 inhibitors (*see* Chapter 26) holds promise for analgesia without respiratory depression. In addition, regional anesthetic techniques are an important part of a perioperative multimodal approach that employs local anesthetic wound infiltration; epidural, spinal, and plexus blocks; and nonsteroidal anti-inflammatory drugs, opioids, α_2 adrenergic receptor agonists, and NMDA receptor antagonists. Patient-controlled administration of intravenous and epidural analgesics makes use of small, computerized pumps activated on demand but programmed with safety limits to prevent overdose. Agents used are intravenous opioids (frequently *morphine*), and opioid, local anesthetic, or both, by the epidural route. These techniques have revolutionized postoperative pain management, can be continued for hours or days, and promote ambulation and improved bowel function until oral pain medications are initiated.

ACTIONS AND MECHANISMS OF GENERAL ANESTHETICS
The Anesthetic State

General anesthetics produce a behavioral state referred to as *general anesthesia*, which can be defined as a global but reversible depression of CNS function resulting in the loss of response to and perception of all external stimuli. However, anesthesia is not simply a deafferented state (*e.g.,* amnesia is an important aspect of the anesthetic state), and not all general anesthetics produce identical patterns of deafferentation.

Components of the anesthetic state include *amnesia, immobility* in response to noxious stimulation, *attenuation of autonomic responses* to noxious stimulation, *analgesia,* and *unconsciousness.* General anesthesia is useful only insofar as it facilitates the performance of surgery or other noxious procedures. The performance of surgery usually requires an immobilized patient who does not have an excessive autonomic response to surgery (blood pressure and heart rate) and who has amnesia for the procedure. Thus, the essential components of the anesthetic state are immobilization, amnesia, and attenuation of autonomic responses to noxious stimulation. If an anesthetic produces profound amnesia, it can be difficult in principle to determine if it also produces either analgesia or unconsciousness.

Anesthetic Potency

The potency of general anesthetics usually is measured by determining the concentration of drug that prevents movement in response to surgical stimulation. For inhalational anesthetics, anesthetic potency is measured in MAC units, with 1 MAC defined as the *minimum alveolar concentration* that prevents movement in response to surgical stimulation in 50% of subjects. The strengths of MAC as a measurement are that (1) alveolar concentrations can be monitored continuously by measuring end-tidal anesthetic concentration using infrared spectroscopy or mass spectrometry; (2) it provides a direct correlate of the free concentration of the anesthetic at its site(s) of action in the CNS; (3) it is a simple-to-measure end point that reflects an important clinical goal. End points other than immobilization also can be used to measure anesthetic potency (*e.g.*, the ability to respond to verbal commands [MAC_{awake}] or to form memories; both are suppressed at a fraction of MAC) (Table 13–1). Potency of intravenous anesthetic agents is defined as the free plasma concentration (at equilibrium) that produces loss of response to surgical incision (or other end points) in 50% of subjects.

Sites and Mechanisms of Anesthesia

The molecular and cellular mechanisms by which general anesthetics produce their effects have remained one of the great mysteries of pharmacology.

SITES OF ACTION

In principle, general anesthetics could interrupt nervous system function at myriad levels, including peripheral sensory neurons, the spinal cord, the brainstem, and the cerebral cortex. Delineation of the precise anatomic sites of action is difficult because many anesthetics diffusely inhibit electrical activity in the CNS. Anesthetics may produce specific components of the anesthetic state via actions at specific sites in the CNS. Inhalational anesthetics produce immobilization in response to a surgical incision (the end point used in determining MAC) by action on the spinal cord. Given that amnesia or unconsciousness cannot result from anesthetic actions in the spinal cord, different components of anesthesia must be produced at different sites in the CNS. Indeed, the sedative effects of pentobarbital and propofol (GABAergic anesthetics) are mediated by $GABA_A$ receptors in the tuberomammillary nucleus, and the sedative effects of the intravenous anesthetic dexmedetomidine (an α_2 adrenergic receptor agonist) are produced via actions in the locus ceruleus, suggesting that the sedative actions of some anesthetics share the neuronal pathways involved in endogenous sleep. Inhalational anesthetics depress the excitability of thalamic neurons, pointing to the thalamus as a potential locus for the sedative effects of inhalational anesthetics, since blockade of thalamocortical communication would produce unconsciousness. Finally, both intravenous and inhalational anesthetics depress hippocampal neurotransmission, a probable locus for their amnestic effects.

CELLULAR MECHANISMS

General anesthetics produce two important physiologic effects at the cellular level. First, inhalational anesthetics hyperpolarize neurons, possibly an important effect on neurons serving a pacemaker role and on pattern-generating circuits and in synaptic communication, since reduced excitability in a postsynaptic neuron diminishes the likelihood that an action potential will be initiated in response to neurotransmitter release. Second, at anesthetizing concentrations, both inhalational and intravenous anesthetics have substantial effects on synaptic transmission and much smaller effects on action-potential generation or propagation. Inhalational anesthetics inhibit excitatory synapses and enhance inhibitory synapses via effects on pre- and postsynaptic sites. The inhalational anesthetic isoflurane clearly can inhibit neurotransmitter release and produce a small reduction in presynaptic action potential amplitude (3% reduction at MAC concentration) that inhibits neurotransmitter release, a significant effect because the reduced action potential is amplified into a larger reduction in presynaptic Ca^{2+} influx, and thence into an even greater reduction in transmitter release. Inhalational anesthetics also can act postsynaptically, to alter the response to released neurotransmitter, probably via actions at neurotransmitter receptors.

Intravenous anesthetics produce a narrower range of physiological effects, predominantly at the synapse, where they have profound and relatively specific effects on the postsynaptic response to released neurotransmitter. Most of the intravenous agents act predominantly by enhancing inhibitory neurotransmission, whereas ketamine predominantly inhibits excitatory neurotransmission at glutamatergic synapses.

MOLECULAR ACTIONS

There is strong evidence that ligand-gated ion channels are important targets for anesthetic action. Chloride channels gated by the inhibitory $GABA_A$ receptors (see Chapters 12 and 16) are sensitive

Table 13–1

Properties of Inhalational Anesthetic Agents

Anesthetic Agent	MAC*(vol %)	MAC_awake† (vol %)	EC_50‡ for Suppression of Memory (vol %)	Vapor Pressure (mm Hg at 20°C)	Partition Coefficient at 37°C			Recovered as Metabolites (%)
					Blood:Gas	Brain:Blood	Fat:Blood	
Halothane	0.75	0.41	—	243	2.3	2.9	51	20
Isoflurane	1.2	0.4	0.24	250	1.4	2.6	45	0.2
Enflurane	1.6	0.4	—	175	1.8	1.4	36	2.4
Sevoflurane	2	0.6	—	160	0.65	1.7	48	3
Desflurane	6	2.4	—	664	0.45	1.3	27	0.02
Nitrous oxide	105	60.0	52.5	Gas	0.47	1.1	2.3	0.004
Xenon	71	32.6	—	Gas	0.12	—	—	0

*MAC (minimum alveolar concentration) values are expressed as vol %, the percentage of the atmosphere that is anesthetic. A value of MAC greater than 100% means that hyperbaric conditions would be required.

†MAC_awake is the concentration at which appropriate responses to commands are lost.

‡EC_50 is the concentration that produces memory suppression in 50% of patients.

—, Not available.

to clinical concentrations of a wide variety of anesthetics, including the halogenated inhalational agents and many intravenous agents (propofol, barbiturates, etomidate, and neurosteroids). At clinical concentrations, general anesthetics increase the sensitivity of the $GABA_A$ receptor to GABA, thus enhancing inhibitory neurotransmission and depressing nervous system activity. This effect probably is mediated by binding of the anesthetics to specific sites on the $GABA_A$ receptor subunits, since point mutations of the receptor eliminate the effects. General anesthetics do not compete with GABA binding to the $GABA_A$ receptor; however, there likely are specific binding sites for several classes of anesthetics, since mutations in various regions (and subunits) of the $GABA_A$ receptor selectively affect the actions of various anesthetics. The capacity of propofol and etomidate to inhibit the response to noxious stimuli is mediated by a specific site on the β_3 subunit of the $GABA_A$ receptor; the sedative effects of these anesthetics are mediated by the same site on the β_2 subunit. These results indicate that two components of anesthesia can be mediated by $GABA_A$ receptors; for anesthetics other than propofol and etomidate, which components of anesthesia are produced by actions on $GABA_A$ receptors remains a matter of conjecture.

Clinical concentrations of inhalational anesthetics enhance the capacity of glycine to activate glycine-gated chloride channels (glycine receptors), which play an important role in inhibitory neurotransmission in the spinal cord and brainstem. Propofol, neurosteroids, and barbiturates also potentiate glycine-activated currents; etomidate and ketamine do not. Subanesthetic concentrations of the inhalational anesthetics inhibit some classes of neuronal nicotinic ACh receptors; these actions do not appear to mediate anesthetic immobilization but could mediate other components of anesthesia such as analgesia or amnesia.

The only general anesthetics that do not have significant effects on $GABA_A$ or glycine receptors are ketamine, nitrous oxide, cyclopropane, and xenon. These agents inhibit a different type of ligand-gated ion channel, the N-methyl-D-aspartate (NMDA) receptor (see Chapter 12). Ketamine inhibits NMDA receptors by binding to the phencyclidine site on the NMDA receptor protein. Nitrous oxide and xenon are potent and selective inhibitors of NMDA-activated currents; perhaps these agents produce unconsciousness via actions on NMDA receptors.

Inhalational anesthetics have two other known molecular targets that may mediate some of their actions. Halogenated inhalational anesthetics activate some members of a class of K^+ channels known as two-pore domain channels; xenon, nitrous oxide, and cyclopropane activate other two-pore domain channel family members. These channels are important in setting the resting membrane potential of neurons and may be the molecular locus through which these agents hyperpolarize neurons. A second target is the molecular machinery involved in neurotransmitter release. In Caenorhabditis elegans, the action of inhalational anesthetics requires a protein complex (syntaxin, SNAP-25, synaptobrevin) involved in synaptic neurotransmitter release. These molecular interactions may explain in part the capacity of inhalational anesthetics to cause presynaptic inhibition in the hippocampus and could contribute to the amnesic effect of inhalational anesthetics.

PARENTERAL ANESTHETICS
Pharmacokinetic Principles

Parenteral anesthetics are small, hydrophobic, substituted aromatic or heterocyclic compounds (Figure 13–1). Hydrophobicity is the key factor governing their pharmacokinetics. After a single intravenous bolus, these drugs preferentially partition into the highly perfused and lipophilic tissues of the brain and spinal cord where they produce anesthesia within a single circulation time. Subsequently, blood levels fall rapidly, resulting in drug redistribution out of the CNS back into the blood. The anesthetic then diffuses into less perfused tissues such as muscle and viscera, and at a slower rate into the poorly perfused but very hydrophobic adipose tissue. Termination of anesthesia after single boluses of parenteral anesthetics primarily reflects redistribution out of the CNS rather than metabolism. After redistribution, anesthetic blood levels fall according to a complex interaction between the metabolic rate and the amount and lipophilicity of the drug stored in the peripheral compartments. Thus, parenteral anesthetic half-lives are "context-sensitive," and the degree to which a $t_{1/2}$ is contextual varies greatly from drug to drug, as might be predicted based on their differing hydrophobicities and metabolic clearances (Table 13–2 and Figure 13–2). Most individual variability in sensitivity to parenteral anesthetics can be accounted for by pharmacokinetic factors. For example, in patients with lower cardiac output, the relative perfusion of and fraction of anesthetic dose delivered to the brain is higher; thus, patients in septic shock or with cardiomyopathy usually require lower doses of anesthetic. The elderly also typically require a smaller anesthetic dose, primarily because of a smaller initial volume of distribution.

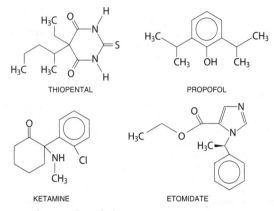

FIGURE 13–1 *Structures of parenteral anesthetics.*

Thiopental and propofol are the two most commonly used parenteral agents. Thiopental has a long-established track record of safety. Propofol is advantageous for procedures where rapid return to a preoperative mental status is desirable. Etomidate usually is reserved for patients at risk for hypotension and/or myocardial ischemia. Ketamine is best suited for patients with asthma or for children undergoing short, painful procedures.

SPECIFIC PARENTERAL AGENTS
Barbiturates
CHEMISTRY AND FORMULATIONS
The three barbiturates used for clinical anesthesia are sodium thiopental *(Figure 13–1),* thiamylal, *and* methohexital. *Thiopental (PENTOTHAL) is most frequently used for inducing anesthesia. Barbiturates are formulated as the sodium salts and reconstituted in water or isotonic saline to produce alkaline solutions (pHs of 10–11). Once reconstituted, thiobarbiturates are stable in solution for up to 1 week.* Mixing with more acidic drugs commonly used during anesthetic induction can result in precipitation of the barbiturate as the free acid; thus, standard practice is to delay the administration of other drugs until the barbiturate has cleared the intravenous tubing.

DOSAGES AND CLINICAL USE   Recommended intravenous dosing for parenteral anesthetics in a healthy young adult is given in Table 13–2.

The typical induction dose (3–5 mg/kg) of thiopental produces unconsciousness in 10–30 seconds with a peak effect in 1 minute and duration of anesthesia of 5–8 minutes. Neonates and infants usually require a higher induction dose (5–8 mg/kg); elderly and pregnant patients require less (1–3 mg/kg). Dosage calculation based on lean body mass reduces individual variation in dosage requirements. Doses can be reduced by 10–50% after premedication with benzodiazepines, opiates, or α_2 adrenergic agonists, because of their additive hypnotic effect. Thiamylal is approximately equipotent with and in all aspects similar to thiopental. Methohexital (BREVITAL) is threefold more potent but otherwise similar to thiopental in onset and duration of action. Thiopental and thiamylal produce little to no pain on injection; methohexital elicits mild pain. Veno-irritation can be reduced by injection into larger non-hand veins and by prior intravenous injection of lidocaine (0.5–1 mg/kg). Intra-arterial injection of thiobarbiturates can induce a severe inflammatory and potentially necrotic reaction and should be avoided. Thiopental often evokes the taste of garlic just prior to inducing anesthesia. Methohexital and to a lesser degree the other barbiturates can produce excitement phenomena such as muscle tremor, hypertonus, and hiccups. For induction of pediatric patients without IV access, all three drugs can be given per rectum at approximately tenfold the IV dose.

PHARMACOKINETICS AND METABOLISM   Pharmacokinetic parameters for parenteral anesthetics are given in Table 13–2. As discussed above, the principal mechanism limiting anesthetic duration after single doses is redistribution of these hydrophobic drugs from the brain to other tissues. However, after multiple doses or infusions, the duration of action of the barbiturates varies considerably depending on their clearances.

Table 13–2

Pharmacological Properties of Parenteral Anesthetics

Drug	Formulation	IV Induction Dose (mg/kg)	Minimal Hypnotic Level (μg/mL)	Induction Dose Duration (min)	$T_{1/2\beta}$ (hours)	CL (mL·min^{-1}·kg^{-1})	Protein Binding (%)	V_{ss} (L/kg)
Thiopental	25 mg/mL in aqueous solution + 1.5 mg/mL Na$_2$CO$_3$; pH = 10–11	3–5	15.6	5–8	12.1	3.4	85	2.3
Methohexital	10 mg/mL in aqueous solution + 1.5 mg/mL Na$_2$CO$_3$; pH = 10–11	1–2	10	4–7	3.9	10.9	85	2.2
Propofol	10 mg/mL in 10% soybean oil, 2.25% glycerol, 1.2% egg PL, 0.005% EDTA or 0.025% Na-MBS; pH = 4.5–7	1.5–2.5	1.1	4–8	1.8	30	98	2.3
Etomidate	2 mg/mL in 35% PG; pH = 6.9	0.2–0.4	0.3	4–8	2.9	17.9	76	2.5
Ketamine	10, 50, or 100 mg/mL in aqueous solution; pH = 3.5–5.5	0.5–1.5	1	10–15	3.0	19.1	27	3.1

ABBREVIATIONS: $t_{1/2\beta}$, β phase half-life; CL, clearance; V_{ss}, volume of distribution at steady state; EDTA, ethylenediaminetetraacetic acid; Na-MBS, Na-metabisulfite; PG, propylene glycol; PL, phospholipid.

227

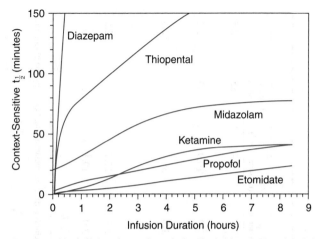

FIGURE 13–2 *Context-sensitive half-time of general anesthetics.* The duration of action of single intravenous doses of anesthetic/hypnotic drugs is similarly short for all and is determined by redistribution of the drugs away from their active sites. However, after prolonged infusions, drug half-lives and durations of action are dependent on a complex interaction between the rate of redistribution of the drug, the amount of drug accumulated in fat, and the drug's metabolic rate. This phenomenon has been termed the *context-sensitive half-time*; that is, the half-time of a drug can be estimated only if one knows the context—the total dose and over what time period it has been given. Note that the half-times of some drugs such as etomidate, propofol, and ketamine increase only modestly with prolonged infusions; others (*e.g.*, diazepam and thiopental) increase dramatically.

All three barbiturates are primarily eliminated by hepatic metabolism and renal excretion of inactive metabolites; a small fraction of thiopental undergoes desulfuration to the longer-acting hypnotic pentobarbital. Each drug is highly protein bound (Table 13–2). Hepatic disease or other conditions that reduce serum protein concentration will decrease the volume of distribution and thereby increase the initial free concentration and hypnotic effect of an induction dose.

SIDE EFFECTS

Nervous System Besides producing general anesthesia, barbiturates reduce the cerebral oxygen consumption (CMR_{O_2}) in a dose-dependent manner. As a consequence, cerebral blood flow and intracranial pressure are similarly reduced.

Because it markedly lowers cerebral metabolism, thiopental has been used as a protectant against cerebral ischemia. At least one human study suggests that thiopental may be efficacious in ameliorating ischemic damage in the perioperative setting. Thiopental also reduces intraocular pressure. Perhaps due to their CNS depressant activity, barbiturates are effective anticonvulsants; thiopental in particular is effective in the treatment of status epilepticus.

Cardiovascular *The anesthetic barbiturates produce dose-dependent decreases in blood pressure* that are due primarily to vasodilation, particularly venodilation, and to a lesser degree to a direct decrease in cardiac contractility. Typically, heart rate increases as a compensatory response to a lower blood pressure, although barbiturates also blunt the baroreceptor reflex.

Thiopental is not contraindicated in patients with coronary artery disease because the ratio of myocardial oxygen supply to demand appears to be adequately maintained within a patient's normal blood pressure range.

Respiratory *Barbiturates are respiratory depressants.* Induction doses of thiopental decrease minute ventilation and tidal volume with a smaller and inconsistent decrease in respiratory rate; reflex responses to hypercarbia and hypoxia are diminished by anesthetic barbiturates; at higher doses or in the presence of other respiratory depressants such as opiates, apnea can result. With the exception of uncommon anaphylactoid reactions, these drugs have little effect on bronchomotor tone and can be used safely in asthmatics.

Other Side Effects

Short-term administration of barbiturates has no clinically significant effect on the hepatic, renal, or endocrine systems. A single induction dose of thiopental does not alter tone of the gravid uterus, but may produce mild transient depression of newborn activity. Drug-induced histamine release is occasionally seen. Barbiturates can induce fatal attacks of porphyria in patients with acute intermittent or variegate porphyria and are contraindicated in such patients. Unlike inhalational anesthetics and succinylcholine, barbiturates and all other parenteral anesthetics apparently do not trigger malignant hyperthermia.

Propofol

CHEMISTRY AND FORMULATIONS

Propofol (DIPRIVAN Figure 13–1) is the most commonly used parenteral anesthetic in the U.S. The drug is insoluble in aqueous solutions and is formulated only for IV administration as a 1% (10 mg/mL) emulsion in 10% soybean oil, 2.25% glycerol, and 1.2% purified egg phosphatide. Significant bacterial contamination of open containers has been associated with serious patient infection; propofol should be either administered or discarded shortly after removal from sterile packaging.

DOSAGE AND CLINICAL USE   The induction dose, onset, and duration of anesthesia are similar to thiopental (Table 13–2). Dosages should be reduced in the elderly and in the presence of other sedatives and increased in young children. Because of its reasonably short elimination $t_{1/2}$, propofol often is used for maintenance of anesthesia as well as for induction. For short procedures, small boluses (10–50% of the induction dose) every 5 minutes or as needed are effective. An infusion of propofol (100–300 μg/kg/min) produces a more stable drug level and is better suited for longer-term anesthetic maintenance. Sedating doses of propofol are 20–50% of those required for general anesthesia. However, even at these lower doses, caregivers should be prepared for all of the side effects of propofol, particularly airway obstruction and apnea. Propofol elicits pain on injection that can be reduced with lidocaine and the use of larger arm and antecubital veins. Excitatory phenomena during induction with propofol occur at about the same frequency as with thiopental.

PHARMACOKINETICS AND METABOLISM

The pharmacokinetics of propofol are summarized in Table 13–2. Propofol's duration after infusion (shorter than that of thiopental) can be explained by its very high clearance, coupled with the slow diffusion of drug from the peripheral to the central compartment. The rapid clearance of propofol explains its less severe hangover compared with barbiturates and may allow for a more rapid discharge from the recovery room. Propofol is metabolized in the liver to less active metabolites that are renally excreted Propofol is highly protein bound, and its pharmacokinetics, like those of the barbiturates, may be affected by conditions that alter serum protein levels.

SIDE EFFECTS

Nervous System   The CNS effects of propofol are similar to those of barbiturates, but, unlike thiopental, propofol is not a proven acute intervention for seizures.

Cardiovascular   Propofol produces a dose-dependent decrease in blood pressure that is significantly greater than that produced by thiopental; the effect is explained by vasodilation and mild depression of myocardial contractility. Propofol appears to blunt the baroreceptor reflex or is directly vagotonic. As with thiopental, propofol should be used with caution in patients at risk for or intolerant of decreases in blood pressure.

Respiratory and Other Side Effects   At equipotent doses, propofol produces a slightly greater degree of respiratory depression than thiopental. Patients given propofol should be monitored to ensure adequate oxygenation and ventilation. Propofol has significant antiemetic action and is a good choice for sedation or anesthesia of patients at high risk for nausea and vomiting. Propofol provokes anaphylactoid reactions and histamine release at about the same low frequency as thiopental. Propofol is considered safe for use in pregnant women, and like thiopental, only transiently depresses activity in the newborn.

Etomidate

CHEMISTRY AND FORMULATION

Etomidate (Figure 13–1) is poorly soluble in water and is formulated as a 2 mg/mL solution in 35% propylene glycol. Unlike thiopental, etomidate does not induce precipitation of neuromuscular blockers or other drugs frequently given during anesthetic induction.

DOSAGE AND CLINICAL USE Etomidate (AMIDATE) is primarily used for anesthetic induction of patients at risk for hypotension.

Induction doses (Table 13–2) are accompanied by a high incidence of pain on injection and myoclonic movements. Lidocaine effectively reduces the pain of injection; myoclonic movements can be reduced by premedication with either benzodiazepines or opiates. Long-term infusions are not recommended for reasons discussed below.

PHARMACOKINETICS AND METABOLISM

An induction dose of etomidate has a rapid onset; redistribution limits the duration of action (Table 13–2). Metabolism occurs in the liver, primarily to inactive compounds. Elimination is both renal (78%) and biliary (22%). Compared to thiopental, the duration of action of etomidate increases less with repeated doses (Figure 13–2).

SIDE EFFECTS

Nervous System The effects of etomidate on cerebral blood flow, metabolism, and intracranial pressure (ICP) and intraocular pressure are similar to those of thiopental. Etomidate is not a proven treatment for seizures.

Cardiovascular Cardiovascular stability after induction is a major advantage of etomidate over either barbiturates or propofol. Induction doses of etomidate typically produce a small increase in heart rate and little or no decrease in blood pressure or cardiac output. Etomidate has little effect on coronary perfusion pressure while reducing myocardial O_2 consumption. Thus, of all induction agents, etomidate is best suited to maintain cardiovascular stability in patients with coronary artery disease, cardiomyopathy, cerebral vascular disease, or hypovolemia.

Respiratory and Other Side Effects The degree of respiratory depression due to etomidate is less than that due to thiopental. Etomidate may induce hiccups but does not significantly stimulate histamine release. Despite minimal cardiac and respiratory effects, etomidate has two major drawbacks: etomidate has been associated with nausea and vomiting; second, the drug inhibits adrenal biosynthetic enzymes required for the production of cortisol and other steroids, possibly inhibiting the adrenocortical stress response. Even single induction doses of etomidate may mildly and transiently reduce cortisol levels. Thus, while etomidate is not recommended for long-term infusion, it appears safe for anesthetic induction and has some unique advantages in patients prone to hemodynamic instability.

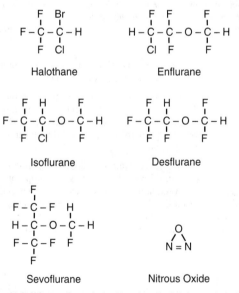

FIGURE 13–3 *Structures of inhaled general anesthetics.* Note that all *inhaled* general anesthetic agents except nitrous oxide and halothane are ethers and that fluorine progressively replaces other halogens in the development of the halogenated agents. All structural differences are associated with important differences in pharmacological properties.

Ketamine

CHEMISTRY AND FORMULATION

Ketamine is a congener of phencyclidine (Figure 13–1). Although more lipophilic than thiopental, ketamine is water soluble.

DOSAGE AND CLINICAL USE

Ketamine (KETALAR, others) has unique properties that make it useful for anesthetizing patients at risk for hypotension and bronchospasm and for certain pediatric procedures. However, significant side effects limit its routine use. Ketamine rapidly produces a hypnotic state quite distinct from that of other anesthetics. Patients have profound analgesia, unresponsiveness to commands, and amnesia, but may have their eyes open, move their limbs involuntarily, and breathe spontaneously, a cataleptic state that has been termed *dissociative anesthesia.*

Ketamine typically is administered intravenously but also is effective by intramuscular, oral, and rectal routes. Ketamine does not elicit pain on injection or true excitatory behavior as described for methohexital, although involuntary movements produced by ketamine can be mistaken for anesthetic excitement.

PHARMACOKINETICS AND METABOLISM

The onset and duration of an induction dose of ketamine (Table 13–2) are determined by the same distribution/redistribution mechanism operant for all the other parenteral anesthetics.

Ketamine is hepatically metabolized to norketamine, which has reduced CNS activity; norketamine is further metabolized and excreted in urine and bile. Ketamine has a large volume of distribution and rapid clearance that make it suitable for continuous infusion without the drastic lengthening in duration of action seen with thiopental (Table 13–2 and Figure 13–2).

SIDE EFFECTS

Nervous System Ketamine has indirect sympathomimetic activity and produces distinct behavioral effects. The ketamine-induced cataleptic state is accompanied by nystagmus with pupillary dilation, salivation, lacrimation, and spontaneous limb movements with increased overall muscle tone. Although ketamine does not produce the classic anesthetic state, patients are amnestic and unresponsive to painful stimuli. Ketamine produces profound analgesia, a distinct advantage over other parenteral anesthetics.

Unlike other parenteral anesthetics, ketamine increases cerebral blood flow and ICP with minimal alteration of cerebral metabolism. These effects can be attenuated by concurrent administration of thiopental and/or benzodiazepines along with hyperventilation. However, given that other anesthetics actually reduce ICP and cerebral metabolism, ketamine is relatively contraindicated for patients with increased ICP or those at risk for cerebral ischemia. The effects of ketamine on seizure activity are mixed. Emergence delirium characterized by hallucinations is a frequent complication of ketamine that can result in serious patient dissatisfaction and can complicate postoperative management. Delirium is most frequent in the first hour after emergence and appear to occur less frequently in children; benzodiazepines reduce the incidence of emergence delirium.

Cardiovascular System Unlike other anesthetics, induction doses of ketamine typically increase blood pressure, heart rate, and cardiac output. The cardiovascular effects are indirect and are most

Table 13–3

Some Pharmacological Effects of Parenteral Anesthetics*

Drug	CBF	CMR_{O_2}	ICP	MAP	HR	CO	RR	$\dot{V}_E$
Thiopental	---	---	---	-	+	-	-	--
Etomidate	---	---	---	0	0	0	-	-
Ketamine	++	0	++	+	++	+	0	0
Propofol	---	---	---	--	+	-	--	---

ABBREVIATIONS: CBF, cerebral blood flow; CMR_{O_2}, cerebral oxygen consumption; ICP, intracranial pressure; MAP, mean arterial pressure; HR, heart rate; CO, cardiac output; RR, respiratory rate; $\dot{V}_E$, minute ventilation.

*Typical effects of a single induction dose in human beings.

Qualitative scale from --- to +++ = slight, moderate, or large decrease or increase, respectively; 0 indicates no significant change.

likely mediated by inhibition of both central and peripheral catecholamine reuptake. Ketamine has direct negative inotropic and vasodilating activity, but these effects usually are overwhelmed by the indirect sympathomimetic action. Thus, ketamine is a useful drug, along with etomidate, for patients at risk for hypotension during anesthesia. Ketamine increases myocardial oxygen consumption and is not an ideal drug for patients at risk for myocardial ischemia.

Respiratory System The respiratory effects of ketamine are perhaps the best indication for its use. Induction doses of ketamine produce small and transient decreases in minute ventilation, but respiratory depression is less severe than with other general anesthetics. Ketamine is a potent bronchodilator and is well-suited for anesthetizing patients at high risk for bronchospasm.

INHALATIONAL ANESTHETICS

Structures of the currently used inhalational anesthetics are shown in Figure 13–3. One of the troublesome properties of the inhalational anesthetics is their low safety margin. The inhalational anesthetics have therapeutic indices (LD_{50}/ED_{50}) that range from 2–4, making these among the most dangerous drugs in clinical use. The toxicity of these drugs is largely a function of their side effects, and each of the inhalational anesthetics has a unique side-effect profile. Hence, the selection of an inhalational anesthetic often is based on matching a patient's pathophysiology with drug side-effect profiles. The inhalational anesthetics also vary widely in their physical properties (Table 13–1), which govern the pharmacokinetics of the inhalational agents. Ideally, an inhalational agent would produce a rapid induction of anesthesia and a rapid recovery following discontinuation.

Pharmacokinetic Principles

The fact that these agents behave as gases rather than as liquids requires that different pharmacokinetic constructs be used in analyzing their uptake and distribution. Inhalational anesthetics distribute between tissues (or between blood and gas) such that equilibrium is achieved when the partial pressure of anesthetic gas is equal in the two tissues. When a person has breathed an inhalational anesthetic for a sufficiently long time that all tissues are equilibrated with the anesthetic, the partial pressure of the anesthetic in all tissues will be equal to the partial pressure of the anesthetic in inspired gas. However, while the partial pressure of the anesthetic may be equal in all tissues, the concentration of anesthetic in each tissue will be different; indeed, anesthetic partition coefficients are defined as the ratio of anesthetic concentrations in two tissues when the partial pressures of anesthetic are equal in the two tissues. Blood:gas, brain:blood, and fat:blood partition coefficients (Table 13–1) show that inhalational anesthetics are more soluble in some tissues (*e.g.,* fat) than they are in others (*e.g.,* blood), and that there is significant range in the solubility of the various inhalational agents.

In clinical practice, one can monitor the equilibration of a patient with anesthetic gas. Equilibrium is achieved when the partial pressure in inspired gas is equal to the partial pressure in end-tidal (alveolar) gas. This defines equilibrium because it is the point at which there is no net uptake of anesthetic from the alveoli into the blood. For inhalational agents that are not very soluble in blood or any other tissue, equilibrium is achieved quickly (*e.g.,* nitrous oxide, Figure 13–4). If an agent is more soluble in a tissue such as fat, equilibrium may take many hours to reach. This occurs because fat represents a huge anesthetic reservoir that will be filled slowly because of the modest blood flow to fat (*e.g.,* halothane, Figure 13–4).

In considering the pharmacokinetics of anesthetics, one important parameter is the speed of anesthetic induction. Anesthesia is produced when anesthetic partial pressure in brain is ≥MAC. Because the brain is well perfused, anesthetic partial pressure in brain becomes equal to the partial pressure in alveolar gas (and in blood) over the course of several minutes. Therefore, anesthesia is achieved shortly after alveolar partial pressure reaches MAC. While the rate of rise of alveolar partial pressure will be slower for anesthetics that are highly soluble in blood and other tissues, this limitation on speed of induction can be overcome largely by delivering higher inspired partial pressures of the anesthetic.

Elimination of inhalational anesthetics is largely the reverse process of uptake. For agents with low blood and tissue solubility, recovery from anesthesia should mirror anesthetic induction, regardless of the duration of administration. For inhalational agents with high blood and tissue solubility, recovery will be a function of the duration of administration, because anesthetic accumulated in the fat reservoir will prevent blood (and therefore alveolar) partial pressures from falling rapidly. Patients will be arousable when alveolar partial pressure reaches MAC_{awake}, a partial pressure somewhat lower than MAC (Table 13–1).

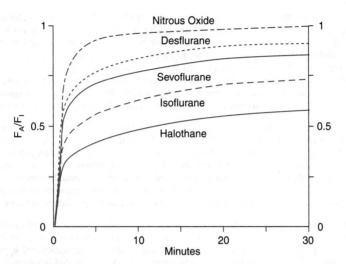

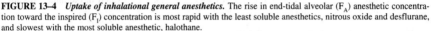

FIGURE 13–4 *Uptake of inhalational general anesthetics.* The rise in end-tidal alveolar (F_A) anesthetic concentration toward the inspired (F_I) concentration is most rapid with the least soluble anesthetics, nitrous oxide and desflurane, and slowest with the most soluble anesthetic, halothane.

Halothane

CHEMISTRY AND FORMULATION

Halothane (FLUOTHANE Figure 13–3) is a volatile liquid at room temperature and must be stored in a sealed container. Because halothane is light-sensitive and subject to spontaneous breakdown, it is marketed in amber bottles with thymol added as a preservative. Mixtures of halothane with oxygen or air are neither flammable nor explosive.

PHARMACOKINETICS

Halothane has a relatively high blood:gas partition coefficient and high fat:blood partition coefficient (Table 13–1). Thus, induction with halothane is relatively slow, and the alveolar halothane concentration remains substantially lower than the inspired halothane concentration for many hours of administration. Since halothane accumulates in tissues during prolonged administration, the speed of recovery from halothane is lengthened as a function of duration of administration.

Approximately 60–80% of halothane taken up by the body is eliminated unchanged via the lungs in the first 24 hours after its administration. A substantial amount of the halothane not eliminated in exhaled gas is biotransformed by hepatic CYPs. Trifluoroacetylchloride, an intermediate in oxidative metabolism of halothane, can trifluoroacetylate several proteins in the liver. An immune reaction to these altered proteins may be responsible for the rare cases of fulminant halothane-induced hepatic necrosis.

CLINICAL USE   Halothane is a potent, nonpungent and well-tolerated agent that usually is used for maintenance of anesthesia and is well tolerated for inhalation induction of anesthesia, most commonly in children, in whom preoperative placement of an intravenous catheter can be difficult. Anesthesia is produced by halothane at end-tidal concentrations of 0.7–1%. The use of halothane in the U.S. has diminished substantially since the introduction of newer inhalational agents with better pharmacokinetic and side-effect profiles.

SIDE EFFECTS

Cardiovascular System   The most predictable side effect of halothane is a dose-dependent reduction in arterial blood pressure. Mean arterial pressure typically decreases ~20–25% at MAC concentrations of halothane, primarily as a result of direct myocardial depression, and perhaps an inability of the heart to respond to the effector arm of the baroreceptor reflex. Halothane-induced reductions in blood pressure and heart rate generally disappear after several hours of constant halothane administration, presumably because of progressive sympathetic stimulation.

Halothane dilates the vascular beds of the skin and brain, whereas autoregulation of renal, splanchnic, and cerebral blood flow is inhibited by halothane, leading to reduced perfusion of these organs in the face of reduced blood pressure. Coronary autoregulation is largely preserved. Halothane inhibits hypoxic pulmonary vasoconstriction, leading to increased perfusion to poorly ventilated regions of the lung and an increased alveolar:arterial oxygen gradient.

Sinus bradycardia and atrioventricular rhythms occur frequently during halothane anesthesia but usually are benign and result mainly from a direct depressive effect of halothane on sinoatrial node discharge. Halothane also can sensitize the myocardium to the arrhythmogenic effects of epinephrine.

Respiratory System   Spontaneous respiration is rapid and shallow during halothane anesthesia. The decreased alveolar ventilation results in an elevation in arterial CO_2 tension from 40 mm Hg to >50 mm Hg at 1 MAC. The elevated CO_2 does not provoke a compensatory increase in ventilation, because halothane causes a concentration-dependent inhibition of the ventilatory response to CO_2. Halothane also inhibits peripheral chemoceptor responses to arterial hypoxemia. Thus, neither hemodynamic (tachycardia and hypertension) nor ventilatory responses to hypoxemia are observed during halothane anesthesia, making it prudent to monitor arterial oxygenation directly.

Nervous System   Halothane dilates the cerebral vasculature, increasing cerebral blood flow under most conditions. This increase in blood flow can increase intracranial pressure in patients with space-occupying intracranial masses, brain edema, or preexisting intracranial hypertension. Thus, halothane is relatively contraindicated in patients at risk for elevated intracranial pressure. Halothane also attenuates autoregulation of cerebral blood flow.

Muscle   Halothane causes some relaxation of skeletal muscle *via* its central depressant effects and potentiates the actions of nondepolarizing muscle relaxants (curariform drugs; *see* Chapter 9), increasing both their duration of action and the magnitude of their effect. Halothane and the other halogenated inhalational anesthetics can trigger malignant hyperthermia; this syndrome frequently is fatal and is treated by immediate discontinuation of the anesthetic and administration of dantrolene.

Halothane relaxes uterine smooth muscle, a useful property for manipulation of the fetus (version) in the prenatal period and for delivery of retained placenta.

Kidney, Liver, and GI Tract   Patients anesthetized with halothane usually produce a small volume of concentrated urine, a consequence of halothane-induced reduction of renal blood flow and glomerular filtration rate. Halothane-induced changes in renal function are fully reversible and are not associated with long-term nephrotoxicity.

Halothane reduces splanchnic and hepatic blood flow. Halothane can produce fulminant hepatic necrosis in a small number of patients, a syndrome characterized by fever, anorexia, nausea, and vomiting, developing several days after anesthesia and sometimes accompanied by a rash and peripheral eosinophilia. There is a rapid progression to hepatic failure, with a fatality rate of ~50%. This syndrome occurs in about 1 in 10,000 patients receiving halothane and is referred to as halothane hepatitis. Halothane hepatitis may be the result of an immune response to hepatic proteins that become trifluoroacetylated as a consequence of halothane metabolism (*see* Pharmacokinetics, above).

Isoflurane

CHEMISTRY AND PHYSICAL PROPERTIES

Isoflurane (FORANE, others Figure 13–3) is a volatile liquid at room temperature and is neither flammable nor explosive in mixtures of air or oxygen.

PHARMACOKINETICS

Isoflurane has a blood:gas partition coefficient substantially lower than that of halothane or enflurane (Table 13–1). Consequently, induction with isoflurane and recovery from isoflurane are relatively rapid. More than 99% of inhaled isoflurane is excreted unchanged via *the lungs. Isoflurane does not appear to be a mutagen, teratogen, or carcinogen.*

CLINICAL USE   Isoflurane is typically used for maintenance of anesthesia *after induction* with other agents because of its pungent odor, but induction of anesthesia can be achieved in <10 minutes with an inhaled concentration of 3% isoflurane in O_2; this concentration is reduced to 1–2% for maintenance of anesthesia. Use of drugs (*e.g.*, opioids, nitrous oxide) reduces the concentration of isoflurane required for surgical anesthesia.

SIDE EFFECTS

Cardiovascular System   Isoflurane produces a concentration-dependent decrease in arterial blood pressure; cardiac output is maintained and hypotension is the result of decreased systemic vascular resistance. Vasodilation occurs in most vascular beds, particularly in skin and muscle. Isoflurane is a potent coronary vasodilator, simultaneously producing increased coronary blood flow and decreased myocardial O_2 consumption. Patients anesthetized with isoflurane generally have mildly elevated heart rates as a compensatory response to reduced blood pressure; however, rapid changes in isoflurane concentration can produce both transient tachycardia and hypertension due to isoflurane-induced sympathetic stimulation.

Respiratory System   Patients spontaneously breathing isoflurane have a normal respiration rate but a reduced tidal volume, resulting in a marked reduction in alveolar ventilation and an increase in arterial CO_2 tension. Isoflurane depresses the ventilatory response to hypercapnia and hypoxia. While an effective bronchodilator, isoflurane also is an airway irritant and can stimulate airway reflexes during induction, producing coughing and laryngospasm.

Nervous System   Isoflurane reduces cerebral metabolic O_2 consumption and causes less cerebral vasodilation than do either enflurane or halothane, making it a preferred agent for neurosurgical procedures. The modest effects of isoflurane on cerebral blood flow can be reversed readily by hyperventilation.

Muscle   Isoflurane produces some relaxation of skeletal muscle *via* its central effects. It also enhances the effects of depolarizing and nondepolarizing muscle relaxants. Isoflurane is more potent than halothane in its potentiation of neuromuscular blocking agents. The drug relaxes uterine smooth muscle and is not recommended for analgesia or anesthesia for labor and vaginal delivery.

Kidney, Liver, and GI Tract

Isoflurane reduces splanchnic and hepatic blood flows and renal blood flow and glomerular filtration rate. There are no reports of toxicities or long-term sequelae.

Enflurane

CHEMICAL AND PHYSICAL PROPERTIES

Enflurane (ETHRANE, others Figure 13–3) is a clear, colorless liquid at room temperature with a mild, sweet odor. It is volatile and must be stored in a sealed bottle but is nonflammable and nonexplosive in mixtures of air or oxygen.

PHARMACOKINETICS

Consistent with its blood: gas partition coefficient, induction of anesthesia and recovery from enflurane are relatively slow (Table 13–1). Enflurane is metabolized to a modest extent (2–8% of absorbed enflurane) by hepatic CYP2E1. Fluoride ions are a by-product of enflurane metabolism, but plasma fluoride levels are low and nontoxic. Patients taking isoniazid exhibit enhanced metabolism of enflurane with a consequent elevation of serum fluoride.

CLINICAL USE   Enflurane is primarily utilized for maintenance rather than induction of anesthesia, although surgical anesthesia can be induced in <10 minutes with an inhaled concentration of 4% in oxygen. Anesthesia can be maintained with concentrations from 1.5% to 3%. Concentrations required to produce anesthesia are reduced when enflurane is coadministered with nitrous oxide or opioids.

SIDE EFFECTS

Cardiovascular System   Enflurane causes a concentration-dependent decrease in arterial blood pressure, due, in part, to depression of myocardial contractility and peripheral vasodilation. Enflurane has minimal effects on heart rate.

Respiratory System   The respiratory effects of enflurane are similar to those of halothane. Enflurane produces a greater depression of the ventilatory responses to hypoxia and hypercarbia than do either halothane or isoflurane and, like other inhalational anesthetics, is an effective bronchodilator.

Nervous System   Enflurane is a cerebral vasodilator that increases intracranial pressure in some patients. The drug reduces cerebral metabolic O_2 consumption and has an unusual property of producing electrical seizure activity. High concentrations of enflurane or profound hypocarbia during enflurane anesthesia result in a characteristic high-voltage, high-frequency EEG pattern that progresses to spike-and-dome complexes punctuated by frank seizure activity that may be accompanied by peripheral motor manifestations. The seizures are self-limited and are not thought to produce permanent damage. Epileptic patients are not particularly susceptible to enflurane-induced seizures; nonetheless, enflurane generally is not used in patients with seizure disorders.

Muscle Enflurane produces significant skeletal muscle relaxation and noticeably enhances the effects of nondepolarizing muscle relaxants. As with other inhalational agents, enflurane relaxes uterine smooth muscle.

Kidney, Liver, and GI Tract

Enflurane reduces renal blood flow, glomerular filtration rate, and urinary output. These effects are rapidly reversed upon drug discontinuation. There is scant evidence of long-term nephrotoxicity following enflurane use, and it is safe to use in patients with renal impairment provided that the depth of enflurane anesthesia and the duration of administration are not excessive. Enflurane reduces splanchnic and hepatic blood flow in proportion to reduced arterial blood pressure but does not appear to alter liver function or to be hepatotoxic.

Desflurane

CHEMISTRY AND PHYSICAL PROPERTIES

Desflurane *(SUPRANE, Figure 13–3) is a highly volatile liquid at room temperature (vapor pressure = 681 mm Hg) and thus must be stored in tightly sealed bottles. Delivery of a precise concentration of desflurane requires the use of a specially heated vaporizer that delivers pure vapor that then is diluted appropriately with other gases (O_2, air, or N_2O). Desflurane is nonflammable and nonexplosive in mixtures of air or oxygen.*

PHARMACOKINETICS

Desflurane partitions poorly into blood, fat, and other peripheral tissues (Table 13–1). Thus, the alveolar and blood concentrations rapidly rise to the level of inspired concentration. Within 5 minutes of administration, the alveolar concentration reaches 80% of the inspired concentration, providing for very rapid induction of anesthesia, rapid changes in depth of anesthesia following changes in the inspired concentration, and rapid emergence from anesthesia. The time to awakening following desflurane is half as long as with halothane or sevoflurane and usually does not exceed 5–10 minutes in the absence of other sedative agents.

Desflurane is minimally metabolized; more than 99% of absorbed desflurane is eliminated unchanged via the lungs.

CLINICAL USE Desflurane is widely used for outpatient surgery because of its fast onset and recovery kinetics. The drug irritates the airway of awake patients, provoking coughing, salivation, and bronchospasm. Anesthesia therefore usually is induced with an intravenous agent, with desflurane subsequently administered for maintenance of anesthesia with inhaled concentrations of 6–8% (or lower if coadministered with nitrous oxide or opioids).

SIDE EFFECTS

Cardiovascular System Desflurane lowers blood pressure—primarily by decreasing systemic vascular resistance—and has a modest negative inotropic effect. Thus, cardiac output is preserved, as is perfusion of major organ beds (*e.g.,* splanchnic, renal, cerebral, and coronary). Marked increases in heart rate often occur during induction of desflurane anesthesia and with abrupt increases in the delivered concentration of desflurane; this results from desflurane-induced stimulation of the sympathetic nervous system. The hypotensive effects of desflurane do not wane with increasing duration of administration.

Respiratory System As with halothane and enflurane, desflurane causes a concentration-dependent increase in respiratory rate and a decrease in tidal volume. At concentrations <1 MAC, the net effect is to preserve minute ventilation at concentrations >1 MAC, minute ventilation is markedly depressed, resulting in elevated arterial CO_2 tension (Pa_{CO_2}). Patients spontaneously breathing desflurane at concentrations greater than 1.5 MAC have extreme elevations of Pa_{CO_2} and may become apneic. Desflurane is a bronchodilator; it also is a strong airway irritant and can cause coughing, breath-holding, laryngospasm, and excessive respiratory secretions. Thus, desflurane is not used for induction of anesthesia.

Nervous System Desflurane decreases cerebral vascular resistance and cerebral metabolic O_2 consumption. Under conditions of normocapnia and normotension, desflurane produces an increase in cerebral blood flow and can increase ICP in patients with poor intracranial compliance. The vasoconstrictive response to hypocapnia is preserved during desflurane anesthesia, and increases in ICP thus can be prevented by hyperventilation.

Muscle, Kidney, Liver, and GI Tract

Desflurane produces direct skeletal muscle relaxation and enhances the effects of nondepolarizing and depolarizing neuromuscular blocking agents. Consistent with its minimal metabolism, desflurane has no reported nephrotoxicity or hepatotoxicity.

Sevoflurane

CHEMISTRY AND PHYSICAL PROPERTIES

Sevoflurane (ULTANE Figure 13–3) is a clear, colorless, volatile liquid at room temperature and must be stored in a sealed bottle. It is nonflammable and nonexplosive in mixtures of air or oxygen. Sevoflurane can undergo an exothermic reaction with desiccated CO_2 absorbent (BARA-LYME) to produce airway burns or spontaneous ignition, explosion, and fire. Care must be taken to ensure that sevoflurane is not used with an anesthesia machine in which the CO_2 absorbent has been dried by prolonged gas flow through the absorbent. Sevoflurane reaction with desiccated CO_2 absorbent also can produce CO, which can result in serious patient injury.

PHARMACOKINETICS

The low solubility of sevoflurane in blood and other tissues provides for rapid induction of anesthesia, rapid changes in anesthetic depth following changes in delivered concentration, and rapid emergence following discontinuation of administration (Table 13–1).

Approximately 3% of absorbed sevoflurane is biotransformed by hepatic CYP2E1, the predominant product being hexafluoroisopropanol; metabolism of sevoflurane also produces inorganic fluoride. Interaction of sevoflurane with soda lime (CO_2 absorbent) produces decomposition products, one of which, compound A (pentafluoroisopropenyl fluoromethyl ether), may have toxicity (see Side Effects: Kidney, Liver, and Gastrointestinal Tract below).

CLINICAL USE   Sevoflurane is widely used, particularly for outpatient anesthesia, because of its rapid recovery profile. It is well-suited for inhalation induction of anesthesia (particularly in children) because it is not irritating to the airway. Induction of anesthesia is rapidly achieved using inhaled concentrations of 2–4%.

SIDE EFFECTS
Cardiovascular System   The hypotensive effect of sevoflurane primarily is due to systemic vasodilation, although sevoflurane also produces a concentration-dependent decrease in cardiac output. Unlike isoflurane or desflurane, sevoflurane does not produce tachycardia and thus may be a preferable agent in patients prone to myocardial ischemia.

Respiratory System   Sevoflurane produces a concentration-dependent reduction in tidal volume and increase in respiratory rate in spontaneously breathing patients. The increased respiratory frequency does not compensate for reduced tidal volume, with the net effect being a reduction in minute ventilation and an increase in Pa_{CO_2}. Sevoflurane is not irritating to the airway and is a potent bronchodilator. Thus, sevoflurane is the most effective clinical bronchodilator of the inhalational anesthetics.

Nervous System   Sevoflurane produces effects on cerebral vascular resistance, cerebral metabolic O_2 consumption, and cerebral blood flow similar to those produced by isoflurane and desflurane. Sevoflurane can increase ICP in patients with poor intracranial compliance. The response to hypocapnia is preserved during sevoflurane anesthesia, and increases in ICP can be prevented by hyperventilation.

Muscle   Sevoflurane produces skeletal muscle relaxation and enhances the effects of nondepolarizing and depolarizing neuromuscular blocking agents.

Kidney, Liver, and GI Tract

Controversy has surrounded the potential nephrotoxicity of compound A (pentafluoroisopropenyl fluoromethyl ether), a chemical produced by interaction of sevoflurane with the CO_2 absorbent soda lime. Although biochemical evidence of transient renal injury has been reported, large clinical studies have shown no evidence of renal impairment following sevoflurane administration. The current FDA recommendation is that sevoflurane be administered with fresh gas flows of at least 2 L/min to minimize accumulation of compound A. *Sevoflurane is not known to cause hepatotoxicity or alterations of hepatic function tests.*

Nitrous Oxide

CHEMICAL AND PHYSICAL PROPERTIES

Nitrous oxide (dinitrogen monoxide; N_2O) is a colorless, odorless gas at room temperature (Figure 13–3). It is sold in steel cylinders and must be delivered through calibrated flow meters provided on all anesthesia machines. Nitrous oxide is neither flammable nor explosive, but it does support combustion as actively as oxygen does when it is present in proper concentration with a flammable anesthetic or material.

PHARMACOKINETICS

Nitrous oxide is very insoluble in blood and other tissues (Table 13–1). This results in rapid equilibration between delivered and alveolar anesthetic concentrations and provides for rapid induction of anesthesia and rapid emergence following discontinuation of administration. The rapid uptake of N_2O from alveolar gas serves to concentrate coadministered halogenated anesthetics; this effect (the "second gas effect") speeds induction of anesthesia. On discontinuation of N_2O administration, nitrous oxide gas can diffuse from blood to the alveoli, diluting O_2 in the lung. This can produce an effect called diffusional hypoxia. To avoid hypoxia, 100% O_2 rather than air should be administered when N_2O is discontinued.

99.9% of absorbed nitrous oxide is eliminated unchanged via the lungs. *Nitrous oxide can interact with vitamin B_{12} resulting in vitamin B_{12} deficiency (megaloblastic anemia and peripheral neuropathy) following long-term nitrous oxide administration. Thus, N_2O is not used as a chronic analgesic or as a sedative in critical care settings.*

CLINICAL USE Nitrous oxide is a weak anesthetic agent and produces reliable surgical anesthesia only under hyperbaric conditions. It does produce significant analgesia at concentrations as low as 20% and usually produces sedation in concentrations between 30% and 80%. It frequently is used in concentrations of ~50% to provide analgesia and sedation in outpatient dentistry. Nitrous oxide cannot be used at concentrations >80% because this limits the delivery of adequate O_2. Consequently, N_2O is used primarily as an adjunct to other anesthetics. Nitrous oxide substantially reduces the requirement for inhalational anesthetics. For example, at 70% nitrous oxide, the MAC for other inhalational agents is reduced by about 60%, allowing for lower concentrations of halogenated anesthetics and a lesser degree of side effects.

One major problem with N_2O is that it will exchange with N_2 in any air-containing cavity in the body. Moreover, because of their differential blood:gas partition coefficients, nitrous oxide will enter the cavity faster than nitrogen escapes, thereby increasing the volume and/or pressure in this cavity. Examples of air collections that can be expanded by nitrous oxide include a pneumothorax, an obstructed middle ear, an air embolus, an obstructed loop of bowel, an intraocular air bubble, a pulmonary bulla, and intracranial air. Nitrous oxide should be avoided in these clinical settings.

SIDE EFFECTS

Cardiovascular System Although N_2O produces a negative inotropic effect on heart muscle *in vitro,* depressant effects on cardiac function generally are not observed in patients because of the stimulatory effects of nitrous oxide on the sympathetic nervous system. When N_2O is coadministered with halogenated inhalational anesthetics, it generally produces an increase in heart rate, arterial blood pressure, and cardiac output. In contrast, when N_2O is coadministered with an opioid, it generally decreases arterial blood pressure and cardiac output. Nitrous oxide also increases venous tone in both the peripheral and pulmonary vasculature. The effects of N_2O on pulmonary vascular resistance can be exaggerated in patients with preexisting pulmonary hypertension, and the drug generally is not used in these patients.

Respiratory System Nitrous oxide causes modest increases in respiratory rate and decreases in tidal volume in spontaneously breathing patients. The net effect is that minute ventilation is not significantly changed and Pa_{CO_2} remains normal. Even modest concentrations of N_2O markedly depress the ventilatory response to hypoxia. Thus, it is prudent to monitor arterial O_2 saturation directly in patients receiving or recovering from nitrous oxide.

Nervous System When administered alone, N_2O can significantly increase cerebral blood flow and ICP. When nitrous oxide is coadministered with intravenous anesthetic agents, increases in cerebral blood flow are attenuated or abolished. When N_2O is added to a halogenated inhalational anesthetic, its vasodilatory effect on the cerebral vasculature is slightly reduced.

Muscle Nitrous oxide does not relax skeletal muscle or enhance the effects of neuromuscular blocking drugs. Unlike the halogenated anesthetics, N_2O does not trigger malignant hyperthermia.

Kidney, Liver, and Gastrointestinal Tract Nitrous oxide is neither nephrotoxic nor hepatotoxic.

Xenon

Xenon is an inert gas that is not approved for use in the U.S. and is unlikely to enjoy widespread use because it is a rare gas that cannot be manufactured and must be extracted from air. This limits its availability and renders xenon very expensive. Despite these shortcomings, xenon has properties that make it a virtually ideal anesthetic gas that ultimately may be used in critical situations.

Xenon is extremely insoluble in blood and other tissues, providing for rapid induction and emergence from anesthesia (Table 13–1). It is sufficiently potent to produce surgical anesthesia when administered with 30% oxygen. Most importantly, xenon has minimal side effects. It has no effects on cardiac output or cardiac rhythm and is not thought to have a significant effect on systemic vascular resistance. It also does not affect pulmonary function and is not known to have any hepatic or renal toxicity. Finally, xenon is not metabolized in the human body. Xenon is an anesthetic that may be available in the future if the limitations of availability and cost can be overcome.

ANESTHETIC ADJUNCTS

A general anesthetic is usually given with adjuncts that augment specific components of anesthesia, permitting lower doses of general anesthetics with fewer side effects.

Benzodiazepines

Benzodiazepines (*see* Chapter 16) can produce anesthesia similar to that of barbiturates, but are more commonly used for sedation rather than anesthesia because prolonged amnesia and sedation may result from anesthetizing doses. As adjuncts, benzodiazepines are used for anxiolysis, amnesia, and sedation prior to induction of anesthesia or for sedation during procedures not requiring general anesthesia. The benzodiazepine most frequently used in the perioperative period is *midazolam* (VERSED) followed distantly by *diazepam* (VALIUM), and *lorazepam* (ATIVAN). Midazolam is water soluble and typically is administered intravenously but also can be given orally, intramuscularly, or rectally; oral midazolam is particularly useful for sedation of young children. Midazolam produces minimal venous irritation as opposed to diazepam and lorazepam, which are formulated in propylene glycol and are painful on injection, sometimes producing thrombophlebitis. Midazolam has the pharmacokinetic advantage, particularly over lorazepam, of more rapid onset and shorter duration of effect. Sedative doses of midazolam (0.01–0.07 mg/kg intravenously) reach peak effect in about 2 minutes and provide sedation for about 30 minutes. Elderly patients tend to be more sensitive to and have a slower recovery from benzodiazepines; thus, titration to the desired effect of smaller doses in this age group is prudent. For either prolonged sedation or general anesthetic maintenance, midazolam is more suitable for infusion than other benzodiazepines, although its duration of action does significantly increase with prolonged infusions (Figure 13–2). Benzodiazepines reduce both cerebral blood flow and metabolism, but at equianesthetic doses are less potent in this respect than are barbiturates. They are effective anticonvulsants and sometimes are given to treat status epilepticus. Benzodiazepines modestly decrease blood pressure and respiratory drive, occasionally resulting in apnea; thus, blood pressure and respiratory rate should be monitored in patients sedated with intravenous benzodiazepines.

α_2 Adrenergic Agonists

The α_2 adrenergic agonist dexmedetomidine (PRECEDEX) is widely used in the intensive care unit setting for short-term sedation of adults. and is beginning to be administered off-label in other clinical scenarios including as an anesthetic adjunct. Activation of the α_{2A} adrenergic receptor by dexmedetomidine produces both sedation and analgesia, but does not reliably provide general anesthesia, even at maximal doses.

Common side effects of dexmedetomidine include hypotension and bradycardia, attributed to decreased catecholamine release mediated by activation of α_{2A} receptors. Nausea and dry mouth also are common. At higher drug concentrations, the α_{2B} subtype is activated, resulting in hypertension and a further decrease in heart rate and cardiac output. Dexmedetomidine produces sedation and analgesia with minimal respiratory depression. Sedation produced by dexmedetomidine is noted to be more akin to natural sleep, with patients relatively easy to arouse. However, dexmedetomidine does not appear to provide reliable amnesia and additional agents may be needed if lack of recall is desirable.

The recommended loading dose is 1 µg/kg given over 10 minutes, followed by infusion at a rate of 0.2–0.7 µg/kg/h. Infusions longer than 24 hours are not recommended because of a potential for rebound hypertension. Reduced doses should be considered in patients with risk factors for severe hypotension.

Analgesics

With the exception of ketamine and nitrous oxide, neither parenteral nor currently available inhalational anesthetics are effective analgesics. Thus, analgesics typically are administered with general anesthetics to reduce anesthetic requirement and minimize hemodynamic changes produced by painful stimuli. Nonsteroidal anti-inflammatory drugs, cyclooxygenase-2 inhibitors, or acetaminophen may provide adequate analgesia for minor surgical procedures. Because they produce rapid and profound analgesia, opioids are the primary analgesics used during the perioperative period.

Fentanyl (SUBLIMAZE), *sufentanil* (SUFENTA), *alfentanil* (ALFENTA), *remifentanil* (ULTIVA), meperidine (DEMEROL), and morphine are the major parenteral opioids used in the perioperative period. The primary analgesic activity of each of these drugs is produced by agonist activity at μ-opioid receptors. Their order of potency (relative to morphine) is: sufentanil (1000x) > remifentanil (300x) > fentanyl (100x) > alfentanil (15x) > morphine (1x) > meperidine (0.1x). Pharmacological properties of these agents are discussed in more detail in Chapter 21.

The choice of a perioperative opioid is based primarily on duration of action, given that at appropriate doses, all produce similar analgesia and side effects. Remifentanil has an ultrashort duration of action (~10 minutes) and accumulates minimally with repeated doses or infusion; it is particularly well suited for procedures that are briefly painful but for which little postoperative analgesia is required. Single doses of fentanyl, alfentanil, and sufentanil all have similar intermediate durations of action (30, 20, and 15 minutes, respectively), but recovery after prolonged administration varies considerably. Fentanyl's duration of action lengthens most with infusion, sufentanil's much less so, and alfentanil's the least. After prolonged administration, morphine metabolites have significant analgesic and hypnotic activity.

During the perioperative period, opioids often are given at induction to preempt responses to predictable painful stimuli (e.g., endotracheal intubation and surgical incision). Subsequent doses either by bolus or infusion are titrated to the surgical stimulus and the patient's hemodynamic response. Marked decreases in respiratory rate and heart rate with much smaller reductions in blood pressure are seen to varying degrees with all opioids. Muscle rigidity that can impair ventilation sometimes accompanies larger doses of opioids. The incidence of sphincter of Oddi spasm is increased with all opioids, although morphine appears to be more potent in this regard. The frequency and severity of nausea, vomiting, and pruritus after emergence from anesthesia are increased by all opioids to about the same degree. A useful side effect of meperidine is its capacity to reduce shivering, a common problem during emergence from anesthesia. Finally, opioids often are administered intrathecally and epidurally for management of acute and chronic pain. Neuraxial opioids with or without local anesthetics can provide profound analgesia for many surgical procedures; however, respiratory depression and pruritus usually limit their use to major operations.

Neuromuscular Blocking Agents

Depolarizing (e.g., succinylcholine) and nondepolarizing muscle relaxants (e.g., pancuronium) often are administered during the induction of anesthesia to relax muscles of the jaw, neck, and airway and thereby facilitate laryngoscopy and endotracheal intubation. Barbiturates will precipitate when mixed with muscle relaxants and should be allowed to clear from the IV line prior to injection of a muscle relaxant. Following induction, continued muscle relaxation is desirable for many procedures to aid surgical exposure and to provide additional insurance of immobility. Note: muscle relaxants are not anesthetics and should not be used in lieu of adequate anesthetic depth. The action of nondepolarizing muscle relaxants usually is antagonized, once muscle paralysis is no longer desired, with an acetylcholinesterase inhibitor such as neostigmine or edrophonium (see Chapter 8) combined with a muscarinic receptor antagonist (e.g., glycopyrolate or atropine) (see Chapter 7) to offset the muscarinic activation resulting from esterase inhibition. Other than histamine release by some agents, nondepolarizing muscle relaxants used in this manner have few side effects. However, succinylcholine has multiple serious side effects (e.g., bradycardia, hyperkalemia, and severe myalgia) including induction of malignant hyperthermia in susceptible individuals. Chapter 9 covers the detailed pharmacology of these agents.

For a complete Bibliographical listing see Goodman & Gilman's *The Pharmacological Basis of Therapeutics*, 11th ed., or Goodman & Gilman Online at www.accessmedicine.com.

14

LOCAL ANESTHETICS

Local anesthetics bind reversibly to a specific receptor site within the pore of the Na^+ channels in nerves and block ion movement through this pore. When applied locally to nerve tissue in appropriate concentrations, local anesthetics can act on any part of the nervous system and on every type of nerve fiber, reversibly blocking the action potentials responsible for nerve conduction. Thus, a local anesthetic in contact with a nerve trunk can cause both sensory and motor paralysis in the area innervated. These effects of clinically relevant concentrations of local anesthetics are reversible with recovery of nerve function and no evidence of damage to nerve fibers or cells in most clinical applications.

CHEMISTRY AND STRUCTURE–ACTIVITY RELATIONSHIP

The typical local anesthetics contain hydrophilic and hydrophobic moieties that are separated by an intermediate ester or amide linkage (Figure 14–1). A broad range of compounds containing these minimal structural features can satisfy the requirements for action as local anesthetics. The hydrophilic group usually is a tertiary amine but also may be a secondary amine; the hydrophobic moiety must be aromatic. The nature of the linking group determines some of the pharmacological properties of these agents. For example, local anesthetics with an ester link are hydrolyzed readily by plasma esterases.

Hydrophobicity increases both the potency and the duration of action of the local anesthetics because association of the drug at hydrophobic sites enhances the partitioning of the drug to its sites of action and decreases the rate of metabolism by plasma esterases and hepatic enzymes. In addition, the receptor site for these drugs on Na^+ channels is thought to be hydrophobic, so that receptor affinity for anesthetic agents is greater for more hydrophobic drugs. Hydrophobicity also increases toxicity, so that the therapeutic index is decreased for more hydrophobic drugs.

Molecular size influences the rate of dissociation of local anesthetics from their receptor sites. Smaller drug molecules can escape from the receptor site more rapidly. This characteristic is important in rapidly firing cells, in which local anesthetics bind during action potentials and dissociate during the period of membrane repolarization. Rapid binding of local anesthetics during action potentials causes the frequency- and voltage-dependence of their action.

MECHANISM OF ACTION Local anesthetics block conduction by decreasing or preventing the large transient increase in the permeability of excitable membranes to Na^+ that normally is produced by a slight depolarization of the membrane (*see* Chapter 12). This action is due to direct interaction with voltage-gated Na^+ channels. As the anesthetic action progressively develops in a nerve, the threshold for electrical excitability gradually increases, the rate of rise of the action potential declines, impulse conduction slows, and nerve conduction eventually fails.

Local anesthetics can block K^+ channels at higher concentrations of drug; thus, blockade of conduction is not accompanied by any large or consistent change in resting membrane potential.

Quaternary analogs of local anesthetics block conduction when applied internally to perfused giant axons of squid but are relatively ineffective when applied externally, suggesting that the site at which local anesthetics act, at least in their charged form, is accessible only from the inner surface of the plasma membrane. Therefore, local anesthetics applied externally first must cross the membrane before they can exert a blocking action.

The major mechanism of action of these drugs involves their interaction with one or more specific binding sites within the Na^+ channel (Figure 14–2).

FREQUENCY- AND VOLTAGE-DEPENDENCE OF LOCAL ANESTHETIC ACTION

The degree of block produced by a given concentration of local anesthetic depends on how the nerve has been stimulated and on its resting membrane potential. Thus, a resting nerve is much less sensitive to a local anesthetic than one that is repetitively stimulated; higher frequency of stimulation and more positive membrane potential cause a greater degree of anesthetic block. These frequency- and voltage-dependent effects of local anesthetics occur because the local anesthetic molecule in its charged form gains access to its binding site within the pore only when the Na^+ channel is in an open state and because the local anesthetic binds more tightly to and stabilizes the inactivated state of the Na^+ channel.

DIFFERENTIAL SENSITIVITY OF NERVE FIBERS TO LOCAL ANESTHETICS

Generally, treatment with local anesthetics causes the sensation of pain to disappear first, followed by loss of the sensations of temperature, touch, deep pressure, and finally motor function (Table 14–1). In general, autonomic fibers, small unmyelinated C fibers (mediating pain sensations), and small

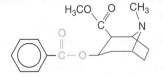

COCAINE

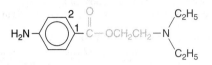

PROCAINE

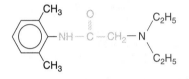

LIDOCAINE

FIGURE 14–1 *Structural formulas of selected local anesthetics.* Most local anesthetics consist of a hydrophobic (aromatic) moiety (black), a linker region (light blue), and a substituted amine (hydrophilic region, in dark blue). The structures above are grouped by the nature of the linker region. Procaine is a prototypic ester-type local anesthetic; esters generally are well hydrolyzed by plasma esterases, contributing to the relatively short duration of action of drugs in this group. Lidocaine is a prototypic amide-type local anesthetic; these structures generally are more resistant to clearance and have longer durations of action. There are exceptions, including benzocaine (poorly water soluble; used only topically) and the structures with a ketone, an amidine, and an ether linkage. See 11th edition of the parent text, Figure 14–1, for additional details and structures.

myelinated $A\delta$ fibers (mediating pain and temperature sensations) are blocked before the larger myelinated $A\gamma$, $A\beta$, and $A\alpha$ fibers (mediating postural, touch, pressure, and motor information). This differential rate of block exhibited by fibers mediating different sensations is of considerable practical importance in the use of local anesthetics; the mechanisms responsible for this apparent specificity are not known.

EFFECT OF pH Local anesthetics tend to be only slightly soluble as unprotonated amines. Therefore, they generally are marketed as water-soluble salts, usually hydrochlorides. Since local anesthetics are weak bases (typical pK_a values range 8–9), their hydrochloride salts are mildly acidic. This property increases the stability of the local anesthetic esters and catecholamines added as vasoconstrictors. Following administration, the pH of the local anesthetic solution rapidly equilibrates to that of the extracellular fluids.

Although the unprotonated species of the local anesthetic is necessary for diffusion across cellular membranes, it is the cationic species that interacts preferentially with Na^+ channels.

PROLONGATION OF ACTION BY VASOCONSTRICTORS The duration of action of a local anesthetic is proportional to the time of contact with nerve. Consequently, maneuvers that keep the drug at the nerve prolong the period of anesthesia. Thus, catecholamines, acting at α-adrenergic receptors in the vasculature, cause vasoconstriction and reduced absorption of local anesthetics in vascular beds where α adrenergic effects predominate (*see* Chapters 6 and 10). In clinical practice, a vasoconstrictor, usually epinephrine, is often added to local anesthetics. The vasoconstrictor performs a dual service. By decreasing the rate of absorption, it not only localizes the anesthetic at the desired site, but reduces systemic toxicity by slowing systemic absorption, thereby favoring metabolism rather than accumulation of absorbed drug. Note, however, that epinephrine dilates skeletal muscle vascular beds through actions at β_2 adrenergic receptors and therefore has the potential to increase systemic toxicity of anesthetic deposited in muscle tissue.

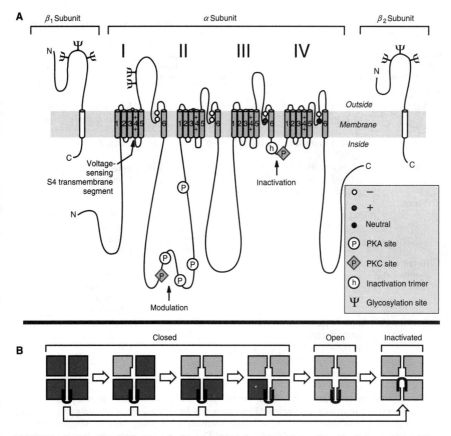

FIGURE 14–2 Structure and function of voltage-gated Na+ channels. A. A two-dimensional representation of the α (center), β_1 (left), and β_2 (right) subunits of the voltage-gated Na+ channel from mammalian brain. The polypeptide chains are represented by continuous lines with length approximately proportional to the actual length of each segment of the channel protein. Cylinders represent regions of transmembrane α helices. ψ indicates sites of demonstrated N-linked glycosylation. Note the repeated structure of the four homologous domains (I through IV) of the α subunit. **Voltage Sensing.** The S4 transmembrane segments in each homologous domain of the α subunit serve as voltage sensors. (+) represents the positively charged amino acid residues at every third position within these segments. Electrical field (negative inside) exerts a force on these charged amino acid residues, pulling them toward the intracellular side of the membrane; depolarization allows them to move outward. **Pore.** The S5 and S6 transmembrane segments and the short membrane-associated loop between them (*P loop*) form the walls of the pore in the center of an approximately symmetrical square array of the four homologous domains (see Panel **B**). The amino acid residues indicated by circles in the P loop are critical for determining the conductance and ion selectivity of the Na+ channel and its ability to bind the extracellular pore-blocking toxins tetrodotoxin and saxitoxin. **Inactivation.** The short intracellular loop connecting homologous domains III and IV serves as the inactivation gate of the Na+ channel. It is thought to fold into the intracellular mouth of the pore and occlude it within a few milliseconds after the channel opens. Three hydrophobic residues (isoleucine–phenylalanine–methionine; IFM) at the position marked **h** appear to serve as an inactivation particle, entering the intracellular mouth of the pore and binding therein to an inactivation gate receptor there. **Modulation.** The gating of the Na+ channel can be modulated by protein phosphorylation. Phosphorylation of the inactivation gate between homologous domains III and IV by protein kinase C slows inactivation. Phosphorylation of sites in the intracellular loop between homologous domains I and II by either protein kinase C ( ) or cyclic AMP–dependent protein kinase (P) reduces Na+ channel activation. **B.** The four homologous domains of the Na+ channel α subunit are illustrated as a square array, as viewed looking down on the membrane. The sequence of conformational changes that the Na+ channel undergoes during activation and inactivation is diagrammed. Upon depolarization, each of the four homologous domains sequentially undergoes a conformational change to an activated state. After all four domains have activated, the Na+ channel can open. Within a few milliseconds after opening, the inactivation gate between domains III and IV closes over the intracellular mouth of the channel and occludes it, preventing further ion conductance.

Table 14–1

Susceptibility to Block of Types of Nerve Fibers

Conduction Biophysical Classification	Anatomic Location	Myelin	Diameter (μm)	Conduction Velocity (m/sec)	Function	Clinical Sensitivity to Block
A fibers						
A α	Afferent to and efferent from	Yes	6–22	10–85	Motor and proprioception	+ ++
A β	muscles and joints					
A γ	Efferent to muscle spindles	Yes	3–6	15–35	Muscle tone	++
A δ	Sensory roots and afferent peripheral nerves	Yes	1–4	5–25	Pain, temperature, touch	+++
B fibers						
	Preganglionic sympathetic	Yes	<3	3–15	Vasomotor, visceromotor, sudomotor, pilomotor	++++
C fibers						
Sympathetic	Postganglionic sympathetic	No	0.3–1.3	0.7–1.3	Vasomotor, visceromotor, sudomotor, pilomotor	++++
Dorsal root	Sensory roots and afferent peripheral nerves	No	0.4–1.2	0.1–2	Pain, temperature, touch	++++

Some of the vasoconstrictor may be absorbed systemically, occasionally to an extent sufficient to cause untoward reactions (*see* below). There also may be delayed wound healing, tissue edema, or necrosis after local anesthesia. These effects seem to occur partly because sympathomimetic amines can cause hypoxia and local tissue damage. The use of vasoconstrictors in local-anesthetic preparations for anatomical regions with limited collateral circulation could produce irreversible hypoxic damage, tissue necrosis, and gangrene, and therefore is contraindicated.

UNDESIRED EFFECTS OF LOCAL ANESTHETICS In addition to blocking conduction in nerve axons in the peripheral nervous system, local anesthetics interfere with the function of all organs in which conduction or transmission of impulses occurs. Thus, they have important effects on the CNS, autonomic ganglia, neuromuscular junctions, and all forms of muscle. The danger of such adverse reactions is proportional to the concentration of local anesthetic achieved in the circulation. In general, in local anesthetics with chiral centers, the *S*-enantiomer is less toxic than the R-enantiomer.

Central Nervous System
Following absorption, local anesthetics may cause central nervous system (CNS) stimulation (presumably due to suppression of inhibitory neurons), producing restlessness and tremor that may progress to clonic convulsions. In general, the more potent the anesthetic, the more readily convulsions may be produced. Alterations of CNS activity are thus predictable from the local anesthetic agent in question and the blood concentration achieved. Central stimulation is followed by depression; death usually is caused by respiratory failure. Airway control and ventilatory support are essential features of treatment in the late stage of intoxication. Benzodiazepines or rapidly acting barbiturates administered intravenously are the drugs of choice for both the prevention and arrest of convulsions (see Chapter 16).

Although drowsiness is the most frequent complaint that results from the CNS actions of local anesthetics, lidocaine may produce dysphoria or euphoria and muscle twitching. Moreover, both lidocaine and procaine may produce a loss of consciousness that is preceded only by symptoms of sedation. Cocaine has a particularly prominent effect on mood and behavior (see Chapter 23).

Cardiovascular System Following systemic absorption, local anesthetics decrease electrical excitability, conduction rate, and force of contraction. Most local anesthetics also cause arteriolar dilation. Untoward cardiovascular effects usually are seen only after high systemic concentrations are attained and effects on the CNS are produced. However, on rare occasions, lower doses of some local anesthetics will cause cardiovascular collapse and death, probably due to either an action on the pacemaker or the sudden onset of ventricular fibrillation. Ventricular tachycardia and fibrillation are relatively uncommon consequences of local anesthetics other than bupivacaine. The use of local anesthetics as antiarrhythmic drugs is discussed in Chapter 34. Untoward cardiovascular effects of local anesthetic agents may result from their inadvertent intravascular administration, especially if epinephrine also is present.

Smooth Muscle Local anesthetics depress contractions in gastrointestinal (GI), vascular, and bronchial smooth muscle, although low concentrations initially may produce contraction. Spinal and epidural anesthesia, as well as instillation of local anesthetics into the peritoneal cavity, cause sympathetic nervous system paralysis, which can result in increased tone of GI musculature (*see* below). Local anesthetics seldom depress uterine contractions directly during intrapartum regional anesthesia.

HYPERSENSITIVITY TO LOCAL ANESTHETICS Rare individuals are hypersensitive to local anesthetics, displaying allergic dermatitis or a typical asthmatic attack. It is important to distinguish allergic reactions from toxic side effects and from effects of coadministered vasoconstrictors. Hypersensitivity seems to occur more frequently with local anesthetics of the ester type and frequently extends to chemically related compounds. Although allergic responses to agents of the amide type are uncommon, solutions of such agents may contain preservatives such as methylparaben that may provoke an allergic reaction. Local anesthetic preparations containing a vasoconstrictor also may elicit allergic responses due to the sulfite added as an antioxidant.

METABOLISM OF LOCAL ANESTHETICS The metabolic fate of local anesthetics is of great practical importance, because their toxicity depends largely on the balance between their rates of absorption and elimination. The rate of absorption of many anesthetics can be reduced by incorporation of a vasoconstrictor in the anesthetic solution. However, the rate of degradation of local anesthetics varies greatly, and this is a major factor in determining the safety of a particular agent. Since toxicity is related to the free concentration of drug, binding of the anesthetic to proteins in the serum and to tissues reduces the concentration of free drug in the systemic circulation, and consequently reduces toxicity.

Some of the common local anesthetics (*e.g.*, tetracaine) are esters; they are hydrolyzed and inactivated primarily by a plasma esterase, probably plasma cholinesterase. Hepatic enzymes also hydrolyze local anesthetic esters. Since spinal fluid contains little or no esterase, anesthesia produced by the intrathecal injection of an anesthetic agent will persist until the local anesthetic agent has been absorbed into the circulation.

The amide-linked local anesthetics are, in general, degraded by the hepatic CYPs, the initial reactions involving *N*-dealkylation and subsequent hydrolysis (*see* Chapter 3). However, with *prilocaine*, the initial step is hydrolytic, forming *o*-toluidine metabolites that can cause methemoglobinemia. The extensive use of amide-linked local anesthetics in patients with severe hepatic disease requires caution. The amide-linked local anesthetics are extensively (55–95%) bound to plasma proteins, particularly α_1-acid glycoprotein. Many factors increase (*e.g.*, cancer, surgery, trauma, myocardial infarction, smoking, and uremia) or decrease (*e.g.*, oral contraceptives) the level of this glycoprotein, thereby changing the amount of anesthetic delivered to the liver for metabolism and thus influencing systemic toxicity. Age-related changes in protein binding of local anesthetics also occur. The neonate is relatively deficient in plasma proteins that bind local anesthetics and thereby is more susceptible to toxicity. Plasma proteins are not the sole determinant of local anesthetic availability. Reduced cardiac output slows delivery of the amide compounds to the liver, reducing their metabolism and prolonging their plasma half-lives (*see* Chapter 34).

COCAINE

Cocaine (Figure 14-1) is an ester of benzoic acid and methylecgonine. The clinically desired actions of cocaine are the blockade of nerve impulses, as a consequence of its local anesthetic properties, and local vasoconstriction, secondary to inhibition of local norepinephrine reuptake. Toxicity and its potential for abuse have steadily decreased the clinical utility of cocaine. Its high toxicity is due to reduced catecholamine uptake in both the central and peripheral nervous systems.

Its euphoric properties are due primarily to inhibition of catecholamine uptake, particularly dopamine, in the CNS. Other local anesthetics do not block the uptake of norepinephrine and do not produce the sensitization to catecholamines, vasoconstriction, or mydriasis characteristic of cocaine. Currently, cocaine is used primarily for topical anesthesia of the upper respiratory tract, where its combination of both vasoconstrictor and local anesthetic properties provide anesthesia and shrinking of the mucosa. Because of its abuse potential, cocaine is listed as a schedule II drug by the U.S. Drug Enforcement Agency.

LIDOCAINE

Lidocaine (XYLOCAINE, others), an aminoethylamide (Figure 14–1), is the prototypical amide local anesthetic.

CLINICAL PHARMACOLOGY

Lidocaine produces faster, more intense, longer lasting, and more extensive anesthesia than does an equal concentration of procaine. Lidocaine is an alternative choice for individuals sensitive to ester-type local anesthetics.

Lidocaine is absorbed rapidly after parenteral administration and from the GI and respiratory tracts. In addition to preparations for injection, an iontophoretic, needle-free drug-delivery system for a solution of lidocaine and epinephrine (IONTOCAINE) is available for dermal procedures and provides anesthesia to a depth of up to 10 mm.

A lidocaine transdermal patch (LIDODERM) is used for relief of pain associated with postherpetic neuralgia. The combination of lidocaine (2.59%) and prilocaine (2.5%) in an occlusive dressing (EMLA ANESTHETIC DISC) is used as an anesthetic prior to venipuncture, skin graft harvesting, and infiltration of anesthetics into genitalia.

Lidocaine is dealkylated by hepatic CYPs to metabolites with local anesthetic activity.

TOXICITY

The side effects of lidocaine seen with increasing dose include drowsiness, tinnitus, dysgeusia, dizziness, and twitching. As the dose increases, seizures, coma, and respiratory depression and arrest will occur. Clinically significant cardiovascular depression usually occurs at serum lidocaine levels that produce marked CNS effects. The active metabolites may contribute to some of these side effects.

CLINICAL USES

Lidocaine has utility in almost any application where a local anesthetic of intermediate duration is needed. Lidocaine also is used as an antiarrhythmic agent (see Chapter 34).

BUPIVACAINE

PHARMACOLOGICAL ACTIONS

Bupivacaine (MARCAINE, SENSORCAINE), is an amide local anesthetic. Levobupivacaine (CHIROCAINE), the S-enantiomer of bupivacaine, also is available. Bupivacaine's long duration of action plus its tendency to provide more sensory than motor block has made it a popular drug for providing prolonged analgesia during labor or the postoperative period. By taking advantage of indwelling catheters and continuous infusions, bupivacaine can be used to provide several days of effective analgesia.

TOXICITY

Bupivacaine is more cardiotoxic than equi-effective doses of lidocaine. Clinically, this is manifested by severe ventricular arrhythmias and myocardial depression after inadvertent intravascular administration of large doses of bupivacaine. Bupivacaine dissociates slowly during diastole, so a significant fraction of Na^+ channels at physiological heart rates remains blocked with bupivacaine at the end of diastole. Thus, the block by bupivacaine is cumulative and substantially more than would be predicted by its local anesthetic potency. Bupivacaine-induced cardiac toxicity can be very difficult to treat, and its severity is enhanced by coexisting acidosis, hypercarbia, and hypoxemia. The S-enantiomer and the racemate are equally efficacious and potent, but levobupivacaine may be less cardiotoxic.

OTHER SYNTHETIC LOCAL ANESTHETICS

The number of synthetic local anesthetics is so large that it is impractical to consider them all here. The use of some is restricted to topical application to the eye (*see* Chapter 63), the mucous membranes, or the skin (*see* Chapter 62). Many local anesthetics are suitable, however, for infiltration or injection to produce nerve block; some of them also are useful for topical application. The main categories of local anesthetics are given below; agents are listed alphabetically.

Local Anesthetics Suitable for Injection

ARTICAINE

Articaine *(SEPTOCAINE) is a recently introduced amino amide, approved in the U.S. for dental and periodontal procedures. It exhibits a rapid onset (1–6 minutes) and duration of action of ~1 hour.*

CHLOROPROCAINE

Chloroprocaine *(NESACAINE), an ester local anesthetic, is a chlorinated derivative of procaine with rapid onset, short duration of action, and reduced acute toxicity due to rapid metabolism (plasma $t_{1/2}$ ~25 seconds). A higher-than-expected incidence of muscular back pain following epidural anesthesia with 2-chloroprocaine has been reported; this back pain is thought to be due to tetany in the paraspinus muscles, which may be a consequence of Ca^{2+} binding by the EDTA included as a preservative; the incidence of back pain appears to be related to the volume of drug injected and its use for skin infiltration.*

ETIDOCAINE

Etidocaine *(DURANEST) is a long-acting amino amide with an onset of action faster than that of bupivacaine and comparable to that of lidocaine, and a duration of action similar to that of bupivacaine. It is no longer marketed in the U.S.*

MEPIVACAINE

Mepivacaine *(CARBOCAINE, POLOCAINE) is an intermediate-acting amino amide pharmacologically similar to lidocaine. Mepivacaine, however, is more toxic to the neonate and thus is not used in obstetrical anesthesia. Mepivacaine is not effective as a topical anesthetic.*

PRILOCAINE

Prilocaine *(CITANEST) is an intermediate-acting amino amide that is pharmacologically similar to lidocaine, except that it causes little vasodilation and thus can be used without a vasoconstrictor if desired, and its increased volume of distribution reduces its CNS toxicity, making it suitable for intravenous regional blocks (see below). As a consequence of the metabolism of the aromatic ring to o-toluidine, prilocaine can cause methehemoglobinemia. Development of methemoglobinemia is dose dependent, usually appearing after a dose of 8 mg/kg. Methemoglobinemia usually is not a problem in healthy adults but is more common in neonates due to decreased resistance of fetal hemoglobin to oxidant stresses and the immaturity of enzymes that convert methemoglobin back to the ferrous state.*

ROPIVACAINE

Ropivacaine *(NAROPIN), an amino ethylamide, is slightly less potent than bupivacaine in producing anesthesia. In clinical studies, ropivacaine appears to be suitable for both epidural and regional anesthesia, with duration of action similar to that of bupivacaine. Interestingly, it seems to be even more motor sparing than bupivacaine.*

PROCAINE

Procaine *(NOVOCAIN), the first synthetic local anesthetic, is an amino ester (see Figure 14–1) with low potency, slow onset, and short duration of action. Its use now is confined to infiltration anesthesia and occasionally for diagnostic nerve blocks. Its hydrolysis in vivo produces para-aminobenzoic acid, which inhibits the action of sulfonamides. Thus, large doses should not be administered to patients taking sulfonamide drugs.*

TETRACAINE

Tetracaine *(PONTOCAINE), a long-acting amino ester, is significantly more potent and has a longer duration of action than procaine. Tetracaine may exhibit increased systemic toxicity because it is more slowly metabolized than the other commonly used ester local anesthetics. It is widely used in spinal anesthesia when a drug of long duration is needed. Tetracaine also is incorporated into several topical anesthetic preparations. Tetracaine is rarely used in peripheral nerve blocks because of the large doses often necessary, its slow onset, and its potential for toxicity.*

Local Anesthetics Used Primarily to Anesthetize Mucous Membranes and Skin

Some anesthetics are either too irritating or too ineffective to be applied to the eye. However, they are useful as topical anesthetic agents on the skin and/or mucous membranes. These preparations are effective in the symptomatic relief of anal and genital pruritus, poison ivy rashes, and numerous *other acute and chronic dermatoses. They sometimes are combined with a glucocorticoid or anti-histamine and are available in a number of proprietary formulations.*

Dibucaine *(NUPERCAINAL) is a quinoline derivative. Because of its toxicity, it is not available in the U.S. as an injectable preparation; it retains wide popularity outside the U.S. as a spinal anesthetic. It currently is available as a cream and an ointment for use on the skin.*

Dyclonine hydrochloride *(DYCLONE) has a rapid onset of action and duration of effect comparable to that of procaine. It is absorbed through the skin and mucous membranes. Marketing of dyclonine solutions for clinical use has been discontinued in the U.S. Dyclonine is an active ingredient of OTC medications including sore throat lozenges (SUCRETS, others), a gel for cold sores (TANAC), and a 0.75% solution (SKIN SHIELD) to protect against contact dermatitis.*

Pramoxine hydrochloride *(ANUSOL, TRONOTHANE, others) is a surface anesthetic agent that is not a benzoate ester. Its distinct chemical structure may help minimize the danger of cross-sensitivity reactions in patients allergic to other local anesthetics. Pramoxine produces satisfactory surface anesthesia and is reasonably well tolerated on the skin and mucous membranes. It is too irritating to be used on the eye or in the nose.*

Anesthetics of Low Solubility

Some local anesthetics are poorly soluble in water, and consequently are too slowly absorbed to be toxic. They can be applied directly to wounds and ulcerated surfaces, where they remain localized for long periods of time, producing a sustained anesthetic action. Chemically, they are esters of para-aminobenzoic acid lacking a terminal amino group common to other local anesthetics. Benzocaine (ethyl aminobenzoate; AMERICAINE ANESTHETIC, others) is the prototype. Benzocaine is structurally similar to procaine, but lacks the terminal diethylamino group. It is used in numerous topical preparations. Benzocaine can cause methemoglobinemia (see text concerning methemoglobinemia caused by prilocaine, above).

Local Anesthetics Largely Restricted to Ophthalmological Use

Anesthesia of the cornea and conjunctiva can be obtained readily by topical application of local anesthetics. Most local anesthetics are too irritating for ophthalmological use. The suitable two compounds are proparacaine *(ALCAINE, OPHTHAINE, others) and* tetracaine. *In addition to being less irritating during administration, proparacaine has the advantage of bearing little antigenic similarity to the other benzoate local anesthetics. For use in ophthalmology, these local anesthetics are instilled a single drop at a time. If anesthesia is incomplete, successive drops are applied until satisfactory conditions are obtained. The duration of anesthesia is determined chiefly by the vascularity of the tissue; thus, it is longest in normal cornea and shortest in inflamed conjunctiva. In the latter case, repeated instillations may be necessary to maintain adequate anesthesia for the duration of the procedure. Long-term administration of topical anesthesia to the eye has been associated with retarded healing, pitting and sloughing of the corneal epithelium, and predisposition of the eye to inadvertent injury. Thus, these drugs should not be prescribed for self-administration. For drug delivery, pharmacokinetic, and toxicity issues unique to drugs for ophthalmic use, see Chapter 63.*

CLINICAL USES OF LOCAL ANESTHETICS

Local anesthesia is the loss of sensation in a body part without the loss of consciousness or the impairment of central control of vital functions. It offers two major advantages. First, physiological perturbations associated with general anesthesia are avoided; second, neurophysiological responses to pain and stress can be modified beneficially. However, local anesthetics can produce deleterious side effects. Proper choice of a local anesthetic and care in its use are the primary determinants in avoiding toxicity. There is a poor relationship between the amount of local anesthetic injected and peak plasma levels in adults. Furthermore, peak plasma levels vary widely depending on the area of injection. They are highest with interpleural or intercostal blocks and lowest with subcutaneous infiltration. Thus, recommended maximum doses serve only as general guidelines.

The following discussion summarizes the pharmacological and physiological consequences of the use of local anesthetics categorized by method of administration.

Topical Anesthesia

Anesthesia of mucous membranes of the nose, mouth, throat, tracheobronchial tree, esophagus, and genitourinary tract can be produced by direct application of aqueous solutions of salts of many local anesthetics or by suspension of the poorly soluble local anesthetics. Tetracaine (2%), lidocaine (2–10%), and cocaine (1–4%) typically are used. Cocaine is used only in the nose, nasopharynx, mouth, throat, and ear, where it uniquely produces vasoconstriction as well as anesthesia.

The shrinking of mucous membranes decreases operative bleeding while improving surgical visualization. Comparable vasoconstriction can be achieved with other local anesthetics by the addition of a low concentration of a vasoconstrictor such as phenylephrine (0.005%). Epinephrine, topically applied, does not prolong the duration of action of local anesthetics applied to mucous membranes because of poor penetration. Maximal safe total dosages for topical anesthesia in a healthy 70-kg adult are 300 mg for lidocaine, 150 mg for cocaine, and 50 mg for tetracaine.

Local anesthetics are absorbed rapidly into the circulation following topical application to mucous membranes or denuded skin. Thus, topical anesthesia always carries the risk of systemic toxic reactions.

The introduction of a eutectic mixture of lidocaine (2.5%) and prilocaine (2.5%) (EMLA) bridges the gap between topical and infiltration anesthesia. The efficacy of this combination lies in the fact that the mixture of prilocaine and lidocaine has a melting point less than that of either compound alone, existing at room temperature as an oil that can penetrate intact skin. EMLA cream produces anesthesia to a maximum depth of 5 mm and is applied as a cream on intact skin under an occlusive dressing, for procedures involving skin and superficial subcutaneous structures (e.g., venipuncture and skin graft harvesting). EMLA must not be used on mucous membranes or abraded skin, as rapid absorption across these surfaces may result in systemic toxicity.

Infiltration Anesthesia

Infiltration anesthesia is the injection of local anesthetic directly into tissue without taking into consideration the course of cutaneous nerves. Infiltration anesthesia can be so superficial as to include only the skin. It also can include deeper structures, including intra-abdominal organs, when these too are infiltrated.

The duration of infiltration anesthesia can be approximately doubled by the addition of epinephrine (5 μg/mL) to the injection solution; epinephrine also decreases peak concentrations of local anesthetics in blood. Epinephrine-containing solutions should not, however, be injected into tissues supplied by end arteries—for example, fingers and toes, ears, the nose, and the penis. The resulting vasoconstriction may cause gangrene.

The local anesthetics used most frequently for infiltration anesthesia are lidocaine (0.5–1%), procaine (0.5–1%), and bupivacaine (0.125–0.25%). When used without epinephrine, up to 4.5 mg/kg of lidocaine, 7 mg/kg of procaine, or 2 mg/kg of bupivacaine can be employed in adults. When epinephrine is added, these amounts can be increased by one-third.

The advantage of infiltration anesthesia and other regional anesthetic techniques is that it can provide satisfactory anesthesia without disrupting normal bodily functions. The chief disadvantage of infiltration anesthesia is that relatively large amounts of drug must be used to anesthetize relatively small areas.

Field Block Anesthesia

Field block anesthesia is produced by subcutaneous injection of a solution of local anesthetic in order to anesthetize the region distal to the injection. For example, subcutaneous infiltration of the proximal portion of the volar surface of the forearm results in an extensive area of cutaneous anesthesia that starts 2–3 cm distal to the site of injection. The same principle can be applied with particular benefit to the scalp, the anterior abdominal wall, and the lower extremity. The drugs, concentrations, and doses recommended are the same as for infiltration anesthesia. The advantage of field block anesthesia is that less drug can be used to provide a greater area of anesthesia than when infiltration anesthesia is used.

Nerve Block Anesthesia

Injection of a local anesthetic into or around individual peripheral nerves or nerve plexuses produces even greater areas of anesthesia than do the techniques described above. Blockade of mixed peripheral nerves and nerve plexuses also usually anesthetizes somatic motor nerves, producing skeletal muscle relaxation, which is essential for some surgical procedures. The areas of sensory and motor block usually start several centimeters distal to the site of injection. Brachial plexus blocks are particularly useful for procedures on the upper extremity and shoulder. Intercostal nerve blocks are effective for anesthesia and relaxation of the anterior abdominal wall. Cervical plexus block is appropriate for surgery of the neck. Sciatic and femoral nerve blocks are useful for surgery distal to the knee. Other useful nerve blocks prior to surgical procedures include blocks of individual nerves at the wrist and at the ankle, blocks of individual nerves such as the median or ulnar at the elbow, and blocks of sensory cranial nerves.

Local anesthetic is never intentionally injected into the nerve; this would be painful and could cause nerve damage. Instead, the anesthetic agent is deposited as close to the nerve as possible. Higher concentrations of local anesthetic will provide a more rapid onset of peripheral nerve block, but the potential for systemic toxicity and direct neural toxicity limits use of high concentrations. Duration of nerve block anesthesia depends on the physical characteristics of the local anesthetic used and the presence or absence of vasoconstrictors. Especially important physical characteristics are lipid solubility and protein binding. Local anesthetics can be broadly divided into three categories: those with a short (20–45 minutes) duration of action in mixed peripheral nerves, such as procaine; those with an intermediate (60–120 minutes) duration of action, such as lidocaine and mepivacaine; and those with a long (400–450 minutes) duration of action, such as bupivacaine, ropivacaine, and tetracaine. Block duration of the intermediate-acting local anesthetics such as lidocaine can be prolonged by the addition of epinephrine (5 μg/mL). The degree of block prolongation in peripheral nerves due to epinephrine appears to be related to the intrinsic vasodilating properties of the local anesthetic and thus is most pronounced with lidocaine.

The types of nerve fibers that are blocked when a local anesthetic is injected about a mixed peripheral nerve depend on the concentration of drug used, nerve-fiber size, internodal distance, and frequency and pattern of nerve-impulse transmission (see above). Anatomical factors are similarly important. Nerves in the outer mantle of the mixed nerve are blocked first. These fibers usually are distributed to more proximal anatomical structures than are those situated near the core of the mixed nerve and often are motor. If the volume and concentration of local anesthetic solution deposited about the nerve are adequate, the local anesthetic eventually will diffuse inward in amounts adequate to block even the most centrally located fibers. Since removal of local anesthetics occurs primarily in the core of a mixed nerve or nerve trunk, where the vascular supply is located, the duration of blockade of centrally located nerves is shorter than that of more peripherally situated fibers.

The choice of local anesthetic and the amount and concentration administered are determined by the nerves and the types of fibers to be blocked, the required duration of anesthesia, and the size and health of the patient. For blocks of 2–4 hours, lidocaine (1–1.5%) can be used in the amounts recommended above (see "Infiltration Anesthesia"). Mepivacaine (up to 7 mg/kg of a 1–2% solution) provides anesthesia that lasts about as long as that from lidocaine. Bupivacaine (2–3 mg/kg of a 0.25–0.375% solution) can be used when a longer duration of action is required. Addition of 5 μg/mL epinephrine slows systemic absorption and, therefore, prolongs duration and lowers the plasma concentration of the intermediate-acting local anesthetics.

Intravenous Regional Anesthesia (Bier's Block)

This technique relies on using the vasculature to bring the local anesthetic solution to the nerve trunks and endings. In this technique, an extremity is exsanguinated with an Esmarch (elastic) bandage, and a proximally located tourniquet is inflated to 100–150 mm Hg above the systolic blood pressure. The Esmarch bandage is removed, and the local anesthetic is injected into a previously cannulated vein. Typically, complete anesthesia of the limb ensues within 5–10 minutes. Pain from the tourniquet and the potential for ischemic nerve injury limits tourniquet inflation to 2 hours or less. However, the tourniquet should remain inflated for at least 15–30 minutes to prevent toxic amounts of local anesthetic from entering the circulation following deflation. Lidocaine, 40–50 mL (0.5 mL/kg in children) of a 0.5% solution without epinephrine is the drug of choice for this technique. The attractiveness of this technique lies in its simplicity. Its primary disadvantages are that it can be used only for a few anatomical regions, sensation (i.e., pain) returns quickly after tourniquet deflation, and premature release or failure of the tourniquet can produce toxic levels of local anesthetic. Thus, the more cardiotoxic local anesthetics, bupivacaine and etidocaine, are not recommended for this technique. Intravenous regional anesthesia is used most often for surgery of the forearm and hand, but can be adapted for the foot and distal leg.

Spinal Anesthesia

Spinal anesthesia follows the injection of local anesthetic into the cerebrospinal fluid (CSF) in the lumbar space. For a number of reasons, including the ability to produce anesthesia of a considerable fraction of the body with a dose of local anesthetic that produces negligible plasma levels, spinal anesthesia remains one of the most popular forms of anesthesia. In most adults, the spinal cord terminates above the second lumbar vertebra; between that point and the termination of the thecal sac in the sacrum, the lumbar and sacral roots are bathed in CSF. Thus, in this region there is a relatively large volume of CSF within which to inject drug, thereby minimizing the potential for direct nerve trauma.

PHARMACOLOGY OF SPINAL ANESTHESIA

In the U.S., the drugs most commonly used in spinal anesthesia are lidocaine, tetracaine, and bupivacaine. General guidelines are to use lidocaine for short procedures, bupivacaine for intermediate to long procedures, and tetracaine for long procedures. The distribution of local anesthetics *determines the height of block. Important pharmacological factors include the amount, and possibly the volume, of drug injected and its baricity. The speed of injection of the local anesthesia solution also may affect the height of the block, just as the position of the patient can influence the rate of distribution of the anesthetic agent and the height of blockade achieved (see below). For a given preparation of local anesthetic, administration of increasing amounts leads to a fairly predictable increase in the level of block attained. For example, 100 mg of lidocaine, 20 mg of bupivacaine, or 12 mg of tetracaine usually will result in a T4 sensory block. More complete tables of these relationships can be found in standard anesthesiology texts. Epinephrine often is added to spinal anesthetics to increase the duration or intensity of block, but the mechanism of action of vasoconstrictors in prolonging spinal anesthesia is uncertain.*

Spinal anesthesia is a safe and effective technique, especially during surgery involving the lower abdomen, the lower extremities, and the perineum. It often is combined with intravenous medication to provide sedation and amnesia. The physiological perturbations associated with low spinal anesthesia often have less potential harm than those associated with general anesthesia. The same does not apply for high spinal anesthesia. The sympathetic blockade that accompanies levels of spinal anesthesia adequate for mid- or upper-abdominal surgery, coupled with the difficulty in achieving visceral analgesia, is such that equally satisfactory and safer operating conditions can be realized by combining the spinal anesthetic with a "light" general anesthetic or by the administration of a general anesthetic and a neuromuscular blocking agent.

Epidural Anesthesia

Epidural anesthesia is administered by injecting local anesthetic into the epidural space—the space bounded by the ligamentum flavum posteriorly, the spinal periosteum laterally, and the dura anteriorly. Epidural anesthesia can be performed in the sacral hiatus (caudal anesthesia) or in the lumbar, thoracic, or cervical regions of the spine. Its current popularity arises from the development of catheters that can be placed into the epidural space, allowing either continuous infusions or repeated bolus administration of local anesthetics. The primary site of action of epidurally administered local anesthetics is on the spinal nerve roots. However, epidurally administered local anesthetics also may act on the spinal cord and on the paravertebral nerves.

The selection of drugs available for epidural anesthesia is similar to that for major nerve blocks. As for spinal anesthesia, the choice of drugs to be used during epidural anesthesia is dictated primarily by the duration of anesthesia desired. However, when an epidural catheter is placed, short-acting drugs can be administered repeatedly, providing more control over the duration of block. Bupivacaine, 0.5–0.75%, is used when a long duration of surgical block is desired. Due to enhanced cardiotoxicity in pregnant patients, the 0.75% solution is not approved for obstetrical use. Lower concentrations—0.25%, 0.125%, or 0.0625%—of bupivacaine, often with 2 μg/mL of fentanyl added, frequently are used to provide analgesia during labor. They also are useful preparations for providing postoperative analgesia in certain clinical situations. Lidocaine 2% is the most frequently used intermediate-acting epidural local anesthetic. The duration of action of epidurally administered local anesthetics frequently is prolonged, and systemic toxicity decreased, by addition of epinephrine. Addition of epinephrine also makes inadvertent intravascular injection easier to detect and modifies the effect of sympathetic blockade during epidural anesthesia.

For each anesthetic agent, a relationship exists between the volume of local anesthetic injected epidurally and the segmental level of anesthesia achieved. For example, in 20- to 40-year-old, healthy, nonpregnant patients, each 1–1.5 mL of 2% lidocaine will give an additional segment of anesthesia. The amount needed decreases with increasing age and also decreases during pregnancy and in children.

The concentration of local anesthetic used determines the type of nerve fibers blocked. The highest concentrations are used when sympathetic, somatic sensory, and somatic motor blockade are required. Intermediate concentrations allow somatic sensory anesthesia without muscle relaxation. Low concentrations will block only preganglionic sympathetic fibers. A significant difference between epidural and spinal anesthesia is that the dose of local anesthetic used can produce high concentrations in blood following absorption from the epidural space.

EPIDURAL AND INTRATHECAL OPIATE ANALGESIA

Small quantities of opioid injected intrathecally or epidurally produce segmental analgesia. Thus, spinal and epidural opioids are used in surgical procedures and for the relief of postoperative and chronic pain. As with local anesthesia, analgesia is confined to sensory nerves that enter the spinal cord dorsal horn in the vicinity of the injection. Presynaptic opioid receptors inhibit the release of substance P and other neurotransmitters from primary afferents, while postsynaptic opioid receptors decrease the activity of certain dorsal horn neurons in the spinothalamic tracts (see Chapters 6 and 21). Since conduction in autonomic, sensory, and motor nerves is not affected by the opioids, blood pressure, motor function, and non-nociceptive sensory perception typically are not influenced by spinal opioids. The volume-evoked micturition reflex is inhibited, as manifested by urinary retention. Other side effects include pruritus and nausea and vomiting in susceptible individuals. Delayed respiratory depression and sedation, presumably from cephalad spread of opioid within the CSF, occurs infrequently with the doses of opioids currently used.

Spinally administered opioids by themselves do not provide satisfactory anesthesia for surgical procedures. Thus, opioids have found the greatest use in the treatment of postoperative and chronic pain. In selected patients, spinal or epidural opioids can provide excellent analgesia following thoracic, abdominal, pelvic, or lower extremity surgery without the side effects associated with high doses of systemically administered opioids. For postoperative analgesia, spinally administered morphine, 0.2–0.5 mg, usually will provide 8–16 hours of analgesia. Placement of an epidural catheter and repeated boluses or an infusion of opioid permits an increased duration of analgesia. Many opioids have been used epidurally. Morphine, 2–6 mg, every 6 hours, commonly is used for bolus injections, while fentanyl, 20–50 μg/hour, often combined with bupivacaine, 5–20 mg/hour, is used for infusions. For cancer pain, repeated doses of epidural opioids can provide analgesia of several months' duration. The dose of epidural morphine, for example, is far less than the dose of systemically administered morphine that would be required to provide similar analgesia. This reduces the complications that usually accompany the administration of high doses of systemic opioids, particularly sedation and constipation. Unfortunately, as with systemic opioids, tolerance will develop to the analgesic effects of epidural opioids, but this usually can be managed by increasing the dose.

For a complete Bibliographical listing see Goodman & Gilman's *The Pharmacological Basis of Therapeutics*, 11th ed., or Goodman & Gilman Online at www.accessmedicine.com.

15

THERAPEUTIC GASES: O_2, CO_2, NO, AND He

OXYGEN

Normal Oxygenation

Oxygen makes up 21% of air, with a partial pressure of 21 kPa (158 mm Hg) at sea level. The partial pressure drives the diffusion of oxygen; thus, ascent to elevated altitude reduces the uptake and delivery of oxygen to the tissues. As air is delivered to the distal airways and alveoli, the P_{O_2} decreases by dilution with carbon dioxide and water vapor and by uptake into the blood. Under ideal conditions, when ventilation and perfusion are well matched, the alveolar P_{O_2} will be ~14.6 kPa (110 mm Hg). The corresponding alveolar partial pressures of water and CO_2 are 6.2 kPa (47 mm Hg) and 5.3 kPa (40 mm Hg), respectively. Under normal conditions, there is complete equilibration of alveolar gas and capillary blood. In some diseases, the diffusion barrier for gas transport may be increased; during exercise, when high cardiac output reduces capillary transit time, full equilibration may not occur, and the alveolar–end-capillary P_{O_2} gradient may be increased.

The P_{O_2} in arterial blood, however, is further reduced by venous admixture (shunt), the addition of mixed venous blood from the pulmonary artery, which has a P_{O_2} of ~5.3 kPa (40 mm Hg). Together, the diffusional barrier, ventilation–perfusion mismatches, and the shunt fraction are the major causes of the alveolar-to-arterial oxygen gradient, which is normally 1.3–1.6 kPa (10–12 mm Hg) when air is breathed and 4.0–6.6 kPa (30–50 mm Hg) when 100% oxygen is breathed.

Oxygen is delivered to the tissue capillary beds by the circulation and again follows a gradient out of the blood and into cells. Tissue extraction of oxygen typically reduces the P_{O_2} of venous blood by an additional 7.3 kPa (55 mm Hg). Although the P_{O_2} at the mitochondria is not known, oxidative phosphorylation can continue at a P_{O_2} of only a few millimeters of mercury.

In the blood, O_2 is carried primarily by hemoglobin and is to a small extent dissolved in solution. The quantity of O_2 combined with hemoglobin depends on the P_{O_2} (Figure 15–1). Hemoglobin is about 98% saturated with oxygen when air is breathed under normal circumstances, and it binds 1.3 mL of oxygen per gram when fully saturated. The steep slope of this curve with falling P_{O_2} facilitates unloading of oxygen from hemoglobin at the tissue level and reloading when desaturated mixed venous blood arrives at the lung. Shifting of the curve to the right with increasing temperature, increasing P_{CO_2}, and decreasing pH, as is found in metabolically active tissues, lowers the oxygen saturation for the same P_{O_2} and thus delivers additional oxygen where and when it is most needed. However, the flattening of the curve with higher P_{O_2} indicates that increasing blood P_{O_2} by inspiring oxygen-enriched mixtures can increase the amount of oxygen carried by hemoglobin only minimally. Further increases in blood O_2 content can occur only by increasing the amount of oxygen dissolved in plasma. Because of the low solubility of oxygen (0.226 mL/L/kPa or 0.03 mL/L/mm Hg at 37°C), breathing 100% O_2 can increase the amount of O_2 dissolved in blood by only 15 mL/L, less than one-third of normal metabolic demands. However, if the inspired P_{O_2} is increased to 3 atm (304 kPa) in a hyperbaric chamber, the amount of dissolved oxygen is sufficient to meet normal metabolic demands even in the absence of hemoglobin (Table 15–1).

Oxygen Deprivation

Classically, there are five causes of hypoxemia: low inspired oxygen fraction (F_{IO_2}), increased diffusion barrier, hypoventilation, ventilation–perfusion ($\dot{V}/\dot{Q}$) mismatch, and shunt or venous admixture.

In addition to failure of the respiratory system to oxygenate the blood adequately, a number of other factors can contribute to hypoxia at the tissue level. These may be divided into categories of oxygen delivery and oxygen utilization. Oxygen delivery decreases globally when cardiac output falls or locally when regional blood flow is compromised, such as from a vascular occlusion (*e.g.*, stenosis, thrombosis, or microvascular occlusion) or increased downstream pressure (*e.g.*, compartment syndrome, venous stasis, or venous hypertension). Decreased oxygen-carrying capacity of the blood likewise will reduce oxygen delivery, such as occurs with anemia, carbon monoxide poisoning, or hemoglobinopathy. Finally, hypoxia may occur when transport of oxygen from the capillaries to the tissues is decreased (edema) or utilization of the oxygen by the cells is impaired (cyanide toxicity). Our understanding of some of the cellular responses to hypoxia has been advanced by studies of hypoxia-inducible factors.

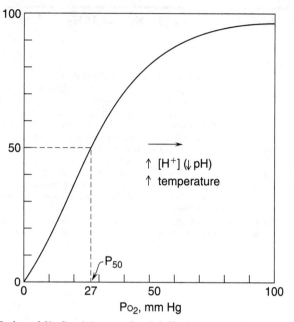

FIGURE 15–1 *Oxyhemoglobin dissociation curve for whole blood.* The relationship between P_{O_2} and hemoglobin (Hb) saturation is shown. The P_{50}, or the P_{O_2} resulting in 50% saturation, is indicated as well. An increase in temperature or a decrease in pH (as in working muscle) shifts this relationship to the right, reducing the hemoglobin saturation at the same P_{O_2} and thus aiding in the delivery of oxygen to the tissues.

Oxygen Inhalation

Oxygen inhalation is used primarily to reverse or prevent the development of hypoxia; other consequences usually are minor. However, when oxygen is breathed in excessive amounts or for prolonged periods, secondary physiological changes and toxic effects can occur.

Respiratory System Inhalation of oxygen at 1 atm or above causes a small degree of respiratory depression in normal subjects, presumably as a result of loss of tonic chemoreceptor activity. However, ventilation typically increases within a few minutes of oxygen inhalation because of a paradoxical increase in the tension of carbon dioxide in tissues, a result of increased oxyhemoglobin in venous blood, which causes less efficient removal of carbon dioxide from the tissues.

In a small number of patients whose respiratory center is depressed by long-term retention of carbon dioxide, injury, or drugs, ventilation is maintained largely by stimulation of carotid and aortic chemoreceptors, commonly referred to as the *hypoxic drive*. The provision of too much oxygen can depress this drive, resulting in respiratory acidosis. In these cases, supplemental oxygen should be titrated carefully to ensure adequate arterial saturation. If hypoventilation results, then mechanical ventilatory support with or without tracheal intubation should be provided.

Expansion of poorly ventilated alveoli is maintained in part by the nitrogen content of alveolar gas; nitrogen is poorly soluble and thus remains in the airspaces while oxygen is absorbed. High oxygen concentrations delivered to poorly ventilated lung regions dilute the nitrogen content and can promote absorption atelectasis, occasionally resulting in an increase in shunt and a paradoxical worsening of hypoxemia after a period of oxygen administration.

Cardiovascular System Aside from reversing the effects of hypoxia, the physiological consequences of oxygen inhalation on the cardiovascular system are of little significance. Heart rate and cardiac output are slightly reduced; blood pressure changes little. While pulmonary arterial pressure changes little in normal subjects with oxygen inhalation, elevated pulmonary artery pressures in patients living at high altitude who have chronic hypoxic pulmonary hypertension may reverse with oxygen therapy or return to sea level. In neonates with congenital heart disease and left-to-right

Table 15–1
The Carriage of Oxygen in Blood*

Arterial Po$_2$, kPa (mm Hg)	Arterial O$_2$ Content (mL O$_2$/L)			Mixed Venous Po$_2$, kPa (mm Hg)	Mixed Venous O$_2$ Content (mL O$_2$/L)			Examples
	Dissolved	Bound to Hemoglobin	Total		Dissolved	Bound to Hemoglobin	Total	
4.0 (30)	0.9	109	109.9	2.7 (20)	0.6	59	59.6	High altitude; respiratory failure breathing air
12.0 (90)	2.7	192	194.7	5.5 (41)	1.2	144	145.2	Normal person breathing air
39.9 (300)	9.0	195	204	5.9 (44)	1.3	153	154.3	Normal person breathing 50% O$_2$
79.7 (600)	18	196	214	6.5 (49)	1.5	163	164.5	Normal person breathing 100% O$_2$
239 (1800)	54	196	250	20.0 (150)	4.5	196	200.5	Normal person breathing hyperbaric O$_2$

*This table illustrates the carriage of oxygen in the blood under a variety of circumstances. As arterial O$_2$ tension increases, the amount of dissolved O$_2$ increases in direct proportion to the Po$_2$, but the amount of oxygen bound to hemoglobin reaches a maximum of 196 mL O$_2$/L (100% saturation of hemoglobin at 15 g/dL). Further increases in O$_2$ content require increases in dissolved oxygen. At 100% inspired O$_2$, dissolved O$_2$ still provides only a small fraction of total demand. Hyperbaric oxygen therapy is required to increase the amount of dissolved oxygen to supply all or a large part of metabolic requirements. Note that, during hyperbaric oxygen therapy, the hemoglobin in the mixed venous blood remains fully saturated with O$_2$.

The figures in this table are approximate and are based on the assumptions of 15 g/dL hemoglobin, 50 mL O$_2$/L whole-body oxygen extraction, and constant cardiac output. When severe anemia is present, arterial Po$_2$ remains the same, but arterial content is lower; oxygen extraction continues, resulting in lower O$_2$ content and tension in mixed venous blood. Similarly, as cardiac output falls significantly, the same oxygen extraction occurs from a smaller volume of blood and results in lower mixed venous oxygen content and tension.

shunting of cardiac output, oxygen supplementation must be regulated carefully because of the risk of further reducing pulmonary vascular resistance and increasing pulmonary blood flow.

Metabolism Inhalation of 100% oxygen does not produce detectable changes in oxygen consumption, carbon dioxide production, respiratory quotient, or glucose utilization.

Oxygen Administration

For safety, oxygen cylinders and piping are color-coded (green in the U.S.), and some form of mechanical indexing of valve connections is used to prevent the connection of other gases to oxygen systems. Oxygen is delivered by inhalation except during extracorporeal circulation, when it is dissolved directly into the circulating blood. Only a closed delivery system with an airtight seal to the patient's airway and complete separation of inspired from expired gases can precisely control FIO_2. In all other systems, the actual delivered FIO_2 will depend on the ventilatory pattern (*i.e.*, rate, tidal volume, inspiratory–expiratory time ratio, and inspiratory flow) and delivery system characteristics.

Low-Flow Systems

Low-flow systems, in which the oxygen flow is lower than the inspiratory flow rate, have a limited ability to raise the FIO_2 because they depend on entrained room air to make up the balance of the inspired gas. The FIO_2 of these systems is extremely sensitive to small changes in the ventilatory pattern. Devices such as face tents are used primarily for delivering humidified gases to patients and cannot be relied on to provide predictable amounts of supplemental oxygen. Nasal cannulae—small, flexible prongs that sit just inside each naris—deliver oxygen at 1–6 L/min. The nasopharynx acts as a reservoir for storing the oxygen, and patients may breathe through either the mouth or nose as long as the nasal passages remain patent. These devices typically deliver 24–28% FIO_2 at 2–3 L/min. Up to 40% FIO_2 is possible at higher flow rates, although this is poorly tolerated for more than brief periods because of mucosal drying. The simple facemask, a clear plastic mask with side holes for clearance of expiratory gas and inspiratory air entrainment, is used when higher concentrations of oxygen delivered without tight control are desired. The maximum FIO_2 of a facemask can be increased from around 60% at 6–15 L/min to >85% by adding a 600- to 1000-mL reservoir bag. With this partial rebreathing mask, most of the inspired volume is drawn from the reservoir, avoiding dilution by entrainment of room air.

High-Flow Systems

The most commonly used high-flow oxygen delivery device is the Venturi mask, which uses a specially designed mask insert to entrain room air reliably in a fixed ratio and thus provides a relatively constant FIO_2 at relatively high flow rates. Typically, each insert is designed to operate at a specific oxygen flow rate, and different inserts are required to change the FIO_2. Lower delivered FIO_2 values use greater entrainment ratios, resulting in higher total (oxygen plus entrained air) flows to the patient, ranging from 80 L/min for 24% FIO_2 to 40 L/min at 50% FIO_2. These flow rates still may be lower than the peak inspiratory flows for patients in respiratory distress, and thus the actual delivered oxygen concentration may be lower than the nominal value. Oxygen nebulizers, another type of Venturi device, provide patients with humidified oxygen at 35–100% FIO_2 at high flow rates. Finally, oxygen blenders provide high inspired oxygen concentrations at very high flow rates. These devices mix high-pressure compressed air and oxygen to achieve any concentration of oxygen from 21–100% at flow rates of up to 100 L/min. Despite the high flows, the delivery of high FIO_2 to an individual patient also depends on maintaining a tight-fitting seal to the airway and/or the use of reservoirs to minimize entrainment of diluting room air.

MONITORING OF OXYGENATION

Monitoring and titration are required to meet the therapeutic goal of oxygen therapy and to avoid complications and side effects. Although cyanosis is a physical finding of substantial clinical importance, it is not an early, sensitive, or reliable index of oxygenation. Noninvasive monitoring of arterial oxygen saturation now is widely available from transcutaneous pulse oximetry, in which oxygen saturation is measured from the differential absorption of light by oxyhemoglobin and deoxyhemoglobin and the arterial saturation determined from the pulsatile component of this signal. Pulse oximetry measures hemoglobin saturation and not PO_2; thus, it is insensitive to increases in PO_2 beyond that required to saturate the blood fully. However, pulse oximetry is very useful for monitoring the adequacy of oxygenation during procedures requiring sedation or anesthesia, rapid evaluation and monitoring of potentially compromised patients, and titrating oxygen therapy in situations where toxicity from oxygen or side effects of excess oxygen are of concern.

COMPLICATIONS OF OXYGEN THERAPY

Administration of supplemental oxygen is not without potential complications. In addition to the potential to promote absorption atelectasis and depress ventilation, high flows of dry oxygen can dry out and irritate mucosal surfaces of the airway and the eyes, as well as decrease mucociliary transport and clearance of secretions. Humidified oxygen thus should be used when prolonged therapy (>1 hour) is required. Finally, any oxygen-enriched atmosphere constitutes a fire hazard, and appropriate precautions must be taken both in the operating room and for patients on oxygen at home. Hypoxemia still can occur despite the administration of supplemental oxygen. Furthermore, when supplemental oxygen is administered, desaturation occurs at a later time after airway obstruction or hypoventilation, potentially delaying the detection of these critical events. Therefore, it is essential that oxygen saturation and adequacy of ventilation be assessed frequently.

Therapeutic Uses of Oxygen

CORRECTION OF HYPOXIA

The primary therapeutic use of oxygen is to correct hypoxia. However, hypoxia is generally a manifestation of an underlying disease, and administration of oxygen thus should be viewed as a symptomatic therapy. Efforts must be directed at correcting the cause of the hypoxia. For example, airway obstruction is unlikely to respond to an increase in inspired oxygen tension without relief of the obstruction. More important, while hypoxemia owing to hypoventilation after a narcotic overdose can be improved with supplemental oxygen administration, the patient remains at risk for respiratory failure if ventilation is not increased through stimulation, narcotic reversal, or mechanical ventilation. The hypoxia that results from most pulmonary diseases can be alleviated at least partially by administration of oxygen, thereby allowing time for definitive therapy to reverse the primary process. Thus, administration of oxygen is used in all forms of hypoxia, with the understanding that the response will vary in a way that generally is predictable from knowledge of the underlying pathophysiology.

REDUCTION OF PARTIAL PRESSURE OF AN INERT GAS

Nitrogen, which constitutes 79% of ambient air, predominates in most gas-filled spaces in the body. In certain situations, such as bowel distension from obstruction or ileus, intravascular air embolism, or pneumothorax, it is desirable to reduce the volume of these air-filled spaces. Since nitrogen is relatively insoluble, inhalation of high concentrations of oxygen (and thus low concentrations of nitrogen) rapidly lowers the total-body partial pressure of nitrogen and provides a substantial gradient for the removal of nitrogen from gas spaces. Administration of oxygen for air embolism is additionally beneficial because it also helps to relieve the localized hypoxia distal to the embolic vascular obstruction. In the case of decompression sickness, *or* bends, *lowering of inert gas tension in blood and tissues by oxygen inhalation prior to or during a barometric decompression can reduce the degree of supersaturation that occurs after decompression so that bubbles do not form. If bubbles do form in either tissues or the vasculature, administration of oxygen is based on the same rationale as that described for gas embolism.*

HYPERBARIC OXYGEN THERAPY

Oxygen is administered at greater than atmospheric pressure for a number of conditions when 100% oxygen at 1 atm is insufficient.

Hyperbaric oxygen therapy has two components: increased hydrostatic pressure and increased oxygen pressure. Both factors are necessary for the treatment of decompression sickness and air embolism. The hydrostatic pressure reduces bubble volume, and the absence of inspired nitrogen increases the gradient for elimination of nitrogen and reduces hypoxia in downstream tissues. Increased oxygen pressure at the tissue level is the primary therapeutic goal for most of the other indications for hyperbaric oxygen. For example, even a small increase in Po_2 in previously ischemic areas may enhance the bactericidal activity of leukocytes and increase angiogenesis. Thus, repetitive brief exposures to hyperbaric oxygen are a useful adjunct in the treatment of chronic refractory osteomyelitis, osteoradionecrosis, or crush injury or for the recovery of compromised skin, tissue grafts, or flaps. Furthermore, increased oxygen tension itself can be bacteriostatic; the spread of infection with Clostridium perfringens *and production of toxin by the bacteria are slowed when oxygen tensions exceed 33 kPa (250 mm Hg), justifying the early use of hyperbaric oxygen in clostridial myonecrosis (gas gangrene).*

Hyperbaric oxygen also is useful in selected instances of generalized hypoxia. In CO poisoning, hemoglobin (Hb) and myoglobin become unavailable for O_2 binding because of the high affinity of these proteins for CO. This affinity is ~250 times greater than the affinity for O_2; thus, an alveolar concentration of CO = 0.4 mm Hg (1/250th that of alveolar O_2, which is ~100 mm Hg), *will compete equally with O_2 for binding sites on Hb. A high P_{O_2} facilitates competition of O_2 for Hb binding sites as CO is exchanged in the alveoli; i.e., the high P_{O_2} increases the probability that O_2 rather than CO will bind to Hb once CO dissociates. In addition, hyperbaric O_2 will increase the availability of dissolved O_2 in the blood (see Table 15–1). The occasional use of hyperbaric oxygen in cyanide poisoning has a similar rationale.*

Oxygen Toxicity

Oxygen toxicity probably results from increased production of hydrogen peroxide and reactive agents such as superoxide anion, singlet oxygen, and hydroxyl radicals that attack and damage lipids, proteins, and other macromolecules, especially those in biological membranes. A number of factors limit the toxicity of oxygen-derived reactive agents, including enzymes such as superoxide dismutase, glutathione peroxidase, and catalase, which scavenge toxic oxygen by-products, and reducing agents such as iron, glutathione, and ascorbate. These factors, however, are insufficient to limit the destructive actions of oxygen when patients are exposed to high concentrations over an extended time period. Tissues show differential sensitivity to oxygen toxicity, which is likely the result of differences in both their production of reactive compounds and their protective mechanisms. Decreases of inspired oxygen concentrations remain the cornerstone of therapy for oxygen toxicity.

The pulmonary system, continuously exposed to the highest O_2 tensions in the body, is usually the first to exhibit toxicity; subtle changes in pulmonary function can occur within 8–12 hours of exposure to 100% oxygen. Increases in capillary permeability and decreased pulmonary function can be seen after only 18 hours of exposure. Serious injury and death require much longer exposures. Pulmonary damage is directly related to the inspired oxygen tension, and concentrations of >0.5 atm appear to be safe over long time periods. The capillary endothelium is the most sensitive tissue of the lung.

Retrolental fibroplasia can occur when neonates are exposed to increased oxygen tensions; these changes can progress to blindness. The incidence of this disorder has decreased with an improved appreciation of the issues and avoidance of excessive inspired oxygen concentrations. Adults do not seem to develop the disease.

CNS problems are rare, and toxicity occurs only under hyperbaric conditions >200 kPa (2 atm). Symptoms include seizures and visual changes, which resolve when oxygen tension is returned to normal. These problems are a further reason to replace oxygen with helium under hyperbaric conditions (*see* below).

CARBON DIOXIDE

Carbon dioxide (CO_2) is produced by the body's metabolism at approximately the same rate as O_2 consumption, about 3 mL/kg/minute at rest, increasing dramatically with heavy exercise. CO_2 diffuses readily from the cells into the bloodstream, where it is carried partly as bicarbonate ion (HCO_3^-), partly in chemical combination with hemoglobin and plasma proteins, and partly in solution at a partial pressure of ~6 kPa (46 mm Hg) in mixed venous blood. CO_2 is transported to the lung, where it is normally exhaled at the same rate at which it is produced, leaving a partial pressure of ~5.2 kPa (40 mm Hg) in the alveoli and in arterial blood. An increase in P_{CO_2} results in a respiratory acidosis and may be due to decreased ventilation or the inhalation of CO_2, whereas an increase in ventilation results in decreased P_{CO_2} and a respiratory alkalosis. Since CO_2 is freely diffusible, changes in blood P_{CO_2} and pH soon are reflected by intracellular changes in P_{CO_2} and pH.

Effects of Carbon Dioxide

Carbon dioxide is a rapid, potent stimulus to ventilation. Inhalation of 10% CO_2 can produce minute volumes of 75 L/min in normal individuals. Carbon dioxide acts at multiple sites to stimulate ventilation. Elevated P_{CO_2} causes bronchodilation, whereas hypocarbia causes constriction of airway smooth muscle; these responses may play a role in matching pulmonary ventilation and perfusion. Circulatory effects of CO_2 result from the combination of direct local effects and centrally mediated effects on the autonomic nervous system. The direct effects are diminished contractility of the heart and vascular smooth muscle (vasodilation). The indirect effects result from the capacity of CO_2 to activate the sympathetic nervous system; these indirect effects generally oppose the local effects of CO_2. Thus, the balance of opposing local and sympathetic effects determines the total circulatory response to CO_2. The net effect of CO_2 inhalation is an increase in cardiac output, heart rate, and blood pressure. In blood vessels, however, the direct vasodilating actions of carbon dioxide appear more important, and total peripheral resistance decreases when the P_{CO_2} is increased. CO_2 also is a potent coronary vasodilator. Cardiac arrhythmias associated with increased P_{CO_2} are due to the release of catecholamines.

Hypocarbia *results in opposite effects: decreased blood pressure and vasoconstriction in skin, intestine, brain, kidney, and heart. These actions are exploited clinically in the use of hyperventilation to diminish intracranial hypertension.*

Hypercarbia depresses the excitability of the cerebral cortex and increases the cutaneous pain threshold through a central action. In patients who are hypoventilating from narcotics or anesthetics, increasing P_{CO_2} may result in further CNS depression, which in turn may worsen the respiratory depression. This positive-feedback cycle can be deadly.

Therapeutic Uses

Inhalation of CO_2 is used less commonly today than in the past because there are now more effective treatments for most indications. Inhalation of carbon dioxide has been used during anesthesia to increase the speed of induction and emergence from inhalational anesthesia by increasing minute ventilation and cerebral blood flow. However, this technique results in some degree of respiratory acidosis. Hypocarbia, with its attendant respiratory alkalosis, still has some uses in anesthesia. It constricts cerebral vessels, decreasing brain size slightly, and thus may facilitate the performance of neurosurgical operations. Although CO_2 stimulates respiration, CO_2 is not useful in situations where respiratory depression has resulted in hypercarbia or acidosis because further depression results.

CO_2 is commonly used for insufflation during endoscopic procedures (e.g., laparoscopic surgery) because CO_2 is highly soluble and does not support combustion. Any inadvertent gas emboli thus are dissolved and eliminated more easily via the respiratory system. CO_2 can be helpful during open cardiac surgery, where the gas is used to flood the surgical field and, because of its density, displaces the air surrounding the open heart, assuring that any gas bubbles trapped are CO_2 rather than insoluble nitrogen. For the same reasons, CO_2 is used to debubble cardiopulmonary bypass and extracorporeal membrane oxygenation (ECMO) circuits. It also can be used to adjust pH during bypass procedures when a patient is cooled.

NITRIC OXIDE

Nitric oxide (NO), a free-radical gas long known as an air pollutant and a potential toxin, is an endogenous cell-signaling molecule of great physiological importance. Endogenous NO is produced from L-arginine by a family of enzymes called *NO synthases*. NO activates the soluble guanyl cyclase, increasing cellular cyclic GMP (*see* Chapter 1). In the vasculature, NO causes relaxation of vascular smooth muscle; basal release of NO by endothelial cells is a primary determinant of resting vascular tone; NO causes vasodilation when synthesized in response to shear stress or a variety of vasodilating agents (*see* Chapter 32). It also inhibits platelet aggregation and adhesion. Impaired NO production has been implicated in diseases such as atherosclerosis, hypertension, cerebral and coronary vasospasm, and ischemia–reperfusion injury. In the immune system, NO serves as an effector of macrophage-induced cytotoxicity, and overproduction of NO is a mediator of inflammation. In neurons, NO acts as a mediator of long-term potentiation, cytotoxicity resulting from *N*-methyl-D-aspartate (NMDA), and nonadrenergic noncholinergic neurotransmission; NO has been implicated in mediating central nociceptive pathways (*see* Chapter 6).

Therapeutic Use of NO

Inhaled NO can selectively dilate the pulmonary vasculature with minimal systemic cardiovascular effects. The lack of effect of inhaled NO on the systemic circulation is due to its strong binding to and inactivation by oxyhemoglobin on exposure to the pulmonary circulation. Ventilation–perfusion matching is preserved or improved by NO because inhaled NO is distributed only to ventilated areas of the lung and dilates only those vessels directly adjacent to the ventilated alveoli. Thus, inhaled NO will decrease elevated pulmonary artery pressure and pulmonary vascular resistance and often improve oxygenation. Therapeutic trials of inhaled NO have confirmed its ability to decrease pulmonary vascular resistance and often increase oxygenation, but have generally not demonstrated long-term improvement in terms of morbidity or mortality. Inhaled NO has been approved by the FDA only for use in newborns with persistent pulmonary hypertension and has become the first-line therapy for this disease. Trials of inhaled NO in adult and pediatric acute respiratory distress syndrome, as well as a recent meta-analysis, demonstrate no impact on outcome. Outside of clinical investigation, therapeutic use and benefit of inhaled NO presently are limited to newborns with persistent pulmonary hypertension.

Diagnostic Uses of NO

Inhaled NO can be used during cardiac catheterization to evaluate safely and selectively the pulmonary vasodilating capacity of patients with heart failure and infants with congenital heart disease. Inhaled NO also is used to determine the diffusion capacity (DL) across the alveolar–capillary unit. NO is more effective than CO_2 in this regard because of its greater affinity for hemoglobin and its higher water solubility at body temperature.

NO is produced from the nasal passages and from the lungs of normal human subjects and can be detected in exhaled gas. Measurement of exhaled NO may prove to be useful in diagnosis and assessment of severity of asthma and in respiratory tract infections.

Toxicity of NO

Administered at low concentrations (0.1–50 ppm), inhaled NO appears to be safe and without significant side effects. Pulmonary toxicity can occur with levels higher than 50–100 ppm. The Occupational Safety and Health Administration places the 7-hour exposure limit at 50 ppm. Part of the toxicity of NO may be related to its further oxidation to NO_2. Even low concentrations of NO_2 (2 ppm) have been shown to be highly toxic in animal models, with observed changes in lung histopathology, including loss of cilia, hypertrophy, and focal hyperplasia in the epithelium of terminal bronchioles. Thus, during NO therapy, it is important to keep NO_2 formation at a low level by using appropriate filters and scavengers and high-quality gas mixtures. Chronic low doses of inhaled NO may cause surfactant inactivation and the formation of peroxynitrite by interaction with superoxide. The capacity of NO to inhibit or alter the function of a number of iron- and heme-containing proteins suggests a need for further investigation of the toxic potential of NO under therapeutic conditions.

The development of methemoglobinemia is a significant complication of inhaled NO at higher concentrations, and rare deaths have been reported with overdoses of NO. The blood content of methemoglobin generally will not increase to toxic levels with appropriate use of inhaled NO. Methemoglobin concentrations should be monitored intermittently during NO inhalation. Inhaled NO can inhibit platelet function and has been shown to increase bleeding time in some clinical studies, although bleeding complications have not been reported.

In patients with impaired function of the left ventricle, NO has a potential to further impair left ventricular performance by dilating the pulmonary circulation and increasing the blood flow to the left ventricle, thereby increasing left atrial pressure and promoting pulmonary edema formation. Careful monitoring of cardiac output, left atrial pressure, or pulmonary capillary wedge pressure is important in this situation.

The most important requirements for safe NO inhalation therapy include (1) continuous measurement of NO and NO_2 concentrations using either chemiluminescence or electrochemical analyzers; (2) frequent calibration of monitoring equipment; (3) intermittent analysis of blood methemoglobin levels; (4) the use of certified tanks of NO; and (5) administration of the lowest NO concentration required for therapeutic effect.

Methods of Administration

Courses of treatment of patients with inhaled NO are highly varied, extending from 0.1–40 ppm in dose and for periods of a few hours to several weeks in duration. The minimum effective inhaled NO concentration should be determined for each patient to minimize the chance for toxicity. Commercial NO systems are available that will accurately deliver inspired NO concentrations between 0.1 and 80 ppm and simultaneously measure NO and NO_2 concentrations. A constant inspired concentration of NO is obtained by administering NO in nitrogen to the inspiratory limb of the ventilator circuit in either a pulse or continuous mode. While inhaled NO may be administered to spontaneously breathing patients via a closely fitting mask, it usually is delivered during mechanical ventilation. Nasal prong administration is being employed in therapeutic trials of home administration for treatment of primary pulmonary hypertension.

Acute discontinuation of NO inhalation can lead to a rebound pulmonary artery hypertension with an increase in right-to-left intrapulmonary shunting and a decrease in oxygenation. To avoid this phenomenon, a graded decrease of inhaled NO concentration is used in weaning a patient from inhaled NO.

HELIUM

Helium (He) is an inert gas whose low density, low solubility, and high thermal conductivity provide the basis for its medical and diagnostic uses; the gas is supplied in brown cylinders. Helium can be mixed with oxygen and administered by mask or tracheal tube. Under hyperbaric conditions, it can be substituted for the bulk of other gases, resulting in a mixture of much lower density that is easier to breathe.

The primary uses of helium are in pulmonary function testing, the treatment of respiratory obstruction, during laser airway surgery, for diving at depth, and most recently, as a label in imaging studies. The determinations of residual lung volume, functional residual capacity, and related lung volumes require a highly diffusible nontoxic gas that is insoluble (and thus does not leave the lung *via* the bloodstream) so that, by dilution, the lung volume can be measured. Helium is well suited to these needs and is much cheaper than alternatives. In these tests, a breath of a known concentration of helium is given, and the concentration of helium then is measured in the mixed expired gas, allowing calculation of the other pulmonary volumes.

Pulmonary gas flow is normally laminar, but with increased flow rate or narrowed flow pathway, a component becomes turbulent. Helium can be added to oxygen to treat the turbulence due to airway obstruction: the density of helium is substantially less than that of air and the viscosity of helium is greater than that of air; addition of helium reduces the Reynolds number of the mixture (the Reynolds number is proportional to density and inversely proportional to viscosity), thereby reducing turbulence. Indeed, flow rates are increased with lower density gases. Thus, with mixtures of helium and oxygen, the work of breathing is less. Several factors limit the utility of this approach, however. Oxygenation is often the principal problem in airway obstruction, and the practical need for increased inspired O$_2$ concentration may limit the fraction of helium that can be used. Furthermore, even though helium reduces the Reynolds number of the gas mixture, the viscosity of helium is higher than that of air, and the increased viscosity increases the resistance to flow according to Poiseuille's law, whereby flow is inversely proportional to viscosity.

Helium has high thermal conductivity, which makes it useful during laser surgery on the airway. This more rapid conduction of heat away from the point of contact of the laser beam reduces the spread of tissue damage and the likelihood that the ignition point of flammable materials in the airway will be reached. Helium's low density improves the flow through the small endotracheal tubes typically used in such procedures.

Recently, laser-polarized helium has been used as an inhalational contrast agent for pulmonary magnetic resonance imaging.

HYPERBARIC APPLICATIONS The depth and duration of diving activity are limited by oxygen toxicity, inert gas (nitrogen) narcosis, and nitrogen supersaturation when decompressing. Oxygen toxicity is a problem with prolonged exposure to compressed air at 500 kPa (5 atm) or more. This problem can be minimized by dilution of oxygen with helium, which lacks narcotic potential even at very high pressures and is quite insoluble in body tissues. This low solubility reduces the likelihood of bubble formation after decompression, which therefore can be achieved more rapidly. The low density of helium also reduces the work of breathing in the otherwise dense hyperbaric atmosphere. The lower heat capacity of helium also decreases respiratory heat loss, which can be significant when diving at depth.

For a complete Bibliographical listing see Goodman & Gilman's *The Pharmacological Basis of Therapeutics*, 11th ed., or Goodman & Gilman Online at www.accessmedicine.com.

16

HYPNOTICS AND SEDATIVES

A *sedative* drug decreases activity, moderates excitement, and calms; a *hypnotic* drug produces drowsiness and facilitates the onset and maintenance of a state of sleep resembling natural sleep and from which the recipient can be aroused easily. The sleep induced by hypnotic drugs does not resemble the artificially induced passive state of suggestibility also called *hypnosis*.

BENZODIAZEPINES

All benzodiazepines in clinical use have the capacity to promote the binding of the major inhibitory neurotransmitter γ-aminobutyric acid (GABA) to $GABA_A$ receptors, thereby enhancing the GABA-induced ionic currents through these channels (*see* Chapter 12). Pharmacological investigations have provided evidence for heterogeneity among sites of binding and action of benzodiazepines and for heterogeneity of subunit composition of the GABA-gated chloride channels of different neurons. A number of distinct mechanisms of action are thought to contribute to the sedative-hypnotic, muscle-relaxant, anxiolytic, and anticonvulsant effects of the benzodiazepines, and specific sub-units of the $GABA_A$ receptor are responsible for specific pharmacological properties of benzodiazepines. Although benzodiazepines exert qualitatively similar clinical effects, quantitative differences in their pharmacodynamic spectra and pharmacokinetic properties have led to varying patterns of therapeutic application.

CHEMISTRY
The basic structure of the benzodiazepines is shown in Table 16–1.

Pharmacological Properties

Virtually all effects of the benzodiazepines result from their actions on the central nervous system (CNS). The most prominent of these effects are sedation, hypnosis, decreased anxiety, muscle relaxation, anterograde amnesia, and anticonvulsant activity. Only two effects of these drugs result from peripheral actions: coronary vasodilation, seen after intravenous administration of therapeutic doses of certain benzodiazepines, and neuromuscular blockade, seen only with very high doses.

A number of benzodiazepine-like effects are classified as *full agonistic effects* (*i.e.*, faithfully mimicking agents such as *diazepam* with relatively low fractional occupancy of binding sites) or *partial agonistic effects* (*i.e.*, producing less intense maximal effects and/or requiring relatively high fractional occupancy compared with agents such as diazepam). Some compounds produce effects opposite to those of diazepam in the absence of benzodiazepine-like agonists and are termed *inverse agonists; partial inverse agonists* also have been recognized (*see* Chapter 1 for a discussion of inverse agonism). The vast majority of effects of agonists and inverse agonists can be reversed or prevented by the benzodiazepine antagonist *flumazenil*, which competes with agonists and inverse agonists for binding to the $GABA_A$ receptor.

CENTRAL NERVOUS SYSTEM While benzodiazepines affect activity at all levels of the neuraxis, some structures are affected preferentially. The benzodiazepines do not produce the same degrees of neuronal depression as do barbiturates and volatile anesthetics. Although the benzodiazepines have similar pharmacological profiles, the drugs differ in selectivity and thus in clinical utility.

As the dose of a benzodiazepine is increased, sedation progresses to hypnosis and then to stupor. The clinical literature often refers to the "anesthetic" effects and uses of certain benzodiazepines, but the drugs do not cause a true general anesthesia because awareness usually persists, and relaxation sufficient to allow surgery cannot be achieved. However, at "preanesthetic" doses, there is amnesia for events subsequent to administration of the drug, possibly creating the illusion of previous anesthesia.

Separating the anxiolytic actions of benzodiazepines from their sedative-hypnotic effects is problematic; measurements of anxiety and sedation are difficult in human beings, and the validity of animal models for anxiety and sedation is uncertain.

Tolerance to Benzodiazepines; Selectivity

Although most patients who ingest benzodiazepines chronically report that drowsiness wanes over a few days, tolerance to the impairment of some measures of psychomotor performance (e.g., visual tracking) usually is not observed. The development of tolerance to the anxiolytic effects of benzodiazepines is a subject of debate. Some benzodiazepines induce muscle hypotonia without

Table 16-1

Benzodiazepines: Names and Structures*

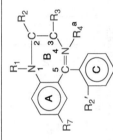

Benzodiazepine	R_1	R_2	R_3	R_7	R_2'
Alprazolam	[Fused triazolo ring][b]		—H	—Cl	—H
Brotizolam[†]	[Fused triazolo ring][b]		—H	[Thieno ring A][c]	—Cl
Chlordiazepoxide[a]	(—)	—NHCH$_3$	—H	—Cl	—H
Clobazam[a,†]	—CH$_3$	=O	—H	—Cl	—H
Clonazepam	—H	=O	—H	—NO$_2$	—Cl
Clorazepate	—H	=O	—COO⁻	—Cl	—H
Demoxepam[a,†,‡]	—H	=O	—H	—Cl	—H
Diazepam	—CH$_3$	=O	—H	—Cl	—H
Estazolam	[Fused triazolo ring][d]		—H	—Cl	—H
Flumazenil[a]	[Fused imidazo ring][e]			—F	[=O at C$_5$][g]
Flurazepam	—CH$_2$CH$_2$N(C$_2$H$_5$)$_2$	=O	—H	—Cl	—F
Lorazepam	—H	=O	—OH	—Cl	—Cl
Midazolam	[Fused imidazo ring][f]		—H	—Cl	—F
Nitrazepam[†]	—H	=O	—H	—NO$_2$	—H
Nordazepam[†,§]	—H	=O	—H	—Cl	—H
Oxazepam	—H	=O	—OH	—Cl	—H
Prazepam[†]	—CH$_2$—CH< (CH$_2$CH$_2$)	=O	—H	—Cl	—H

(Continued)

263

Table 16–1

Benzodiazepines: Names and Structures* (Continued)

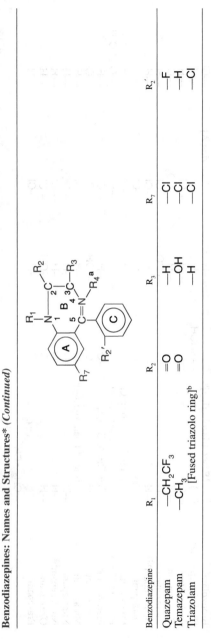

Benzodiazepine	R_1	R_2	R_3	R_7	R_2'
Quazepam	—CH_2CF_3	=O	—H	—Cl	—F
Temazepam	—CH_3	=O	—OH	—Cl	—H
Triazolam	[Fused triazolo ring][b]		—H	—Cl	—Cl

*Alphabetical footnotes refer to alterations of the general formula; symbolic footnotes are used for other comments.
[†]Not available for clinical use in the U.S.
[‡]Major metabolite of chlordiazepoxide.
[§]Major metabolite of diazepam and others; also referred to as nordiazepam and desmethyldiazepam.
[a]No substituent at position 4, except for chlordiazepoxide and demoxepam, which are N-oxides; R_4 is —CH_3 in flumazenil, in which there is no double bond between positions 4 and 5; R_4 is=O in clobazam, in which position 4 is C and position 5 is N.

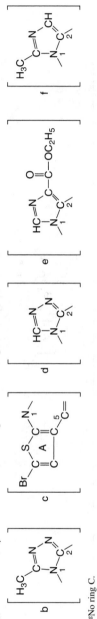

[g]No ring C.

264

interfering with normal locomotion and can decrease rigidity in patients with cerebral palsy. In contrast to effects in animals, there is only a limited selectivity in human beings. Clonazepam *in nonsedative doses does cause muscle relaxation, but diazepam and most other benzodiazepines do not. Tolerance occurs to the muscle relaxant and ataxic effects of these drugs.*

Experimentally, benzodiazepines inhibit some types of seizure activity. Clonazepam, nitrazepam, *and* nordazepam *have more selective anticonvulsant activity than most other benzodiazepines. Benzodiazepines also suppress ethanol-withdrawal seizures in human beings. However, the development of tolerance to the anticonvulsant effects has limited the usefulness of benzodiazepines in the treatment of recurrent seizure disorders* (see Chapter 19).

Only transient analgesia is apparent in humans after intravenous administration of benzodiazepines. Such effects actually may involve the production of amnesia. Unlike barbiturates, benzodiazepines do not cause hyperalgesia.

Effects on the Electroencephalogram and Sleep Stages

The effects of benzodiazepines on the waking electroencephalogram (EEG) resemble those of other sedative-hypnotic drugs. Alpha activity is decreased, but there is an increase in low-voltage fast activity. Tolerance occurs to these effects.

Most benzodiazepines decrease sleep latency, especially when first used, and diminish the number of awakenings and the time spent in stage 0 (a stage of wakefulness). Time in stage 1 (descending drowsiness) usually is decreased, and there is a prominent decrease in the time spent in slow-wave sleep (stages 3 and 4). Most benzodiazepines increase the time from onset of spindle sleep to the first burst of rapid-eye-movement (REM) sleep. The time spent in REM sleep usually is shortened, but the number of cycles of REM sleep cycles usually is increased, mostly late in the sleep time. Zolpidem *and* zaleplon *suppress REM sleep to a lesser extent and thus may be superior to benzodiazepines for use as hypnotics.*

Benzodiazepine administration typically increases total sleep time, largely because of increased time spent in stage 2 (the major fraction of non-REM sleep). The effect is greatest in subjects with the shortest baseline total sleep time. Despite the increased number of REM cycles, the number of shifts to lighter sleep stages (1 and 0) and the amount of body movement are diminished. Nocturnal peaks in the secretion of growth hormone, prolactin, and luteinizing hormone are not affected. During chronic nocturnal use of benzodiazepines, the effects on the various stages of sleep usually decline within a few nights. With discontinuation of drug, the pattern of drug-induced changes in sleep parameters may "rebound," with an increase in the amount and density of REM sleep. If the dosage has not been excessive, patients usually will note only a shortening of sleep time rather than an exacerbation of insomnia.

Benzodiazepine use usually imparts a sense of deep or refreshing sleep. It is uncertain to which effect on sleep parameters this feeling can be attributed. As a result, variations in the pharmacokinetic properties of individual benzodiazepines appear to be much more important determinants of their effects on sleep than are any potential differences in their pharmacodynamic properties.

Molecular Targets for Benzodiazepine Actions in the CNS Benzodiazepines likely exert most of their effects by interacting with inhibitory neurotransmitter receptors directly activated by GABA. Benzodiazepines act at $GABA_A$ (ionotropic) receptors (but not at $GABA_B$ [metabotropic] receptors [GPCRs]) by binding to a specific site that is distinct from that of GABA binding. Unlike barbiturates, benzodiazepines do not activate $GABA_A$ receptors directly but rather require GABA to express their effects; *i.e.*, they only modulate the effects of GABA. Benzodiazepines and related compounds can act as agonists, antagonists, or inverse agonists at the benzodiazepine-binding site on $GABA_A$ receptors. Agonists at the benzodiazepine-binding site shift the GABA concentration–response curve to the left, increasing the amount of chloride current generated by $GABA_A$-receptor activation; inverse agonists shift the curve to the right, reducing the effect of given concentration of GABA. Both these effects are blocked by antagonists at the benzodiazepine-binding site. A pure antagonist (*e.g.*, flumazenil) acting alone at this binding site does not affect $GABA_A$-receptor function but can reverse the effects of high doses of benzodiazepines. The behavioral and electrophysiological effects of benzodiazepines also can be reduced or prevented by prior treatment with antagonists at the GABA-binding site (*e.g.*, bicuculline).

$GABA_A$ Receptor-Mediated Electrical Events: *In Vivo* Properties

The remarkable safety of the benzodiazepines is likely related to the fact that their effects in vivo depend on the presynaptic release of GABA; in the absence of GABA, benzodiazepines have no effects on $GABA_A$ receptor function. Although barbiturates also enhance the effects of GABA at *low concentrations, they directly activate GABA receptors at higher concentrations, which can lead to profound CNS depression (see below). Further, the behavioral and sedative effects of benzodiazepines can be ascribed in part to potentiation of GABA-ergic pathways that serve to regulate the firing of neurons containing various monoamines (see Chapter 12). These neurons are known to promote behavioral arousal and are important mediators of the inhibitory effects of fear and punishment on behavior. Finally, inhibitory effects on muscular hypertonia or the spread of seizure activity can be rationalized by potentiation of inhibitory GABA-ergic circuits at various levels of the neuraxis.*

Molecular Basis for Benzodiazepine Regulation of GABA$_A$ Receptor-Mediated Electrical Events

The enhancement of GABA-induced chloride currents by benzodiazepines results primarily from an increase in the frequency of bursts of chloride channel opening produced by submaximal amounts of GABA. Inhibitory synaptic transmission measured after stimulation of afferent fibers is potentiated by benzodiazepines at therapeutically relevant concentrations. Measurements of GABA$_A$ receptor-mediated currents indicate that benzodiazepines shift the GABA concentration–response curve to the left without increasing the maximum current evoked with GABA, consistent with a model in which benzodiazepines exert their major actions by increasing the gain of inhibitory neurotransmission mediated by GABA$_A$ receptors. Some data are difficult to reconcile with the hypothesis that actions at GABA$_A$ receptors mediate all effects of benzodiazepines. Low concentrations of benzodiazepines that are not blocked by bicuculline or picrotoxin induce depressant effects on hippocampal neurons; the induction of sleep in rats by benzodiazepines also is insensitive to bicuculline or picrotoxin but is prevented by flumazenil. At higher (hypnotic/amnesic) concentrations, actions of the benzodiazepines may involve other mechanisms, including inhibition of the uptake of adenosine and the resulting potentiation of its actions as a neuronal depressant, as well as the GABA-independent inhibition of Ca^{2+} currents, Ca^{2+}-dependent neurotransmitter release, and tetrodotoxin-sensitive Na^+ channels.

The macromolecular complex containing GABA-regulated chloride channels also may be a site of action of general anesthetics, ethanol, inhaled drugs of abuse, and certain metabolites of endogenous steroids.

RESPIRATION Hypnotic doses of benzodiazepines are without effect on respiration in normal adult subjects, but special care must be taken in the treatment of children and individuals with impaired hepatic function (*e.g.*, alcoholics). At higher doses, such as those used for preanesthetic medication or for endoscopy, benzodiazepines slightly depress alveolar ventilation and cause respiratory acidosis as the result of a decrease in hypoxic rather than hypercapnic drive; these effects are exaggerated in patients with chronic obstructive pulmonary disease (COPD), and alveolar hypoxia and/or CO_2 narcosis may result. These drugs can cause apnea during anesthesia or when given with opioids. Patients severely intoxicated with benzodiazepines only require respiratory assistance when they also have ingested another CNS-depressant drug, most commonly ethanol.

In contrast, hypnotic doses of benzodiazepines may worsen sleep-related breathing disorders by adversely affecting control of the upper airway muscles or by decreasing the ventilatory response to CO_2. The latter effect may cause hypoventilation and hypoxemia in some patients with severe COPD, although benzodiazepines may improve sleep and sleep structure in some instances. In patients with obstructive sleep apnea (OSA), hypnotic doses of benzodiazepines may exaggerate the impact of apneic episodes on alveolar hypoxia, pulmonary hypertension, and cardiac ventricular load. Caution should be exercised with patients who snore regularly: partial airway obstruction may be converted to OSA under the influence of these drugs.

CARDIOVASCULAR SYSTEM The cardiovascular effects of benzodiazepines are minor in normal subjects except in severe intoxication. In preanesthetic doses, all benzodiazepines decrease blood pressure and increase heart rate.

GI TRACT Despite anecdotal reports that benzodiazepines improve a variety of "anxiety-related" GI disorders, there is a paucity of evidence. Diazepam markedly decreases nocturnal gastric acid secretion in human beings, but other agents are considerably more effective in acid-peptic disorders (*see* Chapter 36).

ABSORPTION, FATE, AND EXCRETION The physicochemical and pharmacokinetic properties of the benzodiazepines affect their clinical utility. All have high lipid–water distribution coefficients in the nonionized form; nevertheless, lipophilicity varies more than 50-fold according to the polarity and electronegativity of various substituents.

All benzodiazepines are absorbed completely, with the exception of *clorazepate*; this drug is decarboxylated rapidly in gastric juice to *N*-desmethyldiazepam (nordazepam), which subsequently is absorbed completely. Some benzodiazepines (*e.g.*, *prazepam* and *flurazepam*) reach the systemic circulation only in the form of active metabolites.

Drugs active at the benzodiazepine receptor may be divided into four categories based on their elimination half-lives: (1) ultrashort acting; (2) short-acting ($t_{1/2}$ <6 hours): *triazolam*, the non-benzodiazepine *zolpidem* ($t_{1/2}$ ~2 hours), and zopiclone ($t_{1/2}$ = 5–6 hours); (3) intermediate-acting ($t_{1/2}$ = 6–24 hours): *estazolam* and *temazepam*; and (4) long-acting ($t_{1/2}$ >24 hours): flurazepam, diazepam, and *quazepam*.

The extent of binding of benzodiazepines and their metabolites to plasma proteins correlates with lipid solubility and ranges from ~70% (*alprazolam*) to nearly 99% (diazepam). The concentration in the cerebrospinal fluid is approximately equal to the concentration of free drug in plasma. There is rapid uptake of benzodiazepines into the brain and other highly perfused organs after intravenous administration (or oral administration of a rapidly absorbed compound), followed by redistribution into tissues that are less well perfused (*e.g.*, muscle and fat). Redistribution is most rapid for drugs with the highest lipid solubility. In the regimens used for nighttime sedation, the rate of redistribution sometimes can have a greater influence than the rate of biotransformation on the duration of CNS effects. Redistribution kinetics of lipophilic benzodiazepines (*e.g.*, diazepam) is complicated by enterohepatic circulation. The volumes of distribution of the benzodiazepines are large and in many cases are increased in elderly patients. These drugs cross the placental barrier and are secreted into breast milk.

The benzodiazepines are metabolized extensively by CYPs, particularly CYP 3A4 and 2C19. Some benzodiazepines (*e.g.*, *oxazepam*) are conjugated directly. *Erythromycin, clarithromycin, ritonavir, itraconazole, ketoconazole, nefazodone*, and grapefruit juice are inhibitors of CYP 3A4 and can affect the metabolism of benzodiazepines. Because active metabolites of some benzodiazepines are biotransformed more slowly than are the parent compounds, the duration of action of many benzodiazepines bears little relationship to the $t_{1/2}$ of elimination of the drug that has been administered (*e.g.*, the $t_{1/2}$ of flurazepam in plasma is ~2 hours, but that of a major active metabolite *N*-desalkylflurazepam is ~50 hours). Conversely, the rate of biotransformation of agents that are inactivated by the initial reaction is an important determinant of their duration of action; these agents include oxazepam, *lorazepam*, temazepam, triazolam, and midazolam. Metabolism of the benzodiazepines occurs in three major stages. In general terms, the substituent at position 1 (or 2) of the diazepine ring is rapidly removed or modified to form metabolites that frequently are biologically active; then position 3 is more slowly hydroxylated, yielding derivatives that are generally active; finally the 3-OH compounds are conjugated with glucuronic acid to inactive products.

Because benzodiazepines do not significantly induce the synthesis of hepatic CYPs, chronic benzodiazepine administration usually does not result in the accelerated metabolism of benzodiazepines or other substances. Cimetidine *and oral contraceptives inhibit N-dealkylation and 3-hydroxylation of benzodiazepines, as do ethanol, isoniazid, and phenytoin to a lesser degree. These reactions usually are reduced to a greater extent in elderly patients and in patients with chronic liver disease than are those involving conjugation.*

An ideal hypnotic agent would have a rapid onset of action when taken at bedtime, a sufficiently sustained action to facilitate sleep throughout the night, and no residual action by the following morning. Triazolam theoretically fits this description most closely. Because of the slow rate of elimination of *desalkylflurazepam*, flurazepam (or quazepam) might seem to be unsuitable for this purpose. In practice, there appear to be some disadvantages to the use of agents that have a relatively rapid rate of disappearance, including the early-morning insomnia that is experienced by some patients and a greater likelihood of rebound insomnia on drug discontinuation. With careful selection of dosage, flurazepam and other benzodiazepines with slower rates of elimination than triazolam can be used effectively.

Therapeutic Uses

The therapeutic uses and routes of administration of individual benzodiazepines marketed in the U.S. are summarized in Table 16–2. Note that most benzodiazepines can be used interchangeably. Benzodiazepines used as anticonvulsants have a long $t_{1/2}$, and rapid entry into the brain is required for efficacy in treatment of status epilepticus. A short elimination $t_{1/2}$ is desirable for hypnotics,

Table 16-2

Names, Routes of Administration, and Therapeutic Uses of Benzodiazepines

Compound (Trade Name)	Routes of Administration*	Examples of Therapeutic Uses[†]	Comments	$t_{1/2}$, Hours[‡]	Usual Sedative-Hypnotic Hypnotic Dosage, mg[¶]
Alprazolam (XANAX)	Oral	Anxiety disorders, agoraphobia	Withdrawal symptoms may be especially severe	12±2	—
Chlordiazepoxide (LIBRIUM, others)	Oral, IM, IV	Anxiety disorders, management of alcohol withdrawal, anesthetic premedication	Long-acting and self-tapering because of active metabolites	10±3.4	50–100, qd–qid[§]
Clonazepam (KLONOPIN)	Oral	Seizure disorders, adjunctive treatment in acute mania and certain movement disorders	Tolerance develops to anticonvulsant effects	23±5	—
Clorazepate (TRANXENE, others)	Oral	Anxiety disorders, seizure disorders	Prodrug; nordazepam formed by decarboxylation in GI tract	2.0±0.9	3.75–20, bid–qid[§]
Diazepam (VALIUM, others)	Oral, IM, IV, rectal	Anxiety status epilepticus, skeletal muscle relaxation, anesthetic premed	Prototypical benzodiazepine	43±13	5–10, tid–qid[§]
Estazolam (PROSOM)	Oral	Insomnia	Contains triazolo ring; adverse effects may be similar to those of triazolam	10–24	1–2
Flurazepam (DALMANE)	Oral	Insomnia	Active metabolites accumulate with chronic use	74±24	15–30
Lorazepam (ATIVAN)	Oral, IM, IV	Anxiety disorders, preanesthetic medication	Metabolized solely by conjugation	14±5	2–4
Midazolam (VERSED)	IV, IM	Preanesthetic and intraoperative medication	Rapidly inactivated	1.9±0.6	—[#]
Oxazepam (SERAX)	Oral	Anxiety disorders	Metabolized solely by conjugation	8.0±2.4	15–30, tid–qid[§]
Quazepam (DORAL)	Oral	Insomnia	Active metabolites accumulate with chronic use	39	7.5–15
Temazepam (RESTORIL)	Oral	Insomnia	Metabolized mainly by conjugation	11±6	7.5–30
Triazolam (HALCION)	Oral	Insomnia	Rapidly inactivated; may cause disturbing daytime side effects	2.9±1.0	0.125–0.25

*IM, intramuscular injection; IV, intravenous administration; qd, once a day; bid, twice a day; tid, three times a day; qid, four times a day.

[†]The therapeutic uses are identified as examples to emphasize that most benzodiazepines can be used interchangeably. In general, the therapeutic uses of a given benzodiazepine are related to its half-life and may not match the marketed indications. The issue is addressed more extensively in the text.

[‡]Half-life of active metabolite may differ. See Appendix II in the 11th edition of the parent text for additional information.

[¶]For additional dosage information, see Chapter 13 (Anesthesia), Chapter 17 (Anxiety), and Chapter 19 (Seizure Disorders).

[§]Approved as a sedative-hypnotic only for management of alcohol withdrawal; doses in a nontolerant individual would be smaller.

[#]Recommended doses vary considerably depending on specific use, condition of patient, and concomitant administration of other drugs.

although this carries the drawback of increased abuse liability and severity of withdrawal after drug discontinuation. Antianxiety agents should have a long $t_{1/2}$ despite the risk of neuropsychological deficits caused by drug accumulation.

UNTOWARD EFFECTS   At the time of peak concentration in plasma, hypnotic doses of benzodiazepines cause varying degrees of lightheadedness, lassitude, increased reaction time, motor incoordination, impairment of mental and motor functions, confusion, and anterograde amnesia. Cognition appears to be affected less than motor performance. *All these effects can greatly impair driving and other psychomotor skills, especially if combined with ethanol.* These dose-related residual effects can be insidious because most subjects underestimate the degree of their impairment. Residual daytime sleepiness also may occur. The intensity and incidence of CNS toxicity generally increase with age.

Other relatively common side effects are weakness, headache, blurred vision, vertigo, nausea and vomiting, epigastric distress, and diarrhea; joint pains, chest pains, and incontinence are much rarer. Anticonvulsant benzodiazepines sometimes actually increase the frequency of seizures in patients with epilepsy. Possible adverse effects of altered sleep patterns are discussed below.

Adverse Psychological Effects

Benzodiazepines may cause paradoxical effects. Flurazepam occasionally increases the incidence of nightmares—especially during the first week of use—and sometimes causes garrulousness, anxiety, irritability, tachycardia, and sweating. Amnesia, euphoria, restlessness, hallucinations, and hypomanic behavior have been reported to occur during use of various benzodiazepines. The release of bizarre uninhibited behavior occurs in some users; hostility and rage may occur in others; these are referred to as disinhibition or dyscontrol reactions. Paranoia, depression, and suicidal ideation also occasionally may accompany the use of these agents. Such paradoxical or disinhibition reactions are rare and appear to be dose-related. Because of reports of an increased incidence of confusion and abnormal behaviors, triazolam has been banned in the U.K., although the FDA declared triazolam to be safe and effective in low doses of 0.125–0.25 mg. Surveys in the U.K. after the ban found that patients did not have fewer side effects with replacement treatments.

Chronic benzodiazepine use poses a risk for development of dependence and abuse, but not to the same extent as seen with older sedatives and other recognized drugs of abuse. Mild dependence may develop in many patients who have taken therapeutic doses of benzodiazepines on a regular basis for prolonged periods. Withdrawal symptoms may include temporary intensification of the problems that originally prompted their use (e.g., insomnia or anxiety). Dysphoria, irritability, sweating, unpleasant dreams, tremors, anorexia, and faintness also may occur, especially when withdrawal of the benzodiazepine occurs abruptly; it is prudent to taper the dosage gradually to discontinue therapy. Nonetheless, benzodiazepines are relatively safe drugs. Even huge doses are rarely fatal unless other drugs are taken concomitantly, and true coma is uncommon in the absence of another CNS depressant (e.g., ethanol). Although overdosage with a benzodiazepine rarely causes severe cardiovascular or respiratory depression, therapeutic doses can further compromise respiration in patients with COPD or OSA. Abuse of benzodiazepines includes the use of flunitrazepam (ROHYPNOL) as a "date-rape" drug.

Adverse Effects and Drug Interactions

A variety of allergic, hepatotoxic, and hematologic reactions to the benzodiazepines may occur, but the incidence is quite low; these reactions have been associated with the use of flurazepam and triazolam but not with temazepam. Large doses taken just before or during labor may cause hypothermia, hypotonia, and mild respiratory depression in the neonate. Abuse by the pregnant mother can result in a withdrawal syndrome in the newborn.

Except for additive effects with other sedative or hypnotic drugs, reports of clinically important pharmacodynamic interactions between benzodiazepines and other drugs have been infrequent. Ethanol increases both the rate of absorption of benzodiazepines and the associated CNS depression. Valproate and benzodiazepines in combination may cause psychotic episodes.

Novel Benzodiazepine-Receptor Agonists: Zolpidem and Zalephon

Hypnotics that are structurally dissimilar to benzodiazepines include *zolpicone* (not available in the U.S.), zolpidem (AMBIEN), zaleplon (SONATA), and indiplon (under review by the FDA); presumably, their therapeutic efficacies are due to agonist effects at the benzodiazepine site of the GABA$_A$ receptor.

Zaleplon and zolpidem are effective in relieving sleep-onset insomnia. The two drugs have similar efficacies and both display sustained hypnotic efficacy without occurrence of rebound insomnia on abrupt discontinuation. Late-night administration of zolpidem has been associated with morning sedation, delayed reaction time, and anterograde amnesia, whereas zaleplon has no more side effects than placebo. Tolerance to zaleplon does not appear to occur, nor do rebound insomnia or withdrawal symptoms after stopping treatment. Unlike the benzodiazepines, zolpidem has little effect on the stages of sleep in normal human subjects. The drug is as effective as benzodiazepines in shortening sleep latency and prolonging total sleep time in patients with insomnia. After discontinuation of zolpidem, the beneficial effects on sleep reportedly persist for up to 1 week, but mild rebound insomnia on the first night also has occurred. Tolerance and physical dependence develop only rarely. An extended-release formulation of zolpidem (AMBIEN CR) is now marketed in the U.S.

Flumazenil: A Benzodiazepine-Receptor Antagonist

Flumazenil (ROMAZICON) is an imidazobenzodiazepine that behaves as a specific benzodiazepine antagonist. Flumazenil binds with high affinity to specific sites on the $GABA_A$ receptor, where it competitively antagonizes the binding and allosteric effects of benzodiazepines and other ligands. The drug antagonizes both the electrophysiological and behavioral effects of agonist and inverse-agonist benzodiazepines and β-carbolines. Anticonvulsant effects cannot be relied on for therapeutic utility because the administration of flumazenil may precipitate seizures under certain circumstances (see below).

Flumazenil is available only for intravenous administration. Although absorbed rapidly after oral administration, <25% of the drug reaches the systemic circulation owing to extensive first-pass hepatic metabolism; effective oral doses are apt to cause headache and dizziness. On intravenous administration, flumazenil is eliminated almost entirely by hepatic metabolism to inactive products with a $t_{1/2}$ of about 1 hour; the duration of clinical effects usually is only 30–60 minutes.

The primary uses of flumazenil are the management of suspected benzodiazepine overdose and the reversal of sedative effects produced by benzodiazepines administered during either general anesthesia or diagnostic and/or therapeutic procedures.

The administration of a series of small injections is preferred to a single bolus injection. A total of 1 mg flumazenil given over 1–3 minutes usually is sufficient to abolish the effects of therapeutic doses of benzodiazepines; patients with suspected benzodiazepine overdose should respond adequately to a cumulative dose of 1–5 mg given over 2–10 minutes; a lack of response to 5-mg flumazenil strongly suggests that a benzodiazepine is not the major cause of sedation. Additional courses of treatment with flumazenil may be needed within 20–30 minutes should sedation reappear. Flumazenil is not effective in single-drug overdoses with either barbiturates or tricyclic antidepressants. To the contrary, administration of flumazenil in these settings may be associated with the onset of seizures, especially in patients poisoned with tricyclic antidepressants. Seizures or other withdrawal symptoms also may be precipitated in patients who had been taking benzodiazepines for protracted periods and in whom tolerance and/or dependence may have developed.

BARBITURATES

The barbiturates are derivatives of 2,4,6-trioxohexahydropyrimidine (Table 16–3) that reversibly depress the activity of all excitable tissues. The CNS is exquisitely sensitive, and even when barbiturates are given in anesthetic concentrations, direct effects on peripheral excitable tissues are weak. However, serious deficits in cardiovascular and other peripheral functions occur in acute barbiturate intoxication. Except for a few specialized uses, barbiturates have been replaced by the much safer benzodiazepines.

Pharmacological Properties

CENTRAL NERVOUS SYSTEM

Sites and Mechanisms of Action on the CNS

Barbiturates act throughout the CNS; nonanesthetic doses preferentially suppress polysynaptic responses. Facilitation is diminished, and inhibition usually is enhanced. The site of inhibition is either postsynaptic, as at cortical and cerebellar pyramidal cells and in the cuneate nucleus, substantia nigra, and thalamic relay neurons, or presynaptic, as in the spinal cord. Enhancement of inhibition occurs primarily at synapses where neurotransmission is mediated by GABA acting at $GABA_A$ receptors.

Mechanisms underlying the actions of barbiturates on $GABA_A$ receptors appear to be distinct from those of either GABA or the benzodiazepines, a conclusion based on the following observations: (1) barbiturates promote (rather than compete with) the binding of benzodiazepines to $GABA_A$ receptors; (2) barbiturates potentiate GABA-induced chloride currents by prolonging

Structures, Trade Names, and Major Pharmacological Properties of Selected Barbiturates

General Formula:

Compound (Trade Names)	R_3	R_{5a}	R_{5b}	Routes of Administration[†]	$t_{1/2}$ Hours	Therapeutic Uses	Comments
Amobarbital (AMYTAL)	—H	—C_2H_5	—$CH_2CH_2CH(CH_3)_2$	IM, IV	10–40	Insomnia, preoperative sedation, emergency management of seizures	Only Na^+ salt administered parenterally
Butabarbital (BUTISOL, others)	—H	—C_2H_5	—$CH(CH_3)CH_2CH_3$	Oral	35–50	Insomnia, preoperative sedation	Redistribution shortens duration of action of single dose to 8 hours
Butalbital	—H	—$CH_2CH=CH_2$	$CH_2CH(CH_3)_2$	Oral	35–88	Marketed in combination with analgesics	Therapeutic efficacy questionable
Mephobarbital (MEBARAL)	—CH_3	—C_2H_5	(phenyl)	Oral	10–70	Seizure disorders, daytime sedation	Second-line anticonvulsant
Methohexital (BREVITAL)	—CH_3	—$CH_2CH=CH_2$	—$CH(CH_3)C\equiv CCH_2CH_3$	IV	3–5[‡]	Induction and maintenance of anesthesia	Only Na^+ salt is available; single injection provides 5–7 minutes of anesthesia[‡]
Pentobarbital (NEMBUTAL)	—H	—C_2H_5	—$CH(CH_3)CH_2CH_2CH_3$	Oral, IM, IV, rectal	15–50	Insomnia, preoperative sedation, emergency management of seizures	Only Na^+ salt administered parenterally
Phenobarbital (LUMINAL, others)	—H	—C_2H_5	(phenyl)	Oral, IM, IV	80–120	Seizure disorders, status epilepticus, daytime sedation	First-line anticonvulsant; only Na^+ salt administered parenterally
Secobarbital (SECONAL)	—H	—$CH_2CH=CH_2$	—$CH(CH_3)CH_2CH_2CH_3$	Oral	15–40	Insomnia, preoperative sedation	Only Na^+ salt is available
Thiopental (PENTOTHAL)	—H	—C_2H_5	—$CH(CH_3)CH_2CH_2CH_3$	IV	8–10[‡]	Induction/maintenance of anesthesia, preop sedation, emergency management of seizures	Only Na^+ salt is available; single injections provide short periods of anesthesia[‡]

*O except in thiopental, where it is replaced by S. [†]IM, intramuscular injection; IV, intravenous administration.
[‡]Value represents terminal $t_{1/2}$ due to metabolism by the liver; redistribution following parenteral administration produces effects lasting only a few minutes.

271

periods during which bursts of channel opening occur rather than by increasing the frequency of these bursts, as benzodiazepines do; (3) only α and β (not γ) subunits of the receptor/channel are required for barbiturate action; and (4) barbiturate-induced increases in chloride conductance are insensitive to mutations in the β subunit that govern the sensitivity of GABA$_A$ receptors to activation by agonists. In addition, sub-anesthetic concentrations of barbiturates also can reduce glutamate-induced depolarizations of the AMPA subtype of glutamate receptor Thus, the activation of inhibitory GABA$_A$ receptors and inhibition of excitatory AMPA receptors by barbiturates may explain their CNS-depressant effects.

The barbiturates can produce all degrees of depression of the CNS, ranging from mild sedation to general anesthesia. The use of barbiturates for general anesthesia is discussed in Chapter 13. Certain barbiturates, particularly those containing a 5-phenyl substituent (e.g., phenobarbital and mephobarbital), have selective anticonvulsant activity (see Chapter 19). The antianxiety properties of the barbiturates are inferior to those exerted by the benzodiazepines.

Except for the anticonvulsant activities of phenobarbital and its congeners, the barbiturates possess a low degree of selectivity and therapeutic index. Thus, it is not possible to achieve a desired effect without evidence of general depression of the CNS. Pain perception and reaction are relatively unimpaired until the moment of unconsciousness, and in small doses, the barbiturates increase the reaction to painful stimuli. Hence, they cannot be relied on to produce sedation or sleep in the presence of even moderate pain.

Effects on Stages of Sleep

Hypnotic doses of barbiturates increase the total sleep time and alter the stages of sleep in a dose-dependent manner. Like the benzodiazepines, these drugs decrease sleep latency, the number of awakenings, and the durations of REM and slow-wave sleep. During repetitive nightly administration, some tolerance to the effects on sleep occurs within a few days, and the effect on total sleep time may be reduced by as much as 50% after 2 weeks of use. Discontinuation leads to rebound increases in all the parameters decreased by barbiturates.

Tolerance

Pharmacodynamic (functional) and pharmacokinetic tolerance to barbiturates can occur. The former contributes more to the decreased effect than does the latter. With chronic administration of gradually increasing doses, pharmacodynamic tolerance continues to develop over a period of weeks to months, depending on the dosage schedule, whereas pharmacokinetic tolerance reaches its peak in a few days to a week. Tolerance to the effects on mood, sedation, and hypnosis occurs more readily and is greater than that to the anticonvulsant and lethal effects; thus, as tolerance increases, the therapeutic index decreases. Pharmacodynamic tolerance to barbiturates confers tolerance to all general CNS-depressant drugs, including ethanol.

PERIPHERAL NERVOUS STRUCTURES

Barbiturates selectively depress transmission in autonomic ganglia and reduce nicotinic excitation by choline esters, an effect that may account for the fall in blood pressure produced by intravenous oxybarbiturates and by severe barbiturate intoxication. At skeletal neuromuscular junctions, the blocking effects of both tubocurarine and decamethonium are enhanced during barbiturate anesthesia. These actions probably result from the capacity of barbiturates at hypnotic or anesthetic concentrations to inhibit the passage of current through nicotinic cholinergic receptors. Several distinct mechanisms appear to be involved and little stereoselectivity is evident.

RESPIRATION

Barbiturates depress both the respiratory drive and the mechanisms responsible for the rhythmic character of respiration. The neurogenic drive is diminished by hypnotic doses but usually no more so than during natural sleep. However, neurogenic drive is essentially eliminated by a dose three times greater than that used normally to induce sleep. Such doses also suppress the hypoxic drive and, to a lesser extent, the chemoreceptor drive. At still higher doses, the powerful hypoxic drive also fails. However, the margin between the lighter planes of surgical anesthesia and dangerous respiratory depression is sufficient to permit the ultrashort-acting barbiturates to be used, with suitable precautions, as anesthetic agents.

The barbiturates only slightly depress protective reflexes until the degree of intoxication is sufficient to produce severe respiratory depression. Laryngospasm is a major complication of barbiturate anesthesia.

CARDIOVASCULAR SYSTEM

When given orally in sedative or hypnotic doses, the barbiturates do not produce significant overt cardiovascular effects except for a slight decrease in blood pressure and heart rate such as occurs in normal sleep. Cardiovascular reflexes are obtunded by partial inhibition of ganglionic trans-mission; this is most evident in patients with congestive heart failure or hypovolemic shock, whose reflexes already are operating maximally and in whom barbiturates can cause an exaggerated fall in blood pressure. Because barbiturates also impair reflex cardiovascular adjustments to inflation of the lung, positive-pressure respiration should be used cautiously and only when necessary to maintain adequate pulmonary ventilation in patients who are anesthetized or intoxicated with a barbiturate.

Intravenous anesthesia with barbiturates can increase the incidence of ventricular arrhythmias, especially when epinephrine *and* halothane *also are present. Direct depression of cardiac contractility occurs only when doses several times those required to cause anesthesia are administered.*

GI TRACT

Oxybarbiturates tend to decrease the tone of the GI musculature and the amplitude of rhythmic contractions. The locus of action is partly peripheral and partly central, depending on the dose. A hypnotic dose does not significantly delay gastric emptying in human beings. The relief of various GI symptoms by sedative doses is probably largely due to the central-depressant action.

LIVER

The best known effects of barbiturates on the liver are those on the microsomal drug-metabolizing system (see Chapter 3). Acutely, the barbiturates combine with several CYPs and inhibit the biotransformation of a number of other drugs and endogenous substrates, such as steroids; other substrates may reciprocally inhibit barbiturate biotransformations.

Chronic administration of barbiturates markedly induces (approximately doubles) the activities of glucuronyl transferases and CYPs 1A2, 2C9, 2C19, and 3A4, thereby increasing the metabolism of a number of drugs and endogenous substances, including steroid hormones, cholesterol, bile salts, and vitamins K and D, and the barbiturate itself (and thus contributing to tolerance to barbiturates). Many sedative-hypnotics, various anesthetics, and ethanol also are metabolized by and/or induce the microsomal enzymes, and some degree of cross-tolerance therefore can occur. Induction extends to δ-aminolevulinic acid synthetase and can cause dangerous disease exacerbations in persons with acute intermittent porphyria.

KIDNEY

Severe oliguria or anuria may occur in acute barbiturate poisoning, largely as a result of the marked hypotension.

ABSORPTION, FATE, AND EXCRETION For sedative-hypnotic use, the barbiturates usually are administered orally (Table 16–3); absorption is rapid and nearly complete. The onset of action varies from 10–60 minutes, depending on the agent and the formulation, and is delayed by the presence of food in the stomach. When necessary, intramuscular injections of solutions of the sodium salts should be placed deeply into large muscles to avoid the pain and possible necrosis that can result at more superficial sites. The intravenous route usually is reserved for the management of status epilepticus (phenobarbital sodium) or for the induction and/or maintenance of general anesthesia (*e.g.*, thiopental or *methohexital*).

Barbiturates are distributed widely and readily cross the placenta. Following initial distribution to the CNS of an intravenous dose, the highly lipid-soluble barbiturates undergo redistribution to less vascular tissues, especially muscle and fat, leading to a decline in the concentration of barbiturate in the plasma and brain. With thiopental and methohexital, this results in the awakening of patients within 5–15 minutes of the injection of the usual anesthetic doses (*see* Chapter 13).

Except for the less lipid-soluble *aprobarbital* and phenobarbital, nearly complete metabolism and/or conjugation of barbiturates in the liver precedes their renal excretion. The metabolic elimination of barbiturates is more rapid in young people than in the elderly and infants, and half-lives are increased during pregnancy partly because of the expanded volume of distribution. Chronic liver disease, especially cirrhosis, often increases the $t_{1/2}$ of the biotransformable barbiturates. Repeated administration, especially of phenobarbital, shortens the $t_{1/2}$ of barbiturates that are metabolized as a result of the induction of microsomal enzymes (*see* above).

All of these barbiturates will accumulate during repetitive administration unless appropriate adjustments in dosage are made. Furthermore, the persistence of the drug in plasma during the day favors the development of tolerance and abuse.

Therapeutic Uses

The major uses of individual barbiturates are listed in Table 16–3, mostly uses involving CNS actions of these drugs. As with the benzodiazepines, selection of particular barbiturates for a given therapeutic indication is based primarily on pharmacokinetic considerations.

In addition, there are some hepatic metabolic uses. Because hepatic glucuronyl transferase and the bilirubin-binding Y protein are increased by the barbiturates, phenobarbital has been used successfully to treat hyperbilirubinemia and kernicterus in the neonate. The nondepressant barbiturate *phetharbital* (*N*-phenylbarbital) works equally well. Phenobarbital may improve the hepatic transport of bilirubin in patients with hemolytic jaundice.

UNTOWARD EFFECTS

After-Effects   Drowsiness may last for only a few hours after a hypnotic dose of barbiturate, but residual CNS depression sometimes is evident the following day, and subtle distortions of mood and impairment of judgment and fine motor skills may be demonstrable. Residual effects also may take the form of vertigo, nausea, vomiting, or diarrhea or sometimes may be manifested as overt excitement. The user may awaken slightly intoxicated and feel euphoric and energetic; later, as the demands of daytime activities challenge possibly impaired faculties, the user may display irritability and temper.

Paradoxical Excitement   In some persons, barbiturates produce excitement rather than depression, and the patient may appear to be inebriated. This idiosyncrasy is relatively common among geriatric and debilitated patients and occurs most frequently with phenobarbital and *N*-methylbarbiturates. Barbiturates may cause restlessness, excitement, and even delirium when given in the presence of pain and may worsen a patient's perception of pain.

Hypersensitivity   Allergic reactions occur, especially in persons with asthma, urticaria, angioedema, or similar conditions. Hypersensitivity reactions include localized swellings, particularly of the eyelids, cheeks, or lips, and erythematous dermatitis. Rarely, exfoliative dermatitis may be caused by phenobarbital and can prove fatal; the skin eruption may be associated with fever, delirium, and marked degenerative changes in the liver and other parenchymatous organs.

Drug Interactions   Barbiturates combine with other CNS depressants to cause severe depression; ethanol is the most frequent offender, and interactions with first-generation antihistamines also are common. Isoniazid, methylphenidate, and monoamine oxidase inhibitors also increase the CNS-depressant effects. Other prominent drug interactions occur as a result of the induction of hepatic drug-metabolizing enzymes by barbiturates (*see* above).

OTHER UNTOWARD EFFECTS
BARBITURATE POISONING

The lethal dose of barbiturate varies, but severe poisoning is likely to occur when more than 10 times the full hypnotic dose has been ingested at once. If alcohol or other depressant drugs also are present, the concentrations that can cause death are lower.

The treatment of acute barbiturate intoxication is based on general supportive measures, which are applicable in most respects to poisoning by any CNS depressant. Hemodialysis or hemoperfusion is necessary only rarely, and the use of CNS stimulants is contraindicated because they increase the mortality rate (see *Chapter 64*).

MISCELLANEOUS SEDATIVE-HYPNOTIC DRUGS

Structurally diverse agents have been employed for their sedative-hypnotic properties, including paraldehyde, chloral hydrate, ethchlorvynol, glutethimide, methyprylon, ethinamate, and meprobamate. With the exception of meprobamate, the pharmacological actions of these drugs generally resemble those of the barbiturates: they all are general CNS depressants that can produce profound hypnosis with little or no analgesia; their effects on the stages of sleep are similar to those of the barbiturates; their therapeutic index is limited, and acute intoxication, which produces respiratory depression and hypotension, is managed similarly to barbiturate poisoning; their chronic use can result in tolerance and physical dependence; and the syndrome after chronic use can be severe and life-threatening. The use of these drugs is limited.

OTHERS

Etomidate *(AMIDATE) is used as an intravenous anesthetic, often in combination with* fentanyl. *It is advantageous because it lacks pulmonary and vascular depressant activity, although it has a negative inotropic effect on the heart. Its pharmacology and anesthetic uses are described in*

Chapter 13. It also is used in some countries as a sedative-hypnotic drug in intensive care units, during intermittent positive-pressure breathing, in epidural anesthesia, and in other situations. The myoclonus commonly seen after anesthetic doses is not seen after sedative-hypnotic doses.

Clomethiazole *has sedative, muscle relaxant, and anticonvulsant properties. It is used outside the U.S. for hypnosis in elderly and institutionalized patients, for preanesthetic sedation, and especially in the management of withdrawal from ethanol. Given alone, its effects on respiration are slight, and the therapeutic index is high. However, deaths from adverse interactions with ethanol are relatively frequent.*

Propofol *(DIPRIVAN) is a rapidly acting and highly lipophilic di-isopropylphenol used in the induction and maintenance of general anesthesia (see Chapter 13), as well as in the maintenance of long-term sedation. Propofol sedation is of a similar quality to that produced by midazolam. Emergence from sedation occurs quickly owing to its rapid clearance. Propofol has found use in intensive care sedation in adults, as well as for sedation during GI endoscopy procedures and transvaginal oocyte retrieval. Propofol is believed to act primarily through enhancement of* $GABA_A$-*receptor function. Effects on other ligand-gated and G protein–coupled receptors, however, also have been reported.*

NONPRESCRIPTION HYPNOTIC DRUGS

As part of the ongoing systematic review of over-the-counter (OTC) drug products, the FDA has ruled that diphenhydramine is the only ingredient that is recognized as generally safe and effective for use in nonprescription sleep aids. Despite the prominent sedative side effects encountered during the use of antihistamines previously included in OTC sleep aids (e.g., doxylamine and pyrilamine), these agents have been eliminated as ingredients in the OTC nighttime sleep aids marketed in the U.S. With an elimination $t_{1/2}$ *of about 9 hours, diphenhydramine at nighttime is associated with prominent residual daytime sleepiness.*

MANAGEMENT OF INSOMNIA

Adequate sleep improves the quality of daytime wakefulness, and hypnotics should be used judiciously to avoid its impairment. A number of pharmacological agents are available for the treatment of insomnia. The "perfect" hypnotic would allow sleep to occur with normal sleep architecture rather than produce a pharmacologically altered sleep pattern. It would not cause next-day effects, either of rebound anxiety or of continued sedation. It would not interact with other medications. It could be used chronically without causing dependence or rebound insomnia on discontinuation. Regular moderate exercise meets these criteria but often is not effective by itself, and many patients may not be able to exercise. However, even small amounts of exercise often are effective in promoting sleep.

Controversy in the management of insomnia revolves around two issues: pharmacological *versus* nonpharmacological treatment and the use of short-acting *versus* long-acting hypnotics. The side effects of hypnotic medications must be weighed against the sequelae of chronic insomnia, which include a fourfold increase in serious accidents. Two aspects of the management of insomnia traditionally have been underappreciated: a search for specific medical causes and the use of nonpharmacological treatments. In addition to appropriate pharmacological treatment, management of insomnia should correct identifiable causes, address inadequate sleep hygiene, eliminate performance anxiety related to falling asleep, provide entrainment of the biological clock so that maximum sleepiness occurs at the hour of attempted sleep, and suppress the use of alcohol and OTC sleep medications.

CATEGORIES OF INSOMNIA   Like Gaul, insomnia may be divided into three categories:

1. *Transient insomnia* lasts less than 3 days and usually is caused by a brief environmental or situational stressor. It may respond to attention to sleep hygiene rules. Hypnotics, if prescribed, should be used at the lowest dose and for only 2–3 nights. However, benzodiazepines given acutely before important life events, such as examinations, may result in impaired performance.
2. *Short-term insomnia* lasts from 3 days to 3 weeks and usually is caused by a personal stressor such as illness, grief, or job problems. Again, sleep hygiene education is the first step. Hypnotics may be used adjunctively for 7–10 nights. Hypnotics are best used intermittently during this time, with the patient skipping a dose after 1–2 nights of good sleep.
3. *Long-term insomnia* is insomnia that has lasted for more than 3 weeks; no specific stressor may be identifiable. A more complete medical evaluation is necessary in these patients, but most do not need an all-night sleep study.

INSOMNIA ACCOMPANYING MAJOR PSYCHIATRIC ILLNESSES

Insomnia caused by major psychiatric illnesses often responds to specific pharmacological treatment for that illness. In major depressive episodes with insomnia, for example, the selective serotonin reuptake inhibitors, which may cause insomnia as a side effect, usually will result in improved sleep because they treat the depressive syndrome. In patients whose depression is responding to the serotonin reuptake inhibitor but who have persistent insomnia as a side effect of the medication, judicious use of evening trazodone *may improve sleep, as well as augment the antidepressant effect of the reuptake inhibitor. However, the patient should be monitored for priapism, orthostatic hypotension, and arrhythmias.*

Adequate control of anxiety in patients with anxiety disorders often produces adequate resolution of the accompanying insomnia. Sedative use in the anxiety disorders is decreasing because of a growing appreciation of the effectiveness of other agents, such as β-adrenergic receptor antagonists (see Chapter 10) for performance anxiety and serotonin reuptake inhibitors for obsessive-compulsive disorder and perhaps generalized anxiety disorder. The profound insomnia of patients with acute psychosis owing to schizophrenia or mania usually responds to dopamine-receptor antagonists (see Chapter 18); benzodiazepines, often used adjunctively in this situation to reduce agitation, will result in improved sleep.

INSOMNIA ACCOMPANYING OTHER MEDICAL ILLNESSES

For long-term insomnia owing to other medical illnesses, adequate treatment of the underlying disorder, such as congestive heart failure, asthma, or COPD, may resolve the insomnia. Adequate pain management in conditions of chronic pain, including terminal cancer pain, will treat both the pain and the insomnia and may make hypnotics unnecessary. Many patients simply manage their sleep poorly. Adequate attention to sleep hygiene, including reduced caffeine intake, avoidance of alcohol, adequate exercise, and regular sleep and wake times, often will reduce the insomnia.

CONDITIONED (LEARNED) INSOMNIA

In patients without major psychiatric or medical illness and in whom attention to sleep hygiene is ineffective, attention should be directed to conditioned (learned) insomnia. These patients have associated the bedroom with activities consistent with wakefulness rather than sleep. In such patients, the bed should be used only for sex and sleep. All other activities associated with waking, even such quiescent activities as reading and watching television, should be done outside the bedroom.

LONG-TERM INSOMNIA

Nonpharmacological treatments (see above) are important for all patients with long-term insomnia. Side effects of hypnotic agents may limit their usefulness for insomnia management. Long-term hypnotic use leads to a decrease in effectiveness and may produce rebound insomnia on discontinuance. Almost all hypnotics change sleep architecture; while the significance of these findings is not clear, there is an emerging consensus that slow-wave sleep is particularly important for physical restorative processes. REM sleep may also aid in the consolidation of learning. The consensus is that hypnotics should not be given to patients with sleep apnea, especially of the obstructive type, because these agents decrease upper airway muscle tone while also decreasing the arousal response to hypoxia. These individuals benefit from all-night sleep studies to guide treatment.

INSOMNIA IN OLDER PATIENTS The elderly, like the very young, tend to sleep in a *polyphasic* (multiple sleep episodes per day) pattern rather than the *monophasic* pattern characteristic of younger adults. They may have single or multiple daytime naps in addition to nighttime sleep, making assessment of adequate sleep time difficult. Anyone who naps regularly will have shortened nighttime sleep without evidence of impaired daytime wakefulness, regardless of age. This pattern is exemplified in "siesta" cultures and probably is adaptive.

Changes in the pharmacokinetic profiles of hypnotic agents occur in the elderly because of reduced body water, reduced renal function, and increased body fat, leading to a longer $t_{1/2}$ for benzodiazepines. A dose that produces pleasant sleep and adequate daytime wakefulness during week 1 of administration may produce daytime confusion and amnesia by week 3 as the level continues to rise, particularly with long-acting hypnotics. For example, diazepam is highly lipid soluble and is excreted by the kidney; because of the increase in body fat and the decrease in renal excretion that typically occur from age 20–80, the $t_{1/2}$ of the drug may increase fourfold over this span.

Elderly people who are living full lives with relatively unimpaired daytime wakefulness may complain of insomnia because they are not sleeping as long as they did when they were younger. Injudicious use of hypnotics in these individuals can produce daytime cognitive impairment and so impair overall quality of life.

Once an older patient has been taking benzodiazepines for an extended period, whether for daytime anxiety or for nighttime sedation, terminating the drug can be a long, involved process. Since attempts at drug withdrawal may not be successful, it may be necessary to leave the patient on the medication, with adequate attention to daytime side effects.

MANAGEMENT OF PATIENTS AFTER LONG-TERM TREATMENT WITH HYPNOTIC AGENTS If a benzodiazepine has been used regularly for more than 2 weeks, it should be tapered rather than discontinued abruptly. In some patients on hypnotics with a short $t_{1/2}$, it is easier to switch first to a hypnotic with a long $t_{1/2}$ and then to taper.

The onset of withdrawal symptoms from medications with a long $t_{1/2}$ may be delayed. Consequently, the patient should be warned about the symptoms associated with withdrawal effects.

PRESCRIBING GUIDELINES FOR THE MANAGEMENT OF INSOMNIA Hypnotics that act at $GABA_A$ receptors (benzodiazepine hypnotics, zolpidem, zopiclone, and zaleplon) are preferred to barbiturates; the newer agents have a greater therapeutic index, are less toxic in overdose, have smaller effects on sleep architecture, and have less abuse potential. Compounds with a shorter $t_{1/2}$ are favored in patients with sleep-onset insomnia but without significant daytime anxiety who need to function at full effectiveness all day. These compounds also are appropriate for the elderly because of a decreased risk of falls and respiratory depression. However, the patient and physician should be aware that early-morning awakening, rebound daytime anxiety, and amnestic episodes also may occur. These undesirable side effects are more common at higher doses.

Benzodiazepines with longer half-lives are favored for patients who have significant daytime anxiety and who may be able to tolerate next-day sedation but would be impaired further by rebound daytime anxiety. These benzodiazepines also are appropriate for patients receiving treatment for major depressive episodes because the short-acting agents can worsen early-morning awakening. However, longer-acting benzodiazepines can be associated with next-day cognitive impairment or delayed daytime cognitive impairment (after 2–4 weeks of treatment) as a result of drug accumulation with repeated administration.

Older agents such as barbiturates, glutethimide, and meprobamate should be avoided for the management of insomnia; they have high abuse potential and are dangerous in overdose.

For a complete Bibliographical listing see Goodman & Gilman's *The Pharmacological Basis of Therapeutics,* **11th ed., or Goodman & Gilman Online at www.accessmedicine.com.**

DRUG THERAPY OF DEPRESSION AND ANXIETY DISORDERS

Major affective and anxiety disorders represent the most common psychiatric illnesses and are those encountered most often by primary-care clinicians. Major depression may represent a spectrum of disorders, varying in severity from mild and self-limited conditions to extraordinarily severe, psychotic, incapacitating, and deadly diseases. The antipsychotic, antianxiety, antimanic, and antidepressant drugs affect cortical, limbic, hypothalamic, and brainstem mechanisms that are of fundamental importance in the regulation of arousal, consciousness, affect, and autonomic functions. Physiological and pharmacological modifications of these brain regions may have important behavioral consequences and useful clinical effects regardless of the underlying cause of any mental disorder. The lack of diagnostic or even syndromal specificity of most psychotropic drugs tends to reduce the chances of finding a discrete mechanistic correlate for a specific disease based simply on the actions of therapeutic agents. There is no definitive link between discrete biological lesions and the pathogenesis of the most severe mental illnesses (other than delirium and dementias). Nonetheless, we can provide effective medical treatment for most psychiatric patients. It would be clinical folly to underestimate the importance of psychological and social factors in the manifestations of mental illnesses or to overlook psychological aspects of the conduct of biological therapies.

CHARACTERIZATION OF DEPRESSIVE AND ANXIETY DISORDERS

The primary clinical manifestations of major depression are significant depression of mood and impairment of function. Some features of depressive disorders overlap those of the anxiety disorders, including *panic-agoraphobia* syndrome, severe phobias, generalized anxiety disorder, social anxiety disorder, posttraumatic stress disorder, and obsessive-compulsive disorder. Extremes of mood also may be associated with psychosis, as manifested by disordered or delusional thinking and perceptions that often are congruent with the predominant mood. Conversely, secondary changes in mood may be associated with psychotic disorders. This overlap of disorders can lead to errors in diagnosis and suboptimal treatment. Mood and anxiety disorders are the most common mental illnesses, each affecting up to 10% of the general population at some time in their lives.

Clinical depression must be distinguished from normal grief, sadness, disappointment, and the dysphoria or demoralization often associated with medical illness. The condition is underdiagnosed and frequently undertreated. Major depression is characterized by feelings of intense sadness and despair, mental slowing and loss of concentration, pessimistic worry, lack of pleasure, self-deprecation, and variable agitation or hostility. Physical changes also occur, particularly in severe depression, including: insomnia or hypersomnia; altered eating patterns, with anorexia and weight loss or sometimes overeating; decreased energy and libido; and disruption of the normal circadian and ultradian rhythms of activity, body temperature, and many endocrine functions. As many as 10–15% of individuals with severe clinical depression, and up to 25% of those with bipolar disorder, display suicidal behavior at some time. Depressed patients usually respond to antidepressant drugs, or, in severe or treatment-resistant cases, to electroconvulsive therapy (ECT). This method remains the most rapid and effective treatment for severe acute depression and sometimes is life-saving for acutely suicidal patients. Efficacy of other forms of biological treatment of depression (e.g., magnetic stimulation of the brain or electrical stimulation of the vagus nerve) is not well established. The decision to treat with an antidepressant is guided by the presenting clinical syndrome, its severity, and by the patient's personal and family history. The lifetime risk for major depression is ~5% in men and 10% in women.

Anxiety disorders may be acute and transient, or more commonly, recurrent or persistent. Symptoms may include mood changes (fear, panic, or dysphoria) or limited abnormalities of thought (obsessions, irrational fears, or phobias) or of behavior (avoidance, rituals or compulsions, "hysterical" conversion signs, or fixation on imagined or exaggerated physical symptoms). Drugs can be beneficial in such disorders, particularly by modifying associated anxiety and depression to facilitate a more comprehensive program of treatment and rehabilitation. Antidepressants and sedative-antianxiety agents are commonly used to treat anxiety disorder.

Antidepressants

Most antidepressants exert important actions on the metabolism of monoamine neurotransmitters and their receptors, particularly norepinephrine (NE) and serotonin (5-HT) (Table 17–1).

Table 17–1

Antidepressants: Chemical Structures, Dose and Dosage Forms, and Side Effects

Nonproprietary Name (TRADE NAME)	Dose and Dosage Forms			Amine Effects	Side Effects								
	Usual Dose, mg/day	*Extreme Dose, mg/day*	*Dosage Form*		*Agitation*	*Seizures*	*Sedation*	*Hypo-tension*	*Anti-cholinergic Effects*	*Gastro-intestinal Effects*	*Weight Gain*	*Sexual Effects*	*Cardiac Effects*
Norepinephrine Reuptake Inhibitors:													
Tertiary Amine Tricyclics													
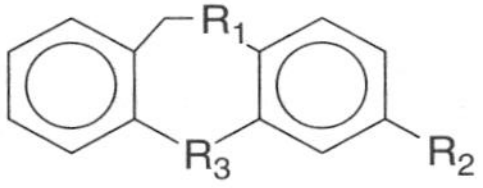													
R_1 R_2 R_3													
Amitriptyline (ELAVIL and others)	100–200	25–300	O, I	NE, 5-HT	0	2+	3+	3+	3+	0/+	2+	2+	3+
C H $C{=}CH(CH_2)_2N(CH_3)_2$													
Clomipramine (ANAFRANIL)	100–200	25–250	O	NE, 5-HT	0	3+	2+	2+	3+	+	2+	3+	3+
C Cl $N{-}(CH_2)_3N(CH_3)_2$													
Doxepin (ADAPIN, SINEQUAN)	100–200	25–300	O	NE, 5-HT	0	2+	3+	2+	2+	0/+	2+	2+	3+
O H $C{=}CH(CH_2)_2N(CH_3)_2$													
Imipramine (TOFRANIL and others)	100–200	25–300	O, I	NE, 5-HT	0/+	2+	2+	2+	2+	0/+	2+	2+	3+
C H $N{-}(CH_2)_3N(CH_3)_2$													
(+)-Trimipramine (SURMONTIL)	75–200	25–300	O	NE, 5-HT	0	2+	3+	2+	3+	0/+	2+	2+	3+
C H $N{-}CH_2CH(CH_3)CH_2N(CH_3)_2$													

(Continued)

Table 17–1

Antidepressants: Chemical Structures, Dose and Dosage Forms, and Side Effects (*Continued*)

Nonproprietary Name (TRADE NAME)	Dose and Dosage Forms			Amine Effects	Side Effects								
	Usual Dose, mg/day	Extreme Dose, mg/day	Dosage Form		Agitation	Seizures	Sedation	Hypotension	Anticholinergic Effects	Gastrointestinal Effects	Weight Gain	Sexual Effects	Cardiac Effects
Norepinephrine Reuptake Inhibitors: **Secondary Amine Tricyclics**													
Amoxapine (ASENDIN) 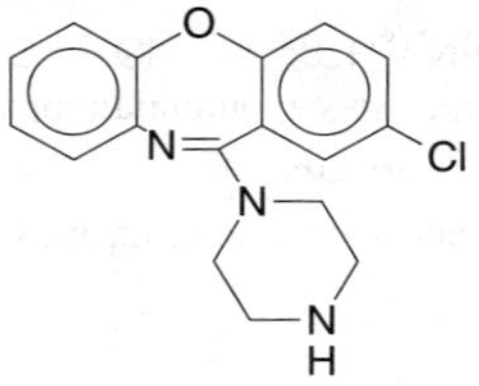	200–300	50–600	O	NE, DA	0	2+	+	2+	+	0/+	+	2+	2+
Desipramine (NORPRAMIN) 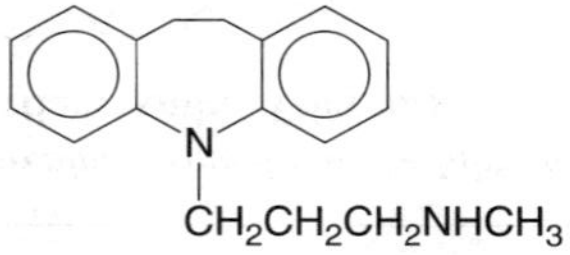	100–200	25–300	O	NE	+	+	0/+	+	+	0/+	+	2+	2+
Maprotiline (LUDIOMIL) 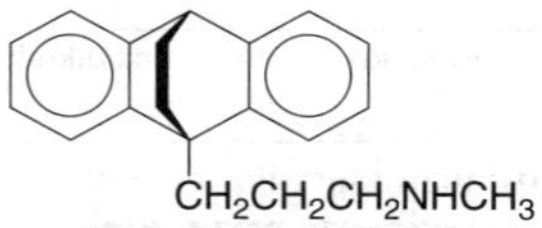	100–150	25–225	O	NE	0/+	3+	2+	2+	2+	0/+	+	2+	2+

Amoxapine (ASENDIN)

Desipramine (NORPRAMIN) — CH$_2$CH$_2$CH$_2$NHCH$_3$

Maprotiline (LUDIOMIL) — CH$_2$CH$_2$CH$_2$NHCH$_3$

280

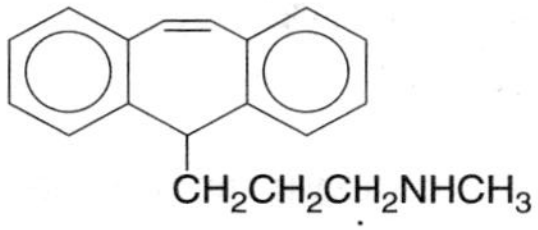

Selective Serotonin Reuptake Inhibitors

Nortriptyline (PAMELOR) — CHCH$_2$CH$_2$NHCH$_3$

Protriptyline (VIVACTIL) — CH$_2$CH$_2$CH$_2$NHCH$_3$

(±)-Citalopram (CELEXA) — N≡C ... F ... (CH$_2$)$_3$N(CH$_3$)$_2$, O

(+)-Escitalopram (LEXAPRO) — NC ... (S) ... O ... (CH$_2$)$_3$NMe$_2$ ... F

Drug												
Nortriptyline (PAMELOR)	75–150	25–250	O	NE	0	+	+	+	0/+	+	2+	2+
Protriptyline (VIVACTIL)	15–40	10–60	O	NE	2+	0/+	+	2+	0/+	+	2+	3+
(±)-Citalopram (CELEXA)	20–40	10–60	O	5-HT	0	0/+	0	0	3+	0	3+	0
(+)-Escitalopram (LEXAPRO)	20–40	10–60	O	5-HT	0	0/+	0	0	3+	0	3+	0

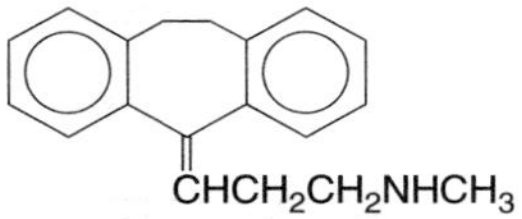

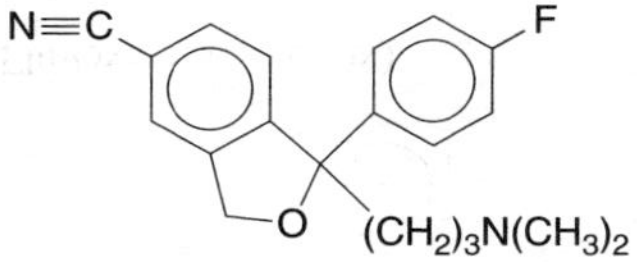

281

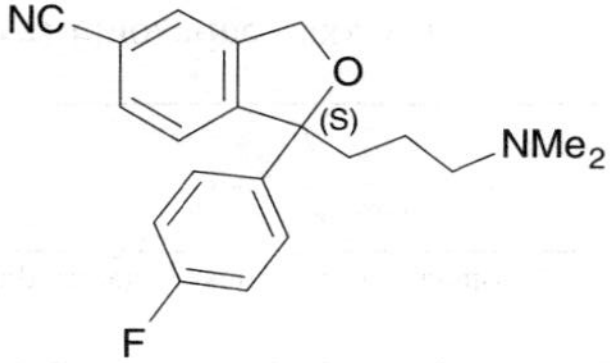

(Continued)

Table 17–1

Antidepressants: Chemical Structures, Dose and Dosage Forms, and Side Effects (Continued)

Nonproprietary Name (TRADE NAME)	Dose and Dosage Forms			Amine Effects	Side Effects								
	Usual Dose, mg/day	Extreme Dose, mg/day	Dosage Form		Agitation	Seizures	Sedation	Hypotension	Anticholinergic Effects	Gastrointestinal Effects	Weight Gain	Sexual Effects	Cardiac Effects
(±)-Fluoxetine (PROZAC) 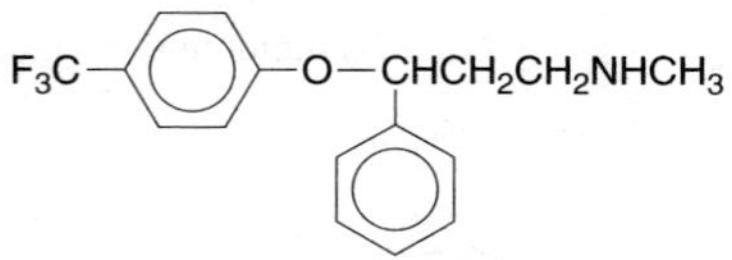	20–40	5–50	O	5-HT	+	0/+	0/+	0	0	3+	0/+	3+	0/+
Fluvoxamine (LUVOX) 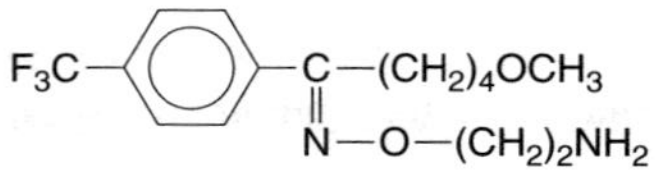	100–200	50–300	O	5-HT	0	0	0/+	0	0	3+	0	3+	0
(−)-Paroxetine (PAXIL) 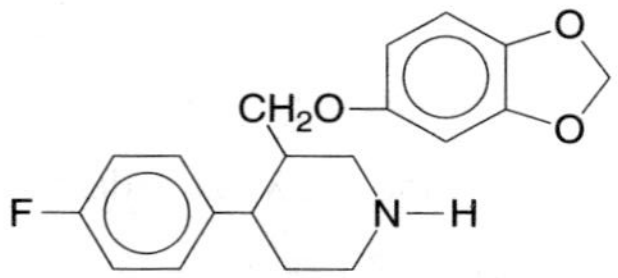	20–40	10–50	O	5-HT	+	0	0/+	0	0/+	3+	0	3+	0

F_3C—○—O—$CHCH_2CH_2NHCH_3$

F_3C—○—$\overset{N-O-(CH_2)_2NH_2}{\underset{}{C}}$—$(CH_2)_4OCH_3$

(structure for (−)-Paroxetine, showing benzodioxole, CH_2O, piperidine N—H, and 4-F-phenyl groups)

(+)-Sertraline (ZOLOFT)   NHCH₃ ... (structure with 3,4-dichlorophenyl tetralin)

100–150	50–200	O	5-HT	+	0	0/+	0	0	3+	0	3+	0

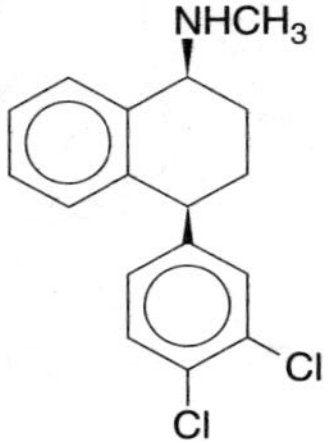

(±)-Venlafaxine (EFFEXOR)   (structure: H₃CO-phenyl, OH, cyclohexyl, CH₂N(CH₃)₂)

| 75–225 | 25–375 | O | 5-HT, NE | 0/+ | 0 | 0 | 0 | 0 | 3+ | 0 | 3+ | 0/+ |

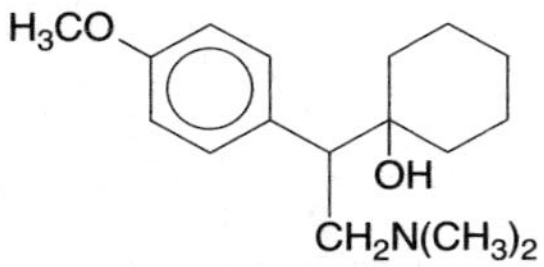

Atypical Antidepressants

(−)-Atomoxetine (STRATTERA)   (structure: H₃C-phenyl-O-CH-phenyl, CH₂CH₂NHC ... · HCl)

| 40–80 | 20–150 (children: 1.0–1.4 mg/kg) | O | NE | 0 | 0 | 0 | 0 | 0 | 0/+ | 0 | 0 | 0 |

283

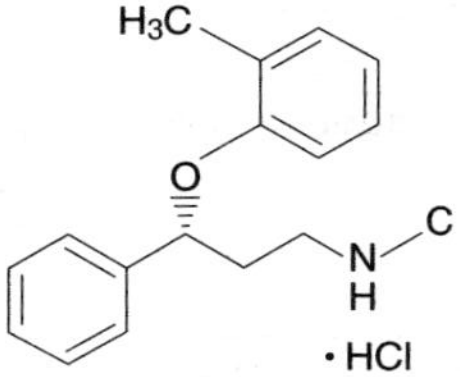

(Continued)

Table 17-1

Antidepressants: Chemical Structures, Dose and Dosage Forms, and Side Effects (*Continued*)

Nonproprietary Name (TRADE NAME)	Dose and Dosage Forms			Amine Effects	Side Effects								
	Usual Dose, mg/day	Extreme Dose, mg/day	Dosage Form		Agitation	Seizures	Sedation	Hypotension	Anti-cholinergic Effects	Gastro-intestinal Effects	Weight Gain	Sexual Effects	Cardiac Effects
Bupropion (WELLBUTRIN)	200–300	100–450	O	DA, ?NE	3+	4+	0	0	0	2+	0	0	0
(+)-Duloxetine (CYMBALTA)	80–100	40–120	O	NE, 5-HT	+	0	0/+	0/+	0	0/+	0/+	0/+	0/+
(±)-Mirtazapine (REMERON)	15–45	7.5–45	O	5-HT, NE	0	0	4+	0/+	0	0/+	0/+	0	0

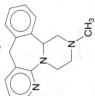

(continued)

Nefazodone* (SERZONE)

Structure: 3-chlorophenyl-piperazine–N–(CH$_2$)$_3$–N triazolone with –(CH$_2$)$_2$O–phenyl and CH$_2$CH$_3$ substituents.

200–400	100–600	O	5-HT	0	0	3+	0	0	2+	0/+	0/+	0/+

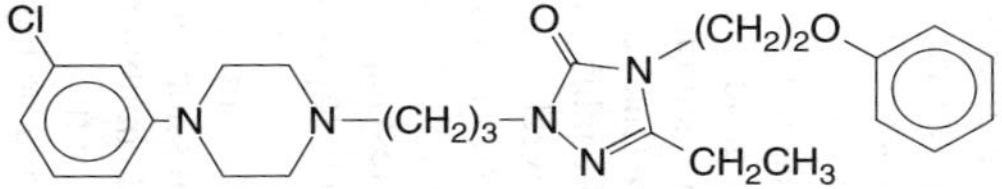

Trazodone† (DESYREL)

Structure: 3-chlorophenyl-piperazine–NCH$_2$CH$_2$CH$_2$N–triazolopyridinone.

150–200	50–600	O	5-HT	0	0	3+	0	0	2+	+	+	0/+

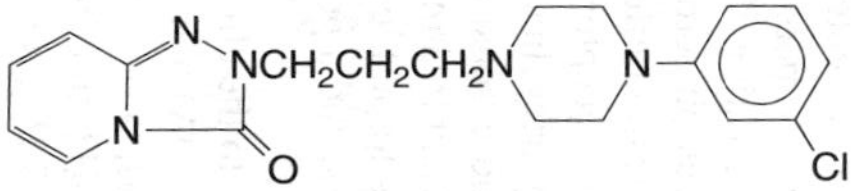

Monoamine Oxidase Inhibitors

Phenelzine (NARDIL)

Structure: benzene–CH$_2$–CH$_2$–NH–NH$_2$

30–60	15–90	O	NE, 5-HT, DA	0/+	0	+	+	0	0/+	+	3+	0

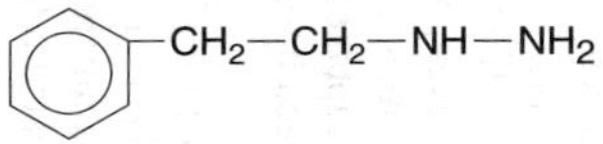

Tranylcypromine (PARNATE)

Structure: benzene–CH–CH–NH$_2$ with CH$_2$ (cyclopropyl).

20–30	10–60	O	NE, 5-HT, DA	2+	0	0	+	0	0/+	+	2+	0

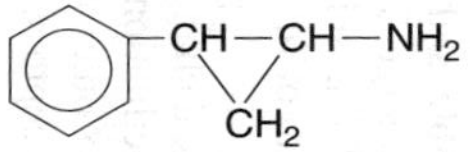

(−)-Selegiline (ELDEPRYL)

Structure: benzene–CH$_2$CH–N(CH$_3$)–CH$_2$C≡CH with CH$_3$.

10	5–20	O	DA, ?NE, ?5-HT	0	0	0	0	0	0	0	+	0

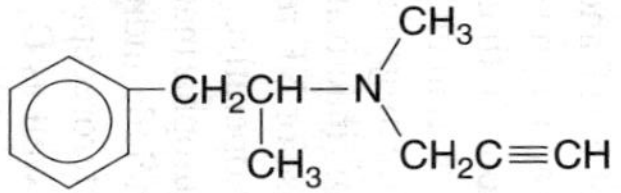

NOTE: Most of the drugs are hydrochloride salts, but SURMONTIL and LUVOX are maleates; CELEXA is a hydrobromide, and REMERON is a free-base. Selegiline is approved for early Parkinson's disease, but may have antidepressant effects, especially at daily doses ≥20 mg, and is under investigation for administration by transdermal patch.

ABBREVIATIONS: O, oral tablet or capsule; I, injectable; NE, norepinephrine; DA, dopamine; 5-HT, 5-hydroxytryptamine, serotonin; 0, negligible; 0/+, minimal; +, mild; 2+, moderate; 3+, moderately severe; 4+, severe. *Nefazodone: additional side effect of impotence (+) and some risk of hepatic toxicity. †Trazodone: additional side effect of priapism (+).

285

PHARMACOLOGICAL PROPERTIES

Tricyclic Antidepressants and Other Norepinephrine-Reuptake Inhibitors Knowledge of the pharmacological properties of antidepressant drugs remains incomplete, and coherent interpretation is limited by a lack of a compelling psychobiological theory of mood disorders. The actions of tricyclic antidepressants include a range of complex, secondary adaptations to their initial and sustained actions as inhibitors of NE neuronal transport (uptake 1, *via* NET; *see* Chapter 2) and variable blockade of 5-HT transport (*via* serotonin transporter [SERT]). Tricyclic antidepressants with secondary-amine side chains or the *N*-demethylated (*nor*) metabolites of agents with tertiary-amine moieties (*e.g.*, amoxapine, desipramine, maprotiline, *norclomipramine, nordoxepin,* and nortriptyline) are relatively selective inhibitors of NE transport. Most tertiary-amine tricyclic antidepressants also inhibit the reuptake of 5-HT. Trimipramine is exceptional among the tricyclic antidepressants in that it lacks prominent inhibitory effects at monoamine transport.

The tricyclic and other NE-active antidepressants do not block dopamine (DA) transport (*via* DAT); they thereby differ from central nervous system (CNS) stimulants, including cocaine, methylphenidate, and amphetamines (*see* Chapter 10). Nevertheless, they may indirectly facilitate effects of DA by inhibiting the nonspecific transport of DA into noradrenergic terminals in the cerebral cortex. Tricyclic antidepressants also can desensitize D_2 autoreceptors through uncertain mechanisms and with uncertain behavioral contributions.

Tricyclic antidepressants variably interact with receptors (*e.g.*, α adrenergic receptor, muscarinic receptor, H_1 histamine receptor). Interactions with the adrenergic receptors apparently are critical for responses to increased availability of extracellular NE in or near synapses. Most tricyclic antidepressants have at least moderate and selective affinity for α_1 adrenergic receptors, much less for α_2, and virtually none for β receptors. The α_2 receptors include presynaptic autoreceptors that limit the neurophysiological activity of noradrenergic neurons ascending from the locus ceruleus in brainstem to supply mid- and forebrain projections. The same noradrenergic neurons provide descending projections to the spinal cord preganglionic cholinergic efferents to the peripheral autonomic ganglia (*see* Chapters 6 and 10). Autoreceptor mechanisms also reduce the synthesis of NE, presumably by attenuation of the cyclic AMP-PKA activation of tyrosine hydroxylase, *via* α_2 adrenergic receptor inhibition of adenylyl cyclase. Activation of these autoreceptors also inhibits transmitter release.

The α_2 receptor–mediated, presynaptic, negative-feedback mechanisms are rapidly activated after administration of tricyclic antidepressants. By limiting synaptic availability of NE, such mechanisms normally tend to maintain functional homeostasis. However, with repeated drug exposure, α_2-receptor responses eventually are diminished, possibly from desensitization secondary to increased exposure to the endogenous agonist (NE) or from prolonged occupation of the NE transporter itself *via* an allosteric effect. Over a period of days to weeks, this adaptation allows the presynaptic production and release of NE to return to, or even exceed, baseline levels. However, long-term treatment eventually can reduce the expression of tyrosine hydroxylase as well as the NE transporter.

The density of functional postsynaptic β adrenergic receptors gradually down-regulates over several weeks of repeated treatment with tricyclics, some selective serotonin reuptake inhibitors (SSRIs), and monoamine oxidase (MAO) inhibitors. Combinations of a 5-HT transport inhibitor with a tricyclic antidepressant may have a more rapid β adrenergic receptor–desensitizing effect. Since β-blockers tend to induce or worsen depression in vulnerable persons, it is unlikely that diminished β-receptor signaling contributes directly to the mood-elevating effects of antidepressant treatment. Nevertheless, loss of inhibitory β adrenergic influences on serotonergic neurons may enhance release of 5-HT and thus contribute indirectly to antidepressant effects (*see* Chapter 10).

With tricyclic antidepressant therapy, postsynaptic α_1 adrenergic receptors may be inhibited initially, probably contributing to early hypotensive effects of many tricyclics. Over weeks of treatment, α_1 receptors remain available and may even become more sensitive to NE as clinical mood-elevating effects gradually emerge. Therefore, as antidepressant treatment gradually becomes clinically effective, inactivation of transmitter reuptake continues to be blocked, presynaptic production and release of NE returns to or may exceed baseline levels, and a postsynaptic α_1 adrenergic mechanism is operative.

Additional neuropharmacological changes that may contribute to the clinical effects of tricyclic antidepressants include indirect facilitation of 5-HT (and perhaps DA) neurotransmission through excitatory α_1 "heteroreceptors" on other monoaminergic neurons, or desensitized, inhibitory α_2 autoreceptors, as well as D_2 autoreceptors. Activated release of 5-HT and DA may, in turn, lead to secondary down-regulation of 5-HT$_1$ autoreceptors, postsynaptic 5-HT$_2$ receptors, and perhaps D_2 autoreceptors and postsynaptic D_2 receptors.

Other adaptive changes observed in response to long-term treatment with tricyclic antidepressants include altered sensitivity of muscarinic acetylcholine receptors and decreases in gamma-aminobutyric acid ($GABA_B$) receptors and possibly N-methyl-D-aspartate (NMDA) glutamate receptors. In addition, the cyclic AMP-PKA pathway is more activated in some cells, with effects on CREB and brain-derived neurotrophic factor (BDNF). Additional changes may reflect indirect effects of antidepressant treatment or recovery from depressive illness; these include normalization of glucocorticoid release and glucocorticoid receptor sensitivity and shifts in the production of prostaglandins and cytokines and in lymphocyte functions.

The neuropharmacology of tricyclic antidepressants is not explained simply by blockade of the transport-mediated removal of NE, even though this effect undoubtedly is a crucial event that initiates a series of important secondary adaptations. Interactions of antidepressants with monoaminergic synaptic transmission are illustrated in Figure 17–1.

Selective Serotonin Reuptake Inhibitors (SSRIs) The late and indirect actions of these antidepressant and antianxiety agents remain less well understood than are those of tricyclic antidepressants, but there are striking parallels between responses in the noradrenergic and serotonergic systems. Like tricyclic antidepressants, which block NE reuptake, the SSRIs block neuronal transport of 5-HT both immediately and chronically, leading to complex secondary responses. Increased synaptic availability of 5-HT results in stimulation of a large number of postsynaptic 5-HT receptor types (*see* Chapter 11), which may contribute to adverse effects characteristic of this class of drugs, including GI effects (nausea and vomiting) and sexual effects (delayed or impaired orgasm). Stimulation of 5-HT_{2C} receptors may contribute to the agitation or restlessness sometimes induced by SSRIs.

In both serotoninergic and noradrenergic neurons, negative feedback mechanisms rapidly emerge to restore homeostasis. In the 5-HT system, 5-HT_1–subtype autoreceptors (types 1A and 7 at raphe cell bodies and dendrites, type 1D at terminals) suppress serotoninergic neurons in the raphe nuclei of the brainstem, inhibiting both tryptophan hydroxylase (probably through reduced phosphorylation-activation) and neuronal release of 5-HT. Repeated treatment leads to gradual down-regulation and desensitization of autoreceptor mechanisms over several weeks (particularly of 5-HT_{1D} receptors at nerve terminals), with a return or increase of presynaptic activity, production, and release of 5-HT. Additional secondary changes include gradual down-regulation of postsynaptic 5-HT_{2A} receptors, which may contribute to antidepressant effects directly and by influencing the function of noradrenergic and other neurons *via* serotonergic heteroreceptors. Many other postsynaptic 5-HT receptors presumably remain available to mediate increased serotonergic transmission and contribute to the mood-elevating and anxiolytic effects of this class of drugs.

Complex late adaptations occur upon repeated treatment with SSRIs, including indirect enhancement of NE output by reduction of tonic inhibitory effects of 5-HT_{2A} heteroreceptors. Finally, similar nuclear and cellular adaptations occur as with the tricyclic antidepressants, including increased intraneuronal cyclic AMP, activation/phosphorylation of transcription factors (*e.g.,* CREB), and increased production of BDNF.

Other Drugs Affecting Monoamine Neurotransmitters

The MAO inhibitor tranylcypromine is amphetamine-like in structure but interacts only weakly at DA transporters. The phenylpiperazine nefazodone, *and to a lesser extent, the structurally related* trazodone *have weak inhibitory actions on 5-HT transport; nefazodone also may have a minor effect on NE transport. This agent also has a prominent direct antagonistic effect at 5-HT_{2A} receptors that may contribute to antidepressant and anxiolytic activity. Both drugs also may inhibit presynaptic 5-HT_1 subtype autoreceptors to enhance neuronal release of 5-HT, though they probably also exert at least partial-agonist effects on postsynaptic 5-HT_1 receptors. Trazodone also blocks cerebral α_1 and H_1 receptors, possibly contributing to its tendency to induce priapism and sedation, respectively.*

Finally, the atypical antidepressants mirtazapine *and* mianserin *are structural analogs of 5-HT with potent antagonistic effects at several postsynaptic 5-HT receptor types (including 5-HT_{2A}, 5-HT_{2C}, and 5-HT_3 receptors) and can produce gradual down-regulation of 5-HT_{2A} receptors. Mirtazapine limits the effectiveness of inhibitory α_2 adrenergic heteroreceptors on serotonergic neurons as well as inhibitory α_2 autoreceptors and 5-HT_{2A} heteroreceptors on noradrenergic neurons. These effects may enhance release of amines and contribute to the antidepressant effects of these drugs. Mirtazapine also is a potent histamine H_1-receptor antagonist and is relatively sedating. Mianserin is not used in the U.S. owing largely to its bone marrow suppression.*

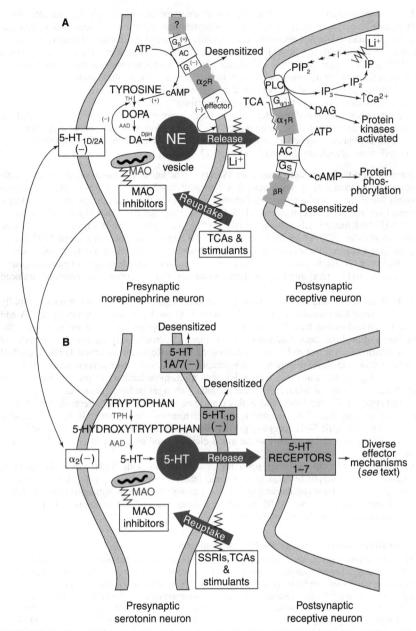

FIGURE 17–1 *Sites of action of antidepressants.* *A.* In varicosities ("terminals") of norepinephrine (NE) neurons projecting from brainstem to forebrain, L-tyrosine is oxidized to dihydroxyphenylalanine (L-DOPA) by tyrosine hydroxylase (TH), then decarboxylated to dopamine (DA) by aromatic L-amino acid decarboxylase (AAD) and stored in vesicles, where side-chain oxidation by dopamine β-hydroxylase (DβH) converts DA to NE. Following exocytotic release by depolarization in the presence of Ca^{2+} (inhibited by lithium), NE interacts with postsynaptic α and β adrenergic receptor (R) subtypes as well as presynaptic α_2 autoreceptors. Regulation of NE release by α_2 receptors is principally through attenuation of Ca^{2+} currents and activation of K^+ currents. Inactivation of trans-synaptic communication occurs primarily by active transport ("reuptake") into presynaptic terminals (inhibited by most tricyclic antidepressants [TCAs] and stimulants), with secondary deamination (by mitochondrial monoamine oxidase [MAO], blocked by MAO inhibitors). Blockade of inactivation of NE by TCAs initially leads to α_2 receptor–mediated inhibition of firing rates, metabolic activity, and transmitter release from NE neurons; gradually, however, α_2 autoreceptor response diminishes and presynaptic activity

Monoamine Oxidase Inhibitors

The MAOs comprise two structurally related flavin-containing enzymes, designated MAO-A and MAO-B, that share ~70% homology but are encoded by distinct genes. They are localized in mitochondrial membranes and widely distributed throughout the body in nerve terminals, the liver, intestinal mucosa, platelets, and other organs. Within the CNS, MAO-A is expressed predominantly in noradrenergic neurons, while MAO-B is expressed in serotonergic and histaminergic neurons. MAO activity is closely linked functionally with an aldehyde reductase and an aldehyde dehydrogenase, depending on the substrate and tissue.

MAO regulates the metabolic degradation of catecholamines, 5-HT, and other endogenous amines in the CNS and peripheral tissues. Hepatic MAO has a crucial defensive role in inactivating circulating monoamines and compounds (e.g., the indirect-acting sympathomimetic tyramine) that are ingested or originate in the gut and get absorbed into the portal circulation. Inhibition of this enzyme system by MAO inhibitors causes a reduction in metabolism and a subsequent increase in the concentrations of biogenic amines. MAO-A preferentially deaminates Epi, NE, and 5-HT and is selectively inhibited by clorgyline, while MAO-B metabolizes phenethylamine and is inhibited by selegiline. DA and tyramine are metabolized by both MAO isozymes and both types are inhibited by phenelzine, tranylcypromine, and isocarboxazid.

Selective MAO-A inhibitors are more effective in treating major depression than type B inhibitors. The MAO-B inhibitor selegiline is approved for treatment of early Parkinson's disease and acts by potentiating remaining DA in degenerating nigrostriatal neurons and possibly by reducing neuronal damage due to reactive products of the oxidative metabolism of DA or other potential neurotoxins (see Chapter 20). Selegiline also has antidepressant effects, particularly at doses >10 mg that also inhibit MAO-A or yield amphetamine-like metabolites. Several short-acting selective inhibitors of MAO-A (e.g., brofaromine and moclobemide) and toloxatone have at least moderate antidepressant effects and are less likely to potentiate the pressor actions of tyramine and other indirect-acting sympathomimetic amines than are the nonselective, irreversible MAO inhibitors.

Although MAO inhibition occurs rapidly and is usually maximal within days, clinical benefits usually are delayed for several weeks, perhaps reflecting down-regulation of serotonergic and adrenergic receptors. Favorable clinical responses occur when human platelet MAO-B is inhibited by at least 85%, suggesting the need to use aggressive dosages to achieve the maximal therapeutic potential of MAO inhibitors. Finally, despite long-lasting inhibition of MAO by the irreversible inhibitors of MAO, optimal therapeutic benefit appears to require daily dosing.

ABSORPTION AND BIOAVAILABILITY Most antidepressants are fairly well absorbed after oral administration; nefazodone is an exception, with a bioavailability of ~20%. The MAO inhibitors are absorbed readily when given by mouth. High doses of the strongly anticholinergic tricyclic antidepressants (Table 17–1) can slow GI activity and gastric emptying time, resulting in slower or erratic drug absorption and complicating management of acute overdosages. Serum concentrations of most tricyclic antidepressants peak within several hours. Injectable formulations of tricyclic antidepressants are not commercially available in the U.S.

DISTRIBUTION AND SERUM LEVEL MONITORING Once absorbed, tricyclic antidepressants are widely distributed. They are relatively lipophilic and strongly bind to plasma proteins and constituents of tissues, leading to apparent volumes of distribution as high as 10–50 L/kg. The tendency of tricyclic antidepressants and their ring-hydroxy metabolites to accumulate in cardiac tissue adds to their cardiotoxicity. Serum concentrations of antidepressants that correlate meaningfully with clinical effects are only established for a few tricyclic antidepressants (particularly amitriptyline,

---

FIGURE 17–1 *(Continued)* returns. Postsynaptically, β adrenergic receptors activate the G_s-adenylyl cyclase (AC)-cyclic AMP (cAMP) pathway. Adrenergic α_1 (and other) receptors activate the phospholipase C-G_q-IP_3 pathway with secondary modulation of intracellular Ca^{2+} and protein kinases. Postsynaptic β receptors also desensitize; α_1 receptors do not. ***B.*** Selective serotonin reuptake inhibitors (SSRIs) have analogous actions to TCAs at 5-HT-containing neurons, and TCAs can interact with serotonergic neurons and receptors. 5-HT is synthesized from L-tryptophan by a relatively rate-limiting tryptophan hydroxylase (TPH); the resulting 5-hydroxytryptophan is deaminated by AAD to 5-hydroxytryptamine (5-HT, serotonin). Following release, 5-HT interacts with a large number of postsynaptic 5-HT receptors that exert their effects through a variety of PLC and AC-mediated mechanisms. Inhibitory autoreceptors include types $5-HT_{1A}$ and perhaps $5-HT_7$ receptor subtypes at cell bodies and dendrites, as well as $5-HT_{1D}$ receptors at the nerve terminals; these receptors probably become desensitized following prolonged treatment with a SSRI antidepressant that blocks 5-HT transporters. The adrenergic and serotonergic systems also influence each other, in part through complementary heteroceptor mechanisms (inhibitory α_2 receptors on 5-HT neurons, and inhibitory $5-HT_{1D}$ and $5-HT_{2A}$ receptors on noradrenergic neurons).

desipramine, imipramine, and nortriptyline), typically at concentrations of ~100–250 ng/mL (Table 17–2). Toxic effects of tricyclic antidepressants can be expected at serum concentrations >500 ng/mL; levels >1 μg/mL can be fatal. Individual variance in tricyclic antidepressant levels in response to a given dose is as high as ten- to thirtyfold, due largely to genetic control of hepatic CYPs, but the utility of therapeutic drug monitoring in the routine clinical use of antidepressants is limited.

METABOLISM, HALF-LIVES, AND DURATION OF ACTION Tricyclic antidepressants are oxidized by hepatic CYPs, followed by conjugation with glucuronic acid. Hydroxy metabolites frequently retain some pharmacological activity. Conjugation of ring-hydroxylated metabolites with glucuronic acid extinguishes any remaining biological activity. The N-demethylated metabolites of several tricyclic antidepressants are pharmacologically active and may accumulate in concentrations approaching or exceeding those of the parent drug and contribute variably to overall

Table 17–2

Disposition of Antidepressants

Drug	Elimination $t_{1/2}$,* Hours, Parent drug (Active Metabolite)	Typical Serum Concentrations, ng/mL	Preferred CYP Isozymes‡
Tertiary-amine tricyclic antidepressants			2D6, 2C19, 3A3/4
Amitriptyline	16 (30)	100–250	
Clomipramine	32 (70)	150–500	
Doxepin	16 (30)	150–250	
Imipramine	12 (30)	175–300	
Trimipramine	16 (30)	100–300	
Secondary-amine tricyclic antidepressants			2D6, 2C19, 3A3/4
Amoxapine	8 (30)	200–500	
Desipramine	30	125–300	
Maprotiline	48	200–400	
Nortriptyline	30	60–150	
Protriptyline	80	100–250	
Selective serotonin reuptake inhibitors			
R,S-Citalopram	36	75–150	3A4, 2C19
S-Citalopram	30	40–80	3A4, 2C19
Fluoxetine	50 (240)	100–500	2D6, 2C9
Fluvoxamine	18	100–200	2D6, 1A2, 3A4, 2C9
Paroxetine	22	30–100	2D6
Sertraline	24 (66)	25–50	2D6
Venlafaxine†	5 (11)	—	2D6, 3A4
Atypical agents			
Atomoxetine	5 (child: 3)	—	2D6, 3A3/4
Bupropion†	14	75–100	2B6
Duloxetine	11	—	2D6
Mirtazapine	16–30	—	2D6
Nefazodone	3	—	3A3/4
Reboxetine	12	—	—
Trazodone	6	800–1600	2D6

*Half-life is the approximate elimination (β) half-life (limited data for newer agents). Half-life values given in parentheses are those of active metabolites (commonly N-demethylated) that contribute to overall duration of action.
†Agents available in slow-release forms that delay absorption but not elimination half-life; venlafaxine also inhibits norepinephrine transport at higher doses.
‡Some serotonin reuptake inhibitors inhibit the hepatic oxidation of other agents: potent inhibition is produced by fluoxetine (2D6 and other CYP isozymes), fluvoxamine (1A2, 2C8, and 3A3/4), paroxetine (2D6), and nefazodone (3A3/4); sertraline produces moderate effects at high doses (2D6 and others); citalopram (2C19) and venlafaxine have weak interactions.

Serum concentrations are levels encountered at typical clinical doses and not intended as guidelines to optimal dosing. Information was obtained from manufacturers' product information summaries.

pharmacodynamic activity. The 8-hydroxy metabolite of amoxapine is pharmacologically active, including antagonistic interactions with D_2 receptors. Amoxapine has some risk of extrapyramidal side effects, including tardive dyskinesia, reminiscent of those of the N-methylated congener loxapine, a typical neuroleptic (*see* Chapter 18).

As occurs with the tertiary-amine tricyclic antidepressants, the N-demethylated metabolites of SSRIs also are eliminated more slowly, and some are pharmacologically active. Norclomipramine contributes noradrenergic activity. Norfluoxetine is a very long-acting inhibitor of 5-HT transport (elimination $t_{1/2}$ ~10 days) (Table 17–2) that requires several weeks for elimination. Norfluoxetine also competes for hepatic CYPs and thereby elevates levels of other agents, including tricyclic antidepressants. These effects can persist for days after administration of the parent drug has been stopped. Norsertraline (elimination $t_{1/2}$ of 60–70 hours) contributes limited pharmacological activity or risk of drug interactions. Nornefazodone contributes little to the biological activity or duration of action of nefazodone.

With some notable exceptions, inactivation and elimination of most antidepressants occurs over a period of several days. Generally, secondary-amine tricyclic antidepressants and the N-demethylated derivatives of SSRIs have elimination half-lives about twice those of the parent drugs. Nevertheless, most tricyclics are almost completely eliminated within 7–10 days; protriptyline is an exception ($t_{1/2}$ ~80 hours). Most MAO inhibitors are long acting, because recovery from their effects requires the synthesis of new enzyme over a period of 1–2 weeks.

At the other extreme, trazodone, nefazodone, and venlafaxine have short half-lives (3–6 hours), as does the active 4-hydroxy metabolite of venlafaxine ($t_{1/2}$ of ~11 hours). The $t_{1/2}$ of bupropion is ~14 hours. Owing to rapid aromatic hydroxylation, the $t_{1/2}$ of nefazodone is very short (~3 hours). The shorter duration of action of these agents usually implies the need for multiple daily doses. Some short-acting antidepressants have been prepared in slow-release preparations (notably bupropion and venlafaxine), to allow less frequent dosing and potentially to temper side effects related to agitation and GI disturbance.

Relative to young adults, antidepressants are metabolized more rapidly by children and more slowly by patients over 60 years of age. Dosages are adjusted accordingly, sometimes to daily doses in children that far exceed those typically given to adults.

The hydrazide MAO inhibitors are thought to be cleaved to liberate pharmacologically active products (e.g., hydrazines) that are inactivated primarily by acetylation. About one-half the population of the U.S. and Europe (and more in certain Asian and Arctic regions) are "slow acetylators" of hydrazine-type drugs, including phenelzine; this genetic trait may contribute to exaggerated effects observed in some patients given standard doses of phenelzine (see Chapters 3 and 4).

INTERACTIONS WITH CYPs   The metabolism of most antidepressants depends greatly on the activity of hepatic CYPs (*see* Table 17–2). In general, CYP1A2 and CYP2D6 mediate aromatic hydroxylation, and CYP3A3/4 mediate N-dealkylation and N-oxidation reactions in the metabolism of antidepressants. Some antidepressants not only are substrates for metabolism by CYPs but also can inhibit the metabolic clearance of other drugs, sometimes producing clinically significant drug interactions. Notable inhibitory interactions include fluvoxamine with CYP1A2; fluoxetine and fluvoxamine with CYP2C9, and fluvoxamine with CYP1A2 and CYP2C19; paroxetine, fluoxetine, and less actively, sertraline with CYP2D6; norfluoxetine with CYP3A4; and fluvoxamine and nefazodone with CYP3A3/4. Citalopram or S-citalopram and venlafaxine interact much less with CYPs. Atomoxetine has weak effects on the metabolism of most other agents, but its clearance is inhibited by some SSRIs, including paroxetine. Duloxetine can inhibit the metabolism of agents such as desipramine that are metabolized extensively through CYP2D6, and its own metabolism is inhibited by some SSRIs (*e.g.,* paroxetine). Potentially significant interactions include the tendency for fluvoxamine to increase circulating concentrations of oxidatively metabolized benzodiazepines, clozapine, theophylline, and warfarin. Sertraline and fluoxetine can increase levels of benzodiazepines, clozapine, and warfarin. Paroxetine increases levels of clozapine, theophylline, and warfarin. Fluoxetine also potentiates tricyclic antidepressants and some antiarrhythmics with a narrow therapeutic index (*e.g., propafenone*; *see* Chapter 34). Nefazodone potentiates benzodiazepines other than *lorazepam* and *oxazepam*.

TOLERANCE AND PHYSICAL DEPENDENCE   Some tolerance to the sedative and autonomic effects of tricyclic antidepressants and to the nausea commonly associated with SSRIs tends to develop with continued drug use. Various antidepressants have been used for months or years by patients with severe recurring depression without obvious loss of efficacy, though some therapeutic tolerance may occur, more often with SSRIs than with older agents. Sometimes, this loss of benefit may be overcome by increasing the dose of antidepressant, by temporary addition of lithium or by a small dose of an antipsychotic agent, or by changing to an antidepressant in a different class. To avoid toxicity and precipitation of "serotonin syndrome" (see Drug Interactions), extreme caution is advised when these strategies are employed.

Occasionally, patients show physical dependence on the tricyclic antidepressants, with malaise, chills, coryza, muscle aches, and sleep disturbance following abrupt discontinuation, particularly of high doses. Similar reactions, along with GI and sensory symptoms (paresthesias) and irritability, also occur with abrupt discontinuation of SSRIs, particularly with paroxetine and venlafaxine. Withdrawal reactions from MAO inhibitors may be severe, commencing 24–72 hours after drug discontinuation; such reactions are more common with tranylcypromine and isocarboxazid when used in excess of the usual therapeutic range. Symptoms range from nausea, vomiting, and malaise to nightmares, agitation, psychosis, and convulsions.

Some withdrawal effects may reflect increased cholinergic activity following its inhibition by such agents as amitriptyline, imipramine, and paroxetine, whereas serotonergic mechanisms may contribute to the effects of abrupt discontinuation of SSRIs. Some of these reactions can be confused with clinical worsening of depressive symptoms. Emergence of agitated or manic reactions also has been observed after abrupt discontinuation of tricyclics, indicating that it is wise to discontinue antidepressants gradually over at least a week, or longer when feasible.

Treatment discontinuation of several psychotropic agents has been proposed to increase the risk of recurrence of morbidity to a degree greater than would be predicted by the natural history of untreated illness; this risk probably extends over several months. Evidence for this phenomenon is particularly strong with lithium in bipolar disorder, is likely with some antipsychotics, and may occur with antidepressants. Such risk may be reduced by gradual discontinuation of long-term medication over at least several weeks (see Chapter 18).

ADVERSE EFFECTS Tricyclic antidepressants routinely produce adverse autonomic responses, in part related to their relatively potent antimuscarinic effects, including dry mouth and a sour or metallic taste, epigastric distress, constipation, dizziness, tachycardia, palpitations, blurred vision (poor accommodation and increased risk of glaucoma), and urinary retention. Cardiovascular effects include orthostatic hypotension, sinus tachycardia, and variable prolongation of cardiac conduction times with the potential for arrhythmias, particularly with overdoses.

In the absence of cardiac disease, the principal problem associated with imipramine-like agents is postural hypotension, probably related to anti-α_1 adrenergic actions. Hypotension can be severe, with falls and injuries. Among tricyclics, nortriptyline may be less likely to induce postural blood pressure changes. Tricyclic antidepressants should be avoided following an acute myocardial infarction; in the presence of defects in bundle-branch conduction or slowed repolarization; or when other cardiac depressants (including other psychotropic agents such as thioridazine) are being administered. They have direct cardiac-depressing actions like those of certain antiarrhythmics, related to actions at fast Na^+ channels (see Chapter 34). Mild congestive heart failure and the presence of some cardiac arrhythmias are not absolute contraindications to the short-term use of a tricyclic antidepressant when depression and its associated medical risks are severe, safer alternatives fail, and appropriate medical care is provided. Nevertheless, modern nontricyclic antidepressants—notably the SSRIs—have less risk and are a prudent choice for cardiac patients. ECT also is an option.

Weakness and fatigue are attributable to central effects of tricyclic antidepressants, particularly tertiary amines (Table 17–1) and mirtazapine, all of which have potent central antihistaminic effects. Trazodone and nefazodone also are relatively sedating. Other CNS effects include variable risk of confusion or delirium, largely due to atropine-like effects of tricyclic antidepressants. Epileptic seizures can occur, especially with daily doses of bupropion >450 mg, maprotiline >250 mg, or acute overdoses of amoxapine or tricyclics. The risk of cerebral or cardiac intoxication can increase if such agents are given in relatively high doses, particularly when combined with SSRIs that inhibit their metabolism (Table 17–2). MAO inhibitors can induce sedation or behavioral excitation and have a high risk of inducing postural hypotension.

Miscellaneous toxic effects of tricyclic antidepressants include jaundice, leukopenia, and rashes, but these are very infrequent. Weight gain is a common adverse effect of many antidepressants but is less likely with the SSRIs and is rare with bupropion (Table 17–1). Excessive sweating also is common.

Newer antidepressants generally present fewer or different side effects and toxic risks than older tricyclics and MAO inhibitors. As a group, the SSRIs have a high risk of nausea and vomiting, headache, and sexual dysfunction, including inhibited ejaculation in men and impaired orgasm in women. Adverse sexual effects also occur with tricyclic antidepressants but are less common with bupropion, nefazodone, and mirtazapine. Trazodone can produce priapism in men, presumably due to antiadrenergic actions. Some SSRIs, and perhaps fluoxetine in particular, have been associated with agitation and restlessness that resembles akathisia (*see* Chapter 18). Bupropion can act as a stimulant, with agitation, anorexia, and insomnia. SSRIs, while generally less likely to produce adverse cardiovascular effects than older antidepressants, can elicit electrophysiological changes in cardiac tissue. SSRIs can also induce the syndrome of inappropriate secretion of antidiuretic hormone with hyponatremia (*see* Chapter 29). Nefazodone has been associated with increased risk of hepatic toxicity that has prompted its removal in some countries. Such reactions also occur with tricyclic and MAO inhibitor antidepressants but only rarely with SSRIs.

Another risk of antidepressants in vulnerable patients (particularly those with unrecognized bipolar depression) is switching, sometimes suddenly, from depression to hypomanic or manic excitement, or mixed, dysphoric-agitated, manic-depressive states. To some extent this effect is dose-related and is somewhat more likely in adults treated with tricyclic antidepressants than with SSRIs, bupropion, and perhaps with MAO inhibitors. Risk of mania with newer sedating antidepressants, including nefazodone and mirtazapine, also may be relatively low, but some risk of inducing mania can be expected with any treatment that elevates mood.

Safety through the Life Cycle   Most antidepressants appear to be safe during pregnancy. Most antidepressants and lithium are secreted in breast milk, at least in small quantities, and their safety in nursing infants is neither firmly established nor safely assumed. For severe depression during pregnancy and lactation, ECT can be a relatively safe and effective alternative.

Major affective disorders are being recognized more often in children, and antidepressants increasingly are used in this age group. Children are vulnerable to the cardiotoxic and seizure-inducing effects of high doses of tricyclic antidepressants. Deaths have occurred in children after accidental or deliberate overdosage with only a few hundred milligrams of drug, and several cases of unexplained sudden death have been reported in preadolescent children treated with desipramine. Most children are relatively protected by vigorous hepatic drug metabolism. Indeed, attaining serum concentrations of desipramine like those encountered in adults (Table 17–2) may require doses of 5 mg/kg of body weight (or more in some school-age children) compared to only 2–3 mg/kg in adults. Note that many trials of tricyclic antidepressants in children have failed to show substantial superiority to placebo, and the efficacy of modern agents, including SSRIs, is not securely established other than for fluoxetine and sertraline. Other antidepressants have received little assessment in juveniles. Antidepressants appear to be more effective in adolescents. In children, they risk inducing agitated states that may represent mania in undiagnosed juvenile bipolar disorder. The possibility of increased suicidal risk in juveniles treated with SSRIs has been suggested, with proposed restrictions and caution on their use.

Among geriatric patients, dizziness, postural hypotension, constipation, delayed micturition, edema, and tremor are found commonly with tricyclic antidepressants. These patients are much more likely to tolerate SSRIs and other modern antidepressants. Risks in geriatric patients are higher due to decreased metabolic clearance of antidepressants and less ability to tolerate them.

Toxic Effects of Acute Overdoses   Acute poisoning with tricyclic antidepressants or MAO inhibitors is potentially life-threatening. Fatalities are much less common since modern antidepressants have widely replaced these drugs; however, suicide rates have not declined consistently as clinical usage of modern antidepressants has increased. Deaths have been reported with acute doses of ~2 g of imipramine, and severe intoxication can be expected at doses >1 g, or about a week's supply. If a patient is severely depressed, potentially suicidal, impulsive, or has a history of substance abuse, prescribing a relatively safe antidepressant agent with close clinical follow-up is appropriate. If a potentially lethal agent is prescribed, it is best dispensed in small, sublethal quantities, with the risk that sustained adherence to recommended treatment may be compromised.

Acute poisoning with a tricyclic antidepressant often is clinically complex: brief excitement and restlessness, sometimes with myoclonus, tonic-clonic seizures, or dystonia, followed by rapid development of coma, often with depressed respiration, hypoxia, depressed reflexes, hypothermia, and hypotension. Antidepressants with strong antimuscarinic potency commonly induce an atropine-like syndrome of mydriasis, flushed dry skin and dry mucosae, absent bowel sounds, urinary retention, and tachycardia or other cardiac arrhythmias. A patient intoxicated with a tricyclic antidepressant must be treated early, ideally in an intensive care unit. Gastric lavage with activated charcoal may be useful, but dialysis and diuresis are ineffective. Coma abates gradually over 1–3 days, and excitement and delirium may reappear. Risk of life-threatening cardiac arrhythmias continues for at least several days, requiring close medical supervision.

Cardiac toxicity and hypotension can be especially difficult to manage in patients with overdoses of tricyclic antidepressants. The most common cardiac effect is sinus tachycardia, due both to anticholinergic effects and diminished uptake of NE. Intravenous sodium bicarbonate can improve hypotension and cardiac arrhythmias, although the precise roles of alkalinization versus increased sodium have not been established. Cardiac glycosides and antiarrhythmic drugs such as quinidine, procainamide, and disopyramide are contraindicated, but phenytoin and lidocaine can be used for ventricular arrhythmias. If the prolonged QT interval results in torsades de pointes, magnesium, isoproterenol, and atrial pacing may be employed. Hypotension that does not respond to alkalinization should be treated with NE and intravenous fluids.

Effects of MAO inhibitor overdosage include agitation, hallucinations, hyperreflexia, fever, and convulsions. Both hypotension and hypertension can occur. Treatment of such intoxication is problematic, but conservative treatment often is successful.

DRUG INTERACTIONS Binding of tricyclic antidepressants to plasma albumin can be reduced by competition with a number of drugs, including phenytoin, aspirin, aminopyrine, scopolamine, and phenothiazines. Barbiturates and many anticonvulsant agents (particularly carbamazepine), as well as cigarette smoking, can increase the hepatic metabolism of antidepressants by inducing CYPs.

Conversely, competition for the metabolism of other drugs by SSRIs can cause significant drug interactions. For example, during the use of combinations of SSRIs with tricyclic antidepressants, serum concentrations of the tricyclic drug may rise to toxic levels. Such an interaction can persist for days after discontinuing fluoxetine due to the prolonged elimination $t_{1/2}$ of norfluoxetine. Several SSRIs are potent inhibitors of hepatic CYPs; venlafaxine, citalopram, and sertraline appear to have relatively low risk of such interactions. Significant interactions may be most likely in persons who are relatively rapid metabolizers through the microsomal oxidase system, including children.

Examples of drug interactions with SSRIs include potentiation of agents metabolized prominently by CYP1A2 (*e.g., β* adrenergic receptor antagonists, caffeine, several antipsychotic agents, and most tricyclic antidepressants); CYP2C9 (carbamazepine); CYP2C19 (barbiturates, imipramine, propranolol, and phenytoin); CYP2D6 (*β* adrenergic receptor antagonists, some antipsychotics, and many antidepressants); and CYP3A3/4 (benzodiazepines, carbamazepine, many antidepressants, and several macrolide antibiotics).

Antidepressants potentiate the effects of alcohol and probably other sedatives. The anticholinergic activity of tricyclic antidepressants can add to that of antiparkinsonism agents, antipsychotic drugs of low potency (especially clozapine and thioridazine), or other compounds with antimuscarinic activity to produce toxic effects. Tricyclic antidepressants have prominent and potentially dangerous potentiative interactions with biogenic amines such as NE, which normally are removed from their site of action by neuronal reuptake. However, these inhibitors of NE transport block the effects of indirectly acting amines such as tyramine, which must be taken up by sympathetic neurons to release NE. Presumably by a similar mechanism, tricyclic antidepressants prevent the antihypertensive action of adrenergic neuron blocking agents such as guanadrel. Tricyclic agents and trazodone also can block the centrally mediated antihypertensive action of clonidine.

SSRIs and other agents with 5-HT-potentiating activity can interact dangerously or even fatally with MAO inhibitors (particularly long-acting MAO inhibitors). The resulting reactions are referred to as "serotonin syndrome" and most commonly occur in patients receiving combination therapy with two or more serotonergic agents. Besides the combination of MAO inhibitors with SSRIs, other drug combinations or conditions that increase 5-HT synthesis (e.g., L-tryptophan [L-Trp]) or release (e.g., amphetamines and cocaine), that act as 5-HT agonists (e.g.., buspirone, dihydroergotamine, and sumatriptan), or that otherwise increase 5-HT activity (e.g., ECT and lithium) all have been implicated in the development of serotonin syndrome. This syndrome typically includes akathisia-like restlessness, muscle twitches and myoclonus, hyperreflexia, sweating, penile erection, shivering, and tremor as a prelude to more severe intoxication, with seizures and coma. The reaction often is self-limiting if the diagnosis is made quickly and the offending agents are discontinued. Selegiline, moclobemide, and perhaps St. John's wort preparations also should be considered to have some risk of such interactions.

To avoid drug toxicity and prevent the precipitation of serotonin syndrome, duration of effect should be considered when switching between antidepressants (e.g., a MAO inhibitor should not be started for 5 weeks after discontinuing fluoxetine; 2–3 weeks should elapse between stopping a nonselective MAO inhibitor and initiating therapy with a tricyclic antidepressant).

The hypertensive interaction of MAO inhibitors with indirectly acting pressor phenethylamines requires scrupulous avoidance of many agents, such as over-the-counter cold remedies containing indirect-acting sympathomimetic drugs (see Chapter 10). Fatal intracranial bleeding has occurred in such hypertensive reactions. Headache is a common symptom, and fever frequently accompanies the hypertensive episode. Meperidine should never be used for such headaches (it could prove to be fatal), and blood pressure should be evaluated immediately when a patient taking an MAO inhibitor reports a severe throbbing headache or a feeling of pressure in the head.

Drug Treatment of Mood Disorders

Disorders of mood (*affective disorders*) are very common, with severity ranging from normal grief reactions and dysthymia to severe, incapacitating psychotic and melancholic illnesses that may result in death. The lifetime risk of suicide in severe forms of major affective disorders requiring hospitalization is 10–15%, but as low at 3–5% in less severely ill outpatients. Probably only 30–40% of cases of clinical depression are diagnosed, and a much smaller number are adequately treated. Not all types of grief and misery call for medical treatment, and even severe mood disorders have a high rate of spontaneous remission in time (often months). Antidepressants generally are reserved for the more severe and incapacitating depressive disorders. The most satisfactory results tend to occur in patients who have moderately severe illnesses with "endogenous" or "melancholic" characteristics without psychotic features. Antidepressant agents clearly are effective for adult major depression, but a number of shortcomings continue to be associated with all drugs used to treat affective disorders.

A major problem with antidepressants is that placebo response rates tend to be as high as 30–40% in subjects diagnosed with major depression; thus, clinical distinctions between active drug and placebo are difficult to prove.

Pediatric studies often have failed to show superiority of antidepressant drugs over placebo, particularly with older antidepressants but also with most SSRIs, and the future of tricyclic antidepressant use in children is uncertain. Finally, evidence concerning clinical dose-response and dose-risk relationships is especially limited with the newer antidepressant drugs. Despite lack of consistency and convincingly demonstrated efficacy, the modern antidepressants have largely replaced the tricyclics as first-line options in children, adolescents, and the elderly, largely owing to their relative safety.

CHOICE OF ANTIDEPRESSANT MEDICATION AND DOSING

The usual dosages and dose ranges of antidepressant medications are listed in Table 17–1, along with the severity of common side effects. Although they usually are used initially in divided doses, transition to a single daily dose usually is possible due to the relatively long half-lives and wide range of tolerated concentrations of most antidepressants. With the tricyclic antidepressants, dosing is most safely done with single doses up to the equivalent of 150 mg of imipramine.

Tricyclic and Selective Serotonin Reuptake Inhibitors

SSRIs and other atypical modern agents now are broadly accepted as drugs of first choice, particularly for medically ill or potentially suicidal patients and in the elderly and young. MAO inhibitors commonly are reserved for patients who fail to respond to vigorous trials of at least one of the newer agents and a standard tricyclic antidepressant, administered alone or with lithium to enhance overall therapeutic effectiveness. The somewhat less anticholinergic secondary-amine tricyclics, particularly nortriptyline and desipramine, are alternatives or a second choices for elderly or medically ill patients, particularly if administered in moderate, divided doses (Table 17–1). Patients with severe, prolonged, disabling, psychotic, suicidal, or bipolar depression require vigorous and prompt medical intervention.

MAO Inhibitors

Indications for the MAO inhibitors are limited and must be weighed against their potential toxicity and their complex interactions with other drugs. Thus, the MAO inhibitors generally are considered drugs of late choice for the treatment of severe depression. Nevertheless, MAO inhibitors sometimes are used when vigorous trials of several standard antidepressants have been unsatisfactory and when ECT is refused. In addition, MAO inhibitors may have selective benefits for conditions other than typical major depression, including illnesses marked by phobias and anxiety or panic as well as dysphoria, and possibly in chronic dysthymic conditions. Similar benefits, however, may be found with imipramine-like agents or SSRIs.

Bipolar Forms of Depression

The safe and effective treatment of bipolar depression is a difficult clinical challenge. This condition sometimes is misdiagnosed in patients with bipolar disorder who present with mixed dysphoric-agitated moods, who then are inappropriately treated with an antidepressant without a mood stabilizing agent to protect against worsening agitation or mania. For this reason, the management of manic, mixed, and depressive mood states in bipolar disorder best relies on lithium or other mood-stabilizing agents, notably the anticonvulsant lamotrigine, as the primary treatment (see Chapter 18). An antidepressant can be added cautiously and temporarily to treat bipolar depression, but the additional benefit and safety of sustained combinations of an antidepressant with a mood stabilizer are unproven. The combination SSRI/atypical antipsychotic (fluoxetine/olanzapine; SYMBYAX) is FDA-approved for treatment of depressive episodes associated with bipolar disorder.

Duration of Treatment

The natural history of major depression (either as unipolar depression or depressive phases of bipolar disorder) is that individual episodes tend to remit spontaneously over 6–12 months; however, there is a high risk of relapse of depression for at least several months after discontinuation of antidepressant treatment. This risk is estimated at 50% within 6 months and 65–70% at 1 year, rising to 85% by 3 years. To minimize this risk, it is best to continue antidepressant medication for at least 6 months following apparent clinical recovery. Continued use of initially therapeutic doses is recommended, although tolerability and acceptance by patients may require flexibility.

Many depressed patients follow a recurring course of episodic illness, often with lesser levels of symptoms and disability between major episodes, and therefore merit consideration of long-term maintenance medication to reduce the risk of recurrence. Such treatment has been tested for as long as 5 years, using relatively high doses of imipramine, with evidence that early dose reduction led to a higher risk of relapse. Long-term supplementation of an antidepressant with lithium may enhance the result. Prolonged maintenance treatment of patients with recurring major depression for more than a year has rarely been evaluated with modern antidepressants, and long-term dose-response data with any antidepressant are very limited. The use of indefinitely prolonged maintenance treatment with an antidepressant is guided by the history of multiple, and especially severe or life-threatening, recurrences and the impression that recurrence risk is greater in older patients. Because rapid discontinuation or sharp reduction in doses of antidepressants and lithium may contribute to excess early recurrence of illness, gradual reduction and close clinical follow-up over at least several weeks are recommended when maintenance treatment is to be discontinued and when stopping continuation therapy within the months following recovery from an acute episode of depression.

PHARMACOTHERAPY OF ANXIETY

Anxiety is a symptom of many psychiatric disorders and an almost inevitable component of many medical and surgical conditions. Symptoms of anxiety commonly are associated with depression and especially with dysthymic disorder (chronic depression of moderate severity), panic disorder, agoraphobia and other specific phobias, obsessive-compulsive disorder, eating disorders, and many personality disorders. Sometimes, no treatable primary illness is found, or if one is found and treated, it may be desirable to deal directly with the anxiety at the same time. In such situations, antianxiety medications are frequently and appropriately used.

Currently, the benzodiazepines and the SSRIs are the most commonly employed pharmacotherapies for common clinical anxiety disorders (*see* Chapter 16). Benzodiazepines sometimes are given to patients presenting with anxiety mixed with symptoms of depression, although their efficacy in altering the core features of severe major depression has not been demonstrated.

The most favorable responses to the benzodiazepines are obtained in situations that involve relatively acute anxiety reactions in medical or psychiatric patients who have either modifiable primary illnesses or primary anxiety disorders. However, this group of anxious patients also has a high response rate to placebo and is likely to undergo spontaneous improvement. Antianxiety drugs also are used in the management of more persistent or recurrent primary anxiety disorders. A particularly controversial aspect of the use of benzodiazepines, especially those of high potency, is in long-term management of patients with sustained or recurring symptoms of anxiety; despite clinical benefit for at least several months, it is unclear if the long-term benefits can be distinguished from nonspecific ("placebo") effects following development of tolerance on the one hand, or prevention of related withdrawal-emergent anxiety on the other.

The antihistamine hydroxyzine *is an effective antianxiety agent, but only at doses (~400 mg/day) that produce marked sedation* (see *Chapter 24*). Propranolol *and* metoprolol, *lipophilic β adrenergic receptor antagonists that enter the CNS, can reduce the autonomic symptoms (nervousness and muscle tremor) associated with specific situational or social phobias but do not appear to be effective in generalized anxiety or panic disorder* (see *Chapter 10*). *Similarly, other antiadrenergic agents, including* clonidine, *may modify autonomic expression of anxiety but are not demonstrably useful in the treatment of severe anxiety disorders.*

The azapirones (azaspirodecanediones) (e.g.,buspirone [*BUSPAR*]) *are useful in anxiety or dysphoria of moderate intensity. The azapirones have limited antidopaminergic actions in vivo, do not induce clinical extrapyramidal side effects, and do not interact with binding sites for benzodiazepines or facilitate the action of GABA. They are not anticonvulsant (and may even lower seizure threshold slightly), do not appear to cause tolerance or withdrawal reactions, and do not show cross-tolerance with benzodiazepines or other sedatives. Buspirone and several experimental congeners* (e.g., gepirone, ipsapirone, *and* tiospirone) *have selective affinity for 5-HT receptors of the 5-HT$_{1A}$ type, for which they appear to be partial agonists* (see *Chapter 11*). *Buspirone lacks beneficial actions in severe anxiety with panic attacks. The risk of suicide with buspirone is very low.*

OTHER THERAPEUTIC USES OF THESE DRUGS The various antidepressant agents have found broad utility in other disorders that may not be related psychobiologically to the mood disorders. Current applications include rapid but temporary suppression of enuresis with low (*e.g.,* 25 mg) pre-bedtime doses of tricyclic antidepressants, including imipramine and nortriptyline, by uncertain mechanisms in children and in geriatric patients, as well as a beneficial effect of duloxetine on urinary stress incontinence. Antidepressants have a growing role in *attention-deficit/hyperactivity disorder* in children and adults, for which imipramine, desipramine, and nortriptyline appear to be effective, even in patients responding poorly to or who are intolerant of the stimulants (*e.g.,* methylphenidate). Newer NE selective reuptake inhibitors also may be useful in this disorder; atomoxetine is approved for this application. Utility of SSRIs in this syndrome is not established, and bupropion, despite its similarity to stimulants, appears to have limited efficacy.

Antidepressants tend to provide a more sustained and continuous improvement of the symptoms of attention-deficit/hyperactivity disorder than do the stimulants and do not induce tics or other abnormal movements sometimes associated with stimulants. Indeed, desipramine and nortriptyline may effectively treat tic disorders, either in association with the use of stimulants or in patients with both attention deficit disorder and Tourette's syndrome. Antidepressants also are leading choices in the treatment of severe anxiety disorders, including panic disorder with agoraphobia, generalized anxiety disorder, social phobia, and obsessive-compulsive disorder, as well as for the common comorbidity of anxiety in depressive illness. Antidepressants, especially SSRIs, also are employed in the management of posttraumatic stress disorder, which is marked by anxiety, startle, painful recollection of the traumatic events, and disturbed sleep. Initially, anxious patients often tolerate nonsedating antidepressants poorly (Table 17–1), requiring slowly increased doses. Their beneficial actions typically are delayed for several weeks in anxiety disorders, just as they are in major depression.

For panic disorder, tricyclic antidepressants and MAO inhibitors, as well as high-potency benzodiazepines (notably alprazolam, clonazepam, and lorazepam) (*see* Chapter 16), are effective in blocking the autonomic expression of panic itself, thereby facilitating a comprehensive rehabilitation program. Imipramine and phenelzine are well-studied antidepressants for panic disorder. SSRIs also may be effective, but β adrenergic receptor antagonists, buspirone, and low-potency benzodiazepines usually are not, and bupropion can worsen anxiety.

SSRIs are agents of choice in obsessive-compulsive disorder and in the syndromes of impulse dyscontrol or obsessive preoccupations (*e.g.,* compulsive gambling, trichotillomania, bulimia, but usually not anorexia nervosa and body dysmorphic disorder). Despite their limited benefits, SSRIs offer an important advance in the medical treatment of these often chronic and sometimes incapacitating disorders. The effectiveness of pharmacological treatment for these disorders is greatly enhanced by use of behavioral treatments.

Several psychosomatic disorders may respond at least partly to treatment with tricyclic antidepressants, MAO inhibitors, or SSRIs; among these are chronic pain disorders, including diabetic and other peripheral neuropathic syndromes (for which tertiary-amine tricyclics probably are superior to fluoxetine, and both duloxetine and venlafaxine also may be effective); fibromyalgia; peptic ulcer and irritable bowel syndrome; hot flashes of menopause; chronic fatigue; cataplexy; tics; migraine; and sleep apnea. These disorders may have some psychobiological relationship to mood or anxiety disorders.

For a complete Bibliographical listing see Goodman & Gilman's *The Pharmacological Basis of Therapeutics*, 11th ed., or Goodman & Gilman Online at www.accessmedicine.com.

18

PHARMACOTHERAPY OF PSYCHOSIS AND MANIA

I. DRUGS USED IN THE TREATMENT OF PSYCHOSES

The psychotic disorders include schizophrenia, the manic phase of bipolar (manic-depressive) illness, acute idiopathic psychotic illnesses, and other conditions marked by severe agitation. All exhibit major disturbances in reasoning, often with delusions and hallucinations. Several classes of drugs are effective for symptomatic treatment. Antipsychotic agents also are useful alternatives to electroconvulsive therapy (ECT) in severe depression with psychotic features, and sometimes are used in the management of patients with psychotic disorders associated with delirium or dementia or induced by other agents (*e.g.*, stimulants or L-DOPA).

The term *neuroleptic* is often applied to drugs that have relatively prominent experimental and clinical evidence of antagonism of D_2 dopamine (DA) receptors, with substantial risk of adverse extrapyramidal neurological effects and increased release of prolactin. The term *atypical antipsychotic* is applied to agents that are associated with substantially lower risks of such extrapyramidal effects. Although the antipsychotic drugs have had a revolutionary, beneficial impact on medical and psychiatric practice, their liabilities, especially of the older typical or neuroleptic agents, must be emphasized. Newer antipsychotics are atypical in having less risk of extrapyramidal side effects, but these agents present their own spectrum of adverse effects, including hypotension, seizures, weight gain, and increased risk of type 2 diabetes mellitus and hyperlipidemia.

The psychoses are among the most severe psychiatric disorders, in which there is not only marked impairment of behavior but also a serious inability to think coherently, to comprehend reality, or to gain insight into the presence of these abnormalities. These common disorders (affecting perhaps 1% of the population at some age) typically include symptoms of false beliefs (delusions) and abnormal sensations (hallucinations). Representative syndromes in this category include schizophrenia, brief psychoses, and delusional disorders. Psychotic features also occur in major mood disorders, particularly mania and severe melancholic depression. Psychotic illnesses are characterized by disordered thought processes (as inferred from illogical or highly idiosyncratic communications) with disorganized or irrational behavior and varying degrees of altered mood that can range from excited agitation to severe emotional withdrawal. Idiopathic psychoses characterized by chronically disordered thinking and emotional withdrawal, and often associated with delusions and auditory hallucinations, are called schizophrenia. *Acute and recurrent idiopathic psychoses that bear an uncertain relationship to schizophrenia or the major affective disorders also occur. Delusions that are more or less isolated are characteristic of* delusional disorder *or* paranoia.

The beneficial effects of antipsychotic drugs are not limited to schizophrenia. They also are employed in disorders ranging from postsurgical delirium and amphetamine intoxication to paranoia, mania, psychotic depression, and the agitation of Alzheimer's dementia (although their efficacy in this disorder in not proven). They are especially useful in severe depression and possibly in other conditions marked by severe turmoil or agitation.

TRICYCLIC ANTIPSYCHOTIC AGENTS

Several dozen phenothiazine antipsychotic drugs and chemically related agents are used worldwide. Other phenothiazines are marketed primarily for their antiemetic, antihistaminic, or anticholinergic effects.

Pharmacological Properties

Antipsychotic drugs share many pharmacological effects and therapeutic applications. Chlorpromazine and haloperidol are prototypic of the older, standard neuroleptic-type agents. Many antipsychotic drugs, especially chlorpromazine and other agents of low potency, have a prominent sedative effect. This is particularly conspicuous early in treatment, although some tolerance typically develops and can be of added value when very agitated psychotic patients are treated. Despite their sedative effects, neuroleptic drugs generally are not used to treat anxiety disorders or insomnia, largely because of their adverse autonomic and neurologic effects, which paradoxically can include severe anxiety and restlessness (akathisia). The risk of developing adverse extrapyramidal effects, including tardive dyskinesia, following long-term administration of neuroleptic drugs makes them less desirable than several alternative treatments for anxiety disorders (*see* Chapter 17).

The term *neuroleptic* was intended to contrast the effects of drugs such as chlorpromazine to those of sedatives and other CNS depressants. The neuroleptic syndrome involves suppression of spontaneous movements and complex behaviors, whereas spinal reflexes and unconditioned nociceptive-avoidance behaviors remain intact. In humans, neuroleptic drugs reduce initiative and interest in the environment as well as manifestations of emotion. In clinical use, there may be some initial drowsiness and slowness in response to external stimuli. However, subjects are easily aroused, can answer questions, and retain intact cognition. Ataxia, incoordination, or dysarthria do not occur at ordinary doses. Typically, psychotic patients soon become less agitated, withdrawn or autistic patients sometimes become more responsive and communicative, and aggressive and impulsive behavior diminishes. Gradually (usually over days), psychotic symptoms of hallucinations, delusions, and disorganized or incoherent thinking ameliorate. Neuroleptic agents also exert characteristic neurological effects—including bradykinesia, mild rigidity, tremor, and akathisia—that resemble the signs of Parkinson's disease.

Although the term *neuroleptic* initially encompassed this whole unique syndrome and is still used as a synonym for *antipsychotic*, it now is used to emphasize the more neurological aspects of the syndrome (*i.e.*, the parkinsonian and other extrapyramidal effects). Except for clozapine, aripiprazole, quetiapine, ziprasidone, and low doses of olanzapine and risperidone, antipsychotic drugs available in the U.S. also have effects on movement and posture and can be called neuroleptic. The more general term *antipsychotic* is preferable, as reinforced by the growing number of modern atypical antipsychotic drugs with little extrapyramidal action.

BEHAVIORAL EFFECTS   A number of effects in animal behavioral models have been used to predict the efficacy or potential adverse effects of antipsychotic agents. Despite their widespread use, these paradigms generally have not provided important insights into the basis for clinical antipsychotic effects.

EXTRAPYRAMIDAL EFFECTS OF ANTIPSYCHOTICS   The acute adverse clinical effects of antipsychotic agents are best mimicked in animals by assessing catalepsy in rats (immobility that allows an animal to be placed in abnormal postures that persist) or dystonia in monkeys. Late dyskinetic effects of antipsychotics are represented by the development of vacuous chewing movements in rats.

A particularly disturbing adverse effect of most antipsychotics is restless activity, termed *akathisia*, which is not readily mimicked by animal behavior. The cataleptic immobility of animals treated with classical antipsychotics resembles the catatonia seen in some psychotic patients and in a variety of metabolic and neurological disorders affecting the CNS. In patients, catatonic signs, along with other features of psychotic illnesses, are sometimes relieved by antipsychotic agents. However, rigidity and bradykinesia, which mimic catatonia, can be induced by administering large doses of potent traditional neuroleptics and by addition of an antimuscarinic-antiparkinson agent.

EFFECTS ON COGNITIVE FUNCTION
Several cognitive functions, including auditory processing and attention, spatial organization, verbal learning, semantic and verbal memory, and executive functions, are impaired in schizophrenia patients. Potent D_2-antagonist neuroleptics have very limited beneficial effects on such functions. Some atypical antipsychotic agents with mixed $D_2/5\text{-}HT_{2A}$ activity (including clozapine, quetiapine, olanzapine, and risperidone), as well as the D_2 partial agonist aripiprazole, seem to improve cognitive functioning in psychotic patients. Nevertheless, significant long-term gains in social and occupational function during long-term treatment of chronically psychotic patients with these drugs are not well documented.

EFFECTS ON SLEEP
Antipsychotic drugs have inconsistent effects on sleep patterns but tend to normalize sleep disturbances characteristic of many psychoses and mania. The capacity to prolong and enhance the effect of opioid and hypnotic drugs appears to parallel the sedative, rather than the neuroleptic, potency of a particular agent; thus, potent, less-sedating antipsychotics do not enhance sleep.

EFFECTS ON SPECIFIC AREAS OF THE NERVOUS SYSTEM   The antipsychotic drugs affect all levels of the CNS. Theories on the actions of antipsychotic agents are based on their ability to antagonize the actions of DA as a neurotransmitter in the basal ganglia and limbic portions of the forebrain. Although supported by a large body of data, these theories reflect a degree of circularity in the consideration of antipsychotic drug candidates for development after identifying their antidopaminergic activity.

Cerebral Cortex   Since psychosis involves disordered thought processes, cortical effects of antipsychotic drugs are of particular interest. Antipsychotic drugs interact with dopaminergic projections to the prefrontal and deep-temporal (limbic) regions of the cerebral cortex, with relative sparing of these areas from adaptive changes in DA metabolism that would suggest tolerance to the actions of neuroleptics.

Seizure Threshold

Many neuroleptic drugs can lower the seizure threshold and induce discharges in the electroencephalogram (EEG) that are associated with epileptic seizure disorders. Clozapine, olanzapine, and aliphatic phenothiazines with low potency (e.g., chlorpromazine) seem particularly able to do this, while the more potent piperazine phenothiazines and thioxanthenes (notably fluphenazine and thiothixene), risperidone, and quetiapine are much less likely to have this effect. The butyrophenones and molindone variably and unpredictably rarely cause seizures. Clozapine has a clearly dose-related risk of inducing seizures in nonepileptic patients. Antipsychotic agents, especially clozapine, olanzapine, and low-potency phenothiazines and thioxanthenes, should be used with extreme caution, if at all, in untreated epileptic patients and in patients undergoing withdrawal from CNS depressants such as alcohol, barbiturates, or benzodiazepines. Most antipsychotic drugs, especially the piperazines, and the newer atypical agents aripiprazole, quetiapine, risperidone, and ziprasidone, can be used safely in epileptic patients if moderate doses are attained gradually and if concomitant anticonvulsant drug therapy is maintained (see Chapter 19).

Basal Ganglia   Because the extrapyramidal effects of many antipsychotic drugs are prominent, a great deal of interest has centered on their actions in the basal ganglia, notably the caudate nucleus, putamen, globus pallidus, and allied nuclei, which play a crucial role in the control of posture and the extrapyramidal aspects of movement. The critical pathogenic role of DA deficiency in this region in Parkinson's disease, the potent activity of neuroleptics as DA receptor antagonists, and the striking resemblance between clinical manifestations of Parkinson's disease and some of the neurological effects of neuroleptic drugs have all focused attention on the role of deficient dopaminergic activity in some of the neuroleptic-induced extrapyramidal effects.

Antagonism of DA-mediated synaptic neurotransmission is an important action of many antipsychotics; this prompted the proposal that many adverse extrapyramidal neurological and neuroendocrinological effects of the neuroleptics are mediated by antidopaminergic effects in the basal ganglia and hypothalamic systems, whereas the antipsychotic effects of neuroleptics are mediated by modification of dopaminergic neurotransmission in the limbic and mesocortical systems. Thus, neuroleptic drugs (but not their inactive congeners) initially increase the rate of production of DA metabolites, the rate of conversion of the precursor amino acid L-tyrosine to L-dihydroxyphenylalanine (L-DOPA) and its metabolites, and initially increase the rate of firing of DA-containing cells in the midbrain. These effects presumably represent adaptive responses of neuronal systems aimed at reducing the impact of impaired synaptic transmission at dopaminergic terminals in the forebrain.

Evidence supporting this interpretation includes the observation that small doses of neuroleptics block behavioral or neuroendocrine effects of systemically administered or intracerebrally injected dopaminergic agonists. Many antipsychotic drugs also block the effects of agonists on DA-sensitive adenylyl cyclase associated with D_1/D_5-receptors in forebrain tissue (Figure 18–1). Atypical antipsychotic drugs such as clozapine and quetiapine are characterized by low affinity or weak actions in such tests. Initially, the standard antipsychotics increase firing and metabolic activity in dopaminergic neurons. These responses eventually are replaced by diminished presynaptic activity ("depolarization inactivation") with reduced firing and production of DA, particularly in the extrapyramidal basal ganglia. The timing of these adaptive changes following the administration of neuroleptics correlates well with the gradual evolution of parkinsonian bradykinesia over several days.

Estimated clinical potencies of most antipsychotic drugs correlate well with their relative potencies in vitro *to inhibit binding of radioligands to D_2 receptors. Almost all clinically effective antipsychotic agents (with the notable exception of clozapine and quetiapine) have high or moderate affinity for D_2 receptors. Although some antipsychotics (especially thioxanthenes, phenothiazines, and clozapine) bind with relatively high affinity to D_1 receptors, they also block D_2 receptors and D_2-like receptors, including the D_3 and D_4 subtypes. Butyrophenones and con-*

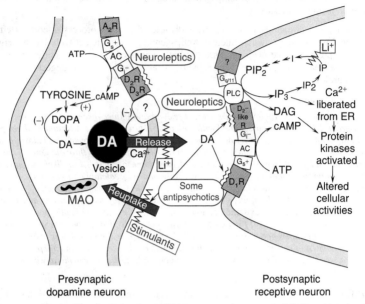

Presynaptic dopamine neuron

Postsynaptic receptive neuron

FIGURE 18–1 *Sites of action of neuroleptics and lithium.* In varicosities ("terminals") along dopamine (DA) neurons projecting from midbrain to forebrain, tyrosine is oxidized to dihydroxyphenylalanine (DOPA) by tyrosine hydroxylase (TH), the rate-limiting step in catecholamine biosynthesis, then decarboxylated to DA by aromatic L-amino acid decarboxylase (AAD) and stored in vesicles. Following exocytotic release (inhibited by Li$^+$) by depolarization in the presence of Ca^{2+}, DA interacts with postsynaptic receptors (R) of D$_1$ and D$_2$ types (and structurally similar but less prevalent D$_1$-like and D$_2$-like receptors), as well as with presynaptic D$_2$ and D$_3$ autoreceptors. Inactivation of transsynaptic communication occurs primarily by active transport ("reuptake" via DAT) of DA into presynaptic terminals (inhibited by many stimulants), with secondary deamination by mitochondrial monoamine oxidase (MAO). Postsynaptic D$_1$ receptors, through G$_s$, activate adenylyl cyclase (AC) to increase cyclic AMP (cAMP), whereas D$_2$ receptors inhibit AC through G$_i$. D$_2$ receptors also activate receptor-operated K$^+$ channels, suppress voltage-gated Ca^{2+} currents, and stimulate phospholipase C (PLC), perhaps *via* the $\beta\gamma$ subunits liberated from activated G$_i$ (*see* Chapter 1), activating the IP$_3$-Ca^{2+} pathway, thereby modulating a variety of Ca^{2+}-dependent activities including protein kinases. Lithium inhibits the phosphatase that liberates inositol (I) from inositol phosphate (IP). Both Li$^+$ and valproate can modify the abundance or function of G proteins and effectors, as well as protein kinases and several cell and nuclear regulatory factors. D$_2$-like autoreceptors suppress synthesis of DA by diminishing phosphorylation of rate-limiting TH, and by limiting DA release (possibly through modulation of Ca^{2+} or K$^+$ currents). In contrast, presynaptic A$_2$ adenosine receptors (A$_2$R) activate AC and, *via* the cyclic AMP–PKA pathway, TH activity. Nearly all antipsychotic agents block D$_2$ receptors and autoreceptors; some also block D$_1$ receptors. Initially in antipsychotic treatment, DA neurons activate and release more DA, but following repeated treatment, they enter a state of physiological depolarization inactivation, with diminished production and release of DA, in addition to continued receptor blockade. ER, endoplasmic reticulum.

geners (e.g., haloperidol, pimozide, N-methylspiperone) and experimental benzamide neuroleptics are relatively selective antagonists of D$_2$ and D$_3$ receptors, with either high (nemonapride) or low (eticlopride, raclopride, remoxipride) D$_4$ affinity.

Many other antipsychotic agents are active α$_1$ adrenergic antagonists. This action may contribute to sedative and hypotensive side effects or may underlie useful psychotropic effects. Many antipsychotic agents (aripiprazole, clozapine, olanzapine, quetiapine, risperidone, and ziprasidone) also have affinity for forebrain 5-HT$_{2A}$ receptors (see Chapter 11). This mixture of moderate affinities for several CNS receptor types (including muscarinic and H$_1$ receptors) may contribute to the distinct pharmacological profiles of the atypical antipsychotic agent clozapine and other newer atypical antipsychotics.

Limbic System Dopaminergic projections from the midbrain terminate on septal nuclei, the olfactory tubercle and basal forebrain, the amygdala, and other structures within the temporal and prefrontal cerebral lobes and the hippocampus. The DA hypothesis has focused considerable attention on the mesolimbic and mesocortical systems as possible sites where antipsychotic effects are mediated. Speculations about the pathophysiology of idiopathic psychoses such as schizophrenia have long centered on dopaminergic functions in the limbic system.

Certain important effects of antipsychotic drugs are similar in extrapyramidal and limbic regions; however, the extrapyramidal and antipsychotic actions of these drugs differ in several ways: while some acute extrapyramidal effects of neuroleptics tend to diminish or disappear with time or with concurrent administration of anticholinergic drugs, antipsychotic effects do not. Moreover, dopaminergic subsystems in the forebrain differ functionally and in their physiological responses to drugs: anticholinergic agents block the increased turnover of DA in the basal ganglia induced by neuroleptic agents, but not in dopaminergic terminals of limbic areas; tolerance to the enhanced DA metabolism by antipsychotics is much less prominent in cortical and limbic areas than in extrapyramidal areas.

Newer Dopaminergic Receptors in Basal Ganglia and Limbic System

The discovery that D_3 and D_4 receptors are preferentially expressed in limbic areas has led to efforts to identify selective inhibitors for these receptors that might have antipsychotic efficacy and low risk of extrapyramidal effects. Clozapine has modest selectivity for D_4 receptors over other DA receptor types. D_4 receptors, preferentially localized in cortical and limbic brain regions in relatively low abundance, are upregulated after repeated administration of most typical and atypical antipsychotic drugs. These receptors may contribute to clinical antipsychotic actions, but agents that are D_4 selective or mixed $D_4/5\text{-}HT_{2A}$ antagonists have not proved effective in the treatment of psychotic patients.

D_3 receptors are unlikely to play a pivotal role in antipsychotic drug actions, perhaps because their avid affinity for endogenous DA prevents their interaction with antipsychotics. The subtle and atypical functional activities of cerebral D_3 receptors suggest that D_3 agonists rather than antagonists may have useful psychotropic effects, particularly in antagonizing stimulant-reward and dependence behaviors.

Hypothalamus and Endocrine Systems Endocrine changes occur because of effects of antipsychotic drugs on the hypothalamus or pituitary, including their antidopaminergic actions. Most older antipsychotics and risperidone increase prolactin secretion, probably due to a blockade of the pituitary actions of the tuberoinfundibular dopaminergic neurons. These neurons project from the arcuate nucleus of the hypothalamus to the median eminence, where they deliver DA to the anterior pituitary *via* the hypophyseoportal blood vessels. D_2 receptors on lactotropes in the anterior pituitary mediate the tonic prolactin-inhibiting action of DA (*see* Chapter 55).

Correlations between the potencies of antipsychotic drugs in stimulating prolactin secretion and causing behavioral effects are excellent for many types of agents. Aripiprazole, clozapine, olanzapine, quetiapine, and ziprasidone are exceptional in having minimal or transient effects on prolactin, while olanzapine produces only minor, transient increases in prolactin levels. Risperidone has an unusually potent prolactin-elevating effect, even at doses with little extrapyramidal impact. Effects of neuroleptics on prolactin secretion generally occur at lower doses than do their antipsychotic effects. This may reflect their action outside the blood–brain barrier in the adenohypophysis, or differences in the regulation of pituitary and cerebral D_2 receptors. Little tolerance develops to the effect of antipsychotic drugs on prolactin secretion, correlating with a relative lack of up- or down-regulation of pituitary D_2 receptors and their relative sensitivity to DA partial agonists. The hyperprolactinemic effect of antipsychotics is rapidly reversible when the drugs are discontinued. This activity is presumed to be responsible for the galactorrhea that may be associated with their use. Perhaps due to the effects of hyperprolactinemia, some antipsychotic drugs reduce the secretion of gonadotropins and sex steroids, which can cause amenorrhea in women and sexual dysfunction or infertility in men.

Other autonomic effects of antipsychotic drugs are probably mediated by the hypothalamus, such as an impairment of the body's ability to regulate temperature. Clozapine can induce moderate elevations of body temperature that can be confusing clinically; central effects on temperature regulation and cardiovascular and respiratory function probably contribute to the features of *neuroleptic malignant syndrome* (*see* Table 18–1).

Brainstem

Clinical doses of antipsychotic agents usually have little effect on respiration. However, vasomotor reflexes mediated by either the hypothalamus or the brainstem are depressed by some antipsychotics, which may lead to hypotension. This risk is associated particularly with older low-potency

Table 18–1

Neurological Side Effects of Neuroleptic Drugs

Reaction	Features	Time of Maximal Risk	Proposed Mechanism	Treatment
Acute dystonia	Spasm of muscles of tongue, face, neck, back; may mimic seizures; *not* hysteria	1–5 days	Unknown	Antiparkinsonian agents are diagnostic and curative*
Akathisia	Motor restlessness; *not* anxiety or "agitation"	5–60 days	Unknown	Reduce dose or change drug; antiparkinsonian agents,[†] benzodiazepines or propranolol[‡] may help
Parkinsonism	Bradykinesia, rigidity, variable tremor, mask facies, shuffling gait	5–30 days; can recur even after a single dose	Antagonism of dopamine	Antiparkinsonian agents helpful[†]
Neuroleptic malignant syndrome	Catatonia, stupor, fever, unstable blood pressure, myoglobinemia; can be fatal	Weeks; can persist for days after stopping neuroleptic	Antagonism of dopamine may contribute	Stop neuroleptic immediately; dantrolene or bromocriptine[§] may help; antiparkinsonian agents not effective
Perioral tremor ("rabbit syndrome")	Perioral tremor (may be a late variant of parkinsonism)	After months or years of treatment	Unknown	Antiparkinsonian agents often help[†]
Tardive dyskinesia	Oral-facial dyskinesia; widespread choreoathetosis or dystonia	After months or years of treatment (worse on withdrawal)	Excess function of dopamine hypothesized	Prevention crucial; treatment unsatisfactory

*Many drugs have been claimed to be helpful for acute dystonia. Among the most commonly employed treatments are diphenhydramine hydrochloride, 25 or 50 mg intramuscularly or benztropine mesylate, 1 or 2 mg intramuscularly or slowly intravenously, followed by oral medication with the same agent for a period of days to perhaps several weeks thereafter.
[†]For details regarding the use of oral antiparkinsonian agents, *see* the text and Chapter 20: Treatment of Central Nervous System Degenerative Disorders.
[‡]Propranolol often is effective in relatively low doses (20–80 mg/day). Selective β_1 adrenergic receptor antagonists are less effective.
[§]Despite the response to dantrolene, there is no evidence of an abnormality of Ca^{2+} transport in skeletal muscle; with lingering neuroleptic effects, bromocriptine may be tolerated in large doses (10–40 mg/day).

antipsychotics and with risperidone. Even in cases of acute overdose with suicidal intent, the antipsychotic drugs usually do not cause life-threatening coma or suppress vital functions.

Chemoreceptor Trigger Zone

Most antipsychotics protect against the nausea- and emesis-inducing effects of apomorphine and certain ergot alkaloids, all of which can interact with central dopaminergic receptors in the chemoreceptor trigger zone (CTZ) of the medulla. The antiemetic effect of most neuroleptics occurs with low doses and can contribute to toxicity of acute overdoses of mixed agents by preventing their elimination by vomiting. Drugs or other stimuli that cause emesis by an action on the nodose ganglion or locally on the GI tract are not antagonized by antipsychotic drugs, but potent piperazines and butyrophenones are sometimes effective against nausea caused by vestibular stimulation.

Autonomic Nervous System

Antipsychotic agents have variable antagonistic interactions at peripheral α, $5\text{-}HT_{2A/2C}$, and H_1 receptors; thus, the drugs' effects on the autonomic nervous system are complex and unpredictable. Chlorpromazine, clozapine, and thioridazine have particularly significant α-adrenergic antagonistic activity. The potent piperazine tricyclic neuroleptics (e.g., fluphenazine, trifluoperazine, haloperidol, and risperidone) have antipsychotic effects even when used in low doses and show little antiadrenergic activity.

The muscarinic-cholinergic blocking effects of most antipsychotic drugs are relatively weak, but the blurred vision commonly associated with chlorpromazine may be due to an anticholinergic action on the ciliary muscle. Chlorpromazine regularly produces miosis, which can be due to α adrenergic blockade. Other phenothiazines can cause mydriasis (especially clozapine and thioridazine, which are potent muscarinic antagonists). Chlorpromazine can cause constipation and decreased gastric acid secretion and motility; clozapine can decrease the efficiency of clearing saliva and severely impair intestinal motility. Decreased sweating and salivation also result from the anticholinergic effects. Acute urinary retention is uncommon but can occur in males with prostatism. Anticholinergic effects are least frequently caused by the potent antipsychotics such as haloperidol and risperidone. However, olanzapine has substantial anticholinergic activity that may tend to offset its considerable D_2 anti-DA effects on the extrapyramidal system. Clozapine is sufficiently anticholinergic to induce an atropine-like poisoning on overdose. The phenothiazines inhibit ejaculation without interfering with erection. Thioridazine produces this effect with some regularity, sometimes limiting its acceptance by men.

Kidney and Electrolyte Balance

Chlorpromazine may have weak diuretic effects because of a depressant action on the secretion of vasopressin (antidiuretic hormone, ADH), inhibition of reabsorption of water and electrolytes by a direct action on the renal tubule, or both. The syndrome of idiopathic polydipsia and hyponatremia sometimes associated with psychotic illness has responded to clozapine, presumably via CNS actions.

Cardiovascular System

Chlorpromazine has complex actions on the cardiovascular system, directly affecting the heart and blood vessels and indirectly acting through CNS and autonomic reflexes. Chlorpromazine and less potent antipsychotic agents, as well as reserpine, risperidone, and olanzapine, can cause orthostatic hypotension, usually with rapid development of tolerance.

Thioridazine, mesoridazine, and other phenothiazines with low potency, as well as ziprasidone, droperidol, and perhaps high doses of haloperidol, have a potentially clinically significant direct negative inotropic action and a quinidine-like effect on the heart (prolongation of the QTc and PR intervals, blunting of T waves, and depression of the ST segment). Thioridazine in particular causes a high incidence of QTc- and T-wave changes and may rarely produce ventricular arrhythmias and sudden death. These effects are less common with potent antipsychotic agents. Ziprasidone also has the propensity to prolong QTc; thus, extra caution is needed when this agent, thioridazine, or mesoridazine are given in combination with other agents that depress cardiac conduction (see Chapter 34).

MISCELLANEOUS PHARMACOLOGICAL EFFECTS

Interactions of antipsychotic drugs with central neurotransmitters other than DA may contribute to their antipsychotic effects or other actions. For example, many antipsychotics enhance the turnover of acetylcholine, especially in the basal ganglia, perhaps secondary to the blockade of inhibitory dopaminergic heteroceptors on cholinergic neurons. In addition, there is an inverse relationship between antimuscarinic potency of antipsychotic drugs in the brain and the likelihood of extrapyramidal effects. Chlorpromazine and low-potency antipsychotic agents, including cloza-pine and quetiapine, have antagonistic actions at histamine receptors that probably contribute to their sedative effects.

ABSORPTION, DISTRIBUTION, FATE, AND EXCRETION Some antipsychotic drugs have erratic and unpredictable patterns of absorption after oral administration. Parenteral (intramuscular) administration increases the bioavailability of active drug 4–10-fold. Most antipsychotic drugs are highly lipophilic, highly membrane- or protein-bound, and accumulate in the brain, lung, and other tissues with a rich blood supply. They also enter the fetal circulation and breast milk. It is virtually impossible to remove these agents by dialysis.

Elimination half-lives with respect to total concentrations in plasma are typically 20–40 hours. However, complex patterns of delayed elimination may occur with some drugs, particularly the butyrophenones and their congeners. Biological effects of single doses of most antipsychotics usu-ally persist for at least 24 hours, permitting once-daily dosing once the patient has adjusted to ini-tial side effects. Elimination from the plasma may be more rapid than from sites of high lipid content and binding, notably in the CNS; metabolites of some agents have been detected in the urine several months after drug administration was discontinued. Slow removal of drug may con-tribute to the typically delayed exacerbation of psychosis after stopping drug treatment. Repository ("depot") preparations of esters of neuroleptic drugs, as well as risperidone incorporated into car-bohydrate microspheres, are absorbed and eliminated much more slowly than are oral prepara-tions. For example, half of an oral dose of fluphenazine hydrochloride is eliminated in ~20 hours, while the decanoate ester injected intramuscularly has a $t_{1/2}$ of 7–10 days. Clearance of fluphena-zine decanoate and normalization of hyperprolactinemia following repeated dosing can require 6–8 months. Effects of long-acting risperidone (RISPERIDAL CONSTA) are delayed for 2–3 weeks because of slow biodegradation of the microspheres and persist for at least 2 weeks after the injec-tions are discontinued.

The antipsychotic drugs are metabolized largely by hepatic CYPs and by glucuronidation, sul-fation, and other conjugation processes. Hydrophilic metabolites of these drugs are excreted in the urine and to some extent in the bile. Most oxidized metabolites of antipsychotic drugs are biologi-cally inactive. Less potent antipsychotic drugs like chlorpromazine may weakly induce their own hepatic metabolism, since their concentrations in blood are lower after several weeks of treatment at the same dosage. Alterations of GI motility also may contribute. The fetus, the infant, and the elderly have diminished capacity to metabolize and eliminate antipsychotic agents; young children tend to metabolize these drugs more rapidly than do adults.

With several antipsychotic agents, bioavailability and drug acceptance by hospitalized patients is somewhat increased with liquid concentrates and rapidly disintegrating tablets that yield peak serum concentrations of chlorpromazine and other phenothiazines within 2–4 hours. Intramuscu-lar administration avoids much of the first-pass enteric metabolism and provides measurable con-centrations in plasma within 15–30 minutes. Bioavailability of chlorpromazine may be increased up to tenfold with injections, but the clinical dose usually is decreased by only three- to fourfold. GI absorption of chlorpromazine is modified unpredictably by food and probably is decreased by antacids. Antipsychotic agents bind significantly to membranes and to plasma proteins. Elimina-tion kinetics can be multiphasic and variable with dose, and termination of action may rely on clearance of both active metabolites and the parent compound. Approximate elimination half-lives of clinically employed antipsychotic agents are provided in Table 18–2; see also Appendix II, Pharmacokinetic Data in the 11th edition of the parent text.

TOLERANCE AND PHYSICAL DEPENDENCE

As defined in Chapter 23, the antipsychotic drugs are not addicting, but some degree of physical dependence may occur, with malaise and difficulty in sleeping developing several days after abrupt drug discontinuation after prolonged use.

Loss of efficacy with prolonged treatment is not known to occur with antipsychotic agents, but some tolerance to sedative effects of antipsychotics usually develops over days or weeks. One correlate of tolerance in forebrain dopaminergic systems is the development of supersen-sitivity, probably mediated by upregulation and sensitization of DA D_2 receptors. These changes may underlie the clinical phenomenon of withdrawal-emergent dyskinesias (e.g., choreoathetosis on abrupt discontinuation of antipsychotic agents, especially following pro-longed use of high doses of potent agents) and may contribute to the pathophysiology of tardive dyskinesias.

Table 18–2

Elimination Half-Lives of Antipsychotic Drugs

Drug	$t_{1/2}$ (Hours)*
Aripiprazole	75
Chlorpromazine	24 (8–35)
Clozapine	12 (4–66)
Fluphenazine	18 (14–24)
Haloperidol	24 (12–36)[†]
Loxapine	8 (3–12)
Mesoridazine	30 (24–48)
Molindone	12 (6–24)
Olanzapine	30 (20–54)
Perphenazine	12 (8–21)
Pimozide	55 (29–111)[†]
Quetiapine	6
Risperidone	20–24[‡]
Thioridazine	24 (6–40)
Thiothixene	34
Trifluoperazine	18 (14–24)[§]
Ziprasidone	7.5

*Average and range.
[†]May have multiphasic elimination with much longer terminal $t_{1/2}$.
[‡]Half-life of the main active metabolite (parent drug $t_{1/2}$ ca. 3–4 hours).
[§]Estimated, assuming similarity to fluphenazine.

Although cross-tolerance may occur among antipsychotic drugs, clinical problems occur in making rapid changes from high doses of one type of agent to another. Sedation, hypotension, and other autonomic effects or acute extrapyramidal reactions can result. Clinical worsening of psychotic symptoms is particularly likely after rapid discontinuation of clozapine and is difficult to control with alternative antipsychotics.

PREPARATIONS AND DOSAGE

Table 18–3 summarizes the large number of drugs currently marketed in the U.S. for the treatment of psychotic disorders or mania.

Prochlorperazine (COMPAZINE) has questionable utility as an antipsychotic agent and frequently produces acute extrapyramidal reactions. It is rarely employed in psychiatry, although it is used as an antiemetic. Thiethylperazine (TORECAN), marketed only as an antiemetic, is a potent dopaminergic antagonist with many neuroleptic-like properties. At high doses, it may be an efficacious antipsychotic agent. In the U.S., only the decanoates of fluphenazine and haloperidol and an injected carbohydrate microsphere preparation of risperidone are commonly employed as long-acting repository preparations.

TOXIC REACTIONS AND ADVERSE EFFECTS Antipsychotic drugs have a high therapeutic index and are generally safe agents. Most phenothiazines, haloperidol, clozapine, and quetiapine can be used over a wide range of dosages (Table 18–3). Although occasional deaths from overdoses have been reported, fatalities are rare in patients given medical care unless the overdose is complicated by concurrent ingestion of alcohol or other drugs. Adverse effects often are extensions of the many pharmacological actions of these drugs. The most important are those on the cardiovascular, central and autonomic nervous systems, and endocrine system. Other dangerous effects are seizures, agranulocytosis, cardiac toxicity, and pigmentary degeneration of the retina, all of which are rare (*see* below). Therapeutic doses of phenothiazines may cause faintness, palpitations, and anticholinergic effects including nasal stuffiness, dry mouth, blurred vision, constipation, worsening of glaucoma, and urinary retention in males with prostatism.

Table 18-3

Selected Antipsychotic Drugs: Classes, Doses and Dosage Forms, and Side Effects*

	Dose and Dosage Forms			Side Effects		
	Adult Antipsychotic Oral Dose Range (Daily)		Single IM Dose[‡]			
Nonproprietary Name (TRADE NAME)	Usual, mg	Extreme,[§] mg	Usual, mg	Sedative	Extra-pyramidal	Hypotensive
Phenothiazines						
Chloropromazine hydrochloride (THORAZINE)	200–800 O, SR, L, I, S	30–2000	25–50	+++	++	IM+++ Oral++
Mesoridazine besylate (SERENTIL)	75–300 O, L, I	30–400	25	+++	+	++
Thioridazine hydrochloride (MELLARIL)	150–600 O, L	20–800		+++	+	+++
Fluphenazine hydrochloride	2–20 O, L, I	0.5–30	1.25–2.5 (decanoate or enanthate: 12.5–50 every 1–4 weeks)	+	+++	+
Fluphenazine enanthate						
Fluphenazine decanoate (PERMITIL and PROLIXIN) (PROLIXIN D)						
Perphenazine (TRILAFON)	8–32 O, L, I	4–64	5–10	++	++	+
Trifluoperazine hydrochloride (STELAZINE)	5–20 O, L, I	2–30	1–2	+	+++	+
Thioxanthenes						
Chlorprothixene (TARACTAN)	50–400 O, L, I	30–600	25–50	+++	++	++
Thiothixene hydrochloride (NAVANE)	5–30 O, L, I	2–30	2–4	+ to ++	+++	++
Other Heterocyclic Compounds						
Aripiprazole (ABILIFY)	10–15 O	5–30		0/+	0	0/+
Clozapine (CLOZARIL)	150–450 O	12.5–900		+++	0	+++

308

Other Heterocyclic Compounds (Continued)

Haloperidol; haloperidol decanoate (HALDOL)	2–20 O, L, I	1–100	2–5 (haloperidol decanoate: 25–250 every 2–4 weeks)	+	+++	+
Loxapine succinate (LOXITANE)	60–100 O, L, I	20–250	12.5–50	+	++	+
Molindone hydrochloride (MOBAN)	50–225 O, L	15–225		++	++	+
Olanzapine (ZYPREXA)	5–10 O, I	2.5–20		+	+	++
Pimozide (ORAP)	2–6 O, I	1–10		+	+++	+
Quetiapine fumarate (SEROQUEL)	300–500 O	50–750		++	0	++
Risperidone (RISPERDAL)	2–8 O, I (long-acting)	0.25–16		++	++	+++
Ziprasidone (GEODON)	80–160 O, I [hydrochloride (O), mesylate (I)]	20–160		+/++	0/+	+

For chemical structures of these agents, see Table 18–1 in the 11th edition of the parent text.

*Antipsychotic agents for use in children under age 12 years include chlorpromazine, chlorprothixene (>6 years), thioridazine, and triflupromazine (among agents of low potency); and prochlorperazine and trifluoperazine (>6 years) (among agents of high potency). Haloperidol (orally) has also been used extensively in children.

†Dosage forms are indicated as follows: I, regular or long-acting injection; L, oral liquid or oral liquid concentrate; O, oral solid; S, suppository; SR, oral, sustained-release.

‡Except for the enanthate and decanoate forms of fluphenazine and haloperidol decanoate, dosage can be given intramuscularly up to every 6 hours for agitated patients. Haloperidol lactate has been given intravenously; this is experimental.

§Extreme dosage ranges are occasionally exceeded cautiously and only when other appropriate measures have failed.

Side effects: 0, absent; +, low; ++, moderate; +++, moderately high; ++++, high

309

Adverse Cardiovascular and Cerebrovascular Effects   The most common adverse cardiovascular effect is orthostatic hypotension, which may result in syncope, falls, and injuries. Hypotension is most likely to occur with administration of the phenothiazines with aliphatic side chains or atypical antipsychotics. Potent neuroleptics generally produce less hypotension.

Some antipsychotic agents depress cardiac repolarization, as reflected in the QT interval corrected for heart rate (QTc). Prolongations above 500 msec can be dangerous clinically, particularly by increasing the risk of *torsades de pointes*, which often is a precursor of fatal cardiac arrest (*see* Chapter 34). Such cardiac depressant effects are especially prominent with thioridazine and its active metabolite, mesoridazine, as well as pimozide, high doses of haloperidol, and ziprasidone. These drugs are used cautiously, if at all, in combination with other agents with known cardiac-depressant effects, including tricyclic antidepressants (*see* Chapter 17), certain antiarrhythmic agents (*see* Chapter 34), other antipsychotics with similar actions (such as pimozide and thioridazine), or specific DA antagonists (cisapride and metoclopramide; *see* Chapter 37). Clozapine has rarely been associated with myocarditis and cardiomyopathy. Some clinical observations have suggested increased risk of stroke among elderly patients treated with risperidone and perhaps olanzapine. The clinical significance of these uncommon cardiac and cerebrovascular events remains uncertain.

Adverse Neurological Effects   Many neurological syndromes, particularly involving the extrapyramidal motor system, occur following the use of most antipsychotic drugs, especially with the high-potency D_2-receptor antagonists (tricyclic piperazines and butyrophenones). Acute adverse extrapyramidal effects are less likely with aripiprazole, clozapine, quetiapine, thioridazine, and ziprasidone, or low doses of olanzapine or risperidone.

Six distinct neurological syndromes are characteristic of older neuroleptic-antipsychotic drugs. Four of these (acute dystonia, akathisia, parkinsonism, and the rare neuroleptic malignant syndrome) usually appear soon after administration of the drug. Two (tardive dyskinesias or dystonias, and rare perioral tremor) are late-appearing syndromes that evolve during prolonged treatment. The clinical features of these syndromes and guidelines for their management are summarized in Table 18–1.

Certain therapeutic guidelines should be followed to minimize the neurological syndromes that complicate the use of antipsychotic drugs. Routine use of antiparkinson agents in an attempt to avoid early extrapyramidal reactions adds complexity, side effects, and expense to the regimen. Antiparkinson agents are best reserved for cases of overt extrapyramidal reactions that respond favorably to such intervention. The need for such agents for the treatment of acute dystonic reactions ordinarily diminishes with time, but parkinsonism and akathisia typically persist. The thoughtful and conservative use of antipsychotic drugs, particularly modern atypical agents, in patients with chronic or frequently recurrent psychotic disorders almost certainly can reduce the risk of tardive dyskinesia. Although reduction of the dose of an antipsychotic agent is the best way to minimize its adverse neurological effects, this may not be practical in a patient with uncontrollable psychotic illness. The best preventive practice is to use the minimum effective dose of an antipsychotic drug. The growing number of modern atypical antipsychotic agents with a low risk of inducing extrapyramidal side effects provides an alternative for many patients.

Weight Gain and Metabolic Effects   Weight gain and its associated long-term complications can occur with extended treatment with most antipsychotic and antimanic drugs. Weight gain is especially prominent with clozapine and olanzapine; somewhat less with quetiapine; even less with fluphenazine, haloperidol, and risperidone; and very low with aripiprazole, molindone, and ziprasidone. Adverse effects of weight gain likely include increased risk of new-onset or worsening of type 2 diabetes mellitus, hypertension, and hyperlipidemia. In some patients with morbid increases in weight, the airway may be compromised (Pickwickian syndrome), especially during sleep (including sleep apnea).

Blood Dyscrasias   Mild leukocytosis, leukopenia, and eosinophilia occasionally occur with antipsychotic treatment, particularly with clozapine and less often with phenothiazines of low potency. It is difficult to determine whether leukopenia that develops during the administration of such agents is a forewarning of impending agranulocytosis. This serious complication occurs in not more than 1 in 10,000 patients receiving chlorpromazine or other low-potency agents (other than clozapine); it usually appears within the first 8–12 weeks of treatment.

Bone marrow suppression, or less commonly agranulocytosis, has been associated with the use of clozapine. The incidence approaches 1% within several months of treatment, independent of dose, without regular monitoring of white blood cell counts. Because blood dyscrasia may develop suddenly, the appearance of fever, malaise, or apparent respiratory infection in a patient being treated with an antipsychotic drug should be followed immediately by a complete blood count. Risk of agranulocytosis is greatly reduced, though not eliminated, by frequent white blood cell counts in patients being treated with clozapine, as is required in the U.S. (weekly for 6 months and biweekly thereafter). The safety of resuming even low doses of clozapine or other antipsychotics following recovery from agranulocytosis should not be assumed.

Skin Reactions

Dermatological reactions to the phenothiazines, including urticaria or dermatitis, occur in ~5% of patients receiving chlorpromazine. Contact dermatitis may occur in personnel who handle chlorpromazine, and there may be a degree of cross-sensitivity to other phenothiazines. Sunburn and photosensitivity resembling severe sunburn occur and require use of an effective sunscreen preparation. Epithelial keratopathy often is observed in patients on long-term therapy with chlorpromazine, and opacities in the cornea and in the lens of the eye have been noted. Pigmentary retinopathy has been reported, particularly following doses of thioridazine in excess of 1000 mg/day. A maximum daily dose of 800 mg currently is recommended. Dermatological reactions to modern atypical antipsychotic agents are uncommon.

GI and Hepatic Effects

A mild jaundice, typically occurring early in therapy, may be seen in some patients receiving chlorpromazine. Pruritus is rare. The reaction probably is a manifestation of hypersensitivity, because eosinophilia and eosinophilic infiltration of the liver occur. For uninterrupted drug therapy in a patient with neuroleptic-induced jaundice, it probably is safest to use low doses of a potent, dissimilar agent. Hepatic dysfunction with other antipsychotic agents is uncommon. Clozapine can cause potentially severe ileus and sialorrhea.

INTERACTIONS WITH OTHER DRUGS The phenothiazines and thioxanthenes, especially those of lower potency, affect the actions of a number of other drugs. Antipsychotic drugs can strongly potentiate the effect of medically prescribed sedatives and analgesics, alcohol, nonprescription sedatives and hypnotics, antihistamines, and cold remedies. Chlorpromazine increases the miotic and sedative effects of morphine and may increase its analgesic actions. The drug markedly increases the respiratory depression produced by meperidine and can be expected to have similar effects when administered concurrently with other opioids. Obviously, neuroleptic drugs inhibit the actions of dopaminergic agonists and levodopa and worsen the neurological symptoms of Parkinson's disease.

The antimuscarinic action of clozapine and thioridazine can cause tachycardia and enhance the peripheral and central effects (confusion, delirium) of other anticholinergic agents, such as the tricyclic antidepressants and antiparkinson agents.

Sedatives or anticonvulsants (e.g., carbamazepine, oxcarbazepine, phenobarbital, and phenytoin, but not valproate) that induce CYPs (see Chapter 3) can enhance the metabolism of antipsychotic and many other agents (including anticoagulants and oral contraceptives), sometimes with significant clinical consequences. Conversely, selective serotonin (5-HT) reuptake inhibitors including fluvoxamine, fluoxetine, paroxetine, venlafaxine, sertraline, and nefazodone (see Chapter 17) compete for these enzymes and can elevate circulating levels of neuroleptics.

DRUG TREATMENT OF PSYCHOSES

SHORT-TERM TREATMENT The antipsychotic drugs are effective in acute psychoses of unknown etiology, including mania, acute idiopathic psychoses, and acute exacerbations of schizophrenia. The best studied indications are for the acute and chronic phases of schizophrenia and in acute mania. Antipsychotic drugs also are used empirically in many other neuromedical and idiopathic disorders with prominent psychotic symptoms or severe agitation.

Neuroleptic agents are effective antipsychotics and are superior to sedatives (*e.g.*, barbiturates and benzodiazepines), or alternatives (*e.g.*, ECT, other medical or psychological therapies). The "target" symptoms for which antipsychotic agents are especially effective include agitation, combativeness, hostility, hallucinations, acute delusions, insomnia, anorexia, poor self-care, negativism, and sometimes withdrawal and seclusiveness. More variable or delayed are improvements in motivation and cognition, including insight, judgment, memory, orientation, and functional recovery. The most favorable prognosis is for patients with acute illnesses of brief duration who had functioned relatively well prior to the illness.

No one drug or combination of drugs selectively affects a particular symptom complex in groups of psychotic patients. Drug responses in individual patients can be determined only by trial and error. Generally, "positive" (irrational thinking, delusions, agitated turmoil, hallucinations) and "negative" symptoms tend to respond (or not) together with overall clinical improvement, a tendency well documented with typical neuroleptics and modern atypical antipsychotic agents. Aripiprazole, clozapine, quetiapine, and ziprasidone induce less bradykinesia and other parkinsonian effects than do typical neuroleptics, and aripiprazole and ziprasidone are minimally sedating. Minimizing such side effects is sometimes interpreted clinically as specific improvement in impoverished affective responsiveness and energy level.

The short-term clinical superiority of modern antipsychotic agents over older neuroleptics has been particularly hard to prove. Nevertheless, in the U.S., the modern atypical agents dominate clinical practice, owing mainly to their perceived superior tolerability and acceptability.

It is important to simplify the treatment regimen and to ensure that the patient is receiving the drug. In cases of suspected severe and dangerous noncompliance or with failure of oral treatment, the patient can be treated with injections of fluphenazine decanoate, haloperidol decanoate, or other long-acting preparations, including risperidone microspheres.

Because the choice of an antipsychotic drug cannot be made reliably on the basis of anticipated therapeutic effect, drug selection often depends on likely tolerability of specific side effects, the need for sedation, or on a previous favorable response. If the patient has a history of cardiovascular disease or stroke and the threat from hypotension is serious, a modern atypical agent or a potent older neuroleptic should be used in the smallest dose that is effective (Table 18–1). For minimizing the risk of acute extrapyramidal symptoms, aripiprazole, clozapine, quetiapine, ziprasidone, or a low dose of olanzapine or risperidone should be considered. If the patient would be seriously discomfited by interference with ejaculation or if there are serious risks of cardiovascular or other autonomic toxicity, low doses of a potent neuroleptic might be preferred. If sedative effects are undesirable, a potent agent (aripiprazole or ziprasidone) is preferable. Small doses of antipsychotic drugs of high or moderate potency may be safest in the elderly, in whom the possible risk of stroke with risperidone and olanzapine must be considered. If hepatic function is compromised or there is a potential threat of jaundice, low doses of a high-potency agent may be used. The physician's experience with a particular drug may outweigh other considerations. Skill in the use of antipsychotic drugs depends on selection of an adequate but not excessive dose, knowledge of what to expect, and judgment as to when to stop therapy or change drugs.

A substantial minority of psychotic patients do poorly with any antipsychotic medicine, including clozapine. If a patient does not improve after a course of seemingly adequate treatment and fails to respond to another drug given in adequate dosage, the diagnosis should be reevaluated.

Usually 2–3 weeks or more are required to demonstrate obvious beneficial effects in schizophrenia patients; maximum benefit in chronically ill patients may require several months. In contrast, improvement of some acutely psychotic or manic patients can be seen within 48 hours. Aggressive dosing with high doses of an antipsychotic drug at the start of an acute episode of psychosis has not been found to increase either the magnitude or the rate of therapeutic responses. However, parenteral agents in moderate doses can bring about rapid sedation and may be useful in acute behavioral control. After the initial response, drugs usually are used in conjunction with psychological, supportive, and rehabilitative treatments.

There is no convincing evidence that combinations of antipsychotic drugs offer clear or consistent advantages. A combination of an antipsychotic drug and an antidepressant may be useful in some cases, especially in depressed psychotic patients or in cases of agitated major depression with psychotic features. The first combination antipsychotic/antidepressant (olanzapine/fluoxetine; SYMBYAX) was approved in the U.S. for treatment of depressive episodes associated with bipolar disorder. However, antidepressants and stimulants are unlikely to reduce apathy and withdrawal in schizophrenia, and they may induce clinical worsening in some cases. Adjunctive addition of lithium or an antimanic anticonvulsant may add benefit in some psychotic patients with prominent affective, aggressive, or resistant symptoms.

Optimal dosage of antipsychotic drugs requires individualization to determine doses that are effective, well tolerated, and accepted by the patient. Dose–response relationships for antipsychotic and adverse effects overlap, and it can be difficult to determine an end-point of a desired therapeutic response. To achieve control of symptoms in the treatment of acute psychoses, the dose of antipsychotic drug is increased as tolerated during the first few days. The dose is then adjusted during the next several weeks as the patient's condition warrants. Severe and poorly controlled agitation usually can be managed safely by use of adjunctive sedation (e.g., with a benzodiazepine such as lorazepam) and close supervision in a secure setting. One must remain alert for acute dystonic reactions, which are especially likely to appear early with aggressive use of potent neuroleptics, and for side effects such as hypotension. After an initial period of stabilization, regimens based on a single daily dose often are effective and safe. The time of administration may be varied to minimize adverse effects.

Table 18–3 gives the usual and extreme ranges of dosage for antipsychotic drugs used in the U.S. The ranges have been established for the most part in the treatment of young and middle-aged adult patients diagnosed with schizophrenia or mania. Acutely disturbed hospitalized patients often require higher doses of an antipsychotic drug than do more stable outpatients. However, the concept that a low or flexible maintenance dose often will suffice during follow-up care of a partially recovered or chronic psychotic patient is well supported by controlled trials.

LONG-TERM TREATMENT

In reviews of nearly 30 controlled prospective studies involving several thousand schizophrenic patients, the mean overall relapse rate was 58% for patients withdrawn from antipsychotic drugs and given a placebo versus only 16% of those who continued on drug therapy. Daily dosage in chronic cases often can be lowered to 50–200 mg of chlorpromazine or its equivalent without signs of relapse, but rapid dose reduction or discontinuation appears to increase risk of exacerbation or relapse. Flexible therapy in which dosage is adjusted to changing current requirements can be useful and can reduce the incidence of adverse effects.

If the modern or atypical antipsychotic agents have superiority to older neuroleptics, this advantage is most important in the long-term treatment of chronic or recurrent psychotic illnesses, where it is standard practice to continue maintenance treatment with moderate and well-tolerated doses of an antipsychotic agent indefinitely, as long as the clinical indications, benefits, and tolerability remain clear. The only agent with securely proven superiority is clozapine. Nevertheless, there is some evidence that modern atypical antipsychotics may yield superior results in long-term treatment, if only due to superior tolerability and adherence to treatment.

Maintenance with injections of the decanoate ester of fluphenazine or haloperidol every 2–4 weeks, or with long-acting risperidone microspheres every 2–3 weeks, can be very effective. However, an expectation of superiority of long-acting injected antipsychotics is not well supported by available studies, most of which involve randomization of patients who already are largely cooperative with long-term oral treatment.

Special Populations

The treatment of some symptoms and behaviors associated with delirium or dementia is another accepted use for the antipsychotic drugs. They may be administered temporarily while a specific and correctable structural, infectious, metabolic, or toxic cause is vigorously sought. They sometimes are used for prolonged periods when no correctable cause can be found. There are no drugs of choice or clearly established dosage guidelines for such indications, although older neuroleptics of high potency are preferred. Modern atypical agents have not established their place in the management of delirium or dementia. In patients with delirium without likelihood of seizures, frequent small doses (e.g., 2–6 mg) of haloperidol or another potent antipsychotic may be effective in controlling agitation. Agents with low potency should be avoided because of their greater tendency to produce sedation, hypotension, and seizures, and those with central anticholinergic effects may worsen confusion and agitation.

A challenging special population is Parkinson's disease patients with psychotic symptoms related to dopaminergic therapy (see Chapter 20). Standard neuroleptics, risperidone (even in small doses), and olanzapine often produce unacceptable worsening of bradykinesia-akinesia. Clozapine is relatively well tolerated and effective, though more complicated to use. Use of moderate doses of newer agents with very low risk of parkinsonism (aripiprazole, quetiapine, ziprasidone) requires further study.

Most antipsychotics are rapidly effective in the treatment of mania and often are used concomitantly with the institution of lithium or anticonvulsant therapy (see below).

Antipsychotic drugs may have a limited role in the treatment of severe depression, especially in patients with striking agitation or psychotic features; addition of an antipsychotic to an antidepressant in this setting may yield results approaching those obtained with ECT. Antipsychotic agents ordinarily are not used for the treatment of anxiety disorders. The use of clozapine in patients with schizophrenia and a high risk of suicidal behavior may reduce the risk of suicide attempts. Clozapine is the first drug to be FDA-approved for an antisuicide indication.

Drug treatment of childhood psychosis and other behavioral disorders of children is confused by diagnostic inconsistencies and a paucity of controlled trials. Antipsychotics can benefit children with disorders characterized by features that occur in adult psychoses, mania, autism, or Tourette's syndrome. Low doses of the more potent or modern atypical agents usually are preferred in an attempt to avoid interference with daytime activities or performance in school. Attention deficit disorder, with or without hyperactivity, responds poorly to antipsychotic agents, but often if the condition is not comorbid with bipolar disorder, responds very well to stimulants and some antidepressants. The recommended doses of antipsychotic agents for school-aged children with moderate degrees of agitation are lower than those for acutely psychotic children, who may require daily doses similar to those used in adults (Table 18–3). Doses of modern atypical antipsychotic agents for children and adolescents with psychotic or manic illness usually are started at the lower end of the range prescribed for adults.

Poor tolerance of the adverse effects of the antipsychotic drugs often limits the dose in elderly patients. One should proceed cautiously, using small, divided doses of agents with moderate or high potency, with the expectation that elderly patients will require doses that are one-half or less of those needed for young adults. The potential risk of stroke associated with risperidone and olanzapine in elderly patients should be considered.

MISCELLANEOUS MEDICAL USES FOR ANTIPSYCHOTIC DRUGS

Many antipsychotic agents can prevent vomiting due to specific etiologies when given in relatively low, nonsedative doses (see Chapter 37). Antipsychotic drugs are useful in the management of several syndromes with psychiatric features that also are characterized by movement disorders (e.g., Tourette's syndrome and Huntington's disease). Haloperidol currently is regarded as a drug of choice for these conditions, although it probably is not unique in its antidyskinetic actions. Pimozide also is used; clonidine and tricyclic antidepressants (e.g., nortriptyline) also may be effective in Tourette's syndrome. Antipsychotic drugs are not useful in the management of withdrawal from opioids, and their use in the management of withdrawal from barbiturates, other sedatives, or alcohol is contraindicated because of the high risk of seizures. These drugs can be used safely and effectively in psychoses associated with chronic alcoholism—especially the syndrome known as alcoholic hallucinosis.

II. TREATMENT OF MANIA

ANTIMANIC MOOD-STABILIZING AGENTS: LITHIUM

Evidence for the safety and the efficacy of lithium salts in the treatment of mania and the prevention of recurrent attacks of bipolar manic-depressive illness is both abundant and convincing. However, the limitations and adverse effects of lithium salts have become increasingly well appreciated, and efforts to find alternative antimanic or mood-stabilizing agents have intensified. The most successful alternatives or adjuncts to lithium to date are the anticonvulsants carbamazepine, lamotrigine, and valproic acid.

Pharmacological Properties

Lithium is the lightest of the alkali metals (group Ia); the salts of this monovalent cation share some characteristics with those of Na^+ and K^+. Traces of the ion occur normally in animal tissues, but Li^+ has no known physiological role. In the U.S., the drug forms are the salts, lithium carbonate and lithium citrate. Therapeutic concentrations of Li^+ have almost no discernible psychotropic effects in normal individuals. Li^+ is not a sedative, depressant, or euphoriant, characteristics that differentiate it from other psychotropic agents. The precise mechanism of action of Li^+ as a mood-stabilizing agent remains unknown.

CENTRAL NERVOUS SYSTEM

A selective action of Li^+ is inhibition of inositol monophosphatase, thereby interfering with the phosphatidylinositol pathway (Figure 18–1). This effect can decrease cerebral inositol concentrations, possibly interfering with neurotransmission mechanisms by affecting the phosphatidylinositol pathway and decreasing the activation of PKC, particularly the α and β isoforms. This effect also is shared by valproic acid (particularly for PKC) but not carbamazepine. A major substrate for cerebral PKC is the myristolated alanine-rich PKC-kinase substrate (MARCKS) protein, which has been implicated in synaptic and neuronal plasticity. The expression of MARCKS protein is reduced by treatment with both Li^+ and valproate but not by carbamazepine or antipsychotic, antidepressant, or sedative drugs. Both Li^+ and valproate treatment inhibit glycogen synthase kinase-3β, which is involved in neuronal and nuclear regulatory processes, including limiting expression of the regulatory protein β-catenin. Both Li^+ and valproic acid affect gene expression, increasing DNA binding of the transcription factor activator protein-1 (AP-1) and altering expression of other transcription factors. Treatment with Li^+ and valproate has been associated *with increased expression of the regulatory protein B-cell lymphocyte protein-2 (bcl-2), which is associated with protection against apoptotic neuronal degeneration.*

ABSORPTION, DISTRIBUTION, AND EXCRETION Li^+ is absorbed readily and almost completely from the GI tract. Complete absorption occurs in ~8 hours, with peak plasma concentrations occurring 2–4 hours after an oral dose. Slow-release preparations of lithium carbonate provide a slower rate of absorption and thereby minimize early peaks in Li^+ plasma concentrations, but absorption can be variable, lower GI tract symptoms may be increased, and elimination rate is not altered with such preparations. Li^+ initially is distributed in the extracellular fluid and then gradually accumulates in various tissues; it does not bind appreciably to plasma proteins. The final volume of distribution (0.7–0.9 L/kg) approaches that of total body water and is much lower than that of most other psychotropic agents, which are lipophilic and protein bound. Passage through the blood–brain barrier is slow, and when a steady state is achieved, the concentration of Li^+ in the cerebrospinal fluid and in brain tissue is ~40–50% of the concentration in plasma. Approximately 95% of a single dose of Li^+ is eliminated in the urine. From one- to two-thirds of an acute dose is excreted during a 6–12-hour initial phase of excretion, followed by slow excretion over the next 10–14 days. The elimination $t_{1/2}$ averages 20–24 hours. With repeated administration, Li^+ excretion increases during the first 5–6 days until a steady state is reached between ingestion and excretion. When Li^+ therapy is stopped, there is a rapid phase of renal excretion followed by a slow 10–14-day phase. Since 80% of the filtered Li^+ is reabsorbed by the proximal tubule, renal clearance of Li^+ is ~20% of that for creatinine, ranging between 15 and 30 mL/min. This rate is somewhat lower in elderly patients (10–15 mL/min). Loading with Na^+ slightly enhances Li^+ excretion, but Na^+ depletion promotes a clinically important degree of retention of Li^+.

A well-established regimen can be complicated by occasional periods of Na^+ loss, as may occur with intercurrent fever, diarrhea, or other medical illness, with losses or restrictions of fluids and electrolytes, or during treatment with a diuretic. Heavy sweating may be an exception due to a preferential secretion of Li^+ over Na^+ in sweat.

Most of the renal tubular reabsorption of Li^+ occurs in the proximal tubule. Nevertheless, Li^+ retention can be increased by any diuretic that leads to depletion of Na^+, particularly the thiazides (see Chapter 28). Renal excretion can be increased by administration of osmotic diuretics, acetazolamide or aminophylline, and triamterene. Spironolactone does not increase the excretion of Li^+. Some nonsteroidal anti-inflammatory agents can facilitate renal proximal tubular resorption of Li^+ and thereby increase concentrations in plasma to toxic levels. This interaction appears to be particularly prominent with indomethacin, but also may occur with ibuprofen, naproxen, and COX-2 inhibitors, and possibly less so with sulindac and aspirin. A potential drug interaction can occur with angiotensin-converting enzyme inhibitors, causing lithium retention (see Chapter 29).

Less than 1% of ingested Li^+ leaves the human body in the feces, and 4–5% is secreted in sweat. Li^+ is secreted in saliva in concentrations about twice those in plasma, while its concentration in tears is about equal to that in plasma. Since the ion also is secreted in human milk, women receiving Li^+ should not breast-feed infants.

Dose; Serum-Level Monitoring   The recommended therapeutic concentration usually is attained by doses of 900–1500 mg of lithium carbonate per day in outpatients and 1200–2400 mg/day in hospitalized manic patients. The optimal dose tends to be larger in younger and heavier individuals. Because of its low therapeutic index, periodic determination of serum concentrations of Li^+ is crucial. Li^+ cannot be used safely in patients who cannot be tested regularly. Concentrations considered to be effective and acceptably safe are between 0.6 and 1.25 mEq/L. The range of 0.9–1.1 mEq/L is favored for treatment of acutely manic or hypomanic patients. Somewhat lower values (0.6–0.75 mEq/L) are considered adequate and are safer for long-term use for prevention of recurrent manic-depressive illness. Some patients may not relapse at concentrations as low as 0.5–0.6 mEq/L, and lower levels usually are better tolerated.

Serum concentrations of Li^+ have been found to follow a clear dose-effect relationship between 0.4 and 0.9 mEq/L, with a corresponding dose-dependent rise in polyuria and tremor as indices of adverse effects, and little gain in benefit at levels above 0.75 mEq/L. This pattern indicates the need for individualization of serum levels to obtain a favorable risk-benefit relationship. The concentration of Li^+ in blood usually is measured at a trough of the daily oscillations that result from repetitive administration (*i.e.*, from samples obtained 10–12 hours after the last oral dose of the day). Peaks can be two or three times higher at a steady state. When the peaks are reached, intoxication may result, even when concentrations in morning samples of plasma at the daily nadir are in the acceptable range of 0.6–1 mEq/L. Because of the low margin of safety of Li^+ and because of its short $t_{1/2}$ during initial distribution, divided daily doses are usually indicated even with slow-release formulations.

TOXIC REACTIONS AND SIDE EFFECTS Toxicity is related to the serum concentration of Li⁺ and its rate of rise following administration. Acute intoxication is characterized by vomiting, profuse diarrhea, coarse tremor, ataxia, coma, and convulsions. Symptoms of milder toxicity are most likely to occur at the absorptive peak of Li⁺ and include nausea, vomiting, abdominal pain, diarrhea, sedation, and fine tremor. The more serious effects involve the nervous system and include mental confusion, hyperreflexia, gross tremor, dysarthria, seizures, and cranial nerve and focal neurological signs, progressing to coma and death. Sometimes both cognitive and motor neurological damage may be irreversible. Other toxic effects are cardiac arrhythmias, hypotension, and albuminuria. Adverse effects common even in therapeutic dose ranges include nausea, diarrhea, daytime drowsiness, polyuria, polydipsia, weight gain, fine hand tremor, and dermatological reactions, including acne.

A small number of patients treated with Li⁺ develop diffuse thyroid enlargement; patients usually remain euthyroid, and overt hypothyroidism is rare. In patients who do develop goiter, discontinuation of Li⁺ or treatment with thyroid hormone results in shrinkage of the gland.

The kidneys' ability to concentrate urine decreases during Li⁺ therapy. Polydipsia and polyuria occur in patients treated with Li⁺, occasionally to a disturbing degree. Acquired nephrogenic diabetes insipidus can occur in patients maintained at therapeutic plasma concentrations (see Chapter 29). Typically, mild polyuria appears early in treatment and then disappears. Late-developing polyuria is an indication to evaluate renal function, lower the dose of Li⁺, or consider adding a potassium-sparing agent such as amiloride to counteract the polyuria. Polyuria disappears with cessation of Li⁺ therapy. Since progressive, clinically significant impairment of renal function is rare, many experts consider these to be incidental findings. Nevertheless, plasma creatinine and urine volume should be monitored during long-term use of Li⁺.

Li⁺ routinely causes EEG changes characterized by diffuse slowing, widened frequency spectrum, and potentiation with disorganization of background rhythm. Seizures have been reported in nonepileptic patients with therapeutic plasma concentrations of Li⁺. Myasthenia gravis may worsen during treatment with Li⁺. A benign, sustained increase in circulating polymorphonuclear leukocytes occurs during the chronic use of Li⁺, which reverses within a week after termination of treatment. Allergic reactions such as dermatitis and vasculitis can occur with Li⁺ administration. Worsening of acne vulgaris is a common problem, and some patients may experience mild alopecia.

In pregnancy, Li⁺ may exacerbate maternal polyuria. Concomitant use of lithium with natriuretics and a low-Na⁺ diet during pregnancy can contribute to maternal and neonatal Li⁺ intoxication. During postpartum diuresis, one can anticipate potentially toxic retention of Li⁺ by the mother. Lithium freely crosses the placenta, and fetal or neonatal lithium toxicity may develop when maternal blood levels are within the therapeutic range. Lithium also is secreted in breast milk of nursing mothers. The use of Li⁺ in pregnancy has been associated with neonatal goiter, CNS depression, hypotonia ("floppy baby" syndrome), and cardiac murmur. All of these conditions reverse with time, and no long-term neurobehavioral sequelae have been observed.

The use of Li⁺ in early pregnancy may be associated with an increase in the incidence of cardiovascular anomalies of the newborn, especially Ebstein's malformation. The antimanic anticonvulsants valproic acid and probably carbamazepine have an associated risk of irreversible spina bifida that may exceed 1/100, and so do not represent a rational alternative for pregnant women. In balancing the risk versus benefit of using Li⁺ in pregnancy, it is important to evaluate the risk of untreated manic-depressive disorder and to consider conservative measures, such as deferring intervention until symptoms arise or using a safer treatment, such as a neuroleptic or ECT.

TREATMENT OF LITHIUM INTOXICATION There is no specific antidote for Li⁺ intoxication, and treatment is supportive. Vomiting induced by rapidly rising plasma Li⁺ may tend to limit absorption, but fatalities have occurred. Care must be taken to assure that the patient is not Na⁺- and water-depleted. Dialysis is the most effective means of removing the ion from the body and is necessary in severe poisonings, *i.e.*, in patients exhibiting symptoms of toxicity or patients with serum Li⁺ concentrations >4 mEq/L in acute overdoses or >1.5 mEq/L in chronic overdoses.

INTERACTIONS WITH OTHER DRUGS

Interactions between Li⁺ and diuretics (especially spironolactone and amiloride) and nonsteroidal anti-inflammatory agents have been discussed above (see Absorption, Distribution, and Excretion and Toxic Reactions and Side Effects). Relative to thiazides and other diuretics that deplete Na⁺, retention of Li⁺ may be limited during administration of the weakly natriuretic agent amiloride as well as the loop diuretic furosemide. Amiloride and other diuretic agents (sometimes with reduced doses of Li⁺) have been used safely to reverse the syndrome of diabetes insipidus occasionally associated with Li⁺ therapy (see Chapter 29).

Li⁺ often is used in conjunction with antipsychotic, sedative, antidepressant, and anticonvulsant drugs. Case reports suggesting a risk of increased CNS toxicity when Li⁺ is combined with haloperidol are at variance with many years of experience with this combination. Antipsychotic drugs may prevent nausea, which can be an early sign of Li⁺ toxicity. There is no absolute contraindication to the concurrent use of Li⁺ and psychotropic drugs. Finally, anticholinergic and other agents that alter GI motility also may alter Li⁺ concentrations in blood over time.

Therapeutic Uses

DRUG TREATMENT OF BIPOLAR DISORDER   Treatment with Li⁺ ideally is conducted in cooperative patients with normal Na⁺ intake and with normal cardiac and renal function. Occasionally, patients with severe systemic illnesses are treated with Li⁺, provided that the indications are compelling. Treatment of acute mania and the prevention of recurrences of bipolar illness in otherwise healthy adults or adolescents currently are the only uses approved by the FDA, even though the primary indication for Li⁺ treatment is for long-term prevention of recurrences of major affective illness, particularly both mania and depression in bipolar I or II disorders.

Li⁺ sometimes is used as an alternative or adjunct to antidepressants in severe, especially melancholic, recurrent depression, as a supplement to antidepressant treatment in acute major depression, including in patients who present clinically with only mild mood elevations or hypomania (bipolar II disorder), or as an adjunct when later response to an antidepressant alone is unsatisfactory. In major affective disorders, Li⁺ has stronger evidence of reduction of suicide risk than any other treatment. Clinical experience also suggests the utility of Li⁺ in the management of childhood disorders that are marked by adult-like manic depression or by severe changes in mood and behavior, which are probable precursors to bipolar disorder in adults. Evidence of efficacy of Li⁺ in many additional episodic disorders (e.g., premenstrual dysphoria, episodic alcohol abuse, and episodic violence) is unconvincing.

FORMULATIONS   Most preparations used in the U.S. are tablets or capsules of lithium carbonate. Slow-release preparations of lithium carbonate also are available, as is a liquid preparation of lithium citrate (with 8 mEq of Li⁺, equivalent to 300 mg of carbonate salt, per 5 mL or 1 teaspoonful of citrate liquid). The carbonate salt is favored for tablets and capsules because it is relatively less hygroscopic and less irritating to the gut than other salts, especially the chloride.

DRUG TREATMENT OF MANIA AND PROPHYLACTIC TREATMENT OF BIPOLAR DISORDER   Lithium is effective in acute mania, but is rarely employed as a sole treatment due to its slow onset of action, need for monitoring blood Li⁺ concentrations, and the difficulties associated with adherence to the therapeutic regimen by highly agitated and uncooperative manic patients. Rather, an antipsychotic or potent sedative benzodiazepine (such as *lorazepam* or *clonazepam*) commonly is used to attain a degree of control of acute agitation. Alternatively, the anticonvulsant sodium valproate can provide rapid antimanic effects, particularly when doses as high as 30 mg/kg and later 20 mg/kg daily are used to rapidly obtain serum concentrations of 90–120 μg/mL. Once patients are stabilized and cooperative, Li⁺ can be introduced for longer-term mood stabilization, or the anticonvulsant may be continued alone (*see* below).

Li⁺ or an alternative antimanic agent usually is continued for at least several months after full recovery from a manic episode, due to a high risk of relapse or of cycling into depression within 12 months. The clinical decision to recommend more prolonged maintenance treatment is based on balancing the frequency and severity of past episodes of manic-depressive illness, the age and estimated reliability of the patient, and the risk of adverse effects. Regardless of the number of previous episodes of mania or depression, or delay in initiating maintenance treatment, Li⁺ remains the best established, long-term treatment to prevent recurrences of mania (and bipolar depression). There is compelling evidence of substantial lowering of risk of suicide and suicide attempts during treatment with lithium but not with either carbamazepine or *divalproex*.

Antimanic anticonvulsants, particularly sodium valproate and carbamazepine, also have been employed prophylactically in bipolar disorder. However, research supporting their long-term use remains limited, and there is growing evidence for the inferiority of carbamazepine compared to lithium (carbamazepine is not FDA-approved for bipolar disorder). Divalproex, the sodium salt of valproic acid, is FDA-approved for mania and is extensively used off-label for long-term prophylactic treatment of bipolar disorder patients. In addition, lamotrigine is the first agent given FDA approval for long-term prophylactic treatment in bipolar disorder without an indication for acute mania; it is particularly effective against bipolar depression with minimal risk of inducing mania. Other anticonvulsants may have utility in bipolar disorder (*topiramate, zonisamide*, and the carbamazepine congener *oxcarbazepine*). Relevant pharmacology and dosing guidelines for anticonvulsants are in Chapter 19.

Antipsychotic drugs commonly have been used empirically to manage manic and psychotic illness in bipolar disorder patients. Indeed, standard neuroleptics are a mainstay of the treatment of acute mania (only chlorpromazine is FDA-approved for this indication, although haloperidol has also been widely used) and for manic episodes that break through prophylactic treatment with Li^+ or an anticonvulsant. However, the older antipsychotics are not used routinely for long-term prophylactic treatment in bipolar disorder because their effectiveness is untested, some may worsen depression, and the risk of tardive dyskinesia in these syndromes may be higher than in schizophrenia.

Several modern, better-tolerated antipsychotic agents (olanzapine, quetiapine, and risperidone) have recently received FDA approval for use in acute mania. There is also evidence of antimanic efficacy for aripiprazole and ziprasidone. Olanzapine is FDA-approved for its long-term effectiveness in bipolar disorder I. Other atypical antipsychotic drugs are under investigation for long-term prophylactic treatment of bipolar disorder.

Discontinuation of maintenance treatment with Li^+ carries a high risk of early recurrence and of suicidal behavior over a period of several months, even if the treatment had been successful for several years. Recurrence is much more rapid than is predicted by the natural history of untreated bipolar disorder, in which cycle lengths average ~1 year. When medically feasible, this risk probably can be moderated by slowing the gradual removal of Li^+. Significant risk also is suspected after rapid discontinuation or even sharp dosage reduction during maintenance treatment with other agents, including antipsychotic, antidepressant, and antianxiety drugs.

Novel Treatments for Bipolar Disorder

For bipolar disorder, a critical challenge is to develop safe and effective antidepressants that do not induce mania and mood-stabilizing agents that consistently outperform lithium in broad effectiveness, with improved safety. The clinical successes of valproate and carbamazepine as antimanic agents, and of lamotrigine as a mood-stabilizing agent, have encouraged exploration of other anticonvulsants (*see* Chapter 19); several anticonvulsants are currently being tested in clinical trials. Aside from extensions of the known principles of applying anticonvulsants and antipsychotics for the treatment of bipolar disorder, some highly innovative concepts have emerged. Given the overlapping actions of lithium and valproate, it may be possible to develop novel antimanic agents that act directly on effector mechanisms that mediate the actions of adrenergic and other neurotransmitter receptors.

For a complete Bibliographical listing see Goodman & Gilman's *The Pharmacological Basis of Therapeutics*, 11th ed., or Goodman & Gilman Online at www.accessmedicine.com.

19

PHARMACOTHERAPY OF THE EPILEPSIES

A *seizure* is a transient alteration of behavior due to the disordered, synchronous, and rhythmic firing of populations of brain neurons. *Epilepsy* refers to a disorder of brain function characterized by the periodic and unpredictable occurrence of seizures. Epileptic seizures have been classified into *partial* seizures, which begin focally in a cortical site, and *generalized* seizures, which involve both hemispheres widely from the outset. The behavioral manifestations of a seizure are determined by the functions normally served by the cortical site at which the seizure arises. For example, a seizure involving motor cortex is associated with clonic jerking of the body part controlled by this region of cortex. A *simple* partial seizure is associated with preservation of consciousness. A *complex* partial seizure is associated with impairment of consciousness. The majority of complex partial seizures originate from the temporal lobe. Examples of generalized seizures include absence, myoclonic, and tonic-clonic.

Classification of epileptic syndromes guides clinical assessment and management, and in some cases, selection of antiseizure drugs (Table 19–1). More than 40 distinct epileptic syndromes have been categorized into partial versus generalized epilepsies. The partial epilepsies may consist of any of the partial seizure types and account for ~60% of all epilepsies; the etiology commonly consists of a lesion in some part of the cortex (e.g., tumor, developmental malformation, damage due to trauma or stroke), but may also be genetic. The generalized epilepsies account for ~40% of all epilepsies and usually are genetic. The most common generalized epilepsy is juvenile myoclonic epilepsy, accounting for ~10% of all epileptic syndromes. This disorder presents in the early teens and is characterized by myoclonic, tonic-clonic, and often absence seizures. Like most generalized-onset epilepsies, juvenile myoclonic epilepsy is probably due to inheritance of multiple susceptibility genes.

NATURE AND MECHANISMS OF SEIZURES AND ANTISEIZURE DRUGS
PARTIAL EPILEPSIES

Either reduction of inhibitory synaptic activity or enhancement of excitatory synaptic activity might trigger a seizure. The neurotransmitters mediating the bulk of synaptic transmission in the mammalian brain are amino acids, with γ-aminobutyric acid (GABA) and glutamate being the principal inhibitory and excitatory neurotransmitters, respectively (see Chapter 12). Pharmacological studies showed that antagonists of the $GABA_A$ receptor or agonists of different glutamate-receptor subtypes (NMDA, AMPA, or kainic acid; see Table 12–1) trigger seizures in experimental animals. Conversely, drugs that enhance GABA-mediated synaptic inhibition or glutamate-receptor antagonists inhibit seizures. Such studies support the concept that pharmacological modulation of synaptic function can affect the propensity for seizures.

Electrophysiological analyses during a partial seizure demonstrate that the individual neurons undergo depolarization and fire action potentials at high frequencies. This pattern of rapid firing is characteristic of a seizure but is uncommon during normal neuronal activity. Thus, selective inhibition of this rapid firing would be expected to reduce seizures with minimal unwanted effects. Inhibition of the high-frequency firing may be mediated by reducing the ability of Na^+ channels to recover from inactivation, thus prolonging the refractory period when another action potential cannot be evoked. Thus, reducing the rate of recovery of Na^+ channels from inactivation would limit the ability of a neuron to fire at high frequencies, an effect that likely underlies the effects of carbamazepine, lamotrigine, phenytoin, topiramate, valproic acid, *and* zonisamide *against partial seizures (Figure 19–1).*

Enhancing GABA-mediated synaptic inhibition may reduce neuronal excitability and raise the seizure threshold. Several drugs may inhibit seizures by regulating GABA-mediated synaptic inhibition. The principal postsynaptic receptor of synaptically released GABA is the $GABA_A$ receptor (see Chapter 16). Activation of the $GABA_A$ receptor inhibits the postsynaptic cell by increasing Cl^- inflow into the cell and hyperpolarizing the neuron. Clinically relevant concentrations of benzodiazepines and barbiturates enhance $GABA_A$ receptor–mediated hyperpolarization through distinct actions on the $GABA_A$ receptor; this enhanced inhibition probably underlies their effectiveness against partial and tonic-clonic seizures (Figure 19–2). At higher concentrations, such as might be used for status epilepticus, these drugs also inhibit high-frequency firing of action potentials. A second mechanism of enhancing GABA-mediated synaptic inhibition is thought to underlie the antiseizure mechanism of tiagabine *which inhibits the GABA transporter GAT-1 and reduces neuronal and glial uptake of GABA and thereby enhancing GABA-mediated neurotransmission (Figure 19–2).*

Table 19–1

Classification of Epileptic Seizures

Seizure Type	Features	Conventional Antiseizure Drugs	Recently Developed Antiseizure Drugs
Partial seizures:			
Simple partial	Diverse manifestations determined by the region of cortex activated by the seizure (*e.g.,* if motor cortex representing left thumb, clonic jerking of left thumb results; if somatosensory cortex representing left thumb, paresthesia of left thumb results), lasting ~20–60 seconds. *Key feature is preservation of consciousness.*	Carbamazepine, phenytoin, valproate	Gabapentin, lamotrigine, levetiracetam, tiagabine, topiramate, zonisamide
Complex partial	Impaired consciousness lasting 30 seconds to 2 minutes, often associated with purposeless movements such as lip smacking or hand wringing.	Carbamazepine, phenytoin, valproate	Gabapentin, lamotrigine, levetiracetam, tiagabine, topiramate, zonisamide
Partial with secondarily generalized tonic-clonic seizure	Simple or complex partial seizure evolves into a tonic-clonic seizure with loss of consciousness and sustained contractions (tonic) of muscles throughout the body followed by periods of muscle contraction alternating with periods of relaxation (clonic), typically lasting 1 to 2 minutes.	Carbamazepine, phenobarbital, phenytoin, primidone, valproate	Gabapentin, lamotrigine, levetiracetam, tiagabine, topiramate, zonisamide
Generalized seizures:			
Absence seizure	Abrupt onset of impaired consciousness associated with staring and cessation of ongoing activities typically lasting <30 seconds.	Ethosuximide, valproate	Lamotrigine
Myoclonic seizure	A brief (perhaps a second), shock-like contraction of muscles which may be restricted to part of one extremity or may be generalized.	Valproate	Lamotrigine, topiramate
Tonic-clonic seizure	As described above for partial with secondarily generalized tonic-clonic seizures except that it is not preceded by a partial seizure.	Carbamazepine, phenobarbital, phenytoin, primidone, valproate	Lamotrigine, topiramate

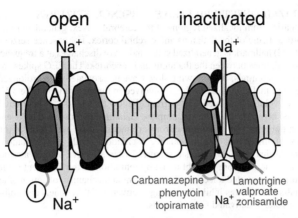

FIGURE 19–1 *Antiseizure drug–enhanced Na+* **channel inactivation.** Some antiseizure drugs (shown in blue text) prolong the inactivation of the Na+ channels, thereby reducing the ability of neurons to fire at high frequencies. Note that the inactivated channel itself appears to remain open, but is blocked by the inactivation gate (I). A, activation gate.

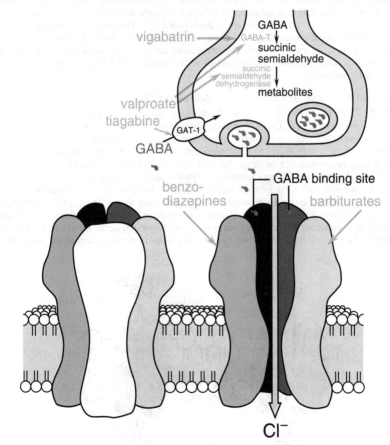

FIGURE 19–2 *Enhanced GABA synaptic transmission.* In the presence of GABA, the GABA$_A$ receptor (structure on left) is opened, allowing an influx of Cl−, which in turn increases membrane polarization (*see* Chapter 16). Some antiseizure drugs (shown in larger blue text) act by reducing the metabolism of GABA. Others act at the GABA$_A$ receptor, enhancing Cl− influx in response to GABA. As outlined in the text, gabapentin acts presynaptically to promote GABA release; its molecular target is currently under investigation. GABA-T, GABA transaminase; GAT-1, GABA transporter.

GENERALIZED-ONSET EPILEPSIES: ABSENCE SEIZURES In contrast to partial seizures, which arise from localized regions of the cerebral cortex, generalized-onset seizures arise from the reciprocal firing of the thalamus and cerebral cortex. For absence seizures, the electroencephalogram (EEG) hallmark is generalized spike-and-wave discharges at a frequency of 3/sec (3 Hz) that represent oscillations between the thalamus and neocortex. The EEG spikes are associated with the firing of action potentials; the following slow wave is associated with prolonged inhibition. One intrinsic property of thalamic neurons that is involved in the generation of the 3-Hz discharges is a particular form of voltage-regulated Ca^{2+} current, the low threshold ("T") current. In contrast to its small size in most neurons, the T current in many thalamic neurons has a large amplitude. Indeed, bursts of action potentials in thalamic neurons are mediated by activation of the T current. The T current plays an amplifying role in thalamic oscillations, with one oscillation being the 3-Hz spike-and-wave discharge of the absence seizure. Drugs effective against absence seizures (*e.g., ethosuximide*, valproic acid) are thought to act by inhibition of the T current (Figure 19–3). Thus, inhibition of voltage-regulated ion channels is a common mechanism of action of antiseizure drugs, with anti–partial-seizure drugs inhibiting voltage-activated Na^+ channels and anti–absence-seizure drugs inhibiting voltage-activated Ca^{2+} channels.

GENETIC APPROACHES TO THE EPILEPSIES Most patients with epilepsy are neurologically normal; elucidating mutant genes underlying familial epilepsy in otherwise normal individuals has led to the identification of genes implicated in distinct, albeit rare, idiopathic epilepsy syndromes that account for <1% of all human epilepsies. Interestingly, almost all of the mutant genes encode ion channels that are gated by voltage or ligands. Mutations have been identified in voltage-gated Na^+ and K^+ channels and in channels gated by GABA and acetylcholine. The cellular electrophysiological consequences of some of these mutations may relate to mechanisms of seizures and antiseizure drugs. For example, generalized epilepsy with febrile seizures is caused by a point mutation in the β subunit of a voltage-gated Na^+ channel (*SCN1B*) that appears to interfere with channel inactivation.

ANTISEIZURE DRUGS: GENERAL CONSIDERATIONS

THERAPEUTIC ASPECTS The ideal antiseizure drug would suppress all seizures without causing any unwanted effects. Drugs used currently not only fail to control seizure activity in some patients, but frequently cause unwanted effects that range in severity from minimal impairment of the central nervous system (CNS) to death from aplastic anemia or hepatic failure. The task is to select the drug or combination of drugs that best controls seizures in an individual patient at an acceptable level of untoward effects. Complete control of seizures can be achieved in up to 50% of patients, while another 25% can be improved significantly. Success varies as a function of seizure type, cause, and other factors. To minimize toxicity, treatment with a single drug is preferred. If seizures are not controlled with the initial agent at adequate plasma concentrations, substitution of a second drug is preferred to concurrent administration of a second agent. However, multiple-drug therapy may be needed, especially when two or more types of seizure occur in the same patient.

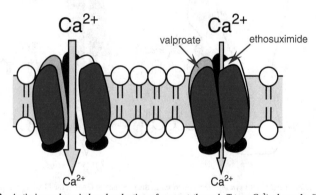

FIGURE 19–3 *Antiseizure drug–induced reduction of current through T-type Ca^{2+} channels.* Some antiseizure drugs (shown in blue text) reduce the flow of Ca^{2+} through T-type Ca^{2+} channels (*see* Chapter 12), thus reducing the pacemaker current that underlies the thalamic rhythm in spikes and waves seen in generalized absence seizures.

Measurement of drug concentrations in plasma facilitates pharmacotherapy, especially when therapy is initiated, after dosage adjustments, in the event of therapeutic failure, when toxic effects appear, or when multiple-drug therapy is instituted. However, clinical effects of some drugs do not correlate well with their plasma concentrations, and recommended concentrations are only guidelines. The ultimate therapeutic regimen must be determined by clinical assessment of efficacy and toxicity.

Phenytoin

Phenytoin (DILANTIN) is effective against all types of partial and tonic-clonic seizures but not absence seizures.

PHARMACOLOGICAL EFFECTS
Central Nervous System   Phenytoin exerts antiseizure activity without causing general CNS depression. In toxic doses, phenytoin may produce excitatory signs and, at lethal levels, a type of decerebrate rigidity.

MECHANISM OF ACTION
Phenytoin limits the repetitive firing of action potentials evoked by a sustained depolarization. This effect is mediated by a slowing of the rate of recovery of voltage-activated Na^+ channels from inactivation. At therapeutic concentrations, the effects on Na^+ channels are selective, without changes in spontaneous activity or in responses to GABA or glutamate. At concentrations five- to tenfold higher, other effects of phenytoin include reduction of spontaneous activity and enhancement of responses to GABA that may underlie some of the toxicity associated with high levels of phenytoin.

PHARMACOKINETIC PROPERTIES   Phenytoin is available in rapid-release and extended-release oral forms; once-daily dosing is possible only with extended-release formulations. Due to differences in dissolution and other formulation-dependent factors, the plasma phenytoin level may change upon conversion from one formulation to the other. Different formulations can include either phenytoin or phenytoin sodium; therefore, comparable doses can be approximated by considering "phenytoin equivalents," but serum level monitoring is necessary to assure therapeutic safety.

Phenytoin is extensively (~90%) bound to serum proteins, mainly albumin. Small variations in the bound fraction dramatically affect the absolute amount of free (active) drug; increased proportions of free drug are evident in the neonate, in patients with hypoalbuminemia, and in uremic patients. Some agents (*e.g.*, valproic acid) can compete with phenytoin for binding sites on plasma proteins; when combined with valproate-mediated inhibition of phenytoin metabolism, marked increases in free phenytoin can result.

Phenytoin's rate of elimination varies as a function of its concentration (*i.e.*, the rate is nonlinear). The plasma $t_{1/2}$ of phenytoin ranges between 6 and 24 hours at plasma concentrations <10 μg/mL but increases with higher concentrations. As a result, plasma concentration increases disproportionately as dosage is increased, even with small adjustments for levels near the therapeutic range.

Phenytoin is largely (95%) metabolized by hepatic CYPs (Table 19–2). The principal metabolite, a parahydroxyphenyl derivative, is inactive. Phenytoin metabolism is saturable, and other substrates of these CYPs can inhibit phenytoin metabolism and increase its plasma concentration. Conversely, phenytoin will reduce the degradation of other drugs that are substrates for these enzymes, such as *warfarin*. The addition of phenytoin to a patient receiving warfarin can lead to bleeding disorders (*see* Chapter 54). Other drug interactions arise from phenytoin's capacity to induce CYPs (*see* Chapter 3 and Table 19–2) and increase the degradation of drugs (*e.g.*, oral contraceptives) metabolized by CYP3A4; treatment with phenytoin could enhance the metabolism of oral contraceptives and lead to unplanned pregnancy. The potential teratogenic effects of phenytoin underscore the importance of attention to this interaction. Carbamazepine, *oxcarbazepine*, phenobarbital, and *primidone* also can induce CYP3A4 and likewise might increase degradation of oral contraceptives.

The low aqueous solubility of phenytoin hindered its intravenous use. Fosphenytoin (CEREBYX), a water soluble prodrug, is rapidly converted into phenytoin by phosphatases in liver and erythrocytes. Fosphenytoin is extensively (95–99%) bound to plasma proteins, primarily albumin. This binding is saturable, and fosphenytoin displaces phenytoin from binding sites. Fosphenytoin is useful for adults with partial or generalized seizures when intravenous or intramuscular administration is indicated.

Table 19–2

Interactions of Antiseizure Drugs with Hepatic Microsomal Enzymes*

Drug	Induces CYP	Induces UGT	Inhibits CYP	Inhibits UGT	Metabolized by CYP	Metabolized by UGT
Carbamazepine	2C9;3A families	Yes			1A2;2C8;2C9;3A4	No
Ethosuximide	No	No	No	No	Uncertain	Uncertain
Gabapentin	No	No	No	No	No	No
Lamotrigine	No	Yes	No	No	No	Yes
Levetiracetam	No	No	No	No	No	No
Oxcarbazepine	3A4/5	Yes	2C19	Weak	No	Yes
Phenobarbital	2C;3A families	Yes	Yes	No	2C9;2C19	No
Phenytoin	2C;3A families	Yes	Yes	No	2C9;2C19	No
Primidone	2C;3A families	Yes	Yes	No	2C9;2C19	No
Tiagabine	No	No	No	No	3A4	No
Topiramate	No	No	2C19	No		
Valproate	No	No	2C9	Yes	2C9;2C19	Yes
Zonisamide	No	No	No	No	3A4	Yes

*CYP, cytochrome P450; UGT, UDP-glucuronosyltransferase.

TOXICITY   The toxic effects of phenytoin depend on the route of administration, the duration of exposure, and the dosage.

When fosphenytoin is administered intravenously at an excessive rate in the emergency treatment of status epilepticus, the most notable toxic signs are cardiac arrhythmias, with or without hypotension, and/or CNS depression. Cardiac toxicity occurs more frequently in older patients and in those with known cardiac disease but also can develop in young, healthy patients. These complications can be minimized by administering fosphenytoin at a rate of <150 mg of phenytoin sodium equivalent per minute. Acute oral overdosage results primarily in signs referable to the cerebellum and vestibular system; high doses have been associated with marked cerebellar atrophy. Toxic effects associated with chronic treatment also are primarily dose-related cerebellarvestibular effects but also include other CNS effects, behavioral changes, increased seizures frequency, gastrointestinal (GI) symptoms, gingival hyperplasia, osteomalacia, and megaloblastic anemia. Hirsutism is an annoying untoward effect in young females. Usually, these phenomena can be diminished by proper adjustment of dosage. Serious adverse effects, including those on the skin, bone marrow, and liver, probably are manifestations of rare drug allergy and necessitate drug withdrawal. Moderate elevation of hepatic transaminases sometimes is observed; since these changes are transient and may result in part from induced synthesis of the enzymes, they do not necessitate drug withdrawal.

Gingival hyperplasia, apparently due to altered collagen metabolism, occurs in ~20% of patients during chronic therapy and is probably the most common toxicity in children and young adolescents. It may be more frequent in individuals who also develop coarsened facial features. Toothless portions of the gums are not affected. The condition does not necessarily require withdrawal of medication and can be minimized by good oral hygiene.

A variety of endocrine effects have been reported. Inhibition of vasopressin release has been observed in patients with inappropriate secretion of this hormone. Hyperglycemia and glycosuria appear to be due to inhibition of insulin secretion. Osteomalacia has been attributed to altered metabolism of vitamin D and the attendant inhibition of intestinal Ca^{2+} absorption. Phenytoin also increases the metabolism of vitamin K and reduces the concentration of vitamin K–dependent proteins that are important for normal Ca^{2+} metabolism in bone, perhaps explaining why the osteomalacia does not always respond to vitamin D.

Hypersensitivity reactions include morbilliform rash in 2–5% of patients and occasionally more serious skin reactions, including Stevens-Johnson syndrome. Systemic lupus erythematosus and potentially fatal hepatic necrosis have been reported rarely. Hematological reactions include neutropenia and leucopenia, or more rarely, red-cell aplasia, agranulocytosis, and thrombocytopenia. Lymphadenopathy is associated with reduced immunoglobulin A (IgA) production. Hypoprothrombinemia and hemorrhage have occurred in the newborns of mothers who received phenytoin during pregnancy; vitamin K is effective treatment or prophylaxis.

PLASMA DRUG CONCENTRATIONS

A good correlation usually is observed between the total concentration of phenytoin in plasma and its clinical effect. Thus, control of seizures generally is obtained with concentrations >10 µg/mL, while toxic effects (e.g., nystagmus) develop at concentrations ~20 µg/mL.

DRUG INTERACTIONS

Concurrent administration of any drug metabolized by CYP2C9 or CYP2C10 can increase the plasma concentration of phenytoin by decreasing its rate of metabolism. Conversely, drugs that induce hepatic CYPs can increase phenytoin catabolism. Thus, carbamazepine causes a decrease in phenytoin concentration and phenytoin reduces the concentration of carbamazepine. Interaction between phenytoin and phenobarbital is variable.

THERAPEUTIC USES

Epilepsy Phenytoin is effective against partial and tonic-clonic but not absence seizures. Phenytoin preparations differ significantly in bioavailability and rate of absorption. In general, patients should consistently be treated with the same drug from a single manufacturer. However, if it becomes necessary to temporarily switch between products, care should be taken to select a therapeutically equivalent product and patients should be monitored for loss of seizure control or onset of new toxicities.

Other Uses

Some cases of trigeminal and related neuralgias appear to respond to phenytoin, but carbamazepine is preferred.

ANTISEIZURE BARBITURATES

Most barbiturates have antiseizure properties. The discussion below is limited to the two barbiturates that exert maximal antiseizure action at doses below those required for hypnosis, a property that determines their clinical utility as antiseizure agents. The pharmacology of barbiturates is considered in Chapter 16.

Phenobarbital

Phenobarbital (LUMINAL, others) was the first effective organic antiseizure agent. It has relatively low toxicity, is inexpensive, and is still an effective and widely used drug for this purpose.

Mechanism of Action

Phenobarbital likely inhibits seizures by potentiation of synaptic inhibition through an action on the $GABA_A$ receptor. At therapeutic concentrations, phenobarbital enhances $GABA_A$ receptor–mediated current by increasing the duration of bursts of current without changing their frequency. At levels exceeding therapeutic concentrations, phenobarbital also limits sustained repetitive firing; this may underlie some of the antiseizure effects of higher concentrations of phenobarbital achieved during therapy of status epilepticus.

PHARMACOKINETIC PROPERTIES Oral absorption of phenobarbital is complete but slow; peak plasma concentrations occur several hours after a single dose. Phenobarbital is 40–60% bound to plasma and tissue proteins. Up to 25% of a dose is eliminated by renal excretion of the unchanged drug; the remainder is inactivated by hepatic CYPs. Phenobarbital induces UGTs and several CYPs, thereby stimulating degradation of drugs cleared by these mechanisms (*see* Table 19–2).

TOXICITY

Sedation, the most frequent undesired effect of phenobarbital, is apparent to some extent in all patients upon drug initiation, but tolerance develops during chronic therapy. Nystagmus and ataxia occur at excessive dosage. Phenobarbital sometimes produces irritability and hyperactivity in children and agitation and confusion in the elderly. Scarlatiniform or morbilliform rash, possibly with other manifestations of drug allergy, occurs in 1–2% of patients. Exfoliative dermatitis is rare. Hypoprothrombinemia with hemorrhage has been observed in the newborns of mothers who have received phenobarbital during pregnancy. As with phenytoin, megaloblastic anemia that responds to folate and osteomalacia that responds to vitamin D occur during chronic phenobarbital therapy.

PLASMA DRUG CONCENTRATIONS

During long-term therapy in adults, the plasma concentration of phenobarbital averages 10 µg/mL per daily dose of 1 mg/kg; in children, the value is 5–7 µg/mL per 1 mg/kg. Although there is no *precise relationship between efficacy and drug concentration, plasma concentrations of 10–35 μg/mL are usually recommended. The relationship between plasma phenobarbital concentration and adverse effects varies with the development of tolerance. Sedation, nystagmus, and ataxia usually are absent at concentrations <30 μg/mL during long-term therapy; adverse effects may be apparent for several days at lower concentrations when therapy is initiated or when dosage is increased. Concentrations >60 μg/mL may be associated with marked intoxication in the nontolerant individual.*

Since significant behavioral toxicity may be present despite the absence of overt signs of toxicity, the tendency to maintain patients, particularly children, on excessively high doses of phenobarbital should be resisted. The plasma phenobarbital concentration should be increased above 30–40 μg/mL only if the increment is adequately tolerated and only if it contributes significantly to seizure control.

DRUG INTERACTIONS

Interactions between phenobarbital and other drugs usually involve induction of the hepatic CYPs by phenobarbital (see Table 19–2). Concentrations of phenobarbital in plasma may be elevated by up to 40% during concurrent administration of valproic acid (see below).

THERAPEUTIC USES Phenobarbital is an effective drug for generalized tonic-clonic and partial seizures. It is efficacious, inexpensive, and has low toxicity. However, its sedative effects and its tendency to disturb behavior in children have reduced its use.

Mephobarbital (MEBARAL) is *N*-methylphenobarbital. It is *N*-demethylated in the liver, and most of its activity during long-term therapy results from the accumulation of phenobarbital. Consequently, the pharmacological properties, toxicity, and clinical uses of mephobarbital are the same as those for phenobarbital.

IMINOSTILBENES
Carbamazepine
PHARMACOLOGICAL EFFECTS

Carbamazepine (TEGRETOL, CARBATROL, others) *is a primary drug for the treatment of partial and tonic-clonic seizures and is also used for the treatment of trigeminal neuralgia. Although effects of carbamazepine resemble those of phenytoin, the drugs exhibit some important differences. For example, carbamazepine will produce therapeutic responses in manic-depressive patients, including some in whom lithium carbonate is not effective. The mechanisms responsible for these effects of carbamazepine are not clearly understood.*

Mechanism of Action

Like phenytoin, carbamazepine appears to limit the repetitive firing of action potentials evoked by a sustained depolarization by slowing the rate of recovery of voltage-activated Na^+ channels. At therapeutic concentrations, carbamazepine is selective in that there are no effects on spontaneous activity or on responses to GABA or glutamate. The carbamazepine metabolite, 10,11-epoxycarbamazepine, has similar effects and may contribute to the antiseizure efficacy of carbamazepine.

PHARMACOKINETIC PROPERTIES Carbamazepine is absorbed slowly and erratically after oral administration. Peak concentrations in plasma usually occur 4–8 hours after oral ingestion but may be delayed by up to 24 hours, especially following the administration of a large dose. The drug distributes rapidly into all tissues. Approximately 75% of carbamazepine binds to plasma proteins, and the drug concentration in the cerebrospinal fluid (CSF) corresponds to the concentration of free drug in plasma.

The predominant pathway of metabolism in humans involves conversion to the 10,11-epoxide. This metabolite is as active as the parent compound, and its concentrations in plasma and brain may reach 50% of those of carbamazepine, especially with concurrent administration of phenytoin or phenobarbital. The 10,11-epoxide is metabolized further to inactive compounds, which are excreted in the urine principally as glucuronides. Carbamazepine also is inactivated by conjugation and hydroxylation. Hepatic CYP3A4 is primarily responsible for biotransformation of carbamazepine. Carbamazepine induces CYP2C, CYP3A4, and UGT, thus enhancing the metabolism of drugs degraded by these enzymes (*e.g.,* oral contraceptives, which are metabolized by CYP3A4).

TOXICITY Acute intoxication with carbamazepine can result in stupor or coma, hyperirritability, convulsions, and respiratory depression. During long-term therapy, untoward effects include drowsiness, vertigo, ataxia, diplopia, and blurred vision. The frequency of seizures may increase, especially with overdosage. Other adverse effects include nausea, vomiting, serious hematological toxicity (aplastic anemia, agranulocytosis), and hypersensitivity reactions (dermatitis, eosinophilia, lymphadenopathy, splenomegaly). A late complication of therapy with carbamazepine is water retention, with decreased osmolality and hyponatremia, especially in elderly patients with cardiac disease.

Some tolerance develops to the neurotoxic effects of carbamazepine, and they can be minimized by gradual increase in dosage. Carbamazepine causes a transient elevation of hepatic transaminases in 5–10% of patients. A transient, mild leukopenia occurs in ~10% of patients during initiation of therapy and usually resolves within the first 4 months of continued treatment; transient thrombocytopenia also has been noted. In ~2% of patients, a persistent leukopenia may develop that requires drug withdrawal. Aplastic anemia occurs in 1 in 200,000 patients who are treated; it is not clear whether periodic blood tests can avert the development of irreversible aplastic anemia. The induction of fetal malformations in pregnant women is discussed below.

PLASMA DRUG CONCENTRATIONS

There is no simple relationship between the dose of carbamazepine and concentrations of the drug in plasma. Therapeutic concentrations are reported to be 6–12 µg/mL, although considerable variation occurs. Side effects referable to the CNS are frequent at concentrations >9 µg/mL.

DRUG INTERACTIONS

Phenobarbital, phenytoin, and valproic acid may increase the metabolism of carbamazepine by inducing CYP3A4; carbamazepine may enhance the biotransformation of phenytoin. Concurrent administration of carbamazepine may lower concentrations of valproic acid, lamotrigine, tiagabine, and topiramate. Carbamazepine reduces both the plasma concentration and therapeutic effect of haloperidol. The metabolism of carbamazepine may be inhibited by propoxyphene, erythromycin, cimetidine, fluoxetine, and isoniazid.

THERAPEUTIC USES Carbamazepine is useful in patients with generalized tonic-clonic and both simple and complex partial seizures. Renal and hepatic function and hematological parameters should be monitored. The therapeutic use of carbamazepine is discussed below.

Carbamazepine is the primary agent for treatment of trigeminal and glossopharyngeal neuralgias. It is also effective for lightning tabetic pain associated with bodily wasting. Most patients with neuralgia benefit initially, but only 70% obtain continuing relief. Adverse effects require discontinuation of medication in 5–20% of patients. The therapeutic range of plasma concentrations for antiseizure therapy serves as a guideline for its use in neuralgia. Carbamazepine also has found use in the treatment of bipolar affective disorders (*see* Chapter 18).

Oxcarbazepine

Oxcarbazepine (TRILEPTAL) (10,11-dihydro-10-oxocarbamazepine) is a keto analog of carbamazepine. Oxcarbazepine is a prodrug: it is rapidly converted to its active metabolite, a 10-monohydroxy derivative, which is inactivated by glucuronidation and eliminated by renal excretion. Its mechanism of action is similar to that of carbamazepine. Oxcarbazepine is a less potent enzyme inducer than is carbamazepine, and substitution of oxcarbazepine for carbamazepine is associated with increased levels of phenytoin and valproic acid, presumably because of reduced induction of hepatic enzymes. Although oxcarbazepine does not appear to reduce the anticoagulant effect of warfarin, it does induce CYP3A4 and thus reduces plasma levels of oral contraceptives. Oxcarbazepine is approved for monotherapy or adjunct therapy for partial seizures in adults and as adjunctive therapy for partial seizures in children ages 4–16.

SUCCINIMIDES
Ethosuximide

PHARMACOLOGICAL EFFECTS Ethosuximide (ZARONTIN) is a primary agent for the treatment of absence seizures.

Mechanism of Action Ethosuximide reduces low threshold Ca^{2+} currents (T currents) in thalamic neurons and thus modulates thalamic 3-Hz spike-and-wave activity. At clinically relevant concentrations, ethosuximide inhibits the T current without modifying the voltage dependence of steady-state inactivation or the time course of recovery from inactivation. Therapeutic concentrations of ethosuximide do not inhibit sustained repetitive firing or enhance GABA responses.

PHARMACOKINETIC PROPERTIES   Absorption of ethosuximide appears to be complete, with peak concentrations in plasma within ~3 hours after a single oral dose. Ethosuximide is not significantly bound to plasma proteins; during long-term therapy, its concentration in the CSF is similar to that in plasma. Approximately 25% of the drug is excreted unchanged in the urine; the remainder is metabolized by hepatic microsomal enzymes. The major metabolite, the hydroxyethyl derivative, accounts for 40% of administered drug, is inactive, and is excreted unchanged and as the glucuronide in urine. The plasma $t_{1/2}$ of ethosuximide is 40–50 hours in adults and ~30 hours in children.

TOXICITY   Common dose-related side effects are GI complaints (nausea, vomiting, and anorexia) and CNS effects (drowsiness, lethargy, euphoria, dizziness, headache, and hiccups); some tolerance to these effects develops. Parkinson-like symptoms and photophobia also have occurred. Restlessness, agitation, anxiety, aggressiveness, inability to concentrate, and other behavioral effects have occurred primarily in patients with a history of psychiatric disturbance. Urticaria and other skin reactions, including Stevens-Johnson syndrome, as well as systemic lupus erythematosus, eosinophilia, leukopenia, thrombocytopenia, pancytopenia, and aplastic anemia have been attributed to the drug, and deaths have resulted from bone marrow depression.

PLASMA DRUG CONCENTRATIONS   During long-term therapy, the plasma concentration of ethosuximide averages ~2 μg/mL per daily dose of 1 mg/kg. A plasma concentration of 40–100 μg/mL usually is required for satisfactory control of absence seizures.

THERAPEUTIC USES

Ethosuximide is effective against absence seizures but not tonic-clonic seizures. An initial daily dose of 250 mg in children (3–6 years old) and 500 mg in older children and adults is increased by 250-mg increments at weekly intervals until seizures are adequately controlled or toxicity intervenes. Divided dosage is required occasionally to diminish nausea or drowsiness. The usual maintenance dose is 20 mg/kg/day. Use caution if the daily dose exceeds 1500 mg in adults or 750–1000 mg in children. The use of ethosuximide is discussed further below.

VALPROIC ACID
PHARMACOLOGICAL EFFECTS   The antiseizure properties of valproic acid (DEPAKENE, others) were discovered serendipitously when it was employed as a vehicle for other compounds that were being screened for antiseizure activity. Its efficacy in animal models parallels its efficacy against absence as well as partial and generalized tonic-clonic seizures in humans.

Mechanism of Action
At therapeutic concentrations, valproic acid inhibits sustained repetitive firing induced by depolarization of mouse cortical or spinal cord neurons, an effect apparently mediated by prolonging the recovery phase of voltage-activated Na^+ channels. Valproic acid does not modify neuronal responses to GABA. Valproic acid also reduces the T Ca^{2+} current at clinically relevant but slightly higher concentrations than those that limit sustained repetitive firing; this effect on T currents in thalamic neurons is similar to that of ethosuximide. Limiting sustained repetitive firing and reducing T currents may contribute to the efficacy of valproic acid against partial and tonic-clonic seizures and absence seizures, respectively.

Another putative antiseizure action of valproic acid involves GABA metabolism. In vitro, valproic acid stimulates the activity of glutamic acid decarboxylase, the GABA synthetic enzyme, and inhibits GABA degradative enzymes.

PHARMACOKINETIC PROPERTIES   Valproic acid is absorbed rapidly and completely after oral administration. Peak concentration in plasma is attained in 1–4 hours, or several hours later if the drug is administered in enteric-coated tablets or ingested with meals. Its extent of binding to plasma proteins is usually ~90%, but the bound fraction is reduced as the total concentration of valproic acid is increased through the therapeutic range. Although CSF concentrations of valproic acid suggest equilibration with free drug in the blood, there is evidence for carrier-mediated transport both into and out of the CSF.

The bulk of valproic acid (95%) undergoes hepatic metabolism (*via* UGTs and β-oxidation), with <5% excreted unchanged in urine. Valproic acid is a substrate for CYP2C9 and CYP2C19, but metabolism by these enzymes accounts for a relatively minor portion of its elimination. The metabolites, 2-propyl-2-pentenoic acid and 2-propyl-4-pentenoic acid, are nearly as potent antiseizure agents as valproate, but only the former significantly accumulates in plasma and brain. The $t_{1/2}$ of valproic acid is ~15 hours but is reduced in patients taking other antiepileptic drugs.

TOXICITY   The most common side effects are transient GI symptoms, including anorexia, nausea, and vomiting in ~16% of patients. CNS effects include sedation, ataxia, and tremor; these symptoms occur infrequently and usually respond to a decrease in dosage. Rash, alopecia, and stimulation of appetite have been observed occasionally, and weight gain has been seen with chronic valproic acid treatment. Elevation of hepatic transaminases is observed in up to 40% of patients and often occurs asymptomatically during the first several months of therapy.

A rare complication is fulminant hepatitis. Children <2 years of age with other medical conditions who were given multiple antiseizure agents were especially likely to suffer fatal hepatic injury; there were no deaths reported for patients >10 years old who received only valproate. Acute pancreatitis and hyperammonemia have been associated with the use of valproic acid. Valproic acid can produce teratogenic effects such as neural tube defects.

PLASMA DRUG CONCENTRATIONS
Therapeutic effects of valproic acid occur with plasma levels of 30–100 μg/mL, but there is a poor correlation between the plasma concentration and efficacy. There appears to be a threshold at ~30–50 μg/mL, the concentration at which binding sites on plasma albumin approach saturation.

DRUG INTERACTIONS
Valproic acid inhibits the metabolism of drugs that are substrates for CYP2C9, including phenytoin and phenobarbital. Valproic acid also inhibits UGT and thus inhibits the metabolism of lamotrigine and lorazepam. Valproic acid is highly bound to albumin and can displace phenytoin and other drugs; this displacement can exacerbate valproic acid's inhibition of phenytoin metabolism. The concurrent administration of valproate and clonazepam rarely has been associated with the development of absence status epilepticus.

THERAPEUTIC USES   Valproate is effective in the treatment of absence, myoclonic, partial, and tonic-clonic seizures. The initial daily dose usually is 15 mg/kg, increased at weekly intervals by 5–10 mg/kg/day to a maximum daily dose of 60 mg/kg. Divided doses should be given when the total daily dose exceeds 250 mg. The therapeutic uses of valproate in epilepsy are discussed further below.

BENZODIAZEPINES

The benzodiazepines are used primarily as sedative-antianxiety drugs (*see* Chapters 16 and 17) but also have broad antiseizure properties. Clonazepam (KLONOPIN) and *clorazepate* (TRANXENE-SD, others) have been approved in the U.S. for the long-term treatment of certain types of seizures. *Diazepam* (VALIUM, DIASTAT; others) and *lorazepam* (ATIVAN) have well-defined roles in the management of status epilepticus.

Mechanism of Action

Antiseizure actions of the benzodiazepines largely result from their capacity to enhance GABA-mediated synaptic inhibition (see Chapter 16). At therapeutic concentrations, benzodiazepines act at GABA$_A$ receptors and increase the frequency, but not duration, of openings at GABA-activated Cl$^-$ channels. At higher concentrations, diazepam and other benzodiazepines can reduce sustained, high-frequency firing of neurons. Although these concentrations correspond to concentrations achieved in patients during treatment of status epilepticus with diazepam, they are considerably higher than those associated with antiseizure or anxiolytic effects in ambulatory patients.

PHARMACOKINETIC PROPERTIES   Benzodiazepines are well absorbed orally, and peak plasma concentrations are usually reached within 1–4 hours. After intravenous administration, they redistribute in a manner typical of highly lipid-soluble agents (*see* Chapters 1 and 16). CNS effects develop rapidly but wane quickly as the drugs move to other tissues. Diazepam redistributes rapidly ($t_{1/2}$ of redistribution, ~1 hour). The extent of binding of benzodiazepines to plasma proteins correlates with lipid solubility, ranging from 99% for diazepam to ~85% for clonazepam.

The major metabolite of diazepam, N-desmethyl-diazepam, is somewhat less active than the parent drug and may act as a partial agonist. This metabolite also is produced by the rapid decarboxylation of clorazepate. Both diazepam and N-desmethyl-diazepam are slowly hydroxylated to other active metabolites such as *oxazepam*. The $t_{1/2}$ of diazepam in plasma is 1–2 days; that of N-desmethyl-diazepam is ~60 hours. Clonazepam is metabolized principally by reduction of the nitro group to produce inactive 7-amino derivatives. Less than 1% of the drug is recovered unchanged in the urine. The $t_{1/2}$ of clonazepam in plasma is 1 day. Lorazepam is metabolized chiefly by conjugation with glucuronic acid; its $t_{1/2}$ in plasma is ~14 hours.

TOXICITY   The principal side effects of long-term oral therapy with clonazepam are drowsiness and lethargy. These occur in ~50% of patients initially, but tolerance often develops with continued administration. Muscular incoordination and ataxia are less frequent. Although these symptoms usually can be kept to tolerable levels by reducing the dosage or the rate at which it is increased, they sometimes force drug discontinuation. Other side effects include hypotonia, dysarthria, and dizziness. Behavioral disturbances (aggression, hyperactivity, irritability, difficulty in concentration), especially in children, can be very troublesome. Anorexia and hyperphagia have been reported. Increased salivary and bronchial secretions may cause difficulties in children. Seizures are sometimes exacerbated and status epilepticus may be precipitated if the drug is discontinued abruptly. Cardiovascular and respiratory depression may occur after the intravenous administration of diazepam, clonazepam, or lorazepam, particularly if other antiseizure agents or central depressants have been administered previously.

PLASMA DRUG CONCENTRATIONS
Because tolerance affects the relationship between drug concentration and drug antiseizure effect, plasma concentrations of benzodiazepines are of limited value.

THERAPEUTIC USES   Clonazepam is useful in the therapy of absence seizures as well as myoclonic seizures in children, but tolerance to its antiseizure effects usually develops within 1–6 months, after which some patients will not respond to clonazepam at any dosage. The initial dose of clonazepam for adults should not exceed 1.5 mg/day and for children 0.01–0.03 mg/kg/day. Dose-dependent side effects are reduced if two or three divided doses are given each day. The dose may be increased every 3 days in amounts of 0.25–0.5 mg/day in children and 0.5–1 mg/day in adults. The maximal recommended dose is 20 mg/day for adults and 0.2 mg/kg/day for children.

Diazepam is an effective agent for treatment of status epilepticus, but its short duration of action is a disadvantage, leading to the more frequent use of lorazepam. Although diazepam is not useful as an oral agent for the treatment of seizure disorders, clorazepate is effective in combination with certain other drugs in the treatment of partial seizures (*see* below). The maximal initial dose of clorazepate is 22.5 mg/day in three portions for adults and 15 mg/day in two doses in children. Clorazepate is not recommended for children under the age of 9.

OTHER ANTISEIZURE DRUGS
Gabapentin

Gabapentin (NEURONTIN) is an antiseizure drug that consists of a GABA molecule covalently bound to a lipophilic cyclohexane ring. Gabapentin was designed to be a centrally active GABA agonist.

PHARMACOLOGICAL EFFECTS AND MECHANISMS OF ACTION   Gabapentin's efficacy in animal models parallels that of valproic acid and distinguishes gabapentin from phenytoin and carbamazepine. Despite its design as a GABA agonist, gabapentin does not mimic GABA when applied to neurons in primary culture. Gabapentin may promote release of GABA. The drug binds a protein in cortical membranes with an amino acid sequence identical to that of the $\alpha 2\delta$ subunit of the L type voltage-sensitive Ca^{2+} channel but does not affect Ca^{2+} currents of the T, N, or L types in dorsal root ganglion cells.

PHARMACOKINETICS   Gabapentin is absorbed after oral administration and excreted unchanged, mainly in the urine. Its $t_{1/2}$, when used as monotherapy, is 4–6 hours. It has no known interactions with other antiseizure drugs.

THERAPEUTIC USES
When combined with other antiseizure drugs, gabapentin is effective for partial seizures, with or without secondary generalization. Gabapentin (900 or 1800 mg/day) monotherapy is equivalent to carbamazepine (600 mg/day) for newly diagnosed partial or generalized epilepsy. Gabapentin also is used off-label for the treatment of migraine, chronic pain, and bipolar disorder. Gabapentin usually is effective at 900–1800 mg daily in three divided doses, although 3600 mg may be required in some patients. Therapy usually is begun with a low dose (300 mg once on the first day), which is increased in daily increments of 300 mg until an effective dose is reached.

TOXICITY   Overall, gabapentin is well tolerated. The most common adverse effects are somnolence, dizziness, ataxia, and fatigue. These effects usually are mild and resolve within 2 weeks of onset during continued treatment.

Lamotrigine

Lamotrigine (LAMICTAL) was developed as an antifolate agent, based on the model that reducing folate would combat seizures. The antiseizure effect of lamotrigine is unrelated to its antifolate properties.

PHARMACOLOGICAL EFFECTS AND MECHANISMS OF ACTION Lamotrigine blocks sustained repetitive firing of neurons and delays recovery from inactivation of recombinant Na^+ channels, mechanisms similar to those of phenytoin and carbamazepine that may explain lamotrigine's actions on partial and secondarily generalized seizures. However, lamotrigine is effective against a broader spectrum of seizures than phenytoin and carbamazepine, suggesting additional actions that may include inhibiting synaptic release of glutamate.

PHARMACOKINETICS AND DRUG INTERACTIONS Lamotrigine is completely absorbed from the GI tract and is metabolized primarily by glucuronidation. The plasma $t_{1/2}$ of a single dose is 15–30 hours. Administration of phenytoin, carbamazepine, or phenobarbital reduces the $t_{1/2}$ and plasma concentrations of lamotrigine. Conversely, addition of valproic acid markedly increases plasma concentrations of lamotrigine, likely by inhibiting glucuronidation. Addition of lamotrigine to valproic acid produces a reduction of valproate concentrations by ~25% over a few weeks. Concurrent use of lamotrigine and carbamazepine may be associated with increased levels of the 10,11-epoxide of carbamazepine and clinical toxicity.

THERAPEUTIC USE Lamotrigine is useful for monotherapy and add-on therapy of partial and secondarily generalized tonic-clonic seizures in adults and Lennox-Gastaut syndrome in both children and adults.

Patients already taking antiseizure drugs that induce hepatic enzymes (e.g., carbamazepine, phenytoin, phenobarbital, or primidone) should be given lamotrigine initially at 50 mg/day for 2 weeks. The dose is increased to 50 mg twice per day for 2 weeks and then increased in increments of 100 mg/day each week up to a maintenance dose of 300–500 mg/day divided into two doses. For patients taking valproic acid in addition to an enzyme-inducing antiseizure drug, the initial dose should be 25 mg every other day for 2 weeks, followed by an increase to 25 mg/day for 2 weeks; the dose then can be increased by 25–50 mg/day every 1–2 weeks up to a maintenance dose of 100–150 mg/day divided into two doses.

TOXICITY Common adverse effects when lamotrigine is added to another antiseizure drug are dizziness, ataxia, blurred or double vision, nausea, vomiting, and rash. A few cases of Stevens-Johnson syndrome and disseminated intravascular coagulation have been reported. The incidence of serious rash in children (~0.8%) is higher than in adults (0.3%).

Levetiracetam

Levetiracetam (KEPPRA) is the S-enantiomer of α-ethyl-2-oxo-1-pyrrolidineacetamide.

PHARMACOLOGICAL EFFECTS AND MECHANISM OF ACTION Levetiracetam exhibits clinical effectiveness against partial and secondarily generalized tonic-clonic seizures. The mechanism by which levetiracetam exerts these antiseizure effects is unknown.

PHARMACOKINETICS AND DRUG INTERACTIONS Levetiracetam is rapidly and almost completely absorbed after oral administration and is not bound to plasma proteins. Ninety-five percent of the drug and its inactive metabolite are excreted in the urine, 65% of which is unchanged drug; 24% of the drug is metabolized by hydrolysis of the acetamide group. Levetiracetam neither induces nor is a high-affinity substrate for CYPs or glucuronidases and thus does not interact with other antiseizure drugs, oral contraceptives, or anticoagulants.

THERAPEUTIC USE; TOXICITY The addition of levetiracetam to other antiseizure medications in adults with refractory partial seizures improved control in one clinical trial. Insufficient evidence is available on use of levetiracetam as monotherapy for partial or generalized epilepsy. The drug is well tolerated; adverse effects include somnolence, asthenia, and dizziness.

Tiagabine

Tiagabine (GABITRIL) is a derivative of nipecotic acid.

PHARMACOLOGICAL EFFECTS AND MECHANISM OF ACTION Tiagabine inhibits the GABA transporter, GAT-1, and thereby reduces GABA uptake into neurons and glia.

As a consequence, tiagabine prolongs the synaptic dwell time of GABA and increases the duration of synaptic inhibition.

PHARMACOKINETICS   Tiagabine is rapidly absorbed after oral administration, extensively bound to serum or plasma proteins, and metabolized in the liver by CYP3A. Its $t_{1/2}$ (~8 hours) is shortened by 2–3 hours when the drug is coadministered with hepatic enzyme–inducers such as phenobarbital, phenytoin, or carbamazepine.

THERAPEUTIC USE   Tiagabine is effective as add-on therapy of refractory partial seizures, with or without secondary generalization. Its efficacy as monotherapy for newly diagnosed or refractory partial and generalized epilepsy has not been established.

TOXICITY   Adverse effects include dizziness, somnolence, and tremor, which are mild to moderate in severity and appear shortly after initiation of therapy. Tiagabine-enhanced effects of synaptically released GABA can facilitate spike-and-wave discharges in animal models of absence seizures, suggesting that tiagabine may be contraindicated in patients with generalized absence epilepsy; patients with a history of spike-and-wave discharges have been reported to have exacerbations of their EEG abnormalities.

Topiramate

Topiramate (TOPAMAX) is a sulfamate-substituted monosaccharide.

PHARMACOLOGICAL EFFECTS AND MECHANISMS OF ACTION   Topiramate reduces voltage-gated Na^+ currents in cerebellar granule cells and may act in a manner similar to phenytoin. In addition, topiramate activates a hyperpolarizing K^+ current, enhances postsynaptic $GABA_A$-receptor currents, and also limits activation of the AMPA-kainate-subtype(s) of glutamate receptor. Topiramate also is a weak carbonic anhydrase inhibitor.

PHARMACOKINETICS   Topiramate is rapidly absorbed after oral administration, exhibits little (10–20%) binding to plasma proteins, and is mainly excreted unchanged in the urine. Its $t_{1/2}$ is ~1 day. Reduced plasma concentrations of estradiol occur with concurrent topiramate, suggesting that low-dose oral contraceptives should be avoided in this setting.

THERAPEUTIC USE   Topiramate is equivalent to valproic acid and carbamazepine in children and adults with newly diagnosed partial and primary generalized epilepsy; the drug is also effective as monotherapy for refractory partial epilepsy and refractory generalized tonic-clonic seizures. Topiramate also is more effective than placebo against both drop attacks and tonic-clonic seizures in patients with Lennox-Gastaut syndrome.

TOXICITY   Topiramate is well tolerated. Common adverse effects are somnolence, fatigue, weight loss, and nervousness. The drug can precipitate renal calculi (probably due to inhibition of carbonic anhydrase). Topiramate has been associated with cognitive impairment; patients may also complain about a change in the taste of carbonated beverages.

Zonisamide

Zonisamide (ZONEGRAN) is a sulfonamide derivative.

PHARMACOLOGICAL EFFECTS AND MECHANISM OF ACTION   Zonisamide inhibits both the T-type Ca^{2+} currents and the sustained, repetitive firing of spinal cord neurons, presumably by prolonging the inactivated state of voltage-gated Na^+ channels in a manner similar to that of phenytoin and carbamazepine.

PHARMACOKINETICS   Zonisamide is almost completely absorbed after oral administration, has a long $t_{1/2}$ (~63 hours), and is ~40% bound to plasma protein. Approximately 85% of an oral dose is excreted in the urine, principally as unmetabolized zonisamide and a glucuronide of the CYP3A4 metabolite, sulfamoylacetyl phenol. Phenobarbital, phenytoin, and carbamazepine decrease the plasma concentration/dose ratio of zonisamide, whereas lamotrigine increases this ratio. Zonisamide has little effect on the plasma concentrations of other antiseizure drugs.

THERAPEUTIC USE   Clinical trials of patients with refractory partial seizures demonstrated that addition of zonisamide to other drugs was superior to placebo. Its efficacy as monotherapy for newly diagnosed or refractory epilepsy remains unproven.

TOXICITY   Zonisamide is well tolerated. Adverse effects include somnolence, ataxia, anorexia, nervousness, and fatigue. Approximately 1% of individuals develop renal calculi during treatment with zonisamide, probably related to its ability to inhibit carbonic anhydrase.

GENERAL PRINCIPLES AND CHOICE OF DRUGS FOR THE THERAPY OF THE EPILEPSIES

Early diagnosis and treatment of seizure disorders with a single appropriate agent offers the best prospect of achieving prolonged seizure-free periods with the lowest risk of toxicity (*see* Table 19–1). A balancing of efficacy and unwanted effects in the individual patient provides the optimal therapeutic choice.

The first consideration is whether to initiate treatment. For example, drug therapy may not be necessary after an isolated tonic-clonic seizure in a healthy young adult who lacks a family history of epilepsy and who has a normal neurological exam, EEG, and brain magnetic resonance imaging (MRI) scan—a setting where the risk of a drug reaction approximates the likelihood of seizure recurrence in the next year (15%). Alternatively, a similar seizure occurring in an individual with a positive family history of epilepsy, an abnormal neurological exam, an abnormal EEG, and an abnormal MRI carries a recurrence risk of 60% that favors initiation of therapy.

Unless extenuating circumstances exist (*e.g.*, status epilepticus), therapy should be initiated with a single drug, typically in dosage expected to provide a plasma concentration in the lower portion of the therapeutic range. To minimize dose-related adverse effects, therapy may be initiated at reduced dosage, increasing dosage at appropriate intervals, as required for control of seizures or as limited by toxicity, preferably assisted by monitoring of plasma drug concentrations.

Faulty compliance is the most frequent cause for failure of therapy with antiseizure drugs; regularity of medication is essential. Compliance with a properly selected, single drug in maximal tolerated dosage results in complete control of seizures in ~50% of patients. If a seizure occurs despite therapeutic drug levels, the physician should assess the presence of potential precipitating factor (*e.g.*, sleep deprivation, concurrent febrile illness, or drugs, including caffeine or over-the-counter medications). If compliance is confirmed yet seizures persist, another drug should be substituted. Unless serious adverse effects of the drug dictate otherwise, dosage always should be reduced gradually when a drug is discontinued to minimize risk of seizure recurrence. In the case of partial seizures in adults, the diversity of available drugs permits selection of a second drug that acts by a distinct mechanism.

In the event that therapy with a second single drug also is inadequate, many physicians resort to treatment with two drugs simultaneously. This decision should not be taken lightly, because most patients obtain optimal seizure control with fewest unwanted effects when taking a single drug. Nonetheless, some patients will not be controlled adequately without the simultaneous use of two or more antiseizure drugs. No properly controlled studies have systematically compared one particular drug combination with another, and the chances of complete control with this approach are not high. It seems wise to select two drugs that act by distinct mechanisms (*e.g.*, one that promotes Na^+ channel inactivation, another that enhances GABA-mediated synaptic inhibition). Additional issues are the unwanted effects of each drug and the potential drug interactions. Many of these drugs induce expression of CYPs and thereby alter the metabolism of themselves and/or other drugs (*see* Table 19–2).

DURATION OF THERAPY

Antiseizure drugs are typically continued for at least 2 years. If the patient is seizure-free after 2 years, consideration should be given to discontinuing therapy. Factors associated with high risk for recurrent seizures following drug discontinuation include EEG abnormalities, a known structural lesion, abnormalities on neurological exam, and history of frequent seizures or medically refractory seizures prior to control. Conversely, factors associated with low risk for recurrent seizures include idiopathic epilepsy, normal EEG, onset in childhood, and seizures easily controlled with a single drug. The risk of recurrent seizures is ~25% in low-risk individuals and >50% in high-risk individuals. Typically, 80% of recurrences occur within 4 months of discontinuing therapy. The clinician and patient must weigh the risk of recurrent seizure and the associated potential deleterious consequences (e.g., loss of driving privileges) against the implications of continuing medication (e.g., cost, unwanted effects, implications of diagnosis of epilepsy). Ideally, tapering is performed over a period of several months.

SIMPLE AND COMPLEX PARTIAL AND SECONDARILY GENERALIZED TONIC-CLONIC SEIZURES

Carbamazepine and phenytoin are the most effective overall drugs for monotherapy of partial or generalized tonic-clonic seizures. The choice between carbamazepine and phenytoin requires assessment of toxic effects of each drug. Decreased libido and impotence were associated with both drugs (carbamazepine 13%, phenytoin 11%). Between carbamazepine and valproic acid, carbamazepine provides superior control of complex partial seizures. Overall, data demonstrate that carbamazepine and phenytoin are preferable for treatment of partial seizures, but phenobarbital and valproic acid are also efficacious. Control of secondarily generalized tonic-clonic seizures does not differ significantly with carbamazepine, phenobarbital, or phenytoin, and valproic acid is as effective as carbamazepine. Since secondarily generalized tonic-clonic seizures usually coexist with partial seizures, these data indicate that among drugs introduced before 1990, carbamazepine and phenytoin are the first-line drugs here.

A key issue is choosing the optimal drug for initiating treatment in the patient newly diagnosed with partial or generalized onset epilepsy. This issue may appear unimportant since ~50% of newly diagnosed patients become seizure free with the first drug, whether old or new drugs are used. However, responsive patients typically receive the initial drug for several years, underscoring the importance of proper drug selection. Phenytoin, carbamazepine, and phenobarbital induce hepatic CYPs, thereby complicating use of multiple antiseizure drugs as well as impacting metabolism of oral contraceptives, warfarin, and others. These drugs also enhance metabolism of endogenous compounds including gonadal steroids and vitamin D, potentially impacting reproductive function and bone density. By contrast, most of the newer drugs have little if any effect on the CYPs. Factors arguing against use of recently introduced drugs include higher costs and less clinical experience with the compounds. Unfortunately, prospective studies comparing newly introduced antiseizure drugs with drugs available before 1990 have not been performed such that one drug can be declared clearly superior. Although many experts advocate the use of gabapentin, lamotrigine, and topiramate as initial therapy for newly diagnosed partial or mixed seizure disorders, none of these drugs is FDA-approved for these indications.

ABSENCE SEIZURES

Data indicate that ethosuximide and valproic acid are equally effective in the treatment of absence seizures; 50–75% of newly diagnosed patients can be rendered free of seizures following therapy with either drug. In the event that tonic-clonic seizures are present or emerge during therapy, valproic acid is the agent of first choice. Lamotrigine is also effective for newly diagnosed absence epilepsy but is not FDA-approved for this indication.

MYOCLONIC SEIZURES

Valproic acid is the drug of choice for myoclonic seizures in juvenile myoclonic epilepsy, in which myoclonic seizures often coexist with tonic-clonic and absence seizures. No trials have examined any of the newly introduced drugs for patients with juvenile myoclonic epilepsy or other idiopathic generalized epilepsy syndromes.

FEBRILE CONVULSIONS

Two to four percent of children experience a convulsion associated with a febrile illness; 25–33% of these will have another febrile convulsion. Only 2–3% become epileptic in later years. Several factors are associated with an increased risk of developing epilepsy: preexisting neurological disorder or developmental delay, a family history of epilepsy, or a complicated febrile seizure (i.e., the febrile seizure lasted more than 15 minutes, was one-sided, or was followed by a second seizure in the same day). If all of these risk factors are present, the risk of developing epilepsy is ~10%. For children at high risk of developing recurrent febrile seizures and epilepsy, rectally administered diazepam at the onset of fever may prevent recurrent seizures and avoid side effects of chronic therapy. Uncertain efficacy and substantial side effects argue against the use of chronic phenobarbital therapy for prophylactic purposes in this condition.

SEIZURES IN INFANTS AND YOUNG CHILDREN

Infantile spasms with hypsarrhythmia are refractory to the usual antiseizure agents; glucocorticoids are commonly used. Vigabatrin (γ-vinyl GABA) is efficacious in comparison to placebo, although constriction of visual fields has been reported in some adults treated with vigabatrin. Vigabatrin has orphan drug status in the U.S. for the treatment of infantile spasms and is available elsewhere.

Lennox-Gastaut syndrome is a severe form of epilepsy that usually begins in childhood and is characterized by cognitive impairments and multiple types of seizures including tonic-clonic, tonic, atonic, myoclonic, and atypical absence seizures. Lamotrigine is an effective and well-tolerated drug for this treatment-resistant form of epilepsy; addition of lamotrigine to other antiseizure drugs may improve seizure control. Topiramate also has demonstrated efficacy in Lennox-Gastaut syndrome.

STATUS EPILEPTICUS AND OTHER CONVULSIVE EMERGENCIES

Status epilepticus is a neurological emergency. Mortality for adults is ~20%. The goal of treatment is rapid termination of behavioral and electrical seizure activity; the longer the episode of status epilepticus is untreated, the more difficult it is to control and the greater the risk of permanent brain damage. Critical to the management are a clear plan, prompt treatment with effective drugs in adequate doses, and attention to hypoventilation and hypotension. Since the high doses of drugs used may cause hypoventilation, it may be necessary to assist respiration temporarily. Drugs should be administered intravenously. Four regimens have similar success rates of 44–65%: diazepam followed by phenytoin; lorazepam; phenobarbital; and phenytoin alone. Studies show no significant differences with respect to recurrences or adverse reactions.

ANTISEIZURE THERAPY AND PREGNANCY

Antiseizure therapy has importance implications for women's health. The efficacy of oral contraceptives is reduced by concomitant use of antiseizure drugs (failure rate of 3.1/100 years versus 0.7/100 years in nonepileptic controls); this may relate to the increased rate of oral contraceptive metabolism caused by antiseizure drugs that induce hepatic enzymes (Table 19–2); particular caution is needed with antiseizure drugs that induce CYP3A4.

Infants of epileptic mothers are at twice the risk of major congenital malformations than offspring of nonepileptic mothers. These malformations include congenital heart defects and neural tube defects. A causal role for antiseizure drugs is suggested by association of congenital defects with higher concentrations of a drug or with polytherapy compared to monotherapy. Phenytoin, carbamazepine, valproate, and phenobarbital all have been associated with teratogenic effects. The antiseizure drugs introduced after 1990 have teratogenic effects in animals but whether such effects occur in humans is uncertain. One consideration for a woman with epilepsy who wishes to become pregnant is a trial period without antiseizure medication; monotherapy with careful attention to drug levels is another alternative. Polytherapy with toxic levels should be avoided. Folate supplementation (0.4 mg/day) is recommended for all women of childbearing age to reduce the likelihood of neural tube defects, and this is appropriate for epileptic women as well.

Antiseizure drugs that induce CYPs are associated with vitamin K deficiency in the newborn, possibly resulting in coagulopathy and intracerebral hemorrhage. Treatment of the mother with vitamin K_1, 10 mg/day during the last 2–4 weeks of gestation, has been recommended for prophylaxis.

For a complete Bibliographical listing see Goodman & Gilman's *The Pharmacological Basis of Therapeutics*, 11th ed., or Goodman & Gilman Online at www.accessmedicine.com.

20

TREATMENT OF CENTRAL NERVOUS SYSTEM DEGENERATIVE DISORDERS

Parkinson's disease (PD), Huntington's disease (HD), Alzheimer's disease (AD), and amyotrophic lateral sclerosis (ALS) are characterized by progressive and irreversible loss of neurons from specific regions of the brain. The pharmacotherapy of these neurodegenerative disorders is limited mostly to symptomatic treatments that do not alter the course of the underlying disease.

SELECTIVE NEURONAL VULNERABILITY

A striking feature of these disease processes is their specificity for particular types of neurons. In PD there is extensive destruction of the dopaminergic neurons of the substantia nigra; neurons in the cortex and many other areas of the brain are unaffected. In contrast, neural injury in AD is most severe in the hippocampus and neocortex, and even varies dramatically in different functional cortical regions. In HD, the mutant gene responsible for the disorder is expressed throughout the brain and in many other organs, yet the pathological changes are most prominent in the neostriatum. In ALS, there is loss of spinal motor neurons and the cortical neurons that provide their descending input. Currently, the processes of neural injury are viewed as the interaction of genetic and environmental influences with the intrinsic physiological characteristics of the affected populations of neurons.

Genetic predisposition plays a role in the etiology of neurodegenerative disorders. HD is transmitted by autosomal dominant inheritance, and the molecular nature of the genetic defect has been defined (*see* below). Most cases of PD, AD, or ALS are sporadic, but familial links occur and studies of familial disease are yielding clues to the pathogenesis of the disorders. Mutations in four different proteins can lead to genetically determined forms of PD: α-synuclein, an abundant synaptic protein; parkin, a ubiquitin hydrolase; UCHL1, which also participates in ubiquitin-mediated degradation of proteins in the brain; and DJ-1, a protein thought to be involved in the neuronal response to stress. Mutations in the genes encoding the amyloid precursor protein (APP) and proteins known as the presenilins, which may be involved in APP processing, lead to inherited forms of AD. Mutations in the gene encoding copper-zinc superoxide dismutase (*SOD1*) account for ~2% of cases of adult-onset ALS.

Apolipoprotein E (apoE) is a genetic risk factor for AD. There are four distinct isoforms of apoE, which is involved in transport of cholesterol and lipids in blood. Although all the isoforms function equally well, individuals who are homozygous for the apoE 4 allele ("4/4") have a much higher lifetime risk of AD than do those homozygous for the apoE 2 allele ("2/2"). The mechanism by which the apoE 4 protein increases the risk of AD is not known.

The decline in metabolic activity with age, oxidative stress, and the local production of oxygen radicals from the metabolism of dopamine via the Fenton reaction (Figure 20–1) may play roles in the etiology of some of these diseases.

PARKINSON'S DISEASE

CLINICAL OVERVIEW AND PATHOPHYSIOLOGY Parkinsonism has four cardinal features: bradykinesia (slowness and poverty of movement), muscular rigidity, resting tremor (which usually abates during voluntary movement), and an impairment of postural balance leading to disturbances of gait and falling. The pathological hallmark of PD is a loss of the pigmented, dopaminergic neurons of the substantia nigra pars compacta (SNpc) that provide dopaminergic innervation to the striatum (caudate and putamen). Progressive loss of dopaminergic neurons is a feature of normal aging; however, symptoms of PD coincide with excessive loss (70–80%) of these neurons. Without treatment, PD progresses over 5–10 years to a rigid, akinetic state in which patients are incapable of caring for themselves. Death frequently results from complications of immobility, including aspiration pneumonia or pulmonary embolism. The availability of effective pharmacological treatment has altered radically the prognosis of PD; in most cases, good functional mobility can be maintained for many years, and the life expectancy increased substantially. Several disorders other than PD also may produce parkinsonism, including some relatively rare neurodegenerative disorders, stroke, and intoxication with dopamine-receptor antagonists. Drugs in common clinical use that may cause parkinsonism include antipsychotics such as *haloperidol* and *thorazine* (*see* Chapter 18) and antiemetics such as *prochloperazine* and *metoclopramide* (*see* Chapter 37). Parkinsonism arising from other causes usually is refractory to all forms of treatment.

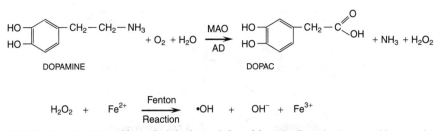

$$H_2O_2 + Fe^{2+} \xrightarrow[\text{Reaction}]{\text{Fenton}} \cdot OH + OH^- + Fe^{3+}$$

FIGURE 20–1 *Production of free radicals by the metabolism of dopamine.* Dopamine is converted by monamine oxidase (MAO) and aldehyde dehydrogenase (AD) to 3,4-dihydroxyphenylacetic acid (DOPAC), producing hydrogen peroxide (H_2O_2). In the presence of ferrous iron, H_2O_2 undergoes spontaneous conversion, forming a hydroxyl-free radical (the Fenton reaction).

DOPAMINE SYNTHESIS, METABOLISM, AND ACTION

Dopamine, a catecholamine, is synthesized in the terminals of dopaminergic neurons from tyrosine and stored, released, and metabolized by processes described in Chapter 6 and summarized in Figures 20–2 and 20–3. The actions of dopamine in the brain are mediated by dopamine receptors, all of which are heptahelical G protein–coupled receptors (GPCRs) (see Chapter 1). The five dopamine receptors can be divided into two groups on the basis of their pharmacological and structural properties (Figure 20–4). The D_1 and D_5 proteins have a long intracellular carboxyterminal tail and are members of the class defined pharmacologically as D_1; they stimulate the formation of cyclic AMP and phosphatidyl inositol hydrolysis. The D_2, D_3, and D_4 receptors share a large third intracellular loop and are of the D_2 class. They decrease cyclic AMP formation and modulate K^+ and Ca^{2+} currents. Each of the five dopamine receptor proteins has a distinct anatomical distribution in the brain. The D_1 and D_2 proteins are abundant in the striatum and are the most important receptor sites with regard to the causes and treatment of PD. The D_4 and D_5 proteins are largely extrastriatal, whereas D_3 expression is low in the caudate and putamen but more abundant in the nucleus accumbens and olfactory tubercle.

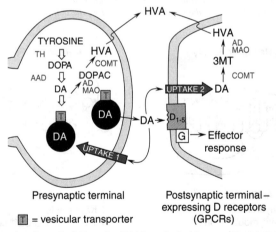

Presynaptic terminal

Postsynaptic terminal– expressing D receptors (GPCRs)

⊤ = vesicular transporter

FIGURE 20–2 *Dopaminergic terminal.* Dopamine (DA) is synthesized in neuronal terminals from tyrosine by the sequential actions of tyrosine hydroxylase (TH), producing the intermediary L-dihydroxyphenylalanine (L-DOPA), and aromatic L-amino acid decarboxylase (AAD). In the terminal, DA is transported into storage vesicles by a vesicular membrane transporter (T). Release, triggered by depolarization and entry of Ca^{2+}, allows dopamine to act on a variety of postsynaptic GPCRs for DA. The D_1 and D_2 receptors are important in brain regions involved in PD. The differential actions of DA on postsynaptic targets bearing different types of DA receptors have important implications for the function of neural circuits. The actions of DA are terminated by reuptake into the nerve terminal (where DA may be restored or metabolized) or uptake into the postsynaptic cell (where DA is metabolized). Metabolism occurs by the sequential actions of the enzymes catechol-O-methyltransferase (COMT), monoamine oxidase (MAO), and aldehyde dehydrogenase (AD). 3MT, 3-methoxytyramine; DOPAC, 3,4-dihydroxyphenylacetic acid; HVA, 3-methoxy-4-hydroxy-phenylacetic acid (see Figure 20–3). In humans, HVA is the principal metabolite of DA. (From Cooper *et al.*, 1996, with permission.)

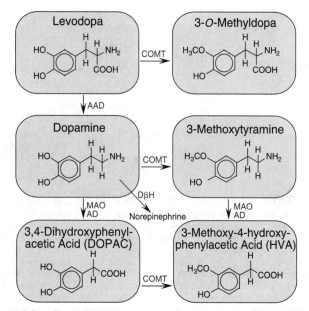

FIGURE 20-3 *Metabolism of levodopa (L-DOPA).* AD, aldehyde dehydrogenase; COMT, catechol-O-methyltransferase; DβH, dopamine βhydroxylase; AAD, aromatic L-amino acid decarboxylase; MAO, monoamine oxidase.

NEURAL MECHANISM OF PARKINSONISM

The basal ganglia can be viewed as a modulatory side loop that regulates the flow of information from the cerebral cortex to the motor neurons of the spinal cord (Figure 20–5). The net effect of stimulation of the direct pathway at the level of the striatum is to increase the excitatory outflow from the thalamus to the cortex; the net effect of stimulating the indirect pathway at the level of

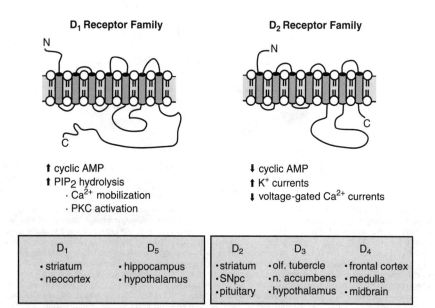

FIGURE 20-4 *Distribution and characteristics of dopamine receptors in the central nervous system.* SNpc, substantia nigra pars compacta.

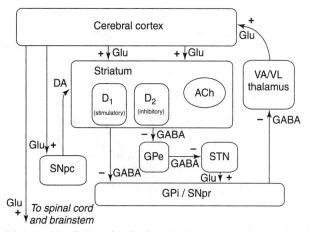

FIGURE 20–5 *Schematic wiring diagram of the basal ganglia.* The striatum is the principal input structure of the basal ganglia and receives excitatory glutamatergic input from many areas of cerebral cortex. The striatum contains projection neurons expressing predominantly D_1 or D_2 dopamine receptors, as well as interneurons that use acetylcholine (ACh) as a neurotransmitter. Outflow from the striatum proceeds along two routes. The direct pathway, from the striatum to the substantia nigra pars reticulata (SNpr) and globus pallidus interna (GPi), uses the inhibitory transmitter GABA. The indirect pathway, from the striatum through the globus pallidus externa (GPe) and the subthalamic nucleus (STN) to the SNpr and GPi consists of two inhibitory GABAergic links and one excitatory glutamatergic projection (Glu). The substantia nigra pars compacta (SNpc) provides dopaminergic innervation to the striatal neurons, giving rise to both the direct and indirect pathways, and regulates the relative activity of these two paths. The SNpr and GPi are the output structures of the basal ganglia and provide feedback to the cerebral cortex through the ventroanterior and ventrolateral nuclei of the thalamus (VA/VL).

the striatum is to reduce the excitatory outflow from the thalamus to the cerebral cortex. The key feature of this model of basal ganglia function that accounts for the symptoms observed in PD as a result of loss of dopaminergic neurons is the differential effect of dopamine on the direct and indirect pathways (Figure 20–6). The striatal neurons of the direct pathway express primarily the excitatory D_1 dopamine receptor protein, whereas the striatal neurons forming the indirect pathway

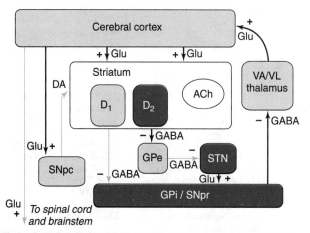

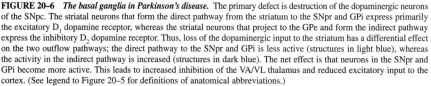

FIGURE 20–6 *The basal ganglia in Parkinson's disease.* The primary defect is destruction of the dopaminergic neurons of the SNpc. The striatal neurons that form the direct pathway from the striatum to the SNpr and GPi express primarily the excitatory D_1 dopamine receptor, whereas the striatal neurons that project to the GPe and form the indirect pathway express the inhibitory D_2 dopamine receptor. Thus, loss of the dopaminergic input to the striatum has a differential effect on the two outflow pathways; the direct pathway to the SNpr and GPi is less active (structures in light blue), whereas the activity in the indirect pathway is increased (structures in dark blue). The net effect is that neurons in the SNpr and GPi become more active. This leads to increased inhibition of the VA/VL thalamus and reduced excitatory input to the cortex. (See legend to Figure 20–5 for definitions of anatomical abbreviations.)

express primarily the inhibitory D_2 *type. Thus, dopamine released in the striatum tends to increase the activity of the direct pathway and reduce the activity of the indirect pathway. The net effect of the reduced dopaminergic input in PD is to increase markedly the inhibitory outflow from the SNpr and globus pallidus interna (GPi) to the thalamus and reduce excitation of the motor cortex. Despite limitations, the model has utility for the rational design and use of pharmacological agents in PD. First, it suggests that to restore the balance of the system through stimulation of dopamine receptors, the complementary effect of actions at both D_1 and D_2 receptors, as well as the possibility of adverse effects that may be mediated by D_3, D_4, or D_5 receptors, must be considered. Second, it explains why replacement of dopamine is not the only approach to the treatment of PD. Drugs that inhibit cholinergic receptors are also effective; although their mechanisms of action are not completely understood, their effects are likely mediated at the level of the striatal projection neurons, which normally receive cholinergic input from striatal cholinergic interneurons. Few clinically useful drugs for parkinsonism are presently available based on actions through γ-aminobutyric acid (GABA) and glutamate receptors.*

TREATMENT OF PARKINSON'S DISEASE

Commonly used medications and their dosage ranges for the treatment of PD are summarized in Table 20–1.

Levodopa

Levodopa (L-DOPA, LARODOPA, L-3,4-dihydroxyphenylalanine), the metabolic precursor of dopamine, is the single most-effective agent in the treatment of PD; the therapeutic and adverse effects of levodopa result from its decarboxylation to dopamine. Oral levodopa is absorbed rapidly from the small bowel by the transport system for aromatic amino acids. Concentrations of the drug in plasma usually peak between 0.5 and 2 hours after an oral dose. The $t_{1/2}$ in plasma is short (1–3 hours). The rate and extent of absorption of levodopa depend on the rate of gastric emptying, the pH of gastric juice, and the length of time the drug is exposed to the degradative enzymes of the gastric and intestinal mucosa. Competition for absorption sites in the small bowel from dietary amino acids also may alter absorption of levodopa; administration of levodopa with meals delays absorption and reduces peak plasma concentrations. A membrane transporter for aromatic amino acids facilitates entry of the drug into the CNS, and competition between dietary protein and levodopa may occur at this level. In the brain, levodopa is converted to dopamine by decarboxylation, primarily within the

Table 20–1

Commonly Used Medications for the Treatment of Parkinson's Disease

Agent	Typical Initial Dose	Total Daily Dose—Useful Range	Comments
Carbidopa/levodopa	25 mg carbidopa + 100 mg levodopa ("25/100" tablet), twice or three times a day	200–1200 mg levodopa	
Carbidopa/levodopa sustained release	50 mg carbidopa + 200 mg levodopa ("50/200 sustained release" tablet) twice a day	200–1200 mg levodopa	Bioavailability 75% of immediate release form
Bromocriptine	1.25 mg twice a day	3.75–40 mg	Titrate slowly
Pergolide*	0.05 mg once a day	0.75–5 mg	Titrate slowly
Ropinirole	0.25 mg three times a day	1.5–24 mg	
Pramipexole	0.125 mg three times a day	1.5–4.5 mg	
Entacapone	200 mg with each dose of levodopa/carbidopa	600–2000 mg	
Tolcapone	100 mg twice a day or three times a day	200–600 mg	May be hepatotoxic; requires monitoring of liver enzymes
Selegiline	5 mg twice a day	2.5–10 mg	
Amantadine	100 mg twice a day	100–200 mg	
Trihexyphenidyl HCl	1 mg twice a day	2–15 mg	

*Withdrawn in U.S. due to reports of cardiac valvular disease associated with long-term use.

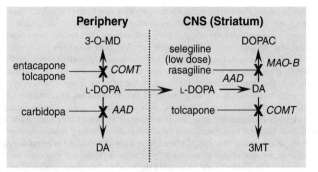

FIGURE 20-7 *Pharmacological preservation of L-DOPA and striatal dopamine.* The principal site of action of inhibitors of catechol-O-methyltransferase (COMT) (such as tolcapone and entacapone) is in the peripheral circulation. They block the O-methylation of levodopa (L-DOPA) and increase the fraction of the drug available for delivery to the brain. Tolcapone also has effects in the CNS. Inhibitors of MAO-B, such as low-dose selegiline and rasagiline, will act within the CNS to reduce oxidative deamination of DA, thereby enhancing vesicular stores. AAD, aromatic L-amino acid decarboxylase; DA, dopamine; DOPAC, 3,4-dihydroxyphenylacetic acid; MAO, monoamine oxidase; 3MT, 3-methoxyltyramine; 3-O-MD, 3-O-methyl DOPA.

presynaptic terminals of dopaminergic neurons in the stratium. The dopamine thus produced is responsible for the therapeutic effectiveness of levodopa in PD; after release, the dopamine is either transported back into dopaminergic terminals or postsynaptic cells, where it may be restored in granules (neurons) or metabolized by MAO and COMT (neurons and nonneurons) (Figure 20-3).

In practice, levodopa is generally administered with a peripherally acting inhibitor of aromatic L-amino acid decarboxylase (AAD) (*e.g.*, carbidopa, benserazide) that does not penetrate well into the CNS. In the absence of decarboxylase inhibition, levodopa is largely decarboxylated in the intestinal mucosa and at other peripheral sites so that little of the parent drug reaches the cerebral circulation and probably <1% penetrates the CNS. Inhibition of peripheral decarboxylase markedly increases the fraction of administered levodopa that remains unmetabolized and available to cross the blood–brain barrier (*see* Figure 20-7) and reduces the incidence of nausea and other GI side effects due to peripheral conversion of the drug to dopamine. Generally, a dose of 75 mg/day of carbidopa is sufficient to prevent the development of nausea. For this reason, the most commonly prescribed form of carbidopa/levodopa (SINEMET, ATAMET) is the *25/100* form, containing 25 mg carbidopa and 100 mg levodopa, 3–4 times daily. Administration of supplemental carbidopa (LODOSYN) may be beneficial in refractory cases.

Levodopa therapy can affect all the signs and symptoms of PD. In early PD, the duration of the beneficial effects of levodopa may exceed the plasma lifetime of the drug, suggesting that the nigrostriatal dopamine system retains some capacity to store and release dopamine. A principal limitation of the long-term use of levodopa therapy is that with time this apparent "buffering" capacity is lost, and the patient's motor state may fluctuate dramatically with each dose of levodopa. A common problem is the development of the "wearing off" phenomenon: each dose of levodopa effectively improves mobility for a period of time, perhaps 1–2 hours, but rigidity and akinesia return rapidly at the end of the dosing interval. Increasing the dose and frequency of administration can improve this situation, but this often is limited by the development of *dyskinesias*, excessive and abnormal involuntary movements that occur most often when the plasma levodopa concentration is high. Dyskinesias or dystonia may be triggered when the level is rising or falling, and these movements can be as uncomfortable and disabling as the rigidity and akinesia of PD. In the later stages of PD, patients may fluctuate rapidly between being "off," having no beneficial effects from their medications, and being "on" but with disabling dyskinesias, a situation called the *on/off phenomenon.*

Due to the on/off phenomena and concerns about the exact role of dopamine's contribution to free radical generation and tissue damage, most practitioners use levodopa only when the symptoms of PD cause functional impairment. When levodopa levels are maintained constant by intravenous infusion, dyskinesias and fluctuations are greatly reduced, and the clinical improvement is maintained for up to several days after returning to oral levodopa dosing. A sustained-release formulation and division of the total daily dose into more frequently administered portions have been used to overcome the on/off phenomenon.

In addition to motor fluctuations and nausea, several other adverse effects may be observed with levodopa treatment. A common and dose-limiting adverse effect is the induction of hallucinations and confusion, particularly in the elderly and in those with preexisting cognitive dysfunction. Conventional antipsychotic agents, such as the phenothiazines, are effective against levodopa-induced psychosis but may cause marked worsening of parkinsonism, probably through actions at the D_2 dopamine receptor. A recent approach has been to use the "atypical" antipsychotic agents (e.g., clozapine and quetiapine), which are effective in the treatment of psychosis but do not cause or worsen parkinsonism. Peripheral decarboxylation of levodopa and release of dopamine into the circulation may activate vascular dopamine receptors and produce orthostatic hypotension. Actions of dopamine at α and β adrenergic receptors may induce cardiac arrhythmias, especially in patients with preexisting conduction disturbances. Administration of levodopa with nonspecific inhibitors of MAO (e.g., phenelzine, tranylcypromine) accentuates the actions of levodopa and may precipitate life-threatening hypertensive crisis and hyperpyrexia; nonspecific MAO inhibitors must be discontinued at least 14 days before levodopa is administered (note that this prohibition does not include the MAO-B subtype-specific inhibitor selegiline, which, as discussed below, often is administered safely in combination with levodopa). Abrupt withdrawal of levodopa or other dopaminergic medications may precipitate the neuroleptic malignant syndrome more commonly observed after treatment with dopamine antagonists.

DOPAMINE-RECEPTOR AGONISTS Direct agonists of striatal dopamine receptors offer several potential advantages. Since enzymatic conversion of these drugs is not required for activity, they do not depend on the functional capacities of the nigrostriatal neurons. Most dopamine-receptor agonists in clinical use have durations of action substantially longer than that of levodopa and are useful in the management of dose-related fluctuations in motor state. Finally, if free radical formation from dopamine metabolism actually contributes to neuronal death, then dopamine-receptor agonists may modify the course of the disease by reducing endogenous release of dopamine as well as the need for exogenous levodopa.

Four orally administered dopamine-receptor agonists are available for treatment of PD: two older agents, *bromocriptine* (PARLODEL) and *pergolide* (PERMAX); and two newer, more selective compounds, *ropinirole* (REQUIP) and *pramipexole* (MIRPEX). Bromocriptine and pergolide are ergot derivatives with similar therapeutic actions and adverse effects. Bromocriptine is a D_2 agonist and a partial D_1 antagonist; pergolide is an agonist of both receptor types. Ropinirole and pramipexole have selective activity at D_2 and D_3 receptors and little or no activity at receptors of the D_1 class. All four drugs are well absorbed orally and can relieve the clinical symptoms of PD. The duration of action of the dopamine agonists (8–24 hours) often is longer than that of levodopa (6–8 hours), and they are particularly effective in the treatment of patients who have developed on/off phenomena. All four also may produce hallucinosis or confusion and may worsen orthostatic hypotension.

The principal distinction between the newer agents and the older ergot derivatives is in their tolerability and speed of titration. Initial treatment with bromocriptine or pergolide may cause nausea, fatigue, and profound hypotension; they should be initiated at low dosage. Symptoms usually are transient, but require slow upward adjustment of the dose over a period of weeks to months. Ropinirole and pramipexole can be initiated more quickly, achieving therapeutically useful doses in a week or less. They generally cause less GI disturbance than do the ergot derivatives, but they can produce nausea and somnolence. The somnolence can be quite severe; and it is prudent to advise patients of this possibility and to switch to another treatment if sleepiness interferes with daily life or poses a hazard (driving, *etc.*). Recent reports have associated long-term use of pergolide with significant cardiac valvular disease, and the drug has been withdrawn from the U.S. market.

The introduction of pramipexole and ropinirole has changed the clinical use of dopamine agonists in PD. These selective agonists are well tolerated and are used increasingly as initial treatment for PD rather than as adjuncts to levodopa. This change has been driven by two factors: (1) the belief that because of their longer duration of action, dopamine agonists may be less likely than levodopa to induce on/off effects and dyskinesias and (2) the concern that levodopa may contribute to oxidative stress, thereby accelerating loss of dopaminergic neurons. Many experts favor dopamine agonists as initial therapy in younger patients with PD and levodopa as the initial treatment in older patients who may be more vulnerable to the adverse cognitive effects of the agonists.

Apomorphine (APOKYN) is a dopaminergic agonist that can be administered by subcutaneous injection. It has high affinity for D_4 receptors; moderate affinity for D_2, D_3, D_5, and adrenergic α_{1D}, α_{2B}, and α_{2C} receptors; and low affinity for D_1 receptors. Apomorphine is used as a "rescue therapy" for the acute intermittent treatment of "off" episodes in patients with a fluctuating response to dopaminergic therapy. Apomorphine shares the side effects of the oral dopamine agonists; it is highly emetogenic and requires pre- and posttreatment antiemetic therapy (generally, oral trimethobenzamide [TIGAN, 300 mg three times daily], started 3 days prior to the initial dose of apomorphine and continued at least during the first 2 months of therapy). Based on reports of profound hypotension and loss of consciousness when apomorphine is administered with ondansetron, the concomitant use of apomorphine with antiemetic drugs of the 5-HT_3 antagonist class is contraindicated. Other potentially serious side effects of apomorphine include QT prolongation, injection-site reactions, and the development of a pattern of abuse characterized by increasingly frequent dosing leading to hallucinations, dyskinesia, and abnormal behavior. Because of these potential adverse effects, use of apomorphine is appropriate only when other measures, such as oral dopamine agonists or COMT inhibitors, have failed to control the "off" episodes. Apomorphine therapy should be initiated in a setting where the patient can be monitored carefully, beginning with a 2-mg test dose. If this is tolerated, apomorphine can be titrated slowly up to a maximum dosage of 6 mg. For effective control of symptoms, patients may require three or more injections daily.

CATECHOL-O-METHYLTRANSFERASE INHIBITORS Catechol-O-Methyltransferase (COMT) metabolizes levodopa as well as dopamine, producing the pharmacologically inactive compounds 3-O-methyl DOPA (from levodopa) and 3-methoxytyramine (from dopamine) (Figure 20–7). Approximately 99% of an orally administered dose of levodopa does not reach the brain but, rather, is decarboxylated to dopamine, which causes nausea and hypotension. Addition of an AAD inhibitor (e.g., carbidopa) reduces the formation of dopamine but increases the fraction of levodopa that is methylated by COMT. COMT inhibitors will block this peripheral conversion of levodopa to 3-O-methyl DOPA, increasing both the plasma $t_{1/2}$ of levodopa as well as the fraction that reaches the CNS.

Two COMT inhibitors are available for this use, *tolcapone* (TASMAR) and *entacapone* (COMTAN). Tolcapone has a relatively long duration of action, allowing for administration two to three times a day, and appears to act by both central and peripheral inhibition of COMT. The duration of action of entacapone is short, around 2 hours, so it usually is administered simultaneously with each dose of levodopa/carbidopa. The action of entacapone is attributable principally to peripheral inhibition of COMT. The common adverse effects of these agents are similar to those observed in patients treated with levodopa/carbidopa alone and include nausea, orthostatic hypotension, vivid dreams, confusion, and hallucinations. An adverse effect associated with tolcapone is hepatotoxicity; tolcapone should be used only in patients who have not responded to other therapies and with appropriate monitoring of hepatic transaminases. Entacapone has not been associated with hepatotoxicity and requires no special monitoring. Entacapone also is available in fixed-dose combinations with levodopa/carbidopa (STALEVO).

SELECTIVE MAO-B INHIBITORS Two isozymes of MAO (MAO-A and MAO-B) oxidize monoamines and both are present in the periphery and GI tract; MAO-B is the predominant form in the striatum and is responsible for most of the oxidative metabolism of dopamine in the brain. At low-to-moderate doses (10 mg/day or less), *selegiline* (ELDEPRYL) selectively and irreversibly inhibits MAO-B. Unlike nonspecific inhibitors of MAO (e.g., phenelzine, tranylcypromine, isocarboxazid), selegiline does not inhibit peripheral metabolism of catecholamines and can be taken safely with levodopa. Selegiline does not cause the lethal potentiation of indirectly acting sympathomimetic amines such as dietary tyramine. Doses of selegiline higher than 10 mg daily can produce inhibition of MAO-A and should be avoided.

Since it may retard dopamine degradation in the striatum, selegiline has been used as a symptomatic treatment for PD, although its benefit is modest. A putative action of selegiline is to retard the metabolism of dopamine, reduce free radical production and oxidative stress, and thereby confer neuroprotective effects. Selegiline is generally well tolerated in patients with early or mild PD. In patients with more advanced PD or underlying cognitive impairment, selegiline may accentuate the adverse motor and cognitive effects of levodopa therapy. Metabolites of selegiline include amphetamine and methamphetamine, which may cause anxiety, insomnia, and other adverse symptoms. A related compound, rasagiline, also acts through inhibition of MAO-B but does not form these undesirable metabolites. Rasagiline shows efficacy in early and advanced PD but is not yet approved for use in the U.S. Selegiline, like the nonspecific MAO inhibitors, can lead to the development of stupor, rigidity, agitation, and hyperthermia after administration of the analgesic meperidine; the basis of this interaction is uncertain. There are reports of adverse effects resulting from interactions between selegiline and tricyclic antidepressants and between selegiline and SSRIs. The combination of selegiline and SSRIs seems well tolerated in patients with PD, but the concomitant administration of selegiline and serotonergic drugs should be done with caution.

MUSCARINIC RECEPTOR ANTAGONISTS Antagonists of muscarinic acetylcholine (ACh) receptors were used widely for the treatment of PD before the discovery of levodopa. The biological basis for the therapeutic actions of anticholinergics is not completely understood. These drugs probably act in the neostriatum through the receptors that normally mediate the response to intrinsic cholinergic innervation of this structure, which arises primarily from cholinergic striatal interneurons. The agents acting as muscarinic antagonists currently used in the treatment of PD include *trihexyphenidyl* (ARTANE, 2–4 mg three times per day), *benztropine mesylate* (COGENTIN, 1–4 mg two times per day), and *diphenhydramine hydrochloride* (BENADRYL, 25–50 mg three to four times per day; *diphenhydramine* also is a histamine H_1 antagonist; *see* Chapter 24). All have modest antiparkinsonian activity that is useful in the treatment of early PD or as an adjunct to dopamimetic therapy. The adverse effects of these drugs are a result of their anticholinergic properties (principally sedation and mental confusion, but also constipation, urinary retention, and blurred vision through cycloplegia); these drugs must be used with caution in patients with narrow-angle glaucoma.

AMANTADINE *Amantadine* (SYMMETREL) is an antiviral agent used for the prophylaxis and treatment of influenza A (*see* Chapter 49). The drug also appears to alter dopamine release in the striatum, has anticholinergic properties, and blocks NMDA glutamate receptors. Presumably through a combination of these mechanisms, amantidine has modest antiparkinsonian activity, and is used as initial therapy of mild PD. Amantadine also may be helpful as an adjunct in patients on levodopa with dose-related fluctuations and dyskinesias. Amantadine usually is administered in a dose of 100 mg twice a day and is well tolerated. Dizziness, lethargy, anticholinergic effects, and sleep disturbance, as well as nausea and vomiting, have been observed occasionally, but these effects are mild and reversible.

ALZHEIMER'S DISEASE

CLINICAL OVERVIEW AD produces an impairment of cognitive abilities that is gradual in onset but relentless in progression. Impairment of short-term memory usually is the first clinical feature; retrieval of distant memories is preserved relatively well. As the condition progresses, additional cognitive abilities are impaired, among them the ability to calculate, exercise visuospatial skills, and use common objects and tools (ideomotor apraxia). The level of arousal or alertness of the patient is not affected until the condition is very advanced, nor is there motor weakness, although muscular contractures are an almost universal feature of advanced stages of the disease. Death, most often from a complication of immobility such as pneumonia or pulmonary embolism, usually ensues within 6–12 years of onset. The diagnosis of AD is based on careful clinical assessment of the patient and appropriate laboratory tests to exclude other disorders that may mimic AD; at present, no direct antemortem confirmatory test exists.

Pathophysiology

AD is characterized by marked atrophy of the cerebral cortex and loss of cortical and subcortical neurons. The pathological hallmarks of AD are senile plaques, which are spherical accumulations of the protein β-amyloid accompanied by degenerating neuronal processes, and abundant neurofibrillary tangles, composed of paired helical filaments and other proteins. In advanced AD, senile plaques and neurofibrillary tangles are most abundant in the hippocampus and associative regions of the cortex, whereas areas such as the visual and motor cortices are relatively spared. This corresponds to the clinical features of marked impairment of memory and abstract reasoning, with preservation of vision and movement.

NEUROCHEMISTRY

Direct analysis of neurotransmitter content in the cerebral cortex shows a reduction of many transmitter substances that parallels neuronal loss, with a striking and disproportionate deficiency of ACh due to atrophy and degeneration of subcortical cholinergic neurons, particularly those in the basal forebrain (nucleus basalis of Meynert) that provide cholinergic innervation to the whole cerebral cortex. Although the conceptualization of AD as a "cholinergic deficiency syndrome" in parallel with the "dopaminergic deficiency syndrome" of PD provides a useful framework, the deficit in AD is far more complex, involving multiple neurotransmitter systems, including serotonin, glutamate, and neuropeptides, with destruction of not only cholinergic neurons but also the cortical and hippocampal targets that receive cholinergic input.

TREATMENT OF ALZHEIMER'S DISEASE The treatment of AD has involved attempts to augment the cholinergic function of the brain. Precursors of ACh synthesis, such as *choline chloride* and *phosphatidyl choline (lecithin)* do not produce clinically significant effects; however, inhibitors of acetylcholinesterase (AChE; *see* Chapter 8) have shown efficacy.

Four inhibitors of AChE currently are approved by the FDA for treatment of AD: *tacrine* (1,2,3,4-tetrahydro-9-aminoacridine; COGNEX), *donepezil* (ARICEPT), *rivastigmine* (EXCELON), and *galantamine* (RAZADYNE). Tacrine is a potent centrally acting inhibitor of AChE. Oral tacrine, in combination with lecithin, produces modest effects on memory performance, and the side effects of tacrine often are significant and dose-limiting; abdominal cramping, nausea, vomiting, and diarrhea are observed in up to one-third of patients receiving therapeutic doses, and elevations of serum transaminases are observed in up to 50% of those treated. Because of significant side effects, tacrine is not used widely clinically. Donepezil is a selective inhibitor of AChE in the CNS with little effect on peripheral AChE. It produces modest improvements in cognitive scores in AD patients and has a long $t_{1/2}$, allowing once-daily dosing. Rivastigmine and galantamine are dosed twice daily and produce a similar degree of cognitive improvement. Adverse effects associated with donepezil, rivastigmine, and galantamine are similar in character but generally less frequent and less severe than those observed with tacrine: nausea, diarrhea, vomiting, and insomnia. Donepezil, rivastigmine, and galantamine are not associated with the hepatotoxicity that limits the use of tacrine.

An alternative strategy for the treatment of AD is the use of the NMDA glutamate-receptor antagonist memantine (NAMENDA). Memantine produces a use-dependent blockade of NMDA receptors. In patients with moderate-to-severe AD, use of memantine is associated with a reduced rate of clinical deterioration. Whether this is due to a true disease-modifying effect, possibly reduced excitotoxicity, or is a symptomatic effect of the drug is unclear. Adverse effects of memantine usually are mild and reversible and may include headache or dizziness.

HUNTINGTON'S DISEASE

CLINICAL FEATURES HD is a dominantly inherited disorder characterized by the gradual onset of motor incoordination and cognitive decline in midlife. Symptoms develop insidiously, either as a movement disorder manifest by brief, jerk-like movements of the extremities, trunk, face, and neck (chorea) or as personality changes or both. Fine motor incoordination and impairment of rapid-eye-movements are early features. Occasionally, choreic movements are less prominent and bradykinesia and dystonia predominate. As the disorder progresses, the involuntary movements become more severe, dysarthria and dysphagia develop, and balance is impaired. The cognitive disorder manifests first as slowness of mental processing and difficulty in organizing complex tasks. Memory is affected, but affected persons rarely lose their memory of family, friends, and the immediate situation. Such persons often become irritable, anxious, and depressed. Less frequently, paranoia and delusional states are manifest. The outcome of HD is invariably fatal; over a course of 15–30 years, the affected person becomes totally disabled and unable to communicate, requiring full-time care; death ensues from the complications of immobility.

PATHOLOGY AND PATHOPHYSIOLOGY

HD is characterized by prominent neuronal loss in the striatum (caudate/putamen). Atrophy of these structures proceeds in an orderly fashion, first affecting the tail of the caudate nucleus and then proceeding anteriorly from mediodorsal to ventrolateral. Other areas of the brain also are affected, although much less severely; one result is a prominent decrease in striatal GABA concentrations, whereas somatostatin and dopamine concentrations are relatively preserved. In most adult-onset cases, the medium spiny neurons that project to the GPi and SNpr (the indirect pathway) appear to be affected earlier than those projecting to the GPe (the direct pathway; see Figure 20–8). The disproportionate impairment of the indirect pathway increases excitatory drive to the neocortex, producing involuntary choreiform movements. In some individuals, rigidity rather than chorea is the predominant clinical feature; this is especially common in juvenile-onset cases. In these cases, the striatal neurons giving rise to both the direct and indirect pathways are impaired to a comparable degree.

GENETICS

HD is an autosomal dominant disorder with nearly complete penetrance. In affected individuals, the short arm of chromosome 4 contains a polymorphic $(CAG)_n$ trinucleotide repeat that is significantly expanded in all individuals with HD; this trinucleotide repeat is the genetic alteration

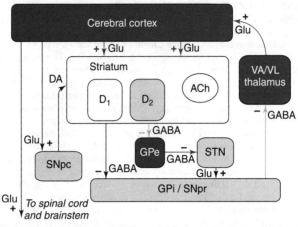

FIGURE 20-8 *The basal ganglia in Huntington's disease. HD* is characterized by loss of neurons from the striatum. The neurons that project from the striatum to the GPe and form the indirect pathway are affected earlier in the course of the disease than those which project to the GPi. This leads to a loss of inhibition of the GPe. The increased activity in this structure, in turn, inhibits the STN, SNpr, and GPi, resulting in a loss of inhibition to the VA/VL thalamus and increased thalamocortical excitatory drive. Structures in light blue have reduced activity in HD, whereas structures in dark blue have increased activity. (*See* legend to Figure 20–5 for definitions of anatomical abbreviations.)

responsible for HD and is increased from the normal range (9–34 triplets) to 40–100 triplets in HD patients. Several other neurodegenerative diseases also arise through expansion of a CAG repeat, including hereditary spinocerebellar ataxias and Kennedy's disease, a rare inherited disorder of motor neurons. The mechanism by which the expanded trinucleotide repeat leads to the clinical and pathological features of HD is unknown. The HD mutation lies within a gene designated IT15 *that encodes a protein of ~348,000 Da. The trinucleotide repeat, which encodes the amino acid glutamine, occurs at the 5′ end of* IT15 *and is followed directly by a second, shorter repeat of* $(CCG)_n$ *that encodes proline. The protein, named* huntingtin, *does not resemble any other known protein, and the normal function of the protein has not been identified. The HD gene is expressed widely throughout the body, with high levels in brain, pancreas, intestine, muscle, liver, adrenals, and testes. Although the striatum is most severely affected, neurons in all regions of the brain express similar levels of* IT15 *mRNA.*

SYMPTOMATIC TREATMENT OF HUNTINGTON'S DISEASE No current treatment slows the progression of HD, and many medications can impair function because of side effects. Treatment is needed for patients who are depressed, irritable, paranoid, excessively anxious, or psychotic. Depression can be treated effectively with standard antidepressant drugs with the caveat that drugs with substantial anticholinergic profiles can exacerbate chorea. *Fluoxetine* (*see* Chapter 17) is effective treatment for both the depression and the irritability manifest in symptomatic HD; *carbamazepine* (*see* Chapter 19) also is effective for depression. Paranoia, delusional states, and psychosis usually require treatment with antipsychotic drugs, but the doses required often are lower than those usually used in primary psychiatric disorders. These agents also reduce cognitive function and impair mobility and thus should be used in the lowest doses possible and should be discontinued when the psychiatric symptoms resolve. In individuals with predominantly rigid HD, *clozapine, quetiapine* (*see* Chapter 18), or carbamazepine may be more effective for treatment of paranoia and psychosis.

The movement disorder of HD *per se* only rarely justifies pharmacological therapy. For those with large-amplitude chorea causing frequent falls and injury, dopamine-depleting agents such as *tetrabenazine* and *reserpine* (*see* Chapter 32) can be tried, although patients must be monitored for hypotension and depression. Antipsychotic agents also can be used, but these often do not improve overall function because they decrease fine motor coordination and increase rigidity. Many HD patients exhibit worsening of involuntary movements as a result of anxiety or stress. In these situations, judicious use of sedative or anxiolytic *benzodiazepines* can be very helpful. In juvenile-onset cases, where rigidity rather than chorea predominates, dopamine agonists variably improve rigidity. These individuals also occasionally develop myoclonus and seizures that can be responsive to *clonazepam, valproic acid,* and other anticonvulsants.

AMYOTROPIIIC LATERAL SCLEROSIS
CLINICAL FEATURES AND PATHOLOGY

ALS is a disorder of the motor neurons of the ventral horn of the spinal cord and the cortical neurons that provide their afferent input, characterized by rapidly progressive weakness, muscle atrophy and fasciculations, spasticity, dysarthria, dysphagia, and respiratory compromise. Sensory function generally is spared, as is cognitive, autonomic, and oculomotor activity. ALS usually is progressive and fatal, with most affected patients dying of respiratory compromise and pneumonia after 2–3 years. The pathology of ALS corresponds closely to the clinical features: prominent loss of the spinal and brainstem motor neurons that project to striated muscles (although the oculomotor neurons are spared), as well as loss of the large pyramidal motor neurons in layer V of motor cortex, which are the origin of the descending corticospinal tracts. In familial cases (FALS, ~10% of cases, usually with an autosomal dominant pattern of inheritance), Clarke's column and the dorsal horns sometimes are affected. Mutations in SOD1 *account for ~20% of cases of FALS; many of the mutations of* SOD1 *associated with the disease do not reduce the capacity of the enzyme to perform its primary function, the catabolism of superoxide radicals. More than 90% of ALS cases are not associated with abnormalities of* SOD1 *or any other known gene. The cause of the motor neuron loss in sporadic ALS is unknown.*

TREATMENT OF ALS WITH RILUZOLE The only currently approved therapy for ALS is *riluzole* (2-amino-6-[trifluoromethoxy]benzothiazole; RILUTEK), an agent with complex actions in the nervous system. Riluzole is absorbed orally and is highly protein bound. It undergoes extensive metabolism in the liver by both CYP–mediated hydroxylation and glucuronidation. Its $t_{1/2}$ is ~12 hours. *In vitro,* riluzole inhibits glutamate release, blocks postsynaptic NMDA- and kainate-type glutamate receptors, and inhibits voltage-dependent Na^+ channels. In clinical trials, riluzole has modest but genuine effects on the survival of patients with ALS. The recommended dose is 50 mg every 12 hours, taken 1 hour before or 2 hours after a meal. Riluzole usually is well tolerated, although nausea or diarrhea may occur. Rarely, riluzole may produce hepatic injury with elevations of serum transaminases; thus, periodic monitoring is recommended. Although the effect of riluzole on ALS is small (mean extension of survival ~60 days), it represents a significant therapeutic advance in the treatment of a disease refractory to all previous drugs.

SYMPTOMATIC THERAPY OF ALS: SPASTICITY Spasticity is a clinical feature of ALS that often leads to considerable pain and discomfort and reduces mobility, which already is compromised by weakness. Furthermore, spasticity is the feature of ALS that is most amenable to present forms of treatment. *Spasticity* is an increase in muscle tone characterized by an initial resistance to passive displacement of a limb at a joint, followed by a sudden relaxation (the so-called clasped-knife phenomenon). Spasticity is the result of the loss of descending inputs to the spinal motor neurons, and the character of the spasticity depends on which nervous system pathways are affected. Whole repertoires of movement can be generated directly at the spinal cord level; it is beyond the scope of this chapter to describe these in detail. In general, pyramidal pathways that use glutamate as a neurotransmitter are impaired, with relative preservation of the other descending pathways, resulting in hyperactive deep-tendon reflexes, impaired fine motor coordination, increased extensor tone in the legs, and increased flexor tone in the arms. The gag reflex often is overactive as well.

The most useful agent for the symptomatic treatment of spasticity in ALS is *baclofen* (LIORESAL), a $GABA_B$ receptor agonist. Initial doses of 5–10 mg/day are recommended, but the dose can be increased to as much as 200 mg/day if necessary. If weakness occurs, the dose should be lowered. In addition to oral administration, baclofen also can be delivered directly into the space around the spinal cord by use of a surgically implanted pump and an intrathecal catheter. This approach minimizes the adverse effects of the drug, especially sedation, but it carries the risk of potentially life-threatening CNS depression and should be only used by physicians trained in delivering chronic intrathecal therapy. *Tizanidine* (ZANFLEX), an agonist of α_2 adrenergic receptors in the CNS, reduces muscle spasticity and is assumed to act by increasing presynaptic inhibition of motor neurons. Tizanidine is used most widely in the treatment of spasticity in multiple sclerosis or after stroke but may be effective in patients with ALS. Treatment should be initiated at a low dose of 2–4 mg at bedtime and titrated upward gradually. Drowsiness, asthenia, and dizziness may limit the dose that can be administered. Benzodiazepines (*see* Chapter 16) such as *clonazepam* (KLONIPIN) are effective antispasmodics but may contribute to respiratory depression in patients with advanced ALS. *Dantrolene* (DANTRIUM), approved in the U.S. for the treatment of muscle spasm, can exacerbate muscular weakness and thus is not used in ALS (*see* Chapter 9).

For a complete Bibliographical listing see Goodman & Gilman's *The Pharmacological Basis of Therapeutics*, 11th ed., or Goodman & Gilman Online at www.accessmedicine.com.

21

OPIOID ANALGESICS

The term opioid *refers broadly to all compounds related to opium, a natural product derived from the poppy.* Opiates *are drugs derived from opium and include the natural products* morphine, codeine, *and* thebaine, *and many semisynthetic derivatives.* Endogenous opioid peptides, *or* endorphins, *are the naturally occurring ligands for opioid receptors. Opiates exert their effects by mimicking these peptides. The term* narcotic *is derived from the Greek word for "stupor"; it originally referred to any drug that induced sleep, but it now is associated with opioids.*

The diverse functions of the endogenous opioid system include the best known sensory role, prominent in inhibiting responses to painful stimuli; a modulatory role in gastrointestinal (GI), endocrine, and autonomic functions; an emotional role, evident in the powerful rewarding and addicting properties of opioids; and a cognitive role in the modulation of learning and memory. The endogenous opioid system has considerable diversity in endogenous ligands (>12) but only 4 major receptor types.

ENDOGENOUS OPIOID PEPTIDES

Three distinct families of classical opioid peptides have been identified: the *enkephalins, endorphins,* and *dynorphins.* Each family derives from a distinct precursor protein, prepro-opiomelanocortin (POMC), preproenkephalin, and preprodynorphin, respectively, which are encoded by distinct genes. Each precursor is subject to complex cleavages and posttranslational modifications that result in the synthesis of multiple active peptides. The opioid peptides share a common amino-terminal sequence of Tyr-Gly-Gly-Phe-(Met or Leu), the *opioid motif.* This motif is followed by C-terminal extensions yielding peptides ranging from 5 to 31 residues (Table 21–1).

The major opioid peptide derived from POMC is β-endorphin. In addition to β-endorphin, the POMC precursor also is processed into the nonopioid peptides adrenocorticotropic hormone (ACTH), melanocyte-stimulating hormone (α-MSH), and β-lipotropin β-LPH). Proenkephalin contains multiple copies of met-enkephalin, as well as a single copy of leu-enkephalin. Prodynorphin contains three peptides of differing lengths that all begin with the leu-enkephalin sequence: dynorphin A, dynorphin B, and neoendorphin (Figure 21–1).

A novel endogenous opioid peptide with significant sequence homology to dynorphin A was alternatively termed nociceptin or orphanin FQ (now termed N/OFQ; Table 21–1). The substitution of Phe for Tyr in the opioid motif is sufficient to abolish interactions with the three classical opioid peptide receptors. N/OFQ has behavioral and pain modulatory properties distinct from those of the three classical opioid peptides.

OPIOID RECEPTORS

Three classical opioid receptor types, μ, δ, and κ, have been studied extensively; the N/OFQ receptor system is still being defined. Highly selective ligands that allowed for type-specific labeling of the three classical opioid receptors (*e.g.,* DAMGO for μ, DPDPE for δ, and U-50,488 and U-69,593 for κ) made possible the definition of ligand-binding characteristics of each of the receptor types and the determination of anatomical distribution of the receptors using autoradiographic techniques. Each major opioid receptor has a unique anatomical distribution in brain, spinal cord, and the periphery.

Receptor-selective antagonists and agonists have aided the study of the biological functions of opioid receptors. Commonly used antagonists are cyclic analogs of *somatostatin* such as CTOP as μ-receptor antagonists, a derivative of naloxone called *naltrindole* as a δ-receptor antagonist, and a bivalent derivative of *naltrexone* called *nor-binaltorphimine* (nor-BNI) as a κ-receptor antagonist. In general, functional studies using selective agonists and antagonists have revealed substantial parallels between μ and δ receptors and dramatic contrasts between μ/δ and κ receptors. *In vivo* infusions of selective antagonists and agonists also were used to establish the receptor types involved in mediating various opioid effects (Table 21–2).

Most of the clinically used opioids are relatively selective for μ receptors, reflecting their similarity to morphine (Tables 21–3 and 21–4). However, drugs that are relatively selective at standard doses may interact with additional receptor subtypes when given at sufficiently high doses, leading to possible changes in their pharmacological profile. This is especially true as doses are escalated to overcome tolerance. Some drugs, particularly mixed agonist–antagonist agents, interact with more than one receptor class at usual clinical doses and may act as an agonist at one receptor and an antagonist at another.

Table 21–1

Endogenous and Synthetic Opioid Peptides

Selected Endogenous Opioid Peptides

[Leu^5]enkephalin	**Tyr-Gly-Gly-Phe-Leu**
[Met^5]enkephalin	**Tyr-Gly-Gly-Phe-Met**
Dynorphin A	**Tyr-Gly-Gly-Phe-Leu**-Arg-Arg-Ile-Arg-Pro-Lys-Leu-Lys-Trp-Asp-Asn-Gln
Dynorphin B	**Tyr-Gly-Gly-Phe-Leu**-Arg-Arg-Gln-Phe-Lys-Val-Val-Thr
α-Neoendorphin	**Tyr-Gly-Gly-Phe-Leu**-Arg-Lys-Tyr-Pro-Lys
β-Neoendorphin	**Tyr-Gly-Gly-Phe-Leu**-Arg-Lys-Tyr-Pro
β-Endorphin	**Tyr-Gly-Gly-Phe-Met**-Thr-Ser-Glu-Lys-Ser-Gln-Thr-Pro-Leu-Val-Thr-Leu-Phe-Lys-Asn-Ala-Ile-Ile-Lys-Asn-Ala-Tyr-Lys-Lys-Gly-Glu

Novel Endogenous Opioid-Related Peptides

Orphanin FQ/Nociceptin	Phe-Gly-Gly-Phe-Thr-Gly-Ala-Arg-Lys-Ser-Ala-Arg-Lys-Leu-Ala-Asn-Gln

Selected Synthetic Opioid Peptides

DAMGO	[D-Ala^2,MePhe^4,Gly(ol)^5]enkephalin
DPDPE	[D-Pen^2,d-Pen^5]enkephalin
DSLET	[D-Ser^2,Leu^5]enkephalin-Thr^6
DADL	[D-Ala^2,D-Leu^5]enkephalin
CTOP	D-Phe-Cys-Tyr-D-Trp-Orn-Thr-Pen-Thr-NH$_2$
FK-33824	[D-Ala^2,N-MePhe^4,Met(O)^5-ol]enkephalin
[D-Ala^2]Deltorphin I	Tyr-D-Ala-Phe-Asp-Val-Val-Gly-NH$_2$
[D-Ala^2,Glu^4]Deltorphin II	Tyr-D-Ala-Phe-Glu-Val-Val-Gly-NH$_2$
Morphiceptin	Tyr-Pro-Phe-Pro-NH$_2$
PL-017	Tyr-Pro-MePhe-D-Pro-NH$_2$
DALCE	[D-Ala^2,Leu^5,Cys^6]enkephalin

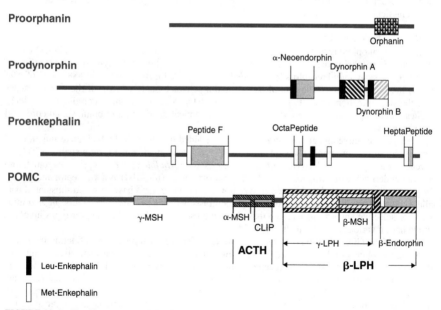

FIGURE 21–1 *Peptide precursors.* POMC, pro-opiomelanocortin; ACTH, adrenocorticotropic hormone; β-LPH, β-lipotropin.

Table 21–2

Classification of Opioid Receptor Subtypes and Actions from Animal Models

Receptor Subtype	Actions of: Agonist	Actions of: Antagonist
Analgesia		
Supraspinal	μ, κ, δ	Analgesic	No effect
Spinal	μ, κ, δ	Analgesic	No effect
Respiratory function	μ	Decrease	No effect
Gastrointestinal tract	μ, κ	Decrease transit	No effect
Psychotomimesis	κ	Increase	No effect
Feeding	μ, κ, δ	Increase feeding	Decrease feeding
Sedation	μ, κ	Increase	No effect
Diuresis	κ	Increase	
Hormone regulation		
Prolactin	μ	Increase release	Decrease release
Growth hormone	μ and/or δ	Increase release	Decrease release
Neurotransmitter release		
Acetylcholine	μ	Inhibit	
Dopamine	μ, δ	Inhibit	
Isolated organ bioassays		
Guinea pig ileum	μ	Decrease contraction	No effect
Mouse vas deferens	δ	Decrease contraction	No effect

The actions listed for antagonists are seen with the antagonist alone. All the correlations in this table are based on studies in rats and mice, which occasionally show species differences. Thus, any extensions of these associations to humans are tentative. Clinical studies do indicate that μ receptors elicit analgesia spinally and supraspinally. Preliminary work with a synthetic opioid peptide, [D-Ala^2,D-Leu^5]enkephalin, suggests that intrathecal δ agonists are analgesic in humans.

Opioid Receptor Signaling and Consequent Intracellular Events

COUPLING OF OPIOID RECEPTORS TO SECOND MESSENGERS

The μ, δ and κ receptors are coupled, via *pertussis toxin–sensitive G proteins, to inhibition of adenylyl cyclase activity, activation of receptor-linked K^+ currents, and suppression of voltage-gated Ca^{2+} currents. The hyperpolarization of membrane potential by K^+-current activation and the limiting of Ca^{2+} entry by suppression of Ca^{2+} currents are tenable but unproven mechanisms for explaining opioid inhibition of neurotransmitter release and pain transmission. Opioid receptors couple to an array of second-messenger systems, including activation of MAP kinases and the phospholipase C (PLC)–mediated cascade. Prolonged exposure to opioids results in adaptations at multiple levels within these signaling cascades that may relate to effects such as tolerance, sensitization, and withdrawal.*

RECEPTOR DESENSITIZATION, INTERNALIZATION, AND SEQUESTRATION AFTER CHRONIC EXPOSURE TO OPIOIDS

Tolerance *refers to a decrease in effectiveness of a drug with its repeated administration (see Chapter 23). Transient administration of opioids leads to a phenomenon called* acute tolerance, *whereas sustained administration leads to the development of* classical *or* chronic tolerance. *Short-term receptor desensitization, which may underlie the development of tolerance, probably involves phosphorylation of the μ and δ receptors by PKC. A number of other kinases have been implicated in desensitization, including PKA and β-adrenergic receptor kinase.*

Long-term tolerance may be associated with increases in adenylyl cyclase activity—a counter-regulation to the decreased cyclic AMP levels seen after acute opioid administration. Chronic treatment with μ-receptor opioids causes superactivation of adenylyl cyclase. This effect is prevented by pretreatment with pertussis toxin, *demonstrating involvement of $G_{i/o}$ proteins, and also by cotransfection with scavengers of G protein–$\beta\gamma$ dimers, indicating a role for this complex in superactivation. Recent data, described in the 11th edition of the parent text, argue that opioid tolerance may be related not to receptor desensitization but rather to a lack of desensitization.*

Table 21–3

Actions and Selectivities of Some Opioids at the Various Opioid Receptor Classes

	Receptors		
	μ	δ	κ
Drugs			
Morphine	+++		+
Methadone	+++		
Etorphine	+++	+++	+++
Levorphanol	+++		
Fentanyl	+++		
Sufentanil	+++	+	+
DAMGO	+++		
Butorphanol	P		+++
Buprenorphine	P		– –
Naloxone	– – –	–	– –
Naltrexone	– – –	–	– – –
CTOP	– – –		
Diprenorphine	– – –	– –	– – –
β-Funaltrexamine	– – –	–	++
Naloxonazine	– – –	–	–
Nalorphine	– – –		+
Pentazocine	P		++
Nalbuphine	– –		++
Naloxone benzoylhydrazone	– – –	–	–
Bremazocine	+++	++	+++
Ethylketocyclazocine	P	+	+++
U50,488			+++
U69,593			+++
Spiradoline	+		+++
nor-Binaltorphimine	–	–	– – –
Naltrindole	–	– – –	–
DPDPE		++	
[D-Ala^2,Glu^4]deltorphin		++	
DSLET	+	++	
Endogenous Peptides			
Met-enkephalin	++	+++	
Leu-enkephalin	++	+++	
β-Endorphin	+++	+++	
Dynorphin A	+		+++
Dynorphin B	+	+	+++
α-Neoendorphin	+	+	+++

Activities of drugs are given at the receptors for which the agent has reasonable affinity. +, agonist; –, antagonist. The number of symbols (+, –) is an indication of potency; the ratio for a given drug denotes selectivity. These values were obtained primarily from animal studies and should be extrapolated to human beings with caution. Both β-funaltrexamine and naloxonazine are irreversible μ antagonists, but β-funaltrexamine also has reversible κ agonist activity. P, partial agonist; DAMGO, CTOP, DPDPE, DSLET, *see* Table 21–1.

EFFECTS OF CLINICALLY USED OPIOIDS

Morphine and most other clinically used opiates exert their effects through μ opioid receptors and affect a wide range of physiological systems. They produce analgesia, affect mood and rewarding behavior (*see* Chapter 23), and alter respiratory, cardiovascular, GI, and neuroendocrine function. δ-Opioid receptor agonists also are potent analgesics in animals and some have proved useful in humans. Agonists selective for κ receptors produce analgesia that is mediated primarily at spinal

Table 21–4

Properties of the Cloned Opioid Receptors

Receptor Subtype	Selective Ligands		Nonselective Ligands		Putative Endogenous Ligands
	Agonists	Antagonists	Agonists	Antagonists	
μ	DAMGO Morphine Methadone Fentanyl Dermorphin	CTOP	Levorphanol Etorphine	Naloxone Naltrexone β-funaltrexamine	Enkephalin Endorphin
κ	Spiradoline U50,488 Dynorphin A	Nor-BNI	Levorphanol Etorphine EKC	Naloxone Naltrexone	Dynorphin A
δ	DPDPE Deltorphin DSLET	Naltrindole NTB BNTX	Levorphanol Etorphine	Naloxone Naltrexone	Enkephalin

BNTX, 7-benzylidenenaltroxone; EKC, ethylketocyclazosine; NTB, benzofuran analog of naltrindole; nor-BNI, norbinaltorphimine. DAMGO, CTOP, DPDPE, DSLET, *see* Table 21–1.

sites. Respiratory depression and miosis may be less severe with κ agonists. Instead of euphoria, κ receptor agonists produce dysphoric and psychotomimetic effects. In neural circuits mediating reward and analgesia, μ and κ agonists have antagonistic effects (*see* below).

Mixed agonist–antagonist compounds were developed in the hope that they would have less addictive potential and respiratory depression than morphine and related drugs. In practice, for the same degree of analgesia, the same intensity of side effects occurs. A "ceiling effect" limits the amount of analgesia attainable with these drugs. Some mixed agonist–antagonist drugs, such as *pentazocine* and *nalorphine,* can produce severe psychotomimetic effects that are not reversible with naloxone (and thus may not be mediated *via* classical opioid receptors): These drugs also can precipitate withdrawal in opioid-tolerant patients, further limiting their clinical use.

Analgesia

Morphine-like drugs produce analgesia, drowsiness, changes in mood, and mental clouding. The analgesia occurs without loss of consciousness. When therapeutic doses of morphine are given to patients with pain, they report that the pain is less intense, less discomforting, or entirely gone; drowsiness commonly occurs. In addition to relief of distress, some patients experience euphoria.

When morphine in the same dose is given to a normal, pain-free individual, the experience may be unpleasant. Nausea is common, and vomiting may occur. There may be feelings of drowsiness, difficulty in mentation, apathy, and lessened physical activity. As the dose is increased, the subjective, analgesic, and toxic effects, including respiratory depression, become more pronounced. Morphine does not have anticonvulsant activity and usually does not cause slurred speech, emotional lability, or significant motor incoordination.

The relief of pain by morphine-like opioids is relatively selective, in that other sensory modalities are not affected. Patients frequently report that the pain is still present, but they feel more comfortable. Continuous dull pain is relieved more effectively than sharp intermittent pain, but sufficient amounts of opioid can relieve even the severe pain associated with renal or biliary colic.

Mood Alterations and Rewarding Properties

The mechanisms by which opioids produce euphoria, tranquility, and other mood alterations (including rewarding properties) are not entirely clear. However, the neural systems that mediate opioid reinforcement are distinct from those involved in physical dependence and analgesia. Behavioral and pharmacological data point to the role of dopaminergic pathways, particularly involving the nucleus accumbens, in drug-induced reward. There is ample evidence for interactions between opioids and *dopamine* in mediating opioid-induced reward (*see* Chapter 23).

Other Central Nervous System Effects

Whereas opioids are used primarily for analgesia, they produce a host of other effects, as summarized below. High doses of opioids can produce muscular rigidity in humans. Chest wall rigidity severe enough to compromise respiration is not uncommon during anesthesia with fentanyl, *alfentanil, remifentanil,* and *sufentanil.*

EFFECTS ON THE HYPOTHALAMUS

Opioids alter the equilibrium point of the hypothalamic heat-regulatory mechanisms such that body temperature usually falls slightly. However, chronic high dosage may increase body temperature.

NEUROENDOCRINE EFFECTS

Morphine acts in the hypothalamus to inhibit the release of gonadotropin-releasing hormone (GnRH) and corticotropin-releasing hormone (CRH), thus decreasing circulating concentrations of luteinizing hormone (LH), follicle-stimulating hormone (FSH), and ACTH. As a result of the decreased concentrations of pituitary trophic hormones, plasma concentrations of sex steroids and cortisol decline. Thyrotropin secretion is relatively unaffected.

The administration of μ agonists increases the concentration of prolactin in plasma, probably by reducing the dopaminergic inhibition of its secretion. The administration of morphine or β-endorphin has little effect on the concentration of growth hormone in plasma. With chronic administration, tolerance develops to the effects of morphine on hypothalamic releasing factors. Patients maintained on methadone *reflect this phenomenon; in women, menstrual cycles that had been disrupted by intermittent use of heroin return to normal; in men, circulating concentrations of LH and testosterone return to the normal range.*

MIOSIS   Morphine and most μ and κ agonists cause constriction of the pupil by an excitatory action on the parasympathetic nerve innervating the pupil. After toxic doses of μ agonists, the miosis is marked, and pinpoint pupils are pathognomonic; however, marked mydriasis occurs if asphyxia intervenes. Some tolerance to the miotic effect develops, but addicts with high circulating levels of opioids continue to have constricted pupils. Therapeutic doses of morphine increase accommodation and lower intraocular pressure in normal and glaucomatous eyes.

CONVULSIONS   In animals, high doses of morphine and related opioids produce convulsions. Several mechanisms appear to be involved, and different types of opioids produce seizures with different characteristics. Morphine-like drugs excite certain groups of neurons, especially hippocampal pyramidal cells; these excitatory effects probably result from inhibition of the release of GABA by interneurons. Selective δ agonists produce similar effects. These actions may contribute to the seizures that are produced by some agents at doses only moderately higher than those required for analgesia, especially in children. With most opioids, however, convulsions occur only at doses far in excess of those required to produce profound analgesia, and seizures are not seen when potent μ agonists are used to produce anesthesia. Naloxone is more potent in antagonizing convulsions produced by some opioids (*e.g.,* morphine, methadone, and *propoxyphene*) than those produced by others (*e.g., meperidine*). The production of convulsant metabolites of the latter drug may be partially responsible (*see* below). Anticonvulsant agents may not always be effective in suppressing opioid-induced seizures (*see* Chapter 19).

RESPIRATION   Morphine-like opioids depress respiration at least partly by a direct effect on the brainstem respiratory centers. This respiratory depression is discernible even with doses too small to disturb consciousness and increases progressively as the dose is increased. In humans, death from morphine poisoning is nearly always due to respiratory arrest. Therapeutic doses of morphine in humans depress all phases of respiratory activity (rate, minute volume, and tidal exchange) and also may produce irregular and periodic breathing. The diminished respiratory volume is due primarily to a slower rate of breathing; with toxic amounts, the rate may fall to three or four breaths per minute. Although effects on respiration are readily demonstrated, clinically significant respiratory depression rarely occurs with standard morphine doses in the absence of underlying pulmonary dysfunction. One important exception is when opioids are administered parenterally to women shortly before delivery, which can lead to transient respiratory depression in the neonate because of transplacental passage of opioids. The combination of opioids with other medications, such as general anesthetics, tranquilizers, alcohol, or sedative-hypnotics, may increase the risk of respiratory depression. Maximal respiratory depression occurs within 5–10 minutes of intravenous administration of morphine or within 30–90 minutes of intramuscular or subcutaneous administration, respectively.

Maximal respiratory depression occur more rapidly with more lipid-soluble agents. After therapeutic doses, respiratory minute volume may be reduced for as long as 4–5 hours. The respiratory depression by opioids involves a reduction in the responsiveness of the brainstem respiratory centers to CO_2. Opioids also depress the pontine and medullary centers involved in regulating respiratory rhythmicity.

COUGH   Morphine and related opioids also depress the cough reflex, at least partly by direct action on a cough center in the medulla. There is no obligatory relationship between depression of respiration and depression of coughing, and antitussive agents are available that do not depress respiration (*see* below). Suppression of cough by such agents appears to involve receptors in the medulla that are less sensitive to naloxone than those responsible for analgesia.

NAUSEANT AND EMETIC EFFECTS   Nausea and vomiting produced by morphine-like drugs are caused by direct stimulation of the chemoreceptor trigger zone in the area postrema of the medulla. Nausea and vomiting are relatively uncommon in recumbent patients given therapeutic doses of morphine, but nausea occurs in ~40% and vomiting in 15% of ambulatory patients given 15 mg of the drug subcutaneously. This suggests that a vestibular component also is operative. All clinically useful μ agonists produce some degree of nausea and vomiting. Antagonists to the 5-HT$_3$ serotonin receptor have supplanted phenothiazines as the drugs of choice for the treatment of opioid-induced nausea and vomiting. Gastric prokinetic agents such as *metoclopramide* also are useful antinausea and antiemetic drugs (*see* Chapter 37).

CARDIOVASCULAR SYSTEM   In the supine patient, therapeutic doses of morphine-like opioids have no major effect on blood pressure or cardiac rate and rhythm. Such doses do produce peripheral vasodilation, reduced peripheral resistance, and an inhibition of baroreceptor reflexes. Therefore, when supine patients assume the upright position, orthostatic hypotension and fainting may occur. The peripheral arteriolar and venous dilation produced by morphine involves several mechanisms. Morphine and some other opioids provoke release of histamine, which sometimes plays a large role in the hypotension. However, vasodilation usually is only partially blocked by H$_1$ antagonists, but it is effectively reversed by naloxone. Morphine also blunts the reflex vasoconstriction caused by increased P_{CO_2} (*see* Chapter 15).

Effects on the myocardium are not significant in normal individuals. In patients with coronary artery disease but no acute medical problems, 8–15 mg morphine administered intravenously produces a decrease in oxygen consumption, left ventricular end-diastolic pressure, and cardiac work; effects on cardiac index usually are slight. In patients with acute myocardial infarction, the cardiovascular responses to morphine may be more variable than in normal subjects, and hypotension may be more pronounced.

Morphine may exert its well-known therapeutic effect in the treatment of angina pectoris and acute myocardial infarction by decreasing preload, inotropy, and chronotropy, thus favorably altering determinants of myocardial O_2 consumption and helping to relieve ischemia. Morphine can mimic the phenomenon of ischemic preconditioning, where a short ischemic episode paradoxically protects the heart against further ischemia. This effect appears to be mediated by δ receptor modulation of a mitochondrial ATP-sensitive K$^+$ channel in cardiac myocytes.

Morphine-like opioids should be used with caution in patients who have a decreased blood volume because the drugs can aggravate hypovolemic shock. Morphine should be used with great care in patients with cor pulmonale because deaths after ordinary therapeutic doses have been reported. The concurrent use of certain phenothiazines may increase the risk of morphine-induced hypotension.

GASTROINTESTINAL TRACT

Stomach   Morphine and other μ agonists usually decrease gastric acid secretion, although stimulation sometimes occurs. Activation of opioid receptors on parietal cells enhances secretion, but indirect effects, including increased secretion of somatostatin from the pancreas and reduced release of acetylcholine, predominate in most circumstances. Low doses of morphine decrease gastric motility, prolonging gastric emptying time; this can increase the likelihood of esophageal reflux. The tone of the antral portion of the stomach and of the first part of the duodenum is increased, which can make therapeutic intubation of the duodenum more difficult. Passage of the gastric contents through the duodenum may be delayed by as much as 12 hours, and the absorption of orally administered drugs is retarded.

Small Intestine   Morphine diminishes biliary, pancreatic, and intestinal secretions and delays digestion of food in the small intestine. Resting tone is increased, and periodic spasms are observed. The amplitude of the nonpropulsive type of rhythmic, segmental contractions usually is enhanced, but propulsive contractions are decreased markedly. The upper part of the small intestine, particularly the duodenum, is affected more than the ileum. A period of relative atony may follow the hypertonicity. Water is absorbed more completely because of the delayed passage of bowel contents, and intestinal secretion is decreased; this increases the viscosity of the bowel contents.

Large Intestine   Propulsive peristaltic waves in the colon are diminished or abolished after administration of morphine, and tone is increased to the point of spasm. The resulting delay in the passage of bowel contents causes considerable desiccation of the feces, which, in turn, retards their advance through the colon. The amplitude of the nonpropulsive type of rhythmic contractions of the colon usually is enhanced. The tone of the anal sphincter is augmented, and reflex relaxation in response to rectal distension is reduced. These actions, combined with inattention to the normal sensory stimuli for defecation reflex owing to the central actions of the drug, contribute to morphine-induced constipation.

BILIARY TRACT   After the subcutaneous injection of 10 mg *morphine sulfate,* the sphincter of Oddi constricts, and the pressure in the common bile duct may rise more than tenfold within 15 minutes; this effect may persist for 2 hours or more. Fluid pressure also may increase in the gallbladder, producing symptoms that vary from epigastric distress to typical biliary colic. All opioids can cause biliary spasm. *Atropine* only partially prevents morphine-induced biliary spasm, but opioid antagonists prevent or relieve it. *Nitroglycerin* (0.6–1.2 mg) administered sublingually also decreases the elevated intrabiliary pressure.

SKIN

Therapeutic doses of morphine cause dilation of cutaneous blood vessels. The skin of the face, neck, and upper thorax frequently becomes flushed. These changes may be due in part to the release of histamine and may be responsible for the sweating and pruritus that occasionally follow the systemic administration of morphine. Histamine release probably accounts for the urticaria commonly seen at the site of injection, which is not mediated by opioid receptors and is not blocked by naloxone. It is seen with morphine and meperidine but not with oxymorphone, methadone, fentanyl, or sufentanil.

Pruritus is a common and potentially disabling complication of opioid use. It can be caused by intraspinal or systemic injections of opioids, but it appears to be more intense after intraspinal administration. The effect appears to be mediated largely by dorsal horn neurons and is reversed by naloxone.

Tolerance and Physical Dependence

The development of tolerance and physical dependence with repeated use is a characteristic feature of all the opioid drugs. *Tolerance* to the effect of opioids or other drugs simply means that the drug loses its effectiveness over time and an increased dose is required to produce the same physiological response. *Dependence* refers to a complex and poorly understood set of changes in the homeostasis of an organism that causes a disturbance of the homeostatic set point of the organism if the drug is stopped. This disturbance often is revealed when administration of an opioid is stopped abruptly, resulting in *withdrawal. Addiction* is a behavioral pattern characterized by compulsive use of a drug and overwhelming involvement with its procurement and use. Tolerance and dependence are physiological responses seen in all patients and are not predictors of addiction (*see* Chapter 23).

MORPHINE AND RELATED OPIOID AGONISTS

Morphine is the standard against which newer analgesics are measured. However, responses of an individual patient may vary dramatically with different μ-opioid receptor agonists. For example, some patients unable to tolerate morphine may have no problems with an equianalgesic dose of methadone, whereas others can tolerate morphine and not methadone. If problems are encountered with one drug, another should be tried.

ABSORPTION, DISTRIBUTION, FATE, AND EXCRETION

Absorption   In general, the opioids are absorbed readily from the GI tract; absorption through the rectal mucosa is adequate, and a few agents (*e.g.,* morphine, hydromorphone) are available in suppositories. The more lipophilic opioids also are absorbed readily through the nasal or buccal mucosa. Those with the greatest lipid solubility also can be absorbed transdermally. Opioids are absorbed readily after subcutaneous or intramuscular injection and can penetrate the spinal cord adequately after epidural or intrathecal administration. Small amounts of morphine introduced epidurally or intrathecally into the spinal canal can produce profound analgesia that may last 12–24 hours. However, because of the hydrophilic nature of morphine, there is rostral spread of the drug in cerebrospinal fluid (CSF), and side effects, especially respiratory depression, can emerge up to 24 hours later as the opioid reaches supraspinal respiratory control centers. With highly lipophilic agents such as hydromorphone or fentanyl, rapid absorption by spinal neural tissues produces very localized effects and segmental analgesia. The duration of action is shorter because of distribution of the drug in the systemic circulation, and the severity of respiratory depression may be more directly proportional to its concentration in plasma owing to a lesser degree of rostral spread. However, patients receiving epidural or intrathecal fentanyl still should be monitored for respiratory depression.

With most opioids, including morphine, the effect of a given dose is less after oral than after parenteral administration because of variable but significant first-pass metabolism in the liver. The bioavailability of oral preparations of morphine is ~25%. The shape of the time–effect curve also varies with the route of administration, so the duration of action often is somewhat longer with the oral route. If adjustment is made for variability of first-pass metabolism and clearance, adequate relief of pain can be achieved with oral administration of morphine. Satisfactory analgesia in cancer patients is associated with a very broad range of steady-state concentrations of morphine in plasma (16–364 ng/mL).

When morphine and most opioids are given intravenously, they act promptly. However, the more lipid-soluble compounds act more rapidly than morphine after subcutaneous administration because of differences in the rates of absorption and entry into the CNS. Compared with more lipid-soluble opioids such as codeine, heroin, and methadone, morphine crosses the blood–brain barrier at a considerably lower rate.

Distribution and Fate About one-third of morphine in the plasma is protein-bound after a therapeutic dose. Morphine itself does not persist in tissues, and 24 hours after the last dose, tissue concentrations are low.

The major pathway for the metabolism of morphine is conjugation with glucuronic acid. The two major metabolites formed are *morphine-6-glucuronide* and *morphine-3-glucuronide*. Small amounts of morphine-3,6-diglucuronide also may be formed. Although the 3- and 6-glucuronides are quite polar, both still can cross the blood–brain barrier to exert significant clinical effects. Morphine-3-glucuronide has little affinity for opioid receptors but may contribute to excitatory effects of morphine. Morphine-6-glucuronide given systemically is about twice as potent as morphine; with chronic administration, it accounts for a significant portion of morphine's analgesic actions. Indeed, with chronic oral dosing, the blood levels of morphine-6-glucuronide typically exceed those of morphine. Morphine-6-glucuronide is excreted by the kidney. In renal failure, morphine-6-glucuronide can accumulate, perhaps explaining morphine's potency and long duration in patients with compromised renal function. In adults, the $t_{1/2}$ of morphine is ~2 hours; the $t_{1/2}$ of morphine-6-glucuronide is somewhat longer. Children achieve adult renal function values by 6 months of age. In elderly patients, lower doses of morphine are recommended based on its smaller volume of distribution and the general decline in renal function in the elderly. N-Dealkylation also is important in the metabolism of some congeners of morphine.

CODEINE In contrast to morphine, codeine is ~60% as effective orally as parenterally as an analgesic and as a respiratory depressant. Codeine analogs such as *levorphanol*, oxycodone, and methadone have a high ratio of oral-to-parenteral potency. The greater oral efficacy of these drugs reflects lower first-pass metabolism. Once absorbed, codeine is metabolized by the liver, and its metabolites are excreted chiefly as inactive forms in the urine. A relatively small fraction (~10%) of administered codeine is O-demethylated to morphine, and free and conjugated morphine can be found in the urine after therapeutic doses of codeine. Codeine has an exceptionally low affinity for opioid receptors, and the analgesic effect of codeine is due to its conversion to morphine. However, its antitussive actions may involve distinct receptors that bind codeine itself. The $t_{1/2}$ of codeine in plasma is 2–4 hours.

The conversion of codeine to morphine is effected by CYP2D6. Genetic polymorphisms in CYP2D6 lead to the inability to convert codeine to morphine, thus making codeine ineffective as an analgesic for ~10% of the Caucasian population. Other polymorphisms can lead to enhanced metabolism and thus increased sensitivity to codeine's effects. Thus, it is important to consider the possibility of metabolic enzyme polymorphism in any patient who does not receive adequate analgesia from codeine or other opioid prodrugs. A genetic test to identify these CYP2D6 polymorphisms is FDA-approved.

TRAMADOL *Tramadol* (ULTRAM) is a synthetic codeine analog that is a weak μ-opioid receptor agonist. Part of its analgesic effect is produced by inhibition of uptake of NE and 5-HT. In the treatment of mild-to-moderate pain, tramadol is as effective as morphine or meperidine. However, for the treatment of severe or chronic pain, tramadol is less effective. Tramadol is as effective as meperidine in the treatment of labor pain and may cause less neonatal respiratory depression.

HEROIN Heroin (diacetylmorphine) is rapidly hydrolyzed to 6-monoacetylmorphine (6-MAM), which, in turn, is hydrolyzed to morphine. Heroin and 6-MAM are more lipid soluble than morphine and enter the brain more readily. Evidence suggests that morphine and 6-MAM are responsible for the pharmacological actions of heroin. Heroin is excreted mainly in the urine largely as free and conjugated morphine.

UNTOWARD EFFECTS AND PRECAUTIONS Morphine and related opioids produce a wide spectrum of unwanted effects, including respiratory depression, nausea, vomiting, dizziness, mental clouding, dysphoria, pruritus, constipation, increased pressure in the biliary tract, urinary retention, hypotension, and rarely delirium. Increased sensitivity to pain after analgesia has worn off also may occur.

A number of factors may alter a patient's sensitivity to opioid analgesics, including the integrity of the blood–brain barrier. For example, when morphine is administered to a newborn infant in weight-appropriate doses extrapolated from adults, unexpectedly profound analgesia and respiratory depression may be observed. This is due to the immaturity of the blood–brain barrier in neonates. Morphine is hydrophilic, so proportionately less morphine normally crosses into the CNS than with more lipophilic opioids. In neonates or when the blood–brain barrier is compromised, lipophilic opioids may give more predictable clinical results than morphine. In adults, the *duration* of the analgesia produced by morphine increases progressively with age, while the *degree* of analgesia for a given dose changes little. Changes in pharmacokinetics only partly explain this. The patient with severe pain may tolerate larger doses of morphine. However, as the pain subsides, the patient may exhibit sedation and even respiratory depression as the stimulatory effects of pain are diminished. The reasons for this effect are unclear.

All opioid analgesics are metabolized by the liver and should be used with caution in patients with hepatic disease because increased bioavailability after oral administration or cumulative effects may occur. Renal disease also significantly alters the pharmacokinetics of morphine, codeine, *dihydrocodeine,* meperidine, and propoxyphene. Although single doses of morphine are well tolerated, the active metabolite, morphine-6-glucuronide, may accumulate with continued dosing, and symptoms of opioid overdose may result. This metabolite also may accumulate during repeated administration of codeine to patients with impaired renal function. When repeated doses of meperidine are given to such patients, the accumulation of normeperidine may cause tremor and seizures. Similarly, the repeated administration of propoxyphene may lead to naloxone-insensitive cardiac toxicity caused by the accumulation of norpropoxyphene.

Morphine and related opioids must be used cautiously in patients with compromised respiratory function (*e.g.,* emphysema, kyphoscoliosis, or severe obesity). In patients with cor pulmonale, death has occurred after therapeutic doses of morphine. Although many patients with such conditions seem to be functioning within normal limits, they are already using compensatory mechanisms, such as increased respiratory rate. Many have chronically elevated levels of plasma CO_2 and may be less sensitive to the stimulating actions of CO_2. The further imposition of the depressant effects of opioids can be disastrous. The respiratory-depressant effects of opioids and the related capacity to elevate intracranial pressure must be considered in the presence of head injury or an already elevated intracranial pressure. While head injury *per se* does not constitute an absolute contraindication to the use of opioids, the possibility of exaggerated depression of respiration and the potential need to control ventilation of the patient must be considered. Finally, since opioids may produce mental clouding and side effects such as miosis and vomiting, which are important signs in following the clinical course of patients with head injuries, the advisability of their use must be weighed carefully against these risks.

Morphine causes histamine release, which can cause bronchoconstriction and vasodilation, and should be avoided in patients with a history of asthma. Other μ-receptor agonists that do not release histamine, such as the fentanyl derivatives, may be better choices for such patients.

Patients with reduced blood volume are considerably more susceptible to the vasodilatory effects of morphine and related drugs, and these agents must be used cautiously in patients with hypotension from any cause.

OTHER μ-RECEPTOR AGONISTS
Levorphanol

Levorphanol (LEVO-DROMORAN) is the only commercially available opioid agonist of the morphinan series. The D-isomer (dextrorphan) is relatively devoid of analgesic action but may have inhibitory effects at NMDA receptors.

The pharmacological effects of levorphanol closely parallel those of morphine, but it may produce less nausea and vomiting. Levorphanol is metabolized less rapidly than morphine and has a $t_{1/2}$ of ~12–16 hours; thus, repeated administration at short intervals may lead to accumulation of the drug in plasma.

Meperidine and Congeners

Meperidine is predominantly a μ-receptor agonist and acts principally on the CNS and the neural elements in the bowel. Meperidine is no longer recommended for the treatment of chronic pain because of concerns over metabolite toxicity. It should not be used for longer than 48 hours or in doses >600 mg/day.

PHARMACOLOGICAL PROPERTIES Meperidine produces a *pattern* of effects similar but not identical to that described for morphine. The analgesic effects of meperidine are detectable ~15 minutes after oral administration, peak in ~1–2 hours, and subside gradually. The onset of analgesic effect is faster (within 10 minutes) after subcutaneous or intramuscular administration, and the effect reaches a peak in ~1 hour that corresponds closely to peak concentrations in plasma. In clinical use, the duration of effective analgesia is ~1.5–3 hours. In general, 75–100 mg meperidine hydrochloride (*pethidine*, DEMEROL) given parenterally is approximately equivalent to 10 mg morphine, and in equianalgesic doses, meperidine produces as much sedation, respiratory depression, and euphoria as does morphine. In terms of total analgesic effect, meperidine is about one-third as effective when given orally as when administered parenterally. A few patients may experience dysphoria.

Meperidine causes less constipation than morphine even when given over prolonged periods of time; this may be related to its greater ability to enter the CNS, thereby producing analgesia at lower systemic concentrations. Clinical doses of meperidine slow gastric emptying sufficiently to delay absorption of other drugs.

Meperidine is metabolized chiefly in the liver, with a $t_{1/2}$ of ~3 hours. In patients with cirrhosis, the bioavailability of meperidine is increased to as much as 80%, and the $t_{1/2}$ of both meperidine and normeperidine are prolonged. Approximately 60% of meperidine in plasma is protein-bound. Only a small amount of meperidine is excreted unchanged.

UNTOWARD EFFECTS, PRECAUTIONS, AND CONTRAINDICATIONS In patients or addicts who are tolerant to the depressant effects of meperidine, large doses repeated at short intervals may produce an excitatory syndrome, including hallucinations, tremors, muscle twitches, dilated pupils, hyperactive reflexes, and convulsions. These excitatory symptoms are due to the accumulation of normeperidine, the demethylated metabolite, which has a $t_{1/2}$ of 15–20 hours compared with 3 hours for meperidine. Opioid antagonists may block the convulsant effect of normeperidine. Since normeperidine is eliminated by the kidney and the liver, decreased renal or hepatic function increases the likelihood of such toxicity.

Meperidine crosses the placental barrier and increases the percentage of babies who exhibit delayed respiration, decreased respiratory minute volume, or decreased oxygen saturation or who require resuscitation; if present, these conditions can be treated with naloxone. Meperidine produces less respiratory depression in the newborn than does an equianalgesic dose of morphine or methadone.

INTERACTIONS WITH OTHER DRUGS
Severe reactions may follow the administration of meperidine to patients being treated with MAO inhibitors. An excitatory reaction ("serotonin syndrome") with delirium, hyperthermia, headache,

hyper- or hypotension, rigidity, convulsions, coma, and death may be due to the ability of meperidine to block neuronal reuptake of 5-HT and the resulting serotonergic overactivity. Therefore, meperidine and its congeners should not be used in patients taking MAO inhibitors. Potentiation owing to inhibition of hepatic CYPs also can be observed in patients taking MAO inhibitors, necessitating a reduction in the doses of opioids.

Chlorpromazine and tricyclic antidepressants increase the respiratory-depressant and sedative effects of meperidine. Increased respiratory depression is not seen with concomitant use of diazepam. Treatment with phenobarbital or phenytoin increases systemic clearance and decreases oral bioavailability of meperidine; this is associated with an elevation of the plasma concentration of normeperidine. Concomitant administration of amphetamine has been reported to enhance the analgesic effects of meperidine and its congeners while counteracting sedation.

THERAPEUTIC USES   Meperidine is used for analgesia. Single doses of meperidine appear to be effective in the treatment of postanesthetic shivering. Meperidine, 25–50 mg, is used frequently with antihistamines, glucocorticoids, *acetaminophen,* or nonsteroidal anti-inflammatory drugs (NSAIDs) to prevent or ameliorate infusion reactions that accompany the intravenous administration of *amphotericin B, aldesleukin* (interleukin-2), *trastuzumab,* and *alemtuzumab.*

CONGENERS OF MEPERIDINE

Diphenoxylate

Diphenoxylate *is a meperidine congener that is approved for the treatment of diarrhea* (see Chapter 37). Diphenoxylate hydrochloride *is available only in combination with atropine sulfate* (LOMOTIL, *others). The recommended daily dosage of diphenoxylate for the treatment of diarrhea in adults is 20 mg in divided doses.* Difenoxin (MOTOFEN), *a metabolite of diphenoxylate, has actions similar to those of the parent compound.*

Loperamide

Loperamide (IMODIUM, *others), like diphenoxylate, is a piperidine derivative; it penetrates poorly into the CNS. Loperamide slows GI motility by effects on the circular and longitudinal muscles of the intestine, presumably via interactions with opioid receptors in the intestine. In controlling chronic diarrhea, loperamide is as effective as diphenoxylate, and little tolerance develops.*

Fentanyl and Congeners

Fentanyl is a synthetic opioid related to the phenylpiperidines. The actions of fentanyl and congeners are similar to those of other μ-receptor agonists. Fentanyl is a popular anesthetic because of its relatively short time to peak analgesic effect, rapid termination of effect after small bolus doses, and cardiovascular safety (see Chapter 13).

PHARMACOLOGICAL PROPERTIES

Fentanyl is ~100 times more potent than morphine, and sufentanil is ~1000 times more potent than morphine. These drugs are most commonly administered intravenously, although both also are commonly administered epidurally and intrathecally for acute postoperative and chronic pain management. Fentanyl and sufentanil are far more lipid soluble than morphine, greatly reducing the risk of delayed respiratory depression from rostral spread of intraspinally administered narcotic to respiratory centers. The time to peak analgesic effect after intravenous administration of fentanyl and sufentanil is less than that for morphine and meperidine, with peak analgesia being reached after 5 minutes, as opposed to 15 minutes. Recovery from analgesic effects also occurs more quickly. However, with larger doses or prolonged infusions, the effects of these drugs become more lasting, with durations of action becoming similar to those of longer-acting opioids (see below).

Fentanyl and its derivatives decrease the heart rate and can mildly decrease blood pressure. However, these drugs do not release histamine and generally provide a marked degree of cardiovascular stability. Direct depressant effects on the myocardium are minimal. For this reason, high doses of fentanyl or sufentanil are commonly used as the primary anesthetic for patients undergoing cardiovascular surgery or for patients with poor cardiac function. Fentanyl and sufentanil undergo hepatic metabolism and renal excretion. Therefore, with the use of higher doses or prolonged infusions, fentanyl and sufentanil become longer acting.

THERAPEUTIC USES

Fentanyl citrate (SUBLIMAZE) *and* sufentanil citrate (SUFENTA) *have gained widespread popularity as anesthetic adjuvants* (see Chapter 13). *They are used commonly either intravenously, epidurally, or intrathecally* (e.g., *epidural use for postoperative or labor analgesia). Epidural and intrathecal infusions, with or without local anesthetic, are used in the management of chronic malignant pain and selected cases of nonmalignant pain. Transdermal patches (DURAGESIC) that provide sustained release of fentanyl for 48 hours or more are available. However, factors promoting increased absorption (e.g., fever) can lead to relative overdosage and increased side effects (see alternative routes of administration, below).*

Methadone and Congeners

Methadone is a long-acting μ-receptor agonist with properties qualitatively similar to those of morphine.

PHARMACOLOGICAL ACTIONS   The outstanding properties of methadone are its analgesic activity, its oral efficacy, extended duration of action in suppressing withdrawal symptoms in physically dependent individuals, and tendency to show persistent effects with repeated administration. Miotic and respiratory-depressant effects can be detected for >24 hours after a single dose, and on repeated administration, marked sedation is seen in some patients. Effects on cough, bowel motility, biliary tone, and the secretion of pituitary hormones are qualitatively similar to those of morphine.

ABSORPTION, FATE, AND EXCRETION   Methadone is absorbed well from the GI tract and can be detected in plasma within 30 minutes of oral ingestion; it reaches peak concentrations at ~4 hours. After therapeutic doses, ~90% of methadone is bound to plasma proteins. Peak concentrations in the brain occur within 1–2 hours of subcutaneous or intramuscular administration, which correlates well with the intensity and duration of analgesia. Methadone also is absorbed from the buccal mucosa.

Methadone undergoes extensive biotransformation in the liver. The major metabolites, the results of *N*-demethylation and cyclization to form pyrrolidines and pyrroline, are excreted in the urine and the bile along with small amounts of unchanged drug. The amount of methadone excreted in the urine is increased when the urine is acidified. The $t_{1/2}$ of methadone is 15–40 hours.

Methadone is firmly bound to protein in various tissues, including brain, and accumulates gradually with repeated administration. When administration is stopped, low plasma concentrations are maintained by slow release from extravascular binding sites; this process probably accounts for the relatively mild but protracted withdrawal syndrome. Rifampin and phenytoin accelerate methadone metabolism and can precipitate withdrawal symptoms.

THERAPEUTIC USES   The primary uses of *methadone hydrochloride* (DOLOPHINE, others) are relief of chronic pain, treatment of opioid abstinence syndromes, and treatment of heroin users. It should not be used in labor.

The onset of analgesia occurs 10–20 minutes after parenteral administration and 30–60 minutes after oral use. The typical oral dose is 2.5–15 mg depending on the severity of the pain and the response of the patient. Care must be taken when escalating the dosage because of the prolonged $t_{1/2}$ of the drug and its tendency to accumulate over a period of several days with repeated dosing. Despite its longer plasma half-life, the duration of the analgesic action of single doses of methadone is essentially the same as that of morphine. With repeated use, cumulative effects are seen, so either lower dosages or longer intervals between doses become possible.

Propoxyphene

PHARMACOLOGICAL ACTIONS

Although slightly less selective than morphine, propoxyphene binds primarily to μ opioid receptors and produces analgesia and other CNS effects that are similar to those seen with morphine-like opioids. It is likely that at equianalgesic doses the incidence of side effects such as nausea, anorexia, constipation, abdominal pain, and drowsiness are similar to those of codeine.

As an analgesic, propoxyphene is about one-half to two-thirds as potent as codeine given orally. A dose of 90–120 mg of propoxyphene hydrochloride *administered orally would equal the analgesic effects of 60 mg codeine, a dose that usually produces about as much analgesia as 600 mg* aspirin. *Combinations of propoxyphene and aspirin, like combinations of codeine and aspirin, afford a higher level of analgesia than does either agent alone.*

After oral administration, concentrations of propoxyphene peak at 1–2 hours. There is great variability between subjects in the rate of clearance; average $t_{1/2}$ of propoxyphene in plasma after a single dose is 6–12 hours, which is longer than that of codeine. In humans, the major route of metabolism is N-demethylation to yield norpropoxyphene, *which has a $t_{1/2}$ of 30 hours and may accumulate to toxic levels with repeated doses.*

THERAPEUTIC USES

Propoxyphene is recommended for the treatment of mild-to-moderate pain. Given acutely, the commonly prescribed combination of 32 mg propoxyphene with aspirin may not produce more analgesia than aspirin alone, and doses of 65 mg of the hydrochloride or 100 mg of the napsylate are suggested. Propoxyphene is given most often in combination with aspirin or acetaminophen. *The wide popularity of propoxyphene is largely a result of unrealistic overconcern about the addictive potential of codeine.*

ACUTE OPIOID TOXICITY

Acute opioid toxicity may result from clinical overdosage, accidental overdosage in addicts, or attempts at suicide. Occasionally, a delayed type of toxicity may occur from the injection of an opioid into chilled skin areas or in patients with low blood pressure and shock. The drug is not fully absorbed, and therefore, a subsequent dose may be given. When normal circulation is restored, an excessive amount may be absorbed suddenly. It is difficult to define the exact amount of any opioid that is toxic or lethal to humans. In nontolerant individuals, serious toxicity may follow the oral ingestion of 40–60 mg of methadone. A normal, pain-free adult is not likely to die after oral doses of morphine of <120 mg or to have serious toxicity with <30 mg parenterally.

SYMPTOMS AND DIAGNOSIS

The triad of coma, pinpoint pupils, and depressed respiration strongly suggests opioid poisoning. A patient who has taken an overdose of an opioid usually is stuporous or, if a large overdose has been taken, may be in a coma. The respiratory rate will be very low, or the patient may be apneic and cyanotic. As the respiratory exchange decreases, blood pressure, at first likely to be near normal, will fall progressively. If oxygenation is restored early, the blood pressure will improve; if hypoxia persists untreated, there may be capillary damage, and measures to combat shock may be required. The pupils will be symmetrical and pinpoint in size; if hypoxia is severe, they may be dilated. Urine formation is depressed, body temperature falls, and the skin becomes cold and clammy. The skeletal muscles are flaccid, the jaw is relaxed, and the tongue may obstruct the airway. Frank convulsions occasionally occur in infants and children. When death ensues, it is nearly always from respiratory failure. Even if respiration is restored, death still may occur as a result of complications that develop during the period of coma, such as pneumonia or shock. Noncardiogenic pulmonary edema is seen commonly with opioid poisoning.

TREATMENT Establish a patent airway and ventilate the patient. Opioid antagonists (*see* below) can produce dramatic reversal of the severe respiratory depression; naloxone is the treatment of choice. The safest approach is to dilute the standard naloxone dose (0.4 mg) and slowly administer it intravenously, monitoring arousal and respiratory function. With care, it usually is possible to reverse the respiratory depression without precipitating a major withdrawal syndrome. If no response is seen with the first dose, additional doses can be given. Patients should be observed for rebound increases in sympathetic nervous system activity, which may result in cardiac arrhythmias and pulmonary edema. For reversing opioid poisoning in children, the initial dose of naloxone is 0.01 mg/kg. If no effect is seen after a total dose of 10 mg, one can reasonably question the accuracy of the diagnosis. Pulmonary edema sometimes associated with opioid overdosage may be countered by positive-pressure respiration. Tonic-clonic seizures, occasionally seen as part of the toxic syndrome with meperidine and propoxyphene, are ameliorated by treatment with naloxone.

OPIOID AGONIST/ANTAGONISTS AND PARTIAL AGONISTS

Drugs such as *nalbuphine* and *butorphanol* are competitive μ-receptor antagonists that exert analgesic actions by acting as agonists at κ receptors. Pentazocine qualitatively resembles these drugs, but it may be a weaker μ-receptor antagonist or partial agonist while retaining its κ-agonist activity. Buprenorphine, in contrast, is a partial agonist at μ receptors. The clinical use of these drugs is limited by undesirable side effects and limited analgesic effects.

Pentazocine

The CNS effects produced by pentazocine generally are similar to those of the morphine-like opioids, including analgesia, sedation, and respiratory depression. The analgesic effects of pentazocine are due to agonistic actions at κ opioid receptors. Higher doses of pentazocine (60–90 mg) elicit dysphoric and psychotomimetic effects; these effects may involve activation of supraspinal κ receptors and sometimes are reversed by naloxone.

The cardiovascular responses to pentazocine differ from those seen with typical μ-receptor agonists, in that high doses cause an increase in blood pressure and heart rate. Pentazocine acts as a weak antagonist or partial agonist at μ-opioid receptors. Pentazocine does not antagonize the respiratory depression produced by morphine. However, when given to patients dependent on morphine or other μ-receptor agonists, pentazocine may precipitate withdrawal. Ceiling effects for analgesia and respiratory depression are observed above 50–100 mg pentazocine.

Tablets for oral use now contain pentazocine hydrochloride *(equivalent to 50 mg of the base) and* naloxone hydrochloride *(equivalent to 0.5 mg of the base;* TALWIN NX*), which reduces the potential use of tablets as a source of injectable pentazocine. After oral ingestion, naloxone is destroyed rapidly by the liver; however, if the material is dissolved and injected, the naloxone produces aversive effects in subjects dependent on opioids. An oral dose of ~50 mg pentazocine results in analgesia equivalent to that produced by 60 mg codeine orally.*

Nalbuphine

Nalbuphine is an agonist–antagonist opioid with a spectrum of effects that qualitatively resembles that of pentazocine; however, nalbuphine is a more potent antagonist at μ receptors and is less likely to produce dysphoria.

PHARMACOLOGICAL ACTIONS AND SIDE EFFECTS

An intramuscular dose of 10 mg nalbuphine is equianalgesic to 10 mg morphine, with similar onset and duration of analgesia. Nalbuphine depresses respiration as much as morphine. However, it exhibits a ceiling effect such that increases in dosage beyond 30 mg produce no further respiratory depression or analgesia. In contrast to pentazocine and butorphanol, 10 mg nalbuphine given to patients with stable coronary artery disease does not increase cardiac index, pulmonary arterial pressure, or cardiac work, and systemic blood pressure is not significantly altered; these indices also are relatively stable when nalbuphine is given to patients with acute myocardial infarction. Nalbuphine produces few side effects at doses of 10 mg or less; sedation, sweating, and headache are most common. At much higher doses (70 mg), psychotomimetic side effects (e.g., dysphoria, racing thoughts, and distortions of body image) can occur. Nalbuphine is metabolized in the liver and has a $t_{1/2}$ in plasma of 2–3 hours. Given orally, nalbuphine is 20–25% as potent as when given intramuscularly.

THERAPEUTIC USES

Nalbuphine hydrochloride *(*NUBAIN*) is used to produce analgesia. Because it is an agonist–antagonist, administration to patients who have been receiving morphine-like opioids may create difficulties unless a brief drug-free interval is interposed. The usual adult dose is 10 mg parenterally every 3–6 hours; this may be increased to 20 mg in nontolerant individuals.*

Butorphanol

Butorphanol is a morphinan congener with a profile of actions similar to that of pentazocine.

PHARMACOLOGICAL ACTIONS AND SIDE EFFECTS

In postoperative patients, a parenteral dose of 2–3 mg butorphanol produces analgesia and respiratory depression approximately equal to that produced by 10 mg morphine or 80–100 mg meperidine; the onset, peak, and duration of action are similar to those that follow the administration of morphine. The plasma $t_{1/2}$ of butorphanol is ~3 hours. Like pentazocine, analgesic doses of butorphanol produce an increase in pulmonary arterial pressure and in the work of the heart; systemic arterial pressure is slightly decreased.

The major side effects of butorphanol are drowsiness, weakness, sweating, feelings of floating, and nausea. While the incidence of psychotomimetic side effects is lower than that with equianalgesic doses of pentazocine, they are qualitatively similar. Physical dependence on butorphanol can occur.

THERAPEUTIC USES

Butorphanol tartrate *(*STADOL*) is better suited for the relief of acute than chronic pain. Because of its side effects on the heart, it is less useful than morphine or meperidine in patients with congestive heart failure or myocardial infarction. The usual dose is 1–4 mg of the tartrate given intramuscularly or 0.5–2 mg given intravenously every 3–4 hours. A nasal formulation (*STADOL NS*) is available and has proven to be effective.*

Buprenorphine

Buprenorphine is a semisynthetic, lipophilic opioid derived from thebaine that is 25–50 times more potent than morphine.

PHARMACOLOGICAL ACTIONS AND SIDE EFFECTS

About 0.4 mg buprenorphine is equianalgesic with 10 mg morphine given intramuscularly. Although variable, the duration of analgesia usually is longer than that of morphine. Some of the subjective and respiratory-depressant effects are unequivocally slower in onset and last longer than those of morphine.

Buprenorphine appears to be a partial μ-receptor agonist and may cause symptoms of abstinence in patients who have been receiving μ-receptor agonists for several weeks. It antagonizes the respiratory depression produced by anesthetic doses of fentanyl about as well as does naloxone without completely reversing opioid pain relief. The respiratory depression and other effects of buprenorphine can be prevented by prior administration of naloxone, but they are not readily reversed by even high doses of naloxone once the effects have been produced due to slow dissociation of buprenorphine from opioid receptors. Therefore, plasma levels of buprenorphine may not parallel clinical effects. Cardiovascular and other side effects (e.g., sedation, nausea, vomiting, dizziness, sweating, and headache) appear to be similar to those of morphine-like opioids.

Administered sublingually, buprenorphine (0.4–0.8 mg) produces satisfactory analgesia in postoperative patients. Concentrations peak within 5 minutes of intramuscular injection and within 1–2 hours of oral or sublingual administration. The $t_{1/2}$ of ~3 hours bears little relationship to the rate of disappearance of effects (see above). Most of the drug is excreted unchanged in the feces. About 96% of the circulating drug is bound to protein.

THERAPEUTIC USES

Buprenorphine (BUPRENEX; SUBUTEX) is used as an analgesic and as a maintenance drug for opioid-dependent subjects. The usual intramuscular or intravenous dose for analgesia is 0.3 mg given every 6 hours. Sublingual doses of 0.4–0.8 mg also produce effective analgesia. Buprenorphine is metabolized to norbuprenorphine by CYP3A4. Thus, care should be taken in treating patients who also are taking known inhibitors of CYP3A4 (e.g., azole antifungals, macrolide antibiotics, and HIV protease inhibitors) or drugs that induce CYP3A4 activity (e.g., anticonvulsants and rifampin).

Buprenorphine is approved by the FDA for the treatment of opioid addiction. Treatment is initiated with buprenorphine alone administered sublingually, followed by maintenance therapy with a combination of buprenorphine and naloxone (SUBOXONE) to minimize abuse potential. The partial agonist properties of buprenorphine limit its usefulness for the treatment of addicts who require high maintenance doses of opioids. However, conversion to maintenance treatment with higher doses of methadone, a full agonist, is possible.

OPIOID ANTAGONISTS

These agents have obvious therapeutic utility in the treatment of opioid overdose. As the understanding of the role of endogenous opioid systems in pathophysiological states (*e.g.*, shock, stroke, spinal cord and brain trauma) increases, additional therapeutic indications for these antagonists may develop.

Pharmacological Properties

If endogenous opioid systems have not been activated, the pharmacological actions of opioid antagonists depend on whether or not an opioid agonist has been administered previously, on the pharmacological profile of that opioid, and on the degree to which physical dependence on an opioid has developed.

EFFECTS IN THE ABSENCE OF OPIOID DRUGS Subcutaneous doses of naloxone (NARCAN) up to 12 mg produce no discernible subjective effects, and 24 mg causes only slight drowsiness. Naltrexone (REVIA) also appears to be a relatively pure antagonist but with higher oral efficacy and a longer duration of action. At doses in excess of 0.3 mg/kg naloxone, normal subjects show increased systolic blood pressure and decreased performance on tests of memory. High doses of naltrexone appeared to cause mild dysphoria in one study but almost no subjective effect in several others.

Although high doses of antagonists might be expected to alter the actions of endogenous opioid peptides, the detectable effects usually are both subtle and limited. This most likely reflects the low levels of tonic activity of the opioid systems. In this regard, analgesic effects can be differentiated from endocrine effects, in which naloxone causes readily demonstrable changes in hormone levels (see below). Interestingly, naloxone appears to block the analgesic effects of placebo medications and acupuncture.

Endogenous opioid peptides participate in the regulation of pituitary secretion by exerting tonic inhibitory effects on the release of certain hypothalamic releasing hormones (see Chapter 55). Thus, the administration of naloxone or naltrexone increases the secretion of GnRH and CRH and elevates the plasma concentrations of LH, FSH, and ACTH, as well as the steroid hormones produced by their target organs. Naloxone stimulates the release of prolactin in women.

ANTAGONISTIC ACTIONS Small doses (0.4–0.8 mg) of naloxone given intramuscularly or intravenously prevent or promptly reverse the effects of μ-receptor agonists. In patients with respiratory depression, an increase in respiratory rate is seen within 1–2 minutes. Sedative effects are reversed, and blood pressure, if depressed, returns to normal. Higher doses of naloxone are required to antagonize the respiratory-depressant effects of buprenorphine; 1 mg naloxone intravenously completely blocks the effects of 25 mg heroin. Naloxone reverses the psychotomimetic and dysphoric effects of agonist–antagonist agents such as pentazocine, but much higher doses (10–15 mg) are required. The duration of antagonistic effects depends on the dose but usually is 1–4 hours. Antagonism of opioid effects by naloxone often is accompanied by "overshoot" phenomena. For example, respiratory rate depressed transiently by opioids becomes higher than that before the period of depression. Rebound release of catecholamines may cause hypertension, tachycardia, and ventricular arrhythmias. Pulmonary edema also has been reported.

EFFECTS IN PHYSICAL DEPENDENCE In subjects who are dependent on morphine-like opioids, small subcutaneous doses of naloxone (0.5 mg) precipitate a moderate-to-severe withdrawal syndrome that is very similar to that seen after abrupt withdrawal of opioids, except that the syndrome appears within minutes of administration and subsides in ~2 hours. The severity and duration of the syndrome are related to the dose of the antagonist and to the degree and type of dependence. Higher doses of naloxone will precipitate a withdrawal syndrome in patients dependent on pentazocine, butorphanol, or nalbuphine. Naloxone produces overshoot phenomena suggestive of early acute physical dependence 6–24 hours after a single dose of a μ agonist.

TOLERANCE AND PHYSICAL DEPENDENCE Even after prolonged administration of high doses, discontinuation of naloxone is not followed by any recognizable withdrawal syndrome, and the withdrawal of naltrexone, another relatively pure antagonist, produces very few signs and symptoms. However, long-term administration of antagonists increases the density of opioid receptors in the brain and causes a temporary exaggeration of responses to the subsequent administration of opioid agonists. Naltrexone and naloxone have little or no potential for abuse.

ABSORPTION, FATE, AND EXCRETION Although absorbed readily from the GI tract, naloxone is almost completely metabolized by the liver before reaching the systemic circulation and thus must be administered parenterally. The $t_{1/2}$ of naloxone is ~1 hour, but its clinically effective duration of action can be even less.

Compared with naloxone, naltrexone retains much more of its efficacy by the oral route, and its duration of action approaches 24 hours after moderate oral doses. Peak concentrations in plasma are reached within 1–2 hours and the $t_{1/2}$ of ~3 hours does not change with long-term use. Naltrexone is much more potent than naloxone, and 100-mg oral doses given to patients addicted to opioids produce concentrations in tissues sufficient to block the euphorigenic effects of 25-mg intravenous doses of heroin for 48 hours.

Therapeutic Uses

Opioid antagonists have established uses in the treatment of opioid-induced toxicity, especially respiratory depression; in the diagnosis of physical dependence on opioids; and as therapeutic agents in the treatment of compulsive users of opioids (Chapter 23). Naltrexone is also FDA-approved for the treatment of alcohol abuse.

TREATMENT OF OPIOID OVERDOSAGE Naloxone hydrochloride should be used cautiously for opiate overdose because it also can precipitate withdrawal in dependent subjects and cause undesirable cardiovascular side effects. By carefully titrating the dose of naloxone, it usually is possible to antagonize the respiratory-depressant actions without eliciting a full withdrawal syndrome. The duration of action of naloxone is relatively short, and it often must be given repeatedly or by continuous infusion. Opioid antagonists also have been employed effectively to decrease neonatal respiratory depression secondary to the intravenous or intramuscular administration of opioids to the mother. In the neonate, the initial dose is 10 μg/kg given intravenously, intramuscularly, or subcutaneously.

CENTRALLY ACTIVE ANTITUSSIVE AGENTS

Cough is a useful physiological mechanism that serves to clear the respiratory passages of foreign material and excess secretions and should not be suppressed indiscriminately. Chronic cough sometimes can prevent rest or sleep or contribute to fatigue, especially in elderly patients. In such situations, the physician should use a drug that will reduce the frequency or intensity of the coughing. The cough reflex is complex, involving the central and peripheral nervous systems and the smooth muscle of the bronchial tree. It has been suggested that irritation of the bronchial mucosa causes bronchoconstriction, which, in turn, stimulates cough receptors (which probably represent a specialized type of stretch receptor) located in tracheobronchial passages. Afferent conduction from these receptors is *via* the vagus nerve; central components of the reflex probably include several mechanisms or centers that are distinct from the mechanisms involved in the regulation of respiration.

The opioid analgesics discussed earlier (codeine and hydrocodone are the opioids most commonly used to suppress cough), as well as a number of nonopioid agents reduce cough as a result of their central actions. Cough suppression often occurs with lower doses of opioids than those needed for analgesia. A 10- or 20-mg oral dose of codeine, although ineffective for analgesia, produces a demonstrable antitussive effect, and higher doses produce even more suppression of chronic cough.

DEXTROMETHORPHAN   Dextromethorphan (D-3-methoxy-N-methylmorphinan) is the D-isomer of the codeine analog methorphan; unlike the L-isomer, it has no analgesic or addictive properties and does not act through opioid receptors. The drug acts centrally to elevate the threshold for coughing; its potency is nearly equal to that of codeine, but it produces fewer subjective and GI side effects. In therapeutic dosages, the drug does not inhibit ciliary activity, and its antitussive effects persist for 5–6 hours. Its toxicity is low, but extremely high doses may produce CNS depression.

THERAPEUTIC USES OF OPIOID ANALGESICS

Opioids remain the mainstay of pain treatment. Useful guidelines for their administration have been developed for a number of clinical situations, including treatment of acute pain, trauma, cancer, nonmalignant chronic pain, and pain in children. In the case of cancer pain, adherence to standardized protocols can improve pain management significantly. Guidelines for the oral and parenteral dosing of opioids are presented in Table 21–5.

In general, it is recommended that opioids always be combined with other analgesic agents, such as NSAIDs or acetaminophen. In this way, one can take advantage of additive analgesic effects and minimize the dose of opioids and thus undesirable side effects. In some situations, NSAIDs can provide analgesia equal to that produced by 60 mg codeine. This "opioid sparing" strategy is the backbone of the "analgesic ladder" for pain management proposed by the WHO. Weaker opioids can be supplanted by stronger opioids in cases of moderate or severe pain. In addition, analgesics always should be dosed in a continuous or "around the clock" fashion rather than on an as-needed basis for chronic severe pain. This provides more consistent analgesic levels and avoids unnecessary suffering.

Factors guiding the selection of specific opioid compounds for pain treatment include potency, pharmacokinetic characteristics, and the routes of administration available. A more potent compound could be useful when high doses of opioid are required so that the medicine can be given in a smaller volume. Duration of action also is an important consideration. In cases where a lower addiction risk is required or in patients unable to tolerate other opioids, a partial agonist or mixed agonist–antagonist compound might be a rational choice.

Morphine is available for oral use in standard and controlled-release preparations. Owing to first-pass metabolism, morphine is two to six times less potent orally than it is parenterally. This is important to remember when converting a patient from parenteral to oral medication. There is wide variability in the first-pass metabolism, and the dose should be titrated to the patient's needs. In children who weigh <50 kg, morphine can be given at 0.1 mg/kg every 3–4 hours parenterally or at 0.3 mg/kg orally.

Codeine is used widely owing to its high oral/parenteral potency ratio. Orally, codeine at 30 mg is approximately equianalgesic to 600 mg aspirin. Combinations of codeine with aspirin or acetaminophen usually provide additive actions, and at these doses, analgesic efficacy can exceed that of 60 mg codeine. Many drugs can be used instead of morphine or codeine, as shown in Table 21–5. Oxycodone (ROXICODINE, others), with its high oral/parenteral potency ratio, is used widely in combination with aspirin (PERCODAN, others) or acetaminophen (PERCOCET 2.5/325, others). Oxycodone also is available in a sustained-release formulation for chronic pain management

Table 21-5

Dosing Data for Opioid Analgesics

Drug (TRADE NAME)	Approximate Equianalgesic Oral Dose	Approximate Equianalgesic Parenteral Dose	Recommended Starting Dose (Adults >50 kg Body Weight)		Recommended Starting Dose (Children and Adults <50 kg Body Weight)[1]	
			Oral	Parenteral	Oral	Parenteral
Opioid Agonist						
Morphine[2]	30 mg q3-4h (continuous dosing) 60 mg q3-4h (single dose, intermittent dosing)	10 mg q3-4h	30 mg q3-4h	10 mg q3-4h	0.3 mg/kg q3-4h	0.1 mg/kg q3-4h
Codeine[3]	130 mg q3-4h	75 mg q3-4h	60 mg q3-4h	60 mg q2h (im/sq)	1 mg/kg q3-4h[4]	Not recommended
Hydromorphone[2] (DILAUDID)	7.5 mg q3-4h	1.5 mg q3-4h	6 mg q3-4h	1.5 mg q3-4h	0.06 mg/kg q3-4h	0.015 mg/kg q3-4h
Hydrocodone (in LORCET, LORTAB, VICODIN, others)	30 mg q3-4h	Not available	10 mg q3-4h	Not available	0.2 mg/kg q3-4h[4]	Not available
Levorphanol	4 mg q6-8h	2 mg q6-8h	4 mg q6-8h	2 mg q6-8h	0.04 mg/kg q6-8h	0.02 mg/kg q6-8h
Meperidine (DEMEROL)	300 mg q2-3h	100 mg q3h	Not recommended	100 mg q3h	Not recommended	0.75 mg/kg q2-3h
Methadone (DOLOPHINE, et al.)	20 mg q6-8h	10 mg q6-8h	20 mg q6-8h	10 mg q6-8h	0.2 mg/kg q6-8h	0.1 mg/kg q6-8h
Oxycodone (ROXICODONE, also in PERCOCET, PERCODAN, TYLOX, et al.)[7]	30 mg q3-4h	Not available	10 mg q3-4h	Not available	0.2 mg/kg q3-4h[4]	Not available
Opioid Agonist–Antagonist or Partial Agonist						
Oxymorphone[2] (NUMORPHAN)	Not available	1 mg q3-4h	Not available	1 mg q3-4h	Not recommended	Not recommended
Propoxyphene (DARVON)	130 mg[5]	Not available	65 mg q4-6h[5]	Not available	Not recommended	Not recommended
Tramadol[6] (ULTRAM)	100 mg[5]	100 mg	50-100 mg q6h[5]	50-100 mg q6h[5]	Not recommended	Not recommended
Buprenorphine (BUPRENEX)	Not available	0.3-0.4 mg q6-8h	Not available	0.4 q6-8h	Not available	0.004 mg/kg q6-8h

(Continued)

Table 21-5

Dosing Data for Opioid Analgesics (Continued)

Drug	Approximate Equianalgesic Oral Dose	Approximate Equianalgesic Parenteral Dose	Recommended Starting Dose (Adults >50 kg Body Weight)		Recommended Starting Dose (Children and Adults <50 kg Body Weight)[1]	
			Oral	Parenteral	Oral	Parenteral
Opioid Agonist–Antagonist or Partial Agonist (continued)						
Butorphanol (STADOL)	Not available	2 mg q3–4h	Not available	2 mg q3–4h	Not available	Not recommended
Nalbuphine (NUBAIN)	Not available	10 mg q3–4h	Not available	10 mg q3–4h	Not available	0.1 mg/kg q3–4h

Published tables vary in the suggested doses that are equianalgesic to morphine. Clinical response is the criterion that must be applied for each patient; titration to clinical response is necessary. Because there is not complete cross tolerance among these drugs, it is usually necessary to use a lower than equianalgesic dose when changing drugs and to retitrate to response.

Caution: Recommended doses do not apply to patients with renal or hepatic insufficiency or other conditions affecting drug metabolism and kinetics.

[1]*Caution:* Doses listed for patients with body weight less than 50 kg cannot be used as initial starting doses in babies less than 6 months of age. Consult the *Clinical Practice Guideline for Acute Pain Management: Operative or Medical Procedures and Trauma* section on management of pain in neonates for recommendations.

[2]For morphine, hydromorphone, and oxymorphone, rectal administration is an alternate route for patients unable to take oral medications, but equianalgesic doses may differ from oral and parenteral doses because of pharmacokinetic differences.

[3]*Caution:* Codeine doses above 65 mg often are not appropriate due to diminishing incremental analgesia with increasing doses but continually increasing constipation and other side effects.

[4]*Caution:* Doses of aspirin and acetaminophen in combination opioid/NSAID preparations must also be adjusted to the patient's body weight. Maximum acetaminophen dose: 4 gm/day in adults, 90 mg/kg/day in children.

[5]Doses for moderate pain not necessarily equivalent to 30 mg oral or 10 mg parenteral morphine.

[6]Risk of seizures: parenteral formulation not available in the U.S.

[7]OXYCONTIN is an extended-release preparation containing up to 160 mg of oxycodone per tablet and recommended for use every 12 hours. It has been subject to substantial abuse.

ABBREVIATIONS: q, every; im, intramuscular; sq, subcutaneous.

368

(OXYCONTIN). Unfortunately, this formulation has been subject to widespread abuse leading to serious consequences, including death, and the FDA has strengthened warnings for this drug (see Chapter 23).

It also may be helpful to employ other drugs that enhance opioid analgesia and that may add beneficial effects of their own. For example, the combination of an opioid with a small dose of amphetamine may augment analgesia while reducing the sedative effects. Certain antidepressants, such as amitriptyline and desipramine, also may enhance opioid analgesia, and they may have analgesic actions in some types of neuropathic pain. Other potentially useful adjuvants include antihistamines, anticonvulsants such as carbamazepine *and phenytoin, and glucocorticoids.*

Alternative Routes of Administration

In addition to the traditional oral and parenteral formulations for opioids, other methods of administration have been developed in an effort to improve therapeutic efficacy while minimizing side effects.

PATIENT-CONTROLLED ANALGESIA (PCA) With this modality, the patient has limited control of the dosing of opioid from an infusion pump within tightly mandated parameters. PCA can be used for intravenous or epidural infusion. This technique avoids any delays in administration and permits greater dosing flexibility than other regimens, better adapting to individual differences in responsiveness to pain and to opioids. It also gives the patient a greater sense of control.

INTRASPINAL INFUSION Administration of opioids into the epidural or intrathecal space provides more direct access to the first pain-processing synapse in the dorsal horn of the spinal cord. This permits the use of doses substantially lower than those required for oral or parenteral administration (Table 21–6), thereby decreasing systemic side effects. However, epidural opioids have their own dose-dependent side effects, such as itching, nausea, vomiting, respiratory depression, and urinary retention. Administration of hydrophilic opioids (DURAMORPH, others) permits more rostral spread of the compound, allowing it to directly affect supraspinal sites. As a consequence, after intraspinal morphine, delayed respiratory depression can be observed for as long as 24 hours after a bolus dose. Nausea and vomiting are more prominent symptoms with intraspinal morphine. However, supraspinal analgesic centers also can be stimulated, possibly leading to synergistic analgesic effects.

Analogous to the relationship between systemic opioids and NSAIDs, intraspinal narcotics often are combined with local anesthetics. This permits the use of lower doses of both agents,

Table 21–6

Intraspinal Opioids for the Treatment of Acute Pain

Drug	Single Dose* (mg)	Infusion Rate† (mg/h)	Onset (Minutes)	Duration of Effect of a Single Dose‡ (Hours)
Epidural				
Morphine	1–6	0.1–1.0	30	6–24
Meperidine	20–150	5–20	5	4–8
Methadone	1–10	0.3–0.5	10	6–10
Hydromorphone	1–2	0.1–0.2	15	10–16
Fentanyl	0.025–0.1	0.025–0.10	5	2–4
Sufentanil	0.01–0.06	0.01–0.05	5	2–4
Alfentanil	0.5–1	0.2	15	1–3
Subarachnoid				
Morphine	0.1–0.3		15	8–24+
Meperidine	10–30		?	10–24+
Fentanyl	0.005–0.025		5	3–6

*Low doses may be effective when administered to the elderly or when injected in the cervical or thoracic region.
†If combining with a local anesthetic, consider using 0.0625% bupivacaine.
‡Duration of analgesia varies widely; higher doses produce longer duration.

minimizing local anesthetic–induced complications of motor blockade and opioid-induced complications. Epidural opioid administration is widely used in the management of postoperative pain and for providing analgesia during labor and delivery. Lower systemic levels are achieved with epidural opioids, leading to less placental transfer and less potential for respiratory depression of the newborn. Intrathecal administration of opioids as a bolus ("spinal" anesthesia) also is popular for acute pain management. Chronic intrathecal infusions generally are reserved for use in chronic pain patients.

Rectal administration is an alternative for patients with difficulty swallowing or oral pathology and who prefer a less invasive route than parenteral. This route is not well tolerated in children. Onset of action is seen within 10 minutes.

CLINICAL SUMMARY

Opioid analgesics provide symptomatic relief of pain, but the underlying disease remains. The clinician must weigh the benefits against any potential risk to the patient, which may be quite different in an acute versus chronic disease.

Acutely, opioids will reduce the intensity of pain; physical signs (*e.g.,* abdominal rigidity) generally will remain. Relief of pain can facilitate history taking, examination, and the patient's ability to tolerate diagnostic procedures. Patients should not be evaluated inadequately because of the physician's unwillingness to prescribe narcotics, or over concerns of obscuring the progression of underlying disease.

The problems that arise in the relief of pain associated with chronic conditions are more complex. Repeated daily administration of opioid analgesics eventually will produce tolerance and some degree of physical dependence. The degree will depend on the particular drug, the frequency of administration, and the quantity administered. The decision to control any chronic symptom, especially pain, by the repeated administration of an opioid must be made carefully. When pain is due to chronic nonmalignant disease, measures other than opioid drugs should be employed if possible. Such measures include the use of NSAIDs, local nerve blocks, antidepressant drugs, electrical stimulation, acupuncture, hypnosis, or behavioral modification. However, highly selected subpopulations of chronic nonmalignant pain patients can be maintained adequately on opioids for extended periods of time.

In the usual doses, morphine-like drugs relieve suffering by altering the emotional component of the painful experience, as well as by producing analgesia. Control of pain, especially chronic pain, must include attention to both psychological factors and the social impact of the illness that sometimes play dominant roles in determining the suffering experienced by the patient. In addition to emotional support, the physician also must consider the substantial variability in the patient's capacity to tolerate pain and the response to opioids. Some patients may require considerably more than the average dose of a drug to experience any relief from pain; others may require dosing at shorter intervals. Some clinicians, out of an exaggerated concern for the possibility of inducing addiction, prescribe initial doses of opioids that are too small or given too infrequently to alleviate pain and then respond to the patient's continued complaints with an even more exaggerated concern about drug dependence. Infants and children may receive inadequate treatment for pain than are adults owing to communication difficulties, lack of familiarity with appropriate pain assessment methodologies, and inexperience with the use of strong opioids in children.

PAIN OF TERMINAL ILLNESS AND CANCER PAIN Opioids are not indicated in all cases of terminal illness, but the analgesia, tranquility, and even euphoria afforded by the use of opioids can make the final days far less distressing for the patient and family. Although physical dependence and tolerance may develop, this possibility should in no way prevent physicians from fulfilling their primary obligation to ease the patient's discomfort. The physician should not wait until the pain becomes agonizing. This sometimes may entail the regular use of opioid analgesics in substantial doses. Such patients, while they may be physically dependent, are not "addicts" even though they require large doses on a regular basis (*see* Chapter 23).

Most experts in pain management recommend that opioids be administered at sufficiently short, fixed intervals so that pain is continually under control and patients do not dread its return. *Less drug is needed to prevent the recurrence of pain than to relieve it.* Morphine remains the opioid of choice in most of these situations, and the route and dose should be adjusted to the needs of the individual patient. Oral morphine is adequate in most situations. Sustained-release preparations of oral morphine and oxycodone are available that can be administered at 8-, 12- or 24-hour intervals (morphine) or 8- to 12-hour intervals (oxycodone). Superior control of pain often can be achieved with fewer side effects using the same daily dose; a decrease in the fluctuation of plasma concentrations of morphine may be partially responsible.

Constipation is exceedingly common with opioids, and stool softeners and laxatives should be initiated early. Amphetamines have demonstrable mood-elevating and analgesic effects and enhance opioid-induced analgesia. However, not all terminal patients require the euphoriant effects of amphetamine, and some experience side effects, such as anorexia. Although tolerance does develop to oral opioids, many patients obtain relief from the same dosage for weeks or months. In cases where one opioid loses effectiveness, switching to another may improve pain relief. "Cross-tolerance" among opioids exists, but cross-tolerance among related μ-receptor agonists is not complete.

For a complete Bibliographical listing see Goodman & Gilman's *The Pharmacological Basis of Therapeutics*, **11th ed., or Goodman & Gilman Online at www.accessmedicine.com.**

22

PHARMACOLOGY AND TOXICOLOGY OF ETHANOL

The two-carbon alcohol *ethanol*, CH_3CH_2OH, is a CNS depressant that is widely available to adults; its use is legal and accepted in many societies, and its abuse is a societal problem. The relevant pharmacological properties of ethanol include effects on the gastrointestinal (GI), cardiovascular, and central nervous systems (CNS), effects on disease processes, and effects on prenatal development. Ethanol disturbs the fine balance between excitatory and inhibitory influences in the brain, producing disinhibition, ataxia, and sedation. Tolerance to ethanol develops after chronic use, and physical dependence is demonstrated on alcohol withdrawal (*see* Chapter 23). Understanding the cellular and molecular mechanisms of these myriad effects of ethanol *in vivo* requires an integration of knowledge from multiple biomedical sciences (the terms *ethanol* and *alcohol* are used interchangeably in this chapter).

Compared with other drugs, surprisingly large amounts of alcohol are required for physiological effects, resulting in its consumption more as a food than a drug. The alcohol content of beverages typically ranges from 4–6% (volume/volume) for beer, 10–15% for wine, and 40% and higher for distilled spirits (the "proof" of an alcoholic beverage is twice its percentage of alcohol; *e.g.*, 40% alcohol is 80 proof). A glass of beer or wine, or a shot of spirits contains ~14 g alcohol, or ~0.3 mol ethanol. Consumption of 1–2 mol over a few hours is not uncommon. Since the ratio of ethanol in end-expiratory alveolar air and ethanol in the blood is relatively consistent, blood alcohol levels (BALs) in human beings can be estimated readily by the measurement of alcohol levels in expired air; the partition coefficient for ethanol between blood and alveolar air is ~2000:1. Because of the causal relationship between excessive alcohol consumption and vehicular accidents, there has been a near-universal adoption of laws attempting to limit the operation of vehicles while under the influence of alcohol. Legally allowed BALs typically are set at or below 80 mg% (80 mg ethanol/100 mL blood; 0.08% w/v), which is equivalent to a concentration of 17 mM ethanol in blood. A 12-oz bottle of beer, a 5-oz glass of wine, and a 1.5-oz "shot" of 40% liquor each contains ~14 g ethanol, and the consumption of one of these beverages by a 70-kg person would produce a BAL of ~30 mg%. Note that this is only an approximation; a number of factors influence the BAL, including the rate of drinking, gender, body weight and water percentage, and the rates of metabolism and stomach emptying (*see* "Acute Alcohol Intoxication" below).

PHARMACOLOGICAL PROPERTIES
Absorption, Distribution, and Metabolism

After oral administration, ethanol is absorbed rapidly into the bloodstream from the stomach and small intestine and distributes into total-body water (0.5–0.7 L/kg). Peak blood levels occur ~30 minutes after ingestion of ethanol when the stomach is empty. Because absorption occurs more rapidly from the small intestine than from the stomach, delays in gastric emptying (owing, for example, to the presence of food) slow ethanol absorption. Because of first-pass metabolism by gastric and liver alcohol dehydrogenase (ADH), oral ingestion of ethanol leads to lower BALs than would be obtained if the same quantity were administered intravenously. Gastric metabolism of ethanol is lower in women than in men, which may contribute to the greater susceptibility of women to ethanol. *Aspirin* increases ethanol bioavailability by inhibiting gastric ADH. Ethanol is metabolized largely by sequential hepatic oxidation, first to acetaldehyde by ADH and then to acetic acid by aldehyde dehydrogenase (ALDH) (Figure 22–1). Each metabolic step requires NAD^+; thus, oxidation of 1 mol ethanol (46 g) to 1 mol acetic acid requires 2 mol NAD^+ (~1.3 kg). This greatly exceeds the supply of NAD^+ in the liver; indeed, NAD^+ availability limits ethanol metabolism to ~8 g (~170 mmol)/hr in a 70-kg adult, or ~120 mg/kg/hr. Thus, hepatic ethanol metabolism functionally saturates at relatively low blood levels compared with the high BALs achieved, and ethanol metabolism is a zero-order process (constant amount per unit time). Small amounts of ethanol are excreted in urine, sweat, and breath, but metabolism to acetate accounts for 90–98% of ingested ethanol, mostly owing to hepatic metabolism by ADH and ADLH. CYP2E1 also can contribute (Figure 22–1), especially at higher ethanol concentrations and when its activity is induced. Catalase also can produce acetaldehyde from ethanol, but hepatic H_2O_2 availability usually is too low to support significant flux of ethanol through this pathway. Although CYP2E1 usually is not a major factor in ethanol metabolism, it can be an important site of interactions of ethanol with other drugs. CYP2E1 is induced by chronic consumption of ethanol, increasing the clearance of its substrates and activating certain toxins such as CCl_4. There can be decreased clearance of the same

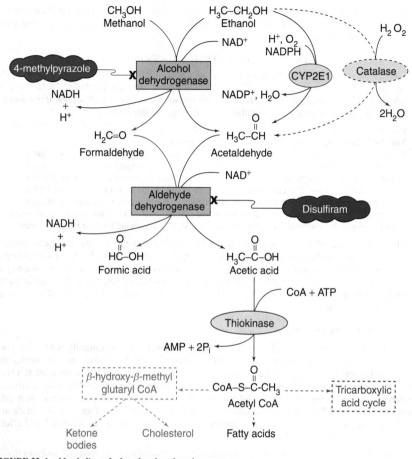

FIGURE 22–1 *Metabolism of ethanol and methanol.*

drugs, however, after acute consumption of ethanol because ethanol competes with them for oxidation by the enzyme system (*e.g.*, *phenytoin* and *warfarin*). The large increase in the hepatic NADH:NAD$^+$ ratio during ethanol oxidation has profound consequences in addition to limiting the rate of ethanol metabolism. Enzymes requiring NAD$^+$ are inhibited; thus, lactate accumulates, activity of the tricarboxylic acid cycle is reduced, and acetyl coenzyme A (acetyl CoA) accumulates (and it is produced in quantity from ethanol-derived acetic acid; Figure 22–1). The combination of increased NADH and elevated acetyl CoA supports fatty acid synthesis and the storage and accumulation of triacylglycerides. Ketone bodies accrue, exacerbating lactic acidosis. Ethanol metabolism by the CYP2E1 pathway produces elevated NADP$^+$, limiting the availability of NADPH for the regeneration of reduced glutathione (GSH), thereby enhancing oxidative stress.

The mechanisms underlying hepatic disease resulting from heavy ethanol use probably reflect a complex combination of these metabolic factors, CYP2E1 induction (and enhanced activation of toxins and production of H$_2$O$_2$ and oxygen radicals), and possibly enhanced release of endotoxin as a consequence of ethanol's effect on gram-negative flora in the GI tract. Effects of heavy ethanol ingestion on various organs are summarized below; damage to tissues very likely reflects the poor nutritional status of alcoholics (malabsorption and lack of vitamins A and D and thiamine), suppression of immune function by ethanol, and a variety of other generalized effects.

The one-carbon alcohol *methanol* also is metabolized by ADH and ALDH, with damaging consequences (*see* below). Competition between methanol and ethanol for ADH forms the basis of the use of ethanol in methanol poisoning. Several drugs inhibit alcohol metabolism, including *4-methylprazole*, an ADH inhibitor useful in ethylene glycol poisoning, and *disulfiram*, an ALDH inhibitor used in treating alcoholism (*see* below). Ethanol also can competitively inhibit the metabolism of other substrates of ADH and CYP2E1, such as methanol and ethylene glycol, and therefore is an effective antidote.

EFFECTS OF ETHANOL ON PHYSIOLOGICAL SYSTEMS

William Shakespeare described the acute pharmacological effects of imbibing ethanol in the Porter scene (Act 2, Scene 3) of *Macbeth*. The Porter, awakened from an alcohol-induced sleep by Macduff, explains three effects of alcohol and then wrestles with a fourth effect that combines the contradictory aspects of soaring overconfidence with physical impairment:

> **Porter:** . . . and drink, sir, is a great provoker of three things.
> **Macduff:** What three things does drink especially provoke?
> **Porter:** Marry, sir, nose-painting *[cutaneous vasodilation]*, sleep *[CNS depression]*, and urine *[a consequence of the inhibition of antidiuretic hormone (vasopressin) secretion, exacerbated by volume loading]*. Lechery, sir, it provokes and unprovokes: it provokes the desire but it takes away] the performance. Therefore much drink may be said to be an equivocator with lechery: it makes him and it mars him; it sets him on and it takes him off; it persuades him and disheartens him, makes him stand to and not stand to *[the imagination desires what the corpus cavernosum cannot deliver]*; in conclusion, equivocates him in a sleep, and, giving him the lie, leaves him.

More recent research has added details to Shakespeare's enumeration—*see* the bracketed additions to the Porter's words above and the section on organ systems below—but the most noticeable consequences of the recreational use of ethanol still are well summarized by the gregarious and garrulous Porter, whose delighted and devilish demeanor demonstrates a frequently observed influence of modest concentrations of ethanol on the CNS. The sections below detail ethanol's effects on physiological systems.

Central Nervous System

Although the public often views alcoholic drinks as stimulating, ethanol primarily is a CNS depressant. Ingestion of moderate amounts of ethanol, like that of other depressants such as barbiturates and benzodiazepines, can have antianxiety actions and produce behavioral disinhibition at a wide range of dosages. Individual signs of intoxication vary from expansive and vivacious affect to uncontrolled mood swings and emotional outbursts that may have violent components. With more severe intoxication, CNS function generally is impaired, and a condition of general anesthesia ultimately prevails. However, there is little margin between the anesthetic actions and lethal effects (usually owing to respiratory depression).

About 10% of alcohol drinkers progress to levels of consumption that are physically and socially detrimental. Chronic abuse is accompanied by tolerance, dependence, and craving for the drug (see below for a discussion of neuronal mechanisms; see also Chapter 23). Alcoholism is characterized by compulsive use despite clearly deleterious social and medical consequences. Alcoholism is a progressive illness, and brain damage from chronic alcohol abuse contributes to the deficits in cognitive functioning and judgment seen in alcoholics. Alcoholism is a leading cause of dementia in the U.S. Chronic alcohol abuse results in shrinkage of the brain owing to loss of both white and gray matter. The frontal lobes are particularly sensitive to damage by alcohol, and the extent of damage is determined by the amount and duration of alcohol consumption, with older alcoholics being more vulnerable than younger ones. Ethanol itself is neurotoxic. Although malnutrition or vitamin deficiencies probably play roles in complications of alcoholism such as Wernicke's encephalopathy and Korsakoff's psychosis, most of the alcohol-induced brain damage in Western countries is due to alcohol itself. In addition to loss of brain tissue, alcohol abuse also reduces brain metabolism (as determined by positron-emission tomography), and this hypometabolic state rebounds to a level of increased metabolism during detoxification. The magnitude of decrease in metabolic state is determined by the number of years of alcohol use and the age of the patients (see "Mechanisms of CNS Actions" below).

Cardiovascular System

SERUM LIPOPROTEINS AND CARDIOVASCULAR EFFECTS In most countries, the risk of mortality due to coronary heart disease (CHD) is correlated with a high dietary intake of saturated fat and elevated serum cholesterol levels. France is an exception to this rule, with relatively low mortality from CHD despite the consumption of high quantities of saturated fats by the French (the "French paradox"). Epidemiological studies suggest that widespread wine consumption

(20–30 g ethanol/day) is one of the factors conferring a cardioprotective effect, with one to three drinks per day resulting in a 10–40% decreased risk of CHD compared to abstainers. In contrast, daily consumption of greater amounts of alcohol leads to an increased incidence of noncoronary causes of cardiovascular failure, such as arrhythmias, cardiomyopathy, and hemorrhagic stroke, offsetting the beneficial effects of alcohol on coronary arteries; *i.e.*, alcohol has a J-shaped dose-mortality curve. Reduced risks for CHD are seen at intakes as low as one-half drink per day. Young women and others at low risk for heart disease derive little benefit from light-to-moderate alcohol intake, whereas those of both sexes who are at high risk and who may have had a myocardial infarction clearly benefit. Data based on a number of prospective, cohort, cross-cultural, and case-control studies in diverse populations consistently reveal lower rates of angina pectoris, myocardial infarction, and peripheral artery disease in those consuming light (1–20 g/day) to moderate (21–40 g/day) amounts of alcohol.

One possible mechanism by which alcohol could reduce the risk of CHD is through its effects on blood lipids. Changes in plasma lipoprotein levels, particularly increases in high-density lipoprotein (HDL; see Chapter 35), have been associated with the protective effects of ethanol. HDL binds cholesterol and returns it to the liver for elimination or reprocessing, decreasing tissue cholesterol levels. Ethanol-induced increases in HDL-cholesterol thus could antagonize cholesterol accumulation in arterial walls, lessening the risk of infarction. Approximately half the risk reduction associated with ethanol consumption is explained by changes in total HDL levels. HDL is found as two subfractions, named HDL_2 and HDL_3. Increased levels of HDL_2 (and possibly also HDL_3) are associated with reduced risk of myocardial infarction. Levels of both subfractions are increased following alcohol consumption and decrease when alcohol consumption ceases. Apolipoproteins A-I and A-II are constituents of HDL; some HDL particles contain only the former, whereas others are composed of both. Increased levels of both apolipoproteins A-I and A-II are associated with individuals who are daily heavy drinkers. In contrast, there are reports of decreased serum apolipoprotein(a) [Apo(a)] levels following acute alcohol consumption. Elevated Apo(a) levels have been associated with an increased risk for the development of atherosclerosis.

Although the cardioprotective effects of ethanol initially were noted in wine drinkers, all forms of alcoholic beverages confer cardioprotection. A variety of alcoholic beverages increase HDL levels while decreasing the risk of myocardial infarction. The flavonoids found in red wine (and purple grape juice) may have an additional antiatherogenic role by protecting low-density lipoprotein (LDL) from oxidative damage. Oxidized LDL has been implicated in several steps of atherogenesis. Another way in which alcohol consumption could play a cardioprotective role is by altering factors involved in blood clotting. Thrombosis is important in the genesis of myocardial infarctions; alcohol consumption elevates the levels of tissue plasminogen activator, a clot-dissolving enzyme (see Chapter 54), decreasing the likelihood of clot formation. Decreased fibrinogen concentrations seen following ethanol consumption also could be cardioprotective, and epidemiological studies have linked the moderate consumption of ethanol to an inhibition of platelet activation.

Should abstainers from alcohol be advised to consume ethanol in moderate amounts? *No.* There have been no randomized clinical trials to test the efficacy of daily alcohol use in reducing rates of CHD and mortality, and it is inappropriate for physicians to advocate alcohol ingestion solely to prevent heart disease. Many abstainers avoid alcohol because of a family history of alcoholism or for other health reasons, and it is imprudent to suggest that they begin drinking. Other lifestyle changes or medical treatments should be encouraged if patients are at risk for the development of CHD.

HYPERTENSION Heavy alcohol use can raise diastolic and systolic blood pressure. Studies indicate a positive, nonlinear association between alcohol use and hypertension that is unrelated to age, education, smoking status, or the use of oral contraceptives. Consumption above 30 g alcohol/day (>two standard drinks) is associated with a 1.5–2.3 mm Hg rise in diastolic and systolic blood pressure. A time effect also has been demonstrated, with diastolic and systolic blood pressure elevation being greatest for persons who consumed alcohol within 24 hours of examination. Women may be at greater risk than men. The mechanism(s) by which alcohol induces hypertension are not well understood.

The prevalence of hypertension attributable to excess alcohol consumption is not known, but studies suggest a range of 5–11%. The prevalence probably is higher for men than for women because they consume more alcohol. A reduction in or cessation of alcohol use in heavy drinkers may *reduce the need for antihypertensive medication or reduce the blood pressure to the normal range. A safe amount of alcohol consumption for hypertensive patients who are light drinkers (1–2 drinks per occasion and <14 drinks per week) has not been determined. Factors to consider are a personal history of ischemic heart disease, a history of binge drinking, or a family history of alcoholism or of cerebrovascular accident. Hypertensive patients with any of these risk factors should abstain from alcohol use.*

CARDIAC ARRHYTHMIAS Alcohol has a number of pharmacological effects on cardiac conduction, including prolongation of ventricular repolarization (as indicated by a prolongation of the QT interval) and sympathetic stimulation. Atrial arrhythmias associated with chronic alcohol use include supraventricular tachycardia, atrial fibrillation, and atrial flutter. Some 15–20% of idiopathic cases of atrial fibrillation may be induced by chronic ethanol use. Ventricular tachycardia may be responsible for the increased risk of unexplained sudden death that has been observed in persons who are alcohol-dependent. During continued alcohol use, treatment of these arrhythmias may be more resistant to cardioversion, digoxin, or Ca^{2+}-channel blocking agents (*see* Chapter 34). Patients with recurrent or refractory atrial arrhythmias should be questioned carefully about alcohol use.

CARDIOMYOPATHY Ethanol is known to have dose-related toxic effects on both skeletal and cardiac muscles. Numerous studies have shown that alcohol can depress cardiac contractility and lead to cardiomyopathy. Echocardiography demonstrates global hypokinesis. Fatty acid ethyl esters (formed from the enzymatic reaction of ethanol with free fatty acids) appear to play a role in the development of this disorder. Approximately half of all patients with idiopathic cardiomyopathy are alcohol-dependent. Although the clinical signs and symptoms of idiopathic and alcohol-induced cardiomyopathy are similar, alcohol-induced cardiomyopathy has a better prognosis if patients are able to stop drinking. Women are at greater risk of alcohol-induced cardiomyopathy than are men. Since 40–50% of persons with alcohol-induced cardiomyopathy who continue to drink die within 3–5 years, abstinence remains the primary treatment. Some patients respond to diuretics, angiotensin-converting enzyme inhibitors, and vasodilators.

STROKE Clinical studies indicate an increased incidence of hemorrhagic and ischemic stroke in persons who drink >40–60 g/day. Many cases of stroke follow prolonged binge drinking, especially when stroke occurs in younger patients. Proposed etiological factors include alcohol-induced (1) cardiac arrhythmias and associated thrombus formation, (2) high blood pressure from chronic alcohol consumption and subsequent cerebral artery degeneration, (3) acute increases in systolic blood pressure and alterations in cerebral artery tone, and (4) head trauma. The effects on hemostasis, fibrinolysis, and blood clotting are variable and could prevent or precipitate acute stroke. The effects of alcohol on the formation of intracranial aneurysms are controversial, but the statistical association disappears when one controls for tobacco use and gender.

Skeletal Muscle

Chronic, heavy, daily alcohol consumption is associated with decreased muscle strength, even when adjusted for other factors such as age, nicotine use, and chronic illness. Heavy doses of alcohol also can cause irreversible damage to muscle, reflected by a marked increase in the activity of creatine kinase in plasma. Muscle biopsies from heavy drinkers also reveal decreased glycogen stores and reduced pyruvate kinase activity. Approximately 50% of chronic heavy drinkers have evidence of type II fiber atrophy. These changes correlate with reductions in muscle protein synthesis and serum carnosinase activities. Most patients with chronic alcoholism show electromyographical changes, and many show evidence of a skeletal myopathy similar to alcoholic cardiomyopathy.

Body Temperature

Ingestion of ethanol causes a feeling of warmth because alcohol enhances cutaneous and gastric blood flow. Increased sweating also may occur. Heat is lost more rapidly, and the internal body temperature falls. After consumption of large amounts of ethanol, the central temperature-regulating mechanism itself becomes depressed, and the fall in body temperature may become pronounced. The action of alcohol in lowering body temperature is greater and more dangerous when the ambient environmental temperature is low. Studies of deaths from hypothermia suggest that alcohol is a major risk factor in these events. Patients with ischemic limbs secondary to peripheral vascular disease are particularly susceptible to cold damage.

Diuresis

Alcohol inhibits the release of vasopressin (antidiuretic hormone; *see* Chapter 29) from the posterior pituitary gland, resulting in enhanced diuresis. The volume loading that accompanies imbibing complements the diuresis that occurs as a result of reduced vasopressin secretion. Alcoholics have less urine output than do control subjects in response to a challenge dose with ethanol, suggesting that tolerance develops to the diuretic effects of ethanol. Alcoholics withdrawing from alcohol exhibit increased vasopressin release and a consequent retention of water, as well as dilutional hyponatremia.

Gastrointestinal System

ESOPHAGUS Alcohol frequently is either the primary etiologic factor or one of multiple causal factors associated with esophageal dysfunction. Ethanol also is associated with the development of esophageal reflux, Barrett's esophagus, traumatic rupture of the esophagus, Mallory-Weiss tears, and esophageal cancer. When compared with nonalcoholic nonsmokers, alcohol-dependent patients who smoke have a tenfold increased risk of developing cancer of the esophagus. There is little change in esophageal function at low blood alcohol concentrations, but at higher blood alcohol concentrations, a decrease in peristalsis and decreased lower esophageal sphincter pressure occur. Patients with chronic reflux esophagitis may respond to proton pump inhibitors (*see* Chapter 36) and abstinence from alcohol.

STOMACH Heavy alcohol use can disrupt the gastric mucosal barrier and cause acute and chronic gastritis. Ethanol appears to stimulate gastric secretions by exciting sensory nerves in the buccal and gastric mucosa and promoting the release of gastrin and histamine. Beverages containing more than 40% alcohol also have a direct toxic effect on gastric mucosa. While these effects are seen most often in chronic heavy drinkers, they can occur after moderate and short-term alcohol use. The diagnosis may not be clear because many patients have normal endoscopic examinations and upper gastrointestinal radiographs. Clinical symptoms include acute epigastric pain that is relieved with antacids or H_2 receptor antagonists (*see* Chapter 36).

Alcohol is not thought to play a role in the pathogenesis of peptic ulcer disease. Unlike acute and chronic gastritis, peptic ulcer disease is not more common in alcoholics. Nevertheless, alcohol exacerbates the clinical course and severity of ulcer symptoms. It appears to act synergistically with Helicobacter pylori *to delay healing. Acute bleeding from the gastric mucosa, while uncommon, can be a life-threatening emergency. Upper GI bleeding is associated more commonly with esophageal varices, traumatic rupture of the esophagus, and clotting abnormalities.*

INTESTINES Many alcoholics have chronic diarrhea as a result of malabsorption in the small intestine. The major symptom is frequent loose stools. The rectal fissures and pruritus ani that frequently are associated with heavy drinking probably are related to chronic diarrhea. The diarrhea is caused by structural and functional changes in the small intestine; the intestinal mucosa has flattened villi, and digestive enzyme levels often are decreased. These changes frequently are reversible after a period of abstinence. Treatment is based on replacing essential vitamins and electrolytes, slowing transit time with an agent such as loperamide (*see* Chapter 38), and abstaining from all alcoholic beverages. Patients with severe magnesium deficiencies (serum Mg^{2+} < 1 mEq/L) or symptomatic patients (a positive Chvostek's sign or asterixis) should receive 1 g magnesium sulfate intravenously or intramuscularly every 4 hours until the serum Mg^{2+} concentration is >1 mEq/L.

PANCREAS Heavy alcohol use is the most common cause of both acute and chronic pancreatitis in the U.S. While pancreatitis can occur after a single episode of heavy alcohol use, prolonged heavy drinking is common in most cases. Acute alcoholic pancreatitis is characterized by the abrupt onset of abdominal pain, nausea, vomiting, and increased levels of serum or urine pancreatic enzymes. Computed tomography is being used increasingly for diagnostic testing. While most attacks are not fatal, hemorrhagic pancreatitis can develop and lead to shock, renal failure, respiratory failure, and death. Management usually involves intravenous fluid replacement—often with nasogastric suction—and opioid pain medication. The etiology of acute pancreatitis probably is related to a direct toxic metabolic effect of alcohol on pancreatic acinar cells. Fatty acid esters and cytokines appear to play a major role.

Two-thirds of patients with recurrent alcoholic pancreatitis will develop chronic pancreatitis. Chronic pancreatitis is treated by replacing the endocrine and exocrine deficiencies that result from pancreatic insufficiency. The development of hyperglycemia often requires insulin for control of blood-sugar levels. Pancreatic enzyme capsules containing lipase, amylase, and proteases may be necessary to treat malabsorption (see Chapter 37). The average lipase dose is 4000–24,000 units with each meal and snack. Many patients with chronic pancreatitis develop a chronic pain syndrome. While opioids may be helpful, non-narcotic methods for pain relief such as anti-inflammatory drugs, tricyclic antidepressants, exercise, relaxation techniques, and self-hypnosis are preferred treatments for this population because cross-dependence to other drugs is common among alcoholics. In particular, for patients receiving chronic opioid therapy for chronic pancreatitis, treatment contracts and frequent assessments for signs of addiction are important.

LIVER Ethanol produces a constellation of dose-related deleterious effects in the liver. The primary effects are fatty infiltration of the liver, hepatitis, and cirrhosis. Because of its intrinsic toxicity, alcohol can injure the liver in the absence of dietary deficiencies. The accumulation of fat in the liver is an early event and can occur in normal individuals after the ingestion of relatively small amounts of ethanol. This accumulation results from inhibition of both the tricarboxylic acid cycle and the oxidation of fat, in part, owing to the generation of excess NADH produced by the actions of ADH and ALDH (*see* Figure 22–1).

Fibrosis, resulting from tissue necrosis and chronic inflammation, is the underlying cause of alcoholic cirrhosis. Alcohol can affect stellate cells in the liver directly; chronic alcohol use is associated with transformation of stellate cells into collagen-producing, myofibroblast-like cells, resulting in deposition of collagen around terminal hepatic venules. The histological hallmark of alcoholic cirrhosis is the formation of Mallory bodies, which are thought to be due to an altered cytokeratin intermediate cytoskeleton. The molecular mechanisms for alcoholic cirrhosis are not well understood but could be due a variety of effects of ethanol and its metabolites on phospholipid peroxidation, GSH metabolism, free radical production and proinflammatory cytokines. In addition, other factors can accelerate or enhance the development of liver cirrhosis.

> Acetaminophen-*induced hepatic toxicity (see Chapter 26) has been associated with alcoholic cirrhosis as a result of alcohol-induced increases in microsomal production of toxic acetaminophen metabolites. Hepatitis C appears to be an important cofactor in the development of end-stage alcoholic liver disease.*
>
> *Several strategies to treat alcoholic liver disease have been evaluated.* Prednisolone *may improve survival in patients with severe alcoholic hepatitis and hepatic encephalopathy. Nutrients such as* S-adenosylmethionine *and polyunsaturated lecithin have been found to have beneficial effects in nonhuman primates and are undergoing clinical trials. Other medications that have been tested include* oxandrolone, propylthiouracil, *and* colchicine. *At present, none of these drugs is approved for use in the U.S. for the treatment of alcoholic liver disease. The current primary treatment for liver failure is transplantation in conjunction with abstinence from ethanol. Long-term outcome studies suggest that patients who are alcohol-dependent have survival rates similar to those of patients with other types of liver disease. Alcoholics with hepatitis C may respond to interferon-2α (see Chapter 52).*

Vitamins and Minerals

The almost complete lack of protein, vitamins, and most other nutrients in alcoholic beverages predisposes those who consume large quantities of alcohol to nutritional deficiencies. Alcoholics often present with these deficiencies owing to decreased intake, decreased absorption, or impaired utilization of nutrients. The peripheral neuropathy, Korsakoff's psychosis, and Wernicke's encephalopathy seen in alcoholics probably are caused by deficiencies of the B complex of vitamins (particularly thiamine), although direct toxicity produced by alcohol itself has not been ruled out. Chronic alcohol abuse decreases the dietary intake of retinoids and carotenoids and enhances the metabolism of retinol by the induction of degradative enzymes. Retinol and ethanol compete for metabolism by ADH; vitamin A supplementation, therefore, should be monitored carefully in alcoholics when they are consuming alcohol to avoid retinol-induced hepatotoxicity. The chronic consumption of alcohol inflicts an oxidative stress on the liver owing to the generation of free radicals, contributing to ethanol-induced liver injury. The antioxidant effects of α-tocopherol (vitamin E) may ameliorate some of this ethanol-induced toxicity in the liver. Plasma levels of α-tocopherol often are reduced in myopathic alcoholics compared with alcoholic patients without myopathy.

Chronic alcohol consumption has been implicated in osteoporosis (*see* Chapter 61). The reasons for this decreased bone mass remain unclear, although impaired osteoblastic activity has been implicated. Acute administration of ethanol produces an initial reduction in serum parathyroid hormone (PTH) and Ca^{2+} levels, followed by a rebound increase in PTH that does not restore Ca^{2+} levels to normal. The hypocalcemia observed after chronic alcohol intake also appears to be unrelated to effects of alcohol on PTH levels, and alcohol likely inhibits bone remodeling by a mechanism independent of Ca^{2+}-regulating hormones. Vitamin D also may play a role. Since vitamin D requires hydroxylation in the liver for activation, alcohol-induced liver damage can indirectly affect the role of vitamin D in intestinal and renal absorption of Ca^{2+}.

Alcoholics tend to have lowered serum and brain levels of magnesium, which may contribute to their predisposition to brain injuries such as stroke. Deficits in intracellular magnesium levels may disturb cytoplasmic and mitochondrial bioenergetic pathways, potentially leading to calcium overload and ischemia. Although there is general agreement that total magnesium levels are decreased in alcoholics, it is less clear that this also applies to ionized Mg^{2+}, the physiologically active form. Magnesium sulfate sometimes is used in the treatment of alcohol withdrawal, but its efficacy has been questioned.

Sexual Function

Despite the widespread belief that alcohol can enhance sexual activities, the opposite effect is noted more often. Many drugs of abuse, including alcohol, have disinhibiting effects that may lead initially to increased libido. With excessive, long-term use, however, alcohol often leads to a deterioration of sexual function. While alcohol cessation may reverse many sexual problems, patients with significant gonadal atrophy are less likely to respond to discontinuation of alcohol consumption.

> *Both acute and chronic alcohol use can lead to impotency in men. Increased blood alcohol concentrations lead to decreased sexual arousal, increased ejaculatory latency, and decreased orgasmic pleasure. Additionally, many chronic alcoholics develop testicular atrophy and decreased fertility; the mechanisms are complex and likely involve altered hypothalamic function and a direct toxic effect of alcohol on Leydig cells. Testosterone levels may be depressed, but many men who are alcohol-dependent have normal testosterone and estrogen levels. Gynecomastia is associated with alcoholic liver disease and is related to increased cellular response to estrogen and to accelerated metabolism of testosterone.*
>
> *Sexual function in alcohol-dependent women is less clearly understood. Many female alcoholics complain of decreased libido, decreased vaginal lubrication, and menstrual cycle abnormalities. Their ovaries often are small and without follicular development. Some data suggest that fertility rates are lower for alcoholic women. The presence of comorbid disorders such as anorexia nervosa or bulimia can aggravate the problem. The prognosis for men and women who become abstinent is favorable in the absence of significant hepatic or gonadal failure.*

Hematological and Immunological Effects

Chronic alcohol use is associated with a number of anemias. Microcytic anemia can occur because of chronic blood loss and iron deficiency. Macrocytic anemias and increases in mean corpuscular volume are common and may occur in the absence of vitamin deficiencies. Normochromic anemias also can occur owing to effects of chronic illness on hematopoiesis. In the presence of severe liver disease, morphological changes can include the development of burr cells, schistocytes, and ringed sideroblasts. Alcohol-induced sideroblastic anemia may respond to vitamin B_6 replacement. Alcohol use also is associated with reversible thrombocytopenia, although platelet counts under 20,000 per mm^3 are rare. Bleeding is uncommon unless there is an alteration in vitamin K_1-dependent clotting factors due to impaired liver function (*see* Chapter 54); other proposed mechanisms for increased bleeding have focused on platelet trapping in the spleen and marrow.

Alcohol also affects granulocytes and lymphocytes. Effects include leukopenia, alteration of lymphocyte subsets, decreased T-cell mitogenesis, and changes in immunoglobulin production. These disorders may play a role in alcohol-related liver disease. In some patients, depressed leukocyte migration into inflamed areas may account in part for the poor resistance of alcoholics to some types of infection (*e.g.*, *Klebsiella* pneumonia, listeriosis, and tuberculosis). Alcohol consumption also may alter the distribution and function of lymphoid cells by disrupting cytokine regulation, in particular regulation involving interleukin 2 (IL-2). Alcohol appears to play a role in the development of infection with the human immunodeficiency virus-1 (HIV). *In vitro* studies with human lymphocytes suggest that alcohol can suppress CD4 T-lymphocyte function and enhance *in vitro* replication of HIV. Moreover, persons who abuse alcohol have higher rates of high-risk sexual behavior.

ACUTE ETHANOL INTOXICATION

An increased reaction time, diminished fine motor control, impulsivity, and impaired judgment become evident when the concentration of ethanol in the blood is 20–30 mg/dL. More than 50% of persons are grossly intoxicated by a concentration of 150 mg/dL. In fatal cases, the average concentration is ~400 mg/dL, although alcohol-tolerant individuals often can withstand comparable BALs. The definition of intoxication varies by state and country. In the U.S., most states set the ethanol level defined as intoxication at 80 mg/dL. There is increasing evidence that lowering the limit to 50–80 mg/dL can reduce motor vehicle injuries and fatalities significantly. While alcohol can be measured in saliva, urine, sweat, and blood, measurement of levels in exhaled air remains the primary method of assessing the level of intoxication.

Many factors, such as body weight and composition and the rate of absorption from the GI tract, determine the concentration of ethanol in the blood after ingestion of a given amount of ethanol. On average, the ingestion of three standard drinks (42 g ethanol) on an empty stomach results in a maximum blood concentration of 67–92 mg/dL in men. After a mixed meal, the maximal blood concentration from three drinks is 30–53 mg/dL in men. Concentrations of alcohol in blood will be higher in women than in men consuming the same amount of alcohol because, on average, women are smaller than men, have less body water per unit of weight into which ethanol can distribute, and have less gastric ADH activity than men. For individuals with normal hepatic function, ethanol is metabolized at a rate of one standard drink every 60–90 minutes.

The characteristic signs and symptoms of alcohol intoxication are well known. Nevertheless, an erroneous diagnosis of drunkenness may occur with patients who appear inebriated but who have not ingested ethanol. Diabetic coma, for example, may be mistaken for severe alcoholic intoxication. Drug intoxication, cardiovascular accidents, and skull fractures also may be confused with alcohol intoxication. The odor of the breath of a person who has consumed ethanol is due not to ethanol vapor but to impurities in alcoholic beverages. Breath odor in a case of suspected intoxication can be misleading because there can be other causes of breath odor similar to that after alcohol consumption. BALs are necessary to confirm the presence or absence of alcohol intoxication.

The treatment of acute alcohol intoxication is based on the severity of respiratory and CNS depression. Acute alcohol intoxication can be a medical emergency, and a number of young people die every year from this disorder. Patients who are comatose and who exhibit evidence of respiratory depression should be intubated to protect the airway and to provide ventilatory assistance. The stomach may be lavaged, but care must be taken to prevent pulmonary aspiration of the return flow. Since ethanol is freely miscible with water, ethanol can be removed from blood by hemodialysis.

Acute alcohol intoxication is not always associated with coma, and careful observation is the primary treatment. Usual care involves observing the patient in the emergency room for 4–6 hours while the patient metabolizes the ingested ethanol. BALs will be reduced at a rate of ~15 mg/dL/hr. During this period, some individuals may display extremely violent behavior. Sedatives and antipsychotic agents have been employed to quiet such patients, but great care must be taken when using sedatives to treat these patients because of possible synergistic CNS depressant effects.

CLINICAL USES OF ETHANOL

Dehydrated alcohol may be injected in close proximity to nerves or sympathetic ganglia to relieve the long-lasting pain related to trigeminal neuralgia, inoperable carcinoma, and other conditions. Epidural, subarachnoid, and lumbar paravertebral injections of ethanol also have been employed for inoperable pain. For example, lumbar paravertebral injections of ethanol may destroy sympathetic ganglia and thereby produce vasodilation, relieve pain, and promote healing of lesions in patients with vascular disease of the lower extremities.

Systemically administered ethanol is confined to the treatment of poisoning by methyl alcohol and ethylene glycol. Treatment consists of sodium bicarbonate to combat acidosis, hemodialysis, and the administration of ethanol, which slows the formation of methanol's metabolites, formaldehyde and formic acid, by competing with methanol for metabolism by ADH (Figure 22–1). Formic acid causes nerve damage; its effects on the retina and optic nerve can cause blindness.

The use of alcohol to treat patients in alcohol withdrawal or obstetrical patients with premature contractions is no longer recommended. Some medical centers continue to use alcohol to prevent or reduce the risk of alcohol withdrawal in postoperative patients, but administering a combination of a benzodiazepine with haloperidol or clonidine may be more appropriate.

MECHANISMS OF CNS EFFECTS OF ETHANOL

Acute Intoxication

Alcohol perturbs the balance between excitatory and inhibitory influences in the brain, resulting in anxiolysis, ataxia, and sedation. This is accomplished by either enhancing inhibitory or antagonizing excitatory neurotransmission. Although ethanol was long thought to act nonspecifically by disordering lipids in cell membranes, ethanol likely produces its effects by simultaneously altering the functioning of a number of proteins that can affect neuronal excitability. A key issue has been to identify proteins that determine neuronal excitability and are sensitive to ethanol at the concentrations (5–20 mM) that produce behavioral effects. Candidate proteins include ion channels in the CNS, and cell signaling enzymes such as protein kinase C-γ and components of signaling pathways such as the MAP kinase and cAMP/PKA pathways. The best studied of these include ligand-gated γ-aminobutyric acid A ($GABA_A$) receptors, whose function is markedly enhanced by a number of classes of sedative, hypnotic, and anesthetic agents, including benzodiazepines, barbiturates, and volatile anesthetics (*see* Chapter 13), neuronal nicotinic acetylcholine receptors (*see* Chapter 8), and excitatory ionotropic glutamate receptors, including *N*-methyl-D-aspartate (NMDA) and non-NMDA receptor classes (*see* Chapter 12).

Tolerance and Dependence

Tolerance is defined as a reduced behavioral or physiological response to the same dose of ethanol (*see* Chapter 23). There is a marked acute tolerance that is detectable soon after administration of ethanol. Acute tolerance can be demonstrated by measuring behavioral impairment at the same BALs on the ascending limb of the absorption phase of the BAL—time curve (minutes after ingestion of alcohol) and on the descending limb of the curve as BALs are lowered by metabolism (one or more hours after ingestion). Behavioral impairment and subjective feelings of intoxication are much greater at a given BAL on the ascending than on the descending limb. There also is a chronic tolerance that develops in the long-term heavy drinker. In contrast to acute tolerance, chronic tolerance often has a metabolic component owing to induction of alcohol-metabolizing enzymes.

Physical dependence is demonstrated by the elicitation of a withdrawal syndrome when alcohol consumption is terminated. The symptoms and severity are determined by the amount and duration of alcohol consumption and include sleep disruption, autonomic nervous system (sympathetic) activation, tremors, and in severe cases, seizures. In addition, two or more days after withdrawal, some individuals experience *delirium tremens*, characterized by hallucinations, delirium, fever, and tachycardia. Delirium tremens can be fatal. Another aspect of dependence is craving and drug-seeking behavior, often termed *psychological dependence*.

Genetic Influences

The acceptance of alcoholism and addiction as "brain diseases" led to a search for biological causes. It has long been appreciated that alcoholism "runs in families"; a series of adoption (cross-fostering) and twin studies showed that human alcohol dependence does, indeed, have a genetic component. Although the genetic contribution varies among studies, it generally is in the range of 40–60%, which means that environmental variables also are critical for individual susceptibility to alcoholism.

The search for the genes and alleles responsible for alcoholism is complicated by the polygenic nature of the disease and the general difficulty in defining multiple genes responsible for complex diseases. One fruitful area of research has been the study of why some populations (mainly Asian) are protected from alcoholism. This has been attributed to genetic differences in alcohol- and aldehyde-metabolizing enzymes. Specifically, genetic variants of ADH that exhibit high activity and variants of ALDH that exhibit low activity protect against heavy drinking. This is so because alcohol consumption by individuals who have these variants results in accumulation of acetaldehyde, which produces a variety of unpleasant effects. These effects are similar to those of disulfiram therapy (see below), but the prophylactic, genetic form of inhibition of alcohol consumption is more effective than the pharmacotherapeutic approach, which is applied after alcoholism has developed.

In contrast to these protective genetic variants, there are little consistent data about genes responsible for increased risk for alcoholism. Several large-scale genetic studies of alcoholism currently are in progress, and these efforts, together with genetic studies in laboratory animals, may lead to identification of genes influencing susceptibility to alcoholism.

TERATOGENIC EFFECTS: FETAL ALCOHOL SYNDROME

Children born to alcoholic mothers display a common pattern of distinct dysmorphology known as *fetal alcohol syndrome* (FAS). The diagnosis of FAS typically is based on the observance of a triad of abnormalities in the newborn, including (1) a cluster of craniofacial abnormalities, (2) CNS dysfunction, and (3) pre- and/or postnatal stunting of growth. Hearing, language, and speech disorders also may become evident as the child ages. Children who do not meet all the criteria for a diagnosis of FAS still may show physical and mental deficits consistent with a partial phenotype, termed *fetal alcohol effects* (FAEs) or *alcohol-related neurodevelopmental disorders.* The incidence of FAS is believed to be in the range of 0.5–1/1000 live births in the general U.S. population, with rates as high as 2–3/1000 in African-American and Native-American populations. A lower socioeconomic status of the mother rather than racial background *per se* appears to be primarily responsible for the higher incidence of FAS observed in those groups. The incidence of FAEs is likely higher than that of FAS, making alcohol consumption during pregnancy a major public health problem. FAS is the most common cause of preventable mental retardation in the Western world, with afflicted children consistently scoring lower than their peers on a variety of IQ tests.

Craniofacial abnormalities commonly observed in the diagnosis of FAS consist of a pattern of microcephaly, a long and smooth philtrum, shortened palpebral fissures, a flat midface, and epicanthal folds. Magnetic resonance imaging studies demonstrate decreased volumes in the basal ganglia, corpus callosum, cerebrum, and cerebellum. The severity of alcohol effects can vary greatly and depends on the drinking patterns and amount of alcohol consumed by the mother. Maternal drinking in the first trimester has been associated with craniofacial abnormalities; facial dysmorphology also is seen in mice exposed to ethanol at the equivalent time in gestation.

CNS dysfunction following in utero *exposure to alcohol manifests in the form of hyperactivity, attention deficits, mental retardation, and learning disabilities. It now is clear that FAS represents the severe end of a spectrum of alcohol effects. A number of studies have documented intellectual deficits, including mental retardation, in children not displaying the craniofacial deformities or retarded growth seen in FAS. Although cognitive improvements are seen with time, decreased IQ scores of FAS children tend to persist as they mature, indicating that the deleterious prenatal effects of alcohol are irreversible. Although a correlation exists between the amount of alcohol consumed by the mother and infant scores on mental and motor performance tests, there is considerable variation in performance on such tests among children of mothers consuming similar quantities of alcohol. The peak BAL reached may be a critical factor in determining the severity of deficits seen in the offspring. Although the evidence is not conclusive, there is a suggestion that even moderate alcohol consumption (2 drinks per day) in the second trimester of pregnancy is correlated with impaired academic performance of offspring at age 6. Maternal age also may be a factor. Pregnant women over age 30 who drink alcohol create greater risks to their children than do younger women who consume similar amounts of alcohol.*

Children exposed prenatally to alcohol most frequently present with attentional deficits and hyperactivity, even in the absence of intellectual deficits or craniofacial abnormalities. Furthermore, attentional problems have been observed in the absence of hyperactivity, suggesting that the two phenomena are not necessarily related. Fetal alcohol exposure also has been identified as a risk factor for alcohol abuse by adolescents. Apart from the risk of FAS or FAEs to the child, the intake of high amounts of alcohol by a pregnant woman, particularly during the first trimester, greatly increases the chances of spontaneous abortion.

PHARMACOTHERAPY OF ALCOHOLISM

Currently, three drugs are approved in the U.S. for treatment of alcoholism: *disulfiram* (ANTABUSE), *naltrexone* (REVIA), and *acamprosate.* Disulfiram has a long history of use but has fallen into disfavor because of its side effects and problems with patient adherence to therapy. Naltrexone and acamprosate were introduced more recently. The goal of these medications is to assist the patient in maintaining abstinence.

Naltrexone

Naltrexone is chemically related to the highly selective opioid-receptor antagonist *naloxone* (NARCAN) but has higher oral bioavailability and a longer duration of action. Neither drug has appreciable opioid-receptor agonist effects. These drugs were used initially in the treatment of opioid overdose and dependence because of their ability to antagonize all the actions of opioids (*see* Chapters 21 and 23). Animal research and clinical experience suggested that naltrexone might reduce alcohol consumption and craving; this was confirmed in clinical trials. There is evidence that naltrexone blocks activation by alcohol of dopaminergic pathways in the brain that are thought to be critical to reward.

Naltrexone helps to maintain abstinence by reducing the urge to drink and increasing control when a "slip" occurs. It is not a "cure" for alcoholism and does not prevent relapse in all patients. Naltrexone works best when used in conjunction with some form of psychosocial therapy, such as cognitive behavioral therapy. It typically is administered after detoxification and given at a dose of 50 mg/day for several months. Adherence to the regimen is important to ensure the therapeutic value of naltrexone and has proven to be a problem for some patients. The most common side effect of naltrexone is nausea, which is more common in women than in men and subsides if the patients abstain from alcohol. When given in excessive doses, naltrexone can cause liver damage. It is contraindicated in patients with liver failure or acute hepatitis and should be used only after careful consideration in patients with active liver disease.

Nalmefene (REVEX) is another opioid antagonist that appears promising in preliminary clinical tests. It has a number of advantages over naltrexone, including greater oral bioavailability, longer duration of action, and lack of dose-dependent liver toxicity.

Disulfiram

Disulfiram (tetraethylthiuram disulfide; ANTABUSE) was taken in the course of an investigation of its potential anthelmintic efficacy by two Danish physicians, who became ill at a cocktail party and were quick to realize that the compound had altered their responses to alcohol. They initiated a series of pharmacological and clinical studies that provided the basis for the use of disulfiram as an adjunct in the treatment of chronic alcoholism. Similar responses to alcohol ingestion are produced by various congeners of disulfiram, namely, *cyanamide*, the fungus *Coprinus atramentarius*, the hypoglycemic *sulfonylureas*, *metronidazole*, certain *cephalosporins*, and animal charcoal.

Disulfiram, given alone, is a relatively nontoxic substance, but it inhibits ALDH activity and causes the blood acetaldehyde concentration to rise to 5–10 times above the level achieved when ethanol is given to an individual not pretreated with disulfiram. Acetaldehyde, produced as a result of the oxidation of ethanol by ADH, ordinarily does not accumulate in the body because it is further oxidized almost as soon as it is formed primarily by ALDH. Following the administration of disulfiram, both cytosolic and mitochondrial forms of ALDH are irreversibly inactivated to varying degrees, and the concentration of acetaldehyde rises. It is unlikely that disulfiram itself is responsible for the enzyme inactivation in vivo; several active metabolites of the drug, especially diethylthiomethylcarbamate, behave as suicide-substrate inhibitors of ALDH in vitro. These metabolites reach significant concentrations in plasma following the administration of disulfiram.

The ingestion of alcohol by individuals previously treated with disulfiram gives rise to marked signs and symptoms of acetaldehyde poisoning. Within 5–10 minutes, the face feels hot and soon afterward becomes flushed and scarlet in appearance. As the vasodilation spreads over the whole body, intense throbbing is felt in the head and neck, and a pulsating headache may develop. Respiratory difficulties, nausea, copious vomiting, sweating, thirst, chest pain, considerable hypotension, orthostatic syncope, marked uneasiness, weakness, vertigo, blurred vision, and confusion are observed. The facial flush is replaced by pallor, and the blood pressure may fall to shock levels.

Alarming reactions may result from the ingestion of even small amounts of alcohol in persons being treated with disulfiram. The use of disulfiram as a therapeutic agent thus is not without danger, and it should be attempted only under careful medical and nursing supervision. Patients must be warned that as long as they are taking disulfiram, the ingestion of alcohol in any form will make them sick and may endanger their lives. Patients must learn to avoid disguised forms of alcohol, as in sauces, fermented vinegar, cough syrups, and even aftershave lotions and back rubs.

The drug never should be administered until the patient has abstained from alcohol for at least 12 hours. In the initial phase of treatment, a maximal daily dose of 500 mg is given for 1–2 weeks. Maintenance dosage then ranges from 125–500 mg daily depending on tolerance to side effects. Unless sedation is prominent, the daily dose should be taken in the morning, the time when the resolve not to drink may be strongest. Sensitization to alcohol may last as long as 14 days after the last ingestion of disulfiram because of the slow rate of restoration of ALDH.

Disulfiram and/or its metabolites can inhibit many enzymes with crucial sulfhydryl groups; thus, disulfiram has a wide spectrum of biological effects. It inhibits hepatic CYPs and thereby interferes with the metabolism of phenytoin, chlordiazepoxide, barbiturates, warfarin, and other drugs.

Disulfiram by itself usually is innocuous, but it may cause acneform eruptions, urticaria, lassitude, tremor, restlessness, headache, dizziness, a garlic-like or metallic taste, and mild GI disturbances. Peripheral neuropathies, psychosis, and ketosis also have been reported.

Acamprosate

Acamprosate (N-acetylhomotaurine, calcium salt), an analog of GABA, is used widely in Europe for the treatment of alcoholism and was approved recently for use in the U.S. A number of double-blind, placebo-controlled studies have demonstrated that acamprosate decreases drinking frequency and reduces relapse drinking in abstinent alcoholics. It acts in a dose-dependent manner (1.3–2 g/day) and appears to have efficacy similar to that of naltrexone. Acamprosate generally is well tolerated, with diarrhea being the main side effect. No abuse liability has been noted. The drug undergoes minimal metabolism in the liver, is excreted primarily by the kidneys, and has an elimination $t_{1/2}$ of 18 hours after oral administration. Concomitant use of disulfiram appears to increase the effectiveness of acamprosate, without any adverse drug interactions being noted. The mechanism of action of acamprosate is obscure, although there is some evidence that it modulates the function of NMDA receptors in brain.

Other Agents

Ondansetron, a 5-HT$_3$-receptor antagonist and antiemetic drug (see Chapters 11 and 37), reduces alcohol consumption in laboratory animals and currently is being tested in humans. Preliminary findings suggest that ondansetron is effective in the treatment of early-onset alcoholics, who respond poorly to psychosocial treatment alone, although the drug does not appear to work well in other types of alcoholics. Ondansetron administration lowers the amount of alcohol consumed, particularly by drinkers who consume <10 drinks per day. It also decreases the subjective effects of ethanol on 6 of 10 scales measured, including the desire to drink, while at the same time not having any effect on the pharmacokinetics of ethanol.

Topiramate, a drug used for treating seizure disorders (see Chapter 19), appears useful for treating alcohol dependence. Compared with the placebo group, patients taking topiramate achieved more abstinent days and a lower craving for alcohol. The mechanism of action of topiramate is not well understood but is distinct from that of other drugs used for the treatment of dependence (e.g., opioid antagonists), suggesting that it may provide a new and unique approach to pharmacotherapy of alcoholism.

For a complete Bibliographical listing see Goodman & Gilman's *The Pharmacological Basis of Therapeutics*, 11th ed., or Goodman & Gilman Online at www.accessmedicine.com.

23

DRUG ADDICTION AND DRUG ABUSE

DRUG DEPENDENCE

Although many physicians are concerned about "creating addicts," relatively few individuals begin their drug addiction problems by misuse of prescription drugs. Confusion exists because the correct use of prescribed medications for pain, anxiety, and even hypertension commonly produces tolerance and physical dependence. These are *normal* physiological adaptations to repeated use of drugs from many different categories. Tolerance and physical dependence are explained in more detail later, but it must be emphasized that they *do not* imply abuse or addiction. This distinction is important because patients with pain sometimes are deprived of adequate opioid medication simply because they have shown evidence of tolerance or they exhibit withdrawal symptoms if the analgesic medication is stopped abruptly.

DEFINITIONS While tolerance and physical dependence are biological phenomena that can be defined precisely in the laboratory and diagnosed accurately in the clinic, there is an arbitrary aspect to the definitions of the overall behavioral syndromes of abuse and addiction. The most influential system of diagnosis for mental disorders is that published by the American Psychiatric Association (APA). The APA diagnostic system uses the term *substance dependence* instead of "addiction" for the overall behavioral syndrome. It also applies the same general criteria to all types of drugs regardless of their pharmacological class. Although accepted widely, this terminology can lead to confusion between *physical dependence* and *psychological dependence*. The term *addiction*, when used here, refers to compulsive drug use, the entire substance-dependence syndrome. This should not be confused with physical dependence alone. *Addiction* is not used as a pejorative term but rather for clarity of communication.

The APA defines *substance dependence* (addiction) as a cluster of symptoms indicating that the individual continues use of the substance despite significant substance-related problems. Evidence of tolerance and withdrawal symptoms are included in the list of symptoms, but neither tolerance nor withdrawal is necessary or sufficient for a diagnosis of substance dependence. Dependence (addiction) requires three or more of the symptoms, whereas abuse can be diagnosed when only one or two symptoms are present. The chronic, relapsing nature of dependence (addiction) fulfills criteria for a chronic disease, but because of the voluntary component at initiation, the disease concept is controversial.

ORIGINS OF SUBSTANCE DEPENDENCE Many variables operate simultaneously to influence the likelihood that a given person will become a drug abuser or an addict. These variables can be organized into three categories: agent (drug), host (user), and environment (Table 23–1).

Agent (Drug) Variables Drugs that reliably produce intensely pleasant feelings (euphoria) are more likely to be taken repeatedly. *Reinforcement* refers to the capacity of drugs to produce effects that make the user wish to take them again. The more strongly reinforcing a drug is, the greater is the likelihood that the drug will be abused.

Reinforcing properties of drugs are associated with their capacity to increase neuronal activity in critical brain areas (see Chapter 12). Cocaine, amphetamine, ethanol, opioids, cannabinoids, and nicotine all reliably increase extracellular fluid dopamine (DA) levels in the ventral striatum, specifically the nucleus accumbens region.

In contrast, drugs that block DA receptors generally produce bad feelings, i.e., dysphoric effects. Despite strong correlative findings, a causal relationship between DA and euphoria/dysphoria has not been established.

The abuse liability of a drug is enhanced by rapidity of onset because effects that occur soon after administration are more likely to initiate the chain of events that leads to loss of control over drug taking. The history of cocaine use illustrates the changes in abuse liability of the same compound, depending on the form and the route of administration (*e.g.*, "crack" cocaine).

Although the drug variables are important, they do not fully explain the development of abuse and addiction. Most people who experiment with drugs that have a high risk of producing addiction (addiction liability) do not intensify their drug use and lose control. The risk for developing addiction among those who try nicotine is about twice that for those who try cocaine (Table 23–2), but this does not imply that the pharmacological addiction liability of nicotine is twice that of cocaine. Rather, there are other variables listed in the categories of host factors and environmental conditions that influence the development of addiction.

Table 23–1

Multiple Simultaneous Variables Affecting Onset and Continuation of Drug Abuse and Addiction

---

Agent (drug)
  Availability
  Cost
  Purity/potency
  Mode of administration
    Chewing (absorption *via* oral mucous membranes)
    Gastrointestinal
    Intranasal
    Subcutaneous and intramuscular
    Intravenous
    Inhalation
  Speed of onset and termination of effects (pharmacokinetics: combination of agent and host)

Host (user)
  Heredity
    Innate tolerance
    Speed of developing acquired tolerance
    Likelihood of experiencing intoxication as pleasure
  Metabolism of the drug
  Psychiatric symptoms
  Prior experiences/expectations
  Propensity for risk-taking behavior

Environment
  Social setting
  Community attitudes
    Peer influence, role models
  Availability of other reinforcers (sources of pleasure or recreation)
  Employment or educational opportunities
  Conditioned stimuli: Environmental cues become associated with drugs after repeated use in the same environment

---

Table 23–2

Dependence Among Users, 1990–1992

Agent	Ever Used* %	Addiction %	Risk of Addiction %
Tobacco	75.6	24.1	31.9
Alcohol	91.5	14.1	15.4
Illicit drugs	51.0	7.5	14.7
Cannabis	46.3	4.2	9.1
Cocaine	16.2	2.7	16.7
Stimulants	15.3	1.7	11.2
Anxiolytics	12.7	1.2	9.2
Analgesics	9.7	0.7	7.5
Psychedelics	10.6	0.5	4.9
Heroin	1.5	0.4	23.1
Inhalants	6.8	0.3	3.7

---

*The ever-used and addiction percentages are those of the general population. The risk of addiction is specific to the drug indicated and refers to the percentage who met criteria for addiction among those who reported having used the agent at least once.

Host (User) Variables In general, effects of drugs vary among individuals. Even blood levels can show wide variation when the same dose of a drug on a milligram per kilogram basis is given to different people. Polymorphism of genes that encode enzymes involved in absorption, metabolism, and excretion and in receptor-mediated responses may contribute to the different degrees of reinforcement or euphoria observed among individuals (*see* Chapters 3 and 4).

Environmental Variables Initiating and continuing illegal drug use appear to be influenced significantly by societal norms and peer pressure. Taking drugs may be seen initially as a form of rebellion against authority. In some communities, drug users and drug dealers are role models who seem to be successful and respected; thus, young people emulate them. There also may be a paucity of other options for pleasure, diversion, or income. These factors are particularly important in communities where educational levels are low and job opportunities scarce.

PHARMACOLOGICAL PHENOMENA

Tolerance While abuse and addiction are complex conditions combining the many variables outlined earlier, there are a number of relevant pharmacological phenomena that occur independently of social and psychological dimensions. First are the changes in the way the body responds to a drug with repeated use. *Tolerance*, the most common response to repetitive use of the same drug, can be defined as the reduction in response to the drug after repeated administrations. Figure 23–1 shows an idealized dose–response curve for an administered drug. As the dose of the drug increases, the observed effect of the drug increases. With repeated use of the drug, however, the curve shifts to the right (tolerance). Thus, a higher dose is required to produce the same effect that once was obtained at a lower dose. As outlined in Table 23–3, there are many forms of tolerance, likely arising *via* multiple mechanisms.

Tolerance develops to some drug effects much more rapidly than to other effects of the same drug. For example, tolerance develops rapidly to the euphoria produced by opioids such as heroin, and addicts tend to increase their dose in order to reexperience that elusive "high." In contrast, tolerance to the gastrointestinal (GI) effects of opiates develops more slowly. The discrepancy between tolerance to euphorigenic effects (rapid) and tolerance to effects on vital functions (slow), such as respiration and blood pressure, can lead to potentially fatal accidents in sedative abusers.

Innate tolerance refers to genetically determined sensitivity (or lack of sensitivity) to a drug that is observed the first time that the drug is administered.

Acquired tolerance can be divided into three major types: pharmacokinetic, pharmacodynamic, and learned tolerance, and includes acute, reverse, and cross-tolerance.

Pharmacokinetic, or dispositional, tolerance refers to changes in the distribution or metabolism of a drug after repeated administrations such that a given dose produces a lower blood concentration than the same dose did on initial exposure (see Chapter 1).

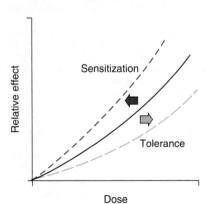

Dose

FIGURE 23–1 *Shifts in a dose–response curve with tolerance and sensitization.* With tolerance, there is a shift of the curve to the right such that doses higher than initial doses are required to achieve the same effects. With sensitization, there is a leftward shift of the dose–response curve such that for a given dose, there is a greater effect than seen after the initial dose.

Table 23–3

Types of Tolerance

Innate (pre-existing sensitivity or insensitivity)
Acquired
    Pharmacokinetic (dispositional or metabolic)
    Pharmacodynamic
    Learned tolerance
        Behavioral
        Conditioned
    Acute tolerance
    Reverse tolerance (sensitization)
    Cross-tolerance

Pharmacodynamic tolerance *refers to adaptive changes that have taken place within systems affected by the drug so that response to a given concentration of the drug is reduced (*see *Chapters 1 and 12).*

Learned tolerance *refers to a reduction in the effects of a drug owing to compensatory mechanisms that are acquired by past experiences. One type of learned tolerance is called* behavioral tolerance. *This simply describes the skills that can be developed through repeated experiences with attempting to function despite a state of mild-to-moderate intoxication.*

Conditioned tolerance *(situation-specific tolerance) develops when environmental cues such as sights, smells, or situations consistently are paired with the administration of a drug. When a drug affects homeostatic balance by producing sedation and changes in blood pressure, pulse rate, gut activity, etc., there is usually a reflexive counteraction or adaptation in the direction of maintaining the* status quo. *If a drug always is taken in the presence of specific environmental cues (e.g., smell of drug preparation and sight of syringe), these cues begin to predict the effects of the drug, and the adaptations begin to occur even before the drug reaches its sites of action. If the drug always is preceded by the same cues, the adaptive response to the drug will be learned, and this will prevent the full manifestation of the drug's effects (tolerance).*

The term acute tolerance *refers to rapid tolerance developing with repeated use on a single occasion.*

Sensitization

With stimulants such as cocaine or amphetamine, reverse tolerance, *or* sensitization, *can occur. This refers to an increase in response with repetition of the same dose of the drug (learned drug effect). Sensitization results in a shift to the left of the dose–response curve (Figure 23–1). Sensitization, in contrast to acute tolerance during a binge, requires a longer interval between doses, usually ~1 day. It has been postulated that stimulant psychosis results from a sensitized response after long periods of use.*

Cross-tolerance *occurs when repeated use of a drug in a given category confers tolerance not only to that drug but also to other drugs in the same structural and mechanistic category. Understanding cross-tolerance is important in the medical management of persons dependent on any drug.* Detoxification *is a form of treatment for drug dependence that involves giving gradually decreasing doses of the drug to prevent withdrawal symptoms, thereby weaning the patient from the drug of dependence (see below).*

Physical Dependence

Physical dependence is a *state* that develops as a result of the adaptation (tolerance) produced by a resetting of homeostatic mechanisms in response to repeated drug use. Drugs can affect numerous systems that previously were in equilibrium; these systems find a new balance in the presence of inhibition or stimulation by a specific drug. A person in this adapted or physically dependent state requires continued administration of the drug to maintain normal function. If administration of the drug is stopped abruptly, there is another imbalance, and the affected systems again must go through a process of readjusting to a new equilibrium without the drug.

WITHDRAWAL SYNDROME The appearance of a withdrawal syndrome when administration of the drug is terminated is the only actual evidence of physical dependence. Withdrawal signs and symptoms occur when drug administration in a physically dependent person is terminated abruptly. Withdrawal symptoms have at least two origins: (1) removal of the drug of dependence and (2) CNS hyperarousal owing to readaptation to the absence of the drug of dependence. Pharmacokinetic variables are of considerable importance in the amplitude and duration of the withdrawal syndrome. Withdrawal symptoms are characteristic for a given category of drugs and tend to be *opposite* to the original effects produced by the drug before tolerance developed. Tolerance, physical dependence, and withdrawal are all biological phenomena. They are the natural consequences of drug use and can be produced in experimental animals and in any human being who takes certain medications repeatedly. These symptoms in themselves do not imply that the individual is involved in abuse or addiction. Patients who take medicine for appropriate medical indications and in correct dosages still may show tolerance, physical dependence, and withdrawal symptoms if the drug is stopped abruptly rather than gradually.

CLINICAL ISSUES

Abuse of combinations of drugs across pharmacologic categories is common. Alcohol is so widely available that it is combined with practically all other categories. Some combinations reportedly are taken because of their interactive effects. An example is the combination of heroin and cocaine ("speedball"). Alcohol and cocaine is another very common combination. When confronted with a patient exhibiting signs of overdose or withdrawal, the physician must be aware of these possible combinations because each drug may require specific treatment.

CNS Depressants

ETHANOL   Experimentation with ethanol is almost universal, and a high proportion of users find the experience pleasant. More than 90% of American adults report experience with ethanol, and ~70% report some level of current use. The lifetime prevalence of alcohol abuse and alcohol addiction (alcoholism) in the U.S. is 5–10% for men and 3–5% for women. Ethanol is classed as a depressant because it indeed produces sedation and sleep. However, the initial effects of alcohol, particularly at lower doses, often are perceived as stimulation owing to a suppression of inhibitory systems (*see* Chapter 22).

Tolerance, Physical Dependence, and Withdrawal   The symptoms of mild intoxication by alcohol vary; some experience motor incoordination and sleepiness, while others initially become stimulated and garrulous. As the blood level increases, the sedating effects increase, with eventual coma and death occurring at toxic levels. The initial sensitivity (innate tolerance) to alcohol varies greatly among individuals and is related to family history of alcoholism. Experience with alcohol can produce greater tolerance (acquired tolerance) such that extremely high blood levels (300–400 mg/dL) can be found in alcoholics who do not appear grossly sedated. In these cases, the lethal dose does not increase proportionately to the sedating dose, and thus the margin of safety (therapeutic index) is decreased.

Heavy consumers of alcohol acquire tolerance and develop a state of physical dependence. This often leads to drinking in the morning to restore blood alcohol levels diminished during the night. Eventually, they may awaken during the night and take a drink to avoid the restlessness produced by falling alcohol levels. The alcohol-withdrawal syndrome (Table 23–4) generally depends on the size of the average daily dose and usually is "treated" by resumption of alcohol ingestion. Withdrawal symptoms are experienced frequently but usually are not severe or life-threatening until they occur in conjunction with other problems, such as infection, trauma, malnutrition, or electrolyte imbalance. In the setting of such complications, the syndrome of *delirium tremens* becomes likely (Table 23–4).

Alcohol produces cross-tolerance to other sedatives such as *benzodiazepines.* This tolerance is operative in abstinent alcoholics, but while the alcoholic is drinking, the sedating effects of alcohol add to those of other sedatives, making the combination more dangerous. This is particularly true for benzodiazepines, which are relatively safe in overdose when given alone but potentially are lethal in combination with alcohol.

The chronic use of alcohol and other sedatives is associated with the development of depression, and the risk of suicide among alcoholics is one of the highest of any diagnostic category. Cognitive deficits have been reported in alcoholics tested while sober. These deficits usually improve after weeks to months of abstinence. More severe recent memory impairment is associated with specific brain damage caused by nutritional deficiencies common in alcoholics, *e.g.*, thiamine deficiency.

Alcohol is toxic to many organ systems. As a result, the medical complications of alcohol abuse and dependence include liver disease, cardiovascular disease, endocrine and GI effects, and

Table 23-4

Alcohol Withdrawal Syndrome

Alcohol craving
Tremor, irritability
Nausea
Sleep disturbance
Tachycardia
Hypertension
Sweating
Perceptual distortion
Seizures (6–48 hours after last drink)
Visual (and occasionally auditory or tactile) hallucinations (12–48 hours after last drink)
Delirium tremens (48–96 hours after last drink; rare in uncomplicated withdrawal)
Severe agitation
Confusion
Fever, profuse sweating
Tachycardia
Nausea, diarrhea
Dilated pupils

---

malnutrition, in addition to the CNS dysfunctions outlined earlier. Ethanol readily crosses the placental barrier, producing the *fetal alcohol syndrome*, a major cause of mental retardation (*see* Chapter 22).

Pharmacological Interventions

Detoxification A patient who presents in a medical setting with an alcohol-withdrawal syndrome should be considered to have a potentially lethal condition. Although most mild cases of alcohol withdrawal never come to medical attention, severe cases require general evaluation; attention to hydration and electrolytes; vitamins, especially high-dose thiamine; and a sedating medication that has cross-tolerance with alcohol. To block or diminish the symptoms described in Table 23-4, a short-acting benzodiazepine such as *oxazepam* (SERAX) can be used at a dose of 15–30 mg every 4–6 hours according to the stage and severity of withdrawal; some authorities recommend a long-acting benzodiazepine unless there is demonstrated liver impairment. When there are complicating medical problems or a history of seizures, hospitalization is required.

Other Measures Detoxification is only the first step of treatment. Complete abstinence is the objective of long-term treatment, and this is accomplished mainly by behavioral approaches. *Disulfiram* (ANTABUSE; *see* Chapter 22) has been useful in some programs that focus behavioral efforts on ingestion of the medication. Disulfiram blocks aldehyde dehydrogenase, the second step in ethanol metabolism, resulting in the accumulation of acetaldehyde, which produces an unpleasant flushing reaction when alcohol is ingested. Knowledge of this unpleasant reaction helps the patient to resist taking a drink. Although quite effective pharmacologically, disulfiram has not been found to be effective in controlled clinical trials because so many patients failed to take it.

Naltrexone (REVIA; *see* Chapter 22) has been shown to block some of the reinforcing properties of alcohol and has resulted in a decreased rate of relapse in the majority of published double-blind clinical trials. It works best in combination with behavioral treatment programs that encourage adherence to medication and to remaining abstinent from alcohol. A depot preparation with a duration of 30 days (VIVITROL) recently received FDA approval and may improve medication adherence, the major problem with the use of medications in alcoholism.

Acamprosate is a competitive inhibitor of the N-methyl-D-aspartate (NMDA)–type glutamate receptor that is proposed to normalize the dysregulated neurotransmission associated with chronic ethanol intake and thereby to attenuate one of the mechanisms that lead to relapse. In several European studies, acamprosate has been shown to promote abstinence, either alone or in combination with naltrexone.

BENZODIAZEPINES Benzodiazepines are among the most commonly prescribed drugs worldwide; they are used mainly for the treatment of anxiety disorders and insomnia (*see* Chapters 16 and 17). Considering their widespread use, intentional abuse of prescription benzodiazepines is

Table 23–5

Benzodiazepine Withdrawal Symptoms

Following moderate dose usage
Anxiety, agitation
Increased sensitivity to light and sound
Paresthesias, strange sensations
Muscle cramps
Myoclonic jerks
Sleep disturbance
Dizziness
Following high-dose usage
Seizures
Delirium

---

relatively rare. When a benzodiazepine is taken for up to several weeks, there is little tolerance and no difficulty in stopping the medication when the condition no longer warrants its use. After several months, the proportion of patients who become tolerant increases, and reducing the dose or stopping the medication produces withdrawal symptoms (Table 23–5). It can be difficult to distinguish withdrawal symptoms from the reappearance of the anxiety symptoms for which the benzodiazepine was prescribed initially. Some patients may increase their dose over time because tolerance definitely develops to the sedative effects. Many patients and their physicians, however, contend that antianxiety benefits continue to occur long after tolerance to the sedating effects. Moreover, these patients continue to take the medication for years according to medical directions without increasing their dose and are able to function very effectively as long as they take the benzodiazepine. The degree to which tolerance develops to the anxiolytic effects of benzodiazepines is a subject of controversy. There is, however, good evidence that significant tolerance does not develop to all benzodiazepine actions because some effects of acute doses on memory persist in patients who have taken benzodiazepines for years. Patients with a history of alcohol- or other drug-abuse problems have an increased risk for the development of benzodiazepine abuse and should rarely, if ever, be treated with benzodiazepines on a chronic basis.

Pharmacological Interventions If patients receiving long-term benzodiazepine treatment by prescription wish to stop their medication, the process may take months of gradual dose reduction. Withdrawal symptoms (Table 23–5) may occur during this outpatient detoxification, but in most cases the symptoms are mild. If anxiety symptoms return, a nonbenzodiazepine such as *buspirone* may be prescribed, but this agent usually is less effective than benzodiazepines for treatment of anxiety in these patients. Some authorities recommend transferring the patient to a long-$t_{1/2}$ benzodiazepine during detoxification; other recommended medications include the anticonvulsants *carbamazepine* and *phenobarbital*.

The specific benzodiazepine receptor antagonist *flumazenil* has been found useful in the treatment of overdose and in reversing the effects of long-acting benzodiazepines used in anesthesia (*see* Chapter 16).

Deliberate abusers of high doses of benzodiazepines usually require inpatient detoxification. Frequently, benzodiazepine abuse is part of a combined dependence involving alcohol, opioids, and cocaine. Detoxification can be a complex clinical pharmacological problem requiring knowledge of the pharmacokinetics of each drug.

BARBITURATES AND NONBENZODIAZEPINE SEDATIVES The use of barbiturates and other nonbenzodiazepine sedating medications has declined greatly in recent years owing to the increased safety and efficacy of newer medications (*see* Chapters 16 and 17). Abuse problems with barbiturates resemble those seen with benzodiazepines. Treatment of abuse and addiction should be handled similarly to interventions for the abuse of alcohol and benzodiazepines. Because drugs in this category frequently are prescribed as hypnotics for patients complaining of insomnia, physicians should be aware of the problems that can develop when the hypnotic agent is withdrawn. Prescription of sedative medications can change the physiology of sleep with subsequent tolerance to these medication effects. When the sedative is stopped, there is a rebound effect with worsened insomnia. This medication-induced insomnia requires detoxification by gradual dose reduction.

Nicotine

Because nicotine (*see* Chapter 9) provides the reinforcement for cigarette smoking, the most common cause of preventable death and disease in the U.S., it is arguably the most dangerous dependence-producing drug. The dependence produced by nicotine can be extremely durable, as exemplified by the high failure rate among smokers who try to quit. Although >80% of smokers express a desire to quit, only 35% try to stop each year, and <5% are successful in unaided attempts to quit.

Cigarette (nicotine) addiction is influenced by multiple variables. Nicotine itself produces reinforcement; users compare nicotine to stimulants such as cocaine or amphetamine, although its effects are of lower magnitude. While there are many casual users of alcohol and cocaine, few individuals who smoke cigarettes smoke a small enough quantity (≤ 5 cigarettes/day) to avoid dependence. Nicotine is absorbed readily through the skin, mucous membranes, and lungs. The pulmonary route produces discernible CNS effects in as little as 7 seconds; each puff producing discrete reinforcement. With 10 puffs per cigarette, the one-pack-per-day smoker reinforces the habit 200 times daily (Table 23–6)

Pharmacological Interventions   The nicotine withdrawal syndrome can be alleviated by nicotine-replacement therapy, available with (*e.g.,* NICOTROL INHALER and NICOTROL NASAL SPRAY) or without (*e.g.,* NICORETTE GUM and others and NICODERM TRANSDERMAL PATCH, NICOTROL TRANSDERMAL PATCH, and others) a prescription. Figure 23–2 shows the blood nicotine concentrations achieved by different methods of nicotine delivery. Because nicotine gum and a nicotine patch do not achieve the *peak levels* seen with cigarettes, they do not produce the same magnitude of subjective effects as nicotine. These methods do, however, suppress the symptoms of nicotine withdrawal. Thus, smokers should be able to transfer their dependence to the alternative delivery system and gradually reduce the daily nicotine dose with minimal symptoms. Although this results in more smokers achieving abstinence, most resume smoking over the ensuing weeks or months. Comparisons with placebo treatment show large benefits of nicotine replacement at 6 weeks, but the effect diminishes with time. The nicotine patch produces a steady blood level (Figure 23–2) and seems to have better patient compliance than that observed with nicotine gum. Verified abstinence rates at 12 months are reported to be in the range of 20%, which is worse than the success rate for any other addiction. The necessary goal of complete abstinence contributes to the poor success rate; when ex-smokers "slip" and begin smoking a little, they usually relapse quickly to their prior level of dependence. A sustained-release preparation of the antidepressant *bupropion* (*see* Chapter 17), improves abstinence rates among smokers. Newer agents such as the cannabinoid (CB-1) receptor antagonist *rimonabant* also have been reported to increase abstinence rates in clinical trials. A combination of behavioral treatment with nicotine replacement to ease withdrawal and an anticraving medication to reduce relapse is currently considered the treatment of choice.

Opioids

Opioid drugs are used primarily for the treatment of pain (see Chapter 21). Some of the CNS mechanisms that reduce the perception of pain also produce a state of well-being or euphoria. Thus, opioid drugs also are taken outside medical channels for the purpose of obtaining the effects on mood. Separating the mechanism of analgesia from that of euphoria has not been achieved, and the standard medications for severe pain remain the opioids.

Heroin is the most important opiate that is abused. There is no legal supply of heroin for clinical use in the U.S., however; heroin is widely available on the illicit market. The purity of illicit street

---

Table 23–6

Nicotine Withdrawal Symptoms

Irritability, impatience, hostility
Anxiety
Dysphoric or depressed mood
Difficulty concentrating
Restlessness
Decreased heart rate
Increased appetite or weight gain

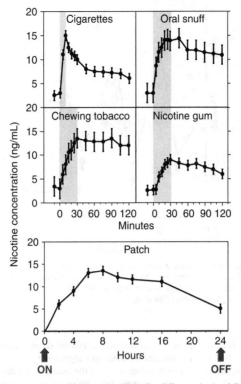

FIGURE 23–2 *Nicotine concentrations in blood resulting from five different nicotine delivery systems.* Shaded areas (upper panel) indicate the periods of exposure to nicotine. Arrows (lower panel) indicate when the nicotine patch was put on and taken off.

heroin in the U.S. has increased from ~4 mg heroin per 100-mg bag (range: 0–8 mg; the rest is filler, such as quinine) to 45–75% purity in many large cities, with some samples testing as high as 90%. This means that the level of physical dependence among heroin addicts is relatively high and that users who interrupt regular dosing will develop more severe withdrawal symptoms. The more potent supplies can be smoked or administered nasally (snorted) rather than injected, thus making the initiation of heroin use accessible to people who would not insert a needle into their veins.

Tolerance, Dependence, and Withdrawal Injection of a heroin solution produces a variety of sensations described as warmth, taste, or high and intense pleasure ("rush") often compared with sexual orgasm. There are some differences among the opioids in their acute effects, with *morphine* producing more of a histamine-releasing effect and *meperidine* producing more excitation or confusion. Even experienced opioid addicts, however, cannot distinguish between heroin and hydromorphone in double-blind tests. Thus, the popularity of heroin may be due to its availability on the illicit market and its rapid onset. After intravenous injection, the effects begin in less than a minute. Heroin has high lipid solubility, crosses the blood–brain barrier quickly, and is deacetylated to the active metabolites 6-monoacetyl morphine and morphine. After the intense euphoria, which lasts from 45 seconds to several minutes, there is a period of sedation and tranquility ("on the nod") lasting up to an hour. The effects of heroin wear off in 3–5 hours, depending on the dose. Experienced users may inject 2–4 times per day. Thus, the heroin addict is constantly oscillating between being "high" and feeling the sickness of early withdrawal (Figure 23–3). This produces many problems in the homeostatic systems regulated at least in part by endogenous opioids. For example, the hypothalamic–pituitary–gonadal axis and the hypothalamic–pituitary–adrenal axis are abnormal in heroin addicts. Women on heroin have irregular menses, and men have a variety of sexual performance

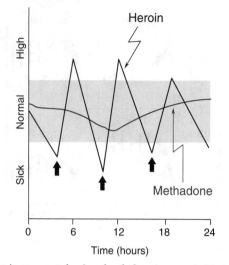

FIGURE 23–3   *Differences in responses to heroin and methadone.* A person who injects heroin (↑) several times per day oscillates between being sick and being high. In contrast, the typical methadone patient remains in the "normal" range (indicated in gray) with little fluctuation after dosing once per day. The ordinate values represent the subject's mental and physical state, not plasma levels of the drug.

problems. Mood also is affected. Heroin addicts are relatively docile and compliant after taking heroin, but during withdrawal, they become irritable and aggressive.

Based on patient reports, tolerance develops early to the euphoria-producing effects of opioids. There also is tolerance to the respiratory depressant, analgesic, sedative, and emetic properties. Heroin users tend to increase their daily dose, depending on their financial resources and the availability of the drug. If a supply is available, the dose can be increased progressively 100 times. Even in highly tolerant individuals, the possibility of overdose remains if tolerance is exceeded. Overdose is likely to occur when potency of the street sample is unexpectedly high or when the heroin is mixed with a far more potent opioid, such as *fentanyl* (SUBLIMAZE, others).

Addiction to heroin or other short-acting opioids produces behavioral disruptions and usually becomes incompatible with a productive life. There is a significant risk for opioid abuse and dependence among physicians and other health care workers who have access to potent opioids, thus tempting them toward unsupervised experimentation.

Opioids frequently are used in combinations with other drugs. A common combination is heroin and cocaine ("speedball"). Users report an improved euphoria because of the combination, and there is evidence of an interaction, because cocaine reduces the signs of opiate withdrawal, and heroin may reduce the irritability seen in chronic cocaine users.

The mortality rate for street heroin users is very high. Early death comes from involvement in crime to support the habit; from uncertainty about the dose, the purity, and even the identity of what is purchased on the street; and from serious infections associated with nonsterile drugs and sharing of injection paraphernalia. Heroin users commonly acquire bacterial infections producing skin abscesses; endocarditis; pulmonary infections, especially tuberculosis; and viral infections producing hepatitis C and acquired immune deficiency syndrome (AIDS).

As with other addictions, the first stage of treatment addresses physical dependence and consists of detoxification. The opioid-withdrawal syndrome (Table 23–7) is very unpleasant but not life-threatening. It begins within 6–12 hours after the last dose of a short-acting opioid and as long as 72–84 hours after a very long-acting opioid medication. Heroin addicts go through early stages of this syndrome frequently when heroin is scarce or expensive. Some therapeutic communities as a matter of policy elect not to treat withdrawal so that the addict can experience the suffering while being given group support. The duration and intensity of the syndrome are related to the clearance of the individual drug. Heroin withdrawal is brief (5–10 days) and intense. *Methadone* withdrawal is slower in onset and lasts longer. Protracted withdrawal also is likely to be longer with methadone.

Table 23–7

Characteristics of Opioid Withdrawal

Symptoms	Signs
Regular withdrawal	
Craving for opioids	Pupillary dilation
Restlessness, irritability	Sweating
Increased sensitivity to pain	Piloerection ("gooseflesh")
Nausea, cramps	Tachycardia
Muscle aches	Vomiting, diarrhea
Dysphoric mood	Increased blood pressure
Insomnia, anxiety	Yawning
	Fever
Protracted withdrawal	
Anxiety	Cyclic changes in weight, pupil size, respiratory center
Insomnia	sensitivity
Drug craving	

Pharmacological Interventions Opioid withdrawal signs and symptoms can be treated by two different pharmacological approaches. The first and most commonly used approach consists of transfer to a prescription opioid medication and then gradual dose reduction. The same principles of detoxification apply as for other types of physical dependence. It is convenient to change the patient to a long-acting drug such as methadone. The initial dose of methadone is typically 20–30 mg. This is a test dose to determine the level needed to reduce observed withdrawal symptoms. The first day's total dose then can be calculated depending on the response and then reduced by 20% per day during the course of detoxification.

A second approach to detoxification involves the use of oral *clonidine* (CATAPRES, others) an α_2 adrenergic agonist that decreases adrenergic neurotransmission from the locus ceruleus. Many of the autonomic symptoms of opioid withdrawal such as nausea, vomiting, cramps, sweating, tachycardia, and hypertension result from the loss of opioid suppression of the locus ceruleus system during the abstinence syndrome. Clonidine can alleviate many of the symptoms of opioid withdrawal except generalized aches and opioid craving. When using clonidine to treat withdrawal, the dose must be titrated according to the stage and severity of withdrawal, beginning with 0.2 mg orally. Postural hypotension commonly occurs when clonidine treatment is used for withdrawal.

Cocaine and Other Psychostimulants

COCAINE Chronic cocaine users total 3.6 million in the U.S. The number of frequent users (at least weekly) has remained steady since 1991 at ~640,000. Not all users become addicts; a key factor is the widespread availability of relatively inexpensive cocaine in the alkaloidal form (free base, "crack") suitable for smoking and the hydrochloride powder form suitable for nasal or intravenous use. Drug abuse in men occurs about twice as frequently as in women. However, smoked cocaine use is particularly common in young women of childbearing age, who may use cocaine in this manner as commonly as do men.

The reinforcing effects of cocaine and cocaine analogs correlate best with their effectiveness in blocking the transporter that recovers DA from the synapse. This leads to increased DA concentrations at critical brain sites. However, cocaine also blocks both norepinephrine (NE) and serotonin (5-HT) reuptake, and chronic use of cocaine produces changes in these neurotransmitter systems.

The general pharmacology and legitimate use of cocaine are discussed in Chapter 14. Cocaine produces a dose-dependent increase in heart rate and blood pressure accompanied by increased arousal, improved performance on tasks of vigilance and alertness, and a sense of self-confidence and well-being. Higher doses produce euphoria, which has a brief duration and often is followed by a desire for more drugs. Involuntary motor activity, stereotyped behavior, and paranoia may occur after repeated doses. Irritability and increased risk of violence are found among heavy chronic users. The $t_{1/2}$ of cocaine in plasma is ~50 minutes, but inhalant ("crack") users typically desire more cocaine after 10–30 minutes. Intranasal and intravenous uses also result in a high of shorter duration than would be predicted by plasma cocaine levels, suggesting that a declining plasma concentration is associated with termination of the high and resumption of cocaine seeking. The major route for cocaine metabolism involves hydrolysis of each of its two ester groups. Benzoylecgonine, produced on loss of the methyl group, represents the major urinary metabolite and can be found in the urine for 2–5 days after a binge. As a result, benzoylecgonine tests are useful for detecting cocaine use; heavy users have detectable amounts of the metabolite in their urine for up to 10 days following a binge. Cocaine frequently is used in combination with other drugs (*see* above). An important metabolic interaction occurs when cocaine and alcohol are taken concurrently. Some cocaine is transesterified to cocaethylene, which is equipotent to cocaine in blocking DA reuptake.

Since cocaine withdrawal is generally mild, treatment of withdrawal symptoms usually is not required (Table 23–8) Rehabilitation programs involving individual and group psychotherapy based on the principles of Alcoholics Anonymous and behavioral treatments based on reinforcing cocaine-free urine tests result in significant improvement in the majority of cocaine users.

AMPHETAMINE AND RELATED AGENTS   Subjective effects similar to those of cocaine are produced by *amphetamine, dextroamphetamine, methamphetamine, phenmetrazine, methylphenidate,* and *diethylpropion.* Amphetamines increase synaptic DA primarily by stimulating presynaptic release rather than by blockade of reuptake. Intravenous or smoked methamphetamine produces an abuse/dependence syndrome similar to that of cocaine, although clinical deterioration may progress more rapidly and methamphetamine is thought to be neurotoxic in DA and 5-HT neurons. Methamphetamine can be produced in small, clandestine laboratories starting with ephedrine, and access to this previously widely available nonprescription stimulant has been restricted.

Caffeine   Caffeine, a mild stimulant, is the most widely used psychoactive drug in the world. It is present in soft drinks, coffee, tea, cocoa, chocolate, and numerous prescription and over-the-counter drugs. It mildly increases NE and DA release and enhances neural activity in numerous brain areas. Caffeine is absorbed from the digestive tract and is distributed rapidly throughout all tissues and easily crosses the placental barrier (*see* Chapter 27). Many of caffeine's effects are believed to occur by means of competitive antagonism at adenosine receptors. Adenosine is a neuromodulator that influences a number of functions in the CNS (*see* Chapters 12 and 27). The mild sedating effects that occur when adenosine activates particular adenosine-receptor subtypes can be antagonized by caffeine.

Tolerance occurs rapidly to the stimulating effects of caffeine. Thus, a mild withdrawal syndrome has been produced in controlled studies by abrupt cessation of as little as 1–2 cups of coffee per day. Caffeine withdrawal consists of feelings of fatigue and sedation. With higher doses, headaches and nausea have been reported during withdrawal; vomiting is rare. Although a withdrawal syndrome can be demonstrated, few caffeine users report loss of control of caffeine intake or significant difficulty in reducing or stopping caffeine, if desired. Thus, caffeine is not listed in the category of addicting stimulants. It is a concern nonetheless that drinks marketed to the young and active are little more that flavored caffeine delivery systems (*e.g.,* caffeinated water).

Cannabinoids (Marijuana)

The cannabis plant has been cultivated for centuries both for the production of hemp fiber and for its presumed medicinal and psychoactive properties. The smoke from burning cannabis contains many chemicals, including 61 different cannabinoids that have been identified. One of these, Δ-9-tetrahydrocannabinol (Δ-9-THC), produces most of the characteristic pharmacological effects of smoked marijuana.

Surveys have shown that marijuana is the most commonly used illegal drug in the U.S. Cannabinoid receptors CB-1 (mainly CNS) and CB-2 (peripheral) have been identified and cloned. An

Table 23–8

Cocaine Withdrawal Symptoms and Signs
Dysphoria, depression
Sleepiness, fatigue
Cocaine craving
Bradycardia

endogenous arachidonic acid derivative *anandamide* is a known agonist ligand. While the physiological function of these receptors and their endogenous ligands are incompletely understood, they are likely to have important functions because they are dispersed widely with high densities in the cerebral cortex, hippocampus, striatum, and cerebellum. Specific CB-1 antagonists have been developed and are in controlled clinical trials. One of these, *rimonabant,* has been reported to reduce relapse in cigarette smokers and to produce weight loss in obese patients.

The pharmacological effects of Δ-9-THC vary with the dose, route of administration, experience of the user, vulnerability to psychoactive effects, and setting of use. Intoxication with marijuana produces changes in mood, perception, and motivation, but the effect sought after by most users is the "high" and "mellowing out." This effect is described as different from the stimulant high and the opiate high. The effects vary with dose, but the typical marijuana smoker experiences a high that lasts ~2 hours. During this time, there is impairment of cognitive functions, perception, reaction time, learning, and memory. Impairments of coordination and tracking behavior have been reported to persist for several hours beyond the perception of the high. These impairments have obvious implications for the operation of a motor vehicle and performance in the workplace or at school.

Marijuana also produces complex behavioral changes such as giddiness and increased hunger. Unpleasant reactions such as panic or hallucinations and even acute psychosis may occur; several surveys indicate that 50–60% of marijuana users have reported at least one anxiety experience. These reactions are seen commonly with higher doses and with oral ingestion rather than smoked marijuana because smoking permits the regulation of dose according to the effects.

One of the most controversial of the reputed effects of marijuana is the production of an "amotivational syndrome"; however, there are no data that demonstrate a causal relationship between marijuana smoking and these behavioral characteristics. There is no evidence that marijuana use damages brain cells or produces any permanent functional changes.

Several medicinal benefits of marijuana have been described. These include antinausea effects that have been applied to the relief of side effects of anticancer chemotherapy, muscle-relaxing effects, anticonvulsant effects, and reduction of intraocular pressure for the treatment of glaucoma. These medical benefits come at the cost of the psychoactive effects that often impair normal activities. Thus, there is no clear advantage of marijuana over conventional treatments for any of these indications.

TOLERANCE, DEPENDENCE, AND WITHDRAWAL

Tolerance to most of the effects of marijuana can develop rapidly after only a few doses, but also disappears rapidly. Withdrawal symptoms and signs typically are not seen. In fact, relative to the number of marijuana smokers, few patients ever seek treatment for marijuana addiction. A withdrawal syndrome in human subjects has been described following close observation of marijuana users given regular oral doses of the agent on a research ward (Table 23–9). This syndrome, however, is only seen clinically in persons who use marijuana on a daily basis and stop abruptly. Compulsive or regular marijuana users do not appear to be motivated by fear of withdrawal symptoms, although this has not been studied systematically.

Psychedelic Agents

Perceptual distortions that include hallucinations, illusions, and disorders of thinking such as paranoia can be produced by toxic doses of many drugs. These phenomena also may be seen during toxic withdrawal from sedatives such as alcohol. There are, however, certain drugs that have as their primary effect the production of disturbances of perception, thought, or mood at low doses with minimal effects on memory and orientation. These are commonly called *hallucinogenic drugs,* but their use does not always result in frank hallucinations. In the late 1990s, the use of "club drugs" at

Table 23–9

Marijuana Withdrawal Syndrome

Restlessness
Irritability
Mild agitation
Insomnia
Sleep EEG disturbance
Nausea, cramping

all-night dance parties became popular. Such drugs include *methylenedioxymethamphetamine* (MDMA, "ecstasy"), *lysergic acid diethylamide* (LSD), *phencyclidine* (PCP), and *ketamine* (KETALAR). They often are used in association with illegal sedatives such as *flunitrazepam* (ROHYP-NOL) or *γ-hydroxybutyrate* (GHB), drugs that have the reputation of being particularly effective in preventing memory storage and have been implicated in "date rape."

While psychedelic effects can be produced by a variety of different drugs, major psychedelic compounds come from two main categories. The indoleamine hallucinogens include LSD, *N,N-dimethyltryptamine* (DMT), and *psilocybin*. The phenethylamines include *mescaline*, *dimethoxymethylamphetamine* (DOM), *methylenedioxyamphetamine* (MDA), and MDMA. Both groups have a relatively high affinity for $5-HT_2$ receptors (*see* Chapter 11), but they differ in their affinity for other subtypes of 5-HT receptors. There is a good correlation between the relative affinity of these compounds for $5-HT_2$ receptors and their potency as hallucinogens in human beings.

LSD LSD is the most potent hallucinogenic drug and produces significant psychedelic effects with a total dose of as little as 25–50 μg. LSD is sold on the illicit market in a variety of forms. A popular contemporary system involves postage stamp-sized papers impregnated with varying doses of LSD (50–300 μg or more).

The effects of hallucinogenic drugs are variable, even in the same individual on different occasions. LSD is absorbed rapidly after oral administration, with effects beginning at 40–60 minutes, peaking at 2–4 hours, and gradually returning to baseline over 6–8 hours. At a dose of 100 μg, LSD produces perceptual distortions and sometimes hallucinations; mood changes, including elation, paranoia, or depression; intense arousal; and sometimes a feeling of panic. Signs of LSD ingestion include pupillary dilation, increased blood pressure and pulse, flushing, salivation, lacrimation, and hyperreflexia. Visual effects are prominent. Colors seem more intense, and shapes may appear altered. The subject may focus attention on unusual items such as the pattern of hairs on the back of the hand.

A "bad trip" usually consists of severe anxiety, although at times it is marked by intense depression and suicidal thoughts. Visual disturbances usually are prominent. Prolonged psychotic reactions lasting 2 days or more may occur after the ingestion of a hallucinogen. Schizophrenic episodes may be precipitated in susceptible individuals, and there is some evidence that chronic use of these drugs is associated with the development of persistent psychotic disorders.

Tolerance, Physical Dependence, and Withdrawal Frequent, repeated use of psychedelic drugs is unusual, and thus tolerance is not commonly seen. Tolerance does develop to the behavioral effects of LSD after 3–4 daily doses, but no withdrawal syndrome has been observed.

Pharmacological Intervention Because of the unpredictability of psychedelic drug effects, any use carries some risk. Dependence and addiction do not occur, but users may require medical attention because of "bad trips." Severe agitation may require medication (*e.g., diazepam*, 20 mg orally), although "talking down" by reassurance has been shown to be effective and is the management of first choice. A particularly troubling after-effect of the use of LSD and similar drugs is the occurrence of episodic visual disturbances in a small proportion of former users. These originally were called "flashbacks" and resembled the experiences of prior LSD trips. There now is an official diagnostic category called the *hallucinogen persisting perception disorder*. The symptoms include false fleeting perceptions in the peripheral fields, flashes of color, geometric pseudohallucinations, and positive afterimages. The visual disorder appears stable in half the cases and represents an apparently permanent alteration of the visual system. Precipitants include stress, fatigue, emergence into a dark environment, marijuana, neuroleptics, and anxiety states.

MDMA ("ECSTASY") AND MDA MDMA and MDA are phenylethylamines that have stimulant as well as psychedelic effects. Acute effects are dose-dependent and include feelings of energy, altered sense of time, and pleasant sensory experiences with enhanced perception. Negative effects include tachycardia, dry mouth, jaw clenching, and muscle aches. At higher doses, visual hallucinations, agitation, hyperthermia, and panic attacks have been reported. A typical oral dose is one or two 100-mg tablets and lasts 3–6 hours, although dosage and potency of street samples are variable (~100 mg/tablet). There is possible neurotoxicity with the use of MDMA.

PHENCYCLIDINE (PCP) PCP was developed originally as an anesthetic in the 1950s and later was abandoned because of a high frequency of postoperative delirium with hallucinations. It was classed as a dissociative anesthetic because, in the anesthetized state, the patient remains conscious with staring gaze, flat facies, and rigid muscles. PCP became a drug of abuse in the 1970s, first in an oral form and then in a smoked version enabling a better regulation of the dose. The effects of PCP have been observed in normal volunteers under controlled conditions. As little as 50 μg/kg produces emotional withdrawal, concrete thinking, and bizarre responses to projective testing. Catatonic posturing also is produced and resembles that of schizophrenia. Abusers taking higher doses may appear to be reacting to hallucinations and exhibit hostile or assaultive behavior. Anesthetic effects increase with dosage; stupor or coma may occur with muscular rigidity, rhabdomyolysis, and hyperthermia. Intoxicated patients in the emergency room may progress from aggressive behavior to coma, with elevated blood pressure and enlarged nonreactive pupils.

PCP binds with high affinity to sites located in the cortex and limbic structures, resulting in blocking of N-methyl-D-aspartate (NMDA)–type glutamate receptors (*see* Chapter 12). LSD and other psychedelics do not bind to NMDA receptors. There is evidence that NMDA receptors are involved in ischemic neuronal death caused by high levels of excitatory amino acids; as a result, there is interest in PCP analogs that block NMDA receptors but with fewer psychoactive effects.

Pharmacological Intervention   Overdose must be treated by life support because there is no antagonist of PCP effects and no proven way to enhance excretion, although acidification of the urine has been proposed. PCP coma may last 7–10 days. The agitated or psychotic state produced by PCP can be treated with *diazepam*. Prolonged psychotic behavior requires neuroleptic medication (*see* Chapter 18), although those with significant anticholinergic effects such as *chlorpromazine* should be avoided.

For a complete Bibliographical listing see Goodman & Gilman's *The Pharmacological Basis of Therapeutics*, 11th ed., or Goodman & Gilman Online at www.accessmedicine.com.

SECTION IV
AUTACOIDS: DRUG THERAPY
OF INFLAMMATION

24

HISTAMINE, BRADYKININ, AND THEIR ANTAGONISTS

HISTAMINE

HISTORY   The discovery of histamine (β-aminoethylimidazole) and the understanding of its actions parallel that of the development of the discipline of pharmacology. A complete description of the history of the discovery of histamine and its actions appears in the 11th Edition of the parent text.

Chemistry

Histamine is a hydrophilic molecule consisting of an imidazole ring and an amino group connected by two methylene groups (Figure 24–1). The pharmacologically active form at all histamine receptors is the monocationic Nγ—H tautomer, i.e., the charged form of the species depicted above, although different chemical properties of this monocation may be involved in interactions with the H_1 and H_2 receptors. The four classes of histamine receptors (H_1–H_4) can be activated differently by analogs of histamine (Table 24–1). Thus, 2-methylhistamine preferentially elicits responses mediated by H_1 receptors, whereas 4(5)-methylhistamine has a preferential effect on H_2 receptors. A chiral analog of histamine with restricted conformational freedom, (R)-α-methylhistamine, is the preferred agonist at H_3-receptor sites, although it is a weak agonist of the H_4 receptor as well. Indeed, a number of compounds have activity at both the H_3 and H_4 receptors.

Distribution and Biosynthesis of Histamine

DISTRIBUTION

Almost all mammalian tissues contain histamine in amounts ranging from <1 to >100 µg/g. Concentrations in plasma and other body fluids generally are very low, but human cerebrospinal fluid (CSF) contains significant amounts. The mast cell is the predominant storage site for histamine in most tissues; in the blood, it is the basophil. The concentration of histamine is particularly high in tissues that contain large numbers of mast cells, such as skin, bronchial tree mucosa, and intestinal mucosa.

SYNTHESIS, STORAGE, AND METABOLISM

Histamine is formed by the decarboxylation of the amino acid histidine by the enzyme L-histidine decarboxylase (Figure 24–1). Every mammalian tissue that contains histamine is capable of synthesizing it from histidine by virtue of its content of L-histidine decarboxylase. Mast cells and basophils synthesize histamine and store it in secretory granules. At the secretory granule pH of ~5.5, histamine is positively charged and complexed with negatively charged acidic groups on proteases and heparin or chondroitin sulfate proteoglycans. The turnover rate of histamine in secretory granules is slow; when tissues rich in mast cells are depleted of their histamine stores, it may take weeks before concentrations return to normal levels. Non–mast cell sites of histamine formation or storage include the epidermis, the gastric mucosa, neurons within the central nervous system (CNS), and cells in regenerating or rapidly growing tissues. Turnover is rapid at these nonmast cell sites because the histamine is released continuously rather than stored. Since L-histidine decarboxylase is an inducible enzyme, the histamine-forming capacity at these sites is subject to regulation. Histamine, in the amounts normally ingested or formed by bacteria in the GI tract, is metabolized rapidly and eliminated in the urine.

Release and Functions of Endogenous Histamine

Histamine has important physiological roles. After its release from storage granules as a result of the interaction of antigen with immunoglobulin E (IgE) antibodies on the mast cell surface, histamine plays a central role in immediate hypersensitivity and allergic responses. The actions of histamine on bronchial smooth muscle and blood vessels account for many of the symptoms of the allergic response. In addition, certain clinically useful drugs can act directly on mast cells to release

HISTAMINE

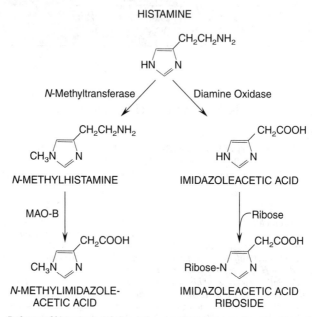

FIGURE 24–1   *Pathways of histamine metabolism in humans.* There are two major paths of histamine metabolism in humans. The more important of these involves ring methylation to form *N*-methylhistamine, catalyzed by histamine-*N*-methyltransferase, which is distributed widely. Most of the *N*-methylhistamine formed is then converted to *N*-methylimidazoleacetic acid by monoamine oxidase (MAO). Alternatively, histamine may undergo oxidative deamination catalyzed mainly by the nonspecific enzyme diamine oxidase (DAO), yielding imidazoleacetic acid, which is then converted to imidazoleacetic acid riboside. These metabolites have little or no activity and are excreted in the urine. Measurement of *N*-methylhistamine in urine affords a more reliable index of histamine production than assessment of histamine itself. Artifactually elevated levels of histamine in urine arise from genitourinary tract bacteria that can decarboxylate histidine.

histamine, thereby explaining some of their untoward effects. Histamine has a major role in the regulation of gastric acid secretion and also modulates neurotransmitter release.

ROLE IN ALLERGIC RESPONSES

The principal target cells of immediate hypersensitivity reactions are mast cells and basophils. As part of the allergic response to an antigen, antibodies (IgE) are generated that bind to the surfaces

Table 24–1

Characteristics of Histamine Receptors

	H_1	H_2	H_3	H_4
Size (amino acids)	487	359	373, 445, 365	390
G protein coupling	$G_{q/11}$	G_s	$G_{i/o}$	$G_{i/o}$
(second messengers)	($\uparrow$Ca^{2+} $\uparrow$cAMP)	($\uparrow$cAMP)	($\downarrow$cAMP)	($\downarrow$cAMP, $\uparrow$Ca^{2+})
Distribution	Smooth muscle, endothelial cells, CNS	Gastric parietal cells, cardiac muscle, mast cells, CNS	CNS: presynaptic, myenteric plexus	Cells of hematopoietic origin
Representative agonist	2-CH$_3$-histamine	Dimaprit	(R)-α-CH$_3$-histamine	Clobenpropit (partial?)
Representative antagonist	Chlorpheniramine	Ranitidine	Thioperamide Clobenpropit	JNJ7777120 Thioperamide

Compounds affecting the H_3 and H_4 receptors exhibit some lack of specificity, although JNJ7777120 seems to be a relatively specific H_4 antagonist. JNJ7777120 is 1-[(5-chloro-1H-indol-2-yl) carbonyl]-4-methylpiperazine.

of mast cells and basophils via high-affinity F_c receptors that are specific for IgE. This receptor, FcεRI, consists of α, β, and two γ chains. The IgE molecules function as receptors for antigens and, via FcεRI, interact with signal-transduction systems in the membranes of sensitized cells (see Chapter 27).

RELEASE OF OTHER AUTACOIDS

The release of histamine only partially explains the biological effects that ensue from immediate hypersensitivity reactions. This is so because a broad spectrum of other inflammatory mediators is released on mast cell activation.

Stimulation of IgE receptors also activates phospholipase A_2 (PLA_2), leading to the production of a host of mediators, including platelet-activating factor (PAF) and metabolites of arachidonic acid. Leukotriene D_4, which is generated in this way, is a potent contractor of the smooth muscle of the bronchial tree (see Chapters 25 and 27). Kinins also are generated during some allergic responses. Thus, the mast cell secretes a variety of inflammatory mediators in addition to histamine, each contributing to the major symptoms of the allergic response (see below).

HISTAMINE RELEASE BY DRUGS, PEPTIDES, VENOMS, AND OTHER AGENTS

Many compounds, including a large number of therapeutic agents, stimulate the release of histamine from mast cells directly and without prior sensitization. Responses of this sort are most likely to occur following intravenous injections of certain substances. Tubocurarine, succinylcholine, morphine, some antibiotics, radiocontrast media, and certain carbohydrate plasma expanders may elicit the response. The phenomenon may account for unexpected anaphylactoid reactions. Vancomycin-induced "red-man syndrome" involving upper body and facial flushing and hypotension may be mediated through histamine release.

Some venoms, such as that of the wasp, contain potent histamine-releasing peptides. Since basic polypeptides are released on tissue injury, they constitute pathophysiological stimuli to secretion for mast cells and basophils. Anaphylatoxins (C3a and C5a), which are low-molecular-weight peptides released during activation of complement, may act similarly.

Within seconds of the intravenous injection of a histamine liberator, human subjects experience a burning, itching sensation. This effect, most marked in the palms of the hand and in the face, scalp, and ears, is soon followed by a feeling of intense warmth. The skin reddens, and the color rapidly spreads over the trunk. Blood pressure falls, the heart rate accelerates, and the subject usually complains of headache. After a few minutes, blood pressure recovers, and crops of hives usually appear on the skin. Colic, nausea, hypersecretion of acid, and moderate bronchospasm also occur frequently.

INCREASED PROLIFERATION OF MAST CELLS AND BASOPHILS; GASTRIC CARCINOID TUMORS

In urticaria pigmentosa (cutaneous mastocytosis), mast cells aggregate in the upper corium and give rise to pigmented cutaneous lesions that urticate (i.e., sting) when stroked. In systemic mastocytosis, overproliferation of mast cells also is found in other organs. Patients with these syndromes suffer a constellation of signs and symptoms attributable to excessive histamine release, including urticaria, dermographism, pruritus, headache, weakness, hypotension, flushing of the face, and a variety of GI effects such as peptic ulceration. Episodes of mast cell activation with attendant systemic histamine release are precipitated by a variety of stimuli, including exertion, emotional upset, exposure to heat, and exposure to drugs that release histamine directly or to which patients are allergic. In myelogenous leukemia, excessive numbers of basophils are present in the blood, raising its histamine content to high levels that may contribute to chronic pruritus. Gastric carcinoid tumors secrete histamine, which is responsible for episodes of vasodilation as part of the patchy "geographical" flush.

GASTRIC ACID SECRETION

Acting at H_2 receptors, histamine is a powerful gastric secretagogue and evokes a copious secretion of acid from parietal cells (see Figure 36–1); it also increases the output of pepsin and intrinsic factor. Although the secretion of gastric acid also is evoked by stimulation of the vagus nerve and by the enteric hormone gastrin, presumably by activation of M_3 and CCK_2 receptors on the parietal cell, acetylcholine and gastrin also stimulate histamine release from the enterochromaffin-like cell. There is no doubt that histamine is the dominant physiological mediator of acid secretion: blockade of H_2 receptors not only eliminates acid secretion in response to histamine but also causes nearly complete inhibition of responses to gastrin and vagal stimulation. The regulation of gastric acid secretion and the clinical utility of H_2 antagonists are discussed in Chapter 36.

CENTRAL NERVOUS SYSTEM

There is substantial evidence that histamine functions as a neurotransmitter in the CNS. Histamine, histidine decarboxylase, and enzymes that catalyze the degradation of histamine are distributed nonuniformly in the CNS and are concentrated in synaptosomal fractions of brain homogenates. H_1 receptors are found throughout the CNS and are densely concentrated in the hypothalamus. Histamine increases wakefulness via H_1 receptors, explaining the potential for sedation by classical antihistamines. Histamine acting through H_1 receptors inhibits appetite. Histamine-containing neurons may participate in the regulation of drinking, body temperature, and the secretion of vasopressin (antidiuretic hormone), as well as in the control of blood pressure and the perception of pain.

Pharmacological Effects

RECEPTOR–EFFECTOR COUPLING AND MECHANISMS OF ACTION Histamine receptors are G protein-coupled receptors (GPCRs) and details of their pharmacodynamic actions and agonist and antagonist ligands are presented in Table 24–1. The pharmacologic definition of H_1, H_2, and H_3 receptors generally is clear: relatively specific agonists and antagonists are available. However, the H_4 receptor exhibits 35–40% homology to the H_3 receptor, and the two are harder to distinguish pharmacologically. High-affinity H_3 agonists interact with H_4 receptors as well, albeit with reduced potency, as do the H_3 antagonists *burimamide* and *clobenpropit*. Several nonimidazole compounds are selective H_3 antagonists. The atypical antipsychotic agent *clozapine* is an effective H_1-receptor antagonist, a weak H_3-receptor antagonist, but a putative H_4-receptor agonist. Many neuroleptics are H_1- and H_2-receptor antagonists, but it is unclear whether interactions with H receptors play a role in the effects of antipsychotic agents. The finding of high constitutive activity of the human H_3 receptor has sparked a reexamination of the potential role of inverse agonists (*see* Chapter 1) of H_3 receptors as therapeutic modulators of H_3-receptor-mediated inhibition of histamine release from histaminergic neurons. H_1 receptors also are reported to express intrinsic or constitutive activity; thus, many H_1 antagonists may function as inverse agonists. H_2-receptor stimulation increases cyclic AMP and leads to feedback inhibition of histamine release from mast cells and basophils. Activation of H_3 and H_4 receptors decreases cellular cyclic AMP; H_3 receptors also may function as presynaptic autoinhibitory receptors on histaminergic neurons.

H_1 AND H_2 RECEPTORS Once released, histamine can exert local or widespread effects on smooth muscles and glands. It contracts many smooth muscles, such as those of the bronchi and gut, but markedly relaxes others, including those in small blood vessels. Histamine also is a potent stimulus of gastric acid secretion (*see* above). Other, less prominent effects include formation of edema and stimulation of sensory nerve endings. Bronchoconstriction and contraction of the gut are mediated by H_1 receptors. Gastric secretion results from the activation of H_2 receptors and, accordingly, can be inhibited by H_2-receptor antagonists (*see* Chapter 36).

H_3 AND H_4 RECEPTORS H_3 receptors are expressed mainly in the CNS, especially in the basal ganglia, hippocampus, and cortex. H_3 receptors function as autoreceptors on histaminergic neurons. H_3 antagonists promote wakefulness; conversely, H_3 agonists promote sleep. H_4 receptors are on immune active cells such as eosinophils and neutrophils, as well as in the GI tract and CNS. Activation of H_4 receptors on eosinophils induces a cellular shape change, chemotaxis, and upregulation of adhesion molecules such as CD11b/CD18 and ICAM-1 suggesting that the histamine released from mast cells acts at H_4 receptors to recruit eosinophils. H_4 antagonists may be useful inhibitors of allergic and inflammatory responses.

CARDIOVASCULAR SYSTEM Histamine characteristically causes dilation of resistance vessels, an increase in capillary permeability, and an overall fall in systemic blood pressure. In some vascular beds, histamine will constrict veins, contributing to the extravasation of fluid and edema formation upstream of the capillaries and postcapillary venules.

Vasodilation Vasodilation, the most important vascular effect of histamine, involves both H_1 and H_2 receptors distributed throughout the resistance vessels in most vascular beds. Activation of either the H_1 or H_2 receptor can elicit maximal vasodilation, but the responses differ. H_1 receptors have a higher affinity for histamine and mediate an endothelium–NO–dependent dilation that is relatively rapid in onset and short-lived. By contrast, activation of H_2 receptors (stimulating the cyclic AMP–PKA pathway in smooth muscle) causes dilation that develops more slowly and is more sustained.

Increased "Capillary" Permeability   This effect of histamine on small vessels results in outward passage of plasma protein and fluid into the extracellular spaces, an increase in the flow of lymph and its protein content, and edema formation. H_1 receptors on endothelial cells are the major mediators of this response.

Increased permeability results mainly from actions of histamine on postcapillary venules, where histamine causes the endothelial cells to contract and separate at their boundaries and thus to expose the basement membrane, which is freely permeable to plasma protein and fluid. The gaps between endothelial cells also may permit passage of circulating cells that are recruited to the tissues during the mast cell response. Recruitment of circulating leukocytes is promoted by H_1-receptor-mediated up-regulation of leukocyte adhesion. This process involves histamine-induced expression of the adhesion molecule P-selectin on the endothelial cells.

Triple Response of Lewis
Intradermal histamine injection elicits a characteristic phenomenon known as the triple response. *This consists of (1) a localized red spot extending for a few millimeters around the site of injection that appears within a few seconds and reaches a maximum in about a minute; (2) a brighter red flush, or "flare," extending about 1 cm or so beyond the original red spot and developing more slowly; and (3) a wheal that is discernible in 1–2 minutes and occupies the same area as the original small red spot at the injection site. The initial red spot results from the direct vasodilating effect of histamine (H_1-receptor-mediated NO production), the flare is due to histamine-induced stimulation of axon reflexes that cause vasodilation indirectly, and the wheal reflects histamine's capacity to increase capillary permeability (edema formation).*

Heart
Histamine affects both cardiac contractility and electrical events directly. It increases the force of contraction of both atrial and ventricular muscle by promoting the influx of Ca^{2+} and speeds heart rate by hastening diastolic depolarization in the sinoatrial (SA) node. It also acts directly to slow atrioventricular (AV) conduction, to increase automaticity, and in high doses especially, to elicit arrhythmias. With the exception of slowed AV conduction, which involves mainly H_1 receptors, all these effects are largely attributable to H_2 receptors and cyclic AMP accumulation. If histamine is given intravenously, direct cardiac effects of histamine are overshadowed by baroreceptor reflexes elicited by the reduced blood pressure. Histamine given in large doses or released during systemic anaphylaxis causes a profound and progressive fall in blood pressure. As the small blood vessels dilate, they trap large amounts of blood, and as their permeability increases, plasma escapes from the circulation. Resembling surgical or traumatic shock, these effects diminish effective blood volume, reduce venous return, and greatly lower cardiac output.

EXTRAVASCULAR SMOOTH MUSCLE   Histamine stimulates or, more rarely, relaxes various extravascular smooth muscles. Contraction is due to activation of H_1 receptors (linked to G_q and Ca^{2+} mobilization); relaxation (for the most part) is due to activation of H_2 receptors. Minute doses of histamine will evoke intense bronchoconstriction in patients with bronchial asthma and certain other pulmonary diseases. Although the spasmogenic influence of H_1 receptors is dominant in bronchial muscle, H_2 receptors with dilator function also are present. Thus, histamine-induced bronchospasm is potentiated slightly by H_2 blockade.

H_1-RECEPTOR ANTAGONISTS
STRUCTURE-ACTIVITY RELATIONSHIP   All the available H_1-receptor antagonists are reversible competitive inhibitors of the interaction of histamine with H_1 receptors. Like histamine, many H_1 antagonists contain a substituted ethylamine moiety. Unlike histamine, which has a primary amino group and a single aromatic ring, most H_1 antagonists have a tertiary amino group linked by a two- or three-atom chain to two aromatic substituents (*e.g.*, diphenhydramine).

DIPHENHYDRAMINE (an ethanolamine)

Pharmacological Properties

Most H_1 antagonists have similar pharmacological actions and therapeutic applications. Their effects are largely predictable from knowledge of the consequences of the activation of H_1 receptors by histamine.

SMOOTH MUSCLE   Within the vascular tree, the H_1 antagonists inhibit both the vasoconstrictor effects of histamine and, to a degree, the more rapid vasodilator effects that are mediated by activation of H_1 receptors on endothelial cells (synthesis/release of NO and other mediators).

CAPILLARY PERMEABILITY H_1 antagonists strongly block the increased capillary permeability and formation of edema and wheal brought about by histamine.

FLARE AND ITCH

H_1 antagonists suppress both the flare component of the triple response and the itching caused by intradermal injection of histamine.

IMMEDIATE HYPERSENSITIVITY REACTIONS: ANAPHYLAXIS AND ALLERGY
During hypersensitivity reactions, histamine is one of the many potent autacoids released (*see* above), and its relative contribution to the ensuing symptoms varies widely with species and tissue. The protection afforded by histamine antagonists thus also varies accordingly.

CENTRAL NERVOUS SYSTEM   The first-generation H_1 antagonists can both stimulate and depress the CNS. Stimulation occasionally is encountered in patients given conventional doses, who become restless, nervous, and unable to sleep. Central excitation is a striking feature of overdose, which commonly results in convulsions, particularly in infants. Central depression, on the other hand, accompanies therapeutic doses of the older H_1 antagonists. Diminished alertness, slowed reaction times, and somnolence are common manifestations. Some of the H_1 antagonists are more likely to depress the CNS than others, and patients vary in their susceptibility and responses to individual drugs. The ethanolamines (*e.g.*, diphenhydramine) are particularly prone to cause sedation and are used as OTC somnolents. Indeed, these drugs cannot be tolerated or used safely by many patients unless given only at bedtime. Patients may experience an antihistamine "hangover" in the morning, resulting in sedation with or without psychomotor impairment.

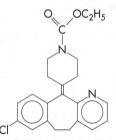

LORATADINE (a tricyclic piperidine)

The second-generation ("nonsedating") H_1 antagonists (*e.g.*, *loratadine*, *cetirizine*, and *fexofenadine*) are largely excluded from the brain when given in therapeutic doses because they do not cross the blood–brain barrier. An interesting and useful property of certain H_1 antagonists is the capacity to counter motion sickness (*see* Chapters 7 and 37). This effect was first observed with *dimenhydrinate* and subsequently with diphenhydramine (the active moiety of dimenhydrinate), various piperazine derivatives, and *promethazine*.

ANTICHOLINERGIC EFFECTS

Many of the first-generation H_1 antagonists tend to inhibit responses to acetylcholine that are mediated by muscarinic receptors. These atropine-like actions are sufficiently prominent in some of the drugs to be manifest during clinical usage (see below). Promethazine has perhaps the strongest muscarinic-blocking activity among these agents and is among the most effective of the H_1 antagonists in combating motion sickness. The second-generation H_1 antagonists have no effect on muscarinic receptors.

ABSORPTION, FATE, AND EXCRETION   The H_1 antagonists are well absorbed from the GI tract. Following oral administration, peak plasma concentrations are achieved in 2–3 hours, and effects usually last 4–6 hours; however, some of the drugs are much longer acting (Table 24–2). Extensive studies of the metabolic fate of the older H_1 antagonists are limited. Diphenhydramine, given orally, reaches a maximal concentration in the blood in about 2 hours, remains at about this level for another 2 hours, and then falls exponentially with a plasma elimination $t_{1/2}$ of ~4–8 hours. The drug is distributed widely throughout the body, including the CNS. Little, if any, is excreted unchanged in the urine; most appears there as metabolites.

Peak concentrations of these drugs are achieved rapidly in the skin and persist after plasma levels have declined. This is consistent with inhibition of "wheal and flare" responses to the intradermal injection of histamine or allergen, which last for 36 hours or more after treatment, even when concentrations in plasma are very low. Such results emphasize the need for flexibility in the interpretation of the recommended dosage schedules (Table 24–2); less frequent dosage may suffice. *Doxepin*, a tricyclic antidepressant (*see* Chapter 17), is one of the most potent antihistamines available; it is ~800 times more potent than diphenhydramine. This may account for the observation that topical doxepin can be effective in the treatment of chronic urticaria when other antihistamines have failed.

H_1 antagonists are eliminated more rapidly by children than by adults (the activity of CYP1A2 and CYP3A4 appears to be greater in infants and children than in adults) and more slowly in those with severe liver disease. H_1-receptor antagonists also induce hepatic CYPs and thus may facilitate their own metabolism.

Many H_1 antihistamines are metabolized by CYPs. Thus, inhibitors of CYP activity such as macrolide antibiotics (*e.g.*, *erythromycin*) or imidazole antifungals (*e.g.*, *ketoconazole*) can increase H_1 antihistamine levels, leading to toxicity. Some newer antihistamines, such as cetirizine, fexofenadine, levocabastine, and acrivastine, are not subject to these drug interactions.

The second-generation H_1 antagonist loratadine is absorbed rapidly from the GI tract and metabolized in the liver to an active metabolite by hepatic CYPs (*see* Chapter 3). Consequently, metabolism of loratadine can be affected by other drugs that compete for metabolism by these enzymes.

SIDE EFFECTS
Common Adverse Effects   The most frequent side effect in the first-generation H_1 antagonists is sedation. Although sedation may be a desirable adjunct in the treatment of some patients, it may interfere with the patient's daytime activities. Concurrent ingestion of alcohol or other CNS depressants produces an additive effect that impairs motor skills. Other untoward central actions include dizziness, tinnitus, lassitude, incoordination, fatigue, blurred vision, diplopia, euphoria, nervousness, insomnia, and tremors.

The next most frequent side effects involve the digestive tract and include loss of appetite, nausea, vomiting, epigastric distress, and constipation or diarrhea. Taking the drug with meals may reduce their incidence. H_1 antagonists appear to increase appetite and cause weight gain in rare patients. Other side effects apparently owing to the antimuscarinic actions of some of the first-generation H_1-receptor antagonists include dryness of the mouth and respiratory passages (sometimes inducing cough), urinary retention or frequency, and dysuria. These effects are not observed with second-generation H_1 antagonists.

Other Adverse Effects   Drug allergy may develop when H_1 antagonists are given orally but results more commonly from topical application. Allergic dermatitis is not uncommon; other hypersensitivity reactions include drug fever and photosensitization. Hematological complications such as leukopenia, agranulocytosis, and hemolytic anemia are very rare. Because H_1 antihistamines cross the placenta, caution must be used when they are taken by women who are or may become pregnant. Several antihistamines (*e.g.*, *azelastine*, *hydroxyzine*, and fexofenadine) showed teratogenic effects in animal studies, whereas others (*e.g.*, chlorpheniramine, diphenhydramine, cetirizine, and loratadine) did not. Antihistamines can be excreted in small amounts in breast milk, and first-generation antihistamines taken by lactating mothers may cause symptoms in the nursing infant such as irritability, drowsiness, or respiratory depression. Since H_1 antagonists interfere with skin tests for allergy, they must be withdrawn well before such tests are performed.

AVAILABLE H_1 ANTAGONISTS   Summarized below are the therapeutic and side effects of a number of H_1 antagonists based on their chemical structures. Representative preparations are listed in Table 24–2.

Table 24–2

Preparations and Dosage of Representative H$_1$-Receptor Antagonists*

Class and Nonproprietary Name	Trade Name	Duration of Action, Hours	Preparations†	Single Dose (Adult)
First-Generation Agents				
Tricyclic Dibenzoxepins				
Doxepin HCl	SINEQUAN	6–24	O, L, T	10–150 mg
Ethanolamines				
Carbinoxamine maleate	RONDEC,¶ others	3–6	O, L	4–8 mg
Clemastine fumarate	TAVIST, others	12	O, L	1.34–2.68 mg
Diphenhydramine HCl	BENADRYL; others	12	O, L, I, T	25–50 mg
Dimenhydrinate	DRAMAMINE; others	4–6	O, L, I	50–100 mg
Ethylenediamines				
Pyrilamine maleate	POLY–HISTINE-D¶	4–6	O, L, T	25–50 mg
Tripelennamine HCl	PBZ	4–6	O	25–50 mg, 100 mg (sustained release)
Tripelennamine citrate	PBZ	4–6	L	37.5–75 mg
Alkylamines				
Chlorpheniramine maleate	CHLOR-TRIMETON; others	24	O, L, I	4 mg 8–12 mg (sustained release) 5–20 mg (injection)
Brompheniramine maleate	BROMPHEN; others	4–6	O, L, I	4 mg 8–12 mg (sustained release) 5–20 mg (injection)
Piperazines				
Hydroxyzine HCl	ATARAX; others	6–24	O, L, I	25–100 mg
Hydroxyzine pamoate	VISTARIL	6–24	O, L	25–100 mg
Cyclizine HCl	MAREZINE	4–6	O	50 mg
Cyclizine lactate	MAREZINE	4–6	I	50 mg
Meclizine HCl	ANTIVERT; others	12–24	O	12.5–50 mg
Phenothiazines				
Promethazine HCl	PHENERGAN; others	4–6	O, L, I, S	12.5–50 mg
Piperidines				
Cyproheptadine HCl§	PERIACTIN	4–6	O, L	4 mg
Phenindamine tartrate	NOLAHIST	4–6	O	25 mg

Second-Generation Agents

Alkylamines				
Acrivastine‡	SEMPREX-D¶	6–8	O	8 mg
Piperazines				
Cetirizine HCl‡	ZYRTEC	12–24	O	5–10 mg
Phthalazinones				
Azelastine HCl‡	ASTELIN	12–24	T	2 sprays per nostril
Piperidines				
Levocabastine HCl	LIVOSTIN	6–12	T	One drop
Loratadine	CLARITIN	24	O, L	10 mg
Desloratadine	CLARINEX, AERIUS	24	O	5 mg
Ebastine	EBASTEL	24	O	10–20 mg
Mizolastine	MIZOLLEN	24	O	10 mg
Fexofenadine	ALLEGRA, TELFAST	12–24	O	60 mg

HCl, hydrochloride.

*For a discussion of phenothiazines, see Chapter 18.

†Preparations are designated as follows: O, oral solids; L, oral liquids; I, Injection; S, suppository; T, topical. Many H_1-receptor antagonists also are available in preparations that contain multiple drugs.

‡Has mild sedating effects.

¶Trade name drug also contains other medications.

§Also has antiserotonin properties.

Dibenzoxepin Tricyclics (Doxepin) Doxepin, the only drug in this class, is marketed as a tricyclic antidepressant (*see* Chapter 17). It also is a remarkably potent H_1 antagonist. Doxepin is much better tolerated by patients who have depression than by those who do not. In nondepressed patients, sometimes even very small doses, *e.g.*, 20 mg may be poorly tolerated because of disorientation and confusion.

Ethanolamines (Prototype: Diphenhydramine) These drugs possess significant antimuscarinic activity and have a pronounced tendency to induce sedation. About half of those treated with conventional doses experience somnolence. The incidence of GI side effects is low.

Ethylenediamines (Prototype: Pyrilamine) These include some of the most specific H_1 antagonists. Although their central effects are relatively feeble, somnolence occurs in a fair proportion of patients. GI side effects are quite common.

Alkylamines (Prototype: Chlorpheniramine) These are among the most potent H_1 antagonists. The drugs are less prone than some H_1 antagonists to produce drowsiness and are more suitable agents for daytime use, but again, a significant proportion of patients do experience sedation. Side effects involving CNS stimulation are more common than with other groups.

First-Generation Piperazines The oldest member of this group, *chlorcyclizine*, has a more prolonged action and produces a comparatively low incidence of drowsiness. Hydroxyzine is a long-acting compound that is used widely for skin allergies; its considerable CNS-depressant activity may contribute to its prominent antipruritic action. *Cyclizine* and *meclizine* have been used primarily to counter motion sickness, although promethazine and diphenhydramine (dimenhydrinate) are more effective (as is scopolamine; *see* below).

Second-Generation Piperazines (Cetirizine) Cetirizine is the only drug in this class. It has minimal anticholinergic effects. It also has negligible penetration into the brain but is associated with a somewhat higher incidence of drowsiness than the other second-generation H_1 antagonists.

Phenothiazines (Prototype: Promethazine) Most drugs of this class are H_1 antagonists and also possess considerable anticholinergic activity. Promethazine, which has prominent sedative effects, and its many congeners are used primarily for their antiemetic effects (*see* Chapter 37).

First-Generation Piperidines (Cyproheptadine, Phenindamine) Cyproheptadine uniquely has both antihistamine and antiserotonin activity. Cyproheptadine and *phenindamine* cause drowsiness and also have significant anticholinergic effects.

Second-Generation Piperidines (Prototype: Loratadine) Current drugs in this class include loratadine, desloratadine, and fexofenadine. These agents are highly selective for H_1 receptors, lack significant anticholinergic actions, and penetrate poorly into the CNS. Taken together, these properties appear to account for the low incidence of side effects of piperidine antihistamines.

Therapeutic Uses

H_1 antagonists have an established and valued place in the symptomatic treatment of various immediate hypersensitivity reactions. In addition, the central properties of some of the series are of therapeutic value for suppressing motion sickness or for sedation.

Allergic Diseases

H_1 antagonists are most useful in acute types of allergy that present with symptoms of rhinitis, urticaria, and conjunctivitis. Their effect is confined to the suppression of symptoms attributable to the histamine released by the antigen-antibody reaction. In bronchial asthma, systemic anaphylaxis and angioedema, histamine antagonists have limited efficacy and are not used as sole therapy.

Other allergies are more amenable to therapy with H_1 antagonists. The best results are obtained in seasonal rhinitis and conjunctivitis (hay fever, pollinosis), in which these drugs relieve the sneezing, rhinorrhea, and itching of eyes, nose, and throat. A gratifying response is obtained in most patients, especially at the beginning of the season when pollen counts are low; however, the drugs are less effective when the allergens are most abundant, when exposure to them is prolonged, and when nasal congestion is prominent. Topical preparations, nasal sprays, or topical ophthalmic preparations of antihistamines have been shown to be effective in allergic conjunctivitis and rhinitis.

Certain allergic dermatoses respond favorably to H_1 antagonists. Benefit is most striking in acute urticaria, although the itching in this condition is perhaps better controlled than are the *edema and the erythema. Chronic urticaria is less responsive, but some benefit may occur in a fair proportion of patients. Furthermore, the combined use of H_1 and H_2 antagonists sometimes is effective when therapy with an H_1 antagonist alone has failed. Doxepin may be effective in the treatment of chronic urticaria that is refractory to other antihistamines.*

H_1 antagonists have a place in the treatment of pruritus. Some relief may be obtained in many patients suffering atopic dermatitis and contact dermatitis (although topical glucocorticoids are more effective) and in such diverse conditions as insect bites and poison ivy. Again, doxepin may be more effective in suppressing pruritus than are other antihistamines. Many drug reactions attributable to allergic phenomena respond to therapy with H_1 antagonists, particularly those characterized by itch, urticaria, and angioedema; serum-sickness reactions also respond to intensive treatment.

Common Cold

Despite persistent popular belief, H_1 antagonists are without value in combating the common cold.

Motion Sickness, Vertigo, and Sedation

Scopolamine, given orally, parenterally, or transdermally, is the most effective of all drugs for the prophylaxis and treatment of motion sickness. Whenever possible, scopolamine should be administered an hour or so before the anticipated motion. Treatment after the onset of nausea and vomiting rarely is beneficial.

Some H_1 antagonists, notably dimenhydrinate and meclizine, often are of benefit in vestibular disturbances such as Meniere's disease and in other types of true vertigo. Only promethazine has usefulness in treating the nausea and vomiting subsequent to chemotherapy or radiation therapy for malignancies; however, other effective antiemetic drugs are available (see Chapter 37).

H_2-RECEPTOR ANTAGONISTS The pharmacology and clinical utility of H_2 antagonists to inhibit gastric acid secretion are described in Chapter 36.

H_3 Receptor and Ligands

The H_3 receptors are localized on terminals as well as on cell bodies/dendrites in the hypothalamic tuberomammillary nucleus on histaminergic neurons. By inhibiting Ca^{2+} conductance, the activated H_3 receptor depresses neuronal firing at the level of cell bodies/dendrites and decreases histamine release from depolarized terminals. Thus, H_3-receptor ligands are unique agents to modify histaminergic neurotransmission in brain; the agonists decrease it, and the antagonists increase it. H_3-receptor ligands currently are research tools to delineate the functional role of cerebral histamine and are drug candidates in neuropsychiatry.

H_4 Receptor and Ligands

The H_4 receptor has considerable sequence similarity with the H_3 receptor and binds many H_3 agonists, although with lower affinity. The H_3 antagonist thioperamide also has significant H_4 antagonistic activity, whereas H_3 antagonists clobenpropit and burimamide are partial agonists of the H_4 receptor. Because the H_4 receptor is expressed primarily on cells of hematopoietic origin (notably mast cells, basophils, and eosinophils) and to a lesser extent in the intestine, there is great interest in the possible role of H_4 receptors in inflammatory processes. H_4 antagonists are promising drug candidates to treat inflammatory conditions involving mast cells and eosinophils, such as allergic rhinitis, asthma, and rheumatoid arthritis.

BRADYKININ, KALLIDIN, AND THEIR ANTAGONISTS

A number of factors, including tissue damage, allergic reactions, viral infections, and other inflammatory events, activate a series of proteolytic reactions that generate bradykinin and kallidin in tissues. These peptides contribute to inflammatory responses as autacoids that act locally to produce pain, vasodilation, and increased vascular permeability. Much of their activity is due to stimulation of the release of potent mediators such as prostaglandins, NO, or endothelium-derived hyperpolarizing factor (EDHF).

The Endogenous Kallikrein–Kininogen–Kinin System

SYNTHESIS AND METABOLISM OF KININS

Bradykinin is a nonapeptide (Table 24–3). Kallidin has an additional lysine residue at the N-terminal position and is sometimes referred to as lysyl-bradykinin. The two peptides are cleaved from α_2 globulins termed kininogens (Figure 24–2). There are two kininogens, high-molecular-weight (HMW) and low-molecular-weight (LMW) kininogen. A number of serine proteases will generate

Table 24–3

Structure of Kinin Agonists and Antagonists

Name	Structure	Function
Bradykinin	Arg-Pro-Pro-Gly-Phe-Ser-Pro-Phe-Arg	Agonist, B_2
Kallidin	Lys-Arg-Pro-Pro-Gly-Phe-Ser-Pro-Phe-Arg	Agonist, B_2
[des-Arg^9]-bradykinin	Arg-Pro-Pro-Gly-Phe-Ser-Pro-Phe	Agonist, B_1
[des-Arg^{10}]-kallidin	Lys-Arg-Pro-Pro-Gly-Phe-Ser-Pro-Phe	Agonist, B_1
des-Arg^9-[Leu^8]-bradykinin	Arg-Pro-Pro-Gly-Phe-Ser-Pro-Leu	Antagonist, B_1
HOE 140	[D-Arg]-Arg-Pro-Hyp-Gly-Thi-Ser-Tic-Oic-Arg	Antagonist, B_2
CP 0127	B(D-Arg-Arg-Pro-Hyp-Gly-Phe-Cys-D-Phe-Leu-Arg)$_2$	Antagonist, B_2

ABBREVIATIONS: Hyp, *trans*-4-hydroxy-Pro; Thi, β-(2-thienyl)-Ala; Tic, [D]-1,2,3,4-tetrahydroisoquinolin-3-yl-carbonyl; Oic, (3as,7as)-octahydroindol-2-yl-carbonyl. B, bissuccimidohexane.

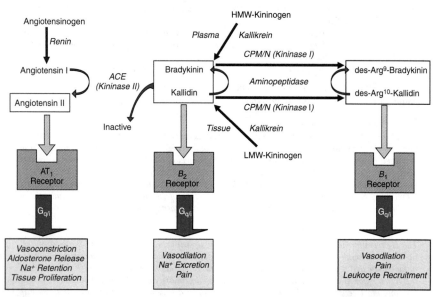

FIGURE 24–2 *Synthesis and receptor interactions of active peptides generated by the kallikrein–kinin and renin–angiotensin systems.* Bradykinin (BK) is generated by the action of *plasma* kallikrein on high-molecular-weight (HMW) kininogen, whereas kallidin (Lys-bradykinin) is synthesized by the hydrolysis of low-molecular-weight (LMW) kininogen by *tissue* kallikrein. Kallidin and BK are natural ligands of the B_2 receptor but can be converted to corresponding agonists of the B_1 receptor by removal of the C-terminal Arg by the action of kininase I–type enzymes: the plasma membrane–bound carboxypeptidase M (CPM) or soluble plasma carboxypeptidase N (CPN). Kallidin or [des-Arg^{10}] kallidin can be converted to the active peptides BK or [des-Arg^9] BK by aminopeptidase removal of the *N*-terminal Lys residue. In a parallel fashion, the inactive decapeptide angiotensin I (Ang I) is generated by the action of renin on the plasma substrate angiotensinogen. By removal of the C-terminal His–Leu dipeptide, angiotensin-converting enzyme (ACE) generates the active peptide Ang II. These two systems have opposing effects. Whereas Ang II is a potent vasoconstrictor that also causes aldosterone release and Na$^+$ retention via activation of the AT$_1$ receptor, BK is a vasodilator that stimulates Na$^+$ excretion by activating the B_2 receptor. ACE generates active Ang II and at the same time inactivates BK and kallidin; thus, its effects are prohypertensive, and ACE inhibitors are effective antihypertensive agents. The B_2 receptor mediates most of BK's effects under normal circumstances, whereas synthesis of the B_1 receptor is induced by inflammatory mediators and plays a major role in chronic inflammatory conditions. Both the B_1 and B_2 receptors couple through G_q to activate PLC and increase intracellular Ca^{2+}; the physiological response depends on receptor distribution on particular cell types and occupancy by agonist peptides. For instance, on endothelial cells, activation of B_2 receptors results in Ca^{2+}–calmodulin–dependent activation of eNOS and generation of NO, which causes cGMP accumulation and relaxation in neighboring smooth muscle cells. On smooth muscle cells, activation of kinin receptor coupling through the same pathway results in an increased [Ca^{2+}]$_i$ and contraction. B_1 and B_2 receptors also can couple through G_i to activate PLA$_2$, causing the release of arachidonic acid and the local generation of prostanoids and other metabolites.

kinins, but the highly specific proteases that release bradykinin and kallidin from the kininogens are termed kallikreins *(see below).*

KALLIKREINS

Bradykinin and kallidin are cleaved from HMW or LMW kininogens by plasma or tissue kallikrein, respectively (Figure 24–2). Plasma kallikrein and tissue kallikrein are distinct enzymes that are activated by different mechanisms. Plasma prekallikrein is an inactive protein that complexes in a 1:1 ratio with its substrate, HMW kininogen. The ensuing proteolytic cascade is restrained by the protease inhibitors present in plasma (e.g., inhibitor of the activated first component of complement [C1-INH] and α_2-macroglobulin). Under experimental conditions, the kallikrein-kinin system is activated by the binding of factor XII, also known as Hageman factor, to negatively charged surfaces. Factor XII, a protease that is common to both the kinin and the intrinsic coagulation cascades (see Chapter 54), undergoes autoactivation and, in turn, activates kallikrein. Importantly, kallikrein further activates factor XII, thereby exerting a positive feedback on the system.

Tissue kallikrein is synthesized as a preproprotein in the epithelial cells or secretory cells of a number of tissues, including salivary glands, pancreas, prostate, and distal nephron. Tissue kallikrein is also expressed in human neutrophils. It acts locally near its sites of origin. The synthesis of tissue prokallikrein is controlled by a number of factors, including aldosterone in the kidney and salivary gland and androgens in certain other glands. The activation of tissue prokallikrein to kallikrein requires proteolytic cleavage to remove a 7-amino acid propeptide.

METABOLISM

The decapeptide kallidin is about as active as the nonapeptide bradykinin even without conversion to bradykinin, which occurs when the N-terminal Lys residue is removed by a plasma aminopeptidase (Figure 24–2). The minimal effective structure required to elicit the classical responses on the B_2 receptor is that of the nonapeptide.

The $t_{1/2}$ of kinins in plasma is ~15 seconds; 80–90% of the kinins may be destroyed in a single passage through the pulmonary vascular bed. Plasma concentrations of bradykinin are difficult to measure because inadequate inhibition of kininogenases or kininases in the blood can lead to artifactual formation or degradation of bradykinin during blood collection. Thus, the reported physiological concentrations of bradykinin range from picomolar to femtomolar.

The principal catabolizing enzyme in the lung and other vascular beds is kininase II, or ACE (Figure 24–2) (see Chapter 30). Removal of the C-terminal dipeptide abolishes kinin-like activity. Neutral endopeptidase 24.11 or neprilysin also inactivates kinins by cleaving off the C-terminal dipeptide. A slower-acting enzyme, carboxypeptidase N (lysine carboxypeptidase, kininase I), releases the C-terminal EF residue, producing [des-Arg^9] bradykinin and [des-Arg^{10}] kallidin (Table 24–3 and Figure 24–2), which are themselves potent B_1-kinin receptor agonists. Carboxypeptidase N is expressed constitutively in blood plasma, where its concentration is about 10^{-7} M. A familial carboxypeptidase N deficiency has been described in which affected individuals with low levels of this enzyme display angioedema or urticaria.

BRADYKININ RECEPTORS

There are at least two distinct receptors for kinins, which have been designated B_1 and B_2. Both are GPCRs, sharing 36% amino acid sequence identity. Bradykinin receptor mechanisms are discussed in the legend to Figure 24–2. The classical bradykinin B_2 receptor is constitutively expressed in most normal tissues, where it selectively binds bradykinin and kallidin (Figure 24–2) and mediates the majority of their effects. The B_1 receptor selectively binds to the C-terminal des-Arg metabolites of bradykinin and kallidin released by carboxypeptidase N or M and is absent or expressed at low levels in most tissues. B_1-receptor expression is up-regulated by inflammation and by cytokines, endotoxins, and growth factors. Under these conditions, B_1-receptor effects may predominate.

Functions and Pharmacology of Kallikreins and Kinins

PAIN The kinins are powerful algesic agents that cause an intense burning pain when applied to the exposed base of a blister. Bradykinin excites primary sensory neurons and provokes the release of neuropeptides such as substance P, neurokinin A, and calcitonin gene-related peptide. Although there is overlap, B_2 receptors generally mediate acute bradykinin algesia, whereas the pain of chronic inflammation appears to involve increased numbers of B_1 receptors.

INFLAMMATION Kinins participate in a variety of inflammatory diseases. Plasma kinins increase permeability in the microcirculation. The effect, like that of histamine and serotonin in some species, is exerted on the small venules and involves separation of the junctions between endothelial cells. This, together with an increased hydrostatic pressure gradient, causes edema. Such edema, coupled with stimulation of nerve endings (*see* below), results in a "wheal and flare" response to intradermal injections in human beings.

In hereditary angioedema, bradykinin is formed, and there is depletion of the components of the kinin cascade during episodes of swelling, laryngeal edema, and abdominal pain. B_1 receptors on inflammatory cells such as macrophages can elicit production of the inflammatory mediators interleukin 1 (IL-1) and tumor necrosis factor-α (TNF-α). Kinin levels are increased in a number of chronic inflammatory diseases, including rhinitis caused by inhalation of antigens and that associated with rhinoviral infection. Kinins may be significant in conditions such as gout, disseminated intravascular coagulation, inflammatory bowel disease, rheumatoid arthritis, and asthma. Kinins also may contribute to the skeletal changes seen in chronic inflammatory states.

RESPIRATORY DISEASE The kinins have been implicated in the pathophysiology of allergic airway disorders such as asthma and rhinitis. Inhalation or intravenous injection of kinins causes bronchospasm in asthmatic patients but not in normal individuals. This bradykinin-induced bronchoconstriction is blocked by anticholinergic agents but not by antihistamines or cyclooxygenase inhibitors. Similarly, nasal challenge with bradykinin is followed by sneezing and serious glandular secretions in patients with allergic rhinitis.

CARDIOVASCULAR SYSTEM Bradykinin causes vasodilation by activating its B_2 receptor on endothelial cells. The endothelium-dependent dilation is mediated by NO, prostacyclin, and a hyperpolarizing epoxyeicosatrienoic acid that is a CYP-derived metabolite of arachidonic acid. The endogenous kallikrein–kinin system plays a minor role in the regulation of blood pressure under normal circumstances, but it may be important in hypertensive states.

The kallikrein–kinin system appears to be cardioprotective. Bradykinin contributes to the beneficial effect of preconditioning the heart against ischemia and reperfusion injury. In the presence of endothelial cells, bradykinin prevents vascular smooth muscle cell growth and proliferation. Bradykinin stimulates tissue plasminogen activator (tPA) release from the vascular endothelium. In this way, bradykinin may contribute to the endogenous defense against cardiovascular events such as myocardial infarction and stroke.

KIDNEY Renal kinins act in a paracrine manner to regulate urine volume and composition. Kallikrein is synthesized and secreted by the connecting cells of the distal nephron. Tissue kininogen and kinin receptors are present in the cells of the collecting duct. Like other vasodilators, kinins increase renal blood flow. Bradykinin also causes natriuresis by inhibiting sodium reabsorption at the cortical collecting duct. Renal kallikreins are increased by treatment with mineralocorticoids, ACE inhibitors, and neutral endopeptidase (neprilysin) inhibitors.

POTENTIAL THERAPEUTIC USES Bradykinin contributes to many of the effects of the ACE inhibitors (Figure 24–2). *Aprotinin*, a kallikrein inhibitor, is administered to patients undergoing coronary bypass to minimize bleeding and blood requirements (*see* below). Kinin agonists potentially may increase the delivery of chemotherapeutic agents past the blood–brain barrier. Based on some of the actions outlined earlier, kinin antagonists are being tested in inflammatory conditions.

KALLIKREIN INHIBITORS Aprotinin (TRASYLOL) is a natural proteinase inhibitor that inhibits mediators of the inflammatory response, fibrinolysis, and thrombin generation following cardiopulmonary bypass surgery, including kallikrein and plasmin. In several clinical studies, administration of aprotinin reduced requirements for blood products in patients undergoing coronary artery bypass grafting. Depending on patient risk factors, aprotinin is given as a loading dose of either 1 or 2 million kallikrein inhibitor units (KIU), followed by continuous infusion of 250,000 or 500,000 KIU/hr during surgery. Hypersensitivity reactions may occur with aprotinin, including anaphylactic or anaphylactoid reactions.

BRADYKININ AND THE EFFECTS OF ACE INHIBITORS ACE inhibitors are used widely in the treatment of hypertension, and they reduce mortality in patients with diabetic nephropathy, left ventricular dysfunction, previous myocardial infarction, or coronary artery disease. ACE inhibitors block the conversion of AngI to AngII, a potent vasoconstrictor and growth promoter (Figure 24–2) (*see* Chapter 30). Studies using the specific bradykinin B_2 antagonist HOE-140 demonstrate that bradykinin also contributes to many of the protective effects of ACE inhibitors. The contribution of bradykinin to the effects of ACE inhibitors may result not only from decreased degradation of bradykinin but also from induction of enhanced receptor sensitivity.

Occasional patients receiving ACE inhibitors have experienced angioedema, which occurs most often shortly after initiating therapy. This is a class effect of ACE inhibitors and is thought to be connected to the inhibition of kinin metabolism by ACE. ACE inhibitor–associated angioedema is more common in blacks than in Caucasians. A common side effect of ACE inhibitors (especially in women) is a chronic nonproductive cough that dissipates when the drug is stopped. The finding that angiotensin AT_1-receptor-subtype antagonists do not cause cough provides presumptive evidence for the role of bradykinin in this effect, but the mechanism and receptor subtype involved have not been clearly defined.

Preliminary data suggest that bradykinin also may contribute to the effects of the AT_1-receptor antagonists. During AT_1-receptor blockade, AngII concentrations increase. Renal bradykinin concentrations also increase through the effects of AngII on the unopposed AT_2-subtype receptor. Whether or not bradykinin contributes to the clinical effects of the AT_1-receptor antagonists remains to be determined.

For a complete Bibliographical listing see Goodman & Gilman's *The Pharmacological Basis of Therapeutics*, 11th ed., or Goodman & Gilman Online at www.accessmedicine.com.

25

LIPID-DERIVED AUTACOIDS: EICOSANOIDS AND PLATELET-ACTIVATING FACTOR

Membrane lipids supply the substrate for the synthesis of eicosanoids and platelet-activating factor (PAF). Eicosanoids—arachidonate metabolites, including prostaglandins, prostacyclin, thromboxane A₂, leukotrienes, lipoxins, and hepoxylins—are not stored but are produced by most cells when a variety of physical, chemical, and hormonal stimuli activate acyl hydrolases that make arachidonate available. Membrane glycerophosphocholine derivatives can be modified enzymatically to produce PAF. PAF is formed by a smaller number of cell types, principally leukocytes, platelets, and endothelial cells. Eicosanoids and PAF lipids contribute to inflammation, smooth muscle tone, hemostasis, thrombosis, parturition, and gastrointestinal (GI) secretion. Several classes of drugs, most notably *aspirin,* the *traditional nonsteroidal anti-inflammatory agents* (tNSAIDs), and the specific inhibitors of cyclooxygenase-2 (COX-2), such as the *coxibs,* owe their principal therapeutic effects to blockade of eicosanoid formation.

EICOSANOIDS

Prostaglandins (PGs), leukotrienes (LTs), and related compounds are called eicosanoids, *from the Greek* eikosi *("twenty"). Precursor essential fatty acids contain 20 carbons and three, four, or five double bonds: 8,11,14-eicosatrienoic acid (dihomo-γ-linolenic acid), 5,8,11,14-eicosatetraenoic acid (arachidonic acid [AA]; Figure 25–1), and 5,8,11,14,17-eicosapentaenoic acid (EPA). AA, the most abundant precursor, is either derived from dietary linoleic acid (9,12-octadecadienoic acid) or ingested directly as a dietary constituent. EPA is a major constituent of oils from fatty fish such as salmon.*

BIOSYNTHESIS

Biosynthesis of eicosanoids is limited by the availability of substrate and depends primarily on the release of AA, esterified in the sn-2 domain of cell membrane phospholipids or other complex lipids, to the eicosanoid-synthesizing enzymes by acyl hydrolases, most notably phospholipase A₂. Chemical and physical stimuli activate the Ca²⁺-dependent translocation of group IV cytosolic PLA₂ (cPLA₂), which has high affinity for AA, to the membrane, where it hydrolyzes the sn-2 ester bond of membrane phospholipids (particularly phosphatidylcholine and phosphatidylethanolamine), releasing arachidonate. Multiple additional PLA₂ isoforms (group IIA secretory [sPLA₂], group V [sPLA₂], group VI Ca²⁺ independent [iPLA₂], and group X [sPLA₂]) have been characterized. Under nonstimulated conditions, AA liberated by iPLA₂ is reincorporated into cell membranes, so there is negligible eicosanoid biosynthesis. While cPLA₂ dominates in the acute release of AA, the inducible sPLA₂ contributes under conditions of sustained or intense stimulation of AA production. Once liberated, a portion of the AA is metabolized rapidly to oxygenated products by several distinct enzyme systems, including cyclooxygenases, lipoxygenases, *and CYPs.*

Products of Prostaglandin G/H Synthases

The prostaglandins prostacyclin and thromboxane, collectively termed prostanoids, *can be considered analogs of unnatural compounds with the trivial names* prostanoic acid *and* thrombanoic acid, *with the structures shown below:*

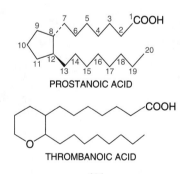

PROSTANOIC ACID

THROMBANOIC ACID

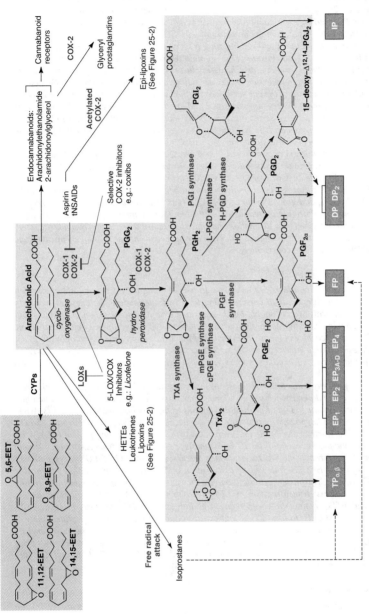

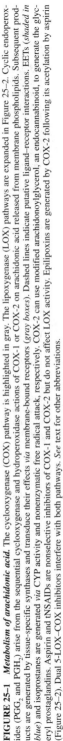

FIGURE 25–1 *Metabolism of arachidonic acid.* The cyclooxygenase (COX) pathway is highlighted in gray. The lipoxygenase (LOX) pathways are expanded in Figure 25–2. Cyclic endoperoxides (PGG_2 and PGH_2) arise from the sequential cyclooxygenase and hydroperoxidase actions of COX-1 or COX-2 on arachidonic acid released from membrane phospholipids. Subsequent products are generated by tissue-specific synthases and transduce their effects *via* membrane-bound receptors (*gray boxes*). Dashed lines indicate putative ligand–receptor interactions. EETs (*shaded in blue*) and isoprostanes are generated *via* CYP activity and nonenzymatic free radical attack, respectively. COX-2 can use modified arachidonoylglycerol, an endocannabinoid, to generate the glyceryl prostaglandins. Aspirin and tNSAIDs are nonselective inhibitors of COX-1 and COX-2 but do not affect LOX activity. Epilipoxins are generated by COX-2 following its acetylation by aspirin (Figure 25–2). Dual 5-LOX–COX inhibitors interfere with both pathways. *See text* for other abbreviations.

417

AA is metabolized successively to the cyclic endoperoxide prostaglandins G (PGG) and H (PGH) (Figure 25–1) by the cyclooxygenase (COX) and hydroperoxidase (HOX) activities of the prostaglandin G/H synthases. Isomerases and synthases effect the transformation of PGH_2 into terminal prostanoids distinguished by substitutions on their cyclopentane rings.

Prostaglandins of the E and D series are hydroxyketones, whereas the F_α prostaglandins are 1,3-diols (Figure 25–1). A, B, and C prostaglandins are unsaturated ketones that arise nonenzymatically from PGE during extraction procedures; it is unlikely that they occur biologically. PGJ_2 and related compounds result from the dehydration of PGD_2. Prostacyclin (PGI_2) has a double-ring structure; in addition to a cyclopentane ring, a second ring is formed by an oxygen bridge between carbons 6 and 9. Thromboxanes (Txs) contain a six-member oxirane ring instead of the cyclopentane ring of the prostaglandins. The main classes are further subdivided in accord with the number of double bonds in their side chains, as indicated by numerical subscripts. Dihomo-γ-linolenic acid is the precursor of the one series, AA for the two series, and EPA for the three series. Prostanoids derived from AA carry the subscript 2 and are the major series in mammals. There is little evidence that one- or three-series prostanoids are made in adequate amounts to be important under normal circumstances. However, the health benefits of dietary supplementation with ω-3 fatty acids remain a focus of investigation.

Synthesis of prostanoids is accomplished in a stepwise manner by a complex of microsomal enzymes. The first enzyme in this synthetic pathway is prostaglandin endoperoxide G/H synthase, which is colloquially called cyclooxygenase, or COX. There are two distinct COX isoforms, COX-1 and COX-2. COX-1 is expressed constitutively in most cells, whereas COX-2 is up-regulated by cytokines, shear stress, and growth factors. Thus, COX-1 is considered to subserve housekeeping functions such as cytoprotection of the gastric epithelium (see Chapter 36). COX-2 is the major source of prostanoids formed in inflammation and cancer. This distinction is overly simplistic: there are physiological and pathophysiological processes in which each enzyme is uniquely involved and others in which they function coordinately.

Products of Lipoxygenases

Lipoxygenases (LOXs) are a family of non-heme iron–containing enzymes that catalyze the oxygenation of polyenic fatty acids to corresponding lipid hydroperoxides. The enzymes require a fatty acid substrate with two cis double bonds separated by a methylene group. AA, which contains several double bonds in this configuration, is metabolized to hydroperoxy eicosatetraenoic acids (HPETEs), which vary in the site of insertion of the hydroperoxy group. Analogous to PGG_2 and PGH_2, these unstable intermediates are further metabolized by a variety of enzymes. HPETEs are converted to their corresponding hydroxy fatty acid (HETE) either nonenzymatically or by a peroxidase.

The 5-LOX pathway leads to the synthesis of the leukotrienes (LTs), which play a major role in the development and persistence of the inflammatory response (Figure 25–2). A nomenclature (LTB_4, LTB_5, etc.) similar to that of prostanoids applies to the subclassification of the LTs. When eosinophils, mast cells, polymorphonuclear leukocytes, or monocytes are activated, 5-LOX translocates to the nuclear membrane and associates with 5-LOX-activating protein (FLAP), an integral membrane protein essential for LT biosynthesis. FLAP may act as an AA transfer protein that presents the substrate to the 5-LOX. A two-step reaction is catalyzed by 5-LOX: oxygenation of AA at C-5 to form 5-HPETE, followed by dehydration of 5-HPETE to an unstable 5,6-epoxide known as LTA_4. LTA_4 is transformed into bioactive eicosanoids by multiple pathways depending on the cellular context: transformation by LTA_4 hydrolase to a 5,12-dihydroxyeicosatetraenoic acid known as LTB_4; conjugation with reduced glutathione by LTC_4 synthase, in eosinophils, monocytes, and mast cells, to form LTC_4; and extracellular metabolism of the peptide moiety of LTC_4, leading to the removal of glutamic acid and subsequent cleavage of glycine, to generate LTD_4 and LTE_4, respectively. LTC_4, LTD_4, and LTE_4, the cysteinyl leukotrienes, were known originally as the slow-reacting substance of anaphylaxis (SRS-A; see Chapter 27). LTB_4 and LTC_4 are actively transported out of the cell.

Products of CYPs P450

Multiple CYPs metabolize arachidonic acid. For instance, epoxyeicosatrienoic acids (EETs) can be formed by CYP epoxygenases, primarily CYP2C and CYP2J. Their biosynthesis can be altered by pharmacological, nutritional, and genetic factors that affect CYP expression (see Chapter 3).

EETs are important modulators of cardiovascular and renal function. They are synthesized in endothelial cells and cause vasodilation in a number of vascular beds by activating the large conductance Ca^{2+}-activated K^+ channels of smooth muscle cells. This results in hyperpolarization of smooth muscle and thus relaxation, leading to reduced blood pressure. Substantial evidence

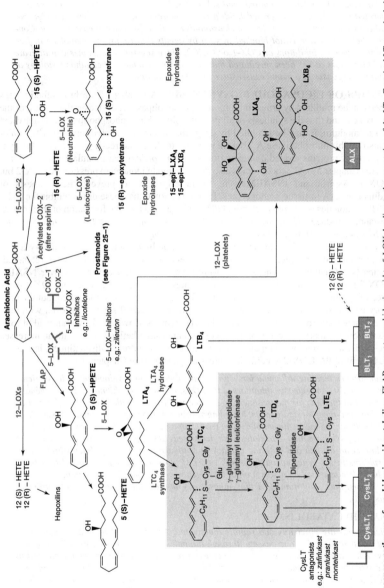

FIGURE 25–2 *Lipoxygenase pathways of arachidonic acid metabolism.* FLAP presents arachidonic acid to 5-LOX, leading to the generation of the LTs. Cysteinyl LTs are shaded in gray. Lipox-ins (*shaded in blue*) are products of cellular interaction *via* a 5-LOX–12-LOX pathway or *via* a 15-LOX–5-LOX pathway. Biological effects are transduced *via* membrane-bound receptors (*dark gray boxes*). Dashed line indicates putative ligand–receptor interactions. Zileuton inhibits 5-LOX but not the COX pathways (expanded in Figure 25–1). Dual 5-LOX–COX pathways interfere with both pathways. CysLT antagonists prevent activation of the CysLT₁ receptor. *See* text for abbreviations.

indicates that EETs may function as endothelium-derived hyperpolarizing factors (EDHFs), particularly in the coronary circulation.

Other Pathways

The isoeicosanoids, a family of eicosanoid isomers, are formed nonenzymatically by direct free radical–based attack on AA and related lipid substrates. Unlike eicosanoids, these compounds are generated initially on the esterified lipid in cell membranes, from which they are cleaved, presumably by phospholipases; the free isoeicosanoids circulate and are excreted in urine. Consequently, their production is not blocked in vivo by agents that suppress metabolism of free arachidonate, such as inhibitors of COX-1 or COX-2. Since several isoprostanes can activate prostanoid receptors, it has been speculated that they may contribute to the pathophysiology of inflammatory responses in a manner insensitive to COX inhibitors.

INHIBITORS OF EICOSANOID BIOSYNTHESIS A number of the biosynthetic steps just described can be inhibited by drugs. Inhibition of phospholipase A_2 decreases the release of the precursor fatty acid and thus the synthesis of all its metabolites. Since phospholipase A_2 is activated by Ca^{2+} and calmodulin, it may be inhibited by drugs that reduce the availability of Ca^{2+}. *Glucocorticoids* also inhibit phospholipase A_2, but they appear to do so indirectly by inducing the synthesis of a group of proteins termed *annexins* (formerly *lipocortins*) that modulate phospholipase A_2 activity (*see* Chapter 59). Glucocorticoids also down-regulate induced expression of COX-2 but not of COX-1. Aspirin and tNSAIDs were found originally to prevent the synthesis of prostaglandins from AA in tissue homogenates. It now is known that these drugs inhibit the COX but not the HOX moieties of the prostaglandin G/H synthases and thus the formation of their downstream prostanoid products. *These drugs do not inhibit LOXs and may result in increased formation of LTs by shunting of substrate to the lipoxygenase pathway.*

COX-1 and COX-2 differ in their sensitivity to inhibition by certain anti-inflammatory drugs. This observation has led to the recent development of agents that selectively inhibit COX-2, including the coxibs (*see* Chapter 26). These drugs were predicted to offer advantages over NSAIDs because COX-2 is the predominant cyclooxygenase at sites of inflammation, whereas COX-1 is the major source of cytoprotective prostaglandins in the GI tract. The matter is not settled, but the anti-inflammatory actions of the coxibs were associated with improved GI safety compared with their nonselective counterparts in at least one trial of clinical outcomes. However, the withdrawal of rofecoxib (VIOXX) from the market because of an association in postmarketing studies with an increased risk of myocardial infarction, which may be present long after the drug is discontinued, leaves the therapeutic benefit of the COX-2-specific inhibitors in question (*see* Chapter 26).

Since leukotrienes mediate inflammation, efforts have focused on development of leukotriene-receptor antagonists and selective inhibitors of the LOXs. Zileuton, an inhibitor of 5-lipoxygenase, was marketed in the U.S. for the treatment of asthma but has been withdrawn. In addition, cysteinyl leukotriene-receptor antagonists, including zafirlukast, pranlukast, and montelukast, have established efficacy in the treatment of asthma (see Chapter 27). A common polymorphism in the gene for LTC_4 synthase that correlates with increased LTC_4 generation is associated with aspirin-intolerant asthma and with the efficacy of antileukotriene therapy. Interestingly, while polymorphisms in the genes encoding 5-LOX or FLAP do not appear to be linked to asthma, studies have demonstrated an association of these genes with myocardial infarction, stroke, and atherosclerosis; thus, inhibition of LT biosynthesis may be useful in the prevention of cardiovascular disease.

EICOSANOID CATABOLISM

Most eicosanoids are efficiently and rapidly inactivated. About 95% of infused PGE_2 (but not PGI_2) is inactivated during one passage through the pulmonary circulation. Broadly speaking, the enzymatic catabolic reactions are of two types: a relatively rapid initial step, catalyzed by widely distributed prostaglandin-specific enzymes, wherein prostaglandins lose most of their biological activity; and a second step in which these metabolites are oxidized, probably by enzymes identical to those responsible for the β-and ω-oxidation of fatty acids.

The degradation of PGI_2 ($t_{1/2}$ of 3 minutes) apparently begins with its spontaneous hydrolysis in blood to 6-keto-$PGF_1\alpha$. The metabolism of this compound involves the same steps as those for PGE_2 and $PGF_{2\alpha}$.

The degradation of LTC_4 occurs in the lungs, kidney, and liver. The initial steps involve its conversion to LTE_4. LTC_4 also may be inactivated by oxidation of its cysteinyl sulfur to a sulfoxide. In leukocytes, LTB_4 is inactivated principally by oxidation by members of the CYP4F subfamily.

Pharmacological Properties of Eicosanoids

CARDIOVASCULAR SYSTEM In most vascular beds, PGE_2 elicits vasodilation and a drop in blood pressure, although vasoconstrictor effects have been reported, depending on which PGE_2 receptor is activated (*see* below). Infusion of PGD_2 results in flushing, nasal stuffiness, and hypotension; subsequent formation of F-ring metabolites may result in hypertension. Responses to $PGF_{2\alpha}$ vary with vascular bed; it is a potent constrictor of both pulmonary arteries and veins but does not alter blood pressure.

PGI_2 relaxes vascular smooth muscle, causing prominent hypotension and reflex tachycardia on intravenous administration. It is about five times more potent than PGE_2 in producing this effect. TxA_2 is a potent vasoconstrictor.

LTC_4 and LTD_4 cause hypotension from a decrease in intravascular volume and also from decreased cardiac contractility secondary to a marked LT-induced reduction in coronary blood flow. Although LTC_4 and LTD_4 have little effect on most large arteries or veins, coronary arteries and distal segments of the pulmonary artery are contracted by nanomolar concentrations of these agents. The renal vasculature is resistant to this constrictor action, but the mesenteric vasculature is not.

The CysLTs have prominent effects on the microvasculature. LTC_4 and LTD_4 appear to act on the endothelial lining of postcapillary venules to cause exudation of plasma; they are more than a 1000-fold more potent than histamine in this regard. At higher concentrations, LTC_4 and LTD_4 constrict arterioles and reduce exudation of plasma.

Isoprostanes usually are vasoconstrictors, although there are examples of vasodilation in pre-constricted vessels.

PLATELETS Low concentrations of PGE_2 enhance and higher concentrations inhibit platelet aggregation. Both PGI_2 and PGD_2 inhibit the aggregation of platelets *in vitro*.

TxA_2, the major product of COX-1 in platelets, induces platelet aggregation. Perhaps more importantly, TxA_2 acts as an amplification signal for other, more potent platelet agonists such as thrombin and adenosine diphosphate (ADP). The actions of TxA_2 on platelets are restrained by PGI_2, which inhibits platelet aggregation by all recognized agonists.

INFLAMMATION AND IMMUNITY Eicosanoids play a major role in the inflammatory and immune responses, as reflected by the clinical usefulness of the NSAIDs. While LTs generally are proinflammatory and lipoxins anti-inflammatory, prostanoids can exert both kinds of activity.

LTB_4 is a potent chemotactic agent for polymorphonuclear leukocytes, eosinophils, and monocytes. In higher concentrations, LTB_4 stimulates the aggregation of polymorphonuclear leukocytes and promotes degranulation and the generation of superoxide. LTB_4 promotes adhesion of neutrophils to vascular endothelial cells and their transendothelial migration and stimulates synthesis of proinflammatory cytokines from macrophages and lymphocytes. Prostaglandins generally inhibit lymphocyte function and proliferation, suppressing the immune response. PGE_2 depresses the humoral antibody response by inhibiting the differentiation of B-lymphocytes into antibody-secreting plasma cells. PGE_2 acts on T-lymphocytes to inhibit mitogen-stimulated proliferation and lymphokine release by sensitized cells. PGE_2 and TxA_2 also may play a role in T-lymphocyte development by regulating apoptosis of immature thymocytes. PGD_2, a major product of mast cells, is a potent chemoattractant for eosinophils and induces chemotaxis and migration of Th2 lymphocytes.

Lipoxins have diverse effects on leukocytes, including activation of monocytes and macrophages and inhibition of the activation of neutrophils, eosinophils, and lymphocytes.

KIDNEY AND URINE FORMATION PGs influence renal salt and water excretion by alterations in renal blood flow and by direct effects on renal tubules. PGE_2 and PGI_2 infused directly into the renal arteries of dogs increase renal blood flow and provoke renal diuresis, natriuresis, and kaliuresis, with little change in glomerular filtration rate. TxA_2 decreases renal blood flow, decreases the rate of glomerular filtration, and participates in tubuloglomerular feedback. PGEs inhibit water reabsorption induced by vasopressin (antidiuretic hormone). PGE_2 also inhibits chloride reabsorption in the thick ascending limb of the loop of Henle in the rabbit. PGI_2, PGE_2, and PGD_2 stimulate renin secretion from the renal cortex, apparently through a direct effect on the granular juxtaglomerular cells.

EYE Although $PGF_{2\alpha}$ induces constriction of the iris sphincter muscle, its overall effect in the eye is to decrease intraocular pressure by increasing the aqueous humor outflow of the eye *via* the uveoscleral and trabecular meshwork pathway. A variety of F prostaglandin-receptor agonists have proven effective in the treatment of open-angle glaucoma, a condition associated with the loss of COX-2 expression in the pigmented epithelium of the ciliary body (*see* Chapter 63).

CENTRAL NERVOUS SYSTEM While effects have been reported following injection of several PGs into discrete brain areas, the best established biologically active mediators are PGE_2 and PGD_2. The induction of fever by a range of endogenous and exogenous pyrogens appears to be mediated by PGE_2. Exogenous $PGF_{2\alpha}$ and PGI_2 induce fever but do not contribute to the pyretic response. PGD_2 and TxA_2 do not induce fever. PGD_2 also appears to act on arachnoid trabecular cells in the basal forebrain to mediate an increase in extracellular adenosine that, in turn, facilitates induction of sleep.

PGs contribute to pain both peripherally and centrally. PLA_2 and COX-2 synthesis are increased at sites of local inflammation that are, in turn, associated with increased central PGE_2 biosynthesis. PGE_2 and PGI_2 sensitize the peripheral nerve endings to painful stimuli by lowering the threshold of nociceptors. Centrally, PGE_2 can increase excitability in pain transmission neuronal pathways in the spinal cord. Hyperalgesia also is produced by LTB_4. The release of these eicosanoids during the inflammatory process thus serves as an amplification system for the pain mechanism (*see* below). The role of PGE_2 and PGI_2 in inflammation is discussed in Chapter 26. COX-2 has been implicated in several neurological diseases, and clinical trials of selective inhibitors of COX-2 are ongoing in the chemoprevention of Alzheimer's disease, Parkinson's disease, and epilepsy.

ENDOCRINE SYSTEM A number of endocrine tissues respond to PGs. In a number of species, the systemic administration of PGE_2 increases circulating concentrations of adrenocorticotropic hormone (ACTH), growth hormone, prolactin, and gonadotropins. Other effects include stimulation of steroid production by the adrenals, stimulation of insulin release, and thyrotropin-like effects on the thyroid. The critical role of $PGF_{2\alpha}$ in parturition relies on its ability to induce an oxytocin-dependent decline in progesterone levels. PGE_2 works as part of a positive-feedback loop to induce oocyte maturation required for fertilization during and after ovulation.

LOX metabolites also have endocrine effects. 12-HETE stimulates the release of aldosterone from the adrenal cortex and mediates part of the aldosterone release stimulated by angiotensin II, but not that occurring in response to ACTH.

BONE PGs are strong modulators of bone metabolism. PGE_2 stimulates bone formation and resorption through osteoblastic and osteoclastic activities affecting bone strength and composition.

MECHANISM OF ACTION OF EICOSANOIDS Many of the responses just described can be understood in light of the distribution of eicosanoid receptors and their coupling to second-messenger systems that modulate cellular activity.

Prostaglandin Receptors PGs act locally near their sites of formation. The diversity of their effects is explained to a large extent by their interaction with a diverse family of distinct receptors (Table 25–1). All eicosanoid receptors are G protein–coupled receptors that interact with G_s, G_i, or G_q to modulate the activities of adenylyl cyclase and phospholipase C (*see* Chapter 1). Single gene products have been identified for the receptors for prostacyclin (the IP receptor), $PGF_{2\alpha}$ (the FP receptor), and TxA_2 (the TP receptor). Four distinct PGE_2 receptors (EP 1–4) and two PGD_2 receptors (DP$_1$ and DP$_2$) have been cloned. Additional isoforms of the TP (α and β), FP (A and B), and EP$_3$ (A–D) receptors can arise through differential mRNA splicing.

Therapeutic Uses

INHIBITORS AND ANTAGONISTS As a consequence of the important and diverse physiological roles of eicosanoids, mimicking their effects with stable agonists, inhibiting eicosanoid formation, and antagonizing eicosanoid receptors produce noticeable and therapeutically useful responses. As outlined earlier and in Chapter 26, the tNSAIDs and their subclass of selective COX-2 inhibitors are used widely as anti-inflammatory drugs, whereas low-dose aspirin is employed frequently for cardioprotection. LT antagonists are useful clinically in the treatment of asthma, and FP agonists are used in the treatment of open-angle glaucoma. EP agonists are used to induce labor and to ameliorate gastric irritation owing to tNSAIDs.

There are as yet no potent selective antagonists of prostanoid receptors in clinical use. TP antagonists are under evaluation in cardiovascular disease, whereas EP agonists and antagonists are under evaluation in the treatment of bone fracture and osteoporosis. Orally active antagonists of LTC_4 and D_4 have been approved for the treatment of asthma (*see* Chapter 27). These agents act by binding to the CysLT$_1$ receptor and include montelukast and zafirlukast. In patients with mild-to-moderately severe asthma, they cause bronchodilation, reduce the bronchoconstriction caused by

Table 25–1

Eicosanoid Receptors

Receptor	Primary Ligand	Secondary Ligand	Primary Coupling	Major Phenotype in Knockout Mice
DP_1	PGD_2		$\uparrow$ cAMP (G_s)	$\downarrow$ Allergic asthma
DP_2/CHRT$_2$	PGD_2	15d-PGJ$_2$?	$\uparrow$ Ca$^{2+}_i$ (G_i)	?
EP_1	PGE_2		G_q	Decreased response of colon to carcinogens
EP_2	PGE_2		$\uparrow$ cAMP	Impaired ovulation and fertilization; salt sensitive hypertension
EP_{3A-D}	PGE_2		$\downarrow$ cAMP (G_i) $\uparrow$ cAMP (G_s) $\uparrow$ PLC (G_q)	Resistance to pyrogens
EP_4	PGE_2		$\uparrow$ cAMP (G_s)	Patent ductus arteriosus
$FP_{A,B}$	$PGF_{2\alpha}$	IsoP?	G_q	Failure of parturition
IP	PGI_2	PGE_2	$\uparrow$ cAMP (G_s)	$\uparrow$ Thrombotic response, $\downarrow$ response to vascular injury
$TP_{\alpha,\beta}$	TxA_2	IsoPs	$\uparrow$ PLC $(G_q, G_i, G_{12/13}, G_{16})$	$\uparrow$ Bleeding time, $\uparrow$ response to vascular injury
BLT_1	LTB_4		G_{16}, G_i	Some suppression of inflammatory response
BLT_2	LTB_4	12(S)-HETE 12(R)-HETE	G_q-like, G_i-like, G_z-like	?
$CysLT_1$	LTD_4	LTC_4/LTE$_4$	$\uparrow$ PLC (G_q)	$\downarrow$ Innate and adaptive immune vascular permeability response, $\uparrow$ pulmonary inflammatory and fibrotic response
$CysLT_2$	LTC_4/LTD$_4$	LTE_4	$\uparrow$ PLC (G_q)	$\downarrow$ Pulmonary inflammatory and fibrotic response

This table lists the major classes of eicosanoid receptors and their signaling characteristics. Splice variants are indicated where appropriate. Major phenotypes in knockout mouse models are listed.

ABBREVIATIONS: Ca$^{2+}_i$, cytosolic Ca^{2+}; cAMP, cyclic AMP; PLC, phospholipase C (activation leads to increased cellular IP$_3$ and diacyl glycerol generation and increased Ca$^{2+}_i$); IsoPs, isopostanes; DP$_2$ is a member of the fMLP receptor superfamily; fMLP, formyl-methionyl-leucyl-phenylalanine. 15d-PGI$_2$, 15 deoxy PGI$_2$.

exercise and exposure to antigen, and decrease the patient's requirement for the use of β_2-adrenergic agonists. Their effectiveness in patients with aspirin-induced asthma also has been shown.

The use of eicosanoids or eicosanoid derivatives themselves as therapeutic agents is limited in part because systemic administration of prostanoids frequently is associated with significant adverse effects and because of their short half-lives in the circulation. Despite these limitations, several prostanoids are of clinical utility.

Therapeutic Abortion

There has been intense interest in the effects of the PGs on the female reproductive system. When given early in pregnancy, their action as abortifacients *may be variable and often incomplete and accompanied by adverse effects. PGs appear, however, to be of value in missed abortion and molar gestation, and they have been used widely for the induction of midtrimester abortion. Systemic or intravaginal administration of the PGE₁ analog* misoprostol *in combination with* mifepristone *(RU486) or* methotrexate *is highly effective in the termination of early pregnancy.*

PGE₂ or PGF₂ₐ are used to facilitate labor by promoting ripening and dilation of the cervix.

Gastric Cytoprotection

The capacity of several PG analogs to suppress gastric ulceration is a property of therapeutic importance. Of these, misoprostol *(CYTOTEC), a* PGE₁ *analog, is approved by the FDA. Misoprostol appears to heal gastric ulcers about as effectively as the* H₂-receptor antagonists *(see Chapter 36);*

however, relief of ulcerogenic pain and healing of duodenal ulcers have not been achieved consistently with misoprostol. This drug currently is used primarily for the prevention of ulcers that often occur during long-term treatment with NSAIDs. In this setting, misoprostol appears to be as effective as the proton pump inhibitor omeprazole.

Impotence

PGE$_1$ (alprostadil) may be used in the treatment of impotence. Intracavernous injection of PGE$_1$ causes complete or partial erection in impotent patients who do not have disorders of the vascular system or cavernous body damage. The erection lasts for 1–3 hours and is sufficient for sexual intercourse. PGE$_1$ is more effective than papaverine. The agent is available as a sterile powder that is reconstituted with water for injections (CAVERJECT), *although it has been superseded largely by the use of PDE5 inhibitors, such as* sildenafil, tadalafil, *and* vardenafil (see *Chapter 31*).

Maintenance of Patent Ductus Arteriosus

The ductus arteriosus in neonates is highly sensitive to vasodilation by PGE$_1$. Maintenance of a patent ductus may be important hemodynamically in some neonates with congenital heart disease. PGE$_1$ (alprostadil, PROSTIN VR PEDIATRIC) *is highly effective for palliative, but not definitive, therapy to maintain temporary patency until surgery can be performed. Apnea is observed in ~10% of neonates so treated, particularly those who weigh <2 kg at birth.*

Pulmonary Hypertension

Primary pulmonary hypertension is a rare idiopathic disease that mainly affects young adults. It leads to right-sided heart failure and frequently is fatal. Long-term therapy with PGI$_2$ (epoprostenol, FLOLAN) *has either delayed or precluded the need for lung or heart–lung transplantation in a number of patients. In addition, many affected individuals have had a marked improvement in symptoms after receiving treatment with PGI$_2$. Epoprostenol also has been used successfully to treat portopulmonary hypertension that arises secondary to liver disease, again with a goal of facilitating ultimate transplantation.*

PLATELET-ACTIVATING FACTOR

Chemistry and Biosynthesis

*PAF is 1-O-alkyl-2-acetyl-*sn-*glycero-3-phosphocholine. Its structure is:*

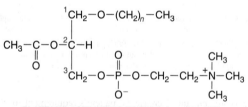

PLATELET-ACTIVATING FACTOR (*n* = 11 to 17)

    PAF contains a long-chain alkyl group joined to the glycerol backbone in an ether linkage at position 1 and an acetyl group at position 2. PAF actually represents a family of phospholipids because the alkyl group at position 1 can vary in length from 12 to 18 carbon atoms. In human neutrophils, PAF consists predominantly of a mixture of the 16- and 18-carbon ethers, but its composition may change when cells are stimulated.

    Like the eicosanoids, PAF is not stored in cells but is synthesized in response to stimulation. The major pathway by which PAF is generated involves the precursor 1-O-alkyl-2-acyl-glycerophosphocholine, a lipid found in high concentrations in the membranes of many types of cells. The 2-acyl substituents include AA. PAF is synthesized from this substrate in two steps (Figure 25–3). The first involves the action of phospholipase A$_2$, the initiating enzyme for eicosanoid biosynthesis, with the formation of 1-O-alkyl-2-lyso-glycerophosphocholine (lyso-PAF) and a free fatty acid (usually AA). Eicosanoid and PAF biosynthesis thus is closely coupled. The second, rate-limiting step is performed by the acetylcoenzyme-A-lyso-PAF acetyltransferase. PAF synthesis also can occur de novo; *a phosphocholine substituent is transferred to alkyl acetyl glycerol by a distinct lysoglycerophosphate acetylcoenzyme-A transferase. This pathway may contribute to physiological levels of PAF for normal cellular functions. The synthesis of PAF may be stimulated during antigen–antibody reactions or by a variety of agents, including chemotactic peptides, thrombin, collagen, and other autacoids; PAF also can stimulate its own formation. Both*

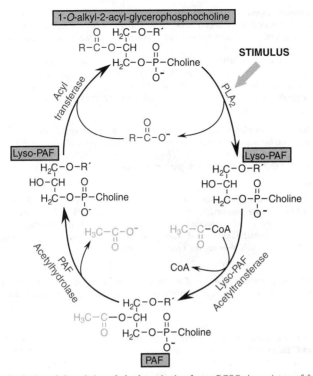

FIGURE 25–3 *Synthesis and degradation of platelet-activating factor.* RCOO⁻ is a mixture of fatty acids but is enriched in arachidonic acid that may be metabolized to eicosanoids. CoA, coenzyme A.

the phospholipase and acetyltransferase are Ca^{2+}-dependent enzymes; thus, PAF synthesis is regulated by the availability of Ca^{2+}.

The inactivation of PAF also occurs in two steps (Figure 25–3). Initially, the acetyl group of PAF is removed by PAF acetylhydrolase to form lyso-PAF; this enzyme, a group VI phospholipase A_2, exists as secreted and intracellular isoforms and has marked specificity for phospholipids with short acyl chains at the sn-2 position. Lyso-PAF is then converted to a 1-O-alkyl-2-acyl-glycerophosphocholine by an acyltransferase.

PAF is synthesized by platelets, neutrophils, monocytes, mast cells, eosinophils, renal mesangial cells, renal medullary cells, and vascular endothelial cells. PAF is released from monocytes but retained by leukocytes and endothelial cells. In endothelial cells, it is displayed on the surface for juxtacrine signaling.

In addition to these enzymatic routes, PAF-like molecules can be formed from the oxidative fragmentation of membrane phospholipids (oxPLs). These compounds are increased in settings of oxidant stress such as cigarette smoking and differ structurally from PAF in that they contain a fatty acid at the sn-1 position of glycerol joined through an ester bond and various short-chain acyl groups at the sn-2 position. OxPLs mimic the structure of PAF closely enough to bind to its receptor (see below) and elicit the same responses. Unlike the synthesis of PAF, which is highly controlled, oxPL production is unregulated; degradation by PAF acetylhydrolase, therefore, is necessary to suppress the toxicity of oxPLs. Levels of PAF acetylhydrolase (also known as lipoprotein-associated phospholipase A_2) *are increased in colon cancer, cardiovascular disease, and stroke; polymorphisms have been associated with altered risk of cardiovascular events. A common missense mutation in Japanese people is associated disproportionately with more severe asthma.*

PHARMACOLOGICAL PROPERTIES
Cardiovascular System

PAF is a potent dilator in most vascular beds; when administered intravenously, it causes hypotension. PAF-induced vasodilation is independent of effects on sympathetic innervation, the renin–angiotensin system, or arachidonate metabolism and likely results from a combination of direct and indirect actions. PAF induces vasoconstriction or vasodilation depending on the concentration, vascular bed, and involvement of platelets or leukocytes. The pulmonary vasculature also is constricted by PAF.

Intradermal injection of PAF causes an initial vasoconstriction followed by a typical wheal and flare. PAF increases vascular permeability and edema in the same manner as histamine and bradykinin. The increase in permeability is due to contraction of venular endothelial cells, but PAF is more potent than histamine or bradykinin by three orders of magnitude.

Platelets

PAF potently stimulates platelet aggregation in vitro. While this is accompanied by the release of TxA_2 and the granular contents of the platelet, PAF does not require the presence of TxA_2 or other aggregating agents to produce this effect. The intravenous injection of PAF causes formation of intravascular platelet aggregates and thrombocytopenia.

Leukocytes

PAF stimulates polymorphonuclear leukocytes to aggregate, to release LTs and lysosomal enzymes, and to generate superoxide. PAF also promotes aggregation of monocytes and degranulation of eosinophils. It is chemotactic for eosinophils, neutrophils, and monocytes and promotes endothelial adherence and diapedesis of neutrophils. When given systemically, PAF causes leukocytopenia, with neutrophils showing the greatest decline.

Stomach

In addition to contracting the fundus of the stomach, PAF is the most potent known ulcerogen. When given intravenously, it causes hemorrhagic erosions of the gastric mucosa that extend into the submucosa.

Kidney

When infused intrarenally in animals, PAF decreases renal blood flow, glomerular filtration rate, urine volume, and excretion of Na^+ without changes in systemic hemodynamics. These effects are the result of a direct action on the renal circulation. PAF exerts a receptor-mediated biphasic effect on afferent arterioles, dilating them at low concentrations and constricting them at higher concentrations. The vasoconstrictor effect appears to be mediated, at least in part, by COX products, whereas vasodilation is a consequence of the stimulation of NO production by endothelium.

MECHANISM OF ACTION OF PAF

Extracellular PAF exerts its actions by stimulating a specific GPCR that is expressed in numerous cell types. The PAF receptor's strict recognition requirements, including a specific head group and specific atypical sn-2 residue, also are met by oxPLs. The PAF receptor couples with G_Q to activate the $PLC–IP_3–Ca^{2+}$ pathway and phospholipases A_2 and D such that AA is mobilized from diacylglycerol, resulting in the synthesis of PGs, TxA_2, or LTs, which may function as extracellular mediators of the effects of PAF. PAF also may exert actions without leaving its cell of origin. For example, PAF is synthesized in a regulated fashion by endothelial cells stimulated by inflammatory mediators. This PAF is presented on the surface of the endothelium, where it activates the PAF receptor on juxtaposed cells, including platelets, polymorphonuclear leukocytes, and monocytes, and acts cooperatively with P-selectin to promote adhesion. Endothelial cells under oxidant stress release oxPLs, which activate leukocytes and platelets and can spread tissue damage.

RECEPTOR ANTAGONISTS

Many compounds have been described that are PAF-receptor antagonists that selectively inhibit the actions of PAF in vivo and in vitro. One would expect a PAF receptor antagonist to be a potent anti-inflammatory agent that might be useful in the therapy of disorders such as asthma, sepsis, and other diseases in which PAF is postulated to play a role. However, trials in humans have been disappointing, and the clinical efficacy of PAF antagonists has yet to be realized.

INFLAMMATORY AND ALLERGIC RESPONSES

The proinflammatory actions of PAF and its elaboration by endothelial cells, leukocytes, and mast cells under inflammatory conditions are well characterized. PAF and PAF-like molecules are thought to contribute to the pathophysiology of inflammatory disorders, including anaphylaxis, bronchial asthma, endotoxic shock, and skin diseases. The plasma concentration of PAF is increased in experimental anaphylactic shock, and the administration of PAF reproduces many of its signs and symptoms, suggesting a role for the autacoid in anaphylactic shock. In addition, mice over expressing the PAF receptor exhibit bronchial hyperreactivity and increased lethality when treated with endotoxin. PAF receptor knockout mice display milder anaphylactic responses to exogenous antigen challenge, including less cardiac instability, airway constriction, and alveolar edema; they are, however, still susceptible to endotoxic shock. Deletion of the PAF receptor augments the lethality of infection with gram-negative bacteria while improving host defense against gram-positive pneumococcal pneumonia.

Despite the broad implications of these observations, the effects of PAF antagonists in the treatment of inflammatory and allergic disorders have been disappointing. Although PAF antagonists reverse the bronchoconstriction of anaphylactic shock and improve survival in animal models, the impact of these agents on animal models of asthma and inflammation is marginal. Similarly, in patients with asthma, PAF antagonists partially inhibit the bronchoconstriction induced by antigen challenge but not by challenges by methacholine, exercise, or inhalation of cold air. These results may reflect the complexity of these pathological conditions and the likelihood that other mediators contribute to the inflammation associated with these disorders.

For a complete Bibliographical listing see Goodman & Gilman's *The Pharmacological Basis of Therapeutics*, 11th ed., or Goodman & Gilman Online at www.accessmedicine.com.

26

ANALGESIC-ANTIPYRETIC AND ANTI-INFLAMMATORY AGENTS; PHARMACOTHERAPY OF GOUT

INFLAMMATION The inflammatory process is the response to an injurious stimulus evoked by a wide variety of noxious agents (*e.g.*, infections, antibodies, or physical injuries). The ability to mount an inflammatory response is essential for survival in the face of environmental pathogens and injury; in some situations and diseases, the inflammatory response may be exaggerated and sustained without apparent benefit and even with severe adverse consequences.

Inflammatory responses occur in three distinct temporal phases, each apparently mediated by different mechanisms: (1) an acute phase characterized by transient local vasodilation and increased capillary permeability; (2) a delayed, subacute phase characterized by infiltration of leukocytes and phagocytic cells; and (3) a chronic proliferative phase, in which tissue degeneration and fibrosis occur.

Many mechanisms are involved in the promotion and resolution of the inflammatory process. Recent work has focused on adhesive interactions, including the E-, P-, and L-selectins, intercellular adhesion molecule-1 (ICAM-1), vascular cell adhesion molecule-1 (VCAM-1), and leukocyte integrins, in the adhesion of leukocytes and platelets to endothelium at sites of inflammation.

Activated endothelial cells play a key role in "targeting" circulating cells to inflammatory sites. Cell adhesion occurs by recognition of cell-surface glycoproteins and carbohydrates on circulating cells due to the augmented expression of adhesion molecules on resident cells. Thus, endothelial activation results in leukocyte adhesion as the leukocytes recognize newly expressed L-selectin and P-selectin. Some, but not all, traditional non-steroidal anti-inflammatory drugs (tNSAIDs) may interfere with adhesion by inhibiting expression or activity of certain of these cell-adhesion molecules.

Recruitment of inflammatory cells to sites of injury involves the concerted interactions of several types of soluble mediators. These include the complement factor C5a, platelet-activating factor, and the eicosanoid LTB_4 (*see* Chapter 25). All can act as chemotactic agonists. Several cytokines also play essential roles in orchestrating the inflammatory process, especially interleukin-1 (IL-1) and tumor necrosis factor-α (TNF-α). IL-1 and TNF are considered principal mediators of the biological responses to bacterial lipopolysaccharide (LPS, also called endotoxin). They are secreted by monocytes and macrophages, adipocytes, and other cells. Working in concert with each other and various cytokines and growth factors (including IL-8 and granulocyte-macrophage colony-stimulating factor; *see* Chapter 53), they induce gene expression and protein synthesis in a variety of cells to mediate and promote inflammation.

Intradermal, intravenous, or intra-arterial injections of small amounts of prostaglandins mimic many components of inflammation. Administration of prostaglandin E_2 (PGE_2) or prostacyclin (PGI_2) causes erythema and an increase in local blood flow. Such effects may persist for up to 10 hours with PGE_2 and include the capacity to counteract the vasoconstrictor effects of substances such as norepinephrine and angiotensin II, properties not generally shared by other inflammatory mediators. In contrast to their long-lasting effects on cutaneous vessels and superficial veins, prostaglandin-induced vasodilation in other vascular beds vanishes within a few minutes.

Although PGE_1 and PGE_2 (but not $PGF_{2\alpha}$) cause edema, it is not clear if they can increase vascular permeability in the postcapillary and collecting venules without the participation of other inflammatory mediators (*e.g.*, bradykinin, histamine, and leukotriene C_4 [LTC_4]). Furthermore, PGE_1 is not produced in significant quantities except under rare circumstances such as essential fatty acid deficiency. Unlike LTs, prostaglandins are unlikely to be involved in chemotactic responses, even though they may promote the migration of leukocytes into an inflamed area by increasing blood flow.

NONSTEROIDAL ANTI-INFLAMMATORY DRUGS

All NSAIDs, including the traditional nonselective drugs and the subclass of selective cyclooxygenase-2 (COX-2) inhibitors, are anti-inflammatory, analgesic, and antipyretic. NSAIDs are a chemically heterogeneous group of organic acids that share certain therapeutic actions and adverse effects. Aspirin also inhibits the COX enzymes but in a manner molecularly distinct from the competitive, reversible, active site inhibitors and is often distinguished from the NSAIDs. Similarly, acetaminophen, which is antipyretic and analgesic but largely devoid of anti-inflammatory activity, also is conventionally segregated from the group despite its sharing NSAID activity with other actions relevant to its clinical action *in vivo*.

Mechanism of Action and Therapeutic Effects of NSAIDs

Prostaglandins are released whenever cells are damaged, and aspirin and tNSAIDs inhibit their biosynthesis in all cell types. However, aspirin and tNSAIDs generally do not inhibit the formation of other inflammatory mediators, including other eicosanoids such as the LTs (see Chapter 25). While the clinical effects of these drugs are explicable in terms of inhibition of prostaglandin synthesis, substantial inter- and intraindividual differences in clinical response are known. At higher concentrations, NSAIDs also are known to reduce production of superoxide radicals, induce apoptosis, inhibit the expression of adhesion molecules, decrease nitric oxide synthase, decrease proinflammatory cytokines (e.g., TNF-α, IL-1), modify lymphocyte activity, and alter cellular membrane functions. However, there are differing opinions as to whether these actions might contribute to the anti-inflammatory activity of NSAIDs at the concentrations attained during treatment.

INHIBITION OF PROSTAGLANDIN BIOSYNTHESIS BY NSAIDS The first enzyme in the prostaglandin synthetic pathway is prostaglandin G/H synthase, also known as COX. This enzyme converts arachidonic acid (AA) to the unstable intermediates PGG_2 and PGH_2 and leads to the production of thromboxane A_2 (TXA_2) and a variety of prostaglandins (*see* Chapter 25).

Therapeutic doses of aspirin and other NSAIDs reduce prostaglandin biosynthesis by blocking COX, and there is a reasonably good correlation between potency as COX inhibitors and anti-inflammatory activity.

There are two forms of COX, COX-1 and COX-2. COX-1 is a primarily constitutive isoform found in most normal cells and tissues, while cytokines and inflammatory mediators that accompany inflammation induce COX-2 production. However, COX-2 also is constitutively expressed in certain areas of kidney and brain, and is induced in endothelial cells by laminar shear forces. Importantly, COX-1, but not COX-2, is expressed as the dominant, constitutive isoform in gastric epithelial cells and is the major source of cytoprotective prostaglandin formation. Inhibition of COX-1 at this site is thought to account largely for the gastric adverse events that complicate therapy with tNSAIDs, thus providing the rationale for the development of NSAIDs specific for inhibition of COX-2.

Aspirin and NSAIDs inhibit the COX enzymes and prostaglandin production; they do not inhibit the lipoxygenase pathways of AA metabolism and hence do not suppress LT formation (*see* Chapter 25). Table 26–1 provides a classification of NSAIDs and other analgesic and antipyretic agents based on their chemical structures.

Aspirin covalently modifies COX-1 and COX-2, irreversibly inhibiting COX activity. This is an important distinction from all the NSAIDs because the duration of aspirin's effects is related to the turnover rate of COX in different target tissues. The duration of effect of nonaspirin NSAIDs, which competitively inhibit the active sites of the COX enzymes, relates more directly to the time course of drug disposition. The importance of enzyme turnover in relief from aspirin action is most notable in platelets, which, being anucleate, have a markedly limited capacity for protein synthesis. Thus, the consequences of inhibition of platelet COX (COX-1) last for the lifetime of the platelet. Inhibition of platelet COX-1–dependent TXA_2 formation, therefore, is cumulative with repeated doses of aspirin (at least as low as 30 mg/day) and takes roughly 8–12 days (the platelet turnover time) to recover once therapy has been stopped.

PAIN NSAIDs usually are classified as mild analgesics. However, consideration of the type of pain, as well as its intensity, is important in the assessment of analgesic efficacy. NSAIDs are particularly effective when inflammation has caused sensitization of pain receptors to normally painless mechanical or chemical stimuli. Pain that accompanies inflammation and tissue injury probably results from local stimulation of pain fibers and enhanced pain sensitivity (hyperalgesia), in part a consequence of increased excitability of central neurons in the spinal cord.

Bradykinin, released from plasma kininogen, and cytokines, such as TNF-α, IL-1, and IL-8, appear to be particularly important in eliciting the pain of inflammation. These agents liberate prostaglandins and probably other mediators that promote hyperalgesia. Neuropeptides, such as substance P and calcitonin gene-related peptide (CGRP), also may be involved in eliciting pain.

The capacity of prostaglandins to sensitize pain receptors to mechanical and chemical stimulation apparently results from a lowering of the threshold of the polymodal nociceptors of C fibers. In general, NSAIDs do not affect either hyperalgesia or pain caused by the direct action of prostaglandins, consistent with the notion that the analgesic effects of these agents are due to inhibition of prostaglandin synthesis.

Table 26–1

Classification and Comparison of Nonsteroidal Analgesics

Class/Drug (Substitution)	Pharmacokinetics	Dosing§	Comments	Compared to Aspirin
Salicylates				
Aspirin (acetyl ester)	Peak C*	Antiplatelet	Permanent platelet COX-1 inhibition (due to acetyl group)	
	Protein^p binding	Pain/fever		
	1 h	40–80 mg/d		
	80–90%	325–650 mg/4–6 h		
	Metabolites† Salicyluric acid		Main side effects: GI, increased bleeding time, hypersensitivity reaction	
	t$_{1/2}$‡	Rheumatic fever		
	Therapeutic 2–3 h	1 g/4–6 h		
	High/toxic 15–30 h	Children	Avoid in children with acute febrile illness	
		10 mg/kg/4–6 h		
Diflunisal (difluorophenyl)	Peak C$_p$ 2–3 h	250–500 mg/8–12 h	Not metabolized to salicylic acid	Analgesic and anti-inflammatory effects 4–5 times more potent
	Protein binding 99%			Antipyretic effect weaker
	Metabolites Glucuronide		Competitive COX inhibitor	
	t$_{1/2}$ 8–12 h Therapeutic		Excreted into breast milk	Fewer platelet and GI side effects
Para-aminophenol derivative				
Acetaminophen	Peak C$_p$ 30–60 min	10–15 mg/kg/4 h (maximum of 5 doses/24 h)	Weak nonspecific inhibitor at common doses	Analgesic and antipyretic effects equivalent to aspirin
	Protien binding 20–50%		Potency may be modulated by peroxides	Anti-inflammatory, GI, and platelet effects less than aspirin at 1000 mg/day
	Metabolites Glucuronide conjugates (60%); sulfuric acid conjugates (35%)		Overdose leads to production of toxic metabolite and liver necrosis	
	t$_{1/2}$ 2 h			

430

Acetic acid derivatives

Drug	Parameter	Value	Dosing	Notes	Efficacy
Indomethacin (methylated indole)	Peak C_p	1–2 h	25 mg 2–3 times/day; 75–100 mg at night	Side effects (3–50% of patients): frontal headache, neutropenia, thrombocytopenia; 20% discontinue therapy	10–40 times more potent; intolerance limits dose
	Protein binding	90%			
	Metabolites	O-demethylation (50%); unchanged (20%)			
	$t_{1/2}$	2½ h			
Sulindac (sulfoxide prodrug)	Peak C_p	1–2 hours; 8 h for sulfide metabolite; extensive enterohepatic cycling	150–200 mg twice/day	20% suffer GI side effects, 10% get CNS side effects	Efficacy comparable to aspirin
	Metabolites	Sulfone and conjugates (30%); sulindac and conjugates (25%)			
	$t_{1/2}$	7 h; 18 h for metabolite			
Etodolac (pyranocarboxylic acid)	Peak C_p	1 h	200–400 mg 3–4 times/day	Some COX-2 selectivity *in vitro*	100 mg etodolac, similar efficacy to aspirin 650 mg, but may be better tolerated
	Protein binding	99%			
	Metabolites	Hepatic metabolites			
	$t_{1/2}$	7 hours			

Femanates (N-phenylanthranilates)

Drug	Parameter	Value	Dosing	Notes	Efficacy
Mefenamic acid	Peak C_p	2–4 h	500-mg load, then 250 mg/6 h	Isolated cases of hemolytic anemia reported; May have some central action	Efficacy similar to aspirin; GI side effects (25%)
	Protein binding	>90%			
	Metabolites	Conjugates of 3-hydroxy and 3-carboxyl metabolites (20% recovered in feces)			
	$t_{1/2}$	3–4 h			
Meclofenamate	Peak C_p	0.5–2 h	50–100 mg 4–6 times/day (maximum of 400 mg/day)		Efficacy similar to aspirin; 25% experience GI side effects
	Protein binding	99%			
	Metabolites	Hepatic metabolism; fecal and renal excretion			
	$t_{1/2}$	2–3 h			

(Continued)

431

Table 26–1

Classification and Comparison of Nonsteroidal Analgesics (*Continued*)

Class/Drug (Substitution)	Pharmacokinetics		Dosing§	Comments	Compared to aspirin
Flufenamic acid	*Not available in U.S.*				
Tolmetin (heteroaryl acetate derivative)	Peak C_p	20–60 min	400–600 mg 3 times/day Children (anti-inflammatory) 20 mg/kg/day in 3–4 divided doses	Food delays and decreases peak absorption May persist longer in synovial fluid to give a biological efficacy longer than its plasma $t_{1/2}$	Efficacy similar 25–40% develop side effects; 5–10% discontinue drug
	Protein binding	99%			
	Metabolites	Oxidized to carboxylic acid/other derivatives, then conjugated			
	$t_{1/2}$	5 h			
Ketorolac (pyrrolizine carboxylate)	Peak C_p	30–60 min after IM route	<65 years: 20 mg (orally), then 10 mg/4–6 h (not to exceed 40 mg/24 h); >65 years: 10 mg/4–6 h (not to exceed 40 mg/24 h)	Commonly given parenterally (60 mg IM followed by 30 mg/6 h or 30 mg IV/6 h) Also available as ocular preparation 0.25%, 1 drop every 6 h	Potent analgesic, poor anti-inflammatory
	Protein binding	99%			
	Metabolites	Glucuronide conjugate (90%)			
	$t_{1/2}$	4–6 h			
Diclofenac (phenylacetate derivative)	Peak C_p	2–3 h	50 mg 3 times/day or 75 mg 2 times/day	Also available as topical gel, ophthalmic solution, and oral tablets combined with misoprostol First-pass effect; oral bioavailability, 50%	More potent; 20% develop side effects, 2% discontinue use,15% develop elevated liver enzymes
	Protein binding	99%			
	Metabolites	Glucuronide and sulfide metabolites (renal 65%, bile 35%)			
	$t_{1/2}$	1–2 h			

432

Proprionic acid derivatives

				Intolerance of one does not preclude use of other proprionate	Usually better tolerated
Ibuprofen	Peak C_p	15–30 min	Analgesia	200–400 mg/4–6 h	Equipotent
	Protein binding	99%	Anti-inflammatory	300 mg/6–8 h or 400–800 mg 3–4 times/day	10–15% discontinue due to adverse effects Children's dosing Antipyretic: 5–10 mg/kg every 6 h (maximum 40 mg/kg/day) Anti-inflammatory: 20–40 mg/kg/day in 3–4 divided doses
	Metabolites	Conjugates of hydroxyl and carboxyl metabolites			
	$t_{1/2}$	2–4 h			
Naproxen	Peak C_p	1 h	250 mg 4 times/day or 500 mg 2 times/day		More potent *in vitro*; usually better tolerated; variably prolonged $t_{1/2}$ may afford cardioprotection in some individuals
	Protein binding	99% (less in elderly)	Children Anti-inflammatory	5 mg/kg twice a day	Peak anti-inflammatory effects may not be seen until 2–4 weeks of use
	Metabolites	6-demethyl and other metabolites			
	$t_{1/2}$	14 h			Decreased protein binding and delayed excretion increase risk of toxicity in elderly
Fenoprofen	Peak C_p	2 h	200 mg 4–6 times/day; 300–600 mg 3–4 times/day		15% experience side effects; few discontinue use
	Protein binding	99%			
	Metabolites	Glucuronide, 4-OH metabolite			
	$t_{1/2}$	2 h			

(Continued)

433

Table 26-1

Classification and Comparison of Nonsteroidal Analgesics (Continued)

Class/Drug (Substitution)	Pharmacokinetics		Dosing§	Comments	Compared to aspirin
Ketoprofen	Peak C_p	1–2 h	Analgesia	25 mg 3–4 times/day;		30% develop side effects (usually GI, usually mild)
	Protein binding	98%			
	Metabolites	Glucuronide conjugates	Anti-inflammatory	50–75 mg 3–4 times/day	
	$t_{1/2}$	2 h			
Flurbiprofen	Peak C_p	1–2 h		200–300 mg/day in 2–4 divided doses	
	Protein binding	99%			
	Metabolites	Hydroxylates and conjugates			
	$t_{1/2}$	6 h			
Oxaprozin	Peak C_p	3–4 h		600–1800 mg/day	Long $t_{1/2}$ allows for daily administration; slow onset of action; inappropriate for fever/acute analgesia	
	Protein binding	99%			
	Major metabolites	Oxidates and glucuronide conjugates			
	$t_{1/2}$	40–60 h			
Enolic acid derivatives					
Piroxicam	Peak [drug]	3–5 h		20 mg/day	May inhibit activation of neutrophils, activity of proteoglycanase, collagenases	
	Protein binding	99%			
	Metabolites	Hydroxylates and then conjugated			
	$t_{1/2}$	45–50 h			
Meloxicam	Peak [drug]	5–10 h		7.5–15 mg/day		Some COX-2 selectivity, especially at lower doses
	Protein binding	99%			
	Metabolites	Hydroxylation			
	$t_{1/2}$	15–20 h			

For Piroxicam "Compared to aspirin": Equipotent; perhaps better tolerated 20% develop side effects; 5% discontinue drug

Drug	Pharmacokinetics	Dosage	Comments	
Nabumetone (naphthyl alkanone)	Peak [drug] 3–6 h Protein binding 99% Major metabolites O-demethylation, then conjugation $t_{1/2}$ 24 h	500–1000 mg 1–2 times/day	A prodrug, rapidly metabolized to 6-methoxy-2-naphthyl-acetic acid; pharmacokinetics reflect active compound *Evidence for cardiovascular adverse events*	Shows some COX-2 selectivity (active metabolite does not) Fewer GI side effects than many NSAIDs *Marked decrease in gastrointestinal side effects and in platelet effects*
COX-2 selective inhibitors				
Celecoxib [diaryl substituted pyrazone; (sulfonamide derivative)]	Peak [drug] 2–4 h Protein binding 97% Metabolites Carboxylic acid and glucuronide conjugates $t_{1/2}$ 6–12 h	100 mg 1–2 times/day	Substrate for CYP2C9; inhibitor of CYP2D6 Coadministration with inhibitors of CYP2C9 or substrates of CYP2D6 should be done with caution	See text for overview of COX-2 inhibitors
	Protein binding 98% Metabolites Hepatic metabolism to hydroxyl derivatives, then renal excretion	Primary dysmenorrhea 10 mg once daily		
Valdecoxib	Peak [drug] 2–4 h, delayed by food Protein binding 98% Metabolites Hepatic metabolism to hydroxyl derivatives, then renal excretion $t_{1/2}$ 7–8 h	Analgesia Primary dysmenorrhea 20 mg twice daily 10 mg once daily	Substrate for CYP2C9 and CYP3A4; weak inhibitor of CYP2C9 and CYP2C19 $t_{1/2}$ longer in elderly or with hepatic impairment	Increased incidence of heart attack and stroke in patients undergoing bypass grafting
Parecoxib Etoricoxib Lumiracoxib	*Not approved for use in the U.S.*			

[*]Time to peak plasma drug concentration (C_p) after a single dose. In general, food delays absorption but does not decrease peak concentration.
[†]The majority of NSAIDs undergo hepatic metabolism, and the metabolites are excreted in the urine. Major metabolites or disposal pathways are listed.
[‡]Typical $t_{1/2}$ is listed for therapeutic doses; if much different with toxic dose, this is given also.
[§]Limited dosing information given. For additional information, refer to text and product information literature.

435

FEVER Regulation of body temperature requires a delicate balance between the production and loss of heat; the hypothalamus regulates the set point at which body temperature is maintained. This set point is elevated in fever (from infection, tissue damage, inflammation, graft rejection, or malignancy), as a result of formation of cytokines such as IL-1β, IL-6, interferons, and TNF-α. The cytokines increase synthesis of PGE_2 in circumventricular organs in and adjacent to the preoptic hypothalamic area; PGE_2, in turn, increases cyclic AMP and triggers the hypothalamus to elevate body temperature by promoting an increase in heat generation and a decrease in heat loss. Aspirin and NSAIDs suppress this response by inhibiting PGE_2 synthesis but do not influence body temperature when it is elevated by factors such as exercise or in response to ambient temperature.

THERAPEUTIC EFFECTS All NSAIDs, including selective COX-2 inhibitors, are antipyretic, analgesic, and anti-inflammatory; the exception is acetaminophen, which is antipyretic and analgesic but is largely devoid of anti-inflammatory activity.

When employed as analgesics, these drugs usually are effective only against pain of low-to-moderate intensity, such as dental pain. Although their maximal efficacy is generally much less than that of the opioids, NSAIDs lack the respiratory depression and the development of physical dependence seen with opiates. NSAIDs do not change the perception of sensory modalities other than pain. Chronic postoperative pain or pain arising from inflammation is controlled particularly well by NSAIDs, whereas pain arising from the hollow viscera usually is not relieved. An exception to this is menstrual pain.

It seems logical to select an NSAID with rapid onset for the management of fever associated with minor illness in adults. Due to the association with Reye's syndrome, aspirin and other salicylates are contraindicated in children and young adults <20 years old with fever associated with viral illness. Reye's syndrome is characterized by the acute onset of encephalopathy, liver dysfunction, and fatty infiltration of the liver and other viscera. The etiology and pathophysiology are not clear. However, the epidemiologic evidence for an association between aspirin use in children and Reye's syndrome was sufficiently compelling that labeling of aspirin and aspirin-containing medications to indicate Reye's syndrome as a risk in children was mandated in 1986. Since then, the use of aspirin in children has declined dramatically, and Reye's syndrome has almost disappeared. Acetaminophen has not been implicated in Reye's syndrome and is the drug of choice for antipyresis in children and teens.

NSAIDs find their chief clinical application as anti-inflammatory agents in the treatment of musculoskeletal disorders, such as rheumatoid arthritis and osteoarthritis. In general, NSAIDs provide only symptomatic relief from pain and inflammation associated with the disease, do not arrest the progression of pathological injury to tissue, and are not considered to be "disease-modifying" (see below). A number of NSAIDs are FDA approved for the treatment of ankylosing spondylitis and gout. The use of NSAIDs for mild arthropathies, together with rest and physical therapy, generally is effective. When the symptoms are limited either to trouble sleeping because of pain or significant morning stiffness, a single NSAID dose given at night may suffice. Patients with more debilitating disease may not respond adequately to full therapeutic doses of NSAIDs and may require aggressive therapy with second-line agents. The choice of drugs for children with juvenile rheumatoid arthritis commonly is restricted to those that have been specifically tested in children, such as aspirin (see discussion of Reye's syndrome, above, under "Fever"), naproxen, or tolmetin.

Prostaglandins also have been implicated in the maintenance of patency of the ductus arteriosus, and indomethacin and other tNSAIDs have been used in neonates to close the inappropriately patent ductus.

OTHER CLINICAL USES

Systemic Mastocytosis Systemic mastocytosis is a condition in which there are excessive mast cells in the bone marrow, reticuloendothelial system, GI system, bones, and skin. In patients with systemic mastocytosis, prostaglandin D_2, released from mast cells in large amounts, has been found to be the major mediator of severe episodes of vasodilation and hypotension; this PGD_2 effect is resistant to antihistamines. The addition of aspirin or *ketoprofen* has provided relief. However, aspirin and tNSAIDs can trigger degranulation of mast cells, so blockade with H_1 and H_2 histamine receptor antagonists should be established before NSAIDs are initiated.

Cancer Chemoprevention Epidemiological studies suggested that frequent use of aspirin is associated with as much as a 50% decrease in the risk of colon cancer and similar observations have been made with other cancers. NSAIDs have been used in patients with familial adenomatous polyposis (FAP), an inherited disorder characterized by multiple adenomatous colon polyps developing during adolescence and the inevitable occurrence of colon cancer by the sixth decade.

Niacin Tolerability   Large doses of niacin (nicotinic acid) effectively lower serum cholesterol levels, reduce LDL, and raise HDL (*see* Chapter 35). However, niacin is tolerated poorly because it induces intense flushing. This flushing is mediated by a release of prostaglandin D_2 from the skin, which can be inhibited by treatment with aspirin.

ADVERSE EFFECTS OF NSAID THERAPY   Common adverse events that complicate therapy with aspirin and NSAIDs are outlined in Table 26–2. Age generally is correlated with an increased probability of developing serious adverse reactions to NSAIDs, and caution is warranted in choosing a lower starting dose for elderly patients.

Gastrointestinal

The most common symptoms associated with these drugs are GI, including anorexia, nausea, dyspepsia, abdominal pain, and diarrhea. These symptoms may be related to the induction of gastric or intestinal ulcers, which is estimated to occur in 15–30% of regular users. Ulceration may range from small superficial erosions to full-thickness perforation of the muscularis mucosa. There may be single or multiple ulcers, and ulceration can be accompanied by gradual blood loss leading to

Table 26–2

Common and Shared Adverse Reactions of NSAIDs

System	Manifestations
GI (adverse effects decreased with COX-2–selective drugs)	Abdominal pain
	Nausea
	Anorexia
	Gastric erosions/ulcers
	Anemia
	GI hemorrhage
	Perforation
	Diarrhea
Renal	Salt and water retention
	Edema, worsening of renal function in renal/cardiac and cirrhotic patients
	Decreased effectiveness of antihypertensive medications
	Decreased effectiveness of diuretic medications
	Decreased urate excretion (especially with aspirin)
	Hyperkalemia
CNS	Headache
	Vertigo
	Dizziness
	Confusion
	Depression
	Lowering of seizure threshold
	Hyperventilation (salicylates)
Platelets (adverse effects decreased with COX-2–selective drugs)	Inhibited platelet activation
	Propensity for bruising
	Increased risk of hemorrhage
Uterus	Prolongation of gestation
	Possible prolongation of labor
Hypersensitivity	Vasomotor rhinitis
	Angioedema
	Asthma
	Urticaria
	Flushing
	Hypotension
	Shock
Vascular	Closure of ductus arteriosus

anemia or by life-threatening hemorrhage. The risk is further increased in those with Helicobacter pylori infection, heavy alcohol consumption, or other risk factors for mucosal injury, including the concurrent use of glucocorticoids.

All of the selective COX-2 inhibitors have been shown to be less prone than equally efficacious doses of tNSAIDs to induce endoscopically visualized gastric ulcers, and this has provided the basis of FDA approval.

Cardiovascular

Given their relatively short half-lives, tNSAIDs, unlike aspirin, are not thought to afford cardio-protection, and most epidemiological overviews are consistent with this likelihood.

Selective inhibitors of COX-2 are thought to be problematic in this regard. They depress PGI_2 formation by endothelial cells without concomitant inhibition of platelet thromboxane. PGI_2 restrains the cardiovascular effects of TXA_2, affording a mechanism by which selective inhibitors might increase the risk of thrombosis; consistent with results from postmarketing trials of rofecoxib.

This mechanism should pertain to individuals otherwise at risk of thrombosis, such as those with rheumatoid arthritis, as the relative risk of myocardial infarction is increased in these patients compared to patients with osteoarthritis or no arthritis. The incidence of myocardial infarction and stroke has diverged in such at-risk patients when COX-2 inhibitors are compared with tNSAIDs. Placebo-controlled trials have now revealed an increased incidence of myocardial infarction and stroke in patients treated with rofecoxib, valdecoxib, and celecoxib, consistent with a mechanism-based cardiovascular hazard for the class. Regulatory agencies in the U.S., Europe, and Australia have concluded that all three drugs increase the risk of heart attack and stroke and will be labeled accordingly and restricted with respect to marketing directly to consumers. Only celecoxib remains on the market in the U.S.

Blood Pressure, Renal, and Renovascular Adverse Events

tNSAIDs and COX-2 inhibitors have been associated with renal and renovascular adverse events. NSAIDs have little effect on renal function or blood pressure in normal subjects. However, in patients with congestive heart failure, hepatic cirrhosis, chronic kidney disease, hypovolemia, and other states of activation of the sympathoadrenal or renin-angiotensin systems, prostaglandin formation becomes crucial. NSAIDs are associated with loss of the prostaglandin-induced inhibition of both the reabsorption of Cl^- and the action of vasopressin, leading to the retention of salt and water. Epidemiological studies suggest hypertensive complications occur more commonly in patients treated with coxibs than with tNSAIDs.

Analgesic Nephropathy

Analgesic nephropathy is a condition of slowly progressive renal failure, decreased concentrating capacity of the renal tubule, and sterile pyuria. Risk factors are the chronic use of high doses of combinations of NSAIDs and frequent urinary tract infections. If recognized early, discontinuation of NSAIDs permits recovery of renal function.

Pregnancy and Lactation

Despite evidence that myometrial COX-2 expression and levels of prostaglandin E_2 and $F_{2\alpha}$ increase in the myometrium during labor, prolongation of gestation by NSAIDs is not useful for the treatment of preterm labor. The use of indomethacin as a tocolytic (preventing uterine contractions) is associated with closure of the ductus arteriosus and impaired fetal circulation in utero, particularly in fetuses older than 32 weeks' gestation. COX-2–selective inhibitors have been associated with stenosis of the ductus arteriosus and oligohydramnios. Finally, the use of NSAIDs and aspirin late in pregnancy may increase the risk of postpartum hemorrhage. Therefore pregnancy, especially close to term, is a relative contraindication to the use of all NSAIDs.

Hypersensitivity

Certain individuals display hypersensitivity to aspirin and NSAIDs, as manifested by symptoms that range from vasomotor rhinitis with profuse watery secretions, angioedema, generalized urticaria, and bronchial asthma to laryngeal edema, bronchoconstriction, flushing, hypotension, and shock. Aspirin intolerance is a contraindication to therapy with any other NSAID because cross-sensitivity can provoke a life-threatening reaction.

Although less common in children, this syndrome may occur in 10–25% of patients with asthma, nasal polyps, or chronic urticaria, and in 1% of apparently healthy individuals. It is provoked by even low doses (<80 mg) of aspirin and apparently involves COX inhibition. Aspirin hypersensitivity is associated with an increase in biosynthesis of LTs, perhaps reflecting diversion of AA to lipoxygenase metabolism.

Drug Interactions

CONCOMITANT NSAIDS AND LOW-DOSE ASPIRIN   Many patients combine either tNSAIDs or COX-2 inhibitors with "cardioprotective" low-dose aspirin. Epidemiological studies suggest that this combination therapy increases significantly the likelihood of GI adverse events over either class of NSAID alone.

OTHER DRUG INTERACTIONS   Angiotensin-converting enzyme (ACE) inhibitors act, at least partly, by preventing the breakdown of kinins that stimulate prostaglandin production. Thus, it is logical that NSAIDs might attenuate the effectiveness of ACE inhibitors by blocking the production of vasodilator and natriuretic prostaglandins. Due to hyperkalemia, the combination of NSAIDs and ACE inhibitors also can produce marked bradycardia leading to syncope, especially in the elderly and in patients with hypertension, diabetes mellitus, or ischemic heart disease. NSAIDs may increase the frequency or severity of GI ulceration when combined with glucocorticoids and augment the risk of bleeding in patients receiving *warfarin*. Many NSAIDs are highly bound to plasma proteins and thus may displace other drugs from their binding sites. Such interactions can occur in patients given salicylates or other NSAIDs together with warfarin, sulfonylurea hypoglycemic agents, or *methotrexate*; the dosage of such agents may require adjustment to prevent toxicity. The problem with warfarin is accentuated, both because almost all NSAIDs suppress normal platelet function and because some NSAIDs also increase warfarin levels by interfering with its metabolism; thus, concurrent administration should be avoided.

PHARMACOKINETICS AND PHARMACODYNAMICS   Most NSAIDs are rapidly and completely absorbed from the GI tract, with peak concentrations occurring within 1–4 hours. Aspirin begins to acetylate platelets within minutes of reaching the presystemic circulation. The presence of food tends to delay absorption without affecting peak concentration. Most NSAIDs are extensively protein bound (95–99%) and undergo hepatic metabolism and renal excretion. In general, NSAIDs are not recommended in the setting of advanced hepatic or renal disease due to their adverse pharmacodynamic effects (*see* below).

OTHER CLINICAL CONSIDERATIONS IN THE RATIONAL SELECTION OF THERAPY

The choice of an agent for use as an antipyretic or analgesic is seldom a problem. Drugs with more rapid onset of action and shorter duration of action probably are preferable for simple fevers accompanying minor viral illnesses or pain after minor musculoskeletal injuries, whereas a longer duration of action may be preferable for postoperative pain management. Sometimes a loading dose of such NSAIDs may be required.

The choice among tNSAIDs for the treatment of chronic arthritic conditions such as rheumatoid arthritis largely is empirical. Substantial differences in response have been noted among individuals treated with the same tNSAID and within an individual treated with different tNSAIDs. It is reasonable to give a drug for two weeks as a therapeutic trial and to continue it if the response is satisfactory. Initially, all patients should be asked about previous hypersensitivity to aspirin or any member of the NSAID class. Thereafter, low doses of the chosen agent should be prescribed to determine initial patient tolerance. Doses then may be adjusted to maximize efficacy or minimize adverse effects.

Adverse effects usually become manifest in the first weeks of therapy, although gastric ulceration and bleeding may present much later. If the patient does not achieve therapeutic benefit from one NSAID, another should be tried. It is best to avoid combination therapy with more than one NSAID. There is little evidence of extra benefit for the patient, and the risk of side effects is at least additive.

Clinical trials have established that at least three selective inhibitors of COX-2—rofecoxib, valdecoxib, and celecoxib—confer an increased risk of heart attack and stroke (*see* above). Of immediate concern are some tNSAIDs, such as meloxicam and diclofenac, which resemble celecoxibs in terms of their selectivity. Evidence for hazard with both drugs has been suggested from observational studies, but controlled trials to address this hypothesis have not been performed. The cardiovascular hazard from both celecoxib and rofecoxib—the two inhibitors for which data are available from placebo-controlled trials lasting more than 1 year—increased with chronicity of dosing. This is consistent with a mechanism-based acceleration of atherogenesis directly *via* inhibition of PGI_2 and indirectly due to the rise in blood pressure consequent to inhibition of COX-2 derived PGE_2 and PGI_2.

If a COX-2 inhibitor is selected, it should be used at the lowest possible dose for the shortest period of time. Patients at risk of cardiovascular disease or prone to thrombosis should not be treated with these drugs. Small absolute risks of thrombosis attributable to these drugs may interact synergistically with absolute risks from genetic variants like factor V Leiden or concomitant therapies, such as oral contraceptives.

The choice of drugs for children is considerably restricted, and only drugs that have been extensively tested in children should be used. This commonly points toward naproxen and ibuprofen.

THE SALICYLATES

Aspirin is the most widely consumed analgesic, antipyretic, and anti-inflammatory agent and is the standard for the comparison and evaluation of the others. Because aspirin is so available, the possibility of misuse and serious toxicity probably is underappreciated.

CHEMISTRY

Salicylic acid is only used externally; therefore various derivatives of this acid have been synthesized for systemic use. These comprise two large classes, namely esters of salicylic acid obtained from substitutions within the carboxyl group and salicylate esters of organic acids, in which the carboxyl group is retained and substitution is made in the hydroxyl group. For example, aspirin is an ester of acetic acid. In addition, there are salts of salicylic acid (Figure 26–1).

Pharmacological Properties of Therapeutic Doses

ANALGESIA

The salicylates are used more widely for pain relief than are any other classes of drugs. The types of pain usually relieved by salicylates are those of low intensity that arise from integumental structures rather than from viscera, especially headache, myalgia, and arthralgia.

ANTIPYRESIS

Salicylates usually lower elevated body temperatures rapidly and effectively. However, moderate doses that produce this effect also increase oxygen consumption and metabolic rate. These compounds have a pyretic effect at toxic doses, and sweating exacerbates the dehydration that occurs in salicylate intoxication (see below).

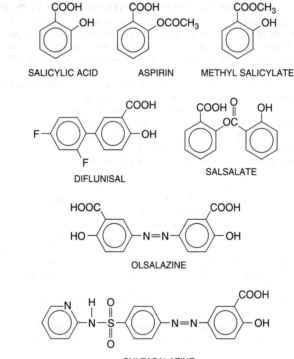

FIGURE 26–1 *Structural formulas of the salicylates.*

RESPIRATION

Salicylates increase oxygen consumption and CO_2 production (especially in skeletal muscle) at full therapeutic doses; these effects are a result of uncoupling oxidative phosphorylation. The increased production of CO_2 stimulates respiration (mainly by an increase in depth of respiration with only a slight increase in rate). The increased alveolar ventilation balances the increased CO_2 production, and thus plasma CO_2 tension (P_{CO_2}) does not change or may decrease slightly.

ACID–BASE AND ELECTROLYTE BALANCE AND RENAL EFFECTS

Therapeutic doses of salicylate produce definite changes in the acid–base balance and electrolyte pattern. Compensation for the initial event, respiratory alkalosis, is achieved by increased renal excretion of bicarbonate, which is accompanied by increased Na^+ and K^+ excretion; plasma bicarbonate is thus lowered, and blood pH returns toward normal. This is the stage of compensatory renal acidosis seen most often in adults given intensive salicylate therapy and seldom proceeds further unless toxicity ensues (see below). Salicylates can cause retention of salt and water, as well as acute reduction of renal function in patients with congestive heart failure, renal disease, or hypovolemia. Although long-term use of salicylates alone rarely is associated with nephrotoxicity, the prolonged and excessive ingestion of analgesic mixtures containing salicylates in combination with other compounds can produce papillary necrosis and interstitial nephritis.

CARDIOVASCULAR EFFECTS

Low doses of aspirin (<100 mg daily) are used widely for their cardioprotective effects (see above). At high therapeutic doses (>3 g daily), as might be given for acute rheumatic fever, salt and water retention can lead to an increase (up to 20%) in circulating plasma volume and decreased hematocrit (via a dilutional effect). There is a tendency for the peripheral vessels to dilate because of a direct effect on vascular smooth muscle. Cardiac output and work are increased. Those with carditis or compromised cardiac function may not have sufficient cardiac reserve to meet the increased demands, and congestive heart failure and pulmonary edema can occur. High doses of salicylates can produce noncardiogenic pulmonary edema, particularly in older patients who ingest salicylates regularly over a prolonged period.

GASTROINTESTINAL EFFECTS

The ingestion of salicylates may result in epigastric distress, nausea, and vomiting. Salicylates also may cause gastric ulceration, exacerbation of peptic ulcer symptoms (heartburn, dyspepsia), GI hemorrhage, and erosive gastritis. These effects occur primarily with aspirin. Because nonacetylated salicylates lack the ability to acetylate COX and thereby irreversibly inhibit its activity, they are weaker inhibitors than aspirin.

Aspirin-induced gastric bleeding sometimes is painless, and if unrecognized may lead to iron-deficiency anemia (see Chapter 53). The daily ingestion of anti-inflammatory doses of aspirin (4 or 5 g) results in an average fecal blood loss of 3–8 mL/day, as compared with ~0.6 mL/day in untreated subjects. Gastroscopic examination of aspirin-treated subjects often reveals discrete ulcerative and hemorrhagic lesions of the gastric mucosa; in many cases, multiple hemorrhagic lesions with sharply demarcated areas of focal necrosis are observed.

HEPATIC EFFECTS

High doses of salicylates can cause hepatic injury. The onset of injury characteristically occurs after several months of treatment. The majority of cases occur in patients with connective tissue disorders. There usually are no symptoms, simply an increase in serum levels of hepatic transaminases, but some patients note right upper quadrant abdominal discomfort and tenderness. Overt jaundice is uncommon. The injury usually is reversible upon discontinuation of salicylates. The use of salicylates is contraindicated in patients with chronic liver disease. Salicylates are associated with the severe hepatic injury and encephalopathy observed in Reye's syndrome.

URICOSURIC EFFECTS

Low doses (1 or 2 g/day) can decrease urate excretion and elevate plasma urate concentrations; intermediate doses (2 or 3 g/day) may not alter urate excretion; large doses (more than 5 g/day) induce uricosuria and lower plasma urate levels. However, such large doses are tolerated poorly. Even small doses of salicylate can block the effects of probenecid and other uricosuric agents that decrease tubular reabsorption of uric acid.

BLEEDING TIME

A single 325-mg dose of aspirin (standard tablet dose) approximately doubles the mean bleeding time of normal persons for a period of 4–7 days. This effect is due to irreversible acetylation of *platelet COX and the consequent reduced formation of TXA_2 until sufficient numbers of new, unmodified platelets are produced and is the mechanistic basis of prophylaxis of thrombogenic myocardial infarction.*

Patients with severe hepatic damage, hypoprothrombinemia, vitamin K deficiency, or hemophilia should avoid aspirin because of the risk of hemorrhage. If possible, aspirin therapy should be stopped one week before surgery; care should be exercised with aspirin in combination with oral anticoagulant agents because of the combined danger of prolongation of bleeding time coupled with blood loss from the gastric mucosa; this is used to advantage coupling patients with bioprosthetic or mechanical heart valves (see *Chapter 54).*

METABOLIC EFFECTS

The uncoupling of oxidative phosphorylation by salicylates may occur with doses of salicylate used in the treatment of rheumatoid arthritis. Salicylates increase O_2 uptake and CO_2 production and in toxic doses may decrease aerobic metabolism and increase the production of strong organic acids.

Large doses of salicylates may cause hyperglycemia and glycosuria and deplete liver and muscle glycogen.

Long-term administration of salicylates decreases thyroidal uptake and clearance of iodine but increases O_2 consumption and the rate of disappearance of thyroxine and triiodothyronine from the circulation. These effects probably are caused by the competitive displacement by salicylate of thyroxine and triiodothyronine from binding proteins in plasma (see *Chapter 56).*

LOCAL IRRITANT EFFECTS

Salicylic acid is irritating to skin and mucosa and destroys epithelial cells. The keratolytic action of the free acid is employed for the local treatment of warts, corns, fungal infections, and certain types of eczematous dermatitis. After treatment with salicylic acid, tissue cells swell, soften, and desquamate. Methyl salicylate (oil of wintergreen) *is used topically as a counter-irritant for the relief of mild musculoskeletal pain.*

PHARMACOKINETICS

Orally ingested salicylates are absorbed rapidly, predominantly from the upper small intestine. Appreciable concentrations are found in plasma in less than 30 minutes; after a single dose, a peak value is reached in ~1 hour and then declines gradually. After absorption, salicylates are distributed throughout most body tissues and transcellular fluids, primarily by pH-dependent passive processes. Salicylates are transported actively by a low-capacity, saturable system out of the cerebrospinal fluid (CSF) across the choroid plexus. The drugs readily cross the placental barrier.

The presence of food delays absorption of salicylates. Rectal absorption of salicylate usually is slower than oral absorption and is incomplete and inconsistent.

Salicylic acid is absorbed rapidly from the intact skin, especially when applied in oily liniments or ointments, and systemic poisoning has occurred from its application to large areas of skin.

The volume of distribution of usual doses of aspirin averages ~170 mL/kg of body weight; at high therapeutic doses, this volume increases to ~500 mL/kg because of saturation of binding sites on plasma proteins. Aspirin can be detected in the plasma only for a short time as a result of hydrolysis in plasma, liver, and erythrocytes.

Roughly 80–90% of the salicylate in plasma is bound to proteins, especially albumin, at concentrations encountered clinically; the proportion of the total that is bound declines as plasma concentrations increase. Hypoalbuminemia, as may occur in rheumatoid arthritis, is associated with a proportionately higher level of free salicylate in the plasma. Salicylate competes with a variety of compounds for plasma protein binding sites; these include thyroxine, triiodothyronine, penicillin, phenytoin, sulfinpyrazone, *bilirubin, uric acid, and other NSAIDs such as naproxen.*

The biotransformation of salicylates takes place in many tissues, but particularly in the liver. The three chief metabolic products are salicyluric acid (the glycine conjugate), the ether or phenolic glucuronide, and the ester or acyl glucuronide.

The plasma $t_{1/2}$ for aspirin is ~20 minutes, and for salicylate 2–3 hours at antiplatelet doses, rising to 12 hours at usual anti-inflammatory doses. The $t_{1/2}$ of salicylate may be as long as 15–30 hours at high therapeutic doses or when there is intoxication. This dose-dependent elimination is the result of the limited capacity of the liver to form salicyluric acid and the phenolic glucuronide, resulting in a larger proportion of unchanged drug being excreted in the urine at higher doses.

Tinnitus may be a reliable index of exceeding the acceptable plasma concentration in patients with normal hearing, but is not a reliable indicator in patients with preexisting hearing loss; thus, surveillance for this symptom is no substitute for periodic monitoring of serum salicylate levels during chronic aspirin treatment.

The plasma concentration of salicylate is increased by conditions that decrease glomerular filtration rate or reduce proximal tubule secretion of salicylates, such as renal disease or the presence of inhibitors that compete for the transport system (e.g., *probenecid*). *Changes in urinary pH also have significant effects on salicylate excretion. For example, the clearance of salicylate is about four times as great at pH 8 as at pH 6, and it is well above the glomerular filtration rate at pH 8. High rates of urine flow decrease tubular reabsorption, whereas the opposite is true in oliguria.*

Therapeutic Uses

SYSTEMIC USES

The two most commonly used preparations of salicylate for systemic effects are aspirin (acetylsalicylic acid) and sodium salicylate. The dose of salicylate depends on the condition being treated.

Other salicylates available for systemic use include salsalate (salicylsalicylic acid; DISALCID, *others), which is hydrolyzed to salicylic acid during and after absorption,* sodium thiosalicylate *(injection;* REXOLATE*),* choline salicylate *(oral liquid;* ARTHROPAN*), and* magnesium salicylate *(tablets;* MAGAN, MOMEMTUM, *others). A combination of* choline and magnesium salicylates (choline magnesium, trisalicylate, TRILISATE, *others) also is available.*

Antipyresis

Antipyretic therapy is reserved for patients in whom fever in itself may be deleterious and for those who experience considerable relief when fever is lowered. The course of the patient's illness may be obscured by the relief of symptoms and the reduction of fever by the use of antipyretic drugs. The antipyretic dose of salicylate for adults is 325–650 mg orally every 4 hours. Salicylates are contraindicated for fever associated with viral infection in children; for nonviral etiologies, 50–75 mg/kg/day has been given in 4–6 divided doses, not to exceed a total daily dose of 3.6 g. The rectal administration of aspirin suppositories may be necessary in infants or when the oral route is unavailable.

Analgesia

Salicylates are valuable for the nonspecific relief of minor aches and pain (e.g., *headache, arthritis, dysmenorrhea, neuralgia, and myalgia). For this purpose, they are prescribed in the same doses and manner as for antipyresis.*

Rheumatoid Arthritis

Although aspirin is regarded as the standard against which other drugs should be compared for the treatment of rheumatoid arthritis, many clinicians favor the use of other NSAIDs perceived to have better GI tolerability, even though this perception remains unproven. Moreover, some patients perceive that aspirin is too commonly available to be effective. Therapy with salicylates produces analgesia adequate to allow more effective movement and physical therapy in osteoarthritis and rheumatoid arthritis. In addition, aspirin therapy is associated with improvement in appetite, a feeling of well-being, and a reduction in the inflammation in joint tissues and surrounding structures.

Inflammatory Bowel Disease

Mesalamine *(5-aminosalicylic acid;* ASACOL, *others) is a salicylate that is used for its local effects in the treatment of inflammatory bowel disease* (see *Chapter 38). It currently is available as a suppository and rectal suspension enema* (ROWASA*) for treatment of mild-to-moderate proctosigmoiditis; a rectal suppository* (CANASA, *others) for the treatment of distal ulcerative colitis, proctosigmoiditis, or proctitis. Oral formulations and controlled-release capsule that deliver drug to the lower intestine are efficacious in treatment of inflammatory bowel disease, in particular ulcerative colitis.* Sulfasalazine *(salicylazosulfapyridine;* AZULFIDINE*) contains mesalamine linked covalently to sulfapyridine* (see *Chapter 38); it is absorbed poorly after oral administration, but it is cleaved to its active components by bacteria in the colon. The drug is of benefit in the treatment of inflammatory bowel disease, principally because of the local actions of mesalamine.*

Salicylate Intoxication

Salicylate poisoning or serious intoxication often occurs in children and sometimes is fatal. Salicylate intoxication should be seriously considered in any young child with coma, convulsions, or cardiovascular collapse. The fatal dose varies with the preparation. Death has followed use of 10–30 g of sodium salicylate or aspirin in adults, but larger amounts have been ingested without a fatal outcome. The lethal dose of methyl salicylate (oil of wintergreen, sweet birch oil, gaultheria oil, betula oil) is considerably less than that of sodium salicylate. As little as 4 mL (4.7 g) of methyl salicylate may be fatal in children.

Mild chronic salicylate intoxication is called salicylism. *When fully developed, the syndrome includes headache, dizziness, tinnitus, difficulty hearing, dimness of vision, mental confusion, lassitude, drowsiness, sweating, thirst, hyperventilation, nausea, vomiting, and occasionally diarrhea.*

NEUROLOGICAL EFFECTS

In high doses, salicylates have toxic effects on the CNS, consisting of stimulation (including convulsions) followed by depression. Confusion, dizziness, tinnitus, high-tone deafness, delirium, psychosis, stupor, and coma may occur. The tinnitus and hearing loss of salicylate poisoning are caused by increased labyrinthine pressure or an effect on the hair cells of the cochlea, perhaps secondary to vasoconstriction in the auditory microvasculature. Tinnitus typically is observed at plasma salicylate concentrations of 200–450 µg/mL, and there is a close relationship between the extent of hearing loss and plasma salicylate concentration. Tinnitus generally resolves within 2 or 3 days after withdrawal of the drug.

RESPIRATION

The respiratory effects of salicylates contribute to the serious acid–base balance disturbances that characterize poisoning. Salicylates stimulate respiration directly and indirectly. Uncoupling of oxidative phosphorylation leads to increased peripheral CO_2 production and a compensatory increase in minute ventilation, usually with no overall change in P_{CO_2}. Uncoupling of oxidative phosphorylation also leads to excessive heat production, and salicylate toxicity is associated with hyperthermia, particularly in children.

Salicylates directly stimulate the respiratory center in the medulla. This is characterized by an increase in depth and a pronounced increase in respiration rate. This can be seen with plasma salicylate concentrations of 350 µg/mL and marked hyperventilation occurs when the level approaches 500 µg/mL. When a barbiturate or opioid (e.g., FIORINAL or DARVON COMPOUND 32) is present, then central respiratory depression will prevent hyperventilation, and the salicylate-induced uncoupling of oxidative phosphorylation will be associated with a marked increase in plasma P_{CO_2} and respiratory acidosis.

Prolonged exposure to high doses of salicylates leads to depression of the medulla, with central respiratory depression and circulatory collapse, secondary to vasomotor depression. Because enhanced CO_2 production continues, respiratory acidosis ensues. Respiratory failure is the usual cause of death in fatal cases of salicylate poisoning.

ACID–BASE BALANCE AND ELECTROLYTES

As described above, high therapeutic doses of salicylate are associated with a primary respiratory alkalosis and compensatory renal acidosis. Subsequent changes in acid–base status generally occur only when toxic doses of salicylates are ingested by infants and children or occasionally after large doses in adults.

The phase of primary respiratory alkalosis rarely is recognized in children with salicylate toxicity. They usually present in a state of mixed respiratory and renal acidosis, characterized by a decrease in blood pH, a low plasma bicarbonate concentration, and normal or nearly normal plasma P_{CO_2}. Direct salicylate-induced depression of respiration prevents adequate respiratory hyperventilation to match the increased peripheral production of CO_2. Consequently, plasma P_{CO_2} increases and blood pH decreases. Because the concentration of bicarbonate in plasma already is low due to increased renal bicarbonate excretion, the acid–base status at this stage essentially is an uncompensated respiratory acidosis. Superimposed, however, is a true metabolic acidosis caused by accumulation of acids as a result of three processes. First, toxic concentrations of salicylates displace ~2–3 mEq/L of plasma bicarbonate. Second, vasomotor depression caused by toxic doses of salicylates impairs renal function, with consequent accumulation of sulfuric and phosphoric acids. Third, salicylates in toxic doses may decrease aerobic metabolism as a result of inhibition of various enzymes. This derangement of carbohydrate metabolism leads to the accumulation of organic acids, especially pyruvic, lactic, and acetoacetic acids.

The low plasma P_{CO_2} leads to decreased renal tubular reabsorption of bicarbonate and increased renal excretion of Na^+, K^+, and water. Water also is lost by salicylate-induced sweating (especially in the presence of hyperthermia) and hyperventilation; dehydration, which can be profound, particularly in children, rapidly occurs. Because more water than electrolyte is lost through the lungs and by sweating, the dehydration is associated with hypernatremia. Prolonged exposure to high doses of salicylate also causes depletion of K^+ due to both renal and extrarenal factors.

TREATMENT

Salicylate poisoning is a medical emergency, and death may result; there is no specific antidote. Management begins with a rapid assessment (see Chapter 64) followed by the "A (airway), B (breathing), C (circulation), D (decontamination)" approach to medical emergencies. Because of the need for respiratory alkalosis to compensate for the metabolic acidosis of salicylate toxicity, intubation should be avoided unless the patient demonstrates hypoventilation or obtundation. High concentrations of inspired oxygen may be required.

Aspirin poisoning leads to inappropriate vasodilation compounded by volume depletion and acidosis, which worsens vasodilation. Aggressive volume repletion with intravenous fluids should be instituted. The aim is to achieve large-volume diuresis to optimize salicylate elimination. If necessary, vasopressors (e.g., norepinephrine, phenylephrine) are added.

Activated charcoal is used to prevent further absorption of aspirin from the GI tract. This is particularly important when enteric-coated aspirin, which has delayed absorption, has been ingested. Sodium bicarbonate should be administered to maintain the pH between 7.5 and 7.55, and if possible, the pH of the urine greater than 8. Forced alkaline diuresis maximizes salicylate elimination. Hemodialysis may be required if the above measures are inadequate, there is clinical deterioration despite therapy, or if plasma salicylate levels are greater than 1000 μg/mL. Plasma salicylate, glucose, pH, and potassium should be monitored frequently and therapy modified accordingly. Decreased CNS glucose levels may occur despite normal plasma glucose levels, and supplemental glucose should be given in cases of altered mental status, regardless of the plasma glucose levels.

Diflunisal

Diflunisal (DOLOBID) is a difluorophenyl derivative of salicylic acid (Figure 26–1). It is almost completely absorbed after oral administration, and peak plasma concentrations occur within 2–3 hours. It is extensively bound to plasma albumin (99%). About 90% of the drug is excreted as glucuronide conjugates, and its rate of elimination is dose-dependent. At the usual analgesic dose (500–750 mg/day), the plasma $t_{1/2}$ averages 8–12 hours. Diflunisal appears in the milk of lactating women.

The drug has been used primarily as an analgesic in the treatment of osteoarthritis and musculoskeletal strains or sprains; in these circumstances it is about three to four times more potent than aspirin. The usual initial dose is 500–1000 mg, followed by 250–500 mg every 8–12 hours. For rheumatoid arthritis or osteoarthritis, 250–500 mg is administered twice daily; maintenance dosage should not exceed 1.5 g/day. Diflunisal does not produce auditory side effects and appears to cause fewer and less intense GI and antiplatelet effects than aspirin.

PARA-AMINOPHENOL DERIVATIVES: ACETAMINOPHEN

Acetaminophen (paracetamol; *N*-acetyl-*p*-aminophenol; TYLENOL, others) is an effective alternative to aspirin as an analgesic–antipyretic agent; however, its anti-inflammatory effects are much weaker. While it is indicated for pain relief in patients with noninflammatory osteoarthritis, it is not a suitable substitute for aspirin or other NSAIDs in chronic inflammatory conditions such as rheumatoid arthritis. Acetaminophen is well tolerated and has a low incidence of GI side effects. It is available without a prescription. Acute overdosage can cause severe hepatic damage, and the number of accidental or deliberate poisonings with acetaminophen continues to grow. Chronic use of less than 2 g/day is not typically associated with hepatic dysfunction.

PHARMACOLOGICAL PROPERTIES

Acetaminophen has only weak anti-inflammatory effects and has been thought to have a generally poor ability to inhibit COX in the presence of high concentrations of peroxides, as are found at sites of inflammation.

Single or repeated therapeutic doses of acetaminophen have no effect on the cardiovascular and respiratory systems, on platelets, or on coagulation. Acid–base changes and uricosuric effects do not occur, nor does the drug produce the gastric irritation, erosion, or bleeding that may occur after salicylate administration.

PHARMACOKINETICS AND METABOLISM

Oral acetaminophen has excellent bioavailability. Peak plasma concentrations occur within 30–60 minutes and the $t_{1/2}$ in plasma is ~2 hours. Binding of the drug to plasma proteins is less than with other NSAIDs. Some 90–100% of the drug may be recovered in the urine within the first day at therapeutic dosing, primarily after hepatic conjugation with glucuronic acid (~60%), sulfuric acid (~35%), or cysteine (~3%); small amounts of hydroxylated and deacetylated metabolites also have been detected (Table 26–1). Children have less capacity for glucuronidation of the drug than do adults. A small proportion of acetaminophen undergoes CYP-mediated N-hydroxylation to form N-acetyl-p-benzoquinoneimine (NAPQI), a highly reactive intermediate (see below).

THERAPEUTIC USES

Acetaminophen is a suitable substitute for aspirin for analgesic or antipyretic uses; it is particularly valuable for patients in whom aspirin is contraindicated (e.g., those with peptic ulcer, aspirin hypersensitivity, children with a febrile illness). The conventional oral dose of acetaminophen is 325–1000 mg (650 mg rectally); total daily doses should not exceed 4000 mg (2000 mg/day for chronic alcoholics). The most common daily dose is 1000 mg, the dose at which epidemiological studies suggest that GI adverse effects are less common than with therapeutic doses of tNSAIDs. Higher doses, which may accomplish complete inhibition of COXs, may approach the adverse effect profile of tNSAIDs. Single doses for children range from 40–480 mg, depending upon age and weight; no more than five doses should be administered in 24 hours. A dose of 10 mg/kg also may be used.

COMMON ADVERSE EFFECTS AND TOXICITY

Acetaminophen usually is well tolerated. Erythematous or urticarial rash may occur and may be accompanied by drug fever and mucosal lesions. Patients who show hypersensitivity reactions to the salicylates only rarely exhibit sensitivity to acetaminophen.

The most serious acute adverse effect of overdosage of acetaminophen is a potentially fatal hepatic necrosis. Renal tubular necrosis and hypoglycemic coma also may occur. The mechanism by which overdosage with acetaminophen leads to hepatocellular injury and death involves its conversion to the toxic NAPQI metabolite (see Chapter 64). The glucuronide and sulfate conjugation pathways become saturated, and increasing amounts undergo CYP-mediated N-hydroxylation to form NAPQI. This is eliminated rapidly by conjugation with GSH and then further metabolized to a mercapturic acid and excreted into the urine. In the setting of acetaminophen overdose, hepatocellular levels of GSH become depleted. The highly reactive NAPQI metabolite binds covalently to cell macromolecules, leading to dysfunction of enzymatic systems and structural and metabolic disarray. Furthermore, depletion of intracellular GSH renders the hepatocytes highly susceptible to oxidative stress and apoptosis.

Management of Acetaminophen Overdose

Acetaminophen overdose constitutes a medical emergency. Severe liver damage occurs in 90% of patients with plasma concentrations of acetaminophen >300 μg/mL at 4 hours or 45 μg/mL at 15 hours after the ingestion of the drug. Early diagnosis and treatment of acetaminophen overdose is essential to optimize outcome. Perhaps 10% of poisoned patients who do not receive specific treatment develop severe liver damage; 10–20% of these eventually die of hepatic failure despite intensive supportive care. Activated charcoal, if given within 4 hours of ingestion, decreases acetaminophen absorption by 50–90% and is the preferred method of gastric decontamination. Gastric lavage is not recommended.

N-acetylcysteine (NAC) (MUCOMYST, MUCOSIL, PARVOLEX) is indicated for those at risk of hepatic injury. NAC therapy should be instituted in suspected cases of acetaminophen poisoning before blood levels become available, with treatment terminated if assay results subsequently indicate that the risk of hepatotoxicity is low.

NAC functions by detoxifying NAPQI. It both repletes GSH stores and may conjugate directly with NAPQI by serving as a GSH substitute. Even in the presence of activated charcoal, there is ample absorption of NAC, and neither should activated charcoal be avoided nor NAC administration be delayed because of concerns of a charcoal-NAC interaction. Adverse reactions to NAC include rash (including urticaria, which does not require drug discontinuation), nausea, vomiting, diarrhea, and rare anaphylactoid reactions.

An oral loading dose of 140 mg/kg is given, followed by the administration of 70 mg/kg every 4 hours for 17 doses. Where available, the intravenous loading dose is 150 mg/kg by intravenous infusion in 100 mL of 5% dextrose over 15 minutes (for those weighing less than 20 kg), followed by 50 mg/kg by intravenous infusion in 250 mL of 5% dextrose over 4 hours, then 100 mg/kg by intravenous infusion in 500 mL of 5% dextrose over 16 hours.

ACETIC ACID DERIVATIVES: INDOMETHACIN, SULINDAC, AND ETODOLAC
Indomethacin
CHEMISTRY

The structural formula of indomethacin, a methylated indole derivative, is:

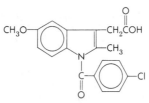

INDOMETHACIN

PHARMACOLOGICAL PROPERTIES

Indomethacin has prominent anti-inflammatory and analgesic–antipyretic properties similar to those of the salicylates. Indomethacin is a more potent inhibitor of COX than is aspirin, but patient intolerance generally limits its use to short-term dosing. Indomethacin has analgesic properties distinct from its anti-inflammatory effects, and there is evidence for central and peripheral actions.

PHARMACOKINETICS AND METABOLISM

Oral indomethacin has excellent bioavailability. Peak concentrations occur 1–2 hours after dosing (Table 26–1). Indomethacin is 90% bound to plasma proteins and tissues. The concentration of the drug in the CSF is low, but its concentration in synovial fluid is equal to that in plasma within 5 hours of administration.

Between 10% and 20% of indomethacin is excreted unchanged in the urine, partly by tubular secretion. The majority is converted to inactive metabolites, including those formed by O-demethylation (~50%), conjugation with glucuronic acid (~10%), and N-deacylation. Free and conjugated metabolites are eliminated in the urine, bile, and feces. There is enterohepatic cycling of the conjugates and probably of indomethacin itself. The $t_{1/2}$ in plasma is variable, perhaps because of enterohepatic cycling, but averages 2.5 hours.

DRUG INTERACTIONS

Indomethacin does not directly modify the effect of warfarin, but platelet inhibition and gastric irritation increase the risk of bleeding; concurrent administration is not recommended. Indomethacin antagonizes the natriuretic and antihypertensive effects of furosemide and thiazide diuretics and blunts the antihypertensive effect of β receptor antagonists, AT_1 receptor antagonists, and ACE inhibitors.

THERAPEUTIC USES

Indomethacin (INDOCIN) is effective for relieving joint pain, swelling, and tenderness, increasing grip strength, and decreasing the duration of morning stiffness. It is estimated to be ~20 times more potent than aspirin. Overall, about two-thirds of patients benefit from treatment with indomethacin, which typically is initiated at 25 mg two or three times daily. In some patients, 100 mg taken at night provides better relief from morning stiffness. Failure to obtain adequate symptom relief with 100 mg within 7–10 days is an indication to try an alternative therapy.

When tolerated, indomethacin often is more effective than aspirin in the treatment of ankylosing spondylitis and osteoarthritis. It also is very effective in the treatment of acute gout pain, although it is not uricosuric.

Indomethacin is FDA approved for closure of persistent patent ductus arteriosus. Successful closure is obtained in >70% of neonates treated with the drug. Such therapy is indicated primarily in premature infants who weigh between 500 and 1750 g, who have a hemodynamically significant patent ductus arteriosus, and in whom other supportive maneuvers have been attempted. Unexpectedly, treatment with indomethacin also may decrease the incidence and severity of intraventricular hemorrhage in low-birth-weight neonates. The principal limitation of treating neonates is renal toxicity, and therapy is stopped if urine output falls to <0.6 mL/kg/h. Renal failure, enterocolitis, thrombocytopenia, or hyperbilirubinemia are contraindications to the use of indomethacin.

COMMON ADVERSE EFFECTS

A high percentage (35–50%) of patients receiving usual therapeutic doses of indomethacin experience untoward symptoms, and ~20% must discontinue its use because of the side effects. Most adverse effects are dose-related.

Gastrointestinal complaints are common and can be serious. Diarrhea may occur and sometimes is associated with ulcerative lesions of the bowel. Underlying peptic ulcer disease is a contraindication to indomethacin use. Acute pancreatitis has been reported, as have rare, but potentially fatal, cases of hepatitis. The most frequent CNS effect (indeed, the most common side effect) is severe frontal headache, occurring in 25–50% of patients who take the drug for long periods. Dizziness, vertigo, light-headedness, and mental confusion may occur. Seizures have been reported, as have severe depression, psychosis, hallucinations, and suicide. Caution is advised when administering indomethacin to elderly patients or to those with underlying epilepsy, psychiatric disorders, or Parkinson's disease, because they are at greater risk for the development of serious CNS adverse effects.

Hematopoietic reactions include neutropenia, thrombocytopenia, and rarely aplastic anemia. As is common with other tNSAIDs, platelet function is impaired transiently during the dosing interval.

Sulindac

CHEMISTRY

Sulindac is related closely to indomethacin; its structure is:

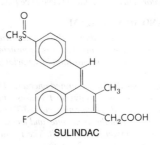

SULINDAC

PHARMACOLOGICAL PROPERTIES

Sulindac, which is less than half as potent as indomethacin, is a prodrug whose anti-inflammatory activity resides in its sulfide metabolite. The same precautions that apply to other NSAIDs regarding patients at risk for GI toxicity or renal impairment also apply to sulindac.

PHARMACOKINETICS AND METABOLISM

About 90% of the drug is absorbed after oral administration (Table 26–1). Peak concentrations of sulindac in plasma are attained within 1–2 hours, while those of the sulfide metabolite occur ~8 hours after the oral administration of sulindac.

Sulindac is oxidized to the sulfone and then reversibly reduced to the active sulfide by the action of bowel microflora on sulindac excreted in the bile.

The $t_{1/2}$ of sulindac is ~7 hours, but the active sulfide has a $t_{1/2}$ as long as 18 hours. Sulindac and its metabolites undergo extensive enterohepatic circulation, and all are bound extensively to plasma protein.

Little of the sulfide (or of its conjugates) is found in urine. The principal components excreted in the urine are the sulfone and its conjugates, which account for nearly 30% of an administered dose; sulindac and its conjugates account for ~20%. Up to 25% of an oral dose may appear as metabolites in the feces.

THERAPEUTIC USES

Sulindac (CLINORIL) has been used mainly for the treatment of rheumatoid arthritis, osteoarthritis, ankylosing spondylitis, and acute gout. Its analgesic and anti-inflammatory effects are comparable to those of aspirin. The most common dosage for adults is 150–200 mg twice a day. The drug usually is given with food to reduce gastric discomfort, although this may delay absorption and reduce its concentration in plasma.

COMMON ADVERSE EFFECTS

Although the incidence of toxicity is lower than with indomethacin, GI side effects (less severe than indomethacin) are seen in nearly 20% of patients. CNS side effects as described above for indomethacin are seen in up to 10% of patients. Rash and pruritus occur in 5% of patients. Transient elevations of hepatic transaminases in plasma are less common.

Etodolac

Etodolac is another acetic acid derivative with some degree of COX-2 selectivity. Thus, at anti-inflammatory doses, the frequency of gastric irritation may be less than with other tNSAIDs.

PHARMACOKINETICS AND METABOLISM

Etodolac is rapidly and well absorbed orally. It is highly bound to plasma protein and undergoes hepatic metabolism and renal excretion (Table 26–1). The drug may undergo enterohepatic circulation in humans; its $t_{1/2}$ in plasma is ~7 hours.

THERAPEUTIC USES

A single oral dose (200–400 mg) of etodolac (LODINE) provides postoperative analgesia that typically lasts for 6–8 hours. Etodolac also is effective in the treatment of osteoarthritis and rheumatoid arthritis and the drug appears to be uricosuric. A sustained-release preparation (LODINE XL) is available, allowing once-a-day administration.

COMMON ADVERSE EFFECTS
Etodolac appears to be relatively well tolerated. About 5% of patients who have taken the drug for up to 1 year discontinue treatment because of side effects, which include GI intolerance, rashes, and CNS effects.

THE FENAMATES
The fenamates include *mefenamic, meclofenamic, and flufenamic acids.*

Therapeutically, they have no clear advantages over several other tNSAIDs and frequently cause GI side effects.

Mefenamic acid (PONSTEL, others) and meclofenamate sodium *(MECLOMEN) have been used mostly in the short-term treatment of pain in soft-tissue injuries, dysmenorrhea, and in rheumatoid and osteoarthritis. These drugs are not recommended for use in children or pregnant women.*

Mefenamic acid and meclofenamate, but not flufenamic acid, are available in the U.S. All three are available in Europe. They are used rarely for chronic therapy of the arthritides.

CHEMISTRY
Mefenamic acid and meclofenamate are N-substituted phenylanthranilic acids.

PHARMACOLOGICAL PROPERTIES
Mefenamic acid has central and peripheral actions, and meclofenamic acid may antagonize directly certain effects of prostaglandins, although it is not clear that receptor blockade is attained at therapeutic concentrations.

PHARMACOKINETIC PROPERTIES
These drugs are absorbed rapidly and have short durations of action. In humans, ~50% of a dose of mefenamic acid is excreted in the urine, primarily as the 3-hydroxymethyl and 3-carboxyl metabolites and their conjugates. About 20% of the drug is recovered in the feces, mainly as the unconjugated 3-carboxyl metabolite.

COMMON ADVERSE EFFECTS AND PRECAUTIONS
Approximately 25% of users develop GI side effects at therapeutic doses. Roughly 5% of patients develop a reversible elevation of hepatic transaminases. Diarrhea, which may be severe and associated with steatorrhea and inflammation of the bowel, also is relatively common. Autoimmune hemolytic anemia is a potentially serious but rare side effect.

The fenamates are contraindicated in patients with a history of GI disease. If diarrhea or rash occur, these drugs should be stopped at once. Vigilance is required for signs or symptoms of hemolytic anemia.

TOLMETIN, KETOROLAC, AND DICLOFENAC
Tolmetin and *ketorolac* are structurally related heteroaryl acetic acid derivatives with different pharmacological features. Diclofenac is a phenylacetic acid derivative that was developed specifically as an anti-inflammatory agent.

Tolmetin
Tolmetin is an anti-inflammatory, analgesic, and antipyretic agent that, in recommended doses (200–600 mg three times a day), appears to be approximately equivalent in efficacy to moderate doses of aspirin. Tolmetin possesses typical tNSAID properties and side effects.

PHARMACOKINETICS AND METABOLISM
Tolmetin demonstrates rapid and complete absorption, extensive plasma protein binding, and a short $t_{1/2}$ (Table 26–1). It undergoes extensive hepatic metabolism, mostly by oxidation of the para-methyl group to a carboxylic acid. Metabolites are excreted in the urine. Accumulation of the drug in synovial fluid begins within 2 hours and persists for up to 8 hours after a single oral dose.

THERAPEUTIC USES
Tolmetin (tolmetin sodium; TOLECTIN) is approved in the U.S. for the treatment of osteoarthritis, rheumatoid arthritis, and juvenile rheumatoid arthritis; it also has been used in the treatment of ankylosing spondylitis. In general, tolmetin is thought to have similar therapeutic efficacy to aspirin. The maximum recommended dose is 2 g/day, typically given in divided doses with meals,

milk, or antacids to lessen abdominal discomfort. Peak plasma concentrations and bioavailability are reduced when the drug is taken with food.

COMMON ADVERSE EFFECTS

Side effects occur in 25–40% of patients who take tolmetin, and 5–10% discontinue use of the drug. Gastrointestinal side effects are the most common (15%) and gastric ulceration has been observed. CNS side effects similar to those seen with indomethacin and aspirin occur, but they are less common and less severe.

Ketorolac

Ketorolac is a potent analgesic but only a moderately effective anti-inflammatory drug. It is one of the few NSAIDs approved for parenteral administration.

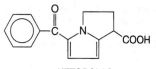

KETOROLAC

PHARMACOLOGICAL PROPERTIES

Ketorolac has greater systemic analgesic than anti-inflammatory activity. Like other tNSAIDs, it inhibits platelet aggregation and promotes gastric ulceration. Ketorolac also has anti-inflammatory activity when topically administered in the eye.

PHARMACOKINETICS AND METABOLISM

Ketorolac has a rapid onset of action, extensive protein binding, and a short duration of action (Table 26–1). Oral bioavailability is ~80%. Urinary excretion accounts for ~90% of eliminated drug, with ~10% excreted unchanged and the remainder as a glucuronidated conjugate. The rate of elimination is reduced in the elderly and in patients with renal failure.

THERAPEUTIC USES

Ketorolac (TORADOL, ULTRAM) has been used as a short-term alternative (<5 days) to opioids for the treatment of moderate-to-severe pain and is administered intramuscularly, intravenously, or orally. Unlike the case with opioids, tolerance, withdrawal, and respiratory depression do not occur. Like other NSAIDs, aspirin sensitivity is a contraindication to the use of ketorolac. Typical doses are 30–60 mg (intramuscular); 15–30 mg (intravenous); and 5–30 mg (oral). Ketorolac is used widely in postoperative patients, but it should not be used for routine obstetric analgesia. Topical (ophthalmic) ketorolac is FDA-approved for the treatment of seasonal allergic conjunctivitis and postoperative ocular inflammation after cataract extraction.

COMMON ADVERSE EFFECTS

Side effects at usual doses include somnolence, dizziness, headache, GI pain, dyspepsia, nausea, and pain at the site of injection.

Diclofenac

Diclofenac is the most commonly used tNSAID in Europe. The selective inhibitor of COX-2 lumiracoxib is an analog of diclofenac.

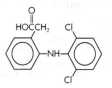

DICLOFENAC

PHARMACOLOGICAL PROPERTIES

Diclofenac has analgesic, antipyretic, and anti-inflammatory activities. Diclofenac appears to reduce intracellular concentrations of free AA in leukocytes, perhaps by altering its release or uptake. The selectivity of diclofenac for COX-2 resembles that of celecoxib. Observational studies have raised the possibility of a cardiovascular hazard from chronic therapy with diclofenac.

PHARMACOKINETICS

Diclofenac has rapid absorption, extensive protein binding, and a short $t_{1/2}$ (Table 26–2). There is a substantial first-pass effect, such that only ~50% of diclofenac is available systemically. Diclofenac accumulates in synovial fluid after oral administration, which may explain why its duration of therapeutic effect is considerably longer than the plasma $t_{1/2}$. Diclofenac is metabolized in the liver by a member of the CYP2C subfamily to 4-hydroxydiclofenac, the principal metabolite, and other hydroxylated forms; after glucuronidation and sulfation the metabolites are excreted in the urine (65%) and bile (35%).

THERAPEUTIC USES

Diclofenac is approved in the U.S. for the long-term symptomatic treatment of rheumatoid arthritis, osteoarthritis, and ankylosing spondylitis (100–200 mg in divided doses). Three formulations are available: an intermediate-release potassium salt (CATAFLAM), a delayed-release form (VOLTARIN, VOLTAROL [UK]), and an extended-release form (VOLTARIN-XR). Diclofenac also is useful for short-term treatment of acute musculoskeletal pain, postoperative pain, and dysmenorrhea. Diclofenac is also available in combination with misoprostol, a PGE_1 analog (ARTHROTEC). An ophthalmic solution of diclofenac is available for treatment of postoperative inflammation following cataract extraction.

COMMON ADVERSE EFFECTS

Diclofenac produces side effects (particularly GI) in ~20% of patients, and ~2% of patients discontinue therapy as a result. Modest reversible elevation of hepatic transaminases in plasma occurs in 5–15% of patients. Transaminases should be measured during the first 8 weeks of therapy with diclofenac, and the drug should be discontinued if abnormal values persist or if other signs or symptoms develop. Other untoward responses to diclofenac include CNS effects, rashes, allergic reactions, fluid retention, and edema, and rarely impairment of renal function. The drug is not recommended for children, nursing mothers, or pregnant women. Consistent with its preference for COX-2, and unlike ibuprofen, diclofenac does not interfere with the antiplatelet effect of aspirin. Given these observations, diclofenac is not a suitable alternative to a selective COX-2 inhibitor in individuals at risk of cardiovascular or cerebrovascular disease.

PROPIONIC ACID DERIVATIVES

Propionic acid derivatives are approved for use in the symptomatic treatment of rheumatoid arthritis, osteoarthritis, ankylosing spondylitis, and acute gouty arthritis; they also are used as analgesics, for acute tendinitis and bursitis, and for primary dysmenorrhea.

Ibuprofen, the most commonly used tNSAID in the U.S., was the first member of the propionic acid class of NSAIDs to come into general use, and it is available without a prescription in the U.S. Naproxen, also available without prescription, has a longer but variable $t_{1/2}$, making twice-daily administration feasible (and perhaps once daily in some individuals). Oxaprozin also has a long $t_{1/2}$ and may possibly be given once daily.

Small clinical studies suggest that the propionic acid derivatives are comparable in efficacy to aspirin for the control of the signs and symptoms of rheumatoid arthritis and osteoarthritis, perhaps with improved tolerability.

Ibuprofen and naproxen are representative of the class and are described individually below.

PHARMACOLOGICAL PROPERTIES The pharmacodynamic properties of the propionic acid derivatives do not differ significantly. All are nonselective COX inhibitors with the effects and side effects common to other tNSAIDs. Some of the propionic acid derivatives, particularly naproxen, have prominent inhibitory effects on leukocyte function, and some data suggest that naproxen may have slightly better efficacy with regard to analgesia and relief of morning stiffness. Epidemiological studies suggest that while the relative risk of myocardial infarction is unaltered by ibuprofen, it is reduced by around 10% by naproxen, compared to a reduction of 20–25% by aspirin. This suggestion of benefit accords with the clinical pharmacology of naproxen that suggests that some but not all individuals dosed with 500 mg twice daily sustain platelet inhibition throughout the dosing interval.

DRUG INTERACTIONS As do other NSAIDs, the propionic acid derivatives may interfere with the action of antihypertensive and diuretic agents, increase the risk of bleeding with warfarin, and increase the risk of bone marrow suppression with methotrexate. Ibuprofen also has been shown to interfere with the antiplatelet effects of aspirin (*see* above). There is also evidence for a similar interaction between aspirin and naproxen.

Ibuprofen

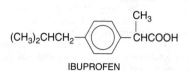

IBUPROFEN

Ibuprofen is supplied as tablets containing 200–800 mg; only the 200-mg tablets (ADVIL, MOTRIN, NUPRIN, others) are available without a prescription.

Doses of up to 800 mg four times daily can be used in the treatment of rheumatoid arthritis and osteoarthritis, but lower doses often are adequate. The usual dose for mild-to-moderate pain, such as that of primary dysmenorrhea, is 400 mg every 4–6 hours as needed.

PHARMACOKINETICS

Ibuprofen is absorbed rapidly, bound avidly to protein, and undergoes hepatic metabolism (90% is metabolized to hydroxylate or carboxylate derivatives) and renal excretion of metabolites. The $t_{1/2}$ is ~2 hours. Slow equilibration with the synovial space means that its antiarthritic effects may persist after plasma levels decline. In experimental animals, ibuprofen and its metabolites readily cross the placenta.

COMMON ADVERSE EFFECTS

Ibuprofen is thought to be better tolerated than aspirin and indomethacin and has been used in patients with a history of gastrointestinal intolerance to other NSAIDs. Nevertheless, 5–15% of patients experience GI side effects. Less frequent adverse effects include thrombocytopenia, rashes, headache, dizziness, blurred vision, and in a few cases toxic amblyopia, fluid retention, and edema. Patients who develop ocular disturbances should discontinue the use of ibuprofen. Ibuprofen can be used occasionally by pregnant women; however, the concerns apply regarding third-trimester effects. Excretion into breast milk is thought to be minimal, so ibuprofen also can be used with caution by women who are breastfeeding.

Naproxen

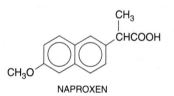

NAPROXEN

PHARMACOKINETICS

Naproxen, (ALEVE, NAPROSYN, others), is absorbed fully when administered orally. Food delays the rate but not the extent of absorption. Peak concentrations in plasma occur within 2–4 hours and are somewhat more rapid after the administration of naproxen sodium. Absorption is accelerated by the concurrent administration of sodium bicarbonate but delayed by magnesium oxide or aluminum hydroxide. Naproxen also is absorbed rectally, but more slowly than after oral administration. The $t_{1/2}$ of naproxen is ~14 hours in the young; it may increase about twofold in the elderly because of age-related decline in renal function (Table 26–1).

Metabolites of naproxen are excreted almost entirely in the urine. About 30% of the drug undergoes 6-demethylation, and most of this metabolite, as well as naproxen itself, is excreted as the glucuronide or other conjugates.

Naproxen is almost completely (99%) bound to plasma proteins after normal therapeutic doses. Naproxen crosses the placenta and appears in the milk of lactating women at ~1% of the maternal plasma concentration.

COMMON ADVERSE EFFECTS

Typical GI adverse effects with naproxen occur at approximately the same frequency as with indomethacin, but perhaps with less severity. CNS side effects range from drowsiness, headache, dizziness, and sweating, to fatigue, depression, and ototoxicity. Less common reactions include pruritus and a variety of dermatological problems. A few instances of jaundice, impairment of renal function, angioedema, thrombocytopenia, and agranulocytosis have been reported.

ENOLIC ACIDS (OXICAMS)

The oxicam derivatives are enolic acids that inhibit COX-1 and COX-2 and have anti-inflammatory, analgesic, and antipyretic activity. In general, they are nonselective COX inhibitors, although one member (meloxicam) shows modest COX-2 selectivity comparable to celecoxib and was approved as a selective COX-2 inhibitor in some countries (*see* below). They are similar in efficacy to aspirin, indomethacin, or naproxen for the long-term treatment of rheumatoid arthritis or osteoarthritis. The main advantage suggested for these compounds is their long $t_{1/2}$, which permits once-a-day dosing.

Piroxicam

PHARMACOLOGICAL PROPERTIES

Piroxicam is effective as an anti-inflammatory agent. It can inhibit activation of neutrophils, apparently independently of its ability to inhibit COX. Approximately 20% of patients experience side effects with piroxicam, and ~5% of patients discontinue use because of these effects.

PHARMACOKINETICS AND METABOLISM

Piroxicam is absorbed completely after oral administration and undergoes enterohepatic recirculation; peak concentrations in plasma occur within 2–4 hours (Table 26–1). Food may delay absorption. Estimates of the $t_{1/2}$ in plasma have been variable; the average is ~50 hours.

After absorption, piroxicam is extensively (99%) bound to plasma proteins. Concentrations in plasma and synovial fluid are similar at steady state (e.g., after 7–12 days). Less than 5% of the drug is excreted into the urine unchanged. The major metabolic transformation is CYP-mediated hydroxylation to an inactive metabolite and its glucuronide conjugate.

THERAPEUTIC USES

Piroxicam (FELDENE) is approved in the U.S. for the treatment of rheumatoid arthritis and osteoarthritis. Due to delayed attainment of steady state (7–12 days), it has slow onset of action and is less suited for acute analgesia, but has been used in acute gout. Piroxicam can reduce the renal excretion of lithium to a clinically significant extent. The usual daily dose is 20 mg.

Meloxicam

Meloxicam (MOBIC) is approved by the FDA for use in osteoarthritis. The recommended dose is 7.5–15 mg once daily for osteoarthritis and 15 mg once daily for rheumatoid arthritis.

Meloxicam demonstrates some COX-2 selectivity, but a clinical advantage or hazard has yet to be established. There is significantly less gastric injury compared to piroxicam (20 mg/day) in subjects treated with 7.5 mg/day of meloxicam, but the advantage is lost with 15 mg/day. Like diclofenac, meloxicam does not offer a desirable alternative to prescribing celecoxib to patients at increased risk of myocardial infarction or stroke.

Nabumetone

Nabumetone is an anti-inflammatory agent with the following structure:

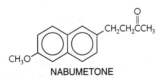

NABUMETONE

Clinical trials with nabumetone (RELAFEN) have indicated substantial efficacy in the treatment of rheumatoid arthritis and osteoarthritis, with a relatively low incidence of side effects. The dose typically is 1000 mg given once daily. The drug also has off-label use in the short-term treatment of soft-tissue injuries.

PHARMACOKINETICS AND METABOLISM

Nabumetone is absorbed rapidly and is converted in the liver to one or more active metabolites, principally 6-methoxy-2-naphthylacetic acid, a potent nonselective inhibitor of COX. This metabolite, inactivated by O-demethylation in the liver, is then conjugated before excretion, and eliminated with a $t_{1/2}$ *of ~24 hours.*

SIDE EFFECTS

Nabumetone is associated with crampy lower abdominal pain and diarrhea, but the incidence of GI ulceration appears to be lower than with other tNSAIDs, although randomized, controlled studies directly comparing tolerability and clinical outcomes have not been performed. Other side effects include rash, headache, dizziness, heartburn, tinnitus, and pruritus.

CYCLCOOXYGENASE-2 SELECTIVE NSAIDS

The therapeutic use of the tNSAIDs has been limited by poor tolerability. Chronic users are prone to experience GI irritation in up to 20% of cases. However, the incidence of these adverse events had been falling sharply in the population prior to the introduction of the coxibs, perhaps reflecting a move away from use of high-dose aspirin as an anti-inflammatory drug strategy. Studies of the immediate early genes induced by inflammation led to the discovery of a gene with significant homology to the original COX enzyme, now designated COX-2. Because expression of this second COX enzyme was regulated by cytokines and mitogens, it was proposed to be the dominant source of prostaglandin formation in inflammation and cancer. It further was proposed that the original, constitutively expressed COX was the predominant source of cytoprotective prostaglandins formed by the gastrointestinal epithelium. Thus, selective inhibition of COX-2 was postulated to afford efficacy similar to tNSAIDs but with better tolerability. Subsequent crystallization of COX-1 and COX-2 revealed remarkable conservation of tertiary structure. However, one difference was in the hydrophobic channel by which the AA substrate gains access to the COX active site, buried deep within the molecule. This channel is more accommodating in the COX-2 structure and consequently exhibits wider substrate specificity than in COX-1. It also contains a side pocket that in retrospect affords a structural explanation for the identification in screens of the two enzymes *in vitro* of small molecule inhibitors that are differentially specific for COX-2. Although there were differences, most tNSAIDs expressed similar selectivity for inhibition of the two enzymes.

Drugs that were developed specifically to favor inhibition of COX-2 are called coxibs. As discussed above, several older drugs (*e.g.*, diclofenac and meloxicam) exhibit relative selectivity for COX-2 inhibition that resembles that of the first-approved specific inhibitor of COX-2, celecoxib.

Three members of the initial class of COX-2 inhibitors, the coxibs, were approved for use in the U.S. and Europe. Both rofecoxib and valdecoxib have now been withdrawn from the market in view of their adverse event profile.

Celecoxib

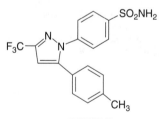

CELECOXIB

PHARMACOKINETICS

*The bioavailability of oral celecoxib (*CELEBREX*) is not known, but peak plasma levels occur at 2–4 hours postdose. Celecoxib is bound extensively to plasma proteins. Little drug is excreted unchanged; most is excreted as carboxylic acid and glucuronide metabolites in the urine and feces. The elimination* $t_{1/2}$ *is ~11 hours. The drug commonly is given once or twice per day during chronic treatment. Renal insufficiency is associated with a modest, clinically insignificant decrease in plasma concentration. Celecoxib has not been studied in patients with severe renal insufficiency. Plasma concentrations are increased by ~40% and 180% in patients with mild and moderate hepatic impairment, respectively, and dosages should be reduced by at least 50% in patients with moderate hepatic impairment. Significant interactions occur with fluconazole and lithium but not with ketoconazole or methotrexate. Celecoxib is metabolized predominantly by*

CYP2C9. Although not a substrate, celecoxib also is an inhibitor of CYP2D6. Clinical vigilance is necessary during coadministration of drugs that are known to inhibit CYP2C9 and drugs that are metabolized by CYP2D6.

PHARMACOLOGICAL PROPERTIES, ADVERSE EFFECTS, AND THERAPEUTIC USES

Effects attributed to inhibition of prostaglandin production in the kidney—hypertension and edema—occur with nonselective COX inhibitors and also with celecoxib. Studies in mice and some epidemiological evidence suggest that the likelihood of hypertension on NSAIDs reflects the degree of inhibition of COX-2 and the selectivity with which it is attained. Thus, the risk of thrombosis, hypertension, and accelerated atherogenesis are mechanistically integrated. The coxibs should be avoided in patients prone to cardiovascular or cerebrovascular disease. None of the coxibs has established clinical efficacy over tNSAIDs, while celecoxib has failed to establish superiority over tNSAIDs in reducing GI adverse events. While selective COX-2 inhibitors do not interact to prevent the antiplatelet effect of aspirin, it now is thought that they lose their GI advantage over a tNSAID alone when used in conjunction with aspirin. Experience with selective COX-2 inhibitors in patients who exhibit aspirin hypersensitivity is limited, and caution should be observed.

Celecoxib is approved in the U.S. for the treatment of osteoarthritis and rheumatoid arthritis. The recommended dose for treating osteoarthritis is 200 mg/day as a single dose or as two 100-mg doses. In the treatment of rheumatoid arthritis, the recommended dose is 100–200 mg twice per day. In the light of recent information on a potential cardiovascular hazard, physicians are advised to use the lowest possible dose for the shortest possible time. Current evidence does not support use of a coxib as a first choice among the NSAIDs.

OTHER NONSTEROIDAL ANTI-INFLAMMATORY DRUGS
Apazone (Azapropazone)

Apazone is a tNSAID that has anti-inflammatory, analgesic, and antipyretic activity and is a potent uricosuric agent. It is available in Europe but not the U.S. Some of its function may arise from its ability to inhibit neutrophil migration, degranulation, and superoxide production.

Apazone has been used for the treatment of rheumatoid arthritis, osteoarthritis, ankylosing spondylitis, and gout but usually is restricted to cases where other tNSAIDs have failed. Typical doses are 600 mg three times per day for acute gout. Once symptoms have abated, or for nongout indications, typical dosage is 300 mg three–four times per day. Clinical experience to date suggests that apazone is well tolerated. Mild GI side effects (nausea, epigastric pain, dyspepsia) and rashes occur in ~3% of patients, while CNS effects (headache, vertigo) are reported less frequently. Precautions appropriate to other nonselective COX inhibitors also apply to apazone.

Nimesulide

Nimesulide is a sulfonanilide compound available in Europe that demonstrates COX-2 selectivity similar to celecoxib in whole blood assays. Additional effects include inhibition of neutrophil activation, decrease in cytokine production, decrease in degradative enzyme production, and possibly activation of glucocorticoid receptors. Its structure is:

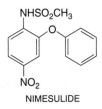

NIMESULIDE

Nimesulide is anti-inflammatory, analgesic, and antipyretic and reportedly is associated with a low incidence of gastrointestinal adverse effects. Given its selectivity profile, it is not a logical alternative for patients switching from the coxibs because of the risk of cardiovascular and cerebrovascular events.

PHARMACOTHERAPY OF GOUT

Gout results from the precipitation of urate crystals in the tissues and the subsequent inflammatory response. Acute gout usually causes an exquisitely painful distal monoarthritis, but it also can cause joint destruction, subcutaneous deposits (tophi), and renal calculi and damage. Gout affects ~0.5–1% of the population of Western countries.

The pathophysiology of gout is understood poorly. While a prerequisite, hyperuricemia does not inevitably lead to gout. Uric acid, the end product of purine metabolism, is relatively insoluble compared to its hypoxanthine and xanthine precursors, and normal serum urate levels approach the limit of solubility. In most patients with gout, hyperuricemia arises from underexcretion rather than overproduction of urate. Urate tends to crystallize in colder or more acidic conditions. Neutrophils ingesting urate crystals secrete inflammatory mediators that lower the local pH and lead to further urate precipitation.

The aims of treatment are to decrease the symptoms of an acute attack, decrease the risk of recurrent attacks, and lower serum urate levels. Therapy of gout focuses on *colchicine, allopurinol,* and the uricosuric agents—probenecid, sulfinpyrazone, and *benzbromarone.*

Treatment of Acute Gout

Several tNSAIDs reportedly are effective in the treatment of acute gout. The specific COX-2 inhibitor etoricoxib has been shown to be effective in gout. When effective, NSAIDs should be given at relatively high doses for 3–4 days and then tapered for a total of 7–10 days. Indomethacin, naproxen, sulindac, and celecoxib all have been found to be effective, although the first three are the only NSAIDs that are FDA-approved for the treatment of gout. Aspirin is not used because it can inhibit urate excretion at low doses, and through its uricosuric actions increase the risk of renal calculi at higher doses. In addition, aspirin can inhibit the actions of uricosuric agents. Likewise, apazone should not be used in acute gout because of the concern that its uricosuric effects may promote nephrolithiasis.

Prevention of Recurrent Attacks

Recurrent attacks of gout can be prevented with the use of colchicine (e.g., 0.6 mg daily or on alternate days). Indomethacin (25 mg/day) also has been used. These agents are used early in the course of uricosuric therapy when mobilization of urate is associated with a temporary increase in the risk of acute gouty arthritis.

ANTIHYPERURICEMIC THERAPY

Isolated hyperuricemia is not necessarily an indication for therapy, as not all of these patients develop gout. Persistently elevated uric acid levels, complicated by recurrent gouty arthritis, nephropathy, or subcutaneous tophi, can be lowered by allopurinol, which inhibits the formation of urate, or by uricosuric agents. Some physicians recommend measuring 24-hour urinary urate levels in patients who are on a low-purine diet to distinguish underexcretors from overproducers. However, tailored and empirical therapies have similar outcomes.

Certain drugs, particularly thiazide diuretics (see Chapter 28) and immunosuppressant agents (especially cyclosporine) may impair urate excretion and thereby increase the risk of gout.

Colchicine

Colchicine is one of the oldest available therapies for acute gout and is considered second-line therapy because it has a narrow therapeutic window and a high rate of side effects, particularly at higher doses.

CHEMISTRY

The structure of colchicine is:

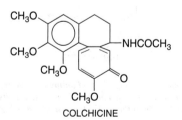

COLCHICINE

MECHANISM OF ACTION

Colchicine exerts a variety of pharmacological effects, but how these occur or how they relate to its activity in gout is not well understood. It has antimitotic effects, arresting cell division in G1 by interfering with microtubule and spindle formation (an effect shared with vinca alkaloids). This effect is greatest on cells with rapid turnover (e.g., neutrophils and GI epithelium). Colchicine renders cell membranes more rigid and decreases the secretion of chemotactic factors by activated neutrophils.

Colchicine inhibits the release of histamine-containing granules from mast cells, the secretion of insulin from pancreatic β cells, and the movement of melanin granules in melanophores; whether this occurs at clinically relevant concentrations is questionable.

Colchicine also exhibits a variety of other pharmacological effects. It lowers body temperature, increases the sensitivity to central depressants, depresses the respiratory center, enhances the response to sympathomimetic agents, constricts blood vessels, and induces hypertension by central vasomotor stimulation. It enhances GI activity by neurogenic stimulation but depresses it by a direct effect, and alters neuromuscular function.

PHARMACOKINETICS AND METABOLISM

Colchicine absorption is rapid but variable. Peak plasma concentrations occur 0.5–2 hours after dosing. In plasma, 50% of colchicine is protein-bound. There is significant enterohepatic circulation. The exact metabolism of colchicine is unknown but seems to involve deacetylation by the liver. Only 10–20% is excreted in the urine, although this increases in patients with liver disease. The kidney, liver, and spleen also contain high concentrations of colchicine, but it apparently is largely excluded from heart, skeletal muscle, and brain. The plasma $t_{1/2}$ of colchicine is ~9 hours, but it can be detected in leukocytes and in the urine for at least 9 days after a single intravenous dose.

TOXIC EFFECTS

Exposure of the GI tract to large amounts of colchicine and its metabolites via enterohepatic circulation and the rapid rate of turnover of the GI mucosa may explain why the GI tract is particularly susceptible to colchicine toxicity. Nausea, vomiting, diarrhea, and abdominal pain are the most common untoward effects of colchicine and the earliest signs of impending toxicity. Drug administration should be discontinued as soon as these symptoms occur. There is a latent period, which is not altered by dose or route of administration, of several hours or more between the administration of the drug and the onset of symptoms. For this reason, adverse effects are common during initial dosing for acute gout. However, since patients often remain relatively consistent in their response to a given dose of the drug, toxicity can be reduced or avoided during subsequent courses of therapy by reducing the dose. Acute intoxication causes hemorrhagic gastropathy. Intravenous colchicine sometimes is used to treat acute gouty arthritis when other medications are not effective, when the patient is unable to take oral medications, or when rapid therapeutic intervention is necessary. The narrow margin of safety for colchicine is even further diminished by intravenous administration because this route obviates early GI side effects that can be a harbinger of serious systemic toxicity. Indiscriminate use of intravenous colchicine has been associated with preventable fatalities. Due to the high rate of serious bone marrow and renal complications (including death from sepsis), this route is not generally recommended.

Colchicine toxicity is associated with bone marrow suppression, particularly from the third to eighth days. There is a tendency toward leukocytosis with appearance of less mature forms. Chronic colchicine use may lead to agranulocytosis. Thrombocytopenia also can occur, and disseminated intravascular coagulation has been reported in cases of severe poisoning.

Chronic use is associated with a proximal myopathy. The associated weakness may go unrecognized, and creatine kinase levels should be monitored in those receiving chronic therapy. Ascending paralysis of the CNS has been reported with acute poisoning.

Proteinuria, hematuria, and acute tubular necrosis have been reported in severely intoxicated patients. Gouty nephropathy may occur in chronically treated patients. Azoospermia has been reported with chronic use.

There is no specific therapy for acute colchicine poisoning. Supportive measures should be used, particularly fluid repletion. Activated charcoal may decrease total colchicine exposure. Hemodialysis does not remove colchicine but may be required as part of supportive care.

THERAPEUTIC USES
Acute Gout

Colchicine dramatically relieves acute attacks of gout. It is effective in roughly two-thirds of patients if given within 24 hours of the onset of the attack. Pain, swelling, and redness abate within 12 hours and are completely gone within 48–72 hours. The typical oral dose is 0.6 mg each hour for a total of three doses. This dose should not be exceeded. Treatment with colchicine should not be repeated within 7 days to avoid cumulative toxicity.

Great care should be exercised in prescribing colchicine for elderly patients. For those with cardiac, renal, hepatic, or GI disease, NSAIDs or glucocorticoids may be preferred.

Prevention of Acute Gout

The main indication for colchicine is in the prevention of recurrent gout, particularly in the early stages of antihyperuricemic therapy. The typical dose is 0.6 mg twice a day, which should be decreased for patients with impaired renal function. One suggestion is 0.6 mg/day for a creatinine clearance of 35–50 mL/min, or in patients younger than 70 years of age, 0.6 mg every 2–3 days for creatinine clearances of 10–35 mL/min, and avoidance in those with creatinine clearance of less than 10 mL/min or with combined hepatic and renal disease.

Allopurinol

Allopurinol inhibits xanthine oxidase and prevents the synthesis of urate from hypoxanthine and xanthine. It is used to treat hyperuricemia in patients with gout and to prevent it in those with hematological malignancies about to undergo chemotherapy (acute tumor lysis syndrome). Even though underexcretion rather than overproduction is the underlying defect in most gout patients, allopurinol remains effective therapy.

CHEMISTRY AND PHARMACOLOGICAL PROPERTIES

Allopurinol, an analog of hypoxanthine, has the following structure:

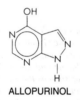

ALLOPURINOL

Both allopurinol and its primary metabolite oxypurinol inhibit xanthine oxidase. Allopurinol competitively inhibits xanthine oxidase at low concentrations and is a noncompetitive inhibitor at high concentrations. Allopurinol also is a substrate for xanthine oxidase; the product of this reaction, oxypurinol, is also a noncompetitive inhibitor of the enzyme. The formation of oxypurinol, together with its long persistence in tissues, is responsible for much of the pharmacological activity of allopurinol.

In the absence of allopurinol, the dominant urinary purine is uric acid. During allopurinol treatment, the urinary purines include hypoxanthine, xanthine, and uric acid. Since each has its independent solubility, the concentration of uric acid in plasma is reduced and purine excretion increased, without exposing the urinary tract to an excessive load of uric acid. Despite their increased concentrations during allopurinol therapy, hypoxanthine and xanthine are efficiently excreted, and tissue deposition does not occur. There is a small risk of xanthine stones in patients with a very high urate load before allopurinol therapy; this can be minimized by liberal fluid intake and urine alkalization.

Allopurinol facilitates the dissolution of tophi and prevents the development or progression of chronic gouty arthritis by lowering the uric acid concentration in plasma below the limit of its solubility. The formation of uric acid stones virtually disappears with therapy, which prevents the development of nephropathy. Once significant renal injury has occurred, allopurinol cannot restore renal function but may delay disease progression. The incidence of acute attacks of gouty arthritis may increase during the early months of allopurinol therapy as a consequence of mobilization of tissue stores of uric acid.

Coadministration of colchicine helps suppress such acute attacks. After reduction of excess tissue stores of uric acid, the incidence of acute attacks decreases and colchicine can be discontinued.

In some patients, the allopurinol-induced increase in excretion of oxypurines is less than the reduction in uric acid excretion; this disparity primarily is a result of reutilization of oxypurines and feedback inhibition of de novo purine biosynthesis.

PHARMACOKINETICS

Allopurinol is absorbed relatively rapidly after oral ingestion, and peak plasma concentrations are reached within 60–90 minutes. About 20% is excreted in the feces in 48–72 hours, presumably as unabsorbed drug, and 10–30% is excreted unchanged in the urine. The remainder undergoes *metabolism, mostly to oxypurinol. Oxypurinol is excreted slowly in the urine by glomerular filtration, counterbalanced by some tubular reabsorption. The plasma $t_{1/2}$ of allopurinol is ~1–2 hours and of oxypurinol ~18–30 hours (longer in those with renal impairment). This allows for once-daily dosing and makes allopurinol the most commonly used antihyperuricemic agent.*

Allopurinol and its active metabolite oxypurinol are distributed in total tissue water, with the exception of brain, where their concentrations are about one-thirds of those in other tissues. Neither compound is bound to plasma proteins. The plasma concentrations of the two compounds do not correlate well with therapeutic or toxic effects.

DRUG INTERACTIONS

Allopurinol increases the $t_{1/2}$ of probenecid and enhances its uricosuric effect, while probenecid increases the clearance of oxypurinol, thereby increasing dose requirements of allopurinol.

Allopurinol inhibits the enzymatic inactivation of mercaptopurine *and its derivative* azathioprine *by* xanthine oxidase*. Thus, when allopurinol is used concomitantly with oral mercaptopurine or azathioprine, dosage of the antineoplastic agent must be reduced by 25–33% (see Chapters 38 and 51). This is of importance when treating gout in the transplant recipient. The risk of bone marrow suppression also is increased when allopurinol is administered with cytotoxic agents that are not metabolized by xanthine oxidase, particularly* cyclophosphamide.

Allopurinol may interfere with the hepatic inactivation of warfarin and increased monitoring of prothrombin activity is recommended in patients receiving both medications.

It remains to be established whether the increased incidence of rash in patients receiving concurrent allopurinol and ampicillin *should be ascribed to allopurinol or to hyperuricemia. Hypersensitivity reactions have been reported in patients with compromised renal function, especially those who are receiving a combination of allopurinol and a thiazide diuretic. The concomitant administration of allopurinol and theophylline leads to increased accumulation of an active metabolite of theophylline, 1-methylxanthine; the concentration of theophylline in plasma also may be increased (see Chapter 27).*

THERAPEUTIC USES

Allopurinol (ZYLOPRIM, ALOPRIM, others) is available for oral use and provides effective therapy for the primary hyperuricemia of gout and the hyperuricemia secondary to polycythemia vera, myeloid metaplasia, other blood dyscrasias, or acute tumor lysis syndrome.

Allopurinol is contraindicated in patients who have exhibited serious adverse effects or hypersensitivity reactions to the medication, and in nursing mothers and children, except those with malignancy or certain inborn errors of purine metabolism (e.g., Lesch-Nyhan syndrome). Allopurinol generally is used in complicated hyperuricemia (see above), to prevent acute tumor lysis syndrome, or in patients with hyperuricemia post-transplantation. If necessary, it can be used in conjunction with uricosuric agents.

The goal of therapy is to reduce the plasma uric acid concentration to <6 mg/dL (360 μmol). In the management of gout, it is customary to antecede allopurinol therapy with colchicine and to avoid starting allopurinol during an acute attack of gouty arthritis. Fluid intake should be sufficient to maintain daily urinary volume of more than 2 L; slightly alkaline urine is preferred. An initial daily dose of 100 mg is increased by 100-mg increments at weekly intervals. Most patients can be maintained on 300 mg/day. Those with more severe gout may require 400–600 mg/day, and those with hematological malignancies may need up to 800 mg/day beginning 2–3 days before the start of chemotherapy. Daily doses in excess of 300 mg should be divided. Dosage must be reduced in patients in proportion to the reduction in glomerular filtration (e.g., 300 mg/day if creatinine clearance is >90 mL/min, 200 mg/day if creatinine clearance is between 60 and 90 mL/min, 100 mg/day if creatinine clearance is 30–60 mL/min, and 50–100 mg/day if creatinine clearance is <30 mL/min).

The usual daily dose in children with secondary hyperuricemia associated with malignancies is 150–300 mg, depending on age.

Allopurinol also is useful in lowering the high plasma concentrations of uric acid in patients with Lesch-Nyhan syndrome and thereby prevents the complications resulting from hyperuricemia; there is no evidence that it alters the progressive neurological and behavioral abnormalities that are characteristic of the disease.

COMMON ADVERSE EFFECTS

Allopurinol is tolerated well by most patients. The most common adverse effects are hypersensitivity reactions that may occur after months or years of medication. The effects usually subside within a few days after medication is discontinued. Serious reactions preclude further use of the drug.

The cutaneous reaction caused by allopurinol is predominantly a pruritic, erythematous, or maculopapular eruption, but occasionally the lesion is urticarial or purpuric. Rarely, toxic epidermal necrolysis or Stevens-Johnson syndrome occurs, which can be fatal. The risk for Stevens-Johnson syndrome is limited primarily to the first 2 months of treatment. Because the rash may precede severe hypersensitivity reactions, patients who develop a rash should discontinue allopurinol. If indicated, desensitization to allopurinol can be carried out starting at 10–25 μg/day, with the drug diluted in oral suspension and doubled every 3–14 days until the desired dose is reached. This is successful in approximately half of patients. Oxypurinol is available for compassionate use in the U.S. for patients intolerant of allopurinol. The safety of oxypurinol in patients with severe allopurinol hypersensitivity is unknown; it is not recommended in this setting.

Fever, malaise, and myalgias also may occur. Such effects are noted in ~3% of patients with normal renal function and more frequently in those with renal impairment.

Transient leukopenia or leukocytosis and eosinophilia are rare reactions that may require cessation of therapy. Hepatomegaly and elevated levels of transaminases in plasma and progressive renal insufficiency also may occur.

Rasburicase

Rasburicase *(ELITEK) is a recombinant urate-oxidase that catalyzes the enzymatic oxidation of uric acid into the soluble and inactive metabolite allantoin. It lowers urate levels more effectively than allopurinol and is indicated for the initial management of elevated plasma uric acid levels in pediatric patients with leukemia, lymphoma, and solid tumor malignancies who are receiving anticancer therapy expected to result in tumor lysis and significant hyperuricemia.*

Produced by a genetically modified Saccharomyces cerevisiae strain, the therapeutic efficacy may be hampered by the production of antibodies against the drug. Hemolysis in glucose-6-phosphate dehydrogenase (G6PD)-deficient patients, methemoglobinemia, acute renal failure, and anaphylaxis all have been associated with the use of rasburicase. Other frequently observed adverse reactions include vomiting, fever, nausea, headache, abdominal pain, constipation, diarrhea, and mucositis. Rasburicase causes enzymatic degradation of the uric acid in blood samples, and special handling is required to prevent spuriously low values for plasma uric acid in patients receiving the drug. The recommended dose of rasburicase is 0.15 mg/kg or 0.2 mg/kg as a single daily dose for 5 days, with chemotherapy initiated 4–24 hours after infusion of the first rasburicase dose.

URICOSURIC AGENTS

Uricosuric agents increase the rate of excretion of uric acid. In humans, urate is filtered, secreted, and reabsorbed by the kidneys. Reabsorption predominates, and the amount excreted usually is ~10% of that filtered. This process is mediated by a specific transporter, which can be inhibited (*see* Chapter 2).

The first step in urate reabsorption is its uptake from tubular fluid by a transporter that exchanges urate for either an organic or an inorganic anion. Uricosuric drugs compete with urate for the brush-border transporter, thereby inhibiting its reabsorption *via* the urate–anion exchanger system. However, transport is bidirectional, and depending on dosage, a drug may either decrease or increase the excretion of uric acid. Decreased excretion usually occurs at a low dosage, while increased excretion is observed at a higher dosage. Not all agents show this phenomenon, and one uricosuric drug may either add to or inhibit the action of another. The biphasic effect may be seen within the normal dosage range with some drugs such as salicylates.

There are two mechanisms by which one drug may nullify the uricosuric action of another. First, the drug may inhibit the secretion of the uricosuric agent, thereby denying it access to its site of action, the luminal aspect of the brush border. Second, the inhibition of urate secretion by one drug may counterbalance the inhibition of urate reabsorption by the other.

Probenecid
CHEMISTRY

Probenecid is a highly lipid-soluble benzoic acid derivative (pK_A 3.4) with the following structure:

$$CH_3CH_2CH_2\diagdown NSO_2-\bigcirc-COOH$$
$$CH_3CH_2CH_2\diagup$$

PROBENECID

PHARMACOLOGICAL ACTIONS
Inhibition of Inorganic Acid Transport

The actions of probenecid are confined largely to inhibition of the transport of organic acids across epithelial barriers. When tubular secretion of a substance is inhibited, its final concentration in the urine is determined by the degree of filtration—which in turn is a function of binding to plasma protein—and by the degree of reabsorption. The significance of each of these factors varies widely with different compounds. Usually, the end result is decreased tubular secretion of the compound, leading to decreased urinary and increased plasma concentration.

Uric acid is the only important endogenous compound whose excretion is known to be increased by probenecid. This results from inhibition of its reabsorption (see above). The uricosuric action of probenecid is blunted by the coadministration of salicylates.

ABSORPTION, FATE, AND EXCRETION

Probenecid is absorbed completely after oral administration. Peak concentrations in plasma are reached in 2–4 hours. The $t_{1/2}$ of the drug in plasma is dose-dependent and varies from <5 hours to >8 hours over the therapeutic range. Between 85% and 95% of the drug is bound to plasma albumin; unbound drug is cleared by glomerular filtration. The majority of the drug is secreted actively by the proximal tubule. The high lipid solubility of the undissociated form results in virtually complete absorption by backdiffusion unless the urine is markedly alkaline. A small amount of probenecid glucuronide appears in the urine. It also is hydroxylated to metabolites that retain their carboxyl function and have uricosuric activity.

COMMON ADVERSE EFFECTS

Probenecid is well tolerated. Approximately 2% of patients develop mild GI irritation. The risk is increased at higher doses, and caution should be used in those with a history of peptic ulcer. It is ineffective in patients with renal insufficiency and should be avoided in those with creatinine clearance of <50 mL/min. Mild hypersensitivity reactions may occur in 2–4% of patients; serious hypersensitivity is extremely rare. The appearance of a rash during the concurrent administration of probenecid and penicillin G presents the physician with an awkward diagnostic dilemma. Substantial overdosage with probenecid results in CNS stimulation, convulsions, and death from respiratory failure.

THERAPEUTIC USE
Gout

Probenecid (BENEMID, others) is marketed for oral administration. The starting dose is 250 mg twice daily, increasing over 1–2 weeks to 500–1000 mg twice daily. Probenecid increases urinary urate levels. Liberal fluid intake therefore should be maintained throughout therapy to minimize the risk of renal stones. Probenecid should not be used in gouty patients with nephrolithiasis or with overproduction of uric acid. Concomitant colchicine or NSAIDs are indicated early in the course of therapy to avoid precipitating an attack of gout, which may occur in up to 20% of gouty patients treated with probenecid alone.

Combination with Penicillin

Probenecid was developed for the purpose of delaying the excretion of penicillin, and it still is used as an adjuvant to prolong penicillin concentrations in patients being treated for specific infections (e.g., syphilis) or in cases where penicillin resistance may be an issue (see Chapter 44).

Benzbromarone

This potent uricosuric agent is used in Europe. It is a potent and reversible inhibitor of the urate–anion exchanger in the proximal tubule. As the micronized powder, it is effective in a single daily dose of 40–80 mg. It is effective in patients with renal insufficiency and may be useful clinically in patients who are either allergic or refractory to other drugs used for the treatment of gout. Preparations that combine allopurinol and benzbromarone lower serum uric acid levels more effectively than either drug alone, despite the fact that benzbromarone lowers plasma levels of oxypurinol, the active metabolite of allopurinol.

For a complete Bibliographical listing see Goodman & Gilman's *The Pharmacological Basis of Therapeutics,* **11th ed., or Goodman & Gilman Online at www.accessmedicine.com.**

27

PHARMACOTHERAPY OF ASTHMA

In the U.S., asthma accounts for 1–3% of all office visits, 500,000 hospital admissions per year, more pediatric hospital admissions than any other single illness, and >5000 deaths annually.

The pharmacotherapy of asthma employs drugs aimed at reducing airway inflammation (*i.e.*, antiinflammatory agents) and drugs aimed more directly at decreasing bronchospasm (*i.e.*, bronchodilators). To these ends, six classes of therapeutic agents are presently indicated for asthma treatment: β adrenergic receptor agonists, glucocorticoids, leukotriene inhibitors, chromones, methylxanthines, and inhibitors of immunoglobulin E (IgE).

ASTHMA AS AN INFLAMMATORY ILLNESS

Asthma is associated with inflammation of the airway wall. Increased numbers of various types of inflammatory cells, most notably eosinophils but also basophils, mast cells, macrophages, and certain types of lymphocytes, can be found in airway wall biopsies and in bronchoalveolar lavage fluid from asthmatic patients. Inflammatory mediators and various cytokines also are increased in the airways of asthmatic subjects compared with healthy control subjects. How bronchial inflammation contributes to the asthmatic condition remains poorly understood. Even asthmatics with normal baseline lung function and no recent exacerbations of their asthma have increased numbers of inflammatory cells in their airways. Conversely, many individuals allergic to inhaled allergens have evidence of lower airway inflammation but suffer only from the symptoms of allergic rhinitis. Many individuals with asthma are atopic and have clearly defined allergen exposures that are partially or substantially responsible for their asthmatic inflammation. Epidemiological studies show a strong correlation between increasing IgE levels and the prevalence of asthma regardless of atopic status. Nonallergic individuals also can suffer from asthma, as is often seen in subjects in whom the onset of disease is later in life.

Although there are subtypes of asthma (allergic *vs.* nonallergic), certain features of airway inflammation are common to all asthmatic airways (Figure 27–1). Airway inflammation presumably is triggered by innate and/or adaptive immune responses. Although there may be multiple "triggers" for an inflammatory response (such as mast cell secretion), there is consensus that a lymphocyte-directed eosinophilic bronchitis is a hallmark of asthma. The lymphocytes that participate in asthma are of the T-helper type 2 (Th2) phenotype, leading to increases in production of interleukin 4 (IL-4), IL-5, and IL-13. IL-4 promotes IgE synthesis in B cells, while IL-5 supports eosinophil survival. The innate or adapted immune response triggers the production of additional cytokines and chemokines, resulting in trafficking of blood-borne cells (*i.e.*, eosinophils, basophils, neutrophils, and lymphocytes) into airway tissues; these cells further generate a variety of autacoids and cytokines. The inflammatory cascade also leads to activation of resident cells within the airways that, in turn, produce a panoply of cytokines, growth factors, chemokines, and autacoids. Over time, the chronic inflammatory response leads to epithelial shedding and reorganization, mucous hypersecretion, and airway wall remodeling most often exemplified by subepithelial fibrosis and smooth muscle hyperplasia. How these processes lead to attacks of asthma, which most often are induced or exacerbated by respiratory viral infections, remains unclear.

In addition to airway inflammation, asthmatics commonly exhibit bronchial hyperreactivity. The concentration of a bronchial spasmogen (*e.g.*, methacholine or histamine) needed to produce a 20% increase in airway resistance in asthmatics is often only 1–2% of the equally effective concentration in healthy control subjects. This bronchial hyperreactivity most often is nonspecific such that the airways are also inordinately reactive to stimuli such as strong odors, cold air, and pollutants.

The pharmacotherapy of asthma centers on controlling the disease with drugs that inhibit airway inflammation. Other drugs that relax bronchial smooth muscle are used for faster, more direct relief of the symptoms of asthma.

TREATMENT OF ASTHMA
Aerosol Delivery of Drugs

Topical delivery of drugs to the lungs can be accomplished by use of aerosols. In theory, this approach should produce a high local concentration in the lungs with a low systemic delivery, thereby significantly minimizing systemic side effects. The drugs used most commonly in the treatment of asthma, β_2 adrenergic receptor agonists and glucocorticoids, have potentially serious side effects when delivered systemically. Since the pathophysiology of asthma appears to involve the

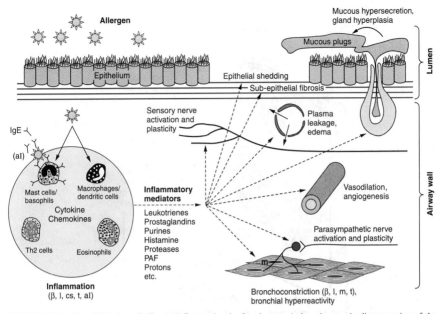

FIGURE 27–1 *Simplified view of allergic inflammation in the airways.* Asthma is an episodic narrowing of the bronchi thought to be caused by an underlying chronic inflammatory disorder. In allergic asthma, inhaled allergen initiates the inflammatory response by interacting with IgE bound to mast cells and basophils. This leads to a cascade of events involving other immune cells and resulting in the release of numerous inflammatory mediators into the interstitial space, where they influence the growth and function of cell types within the airway wall. The drugs available for the treatment of asthma are targeted at inhibiting the inflammatory responses and/or relaxing the bronchial smooth muscle. Letters denote the putative sites of action for the various classes of drugs used in treating asthma. β, β_2 adrenergic agonists; cs, corticosteroids; l, leukotriene modifiers; m, muscarinic receptor antagonists; cr, cromolyn; t, theophylline; aI, anti-IgE therapy. The sunburst (☀) symbolizes an allergen.

respiratory tract alone, the advantages of aerosol treatments with limited systemic effects are substantial. Indeed, in clinical practice, probably >90% of asthmatic patients who are capable of manipulating inhaler devices can be managed by aerosol treatments alone.

Because of the specialized nature of aerosol delivery and the substantial effects that these systems have on the therapeutic index, the principles of this delivery method are important to review (*see* Figure 27–2). Even under ideal circumstances, only a small fraction of the aerosolized drug is deposited in the lungs, typically 2–10%. Most of the remainder is swallowed. To minimize systemic effects, an aerosolized drug should be either poorly absorbed from the gastrointestinal (GI) system or rapidly inactivated *via* first-pass hepatic metabolism. Furthermore, any maneuvers that increase deposition in the lungs or decrease the percentage of drug reaching the GI system should enhance the desired effects and reduce undesired systematic effects. Because >50% of patients using inhalers do not use proper technique and thus deposit too small a fraction of inhaled drug into the lungs, patients should be counseled in the proper use of an inhaler.

β_2 Adrenergic Receptor Agonists

The chemistry, pharmacological properties, and mechanisms of action of the β adrenergic agonists are discussed in Chapter 10. Their discussion here is restricted to their uses in asthma.

MECHANISM OF ACTION AND USE IN ASTHMA The β adrenergic receptor agonists available for the treatment of asthma are selective for the β_2 receptor subtype. With few exceptions, they are delivered directly to the airways *via* inhalation. The agonists can be classified as short- or long-acting. Short-acting agonists are used only for symptomatic relief of asthma, whereas long-acting agonists are used prophylactically in the treatment of the disease.

The mechanism of the antiasthmatic action of β adrenergic receptor agonists is undoubtedly linked to the direct relaxation of airway smooth muscle and consequent bronchodilation. Although

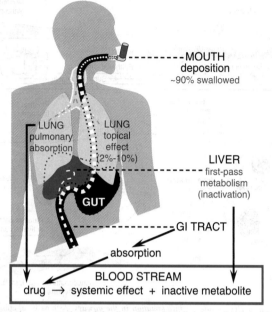

FIGURE 27–2   *Schematic representations of the disposition of inhaled drugs.* Inhalation therapy deposits asthma medications directly, but not exclusively, in the lungs. Distribution of inhaled drug between lungs and esophagus depends on particle size and efficiency of delivery to lungs. Most material, ~90%, will be swallowed and absorbed, entering the systemic circulation. Some drug also will be absorbed from the lungs. Optimal particle size for deposition in small airways is 1–5 μm.

human bronchial smooth muscle receives little or no sympathetic innervation, it nevertheless contains large numbers of β_2 adrenergic receptors. Stimulation of these receptors activates the G_s-adenylyl cyclase–cyclic AMP pathway with a consequent reduction of in smooth muscle tone. β_2 Adrenergic receptor agonists also increase the conductance of Ca^{2+}-sensitive K^+ channels in airway smooth muscle, leading to membrane hyperpolarization and relaxation.

There are β_2 adrenergic receptors on cell types in the airways other than bronchial smooth muscle. Of particular interest, stimulation of β_2 adrenergic receptors inhibits the function of numerous inflammatory cells, including mast cells, basophils, eosinophils, neutrophils, and lymphocytes. In general, stimulating β_2 adrenergic receptors in these cells increase intracellular cyclic AMP, ultimately inhibiting the release of inflammatory mediators and cytokines.

Long-term exposure to β_2 agonists may desensitize some of these receptor-response pathways; thus, there is little evidence that these drugs, used chronically, reduce airway inflammation.

Short-Acting β_2 Adrenergic Receptor Agonists   Drugs in this class include *albuterol* (PROVENTIL, VENTOLIN), *levalbuterol,* the (R)-enantiomer of albuterol (XOPENEX), *metaproterenol* (ALUPENT), *terbutaline* (BRETHAIRE), and *pirbuterol* (MAXAIR). These drugs are used for acute inhalation treatment of bronchospasm. Terbutaline (BRETHINE, BRICANYL), albuterol, and metaproterenol also are available in oral dosage form. Each of the inhaled drugs has an onset of action within 1–5 minutes and produces bronchodilation that lasts for ~2–6 hours. Oral dosage forms have a somewhat longer duration of action (*e.g.,* 4–8 hours for oral terbutaline). Although there are slight differences in the relative β_2/β_1 receptor potency ratios among the drugs, all of them are selective for the β_2 subtype.

The most effective drugs in relaxing airway smooth muscle and reversing bronchoconstriction are short-acting β_2 adrenergic receptor agonists. They are the preferred treatment for rapid symptomatic relief of dyspnea associated with asthmatic bronchoconstriction. Although these drugs are prescribed on an as-needed basis, it is imperative that guidelines be given to the patient so that reliance on relief of symptoms during times of deteriorating asthma does not occur. When the asthma symptoms become persistent, the patient should be reevaluated so that drugs aimed at controlling, in addition to reversing, the disease can be prescribed.

Long-Acting β Adrenergic Receptor Agonists Salmeterol xinafoate (SEREVENT) and *formoterol* (FORADIL) are long-lasting adrenergic agents with very high selectivity for the β_2 receptor subtype; bronchodilation lasts over 12 hours. The mechanism underlying the extended duration of action of salmeterol appears related to its high lipophilicity. After binding the receptor, the less lipophilic, short-acting agonists are removed rapidly from the receptor environment by diffusion in the aqueous phase, while salmeterol persists in the membrane and only slowly dissociates from the environment of the receptor.

Chronic treatment with a receptor agonist often leads to receptor desensitization and diminished effect (see Chapter 1). The β_2 receptors on human bronchial smooth muscle are relatively resistant to desensitization, whereas receptors on mast cells and lymphocytes are desensitized rapidly following agonist exposure. This may help to explain why there is little evidence that these drugs are effective in inhibiting airway inflammation associated with asthma.

ADVERSE DRUG EFFECTS
Owing to their β_2-receptor selectivity and topical delivery, inhaled β adrenergic receptor agonists at recommended doses have relatively few adverse effects. A portion of inhaled drug inevitably is absorbed into the systemic circulation. At higher doses, these drugs may lead to increased heart rate, cardiac arrhythmias, and central nervous system (CNS) effects associated with β adrenergic receptor activation (see Chapter 10). This is of particular concern in patients with poorly controlled asthma, in whom there may be excessive and inappropriate reliance on symptomatic treatment with short-acting β receptor agonists.

Oral Therapy with β Adrenergic Receptor Agonists The use of orally administered β adrenergic agonists for bronchodilation has not gained wide acceptance largely because of the risk of adverse effects, especially tremulousness, muscle cramps, cardiac tachyarrhythmias, and metabolic disturbances (*see* Chapter 10). Brief courses of oral therapy (albuterol or metaproterenol syrups) are well tolerated and effective in young children (<5 years old) who cannot manipulate metered-dose inhalers yet have occasional wheezing with viral upper respiratory infections. In some patients with severe asthma exacerbations, any aerosol, whether delivered *via* a metered-dose inhaler or a nebulizer, can worsen cough and bronchospasm owing to local irritation. In this setting, oral therapy with β_2 adrenergic agonists (*e.g.*, albuterol, metaproterenol, or terbutaline tablets) can be effective. However, the frequency of adverse systemic effects with orally administered agents is higher in adults than in children.

Glucocorticoids
Systemic glucocorticoids long have been used to treat severe chronic asthma or severe acute exacerbations of asthma. The development of aerosol formulations significantly improved the safety of glucocorticoid treatment, allowing it to be used for moderate asthma. Asthmatic subjects who require inhaled β_2 adrenergic agonists four or more times weekly are viewed as candidates for inhaled glucocorticoids.

MECHANISM OF GLUCOCORTICOID ACTION IN ASTHMA
Glucocorticoids do not directly relax airway smooth muscle and thus have little effect on acute bronchoconstriction. Their anti-inflammatory effects in asthma include modulation of cytokine and chemokine production; inhibition of eicosanoid synthesis; marked inhibition of accumulation of basophils, eosinophils, and other leukocytes in lung tissue; and decreased vascular permeability. Because of their profound and generalized anti-inflammatory actions, glucocorticoids are the most effective drugs used in the treatment of asthma.

INHALED GLUCOCORTICOIDS A major advance in asthma therapy was the development of inhaled glucocorticoids that targeted the drug directly to the relevant site of inflammation. These formulations greatly enhance the therapeutic index of the drugs, substantially diminishing the number and degree of side effects without sacrificing clinical utility. There are five glucocorticoids available in the U.S. for inhalation therapy: *beclomethasone dipropionate* (BECLOVENT, VANCERIL), *triamcinolone acetonide* (AZMACORT), *flunisolide* (AEROBID), *budesonide* (PULMICORT), and *fluticasone propionate* (FLOVENT); all are effective in controlling asthma at the appropriate doses.

Inhaled glucocorticoids are used prophylactically to control asthma rather than acutely to reverse asthma symptoms. As with all prophylactic therapies, compliance is a significant concern. Issues relating to drug compliance, therefore, become relevant when choosing among the various steroid formulations. The newer, highly potent drugs (*e.g.*, fluticasone, flunisolide, and budesonide) can be effective with as little as 1–2 puffs administered twice or even once daily. Many patients prefer this more convenient dosage regimen, providing improved compliance and better asthma control. The appropriate dose of steroid must be determined empirically. Important variables that influence the effective dose include the severity of disease, the particular steroid used, and the device used for drug delivery, which determines the actual quantity of drug delivered to the lungs. Maximal improvement in lung function may require several weeks of treatment.

SYSTEMIC GLUCOCORTICOIDS

Systemic glucocorticoids are used for acute asthma exacerbations and chronic severe asthma. Substantial doses of glucocorticoids (e.g., 40–60 mg prednisone or equivalent daily for 5 days; 1–2 mg/kg/day for children) often are used to treat acute exacerbations of asthma. Although an additional week at somewhat reduced dosage may be required, the steroids can be withdrawn once control of the symptoms by other medications has been restored; any suppression of adrenal function dissipates within 1–2 weeks. More protracted bouts of severe asthma may require longer treatment and slower tapering of the dose to avoid exacerbating asthma symptoms and suppressing pituitary/adrenal function. Previously, alternate-day therapy with oral prednisone was employed commonly in persistent asthma. Now, most patients with asthma are better treated with inhaled glucocorticoids.

TOXICITY

Inhaled Glucocorticoids

While inhaled glucocorticoids in asthma are effective, local and systemic adverse effects remain a concern (Table 27–1). Inhaled glucocorticoids have extremely low oral bioavailability owing to extensive first-pass metabolism by the liver and reach the circulation almost exclusively by absorption from the lung. In contrast to the beneficial effects on asthma, which plateau at ~1600 μg/day, the risk of adverse effects continues to increase at higher doses. Oropharyngeal candidiasis and, more frequently, dysphonia can be encountered. The incidence of candidiasis can be reduced substantially by rinsing the mouth and throat with water after each use and by employing spacer or reservoir devices attached to the dispenser to decrease drug deposition in the oral cavity. Appreciable suppression of the hypothalamic-pituitary-adrenal axis is rarely of physiologic importance even at doses up to 1600 μg/day. Modest but statistically significant decreases in bone mineral density do occur in female asthmatics receiving inhaled steroids. While the clinical relevance of these bone metabolism findings remains to be determined, it is argued that inhaled glucocorticoid treatment should be reserved for moderate or severe asthma because such treatment is likely to last for many years. Nonetheless, it has been suggested that the small risk of adverse effects at high doses of inhaled glucocorticoids is outweighed by the risks of inadequately controlling severe asthma.

Table 27–1

Potential Adverse Effects Associated with Inhaled Glucocorticoids

Adverse Effect	Risk
Hypothalamic–pituitary–adrenal axis suppression	No significant risk until dosages of budesonide or beclomethasone increased to >1500 μg/day in adults or >400 μg/day in children
Bone resorption	Modest but significant effects at doses possibly as low as 500 μg/day
Carbohydrate and lipid metabolism	Minor, clinically insignificant changes occur with dosages of beclomethasone >1000 μg/day
Cataracts	Anecdotal reports, risk unproven
Skin thinning	Dosage-related effect with beclomethasone dipropionate over a range of 400 to 2000 μg/day
Purpura	Dosage-related increase in occurrence with beclomethasone over a range of 400 to 2000 μg/day
Dysphonia	Usually of little consequence
Candidiasis	Incidence <5%, reduced by use of spacer device
Growth retardation	Difficult to separate effect of disease from effect of treatment, but no discernible effects on growth when all studies are considered

Systemic Glucocorticoids

The adverse effects of systemic administration of glucocorticoids are well known (see Chapter 59), but treatment for brief periods (5–10 days) causes relatively little dose-related toxicity. The most common adverse effects during a brief course are mood disturbances, increased appetite, impaired glucose control in diabetics, and candidiasis.

Leukotriene Receptor Antagonists and Leukotriene Synthesis Inhibitors

Zafirlukast (ACCOLATE) and *montelukast* (SINGULAIR) are leukotriene receptor antagonists. *Zileuton* (ZYFLO) is an inhibitor of 5-lipoxygenase, which catalyzes the formation of leukotrienes from arachidonic acid.

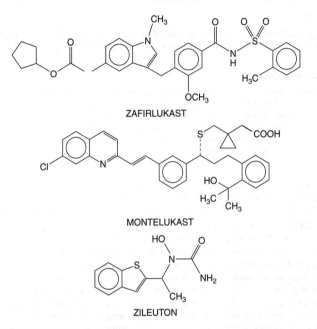

ZAFIRLUKAST

MONTELUKAST

ZILEUTON

PHARMACOKINETICS AND METABOLISM

The leukotriene-modifying drugs are administered orally. Zafirlukast is absorbed rapidly, with >90% bioavailability. At therapeutic plasma concentrations, it is >99% protein-bound. Zafirlukast is metabolized extensively by hepatic CYP2C9. The parent drug is responsible for its therapeutic activity, with metabolites being <10% as effective. The $t_{1/2}$ of zafirlukast is ~10 hours.

Montelukast is absorbed rapidly, with ~60–70% bioavailability. At therapeutic concentrations, it is highly protein-bound (99%). It is metabolized extensively by CYP3A4 and CYP2C9. The $t_{1/2}$ of montelukast is 3–6 hours.

Zileuton is absorbed rapidly on oral administration and is metabolized extensively by CYPs and by UDP-glucuronosyltransferases. The parent molecule is responsible for its therapeutic action. Zileuton is a short-acting drug with a $t_{1/2}$ of ~2.5 hours and also is highly protein-bound (93%).

MECHANISM OF ACTION IN ASTHMA   Leukotriene-modifying drugs act either as competitive antagonists of leukotriene receptors or by inhibiting the synthesis of leukotrienes. The pharmacological properties of leukotrienes are discussed in detail in Chapter 25.

Leukotriene-Receptor Antagonists   Cysteinyl leukotrienes (CysLTs) include leukotriene C4 (LTC$_4$), leukotriene D4 (LTD$_4$), and leukotriene E4 (LTE$_4$). All the CysLTs are potent constrictors of bronchial smooth muscle. On a molar basis, LTD$_4$ is ~1000 times more potent than is histamine as a bronchoconstrictor. The receptor responsible for the bronchoconstrictor effect of leukotrienes is the CysLT$_1$ receptor. Although each of the CysLTs is an agonist at the CysLT$_1$ receptor, LTE4 is less potent than either LTC$_4$ or LTD$_4$. Zafirlukast and montelukast are selective high-affinity competitive antagonists for the CysLT$_1$ receptor. *Pranlukast* is another CysLT$_1$-receptor antagonist used in some countries in the treatment of asthma, but it is not approved for use in the U.S.

Inhibition of CysLT-induced bronchial smooth muscle contraction likely is involved in the therapeutic effects of these agents to relieve the symptoms of asthma.

Leukotriene-Synthesis Inhibitors The formation of leukotrienes depends on lipoxygenation of arachidonic acid by 5-lipoxygenase. Zileuton is a potent and selective inhibitor of 5-lipoxygenase activity and thus blocks the formation of all 5-lipoxygenase products. Thus, in addition to inhibiting the formation of the cys-LTs, zileuton also inhibits the formation of leukotriene B4 (LTB$_4$), a potent chemotactic autacoid, and other eicosanoids that depend on leukotriene A$_4$ (LTA$_4$) synthesis. Logically, the therapeutic effects of a 5-lipoxygenase inhibitor would include all those observed with the CysLT-receptor antagonists, as well as other effects that may result from inhibiting the formation of LTB$_4$ and other 5-lipoxygenase products.

TOXICITY

There are few adverse effects directly associated with inhibition of leukotriene synthesis or function. This likely is due to the fact that leukotriene production is limited predominantly to sites of inflammation.

Zafirlukast and Montelukast

In large clinical studies the adverse-effect profiles of these drugs were similar to that observed with placebo treatment. Very rarely, patients taking these drugs develop systemic eosinophilia and a vasculitis with features similar to Churg-Strauss syndrome. This problem, often associated with a reduction in glucocorticoid therapy, may represent the unmasking of a preexisting disease. Zafirlukast, but not montelukast, may interact with warfarin and increase prothrombin times, which should be monitored in patients subject to this interaction.

Zileuton

In ~4–5% of patients taking zileuton, there is an elevation in hepatic transaminases, generally within the first 2 months of therapy. Zileuton decreases the steady-state clearance of theophylline, substantially increasing its plasma concentrations. Zileuton also decreases warfarin clearance.

USE IN ASTHMA Most clinical trials with these drugs have studied patients with mild asthma who were not taking glucocorticoids. In general, the studies show a modest but significant improvement in pulmonary function and a decrease in symptoms and asthma exacerbations. For those who respond to antileukotriene therapy, the National Heart, Lung, and Blood Institute recognizes these drugs as alternatives to low-dose inhaled steroids for control of mild chronic asthma.

This class of drugs is not indicated for rapid bronchodilator therapy; thus, patients are instructed to have short-acting β adrenergic receptor agonists available as rescue medication. Montelukast and zafirlukast are effective with once- or twice-daily treatment, respectively. In contrast, zileuton is taken 4 times a day. Hepatic transaminases should be monitored in patients beginning zileuton therapy to guard against the potential of liver toxicity.

Anti-IgE Therapy

Omalizumab (XOLAIR) is the first biological agent approved for the treatment of asthma. Omalizumab is a recombinant humanized monoclonal antibody of the IgG1κ subclass, targeted against IgE. IgE bound to omalizumab cannot bind to IgE receptors on mast cells and basophils, thereby preventing the allergic reaction at a very early step in the process (Figure 27–3).

PHARMACOKINETICS AND METABOLISM Omalizumab is delivered as a single subcutaneous injection every 2–4 weeks. It has a bioavailability of ~60%, reaching peak serum levels after 7–8 days. The serum elimination $t_{1/2}$ is 26 days, with a clearance rate of ~2.5 mL/kg/day. The elimination of omalizumab–IgE complexes occurs in the liver reticuloendothelial system at a rate somewhat faster than that of free IgG. Some intact omalizumab is also excreted in the bile. There is little evidence of specific uptake of omalizumab by any tissue.

TOXICITY

Omalizumab generally was well tolerated in several clinical trials. The most frequent adverse effect was injection-site reactions (e.g., redness, stinging, bruising, and induration), but these reactions also were seen at comparable frequencies with placebo. Low titers of antibodies against omalizumab developed in 1 of 1723 treated patients, whereas anaphylaxis was seen in 0.1% of treated patients. Malignancies of various types were observed in 20 of 4127 patients taking omalizumab, a higher frequency than the 5 malignancies in 2236 patients taking other asthma and allergy drugs; additional study is needed to clarify this risk.

Monospecific anti-IgE antibody (Omalizumab)

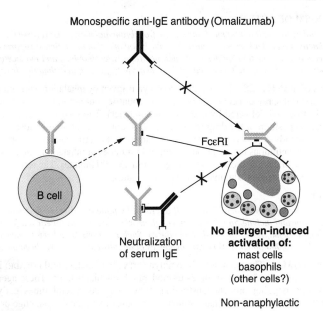

FIGURE 27–3   **Mechanism of Action of Omalizumab.** *Omalizumab is a monospecific anti-IgE antibody.* Specific B lymphocytes produce IgE antibodies. The Fc region of IgE heavy chains binds with high affinity to receptors (FcεRI) in the plasma membranes of mast cells and basophils (and other cells). Allergen interacts with the antigen-binding site of cell-bound IgE, causing FcεRI cross-linking and cell activation. Omalizumab neutralizes the free IgE in the serum by binding to the Fc regions of the heavy chains to form high-affinity IgE-anti–IgE complexes. This prevents the IgE from binding to FcεRI, thereby blocking allergen-induced cell activation.

USE IN ASTHMA   Omalizumab is indicated for adults and adolescents >12 years of age with allergies and moderate-to-severe persistent asthma. In this population, omalizumab has proven to be effective in reducing the dependency on inhaled and oral corticosteroids and in decreasing the frequency of asthma exacerbations. Omalizumab is not an acute bronchodilator and should not be used as a rescue medication or as a treatment of status asthmaticus.

Based on its mechanism of action, omalizumab has been used in the treatment of other allergic disorders, such as nasal allergy and food allergy, but large-scale clinical trials are limited to asthma.

Cromolyn Sodium (disodium cromoglycate) and Nedocromil Sodium

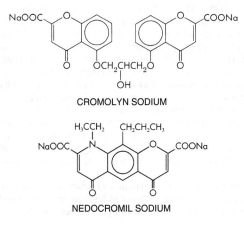

CROMOLYN SODIUM

NEDOCROMIL SODIUM

MECHANISM OF ACTION

Cromolyn and nedocromil inhibit mediator release from bronchial mast cells; reverse the increased functional activation in leukocytes obtained from the blood of asthmatic patients; suppress the activating effects of chemotactic peptides on human neutrophils, eosinophils, and monocytes; inhibit parasympathetic and cough reflexes; and inhibit leukocyte trafficking in asthmatic airways.

PHARMACOKINETICS   For asthma, cromolyn is given by inhalation using either solutions (delivered by aerosol spray or nebulizer) or, in some countries but not in the U.S., powdered drug (mixed with lactose and delivered by a special turboinhaler). The pharmacological effects result from the topical deposition of the drug in the lung, since only ~1% of an oral dose of cromolyn is absorbed. Once absorbed, the drug is excreted unchanged in the urine and bile in about equal proportions. Peak concentrations in plasma occur within 15 minutes of inhalation, and excretion begins after some delay such that the biological $t_{1/2}$ ranges from 45–100 minutes. The terminal $t_{1/2}$ of elimination following intravenous administration is ~20 minutes.

TOXICITY

Cromolyn and nedocromil generally are well tolerated by patients. Adverse reactions are infrequent and minor and include bronchospasm, cough or wheezing, laryngeal edema, joint swelling and pain, angioedema, headache, rash, and nausea. Such reactions have been reported at a frequency of <1 in 10,000 patients. Very rare instances of anaphylaxis also have been documented.

USE IN ASTHMA   The main use of cromolyn (INTAL) and nedocromil (TILADE) is to prevent asthmatic attacks in individuals with mild- to-moderate bronchial asthma. These agents are ineffective in treating ongoing bronchoconstriction. When inhaled several times daily, cromolyn inhibits both the immediate and the late asthmatic responses to antigenic challenge or to exercise. With regular use for >2–3 months, bronchial hyperreactivity is reduced, as measured by response to challenge with histamine or methacholine. Nedocromil is approved for use in asthmatic patients 12 years of age and older; cromolyn is approved for all ages.

Theophylline

Theophylline, a methylxanthine, still is commonly used for asthma pharmacotherapy in many countries. In developed countries, the advent of inhaled glucocorticoids, β adrenergic receptor agonists, and leukotriene-modifying drugs has diminished theophylline use significantly, and it has been relegated to a third- or fourth-line treatment in patients whose asthma is otherwise difficult to control.

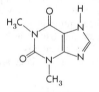

THEOPHYLLINE

MECHANISM OF ACTION   Theophylline inhibits cyclic nucleotide phosphodiesterases (PDEs), thereby preventing hydrolysis of cyclic AMP and cyclic GMP to 5'-AMP and 5'-GMP. Inhibition of PDEs leads to an accumulation of cyclic AMP and cyclic GMP, thereby increasing signal transduction through these pathways. Theophylline and related methylxanthines are relatively nonselective in PDE inhibition. Cyclic nucleotide production is regulated by endogenous receptor–ligand interactions leading to activation of adenylyl cyclase and guanylyl cyclase. Inhibitors of PDEs therefore can be thought of as drugs that enhance the activity of endogenous autacoids, hormones, and neurotransmitters that signal *via* cyclic nucleotides.

Theophylline is also a competitive antagonist at adenosine receptors (*see* Chapter 12). Adenosine can act as an autacoid and transmitter with myriad biological actions. Of particular relevance to asthma are the observations that adenosine can cause bronchoconstriction in asthmatics and potentiate immunologically induced mediator release from lung mast cells. Inhibition of the actions of adenosine therefore also must be considered when attempting to explain the mechanism of action of theophylline.

Theophylline also may owe part of its anti-inflammatory action to its ability to activate histone deacetylases in the nucleus. In theory, the deacetylation of histones could decrease the transcription of several proinflammatory genes and potentiate the effect of corticosteroids.

Pulmonary System

Theophylline effectively relaxes airway smooth muscle; this bronchodilation likely contributes to its acute therapeutic efficacy in asthma. Both adenosine receptor antagonism and PDE inhibition are likely involved in the bronchodilating effect of theophylline. Inhibition of PDE4 and PDE5 effectively relaxes human isolated bronchial smooth muscle, and inhibition of these PDEs likely contributes to the bronchodilating effect of theophylline. Studies with the related methylxanthine enprofylline (3-propylxanthine), which has been investigated extensively for treatment of asthma in Europe, also support a mechanistic role for PDE inhibition in the bronchodilator actions of theophylline.

Theophylline also inhibits synthesis and secretion of inflammatory mediators from numerous cell types, including mast cells and basophils. This effect of theophylline likely is due to PDE inhibition and can be mimicked in large part with drugs that selectively inhibit PDE4.

Absorption, Fate, and Excretion

Theophylline administered in liquids or uncoated tablets is absorbed rapidly and completely. In the absence of food, solutions or uncoated tablets of theophylline produce maximal concentrations in plasma within 2 hours and maximal plasma concentrations are achieved within 1 hour. Numerous sustained-release preparations of theophylline are available, designed for dosing intervals of 8, 12, or 24 hours. There is marked interpatient variability in the rate and extent of absorption, and especially in the effect of food and time of administration on these parameters. Thus, it is necessary to avoid substituting one apparently similar product for another.

Food ordinarily slows the rate of theophylline absorption but does not limit its extent. With sustained-release preparations, food may decrease the bioavailability of theophylline with some products but may increase it with others. Recumbency or sleep also may significantly reduce the rate or extent of absorption. These factors make it difficult to maintain relatively constant concentrations of theophylline in plasma throughout the day. Concentrations required to alleviate asthmatic symptoms do not remain constant, and the emphasis has shifted toward designing dosing regimens that ensure peak concentrations in the early morning hours, when symptoms frequently worsen.

Theophylline is distributed into all body compartments; crossing the placenta and passing into breast milk. Theophylline is eliminated primarily by metabolism in the liver. Less than 15% of administered theophylline is recovered in the urine unchanged. In premature infants, the rate of elimination of theophylline is quite slow; the average $t_{1/2}$ for theophylline ranges between 20 and 36 hours.

There is marked individual variation in the rate of elimination of theophylline owing to both genetic and environmental factors; fourfold differences are not uncommon. The $t_{1/2}$ averages ~3.5 hours in young children, whereas values of 8–9 hours are more typical in adults. In most patients the drug obeys first-order elimination kinetics within the therapeutic range. At higher concentrations, zero-order kinetics become evident because of saturation of metabolic enzymes, prolonging the decline of theophylline concentrations to nontoxic levels.

Hepatic cirrhosis, congestive heart failure, and acute pulmonary edema all increase the $t_{1/2}$ of theophylline, as does concurrent therapy with cimetidine or erythromycin. In contrast, clearance is increased twofold by phenytoin or barbiturates, whereas cigarette smoking, rifampin, and oral contraceptives induce smaller changes.

Although scarcely detectable in adults, the conversion of theophylline to caffeine is significant in preterm infants. In this setting, caffeine accumulates in plasma to a concentration ~25% that of theophylline. About 50% of the theophylline administered to such infants appears in the urine unchanged; the excretion of 1,3-dimethyluric acid, 1-methyluric acid, and caffeine derived from theophylline accounts for nearly all the remainder.

USE IN ASTHMA Theophylline now is relegated to a far less prominent role primarily because of the modest benefits it affords, its narrow therapeutic window, and the required monitoring of drug levels. Nocturnal asthma can be improved with slow-release theophylline preparations, but other interventions such as inhaled glucocorticoids or salmeterol probably are more effective.

Therapy is initiated by the administration of 12–16 mg/kg/day of theophylline (calculated as the free base) up to a maximum of 400 mg/day for at least 3 days. Children <1 year of age require considerably less; the dose in milligrams per kilogram per day may be calculated as 0.2 × (age in weeks) + 5. Starting with these low doses minimizes early side effects of nausea, vomiting, nervousness, and insomnia that often subside with continued therapy and virtually eliminates the possibility of exceeding plasma concentrations of 20 μg/mL in patients older than age 1 year who do not have compromised hepatic or cardiac function. Thereafter, the dosage is increased in two successive stages to between 16 and 20 and, subsequently, 18 and 22 mg/kg/day (up to a maximum of 800 mg/day) depending on the age and clinical response of the patient and allowing at least 3 days between adjustments. The plasma concentration of theophylline is determined before a further adjustment in dosage is made. Although extended-release preparations of theophylline usually allow twice-daily dosing, variations in the rate and extent of absorption of such preparations require individualized calibration of regimens for each patient and preparation.

ADVERSE EFFECTS Adverse CNS effects include headache, anxiety, restlessness, agitation, insomnia, dizziness, and seizures. These reactions are more likely to occur in children than in adults and are also more likely following rapid intravenous administration or in patients with excessive theophylline serum concentrations. Serious reactions can occur without antecedent minor symptoms. A reduction in dosage may eliminate CNS side effects, but if they continue or become severe, theophylline may have to be discontinued.

Urticaria can develop from a hypersensitivity to the ethylenediamine salt in aminophylline. Allergic reactions may not become evident for 12–24 hours after initiation of treatment.

Theophylline decreases peripheral resistance, increases cardiac output, and causes a central vagal effect. Palpitations, sinus bradycardia, extrasystoles, hypotension, ventricular tachycardia, premature ventricular contractions (PVCs), and cardiac arrest have been reported. Although cardiovascular effects are generally mild and transient, serious reactions, such as ventricular arrhythmias, can develop without warning. Patients should be carefully monitored.

In theophylline acute overdose patients are more likely to exhibit hypotension, hypokalemia, and/or metabolic acidosis than are patients receiving chronic overmedication. Patients suffering chronic overmedication can develop seizures and serious arrhythmias with serum concentrations of 28–70 μg/mL. Cardiac arrhythmias include atrial fibrillation or atrial flutter, multifocal atrial tachycardia, sinus tachycardia, supraventricular tachycardia and premature ventricular contractions with hemodynamic instability.

APNEA OF PRETERM INFANTS

In premature infants, episodes of prolonged apnea lasting >15 seconds and accompanied by bradycardia pose the threat of recurrent hypoxemia and neurologic damage. Although they often are associated with serious systemic illness, in many instances no specific cause is found. Methylxanthines have undergone numerous clinical trials for the treatment of apnea of undetermined origin. The oral or intravenous administration of methylxanthines can eliminate episodes of apnea that last >20 seconds and markedly reduces the number of episodes of shorter duration. Satisfactory responses may occur with plasma concentrations of theophylline of 4–8 μg/mL, but concentrations of nearly 13 μg/mL are required more frequently. Still higher concentrations may produce a more regular pattern of respiration without further reduction in the frequency of episodes of apnea and bradycardia, and these usually are associated with a definite tachycardia. Therapeutic concentrations are achieved with loading doses of ~5 mg/kg of theophylline (calculated as the free base) and can be maintained with 2 mg/kg given every 12 or 24 hours.

Anticholinergic Agents

The use of anticholinergic agents in the treatment of asthma is discussed in detail in Chapter 7. With the advent of inhaled β adrenergic agonists, use of anticholinergic agents declined. Renewed interest in anticholinergic agents paralleled the realization that parasympathetic pathways are important in bronchospasm in some asthmatics and the availability of *ipratropium bromide* (ATROVENT), a quaternary muscarinic receptor antagonist that has better pharmacological properties than prior drugs. A particularly good response to ipratropium may be seen in the subgroup of asthmatic patients who experience psychogenic exacerbations.

The cholinergic receptor subtype responsible for bronchial smooth muscle contraction is the muscarinic M_3 receptor. The bronchodilation produced by ipratropium in asthmatic subjects develops more slowly and usually is less intense than that produced by adrenergic agonists. Some asthmatic patients may experience a useful response lasting up to 6 hours. The variability in the response of asthmatic subjects to ipratropium presumably reflects differences in the strength of parasympathetic tone and in the degree to which reflex activation of cholinergic pathways participates in generating symptoms in individual patients. Hence, the utility of ipratropium must be assessed on an individual basis by a therapeutic trial.

Combined treatment with ipratropium and β_2 adrenergic agonists results in slightly greater and more prolonged bronchodilation than with either agent alone in baseline asthma. In acute bronchoconstriction, the combination of a β_2 adrenergic agonist and ipratropium is more effective than either agent alone and more effective than simply giving more β_2 adrenergic agonist. Thus, the combination of a selective β_2 adrenergic agonist and ipratropium should be considered in acute treatment of severe asthma exacerbations. Ipratropium is available in metered-dose inhalers and as a nebulizer solution. A metered-dose inhaler containing a mixture of ipratropium and albuterol (COMBIVENT) also is available in the U.S. In Europe, metered-dose inhalers containing a mixture of ipratropium and fenoterol are available (DUOVENT, BERODUAL).

Recently, tiotropium (SPIRIVA), a structural analogue of ipratropium, has been approved for the treatment of chronic obstructive pulmonary disease (COPD) and emphysema. Like ipratropium, tiotropium has high affinity for all muscarinic receptor subtypes, but it dissociates from the receptors much more slowly that ipratropium. In particular, binding and functional studies indicate that tiotropium dissociates from muscarinic M_3 receptors more slowly than from muscarinic M_2 receptors. The high affinity of tiotropium for muscarinic receptors, combined with its very slow dissociation rate, permits once-daily dosing. The slow dissociation rate also provides a theoretical advantage in that it limits the capacity of large concentrations of the endogenous agonist acetylcholine to surmount the receptor blockade. Tiotropium is provided as a capsule containing a dry-powder formulation that is intended only for oral inhalation using the HandiHaler inhalation device.

PHARMACOGENETICS AND VARIABILITY OF RESPONSE TO ASTHMA MEDICATIONS   There is significant interindividual variability in the response of asthmatic subjects to pharmacotherapy. For example, some individuals benefit dramatically from treatment with leukotriene modifiers, whereas many others are essentially resistant to these treatments. Although more rare, the "steroid resistant" asthmatic receives relatively little benefit from treatment with inhaled corticosteroids. At present, it is impossible to predict who will benefit the most from a given treatment. This unpredictability of response largely reflects our limited understanding of the underlying pathophysiology of asthma. In addition, some component of this variability likely is explained by specific pharmacogenetic factors.

Use of Asthma Drugs in Rhinitis

Seasonal allergic rhinitis (hay fever) is caused by deposition of allergens on the nasal mucosa, resulting in an immediate hypersensitivity reaction. This reaction usually is not accompanied by asthma because the allergenic particles are too large to be inhaled into the lower airways (*e.g.,* pollens). Treatment for allergic rhinitis is similar to that for asthma. Topical glucocorticoids, including *beclomethasone* (BECONASE), *mometasone* (NASONEX), *budesonide* (RHINOCORT), *flunisolide* (NASAREL), *fluticasone* (FLONASE), and *triamcinolone* (NASACORT), can be highly effective with minimal side effects, particularly if treatment is instituted immediately prior to the allergy season. Topical glucocorticoids can be administered twice daily (beclomethasone and flunisolide) or even once daily (budesonide, mometasone, fluticasone, and triamcinolone). Cromolyn usually requires dosing three to six times daily for full effects. Rare instances of local candidiasis have been reported with glucocorticoids and probably can be avoided by rinsing the mouth after use. Unlike in asthma, antihistamines (*see* Chapter 24) afford considerable, though incomplete, symptom relief in allergic rhinitis. Nasal decongestants rely on β adrenergic agonists (*e.g.,* pseudoephedrine and phenylephrine) as vasoconstrictors and are discussed in Chapter 10. Anticholinergic agents such as ipratropium bromide (ATROVENT) are effective in inhibiting parasympathetic reflex–evoked secretions from serous glands lining the nasal mucosa.

Use of Asthma Drugs in COPD

Emphysema can be prevented or its progression slowed if the patient stops smoking. Pharmacological interventions can help patients to stop smoking. *Nicotine gum* (NICORETTE), *nicotine transdermal patches* (NICODERM), and the antidepressant agent *bupropion* (ZYBAN) are moderately useful when combined with other interventions such as support groups and healthcare provider encouragement. Clonidine may be helpful in reducing the craving for cigarettes. Treatment of nicotine addiction is discussed in Chapter 23.

The pharmacological treatment of established emphysema resembles that of asthma largely because the inflammatory/bronchospastic component of a patient's disease is the aspect amenable to therapy. For patients with emphysema who have a significant degree of active inflammation with bronchospasm and excessive mucus production, symptomatic use of inhaled ipratropium or a β_2 adrenergic agonist may be helpful. Ipratropium or tiotropium usually produces about the same modest degree of bronchodilation in patients with COPD as do maximal doses of β_2 adrenergic agonists. As in asthmatic patients, continuous use of bronchodilators is controversial, with some studies suggesting that it is associated with an unfavorable course of COPD. A subgroup of patients may respond favorably to short courses of oral glucocorticoids. Without a treatment trial, it is not possible to predict whether a particular patient will respond to glucocorticoids. Response to oral glucocorticoids may predict those patients who will respond to inhaled glucocorticoids. Except for the treatment of acute bronchospastic episodes, glucocorticoids have given mixed results in the treatment of COPD. In some patients, theophylline may be effective; in others who have a salutary response to β_2 adrenergic agonists, theophylline may provide no additional bronchodilation beyond that already achieved.

In a minority of patients, emphysema results from a genetic deficiency of the plasma proteinase inhibitor α_1-antiproteinase (also called α_1-antitrypsin). Lung tissue destruction is caused by the unopposed action of neutrophil elastase and other proteinases. Purified α_1-*antiproteinase* (PROLASTIN) from human plasma is available for intravenous replacement.

CLINICAL SUMMARY

Bronchodilating drugs, exemplified by the *short-acting β_2 adrenergic receptor agonists,* are used acutely to reverse the bronchospasm of an asthma attack. Anti-inflammatory drugs such as inhaled *glucocorticoids* are used to quell bronchial inflammation in an effort to reduce the severity and frequency of asthma attacks. In hospitalized patients, a short course of systemic steroids often is given, followed by a rapid taper. In patients who remain symptomatic despite inhaled glucocorticoid therapy, *long-acting β_2 adrenergic receptor agonists* may be added to the steroid regimen with good success. Newer agents, directed at specific mechanisms underlying the initiation or progression of asthma, include the *leukotriene receptor antagonists* and the anti-IgE therapy *omalizumab.* The anticholinergic agent *tiotropium* is approved for the treatment of COPD in the U.S.

For a complete Bibliographical listing see Goodman & Gilman's *The Pharmacological Basis of Therapeutics,* 11th ed., or Goodman & Gilman Online at www.accessmedicine.com.

28

DIURETICS

RENAL ANATOMY AND PHYSIOLOGY

The kidney filters large quantities of plasma, reabsorbs substances that the body must conserve, and leaves behind and/or secretes substances that must be eliminated. The two kidneys in humans produce together ~120 mL/min of ultrafiltrate, yet only 1 mL/min of urine is produced. The basic urine-forming unit of the kidney is the nephron, which consists of a filtering apparatus, the glomerulus, connected to a long tubular portion that reabsorbs and conditions the glomerular ultrafiltrate. Each human kidney has ~1 ×10⁶ nephrons. The structure of the nephron and the site of action of different classes of diuretics are shown in Figure 28–1.

The proximal tubule of the nephron is contiguous with Bowman's capsule and takes a tortuous path until finally forming a straight portion that dives into the renal medulla. Normally, ~65% of filtered Na^+ is reabsorbed in the proximal tubule; since this part of the tubule is highly permeable to water, reabsorption is essentially isotonic. Between the outer and inner strips of the outer medulla, the tubule abruptly changes morphology to become the descending thin limb (DTL), which penetrates the inner medulla, makes a hairpin turn, and then forms the ascending thin limb (ATL). At the juncture between the inner and outer medulla, the tubule becomes the thick ascending limb (TAL), which consists of three segments: a medullary portion (MTAL), a cortical portion (CTAL), and a postmacular segment. Together the proximal straight tubule, DTL, ATL, MTAL, CTAL, and postmacular segment are known as the loop of Henle. *The DTL is highly permeable to water but relatively impermeable to NaCl and urea. In contrast, the ATL is permeable to NaCl and urea but impermeable to water. The TAL actively reabsorbs NaCl but is impermeable to water and urea. Approximately 25% of filtered Na^+ is reabsorbed in the loop of Henle, mostly in the TAL, which has a large reabsorptive capacity.*

The TAL passes between the afferent and efferent arterioles and makes contact with the afferent arteriole via *a cluster of specialized columnar epithelial cells known as the* macula densa. *The macula densa is strategically located to sense concentrations of NaCl leaving the loop of Henle. If the concentration of NaCl is too high, the macula densa sends a chemical signal (perhaps adenosine or ATP) to the afferent arteriole of the same nephron, causing it to constrict. This, in turn, causes a reduction in* glomerular filtration rate *(GFR). This homeostatic mechanism, known as* tubuloglomerular feedback *(TGF), serves to protect the organism from salt and volume wasting. The macula densa also regulates renin release from the adjacent juxtaglomerular cells in the wall of the afferent arteriole.*

Approximately 0.2 mm past the macula densa, the tubule becomes the distal convoluted tubule (DCT). The postmacular segment of the TAL and the DCT often are referred to as the early distal tubule. *Like the TAL, the DCT actively transports NaCl and is impermeable to water. Since these characteristics impart the ability to produce a dilute urine, the TAL and the DCT are collectively called the* diluting segment of the nephron, *and the tubular fluid in the DCT is hypotonic regardless of hydration status. However, unlike the TAL, the DCT does not contribute to the countercurrent-induced hypertonicity of the medullary interstitium (see below).*

The collecting duct system (connecting tubule, initial collecting tubule, cortical collecting duct, and outer and inner medullary collecting ducts) is an area of fine control of ultrafiltrate composition and volume and is where final adjustments in electrolyte composition are made. In addition, vasopressin (also called antidiuretic hormone; see Chapter 29) modulates water permeability of this part of the nephron.

The more distal portions of the collecting duct pass through the renal medulla, where the interstitial fluid is markedly hypertonic. In the absence of vasopressin, the collecting duct system is impermeable to water, and a dilute urine is excreted. In the presence of vasopressin, the collecting duct system is permeable to water, which is reabsorbed down a steep concentration gradient that exists between the tubular fluid and the medullary interstitium.

The hypertonicity of the medullary interstitium plays a vital role in the ability to concentrate urine, which is accomplished via a combination of the unique topography of the loop of Henle and the specialized permeability features of the loop's subsegments. The "passive countercurrent

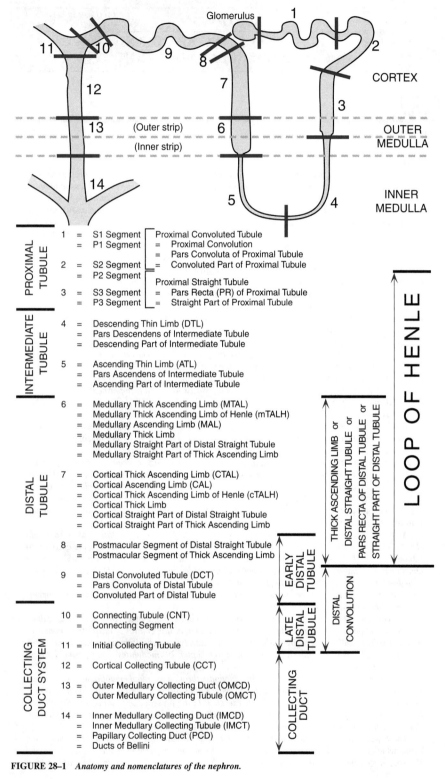

FIGURE 28–1 *Anatomy and nomenclatures of the nephron.*

multiplier hypothesis" proposes that active transport in the TAL concentrates NaCl in the interstitium of the outer medulla, thus generating its hypertonicity. Since this segment of the nephron is impermeable to water, active transport in the ascending limb dilutes the tubular fluid. As the dilute fluid passes into the collecting-duct system, water is extracted if, and only if, vasopressin is present. Since the cortical and outer medullary collecting ducts have a low permeability to urea, urea is concentrated in the tubular fluid. The inner medullary collecting duct, however, is permeable to urea, so urea diffuses into the inner medulla, where it is trapped by countercurrent exchange in the vasa recta. Since the DTL is impermeable to salt and urea, the high urea concentration in the inner medulla extracts water from the DTL and concentrates NaCl in the tubular fluid of the DTL. As the tubular fluid enters the ATL, NaCl diffuses out of the salt-permeable ATL, contributing to the hypertonicity of the medullary interstitium.

In the glomerular capillaries, a portion of the plasma water is forced through a filter that has three basic components: fenestrated capillary endothelial cells, a basement membrane lying just beneath the endothelial cells, and the filtration slit diaphragms formed by the epithelial cells that cover the basement membrane on its urinary space side. Solutes of small size flow with filtered water (solvent drag) into the urinary (Bowman's) space, whereas formed elements and macromolecules are retained by the filtration barrier.

PRINCIPLES OF DIURETIC ACTION

Diuretics are drugs that increase the rate of urine flow; clinically useful diuretics also increase the rate of excretion of Na^+ (natriuresis) and an accompanying anion, usually Cl^-. Most clinical applications of diuretics aim to reduce extracellular fluid volume by decreasing total-body NaCl content. Although continued administration of a diuretic causes a sustained net deficit in total-body Na^+, the time course of natriuresis is finite because renal compensatory mechanisms bring Na^+ excretion in line with Na^+ intake, a phenomenon known as *diuretic braking*. Compensatory mechanisms include activation of the sympathetic nervous system, activation of the renin–angiotensin–aldosterone axis, decreased arterial blood pressure (which reduces pressure natriuresis), hypertrophy of renal epithelial cells, increased expression of renal epithelial transporters, and perhaps alterations in natriuretic hormones such as atrial natriuretic peptide.

Diuretics alter the excretion of Na^+ and also may modify renal handling of other cations (*e.g.*, K^+, H^+, Ca^{2+}, and Mg^{2+}), anions (*e.g.*, Cl^-, HCO_3^-, and $H_2PO_4^-$), and uric acid. In addition, diuretics may alter renal hemodynamics indirectly. Table 28–1 compares the general effects of diuretics classified according to mechanism of action.

INHIBITORS OF CARBONIC ANHYDRASE

The three carbonic anhydrase inhibitors available in the U.S. are *acetazolamide* (DIAMOX), *dichlorphenamide* (DARANIDE), and *methazolamide* (GLAUCTABS). Proximal tubular epithelial cells are richly endowed with the zinc metalloenzyme carbonic anhydrase, which is found in the luminal and basolateral membranes (type IV carbonic anhydrase), as well as in the cytoplasm (type II carbonic anhydrase). Carbonic anhydrase plays a key role in $NaHCO_3$ reabsorption and acid secretion. In the proximal tubule, the free energy in the Na^+ gradient established by the basolateral Na^+ pump is used by a Na^+–H^+ antiporter (also referred to as an Na^+–H^+ exchanger) in the luminal membrane to transport H^+ into the tubular lumen in exchange for Na^+ (Figure 28–1). In the lumen, H^+ reacts with filtered HCO_3^- to form H_2CO_3. Normally, the breakdown of H_2CO_3 to form CO_2 and water occurs slowly, but carbonic anhydrase reversibly accelerates this reaction several thousand times. CO_2 rapidly diffuses across the luminal membrane into the epithelial cell, where it reacts with water to form H_2CO_3, a reaction catalyzed by cytoplasmic carbonic anhydrase. Continued operation of the Na^+–H^+ antiporter maintains a low proton concentration in the cell, so H_2CO_3 ionizes spontaneously to form H^+ and HCO_3^-, creating an electrochemical gradient for HCO_3^- across the basolateral membrane. The electrochemical gradient for HCO_3^- is used by a Na^+–HCO_3^- symporter (also referred to as the Na^+–HCO_3^- cotransporter) in the basolateral membrane to transport $NaHCO_3$ into the interstitial space. The net effect is transport of $NaHCO_3$ from the tubular lumen to the interstitial space, followed by movement of water (isotonic reabsorption). Removal of water concentrates Cl^- in the tubular lumen, and consequently Cl^- diffuses down its concentration gradient into the interstitium *via* the paracellular pathway.

Carbonic anhydrase inhibitors potently inhibit both the membrane-bound and cytoplasmic forms of carbonic anhydrase, resulting in nearly complete abolition of $NaHCO_3$ reabsorption in the proximal tubule (Figure 28–2). Because of the large excess of carbonic anhydrase in proximal tubules, a high percentage of enzyme activity must be inhibited before an effect on electrolyte

Table 28–1

Excretory and Renal Hemodynamic Effects of Diuretics*

	Cations					Anions			Uric Acid		Renal Hemodynamics			
	Na+	K+	H+†	Ca2+	Mg2+	Cl−	HCO3−	H2PO4−	Acute	Chronic	RBF	GFR	FF	TGF
Inhibitors of carbonic anhydrase (primary site of action is proximal tubule)	+	++	−	NC	V	(+)	++	++	I	−	−	−	NC	+
Osmotic diuretics (primary site of action is loop of Henle)	++	+	I	+	++	+	+	+	+	I	+	NC	−	I
Inhibitors of Na+–K+–2Cl− symport (primary site of action is thick ascending limb)	++	++	+	++	++	++	+‡	+‡	+	−	V(+)	NC	V(−)	−
Inhibitors of Na+–Cl− symport (primary site of action is distal convoluted tubule)	+	++	+	V(−)	V(+)	+	+‡	+‡	+	−	NC	V(−)	V(−)	NC
Inhibitors of renal epithelial sodium channels (primary site of action is late distal tubule and collecting duct)	+	−	−	−	−	+	(+)	NC	I	−	NC	NC	NC	NC
Antagonists of mineralocorticoid receptors (primary site of action is late distal tubule and collecting duct)	+	−	−	I	−	+	(+)	I	I	−	NC	NC	NC	NC

*Except for uric acid, changes are for acute effects of diuretics in the absence of significant volume depletion, which would trigger complex physiological adjustments; ++, +, (+), −, NC, V, V(+), V(−) and I indicate marked increase, mild-to-moderate increase, slight increase, decrease, no change, variable effect, variable increase, variable decrease, and insufficient data, respectively. For cations and anions, the indicated effects refer to absolute changes in fractional excretion. RBF, renal blood flow; GFR, glomerular filtration rate; FF, filtration fraction; TGF, tubuloglomerular feedback.

†H+, titratable acid, and NH4+.

‡In general, these effects are restricted to those individual agents that inhibit carbonic anhydrase. However, there are notable exceptions in which symport inhibitors increase bicarbonate and phosphate (e.g., metolazone, bumetanide).

PROXIMAL TUBULE

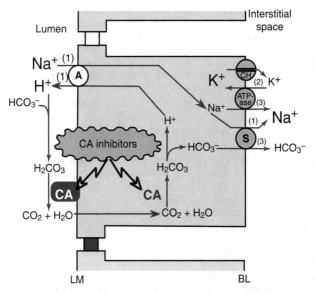

FIGURE 28–2 *NaHCO₃ reabsorption in proximal tubule and mechanism of diuretic action of carbonic anhydrase (CA) inhibitors.* A, antiporter; S, symporter; CH, ion channel. (The actual reaction catalyzed by carbonic anhydrase is $OH^- + CO_2 \rightarrow HCO_3^-$; however, $H_2O \rightarrow OH^- + H^+ \rightarrow$ and $HCO_3^- + H^+ \rightarrow H_2CO_3$, so the net reaction is $H_2O + CO_2 \rightarrow H_2CO_3$.) Numbers in parentheses indicate stoichiometry. BL and LM indicate basolateral and luminal membranes, respectively. The sizes of type for Na^+, K^+, and H^+ reflect relative concentrations.

excretion is observed. Although the proximal tubule is the major site of action of carbonic anhydrase inhibitors, carbonic anhydrase also is involved in secretion of titratable acid in the collecting duct system, which is a secondary site of action for these drugs.

EFFECTS ON URINARY EXCRETION   Inhibition of carbonic anhydrase is associated with a rapid rise in urinary HCO_3^- excretion to ~35% of filtered load. This, along with inhibition of titratable acid and NH_4^+ secretion in the collecting-duct system, results in an increase in urinary pH to ~8 and development of a metabolic acidosis. However, even with a high degree of inhibition of carbonic anhydrase, 65% of HCO_3^- is rescued from excretion by poorly understood mechanisms. Inhibition of the transport mechanism described above results in increased delivery of Na^+ and Cl^- to the loop of Henle, which has a large reabsorptive capacity and captures most of the Cl^- and a portion of the Na^+. Thus, only a small increase in Cl^- excretion occurs, HCO_3^- being the major anion excreted along with the cations Na^+ and K^+. The fractional excretion of Na^+ may be as much as 5%, and the fractional excretion of K^+ can be as much as 70%. The increased excretion of K^+ in part reflects increased delivery of Na^+ to the distal nephron, as described in the section on inhibitors of Na^+ channels. Other mechanisms contributing to enhanced K^+ excretion include flow-dependent enhancement of K^+ secretion by the collecting duct, nonosmotic vasopressin release, and activation of the renin–angiotensin–aldosterone axis. Carbonic anhydrase inhibitors increase phosphate excretion but have little or no effect on the excretion of Ca^{2+} or Mg^{2+}. The effects of carbonic anhydrase inhibitors on renal excretion are self-limiting, probably because the resulting metabolic acidosis decreases the filtered load of HCO_3^- to the point that the uncatalyzed reaction between CO_2 and water is sufficient to achieve HCO_3^- reabsorption.

EFFECTS ON RENAL HEMODYNAMICS   By inhibiting proximal reabsorption, carbonic anhydrase inhibitors increase solute delivery to the macula densa. This triggers TGF, which increases afferent arteriolar resistance and reduces renal blood flow (RBF) and GFR.

OTHER ACTIONS   Carbonic anhydrase is present in a number of extrarenal tissues. Carbonic anhydrase in the ciliary processes of the eye mediates the formation of large amounts of HCO_3^- in aqueous humor. Inhibition of carbonic anhydrase decreases the rate of formation of aqueous humor and consequently reduces intraocular pressure (IOP). Acetazolamide frequently causes paresthesias and somnolence, suggesting a central nervous system (CNS) action of carbonic anhydrase inhibitors. The efficacy of acetazolamide in epilepsy is due in part to the production of metabolic acidosis; however, direct actions of acetazolamide in the CNS also contribute to its anticonvulsant action. Owing to interference with carbonic anhydrase activity in erythrocytes, carbonic anhydrase inhibitors increase CO_2 levels in peripheral tissues and decrease CO_2 levels in expired gas. Large doses of carbonic anhydrase inhibitors reduce gastric acid secretion, but this has no therapeutic applications. Acetazolamide causes vasodilation by opening vascular Ca^{2+}-activated K^+ channels; however, the clinical significance of this effect is unclear.

ABSORPTION AND ELIMINATION The oral bioavailability, plasma $t_{1/2}$, and route of elimination of the three available carbonic anhydrase inhibitors are listed in Table 28–2. Carbonic anhydrase inhibitors bind avidly to the enzyme; thus, tissues rich in this enzyme will have higher concentrations of drug following systemic administration.

TOXICITY, ADVERSE EFFECTS, CONTRAINDICATIONS, DRUG INTERACTIONS Serious toxic reactions to carbonic anhydrase inhibitors are infrequent; however, these drugs are sulfonamide derivatives and, like other sulfonamides, may cause bone marrow depression, skin toxicity, sulfonamide-like renal lesions, and allergic reactions (see Chapter 43). With large doses, many patients exhibit drowsiness and paresthesias. Most adverse effects, contraindications, and drug interactions are secondary to urinary alkalinization or metabolic acidosis, including (1) diversion of ammonia of renal origin from urine into the systemic circulation, a process that may induce or worsen hepatic encephalopathy (the drugs are contraindicated in patients with hepatic cirrhosis); (2) calculus formation and ureteral colic owing to precipitation of calcium phosphate salts in an alkaline urine; (3) worsened metabolic or respiratory acidosis (the drugs are contraindicated in patients with hyperchloremic acidosis or severe chronic obstructive pulmonary disease); and (4) reduced urinary excretion of weak organic bases.

THERAPEUTIC USES The efficacy of carbonic anhydrase inhibitors as single agents for the treatment of edema is low. However, the combination of acetazolamide with diuretics that block Na^+ reabsorption at more distal sites in the nephron causes a marked natriuretic response in patients with low basal fractional excretion of Na^+ (<0.2%), who are resistant to diuretic monotherapy. Even so, the long-term usefulness of carbonic anhydrase inhibitors often is compromised by the development of metabolic acidosis.

Table 28–2

Inhibitors of Carbonic Anhydrase

Drug (TRADE NAME)	Structure	Relative Potency	Oral Availability	$t_{1/2}$ (hours)	Route of Elimination
Acetazolamide (DIAMOX)	CH$_3$CONH — S — SO$_2$NH$_2$ / N — N	1	~100%	6–9	R
Dichlorphenamide (DARAMIDE)	SO$_2$NH$_2$ / Cl — SO$_2$NH$_2$ / Cl	30	ID	ID	ID
Methazolamide (GLAUCTABS)	CH$_3$CON — S — SO$_2$NH$_2$ / N — N / H$_3$C	>1, <10	~100%	~14	~25%R, ~75% M

ABBREVIATIONS: R, renal excretion of intact drug; M, metabolism; ID, insufficient data.

The major indication for carbonic anhydrase inhibitors is open-angle glaucoma. Carbonic anhydrase inhibitors also may be employed for secondary glaucoma and preoperatively in acute angle-closure glaucoma to lower IOP before surgery (*see* Chapter 63). Acetazolamide also is used for the treatment of epilepsy, but the rapid development of tolerance may limit its usefulness. Acetazolamide may provide symptomatic relief in patients with altitude sickness; however, it is more effective when given prophylactically. Acetazolamide also is useful in patients with familial periodic paralysis. The mechanism for the beneficial effects of acetazolamide in altitude sickness and familial periodic paralysis may be related to the induction of a metabolic acidosis. Finally, carbonic anhydrase inhibitors can be useful for correcting metabolic alkalosis, especially that caused by diuretic-induced increases in H^+ excretion.

OSMOTIC DIURETICS

Osmotic diuretics are freely filtered at the glomerulus, undergo limited reabsorption by the renal tubule, and are relatively inert pharmacologically. Osmotic diuretics are administered in sufficient doses to increase significantly the osmolality of plasma and tubular fluid. Table 28–3 gives pharmacokinetic properties of four osmotic diuretics—*glycerin* (OSMOGLYN), *isosorbide* (ISMOTIC), *mannitol* (OSMITROL), and *urea* (UREAPHIL). The major site of action of osmotic diuretics is the loop of Henle.

By extracting water from intracellular compartments, osmotic diuretics expand the extracellular fluid volume, decrease blood viscosity, and inhibit renin release. These effects increase RBF, and the increase in renal medullary blood flow removes NaCl and urea from the renal medulla, thus reducing medullary tonicity. Under some circumstances, prostaglandins may contribute to the renal vasodilation and medullary washout induced by osmotic diuretics. A reduction in medullary tonicity causes a decrease in the extraction of water from the DTL, which limits the concentration of NaCl in the tubular fluid entering the ATL. This latter effect diminishes the passive reabsorption of NaCl in the ATL. In addition, osmotic diuretics may also interfere with transport processes in the TAL.

Table 28–3

Osmotic Diuretics

Drug (TRADE NAME)	Structure	Oral Availability	$t_{1/2}$ (hours)	Route of Elimination
Glycerin (OSMOGLYN)	HO⌒⌒OH / OH	Orally active	0.5–0.75	~80% M / ~20% U
Isosorbide (ISMOTIC)		Orally active	5–9.5	R
Mannitol (OSMITROL)	OH OH OH OH / OH OH	Negligible	0.25–1.7*	~80% R / ~20% M + B
Urea (UREAPHIL)	O ‖ H₂N—C—NH₂	Negligible	ID	R

*In renal failure, 6–36h.

ABBREVIATIONS: R, renal excretion of intact drug; M, metabolism; B, excretion of intact drug into bile; U, unknown pathway of elimination; ID, insufficient data.

EFFECTS ON URINARY EXCRETION Osmotic diuretics increase the urinary excretion of nearly all electrolytes, including Na^+, K^+, Ca^{2+}, Mg^{2+}, Cl^-, HCO_3^-, and phosphate.

EFFECTS ON RENAL HEMODYNAMICS Osmotic diuretics increase RBF by a variety of mechanisms, but total GFR usually is little changed.

ABSORPTION AND ELIMINATION The oral bioavailability, plasma $t_{1/2}$, and route of elimination of the available osmotic diuretics are listed in Table 28–3. Glycerin and isosorbide can be given orally; mannitol and urea must be administered intravenously.

TOXICITY, ADVERSE EFFECTS, CONTRAINDICATIONS, DRUG INTERACTIONS
Osmotic diuretics are distributed in the extracellular fluid and contribute to extracellular osmolality. Thus, water is extracted from intracellular compartments, and the extracellular fluid volume becomes expanded. In patients with heart failure or pulmonary congestion, this may cause frank pulmonary edema. Extraction of water also causes hyponatremia, which may explain the common adverse effects, including headache, nausea, and vomiting. On the other hand, loss of water in excess of electrolytes can cause hypernatremia and dehydration. Osmotic diuretics generally are contraindicated in patients who are anuric owing to renal disease or who are unresponsive to test doses of the drugs. Urea may cause thrombosis or pain if extravasation occurs and should not be administered to patients with impaired liver function because of the risk of elevation of blood ammonia levels. Both mannitol and urea are contraindicated in patients with active intracranial bleeding. Glycerin is metabolized and can cause hyperglycemia.

THERAPEUTIC USES Acute renal failure (ARF) occurs in 5% of hospitalized patients and is associated with a significant mortality rate. Acute tubular necrosis (ATN), *i.e.*, damage to tubular epithelial cells, accounts for most cases of intrinsic ARF. The clinical efficacy of mannitol in attenuating the reduction in GFR due to ischemic or nephrotoxic insults is debated and controlled studies have not shown a benefit over hydration *per se*. In patients with mild-to-moderate renal insufficiency, hydration with 0.45% NaCl is as good as or better than either mannitol or furosemide in protection against decreases in GFR induced by radiocontrast agents. Prophylactic mannitol apparently is effective in jaundiced patients undergoing surgery. However, in vascular and open-heart surgery, prophylactic mannitol maintains urine flow but not GFR. In established ATN, mannitol will increase urine volume in some patients, and patients converted from oliguric to nonoliguric ATN appear to recover more rapidly and require less dialysis compared with patients who do not respond to mannitol. Whether these benefits are due to the diuretic or whether "responders" have lesser degrees of renal damage from the outset compared with "nonresponders" is not clear. Repeated administration of mannitol to nonresponders is not recommended, and loop diuretics are used more frequently to convert oliguric to nonoliguric ATN.

Another use for mannitol and urea is in the treatment of dialysis disequilibrium syndrome. Too rapid removal of solutes from the extracellular fluid by hemo- or peritoneal dialysis reduces the osmolality of the extracellular fluid. Consequently, water moves from the extracellular compartment into the intracellular compartment, causing hypotension and CNS symptoms (*i.e.*, headache, nausea, muscle cramps, restlessness, CNS depression, and convulsions). Osmotic diuretics increase the osmolality of the extracellular fluid compartment and thereby shift water back into the extracellular compartment.

By increasing plasma osmotic pressure, osmotic diuretics extract water from the eye and brain. All four osmotic diuretics are used to control IOP during acute attacks of glaucoma and for short-term reductions in IOP in patients who require ocular surgery. Mannitol and urea also are used to reduce cerebral edema before and after neurosurgery.

INHIBITORS OF NA^+–K^+–$2CL^-$ SYMPORT (LOOP DIURETICS, HIGH-CEILING DIURETICS)

These diuretics inhibit the activity of the Na^+–K^+–$2Cl^-$ symporter in the TAL of the loop of Henle, hence, their designation as *loop diuretics*. Although the proximal tubule reabsorbs ~65% of the filtered Na^+, diuretics acting only in the proximal tubule have limited efficacy because the TAL has the capacity to reabsorb most of the rejectate from the proximal tubule. In contrast, inhibitors of Na^+–K^+–$2Cl^-$ symport in the TAL, sometimes called *high-ceiling diuretics*, are highly efficacious due to a combination of two factors: (1) Approximately 25% of the filtered Na^+ load normally is reabsorbed by the TAL, and (2) nephron segments past the TAL do not possess the reabsorptive capacity to rescue the flood of rejectate exiting the TAL.

Inhibitors of Na+–K+–2Cl− symport are chemically diverse. Furosemide *(LASIX)*, bumetanide *(BUMEX)*, ethacrynic acid *(EDECRIN)*, and torsemide *(DEMADEX) are available in the U.S. Furosemide and bumetanide contain a sulfonamide moiety, ethacrynic acid is a phenoxyacetic acid derivative, and torsemide is a sulfonylurea.*

The flux of Na+, K+, and Cl− from the lumen into the epithelial cells in the TAL is mediated by the Na+–K+–2Cl− symporter (Figure 28–1). This symporter captures the free energy in the Na+ electrochemical gradient established by the basolateral Na+ pump and provides for "uphill" transport of K+ and Cl− into the cell. Hyperpolarization of the luminal membrane due to K+ conductance through apical K+ channels (called *ROMK*) and depolarization of the basolateral membrane due to Cl− conductance through basolateral Cl− channels (called *CLC-Kb*) result in a transepithelial potential difference, with the lumen positive with respect to the interstitial space. This lumen-positive potential difference repels cations (Na+, Ca2+, and Mg2+) and thereby provides an important driving force for the paracellular flux of these cations into the interstitial space.

Inhibitors of the Na+–K+–2Cl− symporter block its function, virtually abolishing salt transport in this segment of the nephron (Figure 28–3). Evidence suggests that these drugs attach to the Cl−-binding site located in the symporter's transmembrane domain. Inhibitors of Na+–K+–2Cl− symport also inhibit Ca2+ and Mg2+ reabsorption in the TAL by abolishing the transepithelial potential difference that is the dominant driving force for reabsorption of these cations.

Na+–K+–2Cl− symporters are found in many secretory and absorbing epithelia and are of two varieties. The "absorptive" symporter (called ENCC2, NKCC2, or BSC1) is expressed only in the kidney, where it is localized to the apical membrane and subapical intracellular vesicles of the TAL and regulated by cyclic AMP-PKA. The "secretory" symporter (called ENCC3, NKCC1, or BSC2) is a widely expressed "housekeeping" protein. The affinity of loop diuretics for the secretory symporter is somewhat less than for the absorptive symporter (e.g., fourfold difference for bumetanide). Mutations in the genes coding for the absorptive Na+–K+–2Cl− symporter, the apical K+ channel, or the basolateral Cl− channel are causes of Bartter's syndrome (inherited hypokalemic alkalosis with salt wasting and hypotension).

THICK ASCENDING LIMB

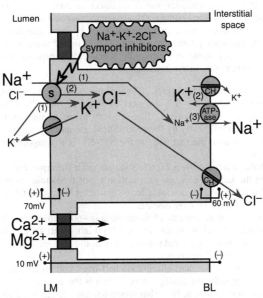

FIGURE 28–3 *NaCl reabsorption in thick ascending limb and mechanism of diuretic action of Na+–K+–2Cl− symport inhibitors.* S, symporter; CH, ion channel. Numbers in parentheses indicate stoichiometry. Designated voltages are the potential differences across the indicated membrane or cell. The mechanisms illustrated here apply to the medullary, cortical, and postmacular segments of the thick ascending limb. BL and LM indicate basolateral and luminal membranes, respectively.

EFFECTS ON URINARY EXCRETION Loop diuretics profoundly increase the urinary excretion of Na^+ and Cl^- (*i.e.*, up to 25% of the filtered load of Na^+) and markedly increase the excretion of Ca^{2+} and Mg^{2+}. Furosemide but not bumetanide also has weak carbonic anhydrase-inhibiting activity that increases the urinary excretion of HCO_3^- and phosphate. All inhibitors of the Na^+-K^+-$2Cl^-$ symporter increase the urinary excretion of K^+ and titratable acid, due in part to increased delivery of Na^+ to the distal tubule. The mechanism by which increased distal delivery of Na^+ enhances excretion of K^+ and H^+ is discussed in the section on inhibitors of Na^+ channels. Other mechanisms contributing to enhanced K^+ and H^+ excretion include flow-dependent enhancement of ion secretion by the collecting duct, nonosmotic vasopressin release, and activation of the renin–angiotensin–aldosterone axis. Loop diuretics acutely increase the excretion of uric acid, whereas their chronic administration reduces uric acid excretion, possibly due to enhanced transport in the proximal tubule secondary to volume depletion or to competition between the diuretic and uric acid for the organic acid secretory mechanism in the proximal tubule.

By blocking active NaCl reabsorption in the TAL, inhibitors of Na^+-K^+-$2Cl^-$ symport interfere with a critical step in the mechanism that produces a hypertonic medullary interstitium. Therefore, loop diuretics block the kidney's ability to concentrate urine. Also, since the TAL is part of the diluting segment, inhibitors of the Na^+-K^+-$2Cl^-$ symporter markedly impair the kidney's ability to excrete a dilute urine during water diuresis.

EFFECTS ON RENAL HEMODYNAMICS If volume depletion is prevented by replacing fluid losses, inhibitors of Na^+-K^+-$2Cl^-$ symport generally increase total RBF and redistribute it to the midcortex. However, these effects are variable. The mechanism of the increase in RBF is not known, but nonsteroidal anti-inflammatory drugs (NSAIDs) attenuate the diuretic response to loop diuretics in part by preventing prostaglandin-mediated increases in RBF. Loop diuretics block TGF by inhibiting salt transport into the macula densa so that the macula densa no longer can detect NaCl concentrations in the tubular fluid. Unlike carbonic anhydrase inhibitors, loop diuretics do not decrease GFR by activating TGF. Loop diuretics stimulate renin release by interfering with NaCl transport by the macula densa and, if volume depletion occurs, by reflex activation of the sympathetic nervous system and stimulation of the intrarenal baroreceptor mechanism. Prostaglandins (*e.g.*, PGI_2) may play a key role in mediating the renin-release response to loop diuretics.

OTHER ACTIONS Loop diuretics may cause direct vascular effects. Loop diuretics, particularly furosemide, acutely increase systemic venous capacitance and thereby decrease left ventricular filling pressure. This effect, which may be mediated by prostaglandins and requires intact kidneys, benefits patients with pulmonary edema even before diuresis ensues. High doses of inhibitors of the Na^+-K^+-$2Cl^-$ symporter can inhibit electrolyte transport in many tissues, but this effect is clinically important only in the inner ear.

ABSORPTION AND ELIMINATION The oral bioavailabilities, plasma $t_{1/2}$, and routes of elimination of inhibitors of Na^+-K^+-$2Cl^-$ symport are listed in Table 28–4. Because these drugs are bound extensively to plasma proteins, their delivery to the tubules by filtration is limited. However, they are secreted efficiently by the organic acid transport system in the proximal tubule and thereby gain access to their binding sites on the Na^+-K^+-$2Cl^-$ symporter in the luminal membrane of the TAL.

Approximately 65% of furosemide is excreted unchanged in the urine, and the rest is conjugated to glucuronic acid in the kidney; thus, the elimination $t_{1/2}$ of furosemide is prolonged in patients with renal disease. Bumetanide and torsemide have significant hepatic metabolism, and their elimination half-lives are prolonged by liver disease.

Although the average oral availability of furosemide is ~60%, this varies from 10–100%; oral availabilities of bumetanide and torsemide are reliably high. Heart failure patients treated with torsemide have fewer hospitalizations and better quality of life than those treated with furosemide, perhaps because of its reliable absorption.

As a class, loop diuretics have short elimination half-lives, and prolonged-release preparations are not available. Consequently, the dosing interval often is too short to maintain adequate levels of loop diuretics in the tubular lumen. Note that torsemide has a longer $t_{1/2}$ than other agents available in the U.S. (Table 28–4). As the concentration of loop diuretic in the tubular lumen declines, nephrons begin to avidly reabsorb Na^+, which often nullifies the overall effect of the loop diuretic on total-body Na^+. This phenomenon of "postdiuretic Na^+ retention" can be overcome by restricting dietary Na^+ intake or by more frequent administration of the loop diuretic.

Table 28-4

Inhibitors of Na$^+$-K$^+$-2Cl$^-$ Symport (Loop Diuretics, High–Ceiling Diuretics)

Drug (TRADE NAME)	Structure	Relative Potency	Oral Availability	$t_{1/2}$ (hours)	Route of Elimination
Furosemide (LASIX)	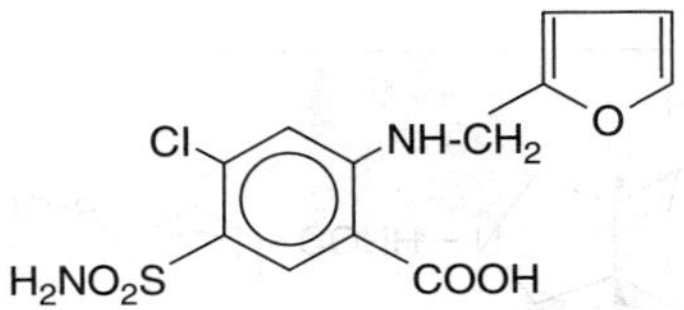	1	~60%	~1.5	~65% R ~35% M‡
Bumetanide (BUMEX)	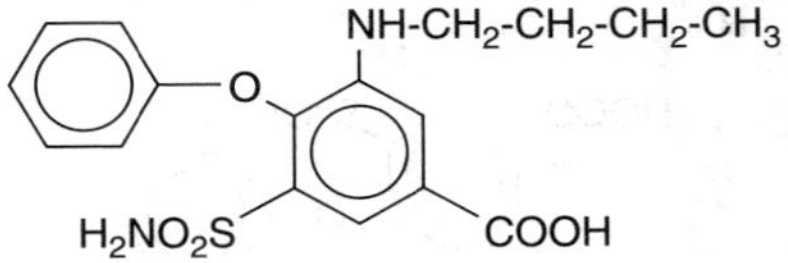	40	~80%	~0.8	~62% R ~38% M
Ethacrynic acid (EDECRIN)	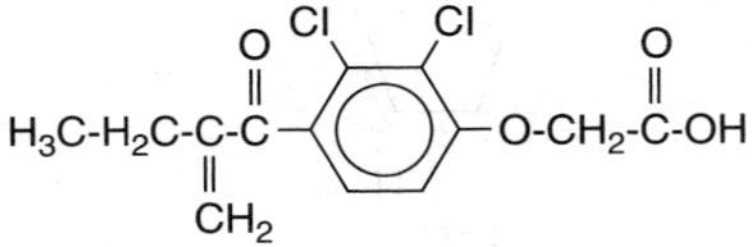	0.7	~100%	~1	~67% R ~33% M
Torsemide (DEMADEX)	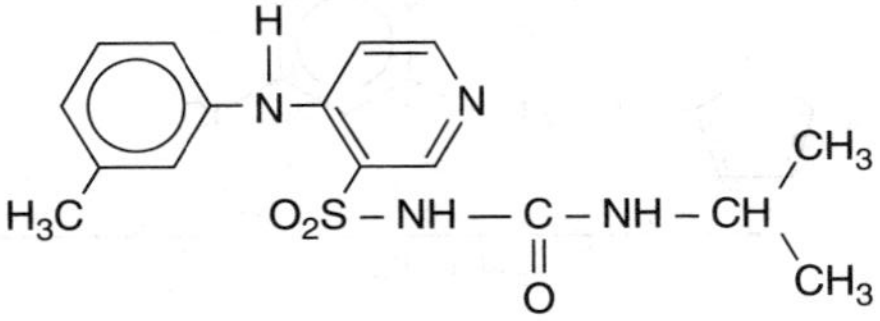	3	~80%	~3.5	~20% R ~80% M

(Continued)

485

Table 28-4

Inhibitors of Na⁺–K⁺–2Cl⁻ Symport (Loop Diuretics, High–Ceiling Diuretics) (*Continued*)

Drug (TRADE NAME)	Structure	Relative Potency	Oral Availability	$t_{1/2}$ (hours)	Route of Elimination
Axosemide*		1	~12%	~2.5	~27% R 63% M
Piretanide*		3	~80%	0.6–1.5	~50% R ~50% M
Tripamide*		ID	ID	ID	ID

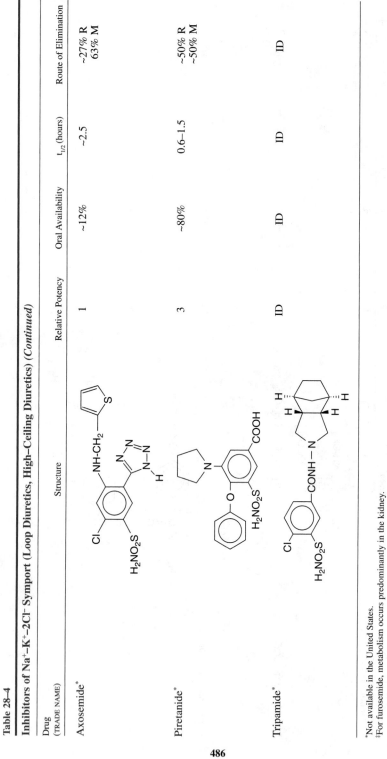

*Not available in the United States.

‡For furosemide, metabolism occurs predominantly in the kidney.

ABBREVIATIONS: R, renal excretion of intact drug; M, metabolism; ID, insufficient data.

TOXICITY, ADVERSE EFFECTS, CONTRAINDICATIONS, DRUG INTERACTIONS

Adverse effects unrelated to diuretic efficacy are rare, and most adverse effects are due to abnormalities of fluid and electrolyte balance. Overzealous use of loop diuretics can seriously deplete total-body Na^+, which may be manifest as hyponatremia and/or extracellular fluid volume depletion associated with hypotension, reduced GFR, circulatory collapse, thromboembolic events, and in patients with liver disease, hepatic encephalopathy. Increased delivery of Na^+ to the distal tubule, particularly when combined with activation of the renin-angiotensin system, leads to increased urinary excretion of K^+ and H^+, causing a hypochloremic alkalosis. If dietary K^+ intake is not sufficient, hypokalemia may develop, and this may induce cardiac arrhythmias, particularly in patients taking cardiac glycosides or antiarrhythmic drugs that prolong repolarization (*see* Chapter 34). Increased Mg^{2+} and Ca^{2+} excretion may result in hypomagnesemia (a risk factor for cardiac arrhythmias) and hypocalcemia (rarely leading to tetany). Recent evidence suggests that loop diuretics should be avoided in postmenopausal osteopenic women, in whom increased Ca^{2+} excretion may have deleterious effects on bone metabolism.

Loop diuretics can cause ototoxicity that manifests as tinnitus, hearing impairment, deafness, vertigo, and a sense of fullness in the ears. Hearing impairment and deafness are usually reversible. Ototoxicity occurs most frequently with rapid intravenous administration and least frequently with oral administration. Ethacrynic acid appears to induce ototoxicity more often than do other loop diuretics and should be used only in patients who cannot tolerate the other drugs. Loop diuretics also can cause hyperuricemia (occasionally leading to gout) and hyperglycemia (infrequently precipitating diabetes mellitus) and can increase plasma levels of low-density lipoprotein (LDL) cholesterol and triglycerides while decreasing plasma levels of high-density lipoprotein (HDL) cholesterol. Other adverse effects include rashes, photosensitivity, paresthesias, bone marrow depression, and GI disturbances.

Contraindications to the use of loop diuretics include severe Na^+ and volume depletion, hypersensitivity to sulfonamides (for sulfonamide-based loop diuretics), and anuria unresponsive to a trial dose of loop diuretic.

Drug interactions may occur when loop diuretics are coadministered with (1) aminoglycosides (synergism of ototoxicity caused by both drugs), (2) anticoagulants (increased anticoagulant activity), (3) cardiac glycosides and antiarrhythmic drugs that prolong repolarization (increased arrhythmias), (4) lithium (increased plasma levels of Li^+), (5) propranolol (increased plasma levels of propranolol), (6) sulfonylureas (hyperglycemia), (7) cisplatin (increased risk of diuretic-induced ototoxicity), (8) NSAIDs (blunted diuretic response and salicylate toxicity when given with high doses of salicylates), (9) probenecid (blunted diuretic response), (10) thiazide diuretics (synergism of diuretic activity of both drugs leading to profound diuresis), and (11) amphotericin B (increased potential for nephrotoxicity and toxicity and intensification of electrolyte imbalance).

THERAPEUTIC USES   A major use of loop diuretics is in the treatment of acute pulmonary edema. A rapid increase in venous capacitance in conjunction with a brisk natriuresis reduces left ventricular filling pressures and thereby rapidly relieves pulmonary edema. Loop diuretics also are used widely for the treatment of chronic congestive heart failure when diminution of extracellular fluid volume is desirable to minimize venous and pulmonary congestion (*see* Chapter 33). In this regard, a meta-analysis of randomized clinical trials demonstrates that diuretics cause a significant reduction in mortality and the risk of worsening heart failure, as well as an improvement in exercise capacity.

Diuretics are used widely for the treatment of hypertension (*see* Chapter 32), and loop diuretics appear to lower blood pressure as effectively as Na^+–Cl^- symporter inhibitors (*e.g.*, thiazides and thiazide-like diuretics) while causing smaller perturbations in the lipid profile. However, the short elimination half-lives of loop diuretics render them less useful for hypertension than thiazide-type diuretics. The edema of nephrotic syndrome often is refractory to other classes of diuretics, and loop diuretics often are the only drugs capable of reducing the massive edema associated with this disease. Loop diuretics also are employed in the treatment of edema and ascites of hepatic cirrhosis; however, care must be taken not to induce encephalopathy or hepatorenal syndrome. In patients with a drug overdose, loop diuretics can be used to induce a forced diuresis to facilitate more rapid renal elimination of the offending drug. Loop diuretics, combined with isotonic saline administration to prevent volume depletion, are used to treat hypercalcemia. Loop diuretics interfere with the kidney's capacity to produce a concentrated urine. Consequently, loop diuretics combined with hypertonic saline are useful for the treatment of life-threatening hyponatremia. Loop diuretics also are used to treat edema associated with chronic renal insufficiency. Most patients with ARF receive a trial dose of a loop diuretic in an attempt to convert oliguric ARF to nonoliguric ARF. However, there is no evidence that loop diuretics prevent ATN or improve outcome in patients with ARF.

INHIBITORS OF Na^+–Cl^- SYMPORT (THIAZIDE AND THIAZIDE-LIKE DIURETICS)

The original inhibitors of Na^+–Cl^- symport were benzothiadiazine derivatives, hence this class of diuretics became known as thiazide diuretics. *Subsequently, drugs that are pharmacologically similar to thiazide diuretics but are not thiazides were developed and are called* thiazide-like diuretics. *The term* thiazide diuretics *is used here to refer to all members of the class of inhibitors of Na^+–Cl^- symport.*

Thiazide diuretics inhibit NaCl transport in the DCT; the proximal tubule may be a secondary site of action. Figure 28–4 illustrates the current model of electrolyte transport in the DCT. Transport is powered by a Na^+ pump in the basolateral membrane. The free energy in the electrochemical gradient for Na^+ is harnessed by a Na^+–Cl^- symporter in the luminal membrane that moves Cl^- into the epithelial cell against its electrochemical gradient. Cl^- then exits the basolateral membrane passively via a Cl^- channel. Thiazide diuretics inhibit the Na^+–Cl^- symporter (Figure 28-4). Na^+ or Cl^- binding to the Na^+–Cl^- symporter modifies thiazide-induced inhibition of the symporter, suggesting that the thiazide-binding site is shared or altered by both Na^+ and Cl^-. The Na^+–Cl^- symporter (called ENCC1) is expressed predominantly in the kidney and is localized to the apical membrane of DCT epithelial cells; its expression is regulated by aldosterone. Mutations in the Na^+–Cl^- symporter cause a familial hypokalemic alkalosis called Gitelman's syndrome.

EFFECTS ON URINARY EXCRETION   Inhibitors of the Na^+–Cl^- symporter increase Na^+ and Cl^- excretion, but are only moderately efficacious (*i.e.*, maximum excretion of filtered load of Na^+ is only 5%) because ~90% of the filtered Na^+ load is reabsorbed before reaching the DCT. Some thiazide diuretics also are weak inhibitors of carbonic anhydrase, an effect that increases HCO_3^- and phosphate excretion and probably accounts for their weak proximal tubular effects. Inhibitors of the Na^+–Cl^- symporter increase the excretion of K^+ and titratable acid by the same mechanisms discussed for loop diuretics. Acute administration of thiazides increases the excretion of uric acid, but uric acid excretion is reduced following chronic administration by the same mechanisms as for loop diuretics. Acute effects of inhibitors of the Na^+–Cl^- symporter on Ca^{2+} excretion are variable; when administered chronically, thiazide diuretics decrease Ca^{2+} excretion. The mechanism involves increased proximal reabsorption owing to volume depletion, as well as direct effects of thiazides to increase Ca^{2+} reabsorption in the DCT. Thiazide diuretics may cause a mild magnesuria by a poorly understood mechanism. Since inhibitors of Na^+–Cl^- symport inhibit transport in the cortical diluting segment, thiazide diuretics attenuate the ability of the kidney to excrete a

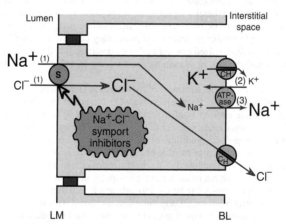

DISTAL CONVOLUTED TUBULE

FIGURE 28–4   *NaCl reabsorption in distal convoluted tubule and mechanism of diuretic action of Na^+–Cl^- symport inhibitors.* S, symporter; CH, ion channel. Numbers in parentheses indicate stoichiometry. BL and LM indicate basolateral and luminal membranes, respectively.

diluted urine during water diuresis. However, since the DCT is not involved in the mechanism that generates a hypertonic medullary interstitium, thiazide diuretics do not alter the kidney's ability to concentrate urine during hydropenia.

In general, inhibitors of Na^+–Cl^- symport do not affect RBF and only variably reduce GFR owing to increases in intratubular pressure. Since thiazides act at a point past the macula densa, they have little or no influence on TGF.

ABSORPTION AND ELIMINATION The relative potency, oral bioavailability, plasma $t_{1/2}$, and route of elimination of inhibitors of Na^+–Cl^- symport are listed in Table 28–5. Of special note is the wide range of half-lives for this class of drugs. Sulfonamides are organic acids and therefore are secreted into the proximal tubule by the organic acid secretory pathway. Since thiazides must gain access to the tubular lumen to inhibit the Na^+–Cl^- symporter, drugs such as probenecid can attenuate the diuretic response to thiazides by competing for transport into the proximal tubule. However, plasma protein binding varies considerably among thiazide diuretics, and this parameter determines the contribution that filtration makes to tubular delivery of a specific thiazide.

TOXICITY, ADVERSE EFFECTS, CONTRAINDICATIONS, DRUG INTERACTIONS Thiazide diuretics rarely cause CNS (*e.g.*, vertigo, headache, paresthesias, and weakness), GI (*e.g.*, anorexia, nausea, vomiting, cramping, diarrhea, constipation, cholecystitis, and pancreatitis), hematological (*e.g.*, blood dyscrasias), and dermatological (*e.g.*, photosensitivity and rashes) disorders. The incidence of erectile dysfunction is greater with the Na^+–Cl^- symporter inhibitors than with several other antihypertensive agents (*e.g.*, β receptor antagonists, Ca^{2+} channel blockers, angiotensin-converting enzyme inhibitors, and α_1 antagonists) but usually is tolerable. Serious adverse effects of thiazides are related to abnormalities of fluid and electrolyte balance, including extracellular volume depletion, hypotension, hypokalemia, hyponatremia, hypochloremia, metabolic alkalosis, hypomagnesemia, hypercalcemia, and hyperuricemia. Thiazide diuretics have caused fatal or near-fatal hyponatremia, and some patients are at recurrent risk of hyponatremia when rechallenged with thiazides.

Thiazide diuretics also decrease glucose tolerance, sometimes unmasking latent diabetes mellitus. The mechanism of the impaired glucose tolerance appears to involve reduced insulin secretion and alterations in glucose metabolism; hyperglycemia is reduced when K^+ is given along with the diuretic. In addition to contributing to hyperglycemia, thiazide-induced hypokalemia compromises the antihypertensive effect and cardiovascular protection afforded by thiazides in patients with hypertension. Thiazide diuretics may increase plasma levels of LDL cholesterol and triglycerides. The drugs are contraindicated in individuals who are hypersensitive to sulfonamides.

Thiazide diuretics may diminish the effects of anticoagulants, uricosuric agents used to treat gout, sulfonylureas, and insulin and increase the effects of anesthetics, diazoxide, cardiac glycosides, lithium, loop diuretics, and vitamin D. The effectiveness of thiazide diuretics may be reduced by NSAIDs and bile acid sequestrants (reduced absorption of thiazides). Amphotericin B and corticosteroids increase the risk of hypokalemia induced by thiazide diuretics.

A potentially lethal drug interaction is that with antiarrhythmic drugs that prolong QT interval (ventricular repolarization) such as quinidine. Prolongation of the QT interval can lead to the development of polymorphic ventricular tachycardia (*torsades de pointes*) owing to triggered activity originating from early after-depolarizations (*see* Chapter 34). Although usually self-limiting, *torsades de pointes* may deteriorate into fatal ventricular fibrillation. Hypokalemia increases the risk of quinidine-induced *torsades de pointes*, and thiazide-induced K^+ depletion may contribute to many cases of quinidine-induced *torsades de pointes*.

THERAPEUTIC USES Thiazide diuretics are used to treat edema associated with heart (congestive heart failure), liver (cirrhosis), and renal (nephrotic syndrome, chronic renal failure, and acute glomerulonephritis) disease. With the possible exceptions of metolazone and indapamide, most thiazide diuretics are ineffective when the GFR is <30–40 mL/min.

Thiazide diuretics decrease blood pressure in hypertensive patients and are used widely for the treatment of hypertension, either alone or in combination with other antihypertensive drugs (*see* Chapter 32). In this regard, thiazide diuretics are inexpensive, as efficacious as other classes of antihypertensive agents, and well tolerated. Thiazides can be administered once daily, do not require dose titration, and have few contraindications; moreover, they have additive or synergistic effects when combined with antihypertensive agents. Although thiazides may marginally increase the risk of sudden death and renal cell carcinoma, they generally are safe and reduce cardiovascular morbidity and mortality in hypertensive patients. Because adverse effects of thiazides

Table 28-5

Inhibitors of Na$^+$–Cl$^-$ Symport (Thiazide and Thiazide-like Diuretics)

Drug (TRADE NAME)	Structure	Relative Potency	Oral Availability	$t_{1/2}$ (hours)	Route of Elimination
Bendroflumethiazide (NATURETIN)	R_2 = H, R_3 = CH$_2$ ⟨phenyl⟩, R_6 = CF$_3$	10	~100%	3–3.9	~30% R ~70% M
Chlorothiazide (DIURIL)	R_2 = H, R_3 = H, R_6 = Cl (Unsaturated between C3 and N4)	0.1	9–56% (dose-dependent)	~1.5	R
Hydrochlorothiazide (HYDRODIURIL)	R_2 = H, R_3 = H, R_6 = Cl	1	~70%	~2.5	R
Hydroflumethiazide (SALURON)	R_2 = H, R_3 = H, R_6 = CF$_3$	1	~50%	~17	40–80% R 20–60% M
Methyclothiazide (ENDURON)	R_2 = CH$_3$, R_3 = CH$_2$Cl, R_6 = Cl	10	ID	ID	M
Polythiazide (RENESE)	R_2 = CH$_3$, R_3 = CH$_2$SCH$_2$CF$_3$, R_6 = Cl	25	~100%	~25	~25% R, ~75% U
Trichlormethiazide (NAQUA)	R_2 = H, R_3 = CHCl$_2$, R_6 = Cl	25	ID	2.3–7.3	R
Chlorthalidone (HYGROTON)		1	~65%	~47	~65% R ~10% B ~25% U

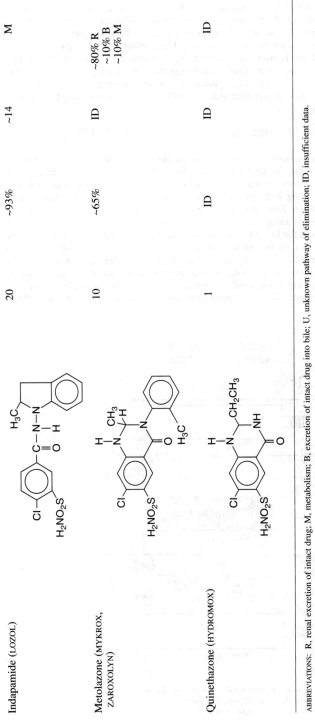

Indapamide (LOZOL)   20   ~93%   ~14   M

Metolazone (MYKROX, ZAROXOLYN)   10   ~65%   ID   ~80% R ~10% B ~10% M

Quinethazone (HYDROMOX)   1   ID   ID   ID

ABBREVIATIONS: R, renal excretion of intact drug; M, metabolism; B, excretion of intact drug into bile; U, unknown pathway of elimination; ID, insufficient data.

491

increase progressively in severity at doses higher than maximally effective antihypertensive doses, only low doses should be prescribed for hypertension. A common dose for hypertension is 25 mg/day of hydrochlorothiazide or the equivalent of another thiazide. Many experts view thiazide diuretics as the best initial therapy for uncomplicated hypertension. Concern regarding the risk of diabetes should not cause clinicians to avoid thiazides in nondiabetic hypertensives.

Thiazide diuretics, which reduce urinary excretion of Ca^{2+}, sometimes are employed to treat calcium nephrolithiasis and may be useful for the treatment of osteoporosis (*see* Chapter 61). Thiazide diuretics also are a mainstay for treatment of nephrogenic diabetes insipidus, reducing urine volume by up to 50%. The mechanism of this paradoxical effect remains unknown. Since other halides are excreted by renal processes similar to those for Cl^-, thiazide diuretics may be useful for the management of Br^- intoxication.

INHIBITORS OF RENAL EPITHELIAL NA⁺ CHANNELS (K⁺-SPARING DIURETICS)

Triamterene (DYRENIUM) and *amiloride* (MID-AMOR) are the two drugs of this class in clinical use. Both drugs cause small increases in NaCl excretion and usually are employed for their antikaliuretic actions to offset the effects of other diuretics that increase K^+ excretion. Consequently, triamterene and amiloride, along with spironolactone (*see* next section), often are classified as *potassium* (K^+)-*sparing diuretics*. Both drugs are organic bases, are transported by the organic base secretory mechanism in the proximal tubule, and act by similar mechanisms. As illustrated in Figure 28–5, principal cells in the late distal tubule and collecting duct have epithelial Na^+ channels in their luminal membranes that provide a conductive pathway for the entry of Na^+ into the cell down the electrochemical gradient created by the basolateral Na^+ pump. The higher permeability of the luminal membrane for Na^+ depolarizes the luminal membrane but not the basolateral membrane, creating a lumen-negative transepithelial potential difference. This transepithelial voltage provides an important driving force for the secretion of K^+ into the lumen *via* K^+ channels (ROMK) in the luminal membrane.

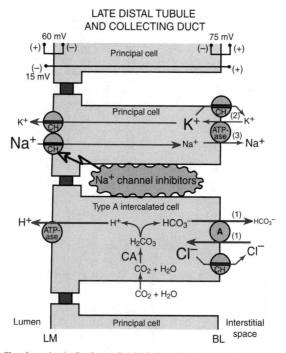

FIGURE 28–5 *NaCl reabsorption in distal convoluted tubule and mechanism of diuretic action of Na^+–Cl^- symport inhibitors.* CA, carbonic anhydrase; S, symporter; CH, ion channel. Numbers in parentheses indicate stoichiometry. BL and LM indicate basolateral and luminal membranes, respectively.

Amiloride and triamterene block epithelial Na$^+$ channels in the luminal membrane of principal cells in the late distal tubule and collecting duct, perhaps by competing with Na$^+$ for negatively charged areas within the pore of the Na$^+$ channel. The amiloride-sensitive Na$^+$ channel (called *ENaC*) consists of three subunits (α, β, and γ). Although the α subunit is sufficient for channel activity, maximal Na$^+$ permeability is induced when all three subunits are coexpressed in the same cell. Liddle's syndrome (pseudohyperaldosteronism) is an autosomal dominant form of low-renin, volume-expanded hypertension that is due to mutations in the β or γ subunits, leading to increased basal activity of ENaC. Amiloride is very effective in treating hypertension in patients carrying these mutations.

EFFECTS ON URINARY EXCRETION Since the late distal tubule and collecting duct have limited capacity to reabsorb solutes, blockade of Na$^+$ channels in this part of the nephron only mildly increases the excretion rates of Na$^+$ and Cl$^-$ (~2% of filtered load). Blockade of Na$^+$ channels hyperpolarizes the luminal membrane, reducing the lumen-negative transepithelial voltage. Since the lumen-negative potential difference normally opposes cation reabsorption and facilitates cation secretion, attenuation of the lumen-negative voltage decreases the excretion rates of K$^+$, H$^+$, Ca^{2+}, and Mg^{2+}. Volume contraction may increase reabsorption of uric acid in the proximal tubule; hence chronic administration of amiloride and triamterene may decrease uric acid excretion. Amiloride and triamterene have little or no effect on renal hemodynamics and do not alter TGF.

ABSORPTION AND ELIMINATION The relative potency, oral bioavailability, plasma $t_{1/2}$, and route of elimination for amiloride and triamterene are listed in Table 28–6. Amiloride is eliminated predominantly by urinary excretion of intact drug. Triamterene is metabolized extensively to an active metabolite, 4-hydroxytriamterene sulfate, and this metabolite is excreted in the urine. Therefore, the toxicity of triamterene may be enhanced in both hepatic disease (decreased metabolism of triamterene) and renal failure (decreased urinary excretion of active metabolite).

TOXICITY, ADVERSE EFFECTS, CONTRAINDICATIONS, DRUG INTERACTIONS The most dangerous adverse effect of Na$^+$-channel inhibitors is hyperkalemia, which can be life-threatening. Consequently, amiloride and triamterene are contraindicated in patients with hyperkalemia, as well as in patients at increased risk of developing hyperkalemia (*e.g.*, patients with renal failure, patients receiving other K$^+$-sparing diuretics, patients taking angiotensin-converting enzyme inhibitors, or patients taking K$^+$ supplements). Even NSAIDs can increase the likelihood of hyperkalemia in patients receiving Na$^+$-channel inhibitors. Pentamidine and high-dose trimethoprim are used often to treat *Pneumocystis carinii* pneumonia in patients with acquired immune deficiency syndrome (AIDS). Because these compounds weakly inhibit ENaC, they too may cause

Table 28–6

Inhibitors of Renal Epithelial Na$^+$ Channels (K$^+$–Sparing Diuretics)

Drug (TRADE NAME)	Structure	Relative Potency	Oral Availability	$t_{1/2}$ (hours)	Route of Elimination
Amiloride (DYRENIUM)		1	15–25%	~21	R
Triamterene (MIDAMOR)		0.1	~50%	~4.2	M

ABBREVIATIONS: R, renal excretion of intact drug; M, metabolism; however, triamterene is transformed into an active metabolite that is excreted in the urine.

hyperkalemia, which may explain the frequent occurrence of hyperkalemia in AIDS patients. Cirrhotic patients are prone to megaloblastosis because of folic acid deficiency, and triamterene, a weak folic acid antagonist, may increase the likelihood of this adverse event. Triamterene also can reduce glucose tolerance and induce photosensitization and has been associated with interstitial nephritis and renal stones. Both drugs can cause CNS, GI, musculoskeletal, dermatological, and hematological adverse effects. The most common adverse effects of amiloride are nausea, vomiting, diarrhea, and headache; those of triamterene are nausea, vomiting, leg cramps, and dizziness.

THERAPEUTIC USES   Because of the mild natriuresis induced by Na^+-channel inhibitors, these drugs seldom are used as sole agents in the treatment of edema or hypertension. Rather, their major utility is in *combination* with other diuretics. Coadministration of a Na^+-channel inhibitor augments the diuretic and antihypertensive response to thiazide and loop diuretics. More important, the ability of Na^+-channel inhibitors to reduce K^+ excretion tends to offset the kaliuretic effects of thiazide and loop diuretics; consequently, the combination of a Na^+-channel inhibitor with a thiazide or loop diuretic tends to result in normal values of plasma K^+. Liddle's syndrome can be treated effectively with Na^+-channel inhibitors. Approximately 5% of people of African origin carry a *T594M* polymorphism in the β subunit of ENaC, and amiloride is particularly effective in lowering blood pressure in hypertensive patients who carry this polymorphism. Aerosolized amiloride improves mucociliary clearance in patients with cystic fibrosis. By inhibiting Na^+ absorption from the surfaces of airway epithelial cells, amiloride augments hydration of respiratory secretions and thereby improves mucociliary clearance. Amiloride also is useful for lithium-induced nephrogenic diabetes insipidus because it blocks Li^+ transport into the cells of the collecting tubules.

ANTAGONISTS OF MINERALOCORTICOID RECEPTORS (ALDOSTERONE ANTAGONISTS, K^+-SPARING DIURETICS)
Mineralocorticoids cause salt and water retention and increase the excretion of K^+ and H^+ by binding to specific mineralocorticoid receptors (MRs). Currently, two MR antagonists are available in the U.S., *spironolactone* and *eplerenone*; two others are available elsewhere (Table 28–7). Epithelial cells in the late distal tubule and collecting duct contain cytosolic MRs that have a high affinity for aldosterone. Aldosterone enters the epithelial cell from the basolateral membrane and binds to MRs; the MR–aldosterone complex translocates to the nucleus, where it regulates the expression of multiple gene products called *aldosterone-induced proteins* (AIPs). Figure 28–6 illustrates some of the proposed effects of AIPs. The net effect of AIPs is to increase Na^+ conductance of the luminal membrane and sodium pump activity of the basolateral membrane. Consequently, transepithelial NaCl transport is enhanced, and the lumen-negative transepithelial voltage is increased. The latter effect increases the driving force for secretion of K^+ and H^+ into the tubular lumen.

Spironolactone and eplerenone competitively inhibit the binding of aldosterone to the MR. Unlike the MR–aldosterone complex, the MR-spironolactone complex is unable to induce the synthesis of AIPs. Since spironolactone and eplerenone block the biological effects of aldosterone, these agents also are referred to as *aldosterone antagonists*. MR antagonists are the only diuretics that do not require access to the tubular lumen to induce diuresis.

EFFECTS ON URINARY EXCRETION   The effects of MR antagonists on urinary excretion are very similar to those induced by renal epithelial Na^+-channel inhibitors. However, unlike that of the Na^+-channel inhibitors, the clinical efficacy of MR antagonists is a function of endogenous levels of aldosterone. The higher the levels of endogenous aldosterone, the greater are the effects of MR antagonists on urinary excretion. MR antagonists have little or no effect on renal hemodynamics and do not alter TGF.

OTHER ACTIONS   Spironolactone has some affinity toward progesterone and androgen receptors and thereby induces side effects such as gynecomastia, impotence, and menstrual irregularities. Owing to the 9,11-epoxide group, eplerenone has very low affinity for progesterone and androgen receptors (<1% and <0.1%, respectively) compared with spironolactone. Therapeutic concentrations of spironolactone block human *ether-a-go-go*-related gene (HERG) K^+ channels, and this may account for the antiarrythmic effects of spironolactone in heart failure. High concentrations of spironolactone can interfere with steroid biosynthesis by inhibiting CYPs (*see* Chapter 59).

ABSORPTION AND ELIMINATION   Spironolactone is absorbed partially (~65%), is metabolized extensively (even during its first passage through the liver), undergoes enterohepatic recirculation, is highly protein-bound, and has a short $t_{1/2}$ (~1.6 hours). However, an active metabolite of spironolactone, canrenone, has a $t_{1/2}$ of ~16.5 hours, which prolongs the biological effects of spironolactone. Although not available in the U.S., canrenone and canrenoate also are in clinical use. Canrenoate is not active *per se* but is converted to canrenone in the body. Eplerenone has good oral availability and is eliminated with a $t_{1/2}$ of ~5 hours, primarily by conversion to inactive metabolites by hepatic CYP3A4.

Table 28–7

Mineralocorticoid Receptor Antagonists (Aldosterone Antagonists, K⁺-Sparing Diuretics)

Drug (TRADE NAME)	Structure	Oral Availability	$t_{1/2}$ (hours)	Route of Elimination
Spironolactone (ALDACTONE)		~65%	~1.6	M
Canrenone*		ID	~16.5	M
Potassium canrenoate*		ID	ID	M
Eplerenone (INSPRA)		ID	~5	M

*Not available in United States.

ABBREVIATIONS: M, metabolism; ID, insufficient data.

LATE DISTAL TUBULE
AND COLLECTING DUCT

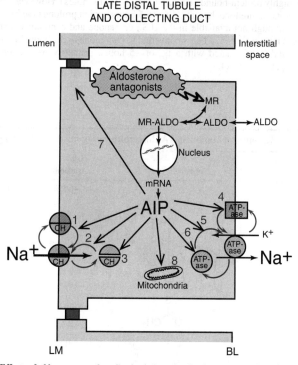

FIGURE 28–6 *Effects of aldosterone on late distal tubule and collecting duct and diuretic mechanism of aldosterone antagonists.* AIP, aldosterone-induced proteins; ALDO, aldosterone; MR, mineralocorticoid receptor; CH, ion channel; 1, activation of membrane-bound Na^+ channels; 2, redistribution of Na^+ channels from cytosol to membrane; 3, *de novo* synthesis of Na^+ channels; 4, activation of membrane-bound Na^+,K^+–ATPase; 5, redistribution of Na^+,K^+–ATPase from cytosol to membrane; 6, *de novo* synthesis of Na^+,K^+–ATPase; 7, changes in permeability of tight junctions; 8, increased mitochondrial production of ATP. BL and LM indicate basolateral and luminal membranes, respectively.

TOXICITY, ADVERSE EFFECTS, CONTRAINDICATIONS, DRUG INTERACTIONS
As with other K^+-sparing diuretics, MR antagonists may cause life-threatening hyperkalemia. Indeed, hyperkalemia is the principal risk of MR antagonists. Therefore, these drugs are contraindicated in patients with hyperkalemia and in those at increased risk of developing hyperkalemia either because of disease or because of administration of other medications. MR antagonists also can induce metabolic acidosis in cirrhotic patients.

Salicylates may reduce the tubular secretion and decrease the diuretic efficacy of spironolactone, and spironolactone may alter the clearance of cardiac glycosides. Owing to its effects on other steroid receptors, spironolactone may cause gynecomastia, impotence, decreased libido, and menstrual irregularities. Spironolactone also may induce diarrhea, gastritis, gastric bleeding, and peptic ulcers (the drug is contraindicated in patients with peptic ulcers). CNS adverse effects include drowsiness, lethargy, ataxia, confusion, and headache. Spironolactone may cause rashes and, rarely, blood dyscrasias. Whether therapeutic doses of spironolactone can induce malignancies remains an open question. Strong inhibitors of CYP3A4 (*see* Chapter 3) may increase plasma levels of eplerenone; such drugs should not be administered to patients taking eplerenone, and *vice versa*. Other than hyperkalemia and GI disorders, the rate of adverse events for eplerenone is similar to that of placebo.

THERAPEUTIC USES Spironolactone often is coadministered with thiazide or loop diuretics in the treatment of edema and hypertension. Such combinations result in increased mobilization of edema fluid with lesser perturbations of K^+ homeostasis. Spironolactone is particularly useful in the treatment of primary hyperaldosteronism (due either to adrenal adenomas or bilateral adrenal hyperplasia) and refractory edema associated with secondary aldosteronism (cardiac failure, hepatic cirrhosis, nephrotic syndrome, and severe ascites). Spironolactone is considered the diuretic of choice in patients with hepatic cirrhosis. Spironolactone, added to standard therapy, substantially reduces morbidity and mortality and ventricular arrhythmias in patients with heart failure (*see* Chapter 34).

Clinical experience with eplerenone is limited; it appears to be a safe and effective antihypertensive drug. In patients with acute myocardial infarction complicated by left ventricular systolic dysfunction, addition of eplerenone to optimal medical therapy significantly reduces morbidity and mortality.

OVERVIEW OF DIURETIC USE

Diuretics are used clinically to treat hypertension (see Chapter 32) and to reduce edema associated with cardiac, renal, and hepatic disorders. Three fundamental strategies exist for mobilizing edema fluid: correct the underlying disease, restrict Na^+ intake, or administer diuretics. The most desirable course of action would be to correct the primary disease; however, this often is impossible. Restriction of Na^+ intake is the favored nonpharmacologic approach to the treatment of edema and hypertension and should be attempted; however, compliance is a major obstacle. Diuretics therefore remain the cornerstone for the treatment of edema or volume overload, particularly that owing to congestive heart failure, ascites, chronic renal failure, or nephrotic syndrome.

The clinical situation dictates whether a patient should receive diuretics and what therapeutic regimen should be used (*i.e.*, type of diuretic, dose, route of administration, and speed of fluid mobilization). Acute pulmonary edema in patients with left-sided heart failure is a medical emergency requiring rapid, aggressive therapy including intravenous administration of a loop diuretic. In this setting, use of oral or less potent diuretics is inappropriate. On the other hand, mild pulmonary and venous congestion associated with chronic heart failure is best treated with an oral loop or thiazide diuretic, the dosage of which should be titrated carefully to maximize the benefit-to-risk ratio. Loop and thiazide diuretics decrease morbidity and mortality in heart failure; MR antagonists also reduce morbidity and mortality in heart failure patients receiving optimal therapy with other drugs. Periodic administration of diuretics to cirrhotic patients with ascites may eliminate the necessity for or reduce the interval between paracenteses, adding to patient comfort and sparing protein reserves that are lost during the paracenteses. Although diuretics can reduce edema associated with chronic renal failure, increased doses of the more powerful loop diuretics usually are required. In the nephrotic syndrome, the response to diuretics often is disappointing. In chronic renal failure and cirrhosis, edema does not pose an immediate health risk. Even so, uncomfortable, oppressive, and/or disfiguring edema can greatly reduce quality of life, and the decision to treat will be based in part on quality-of-life issues. In such cases, only partial removal of edema fluid should be attempted, and the fluid should be mobilized slowly using a diuretic regimen that accomplishes the task with minimal perturbation of normal physiology. Figure 28–7 provides an algorithm for diuretic therapy in patients with edema caused by renal, hepatic, or cardiac disorders.

Diuretic resistance refers to edema that is refractory to a given diuretic. If diuretic resistance develops against a less efficacious diuretic, a more potent diuretic can be substituted (*e.g.*, a loop diuretic for a thiazide). However, resistance to loop diuretics can result from several causes. NSAIDs block prostaglandin-mediated increases in RBF and increase expression of the Na^+–K^+–$2Cl^-$ symporter in the TAL, resulting in resistance to loop diuretics. In chronic renal failure, reduced RBF decreases diuretic delivery to the kidney, and accumulation of endogenous organic acids competes with loop diuretics for transport at the proximal tubule. Consequently, the concentration of diuretic at the active site in the tubular lumen is diminished. In nephrotic syndrome, protein binding of diuretics may limit drug response. In hepatic cirrhosis, nephrotic syndrome, or heart failure, nephrons may have diminished responsiveness to diuretics because of increased proximal tubular Na^+ reabsorption, leading to diminished delivery of Na^+ to the distal nephron.

Faced with resistance to loop diuretics, the clinician has several options. Bed rest may restore drug responsiveness by improving renal circulation. An increase in the dose of loop diuretic may restore responsiveness; however, nothing is gained by increasing the dose above that which causes a near-maximal effect (*i.e.*, the ceiling dose) of the diuretic. Administration of smaller doses more frequently or a continuous intravenous infusion of a loop diuretic will increase the length of time that an effective concentration of the diuretic is present at the site of action. Combination therapy to sequentially block more than one site in the nephron may result in a synergistic interaction between two diuretics. For instance, combining a loop diuretic with a K^+-sparing or a thiazide diuretic may improve therapeutic response; however, nothing is gained by the administration of two

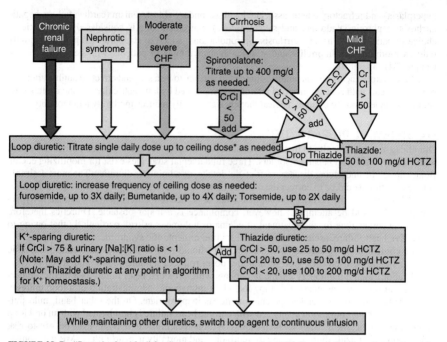

FIGURE 28–7 *"Brater's algorithm" for diuretic therapy of chronic renal failure, nephrotic syndrome, congestive heart failure, and cirrhosis.* Follow algorithm until adequate response is achieved. If adequate response is not obtained, advance to the next step. For illustrative purposes, the thiazide diuretic used in Brater's algorithm is hydrochlorothiazide (HCTZ). An alternative thiazide-type diuretic may be substituted with appropriate dosage adjustment so as to be pharmacologically equivalent to the recommended dose of HCTZ. Do not combine two K^+-sparing diuretics because of the risk of hyperkalemia. CrCl indicates creatinine clearance in mL/min, and ceiling dose refers to the smallest dose of diuretic that produces a near-maximal effect. Ceiling doses of loop diuretics and dosing regimens for continuous intravenous infusions of loop diuretics are disease-state-specific; see Brater (1998) for recommended dosages. Doses are for adults only.

drugs of the same type. Thiazide diuretics with significant proximal tubular effects (*e.g.*, metolazone) are particularly well suited for sequential blockade when coadministered with a loop diuretic. Reducing salt intake will diminish postdiuretic Na^+ retention that can nullify previous increases in Na^+ excretion. Diuretic dosing shortly before eating will provide effective drug concentrations in the tubular lumen when the salt load is highest.

For a complete Bibliographical listing see Goodman & Gilman's *The Pharmacological Basis of Therapeutics,* **11th ed., or Goodman & Gilman Online at www.accessmedicine.com.**

29

VASOPRESSIN AND OTHER AGENTS AFFECTING THE RENAL CONSERVATION OF WATER

Body fluid osmolality is controlled by a homeostatic mechanism that adjusts both the rate of water intake and the rate of solute-free water excretion by the kidneys—*i.e.*, water balance. Abnormalities in this homeostatic system can result from genetic diseases, acquired diseases, or drugs, and may cause serious and potentially life-threatening deviations in plasma osmolality. Arginine vasopressin is the main hormone that regulates body fluid osmolality.

INTRODUCTION TO VASOPRESSIN

Vasopressin is the mediator of a remarkable regulatory system for the conservation of water. The hormone is released by the posterior pituitary whenever water deprivation causes an increased plasma osmolality or whenever the cardiovascular system is challenged by hypovolemia and/or hypotension. In humans, vasopressin acts primarily in the renal collecting duct, increasing the permeability of the cell membrane to water and permitting water to move passively down an osmotic gradient across the collecting duct into the extracellular compartment.

Vasopressin also is a potent vasopressor whose name was chosen in recognition of its vasoconstrictor action. Vasopressin is a neurotransmitter; among its actions in the CNS are apparent roles in the secretion of ACTH and in the regulation of the cardiovascular system, temperature, and other visceral functions. Vasopressin also may play a role in hemostasis by promoting the release of coagulation factors by the vascular endothelium and increasing platelet aggregation.

PHYSIOLOGY OF VASOPRESSIN

The antidiuretic mechanism in mammals involves two anatomical components: a CNS component for the synthesis, transport, storage, and release of vasopressin, and a renal collecting-duct system composed of epithelial cells that respond to vasopressin by increasing their permeability to water. The CNS component of this mechanism, called the hypothalamiconeurohypophyseal system, *consists of neurosecretory neurons with perikarya located predominantly in two specific hypothalamic nuclei, the supraoptic nucleus (SON) and the paraventricular nucleus (PVN). The long axons of magnocellular neurons in the SON and PVN terminate in the neural lobe of the posterior pituitary (neurohypophysis), where they release vasopressin and oxytocin. The relevant anatomy of the renal collecting-duct system is described in Chapter 28.*

Vasopressin is synthesized mainly in the perikarya of magnocellular neurons in the SON and PVN; parvicellular neurons in the PVN also synthesize vasopressin. Vasopressin synthesis is regulated solely at the transcriptional level. In humans, a 168–amino acid preprohormone (Figure 29–1) is synthesized and packaged into membrane-associated granules. The prohormone contains three domains: vasopressin (residues 1–9), vasopressin (VP)–neurophysin (residues 13–105), and VP–glycopeptide (residues 107–145). The vasopressin domain is linked to the VP–neurophysin domain through a Gly-Lys-Arg-processing signal, and the VP–neurophysin is linked to the VP–glycopeptide domain by an Arg-processing signal. In the secretory granules, an endopeptidase, exopeptidase, monooxygenase, and lyase act sequentially on the prohormone to produce vasopressin, VP–neurophysin (sometimes referred to as neurophysin II*), and VP–glycopeptide. The synthesis and transport of vasopressin depend on the conformation of the preprohormone. In particular, VP–neurophysin binds vasopressin and is critical to the correct processing, transport, and storage of vasopressin. Genetic mutations in either the signal peptide or VP–neurophysin give rise to central diabetes insipidus.*

REGULATION OF VASOPRESSIN SECRETION An increase in plasma osmolality is the principal physiological stimulus for vasopressin secretion by the posterior pituitary. Severe hypovolemia/hypotension also is a powerful stimulus for vasopressin release. In addition, pain, nausea, and hypoxia can stimulate vasopressin secretion, and several endogenous hormones and pharmacological agents can modify vasopressin release.

Hyperosmolality The osmolality threshold for secretion of vasopressin is ~280 mOsm/kg. Below this threshold, vasopressin is barely detectable in plasma; above this osmolality, vasopressin levels are a steep and relatively linear function of plasma osmolality. Indeed, a 2% elevation in plasma osmolality causes a 2–3 fold increase in plasma vasopressin levels, which, in turn, causes increased solute-free water reabsorption, with an increase in urine osmolality. Increases in plasma osmolality >290 mOsm/kg lead to an intense desire for water (thirst). Thus, the vasopressin system

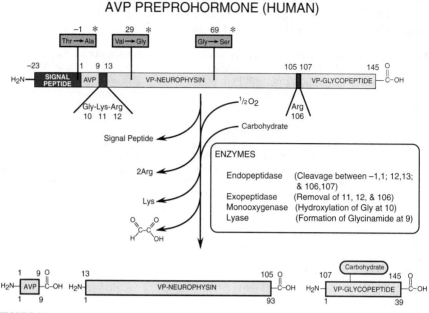

FIGURE 29–1 *Processing of the 168–amino acid human 8-arginine vasopressin (AVP) preprohormone to AVP, vasopressin (VP)–neurophysin, and VP–glycopeptide.* At least 40 mutations in the single gene on chromosome 20 that encodes AVP preprohormone give rise to central diabetes insipidus. *Boxes indicate mutations leading to central diabetes insipidus.

affords the organism longer thirst-free periods and, in the event that water is unavailable, allows the organism to survive longer periods of water deprivation. Above a plasma osmolality of ~290 mOsm/kg, plasma levels of vasopressin exceed 5 pM. Since urinary concentration is maximal (~1200 mOsm/kg) when vasopressin levels exceed 5 pM, further defense against hypertonicity depends entirely on water intake rather than on decreases in water loss.

Hepatic Portal Osmoreceptors An oral salt load activates hepatic portal osmoreceptors, leading to increased vasopressin release. This mechanism augments plasma vasopressin levels even before the oral salt load increases plasma osmolality.

Hypovolemia and Hypotension

Vasopressin secretion also is regulated hemodynamically by changes in effective blood volume and/or arterial blood pressure. Regardless of the cause (e.g., hemorrhage, salt depletion, diuretics, heart failure, cirrhosis with ascites, adrenal insufficiency, or hypotensive drugs), reductions in effective blood volume and/or arterial blood pressure are associated with high circulating concentrations of vasopressin. However, unlike osmoregulation, hemodynamic regulation of vasopressin secretion is exponential; i.e., small decreases (5–10%) in blood volume and/or pressure have little effect on vasopressin secretion, whereas larger decreases (20–30%) can increase vasopressin levels to 20–30 times normal (exceeding the concentration of vasopressin required to induce maximal antidiuresis). Vasopressin is one of the most potent vasoconstrictors known, and the vasopressin response to hypovolemia or hypotension serves as a mechanism to stave off cardiovascular collapse during periods of severe blood loss and/or hypotension. Hemodynamic regulation of vasopressin secretion does not disrupt osmotic regulation; rather, hypovolemia/ hypotension alters the set point and slope of the plasma osmolality–plasma vasopressin relationship.

The neuronal pathways that mediate hemodynamic regulation of vasopressin release are different from those involved in osmoregulation. Baroreceptors in the left atrium, left ventricle, and pulmonary veins sense blood volume (filling pressures), and baroreceptors in the carotid sinus and aorta monitor arterial blood pressure. Nerve impulses reach brainstem nuclei predominantly through the vagal trunk and glossopharyngeal nerve; these signals ultimately are relayed to the SON and PVN.

Hormones and Neurotransmitters

Vasopressin-synthesizing magnocellular neurons have a large array of receptors on both perikarya and nerve terminals; therefore, vasopressin release can be accentuated or attenuated by chemical agents acting at both ends of the magnocellular neuron. Also, hormones and neurotransmitters can modulate vasopressin secretion by stimulating or inhibiting neurons in nuclei that project, either directly or indirectly, to the SON and PVN. Because of these complexities, the physiological relevance of modulation of vasopressin secretion by most hormones and neurotransmitters is unclear.

Several agents are known to stimulate vasopressin secretion, including acetylcholine (via nicotinic receptors), histamine (via H_1 receptors), dopamine (via both D_1 and D_2 receptors), glutamine, aspartate, cholecystokinin, neuropeptide Y, substance P, vasoactive intestinal polypeptide, prostaglandins, and angiotensin II (AngII). Inhibitors of vasopressin secretion include atrial natriuretic peptide, GABA, and opioids (particularly dynorphin via κ receptors). The effects of AngII have received the most attention because AngII synthesized in the brain and circulating angiotensin may stimulate vasopressin release. Inhibition of the conversion of AngII to AngIII blocks AngII–induced vasopressin release, suggesting that AngIII is the main effector peptide of the brain renin–angiotensin system controlling vasopressin release.

Pharmacological Agents

A number of drugs alter urine osmolality by stimulating or inhibiting the secretion of vasopressin. In most cases the mechanism is not known. Stimulators of vasopressin secretion include vincristine, cyclophosphamide, tricyclic antidepressants, nicotine, epinephrine, and high doses of morphine. Lithium, which inhibits the renal effects of vasopressin, also enhances vasopressin secretion. Inhibitors of vasopressin secretion include ethanol, phenytoin, low doses of morphine, glucocorticoids, fluphenazine, haloperidol, promethazine, oxilorphan, and butorphanol. Carbamazepine has a renal action to produce antidiuresis in patients with central diabetes insipidus but actually inhibits vasopressin secretion via a central action.

BASIC PHARMACOLOGY OF VASOPRESSIN

VASOPRESSIN RECEPTORS   The cellular effects of vasopressin are mediated mainly by its interactions with the 3 types of receptors, V_{1a}, V_{1b}, and V_2. The V_{1a} receptor is the most widespread subtype of vasopressin receptor; it is found in vascular smooth muscle, the adrenal gland, myometrium, the bladder, adipocytes, hepatocytes, platelets, renal medullary interstitial cells, vasa recta in the renal microcirculation, epithelial cells in the renal cortical collecting-duct, spleen, testis, and many CNS structures. V_{1b} receptors have a more limited distribution and are found in the anterior pituitary, several brain regions, the pancreas, and the adrenal medulla. V_2 receptors are located predominantly in principal cells of the renal collecting-duct system but also are present on epithelial cells in the thick ascending limb and on vascular endothelial cells. Vasopressin receptors are GPCRs.

V_1 RECEPTOR–EFFECTOR COUPLING

Figure 29–2 summarizes the current model of V_1 receptor–effector coupling. Vasopressin binding to V_1 receptors activates the G_q–PLC pathway, ultimately causing biological effects that include immediate responses (e.g., vasoconstriction, glycogenolysis, platelet aggregation, and ACTH release) and growth of smooth muscle cells.

V_2 RECEPTOR–EFFECTOR COUPLING

Principal cells in the renal collecting duct have V_2 receptors on their basolateral membranes that couple to G_s to stimulate adenylyl cyclase activity (Figure 29–3). The resulting increase in cellular cyclic AMP and PKA activity triggers increased insertion of water channel–containing vesicles (WCVs) into the apical membrane and decreased endocytosis of WCVs from the apical membrane. The distribution of WCVs between the cytosolic compartment and the apical membrane compartment thus is shifted in favor of the apical membrane compartment. Because WCVs contain preformed aquaporin 2 water channels, their net shift into apical membranes in response to V_2-receptor stimulation greatly increases water permeability of the apical membrane.

Aquaporins are a family of water channel proteins that allow water molecules to cross biological membranes. Of the 10 cloned mammalian aquaporins, at least 7 are found in the kidney. Aquaporin 1 is present in the apical and basolateral membrane of the proximal tubule and in the thin descending limb. Aquaporin 2 resides in the apical membrane and WCVs of the collecting-duct principal cells, whereas aquaporins 3 and 4 are present in the basolateral membrane of principal cells. Aquaporin 7 is in the apical brush border of the straight proximal tubule. Aquaporins 6 and 8 are

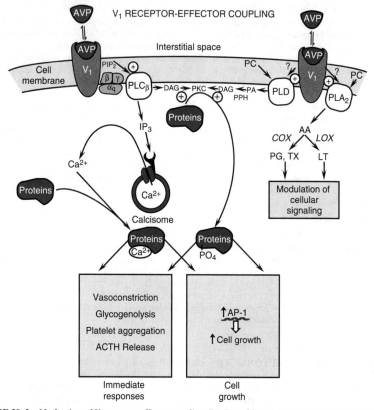

FIGURE 29–2 *Mechanism of V_1 receptor–effector coupling. Binding of 8-arginine vasopressin (AVP) to V_1 vasopressin receptors (V_1) stimulates several membrane-bound phospholipases.* Stimulation of the G_q–PLC_β pathway results in IP_3 formation, mobilization of intracellular Ca^{2+}, and activation of PKC. Activation of V_1 receptors also causes influx of extracellular Ca^{2+} by an unknown mechanism. PKC and Ca^{2+}/calmodulin–activated protein kinases phosphorylate cell-type-specific proteins leading to cellular responses. A further component of the AVP response derives from the production of eicosanoids secondary to the activation of PLA_2; the resulting mobilization of arachidonic acid (AA) provides substrate for eicosanoid synthesis via the cyclooxygenase (COX) and lipoxygenase (LOX) pathways, leading to local production of prostaglandins (PG), thromboxanes (TX), and leukotrienes (LT), which may activate a variety of signaling pathways, including those linked to G_S and G_q. Biological effects mediated by the V_1 receptor include vasoconstriction, glycogenolysis, platelet aggregation, ACTH release, and growth of vascular smooth muscle cells. The effects of vasopressin on cell growth involve transcriptional regulation via the FOS/JUN AP-1 transcription complex.

located intracellularly in the collecting-duct principal cells. In addition to increasing the insertion of aquaporin 2 into apical membranes in collecting-duct principal cells, vasopressin also increases the expression of aquaporin 2 mRNA and protein. Chronic dehydration leads to long-term up-regulation of aquaporin 2 and water transport in the collecting duct.

For maximum concentration of urine, large amounts of urea must be deposited in the interstitium of the inner medullary collecting duct. It is not surprising, therefore, that V_2-receptor activation also increases urea permeability by 400% in the terminal portions of the inner medullary collecting duct by activating a vasopressin-regulated urea transporter (termed VRUT, UT1, or UT-A1), most likely by PKA-induced phosphorylation. The kinetics of vasopressin-induced water and urea permeability differ, and vasopressin-induced regulation of VRUT does not entail vesicular trafficking to the plasma membrane.

In addition to increasing the water permeability of the collecting duct and the urea permeability of the inner medullary collecting duct, V_2-receptor activation also increases Na^+ transport in the thick ascending limb and collecting duct. Na^+ transport in the thick ascending limb is mediated by three mechanisms that affect the Na^+–K^+–$2Cl^-$ symporter: rapid phosphorylation of the symporter, translocation of the symporter into the luminal membrane, and increased

V₂ RECEPTOR-EFFECTOR COUPLING

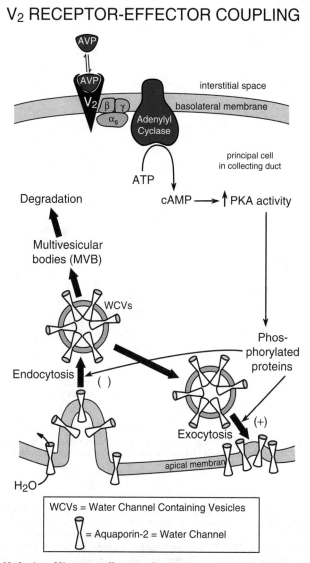

FIGURE 29–3 *Mechanism of V_2 receptor-effector coupling.* Binding of vasopressin (AVP) to the V_2 receptor activates the G_S–adenylyl cyclase–cAMP–PKA pathway and shifts the balance of aquaporin 2 trafficking toward the apical membrane of the principal cell of the collecting duct, thus enhancing water permeability. Although phosphorylation of serine 256 of aquaporin 2 is involved in V_2 receptor signaling, other proteins located both in the water channel–containing vesicles and the apical membrane of the cytoplasm also may be involved.

expression of symporter protein. Enhanced Na^+ transport in the collecting duct is mediated by increased expression of subunits of the epithelial sodium channel. The multiple mechanisms by which vasopressin increases water reabsorption are summarized in Figure 29–4.

RENAL ACTIONS OF VASOPRESSIN Several actions of vasopressin in the kidney involve both V_1 and V_2 receptors. V_1 receptors mediate contraction of mesangial cells in the glomerulus and vascular smooth muscle cells in the vasa recta and efferent arteriole. Indeed, V_1-receptor-mediated reduction of inner medullary blood flow contributes to the maximum concentrating capacity of the kidney (Figure 29–4). V_1 receptors also stimulate prostaglandin synthesis by

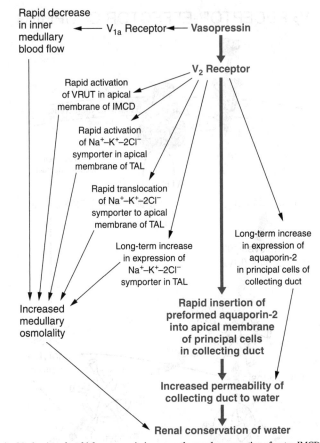

FIGURE 29–4 *Mechanisms by which vasopressin increases the renal conservation of water.* IMCD, inner medullary collecting duct; TAL, thick ascending limb; VRUT, vasopressin-regulated urea transporter. Thick and thin arrows denote major and minor pathways, respectively.

medullary interstitial cells. Since PGE_2 inhibits adenylyl cyclase in the collecting duct, stimulation of prostaglandin synthesis by V_1 receptors may counterbalance V_2-receptor-mediated antidiuresis. V_1 receptors on principal cells in the cortical collecting duct may also inhibit V_2-receptor-mediated water flux *via* activation of PKC. V_2 receptors mediate the most prominent response to vasopressin, increased water permeability of the collecting duct. Indeed, vasopressin can increase water permeability in the collecting duct at concentrations as low as 50 fM. Thus, V_2-receptor-mediated effects of vasopressin occur at concentrations far lower than are required to engage V_1-receptor-mediated actions.

Other renal actions mediated by V_2 receptors include increased urea transport in the inner medullary collecting duct and increased Na^+ transport in the thick ascending limb; both effects contribute to the urine-concentrating ability of the kidney (Figure 29–4). V_2 receptors also increase Na^+ transport in the cortical collecting duct, which may synergize with aldosterone to enhance Na^+ reabsorption during hypovolemia.

PHARMACOLOGICAL MODIFICATION OF THE ANTIDIURETIC RESPONSE TO VASOPRESSIN NSAIDs (*see* Chapter 26), particularly *indomethacin*, enhance the antidiuretic response to vasopressin. Since prostaglandins attenuate antidiuretic responses to vasopressin and NSAIDs inhibit prostaglandin synthesis, reduced prostaglandin production probably accounts for the potentiation of vasopressin's antidiuretic response. *Carbamazepine* and *chlorpropamide* also enhance the antidiuretic effects of vasopressin by unknown mechanisms. Chlorpropamide rarely can induce water intoxication.

A number of drugs inhibit the antidiuretic actions of vasopressin. *Lithium* is of particular importance because of its use in the treatment of manic–depressive disorders. Lithium-induced polyuria is usually reversible. Acutely, lithium appears to reduce V_2-receptor-mediated stimulation of adenylyl cyclase. Also, lithium increases plasma levels of parathyroid hormone, a partial antagonist to vasopressin. In most patients, the antibiotic *demeclocycline* attenuates the antidiuretic effects of vasopressin, probably owing to decreased accumulation and action of cyclic AMP.

NONRENAL ACTIONS OF VASOPRESSIN
Cardiovascular System

The cardiovascular effects of vasopressin are complex. Vasopressin is a potent vasoconstrictor (V_1-receptor-mediated), and resistance vessels throughout the circulation may be affected. Vascular smooth muscle in the skin, skeletal muscle, fat, pancreas, and thyroid gland appear most sensitive, with significant vasoconstriction also occurring in the GI tract, coronary vessels, and brain. Despite the potency of vasopressin as a direct vasoconstrictor, vasopressin-induced pressor responses in vivo are minimal and occur only with vasopressin concentrations significantly higher than those required for maximal antidiuresis. To a large extent, this is due to circulating vasopressin actions on V_1 receptors to inhibit sympathetic efferents and potentiate baroreflexes. In addition, V_2 receptors cause vasodilation in some blood vessels.

Vasopressin appears to help maintain arterial blood pressure during episodes of severe hypovolemia/hypotension. There is no convincing evidence for a role of vasopressin in essential hypertension. The effects of vasopressin on the heart (reduced cardiac output and heart rate) are largely indirect and result from coronary vasoconstriction, decreased coronary blood flow, and alterations in vagal and sympathetic tone. Some patients with coronary insufficiency experience angina even in response to the relatively small amounts of vasopressin required to control diabetes insipidus, and vasopressin-induced myocardial ischemia has led to severe reactions and even death.

Central Nervous System

Vasopressin likely functions as a CNS neurotransmitter and/or neuromodulator, but the physiological relevance of vasopressin's CNS effects is unclear. Although vasopressin is not the principal corticotropin-releasing factor, it may assist in sustained activation of the hypothalamic–pituitary–adrenal axis during chronic stress (see Chapter 59). CNS effects of vasopressin are mediated predominantly by V_1 receptors.

Blood Coagulation

Activation of V_2 receptors by desmopressin or vasopressin increases circulating levels of procoagulant factor VIII and von Willebrand factor. These effects are mediated by extrarenal V_2 receptors. Presumably, vasopressin stimulates the secretion of von Willebrand factor and of factor VIII from storage sites in vascular endothelium. Since release of von Willebrand factor does not occur when desmopressin is applied directly to cultured endothelial cells or to isolated blood vessels, intermediate factors are likely to be involved.

OTHER NONRENAL EFFECTS OF VASOPRESSIN

At high concentrations, vasopressin stimulates contraction of smooth muscle in the uterus (via oxytocin receptors) and GI tract (via V_1 receptors). Vasopressin is stored in platelets, and activation of V_1 receptors stimulates platelet aggregation. Also, activation of V_1 receptors on hepatocytes stimulates glycogenolysis. The physiological significance of these effects of vasopressin in not known.

VASOPRESSIN RECEPTOR AGONISTS AND ANTAGONISTS

The neurohypophyseal vasopressin peptide is 8-arginine vasopressin, and the terms *vasopressin, arginine vasopressin* (AVP), and *antidiuretic hormone* (ADH) are used interchangeably. Arginine vasopressin is a nonapeptide (Cys^1-Tyr^2-Phe^3-Gln^4-Asn^5-Cys^6-Pro^7-Arg^8-Gly^9-NH_2), containing Cys residues in positions 1 and 6 that form an intramolecular disulfide bridge (essential for agonist activity), and an amidated carboxyl terminus. The chemical structure of *oxytocin* is closely related to that of vasopressin: Oxytocin is [Ile^3, Leu^8]AVP. Oxytocin binds to specific oxytocin receptors on myoepithelial cells in the mammary gland (causing milk ejection) and on smooth muscle cells in the uterus (causing contraction). Inasmuch as vasopressin and oxytocin are structurally similar, it is not surprising that vasopressin and oxytocin agonists and antagonists can bind to each other's receptors. Indeed, most of the available peptide vasopressin agonists and antagonists have some affinity for oxytocin receptors; at high doses, they may block or mimic the effects of oxytocin.

Vasopressin analogs with longer duration of action and selectivity for vasopressin receptor subtypes (V_1 vs. V_2 vasopressin receptors, which mediate pressor responses and antidiuretic responses, respectively) have been synthesized. The V_2-selective agonist, 1-deamino-8-D-arginine vasopressin, also called *desmopressin* (DDAVP), has ~3000 times greater antidiuretic-to-vasopressor ratio than vasopressin and is the preferred drug for the treatment of central diabetes insipidus. Substitution of Val for Gln in position 4 further increases the antidiuretic selectivity, and the antidiuretic-to-vasopressor ratio for deamino[Val^4, D-Arg^8]AVP is ~11,000 times greater than vasopressin.

Increasing V_1 selectivity has been more difficult than increasing V_2 selectivity. Vasopressin receptors in the adenohypophysis that mediate vasopressin-induced ACTH release are neither classical V_1 nor V_2 receptors. Since the vasopressin receptors in the adenohypophysis appear to share a common signal-transduction mechanism with classical V_1 receptors, and since many vasopressin analogs with vasoconstrictor activity release ACTH, V_1 receptors have been subclassified into V_{1a} (vascular/hepatic) and V_{1b} (pituitary) receptors. V_{1b} receptors also are called V_3 *receptors*. Vasopressin analogs that are selective agonists for V_{1a} and V_{1b} receptors have been synthesized but are not available clinically.

DISEASES AFFECTING THE VASOPRESSIN SYSTEM

DIABETES INSIPIDUS (DI)   DI is a disease of impaired renal conservation of water owing either to an inadequate secretion of vasopressin from the neurohypophysis (central DI) or to an insufficient renal response to vasopressin (nephrogenic DI). Very rarely, DI can be caused by an abnormally high rate of degradation of vasopressin by circulating vasopressinases. Pregnancy may accentuate or reveal central and/or nephrogenic DI by increasing plasma levels of vasopressinase and by reducing the renal sensitivity to vasopressin. Patients with DI excrete large volumes (>30 mL/kg/day) of dilute (<200 mOsm/kg) urine and, if their thirst mechanism is functioning normally, are polydipsic. The diagnosis of DI rests on demonstrating that the patient is unable to reduce urine volume and increase urine osmolality during a period of carefully observed fluid deprivation. Central DI can be distinguished from nephrogenic DI by administration of desmopressin, which will increase urine osmolality in patients with central DI but have little or no effect in patients with nephrogenic DI. DI can be differentiated from primary polydipsia by measuring plasma osmolality, which will be low to low-normal in patients with primary polydipsia and high to high-normal in patients with DI.

Central DI   Head injury, either surgical or traumatic, in the region of the pituitary and/or hypothalamus may cause central DI. Postoperative central DI may be transient, permanent, or triphasic (recovery followed by permanent relapse). Other causes include hypothalamic or pituitary tumors, cerebral aneurysms, CNS ischemia, and brain infiltrations and infections. Finally, central DI may be idiopathic or familial. Familial central DI usually is autosomal dominant (chromosome 20); vasopressin deficiency occurs several months or years after birth and worsens gradually. Autosomal dominant central DI results from mutations in the vasopressin gene that cause the prohormone to misfold and oligomerize improperly, resulting in accumulation of the mutant vasopressin precursor in the affected neuron and neuronal death. Rarely, familial central DI is autosomal recessive owing to a mutation in the vasopressin peptide itself that gives rise to an inactive vasopressin peptide.

Antidiuretic peptides are the primary treatment for central DI, with desmopressin being the preferred peptide. For patients with central DI who cannot tolerate antidiuretic peptides because of side effects or allergic reactions, other treatment options are available. *Chlorpropamide*, an oral sulfonylurea, potentiates the action of small or residual amounts of circulating vasopressin and will reduce urine volume in more than half of all patients with central DI. A dose of 125–500 mg daily is particularly effective in patients with partial central DI. If polyuria is not controlled satisfactorily with chlorpropamide alone, addition of a thiazide diuretic (*see* Chapter 28) to the regimen usually results in an adequate reduction in the volume of urine. *Carbamazepine* (800–1000 mg daily in divided doses) and *clofibrate* (1–2 g daily in divided doses) also reduce urine volume in patients with central DI. Long-term use of these agents may induce serious adverse effects; therefore, carbamazepine and clofibrate are used rarely to treat central DI. The antidiuretic mechanisms of chlorpropamide, carbamazepine, and clofibrate are not clear. These agents are not effective in nephrogenic DI, which indicates that functional V_2 receptors are required for the antidiuretic effect. Since carbamazepine inhibits and chlorpropamide has little effect on vasopressin secretion, it is likely that carbamazepine and chlorpropamide act directly on the kidney to enhance V_2 receptor-mediated antidiuresis.

Nephrogenic DI Nephrogenic DI may be congenital or acquired. Hypercalcemia, hypokalemia, postobstructive renal failure, lithium, foscarnet, clozapine, demeclocycline, and other drugs can induce nephrogenic DI. As many as 1 in 3 patients treated with lithium may develop nephrogenic DI. X-linked nephrogenic DI is caused by mutations in the gene encoding the V_2 receptor, which maps to Xq28. A number of missense, nonsense, and frame-shift mutations in this gene have been identified in patients with this disorder, causing impaired routing of the V_2 receptor to the cell surface, defective coupling to G proteins, or decreased affinity of the receptor for vasopressin. Autosomal recessive and dominant nephrogenic DI result from inactivating mutations in aquaporin 2. These findings establish that aquaporin 2 is essential for the antidiuretic effect of vasopressin.

Although the mainstay of treatment of nephrogenic DI is assurance of an adequate intake of water, drugs also can be used to reduce polyuria. *Amiloride* blocks the uptake of lithium by the Na⁺ channel in the collecting-duct system and is used off-label for lithium-induced nephrogenic DI. Paradoxically, *thiazide diuretics* reduce the polyuria of patients with DI and often are used to treat non-lithium-induced nephrogenic DI. In infants with nephrogenic DI, thiazides may be crucially important because uncontrolled polyuria may exceed the child's capacity to imbibe and absorb fluids. The natriuretic action of thiazides and resulting depletion of extracellular fluid volume may play an important role in the thiazide-induced antidiuresis since these effects appear to parallel the ability of thiazides to cause natriuresis, and the drugs are given in doses similar to those used to mobilize edema fluid. In patients with DI, a 50% reduction of urine volume is a good response to thiazides. Moderate restriction of sodium intake can enhance the antidiuretic effectiveness of thiazides.

While case reports describe the effectiveness of indomethacin in the treatment of nephrogenic DI, other cyclooxygenase inhibitors (*e.g., ibuprofen*) appear to be less effective. The mechanism of the effect may involve a decrease in glomerular filtration rate, an increase in medullary solute concentration, and/or enhanced proximal reabsorption of fluid. Also, since prostaglandins attenuate vasopressin-induced antidiuresis in patients with at least a partially intact V_2-receptor system, some of the antidiuretic response to indomethacin may be due to diminution of the prostaglandin effect and enhancement of the effects of vasopressin on principal cells of the collecting duct.

SYNDROME OF INAPPROPRIATE SECRETION OF ANTIDIURETIC HORMONE

(SIADH) SIADH is a disease of impaired water excretion with accompanying hyponatremia and hypo-osmolality caused by the *inappropriate* secretion of vasopressin. The clinical manifestations of plasma hypotonicity resulting from SIADH may include lethargy, anorexia, nausea and vomiting, muscle cramps, coma, convulsions, and death. A multitude of disorders can induce SIADH, including malignancies, pulmonary diseases, CNS injuries/diseases (*e.g.*, head trauma, infections, and tumors), and general surgery. The three drug classes most commonly implicated in drug-induced SIADH include psychotropic medications (*e.g., fluoxetine*, haloperidol, and *tricyclic antidepressants*), sulfonylureas (*e.g.*, chloropropamide), and vinca alkaloids (*e.g., vincristine* and *vinblastine*). Other drugs strongly associated with SIADH include thiazide diuretics, clonidine, *enalapril, ifosphamide*, and *methyldopa*. In a normal individual, an elevation in plasma vasopressin *per se* does not induce plasma hypotonicity because the person simply stops drinking owing to an osmotically induced aversion to fluids. Therefore, plasma hypotonicity only occurs when excessive fluid intake (oral or intravenous) accompanies inappropriate secretion of vasopressin. Treatment of hypotonicity in the setting of SIADH includes water restriction, intravenous administration of hypertonic saline, loop diuretics (which interfere with the concentrating ability of the kidneys), and drugs that inhibit the effect of vasopressin to increase water permeability in the collecting ducts. To inhibit vasopressin's action in the collecting ducts, *demeclocycline*, a tetracycline, is the preferred drug.

Although lithium can inhibit the renal actions of vasopressin, it is effective in only a minority of patients, may induce irreversible renal damage when used chronically, and has a low therapeutic index. Therefore, lithium should be considered for use only in patients with symptomatic SIADH who cannot be controlled by other means or in whom tetracyclines are contraindicated, *e.g.*, patients with liver disease. It is important to stress that the majority of patients with SIADH do not require therapy because plasma Na⁺ stabilizes in the range of 125–132 m*M;* such patients usually are asymptomatic. Only when symptomatic hypotonicity ensues, generally when plasma Na⁺ levels drop below 120 m*M,* should therapy with demeclocycline be initiated. Since hypotonicity, which causes an influx of water into cells with resulting cerebral swelling, is the cause of symptoms, the goal of therapy is simply to increase plasma osmolality toward normal.

OTHER WATER-RETAINING STATES   In patients with congestive heart failure, cirrhosis, or nephrotic syndrome, *effective* blood volume often is reduced, and hypovolemia frequently is exacerbated by the liberal use of diuretics. Since hypovolemia stimulates vasopressin release, patients may become hyponatremic owing to vasopressin-mediated retention of water. The development of potent orally active V_2 receptor antagonists and specific inhibitors of water channels in the collecting duct would provide an effective therapeutic strategy not only in patients with SIADH but also in the much more common setting of hyponatremia in patients with heart failure, cirrhosis, or nephrotic syndrome.

CLINICAL USE OF VASOPRESSIN PEPTIDES

THERAPEUTIC USES   Only two antidiuretic peptides are available for clinical use in the U.S. Vasopressin (synthetic 8-L-arginine vasopressin; PITRESSIN) is available as a sterile aqueous solution; it may be administered subcutaneously, intramuscularly, or intranasally. *Desmopressin acetate* (synthetic 1-deamino-8-D-arginine vasopressin; DDAVP, others) is available as a sterile aqueous solution packaged for intravenous or subcutaneous injection, in a nasal solution for intranasal administration with either a nasal spray pump or rhinal tube delivery system, and in tablets for oral administration. Based on the type of vasopressin receptor involved, the therapeutic uses of vasopressin and its congeners can be divided into two main categories.

V_1 receptor-mediated therapeutic applications are based on the rationale that V_1 receptors cause contraction of GI and vascular smooth muscle. V_1 receptor-mediated contraction of GI smooth muscle has been used to treat postoperative ileus and abdominal distension and to dispel intestinal gas before abdominal roentgenography to avoid interfering gas shadows. V_1 receptor-mediated vasoconstriction of the splanchnic arterial vessels reduces blood flow to the portal system and thereby attenuates pressure and bleeding in esophageal varices. Although endoscopic variceal banding ligation is the treatment of choice for bleeding esophageal varices, V_1 receptor agonists have been used emergently until endoscopy can be performed. Simultaneous administration of nitroglycerin with V_1 receptor agonists may attenuate the cardiotoxic effects of V_1 agonists while enhancing their beneficial splanchnic effects. Also, V_1 receptor agonists have been used during abdominal surgery in patients with portal hypertension to diminish the risk of hemorrhage during the procedure. Finally, V_1 receptor-mediated vasoconstriction has been used to reduce bleeding during acute hemorrhagic gastritis, burn wound excision, cyclophosphamide-induced hemorrhagic cystitis, liver transplant, caesarean section, and uterine myoma resection. The applications of V_1 receptor agonists can be accomplished with vasopressin; however, the use of vasopressin for all these indications is no longer recommended because of significant adverse reactions. Although not yet available in the U.S., *terlipressin* (GLYPRESSIN) is preferred for bleeding esophageal varices because of increased safety compared with vasopressin. Terlipressin also is effective in patients with hepatorenal syndrome, particularly when combined with albumin.

Vasopressin levels in patients with vasodilatory shock are inappropriately low, and such patients are extraordinarily sensitive to the pressor actions of vasopressin. The combination of vasopressin and *norepinephrine* is superior to NE alone in the management of catecholamine-resistant vasodilatory shock. Although the efficacy of vasopressin in the resuscitation of patients with ventricular fibrillation or pulseless electrical activity is similar to that of epinephrine, vasopressin followed by Epi appears to be more effective than Epi alone in the treatment of patients with asystole.

V_2 receptor-mediated therapeutic applications are based on the rationale that V_2 receptors cause water conservation and release of blood coagulation factors. Central DI can be treated with V_2 receptor agonists, and polyuria and polydipsia usually are well controlled. While some patients experience transient DI (*e.g.,* in head injury or surgery in the area of the pituitary), therapy for most patients with DI is lifelong. Desmopressin is the drug of choice for the vast majority of patients and is efficacious and well-tolerated in both adults and children. A single intranasal dose lasts from 6 to 20 hours; twice-daily administration is effective in most patients. There is considerable variability in the intranasal dose of desmopressin required to maintain normal urine volume, and the dosage must be tailored individually. The usual intranasal dosage in adults is 10–40 μg/day, either as a single dose or divided into two or three doses. In view of the high cost of the drug and the importance of avoiding water intoxication, the schedule of administration should be adjusted to the minimal amount required. An initial dose of 2.5 μg can be used, with therapy directed toward the control of nocturia. An equivalent or higher morning dose controls daytime polyuria in most patients, although a third dose occasionally may be needed in the afternoon. In some patients, chronic allergic rhinitis or other nasal pathology may preclude reliable absorption of the peptide

following nasal administration. Oral administration of desmopressin in doses 10–20 times the intranasal dose provides adequate blood levels of desmopressin to control polyuria. Daily subcutaneous administration of 1–2 μg of desmopressin also is effective.

Vasopressin has little, if any, place in the long-term therapy of DI because of its short duration of action and V_1 receptor-mediated side effects. Vasopressin can be used as an alternative to desmopressin in the initial diagnostic evaluation of patients with suspected DI and to control polyuria in patients with DI who recently have undergone surgery or experienced head trauma. Under these circumstances, polyuria may be transient, and long-acting agents may produce water intoxication.

V_2 receptor agonists (*e.g.,* desmopressin) are also used in bleeding disorders. In most patients with type I von Willebrand's disease (vWD) and in some with type IIn vWD, desmopressin will elevate von Willebrand factor and shorten bleeding time. However, desmopressin generally is ineffective in patients with types IIa, IIb, and III vWD. Desmopressin may transiently cause a marked thrombocytopenia in individuals with type IIb vWD and is contraindicated in such patients. Desmopressin also increases factor VIII levels in patients with mild-to-moderate hemophilia A. Desmopressin is not indicated in patients with severe hemophilia A, those with hemophilia B, or those with factor VIII antibodies. The response of any given patient with type I vWD or hemophilia A to desmopressin should be determined with a test dose of nasal spray at the time of diagnosis or 1–2 weeks before elective surgery to assess the extent of increase in factor VIII or von Willebrand factor. In patients with renal insufficiency or uremia, desmopressin shortens bleeding time and increases circulating levels of factor VIII coagulant activity, factor VIII-related antigen, and ristocetin cofactor. It also induces the appearance of larger von Willebrand factor multimers. Desmopressin is effective in some patients with cirrhosis- or drug-induced (*e.g., heparin, hirudin,* and *antiplatelet agents*) bleeding disorders. Desmopressin, given intravenously at a dose of 0.3 μg/kg, increases factor VIII and von Willebrand factor for >6 hours. Desmopressin can be given at intervals of 12–24 hours depending on the clinical response and the severity of bleeding. Tachyphylaxis to desmopressin, which usually occurs after several days (owing to depletion of factor VIII and von Willebrand factor storage sites), limits its usefulness to preoperative preparation, postoperative bleeding, excessive menstrual bleeding, and emergency situations.

Another V_2 receptor-mediated application is the use of desmopressin for primary nocturnal enuresis. Bedtime administration of desmopressin intranasal spray or tablets provides a high response rate that is sustained with long-term use, that is safe, and that accelerates the cure rate. Desmopressin also relieves post–lumbar puncture headache, probably by causing water retention and thereby facilitating rapid fluid equilibration in the CNS.

PHARMACOKINETICS When vasopressin and desmopressin are given orally, they are rapidly inactivated by trypsin, which cleaves the peptide bond between amino acids 8 and 9. Inactivation by peptidases in various tissues (particularly the liver and kidneys) results in a plasma $t_{1/2}$ of vasopressin of 17–35 minutes. Following intramuscular or subcutaneous injection, the antidiuretic effects of vasopressin last 2–8 hours. The plasma $t_{1/2}$ of desmopressin has a fast component of 6.5–9 minutes and a slow component of 30–117 minutes. Only 3% and 0.15%, respectively, of intranasally and orally administered desmopressin is absorbed.

TOXICITY, ADVERSE EFFECTS, CONTRAINDICATIONS, DRUG INTERACTIONS Most adverse effects are mediated through the V_1 receptor acting on vascular and GI smooth muscle; such adverse effects are much less common and less severe with desmopressin than with vasopressin. After the injection of large doses of vasopressin, marked facial pallor owing to cutaneous vasoconstriction is observed commonly. Increased intestinal activity is likely to cause nausea, belching, cramps, and an urge to defecate. Most serious, however, is the effect on the coronary circulation. Vasopressin should be administered only at low doses and with extreme caution in individuals suffering from vascular disease, especially coronary artery disease. Other cardiac complications include arrhythmia and decreased cardiac output. Peripheral vasoconstriction and gangrene also have been encountered in patients receiving large doses of vasopressin.

The major V_2 receptor-mediated adverse effect is water intoxication, which can occur with desmopressin or vasopressin. Many drugs, including carbamazepine, chlorpropamide, morphine, tricyclic antidepressants and NSAIDs, can potentiate the antidiuretic effects of these peptides, while lithium, demeclocycline and ethanol can attenuate the antidiuretic response to desmopressin. Desmopressin and vasopressin should be used cautiously when a rapid increase in extracellular water may impose risks (*e.g.,* in angina, hypertension, and heart failure) and should not be used in patients with acute renal failure. Patients receiving desmopressin to maintain hemostasis should be advised to reduce fluid intake. It is imperative that these peptides not be administered to patients with primary or psychogenic polydipsia because severe hypotonic hyponatremia will ensue.

Mild facial flushing and headache are the most common adverse effects associated with desmopressin. Allergic reactions ranging from urticaria to anaphylaxis may occur with desmopressin or vasopressin. Intranasal administration may cause local adverse effects in the nasal passages, such as edema, rhinorrhea, congestion, irritation, pruritus, and ulceration.

Future Directions in Vasopressin Analogs

Nonpeptide vasopressin receptor antagonists and agonists are being developed for a wide range of clinical indications. The V_2 receptor antagonist *conivaptin* (VAPRISOL) is now FDA-approved for the treatment of euvolemic hyponatremia in hospitalized patients who do not have congestive heart failure (*e.g.*, patients with SIADH, or with hypothyroidism or adrenal insufficiency). Conivaptin is contraindicated in patients with volume depletion or those receiving other drugs that inhibit CYP3A4 (*e.g.*, ketoconazole, itraconazole, clarithromycin, indinavir, and ritonavir). Other vasopressin receptor antagonists now in clinical trials, such as *tolvaptan* and *satavaptan*, can be administered orally.

For a complete Bibliographical listing see Goodman & Gilman's *The Pharmacological Basis of Therapeutics*, 11th ed., or Goodman & Gilman Online at www.accessmedicine.com.

30

RENIN AND ANGIOTENSIN

OVERVIEW   Angiotensin II (AngII), the most active angiotensin peptide, is derived from angiotensinogen via two proteolytic steps. First, renin, an enzyme released from the kidneys, cleaves the decapeptide angiotensin I (AngI) from the amino terminus of angiotensinogen (renin substrate). Angiotensin-converting enzyme (ACE) then removes the carboxy-terminal dipeptide of AngI to produce the octapeptide AngII. AngII is degraded subsequently by further proteolysis (see summary, Figure 30–1). AngII acts by binding to two GPCRs (*see* below).

RENIN

The major determinant of the rate of AngII production is the amount of renin released by the kidney. Renin is an aspartyl protease whose principal natural substrate is the circulating α_2-globulin, angiotensinogen, secreted by hepatocytes. Renin is synthesized as a preproenzyme of 406 amino acid residues and processed to prorenin, a mature but inactive form. Prorenin then is activated by proteolytic cleavage to yield the active 340-amino acid renin. Both renin and prorenin are stored in the juxtaglomerular (j-g) cells and, after release, circulate in the blood. The concentration of prorenin in the circulation is approximately tenfold greater than that of the active enzyme. The $t_{1/2}$ of circulating renin is ~15 minutes.

Control of Renin Secretion

Renin secretion from j-g cells is controlled predominantly by three pathways: two acting locally within the kidney, the third acting through the CNS and mediated by norepinephrine (NE) release from renal nerves (Figure 30–2). One intrarenal mechanism controlling renin release is the macula densa pathway *(top of Figure 30–2A). Increased NaCl reabsorption and flux across the macula densa inhibits, while decreased NaCl flux stimulates, renin release. Both adenosine and prostaglandins mediate the macula densa pathway; the former is released when Na^+ transport increases, and the latter is released when NaCl transport decreases. Adenosine, acting via the A_1 adenosine receptor, inhibits renin release, while prostaglandins stimulate renin release. Inducible cyclooxygenase (COX–2) and neuronal nitric oxide synthase (nNOS) also play a role in macula densa–stimulated renin release. Figure 30–2B summarizes possible mechanisms regulating renin release.*

Although a change in NaCl transport is a key modulator, regulation of the macula densa pathway pathway depends more on the luminal concentration of Cl^- than Na^+. Physiological changes in Cl^- concentrations (e.g., from 20 to 60 mEq/L) at the macula densa profoundly affect macula densa–mediated renin release.

The second intrarenal mechanism controlling renin release is the intrarenal baroreceptor pathway *(middle of Figure 30–2A). Increases and decreases in blood pressure in the preglomerular vessels inhibit and stimulate renin release, respectively. The immediate stimulus to secretion is believed to be reduced tension within the wall of the afferent arteriole. Changes in renal prostaglandins may partly mediate the intrarenal baroreceptor pathway, as may biomechanical coupling via stretch-activated ion channels.*

The third mechanism, the β adrenergic receptor pathway (bottom of Figure 30–2A), is mediated by the release of NE from postganglionic sympathetic nerves; activation of β_1 receptors on juxtaglomerular cells enhances renin secretion.

Increased renin secretion enhances the formation of AngII, which stimulates angiotensin subtype 1 (AT_1) receptors on j-g cells to inhibit renin release, an effect termed short-loop negative feedback. *AngII also increases arterial blood pressure via AT_1 receptors. Increases in blood pressure inhibit renin release by (1) activating high-pressure baroreceptors and reducing renal sympathetic tone, (2) increasing pressure in the preglomerular vessels, and (3) reducing NaCl reabsorption in the proximal tubule, which increases tubular delivery of NaCl to the macula densa. The inhibition of renin release by AngII–induced increases in blood pressure has been termed* long-loop negative feedback.

The physiological pathways regulating renin release can be influenced by blood pressure, salt intake, and a number of drugs. In all these cases, renin release is affected by the interplay of mechanisms summarized in Figure 30–2A. Loop diuretics (see Chapter 28) stimulate renin release in part by blocking NaCl reabsorption at the macula densa. Nonsteroidal anti-inflammatory drugs (NSAIDs) (see Chapter 26) inhibit prostaglandin synthesis and thereby decrease renin release. ACE inhibitors, angiotensin receptor blockers (ARBs), and renin inhibitors interrupt both the short- and long-loop negative feedback mechanisms and therefore increase renin release. Chronic administration of ACE inhibitors up-regulates renal COX-2 and nNOS expression. In general, diuretics and vasodilators increase renin release by decreasing arterial blood pressure. Centrally acting sympatholytic drugs and β adrenergic receptor antagonists decrease renin secretion by

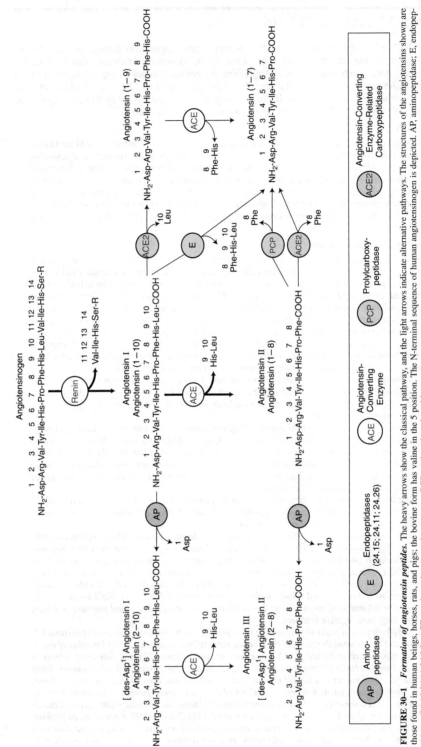

FIGURE 30-1 *Formation of angiotensin peptides.* The heavy arrows show the classical pathway, and the light arrows indicate alternative pathways. The structures of the angiotensins shown are those found in human beings, horses, rats, and pigs; the bovine form has valine in the 5 position. The N-terminal sequence of human angiotensinogen is depicted. AP, aminopeptidase; E, endopeptidases (24.15;24.11;24.26); ACE, angiotensin-converting snzyme; PCP, prolycarboxylpeptidase.

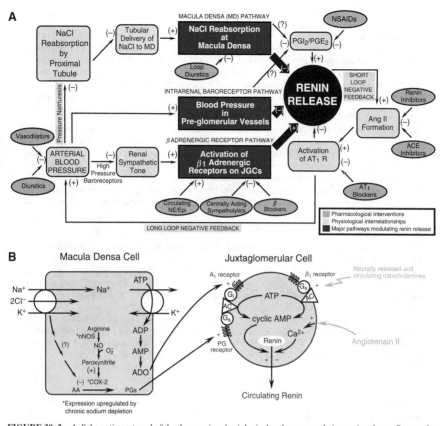

FIGURE 30–2 **A.** Schematic portrayal of the three major physiological pathways regulating renin release. *See* text for details. MD, macula densa; PGI$_2$/PGE$_2$ prostaglandins I$_2$ and E$_2$; NSAIDs, nonsteroidal anti-inflammatory drugs; AngII, angiotensin II; ACE, angiotensin-converting enzyme, AT$_1$ R, angiotensin subtype 1 receptor; NE/Epi, norepinephrine/epinephrine; JGCs, juxtaglomerular cells. **B.** Possible mechanisms by which the macula densa regulates renin release. Both acute changes in tubular delivery of NaCl to the macula densa and chronic changes in dietary sodium intake cause appropriate signals to be conveyed from macula densa to the juxtaglomerular cells. Chronic sodium depletion up-regulates neuronal nitric oxide synthase (nNOS) and inducible cyclooxygenase (COX-2) in the macula densa. nNOS increases nitric oxide (NO) production, and NO reacts with superoxide anion (O$_2^-$) to form peroxynitrite, an activator of COX-2. In addition, COX-2 may be rapidly, although indirectly, inhibited and stimulated by increases and decreases in NaCl transport, respectively, across the macula densa. Arachidonic acid (AA) is converted to prostaglandins (PGs), which diffuse to nearby juxtaglomerular cells to stimulate adenylyl cyclase (AC) *via* prostaglandin receptors, such as EP$_4$ and IP, that couple to G$_s$. Circulating and locally released catecholamines also stimulate adenylyl cyclase via β_1 receptors. Cyclic AMP (cAMP) augments renin release. Increased NaCl transport depletes ATP and increases adenosine (ADO) levels in the macula densa. ADO diffuses to the juxtaglomerular cells and activates the AT$_1$-G$_i$ pathway, inhibiting AC and reducing cellular cAMP. Increased NaCl transport in the macula densa augments the efflux of ATP through basolateral maxi-anion channels, and ATP is converted to adenosine in the extracellular compartment and inhibits adenylyl cyclase *via* A$_1$ receptors. In addition, ATP released from the macula densa may inhibit renin release directly by binding to P2Y receptors coupled to G$_q$ on juxtaglomerular cells. Activation of G$_q$ increases intracellular Ca^{2+}, which inhibits renin release. Circulating AngII binds to AT$_1$ receptors on juxtaglomerular cells and inhibits renin release *via* G$_q$-induced increases in intracellular Ca^{2+}.

reducing activation of β adrenergic receptors on j-g cells. Phosphodiesterase inhibitors stimulate renin release by increasing cyclic AMP in j-g cells.

ANGIOTENSINOGEN

Angiotensinogen is circulating glycoprotein containing 452 amino acids that is synthesized primarily in the liver as preangiotensinogen, (MW = 55,000–60,000). Angiotensinogen synthesis is stimulated by inflammation, insulin, estrogens, glucocorticoids, thyroid hormone, and AngII.

During pregnancy, plasma levels of angiotensinogen increase severalfold owing to increased estrogen.

AngI is cleaved by renin from the amino terminus of angiotensinogen. Circulating levels of angiotensinogen are approximately equal to its K_m for renin cleavage (~1 µM), and the rate of AngII synthesis therefore can be significantly influenced by changes in angiotensinogen levels. For example, estrogen therapy increases circulating levels of angiotensinogen, possibly inducing hypertension, and a missense mutation in the angiotensinogen gene (M235T) that increases circulating angiotensinogen is associated with essential and pregnancy-induced hypertension.

ACE, KININASE II, DIPEPTIDYL CARBOXYPEPTIDASE

The rapid conversion of AngI to AngII in plasma is due to the activity of membrane-bound ACE on the luminal surface of endothelial cells throughout the vasculature. ACE has a large amino-terminal extracellular domain, a short carboxyl-terminal intracellular domain, and a 17–amino acid hydrophobic region that anchors the ectoenzyme to the cell membrane. Circulating ACE represents membrane ACE that has undergone proteolysis. ACE cleaves dipeptides from substrates. Preferred substrates have only one free carboxyl group in the carboxyl-terminal amino acid, and proline must not be the penultimate amino acid; thus, ACE does not degrade AngII. ACE also inactivates bradykinin and other potent vasodilator peptides.

ANGIOTENSIN PEPTIDES

AngI is <1% as potent as AngII on smooth muscle, heart, and the adrenal cortex. Angiotensin III (AngIII), also called [des-Asp¹]AngII or angiotensin (2–8), can be formed either by the action of aminopeptidase on AngII or by the action of ACE on [des-Asp¹]AngI (Figure 30–1). AngIII and AngII have qualitatively similar effects; both stimulate aldosterone secretion with equal potency, but AngIII is only 25% and 10% as potent as AngII in elevating blood pressure and stimulating the adrenal medulla, respectively.

Angiotensin(1–7) is formed by multiple pathways (Figure 30–1). ACE inhibitors increase tissue and plasma levels of angiotensin(1–7), both because AngI levels are increased and diverted away from AngII formation (Figure 30–1) and because ACE contributes importantly to the plasma clearance of angiotensin(1–7). The pharmacological profile of angiotensin(1–7) is distinct from that of AngII: angiotensin(1–7) does not cause vasoconstriction, aldosterone release, or facilitation of noradrenergic neurotransmission. Angiotensin(1–7) releases vasopressin, stimulates prostaglandin biosynthesis, elicits depressor responses when microinjected into certain brainstem nuclei, dilates some blood vessels, and exerts a natriuretic action on the kidneys. Angiotensin(1–7) also inhibits proliferation of vascular smooth muscle cells. The effects of angiotensin(1–7) may be mediated by a specific angiotensin(1–7) receptor; it has been proposed that angiotensin(1–7) serves to counterbalance the actions of AngII. Angiotensin(3–8), also called AngIV, is another biologically active angiotensin peptide that also appears to counteract the effects of AngII.

Various peptidases degrade and inactivate angiotensin peptides, including aminopeptidases, endopeptidases, and carboxypeptidases; none is specific.

LOCAL (TISSUE) RENIN–ANGIOTENSIN SYSTEMS

Circulating renin from the kidney acts on circulating angiotensinogen of hepatic origin to produce AngI in the plasma, circulating AngI is converted by ACE to AngII, and AngII then is delivered to its target organs via the bloodstream to induce a physiological response. This traditional view must be expanded to include local (tissue) renin–angiotensin systems, which consist of extrinsic and intrinsic local renin–angiotensin systems.

Extrinsic Local Renin–Angiotensin Systems

ACE is present on the luminal face of vascular endothelial cells throughout the circulation, and circulating renin of renal origin can be sequestered by the arterial wall and other tissues, permitting the local conversion of precursors to AngII. Indeed, many vascular beds locally produce AngI and II.

Intrinsic Local Renin–Angiotensin Systems

Many tissues (e.g., brain, pituitary, blood vessels, heart, kidney, and adrenal gland) express mRNAs for renin, angiotensinogen, and/or ACE, and can produce renin, angiotensinogen, ACE, and AngI, II, and III. These local renin–angiotensin systems may influence vascular, cardiac, and renal function and structure.

ALTERNATIVE PATHWAYS FOR ANGIOTENSIN BIOSYNTHESIS

Some tissues contain non-renin enzymes that convert angiotensinogen to AngI or directly to AngII (e.g., cathepsin G, tonin) and non-ACE AngI-processing enzymes that convert AngI to AngII (e.g., *cathepsin G, chymostatin-sensitive AngII–generating enzyme, heart chymase). Chymase, possibly derived from mast cells, contributes to the local tissue conversion of AngI to AngII, particularly in the heart and kidneys.*

ANGIOTENSIN RECEPTORS

Angiotensins act through two specific GPCRs, designated AT_1 and AT_2. The AT_1 receptor has a high affinity for losartan, a low affinity for PD 123177, and a low affinity for CGP 42112A (a peptide analog). In contrast, the AT_2 receptor has a high affinity for PD 123177 and CGP 42112A but a low affinity for losartan.

The AT_1 and AT_2 receptors have little sequence homology. Most of the known biological effects of AngII are mediated by the AT_1 receptor. Consistent with its functional preeminence, the AT_1-receptor gene contains a polymorphism (A1166C) that is associated with hypertension, hypertrophic cardiomyopathy, coronary artery vasoconstriction, and aortic stiffness, while preeclampsia is associated with the development of activating autoantibodies against the AT_1 receptor. Potential roles for the AT_2 receptor include antiproliferative, proapoptotic, vasodilatory, and antihypertensive effects.

ANGIOTENSIN RECEPTOR–EFFECTOR COUPLING

AT_1 receptors activate a large array of signal-transduction systems to produce effects that vary with cell type and that are a combination of primary and secondary responses (Figure 30–3). The relative importance of these myriad signal-transduction pathways in mediating biological responses to AngII is tissue-specific. Other receptors may alter the response to AT_1-receptor activation (e.g., AT_1 receptors heterodimerize with bradykinin B_2 receptors, which enhances AngII sensitivity in preeclampsia).

Signaling from AT_2 receptors is mediated largely by G_i. Consequences of AT_2-receptor activation include activation of phosphatases, K^+ channels, and bradykinin and NO production and inhibition of Ca^{2+} channel function.

Functions and Effects of the Renin–Angiotensin System

The renin–angiotensin system plays a major role in the regulation of arterial blood pressure. Modest increases in plasma concentrations of AngII. When a single moderate dose of AngII is injected intravenously, systemic blood pressure begins to rise within seconds, peaks rapidly, and returns to

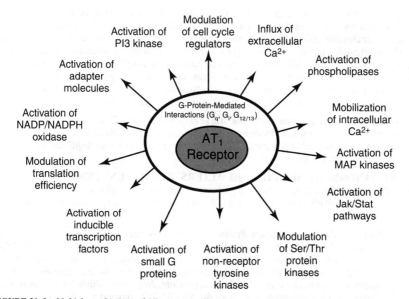

FIGURE 30–3 *Multiple mechanisms of AT_1 receptor–effector coupling.* AT_1 receptors couple to G_q, G_i, and $G_{12/13}$. Through effectors, second messengers, and signaling cascades, a large array of response pathways is subsequently engaged to produce immediate and long-term effects of AngII.

normal within minutes. This *rapid pressor response* to AngII is due to a swift increase in total peripheral resistance—a response that helps to maintain arterial blood pressure in the face of blood loss or vasodilation. Although AngII increases cardiac contractility directly *via* voltage-gated Ca^{2+} channels and increases heart rate indirectly (*via* facilitation of sympathetic tone, enhanced adrenergic neurotransmission, and adrenal catecholamine release), the rapid increase in arterial blood pressure activates a baroreceptor reflex that decreases sympathetic tone and increases vagal tone. Thus, depending on the physiological state, AngII may increase, decrease, or not change cardiac contractility, heart rate, and cardiac output. Changes in cardiac output therefore contribute little, if at all, to the rapid pressor response induced by AngII.

AngII also causes a *slow pressor response* that chronically helps to maintain blood pressure. Continuous infusion of initially subpressor doses of AngII gradually increases blood pressure over a period of days. This slow pressor response probably is mediated by decreases in renal excretion that shift the renal pressure–natriuresis curve to the right (*see* below). AngII stimulates the synthesis of endothelin-1 and superoxide anion, which may contribute to the slow pressor response. In addition to its effects on arterial blood pressure, AngII causes hypertrophy of vascular and cardiac cells and increased collagen deposition by cardiac fibroblasts. The effects of AngII on total peripheral resistance, renal function, and cardiovascular structure are mediated by direct and indirect mechanisms (*see* Figure 30–4).

MECHANISMS BY WHICH ANGII INCREASES TOTAL PERIPHERAL RESISTANCE
AngII increases total peripheral resistance (TPR) by direct and indirect effects on blood vessels.

Direct Vasoconstriction   AngII constricts precapillary arterioles and, to a lesser extent, postcapillary venules by activating AT_1 receptors on vascular smooth muscle cells. AngII has differential effects on vascular beds. The kidneys and splanchnic bed constrict markedly, thereby decreasing blood flow. Blood flow to the brain, lung, and skeletal muscle may actually increase in response to AngII because the elevated systemic blood pressure overcomes the relatively weak vasoconstriction. Nevertheless, high circulating concentrations of AngII may decrease cerebral and coronary blood flow.

Enhancement of Peripheral Noradrenergic Neurotransmission   AngII augments NE release from sympathetic nerve terminals, inhibits the reuptake of NE into nerve terminals, and enhances the vascular response to NE. Intracoronary AngII potentiates sympathetic nervous system–induced coronary vasoconstriction.

Effects on the CNS   Small amounts of AngII infused into the vertebral arteries increases blood pressure. This response—mediated by increased sympathetic outflow—reflects effects of the hormone on circumventricular nuclei that are not protected by the blood–brain barrier. Circulating AngII also attenuates baroreceptor-mediated reductions in sympathetic discharge, thereby increasing arterial pressure. The CNS is affected both by blood-borne AngII and by AngII formed locally. The brain contains all components of a renin–angiotensin system, suggesting that AngII serves as a neurotransmitter or modulator. In addition to increasing sympathetic tone, AngII also causes a centrally mediated dipsogenic effect and enhances the release of vasopressin.

Release of Catecholamines from the Adrenal Medulla   AngII stimulates catecholamine release from the adrenal medulla by depolarizing chromaffin cells. Although this response usually is of minimal physiological importance, dangerous reactions have followed AngII administration to individuals with pheochromocytoma.

MECHANISMS BY WHICH AngII ALTERS RENAL FUNCTION
AngII has pronounced effects on renal function, reducing urinary excretion of Na^+ and water while increasing K^+ excretion. The overall effect of AngII on the kidneys is to shift the renal pressure–natriuresis curve to the right (*see* below).

Direct Effects of AngII on Sodium Reabsorption in the Renal Tubules   Very low concentrations of AngII stimulate Na^+/H^+ exchange in the proximal tubule—an effect that increases Na^+, Cl^-, and bicarbonate reabsorption. Approximately 25% of the bicarbonate handled by the nephron may be affected by this mechanism. AngII also increases the expression of the Na^+–glucose symporter in the proximal tubule. Paradoxically, at high concentrations, AngII may inhibit Na^+ transport in the proximal tubule. AngII also directly stimulates the Na^+–K^+–$2Cl^-$ symporter in the thick ascending limb. The proximal tubule secretes angiotensinogen, and the connecting tubule releases renin, so a paracrine tubular renin–angiotensin system may modulate Na^+ reabsorption.

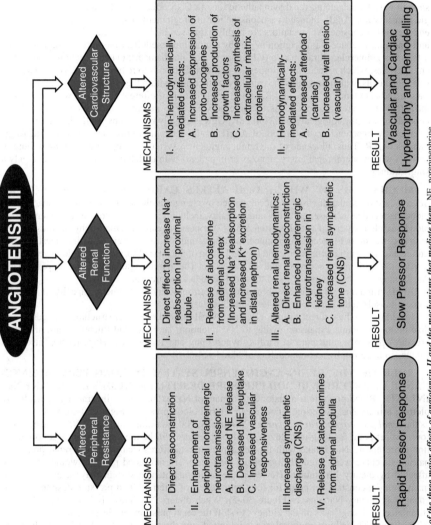

ANGIOTENSIN II

Altered Peripheral Resistance

MECHANISMS

I. Direct vasoconstriction

II. Enhancement of peripheral noradrenergic neurotransmission:
A. Increased NE release
B. Decreased NE reuptake
C. Increased vascular responsiveness

III. Increased sympathetic discharge (CNS)

IV. Release of catecholamines from adrenal medulla

RESULT

Rapid Pressor Response

Altered Renal Function

MECHANISMS

I. Direct effect to increase Na$^+$ reabsorption in proximal tubule.

II. Release of aldosterone from adrenal cortex (Increased Na$^+$ reabsorption and increased K$^+$ excretion in distal nephron)

III. Altered renal hemodynamics:
A. Direct renal vasoconstriction
B. Enhanced noradrenergic neurotransmission in kidney
C. Increased renal sympathetic tone (CNS)

RESULT

Slow Pressor Response

Altered Cardiovascular Structure

MECHANISMS

I. Non-hemodynamically-mediated effects:
A. Increased expression of proto-oncogenes
B. Increased production of growth factors
C. Increased synthesis of extracellular matrix proteins

II. Hemodynamically-mediated effects:
A. Increased afterload (cardiac)
B. Increased wall tension (vascular)

RESULT

Vascular and Cardiac Hypertrophy and Remodelling

FIGURE 30–4 *Summary of the three major effects of angiotensin II and the mechanisms that mediate them.* NE, norepinephrine.

517

Release of Aldosterone from the Adrenal Cortex AngII stimulates the zona glomerulosa of the adrenal cortex to increase the synthesis and secretion of aldosterone and also exerts permissive effects that augment responses to ACTH and K^+. Increased output of aldosterone is elicited by concentrations of AngII that have little or no acute effect on blood pressure. Aldosterone acts on the distal and collecting tubules to cause retention of Na^+ and excretion of K^+ and H^+. AngII-induced stimulation of aldosterone synthesis is enhanced by hyponatremia or hyperkalemia.

Altered Renal Hemodynamics Reduced renal blood flow markedly attenuates renal excretory function, and AngII reduces renal blood flow by directly constricting the renal vascular smooth muscle, enhancing renal sympathetic tone (a CNS effect), and facilitating renal adrenergic transmission. AngII–induced vasoconstriction of preglomerular microvessels is enhanced by endogenous adenosine. AT_1 receptors are highly expressed in the vasa recta of the renal medulla, and AngII may reduce Na^+ excretion in part by diminishing medullary blood flow. AngII variably influences glomerular filtration rate (GFR) *via* several mechanisms: (1) constriction of the afferent arterioles, which reduces intraglomerular pressure and tends to reduce GFR, (2) contraction of mesangial cells, which decreases the capillary surface area within the glomerulus available for filtration and also tends to reduce GFR, and (3) constriction of efferent arterioles, which increases intraglomerular pressure and tends to increase GFR. The outcome of these opposing effects depends on the physiological state. Normally, GFR is slightly reduced by AngII; however, during renal artery hypotension, the effects of AngII on the efferent arteriole predominate and AngII increases GFR. Thus, blockade of the renin–angiotensin system may cause acute renal failure in patients with bilateral renal artery stenosis or in patients with unilateral stenosis who have only a single kidney.

MECHANISMS BY WHICH AngII ALTERS CARDIOVASCULAR STRUCTURE

Several cardiovascular diseases are accompanied by changes in the morphology of the heart and/or blood vessels that increase morbidity and mortality, including: (1) increased wall-to-lumen ratio in blood vessels (associated with hypertension), (2) concentric cardiac hypertrophy (also associated with hypertension), (3) eccentric cardiac hypertrophy and fibrosis (associated with congestive heart failure and myocardial infarction), and (4) thickening of the intimal surface of the blood vessel wall (associated with atherosclerosis and angioplasty). The renin–angiotensin system, particularly AngII, may contribute importantly to these deleterious structural changes.

AngII stimulates migration, proliferation, hypertrophy, and/or synthetic capacity of vascular smooth muscle cells, cardiac myocytes, and fibroblasts.

In addition to these direct cellular effects of AngII on cardiovascular structure, changes in cardiac preload (volume expansion owing to Na^+ retention) and afterload (increased arterial blood pressure) probably contribute to cardiac hypertrophy and remodeling. Hypertension also contributes to hypertrophy and remodeling of blood vessels.

ROLE OF THE RENIN–ANGIOTENSIN SYSTEM IN LONG-TERM MAINTENANCE OF ARTERIAL BLOOD PRESSURE DESPITE EXTREMES IN DIETARY Na^+

INTAKE Blood pressure is a major determinant of Na^+ excretion, as illustrated graphically by plotting urinary Na^+ excretion *versus* mean arterial blood pressure (Figure 30–5), a plot known as the *renal pressure–natriuresis curve*. Chronically, Na^+ excretion must equal Na^+ intake; therefore, the set point for long-term levels of blood pressure will be the intersection of a horizontal line representing Na^+ intake with the renal pressure–natriuresis curve. If the renal pressure–natriuresis curve were fixed, then over the long-term, arterial blood pressure would be greatly affected by dietary Na^+ intake. However, the renin–angiotensin system plays a major role in maintaining a constant set point for long-term levels of arterial blood pressure despite extreme changes in dietary Na^+ intake (Figure 30–5). When dietary Na^+ intake is low, renin release is stimulated, and AngII acts on the kidneys to shift the renal pressure–natriuresis curve to the right; when dietary Na^+ is high, renin release is inhibited, and the withdrawal of AngII shifts the renal pressure–natriuresis curve to the left. Consequently, despite large swings in dietary Na^+ intake, the intersection of salt intake with the renal pressure–natriuresis curve remains near the same set point. When modulation of the renin–angiotensin system is blocked by drugs, changes in salt intake markedly affect blood pressure.

INHIBITORS OF THE RENIN–ANGIOTENSIN SYSTEM

AngII has limited therapeutic utility and is not available for therapeutic use in the U.S. Instead, clinical interest focuses on inhibitors of the renin–angiotensin system.

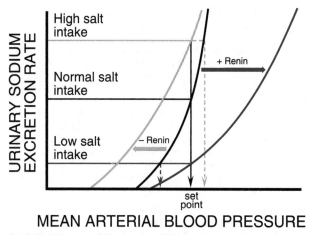

MEAN ARTERIAL BLOOD PRESSURE

FIGURE 30–5 *Interactions among salt intake, the renal pressure-natriuresis mechanism, and the rennin-angiotensin system to stablilize long-term levels of arterial blood pressure despite large variations in dietary sodium intake.*

Renin Inhibitors

The orally active renin inhibitor *aliskiren* (TEKTURNA) is now available for the treatment of hypertension. In studies to date, it has produced a dose-dependent decrease in blood pressure with few adverse effects. Renin inhibitors will likely provide an attractive alterative to current drugs used to inhibit the renin-angiotensin system.

ACE Inhibitors

The essential effect of these agents on the renin–angiotensin system is to inhibit the conversion of AngI to the active AngII (or the conversion of [des-Asp^1]AngI to AngIII). Thus, ACE inhibitors attenuate or abolish responses to AngI but not to AngII (Figure 30–1). They do not interact directly with other components of the renin–angiotensin system, and their principal pharmacological and clinical effects all apparently arise from suppression of AngII synthesis. Nevertheless, ACE is an enzyme with many substrates, and inhibition of ACE may induce effects unrelated to reducing the levels of AngII. Since ACE inhibitors increase bradykinin levels and bradykinin stimulates prostaglandin biosynthesis, bradykinin and/or prostaglandins may contribute to the pharmacological effects of ACE inhibitors. In addition, ACE inhibitors interfere with both short- and long-loop negative feedbacks on renin release (Figure 30–2A). Consequently, ACE inhibitors increase renin release and the rate of formation of AngI. Since the metabolism of AngI to AngII is blocked by ACE inhibitors, AngI is directed down alternative metabolic routes, resulting in increased production of peptides such as Ang(1–7). Whether biologically active peptides such as angiotensin(1–7) contribute to pharmacological effects of ACE inhibitors is unknown.

In a healthy, Na$^+$-replete person, a single oral dose of an ACE inhibitor has little effect on blood pressure, but repeated doses over several days cause a small reduction in blood pressure. By contrast, even a single dose of these inhibitors lowers blood pressure substantially in normal subjects when they have been depleted of Na$^+$.

CLINICAL PHARMACOLOGY ACE inhibitors can be classified into three groups based on structure: (1) sulfhydryl-containing ACE inhibitors related to captopril; (2) dicarboxyl-containing ACE inhibitors related to enalapril (*e.g.*, lisinopril, benazepril, quinapril, moexipril, ramipril, trandolapril, and perindopril); and (3) phosphorus-containing ACE inhibitors related to fosinopril. Many ACE inhibitors are ester-containing prodrugs that are 100–1000 times less potent but have a much better oral bioavailability than the active molecules.

Currently, 11 ACE inhibitors are available for clinical use in the U.S. In general, ACE inhibitors differ with regard to three properties: (1) potency, (2) whether ACE inhibition is primarily a direct effect of the drug itself or the effect of an active metabolite, and (3) pharmacokinetics (*i.e.*, extent of absorption, effect of food on absorption, plasma $t_{1/2}$, tissue distribution, and mechanisms of elimination).

All ACE inhibitors effectively block the conversion of AngI to AngII, and all have similar therapeutic indications, adverse-effect profiles, and contraindications. ACE inhibitors differ markedly in tissue distribution, and this difference might be exploited to inhibit some local renin–angiotensin systems while leaving others relatively intact; possible therapeutic advantages remain to be established.

With the notable exceptions of fosinopril and spirapril (which display balanced elimination by the liver and kidneys), ACE inhibitors are cleared predominantly by the kidneys. Therefore, impaired renal function significantly diminishes the plasma clearance of most ACE inhibitors, and drug dosages should be reduced in patients with renal impairment. *Elevated plasma renin activity (PRA) renders patients hyperresponsive to ACE inhibitor–induced hypotension, and initial dosages of all ACE inhibitors should be reduced in patients with high plasma levels of renin (e.g., patients with heart failure and salt-depleted patients).*

Captopril (*CAPOTEN*)   Captopril is a potent ACE inhibitor (K_i ~1.7 nM). Given orally, captopril is absorbed rapidly and has a bioavailability of ~75%. Peak concentrations in plasma occur within an hour, and the drug is cleared with a $t_{1/2}$ of ~2 hours. Most of the drug is eliminated in urine, 40–50% as captopril and the rest as captopril disulfide dimers and captopril–cysteine disulfide. The oral dose of captopril ranges from 6.25 to 150 mg two to three times daily, with 6.25 mg three times daily or 25 mg twice daily being appropriate for the initiation of therapy for heart failure or hypertension, respectively. Most patients should not receive daily doses in excess of 150 mg. Since food reduces the oral bioavailability of captopril by 25–30%, the drug should be given 1 hour before meals.

Enalapril (*VASOTEC*)   Enalapril maleate is a prodrug that is hydrolyzed by esterases in the liver to produce the active dicarboxylic acid, enalaprilat. *Enalaprilat* is a highly potent inhibitor of ACE with a K_i ~ 0.2 nM. Although it also contains a "proline surrogate," enalaprilat differs from captopril in that it is an analog of a tripeptide rather than a dipeptide. Enalapril is absorbed rapidly when given orally and has an oral bioavailability of about 60% (not reduced by food). Although peak concentrations of enalapril in plasma occur within an hour, enalaprilat concentrations peak only after 3–4 hours. Enalapril has a $t_{1/2}$ of 1.3 hours; enalaprilat, because of tight binding to ACE, has a plasma $t_{1/2}$ of ~11 hours. Nearly all the drug is eliminated by the kidneys as either intact enalapril or enalaprilat. The oral dosage of enalapril ranges from 2.5–40 mg daily (single or divided dosage), with 2.5 and 5 mg daily being appropriate for the initiation of therapy for heart failure and hypertension, respectively. The initial dose for hypertensive patients who are taking diuretics, are water- or Na$^+$-depleted, or have heart failure is 2.5 mg daily.

Enalaprilat (*VASOTEC INJECTION*)   Enalaprilat is not absorbed orally but is available for intravenous administration when oral therapy is not appropriate. For hypertensive patients, the dosage is 0.625–1.25 mg given intravenously over 5 minutes. This dosage may be repeated every 6 hours.

Lisinopril (*PRINIVIL, ZESTRIL*)   Lisinopril is the Lys analog of enalaprilat; unlike enalapril, lisinopril itself is active. Lisinopril is slightly more potent than enalaprilat. Lisinopril is absorbed slowly, variably, and incompletely (about 30%) after oral administration (bioavailability is not reduced by food); peak concentrations in plasma are achieved in ~7 hours. It is cleared intact by the kidney, and its $t_{1/2}$ in plasma is about 12 hours. The oral dosage of lisinopril ranges from 5 to 40 mg daily (single or divided dosage), with 5 and 10 mg daily being appropriate for the initiation of therapy for heart failure and hypertension, respectively. A daily dose of 2.5 mg is recommended for patients with heart failure who are Na$^+$-depleted or have renal impairment.

Benazepril (*LOTENSIN*)   Cleavage of the ester moiety by hepatic esterases transforms benazepril, a prodrug, into benazeprilat, an ACE inhibitor that is more potent than captopril, enalaprilat, or lisinopril. Benazepril is absorbed rapidly but incompletely (37%) after oral administration (only slightly reduced by food). Benazepril is nearly completely metabolized to benazeprilat and to glucuronide conjugates of benazepril and benazeprilat, which are excreted into both the urine and bile; peak concentrations of benazepril and benazeprilat in plasma are achieved in about 0.5–1 hour and 1–2 hours, respectively. Benazeprilat has an effective $t_{1/2}$ in plasma of ~10–11 hours. With the exception of the lungs, benazeprilat does not accumulate in tissues. The oral dosage of benazepril ranges from 5–80 mg daily (single or divided dosage).

Fosinopril (MONOPRIL) Fosinopril contains a phosphinate group that binds to the active site of ACE. Cleavage of the ester moiety by hepatic esterases transforms fosinopril, a prodrug, into fosinoprilat, an ACE inhibitor that is more potent than captopril yet less potent than enalaprilat. Fosinopril is absorbed slowly and incompletely (36%) after oral administration (rate but not extent reduced by food). Fosinopril is largely metabolized to fosinoprilat (75%) and to the glucuronide conjugate of fosinoprilat. These are excreted in urine and bile; peak concentrations of fosinoprilat in plasma are achieved in about 3 hours. Fosinoprilat has an effective $t_{1/2}$ in plasma of about 12 hours, and its clearance is not significantly altered by renal impairment. The oral dosage of fosinopril ranges from 10 to 80 mg daily (single or divided dosage). The dose is reduced to 5 mg daily in patients with Na^+ or water depletion or renal failure.

Trandolapril (MAVIK) Approximately 10% and 70% of an oral dose of trandolapril is bioavailable (absorption rate but not extent is reduced by food) as trandolapril and trandolaprilat, respectively. Trandolaprilat is about eight times more potent than trandolapril as an ACE inhibitor. Trandolapril is metabolized to trandolaprilat and to inactive metabolites (mostly glucuronides of trandolapril and deesterification products), and these are recovered in the urine (33%, mostly trandolaprilat) and feces (66%). Peak concentrations of trandolaprilat in plasma are achieved in 4–10 hours. Trandolaprilat displays biphasic elimination kinetics with an initial $t_{1/2}$ of ~10 hours (the major component of elimination), followed by a more prolonged $t_{1/2}$ owing to slow dissociation of trandolaprilat from tissue ACE. Plasma clearance of trandolaprilat is reduced by both renal and hepatic insufficiency. The oral dosage ranges from 1 to 8 mg daily (single or divided dosage). The initial dose is 0.5 mg in patients who are taking a diuretic or who have renal impairment.

Quinapril (ACCUPRIL) Cleavage of the ester moiety by hepatic esterases transforms quinapril, a prodrug, into quinaprilat, an ACE inhibitor that is about as potent as benazeprilat. Quinapril is absorbed rapidly (peak concentrations are achieved in 1 hour, but the peak may be delayed after food), and the rate but not extent of oral absorption (60%) may be reduced by food. Quinapril is metabolized to quinaprilat and to other minor metabolites, and quinaprilat is excreted in the urine (61%) and feces (37%). Peak concentrations of quinaprilat in plasma are achieved in about 2 hours. Conversion of quinapril to quinaprilat is reduced in patients with diminished liver function. The initial $t_{1/2}$ of quinaprilat is about 2 hours; a prolonged terminal $t_{1/2}$ of ~25 hours may be due to high-affinity binding of the drug to tissue ACE. The oral dosage of quinapril is 5–80 mg daily (single or divided dosage).

Ramipril (ALTACE) Cleavage of the ester moiety by hepatic esterases transforms ramipril into ramiprilat, an ACE inhibitor that is about as potent as benazeprilat and quinaprilat. Ramipril is absorbed rapidly (peak concentrations of ramipril achieved in 1 hour), and the rate but not extent of its oral absorption (50–60%) is reduced by food. Ramipril is metabolized to ramiprilat and to inactive metabolites (glucuronides of ramipril and ramiprilat and the diketopiperazine ester and acid) that predominantly are excreted by the kidneys. Peak concentrations of ramiprilat in plasma are achieved in about 3 hours. Ramiprilat displays triphasic elimination kinetics with $t_{1/2}$ of 2–4 hours, 9–18 hours, and >50 hours. This triphasic elimination is due to extensive distribution to all tissues (initial $t_{1/2}$), clearance of free ramiprilat from plasma (intermediate $t_{1/2}$), and dissociation of ramiprilat from tissue ACE (terminal $t_{1/2}$). The oral dosage of ramipril is 1.25–20 mg daily (single or divided dosage).

Moexipril (UNIVASC) Moexipril is another prodrug whose antihypertensive activity is almost entirely due to its de-esterified metabolite, moexiprilat. Moexipril is absorbed incompletely, with bioavailability as moexiprilat of ~13%. Bioavailability is markedly decreased by food; therefore, the drug should be taken 1 hour before meals. The time to peak plasma concentration of moexiprilat is almost 1.5 hours, and the elimination $t_{1/2}$ is variable (2–12 hours). The recommended dosage range is 7.5–30 mg daily in one or two divided doses. The dosage range is halved in patients who are taking diuretics or who have renal impairment.

Perindopril (ACEON) Perindopril erbumine is a prodrug, and 30–50% of systemically available perindopril is transformed to perindoprilat by hepatic esterases. The oral bioavailability of perindopril (75%) is not affected by food. Perindopril is metabolized to perindoprilat and to inactive metabolites (glucuronides of perindopril and perindoprilat, dehydrated perindopril, and diastereomers of dehydrated perindoprilat) that are excreted predominantly by the kidneys. Peak concentrations of perindoprilat in plasma are achieved in 3–7 hours. Perindoprilat displays biphasic elimination kinetics with half-lives of 3–10 hours (the major component of elimination) and 30–120 hours (owing to slow dissociation of perindoprilat from tissue ACE). The oral dosage ranges from 2 to 16 mg daily (single or divided dosage).

THERAPEUTIC USES OF ACE INHIBITORS AND CLINICAL SUMMARY

ACE Inhibitors in Hypertension   ACE inhibition lowers systemic vascular resistance and mean, diastolic, and systolic blood pressures in various hypertensive states (*see* Chapter 32). ACE inhibitors commonly lower blood pressure in hypertensive subjects, except in those with primary aldosteronism. The initial change in blood pressure is most marked in subjects with high PRA and AngII plasma levels prior to treatment. Several weeks into treatment, additional patients show sizable reductions in blood pressure that correlate poorly or not at all with pretreatment PRA values. It is possible that increased local (tissue) production of AngII and/or increased responsiveness of tissues to normal levels of AngII in some hypertensive patients makes them sensitive to ACE inhibitors despite normal PRA. Regardless of the mechanisms, ACE inhibitors have broad clinical utility as antihypertensive agents.

The long-term fall in systemic blood pressure observed in hypertensive individuals treated with ACE inhibitors is accompanied by a leftward shift in the renal pressure–natriuresis curve (Figure 30–5) and a reduction in total peripheral resistance that varies in different vascular beds. Vasodilation in the kidney is a relatively constant finding that is explained by the exquisite sensitivity of renal vessels to the vasoconstrictor actions of AngII. Increased renal blood flow occurs without an increase in GFR; thus, the filtration fraction is reduced. Both the afferent and efferent arterioles are dilated. Blood flows in the cerebral and coronary beds, where autoregulatory mechanisms are powerful, generally are well maintained.

Besides causing systemic arteriolar dilatation, ACE inhibitors increase the compliance of large arteries, which contributes to a reduction of systolic pressure. Cardiac function in patients with uncomplicated hypertension generally is little changed, although stroke volume and cardiac output may increase slightly with sustained treatment. Baroreceptor function and cardiovascular reflexes are not compromised, and responses to postural changes and exercise are little impaired. Even when a substantial lowering of blood pressure is achieved, heart rate and concentrations of catecholamines in plasma generally increase only slightly, if at all. This perhaps reflects an alteration of baroreceptor function with increased arterial compliance and the loss of the normal tonic influence of AngII on the sympathetic nervous system.

Aldosterone secretion in most hypertensive individuals is reduced, but not seriously impaired, by ACE inhibitors. Aldosterone secretion is maintained at adequate levels by other steroidogenic stimuli, such as ACTH and K^+. The activity of these secretogogues on the zona glomerulosa of the adrenal cortex requires only very small trophic or permissive amounts of AngII, which always are present because ACE inhibition never is complete. Excessive K^+ retention is encountered only in patients taking supplemental K^+, patients with renal impairment, or patients taking other medications that reduce K^+ excretion.

ACE inhibitors alone normalize blood pressure in ~50% of patients with mild-to-moderate hypertension. Ninety percent of patients with mild-to-moderate hypertension will be controlled by the combination of an ACE inhibitor and either a Ca^{2+} channel blocker, a β adrenergic receptor blocker, or a diuretic. Diuretics in particular augment the antihypertensive response to ACE inhibitors by rendering the blood pressure renin-dependent.

There is increasing evidence that ACE inhibitors are superior to many other antihypertensive drugs in hypertensive patients with diabetes, in whom they improve endothelial function and reduce cardiovascular events more so than do Ca^{2+} channel blockers or diuretics and β adrenergic receptor antagonists.

ACE Inhibitors in Left Ventricular Systolic Dysfunction   Left ventricular systolic dysfunction ranges from a modest, asymptomatic reduction in systolic performance to a severe impairment of left ventricular systolic function with florid congestive heart failure (*see* Chapter 33). Unless contraindicated, ACE inhibitors should be given to all patients with impaired left ventricular systolic function whether or not they have symptoms of overt heart failure.

Inhibition of ACE in patients with systolic dysfunction prevents or delays the progression of heart failure, decreases the incidence of sudden death and myocardial infarction, decreases hospitalization, and improves quality of life. The more severe the ventricular dysfunction, the greater is the benefit from ACE inhibition.

Although the mechanisms by which ACE inhibitors improve outcome in patients with systolic dysfunction are not completely understood, the induction of a more favorable hemodynamic state most likely plays an important role. Inhibition of ACE commonly reduces afterload and systolic wall stress, and both cardiac output and cardiac index increase, as do indices of stroke work and stroke volume. In systolic dysfunction, AngII decreases arterial compliance, which is reversed by ACE inhibition. Heart rate generally is reduced. Systemic blood pressure falls, sometimes steeply at the outset, but tends to return toward initial levels. Renovascular resistance falls sharply, and renal blood flow increases. Natriuresis occurs as a result of the improved renal hemodynamics, the reduced stimulus to the secretion of aldosterone by AngII, and the diminished direct effects of AngII on the kidney. The excess volume of body fluids contracts, which reduces venous return to the right side of the heart. A further reduction results from venodilation and an increased capacity of the venous bed, which is somewhat unexpected because AngII has little acute venoconstrictor activity. The response to ACE inhibitors also involves reductions of pulmonary arterial pressure, pulmonary capillary wedge pressure, and left atrial and left ventricular filling volumes and pressures. Consequently, preload and diastolic wall stress are diminished. The better hemodynamic performance results in increased exercise tolerance and suppression of the sympathetic nervous system. Cerebral and coronary blood flows usually are well maintained, even when systemic blood pressure is reduced.

The beneficial effects of ACE inhibitors in systolic dysfunction also involve improvements in ventricular geometry. In heart failure, ACE inhibitors reduce ventricular dilation and tend to restore the heart to its normal elliptical shape. ACE inhibitors may reverse ventricular remodeling *via* changes in preload/afterload, by preventing the growth effects of AngII on myocytes, and by attenuating cardiac fibrosis induced by AngII and aldosterone.

ACE Inhibitors in Acute Myocardial Infarction ACE inhibitors reduce overall mortality when treatment is begun during the peri-infarction period. The beneficial effects of ACE inhibitors in acute myocardial infarction are particularly large in hypertensive and diabetic patients. Unless contraindicated (*e.g.*, cardiogenic shock or severe hypotension), ACE inhibitors should be started immediately during the acute phase of myocardial infarction and can be administered along with thrombolytics, aspirin, and β adrenergic receptor antagonists. After several weeks, ACE-inhibitor therapy should be reevaluated. In high-risk patients (*e.g.*, large infarct, systolic ventricular dysfunction), ACE inhibition should be continued long term.

ACE Inhibitors in Patients Who Are at High Risk of Cardiovascular Events Patients at high risk of cardiovascular events (no left ventricular dysfunction but evidence of vascular disease or diabetes and one other risk factor for cardiovascular disease) benefit considerably from ACE inhibitors, with significant decreases in the rates of myocardial infarction, stroke, and death. The benefits of ACE inhibition in patients at high risk of cardiovascular events persist even after coronary revascularization.

ACE Inhibitors in Chronic Renal Failure Diabetes mellitus is the leading cause of renal disease. In patients with type 1 diabetes mellitus and diabetic nephropathy, ACE inhibitors clearly prevent or delay the progression of renal disease. The renoprotective effects of ACE inhibitors in type 1 diabetes are largely independent of blood pressure reduction. Specific renoprotection by ACE inhibitors is more difficult to demonstrate in type 2 diabetics, with some studies providing positive results, but others failing to demonstrate blood pressure–independent renoprotection. In addition to attenuating diabetic nephropathy, ACE inhibitors also may decrease retinopathy progression in type 1 diabetics. ACE inhibitors also attenuate the progression of renal insufficiency in patients with a variety of nondiabetic nephropathies and may arrest the decline in GFR even in patients with severe renal disease.

Several mechanisms participate in the renal protection afforded by ACE inhibitors. Increased glomerular capillary pressure induces glomerular injury, and ACE inhibitors reduce this parameter both by decreasing arterial blood pressure and by dilating renal efferent arterioles. ACE inhibitors increase the permeability selectivity of the filtering membrane, thereby diminishing exposure of the mesangium to proteinaceous factors that may stimulate mesangial cell proliferation and matrix production, two processes that contribute to expansion of the mesangium in diabetic nephropathy. Since AngII is a growth factor, reductions in the intrarenal levels of AngII may further attenuate mesangial cell growth and matrix production.

ADVERSE EFFECTS OF ACE INHIBITORS Serious untoward reactions to ACE inhibitors are rare, and they generally are well tolerated. Metabolic side effects are not encountered during long-term therapy with ACE inhibitors. The drugs do not alter plasma concentrations of uric acid or Ca^{2+} and actually may improve insulin sensitivity in patients with insulin resistance and decrease cholesterol and lipoprotein(a) levels in proteinuric renal disease.

Hypotension A steep fall in blood pressure may occur following the first dose of an ACE inhibitor in patients with elevated PRA. Special care should be exercised in patients who are salt-depleted, in patients being treated with multiple antihypertensive drugs, and in patients who have congestive heart failure. Such patients should be started on very small doses of ACE inhibitors, or salt intake should be increased and diuretics stopped before beginning therapy.

Cough In 5–20% of patients, ACE inhibitors induce a dry cough; it usually is not dose-related, occurs more frequently in women than men, usually develops between 1 week and 6 months after initiation of therapy, and sometimes requires cessation of therapy. This adverse effect may be mediated by bradykinin, substance P, and/or prostaglandins. Thromboxane antagonism, aspirin, and iron supplementation reduce cough induced by ACE inhibitors. Once ACE inhibitors are stopped, the cough disappears, usually within 4 days.

Hyperkalemia Despite some reduction in the concentration of aldosterone, significant K^+ retention is rarely encountered in patients with normal renal function who are not taking other drugs that cause K^+ retention. However, ACE inhibitors may cause hyperkalemia in patients with renal insufficiency or in patients taking K^+-sparing diuretics, K^+ supplements, β adrenergic receptor antagonists, or NSAIDs.

Acute Renal Failure By constricting the efferent arteriole, AngII helps to maintain adequate glomerular filtration when renal perfusion pressure is low. Consequently, ACE inhibition can induce acute renal insufficiency in patients with bilateral renal artery stenosis, stenosis of the artery to a single remaining kidney, heart failure, or volume depletion owing to diarrhea or diuretics. Older patients with congestive heart failure are particularly susceptible to ACE inhibitor–induced acute renal failure. However, nearly all patients who receive appropriate treatment recover renal function without sequelae.

Fetopathic Potential Administration of ACE inhibitors during the second and third trimesters can cause oligohydramnios, fetal calvarial hypoplasia, fetal pulmonary hypoplasia, fetal growth retardation, fetal death, neonatal anuria, and neonatal death. These fetopathic effects may be due in part to fetal hypotension. While ACE inhibitors are not contraindicated in women of reproductive age, *once pregnancy is diagnosed, it is imperative that ACE inhibitors be discontinued as soon as possible.* If necessary, an alternative antihypertensive regimen should be instituted. The fetus is not at risk of ACE inhibitor–induced pathology if ACE inhibitors are discontinued during the first trimester of pregnancy.

Skin Rash ACE inhibitors occasionally cause a maculopapular rash that may be pruritic. The rash may resolve spontaneously or may respond to a reduced dosage or a brief course of antihistamines. Although initially attributed to the presence of the sulfhydryl group in captopril, a rash also may occur with other ACE inhibitors, albeit less frequently.

Proteinuria ACE inhibitors have been associated with proteinuria (more than 1 g/day); however, a causal relationship has been difficult to establish. In general, proteinuria is not a contraindication for ACE inhibitors because ACE inhibitors are renoprotective in diseases associated with proteinuria, such as diabetic nephropathy.

Angioedema In 0.1– 0.5% of patients, ACE inhibitors induce a rapid swelling in the nose, throat, mouth, glottis, larynx, lips, and/or tongue. This untoward effect, called *angioedema,* apparently is not dose-related, and if it occurs, it does so within the first week of therapy, usually within the first few hours after the initial dose. Airway obstruction and respiratory distress may lead to death. Although the mechanism is unknown, angioedema may involve accumulation of bradykinin or inhibition of complement 1–esterase inhibitor. Once ACE inhibitors are stopped, angioedema disappears within hours; meanwhile, the patient's airway should be protected, and if necessary, epinephrine, an antihistamine, and/or a glucocorticoid should be administered. African Americans have a 4.5 times greater risk of ACE inhibitor–induced angioedema than do Caucasians. Although rare, angioedema of the intestine, characterized by emesis, watery diarrhea, and abdominal pain, also has been associated with ACE inhibitors.

Other Adverse Effects Dysgeusia, an alteration in or loss of taste, can occur. It may be more frequent with captopril and is reversible. Neutropenia is a rare but serious side effect of ACE inhibitors; it occurs predominantly in hypertensive patients with collagen-vascular or renal parenchymal disease. If the serum creatinine concentration is 2 mg/dL or greater, the dose of ACE inhibitor should be kept low, and the patient should be counseled to seek medical evaluation if symptoms (*e.g.*, sore throat, fever) develop. Glycosuria in the absence of hyperglycemia is an exceedingly rare and reversible side effect whose mechanism is unknown. Hepatotoxicity, usually of the cholestatic variety, also is exceedingly rare and reversible. The mechanism again is unknown.

Drug Interactions Antacids may reduce the oral bioavailability of ACE inhibitors; capsaicin may worsen ACE inhibitor–induced cough; NSAIDs, including aspirin, may reduce the antihypertensive response to ACE inhibitors; and K^+-sparing diuretics and K^+ supplements may exacerbate ACE inhibitor–induced hyperkalemia. ACE inhibitors may increase plasma levels of digoxin and lithium and may increase hypersensitivity reactions to allopurinol.

NONPEPTIDE AngII RECEPTOR ANTAGONISTS

The AngII receptor blockers (ARBs) bind to the AT_1 receptor with high affinity and generally are at least 10,000-fold more selective for the AT_1 receptor *versus* the AT_2 receptor. The rank-order affinity of the AT_1 receptor for ARBs is candesartan = omesartan > irbesartan = eprosartan > telmisartan = valsartan = EXP 3174 (the active metabolite of losartan) > losartan. Although binding of ARBs to the AT_1 receptor is competitive, the inhibition often is insurmountable; *i.e.*, the maximal response to AngII cannot be restored in the presence of the ARB.

ARBs potently and selectively inhibit most of the biological effects of AngII, including AngII–induced (1) contraction of vascular smooth muscle, (2) rapid pressor responses, (3) slow pressor responses, (4) thirst, (5) vasopressin release, (6) aldosterone secretion, (7) release of adrenal catecholamines, (8) enhancement of noradrenergic neurotransmission, (9) increases in sympathetic tone, (10) changes in renal function, and (11) cellular hypertrophy and hyperplasia.

A critical issue is whether or not ARBs are equivalent to ACE inhibitors with regard to therapeutic efficacy. Both classes of drugs block the renin–angiotensin system, but ARBs and ACE inhibitors differ in several important aspects: (1) *ARBs reduce activation of AT_1 receptors more effectively than do ACE inhibitors*. ACE inhibitors reduce AngII produced by ACE but do not inhibit alternative non-ACE AngII–generating pathways. Because ARBs block the AT_1 receptor, the actions of AngII via the AT_1 receptor are inhibited regardless of how AngII is formed. (2) In contrast to ACE inhibitors, *ARBs permit activation of AT_2 receptors*. ACE inhibitors increase renin release; however, ACE inhibitors block the conversion of AngI to AngII, resulting in decreased levels of AngII. Blockade of AT_1 receptors by ARBs enhances renin release, which does result in increased circulating levels of AngII. This increased level of AngII is available to activate AT_2 receptors. (3) *ACE inhibitors may increase Ang(1–7) levels more than do ARBs*, since ACE is involved in the clearance of Ang(1–7). (4) *ACE inhibitors increase the levels of a number of ACE substrates, including bradykinin*. ACE processes an array of substrates; inhibiting ACE therefore increases the levels of ACE substrates and decreases the levels of their corresponding products. Whether the pharmacological differences between ARBs and ACE inhibitors result in significant differences in therapeutic outcomes is an open question.

CLINICAL PHARMACOLOGY Oral bioavailability of ARBs generally is low (<50%, except for irbesartan, with 70% available), and protein binding is high (>90%).

Candesartan Cilexetil (ATACAND) Candesartan cilexetil is an inactive ester prodrug that is completely hydrolyzed to the active form, candesartan, during absorption from the GI tract. Peak plasma levels are obtained 3–4 hours after oral administration, and the plasma $t_{1/2}$ is about 9 hours. Plasma clearance of candesartan is due to renal (33%) and biliary (67%) excretion and is affected by renal insufficiency but not by mild-to-moderate hepatic insufficiency. Candesartan cilexetil should be administered orally once or twice daily for a total daily dosage of 4–32 mg.

Eprosartan (TEVETEN) Peak plasma levels are obtained ~1–2 hours after oral administration, and the plasma $t_{1/2}$ varies (5–9 hours). Eprosartan is metabolized in part to the glucuronide conjugate, and the parent compound and its glucuronide conjugate are cleared by renal and biliary elimination such that plasma clearance is affected by both renal and hepatic insufficiency. The recommended dosage of eprosartan is 400–800 mg/day in one or two doses.

Irbesartan (AVAPRO)   Peak plasma levels are obtained approximately 1.5–2 hours after oral administration, and the plasma $t_{1/2}$ ranges (11–15 hours). Irbesartan is metabolized in part to the glucuronide conjugate, and the parent compound and its glucuronide conjugate are cleared by renal elimination (20%) and biliary excretion (80%). The plasma clearance of irbesartan is unaffected by either renal or mild-to-moderate hepatic insufficiency. The oral dosage of irbesartan is 150–300 mg once daily.

Losartan (COZAAR)   Approximately 14% of an oral dose of losartan is converted to the 5-carboxylic acid metabolite EXP 3174, which is more potent than losartan as an AT_1-receptor antagonist. The metabolism of losartan to EXP 3174 and to inactive metabolites is mediated by CYP2C9 and CYP3A4. Peak plasma levels of losartan and EXP 3174 occur ~1–3 hours after oral administration, respectively, and the plasma half-lives are 2.5 and 6–9 hours, respectively. The plasma clearances of losartan and EXP 3174 (600 and 50 mL/min, respectively) are due to renal clearance (75 and 25 mL/min, respectively) and hepatic clearance (metabolism and biliary excretion). The plasma clearance of losartan and EXP 3174 is affected by hepatic but not renal insufficiency. Losartan should be administered orally once or twice daily for a total daily dose of 25–100 mg. In addition to being an ARB, losartan is a competitive antagonist of the thromboxane A_2 receptor and attenuates platelet aggregation. Also, EXP 3179 reduces COX-2 mRNA up-regulation and COX-dependent prostaglandin generation.

Olmesartan Medoxomil (BENICAR)   Olmesartan medoxomil is an inactive ester prodrug that is completely hydrolyzed to the active form, olmesartan, during absorption from the GI tract. Peak plasma levels are obtained 1.4–2.8 hours after oral administration, and the plasma $t_{1/2}$ varies (10–15 hours). Plasma clearance of olmesartan is due to both renal elimination and biliary excretion. Although renal impairment and hepatic disease decrease the plasma clearance of olmesartan, no dose adjustment is required in patients with mild-to-moderate renal or hepatic impairment. The oral dosage of olmesartan medoxomil is 20–40 mg once daily.

Telmisartan (MICARDIS)   Peak plasma levels are obtained ~0.5–1 hour after oral administration, and the plasma $t_{1/2}$ is about 24 hours. Telmisartan is cleared from the circulation mainly by biliary secretion of intact drug and clearance is affected by hepatic but not renal insufficiency. The recommended oral dosage of telmisartan is 40–80 mg once daily.

Valsartan (DIOVAN)   Peak plasma levels occur 2–4 hours after oral administration, and the plasma $t_{1/2}$ is ~9 hours. Food markedly decreases absorption. Valsartan is cleared by the liver (~70%); plasma clearance is affected by hepatic but not renal insufficiency. The oral dosage of valsartan is 80–320 mg once daily.

THERAPEUTIC USES OF AngII RECEPTOR ANTAGONISTS   All ARBs are approved for the treatment of hypertension. In addition, irbesartan and losartan are approved for diabetic nephropathy, losartan is approved for stroke prophylaxis, and valsartan is approved for heart failure patients who are intolerant of ACE inhibitors. The efficacy of ARBs in lowering blood pressure is comparable with that of other established antihypertensive drugs, with an adverse-effect profile similar to that of placebo. ARBs also are available as fixed-dose combinations with hydrochlorothiazide.

Losartan is well tolerated in patients with heart failure and is comparable to enalapril with regard to improving exercise tolerance. Both valsartan and candesartan reduce mortality and morbidity in heart failure patients. Current recommendations are to use ACE inhibitors as first-line agents for the treatment of heart failure and to reserve ARBs for patients who cannot tolerate or have an unsatisfactory response to ACE inhibitors. At present, there is conflicting evidence regarding the benefit of combining an ARB and an ACE inhibitor in heart failure patients.

In part *via* blood pressure–independent mechanisms, ARBs are renoprotective in type 2 diabetes mellitus and many experts now consider them the drugs of choice for renoprotection in diabetic patients. ARBs are superior to β_1 adrenergic receptor antagonists in reducing stroke in hypertensive patients with left ventricular hypertrophy. Irebesartan appears to maintain sinus rhythm in patients with persistent, long-standing atrial fibrillation. Losartan is reported to be safe and highly effective in the treatment of portal hypertension in patients with cirrhosis without compromising renal function.

ADVERSE EFFECTS   The incidence of discontinuation of ARBs owing to adverse reactions is comparable with that of placebo. Unlike ACE inhibitors, ARBs do not cause cough, and the incidence of angioedema with ARBs is much less than with ACE inhibitors. As with ACE inhibitors, *ARBs have teratogenic potential and should be discontinued before the second trimester of pregnancy*. ARBs should be used cautiously in patients whose blood pressure or renal function is highly dependent on the renin–angiotensin system (*e.g.*, renal artery stenosis). In such patients, ARBs can cause hypotension, oliguria, progressive azotemia, or acute renal failure. ARBs may cause hyperkalemia in patients with renal disease or taking K^+ supplements or K^+-sparing diuretics. ARBs enhance the blood pressure–lowering effect of other antihypertensive drugs, a desirable effect but one that may necessitate dosage adjustment.

For a complete Bibliographical listing see Goodman & Gilman's *The Pharmacological Basis of Therapeutics,* **11th ed., or Goodman & Gilman Online at www.accessmedicine.com.**

31

TREATMENT OF MYOCARDIAL ISCHEMIA

PATHOPHYSIOLOGY OF ISCHEMIC HEART DISEASE

Angina pectoris is caused by transient episodes of myocardial ischemia due to an imbalance in myocardial oxygen supply and demand that may result from an increase in myocardial oxygen demand, a decrease in myocardial oxygen supply, or sometimes from both (Figure 31–1). Among the pharmacological agents used in the treatment of angina are nitrovasodilators, β adrenergic receptor antagonists, Ca^{2+} channel antagonists, and antiplatelet agents. All approved antianginal agents improve the balance of myocardial oxygen supply and demand, increasing supply by dilating the coronary vasculature or decreasing demand by reducing cardiac work (Figure 31–1). Drugs used in typical angina function principally by reducing myocardial oxygen demand by decreasing heart rate, myocardial contractility, and/or ventricular wall stress. By contrast, the principal therapeutic goal in unstable angina is to increase myocardial blood flow; strategies include the use of antiplatelet agents and *heparin* to reduce intracoronary thrombosis and coronary stents or coronary bypass surgery to restore flow by mechanical means. The therapeutic aim in variant or Prinzmetal's angina is to prevent coronary vasospasm.

ORGANIC NITRATES

Organic nitrates are polyol esters of nitric acid, whereas organic nitrites are esters of nitrous acid. Nitrate esters (—C—O—NO$_2$) and nitrite esters (—C—O—NO) are characterized by a sequence of carbon–oxygen–nitrogen, whereas nitro compounds possess carbon–nitrogen bonds (C—NO$_2$). Glyceryl trinitrate is not a nitro compound, but the name nitroglycerin *is well entrenched. Organic nitrates of low molecular mass (e.g.* nitroglycerin) *are moderately volatile, oily liquids, whereas the high-molecular-mass nitrate esters* (e.g., erythrityl tetranitrate, isosorbide dinitrate, *and* isosorbide mononitrate) *are solids. The organic nitrates and nitrites, collectively termed* nitrovasodilators, *must be reduced to produce the reactive free radical NO, the active principle of this class of compounds.*

Nitrites, organic nitrates, nitroso compounds, and a variety of other nitrogen oxide–containing substances (including *nitroprusside*) lead to NO formation. NO activates guanylyl cyclase, increases the cellular level of cyclic GMP, activates PKG, and modulates the activities of PDEs 2, 3, and 5 in a variety of cell types. In smooth muscle, NO-mediated increase in intracellular cyclic GMP activate PKG, which leads to reduced phosphorylation of myosin light chain, reduced Ca^{2+} concentration in the cytosol, and vasorelaxation. Although the soluble isoform of guanylyl cyclase remains the most extensively characterized target for NO, NO also forms specific adducts with thiol groups in proteins and with reduced glutathione to form nitrosothiol compounds with distinctive biological properties.

CARDIOVASCULAR EFFECTS

Hemodynamic Effects   Low concentrations of nitroglycerin preferentially dilate the veins more than the arterioles. This venodilation decreases left and right ventricular chamber size and end-diastolic pressures but results in little change in systemic vascular resistance. Systemic arterial pressure may fall slightly, and heart rate is unchanged or may increase slightly in response to a decrease in blood pressure. Pulmonary vascular resistance and cardiac output are slightly reduced. Doses of nitroglycerin that do not alter systemic arterial pressure often produce arteriolar dilation in the face and neck, resulting in a flush, or dilation of meningeal arterial vessels, causing headache.

Higher doses of organic nitrates cause further venous pooling and also may decrease arteriolar resistance, thereby decreasing systolic and diastolic blood pressure and cardiac output and causing pallor, weakness, dizziness, and activation of compensatory sympathetic reflexes. The reflex tachycardia and peripheral arteriolar vasoconstriction tend to restore systemic vascular resistance; this is superimposed on sustained venous pooling. Coronary blood flow may increase transiently as a result of coronary vasodilation but may decrease subsequently if cardiac output and blood pressure decrease sufficiently.

In patients with autonomic dysfunction who cannot increase sympathetic outflow, the fall in blood pressure consequent to the venodilation produced by nitrates cannot be compensated; thus, nitrates may reduce arterial pressure and coronary perfusion pressure significantly, producing potentially life-threatening hypotension and even aggravating angina. The appropriate therapy in patients with orthostatic angina and normal coronary arteries is to correct the orthostatic hypotension by expanding volume (*fludrocortisone* and a high-sodium diet), to prevent venous pooling with

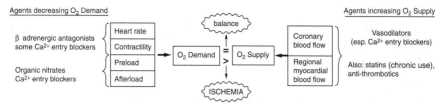

FIGURE 31–1 *Pharmacological modification of the major determinants of myocardial O_2 supply.* When myocardial O_2 requirements exceed O_2 supply, an ischemic episode results. This figure shows the primary hemodynamic sites of actions of pharmacological agents that can reduce O_2 demand (*left side*) or enhance O_2 supply (*right side*). Some classes of agents have multiple effects (*see* text). Stents, angioplasty, and coronary bypass surgery are mechanical interventions that increase O_2 supply. Both pharmacotherapy and mechanotherapy attempt to restore a dynamic balance between O_2 demand and O_2 supply.

fitted support garments, and to carefully titrate use of oral vasopressors. Since patients with autonomic dysfunction occasionally may have coexisting coronary artery disease, the coronary anatomy should be defined before therapy is undertaken.

Effects on Total and Regional Coronary Blood Flow Ischemia is a powerful stimulus to coronary vasodilation, and regional blood flow is adjusted by autoregulatory mechanisms. In the presence of atherosclerotic coronary artery narrowing, ischemia distal to the lesion stimulates vasodilation; if the stenosis is severe, much of the dilatory capacity is needed to maintain resting blood flow and further dilation may not be possible when demand increases. Significant coronary stenoses disproportionately reduce blood flow to the subendocardial regions of the heart, which are subjected to the greatest extravascular compression during systole; organic nitrates tend to restore blood flow in these regions. The hemodynamic mechanisms responsible for the effects on coronary blood flow appear to be due to the ability of organic nitrates to cause dilation and prevent vasoconstriction of large epicardial vessels without impairing autoregulation in the small vessels. By dilating epicardial stenoses and reducing the resistance to flow through such areas, the resulting increase in blood flow would be distributed preferentially to ischemic myocardial regions as a consequence of vasodilation induced by autoregulation. An important indirect mechanism for a preferential increase in subendocardial blood flow is the nitroglycerin-induced reduction in intracavitary systolic and diastolic pressures that oppose blood flow to the subendocardium (*see* below).

Effects on Myocardial Oxygen Requirements By their effects on the systemic circulation, the organic nitrates also can reduce myocardial oxygen demand. The major determinants of myocardial oxygen consumption include left ventricular wall tension, heart rate, and myocardial contractility. Ventricular wall tension is affected by preload and afterload. *Preload* is determined by the diastolic pressure that distends the ventricle (ventricular end-diastolic pressure). Increasing end-diastolic volume augments the ventricular wall tension. Increasing venous capacitance with nitrates decreases venous return to the heart, decreases ventricular end-diastolic volume, and thereby decreases oxygen consumption. An additional benefit of reducing preload is that it increases the pressure gradient for perfusion across the ventricular wall, which favors subendocardial perfusion. *Afterload* is the impedance against which the ventricle must eject, which—in the absence of aortic valvular disease—is related to peripheral resistance. Decreasing peripheral arteriolar resistance reduces afterload and thus myocardial work and oxygen consumption.

Organic nitrates decrease both preload and afterload as a result of dilation of venous capacitance and arteriolar resistance vessels. They do not directly alter the inotropic or chronotropic state of the heart. Since nitrates reduce the primary determinants of oxygen demand, their net effect usually is to decrease myocardial oxygen consumption. Nitrovasodilators also increase cyclic GMP in platelets, with consequent inhibition of platelet function. While this may contribute to their antianginal efficacy, the effect appears to be modest.

Mechanism of Relief of Symptoms of Angina Pectoris The nitrate-induced relief of anginal pain has been ascribed to a decrease in cardiac work secondary to the fall in systemic arterial pressure. The ability of nitrates to dilate epicardial coronary arteries is modest; the bulk of evidence favors a reduction in myocardial work and thus in myocardial oxygen demand as their primary effect in chronic stable angina. Paradoxically, high doses of organic nitrates may reduce blood pressure to such an extent that coronary flow is compromised; reflex tachycardia and adrenergic enhancement of contractility also occur. These effects may override the beneficial action of the drugs on myocardial oxygen demand and can aggravate ischemia. Additionally, sublingual nitroglycerin administration may produce bradycardia and hypotension, probably owing to activation of the Bezold-Jarisch reflex.

ABSORPTION, FATE, AND EXCRETION
NITROGLYCERIN

In humans, peak concentrations of nitroglycerin are found in plasma within 4 minutes of sublingual administration; the drug has a $t_{1/2}$ of 1–3 minutes. The onset of action of nitroglycerin may be even more rapid if it is delivered as a sublingual spray. Anginal pain may be prevented when the drug is used prophylactically immediately prior to exercise or stress. The smallest effective dose should be prescribed. Patients should be instructed to seek medical attention immediately if three tablets taken over a 15-minute period do not relieve a sustained attack because this situation may be indicative of myocardial infarction or another cause of the pain. Patients also should be advised that there is no virtue in trying to avoid taking sublingual nitroglycerin for anginal pain. Application of nitroglycerin ointment (2%) applied to the skin can relieve angina, prolong exercise capacity, and reduce ischemic ST-segment depression with exercise for 4 hours or more. Effects are apparent within 30–60 minutes (although absorption is variable) and last for 4–6 hours. The ointment is particularly useful for controlling nocturnal angina, which commonly develops within 3 hours after the patient goes to sleep. Transdermal nitroglycerin disks use a nitroglycerin-impregnated polymer that permits gradual absorption and a continuous plasma nitrate concentration over 24 hours. The onset of action is slow, with peak effects occurring at 1–2 hours. To avoid tolerance, therapy should be interrupted for at least 8 hours each day. With this regimen, long-term prophylaxis of ischemic episodes often can be attained. Transmucosal or buccal nitroglycerin is inserted under the upper lip above the incisors, where it adheres to the gingiva and dissolves gradually in a uniform manner. Hemodynamic effects are seen within 2–5 minutes, and it is therefore useful for short-term prophylaxis of angina. Nitroglycerin continues to be released into the circulation for a prolonged period, and exercise tolerance may be enhanced for up to 5 hours.

Isosorbide Dinitrate (ISORDIL, SORBITRATE)

Sublingual administration produces maximal plasma concentrations of the drug by 6 minutes, and the fall in concentration is rapid ($t_{1/2}$ of ~45 minutes). The major route of metabolism of isosorbide dinitrate in humans appears to be by enzymatic denitration followed by glucuronide conjugation. The primary initial metabolites, isosorbide-2-mononitrate and isosorbide-5-mononitrate, have longer half-lives (3–6 hours) and presumably contribute to therapeutic efficacy.

Isosorbide-5-Mononitrate (IMDUR)

This agent is available in tablet form. It does not undergo significant first-pass metabolism and so has excellent bioavailability after oral administration. The mononitrate has a significantly longer $t_{1/2}$ than does isosorbide dinitrate and has been formulated as a plain tablet and as a sustained-release preparation; both have longer durations of action than the corresponding dosage forms of isosorbide dinitrate.

Tolerance

Sublingual organic nitrates should be taken at the time of an anginal attack or in anticipation of exercise or stress. Such intermittent treatment provides reproducible cardiovascular effects. However, frequently repeated or continuous exposure to high doses of organic nitrates leads to a marked attenuation in the magnitude of most of their effects. The magnitude of tolerance is a function of dosage and frequency of use.

Tolerance may result from a reduced capacity of the vascular smooth muscle to convert nitroglycerin to NO (*i.e.*, true vascular tolerance), or to the activation of mechanisms extraneous to the vessel wall (*i.e.*, pseudotolerance). Multiple mechanisms are proposed to account for nitrate tolerance, including volume expansion, neurohumoral activation, cellular depletion of sulfhydryl groups, and the generation of free radicals. Inactivation of aldehyde dehydrogenase, a mitochondrial enzyme implicated in nitroglycerin biotransformation, is seen in models of nitrate tolerance. A reactive intermediate formed during the generation of NO from organic nitrates may itself damage and inactivate the enzymes of the activation pathway; tolerance could involve endothelium-derived superoxide.

A more effective approach to restoring responsiveness is to interrupt therapy for 8–12 hours each day, which restores efficacy. It is usually convenient to omit dosing at night in patients with exertional angina, either by adjusting dosing intervals of oral or buccal preparations or by removing cutaneous nitroglycerin. However, patients whose anginal pattern suggests its precipitation by increased left ventricular filling pressures (*i.e.,* occurring in association with orthopnea or paroxysmal nocturnal dyspnea) may benefit from continuing nitrates at night and omitting them during a quiet period of the day. Tolerance also has been seen with *isosorbide-5-mononitrate;* an eccentric twice-daily dosing schedule appears to maintain efficacy.

While these approaches often are effective, some patients develop an increased frequency of nocturnal angina when a nitrate-free interval is employed using nitroglycerin patches; such patients may require another class of antianginal agent during this period. Tolerance is not universal, and some patients develop only partial tolerance. The problem of anginal rebound during nitrate-free intervals is especially problematic in the treatment of unstable angina with intravenous nitroglycerin. As tolerance develops, increasing doses are required to achieve the same therapeutic effects; eventually, despite dose escalation, the drug loses efficacy.

Toxicity and Untoward Responses

Untoward responses to the organic nitrates are almost all secondary to cardiovascular actions. Headache is common and can be severe. It usually decreases over a few days if treatment is continued and often responds to decreasing the dose. Transient episodes of dizziness, weakness, and other manifestations associated with postural hypotension may develop, particularly if the patient is standing immobile, and occasionally may progress to loss of consciousness. This reaction appears to be accentuated by *alcohol,* and also may be seen with very low doses of nitrates in patients with autonomic dysfunction. Even in severe nitrate syncope, positioning and other measures that facilitate venous return are the only therapeutic measures required. All organic nitrates occasionally can produce rash.

INTERACTION OF NITRATES WITH PHOSPHODIESTERASE 5 INHIBITORS
Erectile dysfunction is a frequently encountered problem whose risk factors parallel those of coronary artery disease. Thus, many men desiring therapy for erectile dysfunction already may be receiving antianginal therapy The *phosphodiesterase 5* (PDE5) *inhibitors sildenafil* (VIAGRA), *tadalafil* (CIALIS), and *vardenafil* (LEVITRA) have been developed and widely used for therapy of erectile dysfunction. In the presence of a PDE5 inhibitor, nitrates cause profound increases in cyclic GMP and can dramatically reduce blood pressure. Thus, all three PDE5 inhibitors are contraindicated in patients taking organic nitrate vasodilators, as indicated by a "black box" warning on product labeling. In the event that patients develop significant hypotension following combined administration of PDE5 inhibitor and a nitrate, fluids and α adrenergic receptor agonists, if needed, should be used for support.

Therapeutic Uses

ANGINA Diseases that predispose to angina should be treated as part of a comprehensive therapeutic program with the primary goal being to prolong life. Conditions such as hypertension, anemia, thyrotoxicosis, obesity, heart failure, cardiac arrhythmias, and acute anxiety can precipitate anginal symptoms in many patients. The patient should be asked to stop smoking and overeating; hypertension and hyperlipidemia should be corrected (*see* Chapters 32 and 35); and daily aspirin (or clopidogrel or *ticlopidine* if aspirin is not tolerated) (*see* Chapter 54) should be prescribed. Exposure to sympathomimetic agents (*e.g.,* those in nasal decongestants) should be avoided. The use of drugs that modify the perception of pain is a poor approach to the treatment of angina because the underlying myocardial ischemia is not relieved.

CONGESTIVE HEART FAILURE The utility of nitrovasodilators to relieve pulmonary congestion and to increase cardiac output in congestive heart failure is addressed in Chapter 33.

UNSTABLE ANGINA PECTORIS AND NON-ST-SEGMENT-ELEVATION MYOCARDIAL INFARCTION The term *unstable angina pectoris* has been used to describe a broad spectrum of clinical entities characterized by an acute or subacute worsening in a patient's anginal symptoms. The variable prognosis of unstable angina no doubt reflects the broad range of clinical entities subsumed by the term. More recently, efforts have been directed toward identifying patients with unstable angina on the basis of their risks for subsequent adverse outcomes (*e.g.,* myocardial infarction or death). The term *acute coronary syndrome* is useful in this context: common to most clinical presentations of acute coronary syndrome is disruption of a coronary plaque leading to local platelet aggregation and thrombosis at the arterial wall with subsequent partial or total occlusion of the vessel. There is some variability in the pathogenesis of unstable angina, with gradually progressive atherosclerosis accounting for some cases of new-onset exertional angina. Less commonly, vasospasm in minimally atherosclerotic coronary vessels may account for some cases where rest angina has not been preceded by symptoms of exertional angina. For the most part, the pathophysiological principles that underlie therapy for exertional angina—which are directed at decreasing myocardial oxygen demand—have limited efficacy in the treatment of acute coronary syndromes characterized by an insufficiency of myocardial oxygen (blood) supply.

Drugs that reduce myocardial oxygen consumption by reducing ventricular preload (nitrates) or by reducing heart rate and ventricular contractility (β adrenergic receptor antagonists) are efficacious, but additional therapies are directed at the atherosclerotic plaque itself and the consequences (or prevention) of its rupture. These therapies include combinations of (1) antiplatelet agents, including aspirin and clopidogrel; (2) antithrombin agents such as heparin and the thrombolytics; (3) anti-integrin therapies that directly inhibit platelet aggregation mediated by glycoprotein (GP)IIb/IIIa; (4) mechanopharmacological approaches with percutaneously deployed drug-delivering intracoronary stents; or (5) coronary bypass surgery for selected patients.

Along with nitrates and β adrenergic receptor antagonists, antiplatelet agents represent the cornerstone of therapy for acute coronary syndrome. Aspirin inhibits platelet aggregation and improves survival. Heparin (either unfractionated or low-molecular-weight) also appears to reduce angina and prevent infarction. These and related agents are discussed in detail in Chapters 26 and 54. Anti-integrin agents directed against the platelet integrin GPIIb/IIIa (including abciximab, tirofiban, and eptifibitide) are effective in combination with heparin, as discussed below. Nitrates are useful both in reducing vasospasm and in reducing myocardial oxygen consumption by decreasing ventricular wall stress. Intravenous administration of nitroglycerin allows high concentrations of drug to be attained rapidly. Because nitroglycerin is degraded rapidly, the dose can be titrated quickly and safely using intravenous administration. If coronary vasospasm is present, intravenous nitroglycerin is likely to be effective, although the addition of a Ca^{2+} channel blocker may be required to achieve complete control.

ACUTE MYOCARDIAL INFARCTION Therapeutic maneuvers in myocardial infarction (MI) are directed at reducing the size of the infarct; preserving or retrieving viable tissue by reducing the oxygen demand of the myocardium; and preventing ventricular remodeling that could lead to heart failure.

Nitroglycerin is commonly administered to relieve ischemic pain in patients presenting with MI, but evidence that nitrates improve mortality in MI is sparse. Because they reduce ventricular preload through vasodilation, nitrates are effective in relief of pulmonary congestion. A decreased ventricular preload should be avoided in patients with right ventricular infarction because higher right-sided heart filling pressures are needed in this clinical context. Nitrates are relatively contraindicated in patients with systemic hypotension. According to the American Heart Association/ American College of Cardiology (AHA/ACC) guidelines, "nitrates should not be used if hypotension limits the administration of β blockers, which have more powerful salutary effects."

Since the proximate cause of MI is intracoronary thrombosis, reperfusion therapies are critically important, employing, when possible, direct percutaneous coronary interventions (PCIs) for acute MI, usually using drug-eluting intracoronary stents. Thrombolytic agents are administered at hospitals where emergency PCI is not performed, but outcomes are better with direct PCI than with thrombolytic therapy.

VARIANT (PRINZMETAL) ANGINA

The large coronary arteries normally contribute little to coronary resistance. However, in variant angina, coronary vasoconstriction results in reduced blood flow and ischemic pain. Ca^{2+} channel blockers, but not nitrates, have been shown to influence mortality and the incidence of MI favorably in variant angina and should be included in therapy.

Ca^{2+} CHANNEL ANTAGONISTS

Voltage-sensitive Ca^{2+} channels (L-type or slow channels) mediate the entry of extracellular Ca^{2+} into smooth muscle and cardiac myocytes and sinoatrial (SA) and atrioventricular (AV) nodal cells in response to electrical depolarization. In both smooth muscle and cardiac myocytes, Ca^{2+} is a trigger for contraction. Ca^{2+} channel antagonists, also called *Ca^{2+} entry blockers*, inhibit Ca^{2+} channel function. In vascular smooth muscle, this leads to relaxation, especially in arterial beds. These drugs also may produce negative inotropic and chronotropic effects in the heart.

The Ca^{2+} channel antagonists approved for clinical use in the U.S. have diverse chemical structures, including: phenylalkylamines, dihydropyridines, benzothiazepines, diphenylpiperazines, *and a diarylaminopropylamine. Verapamil (a phenylalkylamine);* diltiazem *(a benzothiazepine);* nifedipine, *amlodipine, felodipine, isradipine, nicardipine, nisoldipine, and* nimodipine *(dihydropyridines); and* bepridil *(a diarylaminopropylamine ether) are approved. Their tissue specificities are shown in Table 31–1. All bind to the a_1 subunit of the L-type Ca^{2+} channels and reduce Ca^{2+} flux through the channel; however, there are fundamental differences amongst verapamil, diltiazem, and the dihydropyridines, especially with respect to pharmacologic characteristics, drug interactions, and toxicities.*

All Ca^{2+} channel blockers relax arterial smooth muscle; they have little effect on most venous beds and hence do not affect cardiac preload significantly. In cardiac muscle, Ca^{2+} channel blockers can produce a negative inotropic effect. Although true for all classes of Ca^{2+} channel blockers, the marked peripheral vasodilation seen with the dihydropyridines is accompanied by a robust baroreflex-mediated increase in sympathetic tone that overcomes the negative inotropic effect.

In the SA and AV nodes, depolarization largely depends on Ca^{2+} movement through the slow L-type channel. The effect of a Ca^{2+} channel blocker on AV conduction and on the rate of the sinus node pacemaker depends on whether the agent delays the recovery of the slow channel. Although nifedipine reduces the slow inward current in a dose-dependent manner, it does not affect the rate of recovery of the slow Ca^{2+} channel. The channel blockade caused by dihydropyridines also shows little dependence on the frequency of stimulation. Thus, at doses used clinically, nifedipine does not affect conduction through the node. In contrast, verapamil not only reduces the magnitude of the Ca^{2+} current through the slow channel but also decreases the rate of channel recovery. In addition, channel blockade caused by verapamil (and to a lesser extent by diltiazem) is enhanced as the frequency of stimulation increases, a phenomenon known as *frequency dependence* or *use dependence.* Thus, verapamil and diltiazem depress the rate of the sinus node pacemaker and slow AV conduction; the latter effect is the basis for their use in the treatment of supraventricular tachyarrhythmias (*see* Chapter 34). Bepridil, like verapamil, inhibits both slow inward Ca^{2+} current and fast inward Na^+ current. It has a direct negative inotropic effect. Its electrophysiological properties lead to slowing of the heart rate, prolongation of the AV nodal effective refractory period, and importantly, prolongation of the Q-Tc interval. Particularly in the setting of hypokalemia, the last effect can be associated with *torsades de pointes,* a potentially lethal ventricular arrhythmia (*see* Chapter 34).

All Ca^{2+} channel blockers approved for clinical use decrease coronary vascular resistance and increase coronary blood flow. The dihydropyridines are more potent vasodilators than verapamil, which is more potent than diltiazem. The hemodynamic effects of these agents vary depending on the route of administration and the extent of left ventricular dysfunction.

Nifedipine, the prototypical dihydropyridine, selectively dilates arterial resistance vessels. The decrease in arterial blood pressure elicits sympathetic reflexes, with resulting tachycardia and positive inotropy. Thus, arteriolar resistance and blood pressure are lowered, contractility and segmental ventricular function are improved, and heart rate and cardiac output are modestly increased. The other dihydropyridines—amlodipine, felodipine, isradipine, nicardipine, nisoldipine, and nimodipine—share many of the cardiovascular effects of nifedipine. There is less reflex tachycardia with amlodipine, possibly because its long $t_{1/2}$ (35–50 hours) produces minimal peaks and troughs in plasma concentrations. Felodipine may have even greater vascular specificity than does nifedipine or amlodipine. At concentrations producing vasodilation, there is no negative inotropic effect. Nicardipine has antianginal properties similar to those of nifedipine and may have selectivity for coronary vessels. Isradipine also produces the typical peripheral vasodilation seen with other dihydropyridines, but because of its inhibitory effect on the SA node, little or no rise in heart rate is seen. This inhibitory effect does not extend to the cardiac myocytes (no cardiodepressant effect is seen). Despite the negative chronotropic effect, isradipine appears to have little effect on the AV node, so it may be used in patients with AV block or combined with a β adrenergic receptor antagonist. In general, because of their lack of myocardial depression and, to a greater or lesser extent, lack of negative chronotropic effect, dihydropyridines are less effective as monotherapy in stable angina than are verapamil, diltiazem, or a β adrenergic receptor antagonist. Nisoldipine is >1000 times more potent in preventing contraction of human vascular smooth muscle than in preventing contraction of human cardiac muscle in vitro, suggesting a high degree of vascular selectivity. Although nisoldipine has a short elimination $t_{1/2}$, a sustained-release preparation is efficacious as an antianginal agent. Nimodipine has high lipid solubility and was developed as an agent to relax the cerebral vasculature. It is effective in inhibiting cerebral vasospasm and has been used primarily to treat patients with neurological defects associated with cerebral vasospasm after subarachnoid hemorrhage.

Table 31–1

Ca^{2+} Channel Blockers: Chemical Structures and Some Relative Cardiovascular Effects*

Chemical Structure (Nonproprietary and TRADE NAMES)	Vasodilation (Coronary Flow)	Suppression of Cardiac Contractility	Suppression of Automaticity (SA Node)	Suppression of Conduction (AV Node)
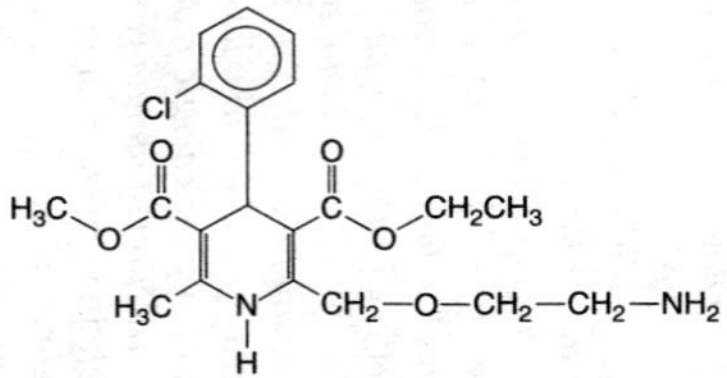 Amlodipine (NORVASC)	5	1	1	0
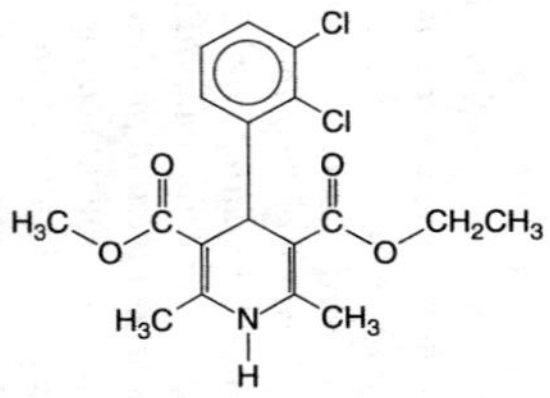 Felodipine (PLENDIL)	5	1	1	0
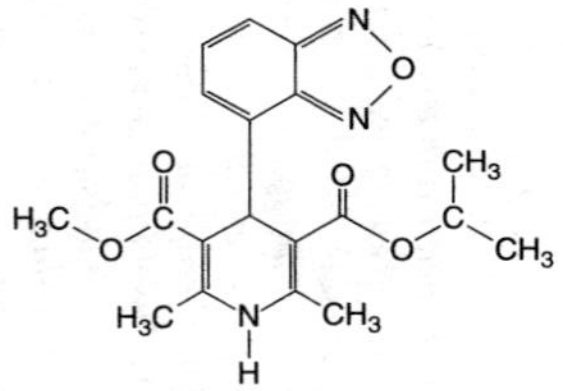 Isradipine (DYNACIRC)	NR	NR	NR	NR

534

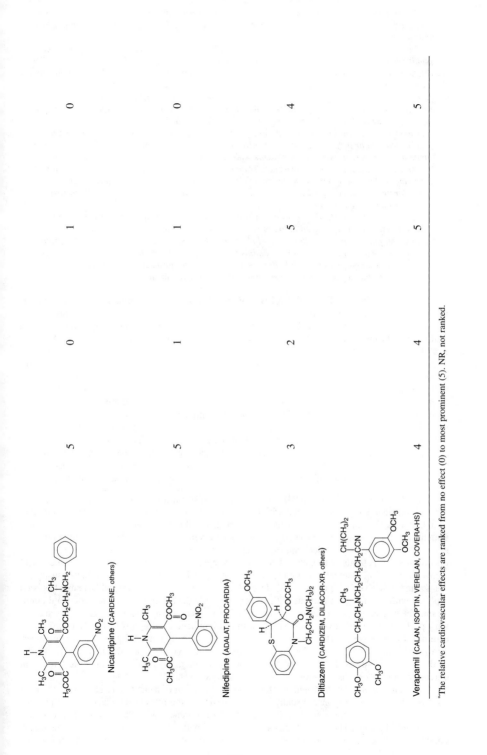

*The relative cardiovascular effects are ranked from no effect (0) to most prominent (5). NR, not ranked.

Bepridil reduces blood pressure and heart rate in patients with stable exertional angina and also produces an increase in left ventricular performance. Its side effects (see below) limit its use to truly refractory patients.

Verapamil is a less potent vasodilator than the dihydropyridines. Like the latter agents, verapamil causes little effect on venous resistance vessels at concentrations that produce arteriolar dilation. With doses of verapamil sufficient to produce peripheral arterial vasodilation, there are more direct negative chronotropic, dromotropic, and inotropic effects than with the dihydropyridines. Intravenous verapamil decreases arterial blood pressure owing to a decrease in vascular resistance, but the reflex tachycardia is blunted or abolished by the direct negative chronotropic effect of the drug. This intrinsic negative inotropic effect is partially offset by both a decrease in afterload and the reflex increase in adrenergic tone. Thus, in patients without congestive heart failure, ventricular performance is not impaired and actually may improve, especially if ischemia limits performance. In contrast, in patients with congestive heart failure, intravenous verapamil can cause a marked decrease in contractility and left ventricular function. Oral administration of verapamil reduces peripheral vascular resistance and blood pressure, often with minimal changes in heart rate. The relief of pacing-induced angina seen with verapamil is due primarily to a reduction in myocardial oxygen demand.

Intravenous administration of diltiazem initially can result in a marked decrease in peripheral vascular resistance and arterial blood pressure, which elicits a reflex increase in heart rate and cardiac output. Heart rate then falls below initial levels because of the direct negative chronotropic effect of the agent. Oral administration of diltiazem decreases both heart rate and mean arterial blood pressure. While diltiazem and verapamil produce similar effects on the SA and AV nodes, the negative inotropic effect of diltiazem is more modest.

ABSORPTION, FATE, AND EXCRETION Although the absorption of these agents is nearly complete after oral administration, their bioavailability is reduced, sometimes markedly, by first-pass hepatic metabolism. The effects of these drugs are evident within 30–60 minutes of an oral dose, with the exception of the more slowly absorbed and longer-acting agents amlodipine, isradipine, and felodipine. For comparison, peak effects of verapamil occur within 15 minutes of its intravenous administration. These agents all are bound extensively to plasma proteins; their elimination half-lives vary widely (*see* Appendix II in the 11th edition of the parent text). During repeated oral administration, bioavailability and $t_{1/2}$ may increase because of saturation of hepatic metabolism. A major metabolite of diltiazem is desacetyldiltiazem, which has about one-half of diltiazem's potency as a vasodilator. N-Demethylation of verapamil results in production of norverapamil ($t_{1/2}$ ~10 hours), which is biologically active but much less potent than the parent compound. Metabolites of dihydropyridines are inactive or weakly active. In patients with cirrhosis, the bioavailabilities and half-lives of the Ca^{2+} channel blockers may be increased, and dosage should be decreased accordingly. The half-lives of these agents also may be longer in older patients. Except for diltiazem and nifedipine, all of the Ca^{2+} channel blockers are administered as racemic mixtures.

TOXICITY AND UNTOWARD RESPONSES The most common side effects caused by the Ca^{2+} channel antagonists, particularly the dihydropyridines, are due to excessive vasodilation. Symptoms include dizziness, hypotension, headache, flushing, digital dysesthesia, and nausea. Patients also may experience constipation, peripheral edema, coughing, wheezing, and pulmonary edema. Nimodipine may produce muscle cramps when given in the large doses required for a beneficial effect in patients with subarachnoid hemorrhage. Less common side effects include rash, somnolence, and occasional minor elevations of liver function tests. These side effects usually are benign and may abate with time or with dose adjustment. Worsened myocardial ischemia has been reported with nifedipine in patients with angiographically demonstrable coronary collateral circulation. The worsening of angina may have resulted from excessive hypotension and decreased coronary perfusion, selective coronary vasodilation in nonischemic regions of the myocardium in a setting where vessels perfusing ischemic regions were already maximally dilated (*i.e.,* coronary steal), or an increase in oxygen demand owing to increased sympathetic tone and excessive tachycardia. Monotherapy with an immediate-release formulation of nisoldipine was associated with a trend toward an increased incidence of serious adverse events.

Although bradycardia, transient asystole, and exacerbation of heart failure have been reported with verapamil, these responses usually have occurred after intravenous administration in patients with disease of the SA node or AV nodal conduction disturbances or in the presence of β adrenergic receptor blockade. The use of intravenous verapamil with a β adrenergic receptor antagonist is contraindicated because of the increased propensity for AV block and/or severe depression of ventricular function. Patients with ventricular dysfunction, SA or AV nodal conduction disturbances, or systolic blood pressures <90 mm Hg should not be treated with verapamil or diltiazem, particularly intravenously. Some Ca^{2+} channel antagonists can cause an increase in the concentration of digoxin in plasma, although toxicity from the cardiac glycoside rarely develops. The use of verapamil to treat digitalis toxicity is contraindicated, as AV nodal conduction disturbances may be exacerbated. Bepridil, because of its ability to prolong the QTc interval, can produce serious arrhythmias. Especially in the setting of hypokalemia and/or bradycardia, polymorphic ventricular tachycardia (*torsades de pointes*) can occur. Agranulocytosis also has been reported. Because of these serious side effects, bepridil should be reserved for patients refractory to all other appropriate medical and surgical therapy.

Several studies have raised concerns about the long-term safety of short-acting nifedipine. The proposed mechanism for this adverse effect lies in abrupt vasodilation with reflex sympathetic activation. There does not appear to be either significant reflex tachycardia or long-term adverse outcomes from treatment with sustained-release forms of nifedipine or with dihydropyridine Ca^{2+} blockers such as amlodipine or felodipine, which have more favorable (slower) pharmacokinetics.

Therapeutic Uses

VARIANT ANGINA Variant angina results from reduced flow rather than increased O_2 demand, and Ca^{2+} channel blockers have proven efficacy. In these patients, these drugs can attenuate *ergonovine*-induced vasospasm, suggesting that protection in variant angina is due to coronary dilation rather than to alterations in peripheral hemodynamics.

EXERTIONAL ANGINA Ca^{2+} channel antagonists also are effective in the treatment of exertional angina. Their utility may result from an increase in blood flow owing to coronary arterial dilation, from a decrease in myocardial O_2 demand (secondary to a decrease in arterial blood pressure, heart rate, or contractility), or both. These drugs decrease the number of anginal attacks and attenuate exercise-induced ST-segment depression.

Ca^{2+} channel antagonists, particularly the dihydropyridines, may aggravate anginal symptoms in some patients when used without a β adrenergic receptor antagonist. This adverse effect is not prominent with verapamil or diltiazem because of their limited ability to induce marked peripheral vasodilation and reflex tachycardia. Concurrent therapy with nifedipine and the β adrenergic receptor antagonist propranolol or with amlodipine and any of several β adrenergic receptor antagonists has proven more effective than either agent given alone in exertional angina, presumably because the β adrenergic receptor antagonist suppresses reflex tachycardia. This concurrent drug therapy is particularly attractive because the dihydropyridines, unlike verapamil and diltiazem, do not delay AV conduction and will not enhance the negative dromotropic effects associated with β adrenergic receptor blockade. Although concurrent administration of verapamil or diltiazem with a β adrenergic receptor antagonist also may reduce angina, the potential for AV block, severe bradycardia, and decreased left ventricular function requires that these combinations be used judiciously, especially if left ventricular function is compromised prior to therapy. Amlodipine produces less reflex tachycardia than does nifedipine, probably because of a flatter plasma concentration profile. Isradipine, approximately equivalent to nifedipine in enhancing exercise tolerance, also produces less rise in heart rate, possibly because of its slow onset of action.

UNSTABLE ANGINA Medical therapy for unstable angina involves the administration of aspirin (which reduces mortality), nitrates, β adrenergic receptor antagonists, and heparin, which are effective in controlling ischemic episodes and angina. Since vasospasm occurs in some patients with unstable angina, Ca^{2+} channel blockers offer an additional approach to this condition. However, there is insufficient evidence to assess whether such treatment decreases mortality except when the underlying mechanism is vasospasm. In contrast, therapy directed toward reducing platelet function and thrombotic episodes clearly decreases morbidity and mortality in patients with unstable angina (*see* Chapters 54).

MYOCARDIAL INFARCTION There is no evidence that Ca^{2+} channel antagonists are beneficial in the early treatment or secondary prevention of acute MI. In several trials, higher doses of the short-acting formulation of the dihydropyridine nifedipine had a detrimental effect on mortality. Diltiazem and verapamil may reduce the incidence of reinfarction in patients with a first non-ST segment elevation infarction who are not candidates for a β adrenergic receptor antagonist, but β blockers remain the preferred drugs.

OTHER USES

Ca²⁺ channel antagonists are also used as antiarrhythmic agents, for the treatment of hypertension, and for the treatment of heart failure. Clinical trials are under way to evaluate the capacity of Ca²⁺ channel blockers to slow the progression of renal failure and to protect the transplanted kidney. Verapamil has been demonstrated to improve left ventricular outflow obstruction and symptoms in patients with hypertrophic cardiomyopathy. Verapamil also has been used in the prophylaxis of migraine headaches. While the dihydropyridines may suppress the progression of mild atherosclerosis, there is no evidence that this alters mortality or reduces the incidence of ischemic events. Nimodipine has been approved for use in patients with neurological deficits secondary to cerebral vasospasm after the rupture of a congenital intracranial aneurysm. Nifedipine, diltiazem, amlodipine, and felodipine appear to provide symptomatic relief in Raynaud's disease. The Ca²⁺ channel antagonists cause relaxation of the myometrium in vitro *and may be effective in stopping preterm uterine contractions in preterm labor (see Chapter 55).*

β ADRENERGIC RECEPTOR ANTAGONISTS

β Adrenergic receptor antagonists are effective in reducing the severity and frequency of attacks of exertional angina and in improving survival in patients after an MI. In contrast, these agents are not useful and may actually exacerbate vasospastic angina. Most β adrenergic receptor antagonists are equally effective in the treatment of exertional angina. *Timolol,* metoprolol, *atenolol,* and propranolol have been shown to exert cardioprotective effects. The effectiveness of β adrenergic receptor antagonists in the treatment of exertional angina is attributable primarily to a fall in myocardial O_2 consumption at rest and during exertion, although there also is some tendency for increased flow toward ischemic regions. The decrease in myocardial O_2 consumption is due to a negative chronotropic effect (particularly during exercise), a negative inotropic effect, and a reduction in arterial blood pressure (particularly systolic pressure) during exercise. Not all actions of β adrenergic receptor antagonists are beneficial in all patients. The decreases in heart rate and contractility cause increases in the systolic ejection period and left ventricular end-diastolic volume; these alterations tend to increase O_2 consumption. However, the net effect of β adrenergic receptor blockade is usually to decrease myocardial O_2 consumption, particularly during exercise. Nevertheless, in patients with limited cardiac reserve who are critically dependent on adrenergic stimulation, β adrenergic receptor blockade can profoundly decrease left ventricular function. Despite this, several β adrenergic receptor antagonists have been shown to reduce mortality in patients with congestive heart failure (*see* Chapter 33). Numerous β adrenergic receptor antagonists are approved for clinical use in the U.S. (*see* Chapter 10).

Therapeutic Uses

UNSTABLE ANGINA

β Adrenergic receptor antagonists are effective in reducing recurrent episodes of ischemia and the risk of progression to acute MI. Clinical trials have lacked sufficient power to demonstrate beneficial effects of β adrenergic receptor antagonists on mortality. On the other hand, if the underlying pathophysiology is coronary vasospasm, nitrates and Ca²⁺ channel blockers may be effective, and β adrenergic receptor antagonists should be used with caution. In some patients, there is a combination of severe fixed disease and superimposed vasospasm; if adequate antiplatelet therapy and vasodilation have been provided by other agents and angina continues, the addition of a β adrenergic receptor antagonist may be helpful.

MYOCARDIAL INFARCTION

β Adrenergic receptor antagonists that lack intrinsic sympathomimetic activity improve mortality in MI. They should be given early and continued indefinitely in patients who can tolerate them.

OVERVIEW OF ANTIANGINAL THERAPEUTIC STRATEGIES

In evaluating trials in which different forms of antianginal therapy are compared, careful attention must be paid to the patient population studied and to the pathophysiology and stage of the disease. The efficacy of antianginal treatment will depend on the severity of angina, the presence of coronary vasospasm, and myocardial O_2 demand. Optimally, the dose of each agent should be titrated to maximum benefit.

Task forces from the ACC and the AHA have published guidelines that are useful in the selection of appropriate initial therapy for patients with chronic stable angina pectoris (www.americanheart.org). Patients with coronary artery disease should be treated with aspirin and a β adrenergic receptor antagonist (particularly if there is a history of prior MI). The guidelines also note that solid data support the use of ACE inhibitors in patients with coronary artery disease who also have left ventricular dysfunction and/or diabetes. Therapy of hypercholesterolemia is also indicated. Nitrates, for treatment of angina symptoms, and Ca^{2+} antagonists also may be used. Table 31–2 summarizes the issues that the ACC/AHA task force considered to be relevant in choosing between β adrenergic receptor antagonists and Ca^{2+} channel blockers in patients with angina and other medical conditions. A meta-analysis comparison of β adrenergic receptor antagonists with Ca^{2+} channel blockers showed that β adrenergic receptor antagonists are associated with fewer episodes of angina per week and a lower rate of withdrawal because of adverse events. However, there were no differences in time to ischemia during exercise or in the frequency of adverse events when Ca^{2+} channel blockers other than nifedipine were compared with β adrenergic receptor antagonists. There were no significant differences in outcome between the studies comparing long-acting nitrates and Ca^{2+} channel blockers and the studies comparing long-acting nitrates with β adrenergic receptor antagonists.

COMBINATION THERAPY

Since the different categories of antianginal agents have different mechanisms of action, it has been suggested that combinations of these agents would allow the use of lower doses, increasing effectiveness and reducing the incidence of side effects. Despite the predicted advantages, combination therapy rarely achieves this potential and may be accompanied by serious side effects. Newer antianginal agents have distinct pharmacological mechanisms to reduce myocardial O_2 consumption (e.g., ranolazine); some studies have suggested that these compounds may have additional efficacy in combination with other antianginal agents. Ranolazine and related compounds (e.g., perhexiline, trimetazidine) are "metabolic" antianginal drugs that shift myocardial metabolism from free fatty acid oxidation to glucose metabolism, resulting in reduced myocardial O_2 consumption. These agents are not FDA-approved, although perhexiline is available in Australia and Europe.

Nitrates and β Adrenergic Receptor Antagonists

The concurrent use of organic nitrates and β adrenergic receptor antagonists can be very effective in the treatment of typical exertional angina. The additive efficacy is primarily a result of the blockade by one drug of a reflex effect elicited by the other. β Adrenergic receptor antagonists can block the baroreceptor-mediated reflex tachycardia and positive inotropic effects that are sometimes associated with nitrates, whereas nitrates, by increasing venous capacitance, can attenuate the increase in left ventricular end-diastolic volume associated with β adrenergic receptor blockade. Concurrent administration of nitrates also can alleviate the increase in coronary vascular resistance associated with blockade of β adrenergic receptors.

Ca^{2+} Channel Blockers and β Adrenergic Receptor Antagonists

Since there is a proven mortality benefit from the use of β adrenergic receptor antagonists in patients with heart disease, they represent the first line of therapy. However, when angina is controlled inadequately by a β adrenergic receptor antagonist plus nitrates, further improvement sometimes can be achieved by the addition of a Ca^{2+} channel blocker, especially if there is a component of coronary vasospasm. The differences among the chemical classes of Ca^{2+} channel blockers can lead to important adverse or salutary drug interactions with β adrenergic receptor antagonists. If the patient already is being treated with maximal doses of verapamil or diltiazem, it is difficult to demonstrate any additional benefit of β adrenergic receptor blockade, and excessive bradycardia, heart block, or heart failure may ensue. However, in patients treated with a dihydropyridine or with nitrates, substantial reflex tachycardia often limits the effectiveness of these agents. A β adrenergic receptor antagonist may be a helpful addition, resulting in a lower heart rate and blood pressure with exercise.

Relative contraindications to the use of β adrenergic receptor antagonists for treatment of angina—bronchospasm, Raynaud's syndrome, or Prinzmetal's angina—may favor initial therapy with a Ca^{2+} channel blocker. Fluctuations in coronary tone are important determinants of variant angina. It is likely that episodes of increased tone, such as those precipitated by cold and by emotion, superimposed on fixed disease have a role in the variable anginal threshold seen in some patients with otherwise chronic stable angina. Increased coronary tone also may be important in the anginal episodes occurring early after MI and after coronary angioplasty and probably accounts for those patients with unstable angina who respond to dihydropyridines. Atherosclerotic arteries have abnormal vasomotor responses to a number of stimuli, including exercise, other forms of sympathetic activation, and cholinergic agonists; in such vessels, stenotic segments actually may become more severely stenosed during exertion. This implies that the normal

Table 31-2

Recommended Drug Therapy for Angina in Patients with Other Medical Conditions

Condition	Recommended Treatment (and Alternatives) for Angina	Drugs to Avoid
Medical Conditions		
Systemic hypertension	β Adrenergic receptor antagonists (Ca^{2+} channel antagonists)	
Migraine or vascular headaches	β Adrenergic receptor antagonists (Ca^{2+} channel antagonists)	
Asthma or chronic obstructive pulmonary disease with bronchospasm	Verapamil or diltiazem	β Adrenergic receptor antagonists
Hyperthyroidism	β Adrenergic receptor antagonists	
Raynaud's syndrome	Long-acting, slow-release Ca^{2+} channel antagonists	
Insulin-dependent diabetes mellitus	β Adrenergic receptor antagonists (particularly if prior MI) or long-acting, slow-release Ca^{2+} channel antagonists	β Adrenergic receptor antagonists
Non-insulin-dependent diabetes mellitus	β Adrenergic receptor antagonists or long-acting, slow-release Ca^{2+} channel antagonists	
Depression	Long-acting, slow-release Ca^{2+} channel antagonists	β Adrenergic receptor antagonists
Mild peripheral vascular disease	β Adrenergic receptor antagonists or Ca^{2+} channel antagonists	
Severe peripheral vascular disease with rest ischemia	Ca^{2+} channel antagonists	β Adrenergic receptor antagonists
Cardiac Arrhythmias and Conduction Abnormalities		
Sinus bradycardia	Dihydropyridine Ca^{2+} channel antagonists	β Adrenergic receptor antagonists, diltiazem, verapamil
Sinus tachycardia (not due to heart failure)	β Adrenergic receptor antagonists	
Supraventricular tachycardia	Verapamil, diltiazem, or β adrenergic receptor antagonists	
Atrioventricular block	Dihydropyridine Ca^{2+} channel antagonists	β Adrenergic receptor antagonists, verapamil, diltiazem
Rapid atrial fibrillation (with digitalis)	Verapamil, diltiazem, or β adrenergic receptor antagonists	
Ventricular arrhythmias	β Adrenergic receptor antagonists	

Left Ventricular Dysfunction

Condition		
Congestive heart failure		
Mild (LVEF ≥ 40%)	β Adrenergic receptor antagonists	
Moderate to severe (LVEF < 40%)	Amlodipine or felodipine (nitrates)	
Left-sided valvular heart disease		
Mild aortic stenosis	β Adrenergic receptor antagonists	
Aortic insufficiency	Long-acting, slow-release dihydropyridines	
Mitral regurgitation	Long-acting, slow-release dihydropyridines	
Mitral stenosis	β Adrenergic receptor antagonists	
Hypertrophic cardiomyopathy	β Adrenergic receptor antagonists, nondihydropyridine Ca^{2+} channel antagonists	Nitrates, dihydropyridine Ca^{2+} channel antagonists

MI, myocardial infarction; LVEF, left ventricular ejection fraction.

541

exercise-induced increase in coronary flow is lost in atherosclerosis. Similar exaggerated vascular contractile responses are seen in hyperlipidemia, even before anatomic evidence of atherosclerosis develops. Because of this, coronary vasodilators (nitrates and/or Ca^{2+} channel blockers) are an important part of the therapeutic program in the majority of patients with ischemic heart disease.

Ca^{2+} Channel Blockers and Nitrates

In severe exertional or vasospastic angina, the combination of a nitrate and a Ca^{2+} channel blocker may provide additional relief over that obtained with either agent alone. Since nitrates primarily reduce preload, whereas Ca^{2+} channel blockers reduce afterload, the net effect on reduction of oxygen demand should be additive. However, excessive vasodilation and hypotension can occur. The concurrent administration of a nitrate and nifedipine has been advocated in particular for patients with exertional angina with heart failure, the sick-sinus syndrome, or AV nodal conduction disturbances, but excessive tachycardia may be seen.

Ca^{2+} Channel Blockers, β Adrenergic Receptor Antagonists, and Nitrates

In patients with exertional angina that is not controlled by the administration of two types of antianginal agents, the use of all three may provide improvement, although the incidence of side effects increases significantly. The dihydropyridines and nitrates dilate epicardial coronary arteries; the dihydropyridines decrease afterload; the nitrates decrease preload; and the β adrenergic receptor antagonists decrease heart rate and myocardial contractility. Therefore, there is theoretical, and sometimes real, benefit with their combination, although adverse drug interactions may lead to clinically important events. For example, combining verapamil or diltiazem with a β adrenergic receptor antagonist greatly increases the risk of conduction system and left ventricular dysfunction–related side effects and should be undertaken with extreme caution.

ANTIPLATELET, ANTI-INTEGRIN, AND ANTITHROMBOTIC AGENTS

Aspirin reduces the incidence of MI and death in patients with unstable angina. In addition, low doses of aspirin appear to reduce the incidence of MI in patients with chronic stable angina. Aspirin, given in doses of 160–325 mg at the onset of treatment, reduces mortality in patients presenting with unstable angina. The addition of clopidogrel to aspirin therapy reduces mortality in patients with acute coronary syndromes. Heparin, in its unfractionated form or as low-molecular-weight heparin, also reduces symptoms and prevents infarction in unstable angina. Thrombin inhibitors, such as *hirudin* or *bivalirudin*, are being investigated; these agents directly inhibit even clot-bound thrombin, are not affected by circulating inhibitors, and function independently of antithrombin III. Thrombolytic agents, on the other hand, are of no benefit in unstable angina. Intravenous inhibitors of the platelet GPIIb/IIIa receptor (abciximab, tirofiban, and eptifibatide) are effective in preventing the complications of PCIs and in the treatment of patients presenting with acute coronary syndromes.

TREATMENT OF CLAUDICATION AND PERIPHERAL VASCULAR DISEASE

Most patients with peripheral vascular disease also have coronary artery disease, and the therapeutic approaches for peripheral and coronary arterial diseases overlap. Mortality in patients with peripheral vascular disease is most commonly due to cardiovascular disease, and treatment of coronary disease remains the central focus of therapy. Many patients with advanced peripheral arterial disease are more limited by the consequences of peripheral ischemia than by myocardial ischemia. In the cerebral circulation, arterial disease may be manifest as stroke or transient ischemic attacks. The painful symptoms of peripheral arterial disease in the lower extremities (claudication) typically are provoked by exertion, with increases in skeletal muscle O_2 demand exceeding blood flow impaired by proximal stenoses. When flow to the extremities becomes critically limiting, peripheral ulcers and rest pain from tissue ischemia can become debilitating.

Most of the therapies shown to be efficacious for treatment of coronary artery disease also have a salutary effect on progression of peripheral artery disease. Reductions in cardiovascular morbidity and mortality in patients with peripheral arterial disease have been documented with antiplatelet therapy using aspirin or with ADP antagonists such as clopidogrel or ticlopidine, administration of ACE inhibitors, and treatment of hyperlipidemia. Interestingly, neither intensive treatment of diabetes mellitus nor antihypertensive therapy appears to alter the progression of symptoms of claudication. Other risk factor and lifestyle modifications remain cornerstones of therapy for patients with claudication: Physical exercise, rehabilitation, and smoking cessation have proven efficacy. Drugs used specifically in the treatment of lower extremity claudication include *pentoxifylline* and *cilostazol*.

Pentoxifylline is a methylxanthine derivative that has been termed a rheologic modifier for its effects on increasing the deformability of red blood cells. The effects of pentoxifylline on lower extremity claudication appear to be modest. Cilostazol is an inhibitor of PDE3 and promotes accumulation of intracellular cyclic AMP in many cells, including blood platelets. Cilostazol-mediated increases in cyclic AMP inhibit platelet aggregation and promote vasodilation. The drug is metabolized by CYP3A4 and has important interactions with other drugs metabolized *via* this pathway (*see* Chapter 3). Cilostazol improves symptoms of claudication but has no effect on cardiovascular mortality. As a PDE3 inhibitor, cilostazol belongs to the same drug class as flosequinan, which was used as an inotropic agent for patients with heart failure. The latter drug was associated with an increase in sudden cardiac death, leading to withdrawal from the market. Cilostazol therefore is contraindicated in patients with heart failure, although it is not clear that it leads to increased mortality in such patients. Cilostazol has been reported to increase nonsustained ventricular tachycardia; headache is the most common side effect. Other treatments for claudication, including *naftidrofuryl, proprionyl levocarnitine,* and *prostaglandins,* may also be efficacious.

MECHANOPHARMACOLOGICAL THERAPY: DRUG-ELUTING ENDOVASCULAR STENTS

Intracoronary stents can ameliorate angina and reduce adverse events in patients with acute coronary syndromes. However, the long-term efficacy of intracoronary stents is limited by subacute luminal restenosis within the stent, which occurs in a substantial fraction of patients. The pathways that lead to "in-stent restenosis" are complex, but smooth muscle proliferation within the lumen of the stented artery is a common pathological finding. Local antiproliferative therapies at the time of stenting have been explored, and the development of drug-eluting stents has had an important impact on clinical practice. Two drugs are currently used in intravascular stents: *paclitaxel* (TAXOL) and *sirolimus* (RAPAMYCIN). Paclitaxel inhibits cellular proliferation by binding to and stabilizing polymerized microtubules. Sirolimus is a macrolide that binds to the cytosolic immunophilin FKBP12; the FKBP12–sirolimus complex inhibits the protein kinase, mammalian target of RAPAMYCIN (mTOR), thereby inhibiting cell cycle progression (*see* Chapter 53). Stent-induced damage to the vascular endothelial cell layer can lead to thrombosis; patients typically are treated with antiplatelet agents, including clopidogrel (for up to 6 months) and aspirin (indefinitely), sometimes in conjunction with intravenously administered GPIIb/IIIa inhibitors. The inhibition of cellular proliferation by paclitaxel and sirolimus not only affects vascular smooth muscle cell proliferation but also attenuates the formation of an intact endothelial layer within the stented artery. Therefore, antiplatelet therapy (typically with clopidogrel) is continued for several months after intracoronary stenting with drug-eluting stents. The rate of restenosis with drug-eluting stents is reduced markedly compared with "bare metal" stents, possibly at the expense of increased risk of thrombosis, especially if antiplatelet therapy is stopped prematurely.

For a complete Bibliographical listing see Goodman & Gilman's *The Pharmacological Basis of Therapeutics,* 11th ed., or Goodman & Gilman Online at www.accessmedicine.com.

32

THERAPY OF HYPERTENSION

Hypertension is the most common cardiovascular disease; its prevalence increases with advancing age. Elevated arterial pressure causes pathological changes in the vasculature and hypertrophy of the left ventricle. Hypertension is the principal cause of stroke, is a major risk factor for coronary artery disease and its complications, and is a major contributor to cardiac failure, renal insufficiency, and dissecting aortic aneurysm. Hypertension is defined as a sustained increase in blood pressure $\geq140/90$ mm Hg, a criterion where risk of hypertension-related cardiovascular disease is high enough to merit medical attention. The risk of fatal and nonfatal cardiovascular disease in adults is lowest with systolic BP <120 mm Hg and diastolic BP <80 mm Hg and increases progressively with higher systolic and diastolic blood pressures. Recognition of this continuously increasing risk provides a simple classification of hypertension (Table 32–1). Isolated systolic hypertension (sometimes defined as systolic BP >140–160 mm Hg with diastolic BP <90 mm Hg) is largely confined to people >60 years of age. At very high blood pressures (systolic ≥210 and/or diastolic ≥120 mm Hg), some patients develop fulminant arteriopathy characterized by endothelial injury and marked intimal proliferation, leading ultimately to arteriolar occlusion and the syndrome of immediately life-threatening hypertension. This is associated with rapidly progressive microvascular occlusive disease in the kidney (with renal failure), brain (hypertensive encephalopathy), congestive heart failure, and pulmonary edema, and typically requires emergent, in-hospital management for prompt lowering of blood pressure.

PRINCIPLES OF ANTIHYPERTENSIVE THERAPY Nonpharmacological therapy is an important component of treatment of all patients with hypertension. In some stage 1 hypertensives, blood pressure may be adequately controlled by a combination of weight loss (in overweight individuals), restricting sodium intake, increasing aerobic exercise, and moderating alcohol consumption. These lifestyle changes may also facilitate pharmacological control of blood pressure.

Drugs lower blood pressure by actions on peripheral resistance, cardiac output, or both. In patients with isolated systolic hypertension, complex hemodynamics in a rigid arterial system contribute to increased blood pressure; drug effects may be mediated by changes in peripheral resistance but also *via* effects on large artery stiffness.

Antihypertensive drugs can be classified according to their sites or mechanisms of action (Table 32–2). The hemodynamic effects of antihypertensive agents (Table 32–3) provide a rationale for potential complementary effects of concurrent therapy with two or more drugs. Concurrent use of drugs from different classes is an effective strategy for achieving effective control of blood pressure while minimizing dose-related adverse effects.

DIURETICS

Diuretic agents (*see* Chapter 28) have antihypertensive effects when used alone and enhance the efficacy of virtually all other antihypertensive drugs; thus, these drugs are very important in the treatment of hypertension.

Benzothiadiazines and Related Compounds

Benzothiadiazines ("thiazides") and related diuretics are the most frequently used class of antihypertensive agents in the U.S. Thiazides block the Na^+-Cl^- symporter and have the same pharmacological effects and are generally interchangeable with appropriate dose adjustment (*see* Chapter 28). Since their pharmacokinetics and pharmacodynamics differ, these drugs do not necessarily have the same clinical efficacy in treating hypertension.

The exact mechanism for reduction of arterial blood pressure by thiazide diuretics is not certain. The drugs decrease extracellular volume by inhibiting the Na-Cl symporter in the distal convoluted tubule, leading to a fall in cardiac output, but the hypotensive effect is maintained during long-term therapy because of reduced vascular resistance; presumably thiazides directly promote vasodilation. *Hydrochlorothiazide* may open Ca^{2+}-activated K^+ channels, leading to hyperpolarization of vascular smooth muscle cells, decreased Ca^{2+} entry through voltage-sensitive L-type Ca^{2+} channels, and ultimately reduced vasoconstriction.

REGIMEN FOR ADMINISTRATION OF THE THIAZIDE-CLASS DIURETICS IN HYPERTENSION When a thiazide diuretic is used as the sole antihypertensive drug (monotherapy), its dose-response curve for lowering blood pressure in patients with hypertension should be

Table 32–1

Criteria for Hypertension in Adults

	Blood Pressure (mm Hg)	
Classification	Systolic	Diastolic
Normal	<120	and <80
Pre-hypertension	120–139	or 80–89
Hypertension, stage 1	140–159	or 90–99
Hypertension, stage 2	≥160	or ≤100

kept in mind. Antihypertensive effects are achieved in many patients with as little as 12.5 mg of chlorthalidone (HYGROTON) or hydrochlorothiazide (HYDRODIURIL) daily. Furthermore, when used as monotherapy, the maximal daily dose of thiazide-class diuretics usually should not exceed 25 mg of hydrochlorothiazide or chlorthalidone (or equivalent). Even though more diuresis can be achieved with higher doses of these diuretics, higher doses generally are not more efficacious in patients with normal renal function. These doses of hydrochlorothiazide are not at the top of the dose-response curve for adverse effects such as K^+ wasting and inhibition of uric acid excretion (see below), emphasizing the importance of the dose-response relationships for both beneficial and adverse effects.

Urinary K^+ loss can be a problem with thiazides. Angiotensin-converting enzyme (ACE) inhibitors and angiotensin receptor antagonists will partly attenuate diuretic-induced loss of K^+, and this is a consideration if a second drug is needed to adequately control blood pressure. Because the diuretic and hypotensive effects of these drugs are greatly enhanced when they are given in combination, care should be taken to initiate combination therapy with low doses of each drug. Administration of ACE inhibitors or angiotensin receptor antagonists together with other K^+-sparing agents or with K^+ supplements requires great caution; combining K^+-sparing agents with each other or with K^+ supplementation can cause potentially dangerous hyperkalemia in some patients.

In contrast to the dose limitations when thiazide diuretics used as monotherapy, the treatment of severe hypertension that is unresponsive to three or more drugs may require larger doses of the thiazide diuretics. Hypertensive patients may become refractory to drugs that block the sympathetic nervous system or to vasodilator drugs because these drugs engender a state in which the blood pressure is very volume-dependent. It therefore is appropriate to consider the use of thiazide diuretics

Table 32–2

Classification of Antihypertensive Drugs by Their Primary Site or Mechanism of Action

Diuretics (Chapter 28)
1. Thiazides and related agents (hydrochlorothiazide, chlorthalidone, *etc.*)
2. Loop diuretics (furosemide, bumetanide, torsemide, ethacrynic acid)
3. K^+-sparing diuretics (amiloride, triamterene, spironolactone)

Sympatholytic drugs (Chapters 9, 10, and 33)
1. β Adrenergic antagonists (metoprolol, atenolol, *etc.*)
2. α Adrenergic antagonists (prazosin, terazosin, doxazosin, phenoxybenzamine, phentolamine)
3. Mixed adrenergic antagonists (labetalol, carvedilol)
4. Centrally acting agents (methyldopa, clonidine, guanabenz, guanfacine)
5. Adrenergic neuron blocking agents (guanadrel, reserpine)

Ca^{2+} channel blockers (Chapters 31 through 34)
(verapamil, diltiazem, nimodipine, felodipine, nicardipine, isradipine, amlodipine)

Angiotensin-converting enzyme inhibitors (Chapters 30 and 31)
(captopril, enalapril, lisinopril, quinapril, ramipril, benazepril, fosinopril, moexipril, perindopril, trandolapril)

Angiotensin II receptor antagonists (Chapters 30 and 33)
(losartan, candesartan, irbesartan, valsartan, telmisartan, eprosartan)

Vasodilators (Chapter 33)
1. Arterial (hydralazine, minoxidil, diazoxide, fenoldopam)
2. Arterial and venous (nitroprusside)

Table 32–3

Hemodynamic Effects of Long-Term Administration of Antihypertensive Agents

Drug Class	Heart Rate	Cardiac Output	Total Peripheral Resistance	Plasma Volume	Plasma Renin Activity
Diuretics	↔	↔	↓	–↓	↑
Sympatholytic agents					
Centrally acting	–↓	–↓	↓	–↑	–↓
Adrenergic neuron blockers	–↓	↓	↓	↑	–↑
α Adrenergic antagonists	–↑	–↑	↓	–↑	↔
β Adrenergic antagonists					
No ISA*	↓	↓	–↓	–↑	↓
ISA	↔	↔	↓	–↑	–↓
Arteriolar vasodilators	↑	↑	↓	↑	↑
Ca^{2+} channel blockers	↓ or ↑	↓ or ↑	↓	–↑	–↑
ACE inhibitors	↔	↔	↓	↔	↑
AT_1 receptor antagonists	↔	↔	↓	↔	↑

Changes are indicated as follows: ↑, increased; ↓, decreased; –↑, increased or no change; –↓, decreased or no change; ↔, unchanged.
*ISA, intrinsic sympathomimetic activity. ACE, angiotensin-converting enzyme; AT_1, the type 1 receptor for AngII.

in doses of 50 mg/day of hydrochlorothiazide or its equivalent when treatment with appropriate combinations and doses of three or more drugs fails to yield adequate blood pressure control. Alternatively, higher-capacity diuretics such as *furosemide* may be needed, especially if renal function is impaired. Dietary Na^+ restriction (*e.g.*, 2 g daily) is a valuable adjunct in such refractory patients that minimizes the dose of diuretic that is required. Since the degree of K^+ loss relates to the amount of Na^+ delivered to the distal tubule, such restriction of Na^+ can minimize the development of hypokalemia and alkalosis. The effectiveness of thiazides as diuretics or antihypertensive agents diminishes progressively when the glomerular filtration rate is <30 mL/min. One exception is *metolazone*, which retains efficacy in patients with this degree of renal insufficiency.

Most patients will respond to thiazide diuretics with a reduction in blood pressure within ~4 weeks, although a minority will not achieve maximum reduction in arterial pressure for up to 12 weeks. Therefore, doses should not be increased more often than every 4–6 weeks. There is no way to predict the antihypertensive response from the duration or severity of the hypertension in a given patient, although diuretics are unlikely to be effective as sole therapy in patients with stage 2 hypertension. Since the effect of thiazide diuretics is additive with that of other antihypertensive drugs, combination regimens that include these diuretics are common and rational. Diuretics also minimize the retention of salt and water that is commonly caused by vasodilators and some sympatholytic drugs. Omitting or underutilizing a diuretic is a frequent cause of "resistant hypertension."

ADVERSE EFFECTS AND PRECAUTIONS Adverse effects of diuretics (*see* Chapter 28) determine tolerance and adherence. Erectile dysfunction is a troublesome adverse effect of thiazide diuretics; physicians should inquire specifically regarding its occurrence. Albeit uncommon, gout may be a consequence of the hyperuricemia induced by these diuretics. Either of these adverse effects is reason to consider alternative therapies. Hydrochlorothiazide may cause rapidly developing, severe hyponatremia in some patients. Thiazides inhibit renal Ca^{2+} excretion, occasionally leading to hypercalcemia; although generally mild, this can be more severe in patients subject to hypercalcemia, such as those with primary hyperparathyroidism. The thiazide-induced decreased Ca^{2+} excretion may be used therapeutically in patients with osteoporosis or hypercalciuria.

The effects of diuretic drugs on several *surrogate markers* merit consideration. The K^+ depletion produced by thiazide diuretics is dose-dependent and variable among individuals, such that some patients may become substantially K^+-depleted on diuretic drugs. Given chronically, even small doses lead to some K^+ depletion. Two types of ventricular arrhythmias may be enhanced by K^+ depletion. One of these is polymorphic ventricular tachycardia (*torsades de pointes; see* Chapter 34), which is initiated by abnormal ventricular repolarization. Because K^+ currents normally mediate repolarization, drugs that produce K^+ depletion potentiate polymorphic ventricular tachycardia. Accordingly, thiazide diuretics should not be given together with drugs that can cause polymorphic ventricular tachycardia (*see* Chapter 34). The more important concern regarding

K^+ depletion is its influence on ischemic ventricular fibrillation, the leading cause of sudden cardiac death and a major contributor to cardiovascular mortality in treated hypertensive patients. Diuretic dose is positively correlated with sudden cardiac death, while there is an inverse correlation between the use of K^+-sparing agents and sudden cardiac death.

Thiazide diuretics have been associated with changes in plasma lipids and glucose tolerance. Nonetheless, clinical studies consistently demonstrate the efficacy of thiazide diuretics in reducing cardiovascular risk. All of the thiazide drugs cross the placenta, but they have not been shown to have direct adverse effects on the fetus. However, if administration of a thiazide is begun during pregnancy, there is a risk of transient volume depletion that may result in placental hypoperfusion. Since the thiazides appear in breast milk, they should be avoided by nursing mothers.

Other Diuretic Antihypertensive Agents

In patients who have normal renal function, the thiazide diuretics are more effective antihypertensive agents than are the loop diuretics, (e.g. furosemide and bumetanide). *This differential effect is most likely related to the short duration of action of loop diuretics, such that a single daily dose does not cause a significant net loss of* Na^+ *throughout the day. Indeed, loop diuretics are frequently and inappropriately prescribed as a once-a-day medication in the treatment of hypertension, congestive heart failure, and ascites. The spectacular efficacy of the loop diuretics in producing a rapid and profound natriuresis can be detrimental for the treatment of hypertension. When a loop diuretic is given twice daily, excessive diuresis can lead to more side effects than occur with a slower-acting, thiazide diuretic. Loop diuretics may be particularly useful in patients with azotemia or with severe edema associated with a vasodilator such as minoxidil.*

Amiloride is a K^+-*sparing diuretic that has some efficacy in lowering blood pressure in patients with hypertension. Spironolactone, a mineralocorticoid receptor antagonist, also lowers blood pressure but has some significant adverse effects, especially in men (e.g., impotence and gynecomastia). Triamterene is a* K^+-*sparing diuretic that decreases the risk of hypokalemia in patients treated with a thiazide diuretic but does not have efficacy in lowering blood pressure by itself. These agents should be used cautiously with frequent measurements of* K^+ *concentrations in plasma in patients predisposed to hyperkalemia. Patients taking spironolactone, amiloride, or triamterene should be cautioned regarding the concurrent use of* K^+-*containing salt substitutes. Renal insufficiency is a relative contraindication to the use of* K^+-*sparing diuretics. Concomitant use of an ACE inhibitor or an angiotensin receptor antagonist magnifies the risk of hyperkalemia with these agents.*

Diuretic-Associated Drug Interactions

Since the antihypertensive effects of diuretics are frequently additive with those of other antihypertensive agents, a diuretic commonly is combined with other drugs. The K^+- *and* Mg^{2+}-*depleting effects of the thiazides and loop diuretics also can potentiate arrhythmias that arise from digitalis toxicity. Corticosteroids can amplify the hypokalemia produced by the diuretics. All diuretics can decrease the clearance of* Li^+, *resulting in increased plasma concentrations of* Li^+ *and potential toxicity. NSAIDs (see Chapter 26), including selective COX-2 inhibitors, that inhibit the synthesis of renal prostaglandins, reduce the antihypertensive effects of diuretics. NSAIDs,* β *adrenergic receptor antagonists, and ACE inhibitors reduce plasma concentrations of aldosterone and can potentiate the hyperkalemic effects of a* K^+-*sparing diuretic.*

SYMPATHOLYTIC AGENTS

α and β adrenergic antagonists are mainstays of antihypertensive therapy (Table 32–2).

β Adrenergic Receptor Antagonists

β receptor antagonists have antihypertensive effects. The pharmacology of these drugs is discussed in Chapter 10. Antagonism of β adrenergic receptors affects blood pressure through a number of mechanisms, including reducing cardiac output. β Adrenergic receptor antagonists also act on the juxtaglomerular complex to reduce renin secretion and thereby diminish production of circulating angiotensin II. Other mechanisms by which β receptor antagonists may lower blood pressure include alteration of the control of the sympathetic nervous system at the level of the CNS, altered baroreceptor sensitivity, altered peripheral adrenergic neuron function, and increased prostacyclin biosynthesis.

PHARMACOLOGICAL EFFECTS The β blockers vary in their lipid solubility, selectivity for the β_1 adrenergic receptor subtype, presence of partial agonist or intrinsic sympathomimetic activity, and membrane-stabilizing properties. While all of the β receptor antagonists are effective as antihypertensive agents, these differences do influence the clinical pharmacokinetics and spectrum of adverse effects of the various drugs. Drugs without intrinsic sympathomimetic activity produce an initial reduction in cardiac output and a reflex-induced rise in peripheral resistance, generally with no net change in arterial pressure; peripheral resistance gradually returns to pretreatment values or less. Persistently reduced cardiac output and possibly decreased peripheral resistance account for the reduced arterial pressure. Drugs with intrinsic sympathomimetic activity produce lesser decreases in resting heart rate and cardiac output; the fall in arterial pressure correlates with a fall in vascular resistance below pretreatment levels, possibly because of stimulation of vascular β_2 adrenergic receptors that mediate vasodilation.

ADVERSE EFFECTS AND PRECAUTIONS The β adrenergic blocking agents should be avoided in patients with asthma, with sinoatrial or atrioventricular (AV) nodal dysfunction, or in combination with other drugs that inhibit AV conduction, such as *verapamil*. Patients with type 1 diabetes mellitus also are better treated with other drugs (*e.g.,* ACE inhibitors).

β Receptor antagonists without intrinsic sympathomimetic activity increase concentrations of triglycerides in plasma and lower those of high-density lipoprotein (HDL) cholesterol. β Adrenergic blocking agents with intrinsic sympathomimetic activity have little or no effect on blood lipids. The long-term consequences of these effects are unknown.

Sudden discontinuation of β adrenergic blockers can produce a withdrawal syndrome that is likely due to up-regulation of β receptors during blockade, causing enhanced tissue sensitivity to endogenous catecholamines; this can exacerbate the symptoms of coronary artery disease. The result, especially in active patients, can be rebound hypertension. Thus, β adrenergic blockers should be tapered over 10–14 days.

NSAIDs such as *indomethacin* can blunt the antihypertensive effect of propranolol and probably other β receptor antagonists. This effect may relate to inhibition of vascular synthesis of prostacyclin, as well as to Na^+ retention.

Epinephrine can produce severe hypertension when used with a nonselective β receptor antagonist due to the unopposed stimulation of α receptors when vascular β_2 receptors are blocked. Such paradoxical hypertensive responses to β adrenergic receptor antagonists have been observed in patients with hypoglycemia or pheochromocytoma, during withdrawal from *clonidine*, following administration of Epi as a therapeutic agent, or in association with the illicit use of cocaine.

THERAPEUTIC USES β receptor antagonists provide effective therapy for all grades of hypertension. Despite marked differences in their pharmacokinetic properties, the antihypertensive effect of all the β blockers is of sufficient duration to permit once or twice daily administration. Populations that tend to have a lesser antihypertensive response to β-blocking agents include the elderly and African Americans. However, this should not discourage the use of these drugs in individual patients, as intraindividual differences in antihypertensive efficacy generally are much larger than differences between racial or age-related groups.

β receptor antagonists do not usually cause salt and water retention, and diuretic administration is not necessary to avoid edema or the development of tolerance. However, diuretics do have additive antihypertensive effects when combined with β blockers. The combination of a β receptor antagonist, a diuretic, and a vasodilator is effective for patients who require a third drug. β Adrenergic receptor antagonists are preferred drugs for hypertensive patients with conditions such as myocardial infarction, ischemic heart disease, or congestive heart failure.

α_1 Adrenergic Antagonists

Drugs that selectively block α_1 adrenergic receptors without affecting α_2 adrenergic receptors also are used in hypertension (Table 32–2). Prazosin (MINIPRESS), terazosin (HYTRIN), and doxazosin (CARDURA) are the agents approved in the U.S. for this indication.

PHARMACOLOGICAL EFFECTS Initially, α_1 adrenergic receptor antagonists reduce arteriolar resistance and increase venous capacitance; this causes a sympathetically mediated reflex increase in heart rate and plasma renin activity. During chronic therapy, vasodilation persists, but cardiac output, heart rate, and plasma renin activity return to normal, and renal blood flow is unchanged. The α_1 adrenergic blockers variably cause postural hypotension, depending on the plasma volume. Retention of salt and water occurs in many patients, which attenuates the postural hypotension. α_1 Receptor antagonists reduce plasma concentrations of triglycerides and total low-density lipoprotein (LDL) cholesterol and increase HDL cholesterol. These potentially favorable effects on lipids persist when a thiazide diuretic is given concurrently. The long-term consequences of these changes in lipids are unknown.

ADVERSE EFFECTS   The use of doxazosin as monotherapy for hypertension increases the risk of developing congestive heart failure. This may be an adverse effect of all of the α_1 adrenergic receptor antagonists.

An important precaution in the use of the α_1 receptor antagonists for hypertension is the so-called first-dose phenomenon, which may occur in up to 50% of patients, especially in patients who are already receiving a diuretic or α receptor antagonist. This effect is characterized by symptomatic orthostatic hypotension within 90 minutes of the initial dose of the drug or after a dosage increase; after the first few doses, patients become tolerant to this marked hypotensive response.

THERAPEUTIC USES α_1 Receptor antagonists are not recommended as monotherapy for hypertensive patients. They rather are used primarily in conjunction with diuretics, β blockers, and other antihypertensive agents. β Receptor antagonists enhance the efficacy of the α_1 blockers. α_1 Receptor antagonists are not the drugs of choice in patients with pheochromocytoma, because a vasoconstrictor response to epinephrine can still result from activation of unblocked vascular α_2 adrenergic receptors. α_1 Receptor antagonists are attractive drugs for hypertensive patients with benign prostatic hyperplasia, since they also improve urinary symptoms.

Combined α_1 and β Adrenergic Receptor Antagonists

Labetalol *(NORMODYNE, TRANDATE) (see Chapter 10) is a mixture of four stereoisomers. One isomer is an α_1 antagonist (like prazosin), another is a nonselective β antagonist with partial agonist activity (like pindolol), and the other two isomers are inactive. Because of its capacity to block α_1 adrenergic receptors, intravenous labetalol can reduce pressure sufficiently rapidly to be useful for the treatment of hypertensive emergencies. Labetalol has efficacy and side effects that would be expected with any combination of β and α_1 receptor antagonists; as with any fixed-dose combination, the relative extents of α receptor and β receptor antagonism vary from patient to patient.*

Carvedilol (COREG) is a β receptor antagonist with α_1 receptor antagonist activity. The drug is approved for the treatment of hypertension and symptomatic heart failure. The ratio of α_1 to β receptor antagonist potency for carvedilol is ~1:10. Carvedilol is oxidized by hepatic CYP2D6 and then glucuronidated. Carvedilol reduces mortality in patients with systolic heart failure when used as an adjunct to therapy with diuretics and ACE inhibitors. It should not be given to those patients with decompensated heart failure who are dependent on sympathetic stimulation. As with labetalol, efficacy and side effects of carvedilol in hypertension are predictable based on its properties as a β and α_1 adrenergic receptor antagonist.

Methyldopa

Methyldopa (ALDOMET) is a centrally acting antihypertensive agent that exerts its antihypertensive action *via* an active metabolite. Methyldopa's significant adverse effects currently limit its use in the U.S. to treatment of hypertension in pregnancy, where it has a record for safety. Methyldopa (α-methyl-3,4-dihydroxy-L-phenylalanine), an analog of 3,4-dihydroxyphenylalanine (DOPA), is metabolized by the L-aromatic amino acid decarboxylase in adrenergic neurons to α-methyldopamine, which then is converted to α-methyl-NE. α-Methylnorepinephrine is stored in the secretory vesicles of adrenergic neurons, substituting for NE. Thus, when adrenergic neurons discharge neurotransmitter, α-methyl-NE is released instead of NE. Because α-methyl-NE is as potent a vasoconstrictor as NE, its substitution for NE in peripheral adrenergic neurosecretory vesicles does not alter the vasoconstrictor response to peripheral adrenergic neurotransmission. Rather, α-methylnorepinephrine acts in the CNS to inhibit adrenergic neuronal outflow from the brainstem. Methylnorepinephrine probably acts as an agonist at presynaptic α_2 adrenergic receptors in the brainstem, attenuating NE release and thereby reducing the output of vasoconstrictor adrenergic signals to the peripheral sympathetic nervous system.

PHARMACOLOGICAL EFFECTS   In younger patients with uncomplicated essential hypertension, methyldopa reduces vascular resistance without much change in cardiac output or heart rate. In older patients, cardiac output may be decreased as a result of decreased heart rate and stroke volume secondary to relaxation of veins and reduced preload. The fall in arterial pressure is maximal 6–8 hours after an oral or intravenous dose. Although the decrease in supine blood pressure is less than that in the upright position, symptomatic orthostatic hypotension is less common with methyldopa than with drugs that act exclusively on peripheral adrenergic neurons or autonomic ganglia; this is because methyldopa attenuates but does not completely block baroreceptor-mediated vasoconstriction. It therefore is well tolerated during surgical anesthesia. Any severe hypotension is reversible with volume expansion. Renal blood flow is maintained and renal function is unchanged during treatment with methyldopa.

Plasma concentrations of NE fall in association with reduction in arterial pressure, reflecting decreased sympathetic tone. Renin secretion also is reduced, but this is not necessary for methyldopa's hypotensive effects. Salt and water often are gradually retained with prolonged use, blunting the antihypertensive effect. This effect, termed "pseudo-tolerance," can be overcome with concurrent use of a diuretic.

ABSORPTION, METABOLISM, AND EXCRETION When administered orally, methyldopa is absorbed by an active amino acid transporter. Peak plasma concentrations occur after 2–3 hours. The drug is eliminated with a $t_{1/2}$ of ~2 hours (prolonged to 4–6 hours in patients with renal failure). Methyldopa transport into the CNS apparently is an active process. Methyldopa is excreted in the urine primarily as the sulfate conjugate (50–70%) and as the parent drug (25%). The remainder is excreted as other metabolites, including methyldopamine, methylnorepinephrine, and O-methylated products of these catecholamines.

In spite of its rapid absorption and short $t_{1/2}$, the peak effect of methyldopa is delayed for 6–8 hours, even after intravenous administration, and the duration of action of a single dose is usually ~24 hours; this permits once- or twice-daily dosing. The discrepancy between the effects and the measured concentrations of the drug in plasma is likely related to the time required for transport into the CNS, conversion to the active metabolite, storage of α-methyl-NE and its subsequent release in the vicinity of relevant α_2 receptors in the CNS.

ADVERSE EFFECTS AND PRECAUTIONS In addition to lowering blood pressure, the active metabolite of methyldopa acts on α_2 adrenergic receptors in the brainstem to inhibit the centers that are responsible for wakefulness and alertness, producing sedation that is largely transient. Decreased mental acuity and lassitude may persist in some patients, and depression occurs occasionally. Medullary centers that control salivation are inhibited by α adrenergic receptors, and methyldopa may produce dry mouth. Other side effects related to pharmacological effects in the CNS include decreased libido, parkinsonian signs, and hyperprolactinemia that may become sufficiently pronounced to cause galactorrhea. In individuals who have sinoatrial node dysfunction, methyldopa may precipitate severe bradycardia and sinus arrest, including that which occurs with carotid sinus hypersensitivity.

Methyldopa also produces adverse effects that are unrelated to its pharmacological action. Hepatotoxicity, sometimes associated with fever, is an uncommon but potentially serious toxic effect. Prompt diagnosis of hepatotoxicity requires a low threshold for considering the drug as a cause for hepatitis-like symptoms (e.g., nausea, anorexia) and screening for hepatotoxicity (e.g., with determination of hepatic transaminases) after 3 weeks and again 3 months after initiation of treatment. The incidence of methyldopa-induced hepatitis is unknown, but ~5% of patients will have transient increases in hepatic transaminases in plasma. Hepatic dysfunction usually is reversible with prompt drug discontinuation but will recur if methyldopa is given again; a few cases of fatal hepatic necrosis have been reported. It is advisable to avoid the use of methyldopa in patients with hepatic disease.

Methyldopa can cause hemolytic anemia. At least 20% of patients who receive methyldopa for a year develop a positive Coombs test due to autoantibodies directed against the Rh antigen on erythrocytes. This does not necessitate drug discontinuation; 1–5% of these patients will develop a hemolytic anemia that mandates prompt drug discontinuation. The Coombs test may remain positive for as long as a year after discontinuation of methyldopa, but the hemolytic anemia usually resolves within a matter of weeks. Severe hemolysis may be attenuated by treatment with glucocorticoids. Rarer adverse effects include leukopenia, thrombocytopenia, red cell aplasia, lupus erythematosus–like syndrome, lichenoid and granulomatous skin eruptions, myocarditis, retroperitoneal fibrosis, pancreatitis, diarrhea, and malabsorption.

THERAPEUTIC USES Methyldopa is a preferred drug for treatment of hypertension during pregnancy based on its effectiveness and safety for both mother and fetus. The usual initial dose of methyldopa is 250 mg twice daily, and there is little additional effect with doses >2 g/day. Administration of a single daily dose of methyldopa at bedtime minimizes sedative effects, but administration twice daily is required for some patients.

Clonidine, Guanabenz, and Guanfacine

The detailed pharmacology of the α_2 adrenergic agonists clonidine (CATAPRES), *guanabenz* (WYTENSIN), and *guanfacine* (TENEX) is discussed in Chapter 10. These drugs stimulate the α_{2A} subtype of α_2 adrenergic receptors in the brainstem, reducing sympathetic outflow from the CNS. Patients who have had a spinal cord transection above the level of the sympathetic outflow tracts do not display a hypotensive response to clonidine. At doses higher than those required to stimulate central α_{2A} receptors, these drugs can activate α_2 receptors of the α_{2B} subtype on vascular smooth muscle cells. This effect accounts for the initial vasoconstriction that is seen when overdoses of these drugs are taken and may be responsible for the loss of therapeutic effect that is observed with high doses.

PHARMACOLOGICAL EFFECTS   The α_2 adrenergic agonists lower arterial pressure by an effect on both cardiac output and peripheral resistance. In the supine position, when the vascular sympathetic tone is low, the major effect is to reduce both heart rate and stroke volume; however, in the upright position, when sympathetic outflow to the vasculature normally increases, these drugs reduce vascular resistance and may lead to postural hypotension. The decrease in cardiac sympathetic tone leads to reduced myocardial contractility and heart rate, possibly promoting congestive heart failure in susceptible patients.

ADVERSE EFFECTS AND PRECAUTIONS   Many patients experience annoying and even intolerable adverse effects with these drugs. Sedation and xerostomia are prominent. The latter may be accompanied by dry nasal mucosa, dry eyes, and parotid gland swelling and pain. Postural hypotension and erectile dysfunction are prominent in some patients. Clonidine may produce a lower incidence of dry mouth and sedation when given transdermally, perhaps because high peak concentrations are avoided. Less common CNS side effects include sleep disturbances with vivid dreams or nightmares, restlessness, and depression. Cardiac effects related to the sympatholytic action of these drugs include symptomatic bradycardia and sinus arrest in patients with dysfunction of the sinoatrial node and AV block in patients with AV nodal disease or in patients taking other drugs that depress AV conduction. Some 15–20% of patients who receive transdermal clonidine may develop contact dermatitis.

Sudden discontinuation of clonidine and related α_2 adrenergic agonists may cause a withdrawal syndrome consisting of headache, apprehension, tremors, abdominal pain, sweating, and tachycardia. The arterial blood pressure may rise to levels above those that were present prior to treatment, but the syndrome may occur in the absence of an overshoot in pressure. Symptoms typically occur 18–36 hours after the drug is stopped and are associated with increased sympathetic discharge, as evidenced by elevated plasma and urine concentrations of catecholamines. The withdrawal syndrome is likely dose related and more dangerous in patients with poorly controlled hypertension. Rebound hypertension also is seen after discontinuation of transdermal administration of clonidine. Treatment of the withdrawal syndrome depends on the urgency of reducing the arterial blood pressure. In the absence of life-threatening target organ damage, clonidine reinitiation may suffice. If a more rapid effect is needed, sodium nitroprusside or a combination of an α and β adrenergic blocker is appropriate. β Adrenergic blocking agents should not be used alone in this setting, since they can accentuate the hypertension by allowing unopposed α adrenergic vasoconstriction caused by activation of the sympathetic nervous system and elevated circulating catecholamines. Because perioperative hypertension has been described when clonidine was withdrawn the night before surgery, surgical patients receiving an α_2 adrenergic agonist either should be switched to another drug prior to elective surgery or should receive their morning dose and/or transdermal clonidine preoperatively. All patients who receive one of these drugs should be warned of the potential danger of discontinuing the drug abruptly; poorly compliant patients should not be given α_2 adrenergic agonists for hypertension.

Adverse drug interactions with α_2 adrenergic agonists are rare. Diuretics predictably potentiate the hypotensive effect of these drugs. Tricyclic antidepressants may inhibit the antihypertensive effect of clonidine by unknown mechanisms.

THERAPEUTIC USES   The CNS effects prevent this class of drugs from being a leading option for monotherapy of hypertension. These drugs effectively lower blood pressure in some patients who have not responded adequately to combinations of other agents. Enthusiasm for these drugs is further diminished by the paucity of evidence demonstrating reduction in risk of adverse cardiovascular events.

Guanadrel

Guanadrel (HYLOREL) specifically inhibits the function of peripheral postganglionic adrenergic neurons. It is an exogenous false neurotransmitter that is accumulated, stored, and released like NE but is inactive at adrenergic receptors. The drug is actively transported into neurons by the same transporter (NET) that mediates NE reuptake (*see* Chapter 6). When given intravenously, guanadrel initially releases NE in an amount sufficient to increase arterial blood pressure. This is not noticeable with oral administration, since NE is released only slowly from the vesicles under this circumstance and is degraded within the neuron by monoamine oxidase. Nonetheless, because of the potential for NE release, guanadrel is contraindicated in patients with pheochromocytoma. During adrenergic neuron blockade with guanadrel, effector cells become supersensitive to NE. The supersensitivity is similar to that produced by postganglionic sympathetic denervation.

PHARMACOLOGICAL EFFECTS

Essentially all of the therapeutic and adverse effects of guanadrel result from functional sympathetic blockade. The antihypertensive effect is achieved by a reduction in peripheral vascular resistance that results from inhibition of α receptor–mediated vasoconstriction. Consequently, arterial pressure is reduced modestly in the supine position when sympathetic activity is usually low, but the pressure can fall considerably when reflex sympathetic activation is needed to maintain arterial pressure, such as assumption of the upright posture, exercise, and depletion of plasma volume. Plasma volume often expands, which may diminish the antihypertensive efficacy of guanadrel and require administration of diuretic to restore the antihypertensive effect.

ABSORPTION, DISTRIBUTION, METABOLISM, AND EXCRETION

Guanadrel is rapidly absorbed, leading to maximal levels in plasma at 1–2 hours. Because guanadrel must be transported into and accumulate in adrenergic neurons, the maximum effect on blood pressure is not seen until 4–5 hours. Although the β phase of its elimination has a $t_{1/2}$ of ~5–10 hours, this almost certainly does not reflect the longer $t_{1/2}$ of drug stored at its site of action in the secretory vesicles of adrenergic neurons. The $t_{1/2}$ of the pharmacological effect of guanadrel is determined by the drug's persistence in this neuronal pool and is probably at least 10 hours. Guanadrel is administered in a regimen of twice-daily doses.

Guanadrel is cleared by both renal and nonrenal disposition. Its elimination is impaired in patients with renal insufficiency; total-body clearance is reduced by four- to fivefold in patients with severe renal dysfunction.

ADVERSE EFFECTS

Guanadrel produces undesirable effects that are related entirely to sympathetic blockade. The lack of sympathetic compensation results in symptomatic hypotension during standing, exercise, ingestion of alcohol, or hot weather. A general feeling of fatigue and lassitude is partially related to postural hypotension. Sexual dysfunction usually presents as delayed or retrograde ejaculation. Diarrhea also may occur.

Because guanadrel is actively transported to its site of action, drugs that block or compete for the catecholamine transporter on the presynaptic membrane will inhibit the effect of guanadrel. Such drugs include the tricyclic antidepressants, cocaine, chlorpromazine, ephedrine, phenylpropanolamine, and amphetamine (see Chapter 6).

THERAPEUTIC USES

Because of the availability of a number of drugs that lower blood pressure without producing this degree of orthostatic hypotension, guanadrel is not employed in the monotherapy of hypertension and only rarely is used as an additional agent in patients who have not achieved a satisfactory antihypertensive effect on multiple other agents. The usual starting dose is 10 mg/day; side effects can be minimized by not exceeding 20 mg/day.

Reserpine

Reserpine is an alkaloid that binds tightly to adrenergic storage vesicles in central and peripheral adrenergic neurons and inhibits the vesicular monoamine transporter (VMAT-2) that facilitates NE storage. Thus, nerve endings lose their capacity to concentrate and store NE and DA. Catecholamines leak into the cytoplasm, where they are metabolized by intraneuronal MAO, such that little or no active transmitter is discharged from nerve endings upon depolarization. The overall result is a pharmacological sympathectomy. A similar process occurs at storage sites for 5-hydroxytryptamine. Recovery of sympathetic function requires synthesis of new storage vesicles, which takes days to weeks after drug discontinuation. Since reserpine depletes amines in the CNS as well as in peripheral adrenergic neurons, its antihypertensive effects probably are related to both central and peripheral actions.

PHARMACOLOGICAL EFFECTS

Both cardiac output and peripheral vascular resistance are reduced during long-term therapy with reserpine. Orthostatic hypotension may occur but does not usually cause symptoms. Heart rate and renin secretion fall. Salt and water are retained, which commonly results in "pseudotolerance."

ABSORPTION, METABOLISM, AND EXCRETION

The amount of drug in plasma is unlikely to bear any consistent relationship to drug concentration at the site of action because of irreversible reserpine binding to storage vesicles. Reserpine is entirely metabolized, and none of the parent drug is excreted unchanged.

TOXICITY AND PRECAUTIONS

Most adverse effects of reserpine are due to its effect on the CNS. Sedation and inability to concentrate or perform complex tasks are the most common adverse effects. More serious is the occasional psychotic depression that can lead to suicide. Depression usually appears insidiously over many weeks or months and may not be attributed to the drug because of the delayed and gradual onset of symptoms. Reserpine must be discontinued at the first sign of depression, which may last several months after the drug is discontinued. The risk of depression is likely dose related. Depression appears to be uncommon, but not unknown, with doses of 0.25 mg/day or less. The drug should never be given to patients with a history of depression. Other adverse effects include nasal stuffiness and exacerbation of peptic ulcer disease, which is uncommon with small oral doses.

THERAPEUTIC USES

With the availability of newer drugs that are both effective and well tolerated, the use of reserpine has diminished because of its CNS side effects. Nonetheless, there has been some interest in using reserpine at low doses, in combination with diuretics, in hypertension therapy, especially in the elderly. Reserpine is used once daily with a diuretic, and several weeks are necessary to achieve a maximum effect. The daily dose should be limited to 0.25 mg or less, and as little as 0.05 mg/day may be effective when a diuretic is also used. Reserpine is considerably less expensive than many other antihypertensive drugs; thus, it is still used in developing nations.

Metyrosine

Metyrosine *(DEMSER) is (−)-α-methyl-L-tyrosine. It inhibits tyrosine hydroxylase, the enzyme that catalyzes the conversion of tyrosine to DOPA, the rate-limiting step in catecholamine biosynthesis (see Chapter 6). At a dose of 1–4 g/day, metyrosine decreases catecholamine biosynthesis by 35–80% in patients with pheochromocytoma. The maximal decrease in synthesis occurs only after several days, as assessed by measurements of urinary catecholamines and their metabolites. Metyrosine is used as an adjunct to phenoxybenzamine and other α adrenergic blocking agents for the management of malignant pheochromocytoma and in the preoperative preparation of patients for resection of pheochromocytoma. Metyrosine carries a risk of crystalluria, which can be minimized by maintaining a daily urine volume of >2 L. Other adverse effects include orthostatic hypotension, sedation, extrapyramidal signs, diarrhea, anxiety, and psychic disturbances. Doses must be titrated carefully to achieve significant inhibition of catecholamine biosynthesis while minimizing these substantial side effects.*

Ca^{2+} CHANNEL ANTAGONISTS

Ca^{2+} channel antagonists are important drugs for the treatment of hypertension. The pharmacology of these drugs is presented in Chapters 31, 33, and 34. The largest chemical class of calcium-channel blockers is the dihydropyridines: *amlodipine, felodipine, isradipine,* and *nifedipine. Diltiazem* and *verapamil* are non-dihydropyridine calcium-channel blockers. All Ca^{2+} channel blockers lower blood pressure by inhibiting Ca^{2+} influx through voltage-sensitive L-type calcium-channels in arteriolar smooth muscle, ultimately leading to smooth muscle relaxation and decreased peripheral vascular resistance. Due to decreased peripheral vascular resistance, the Ca^{2+} channel blockers evoke a baroreceptor-mediated sympathetic discharge. In the case of the dihydropyridines, tachycardia may occur from the adrenergic stimulation of the sinoatrial node; this response is generally quite modest except when drug is administered rapidly. Tachycardia is typically minimal to absent with verapamil and diltiazem because of the direct negative chronotropic effect of these two drugs. All Ca^{2+} channel blockers are effective when used alone for the treatment of mild-to-moderate hypertension; however, these drugs are not considered appropriate for hypertension monotherapy, except in certain situations such as isolated systolic hypertension (*see* below).

The Ca^{2+} channel blockers vary in their adverse reactions. Patients receiving immediate-release capsules of nifedipine develop headache, flushing, dizziness, and peripheral edema. Because of the oscillation in blood pressure and concurrent surges in sympathetic reflex activity within each dosage interval, nifedipine or other dihydropyridine Ca^{2+} channel blockers with short half-lives administered in immediate-release formulation are inappropriate in the long-term treatment of hypertension. Dizziness and flushing are much less of a problem with sustained-release formulations and with dihydropyridines having a long $t_{1/2}$ and relatively constant concentrations of drug in plasma. Peripheral edema is not the result of generalized fluid retention; it most likely results from increased hydrostatic pressure in the lower extremities owing to precapillary dilation and reflex postcapillary constriction. Some other adverse effects of these drugs are due to actions in nonvascular smooth muscle. For example, Ca^{2+} channel blockers can cause or aggravate gastroesophageal reflux by inhibiting contraction of the lower esophageal sphincter. Constipation is a common side effect of verapamil but occurs less frequently with other Ca^{2+} channel blockers. Urinary retention is a rare adverse effect. Inhibition of sinoatrial node function by diltiazem and verapamil can lead to bradycardia and even sinoatrial node arrest, particularly in patients with sinoatrial node dysfunction; this effect is exaggerated by concurrent use of β adrenergic receptor antagonists.

Compared with other classes of antihypertensive agents, there is a greater frequency of achieving blood pressure control with Ca^{2+} channel blockers as monotherapy in elderly subjects and in African Americans, population groups in which the low renin status is more prevalent. Ca^{2+} channel blockers are effective in lowering blood pressure and decreasing cardiovascular events in the elderly with isolated systolic hypertension. Indeed, these drugs may be a preferred treatment in these patients.

Significant drug–drug interactions may be encountered when Ca^{2+} channel blockers are used to treat hypertension. Concurrent use of a β receptor antagonist with a nondihydropyridine drug may magnify negative chronotropic and inotropic effects of these drugs or cause heart block in susceptible patients. Verapamil blocks the P-glycoprotein drug transporter in kidney and liver and inhibits the elimination of digoxin and other drugs (*see* Chapter 2). When used with quinidine, Ca^{2+} channel blockers may cause excessive hypotension, particularly in patients with idiopathic hypertrophic subaortic stenosis.

ANGIOTENSIN-CONVERTING ENZYME INHIBITORS

The ability to reduce levels of angiotensin II (AngII) with orally effective inhibitors of angiotensin-converting enzyme (ACE) represents an important advance in the treatment of hypertension. *Captopril* (CAPOTEN), *enalapril* (VASOTEC), *lisinopril* (PRINIVIL), *quinapril* (ACCUPRIL), *ramipril* (ALTACE), *benazepril* (LOTENSIN), *moexipril* (UNIVASC), *fosinopril* (MONOPRIL), *trandolapril* (MAVIK), and *perindopril* (ACEON) have proven to be very useful for the treatment of hypertension because of their efficacy and their very favorable profile of adverse effects, which enhances patient adherence. Chapter 30 presents the pharmacology of ACE inhibitors in detail.

The ACE inhibitors appear to confer a special advantage in the treatment of patients with diabetes mellitus, slowing the development and progression of diabetic glomerulopathy. They also are effective in slowing the progression of other forms of chronic renal disease, such as glomerulosclerosis, and many of these patients also have hypertension. An ACE inhibitor is the preferred initial agent in these patients. Patients with hypertension and ischemic heart disease are candidates for treatment with ACE inhibitors because administration of ACE inhibitors in the immediate post–myocardial infarction period has been shown to improve ventricular function and reduce morbidity and mortality (*see* Chapter 33).

The decreased biosynthesis of AngII impacts a number of facets of hypertension treatment. Because ACE inhibitors blunt the rise in aldosterone concentrations in response to Na^+ loss, the normal role of aldosterone to oppose diuretic-induced natriuresis is diminished. Consequently, ACE inhibitors tend to enhance the efficacy of diuretics. Thus, even very small doses of diuretics may substantially improve the antihypertensive efficacy of ACE inhibitors, while the use of high doses of diuretics together with ACE inhibitors may lead to excessive blood pressure reduction and volume depletion.

The attenuation of aldosterone production by ACE inhibitors also influences K^+ homeostasis. There is only a very small and clinically unimportant rise in serum K^+ when these agents are used alone in patients with normal renal function. However, substantial K^+ retention can occur in patients with renal insufficiency. Furthermore, the potential for developing hyperkalemia must be considered when ACE inhibitors are used with other drugs that can cause K^+ retention, including K^+-sparing diuretics (amiloride, triamterene, and spironolactone), NSAIDs, K^+ supplements, and β receptor antagonists. Some patients with diabetic nephropathy may be at greater risk of hyperkalemia.

There are several cautions in the use of ACE inhibitors. Angioedema is a rare but potentially fatal adverse effect of the ACE inhibitors. Patients starting treatment with these drugs should be explicitly warned to discontinue their use with the advent of any signs of angioedema. Due to the risk of severe fetal adverse effects, ACE inhibitors are contraindicated during pregnancy, a fact that must be communicated to women of childbearing age.

In most patients there is no appreciable change in glomerular filtration rate following the administration of ACE inhibitors. In renovascular hypertension, however, the glomerular filtration rate generally is maintained by AngII-driven increased resistance in the postglomerular arteriole. Accordingly, in patients with bilateral renal artery stenosis or stenosis in a sole kidney, the administration of an ACE inhibitor will substantially reduce glomerular filtration rate. Similar effects are seen in some patients with preexisting renal disease.

ACE inhibitors decrease blood pressure to some extent in most patients with hypertension. Following the initial dose of an ACE inhibitor, some patients exhibit a considerable fall in blood pressure that is a function of plasma renin activity prior to treatment. Because of this, therapy is initiated with low doses, especially in patients who may have a very active renin-angiotensin system supporting blood pressure (*e.g.*, diuretic-induced volume contraction or congestive heart failure). With continuing treatment, there usually is a progressive fall in blood pressure that often takes several weeks and is not strongly correlated with the pretreatment plasma renin activity. Younger Caucasian patients are more likely to respond to ACE inhibitors, while elderly African American patients generally are more resistant to the hypotensive effect of these drugs. While most ACE inhibitors are approved for once-daily dosing for hypertension, a significant fraction of patients have a response that lasts for less than 24 hours and require twice-daily dosing for optimal blood pressure control.

AT_1 ANGIOTENSIN II RECEPTOR ANTAGONISTS

Nonpeptide antagonists of the AT_1 angiotensin II receptor approved for the treatment of hypertension include *losartan* (COZAAR), *candesartan* (ATACAND), *irbesartan* (AVAPRO), *valsartan* (DIOVAN), *telmisartan* (MICARDIS), and *eprosartan* (TEVETEN). By antagonizing the effects of AngII, these agents relax smooth muscle and thereby promote vasodilation, increase renal salt and water excretion, reduce plasma volume, and decrease cellular hypertrophy (*see* Chapter 30).

Distinct subtypes of AngII receptors are designated as AT_1 and AT_2. The AT_1 receptor subtype is located predominantly in vascular and myocardial tissue and also in brain, kidney, and adrenal glomerulosa cells, which secrete aldosterone (*see* Chapter 30). Because the AT_1 receptor mediates feedback inhibition of renin release, renin and AngII concentrations are increased during AT_1 receptor antagonism. The clinical consequences of increased AngII effects on an uninhibited AT_2 receptor are unknown; emerging data suggest that the AT_2 receptor may elicit antigrowth and antiproliferative responses.

ADVERSE EFFECTS AND PRECAUTIONS Adverse effects of ACE inhibitors that result from inhibiting AngII–related functions also occur with AT_1 receptor antagonists, including hypotension, hyperkalemia, and reduced renal function (especially associated with renal artery stenosis). Hypotension most often occurs in patients in whom the blood pressure is highly dependent on AngII, including those with volume depletion (*e.g.*, with diuretics), renovascular hypertension, cardiac failure, and cirrhosis; in such patients initiation of treatment with low doses and attention to volume status is essential. Hyperkalemia may occur in conjunction with other factors, such as renal insufficiency, ingestion of excess K^+, and the use of drugs that promote K^+ retention. Cough is much less frequent with AngII receptor antagonists, and angioedema occurs very rarely. AT_1 receptor antagonists also should not be administered during pregnancy and should be discontinued as soon as pregnancy is detected.

THERAPEUTIC USES When given in adequate doses, the AT_1 receptor antagonists appear to be as effective as ACE inhibitors in the treatment of hypertension. As with ACE inhibitors, these drugs may be less effective in African Americans and patients with low-renin hypertension. The full effect of AT_1 receptor antagonists on blood pressure typically is not observed until ~4 weeks after initiation of therapy. If blood pressure is not controlled by an AT_1 receptor antagonist alone, a low dose of a thiazide or other diuretic may be added. In patients with mild-to-severe hypertension, the addition of an AT_1 receptor antagonist to a thiazide can produce significant additional reductions in blood pressure in patients who demonstrated an insufficient response to the first agent alone. A smaller initial dosage is preferred for patients who have already received diuretics and therefore have intravascular volume depletion, and for other patients whose blood pressure is highly dependent on AngII. Given their different mechanisms, there is no assurance that the effects of ACE inhibitors and antagonists of the AT_1 receptor will be equivalent in preventing target organ damage in patients with hypertension.

VASODILATORS

Hydralazine

Hydralazine (APRESOLINE) causes direct relaxation of arteriolar smooth muscle, possibly secondary to a fall in intracellular Ca^{2+} concentrations. The drug does not dilate epicardial coronary arteries or relax venous smooth muscle. Hydralazine-induced vasodilation is associated with powerful stimulation of the sympathetic nervous system, likely due to baroreceptor-mediated reflexes, which results in increased heart rate and contractility, increased plasma renin activity, and fluid retention; all of these effects counteract the antihypertensive effect of hydralazine. Although most of the sympathetic activity is due to a baroreceptor-mediated reflex, hydralazine may stimulate NE release from sympathetic nerve terminals and augment myocardial contractility directly. Most of hydralazine's effects are confined to the cardiovascular system; the decrease in blood pressure after administration is associated with a selective decrease in vascular resistance in the coronary, cerebral, and renal circulations, with a smaller effect in skin and muscle. Because of preferential dilation of arterioles, postural hypotension is not common, and hydralazine lowers blood pressure equally in the supine and upright positions.

ABSORPTION, METABOLISM, AND EXCRETION Hydralazine is well absorbed through the gastrointestinal (GI) tract but systemic bioavailability is low (16% in fast acetylators, 35% in slow acetylators). Hydralazine is N-acetylated in the bowel and/or the liver. The $t_{1/2}$ of hydralazine is 1 hour, and systemic clearance of the drug is about 50 mL/kg/min. The rate of acetylation is genetically determined; ~half of all individual in the U.S. are rapid acetylators. The acetylated compound is inactive; thus, the dose necessary to produce a systemic effect is larger in fast acetylators. Since systemic clearance exceeds hepatic blood flow, extrahepatic metabolism must occur. Indeed, hydralazine rapidly combines with circulating α-keto acids to form hydrazones, and the major metabolite recovered from the plasma is hydralazine pyruvic acid hydrazone. This metabolite has a longer $t_{1/2}$ than hydralazine but does not appear to be very active. The rate of acetylation is an important determinant of hydralazine bioavailability but does not play a role in the systemic elimination of the drug, probably because the hepatic clearance is so high that systemic elimination is principally a function of hepatic blood flow. The peak concentration of hydralazine in plasma and its peak hypotensive effect both occur within 30–120 minutes of ingestion. Although its $t_{1/2}$ in plasma is ~1 hour, the duration of the hypotensive effect of hydralazine can last as long as 12 hours. There is no clear explanation for this discrepancy.

TOXICITY AND PRECAUTIONS Extensions of hydralazine's pharmacological effects include headache, nausea, flushing, hypotension, palpitations, tachycardia, dizziness, and angina pectoris. Myocardial ischemia occurs because of the increased O_2 demand induced by the baroreceptor reflex-induced stimulation of the sympathetic nervous system and because hydralazine does not dilate the epicardial coronary arteries; thus, the arteriolar dilation it produces may cause a "steal" of blood flow away from the ischemic region. Following parenteral administration to patients with coronary artery disease, the myocardial ischemia may be sufficiently severe and protracted to cause frank myocardial infarction. For this reason, parenteral administration of hydralazine is not advised in hypertensive patients with coronary artery disease, hypertensive patients with multiple cardiovascular risk factors, or in older patients. In addition, if the drug is used alone, there may be salt retention with development of congestive heart failure. When combined with a β adrenergic receptor blocker and a diuretic, hydralazine is better tolerated, although adverse effects such as headache are still commonly described and may necessitate discontinuation of the drug.

Other adverse effects are caused by immunological reactions, of which the drug-induced lupus syndrome is the most common. Hydralazine also can result in an illness that resembles serum sickness, hemolytic anemia, vasculitis, and rapidly progressive glomerulonephritis; the mechanism of these autoimmune reactions is unknown. The drug-induced lupus syndrome usually occurs after at least 6 months of continuous treatment with hydralazine, and its incidence is related to dose, sex, acetylator phenotype, and race. After 3 years of treatment with hydralazine, drug-induced lupus occurs in 10% of patients who receive 200 mg/day and 5% who receive 100 mg/day. The incidence is four times higher in women than in men, and the syndrome is seen more commonly in Caucasians than in African Americans. The rate of conversion to a positive antinuclear antibody test is faster in slow acetylators than in rapid acetylators, suggesting that the native drug or a nonacetylated metabolite is responsible. However, since the majority of patients with positive antinuclear antibody tests do not develop the drug-induced lupus syndrome, hydralazine need not be discontinued unless clinical features of the syndrome appear. These features are similar to those of other drug-induced lupus syndromes, including arthralgia, arthritis, and fever. Pleuritis and pericarditis may be present, and pericardial effusion can occasionally cause cardiac tamponade. Discontinuation of the drug is all that is necessary for most patients with the hydralazine-induced lupus syndrome; symptoms may persist in a few patients and administration of glucocorticoids may be necessary. Hydralazine also can produce a pyridoxine-responsive polyneuropathy, apparently related to its ability to combine with pyridoxine to form a hydrazone. This side effect is rare with doses $\leq$200 mg/day.

THERAPEUTIC USES   Due to its relatively unfavorable adverse-effect profile, hydralazine is no longer a first-line drug in the treatment of hypertension. It may have utility in patients with congestive heart failure (in combination with nitrates for patients who cannot tolerate ACE inhibitors or AT_1 receptor antagonists), and in the treatment of hypertensive emergencies in pregnant women (especially preeclampsia) on account of extensive experience with the drug in that setting. Hydralazine should be used with great caution if at all in elderly patients and in hypertensive patients with coronary artery disease because of the possibility of precipitation of myocardial ischemia due to reflex tachycardia. The usual oral dosage of hydralazine is 25–100 mg twice daily. Twice-daily administration is as effective as administration four times a day for blood pressure control, regardless of acetylator phenotype. The maximum recommended dose of hydralazine is 200 mg/day to minimize the risk of drug-induced lupus syndrome.

K^+_{ATP} Channel Openers: Minoxidil

Minoxidil (LONITEN) is efficacious in patients with the most severe and drug-resistant forms of hypertension. A small fraction of minoxidil is metabolized by hepatic sulfotransferase to the active molecule, minoxidil N-O sulfate. Minoxidil sulfate activates the ATP-modulated K^+ channel in smooth muscle, causing hyperpolarization and relaxation of arteriolar smooth muscle. Minoxidil produces arteriolar vasodilation with essentially no effect on capacitance vessels. Minoxidil preferentially increases blood flow to skin, skeletal muscle, the GI tract, and the heart. The disproportionate increase in blood flow to the heart may have a metabolic basis, in that administration of minoxidil is associated with a reflex increase in myocardial contractility and in cardiac output. The cardiac output can increase by as much as three- to fourfold, primarily due to enhanced venous return to the heart. The increased venous return probably results from enhanced flow in vascular beds with a fast response for venous return to the heart. The adrenergic increase in myocardial contractility contributes to the increased cardiac output, but is not the predominant factor. The renal effects of minoxidil are complex; it dilates renal arteries, but systemic hypotension produced by the drug actually can decrease renal blood flow. Renal function usually improves in patients who take minoxidil for the treatment of hypertension, especially if renal dysfunction is secondary to hypertension. Minoxidil potently stimulates renin secretion, an effect mediated by renal sympathetic stimulation.

ABSORPTION, METABOLISM, AND EXCRETION   Minoxidil is well absorbed from the GI tract. Although peak concentrations of minoxidil in blood occur 1 hour after oral administration, the maximal hypotensive effect of the drug occurs later, possibly because formation of the active metabolite is delayed. About 20% of the absorbed drug is excreted unchanged in the urine; the main route of elimination is by hepatic metabolism. The major metabolite of minoxidil is the glucuronide conjugate at the N-oxide position. This metabolite is less active than minoxidil but has a long $t_{1/2}$. Minoxidil has a $t_{1/2}$ in plasma of 3–4 hours, but its duration of action is 24 hours or longer.

ADVERSE EFFECTS AND PRECAUTIONS   The adverse effects of minoxidil can be severe and are divided into three major categories: fluid and salt retention, cardiovascular effects, and hypertrichosis.

Salt and water retention result from increased proximal tubular reabsorption due to reduced renal perfusion pressure and reflex stimulation of renal tubular α adrenergic receptors. Similar antinatriuretic effects are observed with other arteriolar dilators (*e.g.,* diazoxide and hydralazine).

Although minoxidil causes increased secretion of renin and aldosterone, this is unimportant for retention of salt and water. Fluid retention usually can be controlled by the administration of a diuretic. However, thiazides may not be sufficiently efficacious, and it may be necessary to use a loop diuretic, especially if the patient has any renal dysfunction. Large doses of loop diuretics may be required to prevent edema formation in some patients.

The cardiac consequences of baroreceptor-mediated activation of the sympathetic nervous system with minoxidil are similar to those with hydralazine; there is an increase in heart rate, myocardial contractility, and myocardial O_2 consumption. Thus, myocardial ischemia can be induced by minoxidil in patients with coronary artery disease. The cardiac sympathetic responses are attenuated by concurrent administration of a β adrenergic blocker. The adrenergically-induced increase in renin secretion also can be ameliorated by a β receptor antagonist or an ACE inhibitor, with enhancement of blood pressure control.

Minoxidil has particularly adverse consequences in hypertensive patients who have left ventricular hypertrophy and diastolic dysfunction. Such poorly compliant ventricles respond suboptimally to increased volume loads, with a resulting increase in left ventricular filling pressure. This likely contributes to the increased pulmonary artery pressure seen with minoxidil therapy in hypertensive patients and is compounded by the drug-induced retention of salt and water. Cardiac failure can result from minoxidil therapy in such patients; the potential for this complication can be reduced but not prevented by effective diuretic therapy. Pericardial effusion is an uncommon but serious complication of minoxidil. Although more commonly described in patients with cardiac failure and renal failure, pericardial effusion can occur in patients with normal cardiovascular and renal function. Mild and asymptomatic pericardial effusion is not an indication for discontinuing minoxidil, but the situation should be monitored closely to avoid progression to tamponade. Effusions usually clear when the drug is discontinued but can recur if treatment with minoxidil is resumed.

Flattened and inverted T waves frequently are observed in the electrocardiogram following the initiation of minoxidil treatment. These are not ischemic in origin and are seen with other drugs that activate K^+ channels; these drugs can accelerate myocardial repolarization, shorten the refractory period, and may lower the ventricular fibrillation threshold in ischemic myocardium. Hypertrichosis occurs in patients who receive minoxidil for extended periods, probably related to K^+ channel activation. Growth of hair occurs on the face, back, arms, and legs and is particularly upsetting to women. Frequent shaving or depilatory agents can be used to manage this problem. Topical minoxidil (ROGAINE) is used for male pattern baldness; it may have cardiovascular effects in some individuals.

Rare side effects of the drug include rashes, Stevens-Johnson syndrome, glucose intolerance, serosanguineous bullae, formation of antinuclear antibodies, and thrombocytopenia.

THERAPEUTIC USES Minoxidil is reserved for the treatment of severe hypertension that responds poorly to other antihypertensive medications, especially in male patients with renal insufficiency. Minoxidil must be given concurrently with a diuretic to avoid fluid retention and with a sympatholytic drug (usually a β receptor antagonist) to control reflex cardiovascular effects. The drug usually is administered either once or twice a day, but some patients may require more frequent dosing for adequate control of blood pressure. The initial daily dose of minoxidil may be as little as 1.25 mg, which can be increased gradually to 40 mg in one or two daily doses.

Sodium Nitroprusside

Sodium nitroprusside is used for the short-term control of severe hypertension and can improve cardiac function in patients with left ventricular failure (*see* Chapter 34). Nitroprusside acts by releasing nitric oxide (NO). NO activates the guanylyl cyclase–cyclic GMP–PKG pathway, leading to vasodilation. The mechanism of release of NO likely involves both enzymatic and nonenzymatic pathways. Tolerance does not develop to nitroprusside. Nitroprusside dilates both arterioles and venules; the hemodynamic response results from a combination of venous pooling and reduced arterial impedance. In subjects with normal left ventricular function, venous pooling affects cardiac output more than does the reduction of afterload; cardiac output thus tends to fall. In patients with severely impaired left ventricular function and diastolic ventricular distention, the reduction of arterial impedance leads to a rise in cardiac output (*see* Chapter 33). Sodium nitroprusside is a nonselective vasodilator, and regional distribution of blood flow is little affected by the drug. In general, renal blood flow and glomerular filtration are maintained, and plasma renin activity increases. Unlike other arteriolar vasodilators, sodium nitroprusside usually causes only a modest increase in heart rate and an overall reduction in myocardial O_2 demand.

ABSORPTION, METABOLISM, AND EXCRETION Sodium nitroprusside is unstable and decomposes under strongly alkaline conditions or when exposed to light. It must be given by continuous intravenous infusion to be effective. Its onset of action is within 30 seconds; the peak hypotensive effect occurs within 2 minutes, and the effect disappears within 3 minutes after the infusion is stopped.

The metabolism of nitroprusside by smooth muscle is initiated by its reduction, followed by the release of cyanide and then nitric oxide. Cyanide is further metabolized by liver rhodanase to thiocyanate, which is eliminated almost entirely in the urine. The mean elimination half-time for thiocyanate is 3 days in patients with normal renal function but can be much longer in patients with renal insufficiency.

TOXICITY AND PRECAUTIONS The short-term adverse effects of nitroprusside are due to excessive vasodilation. Close monitoring of blood pressure and the use of a continuous variable-rate infusion pump will usually prevent an excessive hemodynamic response to the drug. Less commonly, toxicity may result from conversion of nitroprusside to cyanide and thiocyanate. Toxic accumulation of cyanide leading to severe lactic acidosis usually occurs when sodium nitroprusside is infused at a rate >5 μg/kg/min, but also can occur in some patients receiving doses of 2 μg/kg/min for a prolonged period. The limiting factor in the metabolism of cyanide appears to be the availability of sulfur-containing substrates in the body (mainly thiosulfate). The concomitant administration of *sodium thiosulfate* can prevent cyanide accumulation in patients who are receiving higher-than-usual doses of sodium nitroprusside; the efficacy of the nitroprusside is unchanged. The risk of thiocyanate toxicity increases when sodium nitroprusside is infused for >24–48 hours, especially if renal function is impaired. Signs and symptoms of thiocyanate toxicity include anorexia, nausea, fatigue, disorientation, and toxic psychosis. The plasma concentration of thiocyanate should be monitored during prolonged nitroprusside infusions and should not exceed 0.1 mg/mL. Excessive concentrations of thiocyanate rarely may cause hypothyroidism by inhibiting iodine uptake by the thyroid gland. In patients with renal failure, thiocyanate can be removed by hemodialysis.

Nitroprusside can worsen hypoxemia in patients with chronic obstructive pulmonary disease because the drug interferes with hypoxic pulmonary vasoconstriction and thereby promotes ventilation/perfusion mismatch.

THERAPEUTIC USES Sodium nitroprusside is used primarily to treat hypertensive emergencies but can also be used in many situations when short-term reduction of cardiac preload and/or afterload is desired. Nitroprusside has been used to lower blood pressure during acute aortic dissection, to improve cardiac output in congestive heart failure, especially in hypertensive patients with pulmonary edema that does not respond to other treatment (*see* Chapter 33), and to decrease myocardial oxygen demand after acute myocardial infarction. In addition, nitroprusside is used to induce controlled hypotension during anesthesia in order to reduce bleeding in surgical procedures. In the treatment of acute aortic dissection, it is essential to administer a β adrenergic receptor antagonist with nitroprusside, since reduction of blood pressure with nitroprusside alone can increase the rate of rise in pressure in the aorta as a result of increased myocardial contractility, thereby enhancing propagation of the dissection.

Sodium nitroprusside is available in vials that contain 50 mg. The contents of the vial should be dissolved in 2–3 mL of 5% dextrose in water. Addition of this solution to 250–1000 mL of 5% dextrose in water produces a concentration of 50–200 μg/mL. Because the compound decomposes in light, only fresh solutions should be used, and the bottle should be covered with an opaque wrapping. The drug must be administered as a controlled continuous infusion, and the patient must be closely observed. Most hypertensive patients respond to an infusion of 0.25–1.5 μg/kg/min. Higher infusion rates are needed to produce controlled hypotension in normotensive patients under surgical anesthesia. Infusion of nitroprusside at rates >5 μg/kg/min over a prolonged period can cause cyanide and/or thiocyanate poisoning. Patients receiving other antihypertensive medications usually require less nitroprusside to lower blood pressure. If infusion rates of 10 μg/kg/min do not produce adequate reduction of blood pressure within 10 minutes, the rate of administration of nitroprusside should be reduced to minimize potential toxicity.

Diazoxide

Diazoxide (HYPERSTAT IV) is used in the treatment of hypertensive emergencies only if accurate infusion pumps are not available and/or close monitoring of blood pressure is not feasible.

NONPHARMACOLOGICAL THERAPY OF HYPERTENSION

The indications and efficacy of various lifestyle modifications in hypertension are reviewed in a summary statement from the Joint National Committee on Prevention, Detection, Evaluation, and Treatment of High Blood Pressure (www.nhlbi.nih.gov/guidelines/hypertension).

SELECTION OF ANTIHYPERTENSIVE DRUGS IN INDIVIDUAL PATIENTS

Choice of an antihypertensive drug should be driven by likely benefit in an individual patient, taking into account concomitant diseases such as diabetes mellitus, problematic adverse effects of specific drugs, and cost.

Consensus guidelines ((www.nhlbi.nih.gov/guidelines/hypertension) recommend diuretics as preferred initial therapy for most patients with uncomplicated stage 1 hypertension who are unresponsive to nonpharmacological measures. Patients are also commonly treated with other drugs: β receptor antagonists, ACE inhibitors/AT_1 receptor antagonists, and Ca^{2+} channel blockers. Patients with uncomplicated stage 2 hypertension will likely require the early introduction of a diuretic and another drug from a different class. Subsequently, doses can be titrated upward and additional drugs added in order to achieve goals (blood pressure <140/90 mm Hg in uncomplicated patients). Some of patients may require four different drugs to reach their goal.

Some patients with hypertension have compelling indications for specific drugs on account of other underlying serious cardiovascular disease (heart failure, post–myocardial infarction, or with high risk for coronary artery disease), chronic kidney disease, or diabetes. For example, a hypertensive patient with congestive heart failure ideally should be treated with a diuretic, β receptor antagonist, ACE inhibitor/AT_1 receptor antagonist, and spironolactone because of the benefit of these drugs in congestive heart failure, even in the absence of hypertension. Similarly, ACE inhibitors/AT_1 receptor antagonists should be first-line drugs in the treatment of diabetics with hypertension in view of their well-established benefits in diabetic nephropathy.

Other patients may have less serious underlying diseases that could influence choice of antihypertensive drugs. For example, a hypertensive patient with symptomatic benign prostatic hyperplasia might benefit from having an α_1 receptor antagonist as part of this therapeutic program, since α_1 antagonists are efficacious in both diseases. Similarly, a patient with recurrent migraine attacks might particularly benefit from use of a β receptor antagonist since a number of drugs in this class are efficacious in preventing migraine attacks.

Patients with isolated systolic hypertension (systolic blood pressure >160 mm Hg and diastolic blood pressure <90 mm Hg) benefit particularly from diuretics and also from Ca^{2+} channel blockers.

Different considerations are needed for patients in immediately life-threatening settings due to hypertension. Clinical judgment favors rapidly lowering blood pressure in patients with life-threatening complications of hypertension, such as patients with hypertensive encephalopathy or pulmonary edema due to severe hypertension. Rapid reduction in blood pressure has considerable risks for the patients; if blood pressure is decreased too quickly or extensively, cerebral blood flow may diminish due to adaptations in the cerebral circulation that protect the brain from the sequelae of very high blood pressures. The temptation to aggressively treat patients merely on the basis of increased blood pressure should be resisted and therapy should encompass how well the patients' major organs are reacting to the very high blood pressures.

For a complete Bibliographical listing see Goodman & Gilman's *The Pharmacological Basis of Therapeutics,* **11th ed., or Goodman & Gilman Online at www.accessmedicine.com.**

33

PHARMACOTHERAPY OF CONGESTIVE HEART FAILURE

Congestive heart failure (CHF) is a major contributor to morbidity and mortality worldwide. Drug therapies historically have focused on the endpoint components of this syndrome, volume overload (congestion) and myocardial dysfunction (heart failure), with treatment strategies emphasizing the use of diuretics and cardiac glycosides. While effective in relieving symptoms and in stabilizing patients with hemodynamic decompensation, such therapies have not improved survival. Recent work has provided new insights into the induction and propagation of CHF, building a conceptual framework in which heart failure is viewed as a consequence of disordered circulatory dynamics and pathologic cardiac remodeling. These developments have had a major positive impact on the treatment of CHF that has improved survival.

Pathophysiology of Heart Failure

Initially, myocardial dysfunction and the attendant reduction of forward cardiac output lead to expansion of intravascular volume and activation of neurohumoral systems, particularly the sympathetic nervous system and the renin–angiotensin system (Figure 33–1). These compensatory responses maintain perfusion to vital organs by increasing left ventricular preload, stimulating myocardial contractility, and increasing arterial tone. Acutely, these mechanisms help to sustain cardiac output by allowing the heart to operate at higher end-diastolic volumes, leading to increased stroke volume; concomitant peripheral vasoconstriction allows for regional redistribution of the cardiac output to critical organs. Unfortunately, each of these compensatory responses will also promote disease progression. Expansion of the intravascular volume and elevated ventricular chamber volumes lead to increased diastolic and systolic wall stress; these changes in turn impair myocardial energetics and induce hypertrophic remodeling. Neurohumoral activation leads to arterial and venous constriction; the former increases left ventricular afterload (thereby compromising left ventricular stroke volume) and the latter increases preload, thereby exacerbating both diastolic and systolic wall stress. In addition, the neurohumoral effectors (such as norepinephrine [NE] and angiotensin II [AngII]) may act directly on the myocardium to promote unfavorable remodeling by causing myocyte apoptosis, abnormal gene expression, and alterations in the extracellular matrix.

PHARMACOLOGICAL TREATMENT OF HEART FAILURE

The abnormalities of myocardial structure and function that underlie heart failure can activate biological responses that drive disease progression. Drugs that reduce ventricular wall stress or inhibit the renin–angiotensin system (*e.g.*, selected vasodilators, ACE inhibitors, and aldosterone antagonists) or the sympathetic nervous system (*e.g.*, β adrenergic antagonists) can decrease pathological ventricular remodeling, attenuate disease progression, and decrease mortality in patients with heart failure due to systolic dysfunction. As a result, these drugs have become mainstays in the long-term treatment of heart failure. Some of the drugs that slow progression afford an immediate beneficial impact on hemodynamic function and symptoms (*e.g.*, vasodilators and ACE inhibitors). Other agents that attenuate disease progression can adversely affect hemodynamic function and worsen symptoms in the short term and must therefore be used with caution (*e.g.*, β receptor antagonists). Figure 33–1 provides an overview of the pathophysiological mechanisms of heart failure and the sites of action of the major drug classes used in treatment.

The current approach to therapy for CHF involves preload reduction, afterload reduction, and enhancement of inotropic state. A variety of vasodilators will reduce preload and afterload (Table 33–1). Although a vasodilator's more prominent effect may be to reduce either preload or afterload, most agents affect both.

Diuretics

Diuretics retain a central role in the management of the "congestive" symptoms in patients with heart failure. The pharmacological properties of these agents are presented in detail in Chapter 28. Their importance in heart failure management reflects the central role of the kidney in the hemodynamic, hormonal, and autonomic responses to myocardial failure. The net effect of these responses is the retention of Na^+ and water and expansion of the extracellular fluid volume, allowing the heart to operate at higher end-diastolic volumes, and thereby to maintain LV stroke volume. However, this increase in end-diastolic volume results in higher end-diastolic filling pressures,

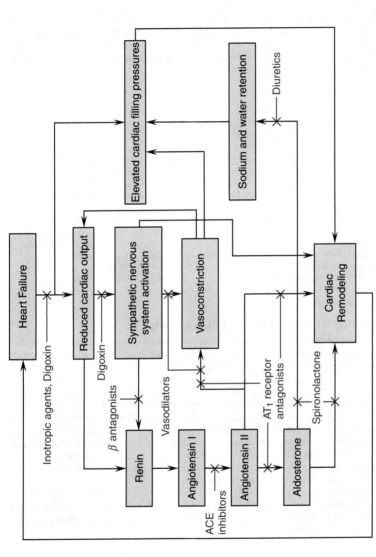

FIGURE 33–1 *Pathophysiological mechanisms of heart failure and major sites of drug action.* Heart failure is accompanied by compensatory neurohormonal responses including activation of the sympathetic nervous and renin–angiotensin systems. Although these responses initially help to maintain cardiovascular function by increasing ventricular preload and systemic vascular tone, with time they contribute to the progression of myocardial failure. Increased ventricular afterload, due to systemic vasoconstriction and chamber dilation, causes a depression in systolic function. In addition, increased afterload and the direct effects of angiotensin and NE on the ventricular myocardium cause pathological remodeling characterized by progressive chamber dilation and loss of contractile function. The figure illustrates several mechanisms that appear to play important roles in the pathophysiology of heart failure, and the sites of action of pharmacological therapies for heart failure.

Table 33–1

Vasodilator Drugs Used to Treat Heart Failure

Drug Class	Examples	Mechanism of Vasodilating Action	Preload Reduction	Afterload Reduction
Organic nitrates	Nitroglycerin, isosorbide dinitrate	NO-mediated vasodilation	+++	+
Nitric oxide donors	Nitroprusside	NO-mediated vasodilation	+++	+++
Angiotensin-converting enzyme inhibitors	Captopril, enalapril, lisinopril	Inhibition of AngII generation, decreased bradykinin degradation	++	++
Angiotensin receptor blockers	Losartan, candesartan	Blockade of AT_1 receptors	++	++
Phosphodiesterase inhibitors	Milrinone, inamrinone	Inhibition of cyclic AMP degradation	++	++
Direct-acting	Hydralazine	Unknown	+	+++
K^+-channel agonist	Minoxidil	Hyperpolarization of vascular smooth muscle cells	+	+++
α_1 Adrenergic antagonists	Doxazosin, prazosin	Selective α_1 adrenergic receptor blockade	+++	++
Nonselective α adrenergic antagonists	Phentolamine	Nonselective α adrenergic receptor blockade	+++	+++
Vasodilating β/α_1 adrenergic antagonists	Carvedilol, labetalol	Selective α_1 adrenergic receptor blockade	++	++
Ca^{2+} channel blockers	Amlodipine, nifedipine, felodipine	Inhibition of L-type Ca^{2+} channels	+	+++
β Adrenergic agonists	Isoproterenol	Stimulation of vascular β_2 adrenergic receptors	+	++

ABBREVIATIONS: AngII, angiotensin II; AT_1, type 1 AngII receptor; NO, nitric oxide.

increased ventricular chamber dimensions, and elevated wall stress. In turn, these changes result in pulmonary venous congestion and peripheral edema, ultimately limiting further augmentation of cardiac output. Elevated filling pressures are associated with enhanced activation of neurohumoral systems that can drive CHF progression.

Diuretics reduce extracellular fluid volume and ventricular filling pressure (or "preload"). Because patients with heart failure often operate on a "plateau" phase of the Starling curve, preload reduction can occur without concomitant reduction in cardiac output. Note that reduction in cardiac output can occur in patients who have had either sustained natriuresis and/or a rapid decline in intravascular volume. In this circumstance, diuretic therapy may augment neurohormonal activation due to volume depletion, with potentially deleterious effects on the progression of heart failure. It therefore is preferable to avoid the use of diuretics in the subset of patients with asymptomatic LV dysfunction and to use the minimal dose necessary to maintain euvolemia in patients with symptoms related to volume retention. Despite the efficacy of diuretics in controlling congestive symptoms and improving exercise capacity, with the exception of aldosterone antagonists, they do not reduce mortality in heart failure.

DIETARY SODIUM RESTRICTION All patients with clinically significant ventricular dysfunction, regardless of symptom status, should be advised to limit dietary intake of NaCl. Most patients will tolerate moderate reductions in salt intake (2–3 g/day total intake). More stringent salt restriction is seldom necessary and may be counterproductive, as it can lead to hyponatremia, hypokalemia, and hypochloremic metabolic alkalosis when combined with loop diuretics.

LOOP DIURETICS *Furosemide* (LASIX), *bumetanide* (BUMEX), and *torsemide* (DEMADEX) are widely used in the treatment of heart failure. Due to the increased risk of ototoxicity, *ethacrynic acid* (EDECRIN) should be reserved for patients who are allergic to sulfonamides or who have developed interstitial nephritis on alternative drugs.

Furosemide and bumetanide are short-acting drugs. The resultant postdose decline in renal tubular diuretic levels leads to avid renal Na^+ retention by all nephron segments. This can limit or prevent negative Na^+ balance and it is a common practice in CHF patients to administer two or more doses daily. In patients with decompensated heart failure of a severity that warrants hospital admission, it is generally desirable to initiate diuresis by intravenous administration of a loop diuretic. This typically provides a more rapid and predictable diuresis than does oral administration. The loop diuretic may be administered as repetitive boluses titrated to achieve the desired response, or by constant infusion. An advantage of infusion is that the same total daily dose of diuretic, given as a continuous infusion, results in a more sustained natriuresis due to maintenance of high drug levels within the lumen of renal tubules. In addition, the risk of ototoxicity is reduced by continuous infusion when compared to repetitive, intermittent intravenous dosing. When there is a poor response to monotherapy, coadministration of a thiazide agent is warranted. If the poor response is due to reduced renal perfusion, short-term administration of sympathomimetic drugs or phosphodiesterase inhibitors to increase cardiac output may be required.

THIAZIDE DIURETICS   The thiazide diuretics (DIURIL, HYDRODIURIL, others) are most frequently used in the treatment of hypertension; they play a more restricted role in the treatment of CHF. Thiazides exhibit true synergism with loop diuretics: the natriuresis that follows coadministration exceeds the summed effects of the drugs administered individually. This synergism is the rationale for combination therapy in patients who appear refractory to loop diuretics. Thiazides are associated with a greater degree of K^+ wasting for comparable volume reduction than are loop diuretics.

K^+-SPARING DIURETICS K^+-sparing diuretics (*see* Chapter 28) act principally in the collecting duct of the nephron and either inhibit apical membrane Na^+ conductance channels in epithelial cells (*e.g., amiloride, triamterene*) or act as aldosterone antagonists (*e.g., spironolactone, eplerenone*). These agents are relatively weak diuretics and therefore are not effective for volume reduction. Historically, these agents have been used to limit renal K^+ and Mg^{2+} wasting and/or to augment the diuretic response to other agents. Aldosterone antagonists improve survival in patients with advanced heart failure *via* a mechanism that is independent of diuresis.

USE OF DIURETICS IN CLINICAL PRACTICE   The majority of patients with heart failure will require chronic administration of a loop diuretic to maintain euvolemia. In patients with clinically evident fluid retention, furosemide typically is started at a dose of 40 mg once or twice/day and increased until an adequate diuresis is achieved. A larger initial dose may be required in patients with more advanced heart failure or with concurrent azotemia. Serum electrolytes and renal function should be monitored frequently in patients with preexisting renal insufficiency or those in whom a rapid diuresis is desirable. Once fluid retention has resolved, the diuretic dose should be reduced to the minimal level necessary to maintain euvolemia. Electrolyte abnormalities and/or worsening azotemia may supervene before euvolemia is achieved. Hypokalemia may be corrected by potassium supplementation or addition of a K-sparing diuretic.

Aldosterone Antagonists

A principal feature of CHF is marked activation of the renin–angiotensin–aldosterone system. In heart failure patients, plasma aldosterone concentrations may increase to as high as 20 times the normal level. Aldosterone has a range of biological effects beyond salt retention (Table 33–2), and antagonism of aldosterone's actions may be beneficial in patients with heart failure. The beneficial effects of spironolactone on mortality appear to be additive to those of ACE inhibitors and β receptor antagonists in patients with symptomatic heart failure; the use of spironolactone should be considered in patients with NYHA Class III and IV heart failure. Caution should be exercised when significant renal impairment is present. Treatment is initiated at a dose of 12.5 or 25 mg daily, as higher doses may lead to hyperkalemia, particularly in patients receiving an ACE inhibitor. Serum K^+ levels and electrolytes should be checked after initiation of treatment, and vigilance is warranted for potential drug interactions and medical disorders that may elevate serum K^+ concentration (e.g., potassium supplements, ACE inhibitors, and worsening renal function).

DIURETIC RESISTANCE IN HEART FAILURE

The response to diuretics is often impaired in patients with CHF. This impaired response may itself be a manifestation of the Na^+ avidity and the volume retention that characterize advanced heart failure. While there may initially be a brisk response to once-daily dosing, a compensatory increase in Na^+ reabsorption during the remainder of the day may prevent effective diuresis; as a result, reduction of the dosing interval may be warranted. In advanced heart failure, edema,

Table 33–2

Potential Roles of Aldosterone in the Pathophysiology of Heart Failure

Mechanism	Pathophysiological Effect
Increased Na^+ and water retention	Edema, elevated cardiac filling pressures
K^+ and Mg^{2+} loss	Arrhythmogenesis and risk of sudden cardiac death
Reduced myocardial norepinephrine uptake	Potentiation of norepinephrine effects: myocardial remodeling and arrhythmogenesis
Reduced baroreceptor sensitivity	Reduced parasympathetic activity and risk of sudden cardiac death
Myocardial fibrosis, fibroblast proliferation	Remodeling and ventricular dysfunction
Alterations in Na^+ channel expression	Increased excitability and contractility of cardiac myocytes

decreased motility of the bowel wall, and reduced splanchnic blood flow can delay or attenuate peak diuretic effect. Patients who have impaired renal function typically require higher doses of diuretic to ensure adequate delivery of the drug to its site of action. Following prolonged administration of a loop diuretic, a process of adaptation can occur in which there is a compensatory increase in Na^+ reabsorption in the distal nephron and blunting of net Na^+ and water loss. The more common causes of diuretic resistance are listed in Table 33–3 and discussed in Chapter 28.

The caveats about concomitant therapy merit particular emphasis when considering coadministration of diuretics and ACE inhibitors or AT_1 receptor antagonists. These inhibitors of the renin–angiotensin system can either augment or reduce the effectiveness of diuretics. A reduced response is observed most commonly in patients with decreased renal arterial perfusion pressure, due either to renal artery stenosis or to reduction of forward cardiac output. In such patients, a high level of AngII–mediated glomerular efferent arteriolar tone is necessary to maintain glomerular filtration pressure. Pharmacologic antagonism of this intrarenal autoregulation may be accompanied by a decline in creatinine clearance and a derivative rise in the serum creatinine. In general, this is readily distinguished from the modest and limited rise in serum creatinine levels that commonly accompanies administration of ACE inhibitors. Diuretic resistance that reflects poor forward cardiac output may require the use of positive inotropic agents (e.g., dobutamine) as vasodilator therapy is initiated.

Decreased responsiveness to loop diuretics in patients with known chronic heart failure should prompt an increase in the dose administered or the dosing frequency. If this is ineffective, a thiazide diuretic (e.g., hydrochlorothiazide or metolazone) administered with the loop diuretic is often effective. However, this combination can result in an unpredictable and sometimes excessive diuresis, leading to intravascular volume depletion and renal K^+ wasting; the combination therefore should be used cautiously. Spironolactone also may be effective in these patients when combined with a loop diuretic.

Table 33–3

Causes of Diuretic Resistance in Heart Failure

Noncompliance with medical regimen; excess dietary Na^+ intake
Decreased renal perfusion and glomerular filtration rate due to:
  Excessive intravascular volume depletion and hypotension due to aggressive diuretic or vasodilator therapy
  Decline in cardiac output due to worsening heart failure, arrhythmias, or other primary cardiac causes
  Selective reduction in glomerular perfusion pressure following initiation (or dose increase) of ACE inhibitor therapy
Nonsteroidal anti-inflammatory drugs
Primary renal pathology (e.g., cholesterol emboli, renal artery stenosis, drug-induced interstitial nephritis, obstructive uropathy)
Reduced or impaired diuretic absorption due to gut wall edema and reduced splanchnic blood flow

METABOLIC CONSEQUENCES OF DIURETIC THERAPY

The side effects of diuretics are discussed in Chapter 28. With regard to diuretic use in heart failure, the most important adverse sequelae of diuretics are electrolyte abnormalities, including hyponatremia, hypokalemia, and hypochloremic metabolic alkalosis. Both hypokalemia and renal Mg^{2+} wasting can be limited by administration of oral KCl supplements or a K^+-sparing diuretic.

Vasodilators

The rationale for the use of oral vasodilator drugs in the pharmacotherapy of CHF derived from the experience with the parenteral agents *phentolamine* and *nitroprusside* in patients with severe heart failure and elevated systemic vascular resistance. Although a number of vasodilators may improve symptoms in heart failure, only the *hydralazine–isosorbide dinitrate* combination and antagonists of the renin–angiotensin system (ACE inhibitors and AT_1 receptor blockers) have been shown to improve survival in prospective randomized trials. Table 33–1 summarizes some properties of vasodilators used to treat heart failure.

Inhibitors of the Renin–Angiotensin System: ACE Inhibitors and AT_1 Receptor Antagonists

RENIN–ANGIOTENSIN SYSTEM ANTAGONISTS The renin–angiotensin system (Figure 33–1; *see* Chapter 30) plays a central role in the pathophysiology of heart failure. Angiotensinogen is cleaved by renin to form the decapeptide angiotensin I (AngI); ACE converts AngI to the octapeptide AngII. AngII is a potent arterial vasoconstrictor and an important mediator of Na^+ and water retention through its effects on glomerular filtration pressure and aldosterone secretion. In addition, AngII potentiates neural catecholamine release, stimulates catecholamine release from the adrenal medulla, is arrhythmogenic, promotes vascular hyperplasia and pathologic myocardial hypertrophy, and stimulates myocyte death. Consequently, the antagonism of AngII is a cornerstone of heart failure management.

ACE inhibitors suppress AngII and aldosterone production, decrease sympathetic nervous system activity, and potentiate the effects of diuretics in heart failure. However, AngII levels frequently return to baseline values following chronic treatment with ACE inhibitors, due in part to production of AngII through ACE-independent enzymes such as chymase, a tissue protease. The sustained clinical effectiveness of ACE inhibitors despite AngII "escape" suggests that there are alternate mechanisms that contribute to the clinical effects of ACE inhibitors in heart failure. ACE also degrades bradykinin and other kinins that stimulate production of NO, cyclic GMP, and vasoactive eicosanoids; these vasodilator substances seem to oppose the effects of AngII on growth of vascular smooth muscle and cardiac fibroblasts and on extracellular matrix production. Thus, increased levels of bradykinin resulting from ACE inhibition may play a role in the hemodynamic and anti-remodeling effects of ACE inhibitors.

ACE inhibitors are more potent arterial than venous dilators. In response to ACE inhibition, mean arterial pressure (MAP) may decrease or be unchanged; the change in MAP will be determined by the stroke volume response to afterload reduction. Heart rate typically is unchanged, even when there is a decrease in systemic arterial pressure, a response that likely reflects a decrease in sympathetic tone in response to ACE inhibition. The decrease in left ventricular afterload results in increased stroke volume and cardiac output. Venodilation results in decreases in right and left heart filling pressures and end-diastolic volumes.

An alternative means of attenuating the hemodynamic and vascular impact of the renin–angiotensin system is through inhibition of angiotensin receptors. Most of the known clinical actions of AngII, including its deleterious effects in heart failure, are mediated through the AT_1 angiotensin receptor. AT_2 angiotensin receptors, also present throughout the cardiovascular system, seem to mediate responses that counterbalance the biological effects of AT_1 receptor stimulation. Due to their more distal site of action, AT_1 receptor antagonists may provide more potent reduction of the effects of AngII than do ACE inhibitors. Furthermore, AT_1 receptor blockade may result in greater AT_2 receptor activation, as AngII levels rise as a consequence of AT_1 receptor blockade. Note that blockade of AT_1 receptors does not alter bradykinin metabolism, which ACE inhibitors reduce.

Angiotensin-Converting Enzyme Inhibitors Six ACE inhibitors-*captopril* (CAPOTEN), *enalapril* (VASOTEC), *ramipril* (ALTACE), *lisinopril* (PRINIVIL, ZESTRIL), *quinapril* (ACCUPRIL), and *fosinopril* (MONOPRIL)—are currently FDA-approved for the treatment of heart failure. Data from numerous clinical trials support the use of ACE inhibitors for the treatment of patients with heart failure of any severity, including patients with asymptomatic left ventricular dysfunction.

ACE-inhibitor therapy should be initiated at a low dose (e.g., 6.25 mg of captopril or 5 mg of lisinopril), as some patients may experience an abrupt drop in blood pressure, particularly in the setting of volume contraction. It is therefore reasonable to consider initiation of these drugs while congestive symptoms are present. ACE-inhibitor doses are customarily increased over several days in hospitalized patients or a few weeks in ambulatory patients, with careful observation of blood pressure, serum electrolytes, and serum creatinine.

There is no precisely defined relationship between dose and long-term clinical effectiveness of these drugs, but it is reasonable to use doses comparable to those used in studies that established efficacy in patients with heart failure. On this basis, target doses of these drugs would be 50 mg three times/day for captopril; 10 mg twice daily for enalapril; 10 mg once daily for lisinopril; or 5 mg twice daily for ramipril. In patients who have not achieved an adequate clinical response at these doses, further increases, as tolerated, may be of value; high-dose lisinopril (32.5 or 35 mg) reduced the combined endpoint of mortality and hospitalization when compared to lower doses of this agent.

In patients with heart failure and reduced renal blood flow, ACE inhibitors limit the kidney's ability to autoregulate glomerular perfusion pressure due to their selective effects on efferent arteriolar tone. If this occurs, the dose of ACE inhibitor should be reduced or another class of vasodilator added or substituted. Rarely, renal function deteriorates following initiation of therapy with an ACE inhibitor, often in patients with bilateral renal artery stenosis. Preferably, the renal artery stenosis should be treated; if this is not feasible, another class of vasodilator should be substituted. Angioedema secondary to ACE inhibition mandates immediate cessation of therapy. A small rise in serum K^+ occurs frequently with ACE inhibitors; this rise can be substantial in patients with renal impairment or in diabetic patients with type IV renal tubular acidosis (hyporeninemic hypoaldosteronism). Mild hyperkalemia is best managed by institution of a low-potassium diet but may require dosage adjustment. A troublesome cough may occur that is likely related to the effects of bradykinin. Substitution of an AT_1 receptor antagonist often alleviates this problem. The inability to use ACE inhibitors as a consequence of cardiorenal side effects (e.g., excessive hypotension, progressive renal insufficiency, or hyperkalemia) is itself a marker of poor prognosis in CHF patients.

Myocardial infarction is the leading cause of heart failure due to systolic dysfunction in industrialized countries. ACE inhibitors prevent the development of clinically significant ventricular dysfunction and mortality following acute infarction, likely by preventing adverse ventricular remodeling. ACE inhibitors are proven effective in specific patient subgroups, including women, African Americans, and the elderly.

AT_1 Receptor Antagonists Activation of the AT_1 receptor mediates most of the deleterious effects of AngII. The receptor blockade provided by AT_1 antagonists provides a pharmacologic means by which to reduce the AngII "escape" that occurs with ACE inhibitors. AT_1 receptor antagonism might also be expected to avoid the bradykinin-mediated side effects of ACE inhibition, principally cough. This side effect, which occurs in >10% of patients, represents an important limitation to the use of ACE inhibitors in clinical practice. Angioedema has been reported with AT_1 receptor antagonists; caution is therefore warranted when prescribing these agents to patients with a history of ACE inhibitor–associated angioedema. AT_1 receptor antagonists provide an alternative to ACE inhibitors in the treatment of heart failure and provide comparable mortality benefits.

The combined use of ACE inhibitors and ARBs in the treatment of heart failure offers the intriguing possibility of additive therapeutic benefit by virtue of distinctive modes of angiotensin antagonism. Some experts suggest that the addition of an AT_1 blocker to a heart failure regimen that includes an ACE inhibitor can be considered in an effort to reduce hospitalizations. AT_1 antagonists also appear to reduce hospitalization in patients with diastolic heart failure.

NITROVASODILATORS Nitrovasodilators have long been used to treat heart failure and remain among the most widely used vasoactive medications. These drugs relax vascular smooth muscle by supplying NO and thereby activating soluble guanylyl cyclase. Thus, they mimic the actions of endogenous NO, an intracellular and paracrine autocoid synthesized from arginine by *NO synthases* in endothelial and smooth muscle cells throughout the vasculature.

Organic Nitrates Organic nitrates are available in a number of formulations that include rapid-acting nitroglycerin tablets or spray for sublingual administration, short-acting oral agents such as isosorbide dinitrate (ISORDIL, SORBITRATE, others), long-acting oral agents such as *isosorbide mononitrate* (IMDUR), topical preparations such as nitroglycerin ointment and transdermal patches, and intravenous nitroglycerin. The nitrates are relatively safe and effective agents whose principal action in the treatment of congestive heart failure is reduction of left ventricular filling pressures. This preload reduction is due to an increase in peripheral venous capacitance. Nitrates will cause a decline in pulmonary and systemic vascular resistance, particularly at higher doses, although this response is less marked and less predictable than with nitroprusside. These drugs have a selective vasodilator effect on the epicardial coronary vasculature and may enhance both systolic and diastolic ventricular function by increasing coronary flow.

Isosorbide dinitrate when administered to patients with CHF is more effective than placebo in improving exercise capacity and reducing symptoms. However, the limited effects of these agents on the systemic vascular resistance and the development of tolerance limit the utility of organic nitrates as monotherapy in the treatment of CHF. An isosorbide dinitrate–hydralazine combination was proven effective in reducing overall mortality in patients with mild-to-moderate heart failure concurrently treated with digoxin *and diuretics. The mononitrate formulation has not been studied in chronic heart failure; the transdermal formulations are infrequently used in the treatment of CHF, reflecting concerns related to perfusion-dependent drug absorption in such patients.*

Tolerance can limit the long-term effectiveness of nitrates in the treatment of CHF. Blood levels of these drugs should be permitted to fall to negligible levels for at least 6–8 hours each day, *which can be adjusted to the patient's symptoms. Patients with recurrent orthopnea or paroxysmal nocturnal dyspnea, for example, would likely benefit most by using nitrates at night.* N-acetylcysteine *(MUCOMYST) may diminish tolerance to the hemodynamic effects of nitrates in heart failure. Likewise, hydralazine may decrease nitrate tolerance by an antioxidant effect that attenuates superoxide formation, thereby increasing NO bioavailability.*

HYDRALAZINE Hydralazine (APRESOLINE) is an effective antihypertensive drug (*see* Chapter 32), particularly when combined with agents that blunt compensatory increases in sympathetic tone and salt and water retention. In heart failure, hydralazine reduces right and left ventricular afterload by reducing pulmonary and systemic vascular resistance. This augments forward stroke volume and reduces ventricular systolic wall stress. Hydralazine also appears to have moderate "direct" positive inotropic activity in cardiac muscle unrelated to afterload reduction. Hydralazine is effective in reducing renal vascular resistance and in increasing renal blood flow to a greater degree than are most other vasodilators, with the exception of ACE inhibitors. Reflecting these aggregate effects, hydralazine may be useful in heart-failure patients with renal dysfunction who cannot tolerate an ACE inhibitor. Hydralazine has minimal effects on venous capacitance and therefore is most effective when combined with agents with venodilating activity (*e.g.*, organic nitrates).

The combination of hydralazine (300 mg/day) and isosorbide dinitrate increased survival when compared to placebo or the α_1 adrenergic antagonist prazosin. Hydralazine, with or without nitrates, may provide additional hemodynamic improvement for patients with advanced heart failure who already are being treated with conventional doses of an ACE inhibitor, digoxin, and diuretics. A combination of isosorbide dinitrate–hydralazine (BIDIL) was most recently investigated in African Americans; when added to standard therapy that included neurohumoral blockade in patients with NYHA Class III or IV heart failure there was a significant reduction in all-cause mortality compared to placebo. This combination preparation is FDA-approved as adjunct to standard therapy for use in CHF patients self-identified as African American. It is the first race-based drug approved by the FDA.

Several important limitations constrain the use of hydralazine in the treatment of CHF. Although hydralazine therapy was associated with a greater increase in ejection fraction and exercise duration when compared to the ACE inhibitor enalapril, the latter was superior with respect to reduction of mortality. Side effects that may necessitate dose adjustment or withdrawal of hydralazine are common. The lupus-like side effects associated with hydralazine are relatively uncommon and may be more likely to occur in patients with the "slow-acetylator" phenotype (see Chapter 3). Finally, compliance with the multidosing regimen may be difficult in CHF patients who often are taking multiple concurrent medications.

The oral bioavailability and pharmacokinetics of hydralazine are not altered significantly by heart failure unless there is severe hepatic congestion or hypoperfusion. Intravenous hydralazine provides little practical advantage over oral formulations except for urgent use during pregnancy, a state in which relative or absolute contraindications exist for most other vasodilators.

β Adrenergic Receptor Antagonists

Heart failure is characterized by sympathetic hyperactivation. Sympathetic activation supports circulatory function by enhancing contractility (inotropy), augmenting ventricular relaxation and filling (lusitropy), and increasing heart rate (chronotropy). For many years, pharmacological approaches to the treatment of heart failure involved the use of drugs that would further stimulate sympathetic responses, reflecting the viewpoint that the fundamental abnormality in CHF is the reduction of stroke volume/cardiac output that occurs as a consequence of myocardial dysfunction. Paradoxically, many of these sympathomimetics increased mortality in CHF patients, while an unexpected mortality benefit was seen with the administration of β adrenergic blocking drugs. The recognition that sustained activation of sympathetic nerves in the context of myocardial injury contributes to the progression of contractile dysfunction is now well established and derives support from the demonstrable adverse consequences of long-term sympathetic stimulation (such as maladaptive proliferative signaling in the myocardium, direct cardiomyocyte toxicity, and myocyte apoptosis).

β Receptor antagonists improve symptoms, exercise tolerance, and measures of ventricular function over a period of several months in patients with heart failure due to idiopathic dilated cardiomyopathy. Serial measurements indicate that a decrease in systolic function does occur immediately after initiation of a β antagonist in CHF patients, but systolic function recovers and improves beyond baseline levels over the ensuing 2–4 months. Improved ventricular function with chronic β receptor antagonist therapy may be due to attenuation or prevention of the β adrenergic receptor–mediated adverse effects of catecholamines on the myocardium.

More important than improving symptoms, β receptor antagonists reduce hospitalization and decrease mortality in patients with mild-to-moderate CHF. A consistent finding is a reduction in the incidence of sudden death, presumably reflecting a decrease in malignant ventricular arrhythmias. Thus, an antiarrhythmic benefit seems likely, possibly reflecting a reduced propensity to develop hypokalemia in the face of systemic β adrenergic blockade, or perhaps a direct consequence of the anti-ischemic effects of these drugs. Another consistent finding with β adrenergic blockade is an improvement in left ventricular structure and function with a decrease in chamber size and an increase in ejection fraction.

METOPROLOL   *Metoprolol* (LOPRESSOR, TOPROL XL, OTHERS) is a β_1-selective antagonist. The 25-mg extended-release tablet formulation is FDA-approved for the management of mild-to-moderate heart failure. A number of clinical trials have demonstrated the beneficial effects of metoprolol therapy in heart failure, with decreased mortality due both to reductions in sudden death and to death from worsening heart failure. These beneficial effects were independent of age, sex, etiology of heart failure, or ejection fraction.

CARVEDILOL   *Carvedilol* (COREG) is a nonselective β receptor antagonist and α_1-selective antagonist that is FDA-approved for the management of mild-to-severe heart failure. Carvedilol, in combination with standard therapy, is associated with significant reductions in all-cause mortality and hospitalization for heart failure exacerbation.

BISOPROLOL   *Bisoprolol* (ZEBETA) is a β_1-selective antagonist that reduces all-cause mortality in CHF patients, due primarily to a decrease in sudden deaths and a lesser decrease in pump failure. The mortality benefit of bisoprolol was independent of the etiology of heart failure and the drug also significant decreased hospitalizations for heart failure. In the U.S., heart failure is an off-label use for bisoprolol.

Clinical Use of β Adrenergic Receptor Antagonists in Heart Failure

The extensive body of data regarding the use of β receptor antagonists in chronic heart failure provides compelling evidence that β antagonists improve symptoms, reduce hospitalization, and decrease mortality in patients with mild and moderate heart failure. Accordingly, β receptor antagonists are now recommended for routine use in patients with an ejection fraction <35% and NYHA Class II or III symptoms in conjunction with ACE inhibitor or angiotensin receptor antagonist, and diuretics as required to palliate symptoms.

This general recommendation should be tempered by certain limitations in the experimental database. First, most of the data that underlie this recommendation were obtained in relatively stable patients with mild-to-moderate symptoms. Therefore, the role of β receptor antagonists in patients with more severe symptoms, or with recent decompensation, is not yet clear. Likewise, the utility of β receptor blockade in patients with asymptomatic left ventricular dysfunction has not been studied. Finally, although it appears likely that the beneficial effects of these drugs are related to β receptor blockade, it cannot be assumed that all β receptor antagonists will exert similar effects. Since β antagonists have the potential to worsen both ventricular function and symptoms in patients with heart failure, several caveats should be considered. β Adrenergic receptor antagonists should be initiated at very low doses, generally less than one-tenth of the final target dose, and the dose should be increased slowly, over the course of weeks and under careful supervision. The rapid institution of the usual β adrenergic receptor–blocking doses used for hypertension or coronary artery disease may cause decompensation in many patients who otherwise would be able to tolerate a slower dose titration. Even when therapy is initiated with low doses of a β antagonist, there may be an increased tendency to retain fluid that will require adjustments in the diuretic regimen. Although limited data suggest that patients with NYHA Class IIIB and IV CHF may tolerate β blockers and benefit from their use, this group of patients should be approached with considerable caution. There is almost no experience in patients with new-onset, recently decompensated heart failure. Such patients should not be treated with β blockers until after they have stabilized for several days to weeks.

Parenteral Vasodilators

The failing left ventricle is characterized by depression of myocardial contractility and increased sensitivity to alterations of left ventricular afterload. This latter attribute of the failing ventricle is manifest by a greater proportional reduction of stroke volume as the impedance to ejection is increased. Conversely, afterload reduction in this setting can be associated with substantial increases in stroke volume. This increased afterload dependence underlies the beneficial effects of load reduction therapy in patients with heart failure due to systolic dysfunction.

SODIUM NITROPRUSSIDE Sodium nitroprusside (NITROPRESS) is a prodrug and potent vasodilator that reduces both ventricular filling pressures and systemic vascular resistance. It has a rapid onset (2–5 minutes) and offset (quickly metabolized to cyanide and NO, the active vasodilator) of action and its dose can be titrated expeditiously to achieve the desired hemodynamic effect. For these reasons, nitroprusside is commonly used in intensive-care settings for rapid control of severe hypertension and for the management of decompensated heart failure. The basic pharmacologic properties of this drug are described in Chapter 32.

Several mechanisms contribute to the reduction of ventricular filling pressures after treatment with nitroprusside. This agent directly increases venous capacitance, redistributing blood volume from the central to the peripheral venous circulation. Nitroprusside also causes a fall in peripheral vascular resistance as well as an increase in aortic wall compliance and improves ventricular–vascular coupling; left ventricular afterload is decreased and cardiac output is thereby increased. This combination of preload and afterload reduction improves myocardial energetics by reducing wall stress. This improvement in myocardial energetics is contingent upon maintenance of a mean arterial pressure sufficient to drive coronary perfusion during diastole. Following the rapid withdrawal of nitroprusside, a transient deterioration in ventricular function associated with a rebound increase in systemic vascular resistance occurs. Nitroprusside is particularly effective in patients with CHF due to elevations of systemic vascular resistance and/or mechanical complications that follow acute myocardial infarction (such as mitral regurgitation or left-to-right shunts through a ventricular septal defect).

The most common adverse effect of nitroprusside is hypotension. In general, nitroprusside initiation in patients with severe heart failure results in increased cardiac output and a parallel increase in renal blood flow, improving both glomerular filtration and diuretic effectiveness. However, excessive reduction of systemic arterial pressure may limit or prevent an increase in renal blood flow in patients with more severe contractile dysfunction. Cyanide produced during the biotransformation of nitroprusside is rapidly metabolized by the liver to thiocyanate, which is cleared by the kidney. Thiocyanate and/or cyanide toxicity is uncommon but may occur in the setting of hepatic or renal failure, or following prolonged, high-dose infusion of the drug. Typical symptoms include unexplained abdominal pain, mental status changes, convulsions, or lactic acidosis. Methemoglobinemia, another unusual complication of prolonged, high-dose nitroprusside infusion, is due to the oxidation of hemoglobin by NO.

INTRAVENOUS NITROGLYCERIN Intravenous nitroglycerin, like nitroprusside, is a vasoactive NO source that is commonly used in intensive care units. Its structure and basic pharmacology are described in Chapter 31. Unlike nitroprusside, nitroglycerin is relatively selective for venous capacitance vessels, particularly at low infusion rates. In patients with CHF, intravenous nitroglycerin is most clearly indicated in the treatment of left heart failure due to acute myocardial ischemia. Parenteral nitroglycerin also is used in the treatment of nonischemic left heart failure when expeditious reduction of ventricular filling pressures is desired; nitroglycerin can be particularly useful in patients with symptomatic volume overload in whom effective diuresis has not been established. At higher infusion rates, this drug can also reduce systemic arterial resistance, although this effect is less predictable. Nitroglycerin therapy may be limited by headache and the development of nitrate tolerance, although the latter is generally overcome by uptitration of the infusion rate to maintain the desired response. Since nitroglycerin is administered in ethanol, high infusion rates can be associated with significant elevation of blood alcohol levels.

NESIRITIDE *Nesiritide* (NATRECOR), a recombinant form of human brain natriuretic peptide (BNP), is FDA-approved for treatment of dyspnea due to congestive heart failure. The natriuretic peptides—atrial natriuretic peptide (ANP), BNP, and C-type natriuretic peptide—are a family of endogenous hormones that possess potent natriuretic, diuretic, and vasodilator properties. BNP is secreted by ventricular cardiac myocytes in response to stretch; circulating levels of BNP correlate with the severity of heart failure. In the setting of heart failure, the effects of BNP counteract the effects of AngII and NE by producing vasodilation, natriuresis, and diuresis.

The BNP receptor is the extracellular domain of type A guanylyl cyclase, GC-A. The active receptor–cyclase complex is a homodimer. Activation of GC-A by nesiritide (BNP) increases cyclic GMP content in target tissues, including vascular, endothelial, and smooth muscle cells. As with nitrovasodilators, elevated cyclic GMP leads to relaxation of vascular smooth muscle and vasodilation in both the venous and arterial systems. BNP is metabolized by specific clearance receptors, which facilitate its internalization and enzymatic degradation. It is also inactivated by neutral endopeptidases (NEP). Dose adjustment is not required in patients with renal dysfunction.

Nesiritide lowers right and left side cardiac filling pressures without a direct chronotropic or inotropic action. The hemodynamic response to nesiritide is characterized by decreased right atrial, pulmonary arterial, and pulmonary capillary wedge pressures; systemic vascular resistance is reduced and cardiac index is increased. Improvement in global clinical status, attenuation of dyspnea and fatigue, and enhanced diuretic responsiveness have been reported. When compared to intravenous nitroglycerin and placebo in the treatment of decompensated heart failure, nesiritide was associated with greater reductions in pulmonary capillary wedge pressure and improvements in dyspnea were comparable to nitroglycerin and better than placebo. In contrast to the effects of parenteral inotropic agents, nesiritide is not associated with increased ventricular or atrial arrhythmias. Thus, nesiritide may be preferable to inotropic drugs when treating refractory heart failure in patients at risk for arrhythmia

Nesiritide therapy is initiated with a loading dose of 2 μg/kg followed by an infusion rate of 0.01 μg/kg/min that can be increased in increments of 0.005 μg/kg/min to a maximum of 0.03 μg/kg/min. The primary side effect is hypotension that is reversible upon discontinuation of the drug. The $t_{1/2}$ of the drug is 18 minutes; however, hypotensive effects may persist for a longer period than would be predicted on the basis of the elimination $t_{1/2}$. Although there is no specific systolic blood pressure below which nesiritide therapy is contraindicated, studies have typically excluded patients with systolic blood pressure ≤90 mm Hg; inotropic support may be preferred in such patients. Also of concern, recent meta-analyses have suggested that nesiritide therapy of CHF is associated with an increased risk of renal dysfunction and death.

VASOPEPTIDASE INHIBITORS AND BNP

Vasopeptidase inhibitors are a novel group of drugs that simultaneously inhibit ACE and neutral endopeptidases (NEPs) and are effective antihypertensive agents. NEPs are responsible for the enzymatic degradation of atrial and brain natriuretic peptides. Inhibitors of NEPs therefore are expected to increase circulating levels of these natriuretic hormones and on this basis have been investigated as therapeutic agents in heart failure. Studies suggest that the vasopeptidase inhibitor omapatrilat is comparable to ACE inhibitors with respect to improving exercise capacity, decreasing symptoms, and reducing the risk of death and hospitalization in chronic heart failure, but is more frequently associated with symptomatic hypotension. Omapatrilat is not approved by the FDA.

Cardiac Glycosides

Beneficial effects of cardiac glycosides in the treatment of heart failure have been attributed to a positive inotropic effect on failing myocardium and efficacy in controlling the ventricular rate response to atrial fibrillation. The cardiac glycosides also modulate autonomic nervous system activity, and it is likely that this mechanism contributes substantially to their efficacy in the management of heart failure. However, the advent of alternative therapies that both palliate symptoms and improve survival has led to a more limited role for the cardiac glycosides in the pharmacotherapy of congestive heart failure. Only digoxin (LANOXIN, LANOXICAPS) is widely used today.

MECHANISM OF THE POSITIVE INOTROPIC EFFECT

All cardiac glycosides are potent and highly selective inhibitors of the active transport of Na^+ and K^+ across cell membranes by their reversible binding to the α subunit of the Na^+, K^+-ATPase. Both Na^+ and Ca^{2+} ions enter cardiac muscle cells during each depolarization (Figure 33–2). Ca^{2+} entry triggers contraction; it then is resequestered by the sarcoplasmic reticular Ca^{2+}-ATPase (SERCA2) and also is removed from the cell by the Na^+-Ca^{2+} exchanger (NCX) and by a sarcolemmal Ca^{2+}-ATPase. Inhibition of the Na^+, K^+-ATPase by cardiac glycosides results in a reduction in the rate of Na^+ extrusion and a rise in cytosolic Na^+, which reduces the ability of the NCX to extrude Ca^{2+} during myocyte repolarization. With reduced Ca^{2+} efflux and repeated entry

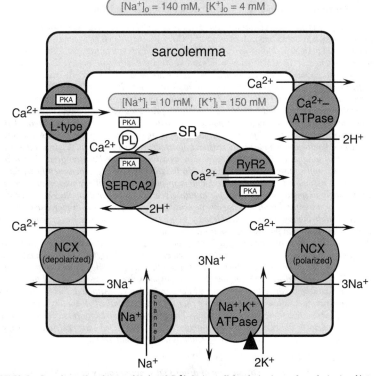

FIGURE 33–2 *Sarcolemmal exchange of Na^+ and Ca^{2+} during cell depolarization and repolarization.* Na^+ and Ca^{2+} enter the cardiac myocyte *via* the Na^+ channel and the L-type Ca^{2+} channel during each cycle of membrane depolarization, triggering the release, through the ryanodine receptor (RyR), of larger amounts of Ca^{2+} from internal stores in the sarcoplasmic reticulum (SR). The resulting increase in intracellular Ca^{2+} interacts with troponin C and activates interactions between actin and myosin that result in sarcomere shortening. The electrochemical gradient for Na^+ across the sarcolemma is maintained by active transport of Na^+ out of the cell by the sarcolemmal Na^+,K^+-ATPase. The bulk of cytosolic Ca^{2+} is pumped back into the SR by a Ca^{2+}-ATPase, SERCA2. The remainder is removed from the cell by either a sarcolemmal Ca^{2+}-ATPase or a high capacity Na^+-Ca^{2+} exchange protein, NCX. NCX exchanges three Na^+ for every Ca^{2+}, using the electrochemical potential of Na^+ to drive Ca^{2+} extrusion. The direction of Na^+–Ca^{2+} exchange may reverse briefly during depolarization, when the electrical gradient across the sarcolemma is transiently reversed. β Receptor agonists and PDE inhibitors, by increasing cellular cyclic AMP levels, activate PKA, which phosphorylates target proteins, including phospholamban, the α subunit of the L-type Ca^{2+} channel and regulatory components of the RyR, as well as TnI, the inhibitory subunit of troponin (not shown). The effect of these phosphorylations is a positive inotropic effect: a faster rate of tension development to a higher level of tension, followed by a faster rate of relaxation. ▲ indicates site of cardiac glycoside binding. *See* text for mechanism of positive inotropic effect of cardiac glycosides.

of Ca²⁺, Ca²⁺ accumulates in the myocyte: Ca²⁺ uptake into the SR is increased; this increased Ca²⁺ becomes available for release from the SR during the next cycle of excitation-contraction coupling and is the penultimate effect by which cardiac glycosides enhance myocardial contractility (Figure 33–2).

ELECTROPHYSIOLOGICAL ACTIONS   At therapeutic concentrations, digoxin decreases automaticity and increases maximal diastolic resting membrane potential in atrial and AV nodal tissues due to an increase in vagal tone and a decrease in sympathetic nervous system activity. This can cause sinus bradycardia and/or prolongation of AV conduction or higher-grade sinus arrest or AV block. At higher concentrations, cardiac glycosides can directly increase automaticity in cardiac tissue, actions that contribute to the genesis of atrial and ventricular arrhythmias. Increased intracellular Ca²⁺ loading and increased sympathetic tone increase the spontaneous (phase 4) rate of diastolic depolarization as well as delayed afterdepolarizations that may trigger generation of a propagated action potential. This simultaneous nonuniform increase in automaticity and depression of conduction in His-Purkinje and ventricular muscle fibers can predispose the heart to serious ventricular arrhythmias (*see* Chapter 34).

PHARMACOKINETICS   The elimination $t_{1/2}$ for digoxin is 36 hours in patients with normal renal function. This permits once-a-day dosing; near steady-state blood levels are achieved one week after initiation of maintenance therapy. Digoxin is excreted by the kidney with a clearance rate that is proportional to the glomerular filtration rate. In patients with congestive heart failure and marginal cardiac reserve, an increase in cardiac output and renal blood flow with vasodilator therapy or sympathomimetic agents may increase renal digoxin clearance, necessitating dosage adjustment. Conversely, the $t_{1/2}$ is increased substantially in patients with advanced renal insufficiency (to ~3.5–5 days); both the volume of distribution and the clearance rate of the drug are decreased in the elderly. Because of its narrow therapeutic index, the drug must be used with caution in patients with renal insufficiency and in the elderly.

Liquid-filled capsules of digoxin (LANOXICAPS) have a higher bioavailability than do tablets (LANOXIN) and require dosage adjustment if a patient is switched from one dosage form to the other. Digoxin is available for intravenous administration, and maintenance doses can be given intravenously when oral dosing is impractical. A number of drug interactions and clinical conditions can alter the pharmacokinetics of digoxin or alter patient susceptibility to its toxic manifestations. For example, chronic renal failure decreases the volume of distribution of digoxin, and therefore requires a decrease in maintenance dosage of the drug. Electrolyte disturbances, especially hypokalemia, acid–base imbalances, and the specific type of underlying heart disease also may alter a patient's susceptibility to toxic manifestations of digoxin.

CLINICAL USE OF DIGOXIN IN HEART FAILURE   There has been controversy surrounding the efficacy of cardiac glycosides in the treatment of patients with heart failure who are in sinus rhythm. It is now recommended that digoxin be reserved for patients with heart failure who are in atrial fibrillation, or for patients in sinus rhythm who remain symptomatic despite maximal therapy with ACE inhibitors and β adrenergic receptor antagonists. Although digoxin is no longer viewed as a first-line agent, it should be emphasized that digoxin—unlike most other inotropic agents—does not have an adverse impact on mortality in CHF. Digoxin may be unique among inotropic drugs by virtue of its neurohumoral effects, which include attenuation of sympathetic activation and reduction of renin release.

DIGOXIN TOXICITY   The incidence and severity of digoxin toxicity have declined substantially, due in part to the development of alternative drugs for the treatment of supraventricular arrhythmias and heart failure, to the increased understanding of digoxin pharmacokinetics, to the monitoring of serum digoxin levels, and to the identification of important interactions between digoxin and other concomitantly administered drugs. Nevertheless, the recognition of digoxin toxicity remains an important consideration in the differential diagnosis of arrhythmias and neurological and GI symptoms in patients receiving cardiac glycosides. Immunotherapy with purified Fab fragments from ovine antidigoxin antisera (DIGIBIND) provides an effective antidote for life-threatening digoxin or *digitoxin* toxicity.

Parenteral Inotropic Agents

GENERAL CONSIDERATIONS   Patients with heart failure are most commonly hospitalized because of fluid retention that results in dyspnea and peripheral edema. Accordingly, relief of congestion through the use of diuretics and venodilators remains a therapeutic priority. A subset of these patients may present with clinical evidence of reduced forward cardiac output, including fatigue, azotemia, and alterations in mental status. Patients who present with more severe decompensation typically require intensive therapy that may include parenteral inotropic agents; in extreme circumstances assisted ventilation and mechanical circulatory support may be required. In the setting of severe decompensation, the principal focus of initial therapy is to increase cardiac output by administration of agents that increase myocardial contractility.

β Adrenergic and Dopaminergic Agonists

Dopamine and dobutamine are the positive inotropic agents most often used for the short-term support of the circulation in advanced heart failure. These drugs act *via* stimulation of the cardiac myocyte dopamine D_1 and β adrenergic receptors, leading to stimulation of the G_s-adenylyl cyclase–cyclic AMP–PKA pathway. *Isoproterenol, epinephrine,* and *norepinephrine,* although useful in specific circumstances, have little role in the treatment of heart failure (*see* Chapter 10).

DOPAMINE (DA)   DA has limited utility in the treatment of most patients with cardiogenic circulatory failure. At *low doses* (≤2 μg/kg lean body mass per minute), DA causes vasodilation by stimulating dopaminergic receptors on smooth muscle (causing cyclic AMP–dependent relaxation) and by stimulating presynaptic D_2 receptors on sympathetic nerves in the peripheral circulation (inhibiting NE release and reducing α adrenergic stimulation of vascular smooth muscle); these receptors are prominent in splanchnic and renal arterial beds. DA infusion at this rate may increase renal blood flow and thereby help to maintain the glomerular filtration rate in patients who are refractory to diuretics. DA also has direct effects on renal tubular epithelial cells that promote diuresis. At *intermediate* infusion rates (2–5 μg/kg/min), DA directly stimulates β receptors on the heart and vascular sympathetic neurons, enhancing cardiac contractility and neural NE release. At *higher* infusion rates (5–15 μg/kg/min), peripheral arterial and venous constriction occur, mediated by α adrenergic receptor stimulation (*see* above). This effect may be desirable for support of a critically reduced arterial pressure in selected patients in whom circulatory failure is the result of vasodilation (*e.g.,* sepsis or anaphylaxis). However, high-dose DA infusion has little role in the treatment of patients with primary contractile dysfunction; in this setting, increased vasoconstriction will lead to increased afterload, further compromising left ventricular stroke volume and forward cardiac output. Tachycardia, which is more pronounced with DA than with dobutamine, may provoke ischemia in patients with coronary artery disease.

DOBUTAMINE   Dobutamine (DOBUTREX) is the preferred β agonist for the management of patients with end-stage systolic dysfunction and CHF. Dobutamine is supplied as a racemic mixture that stimulates both β_1 and β_2 receptor subtypes. In addition, the (–) enantiomer is an agonist for α adrenergic receptors, whereas the (+) enantiomer is a very weak partial agonist. At infusion rates that have a positive inotropic effect in humans, the β_1 adrenergic effect in the myocardium predominates. In the vasculature, the α adrenergic agonist effect of the (–) enantiomer appears to be negated by the partial agonism of the (+) enantiomer and the vasodilator effects of β_2 receptor stimulation. Thus, the principal hemodynamic effect of dobutamine is an increase in stroke volume due to its positive inotropic action. At doses that increase cardiac output, there is relatively little increase in heart rate. Dobutamine infusion generally causes a modest decrease in systemic resistance and intracardiac filling pressures. Dobutamine does not activate dopaminergic receptors. As such, the increase in renal blood flow that occurs in association with dobutamine is proportional to the increase in cardiac output.

> *Continuous infusion of dobutamine for up to several days in patients with severe clinical decompensation has been a common practice; pharmacological tolerance may limit efficacy during longer-term administration. Infusions are typically initiated at 2–3 μg/kg/min, without a loading dose, and increased until the desired hemodynamic response is achieved. The blood pressure response to dobutamine is variable and is dependent on the relative effects of this agent on vascular tone and cardiac output. If cardiac output is significantly increased, heart rate may decline secondary to reflex withdrawal of sympathetic tone. The major side effects of dobutamine are excessive tachycardia and arrhythmias, which may require a reduction in dosage. Tolerance may occur after prolonged use, requiring substitution of an alternative drug such as a PDE3 inhibitor. In patients who have been receiving a β receptor antagonist, the initial response to dobutamine may be attenuated.*

PHOSPHODIESTERASE INHIBITORS

The cyclic AMP–phosphodiesterase (PDE) inhibitors reduce the degradation of cellular cyclic AMP; the consequences are generally those of elevated cyclic AMP, much as would occur in response to a stimulator of adenylyl cyclase activity. In the heart, the result is positive inotropism. In the peripheral vasculature, the result is dilation of both resistance and capacitance vessels, leading to reduction of both afterload and preload. These combined effects on the myocardium and in the periphery underlie the classification of these drugs as "inodilators".

INAMRINONE AND MILRINONE   Parenteral formulations of *inamrinone* (previous name: *amrinone*) and *milrinone* are approved for short-term support of the circulation in advanced heart failure. Both drugs are bipyridine derivatives and relatively selective inhibitors of PDE3, the cyclic GMP–inhibited cyclic AMP PDE. These drugs cause direct stimulation of myocardial contractility and acceleration of myocardial relaxation. In addition, they cause balanced arterial and venous dilation with a consequent fall in systemic and pulmonary vascular resistances, and left and right heart filling pressures. Cardiac output increases due to the stimulation of myocardial contractility and the decrease in left ventricular afterload. As a result of this dual mechanism of action, the increase in cardiac output with milrinone is greater than that seen with nitroprusside at doses that comparably reduce systemic resistance. Conversely, the arterial and venous dilator effects of milrinone are greater than those of dobutamine at doses that produce comparable increases in cardiac output.

Intravenous infusions of either drug should be initiated with a loading dose followed by a continuous infusion. For inamrinone, a 0.75-mg/kg bolus injection administered over 2–3 minutes is followed by a 2- to 20-μg/kg/min infusion. The loading dose of milrinone is usually 50 μg/kg, and the continuous infusion rate ranges from 0.25–1 μg/kg/min. The elimination half-lives of inamrinone and milrinone in healthy subjects are 2–3 hours and 0.5–1 hour, respectively, and are approximately doubled in patients with severe heart failure. Clinically significant thrombocytopenia occurs in 10% of patients receiving inamrinone but is rare with milrinone. Because of its greater selectivity for PDE3 isoenzymes, shorter $t_{1/2}$, and more favorable side-effect profile, milrinone is preferred among currently available PDE inhibitors for short-term, parenteral inotropic support. The vasodilating effects of the drug and its relatively protracted $t_{1/2}$ limit use in patients with low systemic arterial pressure.

Diastolic Heart Failure

Approximately 30–40% of CHF cases occur in patients with normal or preserved left ventricular systolic function. Despite intact systolic function, such patients will present with typical signs and symptoms of heart failure, including dyspnea, impaired functional capacity, and pulmonary/ systemic venous congestion. The pathogenesis of diastolic heart failure includes structural and functional abnormalities of the ventricle that are associated with impaired ventricular relaxation and impaired left ventricular distensibility (*i.e.,* abnormal LV compliance with increased chamber stiffness). Consonant with the definition of heart failure outlined above, the diagnosis of diastolic heart failure is made when the left ventricle is unable to fill to a volume that is sufficient to maintain normal cardiac output without exceeding the upper range of normal diastolic pressure. The underlying problem in diastolic heart failure is the inability to fill (rather than to empty) the ventricle.

There are no definitive trials to guide therapy in patients with diastolic heart failure, and one is therefore unable to initiate treatment in anticipation of attenuating disease progression or reducing mortality. It is, however, possible to make some general comments regarding mechanistic considerations in selecting treatment.

Patients with diastolic heart failure are typically dependent upon preload to maintain adequate cardiac output. While patients with symptomatic volume overload will benefit from careful modulation of intravascular volume, volume reduction should be accomplished gradually and treatment goals reassessed frequently. In addition to cautious volume management, it is important to maintain synchronous atrial contraction in such patients, which maintains adequate left ventricular filling during the latter phase of diastole. Cardiac function is often severely impaired if patients with diastolic heart failure develop atrial fibrillation, particularly in the context of suboptimal ventricular rate control. Meticulous control of the ventricular rate with drugs that slow AV conduction is mandatory (see Chapter 34) and restoration of sinus rhythm should be considered. It is also important to evaluate and treat conditions that are associated with dynamic abnormalities of diastolic function, such as myocardial ischemia and poorly controlled systemic hypertension.

CLINICAL SUMMARY

Heart failure is a chronic illness that begins with a primary myocardial insult (that leads to loss of cardiomyocyte number or function) and that is progressive (through a course that is characterized by a variety of functional and structural compensations). In fact, this temporal progression of disease provides the basis for a revised classification system that is replacing the standard New York Heart Association categories that are based on patient functional status. Under this new construct (Figure 33–3), patients progress from a stage in which they are at risk to develop heart failure (Stage A) to a phase in which structural heart disease is established and demonstrable (Stage B). From this point of asymptomatic ventricular dysfunction, patients progress to a stage in which symptoms of the heart failure syndrome are present (Stage C); a subset of Stage C patients will progress to end-stage status (Stage D) in which symptoms refractory to medical therapy are present. Given that the syndrome of heart failure begins with a primary insult to the myocardium (such as infarction, excessive hemodynamic load, or inflammation), treatment should begin with prevention *via* the identification and remediation of risk factors that predispose to the development of structural heart disease. For example, since coronary artery disease is the most common etiologic basis for systolic dysfunction and CHF, the prevention of myocardial infarction through risk factor modification (*e.g.,* lipid lowering, control of hypertension, and smoking cessation) is a critical therapeutic strategy with substantial public health implications.

Once structural heart disease is established (Stage B), compensatory mechanisms are activated that support cardiovascular function, but that also set the stage for disease progression. This phase can be referred to as the stage of asymptomatic ventricular dysfunction. Treatment in Stage B is directed at attenuation of sustained neurohormonal activation, and target doses of β blockers, ACE inhibitors, or AT_1 receptor antagonists should be selected using the treatment guidelines applied in clinical trials that established the morbidity and mortality benefits of these agents. It is axiomatic that the specific agent selected and the dosing regimen must be individualized.

After an asymptomatic period, heart failure usually progresses to a symptomatic stage. Once symptoms ensue (Stage C), the goals of treatment include both relief of symptoms and prevention of disease progression. In addition to the relief of congestive symptoms with diuretics and load-reducing therapies, antagonism of the renin–angiotensin system and the sympathetic branch of the autonomic nervous system are indicated to prevent further myocardial injury. In the ambulatory patient in a compensated hemodynamic state, diuretics and organic nitrates are used to establish and maintain euvolemia; vasodilators are used to reduce the systemic vascular resistance and optimize forward cardiac output. While maintenance of forward cardiac output will help to attenuate neurohumoral activation, agents that antagonize the effects of AngII and sympathetic stimulation are

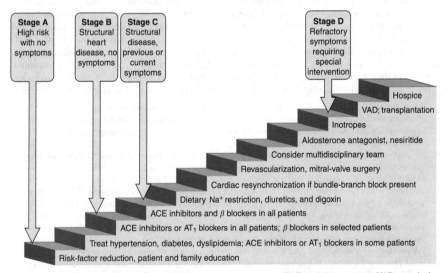

| Stage A
High risk
with no
symptoms | Stage B
Structural
heart
disease, no
symptoms | Stage C
Structural
disease,
previous or
current
symptoms | Stage D
Refractory
symptoms
requiring
special
intervention |

Hospice
VAD; transplantation
Inotropes
Aldosterone antagonist, nesiritide
Consider multidisciplinary team
Revascularization, mitral-valve surgery
Cardiac resynchronization if bundle-branch block present
Dietary Na+ restriction, diuretics, and digoxin
ACE inhibitors and β blockers in all patients
ACE inhibitors or AT_1 blockers in all patients; β blockers in selected patients
Treat hypertension, diabetes, dyslipidemia; ACE inhibitors or AT_1 blockers in some patients
Risk-factor reduction, patient and family education

FIGURE 33–3 *Stages of heart failure.* ACE, Ang-converting enzyme; AT_1,Type 1 Ang receptor; VAD, ventricular assist device.

indicated; ACE inhibitors and AT_1 receptor antagonists are preferred. If neither of these agents is tolerated, treatment with the hydralazine–isosorbide dinitrate combination should be initiated. Treatment with β blockers should be undertaken when hemodynamic stability is established and treatment with aldosterone antagonists considered in patients with preserved renal function. Digoxin is now primarily used for persistent symptoms in the ambulatory patient, and there are no data that cardiac glycosides decrease mortality.

In the symptomatic patient with hemodynamic decompensation, hospitalization may be required, since oral diuretic and vasodilator therapy alone may be inadequate to reestablish euvolemia and adequate peripheral perfusion. In such patients, parenteral vasodilators and inotropic agents may be required to restore forward cardiac output. In designing a treatment regimen, the clinician must consider the hemodynamic status of the individual patient. It is frequently possible to do so by qualitative assessment of the forward cardiac output (normal *vs.* low), systemic vascular resistance (normal *vs.* high), and intracardiac filling pressures (normal *vs.* high).

In patients with elevated systemic vascular resistance and normal-to-elevated systemic blood pressure, afterload reduction with nitroprusside is logical; it should be emphasized that nitroprusside also increases venous capacitance, thereby also decreasing preload. In the context of myocardial dysfunction, afterload reduction will typically lead to improved forward cardiac output. Nitroprusside may also be effective when the systemic vascular resistance is elevated and systemic blood pressure is reduced; the caveat in this more complex hemodynamic setting is that the load reduction produced by nitroprusside must be counterbalanced by an increase in stroke volume. This derivative increase in stroke volume may not occur in the patient with advanced heart failure; rather, the result will be a further reduction in mean arterial pressure and the potential risk of peripheral organ hypoperfusion. An alternative approach would be the use of an inotropic-dilator drug such as milrinone, which will provide both preload and afterload reduction; its concurrent positive inotropic effect may offset the reduction in mean arterial pressure that can occur from vasodilation alone.

In the decompensated patient who presents with heart failure and normal systemic vascular resistance, afterload reduction may be contraindicated, and treatment with a parenteral agent such as dobutamine may be preferable. The risk attendant to treatment with sympathomimetic drugs is related to the increase in myocardial O_2 consumption that may occur; this is of particular concern in patients with left heart failure that occurs as a direct consequence of myocardial ischemia. This clinical quandary has become less common in the era of aggressive myocardial revascularization; when it is encountered, coadministration of dobutamine with parenteral nitroglycerin should be considered.

Therapy in the patient with symptomatic pulmonary congestion generally should include diuresis to alleviate pulmonary and systemic vascular congestion. The administration of an oral or intravenous nitrate preparation may improve pulmonary congestion by increasing venous capacitance. This treatment goal is desirable to reduce patient discomfort; an important ancillary impact of such treatment is the attenuation of the neurohumoral activation that accompanies elevation of intracardiac filling pressures and the attendant dyspnea. Excessive preload reduction should be avoided given the dependence on preload that accompanies advanced myocardial dysfunction.

When advanced heart failure is unresponsive to these standard therapies, invasive hemodynamic monitoring may be required. Effective treatment of these patients is often complicated by concurrent renal insufficiency and hypotension, despite evidence of persistent elevation of intracardiac filling pressures. In patients who remain symptomatic and/or hemodynamically unstable (Stage D), referral to a specialized tertiary center with expertise in the evaluation and management of heart failure should be considered. At this advanced stage of disease, resource-intensive treatment (such as cardiac resynchronization therapy, mechanical assist devices, high-risk surgical interventions, or cardiac transplantation) or investigational therapies can be considered.

For a complete Bibliographical listing see Goodman & Gilman's *The Pharmacological Basis of Therapeutics,* 11th ed., or Goodman & Gilman Online at www.accessmedicine.com.

34

ANTIARRHYTHMIC DRUGS

Cardiac cells undergo depolarization and repolarization ~60 times/min. The shape and duration of each cardiac action potential are determined by the activity of ion channel protein complexes in the membranes of individual cells, and each heartbeat results from the highly integrated electrophysiological behavior of multiple proteins on multiple cardiac cells. Ion channel function can be perturbed by acute ischemia, sympathetic stimulation, or myocardial scarring to create abnormalities of cardiac rhythm, or arrhythmias. Antiarrhythmic drugs suppress arrhythmias by blocking flow through specific ion channels or by altering autonomic function.

Arrhythmias can range from incidental, asymptomatic clinical findings to life-threatening abnormalities. In some arrhythmias, precise mechanisms are known, and treatment can be targeted specifically against those mechanisms. In other cases, the choice of drugs is largely empirical. Antiarrhythmic drug therapy can prevent or terminate an arrhythmia. Unfortunately, antiarrhythmic drugs not only help to control arrhythmias but also can cause them (Table 34–1). Thus, prescribing antiarrhythmic drugs requires that precipitating factors be excluded or minimized, that a precise diagnosis of the type of arrhythmia be made, that the prescriber has reason to believe that drug therapy will be beneficial, and that the risks of drug therapy can be minimized.

PRINCIPLES OF CARDIAC ELECTROPHYSIOLOGY

The normal cardiac cell at rest maintains a transmembrane potential ~80–90 mV negative to the exterior; this gradient is established by pumps, especially the Na^+, K^+–ATPase, and fixed anionic charges within cells. At rest, the normal cardiac cell is permeable to K^+ (because inward rectifier channels are open) and $[K]_o$ is the major determinant of resting potential.

If an atrial or ventricular cell at rest is depolarized above a threshold potential, Na^+ channels change conformation from the "closed" (resting) state to the "open" (conducting) state, allowing up to 10^7 Na^+/second to enter each cell and moving the transmembrane potential toward the equilibrium potential for Na^+, E_{Na} (+65 mV). This surge of Na^+ ions lasts only about a millisecond, after which the Na^+ channel protein rapidly changes conformation from the "open" state to an "inactivated," nonconducting state. The changes in transmembrane potential generated by the inward Na^+ current produce, in turn, a series of openings (and in some cases subsequent inactivation) of other channels (Figure 34–1). For example, when a cell from the epicardium or the His–Purkinje conducting system is depolarized, "transient outward" K^+ channels change conformation to enter an open, or conducting, state; since the transmembrane potential at the end of phase 0 is positive relative to E_K, the opening of transient outward channels results in an outward, or repolarizing, K^+ current (termed I_{TO}), which contributes to the phase 1 "notch" seen in action potentials from these tissues. Transient outward K^+ channels, like Na^+ channels, inactivate rapidly. During the phase 2 plateau of a normal cardiac action potential, inward, depolarizing currents, primarily through Ca^{2+} channels, are balanced by outward, repolarizing currents primarily through K^+ ("delayed rectifier") channels. Delayed rectifier currents (collectively termed I_K) increase with time, whereas Ca^{2+} currents inactivate; as a result, cardiac cells repolarize (phase 3) several hundred milliseconds after the initial Na^+ channel opening.

A common mechanism whereby drugs prolong cardiac action potentials and provoke arrhythmias is through inhibition of a specific delayed rectifier current, I_{Kr}, generated by expression of the human ether-a-go-go related gene (HERG). The ion channel protein generated by HERG expression differs from other ion channels in important structural features that make it much more susceptible to drug block. Avoiding I_{Kr}/HERG channel block has become a major issue in the development of new antiarrhythmic drugs.

Differing Action Potential Behaviors among Cardiac Cells

This general description must be modified for certain cell types (Figure 34–1) presumably because of variability in the ion channel proteins expressed in individual cells. Atrial cells have very short action potentials probably because I_{TO} is larger, and an additional repolarizing K^+ current, activated by acetylcholine, is present. As a result, vagal stimulation further shortens atrial action potentials. Cells of the sinus and atrioventricular (AV) nodes lack substantial Na^+ currents. In addition, these cells, as well as cells from the conducting system, normally display the phenomenon of spontaneous diastolic, or phase 4, depolarization and thus spontaneously reach threshold for regeneration of action potentials. The rate of spontaneous firing usually is fastest in sinus node cells, which therefore serve as the natural pacemaker of the heart. Specialized K^+ channels underlie the pacemaker current in the heart.

Table 34–1

Drug-Induced Cardiac Arrhythmias

Arrhythmia	Drug	Likely Mechanism	Treatment*	Clinical Features
Digoxin	Sinus bradycardia	↑Vagal tone	Antidigoxin antibodies	Atrial tachycardia may also be present
	AV block		Temporary pacing	
Verapamil, Diltiazem	Sinus bradycardia, AV block	Ca^{2+} channel block	Ca^{2+} Temporary pacing	
β-Blockers, Clonidine, Methyldopa	Sinus bradycardia, AV block	Sympatholytic	Isoproterenol Temporary pacing	
β-Blocker withdrawal	Sinus tachycardia Any other tachycardia	Upregulation of β-receptors with chronic therapy; more receptors available for agonist after withdrawal of blocker	β-Blockade	Hypertension, angina also possible
Quinidine, Flecainide, Propafenone	↑ Ventricular rate in atrial flutter	Conduction slowing in atrium, with enhanced (quinidine) or unaltered AV conduction	AV nodal blockers	QRS complexes often widened at fast rates
Digoxin, Verapamil	↑ Ventricular rate in atrial fibrillation in patients with WPW syndrome	↓ Accessory pathway refractoriness	IV procainamide DC cardioversion	Ventricular rate can exceed 300/min
Theophylline	Multifocal atrial tachycardia	?↑ Intracellular Ca^{2+} and DADs	Withdraw theophylline ?Verapamil	Often in advanced lung disease
Quinidine, Sotalol, Procainamide, Disopyramide, Dofetilide, Ibutilide, "Noncardioactive", drugs (see text) Amiodarone (rare)	Polymorphic VT with ↑ QT interval (*torsades de pointes*)	EAD-related triggered activity	Cardiac pacing Isoproterenol Magnesium	Hypokalemia, bradycardia frequent Related to ↑ plasma concentrations, except for quinidine

(Continued)

Table 34-1

Drug-Induced Cardiac Arrhythmias (*Continued*)

Arrhythmia	Drug	Likely Mechanism	Treatment*	Clinical Features
Flecainide, Propafenone, Quinidine (rarer)	Frequent or difficult to terminate VT ("incessant" VT)	Conduction slowing in reentrant circuits	Na$^+$ bolus reportedly effective in some cases	Most often in patients with advanced myocardial scarring
Digoxin	Atrial tachycardia with AV block; ventricular bigeminy and others	DAD-related triggered activity ($\pm\uparrow$ vagal tone)	Antidigoxin antibodies	Coexistence of abnormal impulses with abnormal sinus or AV nodal function
	Ventricular fibrillation	Severe hypotension and/or myocardial ischemia	Cardiac resuscitation (DC cardioversion)	
Inappropriate use of IV verapamil				Misdiagnosis of VT as PSVT → inappropriate use of verapamil

*In each of these cases, recognition and withdrawal of the offending drug(s) are mandatory.

ABBREVIATIONS: AV, atrioventricular; DAD, delayed afterdepolarization; DC, direct current; EAD, early afterdepolarization; WPW, Wolff–Parkinson–White supraventricular tachycardia; IV, intravenous; ↑, increase; ↓, decrease; ?, unclear.

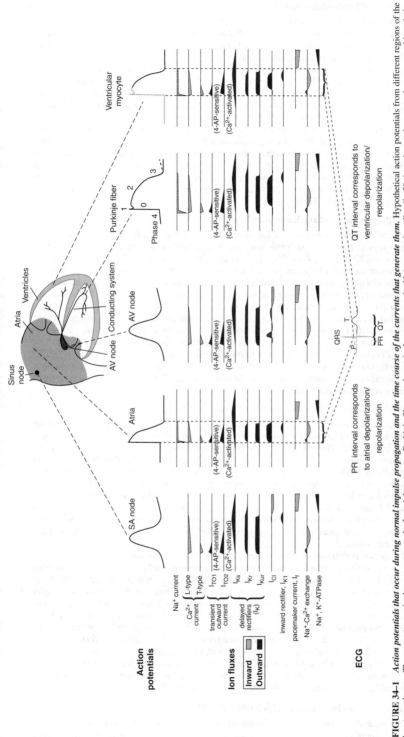

FIGURE 34-1 *Action potentials that occur during normal impulse propagation and the time course of the currents that generate them.* Hypothetical action potentials from different regions of the heart are shown. The current magnitudes are not to scale. In atrial myocytes, Purkinje fibers, and ventricular myocytes the Na$^+$ current is ordinarily 50 times larger than any other current, although the portion that persists into the plateau (phase 2) is small. Multiple types of Ca^{2+} current, transient outward current (I_{TO}), and delayed rectifier (I_K) have been identified. Each represents a different channel protein, usually associated with ancillary (function-modifying) subunits. 4-AP (4-aminopyridine) is a widely used *in vitro* blocker of K$^+$ channels. I_{TO2} may be a Cl$^-$ current in some species. Components of I_K have been separated on the basis of how rapidly they activate: slowly (I_{Ks}), rapidly (I_{Kr}), or ultrarapidly (I_{Kur}). For all currents shown here (with the possible exception of I_{TO2}), the genes encoding the major pore-forming proteins have been cloned.

Maintenance of Intracellular Homeostasis

With each action potential, the cell interior gains Na^+ ions and loses K^+ ions. The Na^+,K^+–ATPase is activated in most cells to maintain intracellular homeostasis, extruding 3 Na^+ ions for every 2 K^+ ions shuttled from the exterior of the cell to the interior; as a result, the act of pumping itself generates a net outward (repolarizing) current.

Normally, intracellular Ca^{2+} is maintained at very low levels (<100 nM). In cardiac myocytes, the entry of Ca^{2+} during each action potential is a signal to the sarcoplasmic reticulum to release its Ca^{2+} stores. The resulting increase in intracellular Ca^{2+} then triggers Ca^{2+}-dependent contraction. Removal of intracellular Ca^{2+} occurs by both an ATP-dependent Ca^{2+} pump (which moves Ca^{2+} ions back to storage sites in the sarcoplasmic reticulum) and an electrogenic Na^+–Ca^{2+} exchange mechanism in the cell membrane, which usually exchanges 3 Na^+ ions from the exterior for each Ca^{2+} ion extruded. Abnormal regulation of intracellular Ca^{2+}, characterized by contractile dysfunction, may contribute to arrhythmias in the setting of heart failure. The initial rise in Ca^{2+}, which serves as the trigger for Ca^{2+} release from intracellular stores, results from the opening of Ca^{2+} channels in the cell membrane or from Ca^{2+} entry through Na^+–Ca^{2+} exchange; i.e., in response to phase 0 entry of Na^+, the Na^+–Ca^{2+} exchange protein may transiently extrude Na^+ ions in exchange for Ca^{2+} ions (Figure 34–1).

Impulse Propagation and the Electrocardiogram

Normal cardiac impulses originate in the sinus node. Once impulses leave the sinus node, they propagate rapidly throughout the atria, resulting in atrial systole and the P wave of the electrocardiogram (ECG; Figure 34–1). Propagation slows markedly through the AV node, where the inward current (through Ca^{2+} channels) is much smaller than the Na^+ current in atria, ventricles, or the subendocardial conducting system. This conduction delay allows the atrial contraction to propel blood into the ventricle, thereby optimizing cardiac output. Once impulses exit the AV node, they enter the conducting system, where Na^+ currents are larger than in any other tissue. Hence propagation is correspondingly faster, up to 0.75 m/s longitudinally, and manifests as the QRS complex on the ECG as impulses spread from the endocardium to the epicardium, stimulating coordinated ventricular contraction. Ventricular repolarization results in the T wave of the ECG.

The ECG can be used as a rough guide to some cellular properties of cardiac tissue: (1) Heart rate reflects sinus node automaticity, (2) PR-interval duration reflects AV nodal conduction time, (3) QRS duration reflects conduction time in the ventricle, and (4) the QT interval is a measure of ventricular action potential duration.

Refractoriness: Fast-Response *versus* Slow-Response Tissue

If a single action potential, such as that shown in Figure 34–1, is restimulated very early during the plateau, no Na^+ channels are available to open, no inward current results, and no action potential is generated: The cell is refractory. On the other hand, if a stimulus occurs after the cell has repolarized completely, Na^+ channels have recovered, and a normal Na^+ channel–dependent upstroke results. When a stimulus occurs during phase 3 of the action potential, the magnitude of the resultant Na^+ current depends on the number of Na^+ channels that have recovered, which depends on the voltage at which the extra stimulus was applied. Thus, in atrial, ventricular, and His–Purkinje cells ("fast-response" cells), refractoriness is determined by the voltage-dependent recovery of Na^+ channels from inactivation. The effective refractory period *is the shortest interval at which a premature stimulus results in a propagated response and often is used to describe drug effects in intact tissue.*

The situation is different in Ca^{2+} channel–dependent ("slow-response") tissue such as the AV node. The major factor controlling recovery from inactivation of Ca^{2+} channels is time. Thus, even after a Ca^{2+} channel–dependent action potential has repolarized to its initial resting potential, not all Ca^{2+} channels are available for reexcitation. Therefore, an extra stimulus applied shortly after repolarization is complete generates a reduced Ca^{2+} current, which may propagate slowly to adjacent cells prior to extinction. An extra stimulus applied later will result in a larger Ca^{2+} current and faster propagation. Thus, in Ca^{2+} channel–dependent tissues, which include not only the AV node but also tissues whose underlying characteristics have been altered by factors such as myocardial ischemia, refractoriness is time-dependent, and propagation occurs slowly. Slow conduction in the heart, a critical factor in the genesis of reentrant arrhythmias (see below), also can occur when Na^+ currents are depressed by disease or membrane depolarization (e.g., elevated $[K]_o$), resulting in decreased steady-state Na^+ channel availability.

MECHANISMS OF CARDIAC ARRHYTHMIAS

When the normal sequence of impulse initiation and propagation is perturbed, an arrhythmia occurs. Failure of impulse initiation may result in slow heart rates (bradyarrhythmias), whereas failure of impulses to propagate normally from atrium to ventricle results in dropped beats (heart block) that usually reflect an abnormality in either the AV node or the His–Purkinje system. These abnormalities may be caused by drugs or by structural heart disease. Abnormally rapid heart rhythms (tachyarrhythmias) are common clinical problems that may be treated with antiarrhythmic drugs. Three major underlying mechanisms have been identified: enhanced automaticity, triggered automaticity, and reentry.

Enhanced Automaticity

Enhanced automaticity may occur in cells that normally display spontaneous diastolic depolarization—the sinus and AV nodes and the His–Purkinje system. β Adrenergic stimulation, hypokalemia, and mechanical stretch of cardiac muscle cells increase phase 4 slope and so accelerate pacemaker rate, whereas acetylcholine *reduces pacemaker rate both by decreasing phase 4 slope and by hyperpolarization (making the maximum diastolic potential more negative). In addition, automatic behavior may occur in sites that ordinarily lack spontaneous pacemaker activity; e.g., depolarization of ventricular cells by ischemia) may produce such "abnormal" automaticity.*

Afterdepolarizations and Triggered Automaticity

Under some pathophysiological conditions, a normal cardiac action potential may be interrupted or followed by an abnormal depolarization. If this abnormal depolarization reaches threshold, it may give rise to secondary upstrokes that can propagate and create abnormal rhythms. These abnormal secondary upstrokes occur only after an initial normal, or "triggering," upstroke and so are termed triggered rhythms.

Under conditions of intracellular Ca^{2+} overload (e.g., myocardial ischemia, adrenergic stress, digitalis intoxication, or heart failure), a normal action potential may be followed by a delayed afterdepolarization (DAD). If this afterdepolarization reaches threshold, a secondary triggered beat or beats may occur. In a second type of triggered activity, the key abnormality is marked prolongation of the cardiac action potential. When this occurs, phase 3 repolarization may be interrupted by an early afterdepolarization (EAD). EAD-mediated triggering clinical arrhythmias are most common when the underlying heart rate is slow, extracellular K^+ is low, and certain drugs that prolong action potential duration are present. EAD-related triggered upstrokes probably reflect inward current through Na^+ or Ca^{2+} channels or Na^+–Ca^{2+} exchange. When cardiac repolarization is markedly prolonged, polymorphic ventricular tachycardia with a long QT interval, known as torsades de pointes, *may occur. This arrhythmia is thought to be caused by EADs, which trigger "functionally defined" reentry owing to heterogeneity of action potential durations across the ventricular wall. Congenital long QT syndrome, a disease in which* torsades de pointes *is common, can be caused by mutations in the genes encoding the Na^+ or Ca^{2+} channels or, more commonly, the channels underlying the repolarizing currents I_{Kr} and I_{Ks}.*

Reentry
ANATOMICALLY DEFINED REENTRY

Reentry can occur when impulses propagate by more than one pathway between two points in the heart, and those pathways have heterogeneous electrophysiological properties. Patients with Wolff–Parkinson–White (WPW) syndrome have accessory connections between the atrium and ventricle. With each sinus node depolarization, impulses can excite the ventricle via the normal structures (AV node) or the accessory pathway. However, the electrophysiological properties of the AV node and accessory pathways are different: Accessory pathways usually consist of fast-response tissue, whereas the AV node is composed of slow-response tissue. Thus, with a premature atrial beat, conduction may fail in the accessory pathway but continue, albeit slowly, in the AV node and then through the His–Purkinje system; there the propagating impulse may encounter the ventricular end of the accessory pathway when it is no longer refractory. The likelihood that the accessory pathway is no longer refractory increases as AV nodal conduction slows. When the impulse reenters the atrium, it then can reenter the ventricle via the AV node, reenter the atrium via the accessory pathway, and so on. Reentry of this type, referred to as AV reentrant tachycardia, *is determined by (1) the presence of an anatomically defined circuit, (2) heterogeneity in refractoriness among regions in the circuit, and (3) slow conduction in one part of the circuit. Similar "anatomically defined" reentry commonly occurs in the region of the AV node (*AV nodal reentrant tachycardia*) and in the atrium (*atrial flutter*). The term* paroxysmal supraventricular tachycardia *(PSVT) includes both AV reentry and AV nodal reentry, which share many clinical features. It now sometimes is possible to identify and ablate critical portions of reentrant pathways (or automatic foci), thus curing the patient and obviating the need for long-term drug therapy.*

FUNCTIONALLY DEFINED REENTRY

Reentry also may occur in the absence of a distinct, anatomically defined pathway. If ischemia or other electrophysiological perturbations result in an area of sufficiently slow conduction in the ventricle, impulses exiting from that area may find the rest of the myocardium reexcitable, in which case fibrillation may ensue. Atrial or ventricular fibrillation is an extreme example of "functionally defined" (or "leading circle") reentry: Cells are reexcited as soon as they are repolarized sufficiently to allow enough Na^+ channels to recover. In this setting, neither organized activation patterns nor coordinated contractile activity is present.

Common Arrhythmias and Their Mechanisms

The primary tool for diagnosis of arrhythmias is the ECG. Table 34–2 lists common arrhythmias, their likely mechanisms, and approaches that should be considered for their acute termination and for long-term therapy to prevent recurrence. Some arrhythmias, notably ventricular fibrillation (VF), are best treated not with drugs but with direct current (dc) cardioversion—the application of a large electric current across the chest. Implantable cardioverter–defibrillators (ICDs), devices that are capable of detecting VF and automatically delivering a defibrillating shock, are used increasingly in patients judged to be at high risk for VF.

MECHANISMS OF ANTIARRHYTHMIC DRUG ACTION

A single arrhythmia may result from multiple mechanisms. Drugs may be antiarrhythmic by suppressing the initiating mechanism or by altering a reentrant circuit. In some cases, drugs may suppress the initiator but nonetheless promote reentry (*see* below).

Drugs may slow automatic rhythms by altering any of the four determinants of spontaneous pacemaker discharge: increase maximum diastolic potential, decrease phase 4 slope, increase threshold potential, or prolong action potential duration. *Adenosine* and acetylcholine may increase maximum diastolic potential, and *β adrenergic receptor antagonists* (β blockers) may decrease phase 4 slope. Block of Na^+ or Ca^{2+} channels usually results in altered threshold, and block of cardiac K^+ channels prolongs the action potential.

Antiarrhythmic drugs may block arrhythmias owing to DADs or EADs by two major mechanisms: (1) inhibition of the development of afterdepolarizations and (2) interference with the inward current (usually through Na^+ or Ca^{2+} channels), which is responsible for the upstroke. Thus, arrhythmias owing to *digitalis*-induced DADs may be inhibited by *verapamil* (which blocks the development of DAD) or by *quinidine* (which blocks Na^+ channels, thereby elevating the threshold required to produce the abnormal upstroke). Similarly, two approaches are used in arrhythmias related to EAD-induced triggered beats (Tables 34–2 and 34–3). EADs can be inhibited by shortening action potential duration; in practice, heart rate is accelerated by *isoproterenol* infusion or by pacing. Triggered beats arising from EADs can be inhibited by Mg^{2+} without normalizing repolarization *in vitro* or QT interval. In patients with congenitally long QT syndrome, *torsades de pointes* often occurs with adrenergic stress; therapies include β adrenergic blockade (which does not shorten the QT interval) and pacing.

In anatomically determined reentry, drugs may terminate the arrhythmia by blocking propagation of the action potential. In the example of the WPW-related arrhythmia described above, drugs that prolong AV nodal refractoriness and slow AV nodal conduction (*e.g.*, Ca^{2+} channel blockers, β adrenergic receptor antagonists, or digoxin) are likely to be effective but should be used with caution. On the other hand, slowing conduction in functionally determined reentrant circuits may change the pathway without extinguishing the circuit. Slow conduction generally promotes the development of reentrant arrhythmias, whereas the most likely approach for terminating functionally determined reentry is prolongation of refractoriness. In fast-response tissues, refractoriness is prolonged by delaying the recovery of Na^+ channels from inactivation. Drugs that block Na^+ channels generally shift the voltage dependence of recovery and so prolong refractoriness. Drugs that increase action potential duration without direct action on Na^+ channels (*e.g.*, by blocking delayed rectifier currents) also will prolong refractoriness. In slow-response tissues, Ca^{2+} channel block prolongs refractoriness.

State-Dependent Ion Channel Block

A key concept is that ion channel–blocking drugs bind to specific sites on ion channel proteins to modify function (*e.g.*, decrease current) and that the affinity of the ion channel protein for the drug on its target site varies as the ion channel protein shuttles among functional conformations (or ion

Table 34-2

A Mechanistic Approach to Antiarrhythmic Therapy

Arrhythmia	Common Mechanism	Acute Therapy[a]	Chronic Therapy[a]
Premature atrial, nodal, or ventricular depolarizations	Unknown	None indicated	None indicated
Atrial fibrillation	Disorganized "functional" reentry	1. Control ventricular response: AV nodal block[b] 2. Restore sinus rhythm: DC cardioversion	1. Control ventricular response: AV nodal block[b] 2. Maintain normal rhythm: K$^+$ channel block Na$^+$ channel block with $\tau_{recovery}$ >1 second
Atrial flutter	Continual AV node stimulation → irregular, often rapid, ventricular rate Stable reentrant circuit in the right atrium Ventricular rate often rapid and irregular	Same as atrial fibrillation	Same as atrial fibrillation AV nodal blocking drugs especially desirable to avoid ↑ ventricular rate Ablation in selected cases[c]
Atrial tachycardia	Enhanced automaticity, DAD-related automaticity, or reentry within the atrium	Same as atrial fibrillation	Same as atrial fibrillation Ablation of tachycardia "focus"[c]
AV nodal reentrant tachycardia (PSVT)	Reentrant circuit within or near AV node	*Adenosine AV nodal block Less commonly: ↑ vagal tone (digitalis, edrophonium, phenylephrine)	*AV nodal block Flecainide Propafenone *Ablation[c]
Arrhythmias associated with WPW syndrome: 1. AV reentry (PSVT)	Reentry	Same as AV nodal reentry	K$^+$ channel block Na$^+$ channel block with $\tau_{recovery}$ > 1 second Ablation[c]
2. Atrial fibrillation with atrioventricular conduction *via* accessory pathway	Very rapid rate due to nondecremental properties of accessory pathway	*DC cardioversion *Procainamide	Ablation[c] K$^+$ channel block Na$^+$ channel block with $\tau_{recovery}$ > 1 second (AV nodal blockers can be harmful)
VT in patients with remote myocardial infarction	Reentry near the rim of the healed myocardial infarction	Lidocaine Amiodarone Procainamide DC cardioversion	*ICD[d] *Amiodarone K$^+$ channel block Na$^+$ channel block

(*Continued*)

585

Table 34-2

A Mechanistic Approach to Antiarrhythmic Therapy *(Continued)*

Arrhythmia	Common Mechanism	Acute Therapy^a	Chronic Therapy^a
VT in patients without structural heart disease	DADs triggered by ↑ sympathetic tone	Adenosine^e Verapamil^e β-Blockers^e DC cardioversion	Verapamil^e β-Blockers^e
VF	Disorganized reentry	*DC cardioversion Lidocaine Amiodarone Procainamide	*ICD^d *Amiodarone K$^+$ channel block Na$^+$ channel block
Torsades de pointes, congenital or acquired; (often drug-related)	EAD-related triggered activity	Pacing Magnesium Isoproterenol	β-Blockade Pacing

*Indicates treatment of choice.

^{a}Acute drug therapy is administered intravenously; chronic therapy implies long-term oral use.

^{b}AV nodal block can be achieved clinically by adenosine, Ca^{2+} channel block, β adrenergic receptor blockade, or increased vagal tone (a major antiarrhythmic effect of digitalis glycosides).

^{c}Ablation is a procedure in which tissue responsible for the maintenance of a tachycardia is identified by specialized recording techniques and then selectively destroyed, usually by high-frequency radio waves delivered through a catheter placed in the heart.

^{d}ICD, implanted cardioverter/defibrillator. A device that can sense VT or VF and deliver pacing and/or cardioverting shocks to restore normal rhythm.

^{e}These may be harmful in reentrant VT and so should be used for acute therapy only if the diagnosis is secure.

ABBREVIATIONS: DAD, delayed afterdepolarization; EAD, early afterdepolarization; WPW, Wolff–Parkinson–White; PSVT, paroxysmal supraventricular tachycardia; VT, ventricular tachycardia; VF, ventricular fibrillation.

Table 34–3

Major Electrophysiological Actions of Antiarrhythmic Drugs

Drug	Na$^+$ Channel Block τ_{RECOVERY} ,[1] Seconds	State Dependence[1]	↑APD	Ca^{2+} Channel Block	Autonomic Effects	Other Effects
Lidocaine	0.1	I > O				
Phenytoin	0.2	I				
Mexiletine*	0.3					
Tocainide*	0.4	O > I				
Procainamide	1.8	O	✓		Ganglionic blockade (especially intravenous)	✓: Metabolite prolongs APD
Quinidine	3	O	✓	(x)	α-Blockade, vagolytic	
Disopyramide†	9	O	✓		Anticholinergic	
Moricizine	~10	O ≈ I				
Propafenone†	11	O ≈ I	✓		β-Blockade (variable clinical effect)	
Flecainide*	11	O	(x)	(x)		
β-Blockers: Propranolol†					β-Blockade	Na$^+$ channel block *in vitro*
Sotalol†			✓		β-Blockade	
Amiodarone	1.6	I	✓	(x)	Noncompetitive β-Blockade	Antithyroid action
Dofetilide			✓			
Ibutilide			✓			
Verapamil*				✓		
Diltiazem*				✓		
Digoxin					✓:Vagal stimulation	✓: Inhibition of Na$^+$, K$^+$–ATPase
Adenosine				✓	✓:Adenosine receptor activation	✓: Activation of outward K$^+$ current
Magnesium			?✓			Mechanism not well understood

✓indicates an effect that is important in mediating the clinical action of a drug.
(x)indicates a demonstrable effect whose relationship to drug action in patients is less well established.
*indicates drugs prescribed as racemates, and the enantiomers are thought to exert similar electrophysiological effects.
†indicates racemates for which clinically relevant differences in the electrophysiological properties of individual enantiomers have been reported (*see text*).
One approach to classifying drugs is:

Class	Major action
I	Na$^+$ channel block
II	β-Blockade
III	action potential prolongation (usually by K$^+$ channel block)
IV	Ca^{2+} channel block

Drugs are listed here according to this scheme. It is important to bear in mind, however, that many drugs exert multiple effects that contribute to their clinical actions. It is occasionally clinically useful to subclassify Na$^+$ channel blockers by their rates of recovery from drug-induced block (τ_{recovery}) under physiological conditions. Since this is a continuous variable and can be modulated by factors such as depolarization of the resting potential, these distinctions can become blurred: class Ib, $\tau_{\text{recovery}} < 1$ s; class Ia, τ_{recovery} 1–10 s; class Ic, $\tau_{\text{recovery}} > 10$ s. These class and subclass effects are associated with distinctive ECG changes, characteristic "class" toxicities, and efficacy in specific arrhythmia syndromes (*see text*).

[1]These data are dependent on experimental conditions, including species and temperature.

ABBREVIATIONS: O, Open state blocker; I, inactivated state blocker; APD, action potential duration.

channel "states"). Most useful antiarrhythmic agents that target Na^+ channels block the open and/or inactivated states and have very little affinity for channels in the resting state. Thus, with each action potential, drugs bind to Na^+ channels and block them, and with each diastolic interval, drugs dissociate, and the block is released. When heart rate increases, the time available for dissociation decreases, and steady-state Na^+ channel block increases. The rate of recovery from block also slows as cells are depolarized, as in ischemia. This explains the finding that Na^+ channel blockers depress Na^+ current, and hence conduction, to a greater extent in ischemic tissues than in normal tissues. Open versus inactivated-state block also may be important in determining the effects of some drugs. Increased action potential duration, which results in a relative increase in time spent in the inactivated state, may increase block by drugs that bind to inactivated channels, such as lidocaine or amiodarone.

The rate of recovery from block often is expressed as a time constant ($\tau_{recovery}$, the time required to complete ~63% of an exponentially determined process to be complete). In the case of drugs such as lidocaine, $\tau_{recovery}$ is so short (<<1 s) that recovery from block is very rapid, and substantial Na^+ channel block occurs only in rapidly driven tissues, particularly in ischemia. Conversely, drugs such as *flecainide* have such long $\tau_{recovery}$ values (>10 s) that roughly the same number of Na^+ channels is blocked during systole and diastole. As a result, marked slowing of conduction occurs even in normal tissues at normal rates.

Classifying Antiarrhythmic Drugs

To the extent that the clinical actions of drugs can be predicted, classifying drugs by common electrophysiological properties is useful. However, differences in pharmacological effects occur even among drugs that share the same classification, some of which may be responsible for the observed clinical differences in responses to drugs of the same broad "class" (Table 34–3). Another way of approaching therapy is to attempt to classify arrhythmia mechanisms and then to target drug therapy to the electrophysiological mechanism most likely to terminate or prevent the arrhythmia (Table 34–2).

Na^+ **CHANNEL BLOCK** The extent of Na^+ channel block depends critically on heart rate, membrane potential, and on drug-specific physicochemical characteristics that determine $\tau_{recovery}$. When Na^+ channels are blocked, threshold for excitability is decreased; *i.e.*, greater membrane depolarization is required to bring Na^+ channels from the rest to open states. This change in threshold probably contributes to the clinical finding that Na^+ channel blockers tend to increase both pacing threshold and the energy required for defibrillation. These deleterious effects may be important if antiarrhythmic drugs are used in patients with pacemakers or implanted defibrillators. Na^+ channel block decreases conduction velocity in fast-response tissue and increases QRS duration. Usual doses of flecainide prolong QRS intervals by 25% or more during normal rhythm, whereas lidocaine increases QRS intervals only at very fast heart rates. Drugs with $\tau_{recovery}$ values greater than 10 s (*e.g.*, flecainide) also tend to prolong the PR interval; it is not known whether this represents additional Ca^{2+} channel block or block of fast-response tissue in the region of the AV node. Drug effects on the PR interval also are highly modified by autonomic effects. For example, quinidine actually tends to shorten the PR interval, largely as a result of its vagolytic properties. Action potential duration is either unaffected or shortened by Na^+ channel block; some Na^+ channel–blocking drugs do prolong cardiac action potentials, but usually by K^+ channel block (Table 34–3).

Na^+ channel block decreases automaticity and can inhibit triggered activity arising from DADs or EADs. Many Na^+ channel blockers also decrease phase 4 slope. In anatomically defined reentry, Na^+ channel blockers may decrease conduction sufficiently to extinguish the propagating reentrant wavefront. However, as described earlier, conduction slowing owing to Na^+ channel block may exacerbate reentry. Thus, whether a given drug exacerbates or suppresses reentrant arrhythmias depends on the balance between its effects on refractoriness and on conduction in a particular reentrant circuit. Lidocaine and *mexiletine* have short $\tau_{recovery}$ values and are not useful in atrial fibrillation or flutter, whereas quinidine, flecainide, *propafenone,* and similar agents are effective in some patients. Many of these agents owe part of their antiarrhythmic activity to blockade of K^+ channels.

Na+ Channel–Blocker Toxicity Conduction slowing in potential reentrant circuits can account for toxicity of drugs that block the Na^+ channel (Table 34–1). For example, Na^+ channel block decreases conduction velocity and hence slows atrial flutter rate. Normal AV nodal function permits a greater number of impulses to penetrate the ventricle, and heart rate actually may increase. Thus, atrial flutter rate may drop from 300/min, with 2:1 or 4:1 AV conduction (*i.e.,* a heart rate of 150 or 75 beats/min), to 220/min, with 1:1 transmission to the ventricle (*i.e.,* a heart rate of 220 beats/min), with potentially disastrous consequences. This form of drug-induced arrhythmia is especially common with quinidine because it also increases AV nodal conduction through its vagolytic properties; flecainide and propafenone also have been implicated. Therapy with Na^+ channel blockers in patients with reentrant ventricular tachycardia after myocardial infarction can increase the frequency and severity of arrhythmic episodes. Slowed conduction allows the reentrant wavefront to persist within the tachycardia circuit. Such drug-exacerbated arrhythmia can be very difficult to manage, and deaths owing to intractable drug-induced ventricular tachycardia have been reported. In this setting, Na^+ infusion may be beneficial.

ACTION POTENTIAL PROLONGATION Most drugs that prolong the action potential do so by blocking K^+ currents, usually I_{Kr}, although enhanced inward Na^+ current also can cause prolongation. Enhanced inward current may underlie QT prolongation (and arrhythmia suppression) by *ibutilide.* Block of cardiac K^+ channels increases action potential duration and reduces normal automaticity. Increased action potential duration, seen as an increase in QT interval, increases refractoriness and therefore should be an effective way of treating reentry. Experimentally, K^+ channel block produces a series of desirable effects: reduced defibrillation energy requirement, inhibition of ventricular fibrillation owing to acute ischemia, and increased contractility. Most K^+ channel blocking drugs also interact with β adrenergic receptors (*sotalol*) or other channels (*e.g.,* amiodarone and quinidine) (*see* Table 34–3). Amiodarone and sotalol appear to be at least as effective as drugs with predominant Na^+ channel–blocking properties in both atrial and ventricular arrhythmias. "Pure" action potential–prolonging drugs (*e.g., dofetilide* and ibutilide) also are available.

Toxicity of Drugs That Prolong QT Interval Most of these agents disproportionately prolong cardiac action potentials when underlying heart rate is slow and can cause *torsades de pointes* (Table 34–1). While this effect usually is seen with QT-prolonging antiarrhythmic drugs, it can occur more rarely with drugs that are used for noncardiac indications. For such agents, the risk of *torsades de pointes* may become apparent only after widespread use postmarketing. For unknown reasons, drug-induced *torsades de pointes* associated with antiarrhythmic drugs is significantly more common in women.

Ca^{2+} CHANNEL BLOCK The major electrophysiological effects resulting from block of cardiac Ca^{2+} channels are in slow-response tissues, the sinus and AV nodes. Dihydropyridines such as *nifedipine,* which are used commonly in angina and hypertension, preferentially block Ca^{2+} channels in vascular smooth muscle; their cardiac effects, such as heart rate acceleration, result principally from reflex sympathetic activation secondary to peripheral vasodilation. Only verapamil, *diltiazem,* and *bepridil* block Ca^{2+} channels in cardiac cells at clinically used doses. These drugs generally slow heart rate, although hypotension can cause reflex sympathetic activation and tachycardia. The velocity of AV nodal conduction decreases, so the PR interval increases. AV nodal block occurs as a result of decremental conduction and increased AV nodal refractoriness, which form the basis for the use of Ca^{2+} channel blockers in reentrant arrhythmias whose circuit involves the AV node, such as AV reentrant tachycardia.

Another important indication for antiarrhythmic therapy is to reduce ventricular rate in atrial flutter or fibrillation. Rare forms of ventricular tachycardia appear to be DAD-mediated and respond to verapamil. Parenteral verapamil and diltiazem are approved for rapid conversion of PSVTs to sinus rhythm and for temporary control of rapid ventricular rate in atrial flutter or fibrillation. Oral verapamil may be used in conjunction with digoxin to control ventricular rate in chronic atrial flutter or fibrillation and for prophylaxis of repetitive PSVT. Unlike β adrenergic receptor antagonists, Ca^{2+} channel blockers have not been shown to reduce mortality after myocardial infarction.

Toxicity of Ca^{2+} Channel Blockers The major adverse effect of intravenous verapamil or diltiazem is hypotension, particularly with bolus administration. This is a particular problem if the drugs are used mistakenly in patients with ventricular tachycardia misdiagnosed as AV nodal reentrant tachycardia. Hypotension also is frequent in patients receiving other vasodilators, including quinidine, and in patients with underlying left ventricular dysfunction, which the drugs can exacerbate. Severe sinus bradycardia or AV block also occurs, especially in patients also receiving β blockers. With oral therapy, these adverse effects tend to be less severe.

Verapamil (CALAN, ISOPTIN, VERELAN, COVERA-HS) is prescribed as a racemate. L-Verapamil is a more potent calcium channel blocker than is D-verapamil. However, with oral therapy, the L-enantiomer undergoes more extensive first-pass hepatic metabolism. For this reason, a given concentration of verapamil prolongs the PR interval to a greater extent when administered intravenously (where concentrations of the L- and D-enantiomers are equivalent) than when administered orally. *Diltiazem* (CARDIZEM, TIAZAC, DILACOR XR, and others) also undergoes extensive first-pass hepatic metabolism, and both drugs have metabolites that exert Ca^{2+} channel–blocking actions. Adverse effects during therapy with verapamil or diltiazem are determined largely by underlying heart disease and concomitant therapy; plasma concentrations of these agents are not measured routinely. Both drugs can increase serum digoxin concentration, although the magnitude of this effect is variable; excess slowing of ventricular response may occur in patients with atrial fibrillation. Constipation can occur with oral verapamil.

BLOCK OF β ADRENERGIC RECEPTORS β Adrenergic stimulation increases the magnitude of the Ca^{2+} current and slows its inactivation, increases the magnitude of repolarizing K^+ and Cl^- currents, increases pacemaker current (thereby increasing sinus rate), and under pathophysiological conditions, can increase both DAD- and EAD-mediated arrhythmias. The increases in plasma Epi associated with severe stress (*e.g.*, acute myocardial infarction or resuscitation from cardiac arrest) lower serum K^+, especially in patients receiving chronic diuretic therapy. β Adrenergic receptor antagonists inhibit these effects and can be antiarrhythmic by reducing heart rate, decreasing intracellular Ca^{2+} overload, and inhibiting afterdepolarization-mediated automaticity. Epi-induced hypokalemia appears to be mediated by β_2 adrenergic receptors and is blocked by "noncardioselective" antagonists such as *propranolol* (*see* Chapter 10). In acutely ischemic tissue, β blockers increase the energy required to fibrillate the heart, an antiarrhythmic action. These effects may contribute to the reduced mortality observed in trials of acute and chronic therapy with β blockers after myocardial infarction.

As with Ca^{2+} channel blockers and digitalis, β blockers slow AV nodal conduction and prolong AV nodal refractoriness; hence, they are useful in terminating reentrant arrhythmias that involve the AV node and in controlling ventricular response in atrial fibrillation or flutter. In some patients, including many with the congenital long QT syndrome, arrhythmias are triggered by physical or emotional stress; β blockers may be useful in these cases. β adrenergic receptor antagonists also reportedly are effective in controlling arrhythmias owing to Na^+ channel blockers; this effect may be due in part to slowing of the heart rate, which then decreases the extent of rate-dependent conduction slowing by Na^+ channel block.

Selected β Adrenergic Receptor Blockers The β antagonists likely share antiarrhythmic properties. Some, such as propranolol, also exert Na^+ channel–blocking ("membrane stabilizing") effects at high concentrations, but the clinical significance of this effect is uncertain. Drugs with intrinsic sympathomimetic activity may be less useful as antiarrhythmics. Sotalol (*see* below) is more effective for many arrhythmias than are other β blockers probably because of its K^+ channel–blocking actions. *Esmolol* is a β_1 selective agent that is metabolized by erythrocyte esterases and so has a very short elimination $t_{1/2}$ (9 minutes). Intravenous esmolol is useful when immediate β adrenergic blockade is desired (*e.g.*, for rate control of rapidly conducted atrial fibrillation). Because of esmolol's very rapid elimination, adverse effects due to β adrenergic blockade—should they occur—dissipate rapidly.

Toxicity of β Adrenergic Blockers Adverse effects of β blockade include fatigue, bronchospasm, hypotension, impotence, depression, aggravation of heart failure, worsening of symptoms owing to peripheral vascular disease, and masking of the symptoms of hypoglycemia in diabetic patients. In patients with arrhythmias owing to excess sympathetic stimulation (*e.g.*, pheochromocytoma or *clonidine* withdrawal), β blockers can cause unopposed α adrenergic stimulation, resulting in severe hypertension and/or α adrenergic-mediated arrhythmias. In such patients, arrhythmias should be treated with both α and β adrenergic antagonists or with a drug such as *labetalol* that combines α and β blocking properties. Abrupt discontinuation of chronic β blocker therapy can lead to "rebound" symptoms, including hypertension, increased angina, and arrhythmias; thus, β receptor antagonist therapy is tapered over 2 weeks.

PRINCIPLES IN THE CLINICAL USE OF ANTIARRHYTHMIC DRUGS

Drugs that modify cardiac electrophysiology often have a narrow therapeutic index. Moreover, antiarrhythmic drugs can induce new arrhythmias with possibly fatal consequences. Nonpharmacological treatments, such as cardiac pacing, electrical defibrillation, or ablation of targeted regions, are indicated for some arrhythmias; in other cases, no therapy is required, even though an arrhythmia is detected. Therefore, the fundamental principles of therapeutics described here must be applied to optimize antiarrhythmic therapy.

1. Identify and Remove Precipitating Factors

Factors that commonly precipitate cardiac arrhythmias include hypoxia, electrolyte disturbances (especially hypokalemia), myocardial ischemia, and certain drugs (Table 34–1). For example, theophylline *can cause multifocal atrial tachycardia, while* torsades de pointes *can arise not only during therapy with action potential–prolonging antiarrhythmics but also with other drugs, including* erythromycin (see *Chapter 46);* pentamidine (see *Chapter 40); and some antipsychotics, notably* thioridazine *(see Chapter 18).*

2. Establish the Goals of Treatment
SOME ARRHYTHMIAS SHOULD NOT BE TREATED: THE *CAST* EXAMPLE

The mere detection of an abnormal cardiac rhythm does not equate with the need for therapy. In the CAST trial, patients convalescing from myocardial infarction whose ventricular ectopic beats were suppressed by the Na$^+$ channel blockers encainide *(no longer marketed) or* flecainide *were randomly assigned to receive those drugs or placebo. Unexpectedly, the mortality rate was two- to threefold higher among patients treated with drugs than those treated with placebo. This pivotal trial reemphasized the concept that therapy should be initiated only when a clear benefit can be identified. When symptoms are obviously attributable to an ongoing arrhythmia, there usually is little doubt that termination of the arrhythmia will be beneficial; when chronic therapy is used to prevent recurrence of an arrhythmia, the risks may be greater.* Among the antiarrhythmic drugs discussed here, only β adrenergic blockers and, to a lesser extent, amiodarone have been shown to reduce mortality during long-term therapy.

SYMPTOMS DUE TO ARRHYTHMIAS

If patients with an arrhythmia are asymptomatic, establishing any benefit for treatment will be very difficult. Some patients may present with presyncope, syncope, or even cardiac arrest, which may be due to brady- or tachyarrhythmias. The sensation of irregular heartbeats (i.e., palpitations) can be minimally symptomatic in some individuals and incapacitating in others. The irregular heartbeats may be due to intermittent premature contractions or to sustained arrhythmias such as atrial fibrillation (which results in an irregular ventricular rate). Finally, arrhythmias in some patients may present with symptoms owing to decreased cardiac output. The most common symptom is breathlessness either at rest or on exertion. Rarely, sustained tachycardias may produce no "arrhythmia" symptoms (such as palpitations) but will depress contractile function; these patients may present with congestive heart failure that can be controlled by treating the arrhythmia.

CHOOSING AMONGST THERAPEUTIC APPROACHES

In choosing among therapeutic options, it is important to establish clear goals. For example, three options are available in patients with atrial fibrillation: (1) Reduce the ventricular response using AV nodal blocking agents such as digitalis, verapamil, diltiazem, or β adrenergic antagonists (Table 34–2); (2) restore and maintain normal rhythm using drugs such as quinidine, flecainide, or amiodarone; or (3) decide not to implement antiarrhythmic therapy, especially if the patient truly is asymptomatic. Most patients with atrial fibrillation also benefit from anticoagulation to reduce stroke incidence regardless of symptoms.

Factors contributing to choice of therapy include not only symptoms but also the type and extent of structural heart disease, the QT interval prior to drug therapy, the coexistence of conduction system disease, and the presence of noncardiac diseases. In the rare patient with the WPW syndrome and atrial fibrillation, the ventricular response can be extremely rapid and can be accelerated paradoxically by AV nodal blocking drugs such as digitalis or Ca^{2+} channel blockers; deaths owing to drug therapy have been reported.

The frequency and reproducibility of arrhythmia should be established prior to initiating therapy because inherent variability in the occurrence of arrhythmias can be confused with a beneficial or adverse drug effect. Techniques for this assessment include recording cardiac rhythm for prolonged periods or evaluating the response of the heart to artificially induced premature beats. It is important to recognize that drug therapy may be only partially effective: A marked decrease in the duration of paroxysms of atrial fibrillation may be sufficient to render a patient asymptomatic even if an occasional episode still can be detected.

3. Minimize Risks
ANTIARRHYTHMIC DRUGS CAN CAUSE ARRHYTHMIAS

One well-recognized risk of antiarrhythmic therapy is the possibility of provoking new arrhythmias, with potentially life-threatening consequences. Antiarrhythmic drugs can provoke arrhythmias by different mechanisms (Table 34–1). These drug-provoked arrhythmias must be recognized because further treatment with antiarrhythmic drugs often exacerbates the problem. Targeting therapies at underlying mechanisms of the arrhythmias may be required.

MONITORING OF PLASMA CONCENTRATION

Some adverse effects of antiarrhythmic drugs result from excessive drug levels. Measuring plasma concentration and adjusting the dose to maintain the concentration within a prescribed therapeutic range may minimize some adverse effects. In many patients, serious adverse reactions relate to interactions involving antiarrhythmic drugs (often at usual plasma concentrations), transient factors such as electrolyte disturbances or myocardial ischemia, and the type and extent of the underlying heart disease.

PATIENT-SPECIFIC CONTRAINDICATIONS

Another way to minimize the adverse effects of antiarrhythmic drugs is to avoid certain drugs in certain patient subsets altogether. In other cases, adverse effects of drugs may be difficult to distinguish from exacerbations of underlying disease. Amiodarone may cause interstitial lung disease; its use therefore is undesirable in a patient with advanced pulmonary disease in whom the development of this potentially fatal adverse effect would be difficult to detect.

ANTIARRHYTHMIC DRUGS

Ca^{2+} channel blockers and β adrenergic antagonists were considered above. The other antiarrhythmic drugs are presented below in alphabetical order, and some pharmacologic properties are summarized in Table 34–4.

ADENOSINE   Adenosine (ADENOCARD) is a nucleoside that is administered as a rapid intravenous bolus for the acute termination of reentrant supraventricular arrhythmias. Rare cases of ventricular tachycardia in patients with otherwise normal hearts are thought to be DAD-mediated and can be terminated by adenosine. Adenosine also has been used to produce controlled hypotension during some surgical procedures and in the diagnosis of coronary artery disease.

Pharmacological Effects   The effects of adenosine are mediated *via* specific GPCRs (*see* Chapter 11). Adenosine activates acetylcholine-sensitive K^+ current in the atrium and sinus and AV nodes, resulting in shortening of action potential duration, hyperpolarization, and slowing of normal automaticity. Adenosine also inhibits the electrophysiological effects of increased cellular cyclic AMP that occur with sympathetic stimulation. Because adenosine thereby reduces Ca^{2+} currents, it can be antiarrhythmic by increasing AV nodal refractoriness and by inhibiting DADs elicited by sympathetic stimulation. Administration of an intravenous bolus of adenosine transiently slows sinus rate and AV nodal conduction velocity and increases AV nodal refractoriness. A bolus of adenosine can produce transient sympathetic activation by interacting with carotid baroreceptors; a continuous infusion can cause hypotension.

Adverse Effects   A major advantage of adenosine therapy is that adverse effects are short-lived because the drug is transported into cells and deaminated so rapidly. Transient asystole is common but usually lasts less than 5 seconds and is in fact the therapeutic goal. Most patients feel a sense of chest fullness and dyspnea when therapeutic doses (6–12 mg) of adenosine are administered. Rarely, an adenosine bolus can precipitate bronchospasm or atrial fibrillation.

Clinical Pharmacokinetics   Adenosine is eliminated with a $t_{1/2}$ of seconds by carrier-mediated uptake in most cell types and subsequent metabolism by adenosine deaminase. Adenosine probably is the only antiarrhythmic drug whose efficacy requires a rapid bolus dose, preferably through a large central intravenous line; slow administration permits elimination of the drug prior to its arrival at the heart. The effects of adenosine are potentiated in patients receiving *dipyridamole,* an adenosine-uptake inhibitor, and in patients with cardiac transplants owing to denervation hypersensitivity. Methylxanthines (*e.g.,* theophylline and caffeine) block adenosine receptors; therefore, larger than usual doses are required to produce an antiarrhythmic effect in patients who have consumed these agents in beverages or as therapy.

Table 34-4

Pharmacokinetic Characteristics and Doses of Antiarrhythmic Drugs

Drug	Bioavailability Reduced: 1st Pass Metabolism	Protein Binding >80%	Elimination Renal	Elimination Hepatic	Elimination Other	Active Metabolite(s)	Therapeutic[+] Plasma Concentration	Usual Doses[‡] Loading Doses	Maintenance Doses
Adenosine[§]					✓				
Amiodarone		✓		✓		✓	0.5–2 μg/mL	6–12 mg (IV only) 800–1600 mg/day × 2–4 weeks (IV: 100–300 mg)	100–400 mg/day
Digoxin	~80%		✓				0.5–2.0 ng/mL	1 mg over 12–24 h	0.125–0.375 mg q24h
Digitoxin	>80%	✓		✓		(Digoxin)	10–30 ng/mL		0.05–0.3 mg q24h
Diltiazem	✓			✓		(x)		0.25–0.35 mg/kg over 10 min (IV)	5–15 mg/h (IV) 30–90 mg q6h 120–300 mg q24h[¶]
Disopyramide	>80%		✓			(x)	2–5 μg/mL		100–200 mg q6h 200–400 mg q12h[¶]
Dofetilide	>80%		✓	(x)					0.25–0.5 mg q12h[¶¶]
Esmolol					✓			0.5 mg/kg/min; may repeat × 2 (IV)	0.05–0.2 mg/kg/min (IV)
Flecainide	>80%			✓			0.2–1 μg/mL		50–200 mg q12h
Ibutilide	✓			✓				1 mg (IV) over 10 min; may repeat once 10 min later	
Lidocaine	✓	✓		✓		(x)	1.5–5 μg/mL	3–4 mg/kg over 20–30 min (IV)	1–4 mg/min (IV)
Mexiletine	>80%			✓			0.5–2 μg/mL		100–300 mg q8h
Moricizine	✓	✓		✓					200–300 mg q8h
Procainamide	>80%		✓	✓		✓	4–8 μg/mL	1 g (IV), given at 20 mg/min	1–4 mg/min (IV) 250–750 mg q3h 500–1000 mg q6h[¶]

Elimination t$_{1/2}$[*]: Adenosine <10 s; Amiodarone Weeks; Digoxin 36 h; Digitoxin 7–9 days; Diltiazem 4 h; Disopyramide 4–10 h; Dofetilide 7–10 h; Esmolol 5–10 min; Flecainide 10–18 h; Ibutilide 6 h; Lidocaine 120 min; Mexiletine 9–15 h; Moricizine 2–3 h; Procainamide 3–4 h.

593

(Continued)

Table 34-4

Pharmacokinetic Characteristics and Doses of Antiarrhythmic Drugs (Continued)

	Bioavailability	Protein Binding >80%	Elimination			Elimination $t_{1/2}$[*]	Active Metabolite(s)	Usual Doses[‡]		
Drug	Reduced: 1st Pass Metabolism		Renal	Hepatic	Other			Therapeutic[†] Plasma Concentration	Loading Doses	Maintenance Doses
(N–Acetyl procainamide)	(>80%)		(✓)			(6–10 h)		(10–20 μg/mL)		150–300 mg q8h
Propafenone	✓			✓		2–32 h	✓	<1 μg/mL	1–3 mg (IV)	10–80 mg q6–8h
Propranolol	✓	✓		✓		4 h				80–240 mg q24h[¶]
Quinidine	>80%	~80%	(x)	✓		4–10 h	✓	2–5 μg/mL		324–648 mg (gluconate) q8h
Sotalol	>80%		✓			8 h		<5 μg/mL (?)		80–320 mg q12h
Tocainide	>80%		✓			15 h		3–11 μg/mL		400–600 mg q8h
Verapamil	✓	✓		✓		3–7 h	✓		5–10 mg (IV)	80–120 mg q8h
										120–240 mg q24h[¶]

(x): metabolite or route of elimination probably of minor clinical importance.

[*]The elimination half-life is one, but not the only, determinant of how frequently a drug must be administered to maintain a therapeutic effect and avoid toxicity (Chapter 5: Principles of Therapeutics). For some drugs with short elimination half-lives, infrequent dosing is nevertheless possible, e.g., propranolol or verapamil. Formulations that allow slow release into the gastrointestinal tract of a rapidly eliminated compound (available for many drugs including procainamide, disopyramide, verapamil, diltiazem, and propranolol) also allow infrequent dosing.

[†]The therapeutic range is bounded by a plasma concentration below which no therapeutic effect is likely, and an upper concentration above which the risk of adverse effects increases. As discussed in the text, many serious adverse reactions to antiarrhythmic drugs can occur at "therapeutic" concentrations in susceptible individuals. When only an upper limit is cited, a lower limit has not been well defined. Variable generation of active metabolites may further complicate the interpretation of plasma concentration data (Chapters 1: Pharmacokinetics: The Dynamics of Drug Absorption, Distribution, and Elimination and 5: Principles of Therapeutics).

[‡]Oral doses are presented unless otherwise indicated. Doses are presented as suggested ranges in adults of average build; lower doses are less likely to produce toxicity. Lower maintenance dosages may be required in patients with renal or hepatic disease. Loading doses are only indicated when a therapeutic effect is desired before maintenance therapy would bring drug concentrations into a therapeutic range, i.e., for acute therapy (e.g., lidocaine, verapamil, adenosine) or when the elimination half-life is extremely long (amiodarone).

[§]Bioavailability reduced by incomplete absorption.

[∥]Indicates suggested dosage using slow-release formulation.

[¶]This drug is available only in a restricted distribution system (see text).

ABBREVIATIONS: IV, intravenous; q, every.

AMIODARONE *Amiodarone* (CORDARONE, PACERONE) exerts multiple pharmacological effects, none of which is clearly linked to its arrhythmia-suppressing properties. Amiodarone is a structural analog of thyroid hormone, and some of its antiarrhythmic actions and its toxicity may be attributable to interaction with thyroid hormone receptors. Amiodarone is highly lipophilic, is concentrated in many tissues, and is eliminated extremely slowly; consequently, adverse effects may resolve very slowly. In the U.S., the drug is indicated for oral therapy in patients with recurrent ventricular tachycardia or fibrillation resistant to other drugs. Oral amiodarone also is effective in maintaining sinus rhythm in patients with atrial fibrillation. An intravenous form is indicated for acute termination of ventricular tachycardia or fibrillation and is supplanting lidocaine as first-line therapy for out-of-hospital cardiac arrest. Oral amiodarone has a modest beneficial effect on mortality after acute myocardial infarction. Despite uncertainties about its mechanisms of action and the potential for serious toxicity, amiodarone now is used very widely in the treatment of common arrhythmias such as atrial fibrillation.

Pharmacological Effects Amiodarone blocks inactivated Na^+ channels and has a relatively rapid rate of recovery ($\tau_{recovery}$ ~1.6 s) from block. It also decreases Ca^{2+} current and transient outward delayed rectifier and inward rectifier K^+ currents and exerts a noncompetitive adrenergic blocking effect. Amiodarone potently inhibits abnormal automaticity and, in most tissues, prolongs action potential duration. Amiodarone decreases conduction velocity by Na^+ channel block and by a poorly understood effect on cell–cell coupling that may be especially important in diseased tissue. Prolongations of the PR, QRS, and QT intervals and sinus bradycardia are frequent during chronic therapy. Amiodarone prolongs refractoriness in all cardiac tissues; Na^+ channel block, delayed repolarization owing to K^+ channel block, and inhibition of cell–cell coupling all may contribute to this effect.

Adverse Effects Hypotension owing to vasodilation and depressed myocardial performance are frequent with the intravenous form of amiodarone. While depressed contractility can occur during long-term oral therapy, it is unusual. Despite administration of high doses that would cause serious toxicity if continued long-term, adverse effects are unusual during oral drug-loading regimens, which typically require several weeks. Occasional patients develop nausea during the loading phase, which responds to a decrease in daily dose. Adverse effects during long-term therapy reflect both the size of daily maintenance doses and the cumulative dose (*i.e.,* duration of therapy), suggesting that tissue accumulation may be responsible. The most serious adverse effect during chronic amiodarone therapy is pulmonary fibrosis, which can be rapidly progressive and fatal. Underlying lung disease, doses of 400 mg/day or more, and recent pulmonary insults such as pneumonia appear to be risk factors. Monitoring plasma concentrations has not been useful; serial chest x-rays or pulmonary function studies may detect early amiodarone toxicity. With low doses, such as 200 mg/day or less used in atrial fibrillation, pulmonary toxicity is unusual. Other adverse effects during long-term therapy include corneal microdeposits (which often are asymptomatic), hepatic dysfunction, neuromuscular symptoms (*e.g.,* peripheral neuropathy or proximal muscle weakness), photosensitivity, and hypo- or hyperthyroidism. Treatment for life-threatening pulmonary toxicity consists of drug withdrawal and supportive measures, including glucocorticoids. Dose reduction may be sufficient if the drug is deemed necessary and the adverse effect is not life-threatening. Despite the marked QT prolongation and bradycardia typical of chronic amiodarone therapy, *torsades de pointes* and other drug-induced tachyarrhythmias are unusual.

Clinical Pharmacokinetics Amiodarone's oral bioavailability, ~30%, must be considered when calculating equivalent dosing regimens in converting from intravenous to oral therapy. After the initiation of amiodarone therapy, increases in refractoriness, a marker of pharmacological effect, require several weeks to develop. Amiodarone undergoes hepatic metabolism by CYP3A4 to desethyl-amiodarone, a metabolite with pharmacological effects similar to those of the parent drug. When amiodarone therapy is withdrawn from a patient who has been receiving therapy for several years, plasma concentrations decline with a $t_{1/2}$ of weeks to months. The mechanism whereby amiodarone and desethyl-amiodarone are eliminated is not well established. A therapeutic plasma amiodarone concentration range of 0.5–2 μg/mL has been proposed. However, efficacy apparently depends as much on duration of therapy as on plasma concentration, and elevated plasma concentrations do not predict toxicity. Because of amiodarone's slow accumulation in tissue, a high-dose oral loading regimen (*e.g.,* 800–1600 mg/day) usually is administered for several weeks before maintenance therapy is started. Maintenance dose is adjusted based on adverse effects and the arrhythmias being treated. If the presenting arrhythmia is life-threatening, dosages of more than

300 mg/day normally are used unless unequivocal toxicity occurs. On the other hand, maintenance doses of 200 mg/day or less are used if recurrence of an arrhythmia would be tolerated, as in patients with atrial fibrillation. Because of its very slow elimination, amiodarone is administered once daily, and omission of one or two doses during chronic therapy rarely results in recurrence of arrhythmia. Dosage adjustments are not required in hepatic, renal, or cardiac dysfunction. Amiodarone potently inhibits the hepatic metabolism or renal elimination of many drugs. Mechanisms include inhibition of CYP3A4, CYP2C9, and P-glycoprotein (*see* Chapter 3). Dosages of warfarin, other antiarrhythmics (*e.g.,* flecainide, procainamide, and quinidine), or digoxin usually require reduction during amiodarone therapy.

CARDIAC GLYCOSIDES

Pharmacological Effects Cardiac glycosides exert positive inotropic effects and thus are also used in heart failure (*see* Chapter 33). Their inotropic action results from increased intracellular Ca^{2+}, which also forms the basis for arrhythmias related to cardiac glycoside intoxication. Cardiac glycosides increase phase 4 slope (*i.e.,* increase the rate of automaticity), especially if $[K]_o$ is low. They also exert prominent vagotonic actions, resulting in inhibition of Ca^{2+} currents in the AV node and activation of acetylcholine-mediated K^+ currents in the atrium. Thus, the major "indirect" electrophysiological effects of cardiac glycosides are hyperpolarization, shortening of atrial action potentials, and increases in AV nodal refractoriness. The latter action accounts for the utility of digitalis in terminating reentrant arrhythmias involving the AV node and in controlling ventricular response in patients with atrial fibrillation. Cardiac glycosides may be especially useful in the latter situation because many such patients have heart failure, which can be exacerbated by other AV nodal blocking drugs such as Ca^{2+} channel blockers or β adrenergic receptor antagonists. However, sympathetic drive is increased markedly in many patients with advanced heart failure, so digitalis is not very effective in decreasing the rate; on the other hand, even a modest decrease in rate can ameliorate heart failure. Similarly, in other conditions in which high sympathetic tone drives rapid atrioventricular conduction (*e.g.,* chronic lung disease and thyrotoxicosis), digitalis therapy may be only marginally effective in slowing the rate. In heart transplant patients, in whom innervation has been ablated, cardiac glycosides are ineffective for rate control. Increased sympathetic activity and hypoxia can potentiate digitalis-induced changes in automaticity and DADs, thus increasing the risk of digitalis toxicity. A further complicating feature in thyrotoxicosis is increased digoxin clearance. The major ECG effects of cardiac glycosides are PR prolongation and a nonspecific alteration in ventricular repolarization (manifested by depression of the ST segment), whose underlying mechanism is not well understood.

Adverse Effects Because of the low therapeutic index of cardiac glycosides, toxicity is common, including arrhythmias, nausea, disturbances of cognitive function, and blurred or yellow vision. Elevated serum concentrations of digitalis, hypoxia, and electrolyte abnormalities (*e.g.,* hypokalemia, hypomagnesemia, and hypercalcemia) predispose patients to digitalis-induced arrhythmias. While digitalis intoxication can cause virtually any arrhythmia, arrhythmias that should raise a strong suspicion of digitalis intoxication are those in which DAD-related tachycardias occur along with impairment of sinus node or AV nodal function. Atrial tachycardia with AV block is classic, but ventricular bigeminy (sinus beats alternating with beats of ventricular origin), "bidirectional" ventricular tachycardia, AV junctional tachycardias, and various degrees of AV block also can occur. With severe intoxication (*e.g.,* with suicidal ingestion), severe hyperkalemia owing to poisoning of Na^+,K^+–ATPase and profound bradyarrhythmias are seen. In patients with elevated serum digitalis levels, the risk of precipitating ventricular fibrillation by DC cardioversion probably is increased; in those with therapeutic blood levels, DC cardioversion can be used safely. Minor forms of cardiac glycoside intoxication may require no specific therapy beyond monitoring cardiac rhythm until symptoms and signs of toxicity resolve. Sinus bradycardia and AV block often respond to intravenous atropine, but the effect is transient. Mg^{2+} has been used successfully in some cases of digitalis-induced tachycardia. Any serious arrhythmia should be treated with antidigoxin Fab fragments (DIGIBIND), which bind digoxin and digitoxin and greatly enhance their renal excretion. Temporary cardiac pacing may be required for advanced sinus node or AV node dysfunction. Digitalis exerts direct arterial vasoconstrictor effects, and mesenteric and coronary ischemia can occur, especially in patients with advanced atherosclerosis who receive intravenous drug.

Clinical Pharmacokinetics The most commonly used digitalis glycoside in the U.S. is *digoxin* (LANOXIN), although *digitoxin* (various generic preparations) also is used. Digoxin tablets are incompletely (75%) bioavailable, but capsules are >90% bioavailable. In some patients, intestinal microflora may metabolize digoxin, markedly reducing bioavailability. In these patients, higher than usual doses are required for clinical efficacy; toxicity is a serious risk if antibiotics such as *tetracycline* or erythromycin are administered because these drugs can destroy intestinal microflora. Inhibition of P-glycoprotein also may play a role. Digoxin is 20–30% protein-bound. The antiarrhythmic effects of digoxin can be achieved with intravenous or oral therapy. However, digoxin undergoes relatively slow distribution to effector site(s); therefore, even with intravenous therapy, there is a lag of several hours between drug administration and the development of measurable antiarrhythmic effects such as PR-interval prolongation or slowing of the ventricular rate in atrial fibrillation. To avoid intoxication, a loading dose of ~1–1.5 mg digoxin is administered over 24 hours. Measurement of postdistribution serum digoxin concentration and adjustment of the daily dose (0.125–0.375 mg) to maintain concentrations of 0.5–2 ng/mL are useful during chronic therapy. Some patients may require and tolerate higher concentrations, but with an increased risk of adverse effects. The elimination $t_{1/2}$ of digoxin ordinarily is ~36 hours, so maintenance doses are administered once daily. Most digoxin is renally excreted as unchanged drug. Digoxin doses should be reduced (or dosing interval increased) and serum concentrations monitored closely in patients with impaired excretion owing to renal failure or in patients who are hypothyroid. Digitoxin undergoes primarily hepatic metabolism and may be useful in patients with fluctuating or advanced renal dysfunction. Digitoxin metabolism is accelerated by drugs such as *phenytoin* and *rifampin* that induce hepatic metabolism. Digitoxin's elimination $t_{1/2}$ is ~7 days; it is highly protein-bound, and its therapeutic range is 10–30 ng/mL. Amiodarone, quinidine, verapamil, diltiazem, *cyclosporine, itraconazole,* propafenone, and flecainide decrease digoxin clearance, likely by inhibiting P-glycoprotein, the major route of digoxin elimination. New steady-state digoxin concentrations are approached in about a week. Digitalis toxicity results so often with quinidine or amiodarone that it is routine to decrease the dose of digoxin if these drugs are started. In all cases, digoxin concentrations should be measured regularly and the dose adjusted if necessary. Hypokalemia will potentiate digitalis-induced arrhythmias.

DISOPYRAMIDE *Disopyramide* (NORPACE, others) exerts electrophysiological effects very similar to those of quinidine, but the drugs have different adverse effects. Disopyramide is used to maintain sinus rhythm in patients with atrial flutter or atrial fibrillation and to prevent recurrence of ventricular tachycardia or ventricular fibrillation.

Pharmacological Actions and Adverse Effects Disopyramide is prescribed as a racemate. The *in vitro* electrophysiological actions of *S*-(+)-disopyramide are similar to those of quinidine. The *R*-(–)-enantiomer produces similar Na⁺ channel block but does not prolong cardiac action potentials. Unlike quinidine, racemic disopyramide is not an α adrenergic receptor antagonist, but it does exert prominent anticholinergic actions that account for many of its adverse effects, including precipitation of glaucoma, constipation, dry mouth, and urinary retention. Disopyramide commonly depresses contractility, which can precipitate heart failure, and also can cause *torsades de pointes*.

Clinical Pharmacokinetics Disopyramide is well absorbed. Binding to plasma proteins is concentration dependent, so a small increase in total concentration may represent a disproportionately larger increase in free drug concentration. Disopyramide is eliminated by both hepatic metabolism (to a weakly active metabolite) and renal excretion of unchanged drug. The dose should be reduced in patients with renal dysfunction. Higher than usual dosages may be required in patients receiving drugs that induce hepatic metabolism, such as phenytoin.

DOFETILIDE *Dofetilide* (TIKOSYN) is a potent and "pure" I_{Kr} blocker that has virtually no extracardiac pharmacological effects. Dofetilide is effective in maintaining sinus rhythm in patients with atrial fibrillation. Dofetilide is available through a restricted distribution system that includes only physicians, hospitals, and other institutions that have received special educational programs covering proper dosing and treatment initiation.

Adverse Effects Torsades de pointes occurred in 1–3% of patients in clinical trials where strict exclusion criteria (*e.g.,* hypokalemia) were applied and continuous ECG monitoring was used to detect marked QT prolongation in the hospital. The incidence of this adverse effect during more widespread use of the drug postmarketing is unknown. Other adverse effects were no more common than with placebo in premarketing trials.

Clinical Pharmacokinetics Most dofetilide is excreted unchanged by the kidneys. In patients with mild-to-moderate renal failure, decreases in dosage based on creatinine clearance are used to minimize the risk of *torsades de pointes*. The drug should not be used in patients with advanced renal failure or with inhibitors of renal cation transport. Dofetilide also undergoes minor hepatic metabolism.

FLECAINIDE   The effects of flecainide (TAMBOCOR) are thought to be attributable to the drug's very long $\tau_{recovery}$ from Na$^+$ channel block. It is approved for the maintenance of sinus rhythm in patients with supraventricular arrhythmias, including atrial fibrillation, in whom structural heart disease is absent.

Pharmacological Effects   Flecainide blocks Na$^+$ current, delayed rectifier K$^+$ current (I_{Kr}), and Ca^{2+} currents. Action potential duration is shortened in Purkinje cells, probably owing to block of late-opening Na$^+$ channels, but prolonged in ventricular cells, probably owing to block of delayed rectifier current. Flecainide does not cause EADs *in vitro* or *torsades de pointes*. In atrial tissue, flecainide disproportionately prolongs action potentials at fast rates, an especially desirable antiarrhythmic drug effect; this effect contrasts with that of quinidine, which prolongs atrial action potentials to a greater extent at slower rates. Flecainide prolongs the PR, QRS, and QT intervals even at normal heart rates.

Adverse Effects   Flecainide usually produces few subjective complaints; dose-related blurred vision is the most common noncardiac adverse effect. It can exacerbate CHF in patients with depressed left ventricular performance. The most serious adverse effects are provocation or exacerbation of potentially lethal arrhythmias. These include acceleration of ventricular rate in patients with atrial flutter, increased frequency of episodes of reentrant ventricular tachycardia, and increased mortality in patients convalescing from myocardial infarction. These effects likely result from Na$^+$ channel block. Flecainide also can cause heart block in patients with conduction system disease.

Clinical Pharmacokinetics   Flecainide is well absorbed. The elimination $t_{1/2}$ (10–18 hours) is sufficiently long to allow dosing twice daily. Elimination occurs by both renal excretion of unchanged drug and hepatic metabolism to inactive metabolites. The latter is mediated by the polymorphically distributed enzyme CYP2D6. However, even in patients in whom this pathway is absent because of genetic polymorphism or inhibition by other drugs (*i.e.*, quinidine and fluoxetine), renal excretion ordinarily is sufficient to prevent drug accumulation. In the rare patient with renal dysfunction and lack of active CYP2D6, flecainide may accumulate to toxic plasma concentrations. Some reports have suggested that plasma flecainide concentrations greater than 1 μg/mL should be avoided to minimize the risk of flecainide toxicity, but the adverse electrophysiological effects of flecainide therapy can occur at therapeutic plasma concentrations.

IBUTILIDE   Ibutilide (CORVERT) is an I_{Kr} blocker that may also activate an inward Na$^+$ current. The action potential–prolonging effect of the drug may arise from either mechanism. Ibutilide is administered as a rapid infusion (1 mg over 10 minutes) for the immediate conversion of atrial fibrillation or flutter to sinus rhythm. The drug's efficacy is higher in patients with atrial flutter (50–70%) than in those with atrial fibrillation (30–50%). In atrial fibrillation, the conversion rate is lower in those in whom the arrhythmia has been present for weeks or months compared with those in whom it has been present for days. The major toxicity with ibutilide is *torsades de pointes,* which occurs in up to 6% of patients and requires immediate cardioversion in up to one-third of these. The drug undergoes extensive first-pass metabolism and so is not used orally. It is eliminated by hepatic metabolism with a $t_{1/2}$ of 2–12 hours (mean, 6 hours).

LIDOCAINE   Lidocaine (XYLOCAINE) is a local anesthetic that also is useful in the acute intravenous therapy of ventricular arrhythmias.

Pharmacological Effects   Lidocaine blocks both open and inactivated cardiac Na$^+$ channels. Recovery from block is very rapid, so lidocaine exerts greater effects in depolarized (*e.g.*, ischemic) and/or rapidly driven tissues. Lidocaine is not useful in atrial arrhythmias, possibly because atrial action potentials are so short that the Na$^+$ channel is in the inactivated state only briefly compared with the long diastolic (recovery) times. Lidocaine can hyperpolarize Purkinje fibers depolarized by low [K]$_o$ or stretch; the resulting increased conduction velocity may inhibit reentry. Lidocaine decreases automaticity by reducing the slope of phase 4 and altering the threshold for excitability. Action potential duration usually is unaffected or shortened; such shortening may be due to block of the few Na$^+$ channels that inactivate late during the cardiac action potential. Lidocaine usually exerts no significant effect on PR or QRS duration; QT is unaltered or slightly shortened. The drug has little effect on hemodynamic function, although rare cases of lidocaine-associated exacerbations of heart failure have been reported in patients with decreased left ventricular function.

Adverse Effects When a large intravenous dose of lidocaine is administered rapidly, seizures can occur. When plasma concentrations of the drug rise slowly above the therapeutic range, as may occur during maintenance therapy, tremor, dysarthria, and altered levels of consciousness are more common. Nystagmus is an early sign of lidocaine toxicity.

CLINICAL PHARMACOKINETICS Lidocaine is well absorbed but undergoes extensive, though variable, first-pass hepatic metabolism; thus, oral use of the drug is inappropriate and the intravenous route is preferred. Lidocaine's metabolites—glycine xylidide (GX) and monoethyl GX—are less potent as Na^+ channel blockers than the parent drug. GX and lidocaine appear to compete for access to the Na^+ channel, suggesting that lidocaine's efficacy may be diminished by GX accumulation. With infusions lasting longer than 24 hours, the clearance of lidocaine falls—which has been attributed to competition between parent drug and metabolites for access to hepatic drug-metabolizing enzymes. The initial drop in plasma lidocaine following intravenous administration occurs rapidly ($t_{1/2}$ of ~8 minutes), and represents distribution from the central compartment to peripheral tissues. The terminal elimination $t_{1/2}$, usually 100–120 minutes, represents drug elimination by hepatic metabolism. Lidocaine's efficacy depends on maintenance of therapeutic plasma concentrations in the central compartment. Therefore, the administration of a single bolus dose of lidocaine can result in transient arrhythmia suppression that dissipates rapidly as the drug is distributed and concentrations in the central compartment fall. To avoid this distribution-related loss of efficacy, a loading regimen of 3–4 mg/kg over 20–30 minutes is used—*e.g.,* an initial 100 mg followed by 50 mg every 8 minutes for three doses. Subsequently, stable concentrations can be maintained in plasma with an infusion of 1–4 mg/min, which replaces drug removed by hepatic metabolism. Routine measurement of plasma lidocaine concentration at the time of expected steady state is useful in adjusting maintenance infusion rate to maintain efficacy and avoid toxicities.

In heart failure, lidocaine clearance is reduced and the total loading dose and the rate of the maintenance infusion must be decreased. Lidocaine clearance also is reduced in hepatic disease, during treatment with *cimetidine* or β blockers, and during prolonged infusions. Frequent measurement of plasma lidocaine concentration and dose adjustment to ensure that the concentrations remain within the therapeutic range (1.5–5 $\mu g/mL$) are necessary to minimize toxicity. Lidocaine is bound to the acute-phase reactant α_1-acid glycoprotein. Diseases such as acute myocardial infarction are associated with increases in α_1-acid glycoprotein and hence a decreased proportion of free drug. These findings may explain why some patients require higher than usual total plasma lidocaine concentrations to maintain antiarrhythmic efficacy.

MEXILETINE *Mexiletine* (MEXITIL) is an analog of lidocaine that has been modified to reduce first-pass hepatic metabolism and permit chronic oral therapy. The electrophysiological actions are similar to those of lidocaine. Tremor and nausea, the major dose-related adverse effects, can be minimized by taking the drugs with food. Mexiletine undergoes hepatic metabolism, which is inducible by drugs such as phenytoin. Mexiletine is approved for treating ventricular arrhythmias; combinations of mexiletine with quinidine or sotalol may increase efficacy while reducing adverse effects. *In vitro* studies and clinical anecdotes have suggested a role for mexiletine in correcting the molecular defect in the form of congenital long QT syndrome caused by abnormal Na^+ channel inactivation.

MORICIZINE *Moricizine* (ETHMOZINE) is a phenothiazine analog with Na^+ channel–blocking properties used in the chronic treatment of ventricular arrhythmias. Moricizine undergoes extensive first-pass hepatic metabolism; despite its short elimination $t_{1/2}$, its antiarrhythmic effect can persist for many hours after a single dose, suggesting that some of its metabolites may be active.

PROCAINAMIDE Procainamide (PROCAN SR, others) is an analog of the local anesthetic procaine. It exerts electrophysiological effects similar to those of quinidine but lacks quinidine's vagolytic and α adrenergic blocking activity. Procainamide is better tolerated than quinidine when given intravenously. Loading and maintenance intravenous infusions are used in the acute therapy of many supraventricular and ventricular arrhythmias. However, long-term oral treatment is poorly tolerated and often is stopped owing to adverse effects.

Pharmacological Effects Procainamide is a blocker of open Na^+ channels with an intermediate time constant of recovery from block. It also prolongs cardiac action potentials, probably by blocking outward K^+ current(s). Procainamide decreases automaticity, increases refractory periods, and slows conduction. Its major metabolite, N-acetyl procainamide, lacks the Na^+ channel–blocking activity of the parent drug but is equipotent in prolonging action potentials. Since the plasma concentrations of N-acetyl procainamide often exceed those of procainamide, increased refractoriness and QT prolongation during chronic procainamide therapy may be partly attributable to the metabolite. However, it is the parent drug that slows conduction and produces QRS-interval prolongation. Hypotension may occur at high plasma concentrations, an effect usually attributable to ganglionic blockade rather than to any negative inotropic effect.

Adverse Effects Hypotension and marked slowing of conduction are major adverse effects of high concentrations (>10 μg/mL) of procainamide, especially during intravenous use. Dose-related nausea is frequent during oral therapy and may be attributable in part to high plasma concentrations of N-acetyl procainamide. *Torsades de pointes* can occur, particularly when plasma concentrations of N-acetyl procainamide exceed 30 μg/mL. Procainamide produces idiosyncratic and potentially fatal bone marrow aplasia in 0.2% of patients. During long-term therapy, most patients will develop circulating antinuclear antibodies. Therapy need not be interrupted merely because of the presence of antinuclear antibodies. However, 25–50% of patients eventually develop symptoms of a drug-induced lupus syndrome, typically rash and arthralgias. Other symptoms of lupus, including pericarditis with tamponade, can occur, although renal involvement is unusual. The lupus-like symptoms resolve on cessation of therapy or during treatment with N-acetyl procainamide (*see* below).

Clinical Pharmacokinetics Procainamide is eliminated rapidly ($t_{1/2}$, 3–4 hours) by both renal excretion of unchanged drug and hepatic metabolism. The major pathway for hepatic metabolism is conjugation by N-acetyl transferase, whose activity is determined genetically, to form N-acetyl procainamide. N-Acetyl procainamide is eliminated by renal excretion ($t_{1/2}$, 6–10 hours) and is not significantly converted back to procainamide. Oral procainamide usually is administered as a slow-release formulation. In patients with renal failure, procainamide and/or N-acetyl procainamide can accumulate to potentially toxic plasma concentrations, and reduction of procainamide dose and dosing frequency and monitoring of plasma concentrations of both compounds are required. Because the parent drug and metabolite exert different pharmacological effects, the practice of using the sum of their concentrations to guide therapy is inappropriate. In individuals who are "slow acetylators," the procainamide-induced lupus syndrome develops more often and earlier during treatment than among rapid acetylators. In addition, the symptoms of procainamide-induced lupus resolve during treatment with N-acetyl procainamide. Both these findings suggest that it is chronic exposure to the parent drug (or an oxidative metabolite) that results in the lupus syndrome.

PROPAFENONE *Propafenone* (RYTHMOL) is a Na^+ channel blocker with a relatively slow time constant for recovery from block. Like flecainide, propafenone may also block K^+ channels. Its major electrophysiological effect is to slow conduction in fast-response tissues. The drug is prescribed as a racemate; while the enantiomers do not differ in their Na^+ channel–blocking properties, S-(+)-propafenone also is a β adrenergic receptor antagonist. Propafenone prolongs PR and QRS durations. Chronic therapy with oral propafenone is used to maintain sinus rhythm in patients with supraventricular tachycardias, including atrial fibrillation; like other Na^+ channel blockers, it also can be used in ventricular arrhythmias but with only modest efficacy. Adverse effects during propafenone therapy include acceleration of ventricular response in patients with atrial flutter, increased frequency or severity of episodes of reentrant ventricular tachycardia, exacerbation of heart failure, and the adverse effects of β adrenergic blockade, such as sinus bradycardia and bronchospasm.

Clinical Pharmacokinetics Propafenone is well absorbed and is eliminated by both hepatic and renal routes. The activity of CYP2D6, functionally absent in ~7% of Caucasians and African Americans (*see* Chapter 3), is a major determinant of plasma propafenone concentration. In most subjects ("extensive metabolizers"), propafenone undergoes extensive first-pass hepatic metabolism to 5-hydroxy propafenone, a metabolite equipotent to propafenone as a Na^+ channel blocker but much less potent as a β adrenergic receptor antagonist. A second metabolite, N-desalkyl propafenone, is formed by non-CYP2D6-mediated metabolism and is a less potent blocker of Na^+ channels and β adrenergic receptors. CYP2D6-mediated metabolism of propafenone is saturable; thus, small increases in dose can increase plasma propafenone concentration disproportionately. In "poor metabolizers" who lack functional CYP2D6, first-pass hepatic metabolism is much less, and plasma propafenone concentrations are much higher after an equal dose. The incidence of adverse effects during propafenone therapy is significantly higher in poor metabolizers. CYP2D6 activity can be inhibited by a number of drugs, including quinidine and fluoxetine. In extensive metabolizers receiving such drugs or in poor metabolizers, plasma propafenone concentrations of more than 1 μg/mL are associated with clinical effects of β adrenergic receptor blockade, such as reduction of exercise heart rate. Patients with moderate-to-severe liver disease should receive ~20–30% of the usual dose, with careful monitoring. It is not known if propafenone doses must be decreased in patients with renal disease. A slow-release formulation allows twice-daily dosing.

QUINIDINE Quinidine, a diastereomer of the antimalarial quinine, is used to maintain sinus rhythm in patients with atrial flutter or atrial fibrillation and to prevent recurrence of ventricular tachycardia or ventricular fibrillation.

Pharmacological Effects Quinidine (various generic preparations) blocks Na^+ current and multiple cardiac K^+ currents. It is an open-state blocker of Na^+ channels, with a $\tau_{recovery}$ in the intermediate (~3 seconds) range; as a consequence, QRS duration increases modestly, usually by 10–20%, at therapeutic dosages. At therapeutic concentrations, quinidine commonly prolongs the QT interval by up to 25%, but the effect is highly variable. At concentrations as low as 1 μM, quinidine blocks Na^+ current and the rapid component of delayed rectifier (I_{Kr}); higher concentrations block the slow component of delayed rectifier, inward rectifier, transient outward current, and L-type Ca^{2+} current. Quinidine's Na^+ channel–blocking properties result in an increased threshold for excitability and decreased automaticity. Due to its K^+ channel–blocking actions, quinidine prolongs action potentials in most cardiac cells, most prominently at slow heart rates. In some cells, such as midmyocardial cells and Purkinje cells, quinidine consistently elicits EADs at slow heart rates, particularly when $[K]_o$ is low. Quinidine prolongs refractoriness in most tissues, probably as a result of both prolongation of action potential duration and Na^+ channel blockade.

Quinidine also produces α adrenergic receptor blockade and vagal inhibition. Thus, the intravenous use of quinidine is associated with marked hypotension and sinus tachycardia. Quinidine's vagolytic effects tend to inhibit its direct depressant effect on AV nodal conduction, so its effect on the PR interval is variable. Moreover, quinidine's vagolytic effect can increase AV nodal transmission of atrial tachycardias such as atrial flutter (Table 34–1).

Adverse Effects

Noncardiac Diarrhea is the most common adverse effect during quinidine therapy, occurring in 30–50% of patients, usually within the first several days of quinidine therapy but sometimes later. Diarrhea-induced hypokalemia may potentiate the risk of *torsades de pointes* due to quinidine. A number of immunological reactions can occur during quinidine therapy. The most common is thrombocytopenia, which can be severe but resolves rapidly with drug discontinuation. Hepatitis, bone marrow depression, and lupus syndrome occur rarely. None of these effects is related to elevated plasma quinidine concentrations. Quinidine also can produce cinchonism, a syndrome that includes headache and tinnitus. In contrast to other adverse responses to quinidine therapy, cinchonism usually is related to elevated plasma quinidine concentrations and can be managed by dose reduction.

Cardiac Between 2% and 8% of patients who receive quinidine therapy will develop marked QT-interval prolongation and *torsades de pointes.* In contrast to sotalol, *N*-acetyl procainamide, and other drugs, quinidine-associated *torsades de pointes* usually occurs at therapeutic or subtherapeutic plasma concentrations. The reasons for individual susceptibility are not known. At high plasma concentrations of quinidine, marked Na^+ channel block can occur, with resulting ventricular tachycardia. Quinidine can exacerbate heart failure or conduction system disease but usually is well tolerated in patients with congestive heart failure, perhaps because of its vasodilating actions.

Clinical Pharmacokinetics Quinidine is well absorbed and is 80% bound to plasma proteins, including albumin and α_1-acid glycoprotein. As with lidocaine, greater than usual doses (and total plasma quinidine concentrations) may be required to maintain therapeutic concentrations of free quinidine in high-stress states such as acute myocardial infarction. Quinidine undergoes extensive hepatic oxidative metabolism, and ~20% is excreted unchanged by the kidneys. One metabolite, 3-hydroxyquinidine, is nearly as potent as quinidine in blocking cardiac Na^+ channels and prolonging cardiac action potentials. Concentrations of unbound 3-hydroxyquinidine equal to or exceeding those of quinidine are tolerated by some patients. Other metabolites are less potent and their plasma concentrations are lower; thus, they are unlikely to contribute significantly to the clinical effects of quinidine. There is substantial individual variability in the range of dosages required to achieve therapeutic plasma concentrations of 2–5 μg/mL. In patients with advanced renal disease or congestive heart failure, quinidine clearance is decreased only modestly. Thus, dosage requirements in these patients are similar to those in other patients.

Drug Interactions Quinidine is a potent inhibitor of CYP2D6, and its administration to patients receiving drugs that undergo extensive CYP2D6-mediated metabolism may result in altered drug effects owing to accumulation of parent drug and failure of metabolite formation. For example, inhibition of CYP2D6-mediated metabolism of *codeine* to its active metabolite *morphine* results in decreased analgesia. On the other hand, inhibition of CYP2D6-mediated metabolism of propafenone results in elevated plasma propafenone concentrations and increased β adrenergic receptor blockade. Quinidine reduces the clearance of digoxin and digitoxin; inhibition of P-glycoprotein–mediated digoxin transport has been implicated. Quinidine metabolism is induced by drugs such as *phenobarbital* and phenytoin. In patients receiving these agents, very high doses of quinidine may be required to achieve therapeutic concentrations. If therapy with the inducing agent is then stopped, quinidine concentrations may rise to very high levels, and its dosage must be adjusted downward. Cimetidine and verapamil also elevate plasma quinidine concentrations, but these effects usually are modest.

SOTALOL *Sotalol* (BETAPACE, BETAPACE AF) is a nonselective β adrenergic receptor antagonist that also prolongs cardiac action potentials by inhibiting delayed rectifier and possibly other K^+ currents. Sotalol is prescribed as a racemate; the L-enantiomer is a much more potent β adrenergic receptor antagonist than the D-enantiomer, but the two are equipotent as K^+ channel blockers. Sotalol is FDA-approved for use in patients with both ventricular tachyarrhythmias and atrial fibrillation or flutter. Clinical trials suggest that it is at least as effective as most Na^+ channel blockers in ventricular arrhythmias. Sotalol prolongs the QT interval, decreases automaticity, slows AV nodal conduction, and prolongs AV refractoriness by blocking both K^+ channels and β adrenergic receptors; it exerts no effect on conduction velocity in fast-response tissue. Sotalol causes EADs and triggered activity *in vitro* and can cause *torsades de pointes,* especially when the serum K^+ concentration is low. Unlike quinidine, the incidence of *torsades de pointes* depends on the dose of sotalol. Because sotalol is eliminated by renal excretion, occasional cases occur at low dosage in patients with renal dysfunction. Other adverse effects of sotalol therapy are those associated with β adrenergic receptor blockade.

MAGNESIUM The intravenous administration of 1–2 g $MgSO_4$ reportedly is effective in preventing recurrent episodes of *torsades de pointes,* even with normal serum Mg^{2+}. The mechanism of action is unknown but may reflect an effect on the inward current, possibly a Ca^{2+} current, responsible for the triggered upstroke arising from EADs. Intravenous Mg^{2+} also has been used successfully in arrhythmias related to digitalis intoxication.

For a complete Bibliographical listing see Goodman & Gilman's *The Pharmacological Basis of Therapeutics,* 11th ed., or Goodman & Gilman Online at www.accessmedicine.com.

35

DRUG THERAPY FOR HYPERCHOLESTEROLEMIA AND DYSLIPIDEMIA

Hyperlipidemia is a major cause of atherosclerosis and atherosclerosis-associated conditions, such as coronary heart disease (CHD), ischemic cerebrovascular disease, and peripheral vascular disease. These conditions account for most morbidity and mortality among middle-aged and older adults. Dyslipidemias, including hyperlipidemia (hypercholesterolemia) and low levels of high-density-lipoprotein cholesterol (HDL-C), are major causes of increased atherogenesis; both genetic disorders and lifestyle (sedentary behavior and diets high in calories, saturated fat, and cholesterol) contribute to the dyslipidemias seen in developed countries.

PLASMA LIPOPROTEIN METABOLISM

Lipoproteins are macromolecular assemblies that contain proteins and lipids, including free and esterified cholesterol, triglycerides, and phospholipids. The protein components, known as apolipoproteins, provide structural stability to the lipoproteins, and also may function as ligands in lipoprotein–receptor interactions or as cofactors in enzymatic processes that regulate lipoprotein metabolism. In all lipoproteins, the most water-insoluble lipids (cholesteryl esters and triglycerides) are core components, and the more polar, water-soluble components (apoproteins, phospholipids, and unesterified cholesterol) are located on the surface. The major classes of lipoproteins and their properties are presented in Table 35–1. Table 35–2 describes apoproteins that have well-defined roles in plasma lipoprotein metabolism.

CHYLOMICRONS   Chylomicrons are synthesized from the fatty acids of dietary triglycerides and cholesterol absorbed from the small intestine by epithelial cells. Intestinal cholesterol absorption is mediated by Niemann-Pick C1–like 1NPC1L1 protein, which appears to be the target of ezetimibe (*see* below). Dietary cholesterol is esterified by the type 2 isozyme of acyl coenzyme A:cholesterol acyltransferase (ACAT). ACAT-2 is found in the intestine and the liver, where cellular free cholesterol is esterified before triglyceride-rich lipoproteins (chylomicrons and very-low-density lipoproteins [VLDL]) are assembled. Chylomicrons are the largest and lowest density plasma lipoproteins. In normal individuals, chylomicrons are present in plasma for 3–6 hours after a fat-containing meal; no chylomicrons remain after 10–12 hours. After entering the circulation *via* the thoracic duct, chylomicrons are metabolized initially at the capillary luminal surface of tissues that synthesize the triglyceride hydrolase lipoprotein lipase (LPL; Figure 35–1), including adipose tissue, skeletal and cardiac muscle, and breast tissue of lactating women. As triglycerides are hydrolyzed by LPL, the resulting free fatty acids are taken up and utilized by adjacent tissues. The interaction of chylomicrons and LPL absolutely requires apolipoprotein (apo) C-II as a cofactor. The absence of functional LPL or functional apoC-II prevents the hydrolysis of triglycerides in chylomicrons and results in severe hypertriglyceridemia and pancreatitis during childhood or even infancy (chylomicronemia syndrome). The chylomicrons can be decreased only by reducing dietary fat consumption. Insulin has a "permissive" effect on LPL-mediated triglyceride hydrolysis.

CHYLOMICRON REMNANTS   After LPL-mediated removal of much of the dietary triglycerides, the chylomicron remnants, which still contain all of the dietary cholesterol, detach from the capillary surface and are removed within minutes from the circulation by the liver in a process mediated by apoE (Figure 35–1). First, the remnants are sequestered by the interaction of apoE with heparan sulfate proteoglycans on the surface of hepatocytes and are processed by hepatic lipase (HL), further reducing the remnant triglyceride content. Next, apoE mediates remnant uptake by interacting with the hepatic low-density lipoproteins (LDL) receptor or the LDL receptor–related protein (LRP). Inherited deficiency of either functional HL (very rare) or functional apoE impedes remnant clearance by the LDL receptor, increasing triglyceride- and cholesterol-rich remnant lipoproteins in the plasma (type III hyperlipoproteinemia).

During the initial hydrolysis of chylomicron triglycerides by LPL, apoA-I and phospholipids are shed from the surface of chylomicrons and remain in the plasma. This is one mechanism by which nascent (precursor) HDL are generated. Chylomicron remnants are not precursors of LDL, but the dietary cholesterol delivered to the liver by remnants increases plasma LDL levels by reducing LDL receptor–mediated catabolism of LDL by the liver.

VERY-LOW-DENSITY LIPOPROTEINS   VLDL are produced in the liver when triglyceride production is stimulated by an increased flux of free fatty acids or by increased hepatic

Table 35-1

Characteristics of Plasma Lipoproteins

Lipoprotein Class	Density of Flotation, g/mL	Major Lipid Constituent	TG:Chol Ratio	Significant Apoproteins	Site of Synthesis	Mechanism(s) of Catabolism
Chylomicrons and remnants	<<1.006	Dietary triglycerides and cholesterol	10:1	B-48, E, A-I, A-IV, C-I, C-II, C-III	Intestine	Triglyceride hydrolysis by LPL ApoE-mediated remnant uptake by liver
VLDL	<1.006	"Endogenous" or hepatic triglycerides	5:1	B-100, E, C-I, C-II, C-III	Liver	Triglyceride hydrolysis by LPL
IDL	1.006–1.019	Cholesteryl esters and "endogenous" triglycerides	1:1	B-100, E, C-II, C-III	Product of VLDL catabolism	50% converted to LDL mediated by HL, 50% apoE-mediated uptake by liver
LDL	1.019–1.063	Cholesteryl esters	NS	B-100	Product of VLDL catabolism	50% apoE-mediated uptake by liver ApoB-100–mediated uptake by LDL receptor (~75% in liver)
HDL	1.063–1.21	Phospholipids, cholesteryl esters	NS	A-I, A-II, E, C-I, C-II, C-III	Intestine, liver, plasma	Complex: Transfer of cholesteryl ester to VLDL and LDL Uptake of HDL cholesterol by hepatocytes
Lp(a)	1.05–1.09	Cholesteryl esters	NS	B-100, apo(a)	Liver	Unknown

ABBREVIATIONS: apo, apolipoprotein; CHOL, cholesterol; HDL, high-density lipoproteins; IDL, intermediate-density lipoproteins; Lp(a), lipoprotein(a); LDL, low-density lipoproteins; NS, not significant (triglyceride is less than 5% of LDL and HDL); TG, triglyceride; VLDL, very-low-density lipoproteins; HL, hepatic lipase; LPL, lipoprotein lipase.

604

Table 35–2

Apolipoproteins

Apolipoprotein	Average Concentration, mg/dL	Chromosome	Molecular Mass, kDa	Sites of Synthesis	Functions
ApoA-I	130	11	~29	Liver, intestine	Structural in HDL; LCAT cofactor; ligand of ABCA1 receptor; reverse cholesterol transport
ApoA-II	40	1	~17	Liver	Forms –S–S– complex with apoE-2 and E-3, which inhibits E-2 and E-3 binding to lipoprotein receptors
ApoA-V	<1	11	~40	Liver	Modulates triglyceride incorporation into hepatic VLDL; activates LPL
ApoB-100	85	2	~513	Liver	Structural protein of VLDL, IDL, LDL; LDL receptor ligand
ApoB-48	Fluctuates according to dietary fat intake	2	~241	Intestine	Structural protein of chylomicrons
ApoC-I	6	19	~6.6	Liver	LCAT activator; modulates receptor binding of remnants
ApoC-II	3	19	8.9	Liver	Lipoprotein lipase cofactor
ApoC-III	12	11	8.8	Liver	Modulates receptor binding of remnants
ApoE	5	19	34	Liver, brain, skin, gonads, spleen	Ligand for LDL receptor and receptors binding remnants; reverse cholesterol transport (HDL with apoE)
Apo(a)	Variable (under genetic control)	6	Variable	Liver	Modulator of fibrinolysis

ABBREVIATIONS: ABCA1, ATP-binding cassette transporter A1; apo, apolipoprotein; HDL, high-density lipoproteins; IDL, intermediate-density lipoproteins; kDa, kilodaltons; LCAT, lecithin:cholesterol acyltransferase; LDL, low-density lipoproteins; LPL, lipoprotein lipase; VLDL, very-low-density lipoproteins.

synthesis of fatty acids. ApoB-100, apoE, and several other lipoproteins are synthesized constitutively by the liver and incorporated into VLDL (Table 35–2). If triglycerides are unavailable, the newly synthesized apoB-100 is degraded by hepatocytes. Small amounts of apoE and the C apoproteins are incorporated into nascent particles within the liver before secretion, but most of the VLDL apoproteins are acquired from plasma HDL after the VLDL are secreted by the liver.

Without the enzyme microsomal triglyceride transfer protein (MTP), hepatic triglycerides cannot be transferred to apoB-100. Patients with dysfunctional MTP fail to make any of the apoB-containing lipoproteins (VLDL, IDL, or LDL). MTP also plays a key role in the synthesis of chylomicrons in the intestine, and mutations of MTP that result in the inability of triglycerides to be transferred to either apoB-100 in the liver or apoB-48 in the intestine prevent VLDL and chylomicron production and cause the genetic disorder abetalipoproteinemia.

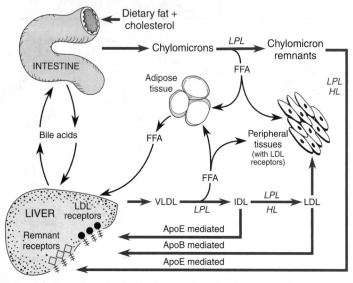

FIGURE 35–1 *The major pathways involved in the metabolism of chylomicrons synthesized by the intestine and VLDL synthesized by the liver.* Chylomicrons are converted to chylomicron remnants by the hydrolysis of their triglycerides by LPL. Chylomicron remnants are rapidly cleared from the plasma by the liver. "Remnant receptors" include the LDL receptor-related protein (LRP), LDL, and perhaps other receptors. FFA released by LPL is used by muscle tissue as an energy source or taken up and stored by adipose tissue. FFA, free fatty acid; HL, hepatic lipase; IDL, intermediate-density lipoproteins; LDL, low-density lipoproteins; LPL, lipoprotein lipase; VLDL, very-low-density lipoproteins.

Plasma VLDL is catabolized by LPL in the capillary beds in a process similar to the lipolytic processing of chylomicrons (Figure 35–1). When triglyceride hydrolysis is nearly complete, the VLDL remnants, usually termed intermediate-density lipoproteins (IDL), are released from the capillary endothelium and reenter the circulation. ApoB-100 containing small VLDL and IDL, which have a $t_{1/2}$ of <30 minutes, have two potential fates: 40–60% are cleared from the plasma by the liver via apoB-100- and apoE-mediated interaction with LDL receptors and LRP; the remainder are converted to LDL by LPL and HL and the C apoproteins and apoE redistribute to HDL. Virtually all LDL particles in the plasma are derived from VLDL.

ApoE plays a major role in the metabolism of triglyceride-rich lipoproteins (chylomicrons, chylomicron remnants, VLDL, and IDL) and in the local redistribution of lipids among cells. About half of the plasma apoE in fasting subjects is associated with triglyceride-rich lipoproteins; the other half is a constituent of HDL.

LOW-DENSITY LIPOPROTEINS   The LDL particles arising from the catabolism of IDL have a $t_{1/2}$ of 1.5–2 days, which accounts for the higher plasma concentration of LDL than of VLDL and IDL. In subjects without hypertriglyceridemia, two-thirds of plasma cholesterol is found in the LDL. Plasma clearance of LDL particles is mediated primarily by LDL receptors. Mutations of the LDL receptor gene cause familial hypercholesterolemia. ApoB-100, the only apoprotein of LDL, is the ligand that binds LDL to its receptor. Mutations in apoB-100 disrupt binding and are a cause of hypercholesterolemia (familial defective apoB-100). Autosomal recessive hypercholesterolemia closely resembles familial hypercholesterolemia, but is not caused by LDL receptor mutations but by mutations in a protein that is required for internalization of LDL receptor complexes on the surface of hepatocytes.

The liver expresses a large complement of LDL receptors and removes ~75% of all LDL from the plasma. Consequently, manipulation of hepatic LDL receptor expression is a most effective way to modulate plasma LDL-C levels. Thyroxine and estrogen enhance LDL receptor gene expression, which explains their LDL-C–lowering effects. The most effective dietary alteration (decreased consumption of saturated fat and cholesterol) and pharmacological treatment (statins) for hypercholesterolemia act by enhancing hepatic LDL receptor expression. *LDL become atherogenic when they are modified by oxidation, a required step for LDL uptake by the scavenger receptors of macrophages. This process leads to foam-cell formation in arterial lesions. Despite the large body of evidence implicating LDL oxidation as a requisite step during atherogenesis, controlled clinical trials have failed to show efficacy of antioxidant vitamins in preventing vascular disease.*

HIGH-DENSITY LIPOPROTEINS

The metabolism of HDL is complex because of the multiple mechanisms by which HDL particles are synthesized and modified plasma. Many factors, including genetic variation, can alter HDL levels and affect CHD risk. ApoA-I is the major HDL apoprotein, and its plasma concentration is a more powerful inverse predictor of CHD risk than is the HDL-C level. Mutations in the apoA-I gene that cause HDL deficiency are variable in their clinical expression and often are associated with accelerated atherogenesis. The membrane transporter ABCA1 facilitates the transfer of free cholesterol from cells to HDL. When ABCA1 is defective, the acquisition of cholesterol by HDL is greatly diminished, and HDL levels are markedly reduced. Loss-of-function mutations of ABCA1 cause Tangier disease, a genetic disorder characterized by extremely low levels of HDL and cholesterol accumulation in the liver, spleen, tonsils, and peripheral nerves.

Mature HDL can be separated by ultracentrifugation into HDL_2, which are larger, more cholesterol-rich lipoproteins, and HDL_3, which are smaller and denser. Newly formed HDL_3 particles are converted to HDL_2 by accepting more free cholesterol, which is then esterified by lecithin: cholesterol acyltransferase (LCAT). As the cholesteryl ester content of the HDL_2 increases, the cholesteryl esters of these particles begin to be exchanged for triglycerides derived from any of the triglyceride-containing lipoproteins (chylomicrons, VLDL, remnant lipoproteins, and LDL). This exchange is mediated by the cholesteryl ester transfer protein (CETP), which in humans accounts for the removal of about two-thirds of the cholesterol associated with HDL. The transferred cholesterol subsequently is metabolized as part of the lipoprotein into which it was transferred. The triglyceride transferred into HDL_2 is hydrolyzed in the liver by HL, regenerating smaller, spherical HDL_3 particles that recirculate and acquire additional free cholesterol from tissues containing excess free cholesterol.

HDL are protective lipoproteins that decrease the risk of CHD; thus, high levels of HDL are desirable. This protective effect may result from the participation of HDL in reverse cholesterol transport, the process by which excess cholesterol is acquired from cells and transferred to the liver for excretion.

HYPERLIPIDEMIA AND ATHEROSCLEROSIS

The major conventional risk factors for CHD are elevated LDL-C, reduced HDL-C, cigarette smoking, hypertension, type 2 diabetes mellitus, advancing age, and a family history of premature (men <55 years; women <65 years) CHD events in a first-degree relative. Control of the modifiable risk factors, which account for 85% of excess risk, is especially important in preventing premature CHD. When total cholesterol levels are <160 mg/dL, CHD risk is markedly attenuated, even in the presence of additional risk factors. This pivotal role of hypercholesterolemia in atherogenesis gave rise to the almost universally accepted cholesterol-diet-CHD hypothesis: elevated plasma cholesterol levels cause CHD; diets rich in saturated fat and cholesterol raise cholesterol levels; and lowering cholesterol levels reduces CHD risk.

Clinical trials with effective cholesterol-lowering drugs, the statins, have documented the safety and efficacy of cholesterol-lowering therapy in preventing CHD. Patients benefit from lowering plasma cholesterol levels regardless of gender, age, or baseline lipid values whether or not they have a prior history of vascular disease. Guidelines based on these clinical trials and were developed in 2001 by the National Cholesterol Education Program (NCEP) Adult Treatment Panel (ATP) III and revised in 2004 (www.nhlbi.nih.gov/guidelines/cholesterol). The key features of the revision include abandoning the concept of a threshold LDL-C level that must be exceeded before initiating cholesterol-lowering drug therapy in CHD or CHD equivalent patients; adopting a new target LDL-C level (<70 mg/dL) for very high-risk patients; and employing a "standard statin dose" (a dosage sufficient to lower LDL-C by 30–40%) as a minimum therapy when initiating cholesterol-lowering therapy with statins (see Table 35–3). Clinical trials suggest that CHD risk is reduced by 1% for every 1% reduction in LDL-C. Current recommendations for statin therapy are that LDL-C levels should be lowered by 30–40% from baseline as well as achieving a specific LDL-C goal.

National Cholesterol Education Program (NCEP) Guidelines for Treatment: Managing Patients with Dyslipidemia

The NCEP guidelines for patient management are of two types. One is a population-based approach to reduce CHD risk, which includes recommendations to increase exercise (to expend ~2000 calories/week)

Table 35–3

Treatment Based on LDL-C Levels (2004 Revision of NCEP Adult Treatment Panel III Guidelines)

		Adults	
Risk Category	LDL-C Goal	Therapeutic Lifestyle Change	Drug Therapy
Very high risk Atherosclerosis-induced CHD plus one of: (a) multiple risk factors, (b) diabetes mellitus, (c) a poorly controlled single factor, (d) acute coronary syndrome, (e) metabolic syndrome	<70 mg/dL[*]	No threshold	No threshold
High risk CHD or CHD equivalent	<100 mg/dL[*]	No threshold	No threshold
Moderately high risk 2+ risk factors 10-year risk: 10–20%	<130 mg/dL (Optional <100 mg/dL)	≥100 mg/dL	≥130 mg/dL (100–129 mg/dL)[†]
Moderate risk 2+ risk factors 10-year risk <10%	<130 mg/dL	≥130 mg/dL	>160 mg/dL
0–1 risk factor	<160 mg/dL	≥160 mg/dL	≥190 mg/dL (Optional: 160–189 mg/dL)[‡]

[*]If pretreatment LDL-C is near or below LDL-C goal value, then a statin dose sufficient to lower LDL-C by 30%–40% should be prescribed.
[†]Patients in this category include those with a 10-year risk of 10%–20% and one of the following: (a) age >60 years; (b) three or more risk factors; (c) a severe risk factor; (d) triglycerides >200 mg/dL and HDL-C <40 mg/dL; (e) metabolic syndrome; (f) highly sensitive C-reactive protein (CRP) >3 mg/L; (g) coronary calcium score (age/gender adjusted) >75th percentile.
[‡]Patients include those with: (a) any severe single risk factor; (b) multiple major risk factors; (c) 10-year risk >8%.

ABBREVIATIONS: CHD, coronary heart disease; CHD equivalent, peripheral vascular disease, abdominal aortic aneurysm, symptomatic carotid artery disease, >20% 10-year CHD risk, or diabetes mellitus; LDL-C, low-density-lipoprotein cholesterol; NCEP, National Cholesterol Education Program.

and to lower blood cholesterol by dietary recommendations: reduce total calories from fat to <30% and from saturated and trans fats to <10%; consume less than 300 mg of cholesterol per day; eat a variety of oily fish twice a week and oils/foods rich in α-linolenic acid (canola, flaxseed, and soybean oils, flaxseed, and walnuts); and maintain desirable body weight. The second is the patient-based approach that focuses on lowering LDL-C levels as the primary goal of therapy.

According to guidelines, all adults >20 years old should have a complete fasting lipoprotein profile (total cholesterol, LDL-C, HDL-C, and triglycerides). The classification of lipid levels is shown in Table 35–4. If the values for total cholesterol, LDL-C, and triglycerides are in the lowest category and the HDL-C level is not low, lifestyle recommendations (diet and exercise) should be made to ensure maintenance of a normal lipid profile. Other vascular disease risk factors (Table 35–5), if present, should be assessed and treated individually. For patients with elevated levels of total cholesterol, LDL-C, or triglycerides, or reduced HDL-C values, further treatment is based on the patient's risk-factor status (Table 35–5), LDL-C levels (Table 35–3), and calculation of the Framingham risk score (Table 35–6) of primary prevention patients with two or more risk factors. A high risk or CHD equivalent status is defined as >20% chance of sustaining a CHD event in the next 10 years.

All patients who meet the criteria for lipid-lowering therapy should receive instruction about therapeutic lifestyle change. Dietary restrictions include <7% of calories from saturated and trans fatty acids, <200 mg of cholesterol daily, up to 20% of calories from monounsaturated fatty acids,

Table 35–4

Classification of Plasma Lipid Levels*

Total cholesterol	
<200 mg/dL	Desirable
200–239 mg/dL	Borderline high
≥240 mg/dL	High
HDL-C	
<40 mg/dL	Low (consider <50 mg/dL as low for women)
>60 mg/dL	High
LDL-C	
<70 mg/dL	Optimal for very high risk (minimal goal for CHD equivalent patients)
<100 mg/dL	Optimal
100–129 mg/dL	Near optimal
130–159 mg/dL	Borderline high
160–189 mg/dL	High
≥190 mg/dL	Very high
Triglycerides	
<150 mg/dL	Normal
150–199 mg/dL	Borderline high
200–499 mg/dL	High
≥500 mg/dL	Very high

ABBREVIATIONS: HDL-C, high-density-lipoprotein cholesterol; LDL-C, low-density-lipoprotein cholesterol.
*2001 National Cholesterol Education Program guidelines.

up to 10% of calories from polyunsaturated fat, and total fat calories ranging between 25–35% of all calories. Two meals of oily fish per week are especially important for patients after myocardial infarction due to a substantial reduction in sudden cardiac death. Patients with CHD or a CHD equivalent (symptomatic peripheral or carotid vascular disease, abdominal aortic aneurysm, >20% 10-year CHD risk, or diabetes mellitus) should immediately start appropriate lipid-lowering drug therapy irrespective of their baseline LDL-C level. Patients without CHD or CHD equivalent

Table 35–5

Risk Factors for Coronary Heart Disease*

Age
Male >45 years or female >55 years

Family history of premature CHD
A first-degree relative (male below 55 years or female below 65 years when the first CHD clinical event occurs)

Current cigarette smoking
Defined as smoking within the preceding 30 days

Hypertension
Blood pressure ≥140/90 or use of antihypertensive medication, irrespective of blood pressure

Low HDL-C
<40 mg/dL (consider <50 mg/dL as "low" for women)

Obesity†
Body mass index >25 kg/m² and waist circumference above 40 inches (men) or 35 inches (women)

ABBREVIATIONS: CHD, coronary heart disease; HDL-C, high-density-lipoprotein cholesterol.
*Diabetes mellitus is considered to be a CHD-equivalent disorder; therefore, the lipid management of diabetes patients is the same as that for patients with established vascular disease (American Diabetes Association, 1999).
†Obesity was returned to the list of CHD risk factors in 1998, although it was not included as a risk factor in the 2001 NCEP guidelines.

Table 35–6

Guidelines Based on LDL-C and Total Cholesterol:HDL-C Ratio for Treatment of Low HDL-C Patients

Risk Category	Goals			Lifestyle Change Initiated for			Drug Therapy Initiated for		
	LDL-C		TC:HDL-C	LDL-C		TC:HDL-C	LDL-C		TC:HDL-C
CHD or equivalent	<100	and	<3.5	≥100	or	≥3.5	≥100	or	≥3.5
2+ risk factors	<130	and	<4.5	≥130	or	≥4.5	≥130	or	≥6.0
0–1 risk factor	<160	and	<5.5	≥160	or	≥5.5	≥160	or	≥7.0

ABBREVIATIONS: CHD, coronary heart disease; HDL-C, high-density lipoprotein cholesterol; LDL-C, low-density-lipoprotein cholesterol; TC, total cholesterol.

should be managed with lifestyle advice (diet, exercise, weight management) for 3–6 months before drug therapy is implemented.

Before drug therapy is initiated, secondary causes of hyperlipidemia should be excluded. Most secondary causes (*e.g.*, diabetes mellitus, nephrotic syndrome, alcohol use, estrogen use, glucocorticoid excess, hypothyroidism, and obstructive liver disease) can be excluded by ascertaining the patient's medication history and by measuring serum creatinine, liver function tests, fasting glucose, and thyroid-stimulating hormone levels. Treatment of the disorder causing secondary dyslipidemia may preclude the necessity of treatment with hypolipidemic drugs.

WHOM AND WHEN TO TREAT   Large-scale trials with statins have provided new insights into which patients with dyslipidemia should be treated and when treatment should be initiated.

Sex   Both men and women benefit from lipid-lowering therapy. Statins are the recommended first-line drug therapy for lowering lipids in postmenopausal women.

Age   Age >45 years in men and >55 years in women is considered to be a CHD risk factor. The statin trials have shown that patients >65 years of age benefit from therapy as much as do younger patients. Thus, old age *per se* is not a reason to withhold drug therapy in an otherwise healthy person.

Cerebrovascular Disease Patients   Plasma cholesterol levels correlate positively with the risk of ischemic stroke and statins reduce stroke and transient ischemic attacks in patients with and without CHD.

Peripheral Vascular Disease Patients   Statins are beneficial in patients with peripheral vascular disease.

Hypertensive Patients and Smokers   The risk reduction for coronary events in hypertensive patients and in smokers is similar to that in subjects without these risk factors.

Type 2 Diabetes Mellitus   Patients with type 2 diabetes benefit very significantly from aggressive lipid lowering (*see* "Treatment of Type 2 Diabetes," below).

Post–Myocardial Infarction or Revascularization Patients

As soon as CHD is diagnosed, it is essential to begin lipid-lowering therapy (NCEP guidelines: LDL-C goal <70 mg/dL for very high-risk patients). Compliance with drug therapy is greatly enhanced if treatment is initiated in the hospital. Statin therapy improves the long-term outcome after bypass surgery; the lower the LDL-C, the better.

CAN CHOLESTEROL LEVELS BE LOWERED TOO MUCH?

There are no significant risks associated with low cholesterol levels.

Treatment of Type 2 Diabetes

Diabetes mellitus is an independent predictor of high risk for CHD. Glucose control is essential but provides only minimal benefit with respect to CHD prevention. Diabetic dyslipidemia typically includes high triglycerides, low HDL-C, and moderate elevations of total cholesterol and LDL-C.

Aggressive treatment of diabetic dyslipidemia through diet, weight control, and drugs is critical in reducing risk. Diabetics without diagnosed CHD have the same level of risk as nondiabetics with established CHD. Thus, the dyslipidemia treatment guidelines for diabetic patients are the same as for patients with CHD, irrespective of whether the diabetic patient has had a CHD event. The first line of treatment for diabetic dyslipidemia usually should be a statin.

Metabolic Syndrome

There is an increased CHD risk associated with the insulin-resistant, prediabetic state described under the rubric of "metabolic syndrome," a constellation of abdominal obesity, hypertension, insulin resistance, hypertriglyceridemia, and low HDL. Treatment should focus on weight loss and increased physical activity, since being overweight or obese usually precludes optimal risk factor reduction. Specific treatment of lipid abnormalities should also be undertaken.

Treatment of Hypertriglyceridemia

There is increased CHD risk associated with the presence of triglyceride levels >150 mg/dL. Three categories of hypertriglyceridemia are recognized (Table 35–4), and treatment depends on the degree of elevation. Weight loss, increased exercise, and alcohol restriction are important for all hypertriglyceridemic patients. The LDL-C goal should be ascertained based on each patient's risk factors or CHD status (Table 35–3). If triglycerides remain >200 mg/dL after the LDL-C goal is reached, further reduction in triglycerides may be achieved by increasing the dose of a statin or of niacin. Combination therapy (statin plus niacin or statin plus fibrate) may be required, but caution is necessary with these combinations to avoid myopathy (*see* below).

TREATMENT OF LOW HDL-C   The most frequent risk factor for premature CHD is low HDL-C. In patients with low HDL-C, the total cholesterol:HDL-C ratio is a particularly useful predictor of CHD risk. A favorable ratio is ≤3.5 and a ratio of >4.5 is associated with increased risk. Patients with low HDL-C may have what are considered to be "normal" total and LDL cholesterol levels; however, because of their low HDL-C levels, such patients may be at high risk based on the total cholesterol:HDL-C ratio (*e.g.,* a total cholesterol, 180 mg/dL; HDL-C, 30 mg/dL; ratio, 6). A desirable total cholesterol level in low–HDL-C patients may be considerably lower than 200 mg/dL, especially since low–HDL-C patients may also have moderately elevated triglycerides, which may reflect increased levels of atherogenic remnant lipoproteins. Patients with average or high LDL-C, low HDL-C, and high total cholesterol:HDL-C ratios have benefited from treatment.

The treatment of low HDL-C patients focuses on lowering LDL-C to the target level based on the patient's risk factor or CHD status (Table 35–4) *and* a reduction of VLDL cholesterol to below 30 mg/dL. Satisfactory treatment results are a ratio of total cholesterol:HDL-C that is 3.5 or less. Patients with total cholesterol:HDL-C ratios >4.5 are at risk even if their "non–HDL-C" levels (LDL-C and VLDL cholesterol) are at the goal values recommended by the NCEP guidelines. Consequently, it is useful to base treatment of patients with low HDL-C levels on both LDL-C levels and the total cholesterol:HDL-C ratio (Table 35–6).

DRUG THERAPY OF DYSLIPIDEMIA
Statins

The statins are the most effective and best-tolerated agents for treating dyslipidemia. These drugs are competitive inhibitors of 3-hydroxy-3-methylglutaryl coenzyme A (HMG-CoA) reductase, which catalyzes an early, rate-limiting step in cholesterol biosynthesis. Higher doses of the more potent statins (*e.g.,* atorvastatin, simvastatin, and rosuvastatin) also can reduce triglyceride levels caused by elevated VLDL levels. Some statins also are indicated for raising HDL-C levels, although the benefits of these effects on HDL-C remain to be proven.

The efficacy and safety of the statins in reducing fatal and nonfatal CHD events, strokes, and total mortality are well established. Rates of non-CHD adverse events in clinical trials were the same in the placebo groups and in the groups receiving the drug, both with regard to noncardiac illness and two laboratory tests, hepatic transaminases and creatine kinase (CK), commonly monitored in patients taking statins.

Pravastatin and simvastatin are chemically modified derivatives of lovastatin. Atorvastatin, *fluvastatin,* and *rosuvastatin* are structurally distinct synthetic compounds. Statins exert their major effect—reduction of LDL levels—through a mevalonic acid–like moiety that competitively inhibits HMG-CoA reductase. By reducing the conversion of HMG-CoA to mevalonate, statins inhibit hepatic cholesterol biosynthesis. In response to the reduced free cholesterol content within hepatocytes, synthesis of LDL receptors is increased and their degradation is reduced. The greater number of LDL receptors on the surface of hepatocytes increases removal of LDL from the blood, thereby lowering LDL-C levels. Statins also can reduce LDL levels by enhancing the removal of LDL precursors (VLDL and IDL) and by decreasing hepatic VLDL production. This mechanism likely accounts for the triglyceride-lowering effect of statins and may account for the reduction (~25%) of LDL-C levels in patients with homozygous familial hypercholesterolemia treated with 80 mg of atorvastatin or simvastatin.

Triglyceride levels >250 mg/dL are reduced substantially by statins, and the percent reduction achieved is similar to that in LDL-C. Accordingly, hypertriglyceridemic patients taking the highest doses of the most potent statins (simvastatin and atorvastatin, 80 mg/day; rosuvastatin, 40 mg/day) experience a 35–45% reduction in LDL-C and a comparable reduction in fasting triglyceride levels. If baseline triglyceride levels are <250 mg/dL, reductions in triglycerides are <25% irrespective of the dose or statin used. Similar reductions (35–45%) in triglycerides can be accomplished with doses of fibrates or niacin (see below), although these drugs do not reduce LDL-C to the same extent as atorvastatin or simvastatin at the 80-mg dose.

Statins lower LDL-C by 20–55%, depending on the dose and statin (Table 35–7). The fractional reductions achieved with the various doses are the same regardless of the absolute value of the baseline LDL-C level. Efficacy of LDL-C lowering is log-linear; LDL-C is reduced by ~6% (from baseline) with each doubling of the dose. Maximal effects on plasma cholesterol levels are achieved within 7–10 days. The statins are effective in almost all patients with high LDL-C levels. Patients with homozygous familial hypercholesterolemia have very attenuated responses to the usual doses of statins because both alleles of the LDL receptor gene encode dysfunctional LDL receptors; the partial response in these patients is due to a reduction in hepatic VLDL synthesis.

Although the statins clearly exert their major effects on CHD by lowering LDL-C and improving the lipid profile (Figure 35–2), a multitude of potentially cardioprotective effects are also ascribed to these drugs. It is not known whether these potential pleiotropic effects represent a class-action effect, differ amongst statins, or are biologically or clinically relevant.

Absorption, Metabolism, and Excretion

After oral administration, intestinal absorption of the statins varies between 30% and 85%. All of the statins, except simvastatin and lovastatin, are administered as active β-hydroxy acids. Simvastatin and lovastatin are administered as inactive lactones that must be transformed in the liver to their respective β-hydroxy acids. There is extensive first-pass hepatic uptake of all statins, but they enter the liver by different mechanisms. Uptake of atorvastatin, pravastatin, and rosuvastatin is mediated by the organic anion transporter 2 (OATP2). The lipophilic lactone forms of simvastatin and lovastatin are thought to enter the liver by simple diffusion. Due to extensive first-pass hepatic uptake, systemic bioavailability of the statins and their hepatic metabolites varies between 5% and 30% of administered doses. Except for fluvastatin and pravastatin, the metabolites of all statins have some HMG-CoA reductase inhibitory activity. Under steady-state conditions, small amounts of the parent drug and its metabolites produced in the liver can be found in the systemic circulation. In the plasma, >95% of statins and their metabolites are protein bound with the exception of pravastatin and its metabolites (50% bound).

After oral dosing, plasma concentrations of statins peak in 1–4 hours. The half-lives of the parent compounds are 1–4 hours, except for atorvastatin and rosuvastatin, which have half-lives of ~20 hours, which may contribute to their greater cholesterol-lowering efficacy. The liver biotransforms all

Table 35–7

Doses (mg) of Statins Required to Achieve Various Reductions in Low-Density-Lipoprotein Cholesterol from Baseline

	20%–25%	26%–30%	31%–35%	36%–40%	41%–50%	51%–55%
Atorvastatin	—	—	10	20	40	80
Fluvastatin	20	40	80			
Lovastatin	10	20	40	80		
Pravastatin	10	20	40			
Rosuvastatin	—	—	—	5	10	20, 40
Simvastatin	—	10	20	40	80	

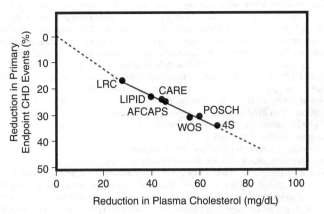

FIGURE 35–2 *Reduction in coronary heart disease events in clinical trials is associated with the extent of plasma cholesterol lowering. As more potent cholesterol-reducing agents become available, will it be possible to reduce events by 50% or more in a typical 5-year trial?* AFCAPS, Air Force/Texas Coronary Atherosclerosis Prevention Study; CARE, Cholesterol and Recurrent Events trial; LIPID, Long-Term Intervention with Pravastatin in Ischaemic Disease (LIPID) study; LRC, Lipid Research Clinics Coronary Primary Prevention Trial; POSCH, Program on the Surgical Control of the Hyperlipidemias; 4S, Scandinavian Simvastatin Survival Study; WOS, West of Scotland Coronary Prevention Study. *(Adapted from Thompson and Barter, 1999, and used by permission of Lippincott Williams & Wilkins.)*

statins, and >70% of statin metabolites are excreted by the liver with subsequent elimination in the feces.

ADVERSE EFFECTS AND DRUG INTERACTIONS

Hepatotoxicity

Serious hepatotoxicity is very rare (~one case per million person-years of use); nonetheless, it is reasonable to measure alanine aminotransferase (ALT) at baseline and thereafter when clinically indicated. Patients taking 80-mg doses (or 40 mg of rosuvastatin) should have their ALT checked after 3 months. If the ALT values are normal, it is not necessary to repeat the ALT test unless clinically indicated.

MYOPATHY

The most significant adverse effect associated with statin use is myopathy. The incidence of myopathy is quite low (~0.01%), but the risk of myopathy and rhabdomyolysis increases in proportion to plasma statin concentrations. Consequently, factors inhibiting statin catabolism are associated with increased myopathy risk, including advanced age (especially >80 years of age), hepatic or renal dysfunction, perioperative periods, multisystem disease (especially in association with diabetes mellitus), small body size, and untreated hypothyroidism. Concomitant use of drugs that diminish statin catabolism is associated with myopathy and rhabdomyolysis in ~50% of cases. The most common statin interactions occurred with fibrates, especially gemfibrozil, *38%;* cyclosporine, *4%;* digoxin, *5%;* warfarin, *4%;* macrolide antibiotics, *3%,* mibefradil, *2%; and* azole antifungals, *1%. Other drugs that increase the risk of statin-induced myopathy include niacin (rare), HIV protease inhibitors,* amiodarone, *and* nefazodone.

There are a variety of pharmacokinetic mechanisms by which these drugs increase myopathy risk when coadministered with statins. Gemfibrozil, the drug most commonly associated with statin-induced myopathy, inhibits uptake of the active hydroxy acid forms of statins into hepatocytes by OATP2 and interferes with the transformation of most statins by CYPs and glucuronidases. Primarily due to inhibition of OATP2-mediated hepatic uptake, coadministration of gemfibrozil nearly doubles the plasma concentration of rosuvastatin. Other fibrates, especially fenofibrate, do not interfere with the glucuronidation of statins and pose less risk of myopathy when combined with statin therapy. Concomitant therapy with simvastatin, 80 mg daily, and fenofibrate, 160 mg daily, results in no clinically significant pharmacokinetic interaction. Similar results were obtained in a study of low-dose rosuvastatin, 10 mg daily, plus fenofibrate, 67 mg three times a day. When statins are administered with niacin, the myopathy is probably caused by an enhanced inhibition of skeletal muscle cholesterol synthesis (a pharmacodynamic interaction).

Other drugs that interfere with statin oxidation are those metabolized primarily by CYP3A4, including certain macrolide antibiotics (e.g., erythromycin); azole antifungals (e.g., itraconazole); cyclosporine; the antidepressant nefazodone; and HIV protease inhibitors. These pharmacokinetic interactions are associated with increased plasma concentrations of statins and their active metabolites. Atorvastatin, lovastatin, and simvastatin are primarily metabolized by CYP3A4. Fluvastatin is mostly (50–80%) metabolized to inactive metabolites by CYP2C9, but CYP3A4 and CYP2C8 also contribute to its metabolism. Pravastatin is not metabolized to any appreciable extent by CYPs and is excreted unchanged in the urine. Because they are not extensively metabolized by CYP3A4, pravastatin, fluvastatin, and rosuvastatin may be less likely to cause myopathy when used with one of the predisposing drugs. However, because myopathy has occurred with all statins, the benefits of combined therapy with any statin should be carefully weighed against the risk of myopathy.

The myopathy syndrome is characterized by intense myalgia, first in the arms and thighs and then in the entire body, along with weakness and fatigue. Symptoms progress as long as the statin is continued. Myoglobinuria, renal failure, and death have been reported. Serum CK levels in affected patients typically are tenfold higher than the upper limit of normal. If myopathy is suspected, a blood sample should be drawn to document the presence of a significantly elevated CK level, since many patients complain of muscle pain unrelated to true statin-induced myopathy. The statin, and any other drug suspected of contributing to myopathy, should be discontinued if true myopathy is suspected, even if it is not possible to measure CK activity to confirm the diagnosis. Rhabdomyolysis should be excluded and renal function monitored.

Since myopathy rarely occurs in the absence of combination therapy, routine CK monitoring is not recommended unless the statins are used with a predisposing drug. Such monitoring is not sufficient to protect patients, as myopathy can occur months to years after combined therapy is initiated. As a rule, statins may be combined with one of these predisposing drugs with reduced risk of myopathy if the statin is administered at no more than 25% of its maximal dose (e.g., 10 mg for rosuvastatin and 20 mg for all other statins).

PREGNANCY

The safety of statins during pregnancy has not been established. *Women wishing to conceive should not take statins. During their childbearing years, women taking statins should use highly effective contraception (see Chapter 57). Nursing mothers also are advised to avoid statins.*

THERAPEUTIC USES   Each statin has a recommended starting dose that reduces LDL-C by 20–30%. Dyslipidemic patients frequently remain on their initial dose and thus remain undertreated. For this reason, it is advisable to start each patient on a dose that will achieve the patient's target goal for LDL-C lowering. For example, a patient with a baseline LDL-C of 150 mg/dL and a goal of 100 mg/dL requires a 33% reduction in LDL-C and should be started on a dose expected to provide it (Table 35–7). Hepatic cholesterol synthesis is maximal between midnight and 2:00 AM. Thus, statins with half-lives of 4 hours or less (all but atorvastatin and rosuvastatin) should be taken in the evening.

The manufacturer's initial recommended dose of lovastatin (MEVACOR) is 20 mg and is slightly more effective if taken with the evening meal than if it is taken at bedtime. The dose of lovastatin may be increased every 3–6 weeks up to a maximum of 80 mg/day. The 80-mg dose is slightly (2–3%) more effective if given as 40 mg twice daily. Lovastatin, at 20 mg, is marketed in combination with 500, 750, or 1000 mg of extended-release niacin (ADVICOR). Few patients are appropriate candidates for this fixed-dose combination. Alternate-day statin therapy has been associated with nearly equivalent efficacy (as judged by serum lipid profiles) and reduced cost, and has been proposed as a means to enhance compliance; clinical trials are needed to evaluate the efficacy of alternate-day dosing with regard to reducing clinical events.

The approved starting dose of simvastatin (ZOCOR) for most patients is 20 mg at bedtime unless the required LDL-C reduction exceeds 45% or the patient is a high-risk secondary prevention patient, in which case a 40-mg starting dose is indicated. The maximal dose is 80 mg, and the drug should be taken at bedtime. In patients taking cyclosporine, fibrates, or niacin, the daily dose should not exceed 20 mg.

Pravastatin (PRAVACHOL) therapy is started with a 20- or 40-mg dose that may be increased to 80 mg; it should be taken at bedtime. Since pravastatin is a hydroxy acid, it is bound by bile-acid sequestrants, which reduce its absorption. This is rarely a problem since the resins should be taken before meals and pravastatin should be taken at bedtime. Pravastatin is also marketed in combination with buffered aspirin (PRAVIGARD). The small advantage of combining these two drugs should be weighed against disadvantages inherent in fixed-dose combinations.

The starting dose of fluvastatin (LESCOL) is 20 or 40 mg, and the maximum is 80 mg/day. Like pravastatin, it is administered as a hydroxy acid and should be taken at bedtime, several hours after ingesting a bile-acid sequestrant (if the combination is used).

Atorvastatin (LIPITOR) has a long $t_{1/2}$, which allows dosing at any time of the day. The starting dose is 10 mg, and the maximum is 80 mg/day. Atorvastatin is marketed in combination with the Ca^{2+}-channel blocker amlodipine (CADUET), for patients with hypertension or angina as well as hypercholesterolemia. The physician should weigh any advantage of combination against the associated risks and disadvantages.

Rosuvastatin (CRESTOR) is available in doses ranging between 5 and 40 mg. It has a $t_{1/2}$ of 20–30 hours and may be taken at any time of day. Since experience with rosuvastatin is more limited, treatment should be initiated with 5–10 mg daily, increasing stepwise if needed. If the combination of gemfibrozil with rosuvastatin is used, the dose of rosuvastatin should not exceed 10 mg. Rosuvastatin at a dose of 80 mg (dose not approved by the FDA) was noted to cause proteinuria and hematuria and isolated cases of renal failure. Other statins have also been observed to cause proteinuria, apparently by inhibiting tubular protein reabsorption. Whether statin-induced proteinuria is harmful or beneficial, especially in patients with chronic kidney disease, remains to be determined.

The choice of statins should be based on efficacy (reduction of LDL-C) and cost. Three drugs (lovastatin, simvastatin, and pravastatin) have been used safely in clinical trials involving thousands of subjects for 5 or more years. The documented safety records of these statins should be considered, especially when initiating therapy in younger patients. Once drug treatment is initiated, it almost always is lifelong. Baseline determinations of alanine aminotransferase (ALT) and repeat testing at 3–6 months are recommended. If ALT is normal after the initial 3–6 months, then it need not be repeated more than once every 6–12 months. CK measurements are not done routinely unless the patient also is taking a drug that enhances the risk of myopathy.

STATIN USE BY CHILDREN Some statins are approved for children with heterozygous familial hypercholesterolemia. Atorvastatin, lovastatin, and simvastatin are indicated for children age 11 or older. Pravastatin is approved for children age 8 or older.

STATINS IN COMBINATION WITH OTHER LIPID-LOWERING DRUGS Statins, in combination with the bile acid–binding resins cholestyramine and colestipol, produce 20–30% greater reductions in LDL-C than statins alone achieve. Preliminary data indicate that colesevelam hydrochloride plus a statin lowers LDL-C by 8–16% more than statins alone. Niacin also can enhance the effect of statins, but the occurrence of myopathy increases when statin doses greater than 25% of maximum are used with niacin. The combination of a fibrate (clofibrate, gemfibrozil, or fenofibrate) with a statin is particularly useful in patients with hypertriglyceridemia and high LDL-C levels. This combination increases the risk of myopathy but usually is safe with a fibrate at its usual maximal dose and a statin at no more than 25% of its maximal dose. Fenofibrate, which is least likely to interfere with statin metabolism, appears to be the safest fibrate to use with statins. Triple therapy with resins, niacin, and statins can reduce LDL-C by up to 70%. VYTORIN, a fixed combination of simvastatin (10, 20, 40, or 80 mg) and ezetimibe (10 mg), decreased LDL-C levels by up to 60% at 24 weeks.

Bile-Acid Sequestrants

The two established bile-acid sequestrants or resins (cholestyramine and colestipol) are most often used as second agents if statin therapy does not lower LDL-C levels sufficiently. When used with a statin, cholestyramine and colestipol usually are prescribed at submaximal doses. Maximal doses can reduce LDL-C by up to 25% but are associated with unacceptable gastrointestinal (GI) side effects (bloating and constipation) that limit compliance. Colesevelam is a newer bile-acid sequestrant that is prepared as an anhydrous gel and taken as a tablet. It lowers LDL-C by 18% at its maximum dose. The safety and efficacy of colesevelam have not been studied in children or pregnant women.

MECHANISM OF ACTION The bile-acid sequestrants are highly positively charged and bind negatively charged bile acids. The resins are not absorbed, and the bound bile acids are excreted in the stool. Since >95% of bile acids are normally reabsorbed, interruption of this process depletes the pool of bile acids and increases hepatic bile-acid synthesis. As a result, hepatic cholesterol content declines, stimulating the production of LDL receptors. The increase in hepatic LDL receptors increases LDL clearance and lowers LDL-C levels, but this effect is partially offset by the enhanced cholesterol synthesis caused by upregulation of HMG-CoA reductase. Inhibition of reductase activity by a statin substantially increases the effectiveness of the resins.

The resin-induced increase in bile-acid production is accompanied by an increase in hepatic triglyceride synthesis, which is of consequence in patients with significant hypertriglyceridemia (baseline triglyceride >250 mg/dL). In such patients, bile-acid sequestrant therapy may increase triglyceride levels; until this issue is resolved, use of colesevelam to lower LDL-C levels in hyper-triglyceridemic patients should be accompanied by frequent (every 1–2 weeks) monitoring of fast-ing triglyceride levels until the triglyceride level is stable, or colesevelam should be avoided in these patients.

EFFECTS ON LIPOPROTEIN LEVELS

The reduction in LDL-C by resins is dose-dependent. Doses of 8–12 g of cholestyramine or 10–15 g of colestipol are associated with 12–18% reductions in LDL-C. Maximal doses (24 g of cholestyramine, 30 g of colestipol) may reduce LDL-C by as much as 25%, but will cause GI side effects that are poorly tolerated by most patients. One to two weeks is sufficient to attain maximal LDL-C reduction by a given resin dose. In patients with normal triglyceride levels, triglycerides may increase transiently and then return to baseline. HDL-C levels increase 4–5%. Statins plus resins or niacin plus resins can reduce LDL-C by as much as 40–60%. Colesevelam, in doses of 3–3.75 g, reduces LDL-C levels by 9–19%.

ADVERSE EFFECTS AND DRUG INTERACTIONS

The resins are generally safe, as they are not systemically absorbed. Since they are adminis-tered as chloride salts, rare instances of hyperchloremic acidosis have occurred. Since they increase triglyceride levels, severe hypertriglyceridemia is a contraindication to the use of cholestyramine and colestipol. At present, there are insufficient data on the effect of colesevelam on triglyceride levels.

Cholestyramine and colestipol both are available as a powder that must be mixed with water and drunk as a slurry. The gritty sensation is unpleasant to patients initially but can be tolerated. Colestipol is available in a tablet that reduces the complaint of grittiness but not the GI symptoms. Colesevelam is available as a hard capsule that absorbs water and creates a soft, gelatinous mate-rial that allegedly minimizes the potential for GI irritation.

Patients taking cholestyramine and colestipol complain of bloating and dyspepsia, which can be substantially reduced if the drug is completely suspended in liquid several hours before inges-tion. Constipation may occur but sometimes can be prevented by adequate daily water intake and psyllium, if necessary. Colesevelam may be less likely to cause the dyspepsia, bloating, and con-stipation observed in patients treated with cholestyramine or colestipol.

Cholestyramine and colestipol interfere with the absorption of many drugs, including some thiazides, furosemide, propranolol, l-thyroxine, *digoxin, warfarin, and some of the statins. It is wise to administer all drugs either 1 hour before or 3–4 hours after a dose of cholestyramine or colestipol. Colesevelam does not appear to interfere with the absorption of fat-soluble vitamins or of drugs such as digoxin, lovastatin, warfarin,* metoprolol, quinidine, *and* valproic acid. *The max-imum concentration and the AUC of sustained-release* verapamil *are reduced by 31% and 11%, respectively, when the drug is coadministered with colesevelam. The effect of colesevelam on the absorption of other drugs has not been tested; prudence suggests that patients take other med-ications 1 hour before or 3–4 hours after a dose.*

THERAPEUTIC USES

The powdered forms of cholestyramine (4 g/dose) and colestipol (5 g/dose) are either mixed with a fluid (water or juice) and drunk as a slurry or mixed with crushed ice in a blender. Ideally, patients should take the resins before breakfast and before supper, starting with one scoop or packet twice daily, and increasing the dosage after several weeks or longer as needed and as tol-erated. Patients generally will not take more than two doses (scoops or packets) twice a day.

*Colesevelam hydrochloride (*WELCHOL*) is available as a solid tablet containing 0.625 g of cole-sevelam. The starting dose is either three tablets taken twice daily with meals or all six tablets taken with a meal. The tablets should be taken with a liquid. The maximum daily dose is 7 tablets (4.375 g).*

Niacin (Nicotinic Acid)

Niacin, *nicotinic acid* favorably affects virtually all lipid parameters. Niacin is a water-soluble B-complex vitamin that functions as a vitamin only after its conversion to NAD or NADP, in which it occurs as an amide. Both niacin and its amide may be given orally for its functions as a vitamin but only niacin affects lipid levels. The hypolipidemic effects of niacin require larger doses than are required for its vitamin effects. Niacin is the best agent available for increasing HDL-C (increments of 30–40%); it also lowers triglycerides by 35–45% (as effectively as fibrates and the more potent statins) and reduces LDL-C levels by 20–30%. Niacin also is the only lipid-lowering drug that reduces Lp(a) levels significantly, by ~40%; however, this is unnecessary because adequate control of other lipid abnormalities mitigates the atherogenic effects of elevated Lp(a). Despite its salutary effect on lipids, niacin use is limited by side effects (*see* below).

In adipose tissue, niacin inhibits the lipolysis of triglycerides by hormone-sensitive lipase, which reduces transport of free fatty acids to the liver and decreases hepatic triglyceride synthesis. Niacin may exert its effects on lipolysis by stimulating a GPCR that couples to G_i to inhibit adenylyl cyclase in adipocytes. In the liver, niacin reduces triglyceride synthesis by inhibiting both the synthesis and esterification of fatty acids, effects that increase apoB degradation. Reduced triglyceride synthesis decreases hepatic VLDL production, which reduces LDL levels. Niacin also enhances LPL activity, promoting the clearance of chylomicrons and VLDL triglycerides. Niacin raises HDL-C levels by decreasing fractional clearance of apoA-I in HDL rather than by enhancing HDL synthesis.

Regular or crystalline niacin in doses of 2–6 g/day reduces triglycerides by 35–50%, and the maximal effect occurs within 4–7 days. Reductions of 25% in LDL-C levels are possible with doses of 4.5–6 g/day, but 3–6 weeks are required for maximal effect. Average increases in HDL-C of 15–30% occur in patients with low HDL-C levels; greater increases may occur in patients with normal HDL-C levels at baseline. Combination therapy with resins can reduce LDL-C levels by as much as 40–60%.

ABSORPTION, FATE, AND EXCRETION

The doses of regular (crystalline) niacin used to treat dyslipidemia are almost completely absorbed, and peak plasma concentrations are achieved within 30–60 minutes. The $t_{1/2}$ is ~60 minutes, which accounts for the necessity of twice- or thrice-daily dosing. At lower doses, most niacin is taken up by the liver; only the major metabolite, nicotinuric acid, is found in the urine. At higher doses, a greater proportion of drug is excreted in the urine as unchanged nicotinic acid.

ADVERSE EFFECTS

Niacin's side effects limit patient compliance. Cutaneous effects include flushing and pruritus of the face and upper trunk, rashes, and acanthosis nigricans. Flushing and associated pruritus are prostaglandin-mediated. Flushing is worse when therapy is initiated or the dosage is increased, but ceases in most patients after 1–2 weeks of a stable dose. Aspirin alleviates the flushing in many patients. Flushing recurs if only one or two doses are missed and is more likely to occur when niacin is consumed with hot beverages (coffee, tea) or with ethanol-containing beverages. Flushing is minimized if therapy is initiated with low doses (100–250 mg twice daily) and if the drug is taken after breakfast or supper. Dry skin, a frequent complaint, can be dealt with by using skin moisturizers, and acanthosis nigricans can be dealt with by using lotions or creams containing salicylic acid. Dyspepsia and rarer episodes of nausea, vomiting, and diarrhea are less likely to occur if the drug is taken at a meal. Patients with any history of peptic ulcer disease should not take niacin because it can reactivate ulcer disease.

The most common serious side effects are hepatotoxicity, manifested as elevated serum transaminases and hyperglycemia. Both regular (crystalline) niacin and sustained-release niacin have been reported to cause severe liver toxicity, and sustained-release niacin can cause fulminant hepatic failure. An extended-release niacin (NIASPAN), appears to be less likely to cause severe hepatotoxicity, perhaps because it is administered only once daily. The incidence of flushing and pruritus with this preparation is not substantially different from that with regular niacin. Severe hepatotoxicity is more likely to occur when patients take >2 g of sustained-release, over-the-counter preparations. Affected patients experience flu-like fatigue and weakness. Usually, serum transaminases are elevated, serum albumin levels decline, and total cholesterol and LDL-C levels decline substantially.

In patients with diabetes mellitus, niacin should be used cautiously, since niacin-induced insulin resistance can cause severe hyperglycemia. Niacin use in patients with diabetes mellitus often mandates a change to insulin therapy. If niacin is prescribed for patients with known or suspected diabetes, blood glucose levels should be monitored at least weekly until proven to be stable. Niacin also elevates uric acid levels; a history of gout is a relative contraindication for niacin use. Rarer reversible side effects include toxic amblyopia and toxic maculopathy. Atrial tachyarrhythmias and atrial fibrillation have been reported, more commonly in elderly patients. Niacin, at doses used in humans, has been associated with birth defects in animal models and should not be taken by pregnant women.

THERAPEUTIC USES

Niacin is indicated for hypertriglyceridemia and elevated LDL-C; it is especially useful in patients with both hypertriglyceridemia and low HDL-C levels. Crystalline niacin (immediate-release or regular) refers to niacin tablets that dissolve quickly after ingestion. Sustained-release niacin refers to preparations that continuously release niacin for 6–8 hours after ingestion. NIASPAN is the only preparation of niacin that is FDA-approved for treating dyslipidemia; it requires a prescription.

Crystalline niacin tablets are available over the counter in a variety of strengths. To minimize the flushing and pruritus, it is best to start with a low dose (e.g., 100 mg twice daily taken after breakfast and supper). The dose may be increased stepwise every 7 days by 100–200 mg to a total daily dose of 1.5–2 g. After 2–4 weeks at this dose, transaminases, serum albumin, fasting glucose, and uric acid levels should be measured. Lipid levels should be checked and the dose increased further until the desired effect on plasma lipids is achieved. After a stable dose is attained, blood should be drawn every 3–6 months to monitor for the various toxicities.

Since concurrent use of niacin and a statin can cause myopathy, the statin should be administered at no more than 25% of its maximal dose. Patients also should be instructed to discontinue therapy if myalgias occur. Routine measurement of CK in patients taking niacin and statins does not assure that severe myopathy will be detected before onset of symptoms, as patients have developed myopathy after several years of concomitant use of niacin with a statin.

Over-the-counter, sustained-release niacin preparations and NIASPAN are effective up to a total daily dose of 2 g/day. All doses of sustained-release niacin, but particularly those >2 g/day, have been reported to cause hepatotoxicity, which may occur soon after beginning therapy or after several years of use. The potential for severe liver damage should preclude its use in most patients. NIASPAN may be less likely to cause hepatotoxicity.

Fibric Acid Derivatives: PPAR Activators

Clofibrate is a halogenated fibric acid derivative. Gemfibrozil is a nonhalogenated compound that is distinct from the halogenated fibrates. A number of fibric acid analogs (e.g., fenofibrate, bezafibrate, and ciprofibrate) have been developed and are used in Europe and elsewhere. The mechanisms by which fibrates lower lipoprotein levels, or raise HDL levels, remain unclear. Many of their effects on blood lipids are mediated by their interaction with peroxisome proliferator activated receptors (PPARs), which regulate gene transcription. Fibrates bind to PPARα, which is expressed primarily in the liver and brown adipose tissue and to a lesser extent in kidney, heart, and skeletal muscle. Fibrates reduce triglycerides through PPARα-mediated stimulation of fatty acid oxidation, increased LPL synthesis, and reduced expression of apoC-III.

LDL levels rise in many patients treated with gemfibrozil, especially those with hypertriglyceridemia. However, LDL levels are unchanged or fall in others, especially those whose triglyceride levels are not elevated or who are taking a second-generation agent e.g., fenofibrate, bezafibrate, or ciprofibrate). The decrease in LDL levels may partly be due to changes in the cholesterol and triglyceride contents of LDL that are mediated by CETP; such changes can alter the affinity of LDL for the LDL receptor.

The effects of the fibrates on lipoprotein levels differ widely, depending on the starting lipoprotein profile, the presence or absence of a genetic hyperlipoproteinemia, the associated environmental influences, and the specific fibrate used. Patients with type III hyperlipoproteinemia (dysbetalipoproteinemia) are among the most sensitive responders to fibrates. Elevated triglyceride and cholesterol levels are dramatically lowered, and xanthomas may regress completely. Angina and intermittent claudication also improve.

In patients with mild hypertriglyceridemia (e.g., triglycerides <400 mg/dL), fibrate treatment decreases triglyceride levels by up to 50% and increases HDL-C concentrations ~15%; LDL-C levels may be unchanged or increase. The second-generation agents, such as fenofibrate, bezafibrate, and ciprofibrate, lower VLDL levels to a degree similar to that produced by gemfibrozil, but they also are more likely to decrease LDL levels by 15–20%. In patients with more marked hypertriglyceridemia (e.g., 400–1000 mg/dl), a similar fall in triglycerides occurs, but LDL increases of 10–30% are seen frequently. Normotriglyceridemic patients with heterozygous familial hypercholesterolemia usually experience little change in LDL levels with gemfibrozil; with the other fibric acid agents, reductions as great as 20% may occur.

Fibrates usually are the drugs of choice for treating severe hypertriglyceridemia and the chylomicronemia syndrome. While the primary therapy is to remove alcohol and as much fat from the diet as possible, fibrates help both by increasing triglyceride clearance and by decreasing hepatic triglyceride synthesis. In patients with chylomicronemia syndrome, fibrate maintenance therapy and a low-fat diet keep triglyceride levels well below 1000 mg/dL and thus prevent episodes of pancreatitis.

ABSORPTION, FATE, AND EXCRETION

All of the fibrates are absorbed rapidly and efficiently (>90%) when given with a meal but less efficiently when taken on an empty stomach. The ester bond is hydrolyzed rapidly, and peak plasma concentrations are attained within 1–4 hours. More than 95% of these drugs are bound to plasma protein, mainly to albumin. The half-lives of fibrates differ significantly, ranging from 1 hour (gemfibrozil) to 20 hours (fenofibrate). The drugs distribute widely throughout the body, and concentrations in liver, kidney, and intestine exceed the plasma level. Gemfibrozil is transferred across the placenta. The fibrate drugs are excreted predominantly as glucuronide conjugates; 60–90% of an oral dose is excreted in the urine, with smaller amounts appearing in the feces. Excretion is impaired in renal failure and fibrates are contraindicated in such patients.

ADVERSE EFFECTS AND DRUG INTERACTIONS

Fibric acid compounds usually are well tolerated. Side effects, most often GI-related, may occur in 5–10% of patients but most often are not sufficient to cause drug discontinuation. Other infrequent side effects include rash, urticaria, hair loss, myalgias, fatigue, headache, impotence, and anemia. Minor increases in liver transaminases and alkaline phosphatase have been reported. Clofibrate, bezafibrate, and fenofibrate reportedly can potentiate the action of oral anticoagulants by displacing them from their binding sites on albumin; thus, monitoring of the prothrombin time and reduction in anticoagulant dosage may be appropriate.

Myopathy occasionally occurs in subjects taking clofibrate, gemfibrozil, or fenofibrate, and may occur in up to 5% of patients treated with a combination of gemfibrozil and higher doses of statins. Statin doses therefore should be reduced when a statin plus a fibrate are combined. Several drug interactions may contribute to this adverse response. Gemfibrozil inhibits hepatic uptake of statins by OATP2 and also competes for the same glucuronosyl transferases that metabolize most statins. Thus, levels of both drugs may increase with coadministration. Patients taking this combination should be told about potential symptoms and followed at 3-month intervals with careful history and determination of CK values until a stable pattern is established. Until there is more experience, patients taking fibrates with rosuvastatin should be followed especially closely even at low doses (5–10 mg) of rosuvastatin. Fenofibrate is glucuronidated by enzymes that are not involved in statin glucuronidation; thus, fenofibrate-statin combinations are less likely to cause myopathy than combination therapy with gemfibrozil and statins.

All fibrates increase the lithogenicity of bile. Clofibrate has been associated with increased risk of gallstone formation; gemfibrozil and fenofibrate reportedly do not increase biliary tract disease. Renal failure and hepatic dysfunction are relative contraindications to fibrate therapy. Combined statin-fibrate therapy should be avoided in patients with impaired renal function. Gemfibrozil should be used with caution and at a reduced dosage to treat the hyperlipidemia of renal failure. Fibrates should not be used by children or pregnant women.

THERAPEUTIC USES Clofibrate is available for oral administration and may be useful in patients who do not tolerate gemfibrozil or fenofibrate. The usual dose is 2 g/day in divided doses. Gemfibrozil (LOPID) is usually administered as a 600-mg dose taken twice a day, 30 minutes before the morning and evening meals. The TRICOR brand of fenofibrate is available in tablets of 48 and 145 mg. The usual daily dose is 145 mg. Generic fenofibrate (LOFIBRA) is available in capsules containing 67, 134, and 200 mg. TRICOR, 145 mg, and LOFIBRA, 200 mg, are equivalent doses.

Fibrates are the drugs of choice for treating hyperlipidemic subjects with type III hyperlipoproteinemia and for subjects with severe hypertriglyceridemia (triglycerides >1000 mg/dL) who are at risk for pancreatitis. Fibrates appear to have an important role in subjects with high triglycerides and low HDL-C levels associated with the metabolic syndrome or type 2 diabetes mellitus. In these settings, the LDL levels should be monitored; if LDL levels rise, the addition of a low dose of a statin may be needed. Many experts now treat such patients first with a statin, and then add a fibrate, based on the reported benefit of gemfibrozil therapy. If this combination is used, there should be careful monitoring for myopathy.

Ezetimibe and the Inhibition of Dietary Cholesterol Uptake

Ezetimibe is the first compound approved for lowering total and LDL-C levels that inhibits cholesterol absorption by enterocytes in the small intestine. It lowers LDL-C levels by 15–20% and is used primarily as adjunctive therapy with statins. Ezetimibe does not affect intestinal triglyceride absorption. In human subjects, ezetimibe reduced cholesterol absorption by 54%, precipitating a compensatory increase in cholesterol synthesis, which can be inhibited with a cholesterol synthesis inhibitor such as a statin. The consequence of inhibiting intestinal cholesterol absorption is a reduction in the incorporation of cholesterol into chylomicrons. The reduced cholesterol content of chylomicrons diminishes the delivery of cholesterol to the liver by chylomicron remnants. The diminished remnant cholesterol content may decrease atherogenesis directly, as chylomicron remnants are very atherogenic lipoproteins.

Reduced delivery of intestinal cholesterol to the liver by chylomicron remnants stimulates expression of the hepatic genes regulating LDL receptor expression and cholesterol biosynthesis. The greater expression of hepatic LDL receptors enhances LDL-C clearance from the plasma.

As monotherapy, ezetimibe is limited to the small group of statin-intolerant patients. The actions of ezetimibe, which inhibits intestinal cholesterol absorption and enhances cholesterol biosynthesis, are complementary to those of statins, and there is a further reduction of 15–20% in LDL-C when ezetimibe is combined with any statin at any dose. Increasing statin dosages from the usual starting dose of 20–80 mg normally yields only an additional 12% reduction in LDL-C, whereas adding ezetimibe, 10 mg daily, to 20 mg of a statin will reduce LDL-C by an additional 18–20%. A combination tablet containing ezetimibe, 10 mg, and various doses of simvastatin (10, 20, 40, and 80 mg) is available (VYTORIN). At the highest simvastatin dose (80 mg), plus ezetimibe (10 mg), average LDL-C reduction was 60%, exceeding that attained with any statin as monotherapy.

ABSORPTION, FATE, AND EXCRETION

Ezetimibe is highly water insoluble. After ingestion, it is glucuronidated in the intestinal epithelium, absorbed, and enters an enterohepatic recirculation. Pharmacokinetic studies indicate that ~70% is excreted in the feces and ~10% in the urine (as a glucuronide conjugate). Bile acid sequestrants inhibit absorption of ezetimibe, and the two agents should not be coadministered. Otherwise, no significant drug interactions have been reported.

ADVERSE EFFECTS AND DRUG INTERACTIONS

Ezetimibe rarely can cause allergic reactions. It has been associated with myopathy, more commonly in association with statins but also when used as monotherapy. The mechanism for this adverse effects is unknown. The safety of ezetimibe during pregnancy has not been established. Since all statins are contraindicated in pregnant and nursing women, combination products containing ezetimibe and a statin should not be used by women in childbearing years in the absence of contraception.

THERAPEUTIC USES

Ezetimibe (ZETIA) is available as a 10-mg tablet that may be taken at any time of day irrespective of food.

For a complete Bibliographical listing see Goodman & Gilman's *The Pharmacological Basis of Therapeutics*, 11th ed., or Goodman & Gilman Online at www.accessmedicine.com.

DRUGS AFFECTING GASTROINTESTINAL FUNCTION

36

PHARMACOTHERAPY OF GASTRIC ACIDITY, PEPTIC ULCERS, AND GASTROESOPHAGEAL REFLUX DISEASE

The acid-peptic diseases are those disorders in which gastric acid and pepsin are necessary, but usually not sufficient, pathogenic factors. Barriers to the reflux of gastric contents into the esophagus comprise the primary esophageal defense. If these protective barriers fail and reflux occurs, dyspepsia and/or erosive esophagitis may result. Therapies are directed at decreasing gastric acidity, enhancing the lower esophageal sphincter pressure, or stimulating esophageal motility (*see* Chapter 37). In the stomach, mucus and bicarbonate, stimulated by the local generation of prostaglandins, protect the gastric mucosa. If these defenses are disrupted, a gastric or duodenal ulcer may form. The treatment and prevention of these acid-related disorders are accomplished either by decreasing the level of gastric acidity or by enhancing mucosal protection. The appreciation that an infectious agent, *Helicobacter pylori*, plays a key role in the pathogenesis of acid-peptic diseases has stimulated new approaches to prevention and therapy.

PHYSIOLOGY OF GASTRIC SECRETION
The regulation of gastric acid secretion is shown in Figure 36-1.

GASTRIC DEFENSES AGAINST ACID
The high [H^+] in the gastric lumen requires defense mechanisms to protect the esophagus and the stomach. The primary esophageal defense is the lower esophageal sphincter, which prevents reflux of acidic gastric contents into the esophagus. The stomach protects itself from acid damage by a number of mechanisms that require adequate mucosal blood flow, perhaps because of the high metabolic activity and oxygen requirements of the gastric mucosa. One key defense is the secretion of a mucus layer that protects gastric epithelial cells. Gastric mucus is soluble when secreted but quickly forms an insoluble gel that coats the mucosal surface of the stomach, slows ion diffusion, and prevents mucosal damage by macromolecules such as pepsin. Mucus production is stimulated by prostaglandins E_2 and I_2, which also directly inhibit gastric acid secretion by parietal cells. Thus, alcohol, aspirin, and other drugs that inhibit prostaglandin formation decrease mucus secretion and predispose to the development of acid-peptic disease. A second important part of the normal mucosal defense is the secretion of bicarbonate ions by superficial gastric epithelial cells. Bicarbonate neutralizes the acid in the region of the mucosal cells, thereby raising pH and preventing acid-mediated damage.

PROTON PUMP INHIBITORS
CHEMISTRY, MECHANISM OF ACTION, AND PHARMACOLOGY The most potent suppressors of gastric acid secretion are inhibitors of the gastric H^+,K^+-ATPase (proton pump) (Figure 36–2A). In typical doses, these drugs diminish the daily production of acid (basal and stimulated) by 80–95%. Five proton pump inhibitors are available for clinical use: *omeprazole* (PRILOSEC, RAPINEX, ZEGERID) and its S-isomer, *esomeprazole* (NEXIUM), *lansoprazole* (PREVACID), *rabeprazole* (ACIPHEX), and *pantoprazole* (PROTONIX). These drugs have different substitutions on their pyridine and/or benzimidazole groups but are remarkably similar in their pharmacological properties. Omeprazole is a racemate; the S-isomer, esomeprazole (S-omeprazole), is eliminated less rapidly than R-omeprazole, which theoretically provides a therapeutic advantage because of the increased $t_{1/2}$. All proton pump inhibitors have equivalent efficacy at comparable doses.

Proton pump inhibitors are prodrugs that require activation in an acid environment. After absorption into the systemic circulation, the prodrug diffuses into the parietal cells of the stomach and accumulates in the acidic secretory canaliculi. Here, it is activated by proton-catalyzed formation of a tetracyclic sulfenamide (Figure 36–2), trapping the drug so that it cannot diffuse back across the

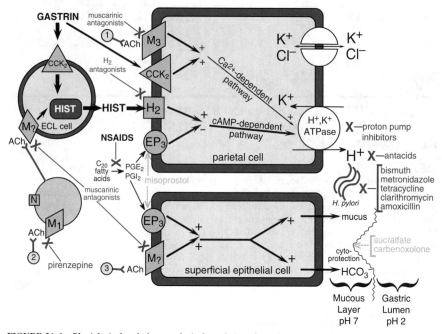

FIGURE 36–1 *Physiological and pharmacological regulation of gastric secretion: the basis for therapy of acid-peptic disorders.* Shown are the interactions among an enterochromaffin-like (ECL) cell that secretes histamine, a parietal cell that secretes acid, and a superficial epithelial cell that secretes cytoprotective mucus and bicarbonate. Physiological pathways, shown in solid black, may be stimulatory (+) or inhibitory (−). 1 and 3 indicate possible inputs from postganglionic cholinergic fibers, while 2 shows neural input from the vagus nerve. Physiological agonists and their respective membrane receptors include: acetylcholine (ACh), muscarinic (M), and nicotinic (N) receptors; gastrin, cholecystokinin receptor 2 (CCK₂); histamine (HIST), H₂ receptor; and prostaglandin E₂ (PGE₂), EP₃ receptor. Drug actions are indicated by dashed lines. A blue X indicates targets of pharmacological antagonism. A light blue dashed arrow indicates a drug action that mimics or enhances a physiological pathway. Shown in blue are drugs used to treat acid-peptic disorders. NSAIDs are nonsteroidal antiinflammatory drugs and are ulcerogenic.

canalicular membrane. The activated form then binds covalently with sulfhydryl groups of cysteines in the H^+,K^+-ATPase, irreversibly inactivating the pump molecule. Acid secretion resumes only after new pump molecules are synthesized and inserted into the luminal membrane, providing a prolonged (up to 24–48 hour) suppression of acid secretion, despite the much shorter plasma half-lives (0.5–2 hours) of the parent compounds. Because they block the final step in acid production, the proton pump inhibitors are effective in acid suppression regardless of other stimulating factors.

To prevent degradation of proton pump inhibitors by acid in the gastric lumen, oral dosage forms are supplied in different formulations: (1) enteric-coated drugs contained inside gelatin capsules (omeprazole, esomeprazole, and lansoprazole); (2) enteric-coated granules supplied as a powder for suspension (lansoprazole); (3) enteric-coated tablets (pantoprazole, rabeprazole, and omeprazole); and (4) powdered drug combined with sodium bicarbonate (omeprazole). The delayed-release and enteric-coated tablets dissolve only at alkaline pH, while admixture of omeprazole with sodium bicarbonate simply neutralizes stomach acid; both strategies substantially improve the oral bioavailability of these acid-labile drugs. In patients for whom the oral route of administration is not available and those requiring immediate acid suppression can be treated parenterally with pantoprazole or lansoprazole. A single intravenous bolus of 80 mg of pantoprazole inhibits acid production by 80–90% within an hour, and this inhibition persists for up to 21 hours, permitting once-daily dosing to achieve the desired degree of hypochlorhydria. The dose of intravenous pantoprazole for gastroesophageal reflux disease is 40 mg daily for up to 10 days. Higher doses (*e.g.*, 160–240 mg in divided doses) are used to manage hypersecretory conditions such as the Zollinger-Ellison syndrome. An intravenous formulation of esomeprazole is available in Europe but not in the U.S.

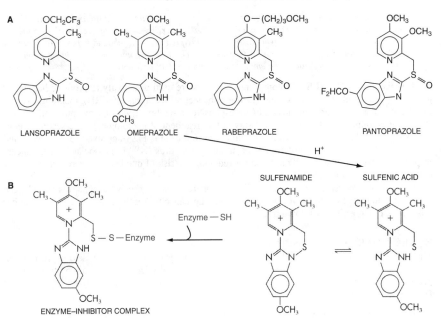

FIGURE 36–2 *Proton pump inhibitors.* **A.** Inhibitors of gastric H^+,K^+-ATPase (proton pump). **B.** Conversion of omeprazole to a sulfenamide in the acidic secretory canaliculi of the parietal cell. The sulfenamide interacts covalently with sulfhydryl groups in the proton pump, thereby irreversibly inhibiting its activity. The other three proton pump inhibitors undergo analogous conversions.

PHARMACOKINETICS

Since an acidic pH in the parietal cell acid canaliculi is required for drug activation, and since food stimulates acid production, these drugs ideally should be given about 30 minutes before meals.

Once in the small bowel, proton pump inhibitors are rapidly absorbed, highly protein bound, and extensively metabolized by hepatic CYPs, particularly CYP2C19 and CYP3A4. Several polymorphic variants of CYP2C19 have been identified. Asians are more likely than Caucasians or African Americans to have the CYP2C19 genotype that correlates with slow metabolism of proton pump inhibitors (23% vs. 3%, respectively), which may contribute to heightened efficacy and/or toxicity in this ethnic group.

It may take 2–5 days of therapy with once-daily dosing to achieve the 70% inhibition of proton pumps that is seen at steady state. Since proton pump inhibition is irreversible, acid secretion is suppressed for 24–48 hours, or more, until new proton pumps are synthesized and incorporated into the luminal membrane of parietal cells.

Chronic renal failure does not lead to accumulation of the proton pump inhibitors with once-a-day dosing. Hepatic disease substantially reduces the clearance of esomeprazole and lansoprazole; thus, in patients with severe hepatic disease, dose reduction is recommended for esomeprazole and should be considered for lansoprazole.

ADVERSE EFFECTS AND DRUG INTERACTIONS

Proton pump inhibitors generally cause remarkably few adverse effects. The most common are nausea, abdominal pain, constipation, flatulence, and diarrhea. Subacute myopathy, arthralgias, headaches, and rashes also have been reported. Proton pump inhibitors can interact with warfarin *(esomeprazole, lansoprazole, omeprazole, and rabeprazole),* diazepam *(esomeprazole and omeprazole), and* cyclosporine *(omeprazole and rabeprazole). Omeprazole inhibits CYP2C19 (thereby decreasing the clearance of* disulfiram, phenytoin, *and other drugs) and induces the expression of CYP1A2 (thereby increasing the clearance of* imipramine, *several antipsychotic drugs,* tacrine, *and* theophylline*).*

Loss of gastric acidity from chronic proton pump inhibitor treatment may affect the bioavailability of such drugs as ketoconazole, ampicillin esters, and iron salts. Chronic therapy, with proton pump inhibitors has been linked to increased frequency of hip fractures, possibly secondary to decreased absorption of calcium.

Hypergastrinemia is more frequent and more severe with proton pump inhibitors than with H_2 receptor antagonists, and gastrin levels of >500 ng/L occur in ~5–10% of users with chronic omeprazole administration. This hypergastrinemia may predispose to rebound hypersecretion of gastric acid upon drug discontinuation (see below). The proton pump inhibitors have a long record of use worldwide without the emergence of major safety concerns.

THERAPEUTIC USES Proton pump inhibitors are used principally to promote healing of gastric and duodenal ulcers and to treat gastroesophageal reflux disease (GERD), including erosive esophagitis, that is either complicated or unresponsive to treatment with H_2 receptor antagonists. Proton pump inhibitors also are the mainstay in the treatment of pathological hypersecretory conditions, such as the Zollinger-Ellison syndrome. Lansoprazole is FDA-approved for treatment and prevention of recurrence of nonsteroidal anti-inflammatory drug (NSAID)-associated gastric ulcers in patients who continue NSAID use and for reducing the risk of duodenal ulcer recurrence associated with *H. pylori* infections.

In children, omeprazole is safe and effective for treatment of erosive esophagitis and GERD. Younger patients generally have increased metabolic capacity, resulting in the need for higher dosages of omeprazole per kilogram in children compared to adults.

H_2 RECEPTOR ANTAGONISTS

The H_2 receptor antagonists were the first truly effective drugs for the therapy of acid-peptic disease, and their long history of safety and efficacy with the eventually led to their availability without a prescription. Increasingly, proton pump inhibitors (some also available OTC) are replacing the H_2 receptor antagonists in clinical practice.

CHEMISTRY; MECHANISM OF ACTION; PHARMACOLOGY The H_2 receptor antagonists inhibit acid production by reversibly competing with histamine for binding to H_2 receptors on the basolateral membrane of parietal cells. Four different H_2 receptor antagonists, which differ mainly in their pharmacokinetics and propensity to cause drug interactions, are available in the U.S. (Figure 36–3): *cimetidine* (TAGAMET), *ranitidine* (ZANTAC), *famotidine* (PEPCID), and *nizatidine* (AXID). These drugs are less potent than proton pump inhibitors but still suppress 24-hour gastric acid secretion by ~70%. The H_2 receptor antagonists predominantly inhibit basal acid secretion, which accounts for their efficacy in suppressing nocturnal acid secretion. Because the most important determinant of duodenal ulcer healing is the level of nocturnal acidity, evening dosing of H_2 receptor antagonists is adequate therapy in most instances.

All four H_2 receptor antagonists are available as prescription and over-the-counter formulations for oral administration. Intravenous and intramuscular preparations of cimetidine, ranitidine, and famotidine also are available. When the oral or nasogastric routes are not an option, these drugs can be given in intermittent intravenous boluses or by continuous intravenous infusion.

PHARMACOKINETICS

The H_2 receptor antagonists are rapidly absorbed after oral administration, with peak serum concentrations within 1–3 hours. Therapeutic levels are achieved rapidly after intravenous dosing and are maintained for 4–5 hours (cimetidine), 6–8 hours (ranitidine), or 10–12 hours (famotidine). Unlike proton pump inhibitors, only a small percentage of H_2 receptor antagonists are protein-bound. Liver disease per se is not an indication for dose adjustment. The kidneys excrete these drugs and their metabolites by filtration and renal tubular secretion, and it is important to reduce doses of H_2 receptor antagonists in patients with decreased creatinine clearance. Neither hemodialysis nor peritoneal dialysis clears significant amounts of the drugs.

ADVERSE REACTIONS AND DRUG INTERACTIONS

The H_2 receptor antagonists generally are well tolerated, with a low (<3%) incidence of adverse effects; including diarrhea, headache, drowsiness, fatigue, muscular pain, and constipation. Less common adverse effects include those affecting the CNS (confusion, delirium, hallucinations, slurred speech, and headaches), which occur primarily with intravenous administration or in elderly subjects. Long-term use of cimetidine at high doses decreases testosterone binding to the androgen receptor and inhibits a CYP that hydroxylates estradiol. Clinically, these effects can cause galactorrhea in women and gynecomastia, reduced sperm count, and impotence in men. Several reports have associated H_2 receptor antagonists with various blood dyscrasias, including thrombocytopenia. H_2 receptor antagonists cross the placenta and are excreted in breast milk.

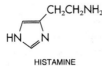

HISTAMINE

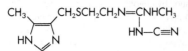

CIMETIDINE

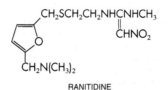

RANITIDINE

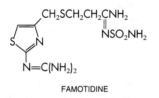

FAMOTIDINE

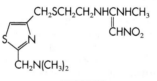

NIZATIDINE

FIGURE 36–3 *Histamine and H₂ receptor antagonists.*

THERAPEUTIC USES   The major therapeutic indications for H₂ receptor antagonists are to promote healing of gastric and duodenal ulcers, to treat uncomplicated GERD, and to prevent the occurrence of stress ulcers.

TOLERANCE AND REBOUND WITH ACID-SUPPRESSING MEDICATIONS

Tolerance to the acid-suppressing effects of H₂ receptor antagonists may account for a diminished therapeutic effect with continued drug administration. Tolerance can develop within 3 days of starting treatment and may be resistant to increased doses. Diminished sensitivity may result from the effect of the secondary hypergastrinemia to stimulate histamine release from ECL cells. Proton pump inhibitors, despite even greater elevations of endogenous gastrin, do not cause this phenomenon, probably because their site of action is distal to the action of histamine on acid release. Rebound increases in gastric acidity can occur when either of these drug classes is discontinued, possibly reflecting changes in function and justifying a gradual drug taper or the substitution of alternatives (*e.g.,* antacids) in at-risk patients.

AGENTS THAT ENHANCE MUCOSAL DEFENSE
Prostaglandin Analogs: Misoprostol

CHEMISTRY; MECHANISM OF ACTION; PHARMACOLOGY PGE_2 and PGI_2 are the major prostaglandins synthesized by the gastric mucosa. They bind to the EP_3 receptor on parietal cells (see Chapter 26) and stimulate the G_i pathway, thereby decreasing intracellular cyclic AMP and gastric acid secretion. PGE_2 also can prevent gastric injury by cytoprotective effects that include stimulation of mucin and bicarbonate secretion and increased mucosal blood flow. Since NSAIDs diminish prostaglandin formation by inhibiting cyclooxygenase, synthetic prostaglandin analogs offer a logical approach to reducing NSAID-induced mucosal damage (see below). Misoprostol (15-deoxy-16-hydroxy-16-methyl-PGE_1; CYTOTEC) is a synthetic analog of PGE_1. The degree of inhibition of gastric acid secretion by misoprostol is directly related to dose; oral doses of 100–200 μg significantly inhibit basal acid secretion (up to 95% inhibition) or food-stimulated acid secretion (up to 85% inhibition). The usual recommended dose for ulcer prophylaxis is 200 μg four times a day.

PHARMACOKINETICS

Misoprostol is rapidly absorbed after oral administration and then is rapidly and extensively de-esterified to form misoprostol acid, the principal and active metabolite of the drug. Some of this conversion may occur in the parietal cells. A single dose inhibits acid production within 30 minutes; the therapeutic effect peaks at 60–90 minutes and lasts for up to 3 hours. Food and antacids decrease the rate of misoprostol absorption, resulting in delayed and decreased peak plasma concentrations of the active metabolite. The free acid is excreted mainly in the urine, with an elimination $t_{1/2}$ of about 20–40 minutes.

ADVERSE EFFECTS

Diarrhea, with or without abdominal pain and cramps, occurs in up to 30% of patients who take misoprostol. Apparently dose-related, it typically begins within the first 2 weeks after therapy is initiated and often resolves spontaneously within a week; more severe or protracted cases may necessitate drug discontinuation. Misoprostol can cause clinical exacerbations of inflammatory bowel disease (see Chapter 38) and should be avoided in patients with this disorder. Misoprostol is contraindicated during pregnancy because it can increase uterine contractility.

THERAPEUTIC USE Misoprostol is FDA-approved to prevent NSAID-induced mucosal injury. However, adverse effects and the inconvenience of four-times-daily dosing limit its use.

SUCRALFATE

CHEMISTRY; MECHANISM OF ACTION; PHARMACOLOGY In the presence of acid-induced damage, pepsin-mediated hydrolysis of mucosal proteins contributes to mucosal erosion and ulcerations. This process can be inhibited by sulfated polysaccharides. *Sucralfate* (CARAFATE) consists of the octasulfate of sucrose to which $Al(OH)_3$ has been added. In an acid environment (pH <4), sucralfate undergoes extensive cross-linking to produce a viscous, sticky polymer that adheres to epithelial cells and ulcer craters for up to 6 hours after a single dose. In addition to inhibiting hydrolysis of mucosal proteins by pepsin, sucralfate may have additional cytoprotective effects, including stimulation of local production of prostaglandins and epidermal growth factor.

THERAPEUTIC USES Because increased gastric pH may be a factor in the development of nosocomial pneumonia in critically ill patients, sucralfate may offer an advantage over proton pump inhibitors and H_2 receptor antagonists for the prophylaxis of stress ulcers (see below). Due to its unique mechanism of action, sucralfate also has been used in several other conditions associated with mucosal inflammation/ulceration that may not respond to acid suppression, including oral mucositis (radiation and aphthous ulcers) and bile reflux gastropathy. Administered by rectal enema, sucralfate also has been used for radiation proctitis and solitary rectal ulcers.

Since it is activated by acid, sucralfate should be taken on an empty stomach 1 hour before meals. The use of antacids within 30 minutes of a dose of sucralfate should be avoided. The usual dose of sucralfate is 1 g four times daily (for active duodenal ulcer) or 1 g twice daily (for maintenance therapy).

ADVERSE EFFECTS

The most common side effect of sucralfate is constipation (~2%). As some aluminum can be absorbed, sucralfate should be avoided in patients with renal failure who are at risk for aluminum overload. Likewise, aluminum-containing antacids should not be combined with sucralfate in these patients. Sucralfate forms a viscous layer in the stomach that may inhibit absorption of other drugs, including phenytoin, digoxin, cimetidine, ketoconazole, and fluoroquinolone antibiotics.

Sucralfate therefore should be taken at least 2 hours after the administration of other drugs. The "sticky" nature of the viscous gel produced by sucralfate in the stomach also may lead to the formation of bezoars in some patients, particularly in those with underlying gastroparesis.

ANTACIDS

Antacids continue to be used by patients for a variety of indications. Many factors, including palatability, determine the effectiveness and choice of antacid (Table 36–1). Although sodium bicarbonate effectively neutralizes acid, it is very water-soluble and rapidly absorbed from the stomach, and the alkali and sodium loads may pose a risk for patients with cardiac or renal failure. Depending on particle size and crystal structure, $CaCO_3$ rapidly and effectively neutralizes gastric H^+, but the release of CO_2 from bicarbonate- and carbonate-containing antacids can cause belching, nausea, abdominal distention, and flatulence. Calcium also may induce rebound acid secretion, necessitating more frequent administration.

Combinations of Mg^{2+} (rapidly reacting) and Al^{3+} (slowly reacting) hydroxides provide a relatively balanced and sustained neutralizing capacity and are preferred by most experts. *Magaldrate* is a hydroxymagnesium aluminate complex that is converted rapidly in gastric acid to $Mg(OH)_2$ and $Al(OH)_3$, which are absorbed poorly and thus provide a sustained antacid effect. Although fixed combinations of magnesium and aluminum theoretically counteract the adverse effects of each other on the bowel (Al^{3+} delays gastric emptying and may cause constipation, while Mg^{2+} exerts the opposite effects), such balance is not always achieved in practice.

Simethicone, a surfactant that may decrease foaming and hence esophageal reflux, is included in many antacid preparations. However, other fixed combinations that are marketed for "acid indigestion", particularly those with aspirin, are potentially unsafe in patients predisposed to gastroduodenal ulcers and should not be used.

The relative effectiveness of antacid preparations is expressed as milliequivalents of acid-neutralizing capacity, but antacid doses in practice are titrated simply to relieve symptoms. For uncomplicated ulcers, antacids are given orally 1 and 3 hours after meals and at bedtime. This regimen, providing ~120 mEq of a Mg-Al combination per dose, may be almost as effective as conventional

Table 36–1

Composition and Neutralizing Capacities of Popular Antacid Preparations

| Product | milligrams per tablet or per 5 mL | | | | Acid Neutralizing Capacity[†] |
	$Al(OH)_3$	$Mg(OH)_2$	$CaCO_3$	Simethicone	
Tablets					
Gelusil	200	200	0	25	10.5
Maalox Quick Dissolve	0	0	600	0	12
Mylanta Double Strength	400	400	0	40	23
Riopan Plus Double Strength	Magaldrate,* 1080			20	30
Calcium Rich Rolaids		80	412	0	11
Tums EX	0	0	750		15
Liquids					
Maalox TC	600	300	0	0	28
Milk of Magnesia	0	400	0	0	14
Mylanta Maximum Strength	400	400	0	40	25
Riopan	Magaldrate,* 540			0	15

[†]Acid-neutralizing capacity, milliequivalents per tablet or per 5 mL.
*magaldrate, a magnesium aluminum hydroxide complex.

The current trend of "reusing" well-known brand names to introduce new products that contain an active ingredient different from expected is a source of confusion that can present a danger to patients.

dosing with an H_2 receptor antagonist. For severe symptoms or uncontrolled reflux, antacids can be given as often as every 30–60 minutes. Antacids generally should be administered in suspension form, as this probably has a greater neutralizing capacity than do powder or tablet dosage forms. If tablets are used, they should be thoroughly chewed for maximum effect.

Antacids are cleared from the empty stomach in ~30 minutes. However, the presence of food is sufficient to elevate gastric pH to about 5 for ~1 hour and to prolong the neutralizing effects of antacids for 2–3 hours.

Antacids vary in the extent to which they are absorbed, and hence in their systemic effects. In general, most antacids can elevate urinary pH by about one pH unit. Antacids that contain Al^{3+}, Ca^{2+}, or Mg^{2+} are absorbed less completely than are those that contain $NaHCO_3$. With normal renal function, the modest accumulations of Al^{3+} and Mg^{2+} do not pose a problem; with renal insufficiency, however, absorbed Al^{3+} can contribute to osteoporosis, encephalopathy, and proximal myopathy. About 15% of orally administered Ca^{2+} is absorbed, causing a transient hypercalcemia. Although this is not a problem in normal patients, the hypercalcemia from as little as 3–4 g of $CaCO_3$ per day can be problematic in patients with uremia. In the past, when large doses of $NaHCO_3$ and $CaCO_3$ were administered with milk or cream for the management of peptic ulcer, the *milk-alkali syndrome* (alkalosis, hypercalcemia, and renal insufficiency) occurred frequently. Today, this syndrome is rare and generally results from the chronic ingestion of large quantities of Ca^{2+} (five to forty 500-mg tablets per day of calcium carbonate) taken with milk. Patients may be asymptomatic or may present with the insidious onset of hypercalcemia, reduced secretion of parathyroid hormone, retention of phosphate, precipitation of Ca^{2+} salts in the kidney, and renal insufficiency.

By altering gastric and urinary pH, antacids may affect a number of drugs (*e.g.,* thyroid hormones, allopurinol, and imidazole antifungals), by altering rates of dissolution and absorption, bioavailability, and renal elimination). Al^{3+} and Mg^{2+} antacids also are notable for their propensity to chelate other drugs present in the gastrointestinal (GI) tract, forming insoluble complexes that pass through the GI tract without absorption. Thus, it generally is prudent to avoid concurrent administration of antacids and drugs intended for systemic absorption. Most interactions can be avoided by taking antacids 2 hours before or after ingestion of other drugs.

OTHER ACID SUPPRESSANTS AND CYTOPROTECTANTS

Rebamipide (2-(4-chlorobenzoylamino)-3-[2(1*H*)-quinolinon-4-yl]-propionic acid) is used for ulcer therapy in parts of Asia. It appears to exert a cytoprotective effect both by increasing prostaglandin generation in gastric mucosa and by scavenging reactive oxygen species. *Ecabet* (GASTROM; 12-sulfodehydroabietic acid monosodium), which appears to increase the formation of PGE_2 and PGI_2, also is used for ulcer therapy, mostly in Japan. *Carbenoxolone*, a derivative of glycyrrhizic acid found in licorice root, has been used with modest success for ulcer therapy in Europe. Its exact mechanism of action is not clear, but it may alter the composition and quantity of mucin. Unfortunately, carbenoxolone inhibits the type 2 isozyme of 11β-hydroxysteroid dehydrogenase, which protects the mineralocorticoid receptor from activation by cortisol in the distal nephron; it therefore causes hypokalemia and hypertension due to excessive mineralocorticoid receptor activation (*see* Chapter 59). *Bismuth compounds* (*see* Chapter 37) may be as effective as cimetidine in patients with peptic ulcers and are frequently prescribed in combination with antibiotics to eradicate *H. pylori* and prevent ulcer recurrence. Bismuth compounds bind to the base of the ulcer, promote mucin and bicarbonate production, and have significant antibacterial effects. Bismuth compounds are an important component of many anti-*Helicobacter* regimens (*see* below); however, bismuth compounds seldom are used alone as cytoprotective agents.

SPECIFIC ACID-PEPTIC DISORDERS AND THERAPEUTIC STRATEGIES

The success of acid-suppressing agents in a variety of conditions is critically dependent upon their ability to keep intragastric pH above a certain target, generally pH 3–5; this target varies to some extent with the disease being treated.

Gastroesophageal Reflux Disease

In the U.S, GERD is common, and it is estimated that one in five adults has symptoms of heartburn or gastroesophageal regurgitation at least once a week. Although most cases follow a relatively benign course, GERD in some individuals can cause severe erosive esophagitis; serious sequelae include stricture formation and Barrett's metaplasia (replacement of squamous by intestinal columnar epithelium), which, in turn, is associated with a small but significant risk of adenocarcinoma. Most of the symptoms of GERD reflect injurious effects of the refluxed gastric content on the esophageal epithelium, providing the rationale for suppression of gastric acid. The goals of GERD therapy are complete resolution of symptoms and healing of esophagitis. Proton pump inhibitors clearly are more effective than H_2 receptor antagonists in achieving these goals. Healing rates after 4 weeks and 8 weeks of therapy with proton pump inhibitors are ~80% and 90%, respectively, while the corresponding healing rates with H_2 receptor antagonists are 50% and 75%, respectively. Indeed, proton pump inhibitors are so effective that their empirical use is advocated as a therapeutic trial in patients in whom GERD is suspected to play a role in the pathogenesis of symptoms. Because of the wide clinical spectrum associated with GERD, the therapeutic approach is best tailored to the level of severity in the individual patient (Figure 36–4). In general, the optimal dose for each patient is determined based upon symptom control, and routine measurement of esophageal pH to guide dosing is not recommended. Strictures associated with GERD also respond better to proton pump inhibitors than to H_2 receptor antagonists. Unfortunately, one of the other complications of GERD, Barrett's esophagus, appears to be more refractory to therapy, as neither acid suppression nor antireflux surgery has been shown convincingly to produce regression of metaplasia or to decrease the incidence of tumors.

Regimens for the treatment of GERD with proton pump inhibitors and histamine H_2 receptor antagonists are listed in Table 36–2. Although some patients with mild GERD symptoms may be managed by nocturnal doses of H_2 receptor antagonists, twice-daily dosing usually is required. Antacids are recommended only for the patient with mild, infrequent episodes of heartburn. Prokinetic agents (*see* Chapter 37) are not particularly useful for GERD, either alone or in combination with acid-suppressant medications.

GERD AND PREGNANCY

Mild cases of GERD during pregnancy should be treated conservatively; antacids or sucralfate are considered the first-line drugs. If symptoms persist, H_2 receptor antagonists can be used, with ranitidine having the most established track record in this setting. Proton pump inhibitors are reserved for women with intractable symptoms or complicated reflux disease. In these situations, lansoprazole is preferred based on animal data and available experience in pregnant women.

Peptic Ulcer Disease

The pathophysiology of peptic ulcer disease is best viewed as an imbalance between mucosal defense factors (bicarbonate, mucin, prostaglandin, nitric oxide, and other peptides and growth factors) and injurious factors (acid and pepsin). On average, patients with duodenal ulcers produce more acid

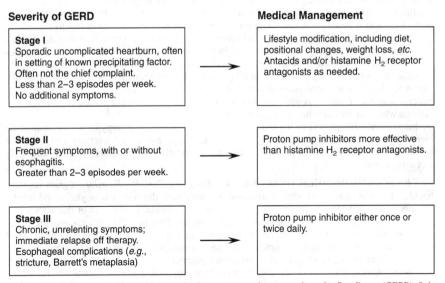

FIGURE 36–4 *General guidelines for the medical management of gastroesophageal reflux disease (GERD).* Only medications that suppress acid production or that neutralize acid are shown.

Table 36–2

Antisecretory Drug Regimens for Treatment and Maintenance of GERD

Drug	Dosage
H₂ Receptor Antagonists	
Cimetidine	400*/800* mg *bid*
Famotidine	20/40 mg *bid*
Nizatidine	150*/300* mg *bid*
Ranitidine	150/300 mg *bid*
Proton Pump Inhibitors	
Esomeprazole	20/40 mg daily/40* mg *bid*
Lansoprazole	30*/60* mg daily/30* mg *bid*
Omeprazole	20/40* mg daily/20* mg *bid*
Pantoprazole	40/80* mg daily/40* mg *bid*
Rabeprazole	20/40* mg daily/20* mg *bid*

bid, twice daily.
*Indicates unlabeled use.

than do control subjects, particularly at night (basal secretion). Although patients with gastric ulcers have normal or even diminished acid production, ulcers rarely if ever occur in the complete absence of acid. Presumably, a weakened mucosal defense and reduced bicarbonate production contribute to the injury from the relatively lower levels of acid in these patients. *H. pylori* and exogenous agents such as NSAIDs interact in complex ways to cause an ulcer. Up to 60% of peptic ulcers are associated with *H. pylori* infection of the stomach. This infection may lead to impaired production of somatostatin by Δ cells, and in time, decreased inhibition of gastrin production, resulting in increased acid production and reduced duodenal bicarbonate production.

NSAIDs also are very frequently associated with peptic ulcers (in up to 60% of patients, particularly those with complications such as bleeding). Topical injury by the luminal presence of the drug appears to play a minor role in the pathogenesis of these ulcers, as evidenced by the fact that ulcers can occur with very low doses of aspirin (10 mg) or with parenteral administration of NSAIDs. The effects of these drugs are instead mediated systemically; the critical element is suppression of COX-1 in the mucosa and decreased production of the cytoprotective prostaglandins PGE_2 and PGI_2.

Table 36–3 summarizes recommendations for drug therapy of gastroduodenal ulcers. Proton pump inhibitors relieve symptoms of duodenal ulcers and promote healing more rapidly than do H_2 receptor antagonists, although both classes of drugs are very effective. Peptic ulcer is a chronic disease, and recurrence within 1 year is expected in the majority of patients who do not receive prophylactic acid suppression. With the appreciation that *H. pylori* plays a major role in the majority of peptic ulcers (*see* below), prevention of relapse is focused on eliminating this organism from the stomach. Chronic acid suppression, once the mainstay of ulcer prevention, now is used mainly in patients who are *H. pylori*–negative or, in some cases, for maximum prevention of recurrence in patients who have had life-threatening complications.

Intravenous pantoprazole or lansoprazole clearly is the preferred therapy in patients with acute bleeding ulcers. The theoretical benefit of maximal acid suppression in this setting is to accelerate healing of the underlying ulcer. In addition, a higher gastric pH enhances clot formation and retards clot dissolution.

TREATMENT OF HELICOBACTER PYLORI INFECTION *H. pylori,* a gram-negative bacillus, has been associated with gastritis and the subsequent development of gastric and duodenal ulcers, gastric adenocarcinoma, and gastric B-cell lymphoma. Eradication of this infection is standard care in patients with gastric or duodenal ulcers. Provided that patients are not taking NSAIDs, this strategy almost completely eliminates the risk of ulcer recurrence. Eradication of *H. pylori* also is indicated in the treatment of mucosa-associated lymphoid tissue lymphomas of the stomach, which can regress significantly after such treatment.

Many regimens for *H. pylori* eradication have been proposed. The ideal regimen in this setting should achieve a cure rate of >80%. Five important considerations influence the selection of an eradication regimen (*see* Table 36–4).

Table 36–3

Recommendations for Treatment of Gastroduodenal Ulcers

Drug	Active Ulcer	Maintenance Therapy
H_2 Receptor Antagonists		
Cimetidine	800 mg at bedtime/400 mg twice daily	400 mg at bedtime
Famotidine	40 mg at bedtime	20 mg at bedtime
Nizatidine/ranitidine	300 mg after evening meal or at bedtime/150 mg twice daily	150 mg at bedtime
Proton Pump Inhibitors		
Lansoprazole	15 mg (DU; NSAID risk reduction) daily 30 mg (GU including NSAID-associated) daily	
Omeprazole	20 mg daily	
Rabeprazole	20 mg daily	
Prostaglandin Analogs		
Misoprostol	200 µg four times daily (NSAID-associated ulcer prevention)*	

DU, duodenal ulcer; GU, gastric ulcer.

*Only misoprostol 800 µg/day has been directly shown to reduce the risk of ulcer complications such as perforation, hemorrhage, or obstruction.

The emergence of resistance to clarithromycin and *metronidazole* increasingly is recognized as an important factor in the failure to eradicate *H. pylori.* Clarithromycin resistance is related to mutations that prevent binding of the antibiotic to the ribosomes of the pathogen and is an all-or-none phenomenon. In contrast, metronidazole resistance is relative rather than absolute and may involve several adaptations by the bacteria. In the presence of *in vitro* evidence of resistance to metronidazole, amoxicillin should be used instead. In areas with a high frequency of resistance to clarithromycin and metronidazole, a 14-day, quadruple-drug regimen (three antibiotics combined with a proton pump inhibitor) generally is effective therapy.

NSAID-RELATED ULCERS

Chronic NSAID users have a 2–4% risk of developing a symptomatic ulcer, GI bleeding, or perforation. Ideally, NSAIDs should be discontinued in patients with an ulcer if at all possible. Healing of ulcers despite continued NSAID use is possible with the use of acid-suppressant agents, usually at higher doses and for a considerably longer duration than standard regimens

Table 36–4

Therapy of *Helicobacter pylori* Infection

Triple therapy × 14 days: [Proton pump inhibitor + clarithromycin 500 mg + (metronidazole 500 mg or amoxicillin 1 g)] twice a day. (Tetracycline 500 mg can be substituted for amoxicillin or metronidazole.)

Quadruple therapy × 14 days: Proton pump inhibitor twice a day + metronidazole 500 mg three times daily + (bismuth subsalicylate 525 mg + tetracycline 500 mg four times daily)

or

H_2 receptor antagonist twice a day + (bismuth subsalicylate 525 mg + metronidazole 250 mg + tetracycline 500 mg) four times daily

Dosages:

Proton pump inhibitors:	H_2 receptor antagonists:
Omeprazole: 20 mg	Cimetidine: 400 mg
Lansoprazole: 30 mg	Famotidine: 20 mg
Rabeprazole: 20 mg	Nizatidine: 150 mg
Pantoprazole: 40 mg	Ranitidine: 150 mg
Esomeprazole: 40 mg	

(e.g., 8 weeks or longer). Again, proton pump inhibitors are superior to H_2 receptor antagonists and misoprostol in promoting the healing of active ulcers (healing rates of 80–90% for proton pump inhibitors versus 60–75% for the H_2 receptor antagonists) and in preventing recurrence of gastric and duodenal ulcers in the setting of continued NSAID administration.

STRESS-RELATED ULCERS

Stress ulcers are ulcers of the stomach or duodenum that occur in the context of a profound illness or trauma requiring intensive care. The etiology of stress-related ulcers differs somewhat from that of other peptic ulcers, involving acid and mucosal ischemia. Because of limitations on the oral administration of drugs in many patients with stress-related ulcers, intravenous H_2 receptor antagonists have been used extensively to reduce the incidence of GI hemorrhage due to stress ulcers. Now that intravenous preparations of proton pump inhibitors are available, it is likely that they will prove to be equally beneficial.

ZOLLINGER-ELLISON SYNDROME

Patients with this syndrome develop pancreatic or duodenal gastrinomas that stimulate the secretion of very large amounts of acid,. This can lead to severe gastroduodenal ulceration and other consequences of uncontrolled hyperchlorhydria. Proton pump inhibitors are the drugs of choice, usually given at twice the routine dosage for peptic ulcers with the therapeutic goal of reducing acid secretion to 1–10 mmol/h.

For a complete Bibliographical listing see Goodman & Gilman's *The Pharmacological Basis of Therapeutics*, 11th ed., or Goodman & Gilman Online at www.accessmedicine.com.

37

TREATMENT OF DISORDERS OF BOWEL MOTILITY AND WATER FLUX; ANTIEMETICS; AGENTS USED IN BILIARY AND PANCREATIC DISEASE

The gastrointestinal (GI) tract is in a continuous contractile, absorptive, and secretory state. The control of this state is complex, with contributions by the muscle itself, local nerves (*i.e.*, the enteric nervous system, ENS), the central nervous system (CNS), and humoral pathways. Of these, perhaps the most important regulator of physiological gut function is the ENS (Figure 37-1), which is an autonomous collection of nerves within the wall of the GI tract, organized into two connected networks of neurons: the *myenteric (Auerbach's) plexus,* found between the circular and longitudinal muscle layers, and the *submucosal (Meissner's) plexus,* found below the epithelium. The former is responsible for motor control, while the latter regulates secretion, fluid transport, and vascular flow.

OVERVIEW OF FUNCTIONAL AND MOTILITY DISORDERS OF THE BOWEL
GI motility disorders include achalasia of the esophagus (impaired relaxation of the lower esophageal sphincter associated with defective esophageal peristalsis that results in dysphagia and regurgitation), gastroparesis (delayed gastric emptying), myopathic, and neuropathic forms of intestinal dysmotility. These disorders can be congenital, idiopathic, or secondary to systemic diseases (*e.g.,* diabetes mellitus or scleroderma). For most of these disorders, treatment remains empirical and symptom-based, reflecting our ignorance of the specific derangements in pathophysiology involved.

PROKINETIC AGENTS AND OTHER STIMULANTS OF GI CONTRACTILITY
Prokinetic agents enhance coordinated GI motility and transit of material in the GI tract. Although ACh, when released from primary motor neurons in the myenteric plexus, is the principal immediate mediator of muscle contractility, most clinically useful prokinetic agents act "upstream" of ACh, at receptor sites on the motor neuron itself, or even more indirectly, on neurons one or two orders removed. These agents appear to enhance the release of excitatory neurotransmitter at the nerve-muscle junction without interfering with the normal physiological pattern and rhythm of motility. Coordination of activity among the segments of the gut, necessary for propulsion of luminal contents, therefore is maintained.

Cholinergic Agents
CHOLINE DERIVATIVES
ACh itself is not used pharmacologically because it affects all classes of cholinergic receptors (nicotinic and muscarinic; see Chapters 6 and 7) and is degraded rapidly by acetylcholinesterase. Modification of the ACh structure has yielded drugs such as bethanechol that have increased receptor selectivity and that resist enzymatic hydrolysis. In addition to its lack of real prokinetic efficacy, bethanechol has significant side effects resulting from its broad muscarinic effects on contractility and secretion in the GI tract and other organs, including bradycardia, flushing, diarrhea and cramps, salivation, and blurred vision.

ACETYLCHOLINESTERASE INHIBITORS
These drugs inhibit the degradation of ACh by its esterase (see Chapter 8), thereby allowing ACh to accumulate at sites of release. Unlike muscarinic receptor agonists, these parasympathomimetic drugs do not stimulate muscle directly, but rather accelerate GI transit times by enhancing the contractile effects of ACh released at synaptic and neuromuscular junctions. Among these cholinergic muscle stimulants, neostigmine methylsulfate has been used off-label for some GI disorders, particularly those associated with acute colonic pseudo-obstruction (Ogilvie's syndrome) and paralytic ileus. The usual dose in the acute setting is 2–2.5 mg of neostigmine administered intravenously over 3 minutes with continuous monitoring of ECG, blood pressure, and O_2 saturation. Atropine should be available in case of severe bradycardia.

Dopamine Receptor Antagonists
Dopamine is present in significant amounts in the GI tract and has several inhibitory effects on motility, including reduction of lower esophageal sphincter and intragastric pressures. These effects, which apparently result from suppression of ACh release from myenteric motor neurons, are mediated by D_2 receptors. By antagonizing the inhibitory effect of dopamine on myenteric motor neurons,

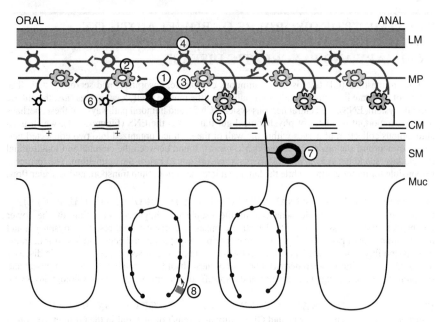

FIGURE 37–1   *The neuronal network that initiates and generates the peristaltic response.* Mucosal stimulation leads to release of serotonin by enterochromaffin cells (8), which excites the intrinsic primary afferent neuron (1), which then communicates with ascending (2) and descending (3) interneurons in the local reflex pathways. The reflex results in contraction at the oral end *via* the excitatory motor neuron (6) and aboral relaxation *via* the inhibitory motor neuron (5). The migratory myoelectric complex (*see* text) is shown here as being conducted by a different chain of interneurons (4). Another intrinsic primary afferent neuron with its cell body in the submucosa also is shown (7). MP, myenteric plexus; CM, circular muscle; LM, longitudinal muscle; SM, submucosa; Muc, mucosa. (*Adapted from Kunze and Furness, 1999, with permission.*)

dopamine receptor antagonists are effective as prokinetic agents; they have the additional advantage of relieving nausea and vomiting by antagonism of dopamine receptors in the chemoreceptor trigger zone (*see* below). Examples of such agents are *metoclopramide* and *domperidone*.

METOCLOPRAMIDE

Chemistry, Mechanism of Action, and Pharmacological Properties   The chemical structure of metoclopramide (REGLAN) is:

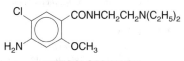

METOCLOPRAMIDE

The mechanisms of action of metoclopramide involve 5-HT$_4$ receptor agonism, vagal and central 5-HT$_3$ antagonism, possible sensitization of muscarinic receptors on smooth muscle, and dopamine receptor antagonism. Metoclopramide, one of the oldest true prokinetic agents, stimulates coordinated contractions that enhance transit. Its effects are confined largely to the upper digestive tract, where it increases lower esophageal sphincter tone and stimulates antral and small intestinal contractions. Metoclopramide has no clinically significant effects on large-bowel motility.

Therapeutic Use and Pharmacokinetics   Metoclopramide is indicated in symptomatic patients with gastroparesis, in whom it may modestly improve gastric emptying. Metoclopramide injection is used as an adjunctive measure in medical or diagnostic procedures such as intestinal intubation or contrast radiography of the GI tract. Although it has been used in patients with postoperative ileus, its ability to improve transit in disorders of small-bowel motility is limited. In general, its greatest utility lies in its ability to ameliorate the nausea and vomiting that often accompany GI dysmotility syndromes.

Metoclopramide is absorbed rapidly after oral ingestion, undergoes sulfation and glucuronide conjugation by the liver, and is excreted principally in the urine, with a $t_{1/2}$ of 4–6 hours. Peak concentrations occur within 1 hour after a single oral dose; the duration of action is 1–2 hours.

Metoclopramide is available for oral and parenteral use. The usual initial oral dose range is 10 mg, 30 minutes before each meal and at bedtime. The onset of action is within 30–60 minutes after an oral dose. In patients with severe nausea, an initial dose of 10 mg can be given intramuscularly (onset of action 10–15 minutes) or intravenously (onset of action 1–3 minutes). For prevention of chemotherapy-induced emesis, metoclopramide can be infused at 1–2 mg/kg of body weight, administered over at least 15 minutes, beginning 30 minutes before the chemotherapy is begun and repeated as needed every 2–3 hours. Alternatively, a continuous intravenous infusion may be given (3 mg/kg of body weight before chemotherapy, followed by 0.5 mg/kg of body weight per hour for 8 hours). The usual pediatric dose for gastroparesis is 0.1–0.2 mg/kg of body weight per dose, given 30 minutes before meals and at bedtime.

Adverse Effects The major side effects of metoclopramide include extrapyramidal effects. Dystonias, usually occurring acutely after intravenous administration, and parkinsonian-like symptoms that may occur several weeks after initiation of therapy generally respond to treatment with anticholinergic or antihistaminic drugs and are reversible upon metoclopramide discontinuation. Tardive dyskinesia also can occur with chronic treatment (months to years) and may be irreversible. Metoclopramide can elevate prolactin levels by blocking the inhibitory effect of dopamine on pituitary lactotropes. Methemoglobinemia has been reported in premature and full-term neonates receiving metoclopramide.

Domperidone; D_2 Receptor Antagonists

In contrast to metoclopramide, domperidone predominantly antagonizes the dopamine D_2 receptor without major involvement of other receptors. It is not available in the U.S. but has been used elsewhere (MOTILIUM, others) and has modest prokinetic activity in doses of 10–20 mg three times a day. Although it does not readily cross the blood–brain barrier to cause extrapyramidal side effects, domperidone exerts effects in the parts of the CNS that lack this barrier, such as those regulating emesis, temperature, and prolactin release.

5-HT Receptor Modulators

5-HT plays an important role in the normal motor and secretory function of the gut (*see* Chapter 11). Indeed, >90% of the total 5-HT in the body exists in the GI tract. The enterochromaffin cell, a specialized cell lining the mucosa of the gut, produces most of this 5-HT and rapidly releases 5-HT in response to chemical and mechanical stimulation (*e.g.,* food boluses; noxious agents such as cisplatin; certain microbial toxins; adrenergic, cholinergic, and purinergic receptor agonists). 5-HT triggers the peristaltic reflex (Figure 37–1) by stimulating intrinsic sensory neurons in the myenteric plexus (*via* variant 5-HT receptors, 5-HT$_{1p}$, and *via* 5-HT$_4$ receptors), as well as extrinsic vagal and spinal sensory neurons (*via* 5-HT$_3$ receptors). Additionally, stimulation of submucosal intrinsic afferent neurons activates secretomotor reflexes resulting in epithelial secretion. 5-HT receptors also are found on other neurons in the ENS, where they can be either stimulatory (5-HT$_3$ and 5-HT$_4$) or inhibitory (5-HT$_{1a}$). In addition, serotonin also stimulates the release of other neurotransmitters, depending upon the receptor subtype. Thus, 5-HT$_1$ stimulation of the gastric fundus results in release of nitric oxide and reduces smooth muscle tone. 5-HT$_4$ stimulation of excitatory motor neurons enhances ACh release at the neuromuscular junction, and both 5-HT$_3$ and 5-HT$_4$ receptors facilitate interneuronal signaling. Developmentally, 5-HT acts as a neurotrophic factor for enteric neurons *via* the 5-HT$_{2B}$ and 5-HT$_3$ receptors.

Reuptake of serotonin by enteric neurons and epithelium is mediated by the same mechanism as 5-HT reuptake by serotonergic neurons in the CNS. This reuptake therefore also is blocked by selective serotonin reuptake inhibitors (*see* Chapter 17), which explains the common side effect of diarrhea that accompanies the use of these agents.

TEGASEROD MALEATE

Chemistry, Mechanism of Action, and Pharmacological Properties *Tegaserod* (ZELNORM), an aminoguanidine indole, is structurally related to serotonin and is a partial 5-HT$_4$ agonist with negligible affinity for other receptor subtypes. Tegaserod has multiple effects on the GI tract. It stimulates motility and accelerates transit in the esophagus, stomach, small bowel, and ascending colon. It also stimulates chloride secretion. The clinical efficacy of tegaserod has been shown for male and female patients with constipation-predominant irritable bowel syndrome (*see* below). In patients with constipation, tegaserod results in mild-to-modest improvement in stool frequency, with less consistent effects on other parameters such as stool form, bloating, and pain. The absolute improvement is modest at best. It is not clear that the drug has any greater efficacy in this regard than other agents used for constipation.

Tegaserod is available for oral administration in 2-mg and 6-mg tablets and is approved for use in women with constipation-dominant irritable bowel syndrome at a dose of 6 mg twice daily. Tegaserod also is approved for the treatment of chronic constipation.

After oral administration, tegaserod is partially absorbed from the gut, reaching peak plasma levels after ~1 hour. Absorption of tegaserod is best on an empty stomach. Once in circulation, tegaserod is ~98% bound to plasma proteins. Tegaserod is degraded by acid hydrolysis before absorption from the stomach, and by oxidation and glucuronidation in the liver to three inactive N-glucuronide metabolites. Approximately two-thirds of the orally administered dose of tegaserod is excreted unchanged in feces, with the remainder excreted in urine; the drug has a $t_{1/2}$ of ~11 hours.

Diarrhea and headache are the most common side effects of tegaserod, occurring in ~10% of patients. Tegaserod does not appear to have any clinically relevant drug-drug interactions. No dosage adjustment is required in elderly patients or those with mild-to-moderate hepatic or renal impairment, but tegaserod should not be used in patients with severe hepatic or renal impairment.

MOTILIN AGONISTS: MACROLIDES AND ERYTHROMYCIN
CHEMISTRY, PHARMACOLOGICAL EFFECTS, AND MECHANISM OF ACTION
Motilin, a 22–amino acid peptide hormone found in the GI M cells and some enterochromaffin cells of the upper small bowel, is a potent contractile agent of the upper GI tract. The effects of motilin can be mimicked by erythromycin *and by other macrolide antibiotics* (see *Chapter 46*), *including* oleandomycin, azithromycin, *and* clarithromycin.

THERAPEUTIC USE
The best-established use of erythromycin as a prokinetic agent is in patients with diabetic gastroparesis, where erythromycin can improve gastric emptying in the short term. Erythromycin-stimulated gastric contractions can be intense and result in "dumping" of relatively undigested food into the small bowel. This potential disadvantage is exploited clinically to clear the stomach of undigestible residue such as plastic tubes or bezoars. Rapid development of tolerance to erythromycin, possibly by down-regulation of the motilin receptor, and undesirable (in this context) antibiotic effects have limited the use of this drug as a prokinetic agent.

A standard dose of erythromycin for gastric stimulation is 3 mg/kg intravenously or 200–250 mg orally every 8 hours. For small-bowel stimulation, a smaller dose (e.g., 40 mg intravenously) may be more useful, as higher doses may actually retard small-bowel motility.

MISCELLANEOUS AGENTS FOR STIMULATING MOTILITY
The GI hormone cholecystokinin (CCK) is released from the intestine in response to meals and delays gastric emptying. Dexloxiglumide *is a CCK_1 (or CCK-A)–receptor antagonist that can improve gastric emptying and is being investigated as a treatment for gastroparesis and constipation-dominant irritable bowel syndrome. Clonidine also may be of benefit in patients with gastroparesis.* Octreotide acetate (*SANDOSTATIN*), *a somatostatin analog, also is used in some patients with intestinal dysmotility* (see *below*).

OTHER AGENTS THAT SUPPRESS MOTILITY
Smooth muscle relaxants such as organic nitrates and Ca^{2+} channel antagonists (see Chapter 31) often produce temporary, if partial, relief of symptoms in motility disorders such as achalasia, in which the lower esophageal sphincter fails to relax, resulting in a functional obstruction to the passage of food and severe difficulty in swallowing. Another approach relies on the use of botulinum toxin, *injected in doses of 80–200 units directly into the lower esophageal sphincter via an endoscope. This agent inhibits ACh release from nerve endings (see Chapter 9) and can produce partial paralysis of the sphincter muscle, with significant improvements in symptoms and esophageal clearance. However, its effects dissipate over a period of several months, requiring repeated injections. Botulinum toxin also is being used increasingly in other GI conditions such as chronic anal fissures.*

LAXATIVES, CATHARTICS, AND THERAPY FOR CONSTIPATION
OVERVIEW OF GI WATER AND ELECTROLYTE FLUX
Fluid content is the principal determinant of stool volume and consistency; water normally accounts for 70–85% of total stool weight. Net stool fluid content reflects a balance between luminal input (ingestion and secretion of water and electrolytes) and output (absorption) along the length of the GI tract. The daily challenge

for the gut is to extract water, minerals, and nutrients from the luminal contents, leaving behind a manageable pool of fluid for proper expulsion of waste material *via* the process of defecation. Normally ~8–9 L of fluid enter the small intestine daily from exogenous and endogenous sources (Figure 37–2). Net absorption of the water occurs in the small intestine in response to osmotic gradients that result from the uptake and secretion of ions and the absorption of nutrients (mainly sugars and amino acids), with only ~1–1.5 L crossing the ileocecal valve. The colon then extracts most of the remaining fluid, leaving ~100 mL of fecal water daily.

Under normal circumstances, these quantities are well within the range of the total absorptive capacity of the small bowel (~16 L) and colon (4–5 L). Neurohumoral mechanisms, pathogens, and drugs can alter these processes, resulting in changes in either secretion or absorption of fluid by the intestinal epithelium. Altered motility also contributes to this process, as the extent of absorption parallels transit time. With decreased motility and excess fluid removal, feces can become inspissated and impacted, leading to constipation. When the capacity of the colon to absorb fluid is exceeded, diarrhea will occur.

CONSTIPATION: GENERAL PRINCIPLES OF PATHOPHYSIOLOGY AND TREATMENT

Patients use the term constipation *not only for decreased frequency, but also for difficulty in initiation or passage, passage of firm or small-volume feces, or a feeling of incomplete evacuation. Constipation has many reversible or secondary causes, including lack of dietary fiber, drugs, hormonal disturbances, neurogenic disorders, and systemic illnesses. In most cases of chronic constipation, no specific cause is found. Up to 60% of patients presenting with constipation will have normal colonic transit. These patients either have irritable bowel syndrome or define constipation in terms other than stool frequency. In the rest, attempts usually are made to categorize the underlying pathophysiology either as a disorder of delayed colonic transit because of an underlying defect in colonic motility, or less commonly, as an isolated disorder of defecation or evacuation (outlet disorder) due to dysfunction of the neuromuscular apparatus of the recto-anal region. Colonic motility is responsible for mixing luminal contents to promote absorption of water and moving them from proximal to distal segments by means of propulsive contractions. In any given patient, the predominant factor underlying constipation (propulsive* vs. *nonpropulsive colonic motility) often is not obvious. Consequently, the pharmacological approach to constipation remains empirical and nonspecific.*

Constipation can be corrected by adherence to a fiber-rich (20–30 g daily) diet, adequate fluid intake, appropriate bowel habits and training, and avoidance of constipating drugs. Constipation related to medications can be corrected by use of alternative drugs where possible, or adjustment of dosage. If nonpharmacological measures alone are inadequate, they may be supplemented with bulk-forming agents or osmotic laxatives. When stimulant laxatives are used, they should be

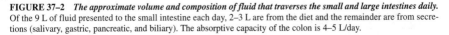

	Rate (L/day)		Ion Concentrations (mEq/L)				Osmolality
	Flow	H_2O Uptake	Na^+	K^+	Cl^-	HCO_3^-	
	9.0		60	15	60	15	variable
		6.0					
	3.0		140	6	100	30	isotonic
		1.5					
	1.5		140	8	60	70	isotonic
		1.4					
	0.1		40	90	15	30	isotonic

FIGURE 37–2 *The approximate volume and composition of fluid that traverses the small and large intestines daily.* Of the 9 L of fluid presented to the small intestine each day, 2–3 L are from the diet and the remainder are from secretions (salivary, gastric, pancreatic, and biliary). The absorptive capacity of the colon is 4–5 L/day.

administered at the lowest effective dosage and for the shortest period of time to avoid abuse. Habitual use of laxatives may lead to excessive loss of water and electrolytes; secondary aldosteronism may occur if volume depletion is prominent. Steatorrhea, protein-losing enteropathy with hypoalbuminemia, and osteomalacia due to excessive loss of calcium in the stool have been reported.

Laxatives are employed before surgical, radiological, and endoscopic procedures where an empty colon is desirable.

The terms *laxatives, cathartics, purgatives, aperients,* and *evacuants* often are used interchangeably. There is a distinction, however, between *laxation* (the evacuation of formed fecal material from the rectum) and *catharsis* (the evacuation of unformed, usually watery fecal material from the entire colon). Most of the commonly used agents promote laxation, but some are cathartics that act as laxatives at low doses.

Laxatives act by: (1) enhancing retention of intraluminal fluid by hydrophilic or osmotic mechanisms, (2) decreasing net absorption of fluid by effects on small- and large-bowel fluid and electrolyte transport, or (3) altering motility by either inhibiting segmenting (nonpropulsive) contractions or stimulating propulsive contractions. Based on their actions, laxatives can be classified as shown in Table 37–1; their known effects on motility and secretion are listed in Table 37–2. A variety of laxatives, both osmotic agents and stimulants, increase the activity of NO synthase and the biosynthesis of platelet-activating factor in the gut. Platelet-activating factor is a phospholipid proinflammatory mediator that stimulates colonic secretion and GI motility. Nitric oxide also may stimulate intestinal secretion and inhibit segmenting contractions in the colon, thereby promoting laxation. Agents that reduce the expression of NO synthase or its activity can prevent the laxative effects of castor oil, cascara, and bisacodyl (but not senna), as well as magnesium sulfate.

Laxatives also can be classed by the pattern of effects produced by the usual clinical dosage (Table 37–3).

Dietary Fiber and Supplements

Bulk, softness, and hydration of feces depend on the fiber content of the diet. Fiber resists enzymatic digestion and reaches the colon largely unchanged. Colonic bacteria ferment fiber to varying degrees, depending on its chemical nature and water solubility. Fermentation of fiber produces short-chain fatty acids that are trophic for colonic epithelium and increases bacterial mass. Although fermentation of fiber generally decreases stool water, short-chain fatty acids also may have a prokinetic effect, and increased bacterial mass may contribute to increased stool volume. Fiber that is not fermented can attract water and increase stool bulk. The net effect on bowel movement therefore varies with different compositions of dietary fiber (Table 37–4). In general, insoluble, poorly fermentable fibers, such as lignin, are most effective in increasing stool bulk and transit.

Bran, the residue left when flour is made from cereals, contains >40% dietary fiber. Wheat bran, with its high lignin content, is most effective at increasing stool weight. Fruits and vegetables contain more *pectins* and *hemicelluloses,* which are more readily fermentable and have less effect on stool transit. *Psyllium husk,* derived from the seed of the plantago herb, is a component of many commercial products for constipation (METAMUCIL, others). Psyllium husk contains a hydrophilic mucilloid that undergoes significant fermentation in the colon, leading to an increase in colonic

---

Table 37–1

Classification of Laxatives

1. Luminally active agents
 a. Hydrophilic colloids; bulk-forming agents (bran, psyllium, *etc.*)
 b. Osmotic agents (nonabsorbable inorganic salts or sugars)
 c. Stool-wetting agents (surfactants) and emollients (docusate, mineral oil)
2. Nonspecific stimulants or irritants (with effects on fluid secretion and motility)
 Diphenylmethanes (bisacodyl)
 Anthraquinones (senna and cascara)
 Castor oil
3. Prokinetic agents (acting primarily on motility)
 5-HT$_4$ receptor agonists
 Opioid receptor antagonists

Table 37–2

Summary of Effects of Some Laxatives on Bowel Function

	Small Bowel		Colon		
Agent	Transit Time	Mixing Contractions	Propulsive Contractions	Mass Actions	Stool Water
Dietary fiber	↓	?	↑	?	↑
Magnesium	↓	—	↑	↑	↑↑
Lactulose	↓	?	?	?	↑↑
Metoclopramide	↓	?	↑	?	—
Cisapride	↓	?	↑	?	↑
Erythromycin	↓	?	?	?	?
Naloxone	↓	↓	—	—	↑
Anthraquinones	↓	↓	↑	↑	↑↑
Diphenylmethanes	↓	↓	↑	↑	↑↑
Docusates	—	?	?	?	—

KEY: ↑, increased; ↓, decreased; ?, no data available; —, no effect on this parameter.
Modified from Kreek, 1994, with permission.

bacterial mass. The usual dose is 2.5–4 g (1–3 teaspoonfuls in 250 mL of fruit juice), titrated upwards until the desired goal is reached. A variety of semisynthetic celluloses—*e.g., methylcellulose* (CITRUCEL, others) and the hydrophilic resin *calcium polycarbophil* (FIBERCON, FIBERALL, others), a polymer of acrylic acid resin—also are available. These poorly fermentable compounds absorb water and increase fecal bulk.

Osmotically Active Agents

SALINE LAXATIVES Laxatives containing magnesium cations or phosphate anions commonly are called *saline laxatives*: magnesium sulfate, magnesium hydroxide, magnesium citrate, sodium phosphate. Their cathartic action is believed to result from osmotically mediated water retention, which then stimulates peristalsis. Magnesium-containing laxatives may stimulate the release of cholecystokinin, which leads to intraluminal fluid and electrolyte accumulation and to increased intestinal motility. For every additional mEq of Mg^{2+} in the intestinal lumen, fecal weight increases by ~7 g. The usual dose of magnesium salts contains 40–120 mEq of Mg^{2+} and produces 300–600 mL of stool within 6 hours.

Table 37–3

Classification and Comparison of Representative Laxatives

Laxative Effect and Latency in Usual Clinical Dosage		
Softening of Feces, 1–3 Days	Soft or Semifluid Stool, 6–8 Hours	Watery Evacuation, 1–3 Hours
Bulk-forming laxatives	*Stimulant laxatives*	*Osmotic laxatives*∗
Bran	Diphenylmethane derivatives	Sodium phosphates
Psyllium preparations	Bisacodyl	Magnesium sulfate
Methylcellulose		Milk of magnesia
Calcium polycarbophil		Magnesium citrate
Surfactant laxatives	*Anthraquinone derivatives*	*Castor oil*
Docusates	Senna	
Poloxamers	Cascara sagrada	
Lactulose		

∗Employed in high dosage for rapid cathartic effect and in lower dosage for laxative effect.

Table 37–4

Properties of Different Dietary Fibers

Type of Fiber	Water Solubility	% Fermented
Nonpolysaccharides		
Lignin	Poor	0
Cellulose	Poor	15
Noncellulose polysaccharides		
Hemicellulose	Good	56–87
Mucilages and gums	Good	85–95
Pectins	Good	90–95

Phosphate salts are better absorbed than magnesium-based agents and therefore need to be given in larger doses to induce catharsis. The most frequently employed preparation of sodium phosphate is an oral solution (FLEET PHOSPHO-SODA), which contains 1.8 g of dibasic sodium phosphate and 4.8 g of monobasic sodium phosphate in 10 mL. The usual adult dose is 20–30 mL taken with ample water. For colonic preparation before a procedure, larger doses are used, typically in the form of two doses of 45 mL each, a few hours apart, the evening before the procedure. A newer preparation of phosphate salts (VISICOL) is available in tablet form, containing 1.5 g total sodium phosphate per tablet. For colon preparation, two doses of 20 tablets each (30 g sodium phosphate) are recommended. Adequate fluid intake (1–3 L) is essential for any oral sodium phosphate regimen used for colonic preparation. Sodium phosphate also can be given as an enema for laxative purposes (*see* below).

Magnesium- and phosphate-containing preparations are tolerated reasonably well by most patients. However, they must be used with caution or avoided in patients with renal insufficiency, cardiac disease, or preexisting electrolyte abnormalities, and in patients on diuretic therapy. Patients taking >45 mL of oral sodium phosphate as a prescribed bowel preparation may experience electrolyte shifts that pose a risk for the development of symptomatic dehydration, renal failure, metabolic acidosis, hypocalcemic tetany, and even death in medically vulnerable populations.

NONDIGESTIBLE SUGARS AND ALCOHOLS *Lactulose* (CEPHULAC, CHRONULAC, others) is a synthetic disaccharide of galactose and fructose that resists intestinal disaccharidase activity. This and other nonabsorbable sugars such as *sorbitol* and *mannitol* are hydrolyzed in the colon to short-chain fatty acids, which stimulate colonic propulsive motility by osmotically drawing water into the lumen. Sorbitol and lactulose are equally efficacious in the treatment of constipation caused by opioids and *vincristine,* of constipation in the elderly, and of idiopathic chronic constipation. They are available as 70% solutions, which are given in doses of 15–30 mL at night, with increases as needed up to 60 mL/day in divided doses. Effects may not be seen for 24–48 hours after dosing is begun. Abdominal discomfort or distention and flatulence are relatively common in the first few days of treatment but usually subside with continued administration.

Lactulose also is used to treat hepatic encephalopathy. Patients with severe liver disease have an impaired capacity to detoxify ammonia produced by bacterial metabolism of urea in the colon. The drop in luminal pH that accompanies hydrolysis to short-chain fatty acids in the colon results in "trapping" of the ammonia by its conversion to the polar ammonium ion. Combined with the increases in colonic transit, this therapy significantly lowers circulating ammonia levels. The therapeutic goal is to give sufficient lactulose (usually 20–30 g, 3–4 times/day) to produce two to three soft stools a day with a pH of 5–5.5.

POLYETHYLENE GLYCOL–ELECTROLYTE SOLUTIONS Long-chain *polyethylene glycols* (PEGs; molecular weight ~3350) are poorly absorbed, and PEG solutions are retained in the lumen by virtue of their high osmotic nature. When used in high volume, aqueous solutions of PEGs (COLYTE, GOLYTELY, others) produce an effective catharsis and are used widely for colonic cleansing for radiological, surgical, and endoscopic procedures (4 L of this solution taken over 3 hours, beginning at least 4 hours before the procedure). To avoid net transfer of ions across the intestinal wall, these preparations contain an isotonic mixture of sodium sulfate, sodium bicarbonate, sodium chloride, and potassium chloride.

Stool-Wetting Agents and Emollients

Docusate salts are anionic surfactants that lower the surface tension of the stool to allow mixing of aqueous and fatty substances, softening the stool, and permitting easier defecation. However, these agents also stimulate intestinal fluid and electrolyte secretion and alter intestinal mucosal permeability. *Docusate sodium* (dioctyl sodium sulfosuccinate; COLACE, DOXINATE, others) and *docusate calcium* (dioctyl calcium sulfosuccinate; SURFAK, others), are available in several dosage forms. Despite their widespread use, these agents have marginal, if any, efficacy in most cases of constipation.

Mineral oil is a mixture of aliphatic hydrocarbons obtained from petrolatum. The oil is indigestible and absorbed only to a limited extent. When mineral oil is taken orally for 2–3 days, it penetrates and softens the stool and may interfere with water resorption. The side effects of mineral oil preclude its regular use and include: interference with absorption of fat-soluble vitamins, elicitation of foreign-body reactions in the intestinal mucosa and other tissues, and leakage of oil past the anal sphincter. Rare complications such as lipid pneumonitis due to aspiration also can occur, so "heavy" mineral oil should not be taken at bedtime and "light" (topical) mineral oil should never be administered orally.

Stimulant (Irritant) Laxatives

Stimulant laxatives have direct effects on enterocytes, enteric neurons, and GI smooth muscle and probably induce a limited low-grade inflammation in the small and large bowel to promote accumulation of water and electrolytes and stimulate intestinal motility. Included in this group are *diphenylmethane derivatives, anthraquinones,* and *ricinoleic acid.*

DIPHENYLMETHANE DERIVATIVES *Sodium picosulfate* (LUBRILAX, SUR-LAX) is widely available outside of the U.S. It is hydrolyzed by colonic bacteria to its active form, and hence acts locally only in the colon. Effective doses vary as much as four- to eightfold in individual patients. Consequently, recommended doses may be ineffective in some patients but may produce cramps and excessive fluid secretion in others.

Bisacodyl *is the only diphenylmethane derivative available in the U.S. It is marketed as an enteric-coated preparation (DULCOLAX, CORRECTOL, others) and as a suppository for rectal administration. The usual oral daily dose of bisacodyl is 10–15 mg for adults and 5–10 mg for children 6–12 years old. The drug requires hydrolysis by endogenous esterases in the bowel for activation, and so the laxative effects after an oral dose usually are not produced in <6 hours; taken at bedtime, it will produce its effect the next morning. Suppositories work within 30–60 minutes. Due to the possibility of developing an atonic nonfunctioning colon, bisacodyl should not be used for more than 10 consecutive days.*

ANTHRAQUINONE LAXATIVES These derivatives of plants such as *aloe, cascara,* and *senna* share a tricyclic anthracene nucleus modified with hydroxyl, methyl, or carboxyl groups to form monoanthrones. For use, monoanthrones are converted to dimeric (dianthrones) or glycoside forms. This process is reversed by bacterial action in the colon to generate the active forms. Senna (SENOKOT, EX-LAX) is obtained from the dried leaflets on pods of *Cassia acutifolia* or *Cassia angustifolia. Cascara sagrada* ("sacred bark"; COLAMIN, SAGRADA-LAX) is obtained from the bark of the buckthorn tree. Aloe and cascara sagrada products sold as laxatives have been withdrawn from the U.S. market.

CASTOR OIL An age-old home remedy seldom recommended now, *castor oil* (PURGE, NEOLOID, others) is derived from the bean of the castor plant, *Ricinus communis,* which contains two well-known noxious ingredients: an extremely toxic protein, *ricin,* and an oil composed chiefly of the triglyceride of ricinoleic acid. The triglyceride is hydrolyzed in the small bowel by the action of lipases into glycerol and the active agent, ricinoleic acid, which acts primarily in the small intestine to stimulate secretion of fluid and electrolytes and speed intestinal transit. When taken on an empty stomach, as little as 4 mL of castor oil may produce a laxative effect within 1–3 hours; however, the usual dose for a cathartic effect is 15–60 mL for adults.

Enemas and Suppositories

Enemas commonly are employed, either by themselves or as adjuncts to bowel preparation regimens, to empty the distal colon or rectum of retained solid material. Bowel distention by any means will produce an evacuation reflex in most people, and almost any form of enema, including normal saline solution, can achieve this. Specialized enemas contain additional substances that either are osmotically active or irritant; however, their safety and efficacy have not been studied in a rigorous manner. Repeated enemas with tap water or other hypotonic solutions can cause hyponatremia; repeated enemas with sodium phosphate–containing solution can cause hypocalcemia.

Glycerin *is a trihydroxy alcohol that acts as a hygroscopic agent and lubricant when given rectally. The resultant water retention stimulates peristalsis and usually produces a bowel movement in less than an hour. Glycerin is for rectal use only and is given in a single daily dose as a 2- or 3-g rectal suppository or as 5–15 mL of an 80% solution in enema form. Rectal glycerin may cause local discomfort, burning, or hyperemia and (minimal) bleeding. Some glycerin suppositories contain sodium stearate, which can cause local irritation.*

ANTIDIARRHEAL AGENTS

DIARRHEA: GENERAL PRINCIPLES AND APPROACH TO TREATMENT   Diarrhea is defined as excessive fluid weight, with 200 g/day representing the upper limit of normal stool water weight for healthy adults. Since stool weight is largely determined by stool water, most cases of diarrhea result from disorders of intestinal water and electrolyte transport.

Diarrhea can be caused by an increased osmotic load within the intestine (resulting in retention of water within the lumen); excessive secretion of electrolytes and water into the intestinal lumen; exudation of protein and fluid from the mucosa; and altered intestinal motility resulting in rapid transit (and decreased fluid absorption). In most instances, multiple processes are affected simultaneously, leading to a net increase in stool volume and weight accompanied by increases in fractional water content.

Many patients with sudden onset of diarrhea have a benign, self-limited illness requiring no treatment or evaluation. In severe cases, dehydration and electrolyte imbalances are the principal risks, particularly in infants, children, and frail elderly patients. *Oral rehydration therapy* therefore is a cornerstone for patients with acute illnesses resulting in significant diarrhea. This is of particular importance in developing countries, where the use of such therapy saves thousands of lives every year. This therapy exploits the fact that nutrient-linked cotransport of water and electrolytes remains intact in the small bowel in most cases of acute diarrhea. Sodium and chloride absorption is linked to glucose uptake by the enterocyte; this is followed by movement of water in the same direction. A balanced mixture of glucose and electrolytes in volumes matched to losses therefore can prevent dehydration. This can be provided by many commercial premixed formulas using glucose-electrolyte or rice-based physiological solutions.

Pharmacotherapy of diarrhea should be reserved for patients with significant or persistent symptoms. Nonspecific antidiarrheal agents typically do not address the underlying pathophysiology responsible for the diarrhea; their principal utility is to provide symptomatic relief in mild cases of acute diarrhea. Many of these agents act by decreasing intestinal motility and should be avoided in acute diarrheal illnesses caused by invasive organisms. In such cases, these agents may mask the clinical picture, delay clearance of organisms, and increase the risk of systemic invasion by the infectious organisms; they also may induce local complications such as toxic megacolon.

BULK-FORMING AND HYDROSCOPIC AGENTS   Hydrophilic and poorly fermentable colloids or polymers such as *carboxymethylcellulose* and calcium polycarbophil absorb water and increase stool bulk. They usually are used for constipation (*see* above) but are sometimes useful in mild chronic diarrhea in patients suffering with irritable bowel syndrome. Clays such as *kaolin* (a hydrated aluminum silicate) and other silicates such as *attapulgite* (magnesium aluminum disilicate; DIASORB) bind water avidly and also may bind enterotoxins. However, this effect is not selective and may involve other drugs and nutrients; hence, these agents are best avoided within 2–3 hours of taking other medications. A mixture of kaolin and pectin (a plant polysaccharide) is a popular over-the-counter remedy (KAOPECTOLIN) and may provide useful symptomatic relief of mild diarrhea.

BILE ACID SEQUESTRANTS   *Cholestyramine, colestipol,* and *colesevelam* effectively bind bile acids and some bacterial toxins. Cholestyramine is useful in the treatment of bile salt–induced diarrhea, as in patients with resection of the distal ileum. In these patients, there is partial interruption of the normal enterohepatic circulation of bile salts, resulting in excessive concentrations reaching the colon and stimulating water and electrolyte secretion (*see* below). Patients with extensive ileal resection (usually >100 cm) eventually develop net bile salt depletion, which can produce steatorrhea because of inadequate micellar formation required for fat absorption. In such patients, the use of cholestyramine will aggravate the diarrhea.

In patients suspected of having bile salt–induced diarrhea, a trial of cholestyramine can be given at a dose of 4 g of the dried resin (contained in either 9 g [QUESTRAN, others] or 5 g [QUESTRAN LIGHT, others] of powder) four times a day. If successful, the dose may be titrated down to achieve the desired stool frequency.

Cholestyramine resin also is helpful for the relief of pruritus associated with partial biliary obstruction and in conditions such as primary biliary cirrhosis. Cholestyramine increases fecal excretion of bile acids and reduces circulating and eventually systemic levels with relief of pruritus in ~1–3 weeks.

BISMUTH   Bismuth compounds have been used to treat a variety of GI diseases and symptoms for centuries. PEPTO-BISMOL (*bismuth subsalicylate*) is an over-the-counter preparation estimated to be used by 60% of U.S. households. It is a crystal complex consisting of trivalent bismuth and salicylate suspended in a mixture of magnesium aluminum silicate clay. In the low pH of the stomach, the bismuth subsalicylate reacts with hydrochloric acid to form bismuth oxychloride and salicylic acid. While 99% of the bismuth passes unaltered and unabsorbed into the feces, the salicylate is absorbed in the stomach and small intestine. Thus, caution should be used in patients taking salicylates for other indications.

Bismuth is thought to have antisecretory, anti-inflammatory, and antimicrobial effects. Nausea and abdominal cramps also are relieved by bismuth. Today, the most common antibacterial use of this agent is in the treatment of Helicobacter pylori *(see Chapter 36). A recommended dose of the bismuth subsalicylate (30 mL of regular strength* PEPTO-BISMOL *liquid or 2 tablets) contains approximately equal amounts of bismuth and salicylate (262 mg each). For control of indigestion, nausea, or diarrhea, the dose is repeated every 30–60 minutes, as needed, up to eight times a day. Bismuth products have a long track record of safety at recommended doses, although impaction may occur in infants and debilitated patients. Dark stools (sometimes mistaken for melena) and black staining of the tongue in association with bismuth compounds are caused by bismuth sulfide formed in a reaction between the drug and bacterial sulfides in the GI tract.*

Antimotility and Antisecretory Agents

OPIOIDS   Opioids continue to be widely used in the treatment of diarrhea. They act principally through either μ- or δ-opioid receptors on enteric nerves, epithelial cells, and muscle (*see* Chapter 21). These mechanisms include effects on intestinal motility (μ receptors), intestinal secretion (δ receptors), or absorption (μ and δ receptors). Commonly used antidiarrheals such as *diphenoxylate, difenoxin,* and *loperamide* act principally *via* peripheral μ-opioid receptors and are preferred over opioids that penetrate the CNS.

Loperamide   Loperamide (IMODIUM, IMODIUM A-D, others), a piperidine butyramide derivative with μ-receptor activity, is an orally active antidiarrheal agent. The drug is 40–50 times more potent than morphine as an antidiarrheal agent and penetrates the CNS poorly. It increases small intestinal and mouth-to-cecum transit times. Loperamide also increases anal sphincter tone, an effect that may be of therapeutic value in some patients who suffer from anal incontinence. In addition, loperamide has antisecretory activity against cholera toxin and some forms of *Escherichia coli* toxin.

Because of its effectiveness and safety, loperamide is marketed for over-the-counter distribution and is available in capsule, solution, and chewable forms. It acts quickly after an oral dose, with peak plasma levels achieved within 3–5 hours. It has a $t_{1/2}$ of ~11 hours and undergoes extensive hepatic metabolism. The usual adult dose is 4 mg initially followed by 2 mg after each subsequent loose stool, up to 16 mg/day. If clinical improvement in acute diarrhea does not occur within 48 hours, loperamide should be discontinued. Recommended maximum daily doses for children are 3 mg for ages 2–5 years, 4 mg for ages 6–8 years, and 6 mg for ages 8–12 years. Loperamide is not recommended for use in children younger than 2 years of age.

Diphenoxylate and Difenoxin   Diphenoxylate and its active metabolite difenoxin (diphenoxylic acid) are related structurally to meperidine. As antidiarrheal agents, diphenoxylate and difenoxin are somewhat more potent than morphine. Both compounds are extensively absorbed after oral administration, with peak levels achieved within 1–2 hours. Diphenoxylate is rapidly deesterified to difenoxin, which is eliminated with a $t_{1/2}$ of ~12 hours. Both drugs can produce CNS effects when used in higher doses (40–60 mg/day) and thus have potential for abuse and/or addiction. They are available in preparations containing small doses of atropine (considered subtherapeutic) to discourage abuse and deliberate overdosage: 25 μg of *atropine sulfate* per tablet with either 2.5 mg diphenoxylate hydrochloride (LOMOTIL) or 1 mg of difenoxin hydrochloride (MOTOFEN). The usual dosage is two tablets initially, then one tablet every 3–4 hours. With excessive use or overdose, constipation and (in inflammatory conditions of the colon) toxic megacolon may develop. In high doses, these drugs cause CNS effects as well as anticholinergic effects from the atropine (*e.g.*, dry mouth, blurred vision) (*see* Chapter 7).

OCTREOTIDE AND SOMATOSTATIN Octreotide (SANDOSTATIN) (*see* Chapter 55) is an octapeptide analog of somatostatin that is effective in inhibiting the severe secretory diarrhea brought about by hormone-secreting tumors of the pancreas and the GI tract. Its mechanism of action appears to involve inhibition of hormone secretion, including serotonin and various other GI peptides (*e.g.*, gastrin, vasoactive intestinal polypeptide, insulin, secretin, *etc.*). Octreotide has been used, with varying success, in other forms of secretory diarrhea such as chemotherapy-induced diarrhea, diarrhea associated with human immunodeficiency virus (HIV), and diabetes-associated diarrhea. Its greatest utility is in the "dumping syndrome" seen in some patients after gastric surgery and pyloroplasty; octreotide inhibits the release of hormones (triggered by rapid passage of food into the small intestine) that are responsible for distressing local and systemic effects.

Standard initial therapy with octreotide is 50–100 µg, given subcutaneously two or three times a day, with titration to a maximum dose of 500 µg three times a day based on clinical and biochemical responses. A long-acting preparation of octreotide acetate enclosed in biodegradable microspheres (SANDOSTATIN LAR DEPOT) is available for monthly use in the treatment of diarrheas associated with carcinoid tumors and vasoactive intestinal peptide–secreting tumors, as well as in the treatment of acromegaly (see Chapter 55). Short-term therapy leads to transient nausea, bloating, or pain at sites of injection. Long-term therapy can lead to gallstone formation and hypo- or hyperglycemia.

Use in Variceal Bleeding

Somatostatin and octreotide reduce hepatic blood flow, hepatic venous wedge pressure, and azygos blood flow. These agents constrict the splanchnic arterioles by a direct action on vascular smooth muscle and by inhibiting the release of peptides contributing to the hyperdynamic circulatory syndrome of portal hypertension. These agents can control bleeding acutely and decrease bleeding-related mortality, with an efficacy comparable to endoscopic therapy or balloon tamponade. The major advantage of somatostatin and octreotide over vasopressin is their safety. For patients with variceal bleeding, octreotide therapy usually is initiated while the patient awaits endoscopy. After a bolus of 100 µg, it is given intravenously as an infusion of 25–50 µg/h for 48 hours. Some clinicians give 100 µg subcutaneously every 6–8 hours for an additional 72 hours until the patient has had the second endoscopic treatment.

IRRITABLE BOWEL SYNDROME

Irritable bowel syndrome (IBS) is a condition that affects up to 15% of the U.S. population. Patients may complain of a variety of symptoms, the most characteristic of which is recurrent abdominal pain associated with altered bowel movements. IBS appears to result from a varying combination of disturbances in visceral motor and sensory function, often associated with significant affective disorders. The disturbances in bowel function can be either constipation or diarrhea or both at different times. Considerable evidence suggests a specific enhancement of visceral (as opposed to somatic) sensitivity to noxious, as well as physiological stimuli in this syndrome.

Many patients can be managed with dietary restrictions and fiber supplementation. Despite these measures, a significant proportion of patients remain plagued by severe symptoms, and drug therapy is attempted almost invariably. However, there are very few effective pharmacological options, a situation that in part reflects our limited understanding of the pathogenesis of this syndrome.

Treatment of bowel symptoms (either diarrhea or constipation) is predominantly symptomatic and nonspecific using agents discussed above.

In recent years, increased emphasis has been placed on the pharmacological treatment of visceral sensitivity in IBS patients. A possible role for serotonin in IBS has been suggested based on its known involvement in sensitization of nociceptor neurons in inflammatory conditions. This has led to the development of specific receptor modulators, such as tegaserod (see above).

The most effective drugs in this regard are the tricyclic antidepressants (see Chapter 17), which have neuromodulatory and analgesic properties. Tricyclic antidepressants have a proven track record in the management of chronic "functional" visceral pain. Effective analgesic doses of these drugs (e.g., 25–75 mg/day of nortryptiline) are significantly lower than those required to treat depression. Although changes in mood usually do not occur at these doses, there may be some diminution of anxiety and restoration of sleep patterns.

a_2 Adrenergic receptor agonists, such as clonidine (see Chapter 10), also can increase visceral compliance and reduce distention-induced pain. The somatostatin analog octreotide has selective inhibitory effects on peripheral afferent nerves projecting from the gut to the spinal cord and has been shown to blunt the perception of rectal distention in patients with irritable bowel syndrome.

Alosetron and Other 5-HT$_3$ Antagonists

The 5-HT$_3$ receptor participates in several important processes in the gut, including sensitization of spinal sensory neurons, vagal signaling of nausea, and peristaltic reflexes. The clinical effect of 5-HT$_3$ antagonism is a general reduction in GI contractility with decreased colonic transit, along with an increase in fluid absorption. In general, effects of these antagonists oppose those seen with 5-HT$_4$ agonists such as tegaserod. The 5-HT$_3$ antagonist alosetron (LOTRONEX) was initially removed from the U.S. market due to an unusually high incidence of ischemic colitis (up to 3 per 1000 patients), leading to surgery and even death in a small number of cases. The mechanism of this effect is not fully established, but may result from the drug's ability to suppress intestinal relaxation, thereby causing severe spasm in segments of the colon in susceptible individuals. The FDA has reapproved alosetron for diarrhea-predominant irritable bowel syndrome under a limited distribution system. The manufacturer requires a prescription program that includes physician certification and an elaborate patient education and consent before dispensing.

Alosetron is rapidly absorbed from the GI tract; its duration of action (~10 hours) is longer than expected from its t$_{1/2}$ of 1.5 hours. It is metabolized by hepatic CYPs. The drug should be started at 1 mg/day for the first 4 weeks, and advanced to a maximum of 1 mg twice daily if an adequate response is not achieved.

Other 5-HT$_3$ antagonists currently available in the U.S. are approved for nausea and vomiting (see below).

ANTISPASMODICS AND OTHER AGENTS

Anticholinergic agents ("spasmolytics" or "antispasmodics") often are used in patients with irritable bowel syndrome. The most common agents of this class available in the U.S. are nonspecific antagonists of the muscarinic receptor (see Chapter 7) and include the tertiary amines dicyclomine (BENTYL) and hyoscyamine (LEVSIN, others) and the quaternary ammonium compounds glycopyrrolate (ROBINUL) and methscopolamine (PAMINE). The advantage of the latter two compounds is that they have a limited propensity to cross the blood–brain barrier and hence a lower risk for neurological side effects such as light-headedness, drowsiness, or nervousness. These agents typically are given either on an as-needed basis (with the onset of pain) or before meals to prevent the pain and fecal urgency that predictably occur in some patients with irritable bowel syndrome.

Dicyclomine is given in doses of 10–20 mg orally every 4–6 hours as necessary. Hyoscyamine is available in many forms, including oral capsules, tablets, elixir, drops, a nonaerosol spray (0.125–0.25 mg every 4 hours as needed), and an extended-release form for oral use (0.375 mg every 12 hours as needed). Glycopyrrolate also comes in extended-release tablets (2 mg once or twice a day), in addition to a standard-release form (1 mg up to three times a day). Methscopolamine is provided as 2.5-mg tablets and the dose is 1 or 2 tablets, three to four times a day.

ANTINAUSEANTS AND ANTIEMETIC AGENTS
Nausea and Vomiting

Nausea and vomiting are protective reflexes that serve to rid the stomach and intestine of toxic substances and prevent their further ingestion. Vomiting is complex, consisting of a preejection phase (gastric relaxation and retroperistalsis), retching (rhythmic action of respiratory muscles preceding vomiting and consisting of contraction of abdominal and intercostal muscles and diaphragm against a closed glottis), and ejection (intense contraction of the abdominal muscles and relaxation of the upper esophageal sphincter). This is accompanied by multiple autonomic phenomena including salivation, shivering, and vasomotor changes. The process appears to be coordinated by a central emesis center in the lateral reticular formation of the mid-brainstem adjacent to both the chemoreceptor trigger zone (CTZ) in the area postrema (AP) at the bottom of the fourth ventricle and the solitary tract nucleus (STN) of the vagus nerve. The lack of a blood–brain barrier allows the CTZ to monitor blood and cerebrospinal fluid constantly for toxic substances and to relay information to the emesis center to trigger nausea and vomiting. The emesis center also receives information from the gut, principally by the vagus nerve (via the STN) but also by splanchnic afferents via the spinal cord. Two other important inputs to the emesis center come from the cerebral cortex (particularly in anticipatory nausea or vomiting) and the vestibular apparatus (in motion sickness). In turn, the center sends out efferents to the nuclei responsible for respiratory, salivary, and vasomotor activity, as well as to striated and smooth muscle involved in the act. The CTZ has high concentrations of receptors for serotonin (5-HT$_3$), dopamine (D$_2$), and opioids, while the STN is rich in receptors for enkephalin, histamine, and ACh, and also contains 5-HT$_3$ receptors. A variety of these neurotransmitters

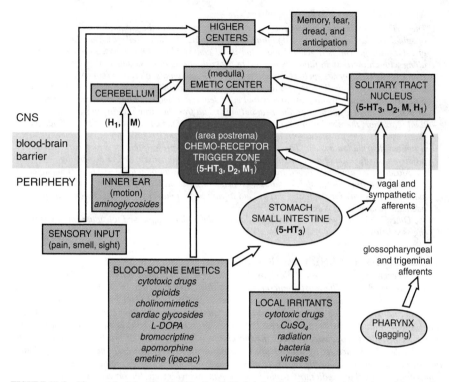

FIGURE 37–3 *Pharmacologist's view of emetic stimuli.* Myriad signaling pathways lead from the periphery to the emetic center. Stimulants of these pathways are noted in *italics*. These pathways involve specific neurotransmitters and their receptors (**bold** type). Receptors are shown for dopamine (D_2), acetylcholine (muscarinic, M), histamine (H_1), and 5-hydroxytryptamine ($5\text{-}HT_3$). Some of these receptors also may mediate signaling in the emetic center.

are involved in nausea and vomiting (Figure 37–3), and an understanding of their nature has allowed a rational approach to pharmacological treatment.

Antiemetics generally are classified according to the predominant receptor on which they are proposed to act (Table 37–5). However, these mechanisms overlap considerably, particularly for the older agents (Table 37–6). For treatment and prevention of the nausea and emesis associated with

Table 37–5

General Classification of Antiemetic Agents

Antiemetic Class	Examples	Type of Vomiting Most Effective Against
5-HT$_3$ receptor antagonists[*]	Ondansetron	Cytotoxic drug-induced emesis
Centrally acting dopamine receptor antagonists	Metoclopramide[*†] Promethazine[‡]	Cytotoxic drug-induced emesis
Histamine H$_1$ receptor antagonists	Cyclizine	Vestibular (motion sickness)
Muscarinic receptor antagonists	Hyoscine (scopolamine)	Motion sickness
Neurokinin receptor antagonists	Investigational	Cytotoxic drug-induced emesis (delayed vomiting)
Cannabinoid receptor agonists	Dronabinol	Cytotoxic drug-induced emesis

[*]The most effective agents for chemotherapy-induced nausea and vomiting are the 5-HT$_3$ antagonists and metoclopramide. In addition to their use as single agents, they are often combined with other drugs to improve efficacy as well as reduce the incidence of side effects.
[†]Also has some peripheral activity at 5-HT$_3$ receptors.
[‡]Also has some antihistaminic and anticholinergic activity.

Table 37–6

Receptor Specificity of Antiemetic Agents

Pharmacologic Class (Drugs in Class)	Dopamine (D$_2$)	Acetylcholine (Muscarinic)	Histamine	Serotonin
Anticholinergics				
Scopolamine	+	++++	+	–
Antihistamines				
Cyclizine	+	+++	++++	–
Dimenhydrinate, diphenhydramine, hydroxyzine	+	++	++++	–
Medizine	+	+++	++++	–
Promethazine	++	++	++++	–
Antiserotonins				
Dolasetron, granisetron, ondansetron, palonosetron, ramosetron	–	–	–	++++
Benzamides				
Domperidone	++++	–	–	+
Metoclopramide	+++	–	–	++
Butyrophenones				
Droperidol	++++	–	+	+
Haloperidol	++++	–	+	–
Phenothiazines				
Chlorpromazine	++++	++	++++	+
Fluphenazine	++++	+	++	–
Perphenazine	++++	+	++	+
Prochlorperazine	++++	++	++	+
Glucocorticoids				
Betamethasone, dexamethasone	–	–	–	–

Plus signs indicate some (+) to considerable (++++) interaction. (–) indicates no effect.

cancer chemotherapy, several antiemetic agents from different pharmacological classes may be combined (Table 37–7).

5-HT$_3$-Receptor Antagonists

CHEMISTRY, PHARMACOLOGICAL EFFECTS, AND MECHANISM OF ACTION

The 5-HT$_3$-receptor antagonists are the most widely used drugs for chemotherapy-induced emesis. Ondansetron (ZOFRAN) is the prototypical drug in this class; other agents include granisetron (KYTRIL), dolasetron (ANZEMET), palonosetron (ALOXI; intravenous use only) and tropisetron (available in some countries but not in the U.S.). Differences among these agents relate mainly to their chemical structures, 5-HT$_3$ receptor affinities, and pharmacokinetic profiles (Table 37–8).

PHARMACOKINETICS

The antiemetic effects of these drugs persist long after they disappear from the circulation, suggesting continued interaction at the receptor level. In fact, all of these drugs can be administered effectively once daily.

These agents are absorbed well from the GI tract. Ondansetron is extensively metabolized in the liver by CYP1A2, CYP2D6, and CYP3A4, followed by glucuronide or sulfate conjugation. Patients with hepatic dysfunction have reduced plasma clearance, and some adjustment in the dosage is advisable. Although ondansetron clearance also is reduced in elderly patients, no adjustment in dosage for age is recommended. Granisetron also is metabolized predominantly by the liver. Dolasetron is converted rapidly by plasma carbonyl reductase to its active metabolite, hydrodolasetron. A portion of this compound then undergoes subsequent biotransformation by CYP2D6 and CYP3A4 in the liver, while about one-third is excreted unchanged in the urine. Palonosetron is metabolized principally by CYP2D6 and excreted in the urine as the metabolized and the unchanged form in about equal proportions.

THERAPEUTIC USE All three agents appear to be equally efficacious in chemotherapy-induced nausea and in treating nausea secondary to upper abdominal irradiation, They also are

Table 37–7

A. Some Antiemetic Regimens Used in Cancer Chemotherapy

Antiemetic Agent	Initial Dose
For Severe Chemotherapy-Induced Emesis (Several Antiemetic Agents Used in Combination)	
⎧Dexamethasone	20 mg IV
⎪Metoclopramide	3 mg/kg body weight IV every 2 h × 2
⎨Diphenhydramine	25–50 mg IV every 2 h × 2
⎩Lorazepam	1–2 mg IV
⎧Dexamethasone	20 mg IV
⎩Ondansetron	32 mg IV daily, in divided doses
For Moderate Chemotherapy-Induced Emesis (Antiemetic Agents Used Singly)	
Prochlorperazine	5–10 mg orally or IV, or 25 mg by rectal suppository
Thiethylperazine	10 mg orally, IM, or by rectal suppository
Dexamethasone	10–20 mg IV
Ondansetron	8 mg orally or 10 mg IV
Dronabinol	10 mg orally

B. Useful Combinations of Antiemetic Agents for Improved Antiemetic Effect

Primary Agent	Supplemental Agent
5-HT$_3$ receptor antagonist	Glucocorticoid, phenothiazine, butyrophenone
Substituted benzamide	Glucocorticoid ± muscarinic receptor antagonist
Phenothiazine/butyrophenone	Glucocorticoid
Glucocorticoid	Benzodiazepine
Cannabinoid	Glucocorticoid

C. Useful Combinations of Antiemetic Agents Providing Decreased Toxicity of the Primary Agent

Primary Agent	Supplemental Agent
Substituted benzamide	H$_1$ receptor antagonist, glucocorticoid, benzodiazepine
Phenothiazine/butyrophenone	H$_1$ receptor antagonist
Cannabinoid	Phenothiazine

ABBREVIATIONS: H, histamine, 5-HT, serotonin; IV, intravenous; IM, intramuscular.
SOURCE: All combination regimens are from Grunberg and Hesketh, 1993, with permission.

effective against hyperemesis of pregnancy, and to a lesser degree, postoperative nausea, but not against motion sickness. Unlike other agents in this class, palonosetron also may be helpful in delayed emesis (*see* below).

These agents are available as tablets, oral solution, and intravenous preparations for injection. For patients on cancer chemotherapy, these drugs can be given in a single intravenous dose (Table 37–8)

Table 37–8

5-HT$_3$ Antagonists in Chemotherapy-Induced Nausea/Emesis

Drug	Chemical Nature	Receptor Interactions	$t_{1/2}$	Dose (IV)
Ondansetron	Carbazole derivative	5-HT$_3$ antagonist and weak 5-HT$_4$ antagonist	3.9 hours	0.15 mg/kg
Granisetron	Indazole	5-HT$_3$ antagonist	9–11.6 hours	10 μg/kg
Dolasetron	Indole moiety	5-HT$_3$ antagonist	7–9 hours	0.6–3 mg/kg
Palonosetron	Isoquinoline	5-HT$_3$ antagonist; highest affinity for 5-HT$_3$ receptor in this class	40 hours	0.25 mg
Ramosetron	Benzidazolyl derivative	5-HT$_3$ antagonist	5.8 hours	300 μg/kg

infused over 15 minutes, beginning 30 minutes before chemotherapy, or in two to three divided doses, with the first usually given 30 minutes before and subsequent doses at various intervals after chemotherapy. The drugs also can be used intramuscularly or orally.

These drugs generally are very well tolerated, with the most common adverse effects being constipation or diarrhea, headache, and light-headedness.

Dopamine Receptor Antagonists

Phenothiazines such as *prochlorperazine, thiethylperazine,* and chlorpromazine (*see* Chapter 18) are among the most commonly used antinauseants and antiemetics. Their principal mechanism of action is dopamine D_2 receptor antagonism at the CTZ. Compared to metoclopramide or ondansetron (*see* above), these drugs do not appear to be as uniformly effective in cancer chemotherapy–induced emesis. On the other hand, they also possess antihistaminic and anticholinergic activities, which are of value in other forms of nausea, such as motion sickness.

Antihistamines

Histamine H_1-receptor antagonists (*see* Chapter 24) are primarily useful for motion sickness and postoperative emesis. They act on vestibular afferents and within the brainstem. *Cyclizine, hydroxyzine, promethazine,* and *diphenhydramine* are examples of this class of agents. Cyclizine has additional anticholinergic effects that may be useful for patients with abdominal cancer.

Anticholinergic Agents

The most commonly used muscarinic receptor antagonist is *scopolamine* (hyoscine), which usually is administered as the free base in the form of a transdermal patch (TRANSDERM-SCOP). Its principal utility is in the prevention and treatment of motion sickness, although it also has some activity in postoperative nausea and vomiting. In general, anticholinergic agents have no role in chemotherapy-induced nausea.

DRONABINOL

Dronabinol (delta-9-tetrahydrocannabinol; MARINOL) is a naturally occurring cannabinoid that can be synthesized chemically or extracted from the marijuana plant, *Cannabis sativa.* The antiemetic action of dronabinol probably relates to stimulation of the CB_1 subtype of cannabinoid receptors on neurons in and around the vomiting center.

PHARMACOKINETICS
Dronabinol is a highly lipid-soluble compound that is absorbed readily after oral administration; its onset of action occurs within an hour, and peak levels are achieved within 2–4 hours. It undergoes extensive first-pass hepatic metabolism with limited systemic bioavailability after single doses (only 10–20%). Metabolites are excreted primarily via the biliary-fecal route, with only 10–15% excreted in the urine. Both dronabinol and its metabolites are highly bound (>95%) to plasma proteins. Because of its large volume of distribution, a single dose of dronabinol can result in detectable levels of metabolites for several weeks.

THERAPEUTIC USE   Dronabinol is a useful prophylactic agent in patients receiving cancer chemotherapy when other antiemetic medications are not effective. It also can stimulate appetite and has been used in patients with AIDS and anorexia. As an antiemetic agent, it is administered at an initial dose of 5 mg/m^2 given 1–3 hours before chemotherapy and then every 2–4 hours afterward for a total of four to six doses. If this is not adequate, incremental increases in dose can be made up to a maximum of 15 mg/m^2. For other indications, the usual starting dose is 2.5 mg twice a day; this can be titrated up to 20 mg a day.

ADVERSE EFFECTS   Dronabinol has complex effects on the CNS, including a prominent central sympathomimetic activity that can lead to palpitations, tachycardia, vasodilation, hypotension, and conjunctival injection (bloodshot eyes). Patient supervision is necessary because marijuana-like "highs" (*e.g.,* euphoria, somnolence, detachment, dizziness, anxiety, nervousness, panic, *etc.*) can occur, as can more disturbing effects such as paranoid reactions and thinking abnormalities. After abrupt withdrawal of dronabinol, an abstinence syndrome manifest by irritability, insomnia, and restlessness can occur. Because of its high affinity for plasma proteins, dronabinol can displace other plasma protein-bound drugs, whose doses may have to be adjusted as a consequence. Dronabinol should be prescribed with great caution to persons with a history of substance abuse because it also may be abused by these patients.

Substance P Receptor Antagonists

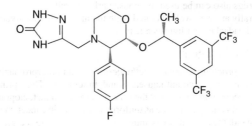

APREPITANT

The nausea and vomiting associated with cisplatin (*see* Chapter 51) has two components: an acute phase within 24 hours after chemotherapy that universally is experienced and a delayed phase on days 2–5 that affects only some patients. 5-HT receptor antagonists are not very effective against delayed emesis. Antagonists of the NK_1 receptors for substance P, such as *aprepitant* (EMEND), have antiemetic effects in delayed nausea and improve the efficacy of standard antiemetic regimens in patients receiving multiple cycles of chemotherapy. Substance P belongs to the tachykinin family of neurotransmitters and is in vagal afferent fibers innervating the STN and area postrema.

After absorption, aprepitant is bound extensively to plasma proteins (>95%); it is extensively metabolized, primarily by hepatic CYP3A4, and is excreted in the stool; its $t_{1/2}$ is 9–13 hours. Aprepitant has the potential to interact with other substrates of CYP3A4, requiring adjustment of other drugs, including dexamethasone, methylprednisolone (whose dose may need to be reduced by 50%), and warfarin. Aprepitant is contraindicated in patients on cisapride (see above) or pimozide, in whom life-threatening ventricular tachyarrthmias has been reported.

Aprepitant is supplied in 80- and 125-mg capsules and is administered for 3 days in conjunction with highly emetogenic chemotherapy along with a 5-HT$_3$-receptor antagonist and a glucocorticoid. The recommended adult dosage of aprepitant is 125 mg administered 1 hour before chemotherapy on day one, followed by 80 mg once daily in the morning on days 2 and 3 of the treatment regimen.

AGENTS USED FOR MISCELLANEOUS GASTROINTESTINAL DISORDERS
Chronic Pancreatitis and Steatorrhea

PANCREATIC ENZYMES Chronic pancreatitis is a debilitating syndrome that results in symptoms from loss of glandular function (exocrine and endocrine) and inflammation (pain). The goals of pharmacological therapy are prevention of malabsorption and palliation of pain. The cornerstone of therapy for malabsorption is the use of pancreatic enzymes.

ENZYME FORMULATIONS
The two common preparations of pancreatic enzymes for replacement therapy are obtained from the pancreas of the hog (Sus scrofa Linne var. domesticus Gray). Pancreatin (DONNAZYME, others) contains amylase, lipase, and protease and has one-twelfth of the lipolytic activity of pancrelipase, on a weight-by-weight basis. Pancrelipase is more commonly used and is available in uncoated forms, as well as capsules containing enteric-coated microspheres and enteric-coated microtablets, which withstand gastric acid (lipase is inactivated by acid) and disintegrate at pH >6 (Table 37–9).

REPLACEMENT THERAPY FOR MALABSORPTION
Fat malabsorption (steatorrhea) and protein maldigestion occur when the pancreas loses >90% of its ability to produce digestive enzymes. The resultant diarrhea and malabsorption can be managed reasonably well if 30,000 USP units of pancreatic lipase are delivered to the duodenum during a 4-hour period with and after meals; this represents ~10% of the normal pancreatic output. Alternatively, the dose can be titrated to the fat content of the diet, with ~8000 USP units of lipase activity required for each 17 g of dietary fat. Available preparations of pancreatic enzymes (Table 37–10) contain up to 20,000 units of lipase and 75,000 units of protease, and the typical dose of pancrelipase is 1–3 capsules or tablets with or just before meals and snacks, adjusted until a satisfactory symptomatic response is obtained. The loss of pancreatic amylase does not present a problem because of other sources of this enzyme (e.g., salivary glands). Patients using uncoated preparations require concomitant pharmacological control of gastric acid production with a proton pump inhibitor (see Chapter 36).

Table 37–9

Comparison of Uncoated and Enteric-Coated Pancreatic Enzyme Preparations[*]

	Uncoated Preparations	Enteric-Coated Preparations
Number of tablets or capsules required per dose	2–8	2–3
Acid suppression required	Yes	No
Site of delivery	Duodenum	More distal small bowel and beyond
Symptoms relieved	Pain; malabsorption	Malabsorption

[*]The major components of these preparations are a lipase and a protease (*see* Table 37–10).

ENZYMES FOR PAIN

Pain is the other cardinal symptom of chronic pancreatitis. The rationale for its treatment with pancreatic enzymes is based on the principle of negative feedback inhibition of the pancreas by the presence of duodenal proteases. The evidence supporting this practice is equivocal at best.

In general, pancreatic enzyme preparations are well tolerated by patients. For patients with hypersensitivity to pork protein, bovine enzymes are available. Hyperuricosuria in patients with cystic fibrosis can occur, and malabsorption of folate and iron has been reported.

BILE ACIDS

Bile acids and their conjugates are essential components of bile that are synthesized from cholesterol in the liver. The major bile acids in human adults are depicted in Figure 37–4. Bile acids induce bile flow, feedback-inhibit cholesterol synthesis, promote intestinal excretion of cholesterol, and facilitate the dispersion and absorption of lipids and fat-soluble vitamins. After secretion into the biliary tract, bile acids are largely (95%) reabsorbed in the intestine (mainly in the terminal ileum), returned to the liver, and then again secreted in bile (enterohepatic circulation). Cholic acid, chenodeoxycholic acid, and deoxycholic acid constitute 95% of bile acids, while lithocholic acid and ursodeoxycholic acid are minor constituents. The bile acids exist largely as glycine and taurine conjugates, the salts of which are called *bile salts*. Colonic bacteria convert primary bile acids (cholic and chenodeoxycholic acid) to secondary acids (mainly deoxycholic and lithocholic acid) by sequential deconjugation and dehydroxylation. These secondary bile acids also are absorbed in the colon and join the primary acids in the enterohepatic pool.

Table 37–10

Pancreatic Enzyme Formulations

Brand Name	Lipase[*]	Protease[*]	Amylase
Conventional (uncoated)			
VIOKASE 8	8,000	30,000	30,000
VIOKASE 16	16,000	60,000	60,000
KUZYME HP	8,000	30,000	30,000
Enteric-coated			
PANCREASE			
MT 4	4,000	12,000	12,000
MT 10	10,000	30,000	30,000
MT 16	16,000	48,000	48,000
CREON			
5	5,000	18,750	16,600
10	10,000	37,500	33,200
20	20,000	75,000	66,400
ULTRASE			
MT 12	12,000	39,000	39,000
MT 18	18,000	58,500	58,500
MT 20	20,000	65,000	65,000

[*]U.S. Pharmacopeia units per tablet or capsule.

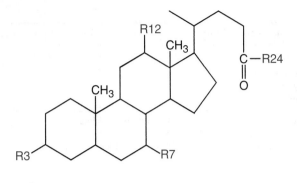

Bile Acid	R3	R7	R12	R24
Cholic acid	–OH	–OH	–OH	
Chenodeoxycholic acid	–OH	–OH	–H	glycine (75%)
Deoxycholic acid	–OH	–H	–OH	taurine (24%)
Lithocholic acid	–SO$_3^-$ / –OH	–H	–H	–OH (<1%)
Ursodeoxycholic acid	–OH	◄OH	–H	

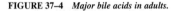

FIGURE 37–4 *Major bile acids in adults.*

Ursodeoxycholic acid *(UDCA; ursodiol, ACTIGALL) (Figure 37–4) is a hydrophilic, dehydroxylated bile acid that is formed by epimerization of chenodeoxycholic acid (CDCA; chenodiol) in the gut by intestinal bacteria; it comprises ~1–3% of the total bile acid pool. When administered orally, litholytic bile acids such as chenodiol and ursodiol can alter relative concentrations of bile acids, decrease biliary lipid secretion, and reduce the cholesterol content of the bile so that it is less lithogenic. Ursodiol also may have cytoprotective effects on hepatocytes and effects on the immune system that account for some of its beneficial effects in cholestatic liver diseases.*

Use of bile acids for gallstone dissolution requires a functional gallbladder because the modified bile must enter the gallbladder to interact with gallstones. To be amenable to dissolution, the gallstones must be composed of cholesterol monohydrate crystals and generally must be <15 mm in diameter. The overall efficacy of litholytic bile acids in the treatment of gallstones has been disappointing (partial dissolution occurs in 40–60% of patients completing therapy and complete dissolution in only 33–50%). Ursodiol is preferred as a single agent because of its greater efficacy and less-frequent side effects (e.g., hepatotoxicity).

Primary biliary cirrhosis is a chronic, progressive, cholestatic liver disease of unknown etiology that typically affects middle-aged to elderly women. Ursodiol (administered at 13–15 mg/kg/day in two divided doses) reduces the concentration of primary bile acids and improves biochemical and histological features of primary biliary cirrhosis.

ANTIFLATULENCE AGENTS

"Gas" is a common but relatively vague GI complaint, used in reference not only to flatulence and eructation, but also bloating or fullness. Although few if any symptoms can be directly attributable to excessive intestinal gas, over-the-counter and herbal preparations that are touted as antiflatulent are very popular. One of these is *simethicone,* a mixture of siloxane polymers stabilized with silicon dioxide.

For a complete Bibliographical listing see Goodman & Gilman's *The Pharmacological Basis of Therapeutics*, 11th ed., or Goodman & Gilman Online at www.accessmedicine.com.

38

PHARMACOTHERAPY OF INFLAMMATORY BOWEL DISEASE

Inflammatory bowel disease (IBD) is a spectrum of chronic idiopathic inflammatory intestinal conditions. IBD causes significant GI symptoms that include diarrhea, abdominal pain, bleeding, anemia, and weight loss. IBD also is associated with a spectrum of extraintestinal manifestations, including arthritis, ankylosing spondylitis, sclerosing cholangitis, uveitis, iritis, pyoderma gangrenosum, and erythema nodosum.

IBD is divided into two major subtypes: ulcerative colitis and Crohn's disease. Ulcerative colitis is characterized by confluent mucosal inflammation of the colon starting at the anal verge and extending proximally for a variable extent (*e.g.*, proctitis, left-sided colitis, or pancolitis). Crohn's disease, by contrast, is characterized by transmural inflammation of any part of the GI tract but most commonly the area adjacent to the ileocecal valve. The inflammation in Crohn's disease is not necessarily confluent, frequently leaving "skip areas" of relatively normal mucosa. The transmural nature of the inflammation may lead to fibrosis and strictures or, alternatively, fistula formation.

Therapy for IBD seeks to dampen the generalized inflammatory response; however, no agent can reliably accomplish this, and the response of an individual patient to a given medicine may be limited and unpredictable. Specific goals of pharmacotherapy in IBD include controlling acute exacerbations of the disease, maintaining remission, and treating specific complications such as fistulas. Specific drugs may be better suited for one or the other of these aims (Table 38–1). For example, *glucocorticoids* remain the treatment of choice for moderate-to-severe flares but are inappropriate for long-term use because of side effects and their inability to maintain remission.

For many years, glucocorticoids and *sulfasalazine* were the mainstays of medical therapy for IBD. More recently, medicines used in other immune/inflammatory conditions, such as azathioprine and *cyclosporine*, have been adapted for IBD therapy. Biological agents have been developed that can target single steps in the immune cascade. Drug delivery to the appropriate site(s) along the GI tract also has been a major challenge, and second-generation agents have been created with improved drug delivery, increased efficacy, and decreased side effects.

PATHOGENESIS OF IBD

A summary of proposed pathogenic events and potential sites of therapeutic intervention in IBD is shown in Figure 38–1. While Crohn's disease and ulcerative colitis share a number of GI and extraintestinal manifestations and can respond to a similar array of drugs, emerging evidence suggests that they result from distinct pathogenetic mechanisms. Histologically, the transmural lesions in Crohn's disease exhibit marked infiltration of lymphocytes and macrophages, granuloma formation, and submucosal fibrosis, whereas the superficial lesions in ulcerative colitis have lymphocytic and neutrophilic infiltrates. Within the diseased bowel in Crohn's disease, the cytokine profile includes increased levels of interleukin-12 (IL-12), interferon-γ, and tumor necrosis factor-α (TNF-α), findings characteristic of T-helper 1 (T_H1)–mediated inflammatory processes. In contrast, the inflammatory response in ulcerative colitis resembles more closely that mediated by the T_H2 pathway.

MESALAMINE (5-ASA)-BASED THERAPY

CHEMISTRY, MECHANISM OF ACTION, AND PHARMACOLOGICAL PROPERTIES First-line therapy for mild-to-moderate ulcerative colitis generally involves *mesalamine* (5-aminosalicylic acid, or 5-ASA). The archetype for this class of medications is sulfasalazine (AZULFIDINE), which consists of 5-ASA linked to *sulfapyridine* by an azo bond. Sulfasalazine represents one of the first examples of an oral drug that is delivered effectively to the distal GI tract. The azo linkage in sulfasalazine prevents absorption in the stomach and small intestine, and the individual components are not liberated for absorption until colonic bacteria cleave the bond. 5-ASA is now regarded as the therapeutic agent, with little, if any, contribution by sulfapyridine.

Although mesalamine is a salicylate, its therapeutic effect does not appear to be related to cyclooxygenase inhibition; indeed, traditional nonsteroidal anti-inflammatory drugs actually may exacerbate IBD. Specific mechanisms of action have not been identified, although a myriad of effects on immune function and inflammation have been shown *in vitro*.

Although not active therapeutically, sulfapyridine causes many of the side effects associated with sulfasalazine. To preserve the therapeutic effect of 5-ASA without the side effects of sulfapyridine, several second-generation 5-ASA compounds have been developed. They are divided into two

Table 38–1

Medications Commonly Used to Treat Inflammatory Bowel Disease

| | Crohn's Disease | | | | | Ulcerative Colitis | | | |
| | Active Disease | | | Maintenance | | Active disease | | | Maintenance |
Class/Drug	Mild–Moderate	Moderate–Severe	Fistula	Medical Remission	Surgical Remission	Distal Colitis	Mild–Moderate	Moderate–Severe	
Mesalamine									
Enema	+[a]	–	–	+/–	–	+	+[b]	–	+
Oral	+	–	–	?	+[c]	+	+	–	+
Antibiotics (metronidazole, ciprofloxacin, others)	+	+	+	?	+[c]	–	–	–	+[c]
Corticosteroids, classic and novel									
Enema, foam, suppository	+[a]	–	–	–	–	+	+[b]	–	–
Oral	+	+	–	–	–	+	+	+	–
Intravenous	–	+	–	–	–	+[d]	–	+	–
Immunomodulators									
6-MP/AZA	–	+	+	+	+[c]	+[d]	–	+[d]	+[d]
Methotrexate	–	+	?	?	?	–	–	–	–
Cyclosporine	–	+[d]	+[d]	–	–	+[d]	–	+[d]	–
Biological response modifiers									
Infliximab	+[d]	+	+	+[c]	?	?	?	?	?

[a]Distal colonic disease only.
[b]For adjunctive therapy.
[c]Some data to support use; remains controversial.
[d]Selected patients.

ABBREVIATIONS: 6-MP, 6-mercaptopurine; AZA, azathioprine.

654

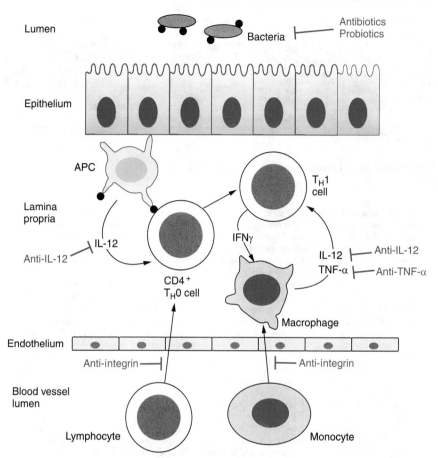

FIGURE 38–1 *Proposed pathogenesis of inflammatory bowel disease and target sites for pharmacological intervention.* Shown are the interactions among bacterial antigens in the intestinal lumen and immune cells in the intestinal wall. If the endothelial barrier is impaired, bacterial antigens (dark circles) can gain access to antigen-presenting cells (APCs) in the lamina propria. These cells then present the antigen(s) to CD4+ lymphocytes and also secrete IL-12, thereby inducing the differentiation of T_H1 cells in Crohn's disease (or type 2 helper T cells in ulcerative colitis). The T_H1 cells produce a characteristic array of lymphokines, including IFN-γ, which in turn activates macrophages. Macrophages positively regulate T_H1 cells by secreting additional IL-12 and TNF-α. In addition to general immunosuppressants that affect multiple sites of inflammation (*e.g.*, glucocorticoids, thioguanine derivatives, methotrexate, and cyclosporine), more specific sites for therapeutic intervention involve the intestinal bacteria (antibiotics and probiotics) and therapy directed at TNF-α (*see* text for further details).

groups: prodrugs and coated drugs. Prodrugs contain the same azo bond as sulfasalazine but replace the linked sulfapyridine with either another 5-ASA (*olsalazine*, DIPENTUM) or an inert compound (*balsalazide*, COLAZIDE). Thus, these compounds act at similar sites along the GI tract as does sulfasalazine. The alternative approaches employ either a delayed-release formulation (PENTASA) or a pH-sensitive coating (ASACOL). Delayed-release mesalamine is released throughout the small intestine and colon, whereas pH-sensitive mesalamine is released in the terminal ileum and colon. These different distributions of drug delivery have potential therapeutic implications (*see* Figure 38–2).

> *Oral sulfasalazine is of proven value in patients with mild or moderately active ulcerative colitis, with response rates of 60–80%. The usual dose is 4 g/day in four divided doses with food; to avoid adverse effects, the dose is increased gradually from an initial dose of 500 mg twice a day. Doses as high as 6 g/day can be used but cause an increased incidence of side effects. For patients with severe colitis, sulfasalazine is of less certain value, even though it is often added as an adjunct to*

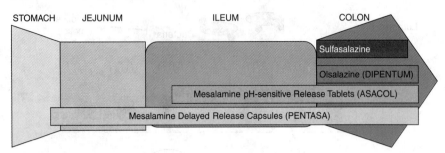

FIGURE 38–2 Sites of release of mesalamine (5-ASA) in the GI tract from different oral formulations.

systemic glucocorticoids. Regardless of disease severity, the drug plays a useful role in preventing relapses once remission has been achieved. Because they lack the dose-related side effects of sulfapyridine, the newer formulations can be used to provide higher doses of mesalamine with some improvement in disease control. The usual doses to treat active disease are 800 mg three times a day for ASACOL and 1 g four times a day for PENTASA. Lower doses are used for maintenance (e.g., ASACOL, 800 mg twice a day).

The efficacy of 5-ASA preparations (e.g., sulfasalazine) in Crohn's disease is less striking, with modest benefit at best. Sulfasalazine has not been shown to be effective in maintaining remission and has been replaced by newer 5-ASA preparations. Some studies have reported that both ASACOL and PENTASA are more effective than placebo in inducing remission in patients with Crohn's disease (particularly colitis), although higher doses than those typically used in ulcerative colitis are required. The role of mesalamine in maintenance therapy for Crohn's disease is controversial, and there is no clear benefit of continued 5-ASA therapy in patients who achieve medical remission. Because they largely bypass the small intestine, the second-generation 5-ASA prodrugs such as olsalazine and balsalazide do not have a significant effect in small bowel Crohn's disease.

Topical preparations of mesalamine suspended in a wax matrix suppository (ROWASA) or in a suspension enema (CANASA) are effective in active proctitis and distal ulcerative colitis, respectively. They appear to be superior to topical hydrocortisone in this setting, with response rates of 75–90%. Mesalamine enemas (4 g/60 mL) should be used at bedtime and retained for at least 8 hours; the suppository (500 mg) should be used two to three times a day with the objective of retaining it for at least 3 hours. Response to local therapy with mesalamine may occur within 3–21 days; however, the usual course of therapy is from 3–6 weeks. Once remission has occurred, lower doses are used for maintenance.

PHARMACOKINETICS

Approximately 20–30% of orally administered sulfasalazine is absorbed in the small intestine. Much of this is taken up by the liver and excreted unmetabolized in the bile; the rest (~10%) is excreted unchanged in the urine. The remaining 70% reaches the colon, where, if cleaved completely by bacterial enzymes, it generates 400 mg mesalamine for every gram of the parent compound. Thereafter, the individual components of sulfasalazine follow different metabolic pathways. Sulfapyridine, which is highly lipid-soluble, is absorbed rapidly from the colon. It undergoes extensive hepatic metabolism, including acetylation and hydroxylation, conjugation with glucuronic acid, and excretion in the urine. The acetylation phenotype of the patient determines plasma levels of sulfapyridine and the probability of adverse effects; rapid acetylators have lower systemic levels of the drug and fewer adverse effects. By contrast, only 25% of mesalamine is absorbed from the colon, and most of the drug is excreted in the stool. Intraluminal concentrations of mesalamine therefore are very high (around 1500 µg/mL or 10 mM in patients taking a typical dose of 3 g/day).

The pH-sensitive coating of ASACOL (EUDAGRIT-S) limits gastric and small intestinal absorption of 5-ASA. The pharmacokinetics of PENTASA differ somewhat. The ethylcellulose-coated microgranules are released in the upper GI tract as discrete, prolonged-release units of mesalamine. Acetylated mesalamine can be detected in the circulation within an hour after ingestion, indicating some rapid absorption, but some intact microgranules also can be detected in the colon. Because it is released in the small bowel, a greater fraction of PENTASA is absorbed systemically compared with the other 5-ASA preparations.

ADVERSE EFFECTS

Side effects of sulfasalazine occur in 10–45% of patients with ulcerative colitis and are related primarily to the sulfa moiety. Some are dose-related, including headache, nausea, and fatigue. These reactions can be minimized by giving the medication with meals or by decreasing the dose. Allergic reactions include rash, fever, Stevens-Johnson syndrome, hepatitis, pneumonitis, hemolytic anemia, and bone marrow suppression. Sulfasalazine reversibly decreases the number and motility of sperm but does not impair female fertility. It also inhibits intestinal folate absorption; therefore, folate usually is given with sulfasalazine.

The newer mesalamine formulations generally are well tolerated, and side effects are relatively infrequent and minor. Headache, dyspepsia, and rash are the most common. Diarrhea appears to be particularly common with olsalazine (occurring in 10–20% of patients); this may be related to its ability to stimulate chloride and fluid secretion in the small bowel. Nephrotoxicity, although rare, is a more serious concern. Mesalamine has been associated with interstitial nephritis; while its pathogenic role is controversial, renal function should be monitored in all patients receiving these drugs. Both sulfasalazine and its metabolites cross the placenta but have not been shown to harm the fetus. Although not studied as thoroughly, the newer formulations also appear to be safe in pregnancy. The risks to the fetus from the consequences of uncontrolled IBD in pregnant women are believed to outweigh the risks associated with the therapeutic use of these agents (see below).

GLUCOCORTICOIDS

The effects of glucocorticoids on the inflammatory response are numerous and well documented (*see* Chapter 59). Although glucocorticoids are universally recognized as effective in acute exacerbations, their use in either ulcerative colitis or Crohn's disease involves considerable challenges and pitfalls, and they are indicated only for moderate-to-severe IBD. Because the same issues impact steroid use in both ulcerative colitis and Crohn's disease, they are discussed together.

The response to glucocorticoids in individual patients with IBD divides them into three general classes: steroid-responsive, steroid-dependent, and steroid-unresponsive. Steroid-responsive patients improve clinically, generally within 1–2 weeks, and remain in remission as the steroids are tapered and then discontinued. Steroid-dependent patients also respond to glucocorticoids but then experience a relapse of symptoms as the steroid dose is tapered. Steroid-unresponsive patients do not improve even with prolonged high-dose glucocorticoids. Approximately 40% of patients are steroid-responsive, 30–40% have only a partial response or become steroid-dependent, and 15–20% of patients do not respond to steroid therapy.

Glucocorticoids sometimes are used for prolonged periods to control symptoms in steroid-dependent patients, but the failure to respond to glucocorticoids with prolonged remission (*i.e.*, a disease relapse) should prompt consideration of alternative therapies, including immunosuppressives and *infliximab* (*see* below). Glucocorticoids are not effective in maintaining remission in either ulcerative colitis or Crohn's disease; thus, their significant side effects have led to increased emphasis on limiting the duration and cumulative dose of steroids in IBD.

Initial doses in IBD are between 40–60 mg prednisone or equivalent per day; higher doses generally are no more effective. The glucocorticoid is tapered over weeks to months. Even with these slow tapers, however, efforts should be made to minimize the duration of steroid therapy. Most patients improve substantially within 5 days of initiating treatment; others require treatment for several weeks before remission occurs. For more severe cases, glucocorticoids (typically methylprednisolone or hydrocortisone) are given intravenously.

Glucocorticoid enemas are useful in patients whose disease is limited to the rectum (proctitis) and left colon. Hydrocortisone is available as a retention enema (100 mg/60 mL), and the usual dose is one 60-mL enema per night for 2 or 3 weeks. When administered optimally, the drug can reach up to or beyond the descending colon. Patients with distal disease usually respond within 3–7 days. Hydrocortisone also can be given once or twice daily as a 10% foam suspension (CORTIFOAM) that delivers 80 mg hydrocortisone per application; this formulation can be useful in patients with very short areas of distal proctitis and difficulty in retaining fluid.

Budesonide (ENTOCORT ER) is an enteric-release form of a synthetic glucocorticoid that is used for ileocecal Crohn's disease. It is proposed to deliver glucocorticoid therapy to a specific portion of inflamed gut while minimizing systemic side effects owing to extensive first-pass hepatic metabolism to inactive derivatives. Topical therapy (e.g., enemas and suppositories) also is effective in treating colitis limited to the left side of the colon. Budesonide (9 mg/day for 10–12 weeks) is effective in the acute management of mild-to-moderate exacerbations of Crohn's disease.

A significant number of patients with IBD fail to respond adequately to glucocorticoids and are either steroid-resistant or steroid-dependent.

IMMUNOSUPPRESSIVE AGENTS
Thiopurine Derivatives

The cytotoxic thiopurine derivatives *mercaptopurine* (6-MP, PURINETHOL) and azathioprine (IMMURAN) (*see* Chapters 51 and 52) are used to treat patients with severe IBD or those who are steroid-resistant or steroid-dependent. These thiopurine antimetabolites impair purine biosynthesis and inhibit cell proliferation. Both are prodrugs: Azathioprine is converted to mercaptopurine, which is subsequently metabolized to 6-thioguanine nucleotides that are the presumed active moiety. These drugs generally are used interchangeably with appropriate dose adjustments, typically azathioprine (2–2.5 mg/kg) or mercaptopurine (1.5 mg/kg). These drugs are considered equally effective in Crohn's disease and ulcerative colitis and can effectively maintain remission in both diseases; they also may prevent (or, more typically, delay) recurrence of Crohn's disease after surgical resection. Finally, they are used successfully to treat fistulas in Crohn's disease. The clinical response to azathioprine or mercaptopurine may take weeks to months, such that other drugs with a more rapid onset of action (*e.g.*, mesalamine, glucocorticoids, or infliximab) are preferred in the acute setting.

PHARMACOGENETICS Favorable responses to azathioprine–mercaptopurine are seen in up to two-thirds of patients. Mercaptopurine has three metabolic fates: (1) conversion by xanthine oxidase to 6-thiouric acid; (2) metabolism by thiopurine methyltransferase (TPMT) to 6-methyl-mercaptopurine (6-MMP); and (3) conversion by hypoxanthine–guanine phosphoribosyl transferase (HGPRT) to 6-thioguanine nucleotides and other metabolites. The relative activities of these different pathways may explain, in part, individual variations in efficacy and side effects of these immunosuppressives. The plasma $t_{1/2}$ of mercaptopurine is limited by its relatively rapid (*i.e.*, within 1–2 hours) uptake into erythrocytes and other tissues. Following this uptake, differences in thiopurine methyltransferase (TPMT) activity determine the drug's fate. Approximately 80% of the U.S. population has what is considered "normal" metabolism, whereas 1 in 300 individuals has minimal TPMT activity. In the latter setting, mercaptopurine metabolism is shifted away from 6-methyl-mercaptopurine and driven toward 6-thioguanine nucleotides, which can severely suppress the bone marrow. About 10% of people have intermediate TPMT activity; given a similar dose, they will tend to have higher 6-thioguanine levels than the normal metabolizers. Finally, ~10% of the population are rapid metabolizers. In these individuals, mercaptopurine is shunted away from 6-thioguanine nucleotides toward 6-MMP, which has been associated with abnormal liver function tests. In addition, relative to normal metabolizers, the 6-thioguanine levels of these rapid metabolizers are lower for an equivalent oral dose, possibly reducing therapeutic response. Pharmacogenetic typing can guide therapy (*see* Chapter 4).

Xanthine oxidase in the small intestine and liver converts mercaptopurine to thiouric acid, which is inactive as an immunosuppressive. Inhibition of xanthine oxidase by allopurinol diverts mercaptopurine to more active metabolites such as 6-thioguanine and increases both immunosuppressive and potential toxic effects. Thus, patients on mercaptopurine should be warned about potentially serious interactions with medications used to treat gout or hyperuricemia, and the dose should be decreased to 25% of the standard dose in subjects who are already taking allopurinol.

Methotrexate

Methotrexate generally is reserved for patients whose IBD is either steroid-resistant or steroid-dependent. In Crohn's disease, it both induces and maintains remission, generally with a more rapid response than that seen with mercaptopurine or azathioprine. Only limited studies have examined the role of methotrexate in ulcerative colitis.

Therapy of IBD with methotrexate differs somewhat from its use in other autoimmune diseases. Most important, higher doses (e.g., 15–25 mg/week) are given parenterally. The increased efficacy with parenteral administration may reflect the unpredictable intestinal absorption at higher doses of methotrexate.

Cyclosporine

Cyclosporine is effective in severe ulcerative colitis that has failed to respond adequately to glucocorticoid therapy. Between 50% and 80% of these severely ill patients improve significantly (generally within 7 days) in response to intravenous cyclosporine (2–4 mg/kg/day), sometimes avoiding emergent colectomy. Careful monitoring of cyclosporine levels is necessary to maintain a therapeutic level in whole blood of 300–400 ng/mL.

Oral cyclosporine is less effective as maintenance therapy in IBD, perhaps because of its limited intestinal absorption. In this setting, long-term therapy with NEORAL (a microemulsion formu-

lation of cyclosporine with increased oral bioavailability) may be more effective. Cyclosporine can be used to treat fistulous complications of Crohn's disease. A significant, rapid response to intravenous cyclosporine has been observed; however, frequent relapses accompany oral cyclosporine therapy, and other medical strategies are required to maintain fistula closure. Thus, calcineurin inhibitors generally are used to treat specific problems over a short term while providing a bridge to longer-term therapy.

ANTI-TNF THERAPY

Infliximab (REMICADE, cA2) is a chimeric immunoglobulin (25% mouse, 75% human) that binds to and neutralizes TNF-α, one of the principal cytokines mediating the T_H1 immune response characteristic of Crohn's disease (*see* Figure 38–1).

Infliximab (5 mg/kg infused intravenously at intervals of several weeks to months) decreases the frequency of acute flares in approximately two-thirds of patients with moderate-to-severe Crohn's disease and also facilitates the closing of enterocutaneous fistulas associated with Crohn's disease. Its role in Crohn's disease is evolving, but emerging evidence supports its efficacy in maintaining remission and in preventing recurrence of fistulas.

The use of infliximab as a biologic response modifier raises several important considerations. Both acute (fever, chills, urticaria, or even anaphylaxis) and subacute (serum sickness–like) reactions may develop after infliximab infusion. Anti–double-stranded DNA antibodies develop in 9% of patients, but a frank lupus-like syndrome occurs only rarely. Antibodies to infliximab can decrease its clinical efficacy; strategies to minimize the development of these antibodies (e.g., treatment with glucocorticoids or other immunosuppressives) may be critical to preserving infliximab efficacy for either recurrent or chronic therapy.

Infliximab therapy is associated with increased incidence of respiratory infections; of particular concern is potential reactivation of tuberculosis or other granulomatous infections with subsequent dissemination. The FDA recommends that candidates for infliximab therapy should be tested for latent tuberculosis with purified protein derivative, and patients who test positive should be treated prophylactically with isoniazid. However, anergy with a false-negative skin test has been noted in some patients with Crohn's disease, and some experts routinely perform chest radiographs to look for active or latent pulmonary disease. Infliximab also is contraindicated in patients with severe congestive heart failure. The significant cost of infliximab is an important consideration in some patients.

ANTIBIOTICS

An emerging concept is that a balance in the GI tract normally exists among the mucosal epithelium, the normal gut flora, and the immune response. Some data suggest that colonic bacteria may either initiate or perpetuate the inflammation of IBD, and specific bacterial antigens in the pathogenesis of Crohn's disease. Thus, certain bacterial strains may be either pro- (*e.g., Bacteroides*) or anti-inflammatory (*e.g., Lactobacillus*), prompting attempts to manipulate the colonic flora in patients with IBD. Traditionally, antibiotics have been used to this end, most prominently in Crohn's disease. More recently, probiotics have been used to treat specific clinical situations in IBD.

Antibiotics can be used as either (1) adjunctive treatment along with other medications for active IBD; (2) treatment for a specific complication of Crohn's disease; or (3) prophylaxis for recurrence in postoperative Crohn's disease. *Metronidazole, ciprofloxacin,* and *clarithromycin* are the antibiotics used most frequently. They are more beneficial in Crohn's disease involving the colon than in disease restricted to the ileum. Specific Crohn's disease–related complications that may benefit from antibiotic therapy include intra-abdominal abscess and inflammatory masses, perianal disease (including fistulas and perirectal abscesses), small bowel bacterial overgrowth secondary to partial small bowel obstruction, secondary infections with organisms such as *Clostridium difficile*, and postoperative complications. Metronidazole may be particularly effective for the treatment of perianal disease. Postoperatively, a 3-month course of metronidazole (20 mg/kg/day) can prolong the time to both endoscopic and clinical recurrence.

Supportive Therapy in IBD

Analgesic, anticholinergic, and antidiarrheal agents play supportive roles in reducing symptoms and improving quality of life. These drugs should be individualized based on a patient's symptoms and are supplementary to anti-inflammatory drugs. Oral iron, folate, and vitamin B$_{12}$ should be administered as indicated. Loperamide or diphenoxylate (see Chapter 37) can be used to reduce the frequency of bowel movements and relieve rectal urgency in patients with mild disease; these agents are contraindicated in severe disease because they may predispose to the development of toxic megacolon.

Cholestyramine *can be used to prevent bile salt–induced colonic secretion in patients who have undergone limited ileocolic resections. Anticholinergic agents (*dicyclomine hydrochloride, *etc.;* see *Chapter 7) are used to reduce abdominal cramps, pain, and rectal urgency. As with the antidiarrheal agents, they are contraindicated in severe disease or when obstruction is suspected. Care should be taken to differentiate exacerbation of IBD from symptoms that may be related to coexistent functional bowel disease (*see Chapter 37).

THERAPY OF IBD DURING PREGNANCY

IBD is a chronic disease that affects women in their reproductive years. In general, decreased disease activity increases fertility and improves pregnancy outcomes. At the same time, limiting medication during pregnancy is always desired but sometimes conflicts with the goal of controlling the disease.

Mesalamine and glucocorticoids are FDA category B drugs that are used frequently in pregnancy and generally are considered safe, whereas methotrexate is clearly contraindicated in pregnant patients. The use of thiopurine immunosuppressives is more controversial. Because these medications are given long term, both their initiation and discontinuation are major management decisions. Although there are no controlled trials of these medications in pregnancy, considerable experience has emerged over the last several years. There does not appear to be an increase in adverse outcomes in pregnant patients maintained on thiopurine-based immunosuppressives. Nonetheless, decisions regarding the use of these medications in patients contemplating pregnancy are complex and necessarily must involve consideration of the risks and benefits involved.

For a complete Bibliographical listing see Goodman & Gilman's *The Pharmacological Basis of Therapeutics,* 11th ed., or Goodman & Gilman Online at www.accessmedicine.com.

39

CHEMOTHERAPY OF PROTOZOAL INFECTIONS
Malaria

BIOLOGY OF MALARIAL INFECTION

Malaria afflicts nearly 500 million people and causes 2 million deaths each year. Infection with *Plasmodium falciparum* is responsible for nearly all this mortality. Human malaria is caused by four species of obligate intracellular protozoa of the genus *Plasmodium*. Infection usually is transmitted by the bite of infected female *Anopheline* mosquitoes. Sporozoites rapidly enter the circulation and localize to hepatocytes, where they transform, multiply, and develop into tissue schizonts (Figure 39–1). This primary asymptomatic stage (pre-erythrocytic or exoerythrocytic) lasts for 5–15 days, depending on the *Plasmodium* species. Tissue schizonts then rupture, releasing merozoites that enter the circulation, invade erythrocytes, and initiate the erythrocytic cycle. Once the tissue schizonts burst in *P. falciparum* and *P. malariae* infections, no parasites remain in the liver. In *P. vivax* and *P. ovale* infections, tissue parasites (hypnozoites) persist and can produce relapses years after the primary attack. Once plasmodia enter the erythrocytic cycle, they cannot reinvade the liver; thus, there is no tissue stage of infection for malaria contracted by transfusion. In erythrocytes, most parasites undergo asexual development from young forms to trophozoites and finally to mature schizonts. Schizont-containing erythrocytes rupture, producing febrile clinical attacks. The merozoites invade more erythrocytes to continue the cycle. The periodicity of parasitemia and fever depends on the timing of generation of erythrocytic parasites. For *P. falciparum*, *P. vivax*, and *P. ovale*, it takes ~48 hours to complete this process; *P. malariae* requires ~72 hours.

Merozoites bind to ligands on the red cell surface. P. falciparum *recognizes a number of molecules and invades all stages of erythrocytes; it therefore can achieve high parasitemia.* P. vivax *recognizes reticulocyte-specific proteins; thus, it only invades reticulocytes and rarely exceeds 1% parasitemia in the bloodstream.* P. ovale *resembles* P. vivax *in its predilection for young red blood cells.* P. malariae *recognizes only senescent red cells, maintains a very low parasitemia, and causes an indolent infection.* P. falciparum *assembles cytoadherence proteins into structures called knobs on the erythrocyte surface, allowing the parasitized erythrocyte to bind the vascular endothelium. This can result in microvascular blockage in the brain and organ beds and local release of vascular mediators, leading to cerebral malaria.*

Some erythrocytic parasites differentiate into sexual forms known as gametocytes. *After a female mosquito ingests infected blood, exflagellation of the male gametocyte is followed by fertilization of the female gametocyte in the insect gut. The resulting zygote, which develops as an oocyst in the gut wall, eventually gives rise to sporozoites, which invade the salivary gland of the mosquito. The insect then can infect a human host by taking a blood meal.*

Malaria is typified by high spiking fevers, chills, headache, myalgias, malaise, and gastrointestinal (GI) symptoms. Each Plasmodium *species causes a distinct illness: (1)* P. falciparum *is the most dangerous. By invading erythrocytes of any age, sequestering in the vasculature, and producing vasoactive products, this species can cause an overwhelming parasitemia, hypoglycemia, and shock with multiorgan failure. Treatment delay may lead to death. If treated early, the infection usually responds within 48 hours. If treatment is inadequate, recrudescence of infection may result. (2)* P. vivax *infection has a low mortality rate in untreated adults and is characterized by relapses due to reactivation of latent tissue forms. (3)* P. ovale *causes infection with a periodicity and relapses similar to those of* P. vivax *but is milder. (4)* P. malariae *causes a generally indolent infection. Clinical attacks may occur years or decades after infection.*

CLASSIFICATION OF ANTIMALARIAL AGENTS

The various stages of the malaria life cycle differ in their drug sensitivity. Thus, the antimalarial drugs are best classified in the context of the life cycle (Figure 39–2). Two generalizations can be made. *Since none of the drugs kills sporozoites, it is not truly possible to prevent infection but only to prevent the development of symptomatic malaria caused by the asexual erythrocytic forms. Also, none of the antimalarials is effective against all liver and red cell stages of the life cycle that may coexist in a patient. Complete cure therefore may require more than one drug.*

Class I agents are directed against the asexual erythrocytic forms and are not reliable against primary or latent liver stages or against *P. falciparum* gametocytes. These drugs will treat, or prevent, clinically symptomatic malaria. When used prophylactically, the class I drugs must be taken for several weeks after exposure until parasites complete the liver phase and become susceptible to therapy. The spectrum is somewhat expanded for the class II agents, which target not only the asexual erythrocytic forms but also the primary liver stages of *P. falciparum.* This additional activity shortens to several days the required period for postexposure prophylaxis. Finally, primaquine is unique in its spectrum of activity, which includes reliable efficacy against primary and latent liver stages as well as gametocytes. Primaquine has no place in the treatment of symptomatic malaria but rather is used most commonly to eradicate the hypnozoites of *P. vivax* and *P. ovale,* which are responsible for relapsing infections.

The use of drugs for prophylaxis or therapy is dictated by their pharmacokinetics and safety. Thus, quinine and primaquine, which have short half-lives and common toxicities, are reserved for

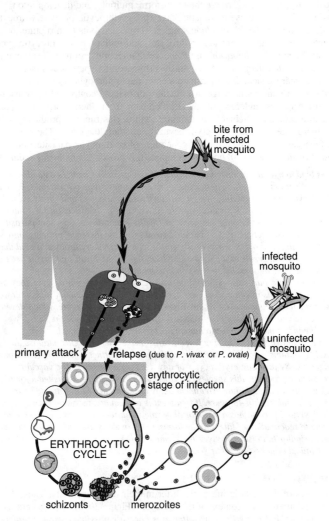

FIGURE 39–1 *Life cycle of malaria parasites. See* text for details.

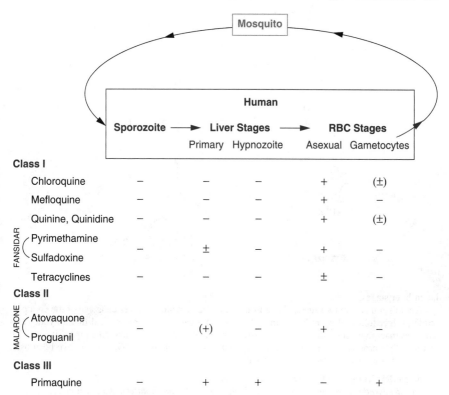

	Sporozoite	Liver Stages		RBC Stages	
		Primary	Hypnozoite	Asexual	Gametocytes
Class I					
Chloroquine	–	–	–	+	(±)
Mefloquine	–	–	–	+	–
Quinine, Quinidine	–	–	–	+	(±)
Pyrimethamine / Sulfadoxine	–	±	–	+	–
Tetracyclines	–	–	–	±	–
Class II					
Atovaquone / Proguanil	–	(+)	–	+	–
Class III					
Primaquine	–	+	+	–	+

FANSIDAR = Pyrimethamine, Sulfadoxine
MALARONE = Atovaquone, Proguanil

FIGURE 39–2 *Spectrum of clinically useful activity for antimalarial drugs.* For atovaquone and proguanil, reliable activity against the primary liver stage has been shown for *P. falciparum* only; for the class I agents, activity against gametocytes does not include *P. falciparum*.

treatment of established infection and not used for prophylaxis in healthy travelers. Chloroquine is relatively safe and has a 1-week $t_{1/2}$ that is convenient for prophylaxis (in those few areas where chloroquine-sensitive malaria persists).

Causal prophylactics act on the initial hepatic stages, drugs for terminal prophylaxis and radical cure target hypnozoites, and agents for suppressive prophylaxis or cure target the asexual red cell forms. Regimens currently recommended for *prophylaxis* in nonimmune individuals are given in Table 39–1, and regimens for the *treatment* of malaria are given in Table 39–2.

ARTEMISININ AND DERIVATIVES

The artemisinins are potent antimalarials with no clinical evidence of resistance. They are particularly well suited for the treatment of severe P. falciparum *malaria and play a key role in combination therapy of drug-resistant infections. They are not FDA approved, and inactive counterfeits are common.*

ANTIPARASITIC ACTIVITY Extensive structure–activity studies have confirmed the requirement for an endoperoxide moiety for antimalarial activity. These drugs act rapidly against the asexual erythrocytic stages of *P. vivax* and *P. falciparum.* Their potency *in vivo* is 10- to 100-fold greater than that of other antimalarials. They are not cross-resistant with other drugs; indeed, sensitivity to the artemisinins may be increased in chloroquine-resistant parasites. When used alone, the artemisinins are associated with a high level of parasite recrudescence, which may be related to their rapid metabolism. They have gametocytocidal activity but do not affect either primary or

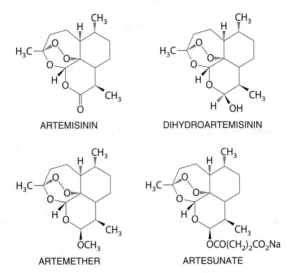

ARTEMISININ

DIHYDROARTEMISININ

ARTEMETHER

ARTESUNATE

latent liver stages.

Artemisinin acts in two steps. Heme iron within the parasite catalyzes cleavage of the endoperoxide bridge, followed by rearrangement to produce a carbon-centered radical that alkylates and damages macromolecules in the parasite. Artemisinin and its derivatives exhibit antiparasitic activity against other protozoa, including *Leishmania major* and *Toxoplasma gondii,* and have been used alone or in combination in patients with schistosomiasis.

ABSORPTION, FATE, AND EXCRETION

The semisynthetic artemisinins are available for oral (dihydroartemisinin, artesunate, and artemether), intramuscular (artesunate and artemether), intravenous (artesunate), and rectal (artesunate) dosing. Absorption after oral dosing typically is <30%. Peak plasma levels occur within minutes with artesunate and at 2–6 hours with artemether. The endoperoxides are not highly bound to plasma proteins. Both artesunate and artemether are converted extensively to dihydroartemisinin, which provides much of their antimalarial activity and has a plasma $t_{1/2}$ of 1–2 hours; its major urinary metabolite is a glucuronide. With repeated dosing, artemisinin and artesunate induce their own CYP–mediated metabolism, which may enhance clearance by up to fivefold.

THERAPEUTIC USES   Given their rapid and potent activity against even multidrug-resistant parasites, the artemisinins are valuable for the initial treatment of severe *P. falciparum* infections. The artemisinins generally are not used alone because of their incomplete efficacy and to avoid selection of resistant parasites. Artemisinin combination treatment (ACT) is preferred because the endoperoxides rapidly and substantially reduce parasite burden, reduce the likelihood of resistance, and may decrease disease transmission by reducing gametocyte carriage. Artemisinins should not be used for prophylaxis because of their short $t_{1/2}$, incompletely characterized safety in healthy subjects, and unreliability when used alone.

TOXICITY AND CONTRAINDICATIONS

The artemisinins enjoy a deserved reputation of safety. The principal targets of toxicity are brain, liver, bone marrow, and fetus. The neurological changes that occur in severe malaria confound the evaluation of neurotoxicity; however, no systematic changes were attributable to treatment in patients >5 years of age. Dose-related and reversible changes also have been seen in reticulocyte and neutrophil counts and in transaminase levels. About 1 in 3000 patients develops an allergic reaction. The artemisinins are potent embryotoxins in animals. Only a few small studies have monitored the outcome of pregnancies in women treated with endoperoxides, but there are no reported increases in congenital or developmental abnormalities. Given the current state of safety information, the artemisinins should be used with caution in very young children and pregnant women.

Table 39-1

Regimens for Malaria Chemoprophylaxis and Self-Treatment in Nonimmune Individuals*

These regimens, based on CDC recommendations current at the time of writing, may change over time. Up-to-date information should be obtained from the CDC at *www.cdc.gov/travel/*. Recommendations and available treatments vary in other countries.

Prophylaxis for infections with chloroquine-sensitive **P. falciparum,**[†] **P. vivax, P. malariae, and P. ovale**

Chloroquine phosphate (ARALEN) is available for oral administration. Adults take 500 mg chloroquine phosphate (300 mg base) weekly starting 1–2 weeks before entering an endemic area and continuing for 4 weeks after leaving. The pediatric dosage is 8.3 mg/kg chloroquine phosphate (5 mg base per kg, up to the maximum adult dose) taken orally by the same schedule. *Note: Primaquine phosphate* is used to eradicate latent tissue forms of *P. vivax* and *P. ovale* and effect a radical cure after individuals leave areas endemic for these infections (*see* Table 39–2 and text).

Prophylaxis for infections with drug-resistant strains of **P. falciparum**[‡] *or* **P. vivax.** *Note:* The choice of regimen depends on the local geographic profile of drug resistance and other factors (*see* text).

Preferred regimens:

Atovaquone–proguanil (MALARONE) is available for oral dosing only as a fixed-combination tablet containing 250 mg atovaquone and 100 mg proguanil hydrochloride (adult tablet) or 62.5 mg atovaquone and 25 g proguanil hydrochloride (pediatric tablet). Adults and children >40 kg should take one adult tablet per day beginning 1–2 days prior to exposure and continuing for 7 days after exposure. Smaller children should be dosed on the same schedule: 11–20 kg, 1 pediatric tablet daily; 21–30 kg, 2 pediatric tablets; 31–40 kg, 3 pediatric tablets. *Note: For P. vivax* malaria, atovaquone–proguanil may not be as effective as mefloquine. Atovaquone–proguanil is not recommended for children <11 kg, pregnant women, or those breast-feeding infants. Contraindicated in persons with severe renal impairment.

Mefloquine hydrochloride (LARIAM) is available for oral administration only. Tablets marketed in the U.S. contain 250 mg mefloquine hydrochloride, equivalent to 228 mg mefloquine base (this may vary in Canada and elsewhere). The dosing below is expressed in mg salt. Adults and children >45 kg body weight take 250 mg weekly starting 1–2 weeks before entering an endemic area and ending 4 weeks after leaving. Pediatric doses, taken by the same schedule, are 5 mg/kg for children up to 15 kg (may have to be prepared by a pharmacist); 62.5 mg (1/4 tablet) for 15–19 kg; 125 mg (1/2 tablet) for 20–30 kg; 187.5 mg (3/4 tablet) for 31–45 kg. *Note:* Mefloquine is *not* recommended for children weighing <5 kg or individuals with a history of seizures, severe neuropsychiatric disturbances, sensitivity to quinoline antimalarials, or cardiac conduction abnormalities.

Doxycycline hyclate (VIBRAMYCIN, others). Formulations of doxycycline are available in capsules, coated tablets, and liquid preparations for oral administration. The adult dose of doxycycline is 100 mg daily. For children >8 years of age, the dosage is 2 mg/kg given once daily, up to the adult dose. Prophylaxis with doxycycline should begin 1 day before travel to an endemic area and end 4 weeks after leaving. This regimen is used in geographical areas where highly multidrug-resistant strains of *P. falciparum* are prevalent. *Note:* Doxycycline should not be given to children <8 years of age or to pregnant women. Doxycycline is contraindicated in individuals who are hypersensitive to any tetracycline. Prophylaxis with doxycycline can be combined with the chloroquine phosphate regimen shown above for chloroquine-sensitive malaria. This strategy often is used in geographic areas where infection with more than one *Plasmodium* species is likely.

Primaquine phosphate USP. Tablets marketed in the U.S. contain 15 mg primaquine base per tablet (this may vary elsewhere); doses below are expressed as primaquine base. Primaquine may be used in special circumstances, such as when preferred agents cannot be tolerated or for multidrug-resistant *P. falciparum.* This should be done with caution and in consultation with malaria experts, such as those available through the CDC. The adult dose is 30 mg base (2 tablets) daily starting several days before exposure and continued for 7 days after exposure. The same regimen at a dose of 0.6 mg/kg base is used for children. Primaquine is contraindicated in G6PD deficiency or pregnancy (*see* text).

(Continued)

Table 39–1

Regimens for Malaria Chemoprophylaxis and Self-Treatment in Nonimmune Individuals* (*Continued*)

Other regimens:
The mefloquine, doxycycline, or chloroquine prophylactic regimens listed above may be used together with a self-treatment regimen. The latter should be used for prompt treatment of presumed malaria if, for example, the traveler is in a very remote area. *Medical attention should be sought immediately.* The preferred regimen is *atovaquone–proguanil* (MALARONE). Adults and children >41 kg should take 4 adult tablets as a single daily dose for three consecutive days; smaller children also should take adult tablets once daily for three consecutive days: 11–20 kg, 1 tablet; 21–30 kg, 2 tablets; 31–40 kg, 3 tablets.

*No chemoprophylactic regimen is always effective in preventing malaria. Recommended drug regimens always should be used in conjunction with other protective measures to avoid mosquito bites (*see* text).
†These strains now exist only in Mexico, Central America west of the Panama Canal Zone, the Caribbean, and parts of South America and the Middle East.
‡These strains exist in other geographical areas endemic for *P. falciparum* malaria.
§Papua New Guinea and Indonesia are the two areas where chloroquine-resistant *P. vivax* are highly prevalent, resulting in a high failure rate with prophylaxis. Resistant *P. vivax* also has been found sporadically in India, Burma, and Central and South America.

ATOVAQUONE

Atovaquone (MEPRON) has potent activity against Plasmodium *species and the opportunistic pathogens* Pneumocystis jirovici *and* Toxoplasma gondii; *it is FDA approved for treatment of* P. jirovici *pneumonia in patients intolerant of* trimethoprim–sulfamethoxazole. *In patients with uncomplicated* P. falciparum *malaria, combination therapy with proguanil and atovaquone evoked high cure rates with few relapses and minimal toxicity. A fixed combination of atovaquone with proguanil (MALARONE) is available in the U.S. for malaria prophylaxis and treatment.*

ANTIPARASITIC EFFECTS, MECHANISM, AND RESISTANCE Atovaquone is a lipophilic drug that has potent activity against blood stages of plasmodia, tachyzoite and cyst forms of *T. gondii*, the fungus *P. jirovici*, and *Babesia* species. It is active against liver stages of *P. falciparum* but not against *P. vivax* hypnozoites. Atovaquone is highly potent against *P. falciparum*. It inhibits electron transport and collapses the mitochondrial membrane potential. Synergism between proguanil and atovaquone may reflect proguanil's action to enhance membrane-potential collapse.

Resistance to atovaquone in P. falciparum *develops readily. Mutations in resistant organisms have been mapped to the mitochondrially encoded cytochrome b gene. Resistance can be prevented by combining proguanil with atovaquone, but it remains to be seen how long this will be effective.*

ABSORPTION, FATE, AND EXCRETION

Absorption is slow and variable after a single oral dose, increased two- to threefold by fatty food, and dose-limited >750 mg. More than 99% of the drug is bound to plasma protein, and cerebrospinal fluid (CSF) levels are <1% of those in plasma. Plasma level–time profiles often show a double peak; the first peak appears in 1–8 hours, whereas the second occurs 1–4 days after a single dose and possibly reflects enterohepatic circulation. Atovaquone has a $t_{1/2}$ of 1.5–3 days and is excreted in bile; >94% of drug is recovered unchanged in feces; its clearance varies among ethnic populations.

THERAPEUTIC USES Atovaquone is used with a biguanide for prophylaxis and treatment of malaria to obtain optimal results and avoid emergence of drug resistance. An oral tablet containing a fixed dose of 250 mg atovaquone and 100 mg proguanil hydrochloride has been highly effective and safe in a 3-day regimen for treating mild-to-moderate attacks of drug-resistant *P. falciparum* malaria. The same regimen followed by primaquine appears to be effective in treatment of *P. vivax* malaria. Experience in treatment of non–*P. falciparum* malaria is limited and should be reserved for chloroquine-resistant *P. vivax* cases in which quinine and mefloquine cannot be used. Atovaquone–proguanil also is useful for malaria prophylaxis, which can be discontinued 1 week after leaving the endemic area because both components have hepatic-phase activity.

Opportunistic infections owing to the fungus P. jiroveci *or the protozoan* T. gondii *are serious threats to patients with acquired immune deficiency syndrome (AIDS). Atovaquone remains an alternative for prophylaxis and treatment of pulmonary* P. jirovecii *infection in patients who can take oral medication but cannot tolerate trimethoprim–sulfamethoxazole or parenteral pentami-*

Table 39–2

Regimens for Treatment of Malaria in the U.S.

These regimens, modified from CDC recommendations current at the time of writing, may change over time. Up-to-date information should be obtained from the CDC at *www.cdc.gov/travel/*. Recommendations and available treatments vary in other countries.

Treatment of severe malarial infections *Note:* Infections with *P. falciparum* in nonimmune or pregnant patients constitute medical emergencies because they can progress rapidly to a fatal outcome.* Chemotherapy should be initiated promptly and not await parasitological confirmation. Parenteral therapy with *quinidine gluconate* is advised for severely ill patients who cannot take oral medication; the regimen is identical for all species of *Plasmodium*. Exchange transfusion may benefit some patients.

Preferred regimen:

Quinidine gluconate is given intravenously to both adults and children starting with a loading dose of 10 mg of the salt per kg dissolved in 300 mL of normal saline and infused over 1–2 hours (maximum dose 600 mg of the salt). This is followed by continuous infusion at the rate of 0.02 mg of the salt per kg per minute for at least 24 hours and until oral therapy with quinine sulfate is feasible. During administration of quinidine gluconate, blood pressure (for hypotension) and ECG (for widening of the QRS complex and lengthening of the QT interval) should be monitored continuously and total blood glucose (for hypoglycemia) periodically. These complications, if severe, may warrant temporary discontinuation of the drug.

Quinine sulfate can be substituted for quinidine gluconate once patients can take oral medication. The dose for adults is 650 mg of the salt given every 8 hours. The pediatric dose is 10 mg of the salt per kg given every 8 hours. Therapy with quinidine/quinine usually is given for 3–7 days depending on the species of *Plasmodium* and geographical profile of drug resistance (7 days for *P. falciparum* in Southeast Asia). Previous use of mefloquine may mandate dosage reduction (*see* text).

Adjunctive therapy:

For optimal clinical response, any one of the following regimens should be used together with oral quinine sulfate therapy. The particular choice depends on the geographical profile of antimalarial drug resistance.

Doxycycline hyclate (VIBRAMYCIN, others). The adult dose is 100 mg taken orally twice a day for 7 days. For children >8 years of age, the dosage is 2 mg/kg, increasing up to the adult dose and given by the same schedule. *Tetracycline* may be substituted if doxycycline hyclate is unavailable. Adults receive 250 mg every 6 hours for 7 days, whereas the pediatric dosage is 6.25 mg/kg every 6 hours for 7 days. *Note:* Because of adverse effects on bones and teeth, tetracyclines should not be given to children <8 years of age or to pregnant women. These drugs are contraindicated in individuals who are hypersensitive to any tetracycline.

Clindamycin. The adult or pediatric dosage is 20 mg (base)/kg/day, orally, divided into 3–4 doses, for 7 days.

Pyrimethamine–sulfadoxine (FANSIDAR). This combination is available for oral use only in tablets containing 25 mg pyrimethamine and 500 mg sulfadoxine. One dose is taken by mouth on the last day of quinine sulfate therapy: Adults take 3 tablets; children 5–10 kg, 0.5 tablet; 11–14 kg, 0.75 tablet; 15–20 kg, 1 tablet; 21–30 kg, 1.5 tablets; 31–40 kg, 2 tablets; 41–50 kg, 2.5 tablets; over 50 kg, 3 tablets. Owing to extensive drug resistance, pyrimethamine–sulfadoxine should be used as an adjunct treatment primarily in young children or women who are not able to tolerate clindamycin.

Other oral treatment regimens for infections with chloroquine-resistant **P. vivax**[†] ***and drug-resistant strains of*** **P. falciparum**

If quinine-based therapy cannot be used, mefloquine currently is the preferred alternative (except for Southeast Asia) but could be supplanted in this role by atovaquone–proguanil once more experience is obtained.

Mefloquine hydrochloride (LARIAM, MEPHAQUINE). The adult dose is 750 mg of the salt taken by mouth followed 6–12 hours later by 500 mg. The corresponding pediatric dose for children weighing less than 45 kg is 15 mg of the salt per kg followed 6–12 hours later by 10 mg of the salt per kg. (*Note:* The pediatric dosage is not approved by the FDA.) The initial dose should be

(*Continued*)

Table 39–2

Regimens for Treatment of Malaria in the U.S. *(Continued)*

repeated *only* if vomiting occurs within the first hour. Therapeutic doses of mefloquine may induce gastrointestinal and neuropsychiatric symptoms. Because of its long $t_{1/2}$ and potential for serious drug interactions, extreme caution is advised in using certain antimalarial agents (*e.g.*, quinine or halofantrine) with or shortly after mefloquine. (*See* text for further details).

Atovaquone–proguanil hydrochloride (MALARONE). A fixed-dose combination of these drugs is available in tablets containing 250 mg atovaquone and 100 mg proguanil hydrochloride. The dose for adults is 1000 mg atovaquone plus 400 mg proguanil hydrochloride taken by mouth once each day for 3 days. The pediatric dose for children weighing 11–20 kg is 250 mg atovaquone plus 100 mg proguanil hydrochloride; 21–30 kg, 500 mg atovaquone plus 200 mg proguanil hydrochloride; 31–40 kg, 750 mg atovaquone plus 300 mg proguanil hydrochloride. These doses are given once daily for 3 days with food to increase drug bioavailability. If vomiting occurs within 30 minutes, the dose should be repeated. If nausea is severe, the dose may be split in half and given twice daily. Experience with children weighing <11 kg is limited, but if necessary, pediatric tablets are available. Consult CDC recommendations for dosages.

Oral treatment of infections with P. vivax, P. malariae, P. ovale, *and chloroquine-sensitive* P. falciparum

Chloroquine phosphate (ARALEN) is available in 250- and 500-mg tablets (equivalent to 150 and 300 mg base, respectively) for oral administration. The adult dosage is two 500-mg tablets immediately, followed by one 500-mg tablet at 6, 24, and 48 hours. The dosage for children is 16.7 mg/kg (10 mg base per kg) immediately, followed by 8.3 mg/kg (5 mg base per kg) at 6, 24, and 48 hours, not to exceed the adult dosage.

Prevention of relapse:

To eradicate latent tissue forms of *P. vivax* and *P. ovale* that persist to cause relapses of infection, primaquine phosphate is supplied in tablets containing either 13.2 or 26.3 mg of the salt (7.5 or 15 mg base, respectively) for oral administration only. Therapy with primaquine is started after the acute attack (about day 4) at doses of 52.6 mg (30 mg base) daily for 14 days. Pediatric doses are 1.06 mg/kg (0.6 mg base per kg) daily, also for 14 days. The same primaquine regimen also can be used during the last 2 weeks of chloroquine phosphate prophylaxis for individuals who have left areas endemic for *P. vivax* or *P. ovale* infection. Alternatively, adults using chloroquine for prophylaxis against *P. vivax* or *P. ovale* may take 500 mg chloroquine phosphate (300 mg base) together with 78.9 mg primaquine phosphate (45 mg base) weekly for 8 weeks starting after leaving an endemic area to achieve a "radical" cure. Primaquine is contraindicated in pregnancy and in severe G6PD deficiency (*see* text).

---

*Emergency advice is available from the Division of Parasitic Diseases, Centers for Disease Control and Prevention (telephone: 770-488-7788).
†Papua New Guinea and Indonesia are the two areas where chloroquine-resistant *P. vivax* are highly prevalent, resulting in a high failure rate. Resistant *P. vivax* also has been found sporadically in India, Burma, and Central and South America. Currently, patients acquiring *P. vivax* infections from regions other than Papua New Guinea and Indonesia should be treated with chloroquine.

dine. T. gondii *infections in these patients, especially cerebral lesions, have shown only limited dose-related positive responses to prolonged regimens of atovaquone.* Toxoplasma *chorioretinitis in immunocompetent patients probably responds better to this drug. Atovaquone also is used in combination with* azithromycin *for infections owing to* Babesia *species.*

TOXICITY

The most common adverse reactions are abdominal pain, nausea, vomiting, diarrhea, headache, and rash. Vomiting and diarrhea may result in therapeutic failure owing to decreased drug absorption. However, readministration of this drug within an hour of vomiting may still evoke a positive therapeutic response in patients with P. falciparum *malaria. Patients treated with atovaquone occasionally exhibit abnormalities of serum transaminase or amylase levels.*

PRECAUTIONS AND CONTRAINDICATIONS

While atovaquone seems remarkably safe, the drug needs further evaluation in pediatric patients weighing <11 kg, pregnant women, and lactating mothers and is not recommended in *these individuals. Atovaquone may compete with certain drugs for binding to plasma proteins, and therapy with* rifampin, *a potent inducer of CYP–mediated drug metabolism, can substan-*

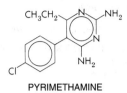

PYRIMETHAMINE

tially reduce plasma levels of atovaquone, whereas plasma levels of rifampin are raised. Coadministration with tetracycline *is associated with a 40% reduction in plasma concentration of atovaquone.*

DIAMINOPYRIMIDINES

ANTIPROTOZOAL EFFECTS

Antimalarial Actions Pyrimethamine is a slow-acting blood schizontocide with antimalarial effects *in vivo* similar to those of proguanil (*see* below). However, pyrimethamine has greater antimalarial potency, and its $t_{1/2}$ is much longer than that of *cycloguanil,* the active metabolite of proguanil. Pyrimethamine's efficacy against hepatic forms of *P. falciparum* is less than that of proguanil, and at therapeutic doses, pyrimethamine fails to eradicate the latent tissue forms of *P. vivax* or gametocytes of any plasmodial species.

Action Against Other Protozoa

High doses of pyrimethamine given concurrently with sulfadiazine *is the preferred therapy for infection with* T. gondii *in infants and immunosuppressed individuals.*

MECHANISMS OF ANTIMALARIAL ACTION AND RESISTANCE The 2,4-diaminopyrimidines inhibit dihydrofolate reductase of plasmodia at concentrations far lower than those required to inhibit the mammalian enzymes. The dihydrofolate reductase in malaria resides on the same polypeptide chain as thymidylate synthase and is not upregulated in the face of inhibition, which contributes to the selective toxicity of the antifolates. Synergism between pyrimethamine and the sulfonamides or sulfones has been attributed to inhibition of two steps in an essential metabolic pathway.

Several factors affect the response to antifolates, including host immunity and dietary p-aminobenzoic acid *or folate, which can reduce efficacy substantially. Pyrimethamine resistance is seen in regions of prolonged or extensive drug use and results from mutations in dihydrofolate reductase–thymidylate synthetase. Several mutations in* P. falciparum *introduce single-amino-acid changes linked to resistance by decreasing the drug's binding affinity for its active site in dihydrofolate reductase.*

ABSORPTION, FATE, AND DISTRIBUTION

Given orally, pyrimethamine is slowly but completely absorbed; it reaches peak plasma levels in about 2–6 hours. The compound binds to plasma proteins and accumulates in kidneys and other organs. Its elimination $t_{1/2}$ in plasma is ~80–95 hours. Concentrations that suppress responsive plasmodial strains remain in the blood for 2 weeks. Pyrimethamine also is excreted in the milk of nursing mothers.

THERAPEUTIC USES Pyrimethamine is almost always given with either a sulfonamide or sulfone to enhance its antifolate activity. It acts slowly relative to the quinoline blood schizontocides, and its prolonged elimination encourages the selection of resistant parasites. The use of pyrimethamine is restricted to the treatment of chloroquine-resistant *P. falciparum* malaria in areas where resistance to antifolates has not yet fully developed. Pyrimethamine together with a short-acting sulfonamide such as sulfadiazine also may be used as an adjunct to quinine to treat an acute malarial attack. Dosage regimens for this indication are given in Table 39–2. Pyrimethamine–sulfadoxine is no longer recommended for prophylaxis because of toxicity owing to the accompanying sulfonamide (*see* below).

High doses of pyrimethamine plus sulfadiazine are the treatment of choice for infections with T. gondii *in immunocompromised adults; without treatment, these infections progress rapidly to death. Initial therapy consists of an oral loading dose of 200 mg followed by 50–75 mg pyrimethamine daily for 4–6 weeks along with 4–6 g sulfadiazine daily in four divided doses.* Leucovorin *(folinic acid), 10–15 mg daily, should also be taken to prevent bone marrow toxicity. For subsequent long-term suppressive therapy, lower doses of pyrimethamine (25–50 mg daily) and sulfadiazine (2–4 g daily) may suffice. Infants with congenital toxoplasmosis usually respond positively to oral pyrimethamine (0.5–1.0 mg/kg daily) and oral sulfadiazine (100 mg/kg daily) given for 1 year.*

TOXICITY, PRECAUTIONS, AND CONTRAINDICATIONS

Antimalarial doses of pyrimethamine alone cause little toxicity except occasional rashes and depression of hematopoiesis. Excessive doses produce a megaloblastic anemia that responds to drug withdrawal or treatment with folinic acid. At high doses, pyrimethamine is teratogenic in animals, and in humans, trimethoprim–sulfamethoxazole therapy is associated with birth defects, but such toxicity has not been studied systematically for pyrimethamine in humans.

Sulfonamides or sulfones usually account for most toxicity associated with coadministration of these antifolate drugs (see Chapter 43). The combination of pyrimethamine (25 mg) and sulfadoxine (500 mg) (FANSIDAR) causes severe and even fatal cutaneous reactions in up to 1 in 5000 people. This combination also has been associated with serum sickness–type reactions, urticaria, exfoliative dermatitis, and hepatitis. Pyrimethamine–sulfadoxine is contraindicated in individuals with previous reactions to sulfonamides, lactating mothers, and infants <2 months of age. Administration of pyrimethamine with dapsone *(MALOPRIM, unavailable in the U.S.), occasionally has been associated with agranulocytosis. Higher doses of pyrimethamine (75 mg daily) used along*

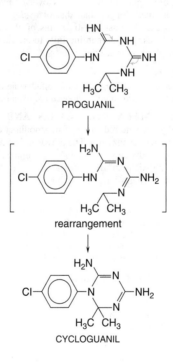

PROGUANIL

rearrangement

CYCLOGUANIL

with sulfadiazine (4–6 g daily) to treat toxoplasmosis produce skin rashes, bone marrow suppression, and renal toxicity in ~40% of immunocompromised patients. Much of this toxicity probably is due to sulfadiazine.

PROGUANIL

Proguanil and its triazine metabolite cycloguanil have the following structures:
Proguanil has the widest margin of safety of a large series of antimalarial biguanide analogs examined. Dihalogen substitution in positions 3 and 4 of the benzene ring yields chlorproguanil (LAPUDRINE), a more potent prodrug that also is used clinically. Cycloguanil is structurally related to pyrimethamine.

ANTIMALARIAL ACTIONS   In sensitive *P. falciparum* malaria, proguanil exerts activity against both the primary liver stages and the asexual red cell stages, thus adequately controlling the acute attack and usually eradicating the infection. Proguanil also is active against acute *P. vivax* malaria, but because the latent tissue stages of *P. vivax* are unaffected, relapses may occur after drug withdrawal. Proguanil treatment does not destroy gametocytes, but fertilized gametes in the gut of the mosquito fail to develop normally.

MECHANISMS OF ANTIMALARIAL ACTION AND RESISTANCE   The active triazine metabolite of proguanil selectively inhibits the bifunctional dihydrofolate reductase–thymidylate synthetase of sensitive plasmodia, inhibiting DNA synthesis and depleting folate cofactors. Certain amino acid changes near the dihydrofolate reductase–binding site are linked to resistance to either cycloguanil, pyrimethamine, or both. Resistance to cycloguanil (and chlorcycloguanil) can be linked to mutations in plasmodial dihydrofolate reductase. This pattern differs from that typically observed for pyrimethamine resistance, but overlapping resistance to cycloguanil and pyrimethamine indicates that resistance mechanisms may be quite complex.

The mechanism of the antimalarial activity of proguanil or chlorproguanil is unknown. Proguanil as the biguanide accentuates the mitochondrial membrane-potential-collapsing action of atovaquone against P. falciparum but displays no such activity by itself (see "Atovaquone," above). In contrast to cycloguanil, resistance to the intrinsic antimalarial activity of proguanil itself, either alone or in combination with atovaquone, has yet to be documented.

ABSORPTION, FATE, AND EXCRETION
Proguanil is slowly but adequately absorbed from the GI tract. After a single oral dose, peak plasma concentrations of the drug usually are attained within 5 hours. The mean plasma elimination $t_{1/2}$ is ~12–20 hours. Metabolism of proguanil cosegregates with CYP2C isoforms that control mephenytoin oxidation. Only ~3% of Caucasians are deficient in this oxidation versus 20% of Asians and Kenyans. Proguanil is oxidized to two major metabolites, cycloguanil and an inactive 4-chlorophenylbiguanide. On a 200-mg daily dosage regimen, extensive metabolizers develop plasma levels of cycloguanil that are above the therapeutic range, whereas poor metabolizers may not. Proguanil does not accumulate appreciably in tissues during long-term administration, except in erythrocytes, where its concentration is about three times that in plasma. The inactive 4-chlorophenyl-biguanide metabolite appears in increased quantities in the urine of poor proguanil metabolizers. In humans, from 40% to 60% of absorbed proguanil is excreted in urine either as the parent drug or as active metabolite.

THERAPEUTIC USES   Proguanil as a single agent is not available in the U.S. but is prescribed in Europe for nonimmune travelers to malarious areas. Strains of *P. falciparum* resistant to proguanil emerge rapidly in areas where the drug is used exclusively, but breakthrough infections also may result from deficient conversion of this compound to its active antimalarial metabolite.

Proguanil is effective and well tolerated when given orally once daily for 3 days in combination with atovaquone for the treatment of malarial attacks owing to chloroquine- and multidrug-resistant strains of *P. falciparum* and *P. vivax* (*see* "Atovaquone," above). Indeed, this drug combination (MALARONE) has been successful in Southeast Asia, where highly drug-resistant strains of *P. falciparum* prevail. *P. falciparum* readily develops clinical resistance to monotherapy with either proguanil or atovaquone, but resistance to the combination is uncommon unless the strain is initially resistant to atovaquone. In contrast, some strains resistant to proguanil do respond to proguanil plus atovaquone.

TOXICITY AND SIDE EFFECTS
In prophylactic doses of 200–300 mg/day, proguanil causes few side effects except occasional nausea and diarrhea. Large doses (1 g or more daily) may cause vomiting, abdominal pain, diarrhea, hematuria, and transient appearance of epithelial cells and casts in the urine. Overdose (up to 15 g) has been followed by complete recovery. Doses as high as 700 mg twice daily have been taken for >2 weeks without serious toxicity. Proguanil is considered safe during pregnancy. It is remarkably safe when coadministered with other antimalarial drugs.

QUINOLINES AND RELATED COMPOUNDS
Chloroquine and Hydroxychloroquine

The structure of chloroquine is shown in Figure 39–3. A chlorine atom attached to position 7 of the quinoline ring confers the greatest antimalarial activity. Hydroxychloroquine (PLAQUENIL) is essentially equivalent to chloroquine against P. falciparum malaria.

PHARMACOLOGICAL EFFECTS

Antimalarial Actions Chloroquine is highly effective against erythrocytic forms of *P. vivax*, *P. ovale*, *P. malariae*, and chloroquine-sensitive strains of *P. falciparum* and is the prophylaxis and treatment of choice for these organisms. It exerts activity against gametocytes of the first three plasmodial species but not against those of *P. falciparum*. The drug has no activity against latent tissue forms of *P. vivax* or *P. ovale*.

Other Effects

Chloroquine or its analogs are used to treat hepatic amebiasis and are secondary drugs for variety of chronic inflammatory diseases, including rheumatoid arthritis, systemic lupus erythematosus, discoid lupus, sarcoidosis, and photosensitivity diseases such as porphyria cutanea tarda.

MECHANISMS OF ANTIMALARIAL ACTION AND RESISTANCE TO CHLOROQUINE AND OTHER ANTIMALARIAL QUINOLINES

Asexual malaria parasites flourish in erythrocytes by digesting hemoglobin; this generates free radicals and heme as highly reactive by-products. Heme is sequestered as an insoluble malarial

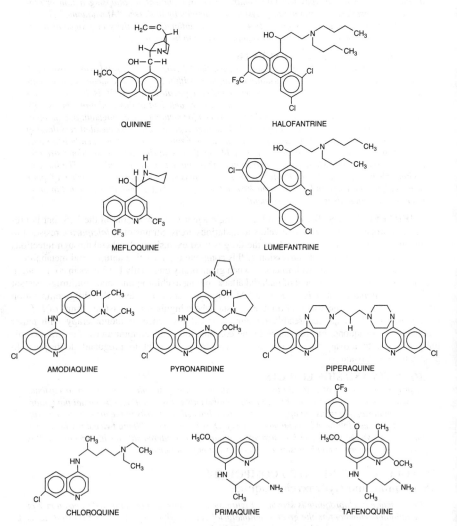

FIGURE 39–3 *Chemical structure of antimalarial quinolines and related compounds.*

pigment termed hemozoin, *and quinolines likely interfere with heme handling. Failure to inactivate heme or even enhanced toxicity of drug–heme complexes is thought to kill the parasites via oxidative damage to membranes.*

Resistance of erythrocytic asexual forms of P. falciparum *to antimalarial quinolines, especially chloroquine, now is common. Chloroquine resistance results from mutations in the gene encoding a chloroquine resistance transporter, designated* crt. *Multiple mutations are needed to confer resistance. Chloroquine-resistant* P. vivax *isolates do not have alterations in their* crt *ortholog and may have a different resistance mechanism. P-glycoprotein and other transporters may modulate chloroquine resistance.*

ABSORPTION, FATE, AND EXCRETION

Chloroquine is well absorbed after oral, intramuscular, and subcutaneous administration. It distributes relatively slowly into a very large apparent volume (over 100 L/kg) and is extensively sequestered in tissues, particularly liver, spleen, kidney, lung, and to a lesser extent, brain and spinal cord. Chloroquine binds moderately (60%) to plasma proteins and is biotransformed via hepatic CYPs to two active metabolites, desethylchloroquine and bisdesethylchloroquine. Renal clearance of chloroquine is about half of total clearance. Unchanged chloroquine and its major metabolites account for >50% and 25% of urinary drug products, respectively, and their renal excretion is increased by urine acidification.

Plasma levels of chloroquine shortly after dosing are determined primarily by the rate of distribution rather than the rate of elimination. Because of extensive tissue binding, a loading dose is used to achieve effective concentrations in plasma. After parenteral administration, rapid entry together with slow exit of chloroquine from a small central compartment can result transiently in potentially lethal drug concentrations in plasma. Hence, parenteral chloroquine is given either by constant intravenous infusion or in small divided doses by the subcutaneous or intramuscular route. Chloroquine is safer when given orally because the rates of absorption and distribution are more closely matched; peak plasma levels are achieved in ~3–5 hours after dosing by this route. The $t_{1/2}$ of chloroquine increases from a few days to weeks as plasma levels decline, reflecting the transition from slow distribution to even slower elimination from extensive tissue stores. The terminal $t_{1/2}$ ranges from 30 to 60 days, and traces of the drug can be found in the urine for years after a therapeutic regimen.

THERAPEUTIC USES Chloroquine is inexpensive and safe, but its usefulness has declined in those parts of the world where strains of *P. falciparum* are resistant. Except in areas where resistant strains of *P. vivax* are reported (Table 39–2), chloroquine is very effective in prophylaxis or treatment of acute attacks of malaria caused by *P. vivax, P. ovale,* and *P. malariae*. Chloroquine has no activity against primary or latent liver stages of the parasite. To prevent relapses in *P. vivax* and *P. ovale* infections, primaquine can be given either with chloroquine or reserved for use until after a patient leaves an endemic area. Chloroquine rapidly controls the clinical symptoms and parasitemia of acute malarial attacks. Most patients become afebrile within 24–48 hours after receiving therapeutic doses. If patients fail to respond by the second day of chloroquine therapy, resistance of *P. falciparum* should be suspected and therapy instituted with quinine or another rapidly acting blood schizontocide. Although parenteral chloroquine can be given safely to comatose or vomiting patients until it can be taken orally, quinidine gluconate usually is given in the U.S. In comatose children, chloroquine is well absorbed when given *via* nasogastric tube. Tables 39–1 and 39–2 provide information about recommended prophylactic and therapeutic dosage regimens for chloroquine.

TOXICITY AND SIDE EFFECTS

Taken in proper doses, chloroquine is an extraordinarily safe drug; however, its safety margin is narrow, and a single dose of 30 mg/kg may be fatal. Acute chloroquine toxicity is encountered most frequently with too rapid administration of parenteral doses. Cardiovascular effects include hypotension, vasodilation, depressed myocardial function, cardiac arrhythmias, and cardiac arrest. Confusion, convulsions, and coma denote central nervous system (CNS) dysfunction. Chloroquine doses of >5 g given parenterally usually are fatal. Prompt treatment with mechanical ventilation, epinephrine, and diazepam may be lifesaving.

Doses of chloroquine used for oral therapy of the acute malarial attack may cause GI upset, headache, visual disturbances, and urticaria. Pruritus also occurs, most commonly among dark-skinned persons. Prolonged medication with suppressive doses occasionally causes side effects such as headache, blurring of vision, diplopia, confusion, convulsions, lichenoid skin eruptions, bleaching of hair, widening of the QRS interval, and T-wave abnormalities. These complications usually disappear soon after the drug is withheld. Rare instances of hemolysis and blood dyscrasias have been reported. Chloroquine may cause discoloration of nail beds and mucous membranes.

Irreversible retinopathy and ototoxicity can result from high daily doses (>250 mg) of chloroquine or hydroxychloroquine that lead to cumulative total doses of more than 1 g of base per kilogram body weight, such as those used for treatment of diseases other than malaria. Retinopathy can be avoided if the daily dose is ≤250 mg. Prolonged therapy with high doses of 4-aminoquinoline also can cause toxic myopathy, cardiopathy, and peripheral neuropathy; these reactions improve if the drug is withdrawn promptly. Rarely, neuropsychiatric disturbances, including suicide, may be related to overdose.

PRECAUTIONS AND CONTRAINDICATIONS
Chloroquine is not recommended for treating individuals with epilepsy or myasthenia gravis. The drug should be used cautiously if at all in the presence of hepatic disease or severe GI, neurological, or blood disorders. The dose must be adjusted in renal failure. In rare cases, chloroquine can cause hemolysis in patients with glucose-6-phosphate dehydrogenase (G6PD) deficiency. Chloroquine should not be used in patients with psoriasis or other exfoliative skin conditions because it causes severe reactions. It should not be used for malaria in patients with porphyria cutanea tarda but is used in smaller doses for treatment of the underlying disease (see Chapter 63). Chloroquine inhibits CYP2D6 and interacts with a variety of drugs. It should not be given with mefloquine because of increased risk of seizures. Most important, this antimalarial opposes the action of anticonvulsants and increases the risk of ventricular arrhythmias from coadministration with amiodarone or halofantrine. By increasing plasma levels of digoxin and cyclosporine, chloroquine can increase the risk of their toxicity. For patients receiving long-term, high-dose therapy, ophthalmological and neurological evaluations are recommended every 3–6 months.

QUININE AND QUINIDINE
Quinine remains a mainstay for treating attacks of chloroquine- and multidrug-resistant P. falciparum malaria (Table 39–2). Multidrug therapy with other antimalarials is supplanting quinine regimens because of increasing resistance of P. falciparum to quinine together with its toxicity. Both quinine and quinidine are obtained from natural sources and contain a quinoline group attached through a secondary alcohol linkage to a quinuclidine ring (Figure 39–3). A methoxy side chain is attached to the quinoline ring and a vinyl to the quinuclidine. They differ only in the steric configuration at two of the three asymmetrical centers. Quinidine is both somewhat more potent as an antimalarial and more toxic than quinine.

PHARMACOLOGICAL EFFECTS
Antimalarial Actions   Quinine acts primarily against asexual erythrocytic forms and has little effect on hepatic forms of malarial parasites. The alkaloid also is gametocidal for *P. vivax* and *P. malariae* but not for *P. falciparum*. Quinine is more toxic and less effective than chloroquine against malarial parasites susceptible to both drugs. However, quinine, along with its stereoisomer quinidine, is especially valuable for the parenteral treatment of severe illness owing to drug-resistant strains of *P. falciparum*, even though these strains have become more resistant to both agents in certain parts of Southeast Asia and South America. Because of its toxicity and short $t_{1/2}$, quinine generally is not used for prophylaxis.

Quinine resistance in P. falciparum more closely resembles resistance to mefloquine and halofantrine than to chloroquine. A number of different transporter genes may confer resistance to quinine.

Action on Skeletal Muscle   Quinine increases the tension response to a single maximal stimulus delivered to muscle, but it also increases the refractory period of muscle so that the response to tetanic stimulation is diminished. The excitability of the motor end-plate region decreases so that responses to repetitive stimulation and to acetylcholine are reduced. Thus, quinine can antagonize the actions of *physostigmine* on skeletal muscle. Quinine also may produce respiratory distress and dysphagia in patients with myasthenia gravis.

ABSORPTION, FATE, AND EXCRETION
Quinine is readily absorbed when given orally or intramuscularly. Oral absorption occurs mainly from the upper small intestine and exceeds 80%, even in patients with marked diarrhea. After an oral dose, plasma levels of quinine reach a maximum in 3–8 hours and, after distributing into an apparent volume of ~1.5 L/kg, decline with a $t_{1/2}$ of ~11 hours after termination of therapy. Quinine pharmacokinetics may change according to the severity of malarial infection. Values for both the apparent volume of distribution and the systemic clearance of quinine decrease, the latter more than the former, so that the average elimination $t_{1/2}$ increases from 11 to 18 hours. After standard therapeutic doses, peak plasma levels of quinine may reach 15–20 mg/L in severely ill patients without causing major toxicity (see below); in contrast, levels >10 mg/L produce severe

drug reactions in self-poisoning. The high levels of plasma α_1-acid glycoprotein in severe malaria may prevent toxicity by binding the drug and reducing its free fraction. Concentrations of quinine are lower in erythrocytes (33–40%) and CSF (2–5%) than in plasma, and the drug readily reaches fetal tissues.

The cinchona alkaloids are metabolized extensively, especially by hepatic CYP3A4, so only ~20% of a dose is excreted unaltered in the urine. The major metabolite of quinine, 3-hydroxyquinine, retains some antimalarial activity and can accumulate and possibly cause toxicity in patients with renal failure. Renal excretion of quinine itself is more rapid when the urine is acidic.

THERAPEUTIC USES

Treatment of Malaria Quinine is the drug of choice for drug-resistant *P. falciparum* malaria. In severe illness, the prompt use of loading doses of intravenous quinine (or quinidine, where IV quinine is not available, as in the U.S.) can be lifesaving. Oral medication to maintain therapeutic concentrations then is given as soon as tolerated and continued for 5–7 days. Especially for treatment of infections with multidrug-resistant strains of *P. falciparum*, slower-acting blood schizontocides such as a sulfonamide or a tetracycline are given concurrently to enhance the efficacy of quinine. Formulations of quinine and quinidine and specific regimens for the treatment of *P. falciparum* malaria are shown in Table 39–2.

The therapeutic range for "free" quinine is 0.2–2.0 mg/L. Regimens to achieve this target may vary based on patient age, severity of illness, and the drug responsiveness of *P. falciparum*. Lower doses are more effective in treating children in Africa than adults in Southeast Asia because quinine pharmacokinetics differ in these populations, as does the susceptibility of *P. falciparum* to the drug. Regimens for quinidine are similar to those for quinine, although quinidine binds less to plasma proteins and has a larger volume of distribution, greater systemic clearance, and shorter terminal elimination $t_{1/2}$ than quinine. The dose of quinidine currently recommended by the Centers for Disease Control and Prevention (CDC), 10 mg salt per kilogram initially, followed by 0.02 mg salt per kilogram per minute, perhaps should be modified to 10 and 0.02 mg of base (60% of the salt is base).

TOXICITY AND SIDE EFFECTS

The fatal oral dose of quinine for adults is ~2–8 g. Quinine is associated with a triad of dose-related toxicities when it is given at full therapeutic or excessive doses. These are cinchonism, hypoglycemia, and hypotension. Mild forms of cinchonism—consisting of tinnitus, high-tone deafness, visual disturbances, headache, dysphoria, nausea, vomiting, and postural hypotension— occur very frequently and disappear soon after the drug is withdrawn. Hypoglycemia can be life-threatening if not treated promptly with intravenous glucose. Hypotension is rare and most often is associated with excessively rapid intravenous infusions of quinine or quinidine. Prolonged medication or high single doses also may produce GI, cardiovascular, and dermal manifestations.

Hearing and vision are particularly affected. Functional impairment of the eighth nerve results in tinnitus, decreased auditory acuity, and vertigo. Visual symptoms also are common. The visual and auditory effects probably reflect direct neurotoxicity, although secondary vascular changes may have a role. Marked spastic constriction of the retinal vessels occurs. In severe cases, optic atrophy results.

GI symptoms (e.g., nausea, vomiting, abdominal pain, and diarrhea) result from the local irritant action of quinine; the nausea and emesis also have a central basis. The skin often is hot and flushed, and sweating is prominent. Rashes appear frequently. Angioedema, especially of the face, is observed occasionally.

Quinine and quinidine, even at therapeutic doses, may cause hyperinsulinemia and severe hypoglycemia through their powerful stimulatory effect on pancreatic beta cells. Despite treatment with glucose infusions, this complication can be life threatening, especially in pregnancy and prolonged severe infection.

Quinine rarely causes cardiovascular complications unless target plasma concentrations are exceeded. QTc prolongation is mild and does not appear to be affected by concurrent mefloquine treatment. However, severe hypotension is predictable when quinine is administered too rapidly intravenously. Acute overdosage also may cause serious and even fatal cardiac dysrhythmias. Quinidine is even more cardiotoxic than quinine. Cardiac monitoring of patients on intravenous quinidine is advisable where possible.

Toxic manifestations of small doses of cinchona alkaloids usually result from drug hypersensitivity. Flushing and pruritus, often accompanied by rashes, fever, gastric distress, dyspnea, ringing in the ears, and visual impairment, are the usual expressions. Hemoglobinuria and asthma from quinine may occur more rarely. "Blackwater fever"—massive hemolysis, hemoglobinemia, and hemoglobinuria leading to anuria, renal failure, and even death—is a rare hypersensitivity reaction to quinine. Quinine occasionally may cause milder hemolysis, especially in people with G6PD deficiency. Immune thrombocytopenic purpura also is rare but can occur even in response to ingestion of tonic water, which has about one-twenty-fifth the therapeutic oral dose per 12 oz. Other rare reactions to the drug include hypoprothrombinemia, leukopenia, and agranulocytosis.

PRECAUTIONS, CONTRAINDICATIONS, AND INTERACTIONS

Quinine must be used with considerable caution, if at all, in patients who manifest drug hypersensitivity. Quinine should be discontinued immediately if evidence of hemolysis appears. The drug should not be used in patients with tinnitus or optic neuritis. In patients with cardiac dysrhythmias, the administration of quinine requires the same precautions as for quinidine. Quinine appears to be fairly safe and is used commonly for treatment of malaria during pregnancy, but caution must be used to avoid hypoglycemia.

Concentrated solutions of quinine may cause abscesses when injected intramuscularly or thrombophlebitis when infused intravenously. GI absorption of quinine can be delayed by antacids containing aluminum. Quinine and quinidine can elevate plasma levels of digoxin. Likewise, the alkaloid may raise plasma levels of warfarin. The action of quinine at neuromuscular junctions will enhance the effect of neuromuscular blocking agents and oppose the action of acetylcholinesterase inhibitors. Prochlorperazine can amplify quinine's cardiotoxicity, as can halofantrine. The clearance of quinine is decreased by cimetidine and increased by acidification of the urine by and rifampin.

Mefloquine

Mefloquine (LARIAM) is 4-quinoline methanol (Figure 39–3) that emerged from clinical trials as safe and highly effective against drug-resistant strains of P. falciparum. Mefloquine was first used to treat chloroquine-resistant P. falciparum malaria in a coformulation with pyrimethamine–sulfadoxine (FANSIMEF) to delay development of resistance. This strategy failed, largely because slow elimination of mefloquine fostered the selection of resistant parasites at subtherapeutic drug concentrations. Mefloquine is used for prophylaxis and chemotherapy of drug-resistant P. falciparum and P. vivax malaria.

ANTIMALARIAL ACTIONS Mefloquine is a highly effective blood schizontocide but has no activity against early hepatic stages and mature gametocytes of *P. falciparum* or latent tissue forms of *P. vivax*. The drug may have some sporontocidal activity but is not used clinically for this purpose.

Mechanisms of Antimalarial Action and Resistance

The mechanism of action of mefloquine is unknown but may be similar to that of chloroquine. Certain isolates of P. falciparum exhibit resistance to mefloquine via unknown mechanisms. Chloroquine-resistant alleles of the crt gene actually confer increased sensitivity to mefloquine and some other quinolines. Amplification of the pfmdr1 gene is associated with resistance to mefloquine and quinine.

Absorption, Fate, and Excretion

Mefloquine is taken orally because parenteral preparations cause severe local reactions. The drug is well absorbed, a process enhanced by food. Probably owing to extensive enterogastric and enterohepatic circulation, plasma levels of mefloquine rise biphasically to peak in ~17 hours. The drug is widely distributed, highly bound (~98%) to plasma proteins, and slowly eliminated with a terminal $t_{1/2}$ of ~20 days. Several mefloquine metabolites are formed. Plasma levels of the inactive mefloquine 4-carboxylic acid exceed those of mefloquine itself and decline at about the same rate. Excretion is mainly by the fecal route; ~10% of mefloquine appears unchanged in the urine.

Therapeutic Uses

Mefloquine should be reserved for the prevention and treatment of malaria caused by drug-resistant *P. falciparum* and *P. vivax*. The drug is especially useful as a prophylactic agent for nonimmune travelers who stay for only brief periods in areas where these infections are endemic (Table 39–1). In areas where malaria is due to drug-resistant strains of *P. falciparum*, mefloquine is more effective when used in combination with an artemisinin compound.

TOXICITY AND SIDE EFFECTS

Mefloquine given orally usually is well tolerated, particularly at prophylaxis dosages. Vomiting occurs more frequently at treatment dosages. Dividing the dose improves tolerance. The full dose should be repeated if vomiting occurs within the first hour. Nausea, vomiting, dizziness, and neuropsychiatric side effects are increased at treatment dosages. CNS manifestations approach 0.5% and include seizures, confusion or decreased sensorium, acute psychosis, and vertigo. Such symptoms generally remit on drug discontinuation. At prophylactic doses, the risk of serious neuropsychiatric effects is ~0.01%. Milder toxicities (e.g., disturbed sleep, dysphoria, headache, GI disturbances, and dizziness) occur even at prophylactic dosages. Adverse effects usually appear after the first to third doses and often abate even with continued treatment. Cardiac abnormalities, hemolysis, and agranulocytosis are rare.

CONTRAINDICATIONS AND INTERACTIONS

At very high doses, mefloquine causes teratogenesis and developmental abnormalities in rodents. Mefloquine is approved for use during pregnancy by the CDC and after the first trimester by the World Health Organization (WHO). However, there have been studies suggesting an increased rate of fetal loss with mefloquine use, especially during the first trimester. The evidence for mefloquine's safety in pregnancy is not fully convincing, and alternatives should be sought. Pregnancy also should be avoided for 3 months after mefloquine use because of its prolonged $t_{1/2}$. The drug is contraindicated for patients with a history of seizures, severe neuropsychiatric disturbances, or adverse reactions to quinoline antimalarials. Although mefloquine can be taken safely 12 hours after a last dose of quinine, taking quinine shortly after mefloquine can be very hazardous because the latter is eliminated so slowly. Treatment with or after halofantrine or within 2 months of prior mefloquine administration is contraindicated. Mefloquine reportedly increases the risk of seizures in epileptic patients controlled by valproate *and may compromise adequate immunization by live typhoid vaccine. Caution is advised for use of mefloquine along with drugs that can perturb cardiac conduction. The WHO advises against mefloquine use for patients in occupations that require great dexterity, such as pilots.*

Primaquine

Primaquine, in contrast with other antimalarials, acts on tissue stages (exoerythrocytic) of plasmodia in the liver to prevent and cure relapsing malaria. The structure of primaquine is shown in Figure 39–3.

ANTIMALARIAL ACTIONS   Primaquine destroys primary and latent hepatic stages of *P. vivax* and *P. ovale* and thus has great clinical value for preventing relapses of *P. vivax* or *P. ovale* malaria. The drug will not treat ongoing attacks of malaria, even though it displays some activity against the erythrocytic stages. The 8-aminoquinolines exert a marked gametocidal effect against all four species of plasmodia that infect humans, especially *P. falciparum*. Some strains of *P. vivax* exhibit partial resistance to the action of primaquine, which makes it imperative that strict adherence to drug regimen be maintained.

MECHANISM OF ANTIMALARIAL ACTION   Little is known about the antimalarial action of the 8-aminoquinolines. Primaquine may be converted to electrophiles that act as oxidation–reduction mediators, which may be the toxic moiety.

ABSORPTION, FATE, AND EXCRETION   *Primaquine is only given orally. Absorption from the GI tract is nearly complete. After a single dose, the plasma concentration peaks within 3 hours and then falls with an elimination $t_{1/2}$ of 6 hours. The apparent volume of distribution is several times that of total-body water. Primaquine is metabolized rapidly; only a small fraction is excreted as the parent drug. The major metabolite in human plasma is 8-(3-carboxyl-1-methylpropylamino)-6-methoxyquinoline, which is eliminated more slowly and accumulates with multiple doses.*

THERAPEUTIC USES   Primaquine is used primarily for the terminal prophylaxis and radical cure of *P. vivax* and *P. ovale* (relapsing) malarias because of its high activity against their latent tissue forms. The compound is given together with a blood schizontocide, usually chloroquine, to eradicate erythrocytic stages of these plasmodia and reduce the possibility of emerging drug resistance. For terminal prophylaxis, primaquine regimens are initiated shortly before or immediately after leaving an endemic area (Table 39–1). Radical cure of *P. vivax* or *P. ovale* malaria can be achieved if the drug is given either during the long-term latent period of infection or during an acute attack. Studies also have shown efficacy in prevention of *P. falciparum* and *P. vivax* malaria when primaquine is taken prophylactically. The drug generally is well tolerated when taken for up to 1 year.

TOXICITY AND SIDE EFFECTS

Primaquine is fairly innocuous when given to most Caucasians in the usual therapeutic doses. Primaquine can cause mild-to-moderate abdominal distress, which can be alleviated by taking the drug with food. Mild anemia, cyanosis (methemoglobinemia), and leukocytosis are less common. High doses (60–240 mg/day) accentuate the abdominal symptoms and cause methemoglobinemia in most subjects. Methemoglobinemia can be severe in individuals with congenital deficiency of nicotinamide adenine dinucleotide (NADH) methemoglobin reductase. Chloroquine and dapsone may be synergistic with primaquine in producing methemoglobinemia in these patients. Granulocytopenia and agranulocytosis are rare complications of therapy and usually are associated with overdosage. Also rare are hypertension, arrhythmias, and symptoms referable to the CNS.

Therapeutic or higher doses of primaquine may cause hemolytic anemia in humans with G6PD deficiency. This condition affects >200 million people worldwide. About 11% of African Americans have a G6PD variant that makes them vulnerable to hemolysis caused by oxidant drugs such as primaquine. Erythrocyte sensitivity to primaquine can be more severe in Sardinians, Sephardic Jews, Greeks, and Iranians. Because primaquine sensitivity is X-linked, hemolysis is of intermediate severity in heterozygous females who have two red cell populations, one normal and the other deficient in G6PD.

PRECAUTIONS AND CONTRAINDICATIONS

Patients should be tested for G6PD deficiency before they receive primaquine. Primaquine has been used cautiously in African American subjects with G6PD deficiency, although benefits of treatment may not necessarily outweigh the risks, but should not be used in patients with more severe deficiency. The CDC recommends use only when a normal G6PD level has been documented. If a daily dose >30 mg of primaquine base (>15 mg in possibly sensitive patients) is given, repeated blood counts and at least gross examination of the urine for hemoglobin should be undertaken. Primaquine should not be used in pregnant women and can be used only in lactating mothers whose infants have a normal G6PD level.

Primaquine is contraindicated in acutely ill patients with diseases that predispose to granulocytopenia (e.g., rheumatoid arthritis and systemic lupus erythematosus). Primaquine should not be given to patients receiving other potentially hemolytic drugs or agents capable of depressing the myelopoiesis.

SULFONAMIDES AND SULFONES

The sulfonamides and sulfones have antimalarial activity. The sulfonamides are used together with pyrimethamine and often in addition to quinine to treat chloroquine-resistant *P. falciparum* malaria, especially in parts of Africa. The sulfonamides and sulfones are slow-acting blood schizontocides that are more active against *P. falciparum* than *P. vivax*. The sulfonamides are used together with inhibitors of parasite dihydrofolate reductase to enhance their antiplasmodial action. The synergistic "antifolate" combination of sulfadoxine, a long-acting sulfonamide, with pyrimethamine (FANSIDAR) is used to treat malarial attacks. The sulfone dapsone given with the biguanide chlorproguanil also has been effective for therapy of chloroquine-resistant *P. falciparum* malaria.

TETRACYCLINES

The tetracyclines are slow-acting blood schizontocides that are used for short-term prophylaxis in areas with chloroquine and mefloquine resistance. Tetracyclines are particularly useful for the treatment of the acute malarial attack owing to multidrug-resistant strains of *P. falciparum* that also show partial resistance to quinine. Their relative slowness of action makes them ineffective as single agents for malaria treatment. *Tetracycline* or *doxycycline* usually is recommended. Tetracyclines have marked activity against primary tissue schizonts of chloroquine-resistant *P. falciparum*. Doxycycline is used by travelers for short-term prophylaxis of multidrug-resistant strains. Regimens for tetracycline and doxycycline are listed in Tables 39–1 and 39–2. Because of their adverse effects on bones and teeth, tetracyclines should not be given to pregnant women or children <8 years of age. Photosensitivity reactions or drug-induced superinfections may mandate their discontinuation.

PRINCIPLES AND GUIDELINES FOR PROPHYLAXIS AND CHEMOTHERAPY OF MALARIA

Pharmacological control of malaria poses a difficult challenge because *P. falciparum*, which causes nearly all the deaths from human malaria, has become progressively more resistant to available antimalarial drugs. Fortunately, chloroquine still is effective against malarias caused by *P. ovale*, *P. malariae*, most strains of *P. vivax*, and chloroquine-sensitive strains of *P. falciparum* found in some geographic areas. However, chloroquine-resistant strains of *P. falciparum* now prevail in most endemic areas. Extensive geographic overlap also exists between chloroquine resistance and resistance to pyrimethamine–sulfadoxine, a combination of antifolate drugs used widely for the treatment of *P. falciparum* malaria. Multidrug-resistant *P. falciparum* malaria, especially prevalent and severe in Southeast Asia and Oceania, now is well established in many areas. These infections may not respond adequately even to mefloquine or quinine.

Isolates of P. falciparum *from patients in highly endemic areas contain many parasite clones with different drug-resistance phenotypes. A patient with severe malaria may have 10^{12} parasites, so it is easy to understand how mutations conferring resistance can arise in virtually every patient and double mutations can arise occasionally. Therefore, drugs or drug combinations must not be susceptible to single-point-mutation resistance. Intense chloroquine use for decades preceded development of resistance to this agent, likely because multiple mutations are necessary to confer resistance. Resistance also can be promoted by free radicals generated by atovaquone treatment in the mitochondria of the parasite; this is thought to promote development of resistance to this drug. Drugs with a long $t_{1/2}$ are more likely to select out resistant parasites. On a population level, the fitness of resistant parasites is an important parameter—if mutation causes a reduced ability to survive or grow, the parasites are less likely to spread. In the case of antifolates, treatment actually induces gametocytogenesis, which promotes propagation and may explain the sweep of resistance alleles across Africa. These considerations strongly suggest using regimens with two or more agents to treat drug-resistant* P. falciparum *malaria; such regimens include artemisinin combination treatment and proguanil together with atovaquone. Recommendations for the prophylaxis and therapy of malaria in nonimmune individuals are shown in Tables 39–1 and 39–2. These should serve only as general guidelines. Importantly, drugs should not replace simple, inexpensive measures for malaria prevention. Individuals visiting malarious areas should take appropriate steps to prevent mosquito bites.*

A number of regimens are available for malaria chemoprophylaxis. Dosing should be started before exposure, ideally before the traveler leaves home, to establish therapeutic blood levels and to detect early signs of intolerance so that the regimen can be modified before departure. The duration of postexposure dosing is dictated by the spectrum of drug action (Figure 39–2). In those few areas where chloroquine-sensitive strains of *P. falciparum* are found, chloroquine still is suitable for prophylaxis. It remains the drug of choice for prophylaxis and control of infections due to *P. vivax*, *P. ovale*, and *P. malariae*. In areas where chloroquine-resistant malaria is endemic, mefloquine and atovaquone–proguanil are preferred for prophylaxis. There is more experience with mefloquine and more evidence for its efficacy against *P. vivax* but also more contraindications and perhaps more toxicity. Doxycycline is an alternative chemoprophylactic agent. In cases where mefloquine, atovaquone–proguanil, and doxycycline all are contraindicated, primaquine is a possibility for prophylaxis. Primaquine, like atovaquone–proguanil, is active against liver stages and can be discontinued shortly after leaving the endemic area. Attempts at radical cure of *P. vivax* malaria with primaquine should be delayed until the patient leaves an endemic area.

A malarial attack is a medical emergency, especially for nonimmune travelers, pregnant women, and young children. Treatment with a rapidly acting blood schizontocide must be instituted promptly if *P. falciparum* malaria is suspected from travel history and clinical findings. One should not wait for a definitive parasitological diagnosis because the clinical status may deteriorate rapidly. Moreover, the clinical presentation may be atypical, and thick blood smears may fail to reveal plasmodia in early stages of this infection. Chloroquine is the drug of choice for *P. vivax*, *P. ovale*, *P. malariae*, and chloroquine-sensitive strains of *P. falciparum*. Oral administration is used whenever possible, but chloroquine can be given intramuscularly or even intravenously with suitable precautions, although quinine and quinidine usually are the parenteral drugs of choice. Within 48–72 hours of initiating therapy, patients should show marked clinical improvement and a substantial decrease in parasitemia. Lack of such a response or failure to clear parasites from the blood by 7 days is indicative of drug resistance. If chloroquine-resistant *P. falciparum* malaria is suspected, either from the travel history or from lack of response to chloroquine, the preferred treatment is quinine. For multidrug-resistant *P. falciparum* malaria, quinine is given together with other effective but slower-acting blood schizontocides such as antifolates or tetracyclines (Table 39–2). Again, the oral route is preferred, but intravenous preparations should be given until oral medication can be taken. For parenteral therapy in the U.S., quinidine gluconate must be substituted for quinine dihydrochloride. Exchange transfusion may be of value in severe *P. falciparum* malaria.

Malarial attacks may recur during or after a course of chemotherapy, even in the absence of reinfection. Recurrent attacks by P. vivax, P. ovale, or P. malariae usually are well controlled by another course of chloroquine combined with or followed by a course of primaquine in the case of P. vivax or P. ovale. Some patients with P. vivax infection may require more than one course of primaquine for cure. Recrudescence of P. falciparum malarial attacks or parasitemia after appropriate treatment with chloroquine usually denotes infection with chloroquine-resistant plasmodia. Quinine together with a slower-acting drug such as doxycycline in Southeast Asia or with antifolate antimalarials (e.g., pyrimethamine–sulfadoxine) in Africa has been successful (Table 39–2). However, the 7-day course of treatment that often is required, the toxic doses of quinine needed to overcome increasingly drug-resistant parasites, and poor patient compliance compromise the utility of these regimens. Mefloquine is a good alternative to quinine in geographical areas where resistance is lacking but cannot be given parenterally. Moreover, toxic doses of mefloquine may be needed to eradicate parasites that exhibit cross-resistance to quinine. Especially promising compounds for treatment of multidrug-resistant P. falciparum malaria are the artemisinin compounds. As the most rapidly acting and potent blood schizontocides, these drugs markedly reduce parasite burden in a single life cycle and, when used to initiate therapy, make ideal partners for other drugs such as quinolines or antifolates. Parasite resistance has not yet been seen, probably because of their rapid action and very short half-lives. Success against multidrug-resistant P. falciparum malaria also has been achieved with atovaquone–proguanil. This combination is relatively expensive, and treatment failure owing to resistance already is being reported.

Malarial infection, especially with *P. falciparum*, is a severe threat to children and pregnant women. With appropriate adjustments and safety precautions, the treatment of children generally is the same as for adults. Tetracyclines should not be given except in an emergency to children <8 years of age, and atovaquone–proguanil has been approved only for children weighing >11 kg. Pregnant women should be urged to avoid endemic areas if possible. While chloroquine and proguanil may be used during pregnancy, safety documentation is incomplete. Antifolates, tetracyclines, the artemisinins, atovaquone, and primaquine should be avoided. Quinine and quinidine can be used with appropriate caution given to the frequently accompanying hypoglycemia. Mefloquine can be used if necessary, but safety data are not quite reassuring.

In lactating mothers, atovaquone–proguanil is not recommended. Also, the infant must be shown to have a normal G6PD level before using primaquine. For prophylaxis in long-term travelers, chloroquine is safe at the doses used, but may necessitate yearly retinal examinations. Mefloquine and doxycycline are well tolerated. Atovaquone–proguanil has been studied for up to 20 weeks but probably is acceptable for years based on experience with the individual components.

For a complete Bibliographical listing see Goodman & Gilman's *The Pharmacological Basis of Therapeutics*, 11th ed., or Goodman & Gilman Online at www.accessmedicine.com.

40

CHEMOTHERAPY OF PROTOZOAL INFECTIONS

Amebiasis, Giardiasis, Trichomoniasis, Trypanosomiasis, Leishmaniasis, and Other Protozoal Infections

INTRODUCTION TO HUMAN PROTOZOAL INFECTIONS

AMEBIASIS

Amebiasis affects ~10% of the world's population. In the U.S., amebiasis is usually seen in those living in crowded, unsanitary conditions. Entamoeba dispar *accounts for ~90% of human infections and* E. histolytica *for only 10%, but only* E. histolytica *causes human disease. Humans are the only known hosts for these protozoa, which are transmitted almost exclusively by the fecal–oral route.* E. histolytica *cysts ingested from contaminated food or water transform into trophozoites that reside in the large intestine. Many individuals infected with* E. histolytica *are asymptomatic but excrete infectious cysts, making them a source for further infections. In others,* E. histolytica *trophozoites invade the colonic mucosa with resulting colitis and bloody diarrhea (amebic dysentery). Rarely,* E. histolytica *trophozoites invade through the colonic mucosa and reach the liver* via *the portal circulation, where they establish an amebic liver abscess.*

Metronidazole or its analogs tinidazole *and* ornidazole *are the cornerstone of therapy. Metronidazole and tinidazole are the drugs of choice for amebic colitis, amebic liver abscess, and other extraintestinal form of amebiasis. Because metronidazole is so well absorbed in the gut, levels may not be therapeutic in the colonic lumen, and it is less effective against cysts. Patients with amebiasis (amebic colitis or amebic liver abscess) therefore also should receive a luminal agent to eradicate any residual trophozoites. Luminal agents are also used to treat asymptomatic individuals infected with* E. histolytica. *The nonabsorbed aminoglycoside* paromomycin *and the 8-hydroxyquinoline compound* iodoquinol *are effective luminal agents. Nitazoxanide (ALINIA), a drug approved in the U.S. for the treatment of cryptosporidiosis and giardiasis, is also active against* E. histolytica.

GIARDIASIS

Giardiasis, caused by Giardia intestinalis, *is the most commonly reported intestinal protozoal infection in the U.S. Infection results from ingestion of cysts in fecally contaminated water or food. Human-to-human transmission via the fecal–oral route is especially common among children in day-care centers and nurseries, institutionalized individuals, and male homosexuals.*

Infection with Giardia *results in an asymptomatic carrier state, acute self-limited diarrhea, or chronic diarrhea. Asymptomatic infection is most common; these individuals excrete* Giardia *cysts and are a source for new infections. Most adults with symptoms develop an acute self-limited illness, with watery, foul-smelling stools and abdominal distension. Some individuals develop a chronic diarrhea syndrome with malabsorption and weight loss.*

The diagnosis of giardiasis is made by identification of cysts or trophozoites in fecal specimens or of trophozoites in duodenal contents. Chemotherapy with a 5-day course of metronidazole usually is successful, although therapy may need to be repeated or prolonged. A single dose of tinidazole (TINDAMAX) probably is superior to metronidazole for giardiasis. Paromomycin has been used to treat pregnant women to avoid any possible mutagenic effects of the other drugs. Nitazoxanide and tinidazole are FDA-approved for the treatment of giardiasis in immune-competent adults and children >1 year of age.

TRICHOMONIASIS

Trichomoniasis is caused by Trichomonas vaginalis, *which inhabits the genitourinary tract and causes vaginitis in women and, uncommonly, urethritis in men. Trichomoniasis is sexually transmitted, with more than 200 million people infected worldwide and ~3 million women infected in the U.S. annually. The lack of symptoms in many men hinders effort to eradicate the disease.*

Only trophozoite *forms of* T. vaginalis *are found in infected secretions. Metronidazole is the drug of choice for trichomoniasis, but treatment failures owing to resistant organisms are increasing. Tinidazole has been used successfully at higher doses to treat metronidazole-resistant* T. vaginalis. *Nitazoxanide shows activity against* T. vaginalis *but is not approved for trichomoniasis.*

TOXOPLASMOSIS

Toxoplasmosis is caused by the obligate intracellular protozoan Toxoplasma gondii. *Although cats are the natural hosts, tissue cysts have been recovered from all mammalian species examined. Common routes of human infection are (1) ingestion of undercooked meat containing tissue cysts; (2) ingestion of vegetable matter contaminated with soil containing infective* oocysts; *(3) direct* oral contact with feces of cats shedding oocysts; and (4) transplacental fetal infection with tachyzoites from acutely infected mothers.

Primary infection with T. gondii produces clinical symptoms in ~10% of immunocompetent individuals. The acute illness is usually self-limiting and rarely requires treatment. It can cause serious disease in pregnant women, often leading to abortion. Immunocompromised individuals may develop toxoplasmic encephalitis from reactivation of tissue cysts deposited in the brain. Toxoplasmic encephalitis typically is seen in patients with AIDS and can be fatal. Clinical manifestations of congenital toxoplasmosis vary widely, but chorioretinitis is the most common finding. The primary treatment for toxoplasmic encephalitis is the antifolates pyrimethamine and sulfadiazine. Therapy must be discontinued in ~40% of cases because of toxicity, primarily of the sulfa drug; clindamycin can be substituted for sulfadiazine without loss of efficacy. Alternative regimens combining azithromycin, clarithromycin, atovaquone, or dapsone with either trimethoprim–sulfamethoxazole or pyrimethamine and folinic acid are less toxic but also less effective than the combination of pyrimethamine and sulfadiazine.

Spiramycin, which concentrates in placental tissue, is used to treat acute acquired toxoplasmosis in pregnancy to prevent transmission to the fetus. If fetal infection is detected, the combination of pyrimethamine and sulfadiazine is administered to the mother (only after the first 12–14 weeks of pregnancy) and to the newborn in the postnatal period.

CRYPTOSPORIDIOSIS

Cryptosporidia are protozoan parasites that cause diarrhea in many species, including humans. Cryptosporidium parvum and C. hominis account for almost all human infections. Infectious oocysts in feces may be spread either by direct human-to-human contact or by contaminated water supplies. Groups at risk include travelers, children in day-care facilities, male homosexuals, animal handlers, veterinarians, and other healthcare personnel. Immunocompromised individuals are especially vulnerable. After ingestion, the mature oocyte releases sporozoites that invade host epithelial cells, Infection usually is self-limited. In AIDS patients and other immunocompromised individuals, severe secretory diarrhea may require hospitalization and supportive therapy.

The most effective therapy for cryptosporidiosis in AIDS patients is immune restoration with highly active antiretroviral therapy (HAART). Nitazoxanide has shown activity in treating cryptosporidiosis in immunocompetent children and may also be effective in adults. Its efficacy in children and adults with AIDS is not clearly established; the lower the CD4 count, the less likely a patient is to respond. Nevertheless, nitazoxanide is the only drug approved for cryptosporidiosis in the U.S.

TRYPANOSOMIASIS

African trypanosomiasis, or "sleeping sickness," is caused by Trypanosoma brucei subspecies that are transmitted by tsetse flies. It causes serious human illness that is fatal unless treated. An estimated 300,000–500,000 Africans carry the infection, and over 60 million people are at risk. It is extremely rare in the U.S. The parasite is entirely extracellular, and early infection is characterized by the presence of replicating parasites in the bloodstream or lymph without central nervous system (CNS) involvement (stage 1). Manifestations of early stage disease include fever, lymphadenopathy, splenomegaly, and occasional myocarditis that result from systemic dissemination of the parasites. Stage 2 is characterized by CNS involvement. There are two types of African trypanosomiasis, the East African and West African, caused by T. brucei rhodesiense and T. brucei gambiense, respectively. T. brucei rhodesiense produces a progressive, rapidly fatal disease marked by early CNS involvement and frequent terminal cardiac failure; T. brucei gambiense causes illness that is characterized by later CNS involvement and a prolonged course that progresses to the classical symptoms of sleeping sickness over months to years. Neurological symptoms include confusion, poor coordination, sensory deficits, an array of psychiatric signs, and eventual progression to coma and death.

Standard therapy for early-stage disease is pentamidine for T. brucei gambiense and suramin for T. brucei rhodesiense. These agents are not effective against late-stage disease, and standard treatment of the CNS phase is melarsoprol. All three compounds must be given parenterally over long periods. Eflornithine offers the only alternative for the treatment of late-stage disease; it has marked efficacy against early and late stages of human T. brucei gambiense infection. It has significantly fewer side effects than melarsoprol but is expensive, difficult to administer, and ineffective as monotherapy for infections of T. brucei rhodesiense.

American trypanosomiasis, or Chagas' disease, is caused by Trypanosoma cruzi. It affects ~20 million people from Mexico to South America, where the chronic form of the disease is a major cause of cardiomyopathy, megaesophagus, megacolon, and death. Bloodsucking triatomid bugs most commonly transmit this infection to young children; transplacental transmission also may occur in endemic areas.

Reactivation also may occur in patients who are immunosuppressed after organ transplantation or because of other conditions (e.g., AIDS, leukemia, and other neoplasias). Occurrences of T. cruzi *infection in transplant patients or through blood transfusions have been reported in the* U.S. *Acute infection is evidenced by a raised tender skin nodule* (chagoma) *at the site of inoculation; other signs may range from fever, adenitis, skin rash, and hepatosplenomegaly to, rarely, acute myocarditis and death. Invading metacyclic* trypomastigotes *penetrate host cells, especially macrophages, where they proliferate as* amastigotes *and then differentiate into trypomastigotes that enter the bloodstream. After recovery from the acute infection, individuals usually remain asymptomatic for years despite sporadic parasitemia. An increasing fraction of adults develops overt cardiac and GI chronic disease as they age. Progressive destruction of myocardial cells and neurons of the myenteric plexus results from the tropism of* T. cruzi *for muscle cells. Two nitroheterocyclic drugs, nifurtimox and benznidazole, are used to treat this infection. Both agents suppress parasitemia and can cure the acute phase of Chagas' disease in 60–80% of cases. Current recommendations are that patients with either acute- or recent chronic-phase disease should be treated. For patients with late chronic-phase disease (>10 years), parasitological cure is less likely, and there is no consensus on management. Both drugs are toxic and must be taken for long periods. Isolates vary with respect to their susceptibility to nifurtimox and benznidazole. In the absence of new drugs, alternative measures such as improved vector control and housing accommodations have reduced the transmission of Chagas' disease substantially.*

LEISHMANIASIS

Leishmaniasis is caused by ~20 different species of protozoa of the genus Leishmania. *Small mammals and canines serve as reservoirs for these pathogens, which can be transmitted to humans by the bites of female sandflies. Various forms of leishmaniasis affect people in southern Europe and many tropical and subtropical regions throughout the world. Flagellated extracellular free* promastigotes, *regurgitated by feeding flies, enter the host, where they are phagocytized by tissue macrophages and transform into* amastigotes, *which multiply within phagolysosomes until the cell bursts. Released amastigotes then propagate the infection by invading more macrophages. Amastigotes taken up by feeding sandflies transform back into promastigotes, thereby completing the life cycle. The particular localized or systemic disease syndrome caused by* Leishmania *depends on the species of infecting parasite, the distribution of infected macrophages, and especially the host's immune response. In increasing order of severity, human leishmaniasis has been classified into cutaneous, mucocutaneous, diffuse cutaneous, and visceral forms. Leishmaniasis increasingly occurs as an AIDS-associated infection.*

Cutaneous forms of leishmaniasis generally are self-limiting, with cures occurring within 3–18 months after infection, but can leave disfiguring scars. The mucocutaneous, diffuse cutaneous, and visceral forms of the disease do not resolve without therapy. Visceral leishmaniasis caused by L. donovani *is fatal unless treated. The classic therapy for all species of* Leishmania *is* pentavalent antimony, *but increasing resistance to this compound has been encountered. Liposomal* amphotericin B *is highly effective for visceral leishmaniasis, and is currently the drug of choice for antimony-resistant disease. Miltefosine, an orally active agent, shows considerable promise for the treatment of leishmaniasis. Paromomycin and pentamidine both have been used successfully as parenteral agents for visceral disease, although pentamidine's usefulness is limited by toxicity. Topical formulations of paromomycin, recently combined with* gentamicin, *also have been effective for cutaneous disease.*

OTHER PROTOZOAL INFECTIONS

Babesiosis *is a tick-borne zoonosis caused by parasites that invade erythrocytes, producing a febrile illness, hemolysis, and hemoglobinuria. Infection usually is self-limiting but can be severe or even fatal in asplenic or severely immunocompromised individuals. Standard therapy is a combination of* clindamycin *and* quinine, *but azithromycin plus atovaquone was as effective with fewer adverse effects.*

Microsporidia are unicellular eukaryotic fungal parasites that cause a number of disease syndromes, including diarrhea in immunocompromised individuals. Infections with microsporidia have been treated successfully with albendazole. *Immunocompromised individuals with intestinal microsporidiosis owing to E. bieneusi (which does not respond to albendazole) have been treated with* fumagillin.

AMPHOTERICIN

Liposomal amphotericin B (AMBISOME) *cures nearly 100% of cases of visceral leishmaniasis and has become the drug of choice for antimonial-resistant disease. Likely due to pharmacokinetic considerations, it is not useful against cutaneous or mucosal leishmaniasis. The recommended dose for the treatment of visceral leishmaniasis is 3 mg/kg/day intravenously for days 1–5, 14, and 21, with the dose being increased to 4 mg/kg and extended to days 1–5, 10, 17, 24, 31, and 38 for immunosuppressed patients. Shorter courses of the drug provide a lower-cost alternative. Cure rates are ~90% with either regimen.*

CHLOROQUINE

Chloroquine is directly toxic to E. histolytica *trophozoites and is highly concentrated within the liver, making it effective for amebic liver abscess. It is used only when metronidazole or another nitroimidazole is either contraindicated or unavailable. Chloroquine is not effective against intestinal amebiasis because it only attains low concentrations in the colon; patients receiving chloroquine for amebic liver abscess also should receive paromomycin or iodoquinol to eliminate intestinal colonization.*

The conventional course of treatment with chloroquine for extraintestinal amebiasis in adults is 1 g/day for 2 days, followed by 500 mg/day for at least 2–3 weeks. Because of its low toxicity, this dose can be increased or the schedule can be repeated if necessary.

EFLORNITHINE

Eflornithine (α-difluoromethylornithine, DFMO, ORNIDYL) *is an irreversible suicide inhibitor of ornithine decarboxylase, which catalyzes the rate-limiting step in the biosynthesis of polyamines. Polyamines are required for cell division and normal cell differentiation. In trypanosomes, spermidine also is required for the synthesis of trypanothione, a conjugate of spermidine and glutathione that replaces many functions of glutathione in the parasite. Eflornithine is used to treat trypanosomiasis caused by* T. brucei gambiense. *The drug usually is curative even for late CNS stages of infection resistant to arsenicals but is largely ineffective for East African trypanosomiasis. Its high cost, production shortages, and difficult treatment regimen have limited use. Eflornithine is no longer available for systemic use in the U.S. but is available for treatment of Gambian trypanosomiasis by special request. The structure of eflornithine is:*

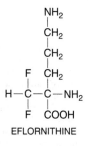

EFLORNITHINE

ANTITRYPANOSOMAL EFFECTS

Eflornithine inhibits ornithine decarboxylase; it irreversibly inhibits both mammalian and trypanosomal enzymes, thereby preventing the synthesis of polyamines needed for cell division. The parasite and human enzymes are equally susceptible to eflornithine, but the mammalian enzyme is turned over rapidly, whereas the parasite enzyme is stable. T. brucei rhodesiense *cells are less sensitive to eflornithine inhibition than* T. brucei gambiense *cells, and effective levels generally cannot be achieved clinically.*

ABSORPTION, FATE, AND EXCRETION

Eflornithine is given intravenously. Peak plasma levels are achieved ~4 hours after an oral dose, and the elimination $t_{1/2}$ averages 200 minutes. The drug does not bind to plasma proteins. It is well distributed and readily penetrates into the cerebrospinal fluid (CSF), which is especially important in late-stage West African trypanosomiasis. Over 80% of eflornithine is cleared by the kidney, largely in unchanged form.

THERAPEUTIC USES In patients with West African trypanosomiasis due to *T. brucei gambiense*, the preferred regimen for adult patients is 100 mg/kg given intravenously every 6 hours for 14 days as a 2-hour infusion. Response rates exceed 90% even in late-stage patients. A higher risk of treatment failure overall was found in patients who were stuporous on admission or were older. Children younger than 12 years of age required higher doses of eflornithine, probably because they clear the drug more rapidly such that the drug does not reach the CNS. To avoid early convulsions, a proposed regimen uses the current intravenous dosage (400 mg/kg/day) in the first few days, followed by an increase for the second part of therapy. Eflornithine and melarsoprol may act synergistically.

Eflornithine has been less successful for AIDS patients with West African trypanosomiasis, presumably because host defenses play a critical role in clearing drug-treated pathogen from the bloodstream. Eflornithine failed to improve treatment of East African trypanosomiasis owing to *T. brucei rhodesiense*, consistent with the relatively short $t_{1/2}$ and high activity of ornithine decarboxylase in these parasites.

TOXICITY AND SIDE EFFECTS Eflornithine causes adverse effects that are generally reversible on drug withdrawal. Anemia (48%), diarrhea (39%), and leukopenia (27%) are the most common complications in patients receiving intravenous drug. Diarrhea is both dose-related and dose-limiting, especially after oral administration. Convulsions occur early in ~7% of treated patients but do not recur despite continuation of therapy. Other complications—such as thrombocytopenia, alopecia, vomiting, abdominal pain, dizziness, fever, anorexia, and headache—occur in <10% of treated patients. Reversible hearing loss can occur after prolonged therapy. Therapeutic doses of eflornithine require coadministration of substantial volumes of intravenous fluid, which poses practical limitations in remote settings and causes fluid overload in susceptible patients.

Fumagillin

Fumagillin (FUMIDIL B, others) is an acyclic polyene macrolide.

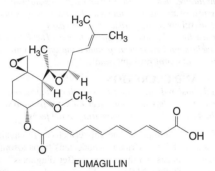

FUMAGILLIN

Fumagillin is toxic to microsporidia and also has some activity against E. histolytica. *Fumagillin is used topically to treat keratoconjunctivitis caused by* E. hellem *at a dose of 3–10 mg/mL in suspension. For intestinal microsporidiosis caused by* E. bieneusi, *fumagillin was used at a dose of 20 mg orally three times daily for 2 weeks. Adverse effects of fumagillin include abdominal cramps, nausea, vomiting, and diarrhea. Reversible thrombocytopenia and neutropenia also have been reported. Fumagillin is not approved for the systemic treatment of microsporidia infection in the U.S.*

8-Hydroxyquinolines

The halogenated 8-hydroxyquinolines iodoquinol *(diiodohydroxyquin) and* clioquinol *(iodochlorhydroxyquin) have been used to eliminate intestinal colonization with* E. histolytica. *Iodoquinol (YODOXIN) is safer and is available for oral use in the U.S. Adverse effects are unusual when used at appropriate doses (never to exceed 2 g/day) and duration of therapy (<20 days in adults). The use of these drugs, especially at doses >2 g/day, for long periods is associated with significant risk. The most important toxic reaction, ascribed primarily to clioquinol, is subacute myelo-optic neuropathy. Peripheral neuropathy is a milder manifestation of neurotoxicity. Administration of iodoquinol in high doses to children has been associated with optic atrophy and permanent loss of vision. Because of its superior safety, paromomycin is preferred as the luminal agent for amebiasis; however, iodoquinol is a reasonable alternative. Iodoquinol is used in combination with metronidazole to treat individuals with amebic colitis or amebic liver abscess but may be used as a single agent for asymptomatic individuals found to be infected with* E. histolytica. *For adults, the recommended dose of iodoquinol is 650 mg orally three times daily for 20 days, whereas children receive 10 mg/kg of body weight orally three times a day (not to exceed 2 g/day) for 20 days.*

MELARSOPROL

Melarsoprol (Mel B; ARSOBAL) is supplied as a 3.6% (w/v) solution in propylene glycol for intravenous administration. It is available in the U.S. only from the CDC.

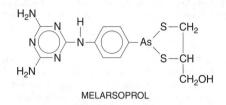

MELARSOPROL

ANTIPROTOZOAL EFFECTS   Melarsoprol is a prodrug that is metabolized rapidly ($t_{1/2}$ of 30 minutes) to melarsen oxide, the active form. Arsenoxides react avidly and reversibly with sulfhydryl groups and thereby inactivate many enzymes. Melarsoprol reacts with trypanothione to form melarsen oxide–trypanothione adduct, which potently inhibits trypanothione reductase. Both the sequestering of trypanothione and the inhibition of trypanothione reductase are expected to have lethal consequences to the cell, but this remains unproven.

The number of treatment failures has risen sharply and some resistant strains are tenfold less sensitive to the drug than sensitive strains. It is not clear that the lack of patient response to the drug correlates with reduced sensitivity of the parasite in most cases.

Melarsoprol resistance likely involves transport defects. The P2 adenine–adenosine transporter has activity on melarsoprol as well as pentamidine and berenil; point mutations in this transporter are found in melarsoprol-resistant isolates.

ABSORPTION, FATE, AND EXCRETION
Melarsoprol is always administered intravenously. A small but therapeutically significant amount of the drug enters the CSF and has a lethal effect on CNS trypanosomes. The compound is excreted rapidly, with 70–80% of the arsenic appearing in the feces.

THERAPEUTIC USES   Melarsoprol is the only effective drug available for treatment of the late meningoencephalitic stage of East African (Rhodesian) trypanosomiasis. Melarsoprol treatment of East African trypanosomiasis is initiated soon after diagnosis because CNS involvement occurs early in this aggressive infection. Melarsoprol is not used for prophylaxis because of its toxicity and rapid elimination.

The pattern of resistance to melarsoprol differs between the two subspecies of *T. brucei.* Patients infected with *T. brucei rhodesiense* who relapse after a course of melarsoprol usually respond to a second course of the drug. In contrast, patients infected with *T. brucei gambiense* who are not cured with melarsoprol rarely benefit from repeated treatment with this drug but often respond to eflornithine.

Melarsoprol is administered by slow intravenous injection, with care to avoid tissue extravasation. A typical course of treatment is three 3- to 4-day courses of 2–3.6 mg/kg with 7-day intervals between courses. Lesser doses should be given to children and debilitated patients. A continuous 10-day course of 2.2 mg/kg/day also is effective and will likely become standard. Unless contraindicated, glucocorticoids should be given to decrease the incidence of reactive encephalopathy.

TOXICITY AND SIDE EFFECTS   Toxicity is common during treatment with melarsoprol. A febrile reaction often occurs soon after drug injection, especially if parasitemia is high. Reactive encephalopathy occurs in ~5–10% of patients, leading to fatality in perhaps half of these. Encephalopathy, when it occurs, typically develops between the two courses of therapy. It is more common in East African than in West African trypanosomiasis and is more likely to develop in patients whose CSF contains many cells and trypanosomes. Manifestations include convulsions associated with acute cerebral edema, rapidly progressive coma, and acute mental disturbances; this likely represents a reaction to trypanosomal antigens. Coadministration of glucocorticoids reduces the frequency of reactive encephalopathy and also can help to control hypersensitivity reactions during the second or subsequent courses of therapy. Peripheral neuropathy, noted in ~10% of patients, probably is a direct toxic effect of the drug. Hypertension and myocardial damage are not uncommon, although shock is rare. Proteinuria occurs frequently, and evidence of renal or hepatic dysfunction may necessitate treatment modification. Vomiting and abdominal colic are reduced by injecting melarsoprol slowly into the supine, fasting patient.

PRECAUTIONS AND CONTRAINDICATIONS Melarsoprol should be given to patients only under hospital supervision. The initial dose must be based on clinical assessment rather than body weight. Initiation of therapy during a febrile episode is associated with an increased incidence of reactive encephalopathy. Administration of melarsoprol to leprous patients may precipitate erythema nodosum. The drug is contraindicated during epidemics of influenza. Severe hemolytic reactions have been reported in patients with glucose-6-phosphate dehydrogenase deficiency.

METRONIDAZOLE

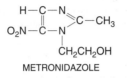

METRONIDAZOLE

ANTIPARASITIC AND ANTIMICROBIAL EFFECTS Metronidazole and related nitroimidazoles are active *in vitro* against a wide variety of anaerobic protozoal parasites and anaerobic bacteria. The drug also has potent amebicidal activity against *E. histolytica*.

Metronidazole has antibacterial activity against all anaerobic cocci and both anaerobic gram-negative bacilli, including *Bacteroides* spp., and anaerobic spore-forming gram-positive bacilli. Metronidazole is clinically effective in trichomoniasis, amebiasis, and giardiasis, and in a variety of infections caused by obligate anaerobic bacteria, including *Bacteroides, Clostridium,* and microaerophilic bacteria such as *Helicobacter* and *Campylobacter* spp.

MECHANISM OF ACTION AND RESISTANCE

Metronidazole is a prodrug that is activated by reduction of the nitro group by susceptible organisms. Unlike their aerobic counterparts, anaerobic and microaerophilic pathogens such as T. vaginalis, E. histolytica, *and* G. lamblia *and anaerobic bacteria contain electron transport components that have a sufficiently negative redox potential to donate electrons to metronidazole. Electron transfer forms a highly reactive nitro radical anion that kills susceptible organisms by radical-mediated mechanisms that target DNA. Metronidazole is catalytically recycled; loss of the active metabolite's electron regenerates the parent compound. Increasing levels of O_2 inhibit metronidazole-induced cytotoxicity because O_2 competes with metronidazole for electrons generated by energy metabolism. Thus, O_2 can both decrease reductive activation of metronidazole and increase recycling of activated drug. In susceptible organisms, pyruvate decarboxylation, catalyzed by pyruvate:ferredoxin oxidoreductase (PFOR), produces electrons that reduce ferredoxin, which then catalytically donates electrons to biological electron acceptors or to metronidazole.*

Clinical resistance to metronidazole is well documented for T. vaginalis, G. lamblia, *and a variety of anaerobic and microaerophilic bacteria. Resistance correlates with impaired oxygen-scavenging capabilities, leading to higher local O_2 concentrations, decreased metronidazole activation, and futile recycling of the activated drug. Other resistant strains have lowered but detectable levels of PFOR and ferredoxin, perhaps explaining why they may still respond to higher levels of drug. In the case of* Bacteroides *spp., metronidazole resistance is linked to a family of nitroimidazole (nim) resistance genes that can be encoded chromosomally or episomally. These nim genes encode nitroimidazole reductases capable of converting a 5-nitroimidazole to a 5-aminoimidazole, thus blocking formation of the reactive nitroso group responsible for microbial killing.*

ABSORPTION, FATE, AND EXCRETION

Metronidazole is supplied for oral, intravenous, intravaginal, and topical administration. It usually is absorbed completely after oral intake. A linear relationship between dose and plasma concentration pertains for doses of 200–2000 mg. Repeated doses every 6–8 hours result in some drug accumulation. The $t_{1/2}$ of metronidazole in plasma is ~8 hours, and its volume of distribution is approximately that of total-body water. Less than 20% of the drug is bound to plasma proteins. With the exception of the placenta, metronidazole penetrates well into body tissues and fluids, including vaginal secretions, seminal fluid, saliva, and breast milk. Therapeutic concentrations also are achieved in CSF.

After an oral dose, >75% of labeled metronidazole is eliminated in the urine largely as metabolites; only ~10% is recovered as unchanged drug. The liver accounts for >50% of the systemic clearance of metronidazole. Two principal metabolites result from side-chain oxidation: a hydroxy derivative and an acid. The hydroxy metabolite has a longer $t_{1/2}$ (~12 hours) and contains nearly 50% of the antitrichomonal activity of metronidazole. Glucuronidation also is observed. Small amounts of reduced metabolites, including ring-cleavage products, are formed by gut flora. The urine of some patients may be reddish brown due to pigments derived from the drug. Oxidative metabolism of metronidazole is induced by phenobarbital, prednisone, rifampin, *and possibly* ethanol *and is inhibited by* cimetidine.

THERAPEUTIC USES Metronidazole cures genital infections with *T. vaginalis* in >90% of cases. The preferred regimen is 2 g metronidazole as a single oral dose for both males and females. For patients who cannot tolerate a single 2-g dose, an alternative is a 250-mg dose given three times daily or a 375-mg dose given twice daily for 7 days. When repeated courses or higher doses of the drug are required for uncured or recurrent infections, it is recommended that intervals of 4–6 weeks elapse between courses. In such cases, leukocyte counts should be carried out before, during, and after each course of treatment.

Treatment failures owing to metronidazole-resistant strains of T. vaginalis *are increasingly common. Most cases can be treated successfully by giving a second 2-g dose to both patient and sexual partner. In addition to oral therapy, the use of a topical gel containing 0.75% metronidazole or a 500- to 1000-mg vaginal suppository may be beneficial in refractory cases.*

Metronidazole is the agent of choice for all symptomatic forms of amebiasis, including colitis and liver abscess. The recommended dose is 500–750 mg metronidazole taken orally three times daily for 7–10 days. The daily dose for children is 35–50 mg/kg, given in three divided doses, for 7–10 days.

While standard recommendations are for 7–10 days' duration of therapy, amebic liver abscess has been treated successfully by short courses (2.4 g daily as a single oral dose for 2 days) of metronidazole or tinidazole. E. histolytica *persist in most patients who recover from acute amebiasis after metronidazole therapy, so it is recommended that all such individuals also be treated with a luminal amebicide.*

Metronidazole is not approved for treatment of giardiasis in the U.S., but favorable responses have been noted with doses similar to or lower than those used for trichomoniasis; the usual regimen is 250 mg given three times daily for 5 days for adults and 15 mg/kg given three times a day for 5 days for children. A daily dose of 2 g for 3 days also has been used successfully.

Metronidazole is used for the treatment of serious infections owing to susceptible anaerobic bacteria, including Bacteroides, Clostridium, Fusobacterium, Peptococcus, Peptostreptococcus, Eubacterium, *and* Helicobacter. *The drug is also given in combination with other antimicrobial agents to treat polymicrobial infections with aerobic and anaerobic bacteria. Metronidazole achieves clinically effective levels in bones, joints, and the CNS and can be given intravenously when oral administration is not possible. A loading dose of 15 mg/kg is followed 6 hours later by a maintenance dose of 7.5 mg/kg every 6 hours, usually for 7–10 days. Metronidazole is used as a component of prophylaxis of postoperative mixed bacterial infections and is used as a single agent to treat bacterial vaginosis.*

Metronidazole is used increasingly as primary therapy for pseudomembranous colitis due to Clostridium difficile *infection. At doses of 250–500 mg orally three times daily for 7–14 days, metronidazole is effective and less expensive than oral* vancomycin. *Metronidazole also is used in patients with Crohn's disease who have perianal fistulas or significant colonic disease (see Chapter 38).*

TOXICITY, CONTRAINDICATIONS, AND DRUG INTERACTIONS Side effects rarely are severe enough to discontinue therapy. The most common are headache, nausea, dry mouth, and a metallic taste. Vomiting, diarrhea, and abdominal distress are experienced occasionally. Neurotoxic side effects (*e.g.*, dizziness, vertigo, and very rarely, encephalopathy, convulsions, incoordination, and ataxia) mandate metronidazole discontinuation. The drug also should be withdrawn if numbness or paresthesias occur. Reversal of serious sensory neuropathies may be slow or incomplete. Urticaria, flushing, and pruritus are indications of drug sensitivity. Metronidazole rarely causes toxic epidermal necrolysis, which may be more common in individuals receiving high doses of metronidazole and concurrent therapy with *mebendazole*.

Dysuria, cystitis, and a sense of pelvic pressure have been reported. Metronidazole has a disulfiram-like effect, and some patients will experience abdominal distress, vomiting, flushing, or headache if they drink alcoholic beverages during or within 3 days of therapy. Metronidazole and *disulfiram* or any disulfiram-like drug should not be taken together because confusional and psychotic states may occur.

Metronidazole should be used with caution in patients with active CNS disease because of its potential neurotoxicity. The drug also may precipitate CNS signs of *lithium* toxicity in patients receiving this agent. Metronidazole can prolong the prothrombin time of patients receiving *coumadin* anticoagulants. The dosage of metronidazole should be reduced in patients with severe hepatic disease.

There are conflicting data about the teratogenicity of metronidazole in animals. While metronidazole has been taken during all stages of pregnancy with no apparent adverse effects, its use during the first trimester generally is not advised.

MILTEFOSINE

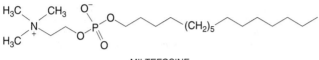

MILTEFOSINE

ANTIPROTOZOAL EFFECTS Miltefosine is the first orally available therapy for leishmaniasis. It is safe and effective treatment for visceral leishmaniasis and has also shown >95% efficacy against cutaneous leishmaniasis. In *Leishmania*, the drug may alter ether–lipid metabolism, cell signaling, or glycosylphosphatidylinositol anchor biosynthesis. Mutations in a P-type ATPase of the aminophospholipid translocase subfamily apparently decrease drug uptake and thereby confer resistance.

ABSORPTION, FATE, AND EXCRETION
Miltefosine is well absorbed orally and distributed throughout the body. Plasma concentrations are proportional to the dose.

THERAPEUTIC USES Oral miltefosine is registered in India for use in the treatment of visceral leishmaniasis in adults at a dose of 100 mg/kg daily (for patients weighing more than 25 kg) for 28 days. A similar dosing schedule has shown efficacy against cutaneous disease. Children should be given 2.5 mg/kg/day. The compound cannot be given intravenously because of hemolysis.

TOXICITY AND SIDE EFFECTS Vomiting and diarrhea have been reported in up to 60% of patients. Elevations in hepatic transaminases and serum creatinine also have been reported. These are typically mild and resolve quickly once the drug is withdrawn. The drug is contraindicated in pregnant women. Women should receive a negative pregnancy test prior to treatment, and birth control is required during and for at least 2 months after treatment.

NIFURTIMOX
ANTIPROTOZOAL EFFECTS Nifurtimox and benznidazole are trypanocidal against both the trypomastigote and amastigote forms of *T. cruzi*. Nifurtimox also has activity against *T. brucei* and can cure early- and late-stage disease.

The trypanocidal action of nifurtimox derives from its ability to undergo activation by partial reduction to nitro radical anions. Transfer of electrons from the activated drug then forms superoxide radical anions and other reactive oxygen species. Reaction of free radicals results in lipid peroxidation and membrane injury, enzyme inactivation, and DNA damage. Benznidazole also requires a one-electron transfer that generates nitro anion radicals, leading to cellular damage that kills the parasites.

ABSORPTION, FATE, AND EXCRETION
Nifurtimox is well absorbed after oral administration, with peak plasma levels observed after ~3.5 hours. Less than 0.5% of the dose is excreted in urine. The elimination $t_{1/2}$ is ~3 hours. High concentrations of several unidentified metabolites are found, and nifurtimox undergoes rapid biotransformation, probably via a presystemic first-pass effect. Whether the metabolites have any trypanocidal activity is unknown.

THERAPEUTIC USES
Nifurtimox and benznidazole are used to treat American trypanosomiasis (Chagas' disease) caused by T. cruzi. *Because of toxicity, benznidazole is preferred. Both drugs markedly reduce the parasitemia, morbidity, and mortality of acute Chagas' disease, producing parasitological cures*

in 80% of cases. In the chronic disease, parasitological cures are still possible in up to 50% of patients. Even without a complete parasitological cure, treatment also reduces clinical symptoms. Treatment with nifurtimox or benznidazole has no effect on irreversible organ lesions. While part of tissue destruction may be autoimmune in nature, the continued presence of parasites in the infected organs of patients with chronic disease argues that Chagas' disease should be treated as a parasitic disease. The clinical response of the acute illness to drug therapy varies with geographical region. Treatment of all seropositive individuals is recommended and should be initiated as soon as possible. Therapy with nifurtimox or benznidazole should start promptly after exposure for persons at risk of T. cruzi infection from laboratory accidents or blood transfusions.

Both drugs are given orally. For nifurtimox, adults with acute infection should receive 8–10 mg/kg/day in four divided doses for 90–120 days. Children 1–10 years of age with acute Chagas' disease should receive 15–20 mg/kg/day in four divided doses for 90 days; for individuals 11–16 years old, the daily dose is 12.5–15 mg/kg given according to the same schedule. For benznidazole, the recommended treatment is 5–7 mg/kg/day in two divided doses for 30–90 days, with children up to 12 years receiving 10 mg/kg/day. Gastric upset and weight loss can occur during treatment. If the latter occurs, dosage should be reduced. The ingestion of alcohol should be avoided.

TOXICITY AND SIDE EFFECTS   Drug-related side effects range from hypersensitivity reactions (*e.g.*, dermatitis, fever, icterus, pulmonary infiltrates, and anaphylaxis) to dose- and age-dependent complications of the GI tract and the peripheral and CNS. Nausea and vomiting, myalgia, and weakness are common. Peripheral neuropathy and GI symptoms are especially common after prolonged treatment. Headache, psychiatric disturbances, paresthesias, polyneuritis, and CNS excitability are less frequent. Leukopenia and decreased sperm counts also have been reported. Because of the seriousness of Chagas' disease and the lack of superior drugs, there are few absolute contraindications to the use of these drugs.

NITAZOXANIDE

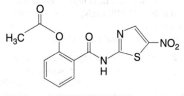

NITAZOXANIDE

ANTIMICROBIAL EFFECTS

Nitazoxanide and its active metabolite tizoxanide inhibit the growth of sporozoites and oocytes of C. parvum *and inhibit the growth of the trophozoites of* G. intestinalis, E. histolytica, *and* T. vaginalis *in vitro. Nitazoxanide also demonstrated activity against intestinal helminths.*

MECHANISM OF ACTION AND RESISTANCE

Nitazoxanide appears to interfere with the PFOR enzyme-dependent electron-transfer reaction, which is essential in anaerobic metabolism. No resistance to nitazoxanide in infectious agents previously known to be susceptible to the drug has yet been reported.

ABSORPTION, FATE, AND EXCRETION

Following oral administration, nitazoxanide is hydrolyzed rapidly to its active metabolite tizoxanide, which undergoes conjugation primarily to tizoxanide glucuronide. Bioavailability after an oral dose is excellent, and maximum plasma concentrations of metabolites are detected within 1–4 hours of administration of the parent compound. Tizoxanide is >99.9% bound to plasma proteins. Tizoxanide is excreted in the urine, bile, and feces, whereas tizoxanide glucuronide is excreted in urine and bile.

THERAPEUTIC USES   In the U.S., nitazoxanide (ALINIA) is available as an oral suspension and as tablets. It is approved for the treatment of *G. intestinalis* infections in adults and in children and for the treatment of diarrhea in children under 12 caused by cryptosporidia. The efficacy of nitazoxanide in children (or adults) with cryptosporidia infection and AIDS is not clearly established. For children between the ages of 12 and 47 months, the recommended dose is 100 mg every 12 hours for 3 days; for children between 4 and 11 years of age, the dose is 200 mg every 12 hours for 3 days. A 500-mg nitazoxanide tablet, suitable for adult dosing (every 12 hours), is not available in the U.S.

Nitazoxanide has been used as a single agent to treat mixed infections with intestinal parasites (protozoa and helminths). Effective parasite clearance after nitazoxanide treatment was shown for G. intestinalis, E. histolytica/E. dispar, B. hominis, C. parvum, C. cayetanensis, I. belli, H. nana, T. trichura, A. lumbricoides, *and* E. vermicularis, *although more than one course of therapy was sometimes required. Nitazoxanide has been used to treat infections with* G. intestinalis *that are resistant to metronidazole and albendazole.*

TOXICITY AND SIDE EFFECTS   Adverse effects are rare with nitazoxanide. A greenish tint to the urine is seen in most individuals taking nitazoxanide. Nitazoxanide is a category B agent for use in pregnancy based on animal studies, but there is no clinical experience with its use in pregnant women or nursing mothers.

PAROMOMYCIN

Paromomycin (aminosidine, HUMATIN) *is an aminoglycoside given orally to treat* E. histolytica, *cryptosporidiosis, and giardiasis. A topical formulation is used to treat trichomoniasis and cutaneous leishmaniasis, and parenteral administration has been used for visceral leishmaniasis.*

Paromomycin shares the same mechanism of action as other aminoglycosides and has the same spectrum of antibacterial activity and toxicity (see Chapter 45). Paromomycin is available only for oral use in the U.S. Following oral administration, 100% of the drug is recovered in the feces, even with compromised gut integrity.

Paromomycin is the drug of choice for intestinal colonization with E. histolytica *and is used in combination with metronidazole to treat amebic colitis and amebic liver abscess. Dosing for adults and children is 25–35 mg/kg/day orally in three divided doses. Adverse effects are rare, but include abdominal pain and cramping, epigastric pain, nausea and vomiting, steatorrhea, and diarrhea. Rarely, rash and headache have been reported. Paromomycin has been used to treat cryptosporidiosis in AIDS patients both as a single agent (oral doses of 500 mg three times daily or 1 g orally twice daily for 14–28 days followed by 500 mg orally twice daily) and in combination with azithromycin (paromomycin 1 g orally twice daily plus azithromycin 600 mg orally once daily for 4 weeks, followed by paromomycin alone for 8 weeks). Paromomycin has been advocated as a treatment for giardiasis in pregnant women, especially during the first trimester when metronidazole is contraindicated, and as an alternative agent for metronidazole-resistant isolates of* G. intestinalis. *Response rates of 55–90% have been reported. Dosing in adults is 500 mg orally three times daily for 10 days, whereas children have been treated with 25–30 mg/kg/day in three divided oral doses. Paromomycin formulated as a 6.25% cream has been used to treat vaginal trichomoniasis in patients who failed or could not receive metronidazole therapy. Cures have been reported, but vulvovaginal ulcerations and pain have complicated treatment.*

Paromomycin as a topical formulation containing 15% paromomycin in combination with either a patented base or 12% methylbenzonium chloride *has shown variable efficacy for the treatment of cutaneous leishmaniasis. Paromomycin has been administered parenterally (doses of 16–18 mg/kg/day) alone or in combination with antimony to treat visceral leishmaniasis. In one study, cure rates of 89% with paromomycin alone were reported, and cure rates of 94% were seen with combination therapy. These results compared favorably with those with antimony alone in areas where antimony resistance is common.*

PENTAMIDINE

Pentamidine is a positively charged aromatic diamidine:

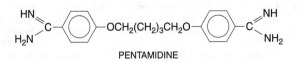

PENTAMIDINE

*Pentamidine isethionate is marketed for injection (*PENTAM 300) *or for use as an aerosol (*NEBU-PENT). *One milligram of pentamidine base is equivalent to 1.74 mg of the pentamidine isethionate. The isethionate salt is highly water soluble. Solutions should be used promptly because pentamidine is unstable in solution.*

ANTIPROTOZOAL EFFECTS   The diamidines are effective for the treatment of *T. brucei gambiense* sleeping sickness but not *T. brucei rhodesiense* or *T. cruzi* infections. They also are useful for treating antimony-resistant leishmania.

MECHANISM OF ACTION AND RESISTANCE

The diamidines display multiple effects on any given parasite and act by disparate mechanisms in different parasites. In T. brucei, *for example, the diamidines are concentrated* via *an energy-dependent uptake system to millimolar concentrations that are essential for efficacy. The best-characterized diamidine transporter is a purine (P2) adenine and adenosine transporter that also is used by the melamine-based arsenicals, which explains the cross-resistance to diamidines exhibited by certain arsenical-resistant strains of* T. brucei. *Multiple transporters mediate pentamidine uptake, which may account for the fact that little resistance to this drug is observed despite years of prophylactic use. The diamidines may exert their trypanocidal effects by reacting with a variety of negatively charged intracellular targets such as membrane phospholipids, enzymes, RNA, and DNA. In* Leishmania, *pentamidine accumulates within mitochondria and causes early disintegration of the kinetoplast and collapse of the mitochondrial membrane potential. Moreover, pentamidine resistance is linked to decreased drug concentration within mitochondria, again implicating this organelle in drug action.*

ABSORPTION, FATE, AND EXCRETION

The pharmacokinetics and biodisposition of pentamidine isethionate have been studied most extensively in AIDS patients with P. jiroveci *infections. Pentamidine isethionate is fairly well absorbed from parenteral sites of administration. Following a single intravenous dose, the drug disappears from plasma with an apparent $t_{1/2}$ of several minutes to a few hours and maximum plasma concentrations after intramuscular injection occur at 1 hour. The drug is highly protein bound and has an elimination $t_{1/2}$ of weeks to months. This highly charged compound does not cross the blood–brain barrier, explaining why it is ineffective against late-stage trypanosomiasis.*

Inhalation of pentamidine aerosols is used for prophylaxis of Pneumocystis pneumonia; *delivery of drug by this route results in little systemic absorption and decreased toxicity compared with intravenous administration in both adults and children.*

THERAPEUTIC USES   For sleeping sickness, pentamidine isethionate usually is given by intramuscular injection in single daily doses of 4 mg/kg/day for a series of 7 days. Because of failure to penetrate the CNS, pentamidine is ineffective against late stage disease and appears to have reduced efficacy against *T. brucei rhodesiense*. Thus, pentamidine is limited to use in early stage *T. brucei gambiense* infections.

Pentamidine has been used successfully in courses of 12–15 intramuscular doses of 2–4 mg/kg either daily or every other day to treat visceral leishmaniasis. It provides an alternative to antimonials or lipid formulations of amphotericin B for patients who cannot tolerate these agents.

Pentamidine is one of several drugs used to treat or prevent Pneumocystis *infection. Pneumocystis pneumonia (PCP) is a major cause of mortality in individuals with AIDS and can occur in patients who are immunosuppressed by other mechanisms. Trimethoprim–sulfamethoxazole is the drug of choice for the treatment and prevention of PCP (see Chapter 43). Pentamidine given intravenously as a 4 mg/kg single daily dose for 21 days is used to treat severe PCP in individuals who cannot tolerate trimethoprim–sulfamethoxazole and are not candidates for alternative agents such as atovaquone or the combination of clindamycin and* primaquine. *Pentamidine has been recommended as a "salvage" agent for individuals with PCP who failed to respond to initial therapy (usually trimethoprim–sulfamethoxazole) but may be less effective than the combination of clindamycin and primaquine or atovaquone for this indication. Pentamidine administered as an aerosol preparation is used to prevent PCP in at-risk individuals who cannot tolerate trimethoprim–sulfamethoxazole and are not deemed candidates for either dapsone (alone or in combination with pyrimethamine) or atovaquone. Candidates for PCP prophylaxis are individuals with HIV infection and a CD4 count of <200 per mm^3 and individuals with HIV infection and persistent unexplained fever or oropharyngeal candidiasis. Secondary prophylaxis is recommended after any documented PCP episode. For prophylaxis, pentamidine isethionate is given monthly as a 300-mg dose in a 5–10% nebulized solution over 30–45 minutes. Although convenient, aerosolized pentamidine has several disadvantages, including its failure to treat any extrapulmonary sites of* Pneumocystis, *the lack of efficacy against any other potential opportunistic pathogens, and a slightly increased risk for pneumothorax. For individuals who receive HAART and achieve CD4 counts persistently >200 per mm^3 for 3 months, primary or secondary PCP prophylaxis can be stopped.*

TOXICITY AND SIDE EFFECTS   Approximately 50% of individuals given pentamidine at recommended doses will show some adverse effect. Intravenous administration may be associated with hypotension, tachycardia, and headache, probably secondary to the ability of pentamidine to bind imidazoline receptors, which can be ameliorated by slowing the infusion rate. Hypoglycemia, which can be life threatening, may occur at any time during pentamidine treatment. Careful monitoring of blood glucose is the key. Paradoxically, pancreatitis, hyperglycemia, and insulin-dependent diabetes also may occur. Pentamidine is nephrotoxic (~25% of treated patients will show signs of renal dysfunction), and if the serum creatinine concentration rises significantly, it may be necessary to withhold the drug temporarily or change to an alternative agent. Individuals developing pentamidine-induced renal dysfunction are at higher risk for hypoglycemia. Other adverse effects include rashes, thrombophlebitis, anemia, neutropenia, and elevated hepatic enzymes. Intramuscular administration of pentamidine can cause sterile abscesses at the injection site, and most authorities prefer intravenous administration. Aerosolized pentamidine has few adverse events.

SODIUM STIBOGLUCONATE

Sodium stibogluconate *(sodium antimony gluconate, PENTOSTAM) is a pentavalent antimonial that has been a mainstay for the treatment of leishmaniasis. In the U.S., sodium stibogluconate is no longer available. Increasing resistance to antimonials has reduced their efficacy, and both lipid-based amphotericin and miltefosine are increasinglyly used.*

The relatively nontoxic pentavalent antimonials are prodrugs that are reduced to the more toxic Sb^{3+} species within the phagolysosomes of macrophages. Following reduction, the drug interferes with the trypanothione redox system, inducing a rapid efflux of trypanothione and glutathione from the cells, and inhibiting trypanothione reductase to deplete the thiol reduction potential.

Most of a single dose of sodium stibogluconate is excreted in the urine within 24 hours. The agent is absorbed rapidly, distributed in an apparent volume of ~0.22 L/kg, and eliminated in two phases. The first has a short $t_{1/2}$ of ~2 hours, and the second is much slower. The prolonged terminal elimination phase ($t_{1/2} = 33$–76 hours) may reflect conversion of the pentavalent antimonial (Sb^{5+}) to the more toxic trivalent (Sb^{3+}) form that is slowly released from tissues.

Sodium stibogluconate is given parenterally. The standard course is 20 mg/kg/day for 20 days for cutaneous disease and for 28 days for visceral disease. Increased resistance has compromised the effectiveness of these drugs, and treatment failure rates of up to 60% have been observed in India. Amphotericin B is the recommended alternative for treatment of either visceral leishmaniasis in India or mucosal leishmaniasis in general, although the newly approved orally active compound miltefosine is likely to see much wider use.

Children usually tolerate the drug well, and the dose per kilogram is the same as for adults. Patients who respond favorably show clinical improvement within 1–2 weeks of initiation of therapy. The drug may be given on alternate days or for longer intervals if unfavorable reactions occur in especially debilitated individuals. Patients infected with HIV typically relapse after successful initial therapy with either pentavalent antimonials or amphotericin B.

Adverse effects noted most commonly include pain at the injection site; chemical pancreatitis in nearly all patients; elevation of serum hepatic transaminases; bone marrow suppression manifested by decreased red cell, white cell, and platelet counts in the blood; muscle and joint pain; weakness and malaise; headache; nausea and abdominal pain; and rashes. Reversible polyneuropathy has been reported. Hemolytic anemia and renal damage are rare manifestations of toxicity, as are shock and sudden death.

SURAMIN

Suramin (BAYER 205) is used primarily for treatment of African trypanosomiasis.

Suramin is a relatively slowly acting trypanocide (>6 hours *in vitro*) with high clinical activity against both *T. brucei gambiense* and *T. brucei rhodesiense*. Selective toxicity likely results from the ability of the parasite to take up the drug by receptor-mediated endocytosis of the protein-bound drug, especially low-density lipoproteins. Suramin inhibits many trypanosomal and mammalian enzymes and receptors unrelated to its antiparasitic effects. The synergism between eflornithine and suramin has led to speculation that it may inhibit polyamine biosynthesis. Suramin is the only microfilaricide used clinically, albeit rarely now, for the treatment of human onchocerciasis.

Suramin is given intravenously. The drug is highly protein bound and has a terminal elimination $t_{1/2}$ of ~90 days. Renal clearance accounts for elimination of ~80% of the compound. Very little suramin penetrates the CSF, consistent with its lack of efficacy once the CNS has been invaded by trypanosomes.

Suramin is the first-line therapy for early-stage *T. brucei rhodesiense* infection but generally is not used for early-stage *T. brucei gambiense*. Because only small amounts of the drug enter the brain, suramin is used primarily to treat early stages (before CNS involvement) of African trypanosomiasis.

For therapy of early West African infections, this drug is more effective when given by intravenous regimens that also include intramuscular injections of pentamidine. In contrast, suramin alone is superior for therapy of early East African disease. Suramin will clear the hemolymphatic system of trypanosomes even in late-stage disease, so it is often administered before initiating melarsoprol to reduce the risk of reactive encephalopathy associated with arsenical administration (*see* above). For adults with *T. brucei rhodesiense*, a test dose of 200 mg is given initially to detect sensitivity, after which the normal 1 g dose is given on days 1, 3, 7, 14, and 21. The pediatric dose is 20 mg/kg, given on the same schedule. Debilitated patients should be treated with lower doses during the first week. A serious immediate reaction consisting of nausea, vomiting, shock, and loss of consciousness occurs rarely. Malaise, nausea, and fatigue are more common immediate reactions. Parasite destruction may cause febrile episodes and rash; concomitant onchocerciasis optimally should be treated first with ivermectin to minimize these reactions (*see* Chapter 41). The most common problems encountered after several doses of suramin are renal toxicity and delayed neurological complications, including headache and peripheral neuropathy; these usually disappear despite continued therapy. The drug should be employed with great caution in individuals with renal insufficiency or if significant proteinuria develops.

For a complete Bibliographical listing see Goodman & Gilman's *The Pharmacological Basis of Therapeutics*, 11th ed., or Goodman & Gilman Online at www.accessmedicine.com.

41

CHEMOTHERAPY OF HELMINTH INFECTIONS

Infections with helminths, or parasitic worms, affect more than two billion people worldwide. Pathogenic worms are classified into roundworms (nematodes) and two types of flatworms, flukes (trematodes) and tapeworms (cestodes). Immature forms invade humans *via* the skin or gastrointestinal (GI) tract and mature into adult worms with characteristic tissue distributions. With few exceptions, such as *Strongyloides* and *Echinococcus*, they cannot complete their life cycle and replicate themselves within the human host.

Anthelmintics are drugs that act locally to expel worms from the GI tract or systemically to eradicate adult helminths or developmental forms that invade organs and tissues. Because metazoan parasites generally are long-lived and have relatively complex life cycles, acquired resistance to anthelmintics in humans is not a major factor limiting clinical efficacy. The extensive use of anthelmintics in veterinary medicine ensures that the potential of drug resistance among helminths in humans cannot be discounted.

TREATMENT OF HELMINTH INFECTIONS
Nematodes (Roundworms)

The major nematode parasites of humans include the soil-transmitted helminths (STHs) and the filarial nematodes. The STH infections, which include ascariasis, trichuriasis, and hookworm infection, are among the most prevalent infections in developing countries. Eradication programs use schools to administer broad-spectrum anthelmintics on a periodic and frequent basis. The most widely used agents for reducing morbidity are the benzimidazole anthelmintics (BZAs), either *albendazole* (ALBENZA and ZENTEL) or *mebendazole* (VERMOX) (*see* Table 41–1).

In addition to targeting STH infections among school-aged children, there is an ongoing attempt to employ anthelmintics that eliminate lymphatic filariasis (LF) and onchocerciasis (river blindness). The goal is to interrupt arthropod-borne transmission by administering combination therapy with either *diethylcarbamazine* and albendazole (in LF-endemic regions such as India and Egypt), or *ivermectin* and albendazole (in LF regions where onchocerciasis and/or loiasis are co-endemic). These drugs target the microfilarial stages of the parasite, which circulate in blood and are taken up by arthropod vectors where further parasite development occurs.

ASCARIS LUMBRICOIDES *AND* TOXOCARA CANIS

A. lumbricoides, *known as the "roundworm," affects up to 90% of persons in some tropical regions but also is seen in temperate climates.*

Mebendazole, albendazole, and pyrantel pamoate *(ANTIMINTH, others) are preferred drugs; all infected persons should be treated. Mebendazole and albendazole are preferred for therapy of asymptomatic-to-moderate ascariasis. Both compounds should be used with caution to treat heavy* Ascaris *infections, alone or with hookworms. Rarely, hyperactive ascarids may migrate to cause complications such as appendicitis, biliary or intestinal obstruction, and intestinal perforation— sometimes requiring surgery. Pyrantel is safe for use in pregnancy, whereas BZAs should be avoided during the first trimester (see below).*

Toxocariasis is common in North America and Europe. Major syndromes caused by T. canis *infection are visceral larva migrans (VLM), ocular larva migrans (OLM), and covert toxocariasis (CT). Treatment of VLM is reserved for patients with severe, persistent, or progressive symptoms. Albendazole is the drug of choice. The role of anthelmintic drugs for OLM and CT is controversial and surgical management often is indicated, sometimes accompanied by glucocorticoids.*

HOOKWORM
Necator americanus, Ancylostoma duodenale

Hookworm species infect 740 million people. N americanus *is the predominant hookworm worldwide, whereas* A. duodenale *is focally endemic in Egypt, India, and China. Hookworm larvae live in the soil and penetrate exposed skin. After reaching the lungs, larvae migrate to the oral cavity and are swallowed. After attaching to the jejunal mucosa, the adult worms feed on host blood. There is a direct correlation between the hookworm burden and fecal blood loss. Unlike heavy* Ascaris *and* Trichuris *infections, which occur mostly in children, heavy hookworm infections also occur in adults.*

The major treatment goal is to remove blood-feeding adult hookworms from the intestines. Albendazole and mebendazole are preferred agents against both A. duodenale *and* N. americanus.

Table 41–1

Structure of the Benzimidazoles

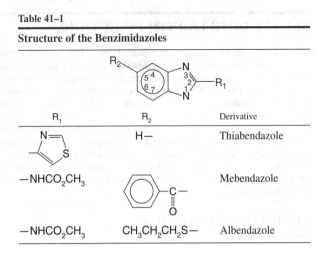

R₁	R₂	Derivative
(thiazole ring structure)	H—	Thiabendazole
—NHCO₂CH₃	(benzoyl structure)	Mebendazole
—NHCO₂CH₃	CH₃CH₂CH₂S—	Albendazole

As a single dose, albendazole is superior to mebendazole at removing adult hookworms from the GI tract. Oral albendazole is the drug of choice for treating cutaneous larva migrans *or "creeping eruption," due most often to skin migration by larvae of the dog hookworm.*

Strongyloides Stercoralis

S. stercoralis, *sometimes called the threadworm, can replicate and cause cycles of larval reinfection entirely within the human host. The organism infects more than 200 million people worldwide, most frequently in the tropics. In the U.S., strongyloidiasis is endemic in Appalachia and also is found in institutionalized individuals living in unsanitary conditions and in immigrants, travelers, and military personnel who lived in endemic areas. Infective larvae in contaminated soil penetrate the skin or mucous membranes, travel to the lungs, and ultimately mature into adult worms in the small intestine, where they reside. Most infected individuals are asymptomatic, while some experience rash and GI symptoms. Life-threatening disease due to massive larval hyperinfection can occur in immunosuppressed persons, even decades after the initial infection. Most deaths caused by parasites in the U.S. probably are due to* Strongyloides *hyperinfection. Ivermectin is the best drug for treating intestinal strongyloidiasis.*

Enterobius Vermicularis

Enterobius, *probably the most common helminth infections in temperate climates, typically causes pruritus in the perianal and perineal regions. Because the infection is easily spread, the clinician must decide whether to treat all close contacts and more than one course of therapy may be required.*

Pyrantel, mebendazole, and albendazole are highly effective. Single oral doses of each should be repeated after 2 weeks. When combined with fastidious personal hygiene, a high cure rate can be obtained.

Trichinella Spiralis

T. spiralis *infection results from eating insufficiently cooked flesh of infected animals, especially pigs. When released, encysted larvae mature into adult worms in the intestine, which then produce infectious larvae that invade tissues, especially skeletal muscle and heart. Severe infection cause marked muscle pain and cardiac complications.*

Albendazole and mebendazole appear to be effective against the intestinal forms of T. spiralis *that are present early in infection. Their efficacy on larvae that have migrated to muscle is questionable. Glucocorticoids are of considerable value in controlling the acute manifestations of infection.*

Wuchereria Bancrofti *and* Brugia Species (Lymphatic Filariasis)

Adult worms that cause human filariasis dwell either in the lymphatics or other tissues. Spread by the bites of infected mosquitoes, lymphatic filariasis (LF) affects ~120 million people in sub-Saharan Africa, India, Southeast Asia, the Pacific region, and tropical America. In LF, host reactions to adult worms initially cause lymphatic inflammation manifested by fever, lymphangitis, and lymphadenitis; this can progress to lymphatic obstruction. A reaction to microfilariae, tropical pulmonary eosinophilia, *may occur. In most countries, the World Health Organization (WHO) recommends yearly combined therapy with albendazole and diethylcarbamazine, which clears circulating microfilariae from infected subjects, thereby reducing the likelihood that mosquitoes will transmit LF to other individuals.*

Diethylcarbamazine is the drug of choice for the treatment of LF adult worms, but the effect is variable; best results are achieved if therapy is started before lymphatic obstruction has occurred.

Loa Loa (*Loiasis*)

L. loa is a tissue-migrating filarial parasite found in river regions of Central and West Africa. Adult worms in subcutaneous tissues typically cause episodic swellings and allergic reactions. Rarely, encephalopathy, cardiomyopathy, or nephropathy occurs. Diethylcarbamazine is the best single drug for the treatment of loiasis, initially in small initial doses to diminish host reactions that result from destruction of microfilariae. Glucocorticoids often are required to control acute reactions.

Onchocerca Volvulus (*Onchocerciasis or River Blindness*)

Transmitted by blackflies, O. volvulus *infects ~17 million people in sub-Saharan Africa, and <100,000 people in parts of Mexico, Guatemala, and South America. Inflammatory reactions, primarily to microfilariae rather than adult worms, affect the subcutaneous tissues, lymph nodes, and eyes. Onchocerciasis is a leading cause of infectious blindness worldwide. Ivermectin is the best single drug for control and treatment of onchocerciasis. It kills only microfilariae of* O. volvulus, *while producing few if any ocular complications.*

Cestodes (Flatworms)

Taenia Saginata

Humans are the definitive hosts for T. saginata, *the beef tapeworm. This most common tapeworm usually is detected after passage of proglottids from the intestine. It is cosmopolitan, occurring most commonly in sub-Saharan Africa and the Middle East, where undercooked beef is consumed.* Praziquantel *is the drug of choice for* T. saginata *infection.*

Taenia Solium

T. solium, *or pork tapeworm, causes two types of infection. The intestinal form with adult tapeworms results from eating undercooked meat containing cysticerci. Invasive larval forms cause* Cysticercosis, *the more dangerous systemic infection. Invasion of the brain (neurocysticercosis) can result in epilepsy, meningitis, and increased intracranial pressure. Praziquantel is preferred for intestinal infections with* T. solium, *while albendazole is the drug of choice for cysticercosis. Chemotherapy is appropriate only when it is directed at live cysticerci causing pathology; pretreatment with glucocorticoids is advised.*

Diphyllobothrium Latum

D. latum, *the fish tapeworm, is acquired by eating inadequately cooked, infested fish. Most infected individuals are asymptomatic; frequent manifestations include abdominal symptoms and weight loss; megaloblastic anemia may occur due to vitamin B_{12} deficiency. Praziquantel eliminates the worm.*

Hymenolepis Nana

H. nana, *the dwarf tapeworm, is the most common tapeworm parasitizing humans. Infection is more prevalent in tropical than temperate climates and most common among institutionalized children, including those in the southern U.S. Cysticerci develop in the villi of the intestine and then regain access to the intestinal lumen where larvae mature into adults. Praziquantel is effective against* H. nana *infections; relatively high doses usually are required, and therapy may need to be repeated.*

Echinococcus *Species*

Humans are one of several intermediate hosts for larval forms of Echinococcus *species that cause "cystic" (*E. granulosus*) and "alveolar" (*E. multilocularis *and* E. vogeli*) hydatid disease. Parasite eggs from canine stools are a major source in associated livestock (e.g., sheep and goats).* E. granulosus *produces unilocular, slowly growing cysts, most often in liver and lung, and* E. multilocularis *creates multilocular invasive cysts in the same organs. Surgical removal of the cyst is the preferred treatment, but leakage may spread disease to other organs. Prolonged regimens of albendazole, either alone or combined with surgery, may be beneficial, but some patients are not cured despite multiple courses of therapy. Adjunct treatment with BZAs is the cornerstone of the interdisciplinary approach to controlling cystic echinococcosis.*

Trematodes (Flukes)

Schistosoma Haematobium, Schistosoma Mansoni, Schistosoma Japonicum

These are the main species of blood flukes that cause human schistosomiasis, which affects about 200 million people. Schistosomiasis is widely distributed over South America (S. mansoni), much of Africa and the Arabian Peninsula (S. mansoni and S. haematobium), and China and Southeast Asia (S. japonicum). Infected snails are intermediate hosts for freshwater transmission. Schistosomiasis primarily involves the liver, spleen, and GI tract (S. mansoni and S. japonicum) or the lower genitourinary tract (S. haematobium). Heavy infections with S. haematobium are associated with bladder carcinoma. Chronic infections can cause portosystemic shunting due to periportal fibrosis in the liver.

Praziquantel is the drug of choice for schistosomes. The artemisinin derivative artemether (see Chapter 39) targets the larval schistosomula stages of the parasite. Combined treatment of animals harboring juvenile and adult schistosome worms with artemether and praziquantel resulted in significantly higher worm burden reductions than either drug administered singly.

Paragonimus westermani *and Other* Paragonimus *Species*

Called lung flukes, a number of Paragonimus *species, of which P. westermani is the most common, are pathogenic for humans. Found in the Far East and on the African and South American continents, these parasites have two intermediate hosts: snails and crustaceans. Humans become infected by eating raw or undercooked crabs or crayfish. Disease is caused by reactions to adult worms. Although these flukes are rather refractory to praziquantel, the drug is effective when used clinically. Bithionol is considered a second-line agent. Triclabendazole also recently was shown to be efficacious.*

Clonorchis sinensis, Opisthorchis viverrini, Opisthorchis felineus

These closely related trematodes exist in the Far East (C. sinensis, "the Chinese liver fluke," and O. viverrini) and parts of Eastern Europe (O. felineus). Metacercariae released from poorly cooked infected fish mature into adult flukes that inhabit the human biliary system. Heavy infections can cause obstructive liver disease, inflammatory gallbladder pathology associated with cholangiocarcinoma, and obstructive pancreatitis. One-day therapy with praziquantel is highly effective.

ANTHELMINTIC DRUGS

Benzimidazoles (BZAs)

The BZAs have been developed as broad-spectrum anthelmintic agents. The most useful have modifications at the 2 and/or 5 positions of the benzimidazole ring system (Table 41–1). Thiabendazole, mebendazole, and albendazole have been used extensively for the treatment of human helminth infections.

Thiabendazole is active against a wide range of nematodes that infect the GI tract, but its clinical use has declined markedly because of its toxicity relative to other equally effective drugs. Mebendazole has supplanted thiabendazole for the treatment of intestinal roundworm infections. Albendazole is used primarily against a variety of intestinal and tissue nematodes but also against larval forms of certain cestodes. Albendazole is the drug of choice for cysticercosis and cystic hydatid disease. When used yearly in conjunction with either ivermectin or diethylcarbamazine, single doses of albendazole have shown considerable promise for global control of LF and other filarial infections.

ANTHELMINTIC ACTION

The BZAs inhibit microtubule polymerization by binding to β-tubulin. The selective toxicity of these agents likely results because the BZAs bind parasite β-tubulin with much higher affinity than they do the mammalian protein. Drug resistance in nematodes may involve expression of a mutated β-tubulin. There is no evidence of emerging resistance among human nematodes.

The BZAs are versatile anthelmintic agents, particularly against GI nematodes, where their action is not dictated by systemic drug concentration. Mebendazole and albendazole are highly effective in treating the major STH infections (ascariasis, enterobiasis, trichuriasis, and hookworm) as well as less common human nematode infections. These drugs are active against both larval and adult stages of nematodes, and they are ovicidal for Ascaris and Trichuris. Immobilization and death of susceptible GI parasites occur slowly, and their clearance from the GI tract may not be complete until several days after treatment.

Albendazole is more effective than mebendazole against strongyloidiasis, cystic hydatid disease caused by E. granulosus, and neurocysticercosis caused by larval forms of T. solium. The BZAs probably are active against the intestinal stages of T. spiralis, but likely do not affect the larval stages in tissues. Albendazole is highly effective against the migrating forms of dog and cat *hookworms that cause cutaneous larval migrans. Regimens in which albendazole with either ivermectin or diethylcarbamazine are given as single annual doses show great promise for the elimination of LF. Certain microsporidia that cause intestinal infections in human immunodeficiency virus (HIV)-infected individuals respond partially (*Enterocytozoon bieneusi*) or completely (*Enterocytozoon intestinalis and related species) to albendazole.*

ABSORPTION, FATE, AND EXCRETION Thiabendazole is absorbed rapidly after oral ingestion and reaches peak plasma concentrations after 1 hour. Most of the drug is excreted in the urine within 24 hours as 5-hydroxythiabendazole, conjugated either as the glucuronide or the sulfate. Tablet formulations of mebendazole are poorly and erratically absorbed, and plasma concentrations are low. The low systemic bioavailability (22%) of mebendazole results from a combination of poor absorption and rapid first-pass hepatic metabolism. Mebendazole is ~95% bound to plasma proteins and is extensively metabolized. The major metabolites have lower rates of clearance than does mebendazole and apparently are inactive. Conjugates of mebendazole and its metabolites have been found in bile, but little unchanged mebendazole appears in the urine.

Albendazole is variably absorbed after oral administration. A fatty meal enhances absorption. After a 400-mg oral dose, albendazole cannot be detected in plasma, because the drug is rapidly metabolized in the liver to its sulfoxide, which has potent anthelmintic activity. Both the (+) and (–) enantiomers of albendazole sulfoxide are formed; the (+) enantiomer reaches much higher peak plasma concentrations and is cleared much more slowly. Albendazole sulfoxide is ~70% bound to plasma proteins and has a variable plasma $t_{1/2}$ (~4–15 hours). It is well distributed into various tissues including hydatid cysts, probably explaining its greater efficacy for tissue-dwelling helminths. Formation of albendazole sulfoxide is catalyzed by both microsomal flavin monooxygenase and CYP isoforms in the liver. Albendazole metabolites are excreted mainly in the urine.

THERAPEUTIC USES Thiabendazole (MINTEZOL) generally has been replaced by newer agents. Mebendazole is highly effective against GI nematodes and is particularly valuable for mixed infections. Mebendazole always is taken orally, and the same dosage schedule applies to adults and children >2 years of age. For treatment of enterobiasis, a single 100-mg tablet is taken, repeated after 2 weeks. For control of ascariasis, trichuriasis, or hookworm infections, the recommended regimen is 100 mg of mebendazole taken in the morning and evening for 3 consecutive days (or a single 500-mg tablet administered once). If the patient is not cured 3 weeks after treatment, a second course should be given. The 3-day mebendazole regimen is more effective than single doses of either mebendazole (500 mg) or albendazole (400 mg).

Like mebendazole, albendazole provides safe and effective therapy against infections with GI nematodes, including mixed infections of *Ascaris*, *Trichuris*, and hookworms. For treatment of enterobiasis, ascariasis, trichuriasis, and hookworm, albendazole is taken as a single 400-mg dose by adults and children >2 years of age. In children between the ages of 12 and 24 months, the WHO recommends a reduced dose of 200 mg. Cure rates for light-to-moderate *Ascaris* infections typically are >97%, although heavy infections may require therapy for 2–3 days. A 400-mg dose of albendazole appears to be superior to a 500-mg dose of mebendazole for curing hookworm infections.

Albendazole is the drug of choice for cystic hydatid disease due to *E. granulosus*. While the drug provides only a modest cure rate when used alone, it produces superior results when used in conjunction with either surgery to remove cysts or aspiration/injection of cysts with protoscolicidal agents. A typical dosage regimen for adults is 400 mg given twice a day (for children 15 mg/kg/day with a maximum of 800 mg) for 1–6 months. While the best drug available, albendazole is only marginally effective for alveolar echinococcosis caused by *E. multilocularis*, and surgical intervention often is needed.

Albendazole also is the preferred treatment of neurocysticercosis caused by larval forms of *T. solium*. The recommended dose is 400 mg given twice a day for adults for 8–30 days, depending on the number, type, and location of the cysts. For children, the dose is 15 mg/kg/day (maximum 800 mg) in two doses for 8–30 days. The course can be repeated as necessary, as long as liver and bone marrow toxicities are monitored. To reduce inflammatory side effects, glucocorticoids are usually given for several days before initiating albendazole therapy. Such pretreatment also increases plasma levels of albendazole sulfoxide. Therapy with either albendazole or praziquantel should include consideration of anticonvulsant therapy, the possible development of complications of arachnoiditis, vasculitis, or cerebral edema, and the need for surgical intervention should obstructive hydrocephalus occur. Albendazole, 400 mg/day, also has shown efficacy for therapy of microsporidial intestinal infections in patients with AIDS.

Albendazole is combined with either diethylcarbamazine or ivermectin in programs directed toward controlling LF. By annual dosing with combination therapy for 4–6 years, the goal is to maintain the microfilaremia at such low levels that transmission cannot occur for a period that corresponds to the duration of fecundity of adult worms. Albendazole is given with diethylcarbamazine to control LF in most parts of the world. To avoid serious reactions to dying microfilariae, an albendazole/ivermectin combination is recommended in locations where filariasis coexists with either onchocerciasis or loiasis.

TOXICITY, SIDE EFFECTS, PRECAUTIONS, AND CONTRAINDICATIONS The BZAs generally have excellent safety profiles. Side effects, primarily mild GI symptoms, occur in ~1% of treated children.

The clinical utility of thiabendazole in adults is compromised by its toxicity, which has diminished its clinical use. Frequent side effects include GI upset, fatigue, drowsiness, and headache. Occasional fever, rash, erythema multiforme, hallucinations, and sensory disturbances have been reported. Angioedema, shock, tinnitus, convulsions, and intrahepatic cholestasis, and crystalluria are rare complications. Transient leukopenia has been noted. Thiabendazole is hepatotoxic and should be used with caution in patients with hepatic disease. The effects of thiabendazole in pregnant women have not been studied adequately, so it should be used in pregnancy only when the potential benefit justifies the risk.

Mebendazole does not routinely cause significant systemic toxicity, even in the presence of anemia and malnutrition. Transient symptoms of abdominal pain, distention, and diarrhea have occurred with massive infestation and expulsion of GI worms. Rare side effects in patients treated with high doses of mebendazole include allergic reactions, alopecia, reversible neutropenia, agranulocytosis, and oligospermia. Reversible elevation of serum transaminases may occur. Mebendazole may be associated with occipital seizures. It should not be used in patients who have experienced allergic reactions to the agent.

Albendazole also produces few side effects when used for short-term therapy of GI helminthiasis, even in patients with heavy worm burdens. Transient mild GI symptoms (epigastric pain, diarrhea, nausea, and vomiting) occur in ~1% of treated individuals. Dizziness and headache occur on occasion. In school-age mass treatments, the incidence of side effects with albendazole is very low. Allergic phenomena rarely occur and usually resolve after 48 hours.

Even in long-term therapy of cystic hydatid disease and neurocysticercosis, albendazole is well tolerated by most patients. The most common side effect is an increase in serum aminotransferases, which return to normal upon drug cessation; rarely jaundice or cholestasis may occur. Liver function tests should be monitored during protracted albendazole therapy, and the drug is not recommended for patients with cirrhosis. Especially if not pretreated with glucocorticoids, some patients with neurocysticercosis may experience serious neurological sequelae. Other side effects during extended therapy include GI pain, severe headaches, fever, fatigue, alopecia, leukopenia, and thrombocytopenia.

The BZAs display remarkably few interactions with other drugs. The most versatile member of this family, albendazole, probably induces its own metabolism, and plasma levels of its sulfoxide metabolites can be increased by coadministration of glucocorticoids and possibly praziquantel. Caution is advised when using high doses of albendazole together with general inhibitors of hepatic CYPs.

Use in Pregnancy Both albendazole and mebendazole are embryotoxic and teratogenic in rats. In postmarketing surveys of women who inadvertently consumed mebendazole during the first trimester, the incidence of spontaneous abortion and malformations did not exceed that of the general population; comparable studies with albendazole are not available. A review of the risk of congenital abnormalities from BZAs concluded that their use during pregnancy is not associated with an increased risk of major congenital defects; nonetheless, it is recommended that treatment should be avoided during the first trimester of pregnancy.

Use in Young Children The WHO concluded that the BZAs may be used to treat children past the first year who are at risk for adverse consequences caused by STHs; a reduced dose of albendazole (200 mg) is used in children between the ages of 12–24 months.

DIETHYLCARBAMAZINE Diethylcarbamazine is a first-line agent for control and treatment of lymphatic filariasis and for therapy of tropical pulmonary eosinophilia caused by *W. bancrofti* and *Brugia malayi*. Although partially effective against onchocerciasis and loiasis, it can cause serious reactions to affected microfilariae. For this reason, ivermectin has replaced diethylcarbamazine for onchocerciasis. Despite its toxicity, diethylcarbamazine remains the best drug available to treat loiasis.

Annual single doses of both diethylcarbamazine and albendazole show considerable promise for the control of lymphatic filariasis in regions where onchocerciasis and loiasis are not endemic.

Diethylcarbamazine (HETRAZAN) is formulated as the water-soluble citrate salt.

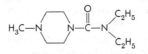

DIETHYLCARBAMAZINE

ANTHELMINTIC ACTION

Microfilarial forms of susceptible species are most affected by diethylcarbamazine, which elicits rapid disappearance from blood for W. bancrofti, B. malayi, and L. loa. The drug kills microfilariae of O. volvulus in skin but not in nodules that contain the adult (female) worms. It does not affect the microfilariae of W. bancrofti in a hydrocele. Diethylcarbamazine appears to exert a direct toxic effect on W. bancrofti microfilariae; it also kills worms of adult L. loa and probably adult W. bancrofti and B. malayi. Diethylcarbamazine may impair intracellular processing and transport of certain macromolecules to the helminth plasma membrane. The drug also may affect specific immune responses of the host.

ABSORPTION, FATE, AND EXCRETION   Diethylcarbamazine is absorbed rapidly from the GI tract. Peak plasma levels occur within 1–2 hours, and the plasma $t_{1/2}$ varies from 2 to 10 hours, depending on urinary pH. Metabolism is rapid and extensive. A major metabolite, diethylcarbamazine-N-oxide, is bioactive. Diethylcarbamazine is excreted by both urinary and extraurinary routes. Alkalinizing the urine can elevate plasma levels, prolong the plasma $t_{1/2}$, and increase both therapeutic effect and toxicity of diethylcarbamazine. Dosage reduction may be required in people with renal dysfunction or sustained alkaline urine.

THERAPEUTIC USES   Recommended regimens for filarial infections differ according to whether the drug is used for population-based chemotherapy, control of filarial disease, or prophylaxis against infection.

W. Bancrofti, B. Malayi, **and** *B. Timori*   The standard regimen for LF has been a 12-day, 72-mg/kg (6 mg/kg/day) course of diethylcarbamazine. A single dose of 6 mg/kg had comparable macrofilaricidal and microfilaricidal efficacy to previous regimens. Single-dose therapy may be repeated every 6–12 months, as necessary.

Although diethylcarbamazine does not usually reverse existing lymphatic damage, early treatment of asymptomatic individuals may prevent progression. Repeat treatment sometimes is recommended if microfilariae remain in the circulation or adult worms are seen on ultrasound. During acute episodes of lymphangitis, diethylcarbamazine is not recommended until acute symptoms subside. Supportive treatment is critical, including prevention of secondary bacterial infections by attention to hygiene, wearing shoes to prevent foot injury, and avoidance of lymphostasis by exercise and limb elevation.

For mass treatment programs, the introduction of diethylcarbamazine into table salt (0.2–0.4% by weight of the base) has markedly reduced the prevalence, severity, and transmission of lymphatic filariasis in many endemic areas. Diethylcarbamazine given annually as a single oral dose of 6 mg/kg is most effective in reducing microfilaremia when coadministered with either albendazole (400 mg) or ivermectin (0.2–0.4 mg/kg). Adverse reactions to microfilarial destruction usually are well tolerated. However, mass chemotherapy with diethylcarbamazine should not be used in regions where onchocerciasis or loiasis coexist because it may induce severe reactions related to parasite burden in these infections.

O. Volvulus **and** *L. Loa*   Diethylcarbamazine is contraindicated for onchocerciasis because it causes severe reactions related to microfilarial destruction, including worsening ocular lesions. For purposes of LF control, ivermectin is preferred in areas where onchocerciasis is endemic. Diethylcarbamazine remains the best drug for therapy of loiasis. Treatment is initiated with test doses of 50 mg (1 mg/kg in children) daily for 2–3 days, escalating as tolerated to daily doses of 9 mg/kg in three doses for a total of 2–3 weeks.

Low test doses are used, often with glucocorticoid or antihistamine pretreatment to minimize reactions to dying microfilariae and adult worms. Repeated courses of diethylcarbamazine treatment, separated by 3–4 weeks, may be required. Ivermectin is not a good alternative for treatment of loiasis, but albendazole may prove to be useful in patients who either fail therapy with diethyl-carbamazine or who cannot tolerate the drug.

TOXICITY AND SIDE EFFECTS At <8–10 mg/kg/day, direct toxic reactions to diethyl-carbamazine, including anorexia, nausea, headache, and vomiting, are rarely severe and usually disappear within a few days despite continued therapy. Major adverse effects result from host response to destruction of parasites, primarily microfilariae.

Reactions typically are most severe in patients heavily infected with O. volvulus, less serious in B. malayi or L. loa infections, and mild in bancroftian filariasis, but the drug occasionally induces retinal hemorrhages and severe encephalopathy in patients heavily infected with L. loa. In patients with onchocerciasis, reactions typically occur within a few hours after the first dose and include intense itching, tender lymphadenitis, and sometimes a papular rash, fever, tachycardia, arthralgias, and headache. This reaction persists for 3–7 days and then subsides, after which high doses sometimes can be tolerated. Ocular complications include limbitis, keratitis, uveitis, and atrophy of the retinal pigment epithelium. In patients with bancroftian or brugian filariasis, nodular swellings may occur along the course of the lymphatics, often with an accompanying lymphadenitis that also subsides within a few days. Almost all patients receiving therapy exhibit a leukocytosis Reversible proteinuria may occur, and the eosinophilia so frequently observed in patients with filariasis can be intensified by diethylcarbamazine. Delayed reactions include lymphangitis, swelling and lymphoid abscesses in bancroftian and brugian filariasis, and small skin wheals in loiasis. Diethylcarbamazine appears to be safe during pregnancy.

PRECAUTIONS AND CONTRAINDICATIONS Population-based therapy with diethylcarbamazine should be avoided in areas where onchocerciasis or loiasis is endemic, although the drug can be used to protect foreign travelers from these infections. Pretreatment with glucocorticoids and antihistamines often is given to minimize indirect reactions to diethylcarbamazine that result from dying microfilariae.

Ivermectin

The *avermectins* are a novel class of 16-membered lactones. Ivermectin (MECTIZAN; STROMECTOL; 22,23-dihydroavermectin B_{1a}) is FDA-approved for treatment of onchocerciasis and for therapy of intestinal strongyloidiasis. Ivermectin taken as a single oral dose every 6–12 months continues to serve as the mainstay of major programs to control onchocerciasis. In addition, annual oral doses of ivermectin, either taken alone or combined with annual oral doses of albendazole, markedly reduce microfilaremia in lymphatic filariasis due to W. bancrofti or B. malayi. Current recommendations advocate diethylcarbamazine (6 mg/kg) plus albendazole (400 mg). The two-drug regimen is preferred in regions where LF coexists with either onchocerciasis or loiasis. Ivermectin is the drug of choice against intestinal strongyloidiasis and is effective against several other human infections caused by intestinal nematodes.

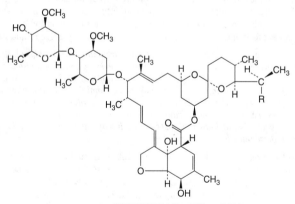

IVERMECTIN (R = CH_3 or C_2H_5)

ANTIPARASITIC ACTIVITY AND RESISTANCE

Ivermectin is effective and highly potent against at least some stages of many parasitic nematodes that affect animals and humans. Avermectins affect a group of glutamate-gated Cl^- channels found in nematode nerve or muscle cells, causing hyperpolarization and paralysis by increasing Cl^- permeability *of the cell membrane. Alterations in genes encoding P-glycoprotein transporters that bind avermectins and in those encoding components of the glutamate-gated Cl⁻ channel have been associated with the development of resistance. Avermectins also interact with γ-aminobutyric acid (GABA) receptors in mammalian brain, but their affinity for invertebrate receptors is ~100-fold higher.*

In humans infected with O. volvulus, ivermectin causes a rapid, marked decrease in microfilarial counts in the skin and ocular tissues that lasts for 6–12 months. The drug has little discernible effect on adult parasites, even at doses as high as 800 µg/kg, but affects developing larvae and blocks egress of microfilariae from the uterus of adult female worms. Regular treatment with ivermectin also may act prophylactically against the development of Onchocerca infection.

Ivermectin also is effective against microfilaria but not adult worms of W. bancrofti, B. malayi, L. loa, *and* M. ozzardi. *It exhibits excellent efficacy against* A. lumbricoides, S. stercoralis, *and cutaneous larva migrans.*

ABSORPTION, FATE, AND EXCRETION Peak plasma levels of ivermectin are achieved within 4–5 hours after oral administration. The long terminal $t_{1/2}$ of ~57 hours primarily reflects a low systemic clearance and a large apparent volume of distribution. Ivermectin is ~93% bound to plasma proteins. The drug is extensively converted by hepatic CYP3A4 to at least 10 metabolites, mostly hydroxylated and demethylated derivatives. Virtually no ivermectin appears in human urine in either unchanged or conjugated form. Highest tissue concentrations occur in liver and fat. Extremely low levels are found in brain; a P-glycoprotein efflux pump in the blood–brain barrier prevents ivermectin from entering the central nervous system (CNS).

THERAPEUTIC USES

Onchocerciasis Single oral doses of ivermectin (150 µg/kg) given every 6–12 months are considered effective, safe, and practical for reducing the number of circulating microfilariae in adults and children 5 years of age or older; widespread use of ivermectin is a mainstay of onchocerciasis control programs. Equally important, such therapy reverses lymphadenopathy and acute inflammatory changes in ocular tissues and arrests the progression of ocular pathology. Marked reduction of microfilariae in the skin and ocular tissues is noted within a few days and lasts for 6–12 months; the dose then should be repeated. Cure is not attained, because ivermectin has little effect on adult O. volvulus. Ivermectin has been widely used for onchocerciasis control programs in Africa, the Middle East, and Latin America.

Lymphatic Filariasis Single annual doses of ivermectin (400 µg/kg) are effective and safe for mass therapy of infections with W. bancrofti and B. malayi. Ivermectin is as effective as diethylcarbamazine for controlling lymphatic filariasis and can be used in regions where onchocerciasis, loiasis, or both are endemic. Although ivermectin as a single agent can reduce W. bancrofti microfilaremia, the duration of treatment required to eliminate LF presumably would be >6 years. A single dose of ivermectin (200 µg/kg) and a single dose of albendazole (400 mg) annually are even more effective in controlling lymphatic filariasis. The duration of treatment is for at least 5 years based on the estimated fecundity of the adult worms. This dual-drug regimen also reduces infections with intestinal nematodes.

Infections with Intestinal Nematodes The finding that a single dose of 150–200 µg/kg of ivermectin can cure strongyloidiasis is encouraging, because this drug also is effective against coexisting ascariasis, trichuriasis, and enterobiasis. A single dose of 100 µg/kg of ivermectin is as effective as traditional treatment of intestinal strongyloidiasis with thiabendazole, and less toxic. In Japan, almost all S. stercoralis–infected patients were cured by 200 µg/kg of ivermectin orally twice at an interval of 2 weeks. In *Strongyloides* hyperinfection syndrome, ivermectin has been used successfully, including cases unresponsive to thiabendazole.

Other Indications

Taken as a single 200-µg/kg oral dose, ivermectin is a first-line drug for treatment of cutaneous larva migrans. Similar doses also are safe and highly effective against human head lice and scabies, even in HIV-infected individuals.

Toxicity, Side Effects, and Precautions Ivermectin generally is well tolerated. In infected humans, ivermectin toxicity nearly always results from reactions to dying microfilariae; the intensity and nature of these reactions relate to the microfilarial burden and the duration and type of filarial infection.

After treatment of O. volvulus *infections with ivermectin, side effects usually are limited to pruritus and swollen, tender lymph nodes, these occur in 5–35% of people, last a few days, and are relieved by aspirin and antihistamines. Rarely, more severe reactions include high fever, tachycardia, hypotension, prostration, dizziness, headache, myalgia, arthralgia, diarrhea, and edema; these may respond to glucocorticoids. Ivermectin induces milder side effects than does diethylcarbamazine, and unlike the latter, seldom exacerbates ocular lesions in onchocerciasis. Serious side effects include marked disability and encephalopathies in patients coinfected with heavy burdens of* L. loa *microfilaria. Loa encephalopathy is associated with ivermectin treatment of individuals with high levels of* Loa *microfilaremia (≥30,000 microfilariae). There is little evidence that ivermectin is teratogenic or carcinogenic.*

Because of its effects on GABA receptors in the CNS, ivermectin is contraindicated in conditions associated with an impaired blood–brain barrier (*e.g.,* African trypanosomiasis and meningitis). Caution also is advised about coadministration of ivermectin with other CNS depressants, but epileptics should not be excluded from onchocerciasis treatment programs. Possible adverse interactions of ivermectin with other substrates for CYP3A4 have yet to be evaluated. Ivermectin is not approved for use in children <5 years old or in pregnant women, but both populations undoubtedly have been exposed to the drug in mass treatment programs. Lactating women taking the drug secrete low levels in their milk; the consequences for nursing infants are unknown.

Metrifonate

Metrifonate (trichlorfon; BILARCIL) *is an organophosphorus compound used as an insecticide and then as an anthelmintic, especially for* S. haematobium. *Metrifonate is a prodrug that is converted nonenzymatically to* dichlorvos *(2,2-dichlorovinyl dimethyl phosphate, DDVP), a potent cholinesterase inhibitor.*

Oxamniquine

*Oxamniquine (*VANSIL) *is a second-line drug to praziquantel for the treatment of schistosomiasis. Most strains of* S. mansoni *are highly susceptible to oxamniquine, but* S. haematobium *and* S. japonicum *are virtually unaffected by therapeutic doses. Because of a low incidence of mild side effects together with normally high efficacy after a single oral dose, oxamniquine continues to be used in* S. mansoni *control programs, especially in South America.*

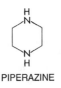

PIPERAZINE

Piperazine

A number of substituted piperazine derivatives have anthelmintic activity, but none apart from diethylcarbamazine has found a place in human therapeutics.
Piperazine is highly effective against A. lumbricoides *and* E. vermicularis. *The predominant effect of piperazine on* Ascaris *is a temporary paralysis that results in expulsion of the worm by peristalsis. Piperazine acts as a GABA-receptor agonist. By increasing Cl⁻ conductance of the* Ascaris *muscle membrane, the drug produces hyperpolarization that leads to flaccid paralysis.*

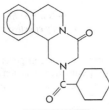

PRAZIQUANTEL

Praziquantel

Praziquantel (BILTRICIDE, DISTOCIDE) is a pyrazinoisoquinoline derivative. Infections with many different cestodes and trematodes respond favorably to this agent, whereas nematodes generally are unaffected. Praziquantel treatment of patients coinfected with schistosomes and hookworms reduces hookworm prevalence and infection intensities (egg counts) significantly.

ANTHELMINTIC ACTION

After rapid and reversible uptake, praziquantel has two major effects on adult schistosomes. At low concentrations, it causes increased muscular activity, followed by contraction and spastic paralysis. Affected worms detach from blood vessel walls, resulting in a rapid shift from the mesenteric veins to the liver. At slightly higher concentrations, praziquantel causes tegumental damage, which exposes a number of tegumental antigens. The tegument of schistosomes seems to be the primary site of action; the drug causes an influx of Ca^{2+} across the tegument via unknown mechanisms.

ABSORPTION, FATE, AND EXCRETION Praziquantel is readily absorbed after oral administration, and maximal levels in human plasma occur in 1–2 hours. Extensive first-pass metabolism to inactive hydroxylated and conjugated products limits drug bioavailability and results in plasma concentrations of metabolites at least 100-fold higher than that of praziquantel. The drug is ~80% bound to plasma proteins. Its plasma $t_{1/2}$ is 1–3 hours but may be prolonged in patients with severe liver disease, including those with hepatosplenic schistosomiasis. About 70% of an oral dose of praziquantel is recovered as metabolites in the urine within 24 hours; most of the remainder is metabolized in the liver and eliminated in the bile.

THERAPEUTIC USES Praziquantel is FDA approved for therapy of schistosomiasis and liver fluke infections, but also is used to treat infections with many other trematodes and cestodes. Praziquantel is the drug of choice for schistosomiasis caused by all *Schistosoma* species. Although dosage regimens vary, a single oral dose of 40 mg/kg or three doses of 20 mg/kg each, given 4–6 hours apart, generally produce cure rates of 70–95% and consistent reductions (>85%) in egg counts. Tablets of 600 mg are available.

Decreased clinical efficacy of praziquantel against infections with S. mansoni *has been reported. However, praziquantel-tolerant or -resistant schistosomes currently do not limit its clinical usefulness.*

Three doses of 25 mg/kg taken 4–8 hours apart on the same day yield high cure rates of infections with either the liver flukes C. sinensis *and O.* viverrini, *or the intestinal flukes Fasciolopsis buski, Heterophyes heterophyes, and Metagonimus yokogawai. The same three-dose regimen used for 2 days is highly effective against lung fluke infections. Infections with Fasciola hepatica are unresponsive to high doses, even though praziquantel penetrates this trematode. Low doses of praziquantel can be used successfully to treat intestinal infections with adult cestodes (e.g., a single oral dose of 25 mg/kg for H.* nana *and 10–20 mg/kg for D.* latum, T. *saginata, or T.* solium*). Retreatment after 7–10 days is advised for individuals heavily infected with H.* nana. *While albendazole is preferred for therapy of human cysticercosis, the tissue infection with intermediate cyst larvae of T.* solium, *prolonged high-dose therapy with praziquantel remains an alternative treatment. Neither the "cystic" nor "alveolar" hydatid diseases caused by larval stages of Echinococcus tapeworms respond to praziquantel; here, too, albendazole is effective.*

TOXICITY, PRECAUTIONS, AND INTERACTIONS Abdominal discomfort, nausea, diarrhea, headache, dizziness, and drowsiness may occur shortly after taking praziquantel; these direct effects are transient and dose-related. Indirect effects such as fever, pruritus, urticaria, rashes, arthralgia, and myalgia are noted occasionally and are related to parasite burden. In neurocysticercosis, inflammatory reactions to praziquantel may produce meningismus, seizures, mental changes, and CSF pleocytosis. These effects usually are delayed in onset, last 2–3 days, and respond to symptomatic therapy such as analgesics and anticonvulsants.

Praziquantel is considered safe in children >4 years of age, who probably tolerate the drug better than do adults. Low levels of the drug appear in breast milk. High doses of praziquantel increase abortion rates in rats, but one study showed that treatment of pregnant women resulted in no significant differences between treated and untreated women in the rates of abortion or preterm deliveries. No congenital abnormalities were noted by clinical examination in any of the babies born to either group.

Inducers of hepatic CYPs such as carbamazepine and phenobarbital reduce the bioavailability of praziquantel. Dexamethasone reduces the bioavailability of praziquantel, but the mechanism is not understood. Under certain conditions, praziquantel may increase the bioavailability of albendazole.

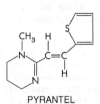

PYRANTEL

Praziquantel is contraindicated in ocular cysticercosis because the host response can irreversibly damage the eye. Tasks requiring mental alertness (*e.g.*, driving, operating machinery) should be avoided shortly after taking the drug. The $t_{1/2}$ of praziquantel can be prolonged in patients with severe hepatic disease, and dosage adjustment may be required.

Pyrantel Pamoate

Pyrantel is a broad-spectrum anthelmintic directed against pinworm, roundworm, and hookworm infections. Pyrantel is given as the pamoate salt and has the following structure:

Pyrantel is a depolarizing neuromuscular blocking agent that opens nonselective cation channels and induces marked, persistent activation of nicotinic acetylcholine receptors, which results in spastic paralysis of the worm. Pyrantel is effective against hookworm, pinworm, and roundworm; unlike its analog oxantel, it is ineffective against Trichuris trichiura.

Pyrantel pamoate is poorly absorbed from the GI tract, a property that contributes to its selective action on GI nematodes. Less than 15% is excreted in the urine as parent drug and metabolites. Most of an administered dose is recovered in the feces.

Pyrantel pamoate is an alternative to mebendazole in the treatment of ascariasis and enterobiasis. High cure rates have been achieved after a single oral dose of 11 mg/kg (maximum of 1 g). Pyrantel also is effective against hookworm infections caused by A. duodenale *and* N. americanus, *although repeated doses are needed to cure heavy infections with the latter organism. The drug is combined with oxantel for mixed infections with* T. trichiura. *For pinworm, treatment should be repeated after an interval of 2 weeks. In the U.S., pyrantel is sold over-the-counter for pinworm treatment (PIN-X).*

Transient and mild GI symptoms occasionally are observed, as are headache, dizziness, rash, and fever. Pyrantel pamoate use in pregnant patients and children <2 years of age is not recommended. Because pyrantel pamoate and piperazine are mutually antagonistic in their neuromuscular effects on parasites, they should not be used together.

For a complete Bibliographical listing see Goodman & Gilman's *The Pharmacological Basis of Therapeutics*, 11th ed., or Goodman & Gilman Online at www.accessmedicine.com.

CHEMOTHERAPY OF MICROBIAL DISEASES

42

GENERAL PRINCIPLES OF ANTIMICROBIAL THERAPY

Antimicrobial agents are among the most commonly used and misused of all drugs. The inevitable consequence of their widespread use has been the emergence of antibiotic-resistant pathogens, fueling an ever-increasing need for new drugs at a time when the pace of antimicrobial drug development has slowed dramatically. Reducing inappropriate antibiotic use is thought to be the best way to control resistance.

CLASSIFICATION AND MECHANISM OF ACTION Antimicrobial agents are classified based on proposed mechanism of action as follows: (1) agents that inhibit synthesis of bacterial cell walls, including the β-lactam class and other agents such as *vancomycin;* (2) agents that act directly on the cell membrane to increase permeability and cause leakage of intracellular compounds; (3) agents that disrupt function of ribosomal subunits to reversibly inhibit protein synthesis *(e.g., chloramphenicol,* the *tetracyclines, erythromycin,* and *clindamycin);* (4) agents that bind to the 30S ribosomal subunit and alter protein synthesis *(e.g.,* the *aminoglycosides);* (5) agents that affect bacterial nucleic acid metabolism by inhibiting RNA polymerase *(e.g., rifampin)* or topoisomerase *(e.g.,* the *quinolones);* (6) the antimetabolites, including *trimethoprim* and the *sulfonamides,* which block essential enzymes of folate metabolism. Classes of antiviral agents include: (1) nucleic acid analogs that selectively inhibit viral DNA polymerase or HIV reverse transcriptase; (2) nonnucleoside HIV reverse transcriptase inhibitors; (3) inhibitors of other essential viral enzymes; (4) fusion inhibitors.

FACTORS THAT DETERMINE THE SUSCEPTIBILITY AND RESISTANCE OF MICROORGANISMS TO ANTIMICROBIAL AGENTS Successful antimicrobial therapy of an infection ultimately depends on the concentration of the antibiotic at the site of infection, which must be sufficient to inhibit growth of the offending microorganisms. If host defenses are intact, agents that interfere with growth or replication of the microorganism but do not kill it (*i.e., bacteriostatic* agents) may suffice. If host defenses are impaired, antibiotic-mediated killing (*i.e.,* a *bactericidal* effect) may be required. The drug concentration at the site of infection must inhibit the organism but also must remain below the level that is toxic to human cells. If this can be achieved, the microorganism is considered sensitive; if not, the microorganism is considered resistant to the drug.

The achievable serum concentration for an antibiotic generally is used to guide decisions on sensitivity or resistance of a microorganism to that drug. However, the concentration at the infection site may be considerably lower than serum concentrations. Local factors (*e.g.,* low pH, high protein concentration, anaerobic conditions) also may impair drug activity.

The emergence of antibiotic resistance in bacterial pathogens is a serious development that threatens the end of the antibiotic era. More than 70% of the bacteria associated with hospital-acquired infections in the U.S. are resistant to one or more of the drugs previously used to treat them. This rampant spread of antibiotic resistance mandates a more responsible approach to antibiotic use. The Centers for Disease Control and Prevention (CDC) has outlined a series of steps to diminish antibiotic resistance, including appropriate use of vaccination, judicious and proper use of indwelling catheters, early involvement of infectious disease experts, antibiotic selection based on local patterns of susceptibility, proper antiseptic technique to ensure infection rather than contamination, appropriate use of prophylactic antibiotics in surgical procedures, infection control procedures to isolate the pathogen, and strict compliance to hand hygiene.

To be effective, an antibiotic must reach its target in an active form, bind to the target, and interfere with its function. Bacterial resistance to an antimicrobial agent is attributable to three general mechanisms: (1) the drug does not reach its target; (2) the drug is not active; or (3) the target is altered.

Failure of the drug to reach its target. The outer membrane of gram-negative bacteria is a barrier that excludes large polar molecules from entering the cell. Small polar molecules, including many antibiotics, enter the cell through protein channels called porins. Absence of, mutation in, or loss of a favored porin can slow drug entry into a cell or prevent entry altogether, effectively reducing drug concentration at its active site. If the target is intracellular and the drug requires active transport across the

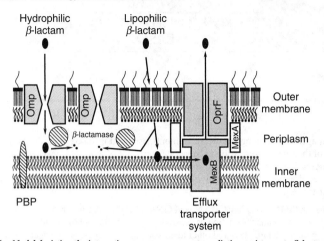

FIGURE 42–1 *Model depicting the interaction among components mediating resistance to β-lactam antibiotics in Pseudomonas aeruginosa. (Courtesy of Hiroshi Nikaido.)* Most β-lactam antibiotics are hydrophilic and must cross the outer membrane barrier of the cell *via* outer membrane protein (Omp) channels, or porins. The channel has size and charge selectivity such that some Omps slow or block transit of the drug. If an Omp permitting drug entry is altered by mutation, is missing, or is deleted, then drug entry is slowed or prevented. β-Lactamase concentrated between the inner and outer membranes in the periplasmic space constitutes an enzymatic barrier that works in concert with the porin permeability barrier. If the antibiotic is a good substrate for β-lactamase, it will be destroyed rapidly even if the outer membrane is relatively permeable to the drug. If the rate of drug entry is slow, then a relatively inefficient β-lactamase with a slow turnover rate can hydrolyze just enough drug that an effective concentration cannot be achieved. If the target (PBP, penicillin-binding protein) has low binding affinity for the drug or is altered, then the minimum concentration for inhibition is elevated, further contributing to resistance. Finally, β-lactam antibiotics (and other polar antibiotics) that enter the cell and avoid β-lactamase destruction can be taken up by an efflux transporter system (*e.g.*, MexA, MexB, and OprF) and pumped across the outer membrane, further reducing the intracellular concentration of active drug.

cell membrane, resistance can result from mutations that inhibit this transport mechanism. For example, gentamicin, which targets the ribosome, is actively transported across the cell membrane using energy provided by the membrane electrochemical gradient. This gradient is generated by respiratory enzymes that couple electron transport and oxidative phosphorylation. A mutation in this pathway or anaerobic conditions slows entry of gentamicin into the cell, resulting in resistance. Bacteria also have efflux pumps that can transport drugs out of cells. Resistance to numerous drugs (*e.g.*, tetracycline, chloramphenicol, fluroquinolones, macrolides, and β-lactam antibiotics) is mediated by an efflux pump mechanism. Figure 42–1 depicts the multiple membrane and periplasm components that reduce the intracellular concentrations of β-lactam antibiotics and cause resistance.

Drug inactivation. Bacterial resistance to aminoglycosides and β-lactam antibiotics usually results from production of enzymes that modify or destroy the antibiotic, respectively. A variation in this mechanism—the failure of bacteria to activate a prodrug—commonly underlies resistance of *Mycobacterium tuberculosis* to *isoniazid*.

Target alteration. This can include mutation of the natural target (*e.g.*, fluoroquinolone resistance), target modification (*e.g.*, ribosomal protection from macrolides and tetracyclines), or acquisition of a resistant form of the susceptible target (*e.g.*, staphylococcal resistance to methicillin caused by production of a low-affinity variant of penicillin-binding protein).

ACQUISITION OF DRUG RESISTANCE Drug resistance may be acquired by *mutation and selection*, with passage of the trait vertically to daughter cells, or by *horizontal transfer* of resistance determinants. For mutation and selection to generate resistance, the mutation cannot be lethal, should not appreciably impair virulence, and the cell carrying the mutation must disseminate and replicate. Resistance acquired by horizontal transfer of resistance determinants can disseminate rapidly either by clonal spread of the resistant strain or by subsequent transfers to other susceptible recipient strains. Horizontal transfer offers several advantages over mutation-selection. Lethal mutation of an essential gene is avoided; the level of resistance often is higher than that produced by mutation, which tends to yield incremental changes; the gene can be mobilized and rapidly amplified within a population by transfer to susceptible cells; and the resistance gene can be eliminated when no longer required.

Mutation-Selection. Mutation and antibiotic selection of the resistant mutant are the molecular basis for resistance to *streptomycin* (ribosomal mutation) quinolones (gyrase or topoisomerase IV mutations) rifampin (RNA polymerase mutation), and *linezolid* (ribosomal RNA mutation). This mechanism underlies all drug resistance in *M. tuberculosis*. The mutations are not caused by drug exposure *per se*, but are random events that confer a survival advantage when the drug is present. High-level resistance can either emerge from a sequential series of mutations that alter susceptibility incrementally (more commonly) or from a mutation that confers high-level resistance in a single step.

Horizontal Gene Transfer. Horizontal gene transfer of resistance genes is greatly facilitated by and is largely dependent on mobile genetic elements. Of these, plasmids play the most important role, with lesser importance of transposable elements, integrons, and gene cassettes. Other mechanisms may play important roles in the horizontal transfer of resistance in certain bacteria. Conjugation, the direct transfer of genes by cell-to-cell contact though a sex pilus or bridge, is an extremely important mechanism because multiple resistance genes can be transferred in a single event. Genetic transfer by conjugation is common among gram-negative bacilli and resistance is conferred on a susceptible cell in a single event. Enterococci and staphylococci are gram-positive bacteria that also transfer antibiotic resistance by conjugative transfer.

Selection of an Antimicrobial Agent

Optimal selection of antimicrobial agents requires clinical judgment and detailed knowledge of pharmacological and microbiological factors. Antibiotics have three general uses: empirical therapy, definitive therapy, and phophylactic therapy. When used as empirical therapy, the antibiotic(s) should cover all the likely pathogens, because the infecting organism has not been identified. Either combination therapy or, preferably, treatment with a single broad-spectrum agent may be employed. Once the infecting microorganism is identified, the course is completed with a narrow-spectrum, low-toxicity drug. Failures to identify the infecting microorganism and to narrow the antibiotic spectrum thereafter are common misuses of antibiotics.

The first consideration in selecting an antibiotic is whether it is even indicated. *The reflex action to associate fever with treatable infections and prescribe antimicrobial therapy without further evaluation is irrational and potentially dangerous.* The diagnosis may be masked if therapy is started before appropriate cultures are obtained. Antibiotics are potentially toxic, and may promote selection of resistant microorganisms. Of course, definitive identification of a bacterial infection before treatment is initiated often is not possible. In the absence of a clear indication, antibiotics often may be used if disease is severe and it seems likely that withholding therapy will result in failure to manage a serious or life-threatening infection.

Initiation of optimal empiric antibiotic therapy requires knowledge of the most likely infecting organisms and their antibiotic susceptibilities. Selection of an antibiotic regimen should rely on the clinical presentation, which may suggest a specific microorganism, and knowledge of the microorganisms most likely to cause a specific infection in a given host. In addition, simple and rapid laboratory tests may provide important clues to the possible infectious microorganism (*e.g.*, Gram's stain of infected secretion or body fluid), thereby permitting more rational selection of initial antibiotic therapy. In many situations, it is not possible to arrive at a specific bacteriological diagnosis, and the selection of a single narrow-spectrum antibiotic may be inappropriate, particularly if the infection is severe. Broad-spectrum antibiotic coverage is then indicated, pending isolation and identification of the microorganism. *Whenever the clinician is faced with initiating therapy on a presumptive bacteriological diagnosis, cultures of the presumed site of infection and blood should be taken prior to the institution of drug therapy.* For definitive therapy, the regimen should be changed to a more specific and narrow-spectrum antibiotic once an organism has been identified and its susceptibility is known.

TESTING FOR MICROBIAL SENSITIVITY TO ANTIMICROBIAL AGENTS Bacterial strains, even from the same species, may vary widely in sensitivity to antibiotics. Information about the antibiotic sensitivity of the infecting microorganism is important for appropriate drug selection. Various methods are used to assess susceptibility, including disk-diffusion, dilution test, and automated broth dilution. The results are either reported on a semi-quantitative scale (*i.e.*, resistant, intermediate, or susceptible) or in terms of the minimal inhibitory concentration (MIC).

PHARMACOKINETIC FACTORS *In vitro* activity, although critical, is only a guide to whether an antibiotic is likely to be effective, and successful therapy also depends on achieving a drug concentration sufficient to inhibit or kill bacteria at the site of infection without harming the host.

The location of the infection may dictate the choice of drug and the route of administration. The minimal drug concentration achieved at the infected site should be approximately equal to the MIC for the infecting organism, although it usually is advisable to achieve multiples of the MIC if possible. Even subinhibitory concentrations of antibiotics may be effective, perhaps by enhancing phagocytosis. Nonetheless, the aim of antibiotic therapy always should be to produce antibacterial concentrations of the drug at the site of the infection during the dosing interval.

Antibiotic access to sites of infection depends on multiple factors. If the infection is in the central nervous system (CNS), the drug must pass the blood–brain barrier. Antibiotics that are polar at physiological pH generally penetrate poorly; some, such as penicillin G, are actively transported out of the cerebrospinal fluid (CSF) by an anion transport mechanism in the choroid plexus. The concentrations of penicillins in the CSF usually are only 0.5–5% of those determined simultaneously in plasma. If the integrity of the blood–brain barrier is diminished by active bacterial infection, antibiotic penetration is increased considerably, permitting the use of penicillins in infectious meningitis. As the inflammatory reactions subside, penetration returns to normal; the drug dosage therefore should not be decreased as the patient improves. In a similar manner, antibiotics that are highly protein bound may penetrate less well into the site of infection than those that are largely unbound.

The dose and dosing frequency of antibiotics traditionally have been selected to achieve antibacterial activity at the site of infection for most of the dosing interval. This may not always be necessary, and superior results may even be obtained with high peak concentrations followed by periods of subinhibitory activity. For example, aminoglycosides are at least as efficacious and less toxic when given in a single large daily dose than when given more frequently in divided doses.

Knowledge of an individual patient's renal and hepatic function also is essential, as the dose of certain antibiotics must be adjusted to avoid toxicity when their elimination is impaired.

HOST FACTORS A critical determinant of antibiotic efficacy is the status of the host humoral and cellular defense mechanisms. In the immunocompetent host, merely halting the multiplication of the microorganism with a bacteriostatic agent frequently is sufficient to cure the infection. If host defenses are impaired, bacteriostatic activity may be inadequate and a bactericidal agent is required for cure. Examples where this applies include bacterial endocarditis, bacterial meningitis, and disseminated bacterial infections in neutropenic patients. Patients with HIV-1 infection and acquired immunodeficiency syndrome have impaired cellular immune responses. Therapy for opportunistic infection therefore often is suppressive but not curative; disseminated infections with *Salmonella* or atypical mycobacteria typically require prolonged antibiotic therapy to prevent relapse.

LOCAL FACTORS Antibiotic activity may be reduced significantly in pus, which contains phagocytes, cellular debris, and proteins that can bind drugs or create conditions unfavorable to drug action. The low pH that is characteristically found in abscesses and many confined infected sites can markedly reduce the activity of some agents, particularly the aminoglycosides.

The presence of a foreign body in an infected site markedly reduces the likelihood for successful antibiotic therapy. Prosthetics such as cardiac valves, artificial joints, pacemakers, vascular grafts, and various shunts promote the formation of a bacterial biofilm that impairs phagocytosis; within the film, the slower growth of bacteria may also reduce antibiotic activity and favor bacterial persistence. Infections associated with foreign bodies thus are characterized by frequent relapses and failure, even with long-term antibiotic therapy. Successful therapy usually requires removal of the foreign material.

Intracellular pathogens (*e.g.*, *Salmonella*, *Brucella*, *Toxoplasma*, *Listeria*, and *M. Tuberculosis*) are protected from the action of antibiotics that penetrate into cells poorly. Certain antibiotics (*e.g.*, fluoroquinolones, isoniazid, trimethoprim-sulfamethoxazole, and rifampin) penetrate cells well and can achieve intracellular concentrations that inhibit or kill pathogens residing within cells.

OTHER FACTORS *Age* may play an important role in antibiotic therapy; newborn babies and the elderly often have impaired mechanisms of elimination of antibiotics and thus are uniquely susceptible to certain drug toxicities. *Genetic polymorphisms* that affect drug metabolism are increasingly appreciated as important factors in interindividual differences in toxic effects of many drugs, including antibiotics. *Pregnancy* may impose an increased risk of reaction to antibiotics for both mother and fetus. Similarly, lactating females can pass antibiotics to nursing babies, sometimes with adverse effects. *Drug allergy* is a common event with many antibiotics, especially β-lactam antibiotics.

Therapy with Combined Antimicrobial Agents

The simultaneous use of two or more antibiotics is recommended in specifically defined situations based on pharmacological rationale. Such combination therapy requires an understanding of the potential for interaction between the antibiotics. For example, vancomycin given alone typically has minimal nephrotoxicity, but it may be nephrotoxic when combined with an aminoglycoside.

To determine the antiomicrobial activity of drug combinations, bacteria are incubated in broth with serial dilutions of antibiotics, either individually or in combination. *Synergism* of the antibiotics is defined as inhibition of growth by the drug combination at concentrations less than or equal to 25% of the MIC of each drug acting alone. This finding implies that one drug is affecting the microorganism so as to increase the susceptibility to the other antibiotic. If one half of the inhibitory concentration of each drug is required to produced inhibition, the result is called additive, suggesting that the two drugs are working independently of each other. If more than one-half of the MIC of each drug is necessary to produce an inhibitory effect, the drugs are said to be antagonistic.

Bacteriostatic antibiotics (*e.g.*, tetracyclines, erythromycin, and chloramphenicol) frequently antagonize the action of bactericidal drugs (*e.g.*, β-lactam antibiotics, vancomycin, and aminoglycosides); this probably is because they inhibit cell division and protein synthesis, which are required for the effect of most bactericidal drugs. Bactericidal drugs from different classes in combination tend to be additive or synergistic. For example, an inhibitor of cell wall synthesis and an aminoglycoside are synergistic against many bacterial species, and such combinations are frequently used. It is important to remember that these antibiotic sensitivities are determined *in vitro*, and the clinical relevance of synergy and antagonism *in vivo* is often much less clearly defined.

INDICATIONS FOR THE CLINICAL USE OF COMBINATIONS OF ANTIMICROBIAL
AGENTS Use of antibiotics in combination may be justified: (1) for empirical therapy of an infection for which the cause is unknown; (2) for treatment of polymicrobial infections; (3) to enhance antimicrobial activity for a specific infection (*i.e.*, for synergy); or (4) to prevent emergence of resistance.

Empirical Therapy of Severe Infections in Which a Cause is Unknown. Empirical therapy of infection is the most common reason for using a combination of antibiotics. Severe illness and less certainty as to the particular infection or causative agent may mandate broad coverage initially, and more than one agent may be required to ensure that the regimen includes a drug that is active against the potential pathogens. In the treatment of community-acquired pneumonia, a macrolide may be used for atypical organisms such as *Mycoplasma* in combination with *cefuroxime* for pneumococci and gramnegative pathogens. Prolonged administration of empirical broad-spectrum coverage or multiple antibiotics should be avoided because it often is unnecessary, is expensive, may select for antibiotic resistance against multiple agents, and may cause additional adverse effects due to the multiple agents. Inappropriately broad coverage often is continued because adequate cultures were not obtained prior to the initiation of therapy or because of the misconception that a broad-spectrum regimen is superior to a narrow-spectrum regimen. Although reluctance to narrow therapy after a favorable initial response has occurred is understandable, *the goal should be to use the most selectively active drug that produces the fewest adverse effects, which includes adverse effects on normal host flora.*

Treatment of Polymicrobial Infections. Treatment of intra-abdominal, hepatic, and brain abscesses, and some genital tract infections may require the use of a drug combination to eradicate these typically mixed aerobic-anaerobic infections. These and other mixed infections may be caused by two or more different microorganisms that are sufficiently different in antibiotic sensitivity that no single agent can provide the required coverage.

Enhancement of Antibacterial Activity in the Treatment of Specific Infections. Antibiotics administered together may produce a synergistic effect. Such synergistic combinations have been shown to be better than single-agent therapy in relatively few infections. Perhaps the best-documented example of the utility of synergistic combinations is in the treatment of enterococcal endocarditis. The clinical outcome clearly is better in patients treated with a combination of penicillin and streptomycin or gentamicin *versus* treatment with penicillin alone. The same combination has shown clinical benefit in the treatment of endocarditis caused by strains of *viridans* streptococci, with more rapid eradication of bacteria. Combinations of β-lactam antibiotics and aminoglycosides also have been recommended for the treatment of serious infections with gram-negative rods, especially *Pseudomonas aeruginosa;* the benefits of these combinations *in vivo* are less well established.

Another frequently employed combination is that of a sulfonamide and an inhibitor of dihydrofolate reductase, such as trimethoprim; this combination is synergistic because the drugs block sequential steps in microbial folate synthesis.

Finally, the combination of flucytosine and amphotericin B is synergistic against *Cryptococcus neoformans* and is often employed in AIDS patients with cryptococcal meningitis.

Prevention of the Emergence of Resistant Microorganisms. The theoretical basis for combination therapy of tuberculosis is to prevent the emergence of resistant mutants that might result from monotherapy; clinical experience amply documents the utility of concomitant use of two or more agents in this setting. Combination therapy to prevent the emergence of resistance also frequently is used when rifampin is used in other infections.

DISADVANTAGES OF COMBINATIONS OF ANTIMICROBIAL AGENTS Disadvantages of antibiotic combinations include increased risk of toxicity, selection of multiple-drug-resistant microorganisms, eradication of normal host flora with subsequent superinfection, and increased cost. Although antibiotic antagonism is frequently observed *in vitro*, well-documented clinical examples are relatively rare; the most notable is pneumococcal meningitis, where penicillin alone is much more effective than a penicillin-tetracycline combination. Concerns of antagonism are most important in situations where achieving a bactericidal effect is critical for cure of the infection (*e.g.*, meningitis, endocarditis, and gram-negative infections in neutropenic patients).

Antibiotic Prophylaxis

In general, if a single, effective, nontoxic drug is used to prevent infection by a specific microorganism or to eradicate an early infection, then chemoprophylaxis frequently is successful. On the other hand, if the aim of prophylaxis is to prevent colonization or infection by any or all organisms present in the environment of the patient, then prophylaxis often fails.

Prophylaxis may be used to protect healthy persons from acquisition of or invasion by specific microorganisms to which they are exposed. Successful examples of this practice include rifampin administration to prevent meningococcal meningitis in close contacts of a known case, prevention of gonorrhea or syphilis after contact with an infected person, and the intermittent use of trimethoprim-sulfamethoxazole to prevent recurrent urinary tract infections.

Antibiotic prophylaxis, often with an oral fluoroquinolone, is used to prevent a variety of infections in patients undergoing organ transplantation or receiving cancer chemotherapy. Prophylaxis is recommended for primary and secondary prevention of opportunistic infections in AIDS patients whose CD4 counts are below certain thresholds (*e.g.*, <200 cell/mm^3 for the prevention of *Pneumocystis* pneumonia and <50 cells/mm^3 for prevention of atypical mycobacterial infections).

Chemoprophylaxis against endocarditis is recommended for patients with valvular or other structural lesions of the heart who are undergoing dental, surgical, or other procedures that may produce a high incidence of bacteremia. Therapy, generally as a single dose, should begin 1 hour before the procedure for oral drugs and 30 minutes before for parenteral drugs. Criteria are established for the selection of specific drugs and patients who should relieve prophylaxis for various procedures (Table 42–1).

The most extensive and probably best-studied use of chemoprophylaxis is to prevent wound infections after various surgical procedures (Table 42–1). Wound infections occur when a critical number of bacteria are present in the wound at the time of closure; factors that influence the size of innoculum needed include: virulence of the bacteria, the presence of devitalized or poorly vascularized tissue, the presence of a foreign body, and the status of the host. Antibiotic agents directed against the invading microorganism may prevent infection by reducing the number of viable bacteria below the critical level.

Several factors are important for effective chemoprophylaxis in surgical procedures. Antimicrobial activity must be present at the wound site at the time of closure. Thus, the drug should be given preoperatively (and perhaps intraoperatively for prolonged procedures) to ensure that therapeutic levels are maintained throughout the procedure. The antibiotic, often a cephalosporin, must be active against the most likely contaminating microorganisms. Prolonged administration of the drug after the surgical procedure is unwarranted, and no data support a lower incidence of wound infections if antibiotics are continued after the day of surgery. Clinical trials support chemoprophylaxis for dirty or contaminated surgical procedures (*e.g.*, resection of the colon) but not for clean surgical procedures. When the surgery involves insertion of a prosthetic implant (*e.g.*, prosthetic valve, vascular grant, prosthetic joint), cardiac surgery, or neurosurgical procedures, the complications of infection are so drastic that most authorities currently advocate antibiotic prophylaxis.

Table 42–1

Guidelines for Prophylactic Antibiotics in Surgical Procedures

Antibiotics should be administered 30–60 minutes prior to incision and may need to be readministered to maintain effective serum drug concentrations during prolonged procedures. A single preoperative antibiotic dose is usually sufficient prophylaxis. Continuation of antibiotics for up to 24 hours may be considered in some cases (e.g., contaminated cases, surgery of long duration, implantation of prosthetic material).

Nature of Surgery	Probable Pathogen(s)	Recommended Drug(s) (Adult Dosage)	Time of Administration
I. Clean			
A. Thoracic, cardiac, vascular, and orthopedic; neurosurgery	*S. aureus**, coagulase-negative staphylococci, gram-negative bacilli, *Pseudomonas*	Cefazolin (1 g IV) Vancomycin* (1 g IV)	At induction of anesthesia
B. Ophthalmic		Gentamicin or neomycin-gramicidin-polymyxin B ophthalmic drops; multiple drugs at intervals for first 24 hours	
II. Clean-Contaminated			
A. Head and neck (potentially entering esophageal lumen)	*S. aureus* and oral anaerobes	Cefazolin (1–2 g IV) or clindamycin (600 mg IV) ± gentamicin (1.5 mg/kg IV)	At induction of anesthesia
B. Abdominal—cholecystectomy and high-risk gastroduodenal or biliary		Cefazolin (1 g IV)	At induction of anesthesia
C. Abdominal—appendectomy		Cefoxitin or cefotetan (1 g IV)	At induction of anesthesia
D. Colorectal		Go-Lytely electrolyte solution (4 liters)	Preoperative day
Preoperative lavage recommended, plus antimicrobial treatment			
1. Oral antimicrobial prophylaxis		Erythromycin stearate (1 g PO) *or* metronidazole (500 mg PO) *plus* neomycin (1 g PO)	At 1 PM, 2 PM, and 11 PM on the preoperative day
2. Parenteral antimicrobial prophylaxis	Patients who have not received lavage and oral prophylaxis should receive parenteral antibiotics for ≤24 hours to cover enteric aerobes (including *Escherichia coli*, *Klebsiella* spp.) and enteric anaerobes (including *Bacterodes fragilis*, *Clostridium* spp., anaerobic cocci, and *Fusobacterium* spp.)	Cefotetan (1 g every 12 hours for 2 doses) Ceftizoxime (1 g every 12 hours for 2 doses) Cefoxitin (1 g every 4–8 hours for 3 doses)	

(Continued)

713

Table 42–1

Guidelines for Prophylactic Antibiotics in Surgical Procedures (*Continued*)

Nature of Surgery	Probable Pathogen(s)	Recommended Drug(s) (Adult Dosage)	Time of Administration
II. Clean-Contaminated			
E. Gynecological			
1. Vaginal or abdominal hysterectomy and high-risk cesarean section (following labor or ruptured membrane only)		Cefazolin (1 g IV)	At induction of anesthesia or postcord clamp
2. High-risk abortion, first trimester		Penicillin G (2 million units IV) *or* doxycycline (300 mg PO)	
3. High-risk abortion, second trimester		Cefazolin (1 g IV)	
F. Urology		Prophylactic antibiotics not shown to reduce incidence of wound infection after urological procedures. Bacteriuria is most common postoperative complication; only patients with evidence of infected urine should be treated with antibiotics directed against the specific pathogens isolated.	
III. Trauma-Contaminated Wounds			
A. Extremity	Antimicrobial coverage for Group A streptococci, staphylococci, and *Clostridium* spp.	Cefazolin (1 g every 8 hours IV) Vancomycin (1 g every 12 hours IV)[†]	
B. Ruptured *viscus*—abdomen/bowel injury		Cefotetan (1 g every 12 hours) *or* ceftizoxime (1 g every 12 hours) *or* cefoxitin (1 g every 6 hours) *or* clindamycin (600 mg IV every 8 hours) + gentamicin (1.5 mg/kg IV every 8 hours)[†] for ≤ 5 days	
C. Bites (cats and human)	Aerobic and anaerobic streptococci from skin and oral flora. Infection of animal bites additionally may be caused by *Pasteurella multocida*, which is penicillin-sensitive	Amoxicillin/clavulanate (750/125 mg twice a day for 5 days *or* doxycycline 100 mg PO twice a day for 5 days)	

[*]Recommended for hospitals with a high prevalence of infections caused by methicillin-resistant staphylococci or for serious allergy to β-lactams.

[†]For serious β-lactam allergy.

ABBREVIATIONS: IV, intravenous administration; PO, oral administration.

714

Superinfections

All individual who receive therapeutic doses of antibiotics undergo alterations in the normal microbial population of the GI, upper respiratory, and genitourinary tracts; as a result, some develop *superinfection*, or the appearance of bacteriological and clinical evidence of a new infection during the chemotherapy of a primary one. Such superinfection is due to the removal of the normal flora, which produces antibacterial substances and competes for essential nutrients. Of concern, the microorganisms responsible for the new infection can be drug-resistant strains of bacteria or fungi. The broader the spectrum and the longer the period of antibiotic treatment, the greater the risk of superinfection. *The most specific and narrowest spectrum antibiotics should be chosen to treat infections whenever feasible.*

Misuses of Antibiotics

TREATMENT OF NONRESPONSIVE INFECTIONS Most viral diseases are self-limited and do not respond to any of the currently available anti-infective compounds. Thus, antibiotic therapy of at least 90% of infections of the upper respiratory tract and many GI infections is ineffective.

THERAPY OF FEVER OF UNKNOWN ORIGIN Fever of short duration in the absence of localizing signs usually is associated with undefined viral infections. Antimicrobial therapy is unnecessary, and resolution of fever usually occurs spontaneously within a week. Fever persisting for 2 or more weeks, commonly referred to as *fever of unknown origin*, has a variety of causes; only about one quarter of these are infections. Moreover, some of these infections (*e.g.*, tuberculosis, disseminated fungal infections) may require antibiotics that are not typically used for bacterial infections. Inappropriately administered antibiotics may mask an underlying infection, delay the diagnosis, and prevent the identification of the infectious pathogen by culture.

IMPROPER DOSAGE Dosing errors with antibiotics are common. Excessive dosing can result in significant toxicities, while too low a dose may result in treatment failure and is most likely to select for antibiotic resistance.

INAPPROPRIATE RELIANCE ON CHEMOTHERAPY ALONE Infections complicated by abscess formation or the presence of necrotic tissue or a foreign body often cannot be cured by antibiotic therapy alone. Drainage, debridement, and removal of the foreign body are at least as important as the choice of antibiotic agent. As a general rule, when an appreciable quantity of pus, necrotic tissue, or a foreign body is present, the most effective therapy is an antimicrobial agent given in adequate dose plus a properly performed surgical procedure.

LACK OF ADEQUATE BACTERIOLOGICAL INFORMATION Antibiotic therapy too often is given in the absence of supporting microbiological data. Bacterial cultures and Gram stains of infected material are obtained too infrequently, and, when available, the results often are disregarded in the selection and application of drug therapy. *Frequent use of drug combinations or drugs with broadest spectra is a cover for diagnostic imprecision.*

For a complete Bibliographical listing see Goodman & Gilman's *The Pharmacological Basis of Therapeutics,* 11th ed., or Goodman & Gilman Online at www.accessmedicine.com.

43

SULFONAMIDES, TRIMETHOPRIM–SULFAMETHOXAZOLE, QUINOLONES, AND AGENTS FOR URINARY TRACT INFECTIONS

SULFONAMIDES

CHEMISTRY

Sulfonamides *are derivatives of* para-*aminobenzenesulfonamide (sulfanilamide); the structures of selected members are shown in Figure 43–1. Most are relatively insoluble in water, but their sodium salts are readily soluble. The minimal structural prerequisites for antibacterial action are embodied in sulfanilamide itself. The sulfur must be linked directly to the benzene ring. The para-*NH_2 *group (the N of which is designated N4) can be replaced only by moieties that can be converted* in vivo *to a free amino group. Substitutions in the amide NH_2 group (N1) have variable effects on antibacterial activity of the molecule, but substitution of heterocyclic aromatic nuclei at N1 yields highly potent compounds.*

Effects on Microbes

Sulfonamides have wide antimicrobial activity, but their usefulness has diminished as resistant strains have emerged. These drugs are bacteriostatic, and host defenses are essential for eradication of the infection.

ANTIBACTERIAL SPECTRUM
MECHANISM OF ACTION

Sulfonamides competitively inhibit dihydropteroate synthase, the bacterial enzyme responsible for the incorporation of para-*aminobenzoic acid (PABA) into dihydropteroic acid, the immediate precursor of folic acid (Figure 43–2). Sensitive microorganisms must synthesize their own folic acid, while bacteria that can use preformed folate are not affected. Mammalian cells require preformed folic acid and are not affected by sulfonamides.*

SYNERGISTS OF SULFONAMIDES

Trimethoprim *exerts a synergistic effect with sulfonamides. It potently and selectively inhibits microbial dihydrofolate reductase, the enzyme that reduces dihydrofolate to tetrahydrofolate—the form required for one-carbon transfer reactions. Coadministration of a sulfonamide and trimethoprim thus introduces sequential blocks in the biosynthetic pathway for tetrahydrofolate (Figure 43–2).*

ACQUIRED BACTERIAL RESISTANCE TO SULFONAMIDES

Bacterial resistance to sulfonamides can originate by random mutation and selection or by plasmid transfer of resistance; it usually does not confer cross-resistance to other classes of antibiotics. Resistance to sulfonamide results from altered constitution of the bacterial cell that causes (1) a lower affinity for sulfonamides by dihydropteroate synthase, (2) decreased bacterial permeability or active efflux of the drug, (3) an alternative metabolic pathway for synthesis of an essential metabolite, or (4) an increased production of an essential metabolite or drug antagonist. Plasmid-mediated resistance is due to plasmid-encoded, drug-resistant dihydropteroate synthetase.

Absorption, Fate, and Excretion

Except for drugs especially designed for local gastrointestinal (GI) effects (*see* Chapter 38), the sulfonamides are absorbed rapidly and well from the GI tract. Peak plasma levels are achieved in 2–6 hours, depending on the drug. Absorption from sites such as the vagina, respiratory tract, or abraded skin is unreliable, but sufficient drug may enter the body to cause toxic reactions in susceptible persons or to produce sensitization.

All sulfonamides are bound in varying degree to plasma proteins, particularly albumin. The extent is determined by the hydrophobicity of a particular drug and its pK_a; at physiological pH, drugs with a high pK_a exhibit a low degree of protein binding and *vice versa.*

Sulfonamides are widely distributed. The diffusible fraction of sulfadiazine is distributed uniformly throughout the total-body water, whereas *sulfisoxazole* is confined largely to the extracellular space. The sulfonamides readily enter body fluids and may reach concentrations therein that are 50–80% of the simultaneously determined serum concentration. Since the protein content of such fluids usually is low, the drug is present in the unbound active form.

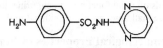

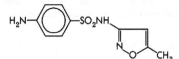

SULFANILAMIDE

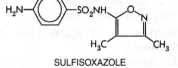

SULFADIAZINE

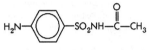

SULFAMETHOXAZOLE

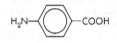

SULFISOXAZOLE

SULFACETAMIDE

PARA-AMINOBENZOIC ACID

FIGURE 43–1 *Structural formulas of selected sulfonamides and para-aminobenzoic acid.* The N of the *para*-NH$_2$ group is designated as N4; that of the amide NH$_2$, as N1.

After systemic administration, *sulfadiazine* and sulfisoxazole attain concentrations in cerebrospinal fluid (CSF) that may be effective in meningitis. Sulfonamides readily cross the placenta to reach the fetal circulation, potentially exerting both antibacterial and toxic effects.

The sulfonamides are metabolized in the liver. The major derivative is the N4-acetylated sulfonamide. Acetylation, which occurs to a varying extent with each agent, is disadvantageous because the resulting products have no antibacterial activity yet retain the toxic potential of the parent substance. Sulfonamides are eliminated partly as the unchanged drug and partly as metabolic products. The largest fraction is excreted in the urine, and the t$_{1/2}$ of sulfonamides in the body thus

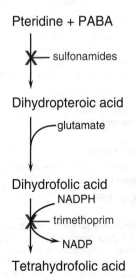

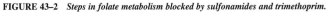

FIGURE 43–2 *Steps in folate metabolism blocked by sulfonamides and trimethoprim.*

depends on renal function. In acid urine, the older sulfonamides are insoluble and crystalluria may result. Small amounts are eliminated in the feces, bile, milk, and other secretions.

Pharmacological Properties of Individual Sulfonamides

The sulfonamides are classed based on the extent or rapidity with which they are absorbed and excreted: (1) agents that are absorbed and excreted rapidly, such as sulfisoxazole and sulfadiazine; (2) agents that are absorbed very poorly when administered orally and hence are active in the bowel lumen, such as *sulfasalazine*; (3) agents that are used mainly topically, such as *sulfacetamide, mafenide,* and *silver sulfadiazine*; and (4) long-acting sulfonamides, such as *sulfadoxine*, that are absorbed rapidly but excreted slowly.

RAPIDLY ABSORBED AND ELIMINATED SULFONAMIDES
Sulfisoxazole

*Sulfisoxazole (*GANTRISIN*, others) is rapidly absorbed and excreted. Its high solubility eliminates much of the renal toxicity inherent in the use of older sulfonamides. Sulfisoxazole is bound extensively to plasma proteins. From 28% to 35% of sulfisoxazole in the blood and ~30% in the urine is in the acetylated form. It has a serum $t_{1/2}$ of 5–6 hours and ~95% of a single dose is excreted by the kidney in 24 hours. Drug concentrations in urine greatly exceed those in blood and may be bactericidal. The CSF concentration is ~33% of that in the blood. Sulfisoxazole acetyl is tasteless and hence preferred for oral use in children; it is marketed in combination with* erythromycin (PEDIAZOLE, *others) for use in children with otitis media.*

The untoward effects of sulfisoxazole are similar to those of other sulfonamides. Because of its relatively high solubility, sulfisoxazole rarely produces hematuria or crystalluria (0.2–0.3%). Patients still should ingest an adequate quantity of water. Sulfisoxazole must be used with caution in patients with impaired renal function. Like all sulfonamides, sulfisoxazole may produce hypersensitivity reactions, some of which are potentially lethal. Sulfisoxazole generally is preferred over other sulfonamides when a rapidly absorbed and excreted sulfonamide is indicated.

Sulfamethoxazole

Sulfamethoxazole is a close congener of sulfisoxazole, but its rates of enteric absorption and urinary excretion are slower; it has a serum $t_{1/2}$ of 11 hours. It is administered orally and employed for both systemic and urinary tract infections. Precautions must be observed to avoid crystalluria because of the high percentage of the acetylated, relatively insoluble form of the drug in urine. The clinical uses of sulfamethoxazole are the same as those for sulfisoxazole. It also is marketed in fixed-dose combinations with trimethoprim (see *below*).

Sulfadiazine

Sulfadiazine given orally is absorbed rapidly, and peak blood concentrations are reached within 3–6 hours after a single dose; the serum $t_{1/2}$ is 10 hours. About half of the drug is bound to plasma protein. Therapeutic concentrations are attained in CSF within 4 hours of a single oral dose.

Sulfadiazine is readily excreted by the kidney in both the free and acetylated forms, rapidly at first and then more slowly over a period of 2–3 days. About 15–40% of the excreted sulfadiazine is acetylated. This form is excreted more readily than the free fraction, and alkalinization of the urine accelerates the renal clearance of both forms by further diminishing their tubular reabsorption.

In adults and children who are treated with sulfadiazine, every precaution must be taken to ensure fluid intake adequate to produce a urine output of at least 1200 mL in adults and a corresponding quantity in children. If this cannot be accomplished, sodium bicarbonate may reduce the risk of crystalluria.

POORLY ABSORBED SULFONAMIDES

*Sulfasalazine (*AZULFIDINE*) is very poorly absorbed from the GI tract and is used in the therapy of ulcerative colitis and Crohn's disease* (see *Chapter 38*).

SULFONAMIDES FOR TOPICAL USE
Sulfacetamide

Sulfacetamide is the N1-acetyl-substituted derivative of sulfanilamide. *Its aqueous solubility is ~90 times that of sulfadiazine. This drug (*ISOPTO-CETAMIDE, *others) is employed extensively for ophthalmic infections. Very high aqueous concentrations are not irritating to the eye and are effective against susceptible microorganisms. The drug penetrates readily into ocular fluids and tissues. Sensitivity reactions to sulfacetamide are rare, but it should not be used in patients with known sulfonamide hypersensitivity.*

Silver Sulfadiazine

Silver sulfadiazine (SILVADENE, others) inhibits the growth of nearly all pathogenic bacteria and fungi, including some species resistant to sulfonamides. The compound is used topically to reduce microbial colonization and the incidence of infections in burn patients. It is not used to treat an established deep infection. Silver is released slowly in concentrations that are selectively toxic to microorganisms. However, bacteria may develop resistance to silver sulfadiazine. The plasma concentration of sulfadiazine may approach therapeutic levels if a large surface area is involved. Adverse reactions—burning, rash, and itching—are infrequent. Silver sulfadiazine is considered one of the agents of choice for the prevention of burn infection.

Mafenide

This sulfonamide (α-amino-p-toluene-sulfonamide) is marketed as mafenide acetate *(SULFAMYLON). It is used topically to prevent colonization of burns by a large variety of gram-negative and gram-positive bacteria. It is associated with significant adverse effects, including intense pain at sites of application, allergic reactions, loss of fluid by evaporation from the burn surface, and metabolic acidosis secondary to inhibition of carbonic anhydrase.*

LONG-ACTING SULFONAMIDES

Sulfadoxine *has a particularly long* $t_{1/2}$ *(7–9 days). In combination with* pyrimethamine *(500 mg sulfadoxine plus 25 mg pyrimethamine as FANSIDAR), it is used for prophylaxis and treatment of malaria caused by* mefloquine-*resistant strains of* Plasmodium falciparum *(see Chapter 39). Because of severe adverse reactions (e.g., Stevens-Johnson syndrome), the drug should be used for prophylaxis only where the risk of resistant malaria is high.*

Sulfonamide Therapy

URINARY TRACT INFECTIONS

Many urinary tract infections are caused by sulfonamide-resistant microorganisms. Trimethoprim–sulfamethoxazole, a quinolone, trimethoprim, fosfomycin, *or* ampicillin *are the preferred agents. Sulfisoxazole may be used in areas where the prevalence of resistance is not high or when the organism is known to be sensitive. The usual dose is 2–4 g initially, followed by 1–2 g, orally four times a day for 5–10 days. Patients with acute pyelonephritis should not be treated with a sulfonamide.*

Nocardiosis

Sulfonamides are of value in treating infections due to Nocardia *spp. Sulfisoxazole or sulfadiazine may be given in dosages of 6–8 g daily and is continued for several months after all manifestations have resolved. The administration of a sulfonamide together with a second antibiotic has been recommended, especially for advanced cases, and ampicillin, erythromycin, and* streptomycin *have been suggested for this purpose. The clinical response and the results of sensitivity testing may be helpful in choosing a companion drug. Some experts consider trimethoprim–sulfamethoxazole to be the drug of choice.*

TOXOPLASMOSIS

The combination of pyrimethamine *and sulfadiazine is the treatment of choice for toxoplasmosis (see Chapter 40). Pyrimethamine is given as a loading dose of 75 mg followed by 25 mg orally per day, with sulfadiazine 1 g orally every 6 hours, plus folinic acid 10 mg orally each day for at least 3–6 weeks. Patients should receive at least 2 L of fluid intake daily to prevent crystalluria.*

USE OF SULFONAMIDES FOR PROPHYLAXIS

The sulfonamides are as efficacious as oral penicillin in preventing streptococcal infections and recurrence of rheumatic fever in susceptible subjects and are used in patients who are hypersensitive to penicillin. Untoward responses usually occur during the first 8 weeks; serious reactions after this time are rare. White blood cell counts should be checked weekly during the first 8 weeks.

Untoward Reactions to Sulfonamides

DISTURBANCES OF THE URINARY TRACT

The incidence of crystalluria is low with more soluble agents (e.g., sulfisoxazole). Crystalluria has occurred in volume-depleted patients with the acquired immune deficiency syndrome (AIDS) who were given sulfadiazine for Toxoplasma encephalitis. Fluid intake should be sufficient to ensure a daily urine volume of at least 1.2 L (in adults). Urinary alkalinization may be helpful if urine volume or pH is unusually low.

DISORDERS OF THE HEMATOPOIETIC SYSTEM

Although rare, acute hemolytic anemia can occur. This may reflect an immune reaction or may be due to glucose-6-phosphate dehydrogenase deficiency. Agranulocytosis occurs in ~0.1% of patients who receive sulfadiazine and also can occur with other sulfonamides. Although neutropenia may persist for weeks or months after sulfonamide is withdrawn, most patients recover spontaneously with supportive care. Pancytopenia with complete suppression of bone-marrow activity is extremely rare. It probably results from a direct myelotoxic effect and may be fatal. Reversible suppression of the bone marrow is quite common in patients with limited bone marrow reserve (e.g., patients with AIDS or those receiving myelosuppressive chemotherapy).

HYPERSENSITIVITY REACTIONS

The sulfonamides are associated with a number of skin and mucous membrane manifestations attributed to sensitization to sulfonamide, including various rashes, erythema nodosum, erythema multiforme of the Stevens-Johnson type, Behçet's syndrome, exfoliative dermatitis, and photosensitivity. These hypersensitivity reactions usually occur after the first week of therapy but may appear earlier in previously sensitized individuals. Fever, malaise, and pruritus frequently are present simultaneously. The incidence of untoward dermal effects is ~2% with sulfisoxazole, although a higher frequency is seen in patients with AIDS. A syndrome similar to serum sickness may appear after several days of sulfonamide therapy. Drug fever occurs in ~3% of patients treated with sulfisoxazole.

Focal or diffuse necrosis of the liver owing to direct drug toxicity or sensitization occurs in <0.1% of patients and rarely may progress to fulminant hepatic failure and death. Hepatomegaly, jaundice, and laboratory evidence of hepatocellular dysfunction usually appear 3–5 days after sulfonamide administration is started.

MISCELLANEOUS REACTIONS

Anorexia, nausea, and vomiting occur in 1–2% of persons receiving sulfonamides. The administration of sulfonamides to newborn infants, especially if premature, may lead to the displacement of bilirubin from albumin, potentially causing kernicterus. Sulfonamides should not be given to pregnant women near term because these drugs cross the placenta and are secreted in milk.

DRUG INTERACTIONS

Important drug interactions of the sulfonamides are seen with the oral anticoagulants, the sulfonylureas, and phenytoin. *In each case, sulfonamides can potentiate the effects of the other drug, either by inhibiting its metabolism or by displacing it from albumin. Dosage adjustment may be necessary.*

TRIMETHOPRIM–SULFAMETHOXAZOLE

The introduction of trimethoprim in combination with sulfamethoxazole constitutes an important advance in the development of clinically effective antimicrobial agents. In addition to its combination with sulfamethoxazole (BACTRIM, SEPTRA, others), trimethoprim also is available as a single-entity preparation (PROLOPRIM, others). It is a diaminopyramidine.

ANTIBACTERIAL SPECTRUM

The antibacterial spectrum of trimethoprim resembles that of sulfamethoxazole. Most gram-negative and gram-positive microorganisms are sensitive to trimethoprim, but there is significant regional variation in the susceptibility of Enterobacteriaceae *to trimethoprim because of the spread of resistance.*

Efficacy of Trimethoprim–Sulfamethoxazole in Combination

A synergistic interaction between these drugs is apparent even when microorganisms are resistant to sulfonamide, but maximal synergism occurs when microorganisms are sensitive to both drugs.

MECHANISM OF ACTION

The antimicrobial activity of the trimethoprim/sulfamethoxazole combination results from actions on two steps of the biosynthetic pathway for tetrahydrofolic acid. Trimethoprim prevents the reduction of dihydrofolate to tetrahydrofolate (Figure 43–2). Mammalian cells use preformed folates from the diet and do not synthesize the compound. Trimethoprim is a highly selective inhibitor of dihydrofolate reductase of lower organisms; ~100,000 times more drug is required to inhibit human reductase than the bacterial enzyme. This relative selectivity is vital because the enzyme is essential to all species.

The synergistic interaction between sulfonamide and trimethoprim is predictable from their respective mechanisms. The most effective ratio of these two drugs for the greatest number of microorganisms is 20 parts sulfamethoxazole to 1 part trimethoprim. The combination thus is formulated to achieve a sulfamethoxazole concentration in vivo *that is 20 times greater than that of trimethoprim.*

BACTERIAL RESISTANCE

Bacterial resistance increasingly complicates treatment and often results from the acquisition of a plasmid that encodes an altered dihydrofolate reductase. Emergence of trimethoprim–sulfamethoxazole–resistant Staphylococcus aureus *and* Enterobacteriaceae *is a special problem in AIDS patients receiving the drug for prophylaxis of* Pneumocystis jiroveci *(formerly called* Pneumocystis carinii*) pneumonia.*

ABSORPTION, DISTRIBUTION, AND EXCRETION The pharmacokinetic profiles of sulfamethoxazole and trimethoprim are closely but not perfectly matched to achieve a constant ratio of 20:1 in their concentrations in blood and tissues. The ratio in blood is often greater than 20:1, while that in tissues is frequently less. After a single oral dose of the combined preparation, peak blood concentrations of trimethoprim usually occur by 2 hours, whereas peak concentrations of sulfamethoxazole require 4 hours. The half-lives of trimethoprim and sulfamethoxazole are ~11 and 10 hours, respectively.

When 800 mg sulfamethoxazole is given with 160 mg trimethoprim (the conventional 5:1 ratio) twice daily, the peak concentrations of the drugs in plasma approximate the optimal ratio. Peak concentrations are similar after intravenous infusion of 800 mg sulfamethoxazole/160 mg trimethoprim over a period of 1 hour.

Trimethoprim is distributed and concentrated rapidly in tissues, and ~40% is bound to plasma protein in the presence of sulfamethoxazole. The volume of distribution of trimethoprim is almost nine times that of sulfamethoxazole. The drug readily enters CSF and sputum. High concentrations of each component also are found in bile. About 65% of sulfamethoxazole is bound to plasma protein.

About 60% of administered trimethoprim and from 25% to 50% of administered sulfamethoxazole are excreted in the urine in 24 hours. Two-thirds of the sulfonamide is unconjugated. Metabolites of trimethoprim also are excreted. The rates of excretion and the concentrations of both compounds in the urine are reduced significantly in patients with uremia.

THERAPEUTIC USES

Urinary Tract Infections

Treatment of uncomplicated lower urinary tract infections with trimethoprim–sulfamethoxazole often is highly effective for sensitive bacteria, usually for a minimum of 3 days. The combination is especially useful in chronic and recurrent infections of the urinary tract. Trimethoprim also is found in therapeutic concentrations in prostatic secretions, and trimethoprim–sulfamethoxazole is often effective for bacterial prostatitis.

Bacterial Respiratory Tract Infections

Trimethoprim–sulfamethoxazole is effective for acute exacerbations of chronic bronchitis. Administration of 800–1200 mg sulfamethoxazole plus 160–240 mg trimethoprim twice a day appears to be effective in decreasing fever, purulence and volume of sputum, and sputum bacterial count. Trimethoprim–sulfamethoxazole should not *be used to treat streptococcal pharyngitis because it does not eradicate the microorganism. It is effective for acute otitis media in children and acute maxillary sinusitis in adults caused by susceptible strains of* Haemophilus influenzae *and* Streptococcus pneumoniae.

Gastrointestinal Infections

The combination is an alternative to fluoroquinolone *for treatment of shigellosis, but resistance to trimethoprim–sulfamethoxazole is increasingly common.*

Trimethoprim–sulfamethoxazole appears to be effective in the management of carriers of sensitive strains of Salmonella typhi *and other* Salmonella spp., *but failures have occurred. Chronic disease of the gallbladder may be associated with a high incidence of failure to clear the carrier state. Acute diarrhea owing to sensitive strains of enteropathogenic* Escherichia coli *can be treated or prevented with either trimethoprim or trimethoprim plus sulfamethoxazole. However, antibiotic treatment (either trimethoprim–sulfamethoxazole or* cephalosporin*) of diarrheal illness due to enterohemorrhagic* E. coli *O157:H7 may increase the risk of hemolytic-uremic syndrome, perhaps by increasing the release of Shiga toxin.*

Infection by Pneumocystis jiroveci

High-dose therapy (trimethoprim 15 mg/kg/day plus sulfamethoxazole 100 mg/kg/day in three or four divided doses) is effective for this severe infection in patients with AIDS. Adjunctive glucocorticoids *should be given in patients with a Po_2 of <70 mm Hg or an alveolar–arterial gradient of >35 mm Hg. The incidence of side effects is high. Lower-dose oral therapy with 800 mg sulfamethoxazole plus 160 mg trimethoprim (given twice daily) has been used successfully in AIDS patients with less severe pneumonia (Po_2 >70 mm Hg). Prophylaxis with 800 mg sulfamethoxazole and 160 mg trimethoprim once daily or three times a week is effective in preventing pneumonia caused by this organism in patients with AIDS. Adverse reactions are less frequent with the lower prophylactic doses of trimethoprim–sulfamethoxazole. The most common problems are rash, fever, leukopenia, and hepatitis.*

Prophylaxis in Neutropenic Patients

Low-dose therapy (i.e., 150 mg/m^2 of body surface area of trimethoprim and 750 mg/m^2 of body surface area of sulfamethoxazole) is effective for the prophylaxis of infection by P. jiroveci. Significant protection against sepsis caused by gram-negative bacteria also was noted when 800 mg sulfamethoxazole and 160 mg trimethoprim were given twice daily to severely neutropenic patients. The emergence of resistant bacteria may limit the usefulness of trimethoprim– sulfamethoxazole for prophylaxis.

Miscellaneous Infections

Nocardia *infections have been treated successfully, but failures also have been reported. Although a combination of doxycycline and streptomycin or gentamicin is considered the treatment of choice for brucellosis, trimethoprim–sulfamethoxazole may be an effective substitute for the doxycycline combination. Trimethoprim–sulfamethoxazole also has been used successfully for Whipple's disease,* Stenotrophomonas maltophilia *infection, and infection by the intestinal parasites* Cyclospora *and* Isospora.

UNTOWARD EFFECTS The margin between toxicity for bacteria and that for human beings may be narrowed when the patient is folate deficient. In such cases, trimethoprim–sulfamethoxazole may cause or precipitate megaloblastosis, leukopenia, or thrombocytopenia. About 75% of the untoward effects involve the skin. Trimethoprim–sulfamethoxazole has been reported to cause up to three times as many dermatological reactions as does sulfisoxazole when given alone (5.9% vs. 1.7%). Severe dermatologic reactions primarily occur in older individuals. Nausea and vomiting constitute the bulk of GI reactions; diarrhea is rare. Glossitis and stomatitis are relatively common. Transient jaundice with histological features of allergic cholestatic hepatitis has been noted. CNS reactions consist of headache, depression, and hallucinations. Hematological reactions include various anemias (including aplastic, hemolytic, and macrocytic), coagulation disorders, granulocytopenia, agranulocytosis, purpura, and sulfhemoglobinemia. Permanent impairment of renal function may follow the use of trimethoprim–sulfamethoxazole in patients with renal disease, and a reversible decrease in creatinine clearance has been noted in patients with normal renal function.

Patients with AIDS frequently have hypersensitivity reactions to trimethoprim–sulfamethoxazole, including rash, neutropenia, Stevens-Johnson syndrome, Sweet's syndrome, and pulmonary infiltrates. It may be possible to continue therapy in such patients following rapid oral desensitization.

THE QUINOLONES

The fluorinated 4-quinolones, such as *ciprofloxacin* (CIPRO), *moxifloxacin* (AVELOX), and *gatifloxacin* (TEQUIN), are orally effective for the treatment of a wide variety of infectious diseases (Table 43–1) and have relatively few side effects.

CHEMISTRY

Compounds available in the U.S. contain a carboxylic acid moiety at position 3 of the primary ring structure. Many newer fluoroquinolones also contain a fluorine substituent at position 6 and a piperazine moiety at position 7 (Table 43–1).

MECHANISM OF ACTION

The quinolone antibiotics target bacterial DNA gyrase and topoisomerase IV. For many grampositive bacteria, topoisomerase IV is the primary target. For many gram-negative bacteria, DNA gyrase is the primary quinolone target, as illustrated in Figure 43–3. The quinolones inhibit gyrase-mediated DNA supercoiling at concentrations that correlate well with their effective antibacterial actions. Mutations of gyrA *can confer resistance to these drugs. Topoisomerase IV separates catenated DNA molecules that result from DNA replication, and also is a target for quinolones.*

ANTIBACTERIAL SPECTRUM

The fluoroquinolones are potent bactericidal agents against a broad variety of microorganisms, as outlined under Therapeutic Uses. Fluoroquinolones have good activity against staphylococci but

Table 43–1

Structural Formulas of Selected Quinolones and Fluoroquinolones

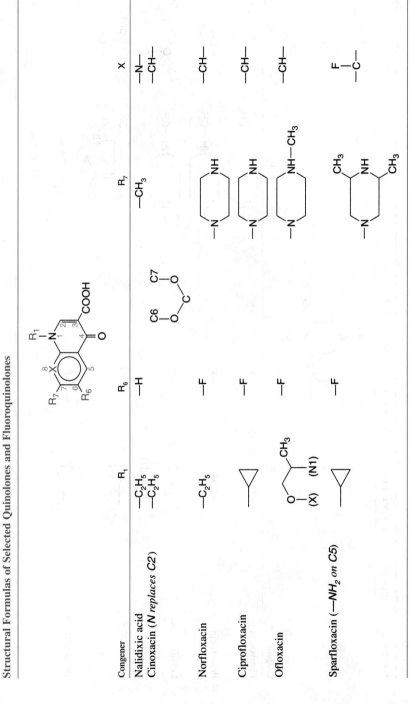

Congener	R_1	R_6	R_7	X
Nalidixic acid	$-C_2H_5$	$-H$	$-CH_3$	$-N-$
Cinoxacin (*N replaces C2*)	$-C_2H_5$			$-CH$
Norfloxacin	$-C_2H_5$	$-F$		$-CH$
Ciprofloxacin		$-F$		$-CH$
Ofloxacin		$-F$		$-CH$
Sparfloxacin (*—NH₂ on C5*)		$-F$		$F-C$

(Continued)

Table 43–1

Structural Formulas of Selected Quinolones and Fluoroquinolones *(Continued)*

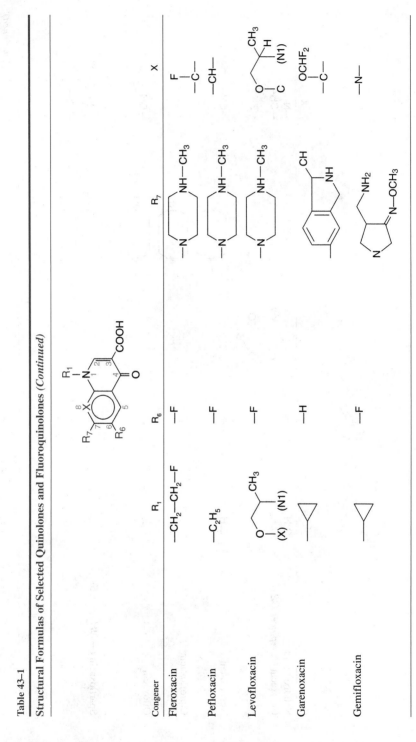

Congener	R_1	R_6	R_7	X
Fleroxacin	—CH₂—CH₂—F	—F	N—NH—CH₃	F—C—
Pefloxacin	—C₂H₅	—F	N—NH—CH₃	—CH—
Levofloxacin	CH₃ O—(X) (N1)	—F	N—NH—CH₃	O—C CH₃ H (N1)
Garenoxacin	(cyclopropyl)	—H	NH CH	OCHF₂ —C—
Gemifloxacin	(cyclopropyl)	—F	N NH₂ N—OCH₃	—N—

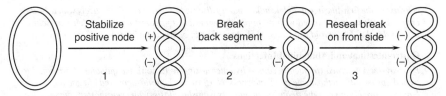

FIGURE 43–3 *Model of the formation of negative DNA supercoils by DNA gyrase.* The enzyme binds to two segments of DNA (1), creating a node of positive (+) superhelix. The enzyme then introduces a double-strand break in the DNA and passes the front segment through the break (2). The break is then resealed (3), creating a negative (–) supercoil. Quinolones inhibit the nicking and closing activity of the gyrase and also block the decatenating activity of topoisomerase IV.

not against methicillin-resistant strains. Activity against streptococci is limited to a subset of the quinolones, including levofloxacin *(LEVAQUIN),* gatifloxacin *(TEQUIN), and* moxifloxacin *(AVELOX). Several intracellular bacteria are inhibited by fluoroquinolones; these include species of* Chlamydia, Mycoplasma, Legionella, Brucella, *and* Mycobacterium *(including* Mycobacterium tuberculosis). Ciprofloxacin, *ofloxacin (FLOXIN), and* pefloxacin *inhibit* M. fortuitum, M. kansasii, *and* M. tuberculosis.

Resistance to quinolones may develop via *mutations in the bacterial chromosomal genes encoding DNA gyrase or topoisomerase IV or by active transport of the drug out of the bacteria. No quinolone-inactivating mechanisms have been identified. Resistance has increased, especially in* Pseudomonas *and staphylococci. Fluoroquinolone resistance also is increasing in* C. jejuni, Salmonella, Neisseria gonorrhoeae, *and* S. pneumoniae.

ABSORPTION, FATE, AND EXCRETION The quinolones are well absorbed after oral administration and are widely distributed. Peak serum levels of the fluoroquinolones occur within 1–3 hours of an oral dose of 400 mg. Relatively low serum levels are reached with norfloxacin and limit its usefulness to the treatment of urinary tract infections. Food does not impair oral absorption but may delay the time to peak serum concentrations. Oral doses in adults are 200–400 mg every 12 hours for ofloxacin, 400 mg every 12 hours for norfloxacin and pefloxacin, and 250–750 mg every 12 hours for ciprofloxacin. Bioavailability of the fluoroquinolones exceeds 50% for all agents and 95% for several. The serum half-lives range from 3 to 5 hours for norfloxacin and ciprofloxacin to 20 hours for sparfloxacin. The volume of distribution of quinolones is high, with concentrations in urine, kidney, lung and prostate tissue, stool, bile, and macrophages and neutrophils higher than serum levels. Quinolone concentrations in CSF, bone, and prostatic fluid are lower than in serum. Pefloxacin and ofloxacin levels in ascites fluid approach serum levels, and ciprofloxacin, ofloxacin, and pefloxacin have been detected in human breast milk.

Most quinolones are cleared predominantly by the kidney, and dose must be adjusted for renal failure. Pefloxacin and moxifloxacin are metabolized predominantly by the liver and should not be used in patients with hepatic failure. None is removed efficiently by peritoneal or hemodialysis.

THERAPEUTIC USES

Urinary Tract Infections

Norfloxacin is approved for use in the U.S. only for urinary tract infections. The fluoroquinolones are more efficacious than trimethoprim–sulfamethoxazole for the treatment of urinary tract infections.

Prostatitis

Norfloxacin, ciprofloxacin, and ofloxacin are effective for the treatment of prostatitis caused by sensitive bacteria. Fluoroquinolones administered for 4–6 weeks appear to be effective in patients not responding to trimethoprim–sulfamethoxazole.

Sexually Transmitted Diseases

The quinolones are contraindicated in pregnancy. Fluoroquinolones lack activity for Treponema pallidum *but have activity* in vitro *against* N. gonorrhoeae, Chlamydia trachomatis, *and* Haemophilus ducreyi. *For chlamydial urethritis/cervicitis, a 7-day course of ofloxacin or sparfloxacin is an alternative to a 7-day course with doxycycline or a single dose of azithromycin. A single oral dose of a fluoroquinolone such as ofloxacin or ciprofloxacin is effective treatment for sensitive strains of* N. gonorrhoeae, *but increasing resistance to fluoroquinolones has made ceftriaxone the first-line agent. Pelvic inflammatory disease has been treated effectively with a 14-day course of ofloxacin combined with an antibiotic with activity against anaerobes (clindamycin or metronidazole). Chancroid (infection by* H. ducreyi*) can be treated with 3 days of ciprofloxacin.*

Gastrointestinal and Abdominal Infections

For traveler's diarrhea (frequently caused by enterotoxigenic E. coli*), the quinolones are equal to trimethoprim–sulfamethoxazole in effectiveness. Norfloxacin, ciprofloxacin, and ofloxacin given for 5 days all are effective in the treatment of patients with shigellosis, with even shorter courses effective in many cases. Norfloxacin is superior to tetracyclines in decreasing the duration of diarrhea in cholera. Ciprofloxacin and ofloxacin cure most patients with enteric fever caused by* S. typhi, *as well as bacteremic nontyphoidal infections in AIDS patients. Shigellosis is treated effectively with either ciprofloxacin or* azithromycin. *The in vitro ability of the quinolones to induce the Shiga toxin (the cause of the hemolytic-uremic syndrome) in* E. coli *suggests that the quinolones should not be used for Shiga toxin–producing* E. coli. *Ciprofloxacin and ofloxacin are less effective in treating episodes of peritonitis occurring in patients on chronic ambulatory peritoneal dialysis, likely owing to their higher MICs for coagulase-negative staphylococci commonly seen in this setting.*

Respiratory Tract Infections

The major limitation to the use of quinolones for the treatment of community-acquired pneumonia and bronchitis was the poor activity against S. pneumoniae *and anaerobic bacteria. Many of the newer fluoroquinolones, including gatifloxacin and moxifloxacin, have excellent activity against* S. pneumoniae *and have shown efficacy comparable to β-lactam antibiotics. The fluoroquinolones have activity against the rest of the common respiratory pathogens, including* H. influenzae, Moraxella catarrhalis, S. aureus, Mycoplasma pneumoniae, Chlamydia pneumoniae, *and* Legionella pneumophila. *Either a fluoroquinolone (ciprofloxacin or levofloxacin) or azithromycin is the antibiotic of choice for* L. pneumophila. *Fluoroquinolones can effectively eradicate both* H. influenzae *and* M. catarrhalis *from sputum. Mild-to-moderate respiratory exacerbations owing to* P. aeruginosa *in patients with cystic fibrosis have responded to oral fluoroquinolones.*

Bone, Joint, and Soft Tissue Infections

The treatment of chronic osteomyelitis requires prolonged antimicrobial therapy with agents active against S. aureus *and gram-negative rods. The fluoroquinolones, by virtue of their oral administration and antibacterial spectrum, may appropriately be used in some cases; recommended doses are 500 mg every 12 hours or, if severe, 750 mg twice daily. Bone and joint infections may require treatment for 4–6 weeks or more. Dosage should be reduced for patients with severely impaired renal function. Ciprofloxacin should not be given to children or pregnant women. Clinical cures have been as high as 75% in chronic osteomyelitis in which gram-negative rods predominated. Failures have been associated with the development of resistance in* S. aureus, P. aeruginosa, *and* Serratia marcescens. *In diabetic foot infections, which commonly are polymicrobial, the fluoroquinolones in combination with an agent with antianaerobic activity are a reasonable choice. Ciprofloxacin as sole therapy is effective in ~50% of diabetic foot infections.*

Other Infections

Ciprofloxacin received wide usage for the prophylaxis of anthrax and is effective for the treatment of tularemia. The quinolones may be used as part of multiple-drug regimens for the treatment of multidrug-resistant tuberculosis and for the treatment of atypical mycobacterial infections and Mycobacterium avium *complex infections in AIDS (see Chapter 47). In neutropenic cancer patients with fever, the combination of a quinolone with an* aminoglycoside *is comparable to β-lactam–aminoglycoside combinations; quinolones are less effective when used alone. Quinolones, when used prophylactically in neutropenic patients, have decreased the incidence of gram-negative rod bacteremias. Ciprofloxacin plus* amoxicillin–clavulanate *is effective as an oral empirical therapy for fever in low-risk patients with granulocytopenia secondary to cancer chemotherapy.*

ADVERSE EFFECTS

The most common adverse reactions involve the GI tract, with 3–17% of patients reporting mostly mild nausea, vomiting, and/or abdominal discomfort. Diarrhea and antibiotic-associated colitis have been unusual. CNS side effects, predominately mild headache and dizziness, have been seen in 1–10% of patients. Rarely, hallucinations, delirium, and seizures have occurred, predominantly in patients who also were receiving theophylline *or a nonsteroidal anti-inflammatory drug. Ciprofloxacin and pefloxacin inhibit the metabolism of theophylline and may induce toxic levels. Nonsteroidal anti-inflammatory drugs may augment displacement of γ-aminobutyric acid (GABA) from its receptors by the quinolones. Rashes, including photosensitivity reactions, also can occur.*

Achilles tendon rupture or tendinitis has occurred rarely. Renal disease, hemodialysis, and glucocorticoid use may be predisposing factors. Traditionally, the use of quinolones in children has been contraindicated because they have produced arthropathy in animal models. However, children with cystic fibrosis given ciprofloxacin, norfloxacin, and nalidixic acid have had few, and reversible, joint symptoms. Therefore, the benefits may outweigh the risks in some children.

Leukopenia, eosinophilia, and mild elevations in serum transaminases occur rarely. Prolongation of the QT_c interval has been observed with sparfloxacin and to a lesser extent with gatifloxacin and moxifloxacin. Quinolones probably should be used only with caution in patients who are taking certain antiarrhythmics, including amiodarone, quinidine, *and* procainamide *(see Chapter 34).*

The prescribing information for gatifloxacin includes a contraindication in diabetic patients due to serious reports of hypoglycemia and hyperglycemia. Risk factors for this adverse effect include older age, renal insufficiency, and concomitant therapy with glucose-altering medications.

ANTISEPTIC AND ANALGESIC AGENTS FOR URINARY TRACT INFECTIONS

The urinary tract antiseptics inhibit the growth of many species of bacteria and can be used therapeutically because they are concentrated in the renal tubules. Effective antibacterial concentrations also reach the renal pelves and bladder.

METHENAMINE

Methenamine *is a urinary tract antiseptic and prodrug that owes its activity to its capacity to generate formaldehyde. It is bactericidal for gram-positive and gram-negative microorganisms and is more effective in an acid urine.*

NITROFURANTOIN

Nitrofurantoin *(FURADANTIN, MACROBID, others) is a synthetic nitrofuran that is used to prevent and treat urinary tract infections. Bacteria reduce nitrofurantoin to toxic products that apparently mediate cell damage. The antibacterial activity is higher in acidic urine.*

Pharmacology and Toxicity

Nitrofurantoin is absorbed rapidly and completely from the GI tract. Antibacterial concentrations are not achieved in plasma at recommended doses because the drug is eliminated rapidly. The plasma $t_{1/2}$ is <1 hour; ~40% is excreted unchanged in the urine. The urine should not be alkalinized because this reduces antimicrobial activity. Nitrofurantoin colors the urine brown.

The most common side effects are anorexia, nausea and vomiting, and diarrhea. Hypersensitivity reactions occur occasionally, including fever, leukopenia, granulocytopenia, hemolytic anemia associated with glucose-6-phosphate dehydrogenase deficiency, cholestatic jaundice, and hepatitis. Acute pneumonitis may occur acutely; the symptoms usually resolve quickly after drug discontinuation. Subacute reactions also may occur, including interstitial pulmonary fibrosis. Elderly patients are especially susceptible to the pulmonary toxicity. Severe polyneuropathies affecting both sensory and motor nerves also have been reported, most often in patients with impaired renal function and in persons on long-term treatment.

The oral dosage of nitrofurantoin for adults is 50–100 mg four times a day with meals and at bedtime. A single 50- to 100-mg dose at bedtime may be sufficient to prevent recurrences. A course of therapy should not exceed 14 days. Pregnant women, individuals with impaired renal function (creatinine clearance <40 mL/min), and children <1 month of age should not receive nitrofurantoin.

Nitrofurantoin is approved only for the treatment of urinary tract infections caused by microorganisms known to be susceptible to the drug. Nitrofurantoin is not recommended for treatment of pyelonephritis or prostatitis but is effective for prophylaxis of recurrent urinary tract infections.

For a complete Bibliographical listing see Goodman & Gilman's *The Pharmacological Basis of Therapeutics*, 11th ed., or Goodman & Gilman Online at www.accessmedicine.com.

44

PENICILLINS, CEPHALOSPORINS, AND OTHER β-LACTAM ANTIBIOTICS

PENICILLINS

Penicillins consist of a thiazolidine ring (A) connected to a β-lactam ring (B), to which is attached a side chain (R) (Figure 44–1). The penicillin nucleus itself is the chief structural requirement for biological activity. The discovery that 6-aminopenicillanic acid could be obtained from cultures that were depleted of side-chain precursors led to the development of the semisynthetic penicillins, which have side chains that alter the susceptibility of the resulting compounds to inactivating enzymes (β-lactamases) and that change the antibacterial activity and pharmacological properties of the drug (Table 44–1).

The international unit of penicillin is the specific penicillin activity contained in 0.6 μg of the crystalline sodium salt of penicillin G. Doses of semisynthetic penicillins are expressed by weight.

MECHANISM OF ACTION OF THE PENICILLINS AND CEPHALOSPORINS

Peptidoglycan is a heteropolymer that provides rigid mechanical stability to the bacterial cell wall by virtue of its highly cross-linked structure (Figure 44–2). In gram-positive bacteria, the cell wall is 50–100 molecules thick; it is only 1 or 2 molecules thick in gram-negative bacteria (Figure 44–3). The peptidoglycan is composed of glycan chains, which are linear strands of two alternating amino sugars (N-acetylglucosamine and N-acetylmuramic acid) cross-linked by peptide chains.

Peptidoglycan precursor formation takes place in the cytoplasm. The synthesis of UDP-acetylmuramyl-pentapeptide is completed with the addition of the dipeptide, D-Ala-D-Ala (formed by racemization and condensation of L-Ala). UDP-acetylmuramyl-pentapeptide and UDP-acetylglucosamine are linked to form a long polymer. The cross-link is completed by a transpeptidation reaction that occurs outside the cell membrane (Figure 44–2). The β-lactam antibiotics inhibit this last step in peptidoglycan synthesis, presumably by acylating the transpeptidase via cleavage of the—CO—N—bond of the β-lactam ring.

Although inhibition of the transpeptidase is demonstrably important, there are additional targets for the actions of penicillins and cephalosporins; these collectively are termed penicillin-binding proteins (PBPs). The transpeptidase responsible for peptidoglycan synthesis is one of these PBPs. Other PBPs are necessary for cell division and cell shape and other essential processes; thus, the lethality of penicillin for bacteria involves both lytic and nonlytic mechanisms.

MECHANISMS OF BACTERIAL RESISTANCE TO PENICILLINS AND CEPHALO-SPORINS
A sensitive strain may acquire resistance by mutations that decrease the affinity of PBPs for the antibiotic. Because β-lactam antibiotics inhibit many different PBPs, their affinity for several PBPs must decrease to confer resistance. Methicillin-resistant *S. aureus* are resistant *via* acquisition of an additional high-molecular-weight PBP (*via* a transposon) with a very low affinity for all β-lactam antibiotics; this mechanism is responsible for methicillin resistance in the coagulase-negative staphylococci.

Bacterial resistance to β-lactam antibiotics also results from the inability of the drug to penetrate to its site of action (Figure 44–3). In gram-positive bacteria, the peptidoglycan polymer is very near the cell surface and antibiotic penetration is not a problem. In gram-negative bacteria, the inner membrane is covered by the outer membrane, lipopolysaccharide, and capsule, which block access of some antibiotics. Some small hydrophilic antibiotics, including β-lactam antibiotics, diffuse through aqueous channels in the outer membrane formed by proteins called *porins*. These porins vary among different gram-negative bacteria, thereby providing greater or lesser antibiotics access to site of action. Active efflux pumps also can remove the antibiotic before it can act.

Bacteria also can destroy β-lactam antibiotics enzymatically via the actions of β-lactamases (Figures 44–1 and 44–3). The substrate specificities of some of these enzymes are relatively narrow; such enzymes are sometimes referred to as penicillinases or cephalosporinases. Other "extended-spectrum" enzymes can hydrolyze a variety of β-lactam antibiotics.

In general, gram-positive bacteria produce and secrete large amounts of β-lactamase (Figure 44–3). Most of these enzymes are penicillinases. The staphylococcal penicillinase is encoded in a plasmid that may be transferred to other bacteria and is inducible by substrate. In gram-negative bacteria, β-lactamases are strategically located in the periplasmic space between the inner and outer cell membranes for maximal protection of the microbe (Figure 44–3). β-lactamases of gram-negative bacteria are encoded either in chromosomes or plasmids, and may be constitutive or inducible. The

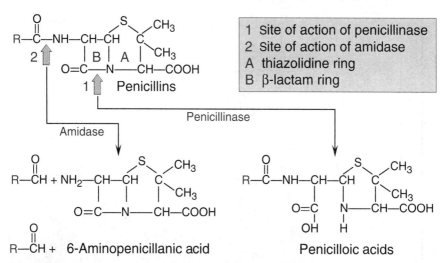

1 Site of action of penicillinase
2 Site of action of amidase
A thiazolidine ring
B β-lactam ring

FIGURE 44–1 *Structure of penicillins and products of their enzymatic hydrolysis.*

plasmids can be transferred between bacteria by conjugation. These enzymes can hydrolyze penicillins, cephalosporins, or both.

OTHER FACTORS THAT INFLUENCE THE ACTIVITY OF β-LACTAM ANTIBIOTICS
Microorganisms adhering to implanted prosthetic devices (e.g., catheters, artificial joints, prosthetic heart valves) produce biofilms. Bacteria in biofilms are much less sensitive to antibiotic therapy, in part owing to decreased growth rates. The β-lactam antibiotics are most active against bacteria in the logarithmic phase of growth and have little effect on microorganisms in the stationary phase. Similarly, intracellular bacteria that survive inside host cells generally are protected from the action of the β-lactam antibiotics.

Classification of the Penicillins and Summary of Their Pharmacological Properties
Penicillins are classified according to their spectra of antimicrobial activity (Table 44–1).

1. *Penicillin G* and its close congener *penicillin V* are highly active against sensitive strains of gram-positive cocci but are readily hydrolyzed by penicillinase and therefore ineffective against most strains of *S. aureus.*
2. The penicillinase-resistant penicillins (*methicillin* [discontinued in the U.S.], *nafcillin, oxacillin, cloxacillin* [not marketed in the U.S.], and *dicloxacillin*) have less potent antimicrobial activity against microorganisms that are sensitive to penicillin G but are the agents of first choice for treatment of penicillinase-producing *S. aureus* and *S. epidermidis* that are not methicillin-resistant.
3. *Ampicillin, amoxicillin,* and others comprise a group of penicillins whose antimicrobial activity is extended to include such gram-negative microorganisms as *Haemophilus influenzae, Escherichia coli,* and *Proteus mirabilis.* Frequently these drugs are administered with a β-lactamase inhibitor to prevent hydrolysis by broad-spectrum β-lactamases that are found with increasing frequency in clinical isolates of these gram-negative bacteria.
4. The antimicrobial activity of *carbenicillin* (discontinued in the U.S.), its indanyl ester (*carbenicillin indanyl*), and *ticarcillin* includes *Pseudomonas, Enterobacter,* and *Proteus* spp. These agents are inferior to ampicillin against gram-positive cocci and *Listeria monocytogenes* and are less active than piperacillin against *Pseudomonas.*
5. *Mezlocillin, azlocillin* (both discontinued in the U.S.), and *piperacillin* have excellent antimicrobial activity against *Pseudomonas, Klebsiella,* and certain other gram-negative microorganisms. Piperacillin retains the activity of ampicillin against gram-positive cocci and *L. monocytogenes.*

Certain useful generalizations can be made. Following oral or parenteral administration, these agents distribute widely throughout the body. Therapeutic concentrations of penicillins are achieved

Table 44-1

Chemical Structures and Major Properties of Various Penicillins

$$R-C-NH_2-CH-CH \quad \overset{S}{\underset{}{C}} \overset{CH_3}{\underset{CH_3}{C}}$$
$$\overset{O}{\overset{\|}{ }} \qquad O=C-N-CH-COOH$$

Penicillins are substituted 6-aminopenicillanic acids

Nonproprietary Name	R	Major Properties		
		Absorption after Oral Administration	Resistance to Penicillinase	Useful Antimicrobial Spectrum
Penicillin G	⬡—CH₂—	Variable (poor)	No	*Streptococcus* species, * Enterococci,* *Listeria, Neisseria meningitidis,* many anaerobes (not *Bacteroides fragilis*),* spirochetes, *Actinomyces, Erysipelothrix* spp., *Pasteurella multocida***
Penicillin V	⬡—OCH₂—	Good	No	
Methicillin	dimethoxyphenyl (OCH₃, OCH₃)	Poor (not given orally)	Yes	
Oxacillin (R₁ = R₂ = H) Cloxacillin (R₁ = Cl; R₂ = H) Dicloxacillin (R₁ = R₂ = Cl)	isoxazolyl-substituted phenyl (R₁, R₂, CH₃)	Good	Yes	Indicated only for non-methicillin-resistant strains of *Staphylococcus aureus* and *Staphylococcus epidermidis.* Compared to other penicillins, these penicillinase-resistant penicillins lack activity against *Listeria monocytogenes* and *Enterococcus* spp.

730

Structure	Name			Spectrum
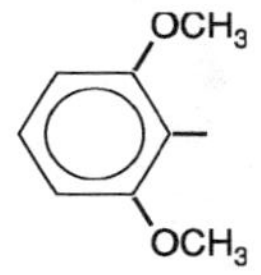 (2,6-dimethoxyphenyl, OCH₃ / OCH₃)	Nafcillin	Variable	Yes	
(phenyl-CH(R₁)-NH₂)	Ampicillin† (R₁ = H)	Good	No	Extends spectrum of penicillin to include sensitive strains of Enterobacteriaceae*** *Escherichia coli*, *Proteus mirabilis*, *Salmonella*, *Shigella*, *Haemophilus influenzae*,*** and *Helicobacter pylori*.
	Amoxicillin (R₁ = OH)	Excellent		Superior to penicillin for treatment of *Listeria monocytogenes* and sensitive enterococci. Amoxicillin most active of all oral β-lactams against penicillin-resistant *Streptococcus pneumoniae*
(phenyl-CH(COOR₁)-)	Carbenicillin (R₁ = H)	Poor (not given orally)	No	Good
	Carbenicillin indanyl (R₁ = 5-indanol)	Good	No	Less active than ampicillin against *Streptococcus* species, *Enterococcus faecalis*, *Klebsiella*, and *Listeria monocytogenes*. Activity against *Pseudomonas aeruginosa* is inferior to that of mezlocillin and piperacillin
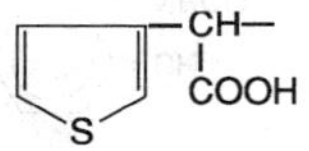 (thiophene-CH(COOH)-)	Ticarcillin	Poor (not given orally)	No	
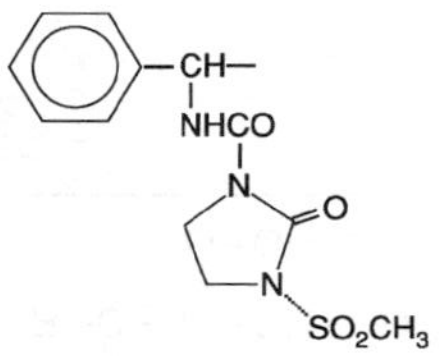 (phenyl-CH(NHCO)- with N-substituted oxo-pyrrolidinone-SO₂CH₃)	Mezlocillin	Poor (not given orally)	No	

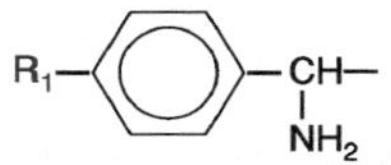

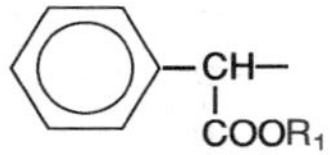

(Continued)

731

Table 44-1

Chemical Structures and Major Properties of Various Penicillins *(Continued)*

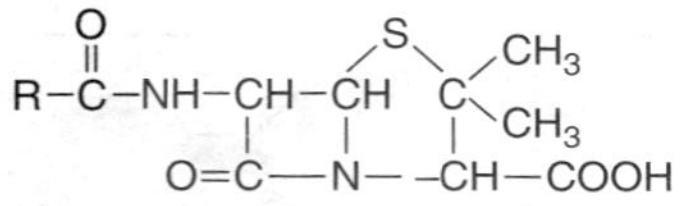

Penicillins are substituted 6-aminopenicillanic acids

$$
\begin{array}{c}
\text{O} \\
\parallel \\
\text{R}-\text{C}-\text{NH}-\text{CH}-\text{CH} \quad \overset{\text{S}}{\diagdown} \quad \text{C} \overset{\diagup \text{CH}_3}{\diagdown \text{CH}_3} \\
\mid \quad\quad\quad\quad\quad \mid \\
\text{O}=\text{C}-\text{N}--\text{CH}-\text{COOH}
\end{array}
$$

		Major Properties	
Nonproprietary Name	Absorption after Oral Administration	Resistance to Penicillinase	Useful Antimicrobial Spectrum
R			
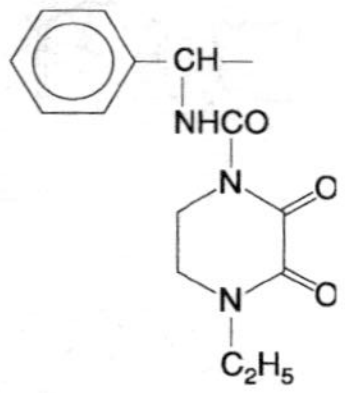 Piperacillin	Poor (not given orally)	No	Extends spectrum of ampicillin to include *Pseudomonas aeruginosa*,[‡] Enterobacteriaceae,** Bacteroides species**

[*]Many strains are resistant due to altered penicillin-binding proteins.
[**]Many strains are resistant due to production of β-lactamases.
[†]There are other congeners of ampicillin; *see* the text.
[‡]Some strains are resistant due to decreased entry or active efflux.

732

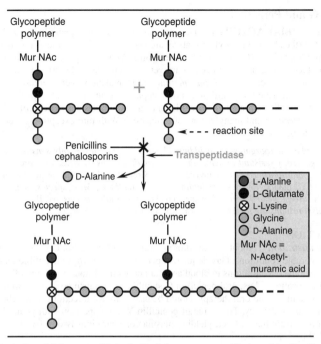

FIGURE 44–2 *Action of β-lactam antibiotics in Staphylococcus aureus.* The bacterial cell wall consists of glycopeptide polymers linked via bridges between amino acid side chains. In *S. aureus*, the bridge is $(Gly)_5$-D-Ala between lysines. The cross-linking is catalyzed by a transpeptidase, the enzyme that penicillins and cephalosporins inhibit.

readily in tissues and in many secretions. Penicillins do not significantly penetrate living phagocytic cells, and only low concentrations are found in prostatic secretions, brain, and intraocular fluid. Concentrations of penicillins in cerebrospinal fluid (CSF) are <1% of those in plasma when the meninges are normal. With inflammation, CSF concentrations may increase to 5% of the plasma value. Penicillins are eliminated rapidly by the kidney; their half-lives in the body are short (typically 30–90 minutes) and their urine concentrations are high.

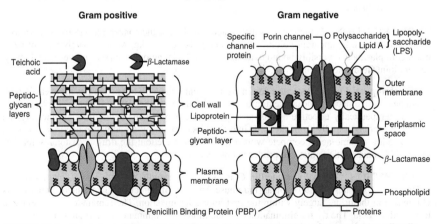

FIGURE 44–3 *Comparison of the structure and composition of gram-positive and gram-negative cell walls.*

Penicillin G and Penicillin V

ANTIMICROBIAL ACTIVITY The antimicrobial spectra of penicillin G *(benzylpenicillin)* and penicillin V (the phenoxymethyl derivative) are very similar for aerobic gram-positive microorganisms. Penicillin G is 5–10 times more active against *Neisseria* spp. and certain anaerobes. Most streptococci (but not enterococci) are very susceptible to the drug. However, penicillin-resistant *viridans* streptococci and *S. pneumoniae* are increasingly seen. Penicillin-resistant pneumococci also are resistant to third-generation cephalosporins and are especially common in children. More than 90% of staphylococcal isolates are now resistant to penicillin G, as are most strains of *S. epidermidis* and many strains of gonococci. With rare exceptions, meningococci are quite sensitive to penicillin G.

Most anaerobic microorganisms, including Clostridium *spp., are highly sensitive.* Bacteroides fragilis *is generally resistant to penicillins and cephalosporins by virtue of expressing a broad-spectrum cephalosporinase.* Actinomyces israelii, Streptobacillus moniliformis, Pasteurella multocida, *and* L. monocytogenes *are inhibited by penicillin G. Most species of* Leptospira *are moderately susceptible to the drug.* Treponema pallidum *is exquisitely sensitive.* Borrelia burgdorferi, *the organism responsible for Lyme disease, also is susceptible.*

ABSORPTION

Oral Administration About one-third of an oral dose of penicillin G is absorbed from the GI tract under favorable conditions. Gastric juice at pH 2 rapidly destroys the antibiotic. Absorption is rapid, and maximal concentrations in blood are attained within 1 hour. Ingestion of food may interfere with GI absorption. Thus, oral penicillin G should be administered at least 30 minutes before or 2 hours after a meal, and oral therapy should be used only for infections in which clinical experience has proven its efficacy. The virtue of penicillin V in comparison with penicillin G is that it is better absorbed from the GI tract, yielding plasma concentrations two to five times greater than those provided by penicillin G.

Parenteral Administration of Penicillin G After intramuscular injection, peak concentrations in plasma are reached within 15–30 minutes. This value declines rapidly ($t_{1/2}$ of 30 minutes). Repository preparations of penicillin G increase the duration of its effect. Such compounds include *penicillin G procaine* (WYCILLIN, others) and *penicillin G benzathine* (BICILLIN L-A, PERMAPEN), which produce relatively low but persistent levels of penicillin in the blood.

Penicillin G procaine suspension combines procaine with penicillin in equimolar ratios; a dose of 300,000 units contains ~120 mg procaine, which exerts local anesthetic effects when injected. If the patient is believed to be hypersensitive to procaine, a test dose of 0.1 mL of 1% solution of procaine should be injected first.

Penicillin G benzathine suspension is the aqueous suspension of the salt obtained by combining 1 mol of an ammonium base and 2 mol of penicillin G; this provides a very slow release. The persistence of penicillin in the blood after an intramuscular dose reduces cost, need for repeated injections, and local trauma. The average duration of demonstrable antimicrobial activity in the plasma is 26 days.

DISTRIBUTION Penicillin G is distributed widely, but the concentration differs in various fluids and tissues. Its apparent volume of distribution is ~0.35 L/kg. Approximately 60% of penicillin G in plasma is reversibly bound to albumin. Significant amounts appear in liver, bile, kidney, semen, joint fluid, and lymph.

Cerebrospinal Fluid Penicillin does not readily enter the CSF but penetrates more easily with meningeal inflammation. The concentration attained usually reaches 5% of the value in plasma and thus is therapeutically effective against susceptible microorganisms. Penicillin and other organic acids are secreted rapidly from the CSF into the bloodstream by an active transport process. In uremia, other organic acids compete with penicillin for secretion; the drug occasionally reaches toxic CNS concentrations that can produce convulsions.

EXCRETION Normally, penicillin G is eliminated rapidly from the body, mainly by the kidney. Approximately 60–90% of an intramuscular dose of penicillin G in aqueous solution is eliminated in the urine, largely within the first hour after injection. The remainder is metabolized to penicilloic acid. The $t_{1/2}$ for elimination of penicillin G is ~30 minutes in normal adults. Approximately 10% of the drug is eliminated by glomerular filtration and 90% by tubular secretion.

Clearance values are considerably lower in neonates and infants because of incomplete development of renal function; thus, penicillin persists in the blood for several times as long in premature infants as in children and adults. After renal function is fully established in young children, renal excretion is considerably more rapid than in adults.

Anuria increases the $t_{1/2}$ of penicillin G to ~10 hours. The dose of the drug must be readjusted during dialysis and the period of progressive recovery of renal function. If hepatic insufficiency also is present, the $t_{1/2}$ is prolonged even further.

THERAPEUTIC USES

Pneumococcal Infections

Penicillin G is the drug of choice for infections caused by sensitive strains of S. pneumoniae, but resistance is an increasing problem. Thus, for pneumococcal pneumonia, a third-generation cephalosporin or high-dose penicillin G (i.e., 20–24 million units daily by continuous intravenous infusion or in divided boluses every 2–3 hours) should be used until sensitivities are determined. For parenteral therapy of sensitive isolates, penicillin G or penicillin G procaine is favored. Therapy should be continued for 7–10 days, including 3–5 days after the patient is afebrile. Similarly, pneumococcal meningitis initially should be treated with a combination of vancomycin and a third-generation cephalosporin until it is established that the infecting pneumococcus is penicillin-sensitive. Recommended therapy is 20–24 million units of penicillin G daily by constant intravenous infusion or divided into boluses given every 2–3 hours for 14 days.

Streptococcal Infections

Pharyngitis is the most common disease produced by S. pyogenes. Penicillin-resistant isolates of this organism have yet to be observed. The preferred oral therapy is with penicillin V, 500 mg every 6 hours for 10 days. Equal results are produced by the administration of 600,000 units of penicillin G procaine intramuscularly once daily for 10 days or by a single injection of 1.2 million units of penicillin G benzathine. Parenteral therapy is preferred if there are questions of patient compliance. Penicillin therapy of streptococcal pharyngitis reduces the risk of subsequent acute rheumatic fever but not of post-streptococcal glomerulonephritis.

Streptococcal Toxic Shock and Necrotizing Fasciitis

These life-threatening infections are best treated with penicillin plus clindamycin *(to decrease toxin synthesis).*

Streptococcal Pneumonia, Arthritis, Meningitis, and Endocarditis

These uncommon conditions should be treated with penicillin G; daily doses of 12–20 million units are administered intravenously for 2–4 weeks (4 weeks for endocarditis).

Infections Caused by Other Streptococci

Viridans *streptococci, the leading cause of infectious endocarditis, increasingly are resistant to penicillin G; quantitative microbial sensitivities therefore should be determined in patients with endocarditis. Patients with penicillin-sensitive S. viridans endocarditis are treated successfully with 1.2 million units of procaine penicillin G four times daily for 2 weeks or with daily doses of 12–20 million units of intravenous penicillin G for 2 weeks, both regimens in combination with streptomycin or gentamicin.*

Recommended therapy for penicillin- and aminoglycoside-sensitive enterococcal endocarditis is 20 million units of penicillin G or 12 g ampicillin *daily administered intravenously in combination with low-dose gentamicin. Therapy usually should be continued for 6 weeks, but selected patients with a short duration of illness (<3 months) have been treated successfully in 4 weeks.*

Infections with Anaerobes

Many anaerobic infections are polymicrobial, and most of the organisms are sensitive to penicillin G. An exception is the B. fragilis group, 75% of which may be resistant. Pulmonary and periodontal infections usually respond well to penicillin G. Mild-to-moderate infections at these sites may be treated with oral medication (either penicillin G or penicillin V 400,000 units four times daily). More severe infections should be treated with 12–20 million units of penicillin G intravenously. Brain abscesses also frequently contain several species of anaerobes, and most experts use high doses of penicillin G (20 million units per day) plus metronidazole *or* chloramphenicol.

Staphylococcal Infections

The vast majority of staphylococcal infections involve penicillinase-producing organisms. Patients with staphylococcal infection should receive penicillinase-resistant penicillins (e.g., nafcillin or oxacillin). Staphylococcal infections increasingly involve methicillin-resistant staphylococci, which are resistant to penicillin G, all the penicillinase-resistant penicillins, and the cephalosporins. Vancomycin, linezolid, quinupristin–dalfopristin, *and* daptomycin *are active against these bacteria (see Chapter 46).*

Meningococcal Infections

Penicillin G is the drug of choice for meningococcal disease. Patients should be treated with high doses of penicillin given intravenously (see above). *The rare penicillin-resistant strains should be considered in patients who are slow to respond to treatment. Penicillin G does not eliminate the meningococcal carrier state and is ineffective for prophylaxis.*

Syphilis

Therapy of syphilis with penicillin G is highly effective. Primary, secondary, and latent syphilis of <1 year's duration may be treated with penicillin G procaine (2.4 million units per day intramuscularly), plus probenecid (1.0 g/day orally) to prolong the $t_{1/2}$, for 10 days or with 1–3 weekly intramuscular doses of 2.4 million units of penicillin G benzathine (three doses in patients with HIV infection). Patients with neurosyphilis or cardiovascular syphilis typically receive intensive therapy with 20 million units of penicillin G daily for 10 days. Since there are no proven alternatives for treating syphilis in pregnant women, penicillin-allergic individuals must be acutely desensitized to prevent anaphylaxis.

Infants with congenital syphilis discovered at birth or during the postnatal period should be treated for at least 10 days with 50,000 units per kg daily of aqueous penicillin G in two divided doses or 50,000 units per kg of procaine penicillin G in a single daily dose.

Most patients with secondary syphilis develop the Jarisch-Herxheimer reaction, including chills, fever, headache, myalgias, and arthralgias occurring several hours after the first dose of penicillin. This is likely due to release of spirochetal antigens that induce a host reaction. Reactions usually persist for a few hours to days but do not recur with subsequent penicillin injections; penicillin therapy should not be stopped.

Other Infections

Penicillin G is the drug of choice for all forms of actinomycosis. *The dose should be 12–20 million units of penicillin G intravenously per day for 6 weeks. Surgical drainage also may be needed.*

Neither penicillin nor any other antibiotic alters the incidence or the outcome of diphtheria; *specific antitoxin is the only effective treatment. Penicillin G can eliminate the carrier state. The parenteral administration of 2–3 million units per day in divided doses for 10–12 days eliminates the diphtheria bacilli from the pharynx and other sites in ~100% of patients. A single daily injection of penicillin G procaine for the same period produces comparable results.*

Penicillin G is the drug of choice for gas gangrene due to clostridia; *the dose is 12–20 million units per day given parenterally. Adequate débridement of the infected areas is essential. Antibiotics probably have no effect on the outcome of tetanus. Débridement and administration of human tetanus immune globulin may be indicated.*

Gingivostomatitis, produced by the synergistic action of Leptotrichia buccalis *and* fusospirochetes *that are present in the mouth, is readily treatable with penicillin. For simple "trench mouth," 500 mg penicillin V given every 6 hours for several days is usually sufficient.*

The two microorganisms responsible for rat-bite fever, Spirillum minor *and* Streptobacillus moniliformis, *are sensitive to penicillin G, the drug of choice. Since most cases due to* Streptobacillus *are complicated by bacteremia and often by infections of the synovia and endocardium, a daily dose of 12–15 million units given parenterally for 3–4 weeks is used.*

Ampicillin (with gentamicin for immunosuppressed patients with meningitis) and penicillin G are the drugs of choice for infections with L. monocytogenes. *The dose of penicillin G is 15–20 million units parenterally per day for at least 2 weeks. With endocarditis, treatment is for at least 4 weeks.*

Severe Lyme disease may be treated with 20 million units of intravenous penicillin G daily for 14 days. The causative agent of erysipeloid, Erysipelothrix rhusiopathiae, *is sensitive to penicillin. Uncomplicated infection responds to a single injection of 1.2 million units of penicillin G benzathine. If endocarditis is present, penicillin G, 12–20 million units per day for 4–6 weeks is required.*

PROPHYLACTIC USES OF THE PENICILLINS

Streptococcal Infections

The administration of penicillin to individuals exposed to S. pyogenes *protects against infection. The oral ingestion of 200,000 units of penicillin G or penicillin V twice a day or a single injection of 1.2 million units of penicillin G benzathine is effective. Indications for prophylaxis include outbreaks of streptococcal disease in closed populations* (e.g., *boarding schools or military bases).*

The oral administration of 200,000 units of penicillin G or penicillin V every 12 hours markedly decreases the incidence of recurrences of rheumatic fever in susceptible individuals. Intramuscular injection of 1.2 million units of penicillin G benzathine once monthly also yields excellent results. Because acute rheumatic fever has been observed in the fifth decade, some advocate that prophylaxis should be continued for life.

Syphilis

Prophylaxis for a contact with syphilis consists of a course of therapy as described for primary syphilis. Serologies for syphilis should be tested monthly for at least 4 months thereafter.

Penicillinase-Resistant Penicillins

These penicillins resist hydrolysis by staphylococcal penicillinase. Their appropriate use is restricted to the treatment of infections that are known or suspected to be caused by staphylococci that elaborate the enzyme, including the vast majority of strains that are encountered clinically. These drugs are much less active than penicillin G against other penicillin-sensitive microorganisms.

The role of the penicillinase-resistant penicillins for most staphylococcal disease is decreasing with the increasing frequency of so-called methicillin-resistant microorganisms. Both *S. aureus* and *S. epidermidis* increasingly are resistant. Vancomycin is the drug of choice for serious infection caused by methicillin-resistant variants of these strains; rifampin is given concurrently when a foreign body is present.

ISOXAZOLYL PENICILLINS: OXACILLIN, CLOXACILLIN, AND DICLOXACILLIN These semisynthetic penicillins are similar structurally and pharmacologically (Table 44–1). All are relatively stable in an acid medium and are absorbed adequately after oral administration. All are markedly resistant to cleavage by penicillinase. These drugs are not substitutes for penicillin G in the treatment of diseases amenable to it and are not active against enterococci or *Listeria.* Oral administration is not a substitute for the parenteral route in the treatment of serious staphylococcal infections.

Pharmacological Properties

The isoxazolyl penicillins potently inhibit the growth of most penicillinase-producing staphylococci. Dicloxacillin is the most active. They are less effective against microorganisms susceptible to penicillin G and are not useful against gram-negative bacteria.

These agents are rapidly but incompletely absorbed from the GI tract (30–80%). As absorption is more efficient on an empty stomach, they ideally are administered 1 hour before or 2 hours after meals. Peak concentrations in plasma are attained by 1 hour. They all are highly bound to plasma albumin (>90%); none is removed from the circulation to a significant degree by hemodialysis.

The isoxazolyl penicillins are excreted rapidly by the kidney. Normally, ~50% of these drugs are excreted in the urine within 6 hours of an oral dose. They also are eliminated in the bile. Their half-lives are between 30 and 60 minutes. Intervals between doses are unchanged for patients with renal failure.

NAFCILLIN

Nafcillin (see Table 44–1) is highly resistant to penicillinase and has proven effective against infections caused by penicillinase-producing strains of S. aureus.

Pharmacological Properties

Nafcillin is slightly more active than oxacillin against penicillin G–resistant S. aureus. *While it is the most active of the penicillinase-resistant penicillins for most microorganisms, it is not as potent as penicillin G.*

Oral absorption of nafcillin is irregular, and injectable preparations should be used. Nafcillin is ~90% bound to plasma protein. Peak concentrations of nafcillin in bile exceed those found in plasma. Drug concentrations in CSF are adequate for therapy of staphylococcal meningitis.

Aminopenicillins: Ampicillin, Amoxicillin, and Their Congeners

ANTIMICROBIAL ACTIVITY

Ampicillin and the related aminopenicillins are bactericidal for both gram-positive and gram-negative bacteria. The meningococci and L. monocytogenes *are sensitive to this class of drugs.*

Many pneumococcal isolates have varying levels of resistance to ampicillin. Penicillin-resistant strains should be considered ampicillin/amoxicillin-resistant. H. influenzae *and the* viridans *group of streptococci exhibit varying degrees of resistance.* Enterococci *are twice as sensitive to ampicillin as they are to penicillin. From 30% to 50% of E.* coli, *a significant number of P.* mirabilis, *and practically all species of* Enterobacter *are insensitive. Resistant strains of Salmonella are recovered with increasing frequency. Most strains of* Shigella, Pseudomonas, Klebsiella, Serratia, Acinetobacter, *and indole-positive* Proteus *are resistant to this group of penicillins; these antibiotics are less active against* B. fragilis *than is penicillin G. Concurrent administration of β-lactamase inhibitors markedly expands their spectrum of activity (see below).*

AMPICILLIN This drug is the prototype of the group (see structure in Table 44–1).

Pharmacological Properties Ampicillin (PRINCIPEN, others) is well absorbed after oral administration. Intake of food prior to ampicillin ingestion diminishes absorption. Severe renal impairment markedly prolongs the $t_{1/2}$ of ampicillin in the plasma. Peritoneal dialysis does not remove the drug from the blood, but hemodialysis removes ~40% of the body store in 7 hours. Ampicillin doses must be decreased in the setting of renal dysfunction. Ampicillin undergoes enterohepatic circulation and is excreted in appreciable quantities in the feces.

AMOXICILLIN This penicillinase-susceptible penicillin is closely related to ampicillin (Table 44–1). The drug is absorbed more rapidly and completely from the GI tract than is ampicillin. The antimicrobial spectrum of amoxicillin is essentially identical to that of ampicillin, except that amoxicillin is less effective for shigellosis.

Peak plasma concentrations of amoxicillin (AMOXIL, others) are twice those of ampicillin after oral administration of the same dose. Food does not interfere with absorption. Perhaps because of its more complete absorption, the incidence of diarrhea with amoxicillin is less than that with ampicillin. The incidence of other adverse effects is similar. While the $t_{1/2}$ of amoxicillin is similar to that for ampicillin, effective concentrations of orally administered amoxicillin are detectable in the plasma for twice as long as with ampicillin because of its more complete absorption. About 20% of amoxicillin is protein-bound in plasma. Most of the antibiotic is excreted in an active form in the urine.

THERAPEUTIC INDICATIONS FOR THE AMINOPENICILLINS

Upper Respiratory Infections Ampicillin and amoxicillin are active against *S. pyogenes* and many strains of *S. pneumoniae* and *H. influenzae*, which are major upper respiratory pathogens. The drugs are effective for sinusitis, otitis media, acute exacerbations of chronic bronchitis, and epiglottitis caused by sensitive strains of these organisms. Amoxicillin is the most active of the oral β-lactam antibiotics against both penicillin-sensitive and penicillin-resistant *S. pneumoniae*. Based on the increasing prevalence of pneumococcal resistance to penicillin, an increase in dose of oral amoxicillin (from 40–45 to 80–90 mg/kg/day) for empirical treatment of acute otitis media in children is recommended. Ampicillin-resistant *H. influenzae* also is a problem in many areas. The addition of a β-lactamase inhibitor (amoxicillin–clavulanate or ampicillin–sulbactam) extends the spectrum to β-lactamase-producing *H. influenzae* and Enterobacteriaceae. Bacterial pharyngitis should be treated with penicillin G or penicillin V because *S. pyogenes* is the major pathogen.

Urinary Tract Infections Most uncomplicated urinary tract infections are caused by Enterobacteriaceae, and *E. coli* is the most common species; ampicillin often is an effective agent, although resistance is increasing. Enterococcal urinary tract infections are treated effectively with ampicillin alone.

Meningitis Ampicillin is not indicated for single-agent treatment of acute bacterial meningitis in children. Ampicillin has excellent activity against *L. monocytogenes*, which causes meningitis in immunocompromised persons. Thus, the combination of ampicillin and vancomycin plus a third-generation cephalosporin is a rational regimen for empirical treatment of suspected bacterial meningitis.

Salmonella Infections High doses of ampicillin (12 g/day for adults) are often effective, but resistance is common. The typhoid carrier state has been eliminated successfully in patients without gallbladder disease with ampicillin.

Antipseudomonal Penicillins: Carboxypenicillins and Ureidopenicillins

The carboxypenicillins, *carbenicillin* and *ticarcillin*, are active against some isolates of *P. aeruginosa* and certain indole-positive *Proteus* spp. that are resistant to ampicillin and its congeners. They are ineffective against most strains of *S. aureus, Enterococcus faecalis, Klebsiella,* and

L. monocytogenes. B. fragilis is susceptible to high concentrations of these drugs, but penicillin G is more active. The ureidopenicillins, *mezlocillin* and *piperacillin*, have superior activity against *P. aeruginosa* compared with carbenicillin and ticarcillin. Mezlocillin and piperacillin also are useful for *Klebsiella* infections. The carboxypenicillins and the ureidopenicillins are sensitive to destruction by β-lactamases.

CARBENICILLIN INDANYL (GEOCILLIN)
This indanyl ester of carbenicillin is excreted rapidly in the urine; its only use is for the management of urinary tract infections caused by Proteus spp. *other than* P. mirabilis *and by* P. aeruginosa.

TICARCILLIN (TICAR)
This semisynthetic penicillin (Table 44–1) is similar to carbenicillin but two to four times more active against P. aeruginosa. *Ticarcillin is inferior to piperacillin for serious infections caused by* Pseudomonas.

MEZLOCILLIN
This ureidopenicillin is more active against Klebsiella *than is carbenicillin; its activity against* Pseudomonas *is similar to that of ticarcillin. It is more active than ticarcillin against* E. faecalis. Mezlocillin sodium (MEZLIN) *has been discontinued in the U.S.*

PIPERACILLIN (PIPRACIL) Piperacillin (PIPRACIL) extends the spectrum of ampicillin to include most strains of *P. aeruginosa*, Enterobacteriaceae (non-β-lactamase-producing), many *Bacteroides* spp. and *E. faecalis*. In combination with a β-lactamase inhibitor (*piperacillin– tazobactam,* ZOSYN), it has the broadest antibacterial spectrum of the penicillins. Pharmacokinetic properties are reminiscent of the other ureidopenicillins. High biliary concentrations are achieved.

THERAPEUTIC INDICATIONS Piperacillin and related agents are important drugs for the treatment of serious infections caused by gram-negative bacteria, including infections acquired in the hospital. These penicillins find their greatest use in treating bacteremias, pneumonias, infections following burns, and urinary tract infections owing to microorganisms resistant to penicillin G and ampicillin; the bacteria especially responsible include *P. aeruginosa*, indole-positive strains of *Proteus*, and *Enterobacter* spp. Since *Pseudomonas* infections are common in neutropenic patients, therapy for severe bacterial infections in such individuals should include a β-lactam antibiotic such as piperacillin with good activity against these bacteria.

Untoward Reactions to Penicillins

HYPERSENSITIVITY REACTIONS Hypersensitivity reactions complicate 0.7–4% of all treatment courses: rash, urticaria, fever, bronchospasm, vasculitis, serum sickness, exfoliative dermatitis, and anaphylaxis. Allergy to one penicillin increases the risk of reaction if another penicillin is given. Hypersensitivity reactions may appear in the absence of previous known exposure to the drug. In some cases, the reaction is mild and disappears even when the penicillin is continued; in others, immediate cessation of penicillin is required. In a few instances, it is necessary to interdict the future use of penicillin because of the risk of death, and the patient should be so warned.

Penicillins and their breakdown products act as haptens after covalent reaction with proteins. The most abundant breakdown product is the penicilloyl (major) moiety. A large percentage of IgE-mediated reactions are to this derivative, but at least 25% of reactions are to other breakdown products. The terms *major* and *minor determinants* refer to the frequency with which antibodies to these haptens appear to form rather than the severity of the reaction that may result, and anaphylactic reactions to penicillin usually are mediated by IgE antibodies against minor determinants.

Antipenicillin antibodies are detectable in virtually all patients who have received the drug (and in many who deny previous exposure). Immediate allergic reactions are mediated by skin-sensitizing or IgE antibodies, usually of minor-determinant specificities. Accelerated and late urticarial reactions usually are mediated by major-determinant–specific skin-sensitizing antibodies. Some reactions may be due to toxic antigen–antibody complexes of major-determinant-specific IgM antibodies.

Rashes of all types may be caused by allergy to penicillin. Henoch–Schönlein purpura with renal involvement has been a rare complication. Contact dermatitis is observed occasionally in pharmacists, nurses, and physicians who prepare penicillin solutions. Fixed-drug reactions also have occurred. More severe reactions involving the skin are exfoliative dermatitis and exudative erythema multiforme. The incidence of rashes appears to be highest following the use of ampicillin (~9%); rash follows the administration of ampicillin in nearly all patients with infectious mononucleosis.

The most serious hypersensitivity reactions produced by the penicillins are angioedema and anaphylaxis. Acute anaphylactic or anaphylactoid reactions to the penicillins constitute the most important immediate danger connected with their use. *Among all drugs, the penicillins are most often responsible for this type of untoward effect.* Anaphylactoid reactions to penicillins may occur at any age; their incidence is thought to be 0.004–0.04%. About 0.001% of patients treated with these agents die from anaphylaxis. Anaphylaxis most often has followed parenteral use but also has been observed after oral or intradermal administration. The most dramatic reaction is sudden hypotension and death. In other instances, bronchoconstriction with severe asthma; abdominal pain, nausea, and vomiting; extreme weakness; or diarrhea and purpuric skin eruptions have characterized the anaphylactic episodes.

Serum sickness reactions mediated by IgG antibodies can rarely appear after penicillin treatment has been continued for 1 week or more; they may be delayed until 1 or 2 weeks after the drug has been stopped and may persist for a week or longer.

Vasculitis may be related to penicillin hypersensitivity. The Coombs reaction frequently becomes positive during prolonged therapy, but hemolytic anemia is rare. Reversible neutropenia has been noted, occurring in up to 30% of patients treated with 8–12 g nafcillin for longer than 21 days. Eosinophilia occasionally accompanies other allergic reactions to penicillin.

Fever may be the only evidence of a hypersensitivity reaction to the penicillins. The febrile reaction usually disappears within 24–36 hours after drug administration is stopped but may persist for days. Penicillins rarely cause interstitial nephritis; methicillin has been implicated most frequently.

MANAGEMENT OF THE PATIENT POTENTIALLY ALLERGIC TO PENICILLIN

Evaluation of the patient's history is the most practical way to identify patients at greatest risk of allergic reaction. Most patients with a history of penicillin allergy should be treated with another antibiotic. There is no totally reliable means to confirm a history of penicillin allergy. Skin testing using major and minor penicillin determinants is useful if available. Occasionally, *desensitization* is recommended for penicillin-allergic patients who must receive the drug. Gradually, increasing doses of penicillin are administered in the hope of binding all of the IgE without provoking anaphylaxis. When full doses are reached, penicillin should not be stopped and then restarted, as immediate reactions may recur. This procedure should be performed only in an intensive care setting, and its efficacy is unproven.

Patients with life-threatening infections (*e.g.*, endocarditis or meningitis) may be continued on penicillin despite the development of a maculopapular rash, although alternative antibiotics should be used whenever possible. The rash often resolves as therapy is continued, perhaps owing to the development of blocking antibodies of the IgG class. Rarely, exfoliative dermatitis, with or without vasculitis, develops in these patients if therapy with penicillin is continued.

OTHER ADVERSE REACTIONS

Apparent toxic effects include bone marrow depression, granulocytopenia, and hepatitis; the latter is rare but is seen most commonly following the administration of oxacillin and nafcillin. Penicillin G, carbenicillin, piperacillin, or ticarcillin has been associated with impaired hemostasis due to defective platelet aggregation.

Most common among the irritative responses to penicillin are pain and sterile inflammation at sites of intramuscular injection. Phlebitis or thrombophlebitis develops in some individuals who receive penicillin intravenously. Many persons who take various penicillin preparations orally experience nausea, with or without vomiting, and some have mild-to-severe diarrhea. These manifestations often are dose related. Injection of penicillin G procaine may result in an immediate procaine reaction, with dizziness, tinnitus, headache, hallucinations, and sometimes seizures. Accidental injection of penicillin into the sciatic nerve causes severe local pain and dysfunction. Intrathecal injection of penicillin may produce arachnoiditis or encephalopathy and should be avoided. The parenteral administration of large doses of penicillin G (>20 million units per day, or less with renal insufficiency) may produce lethargy, confusion, twitching, multifocal myoclonus, or localized or generalized epileptiform seizures. These are most apt to occur in the presence of renal insufficiency, localized lesions of the CNS, or hyponatremia. When the CSF concentration of penicillin G exceeds 10 μg/mL, significant CNS dysfunction is frequent. The injection of 20 million units of penicillin G potassium, which contains 34 mEq of K^+, may lead to severe hyperkalemia in persons with renal dysfunction.

REACTIONS UNRELATED TO HYPERSENSITIVITY OR TOXICITY

Penicillin changes the composition of the microflora. This phenomenon is usually of no clinical significance, and the normal microflora are reestablished shortly after therapy is stopped. In some persons, superinfection results. Pseudomembranous colitis, related to overgrowth and production of a toxin by Clostridium difficile, *has followed oral and, less commonly, parenteral administration of penicillins.*

CEPHALOSPORINS

CHEMISTRY

Cephalosporins are produced from 7-aminocephalosporanic acid by the addition of different side chains (Table 44–2). Modifications at position 7 of the β-lactam ring alter antibacterial activity, while substitutions at position 3 of the dihydrothiazine ring alter the metabolism and pharmacokinetic properties. The cephamycins *are similar to the cephalosporins but have a methoxy group at position 7 of the β-lactam ring of the 7-aminocephalosporanic acid nucleus.*

MECHANISM OF ACTION

Cephalosporins and cephamycins inhibit bacterial cell wall synthesis in a manner similar to that of penicillin.

CLASSIFICATION Cephalosporins are classified by generations. The *first-generation* cephalosporins (*e.g.*, *cephalothin* and *cefazolin*) have good activity against gram-positive bacteria and relatively modest activity against gram-negative microorganisms. Most gram-positive cocci (with the exception of enterococci, methicillin-resistant *S. aureus*, and *S. epidermidis*) are susceptible. Most mouth anaerobes are sensitive, but the *B. fragilis* group is resistant. *Second-generation* cephalosporins have somewhat increased activity against gram-negative microorganisms but are much less active than the third-generation agents. A subset of second-generation drugs (*e.g.*, *cefoxitin, cefotetan*, and *cefmetazole*) also is active against *B. fragilis. Third-generation* cephalosporins generally are less active than first-generation agents against gram-positive cocci but are much more active against the Enterobacteriaceae, including β-lactamase-producing strains. A subset of third-generation agents (*e.g.*, *ceftazidime* and *cefoperazone*) also is active against *P. aeruginosa* but less active than other third-generation agents against gram-positive cocci. *Fourth-generation* cephalosporins, such as *cefepime*, have an extended activity spectrum compared with the third generation and resist hydrolysis by β-lactamases. Fourth-generation drugs are particularly useful for the empirical treatment of serious infections in hospitalized patients when gram-positive microorganisms, Enterobacteriaceae, and *Pseudomonas* all are potential etiologies. None of the cephalosporins has reliable activity against penicillin-resistant *S. pneumoniae*, methicillin-resistant *S. aureus*, methicillin-resistant *S. epidermidis*, and other coagulase-negative staphylococci, *Enterococcus, L. monocytogenes, Legionella pneumophila, L. micdadei, C. difficile, Xanthomonas maltophilia, Campylobacter jejuni*, and *Acinetobacter* spp.

MECHANISMS OF BACTERIAL RESISTANCE TO THE CEPHALOSPORINS

Cephalosporin resistance may be related to the inability of the antibiotic to reach its sites of action or to alterations in the PBPs that are their targets. Alterations in two PBPs that decrease their affinity for cephalosporins render pneumococci resistant to third-generation cephalosporins because the other three PBPs have inherently low affinity.

Cephalosporin resistance usually reflects hydrolysis of the β-lactam ring. The cephalosporins are variably susceptible to β-lactamase. Of the first-generation agents, cefazolin is more susceptible to hydrolysis by β-lactamase from S. aureus *than is cephalothin. Cefoxitin, cefuroxime, and the third-generation cephalosporins are more resistant to hydrolysis by the β-lactamases produced by gram-negative bacteria than first-generation cephalosporins. Third-generation cephalosporins are susceptible to hydrolysis by inducible, chromosomally encoded β-lactamases. Induction of β-lactamases by treatment of infections owing to aerobic gram-negative bacilli with second- or third-generation cephalosporins and/or imipenem may result in resistance to all third-generation cephalosporins. Fourth-generation cephalosporins (e.g., cefepime) are poor inducers of β-lactamases and are less susceptible to hydrolysis than the third-generation agents.*

GENERAL FEATURES OF THE CEPHALOSPORINS Cephalosporins are excreted primarily by the kidney, and dosage should be decreased in patients with renal insufficiency. *Cefpiramide* (not available in U.S.) and cefoperazone are excreted predominantly in the bile. *Cefotaxime* is deacetylated to a metabolite with less antimicrobial activity than the parent compound and excreted by the kidneys. The other cephalosporins do not undergo appreciable metabolism.

Several cephalosporins (*e.g.*, cefotaxime, ceftriaxone, and cefepime) penetrate into CSF in sufficient concentration to be useful for the treatment of meningitis. Cephalosporins also cross the pla-

Table 44-2

Names, Structural Formulas, Dosage, and Dosage Forms of Selected Cephalosporins and Related Compounds

Cephem nucleus

Compound (TRADE NAMES)	R_1	R_2	Dosage Forms,* Adult Dosage for Severe Infection, and $t_{1/2}$
First-generation Cefazolin (ANCEF, KEFZOL, others)		$-CH_2S$	I: 1–1.5 g every 6 hours $t_{1/2}$ = ~2 hours
Cephalexin (KEFLEX, others)		$-CH_3$	O: 1 g every 6 hours $t_{1/2}$ = 0.9 hour
Cefadroxil (DURICEF)		$-CH_3$	O: 1 g every 12 hours $t_{1/2}$ = 1.1 hours
Second-generation Cefoxitin[†] (MEFOXIN)		$-CH_2OC(=O)NH_2$	I: 2 g every 4 hours or 3 g every 6 hours $t_{1/2}$ = 0.7 hours
Cefaclor (CECLOR)		$-Cl$	O: 1 g every 8 hours $t_{1/2}$ = 0.7 hours

Drug	Structure	Dosing
Cefprozil (CEFZIL)	HO — with CH(NH₂) group; $-CH=CH-CH_2$	O: 500 mg every 12 hours $t_{1/2} = 1.3$ hours
Cefuroxime (ZINACEF)	furan ring with $C=N-OCH_3$; $-CH_2OC(=O)NH_2$	I: up to 3 g every 8 hours $t_{1/2} = 1.7$ hours
Cefuroxime acetil‡ (CEFTIN)		T: 500 mg every 12 hours
Loracarbef‖ (LORABID)	$-CH(NH_2)-$ phenyl; $-Cl$	O: 200–400 mg every 12 hours $t_{1/2} = 1.1$ hours
Cefotetan (CEFOTAN)	$H_2NC(=O)$, HOOC, thiazole; $-CH_2S$ tetrazole $-CH_3$	I: 2–3 g every 12 hours $t_{1/2} = 3.3$ hours
Ceforanide (PRECEF)	$-CH_2-$, $-CH_2NH_2$ phenyl	I: 1 g every 12 hours $t_{1/2} = 2.6$ hours
Third-generation Cefotaxime (CLAFORAN)	H_2N thiazole $C=N-OCH_3$; $-CH_2OC(=O)CH_3$	I: 2 g every 4–8 hours $t_{1/2} = 1.1$ hours

(Continued)

Table 44–2

Names, Structural Formulas, Dosage, and Dosage Forms of Selected Cephalosporins and Related Compounds (*Continued*)

Cephem nucleus

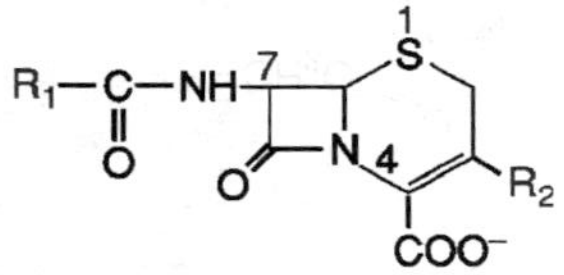

$R_1-\overset{\overset{\textstyle O}{\|}}{C}-NH-$ [cephem nucleus with positions 7, 1(S), 4(N), COO⁻, and R_2]

Compound (TRADE NAMES)	R_1	R_2	Dosage Forms,* Adult Dosage for Severe Infection, and $t_{1/2}$
Cefpodoxime proxetil§ (VANTIN)	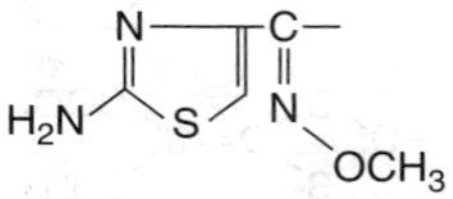 [aminothiazole–C(=N–OCH₃)–]	$-CH_2OCH_3$	O: 200–400 mg every 12 hours $t_{1/2}$ = 2.2 hours
Cefibuten (CEDAX)	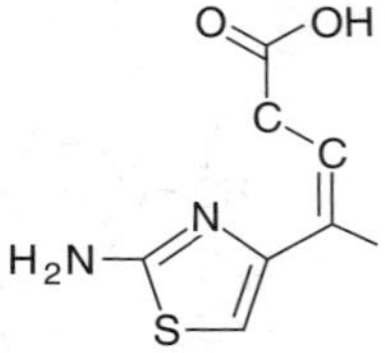 [aminothiazole with =C(COOH)O–C]	$-H$	O: 400 mg every 24 hours $t_{1/2}$ = 2.4 hours
Cefdinir (OMNICEF)	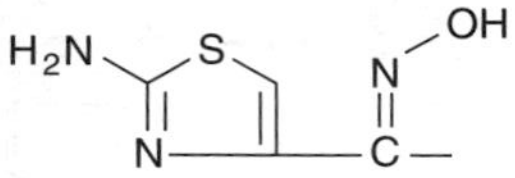 [aminothiazole–C(=N–OH)–]	$-CH=CH_2$	O: 300 mg every 12 hours or 600 mg every 24 hours $t_{1/2}$ = 1.7 hours
Cefditoren pivoxil (SPECTRACEF)	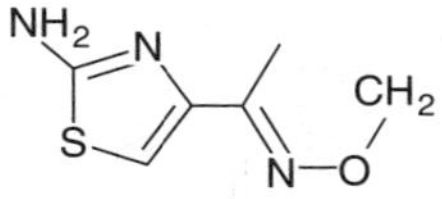 [aminothiazole–C(=N–O–CH₂)–]	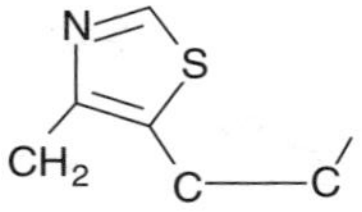 [methylthiazole–CH₂–]	O: 400 mg every 12 hours $t_{1/2}$ = 1.6 hours

744

Ceftizoxime (CEFIZOX)

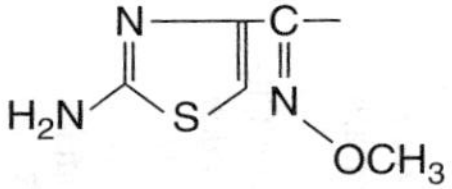

—H

I: 3–4 g every 8 hours
$t_{1/2} = 1.8$ hours

Ceftriaxone (ROCEPHIN)

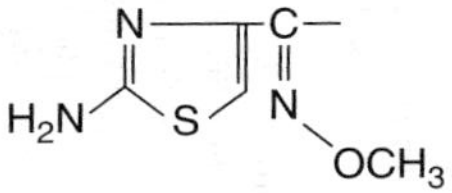

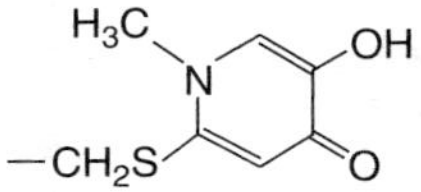

I: 2 g every 12–24 hours
$t_{1/2} = 8$ hours

Cefoperazone (CEFOBID)

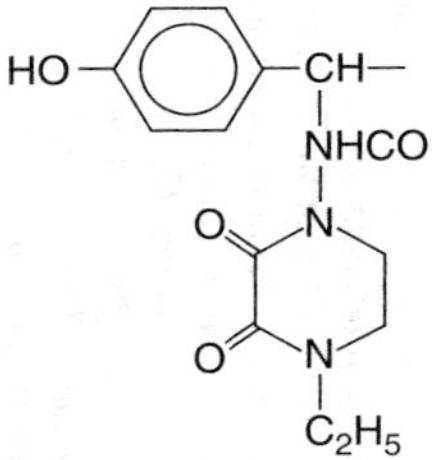

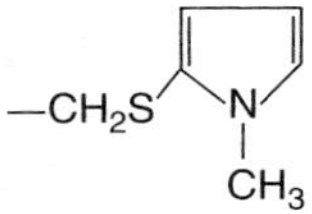

I: 1.5–4 g every 6–8 hours
$t_{1/2} = 2.1$ hours

Ceftazidime (HORTAZ, others)

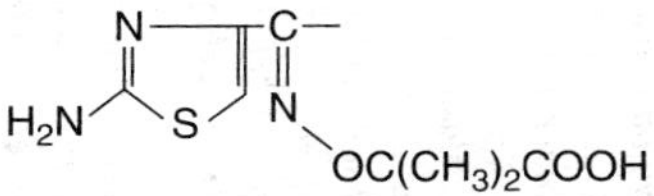

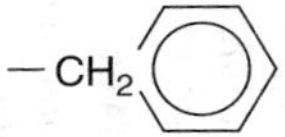

I: 2 g every 8 hours
$t_{1/2} = 1.8$ hours

Fourth-generation
Cefepime (MAXIPIME)

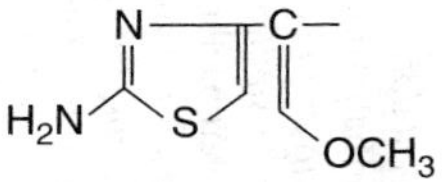

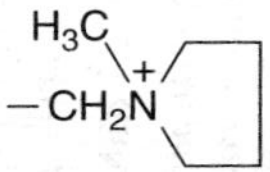

I: 2 g every 8 hours
$t_{1/2} = 2$ hours

---

*T, tablet; C, capsule; O, oral suspension; I, injection.
†Cefoxitin, a cephamycin, has a $-OCH_3$ group at position 7 of cephem nucleus.
‡Cefuroxime axetil is the acetyloxyethyl ester of cefuroxime.
‡Loracarbef, a carbacephem, has a carbon instead of sulfur at position 1 of cephem nucleus.
§Cefpodoxime proxetil has a $-COOCH(CH_3)OCOOCH(CH_3)_2$ group at position 4 of cephem nucleus.

centa and are found in high concentrations in synovial and pericardial fluids. Penetration into the aqueous humor of the eye is relatively good after systemic administration of third-generation agents, but penetration into the vitreous humor is poor. Concentrations sufficient for therapy of ocular infections owing to gram-positive and certain gram-negative microorganisms likely can be achieved after systemic administration. Concentrations in bile usually are high, especially with cefoperazone and cefpiramide.

Specific Agents
FIRST-GENERATION CEPHALOSPORINS

The antibacterial spectrum of cefazolin is typical of first-generation cephalosporins except that it has activity against some Enterobacter *spp. Cefazolin is relatively well tolerated; it is excreted by glomerular filtration and is ~85% bound to plasma proteins. Cefazolin usually is preferred among the first-generation cephalosporins because it can be administered less frequently owing to its longer $t_{1/2}$.*

Cephalexin has the same antibacterial spectrum as the other first-generation cephalosporins. It is somewhat less active against penicillinase-producing staphylococci. Oral therapy with cephalexin provides peak plasma concentrations adequate to inhibit many gram-positive and gram-negative pathogens. The drug is not metabolized and 70–100% is excreted in the urine.

Cephradine is similar in structure to cephalexin and almost identical in its clinical use. Cephradine is not metabolized and, after rapid absorption from the GI tract, is excreted unchanged in the urine. Because cephradine is so well absorbed, concentrations in plasma are nearly equivalent after oral or intramuscular administration.

Cefadroxil is the para-hydroxy analog of cephalexin. Concentrations of cefadroxil in plasma and urine are somewhat higher than are those of cephalexin. The drug is given orally once or twice a day for the treatment of urinary tract infections. Its activity is similar to that of cephalexin.

SECOND-GENERATION CEPHALOSPORINS

Second-generation cephalosporins have a broader spectrum than first-generation agents and are active against Enterobacter *spp.,* indole-positive Proteus *spp., and* Klebsiella *spp. Their serum half-lives are generally ~1–2 hours.*

Cefoxitin is resistant to some β-lactamases produced by gram-negative rods. This antibiotic is less active than the first-generation cephalosporins against gram-positive bacteria, but is more active against anaerobes, especially B. fragilis. *Cefoxitin's special role is for treatment of certain anaerobic and mixed aerobic-anaerobic infections, such as pelvic inflammatory disease and lung abscess.*

Cefaclor's concentration in plasma after oral administration is ~50% of that achieved after an equivalent oral dose of cephalexin. However, cefaclor is more active against H. influenzae *and* Moraxella catarrhalis, *although some β-lactamase-producing strains may be resistant. Loracarbef is similar in activity to cefaclor, which is more stable against some β-lactamases.*

Cefuroxime is similar to loracarbef with broader gram-negative activity against some Citrobacter *and* Enterobacter *spp. Unlike cefoxitin, cefmetazole, and cefotetan, cefuroxime lacks activity against* B. fragilis. *The drug can be given every 8 hours. Concentrations in CSF are ~10% of those in plasma; the drug is effective (but inferior to ceftriaxone) for treatment of meningitis owing to* H. influenzae *(including strains resistant to ampicillin),* N. meningitidis, *and* S. pneumoniae.

Cefuroxime axetil is the 1-acetyloxyethyl ester of cefuroxime. Between 30% and 50% of an oral dose is absorbed and then hydrolyzed to cefuroxime; resulting concentrations in plasma are variable.

Cefotetan, like cefoxitin, has good activity against B. fragilis *and several other species of* Bacteroides *and is slightly more active than cefoxitin against gram-negative aerobes. Hypoprothrombinemia and inhibition of vitamin K activation with bleeding have occurred in malnourished patients receiving cefotetan; this is preventable if vitamin K is also administered.*

Cefprozil is an orally administered agent that is more active than first-generation cephalosporins against penicillin-sensitive streptococci, E. coli, P. mirabilis, Klebsiella *spp., and* Citrobacter *spp.*

THIRD-GENERATION CEPHALOSPORINS

Cefotaxime is highly resistant to many β-lactamases and has good activity against many bacteria; activity against B. fragilis *is poor compared with clindamycin or metronidazole. Cefotaxime should be administered every 4–8 hours for serious infections. The drug is metabolized* in vivo *to desacetylcefotaxime, which is less active against most microorganisms than the parent compound but acts synergistically with the parent compound against certain microbes. Cefotaxime has been used effectively for meningitis caused by* H. influenzae, *penicillin-sensitive* S. pneumoniae, *and* N. meningitides.

Ceftizoxime has a spectrum of activity that is very similar to that of cefotaxime, except that it is less active against S. pneumoniae *and more active against* B. fragilis. *The drug can be administered every 8–12 hours for serious infections. Ceftizoxime is not metabolized, and 90% is recovered in urine.*

Ceftriaxone has activity very similar to that of ceftizoxime and cefotaxime but a $t_{1/2}$ *of ~8 hours. Administration of the drug once or twice daily has been effective for patients with meningitis, and dosage once a day is effective for other infections. About half the drug can be recovered in the urine; the remainder is eliminated by biliary secretion. A single dose of ceftriaxone (125–250 mg) is effective in the treatment of urethral, cervical, rectal, or pharyngeal gonorrhea, including penicillinase-producing microorganisms.*

Cefpodoxime proxetil is an orally administered third-generation agent that is very similar in activity to the fourth-generation agent cefepime (see below) except that it is not more active against Enterobacter *or* Pseudomonas *spp.*

Cefditoren pivoxil is a prodrug that is hydrolyzed by esterases during absorption to the active drug, cefditoren. Cefditoren is eliminated unchanged in the urine. The drug is active against methicillin-susceptible strains of S. aureus, *penicillin-susceptible strains of* S. pneumoniae, S. pyogenes, H. influenzae, H. parainfluenzae, *and* Moraxella catarrhali. *Cefditoren pivoxil is only indicated for the treatment of mild-to-moderate pharyngitis, tonsillitis, uncomplicated skin and skin structure infections, and acute exacerbations of chronic bronchitis.*

Ceftibuten is an orally effective drug that is less active against gram-positive and gram-negative organisms than cefixime, with activity limited to S. pneumonia *and* S. pyogenes, H. influenzae, *and* M. catarrhalis. *Ceftibuten is only indicated for acute bacterial exacerbations of chronic bronchitis, acute bacterial otitis media, pharyngitis, and tonsillitis.*

Cefdinir is effective orally; it is eliminated primarily unchanged in the urine. Cefdinir has a spectrum of activity similar to cefixime. It is inactive against Pseudomonas *and* Enterobacter *spp.*

Third-Generation Cephalosporins with Good Activity Against Pseudomonas

Ceftazidime is one-quarter to one-half as active against gram-positive microorganisms as cefotaxime. Its activity against the Enterobacteriaceae is very similar; its major distinguishing feature is excellent activity against Pseudomonas *and other gram-negative bacteria. Ceftazidime has poor activity against* B. fragilis. *The drug is not metabolized.*

FOURTH-GENERATION CEPHALOSPORINS

Cefepime and cefpirome *(not available in U.S.) are fourth-generation cephalosporins. Cefepime resists hydrolysis by many of the plasmid-encoded β-lactamases. It is a poor inducer of, and is relatively resistant to, chromosomally encoded and some extended-spectrum β-lactamases. Thus, it is active against many Enterobacteriaceae that are resistant to other cephalosporins via induction of β-lactamases but remains susceptible to many bacteria expressing extended-spectrum β-lactamases. Against* H. influenzae, N. gonorrhoeae, *and* N. meningitidis, *cefepime has comparable or greater activity than cefotaxime. For* P. aeruginosa, *cefepime has comparable activity to ceftazidime, although it is less active for other* Pseudomonas *spp. and* X. maltophilia. *Cefepime has higher activity than ceftazidime and is comparable to cefotaxime for streptococci and methicillin-sensitive* S. aureus. *It is inactive against methicillin-resistant* S. aureus, *penicillin-resistant pneumococci, enterococci,* B. fragilis, L. monocytogenes, Mycobacterium avium *complex, or* M. tuberculosis. *Cefepime is excreted renally, and doses should be adjusted for renal failure. Cefepime has excellent penetration into the CSF. The recommended dosage for adults is 2 g intravenously every 12 hours.*

ADVERSE REACTIONS Hypersensitivity reactions are the most common side effects of cephalosporins; they are identical to those caused by the penicillins, perhaps related to their shared β-lactam structure. Patients who are allergic to one drug class may manifest cross-reactivity to a member of the other class. There is no skin test that can reliably predict whether a patient will manifest an allergic reaction to the cephalosporins.

Patients with a history of a mild or a temporally distant penicillin reaction appear to be at low risk of allergic reaction following cephalosporin administration. However, patients who have had a recent severe, immediate reaction to a penicillin should be given a cephalosporin with great caution, if at all. A positive Coombs' reaction appears frequently in patients who receive large doses of a cephalosporin, but hemolysis is rare. Cephalosporins rarely have produced bone marrow depression characterized by granulocytopenia.

Acute tubular necrosis has followed the administration of *cephaloridine* in doses greater than 4 g/day; this agent is no longer available in the U.S. Other cephalosporins, when used by themselves in recommended doses, rarely produce significant renal toxicity. High doses of cephalothin (no longer available in U.S.) have produced acute tubular necrosis, and usual doses (8–12 g/day) have caused nephrotoxicity in patients with preexisting renal disease. Diarrhea can result from the administration of cephalosporins and may be more frequent with cefoperazone, perhaps because of its greater biliary excretion. Intolerance to alcohol has been noted. Serious bleeding related either to hypoprothrombinemia, thrombocytopenia, and/or platelet dysfunction has been reported.

THERAPEUTIC USES First-generation cephalosporins are excellent agents for skin and soft tissue infections owing to *S. aureus* and *S. pyogenes*. A single dose of cefazolin just before surgery is the preferred prophylaxis for procedures in which skin flora are the likely pathogens. For colorectal surgery, where prophylaxis for intestinal anaerobes is desired, the second-generation agents, cefoxitin or cefotetan, are preferred.

Second-generation cephalosporins generally have been displaced by third-generation agents. The oral second-generation cephalosporins can be used to treat respiratory tract infections, although they are inferior to amoxicillin for treatment of penicillin-resistant *S. pneumoniae* pneumonia and otitis media. Cefoxitin and cefotetan both are effective in situations where facultative gram-negative bacteria and anaerobes are involved (*e.g.*, intra-abdominal infections, pelvic inflammatory disease, and diabetic foot infection).

Third-generation cephalosporins are the drugs of choice for serious infections caused by *Klebsiella, Enterobacter, Proteus, Providencia, Serratia,* and *Haemophilus* spp. Ceftriaxone is the drug of choice for all forms of gonorrhea and for severe forms of Lyme disease. Third-generation cephalosporins (*e.g.*, cefotaxime or ceftriaxone) are used for initial treatment of meningitis in immunocompetent adults and children older than 3 months of age (in combination with vancomycin and ampicillin until the causative agent is identified). They are the drugs of choice for meningitis caused by *H. influenzae*, sensitive *S. pneumoniae, N. meningitidis*, and gram-negative enteric bacteria. Cefotaxime has failed in the treatment of meningitis owing to resistant *S. pneumoniae*; thus, vancomycin should be added. Ceftazidime plus an aminoglycoside is the treatment of choice for *Pseudomonas* meningitis. Third-generation cephalosporins lack activity against *L. monocytogenes* and penicillin-resistant pneumococci, which may cause meningitis. The antimicrobial spectrum of cefotaxime and ceftriaxone is excellent for the treatment of community-acquired pneumonia.

The fourth-generation cephalosporins are indicated for the empirical treatment of nosocomial infections where antibiotic resistance owing to extended-spectrum β-lactamases or chromosomally induced β-lactamases is anticipated. For example, cefepime is superior to ceftazidime and piperacillin for nosocomial isolates of *Enterobacter, Citrobacter,* and *Serratia spp.*

OTHER β-LACTAM ANTIBIOTICS
Carbapenems

Carbapenems are β-lactams that have a broader spectrum of activity than most other β-lactam antibiotics.

IMIPENEM
Source and Chemistry
Imipenem is an N-formimidoyl derivative of thienamycin. Its structure is:

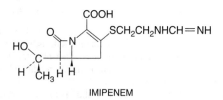

IMIPENEM

Antimicrobial Activity

Imipenem, like other β-lactam antibiotics, binds to PBPs, disrupts bacterial cell wall synthesis, and causes death of susceptible microorganisms. It is very resistant to hydrolysis by most β-lactamases.

The activity of imipenem is excellent for a wide variety of aerobic and anaerobic microorganisms. Streptococci (including penicillin-resistant S. pneumoniae*), enterococci (excluding* E. faecium *and non-β-lactamase-producing penicillin-resistant strains), staphylococci (including* *penicillinase-producing strains), and* Listeria *are all susceptible. Although some strains of methicillin-resistant staphylococci are susceptible, many are not. Activity is excellent against the Enterobacteriaceae, including organisms that are cephalosporin-resistant by virtue of expression of extended-spectrum β-lactamases. Most strains of* Pseudomonas *and* Acinetobacter *are inhibited. Anaerobes, including* B. fragilis, *are highly susceptible.*

Pharmacokinetics and Adverse Reactions

Imipenem is hydrolyzed by a dipeptidase found in the brush border of the proximal tubule. To prolong drug activity, imipenem is combined with cilastatin, an inhibitor of the dehydropeptidase; the combined formulation is available as PRIMAXIN. *Both imipenem and cilastatin have a* $t_{1/2}$ *of ~1 hour. When administered with cilastatin, ~70% of administered imipenem is recovered in the urine as the active drug. Dosage should be reduced for patients with renal insufficiency.*

Nausea and vomiting are the most common side effects. Seizures have been noted in up to 1.5% of patients, especially when high doses are given to patients with CNS lesions or with renal insufficiency. Patients who are allergic to other β-lactam antibiotics may have hypersensitivity reactions to imipenem.

Therapeutic Uses

Imipenem–cilastatin is effective for a wide variety of infections, including urinary tract and lower respiratory infections; intra-abdominal and gynecological infections; and skin, soft tissue, bone, and joint infections. The combination appears to be especially useful for the treatment of serious infections caused by cephalosporin-resistant nosocomial bacteria, as may be seen in hospitalized patients who have recently received other β-lactam antibiotics. Imipenem should not be used as monotherapy for infections with P. aeruginosa *because of the risk of developing resistance during therapy.*

MEROPENEM *Meropenem* (MERREM IV) is a derivative of *thienamycin* that does not require coadministration with cilastatin because it is not sensitive to renal dipeptidase. Its toxicity and clinical efficacy are similar to imipenem, except that it may be less likely to cause seizures.

ERTAPENEM *Ertapenem* (INVANZ) differs from imipenem and meropenem by having a longer serum $t_{1/2}$ that allows once-daily dosing and by having inferior activity against *P. aeruginosa* and *Acinetobacter* spp. Its spectrum of activity against gram-positive organisms, Enterobacteriaceae, and anaerobes makes it attractive for use in intra-abdominal and pelvic infections.

AZTREONAM *Aztreonam* (AZACTAM) is a monocyclic β-lactam. Its structural formula is:

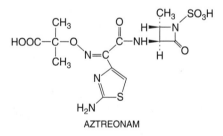

AZTREONAM

Aztreonam is resistant to the β-lactamases that are elaborated by most gram-negative bacteria. The antimicrobial activity of aztreonam differs from those of other β-lactam antibiotics and resembles that of an aminoglycoside. Aztreonam has activity only against gram-negative bacteria; it has no activity against gram-positive bacteria and anaerobic organisms. Activity against Enterobacteriaceae is excellent, as is that against *P. aeruginosa*. It is also highly active against *H. influenzae* and gonococci.

Aztreonam is administered intramuscularly or intravenously. The elimination $t_{1/2}$ *is 1.7 hours, and most drug is excreted unaltered in the urine. The* $t_{1/2}$ *is prolonged to 6 hours in anephric patients. The usual dose of aztreonam for severe infections is 2 g every 6–8 hours (reduced in patients with renal insufficiency). A notable feature is that there is little cross-reactivity with most other β-lactam antibiotics. Aztreonam is therefore used to treat gram-negative infections that normally would be treated with a β-lactam antibiotic were it not for a prior allergic reaction.*

β-LACTAMASE INHIBITORS

Certain molecules can inactivate β-lactamases, thereby protecting β-lactam antibiotics that are their substrates. These β-lactamase inhibitors are most active against plasmid-encoded β-lactamases (including those that hydrolyze ceftazidime and cefotaxime) but are inactive against the chromosomal β-lactamases induced in gram-negative bacilli (such as *Enterobacter, Acinetobacter,* and *Citrobacter*) by treatment with second- and third-generation cephalosporins.

Clavulanic acid is a "suicide" inhibitor that irreversibly binds β-lactamases from a wide range of gram-positive and gram-negative microorganisms. It is combined with amoxicillin for oral administration (AUGMENTIN) and with ticarcillin for parenteral administration (TIMENTIN).

Amoxicillin plus clavulanate is effective for β-lactamase-producing strains of staphylococci, H. influenzae, gonococci, and E. coli. It also is effective in the treatment of acute otitis media in children, sinusitis, animal or human bite wounds, cellulitis, and diabetic foot infections. The addition of clavulanate to ticarcillin (TIMENTIN) extends its spectrum to include aerobic gram-negative bacilli, S. aureus, and Bacteroides spp. There is no increased activity against Pseudomonas spp. The combination is especially useful for mixed nosocomial infections and often is used with an aminoglycoside. The dosage should be adjusted in patients with renal insufficiency.

Sulbactam is combined with ampicillin for intravenous or intramuscular use (UNASYN). The combination has good activity against gram-positive cocci, including β-lactamase-producing strains of S. aureus, gram-negative aerobes (but not Pseudomonas), and anaerobes; it has been used for the treatment of mixed intra-abdominal and pelvic infections. Dosage must be adjusted in patients with impaired renal function.

Tazobactam is a penicillanic acid sulfone β-lactamase inhibitor that has good activity against many of the plasmid β-lactamases, including some of the extended-spectrum class. It has been combined with piperacillin as a parenteral preparation (ZOSYN).

For a complete Bibliographical listing see Goodman & Gilman's *The Pharmacological Basis of Therapeutics,* 11th ed., or Goodman & Gilman Online at www.accessmedicine.com.

45

AMINOGLYCOSIDES

The aminoglycosides are first-line therapy for a limited number of very specific, often historically prominent infections, such as plague, tularemia, and tuberculosis; they also are frequently used to treat infections caused by aerobic gram-negative bacteria. Their clinical roles have diminished as less toxic alternatives have become available. Unlike most inhibitors of microbial protein synthesis, which are bacteriostatic, the aminoglycosides are bactericidal. Resistance most commonly arises from acquisition of plasmids or transposons encoding genes for aminoglycoside-metabolizing enzymes or from impaired transport of drug into the cell; cross-resistance is common.

These agents are polycations whose polarity affects their shared pharmacokinetic properties: none is absorbed adequately after oral administration, inadequate concentrations are found in cerebrospinal fluid (CSF), and all are excreted relatively rapidly by the normal kidney. All members of the group also share the same spectrum of toxicity, most notably nephrotoxicity and ototoxicity.

The aminoglycosides consist of two or more amino sugars joined in glycosidic linkage to a hexose nucleus (Figure 45–1). Different aminoglycosides are distinguished by the amino sugars attached to the aminocyclitol. Streptomycin differs from the other aminoglycoside antibiotics in that it contains streptidine rather than 2-deoxystreptamine, and the aminocyclitol is not in a central position.

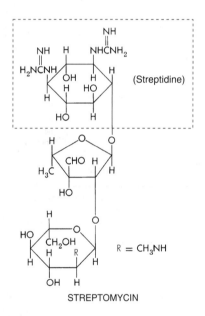

STREPTOMYCIN

MECHANISM OF ACTION The aminoglycoside antibiotics are rapidly bactericidal. Bacterial killing is concentration-dependent, but residual bactericidal activity persists even after the serum concentration has fallen below the minimum inhibitory concentration. These properties account for the efficacy of once-daily dosing regimens.

Driven by the membrane electrical potential (interior negative), aminoglycosides diffuse through aqueous channels formed by porin proteins in the outer membrane of gram-negative bacteria and enter the periplasmic space. This rate-limiting process (and thus the antimicrobial efficacy of aminoglycosides) can be blocked or inhibited by a reduction in pH or anaerobic conditions, as in an abscess. Once inside the cell, aminoglycosides bind to polysomes and interfere with protein synthesis by causing misreading and premature termination of mRNA translation (Figure 45–2). The resulting aberrant proteins may be inserted into the cell membrane, altering permeability and further stimulating aminoglycoside transport.

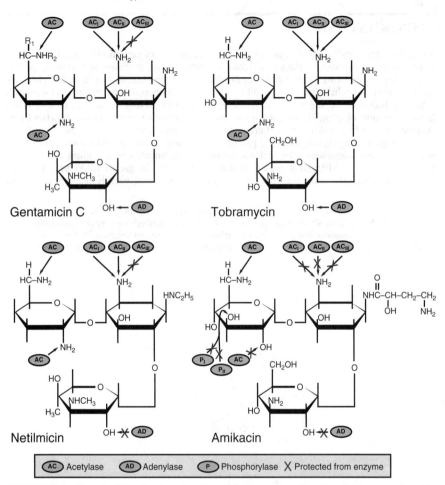

FIGURE 45–1 *Sites of activity of various plasmid-mediated enzymes capable of inactivating aminoglycosides.* The symbol X indicates regions of the molecules that are protected from the designated enzyme. In gentamicin C_1, $R_1=R_2=CH_3$; in gentamicin C_2, $R_1=CH_3$, $R_2=H$; in gentamicin C_{1a}, $R_1=R_2=H$.

The primary site of action of the aminoglycosides is the 30S ribosomal subunit; some aminoglycosides also bind to several sites on the 50S ribosomal subunit. Aminoglycosides disrupt the normal cycle of ribosomal function by interfering with the initiation of protein synthesis, leading to the accumulation of abnormal initiation complexes (Figure 45–2). Aminoglycosides also cause misreading of the mRNA template and incorporation of incorrect amino acids into the growing polypeptide chains. Aminoglycosides vary in their capacity to cause misreading, presumably owing to differences in their affinities for specific ribosomal proteins; bactericidal activity and the ability to induce misreading are strongly correlated.

MICROBIAL RESISTANCE TO THE AMINOGLYCOSIDES Bacteria may be resistant to aminoglycosides because of failure of the antibiotic to penetrate intracellularly, low affinity of the drug for the bacterial ribosome, or—most commonly—drug inactivation by modifying enzymes acquired by conjugative transfer of resistance plasmids. These enzymes phosphorylate, adenylate, or acetylate specific hydroxyl or amino groups (Figure 45–1), preventing binding to ribosomes. Amikacin is modified by only a few of these inactivating enzymes; thus, strains that are resistant to other aminoglycosides may remain susceptible to amikacin.

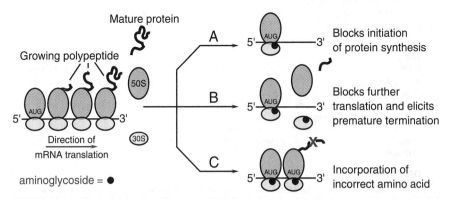

FIGURE 45–2 *Effects of aminoglycosides on protein synthesis.* **A.** Aminoglycoside (represented by closed circles) binds to the 30S ribosomal subunit and interferes with initiation of protein synthesis by fixing the 30S–50S ribosomal complex at the start codon (AUG) of mRNA. As 30S–50S complexes downstream complete translation of mRNA and detach, the abnormal initiation complexes, so-called streptomycin monosomes, accumulate, blocking further translation of the message. Aminoglycoside binding to the 30S subunit also causes misreading of mRNA, leading to **B.** premature termination of translation with detachment of the ribosomal complex and incompletely synthesized protein or **C.** incorporation of incorrect amino acids (indicated by the X), resulting in the production of abnormal or nonfunctional proteins.

Many clinical isolates of *Enterococcus faecalis* and *E. faecium* are highly resistant to all aminoglycosides. Infections caused by aminoglycoside-resistant strains of enterococci can be especially difficult to treat because of the loss of the synergistic bactericidal activity between a *penicillin* or *vancomycin* and an aminoglycoside and because these strains often also are cross-resistant to vancomycin and penicillin. Resistance to gentamicin indicates cross-resistance to tobramycin, amikacin, kanamycin, and netilmicin because one enzyme inactivates all of these drugs; this enzyme does not modify streptomycin, which is inactivated by another enzyme; consequently, gentamicin-resistant strains of enterococci may be susceptible to streptomycin. Natural resistance to aminoglycosides may be caused by failure of the drug to penetrate the cytoplasmic (inner) membrane. Penetration of drug across the outer membrane of gram-negative microorganisms into the periplasmic space can be slow, but resistance on this basis is unimportant clinically. Transport of aminoglycosides across the cytoplasmic membrane is an oxygen-dependent active process. Strictly anaerobic bacteria thus are resistant to these drugs because they lack the necessary transport system. Similarly, facultative bacteria are resistant when grown under anaerobic conditions. Resistance owing to mutations that alter ribosomal structure is relatively uncommon. Missense mutations in *Escherichia coli* that substitute a single amino acid in a crucial ribosomal protein may prevent streptomycin binding. Although highly resistant to streptomycin, these strains are not widespread in nature. Similarly, only 5% of strains of *Pseudomonas aeruginosa* exhibit such ribosomal resistance to streptomycin. It has been estimated that ~50% of the streptomycin-resistant strains of enterococci are ribosomally resistant. Because ribosomal resistance usually is specific for streptomycin, these strains remain sensitive to a combination of penicillin and gentamicin.

ANTIBACTERIAL SPECTRUM OF THE AMINOGLYCOSIDES The antibacterial activity of most aminoglycosides is directed primarily against aerobic gram-negative bacilli. Kanamycin, like streptomycin, has a more limited spectrum than the other aminoglycosides. Aminoglycosides have little activity against anaerobic microorganisms or facultative bacteria under anaerobic conditions. They should not be used as single agents for infections caused by gram-positive bacteria. Combined with a cell wall–active agent, such as a penicillin or vancomycin, aminoglycosides produce synergistic bactericidal effects against enterococci, streptococci, and staphylococci.

Aerobic gram-negative bacilli vary in their susceptibility to the aminoglycosides. Tobramycin and gentamicin exhibit similar activity against most gram-negative bacilli, although tobramycin usually is more active against *P. aeruginosa* and some *Proteus* spp. Many gram-negative bacilli that are resistant to gentamicin because of plasmid-mediated inactivating enzymes also are resistant to tobramycin. Amikacin, and in some instances netilmicin, retain their activity against gentamicin-resistant strains because they are a poor substrate for many of the aminoglycoside-inactivating enzymes.

ABSORPTION, DISTRIBUTION, DOSING, AND ELIMINATION OF THE AMINOGLYCOSIDES

ABSORPTION

The aminoglycosides are highly polar and, thus, poorly absorbed from the gastrointestinal (GI) tract. Instillation of these drugs into body cavities with serosal surfaces may result in rapid absorption and unexpected toxicity (e.g., neuromuscular blockade). Toxic levels also may result from sustained topical application to large wounds, burns, or cutaneous ulcers, particularly with renal insufficiency. Long-term oral or rectal administration of aminoglycosides may result in accumulation to toxic concentrations in patients with renal impairment.

Aminoglycosides are absorbed rapidly after intramuscular injection. In critically ill patients, especially those in shock, drug absorption from intramuscular sites may be reduced by poor perfusion.

DISTRIBUTION

These polar drugs do not penetrate into most cells, central nervous system (CNS), and the eye. Except for streptomycin, there is negligible binding of aminoglycosides to plasma proteins. The volume of distribution of these drugs approximates the volume of extracellular fluid.

Concentrations of aminoglycosides in secretions and tissues are low. High concentrations are found only in the renal cortex and the inner ear, likely contributing to the aminoglycosides' nephrotoxicity and ototoxicity. Due to active hepatic secretion, concentrations in bile approach 30% of those found in plasma, but this represents a very minor excretory route. Penetration into respiratory secretions is poor. Diffusion into pleural and synovial fluid is relatively slow, but concentrations that approximate those in the plasma may be achieved after repeated administration. Inflammation increases aminoglycoside penetration into peritoneal and pericardial cavities.

Aminoglycoside concentrations in CSF following parenteral administration are <10% of those in plasma (~25% with meningitis). Thus, CSF levels are usually subtherapeutic unless delivered intrathecally. Similarly, effective therapy of bacterial endophthalmitis requires periocular and intraocular injections.

Administration of aminoglycosides to pregnant women may result in drug accumulation in fetal plasma and amniotic fluid. Streptomycin and tobramycin can cause hearing loss in children born to women who receive the drug during pregnancy. Aminoglycosides should be used with caution during pregnancy and only in the absence of suitable alternatives.

DOSING

Current practice is to administer the total daily dose as a single injection, which is associated with less toxicity and equal efficacy as multiple-dose regimens. This diminished toxicity is probably due to a threshold effect from accumulation of drug in the inner ear or in the kidney. Despite the higher peak concentration, a once-daily dosing regimen provides a longer period when concentrations fall below the threshold for toxicity than does a multiple-dose regimen (12 hours vs. less than 3 hours total in Figure 45–3), accounting for its lower toxicity. Aminoglycoside bactericidal activity, on the other hand, is related directly to the peak concentration achieved because of concentration-dependent killing and a concentration-dependent postantibiotic effect.

Once-daily regimens are safer with equal efficacy, cost less, and are administered more easily. Exceptions include use in pregnancy, neonatal and pediatric infections, and low-dose combination therapy of bacterial endocarditis. Once-daily dosing also should be avoided in patients with creatinine clearances of <20–25 mL/min, where dosing every 48 hours is more appropriate.

Whether once-daily or multiple-daily dosing is used, the dose must be adjusted for patients with creatinine clearances of <80–100 mL/min, and plasma concentrations must be monitored. Nomograms may be helpful in selecting initial doses, but variability in aminoglycoside clearance among patients is too large for these to be relied on for more than a few days. If a patient likely will be treated with an aminoglycoside for more than 3–4 days, then plasma concentrations should be monitored.

For twice- or thrice-daily dosing regimens, both peak (30 minutes after dosing) and trough (immediately before the next dose) plasma concentrations are determined. The peak concentration documents that the dose produces therapeutic concentrations, while the trough concentration is used to avoid toxicity. With once-daily regimens, the trough concentration is either measured directly or estimated using various nomograms; a trough concentration >2 µg/mL predicts toxicity.

ELIMINATION

The aminoglycosides are excreted almost entirely by glomerular filtration, and urine concentrations of 50–200 µg/mL are achieved. The plasma half-lives of the aminoglycosides vary between 2 and 3 hours in patients with normal renal function.

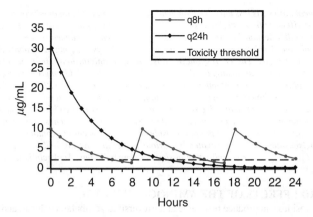

FIGURE 45–3 *Plasma concentrations (μg/mL) after administration of 5.1 mg/kg of gentamicin intravenously to a hypothetical patient either as a single dose (q24h) or as three divided doses (q8h).* The threshold for toxicity has been chosen to correspond to a plasma concentration of 2 μg/mL, the maximum recommended. The once-daily regimen produces a threefold higher plasma concentration, which enhances efficacy that otherwise might be compromised due to prolonged sub-MIC concentrations later in the dosing interval compared with the every-8-hours regimen. The once-daily regimen provides a 12-hour period during which plasma concentrations are below the threshold for toxicity, thereby minimizing the toxicity that otherwise might result from the high plasma concentrations early on. The every-8-hours regimen, in contrast, provides only a brief period during which plasma concentrations are below the threshold for toxicity.

Since aminoglycoside elimination depends almost entirely on the kidney, a linear relationship exists between the serum creatinine and the $t_{1/2}$ of all aminoglycosides in patients with moderately compromised renal function. Because the incidence of nephrotoxicity and ototoxicity is related to the concentration to which an aminoglycoside accumulates, it is critical to reduce the maintenance dosage of these drugs in patients with impaired renal function. The size of the individual dose, the interval between doses, or both can be altered. Determination of drug concentration in plasma is essential for the proper administration of aminoglycosides. In patients with life-threatening systemic infections, aminoglycoside concentrations should be determined several times per week (more frequently if renal function is changing) and should be determined within 24–48 hours of a change in dosage.

Aminoglycosides can be removed from the body by either hemodialysis or peritoneal dialysis. Approximately 50% of the administered dose is removed in 12 hours by hemodialysis. As a general rule, a dose equal to half the loading dose administered after each hemodialysis should maintain the plasma concentration in the desired range, but a number of variables make this a rough approximation at best. The amount of aminoglycoside removed can be replaced by administering ~15–30% of the maximum daily dose (Table 45–1) each day. Frequent monitoring of plasma drug concentrations is crucial.

Table 45–1

Algorithm for Dose Reduction of Aminoglycosides Based on Calculated Creatinine Clearance

Creatinine Clearance, mL/min	% of Maximum Daily Dose*	Frequency of Dosing
100	100	
75	75	Every 24 hours
50	50	
25	25	
20	80	
10	60	Every 48 hours
<10	40	

*The maximum adult daily dose for amikacin, kanamycin, and streptomycin is 15 mg/kg; for gentamicin and tobramycin, 5.5 mg/kg; and for netilmicin, 6.5 mg/kg.

Peritoneal dialysis is less effective than hemodialysis in removing aminoglycosides. Clearance rates are ~5–10 mL/min but highly variable. If a patient who requires dialysis has bacterial peritonitis, the antibiotic can be added to the dialysate to achieve concentrations equal to those desired in plasma. For intermittent dosing via peritoneal dialysate, 2 mg/kg of amikacin is added to the bag once a day. The corresponding dose for gentamicin, netilmicin, or tobramycin is 0.6 mg/kg. For continuous dosing, the dose for amikacin is 12 mg/L (25 mg/L loading dose in the first bag), and the dose for gentamicin, netilmicin, or tobramycin is 4 mg/L in each bag (8 mg/L loading dose). This should be preceded by a loading dose, either parenterally or in dialysis fluid.

Although excretion of aminoglycosides is similar in adults and children >6 months of age, half-lives of the drugs may be prolonged significantly in the newborn. Thus, it is critically important to monitor concentrations of aminoglycosides during treatment of neonates.

Aminoglycosides can be inactivated by various penicillins in vitro and in patients with end-stage renal failure, further complicating dosage recommendations. Amikacin is least affected by this interaction.

UNTOWARD EFFECTS OF THE AMINOGLYCOSIDES

All aminoglycosides can produce reversible and irreversible vestibular, cochlear, and renal toxicity.

OTOTOXICITY Vestibular and auditory dysfunction can follow the administration of any of the aminoglycosides. Aminoglycosides progressively accumulate in the inner ear, and toxicity is more likely to occur in patients with persistently elevated plasma drug concentrations. Ototoxicity is largely irreversible and results from progressive destruction of vestibular or cochlear sensory cells, which are highly sensitive to damage by aminoglycosides. The degree of permanent dysfunction correlates with the number of damaged sensory hair cells. Repeated courses of aminoglycosides, each probably resulting in the loss of more cells, are more likely to cause deafness. Loop diuretics such as *ethacrynic acid* and *furosemide* may potentiate the ototoxic effects of the aminoglycosides and should be avoided when possible. Hearing loss following exposure to aminoglycosides is more likely to develop in patients with preexisting auditory impairment. Neomycin, kanamycin, and amikacin are most likely to cause hearing loss; streptomycin and gentamicin are the most vestibulotoxic aminoglycosides. Since the initial symptoms may be reversible, patients receiving high doses and/or prolonged courses of aminoglycosides should be monitored carefully, but deafness may occur even after therapy is discontinued.

Clinical Symptoms of Cochlear Toxicity

A high-pitched tinnitus often is the first symptom of toxicity and can persist for days to weeks. It is followed in a few days by auditory impairment. Since high-frequency hearing is lost first, the patient may be unaware of the difficulty unless audiometric examination is performed.

Clinical Symptoms of Vestibular Toxicity

Headache may precede the onset of labyrinthine dysfunction, followed immediately by nausea, vomiting, and difficulty with balance, which develop acutely and persist for 1–2 weeks. The acute stage is followed by manifestations of chronic labyrinthitis, in which the patient has difficulty when attempting to walk or make sudden movements; ataxia is prominent. The chronic phase persists for ~2 months. Recovery may require 12–18 months; most patients have some permanent residual damage. Although there is no specific treatment for the vestibular deficiency, early drug discontinuation may permit recovery before irreversible damage of the hair cells.

NEPHROTOXICITY Approximately 8–26% of patients who receive an aminoglycoside for more than several days will develop mild renal impairment that almost always is reversible. The most nephrotoxic aminoglycosides are neomycin, gentamicin, and tobramycin. The toxicity results from accumulation and retention of aminoglycoside in the proximal tubular cells. The initial manifestation is excretion of enzymes of the renal tubular brush border, followed by a defect in renal concentrating ability, mild proteinuria, and the appearance of hyaline and granular casts. The glomerular filtration rate is reduced after several additional days. The nonoliguric phase of renal insufficiency is thought to be due to the effects of aminoglycosides on the distal portion of the nephron that reduce sensitivity to endogenous vasopressin. While severe acute tubular necrosis may occur rarely, the most common finding is a mild rise in plasma creatinine. The impairment in renal function is almost always reversible because the proximal tubular cells can regenerate.

Toxicity correlates with the total amount of drug administered and is more likely to be encountered with longer courses of therapy. Constantly elevated concentration of drug in plasma above a critical level (*i.e.*, an elevated trough concentration) correlates with toxicity. The most important result of this toxicity may be reduced excretion of the drug, which, in turn, predisposes to ototoxicity. Other drugs, such as *amphotericin B, vancomycin, angiotensin-converting enzyme inhibitors, cisplatin,* and *cyclosporine,* may potentiate aminoglycoside-induced nephrotoxicity. Volume depletion and hypokalemia also have been implicated.

NEUROMUSCULAR BLOCKADE

Acute neuromuscular blockade and apnea have been attributed to the aminoglycosides; patients with myasthenia gravis are particularly susceptible. In humans, neuromuscular blockade generally has occurred after intrapleural or intraperitoneal instillation of large doses of an aminoglycoside, but the reaction can follow intravenous, intramuscular, and even oral administration. Neuromuscular blockade may be reversed with calcium gluconate infusion.

OTHER EFFECTS ON THE NERVOUS SYSTEM

The administration of streptomycin may produce dysfunction of the optic nerve, including scotomas, presenting as enlargement of the blind spot, and (rarely) peripheral neuritis. Paresthesia occasionally follows streptomycin use, usually within 30–60 minutes, and can persist for several hours.

OTHER ADVERSE EFFECTS

In general, aminoglycosides have little allergenic potential; anaphylaxis and rash are unusual. Parenterally administered aminoglycosides are not associated with pseudomembranous colitis.

STREPTOMYCIN

Streptomycin is used for the treatment of certain unusual infections usually in combination with other antimicrobial agents. Because it is less active than other members of the class against aerobic gram-negative rods, it has fallen into disuse. Streptomycin may be administered by deep intramuscular injection or intravenously. The dose of streptomycin is 15 mg/kg/day for patients with creatinine clearances above 80 mL/min. It typically is administered as a 1000-mg single daily dose or 500 mg twice daily. The daily dose should be reduced in proportion to creatinine clearance for creatinine clearances >30 mL/min (Table 45–1).

THERAPEUTIC USES

Bacterial Endocarditis   Streptomycin and penicillin in combination are synergistically bactericidal *in vitro* against strains of enterococci, group D streptococci, and the various oral streptococci of the *viridans* group. A combination of penicillin G and streptomycin may be indicated for treatment of streptococcal or enterococcal endocarditis. Streptomycin largely has been replaced by gentamicin but may still be used when the strain is resistant to gentamicin and susceptible to streptomycin.

Tularemia   Streptomycin (or gentamicin) is the drug of choice for the treatment of tularemia. Most cases respond to the administration of 1 g (15–25 mg/kg) streptomycin per day (in divided doses) for 7–10 days. Fluoroquinolones and tetracyclines also are effective.

Plague   Streptomycin is effective for the treatment of all forms of plague. The recommended dose is 2 g/day in two divided doses for 7–10 days. Gentamicin is probably as efficacious.

Tuberculosis   In the treatment of tuberculosis, streptomycin always should be used in combination with at least one or two other drugs to which the causative strain is susceptible (*see* Chapter 47).

GENTAMICIN

Gentamicin is an important drug for the treatment of many serious gram-negative bacillary infections and usually is the aminoglycoside of first choice because of its low cost and reliable activity against all but the most resistant gram-negative aerobes. Gentamicin is given parenterally, ophthalmically, and topically.

THERAPEUTIC USES OF GENTAMICIN AND OTHER AMINOGLYCOSIDES   Gentamicin, tobramycin, amikacin, and netilmicin can be used interchangeably for most infections; gentamicin usually is the preferred agent. Many different types of infections can be treated successfully with these aminoglycosides; however, owing to their toxicities, prolonged use should be restricted to life-threatening infections and those for which a less toxic agent is contraindicated or less effective.

The recommended intramuscular or intravenous dose of gentamicin sulfate (GARAMYCIN) for adults is a loading dose of 2 mg/kg and then 3–5 mg/kg/day, one-third being given every 8 hours when *administered as a multiple-daily-dosing regimen. The once-daily dose is 5–7 mg/kg given over 30–60 minutes for patients with normal renal function (lower if renal function is impaired). The upper limit of this dose range may be required to achieve therapeutic levels for trauma or burn patients, those with septic shock, and others in whom drug clearance is more rapid or volume of distribution is larger than normal. Several dosage schedules have been suggested for newborns and infants: 3 mg/kg once daily for preterm newborns <35 weeks' gestation; 4 mg/kg once daily for newborns older than 35 weeks' gestation; 5 mg/kg daily in two divided doses for neonates with severe infections; and 2–2.5 mg/kg every 8 hours for children up to 2 years of age. Peak plasma concentrations range from 4–10 μg/mL (dosing: 1.7 mg/kg every 8 hours) and 16–24 μg/mL (dosing: 5.1 mg/kg once daily). It should be emphasized that the recommended doses of gentamicin do not always yield desired concentrations. Periodic determinations of the plasma concentration of aminoglycosides are recommended strongly; trough concentrations consistently >2 μg/mL are associated with toxicity.*

Aminoglycosides often are combined with a penicillin or cephalosporin for the therapy of proven or suspected serious gram-negative infections, especially those due to P. aeruginosa, Enterobacter, Klebsiella, Serratia, and other species resistant to less toxic antibiotics, including urinary tract infections, bacteremia, infected burns, osteomyelitis, pneumonia, peritonitis, and otitis. With few exceptions (e.g., enterococcal endocarditis), the superiority of aminoglycoside combination therapy over an effective single drug has not been demonstrated. Because of their toxicity, aminoglycosides should not be used for more than a few days unless deemed essential. Aminoglycosides should never be mixed in the same solution with penicillins because they are inactivated by penicillin. Similar incompatibilities exist in vitro to different degrees between gentamicin and heparin, amphotericin B, and the cephalosporins.

Urinary Tract Infections

Aminoglycosides usually are not indicated for the treatment of uncomplicated urinary tract infections, although a single intramuscular dose of gentamicin (5 mg/kg) can cure more than 90% of uncomplicated infections of the lower urinary tract. As strains of E. coli acquire resistance to other drugs, aminoglycoside use may increase. In the seriously ill patient with pyelonephritis, an aminoglycoside alone or in combination with a β-lactam antibiotic offers broad and effective initial coverage. Once the microorganism is isolated and its antibiotic sensitivities determined, the aminoglycoside is discontinued if the infecting microorganism is sensitive to less toxic drugs.

Pneumonia

Organisms that cause community-acquired pneumonia will be susceptible to broad-spectrum β-lactam antibiotics, macrolides, or a fluoroquinolone, and usually it is not necessary to add an aminoglycoside. Gentamicin (or other aminoglycosides) never should be used as the sole agent to treat pneumonia acquired in the community or as the initial treatment for pneumonia acquired in the hospital.

An aminoglycoside in combination with a β-lactam antibiotic may be used for empirical therapy of hospital-acquired pneumonia in which multiple-drug-resistant gram-negative aerobes are a likely causative agent. However, provided the companion drug is active against the causative agent, there is generally no benefit from adding an aminoglycoside. One exception may be the treatment of pneumonia caused by P. aeruginosa, for which combination therapy generally is recommended, with the goal of preventing the emergence of resistance.

Meningitis

The availability of third-generation cephalosporins has reduced the need for aminoglycoside treatment in most cases of meningitis, except for infections caused by gram-negative organisms that are resistant to β-lactam antibiotics (e.g., species of Pseudomonas and Acinetobacter). If therapy with an aminoglycoside is necessary, in adults, 5 mg of a preservative-free formulation of gentamicin (or equivalent dose of another aminoglycoside) is administered intrathecally once daily.

Peritoneal Dialysis–Associated Peritonitis

Patients who develop peritonitis during peritoneal dialysis may be treated with an aminoglycoside diluted into the dialysis fluid to a concentration of 4–8 mg/L for gentamicin, netilmicin, or tobramycin or 6–12 mg/L for amikacin.

Bacterial Endocarditis

"Synergistic" or low-dose gentamicin (3 mg/kg/day in three divided doses) in combination with a penicillin or vancomycin has been recommended in some circumstances for treating bacterial endocarditis. There is good evidence that penicillin and gentamicin in combination are effective

as a short-course (i.e., 2-week) regimen for uncomplicated native-valve streptococcal endocarditis. In cases of enterococcal endocarditis, concomitant administration of penicillin and gentamicin for 4–6 weeks has been recommended because of an unacceptably high relapse rate with penicillin alone. A 2-week regimen of gentamicin or tobramycin in combination with nafcillin *is effective for selected cases of staphylococcal tricuspid valve endocarditis in injection drug users, although the benefit of including an aminoglycoside is unproven.*

Aminoglycosides have no clinically proven benefit in treatment of staphylococcal mitral or aortic valve endocarditis. Because of toxicity and limited clinical benefit, aminoglycoside combination therapy has fallen from favor as a first-line regimen for treatment of endocarditis.

Sepsis

In febrile patients with granulocytopenia and in infections suspected to be caused by P. aeruginosa, *numerous studies using potent broad-spectrum β-lactams (e.g., carbapenems and antipseudomonal cephalosporins) have demonstrated no benefit of adding an aminoglycoside to the regimen. Most experts recommend combination therapy of documented non–urinary tract* P. aeruginosa *infections, particularly pneumonia with bacteremia. If there is concern that an infection may be caused by a multiple-drug-resistant organism that may be susceptible only to an aminoglycoside, then adding this antibiotic to the regimen is reasonable. Evidence that aminoglycosides are beneficial for other gram-negative infections is weak. To avoid toxicity, aminoglycosides should be used briefly and sparingly as long as other alternatives are available.*

Topical Applications

Gentamicin is absorbed slowly when it is applied topically in an ointment and somewhat more rapidly when it is applied as a cream. When the antibiotic is applied to large areas of denuded body surface (e.g., in burn patients), plasma concentrations can reach 4 μg/mL, and 2–5% of the drug may appear in the urine.

UNTOWARD EFFECTS

The most important and serious side effects of gentamicin are nephrotoxicity and irreversible ototoxicity. Intrathecal or intraventricular administration may cause local inflammation and can result in radiculitis and other complications.

TOBRAMYCIN

The antimicrobial activity, pharmacokinetic properties, and toxicity profile of tobramycin (NEBCIN) are very similar to those of gentamicin. Dosages and serum concentrations are identical with those for gentamicin. Tobramycin (TOBREX) also is available in ophthalmic ointments and solutions.

THERAPEUTIC USES

Indications for tobramycin are the same as those for gentamicin. The superior activity of tobramycin against P. aeruginosa *makes it the preferred aminoglycoside for treatment of serious infections caused by this organism, usually in conjunction with an antipseudomonal β-lactam antibiotic. In contrast to gentamicin, tobramycin shows poor activity in combination with penicillin against enterococci.*

UNTOWARD EFFECTS

Tobramycin causes nephrotoxicity and ototoxicity.

AMIKACIN

The spectrum of antimicrobial activity of amikacin (AMIKIN) is the broadest of the group. Because of its resistance to many aminoglycoside-inactivating enzymes, it has a special role in hospitals where gentamicin- and tobramycin-resistant organisms are prevalent.

The recommended dose of amikacin is 15 mg/kg/day as a single daily dose or divided into two or three equal portions, which must be reduced for patients with renal failure. The drug is absorbed rapidly after intramuscular injection but is usually given intravenously.

THERAPEUTIC USES

Amikacin is preferred for the initial treatment of serious nosocomial gram-negative bacillary infections in hospitals where gentamicin and tobramycin resistance is prevalent. Amikacin is active against the vast majority of aerobic gram-negative bacilli, including most strains of Serratia, Proteus, *and* P. aeruginosa. *It is active against nearly all strains of* Klebsiella, Enterobacter, *and* E. coli *that are resistant to gentamicin and tobramycin. Most resistance to amikacin is found among strains of* Acinetobacter, Providencia, *and* Flavobacter *and strains of* Pseudomonas other *than P. aeruginosa; these all are unusual pathogens. Amikacin is less active than gentamicin against enterococci and should not be used. Amikacin is not active against the majority of gram-positive anaerobic bacteria. It is active against M. tuberculosis, including streptomycin-resistant strains, and atypical mycobacteria. It has been used in the treatment of disseminated atypical mycobacterial infection in acquired immunodeficiency syndrome (AIDS) patients.*

UNTOWARD EFFECTS

Amikacin causes ototoxicity and nephrotoxicity. Auditory deficits are produced most commonly.

NETILMICIN

Netilmicin (NETROMYCIN) is similar to gentamicin and tobramycin in its pharmacokinetic properties and dosage. Its antibacterial activity is broad against aerobic gram-negative bacilli. Like amikacin, it is not metabolized by most of the aminoglycoside-inactivating enzymes and therefore may be active against certain bacteria that are resistant to gentamicin.

The recommended dose of netilmicin for complicated urinary tract infections in adults is 1.5–2 mg/kg every 12 hours. For other serious systemic infections, a total daily dose of 4–7 mg/kg is given as a single dose or two to three divided doses. Children should receive 3–7 mg/kg/day in two to three divided doses; neonates receive 3.5–5 mg/kg/day as a single daily dose.

THERAPEUTIC USES

Netilmicin is useful for serious infections owing to susceptible Enterobacteriaceae and other aerobic gram-negative bacilli. It is effective against some gentamicin-resistant pathogens, with the exception of enterococci.

UNTOWARD EFFECTS

Netilmicin produces ototoxicity and nephrotoxicity. It may be less toxic than other aminoglycosides.

KANAMYCIN

The use of kanamycin has declined markedly because its spectrum of activity is limited compared with other aminoglycosides, and it is among the most toxic.

NEOMYCIN

Neomycin is a broad-spectrum antibiotic. Gram-negative species that are highly sensitive are *E. coli, Enterobacter aerogenes, Klebsiella pneumoniae,* and *Proteus vulgaris.* Gram-positive microorganisms that are inhibited include *S. aureus* and *E. faecalis. M. tuberculosis* also is sensitive to neomycin. Strains of *P. aeruginosa* are resistant to neomycin.

Neomycin sulfate is available for topical and oral administration. Neomycin and polymyxin B have been used for irrigation of the bladder. For this purpose, 1 mL of a preparation (NEOSPORIN G.U. IRRIGANT) containing 40 mg neomycin and 200,000 units polymyxin B per milliliter is diluted in 1 L of 0.9% NaCl solution and is used for continuous irrigation of the urinary bladder through appropriate catheter systems. The goal is to prevent bacteriuria and bacteremia associated with the use of indwelling catheters.

Neomycin is available in many brands of creams, ointments, and other products alone and in combination with polymyxin, bacitracin, other antibiotics and a variety of glucocorticoids. There is no evidence that these topical preparations shorten the time required for healing of wounds.

THERAPEUTIC USES

Neomycin has been used widely for topical application in a variety of infections of the skin and mucous membranes, including those associated with burns, wounds, ulcers, and infected dermatoses. Such treatment does not eradicate bacteria from the lesions.

For hepatic encephalopathy, a daily dose of 4–12 g (in divided doses) by mouth is given, provided that renal function is normal. Because renal insufficiency is a complication of hepatic failure and neomycin is nephrotoxic, it is used rarely for this indication. Lactulose is a much less toxic agent and is preferred.

ABSORPTION AND EXCRETION

Neomycin is poorly absorbed from the GI tract and is excreted by the kidney. Patients with renal insufficiency may accumulate the drug. About 97% of an oral dose of neomycin is not absorbed and is eliminated unchanged in the feces.

UNTOWARD EFFECTS

Hypersensitivity reactions, primarily rashes, occur in 6–8% of patients when neomycin is applied topically. Individuals sensitive to this agent may develop cross-reactions when exposed to other aminoglycosides. The most important toxic effects of neomycin are renal damage and deafness. Toxicity has been reported in patients with normal renal function after topical application or irrigation of wounds with 0.5% neomycin solution. Neuromuscular blockade with respiratory paralysis also has occurred after irrigation of wounds or serosal cavities. The most important adverse effects resulting from the oral administration of neomycin are intestinal malabsorption and superinfection.

For a complete Bibliographical listing see Goodman & Gilman's *The Pharmacological Basis of Therapeutics,* **11th ed., or Goodman & Gilman Online at www.accessmedicine.com.**

46

PROTEIN SYNTHESIS INHIBITORS AND MISCELLANEOUS ANTIBACTERIAL AGENTS

TETRACYCLINES

Tetracyclines (Table 46–1) are inhibitors of bacterial protein synthesis.

EFFECTS ON PATHOGENIC MICROORGANISMS These drugs are bacteriostatic antibiotics with activity against a wide range of aerobic and anaerobic gram-positive and gram-negative bacteria. They intrinsically are more active against gram-positive than gram-negative microorganisms but also are effective against microorganisms such as *Rickettsia, Coxiella burnetii, Mycoplasma pneumoniae, Chlamydia* spp., *Legionella* spp., Ureaplasma, some atypical mycobacteria, and *Plasmodium* spp. that are resistant to cell-wall-active antimicrobial agents. Resistance of a bacterial strain to any one member may result in cross-resistance to other tetracyclines.

Tetracyclines are active against many spirochetes, including Borrelia burgdorferi (Lyme disease) and Treponema pallidum (syphilis). Tetracyclines are active against *Chlamydia* and *Mycoplasma*.

Effects on Intestinal Flora

Many tetracyclines can markedly alter enteric flora. Sensitive aerobic and anaerobic microorganisms are suppressed markedly during long-term tetracycline regimens and overgrowth of tetracycline-resistant microorganisms occurs, particularly yeasts (Candida *spp.*), *enterococci,* Proteus, *and* Pseudomonas. Tetracyclines *occasionally cause pseudomembranous colitis due to* Clostridium difficile.

MECHANISM OF ACTION AND RESISTANCE Tetracyclines inhibit bacterial protein synthesis by binding to the 30S bacterial ribosome and preventing access of aminoacyl tRNA to the acceptor (A) site on the mRNA-ribosome complex (Figure 46–1). They enter gram-negative bacteria by passive diffusion through channels formed by porins in the outer cell membrane and by active transport that pumps tetracyclines across the cytoplasmic membrane.

Resistance is widespread and often is inducible. The three main resistance mechanisms are: (1) decreased accumulation of tetracycline (decreased antibiotic influx or acquisition of an energy-dependent efflux pathway); (2) production of a ribosomal protein that displaces tetracycline from its target, a "protection" that also may occur by mutation; and (3) enzymatic inactivation of tetracyclines. Cross-resistance amongst tetracyclines depends on which mechanism is operative. Tetracycline resistance due to a ribosomal protection mechanism produces cross-resistance to doxycycline and minocycline because the target site protected is the same for all tetracyclines.

ABSORPTION, DISTRIBUTION, AND EXCRETION

Absorption Oral absorption of most tetracyclines is incomplete and the percentage of unabsorbed drug rises as the dose increases. Tetracycline absorption is impaired by concurrent ingestion of dairy products; aluminum hydroxide gels; calcium, magnesium, iron or zinc salts; and bismuth subsalicylate. After a single oral dose, peak plasma concentrations of oxytetracycline and tetracycline are attained in 2–4 hours. These drugs have half-lives in the range of 6–12 hours and often are given two to four times daily. Demeclocycline also is incompletely absorbed but can be administered in lower daily dosages because its $t_{1/2}$ of 16 hours provides effective plasma concentrations for 24–48 hours.

After oral dosing, doxycycline and minocycline are almost completely absorbed and have half-lives of 16–18 hours; they therefore are administered less frequently and at lower doses than tetracycline, oxytetracycline, or demeclocycline. Plasma concentrations are equivalent whether doxycycline is given orally or parenterally. Food, including dairy products, does not interfere with the absorption of doxycycline or minocycline.

Distribution Tetracyclines distribute widely throughout the body, including urine and prostate. They accumulate in reticuloendothelial cells of the liver, spleen, and bone marrow, and in bone, dentine, and enamel of unerupted teeth (*see* below). Meningeal inflammation is not required for passage of tetracyclines into the cerebrospinal fluid (CSF). Tetracyclines cross the placenta and enter the fetal circulation and amniotic fluid. Relatively high concentrations are found in breast milk.

Excretion Except for doxycycline, most tetracyclines are primarily eliminated by the kidney, although they also are concentrated in the liver, excreted in bile, and partially reabsorbed *via* enterohepatic recirculation. Minocycline is significantly metabolized by the liver. Comparable amounts of tetracycline (*i.e.*, 20–60%) are excreted in the urine within 24 hours following oral or intra-

Table 46–1

Structural Formulas of the Tetracyclines

Tetracycline

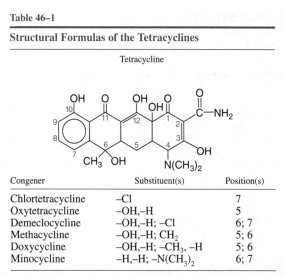

Congener	Substituent(s)	Position(s)
Chlortetracycline	–Cl	7
Oxytetracycline	–OH,–H	5
Demeclocycline	–OH,–H; –Cl	6; 7
Methacycline	–OH,–H; CH_2	5; 6
Doxycycline	–OH,–H; –CH_3, –H	5; 6
Minocycline	–H,–H; –$N(CH_3)_2$	6; 7

venous administration. Approximately 10–35% of a dose of oxytetracycline is excreted in active form in the urine, where it can be detected within 30 minutes and peaks ~5 hours after administration. The rate of renal clearance of demeclocycline is less than half that of tetracycline. Decreased hepatic function or biliary obstruction reduces excretion of these drugs, prolonging half-lives and raising plasma concentrations.

Minocycline is metabolized to a considerable extent and is recovered from urine and feces in lower amounts than other tetracyclines. The drug persists in the body long after its administration is stopped. The $t_{1/2}$ of minocycline is not prolonged in patients with hepatic failure.

Doxycycline at recommended doses does not accumulate significantly in patients with renal failure and thus is one of the safest of the tetracyclines in this setting. The drug is excreted in the feces. Its $t_{1/2}$ may be significantly shortened by concurrent therapy with barbiturates, phenytoin, rifampin, or other inducers of hepatic CYPs.

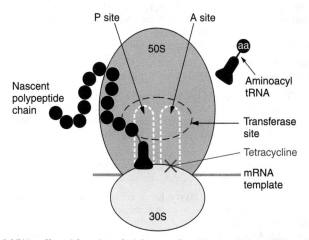

FIGURE 46–1 *Inhibition of bacterial protein synthesis by tetracyclines.* Messenger RNA (mRNA) attaches to the 30S subunit of bacterial ribosomal RNA. The P (peptidyl) site of the 50S ribosomal RNA subunit contains the nascent polypeptide chain; normally, the aminoacyl tRNA charged with the next amino acid (aa) to be added to the chain moves into the A (acceptor) site, with complementary base pairing between the anticodon sequence of tRNA and the codon sequence of mRNA. *Tetracyclines* inhibit bacterial protein synthesis by binding to the 30S subunit and blocking tRNA binding to the A site.

ROUTES OF ADMINISTRATION AND DOSAGE A variety of tetracyclines are available for oral, parenteral, and topical administration. Tetracycline, oxytetracycline (TERRAMYCIN, others), demeclocycline (DECLOMYCIN), minocycline (MINOCIN, others), and doxycycline (VIBRAMYCIN, others) are available in the U.S.

Oral Administration The oral dose of tetracycline ranges from 1 to 2 g/day in adults. Children older than 8 years of age should receive 25–50 mg/kg/day in 2–4 divided doses. The dose of doxy-cycline for adults is 100 mg 12 hours apart on the first day and then 100 mg once a day, or twice daily when severe infection is present; for children older than 8 years of age, the dose is 4–5 mg/kg/day in two divided doses the first day, then 2–2.5 mg/kg given once or twice daily. The dose of minocy-cline for adults is 200 mg initially, followed by 100 mg every 12 hours; for children, it is 4 mg/kg initially followed by 2 mg/kg every 12 hours.

GI distress, nausea, and vomiting can be minimized by administration of tetracyclines with food. Cholestyramine and colestipol can bind orally administered tetracyclines and interfere with their absorption. Generally, tetracyclines should be administered 2 hours before or 2 hours after meals and other drugs that interfere with their absorption.

Parenteral Administration Doxycycline, the preferred parenteral tetracycline in the U.S., is indicated in severe illness, in patients unable to ingest medication, or when the oral drug causes nausea and vomiting. Tetracyclines should not be given intramuscularly because of local irritation and poor absorption.

The usual intravenous dose of doxycycline is 200 mg in one or two infusions on the first day and 100 mg once or twice daily subsequently. For children who weigh <45 kg, the dose is 4.4 mg/kg on the first day and then 2.2 mg/kg/day thereafter. The intravenous dose of minocycline for adults is 200 mg, followed by 100 mg every 12 hours. Children older than 8 years of age should receive an initial dose of 4 mg/kg, followed by 2 mg/kg every 12 hours. Each 100 mg of minocycline must be diluted with 500–1000 mL of compatible fluid and slowly infused over 6 hours to minimize toxicity.

Local Application Except for local use in the eye, topical use of the tetracyclines is not rec-ommended. Minocycline sustained-release microspheres for subgingival administration are used in dentistry as an adjunct in patients with adult periodontitis.

THERAPEUTIC USES The tetracyclines have been used extensively to treat infectious dis-eases and as food additives in animals, leading to widespread resistance. They remain useful for infections caused by rickettsiae, mycoplasmas, and chlamydiae; doxycycline is used for respiratory infections that increasingly are resistant to other drugs.

Rickettsial Infections Tetracyclines may be life-saving in rickettsial infections, including Rocky Mountain spotted fever, recrudescent epidemic typhus, scrub typhus, rickettsialpox, and Q fever. Improvement often is evident within 24 hours. Doxycycline is the drug of choice for suspected or proven Rocky Mountain spotted fever in adults and children, including those <9 years of age, in whom the risk of staining of teeth is outweighed by the seriousness of the potentially fatal infection.

Mycoplasma Infections *Mycoplasma pneumoniae* is sensitive to tetracyclines, which shorten the duration of clinical manifestations in atypical pneumonia.

Chlamydia Doxycycline (100 mg twice daily for 21 days) is first-line therapy for *Lymphogranu-loma Venereum.* If relapse occurs, treatment is resumed with full doses and continued for longer periods. Pneumonia, bronchitis, or sinusitis caused by *Chlamydia pneumoniae* responds to tetracycline ther-apy. The tetracyclines also are of value in psittacosis. Drug therapy for 10–14 days usually is adequate.

Trachoma Doxycycline (100 mg twice daily for 14 days) or tetracycline (250 mg four times daily for 14 days) is effective for Trachoma. This disease is important in early childhood before the complete calcification of permanent teeth, and tetracyclines therefore often are contraindicated.

Sexually Transmitted Diseases Doxycycline is not recommended for gonococcal infections. C. trachomatis often is a coexistent pathogen in acute pelvic inflammatory disease. Doxycycline, 100 mg intravenously twice daily, is recommended for at least 48 hours after substantial clinical improvement, followed by oral therapy at the same dosage to complete a 14-day course. Doxycy-cline usually is combined with a cephalosporin to cover anaerobes and facultative aerobes.

Acute epididymitis in men <35 years old is caused by *C. trachomatis* or *Neisseria gonorrhoeae.* Effective regimens include a single injection of ceftriaxone (250 mg) plus doxycycline, 100 mg orally twice daily for 10 days. Sexual partners also should be treated.

Nonpregnant, penicillin-allergic patients who have primary, secondary, or latent syphilis can be treated with a tetracycline (*e.g.*, doxycycline, 100 mg orally twice daily for 2 weeks). Tetracyclines should not be used for neurosyphilis.

Anthrax   Doxycycline 100 mg every 12 hours (2.2 mg/kg every 12 hours for children weighing <45 kg) is indicated for prevention or treatment of anthrax. It should be combined with another agent when treating inhalational or GI infection. The recommended duration of therapy is 60 days for bioterrorism exposures.

Bacillary Infections
Brucellosis   Tetracyclines in combination with rifampin or streptomycin are effective for infections caused by *Brucella* spp. Effective regimens are doxycycline, 200 mg/day, plus rifampin, 600–900 mg/day for 6 weeks, or the usual dose of doxycycline plus streptomycin 1 g/day, intramuscularly.

Tularemia   Although streptomycin is preferable, tetracyclines also are effective for both ulceroglandular and typhoidal types of tularemia.

Cholera   Doxycycline (300 mg as a single dose) is effective in reducing stool volume and eradicating *Vibrio cholerae* from the stool within 48 hours. Antimicrobial agents are not substitutes for fluid and electrolyte replacement in this disease, and some strains of *V. cholerae* are resistant to tetracyclines.

Other Bacillary Infections   Tetracycline therapy often is ineffective in infections caused by Shigella, Salmonella, or other Enterobacteriaceae because of a high prevalence of drug-resistant strains. Resistance similarly limits usefulness for travelers' diarrhea.

Coccal Infections   Community strains of methicillin-resistant *S. aureus* often are susceptible to tetracycline, doxycycline, or minocycline, which can be effective for uncomplicated skin and soft-tissue infections. Approximately 85% of strains of *S. pneumoniae* are susceptible to tetracyclines, and doxycycline remains effective for empirical therapy of community-acquired pneumonia.

Other Infections   Actinomycosis, although most responsive to penicillin G, may be successfully treated with a tetracycline. Minocycline is an alternative for the treatment of nocardiosis, but a sulfonamide should be used concurrently. Tetracyclines are useful in the acute treatment and for prophylaxis of leptospirosis. *Borrelia* spp., including *B. recurrentis* (relapsing fever) and *B. burgdorferi* (Lyme disease), respond to tetracyclines. The tetracyclines have been used to treat susceptible atypical mycobacteria.

Acne   Tetracyclines (250 mg orally twice a day) have been used to treat acne.

UNTOWARD EFFECTS
Toxic Effects
Gastrointestinal   All tetracyclines can produce GI irritation, typically after oral administration. Tolerability can be improved by administering the drug with food, but *tetracyclines should not be taken with dairy products or antacids*. Tetracycline has been associated with esophagitis and pancreatitis. *Pseudomembranous colitis caused by overgrowth of C. difficile is a potentially life-threatening complication.*

Photosensitivity   Demeclocycline, doxycycline, and other tetracyclines to a lesser extent may produce photosensitivity reactions in treated individuals exposed to sunlight.

Hepatic Toxicity   Hepatic toxicity typically develops in patients receiving 2 g or more of drug per day parenterally but also may occur when large quantities are administered orally. Pregnant women are particularly susceptible.

Renal Toxicity   Tetracyclines may aggravate azotemia in patients with renal disease because of their catabolic effects. Doxycycline has fewer renal side effects than do other tetracyclines. Nephrogenic diabetes insipidus has been observed in some patients receiving demeclocycline, and this effect has been exploited to treat the syndrome of inappropriate secretion of antidiuretic hormone (*see* Chapter 29). Fanconi syndrome has occurred in patients taking outdated tetracycline, presumably due to toxic effects on the proximal tubule.

Effects on Teeth   Children treated with a tetracycline may develop permanent brown discoloration of the teeth. The duration of therapy appears to be less important than the total quantity of antibiotic administered. The risk is highest when given before the first dentition but may develop if the drug between the ages of 2 months and 5 years, Tetracycline treatment of pregnant patients may produce tooth discoloration in their children.

Miscellaneous Effects

Tetracyclines are deposited in the skeleton during gestation and throughout childhood and may depress bone growth in premature infants. This is readily reversible if the drug exposure is short. Thrombophlebitis frequently follows intravenous administration. This irritative effect of tetracyclines has been used for pleurodesis of malignant pleural effusions. Long-term tetracycline therapy may produce leukocytosis, atypical lymphocytes, toxic granulation, and thrombocytopenic purpura. Tetracyclines may cause increased intracranial pressure (pseudotumor cerebri) in young infants, even at the usual doses. Patients receiving minocycline may experience vestibular toxicity, manifested by dizziness, ataxia, nausea, and vomiting. Symptoms occur soon after the initial dose and usually disappear within 1–2 days after drug cessation.

Hypersensitivity Reactions

Various skin reactions rarely may follow the use of any of the tetracyclines. More severe allergic responses are angioedema and anaphylaxis; anaphylactoid reactions can occur even with oral administration. Other hypersensitivity reactions are burning of the eyes, cheilosis, glossitis, pruritus ani or vulvae, and vaginitis, which can persist for months after cessation of therapy. Fever, eosinophilia, and asthma also have been observed. Cross-sensitization among the various tetracyclines is common.

Biological Effects Other Than Allergic or Toxic

The tetracyclines administered orally or parenterally may lead to the development of superinfections caused by strains of bacteria or fungi resistant to these agents. Pseudomembranous colitis due to overgrowth of toxin-producing C. difficile *presents with severe diarrhea, fever, and stools containing mucous membrane neutrophils. Discontinuation of the drug, combined with the oral administration of metronidazole or vancomycin, usually is curative.*

GLYCYLCYCLINES

The glycylcyclines are tetracycline analogs that retain activity against tetracycline-resistant organisms containing genes mediating drug efflux or ribosomal protection. The drug tigecycline (TIGACYL) is FDA approved for the treatment of skin and soft tissue infections.

CHLORAMPHENICOL

Chloramphenicol has the following structure:

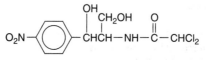

CHLORAMPHENICOL

MECHANISM OF ACTION Chloramphenicol inhibits protein synthesis in bacteria, and to a lesser extent, in eukaryotic cells. It binds reversibly to the 50S ribosomal subunit (near the binding site for the macrolide antibiotics and clindamycin). The drug prevents the binding of the amino acid–containing end of the aminoacyl tRNA to the acceptor site on the 50S ribosomal subunit. The interaction between peptidyltransferase and its amino acid substrate is blocked, inhibiting peptide bond formation (Figure 46–2).

Chloramphenicol also inhibits protein synthesis in mammalian mitochondria *via* a similar mechanism, perhaps because their ribosomes somewhat resemble bacterial ribosomes; erythropoietic cells are particularly sensitive.

ANTIMICROBIAL ACTIONS AND RESISTANCE

Chloramphenicol is bacteriostatic against a broad spectrum of bacteria and may be bactericidal against H. influenzae, Neisseria meningitidis, *and* S. pneumoniae. *Many gram-negative bacilli and most anaerobes are inhibited* in vitro. *Some aerobic gram-positive cocci, including* Streptococcus pyogenes, *S.* agalactiae *(group B streptococci), and* S. pneumoniae, *are sensitive.* S. aureus *tends to be less susceptible. Chloramphenicol is active against* Mycoplasma, Chlamydia, *and* Rickettsia.

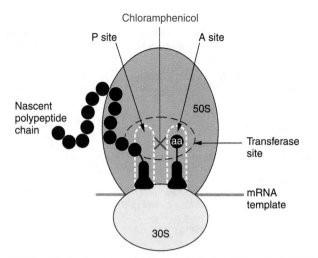

FIGURE 46–2 *Inhibition of bacterial protein synthesis by chloramphenicol.* Chloramphenicol binds to the 50S ribosomal subunit at the peptidyltransferase site and inhibits the transpeptidation reaction. Chloramphenicol binds to the 50S ribosomal subunit near the site of action of clindamycin and the macrolide antibiotics. These agents interfere with the binding of chloramphenicol and thus may interfere with each other's actions if given concurrently. *See* Figure 46–1 and its legend for additional information.

The Enterobacteriaceae are variably sensitive to chloramphenicol. P. aeruginosa *is resistant to even very high concentrations of chloramphenicol. Strains of* V. cholerae *have remained largely susceptible to chloramphenicol. Prevalent strains of* Shigella *and* Salmonella *are resistant to multiple drugs, including chloramphenicol.*

Resistance to chloramphenicol usually is caused by a plasmid-encoded acetyltransferase that inactivates the drug by preventing its binding to bacterial ribosomes. Resistance also can result from decreased permeability or ribosomal mutation.

ABSORPTION, DISTRIBUTION, FATE, AND EXCRETION Chloramphenicol (CHLORO- MYCETIN) is absorbed rapidly from the GI tract. For intravenous or intramuscular use, chloramphenicol succinate is a prodrug that is hydrolyzed by esterases to chloramphenicol *in vivo.* Chloramphenicol succinate is rapidly cleared from plasma by the kidneys; this may reduce bioavailability, since up to 30% of the dose may be excreted before hydrolysis. Poor renal function in the neonate and other states of renal insufficiency result in increased plasma concentrations of chloramphenicol succinate. Decreased esterase activity has been observed in the plasma of neonates and infants, prolonging time to peak concentrations of active chloramphenicol (up to 4 hours) and extending the period over which renal clearance of chloramphenicol succinate can occur.

Chloramphenicol is widely distributed in body fluids and achieves therapeutic concentrations in CSF. Chloramphenicol is present in bile, milk, and placental fluid. It also is found in the aqueous humor after subconjunctival injection.

Hepatic metabolism to the inactive glucuronide is the major route of elimination. This metabolite and chloramphenicol are excreted in the urine. Patients with impaired liver function have decreased metabolic clearance, and dose should be decreased. About 50% of chloramphenicol is bound to plasma proteins; this is reduced in cirrhotic patients and in neonates. Half-life is not altered significantly by renal insufficiency or hemodialysis, and dose adjustment usually is not required. However, if the dose of chloramphenicol has been reduced because of cirrhosis, clearance by hemodialysis may be significant. Drug administration after hemodialysis minimizes this effect. Variability in the metabolism and pharmacokinetics of chloramphenicol in neonates, infants, and children necessitates monitoring of plasma drug levels.

THERAPEUTIC USES Therapy with chloramphenicol must be limited to infections for which its benefits outweigh the risks of the potential toxicities. When other antimicrobial drugs that are equally effective and potentially less toxic are available, they should be used instead of chloramphenicol.

Typhoid Fever

Third-generation cephalosporins and quinolones are drugs of choice for the treatment of typhoid fever. The adult dose of chloramphenicol for typhoid fever is 1 g every 6 hours for 4 weeks.

Bacterial Meningitis

Chloramphenicol is an alternative drug for meningitis caused by H. influenzae, N. meningitidis, *and* S. pneumoniae *in patients who have severe allergy to β-lactams and in developing countries. The total daily dose for children should be 50–75 mg/kg of body weight, divided into equal doses given intravenously every 6 hours for 2 weeks.*

Rickettsial Diseases

Tetracyclines usually are the preferred agents for the treatment of rickettsial diseases. In patients allergic to these drugs, in those with reduced renal function, in pregnant women, and in children <8 years of age who require prolonged or repeated courses of therapy, chloramphenicol may be the drug of choice. Rickettsial diseases, such as Rocky Mountain spotted fever, respond well to chloramphenicol. For adults, a dose of 50 mg/kg/day is recommended for all the rickettsial diseases. The daily dose of chloramphenicol for children with these diseases is 75 mg/kg, divided into equal portions and given every 6–8 hours. Therapy should be continued until the patient has improved and is afebrile for 24–48 hours.

Brucellosis

If tetracyclines are contraindicated, 750–1000 mg of chloramphenicol orally every 6 hours is recommended.

UNTOWARD EFFECTS Chloramphenicol inhibits the synthesis of proteins of the inner mitochondrial membrane, probably by inhibiting the ribosomal peptidyltransferase. Much of its toxicity can be attributed to these effects.

Hypersensitivity Reactions Rashes may result from chloramphenicol hypersensitivity. Fever may appear simultaneously or be the sole manifestation. Angioedema is a rare complication. Jarisch-Herxheimer reactions may occur after institution of chloramphenicol therapy for syphilis, brucellosis, and typhoid fever.

Hematological Toxicity Chloramphenicol causes a dose-related toxicity presenting as anemia, leukopenia, or thrombocytopenia and an idiosyncratic response manifested by aplastic anemia, often leading to fatal pancytopenia. Pancytopenia occurs more commonly in individuals who undergo prolonged therapy and especially in those who are exposed to the drug on multiple occasions. Although the estimated incidence is only 1 in 30,000 courses of therapy, the fatality rate is high with complete bone-marrow aplasia, and there is an increased incidence of acute leukemia in those who recover. Aplastic anemia accounts for ~70% of cases of blood dyscrasias due to chloramphenicol, while hypoplastic anemia, agranulocytosis, and thrombocytopenia make up the remainder. The proposed mechanism involves conversion of the nitro group to a toxic intermediate by intestinal bacteria.

Dose-related erythroid suppression probably reflects inhibition of mitochondrial protein synthesis in erythroid precursors, which impairs iron incorporation into heme. Bone marrow suppression occurs regularly with plasma concentrations >25 μg/mL and is observed with large doses of chloramphenicol, prolonged treatment, or both. Dose-related bone marrow suppression may progress to aplasia if treatment is continued, but most cases of aplasia develop without prior dose-related marrow suppression.

The risk of aplastic anemia does not contraindicate the use of chloramphenicol in situations in which it may be life-saving. The drug should never be used in undefined situations or in diseases readily, safely, and effectively treated with other antimicrobial agents.

Toxic and Irritative Effects Nausea and vomiting, unpleasant taste, diarrhea, and perineal irritation may follow oral administration of chloramphenicol. Rare toxic effects are blurred vision and digital paresthesias. Tissues with high oxygen consumption (*e.g.*, brain, heart) may be particularly susceptible to chloramphenicol's effects on mitochondrial enzymes.

Neonates, especially if premature, may develop a serious illness termed *gray baby syndrome* if exposed to excessive doses of chloramphenicol. This syndrome usually begins several days after treatment is started. Within 24 hours, vomiting, refusal to suck, irregular and rapid respiration, abdominal distention, periods of cyanosis, and passage of loose, green stools occur. The children are severely ill by the end of the first day. Over the next 24 hours, they turn an ashen-gray color and become flaccid and hypothermic. A similar syndrome has occurred in adults who were accidentally overdosed with the drug. Death occurs in ~40% of patients within 2 days of initial symptoms. Those who recover usually exhibit no sequelae.

Two mechanisms contribute to chloramphenicol toxicity in neonates: (1) a developmental deficiency of glucuronyl transferase, the hepatic enzyme that metabolizes chloramphenicol; and (2) inadequate renal excretion of unconjugated drug. At the onset, plasma chloramphenicol concentrations usually exceed 100 μg/mL but may be only 75 μg/mL. For children under 2 weeks of age, the maximum daily chloramphenicol dose is 25 mg/kg of body weight; thereafter, full-term infants may receive up to 50 mg/kg daily.

DRUG INTERACTIONS Chloramphenicol inhibits hepatic CYPs and thereby prolongs the half-lives of CYP substrates, including *coumadin, phenytoin, chlorpropamide,* HIV protease inhibitors, *rifabutin,* and *tolbutamide.* Severe toxicity and death have occurred due to these drug interactions. Concurrent administration of *phenobarbital* or *rifampin,* which potently induce CYPs, shortens chloramphenicol's $t_{1/2}$ and may result in subtherapeutic drug concentrations.

MACROLIDES (ERYTHROMYCIN, CLARITHROMYCIN, AND AZITHROMYCIN)

Macrolide antibiotics inhibit bacterial protein synthesis (Figure 46–3). Macrolides contain a many-membered lactone ring (14 for erythromycin and clarithromycin and 15 for azithromycin) to which are attached one or more deoxy sugars. Azithromycin has an additional methyl-substituted nitrogen in the lactone ring that improves acid stability and tissue penetration and broadens the activity spectrum.

ANTIBACTERIAL ACTIVITY

Erythromycin usually is bacteriostatic. It is most active in vitro *against aerobic gram-positive cocci and bacilli. Cross-resistance is complete. The prevalence of macrolide resistance among group A streptococcal isolates is related to consumption of macrolide antibiotics within the population. Only 5% of penicillin-susceptible strains are macrolide-resistant, whereas 50% or more of penicillin-resistant strains may be macrolide-resistant. Staphylococci are not reliably sensitive to erythromycin. Macrolide-resistant strains of* S. aureus *are potentially also resistant to clindamycin and streptogramin B (quinupristin). Gram-positive bacilli are sensitive to erythromycin, including* Clostridium perfringens, Corynebacterium diphtheriae, *and* Listeria monocytogenes.

Erythromycin is inactive against most aerobic enteric gram-negative bacilli but has modest activity in vitro *against other gram-negative organisms, including* H. influenzae *and* N. meningitidis, *and good activity against most strains of* N. gonorrhoeae. *Useful antibacterial activity also is observed against* Pasteurella multocida, Borrelia spp., *and* Bordetella pertussis. *Resistance is*

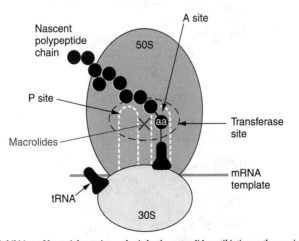

FIGURE 46–3 *Inhibition of bacterial protein synthesis by the macrolide antibiotics erythromycin, clarithromycin, and azithromycin.* Macrolide antibiotics are bacteriostatic agents that inhibit protein synthesis by binding reversibly to the 50S ribosomal subunits of sensitive organisms. Erythromycin apparently inhibits the translocation step wherein the nascent peptide chain temporarily residing at the A site of the transferase reaction fails to move to the P, or donor, site. Alternatively, macrolides may bind and cause a conformational change that terminates protein synthesis by indirectly interfering with transpeptidation and translocation. *See* Figure 46–1 and its legend for additional information.

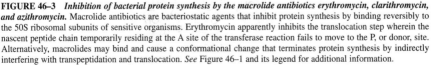

common for B. fragilis. *Macrolides are usually active against* Campylobacter jejuni. *Erythromycin is active against* M. pneumoniae *and* Legionella pneumophila. *Most strains of* C. trachomatis *are inhibited by erythromycin.*

Clarithromycin is slightly more potent than erythromycin against sensitive strains of streptococci and staphylococci and has modest activity against H. influenzae *and* N. gonorrhoeae. *Clarithromycin has good activity against* M. catarrhalis, Chlamydia *spp.,* L. pneumophila, B. burgdorferi, Mycoplasma pneumoniae, *and* H. pylori.

Azithromycin generally is less active than erythromycin against gram-positive organisms and slightly more active than either erythromycin or clarithromycin against H. influenzae *and* Campylobacter *spp.* Azithromycin is very active against M. catarrhalis, P. multocida, Chlamydia spp., M. pneumoniae, L. pneumophila, B. burgdorferi, Fusobacterium spp., *and* N. gonorrhoeae.

Azithromycin and clarithromycin have enhanced activity against M. avium-intracellulare, *as well as against some protozoa (e.g.,* Toxoplasma gondii, Cryptosporidium, *and* Plasmodium spp.*). Clarithromycin has good activity against* Mycobacterium leprae *(see Chapter 47).*

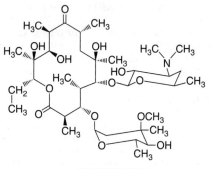

ERYTHROMYCIN

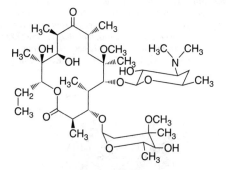

CLARITHROMYCIN

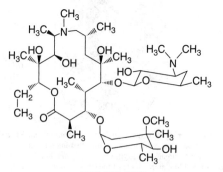

AZITHROMYCIN

MECHANISM OF ACTION   Macrolide antibiotics are bacteriostatic agents that inhibit protein synthesis by binding reversibly to 50S ribosomal subunits of sensitive microorganisms (Figure 46–3) at or very near the site that binds chloramphenicol (Figure 46–2). Erythromycin does not inhibit peptide bond formation *per se*, but rather inhibits the translocation step wherein a newly synthesized peptidyl tRNA molecule moves from the acceptor site on the ribosome to the peptidyl donor site. Gram-positive bacteria accumulate ~100 times more erythromycin than do gram-negative bacteria.

Resistance to macrolides can result from: (1) drug efflux by an active pump mechanism; (2) ribosomal protection by inducible or constitutive production of methylase enzymes that modify the ribosomal target and decrease drug binding; (3) macrolide hydrolysis by esterases produced by Enterobacteriaceae; and (4) chromosomal mutations that alter a 50S ribosomal protein (found in *B. subtilis, Campylobacter* spp., mycobacteria, and gram-positive cocci).

ABSORPTION, DISTRIBUTION, AND EXCRETION
Absorption   Erythromycin base is incompletely but adequately absorbed from the upper small intestine. Because it is inactivated by gastric acid, the drug is administered as enteric-coated tablets, as capsules containing enteric-coated pellets that dissolve in the duodenum, or as an ester. Food may impair absorption. Esters of erythromycin base (*e.g.*, stearate, estolate, and ethylsuccinate) have improved acid stability and are less affected by food. Higher erythromycin concentrations can be achieved by intravenous administration.

Clarithromycin is absorbed rapidly from the GI tract after oral administration, but hepatic first-pass metabolism reduces bioavailability to ~50%. Peak concentrations occur 2 hours after drug administration. Clarithromycin may be given with or without food, but the extended-release form should be administered with food to improve bioavailability.

Azithromycin administered orally is absorbed rapidly and distributed widely throughout the body, except to the brain and CSF. Azithromycin should not be given with food. Azithromycin also can be given intravenously.

Distribution   Erythromycin diffuses readily into intracellular fluids, achieving antibacterial activity in essentially all sites except the brain and CSF. Concentrations in the middle ear may be inadequate for the treatment of otitis media caused by *H. influenzae*. Protein binding is ~70–80% for erythromycin base and even higher for the estolate. Erythromycin crosses the placenta, and drug concentrations in fetal plasma are ~5–20% of those in maternal circulation. Concentrations in breast milk are 50% of those in serum.

Clarithromycin and its active metabolite, 14-hydroxyclarithromycin, achieve high intracellular concentrations throughout the body. Tissue concentrations, including the middle ear, generally exceed serum concentrations. Protein binding ranges from 40–70% and is concentration dependent.

Azithromycin's unique pharmacokinetic properties include extensive tissue distribution and high drug concentrations within cells (including phagocytes), resulting in much greater concentrations of drugs in tissue or secretions compared to simultaneous serum concentrations. Protein binding is 50% at low plasma concentrations and less at higher concentrations.

Elimination   Only 2–5% of orally administered erythromycin is excreted in active form in the urine; this value is from 12–15% after intravenous infusion. The antibiotic is concentrated in the liver and is excreted in the bile. The serum $t_{1/2}$ of erythromycin is ~1.6 hours; although this may be prolonged in patients with anuria, dosage reduction is not routinely recommended in renal insufficiency. The drug is not removed significantly by peritoneal or hemodialysis.

Clarithromycin is metabolized in the liver to several metabolites. Primary metabolic pathways are oxidative *N*-demethylation and hydroxylation at the 14 position to form an active metabolite. The elimination half-lives are 3–7 hours for clarithromycin and 5–9 hours for 14-hydroxyclarithromycin. Metabolism is saturable, resulting in nonlinear pharmacokinetics, and longer half-lives are observed after larger doses. The amount of clarithromycin excreted unchanged in the urine ranges from 20–40%, depending on the dose and the formulation (tablet *vs.* oral suspension). An additional 10–15% of a dose is excreted in the urine as 14-hydroxyclarithromycin. Dose adjustment is not needed unless the creatinine clearance is <30 mL/min.

Azithromycin undergoes some hepatic metabolism to inactive metabolites, but biliary excretion is the major route of elimination. Only 12% of drug is excreted unchanged in the urine. The $t_{1/2}$, 40–68 hours, is prolonged because of extensive tissue sequestration and binding.

DOSAGE   The usual oral dose of erythromycin (*erythromycin base;* E-MYCIN, others) for adults ranges from 1 to 2 g/day, in divided doses, usually given every 6 hours. Daily doses of erythromycin as large as 8 g have been well tolerated. Food ideally should not be taken concurrently with erythromycin base or the stearate formulations but is acceptable with *erythromycin estolate* or *erythromycin ethylsuccinate* (E.E.S., others). The oral dose of erythromycin for children is 30–50 mg/kg/day, divided into four portions; this dose may be doubled for severe infections. Intravenous administration is reserved for the therapy of severe infections, such as legionellosis. The usual dose is 0.5–1 g every 6 hours; 1 g of erythromycin glucoptate has been given intravenously every 6 hours for up to 4 weeks with no adverse effects except for local thrombophlebitis. *Erythromycin lactobionate* (ERYTHROCIN LACTOBIONATE-I.V.) is available for intravenous injection.

Clarithromycin (BIAXIN FILMTABS, BIAXIN XL FILMTABS, and BIAXIN granules for suspension) usually is given twice daily at a dose of 250 mg for children older than 12 years and adults with mild-to-moderate infection. Larger doses (*e.g.*, 500 mg twice daily) are indicated for serious infections such as pneumonia or when infection is caused by organisms such as *H. influenzae*. Children younger than 12 years old should receive 7.5 mg/kg twice daily. The 500-mg, extended-release formulation is given as two tablets once daily. Clarithromycin (500 mg) is also packaged with *lansoprazole* (30 mg) and *amoxicillin* (1 g) as a combination regimen (PREVPAC) administered twice daily for 14 days to eradicate *H. pylori*.

Azithromycin (ZITHROMAX tablet, oral suspension, and powder for intravenous injection) should be given 1 hour before or 2 hours after meals when administered orally. For outpatient therapy of community-acquired pneumonia, pharyngitis, or skin and skin-structure infections, a loading dose of 500 mg is given on the first day, followed by 250 mg/day for 4 additional days. Treatment or prophylaxis of *M. avium-intracellulare* infection in AIDS patients requires 500 mg daily in combination with other agents for treatment; or 1200 mg once weekly for primary prevention. Azithromycin is useful in treatment of sexually transmitted diseases, especially during pregnancy when tetracyclines are contraindicated. Uncomplicated nongonococcal urethritis presumed to be due to *C. trachomatis* is treated with a single 1-g dose of azithromycin, which also is effective for chancroid. Azithromycin (1 g/week for 3 weeks) is an alternative drug for granuloma inguinale or lymphogranuloma venereum.

In children, the recommended dose of azithromycin oral suspension for acute otitis media and pneumonia is 10 mg/kg on the first day (maximum 500 mg) and 5 mg/kg (maximum 250 mg/day) on days 2–5. The dose for tonsillitis or pharyngitis is 12 mg/kg/day, up to 500 mg total, for 5 days.

THERAPEUTIC USES

Mycoplasma pneumoniae Infections

A macrolide is one drug of choice for mycoplasma infections.

Legionnaires' Disease

Because of excellent in vitro *activity, superior tissue concentration, convenience of once-daily dosing, and better tolerability, azithromycin has supplanted erythromycin as the first-line drug for legionellosis. The recommended dose is 500 mg daily, intravenously or orally, for 10–14 days.*

Chlamydial Infections

Chlamydial infections can be treated effectively with any of the macrolides. A single 1-g dose of azithromycin is recommended for patients with uncomplicated urethral, endocervical, rectal, or epididymal infections because of the ease of compliance. During pregnancy, erythromycin base, 500 mg four times daily for 7 days, is recommended as first-line therapy for chlamydial urogenital infections. Azithromycin is a suitable alternative. Erythromycin base is preferred for chlamydial pneumonia of infancy and ophthalmia neonatorum (50 mg/kg/day in four divided doses for 10–14 days).

Pneumonia caused by Chlamydia pneumoniae *responds to macrolides, fluoroquinolones, and tetracyclines in standard doses. A specific etiological diagnosis in community-acquired pneumonia rarely is made, and length of treatment (typically 7–10 days) is based on clinical response.*

Diphtheria

Erythromycin 250 mg four times daily for 7 days is very effective for acute infections or for eradicating the carrier state. Other macrolides likely are also effective but are not FDA-approved for this indication. Antibiotics do not alter the course of an acute infection with diphtheria or decrease the risk of complications. Antitoxin is indicated in the treatment of acute infection.

Pertussis

Erythromycin is the drug of choice for treating persons with B. pertussis disease and for postexposure prophylaxis of household members and close contacts. A 7-day regimen of erythromycin estolate (40 mg/kg/day, maximum 1 g/day) is sufficient. Clarithromycin and azithromycin also are effective. If administered early in the course of whooping cough, erythromycin may shorten the duration of illness; it has little influence on the disease once the paroxysmal stage is reached. Nasopharyngeal cultures should be obtained if pertussis does not improve with erythromycin therapy, since resistance has been reported.

Streptococcal Infections

The macrolides are valuable alternatives for treatment of patients who have a serious allergy to penicillin. Unfortunately, macrolide-resistant strains are increasingly encountered.

Staphylococcal Infections

Macrolides no longer can be relied upon unless in vitro *susceptibility has been documented.*

Campylobacter Infections

Fluroquinolones largely have replaced erythromycin for this disease in adults. Erythromycin remains useful for treatment of Campylobacter gastroenteritis in children.

Helicobacter pylori Infection

Clarithromycin 500 mg, in combination with omeprazole, 20 mg, and amoxicillin, 1 g, each administered twice daily for 10–14 days, is effective for treatment of peptic ulcer disease caused by H. pylori.

Tetanus

Erythromycin (500 mg orally every 6 hours for 10 days) may be given to eradicate C. tetani *in patients with tetanus who are allergic to penicillin. The mainstays of therapy are débridement, physiological support, tetanus antitoxin, and anticonvulsants.*

Mycobacterial Infections

The use of these drugs in the treatment and prevention of mycobacterial infections is described in Chapter 47.

PROPHYLACTIC USES

Erythromycin is an effective alternative for the prophylaxis of recurrences of rheumatic fever in individuals who are allergic to penicillin.

UNTOWARD EFFECTS   Erythromycin rarely causes serious side effects. Allergic reactions include fever, eosinophilia, and rash, either alone or in combination; these manifestations resolve after therapy is stopped. Cholestatic hepatitis, the most striking side effect, is caused primarily by erythromycin estolate and rarely by the ethylsuccinate or the stearate and may be a hypersensitivity reaction to the estolate ester. The illness starts after 1–3 weeks of treatment and presents with nausea, vomiting, and abdominal cramps. These symptoms soon are followed by jaundice, fever, leukocytosis, eosinophilia, and elevated plasma transaminases. Liver biopsy reveals cholestasis and periportal inflammation, sometimes with necrosis of neighboring parenchymal cells. Findings usually resolve within a few days after drug cessation and rarely are prolonged.

Oral or intravenous administration of erythromycin, especially in large doses, frequently is accompanied by epigastric distress. Erythromycin stimulates GI motility by acting on motilin receptors and is used postoperatively to promote peristalsis and in patients with gastroparesis to speed gastric emptying (see Chapter 37). These dose-related GI symptoms occur more commonly in children and young adults; they may be reduced by prolonging the infusion time to 1 hour or by pretreatment with glycopyrrolate. Intravenous infusion of 1-g doses, even when dissolved in a large volume, often is followed by thrombophlebitis, which can be minimized by slow rates of infusion.

Erythromycin can cause cardiac arrhythmias, including QT prolongation with polymorphic ventricular tachycardia. Most patients have had underlying cardiac disease, or the arrhythmias were seen in combination with other drugs (see Chapter 34).

DRUG INTERACTIONS   Erythromycin and clarithromycin inhibit CYP3A4 and cause significant drug interactions. Erythromycin potentiates the effects of *carbamazepine*, glucocorticoids, *cyclosporine, digoxin,* ergot alkaloids, *theophylline, triazolam, valproate,* and coumadin, probably by interfering with their CYP-mediated metabolism (*see* Chapter 3). Clarithromycin has a similar drug interaction profile. Azithromycin lacks these drug interactions, but caution still is advised when using azithromycin in conjunction with drugs that interact with erythromycin.

VANCOMYCIN

Vancomycin is a complex tricyclic glycopeptide (MW ~1500 Da). It acts by inhibiting cell wall synthesis (Figure 46–4).

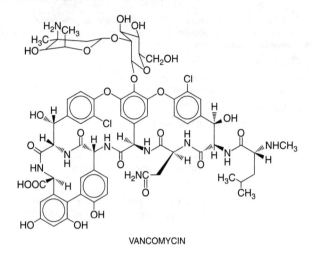

VANCOMYCIN

ANTIBACTERIAL ACTIVITY Vancomycin is primarily active against gram-positive bacteria. *S. aureus* and *S. epidermidis*, including strains resistant to methicillin, usually are inhibited. *S. pyogenes, S. pneumoniae,* and viridans streptococci are highly susceptible to vancomycin. *Bacillus* spp., including *B. anthracis*, are highly sensitive. Essentially all species of gram-negative bacilli and mycobacteria are resistant to vancomycin.

MECHANISMS OF ACTION AND RESISTANCE Vancomycin inhibits cell wall synthesis by binding with high affinity to the D-Ala-D-Ala terminus of precursor units (Figure 46–4). It is bactericidal for dividing microorganisms.

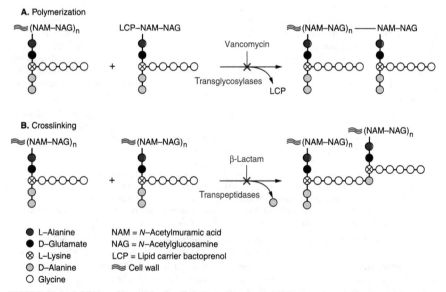

FIGURE 46–4 *Inhibition of bacterial cell wall synthesis.* Vancomycin inhibits the polymerization or transglycosylase reaction (*A*) by binding to the D-Ala-D-Ala terminus of the cell wall precursor unit attached to its lipid carrier and blocks linkage to the glycopeptide polymer (indicated by the subscript n). These (NAM–NAG)n peptidoglycan polymers are located within the cell wall. *Van A*-type resistance is due to expression of enzymes that modify cell wall precursor by substituting a terminal D-lactate for D-Ala, reducing vancomycin-binding affinity by 1000 times. β-Lactam antibiotics inhibit the cross-linking or transpeptidase reaction (*B*) that links glycopeptide polymer chains by formation of a cross-bridge with the stem peptide (the five Glys in this example) of one chain, displacing the terminal D-Ala of an adjacent chain.

Vancomycin-resistant strains of enterococci have emerged as major nosocomial pathogens in the U.S. Vancomycin resistance determinants in *E. faecium* and *E. faecalis* are located on a transposon that is readily transferred among enterococci, and potentially other gram-positive bacteria. These strains typically are resistant to multiple antibiotics, including *streptomycin, gentamicin,* and *ampicillin.* Resistance to streptomycin and gentamicin is of special concern, because the combination of an aminoglycoside with a cell-wall-synthesis inhibitor is the only reliably bactericidal regimen for enterococcal endocarditis.

Enterococcal resistance to vancomycin is the result of alteration of the D-Ala-D-Ala target to D-Ala-D-lactate or D-Ala-D-Ser, which bind vancomycin poorly. Several mutations are required for this target alteration and distinct phenotypes have been described. The *Van A* phenotype confers inducible resistance to teicoplanin and vancomycin in *E. faecium* and *E. faecalis.* The *Van B* phenotype, which tends to be a lower level of resistance, also has been identified in *E. faecium* and *E. faecalis.* The trait is inducible by vancomycin but not teicoplanin, and consequently, many strains remain susceptible to teicoplanin.

S. aureus and coagulase-negative staphylococci may express reduced or "intermediate" susceptibility to vancomycin or high-level resistance. Intermediate resistance is associated with (and may be preceded by) a heterogeneous phenotype in which a small proportion of cells within the population (~1 in 10^6) will grow in the presence of vancomycin concentrations above 4 µg/mL. The basis of the intermediate phenotype is not well understood.

High-level vancomycin-resistance in S. aureus *(MIC ≥32 µg/mL) has resulted from a conjugative plasmid into which the* Van A *transposon was integrated by an interspecies horizontal gene transfer from* E. faecalis *to a methicillin-resistant strain of* S. aureus.

Infections caused by intermediate strains have failed to respond to vancomycin. Prior treatment courses and low vancomycin levels may predispose patients to infection with such vancomycin-intermediate strains, which typically are resistant to methicillin and multiple other antibiotics. Their emergence is a major concern because vancomycin has been the only antibiotic to which staphylococci were reliably susceptible.

ABSORPTION, DISTRIBUTION, AND EXCRETION Vancomycin is poorly absorbed after oral administration. For parenteral therapy, the drug should be administered intravenously. The drug has a serum elimination $t_{1/2}$ of ~6 hours. Approximately 30% of vancomycin is bound to plasma protein. Vancomycin appears in various body fluids, including the CSF when the meninges are inflamed, bile, and pleural, pericardial, synovial, and ascitic fluids. About 90% of an injected dose is excreted by glomerular filtration.

THERAPEUTIC USES Vancomycin (VANCOCIN, others) is marketed for intravenous use as a sterile powder. It should be diluted and infused over at least 60 minutes to avoid infusion-related adverse reactions. The usual dose of vancomycin for adults is 30 mg/kg/day in 2–3 divided doses. A trough serum concentration of 5–15 µg/mL (10–20 µg/mL for serious infections such as endocarditis or meningitis) is recommended. Doses above 30 mg/kg/day may be required to achieve these trough concentrations, and up to 60 mg/kg/day has been suggested for meningitis. The "peak" concentration is not monitored routinely but should generally remain below 60 µg/mL to avoid ototoxicity.

Pediatric doses are as follows: for newborns during the first week of life, 15 mg/kg initially, followed by 10 mg/kg every 12 hours; for infants 8–30 days old, 15 mg/kg followed by 10 mg/kg every 8 hours; for older infants and children, 10 mg/kg every 6 hours.

Dosage alteration is required for patients with impaired renal function. The drug has been used effectively in functionally anephric and dialysis patients by the administration of 1 g (~15 mg/kg) every 5–7 days. Because there is considerable variation in how well vancomycin is dialyzed with different membranes, blood levels should be monitored to guide dose adjustments.

Vancomycin can be administered orally to patients with pseudomembranous colitis, although metronidazole is preferred. The dose for adults is 125–250 mg every 6 hours; the total daily dose for children is 40 mg/kg, given in three to four divided doses.

Vancomycin should be used only to treat serious infections and is particularly useful in the management of infections due to methicillin-resistant staphylococci and in severe staphylococcal infections in patients who are allergic to penicillins and cephalosporins. Vancomycin is less rapidly bactericidal than the antistaphylococcal β-lactams (e.g., nafcillin or cefazolin) and may be less efficacious. Treatment with vancomycin is effective and convenient when there is disseminated staphylococcal infection or localized shunt infection in a patients receiving hemodialysis or peritoneal dialysis, because the drug can be administered once weekly or in the dialysis fluid.

Intraventricular administration of vancomycin (via a shunt or reservoir) has been necessary in a few cases of CNS infections due to susceptible microorganisms that did not respond to intravenous therapy alone.
  In penicillin-allergic patients, vancomycin is an effective alternative for the treatment of endocarditis caused by viridans streptococci or, combined with an aminoglycoside, for enterococcal endocarditis. Vancomycin has become an important antibiotic in the management of known or suspected penicillin-resistant pneumococcal infections.

UNTOWARD EFFECTS   Among the hypersensitivity reactions produced by vancomycin are rashes and anaphylaxis. Chills and fever may occur. Rapid intravenous infusion may cause erythematous or urticarial reactions, flushing, tachycardia, and hypotension. The extreme flushing that can occur is called "red-neck" or "red-man" syndrome. This results from a direct toxic effect of vancomycin on mast cells to induce histamine release.

Auditory impairment, sometimes permanent, is associated with excessive plasma concentrations of the drug (60–100 μg/mL). Nephrotoxicity is unusual when appropriate doses are used, as judged by renal function and determinations of blood levels of the drug. Caution must be exercised when ototoxic or nephrotoxic drugs (*e.g.*, aminoglycosides) are coadministered or in patients with impaired renal function.

KETOLIDES (TELITHROMYCIN)

Telithromycin (KETEK) is a semisynthetic derivative of erythromycin with modifications that render it less susceptible to methylase- and efflux-mediated resistance, increasing activity against many macrolide-resistant gram-positive strains. The structure of telithromycin is:

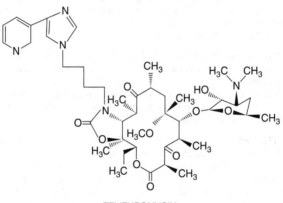

TELITHROMYCIN

ANTIBACTERIAL ACTIVITY   Telithromycin is active against staphylococci, streptococci, *S. pneumoniae, Haemophilus* spp., *Moraxella catarrhalis*, mycoplasma, chlamydia, and *Legionella*. It is slightly more potent than erythromycin.

MECHANISM OF ACTION AND RESISTANCE   Ketolides and macrolides have the same ribosomal target site, but structural modifications within ketolides neutralize the common mechanisms that confer macrolide resistance. Introduction of the 3-keto function converts a methylase-inducing macrolide into a noninducing ketolide. This moiety also prevents drug efflux. The carbamate substitution at C11-C12 enhances binding to the ribosomal target site, even when the site is methylated, by introducing an extra interaction of the ketolide with the ribosome. Inducible and constitutive methylase-producing strains of *S. pneumoniae* are therefore telithromycin-susceptible. However, constitutive methylase-producing strains of *S. aureus* and *S. pyogenes* are telithromycin-resistant because the strength of the ketolide interaction with the fully methylated ribosomal binding site is insufficient to overcome resistance.

ABSORPTION, DISTRIBUTION, AND EXCRETION   Telithromycin is formulated as a 400-mg tablet for oral dosing. It is well absorbed with ~60% bioavailability. Peak serum concentrations are achieved within 30 minutes to 4 hours. With a $t_{1/2}$ of 9.8 hours, the drug can be given once daily. It is 60–70% bound by serum protein, principally albumin. It penetrates well into most tissues, exceeding plasma concentrations by approximately two- to tenfold or more. Telithromycin is concentrated in macrophages and leukocytes, where high concentrations are maintained 24 hours after dosing. The drug is cleared primarily by hepatic metabolism, 50% by CYP3A4 and 50% by CYP-independent metabolism. No dose adjustment is required for hepatic failure or mild-to-moderate renal failure, but dose reduction is advised when the creatinine clearance is <30 mL/min.

THERAPEUTIC USES Telithromycin is approved for treatment of community-acquired pneumonia of mild-to-moderate severity in patients ≥18 years old. Although telithromycin is not indicated for treatment of severe pneumonia or bacteremia, almost 90% of patients who proved to have pneumococcal bacteremia were clinically cured after taking it. In premarketing trials of telithromycin on patients with community-acquired pneumonia caused by multiple-drug-resistant strains of *S. pneumoniae*, over 90% of patients were cured.

UNTOWARD EFFECTS Telithromycin generally is well tolerated. Nausea, vomiting, and diarrhea occur in 3–10% of treatment courses. Slowed accommodation can cause visual symptoms. Reversible hepatic dysfunction with elevated transaminases or hepatitis and pseudomembranous colitis has been reported; in some cases, the hepatotoxicity has been severe and even fatal. Telithromycin is not recommended for routine use in patients with myasthenia gravis due to possible disease exacerbation.

Telithromycin may cause clinically significant QTc prolongation and increased risk of ventricular arrhythmia in predisposed patients (*see* Chapter 34). It should not be used in patients with long QT syndrome, uncorrected hypokalemia or hypomagnesemia, profound bradycardia, or in patients receiving certain antiarrhythmics (*e.g.*, *quinidine, procainamide, amiodarone*) or other agents that prolong QTc (*e.g.*, cisapride, *pimozide*).

Telithromycin is both a substrate and a strong inhibitor of CYP3A4. Coadministration of rifampin, a potent CYP inducer, decreases the serum concentrations of telithromycin by 80%, while CYP3A4 inhibitors (*e.g.*, *itraconazole*) increase peak serum concentrations. Serum concentrations of CYP3A4 substrates (*e.g.*, pimozide, cisapride, *midazolam*, statins, cyclosporine, phenytoin) are increased by telithromycin. Telithromycin also increases peak serum concentrations of *metoprolol* and digoxin.

CLINDAMYCIN

Clindamycin is a congener of *lincomycin*.

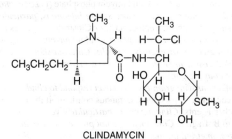

CLINDAMYCIN

MECHANISM OF ACTION Clindamycin binds to the 50S subunit of bacterial ribosomes and suppresses protein synthesis. Although clindamycin, erythromycin, and chloramphenicol are not structurally related, they act at sites in close proximity (Figures 46–2 and 46–3), and ribosome binding by one of these drugs may inhibit the interaction of the others. Macrolide resistance due to ribosomal methylation also may produce resistance to clindamycin. Because clindamycin does not induce the methylase, there is cross-resistance only if the enzyme is produced constitutively. Clindamycin is not a substrate for macrolide efflux pumps; thus, strains that are resistant to macrolides by this mechanism are susceptible to clindamycin.

ANTIBACTERIAL ACTIVITY Clindamycin resembles erythromycin in its *in vitro* activity against susceptible strains of pneumococci, *S. pyogenes*, and viridans streptococci. Ninety percent or more of strains of streptococci, including some that are macrolide-resistant, remain susceptible to clindamycin. Methicillin-susceptible strains of *S. aureus* usually are susceptible to clindamycin, but methicillin-resistant strains of *S. aureus* and coagulase-negative staphylococci frequently are resistant.

Clindamycin is more active than erythromycin or clarithromycin against anaerobic bacteria, especially B. fragilis, *but resistance increasingly is encountered. Between 10–20% of clostridial species other than* C. perfringens *are resistant. Strains of* Actinomyces israelii *and* Nocardia asteroides *are sensitive. Essentially all aerobic gram-negative bacilli are resistant.* M. pneumoniae *is resistant. Clindamycin plus primaquine and clindamycin plus pyrimethamine are second-line regimens for* Pneumocystis jiroveci *pneumonia and* T. gondii *encephalitis, respectively.*

ABSORPTION, DISTRIBUTION, AND EXCRETION

Absorption   Clindamycin is nearly completely absorbed following oral administration. Food does not affect absorption significantly. The $t_{1/2}$ of the antibiotic is ~3 hours.

Clindamycin palmitate, an oral prodrug, is hydrolyzed rapidly *in vivo*. Its absorption is similar to clindamycin. The phosphate ester of clindamycin, given parenterally, also is rapidly hydrolyzed to the active parent compound.

Distribution   Clindamycin is widely distributed in many fluids and tissues, including bone. Significant concentrations are not attained in CSF, but concentrations sufficient to treat cerebral toxoplasmosis are achieved. The drug readily crosses the placenta. Ninety percent or more of clindamycin is bound to plasma proteins. Clindamycin accumulates in polymorphonuclear leukocytes and alveolar macrophages and in abscesses.

Excretion   Only ~10% of clindamycin is excreted unaltered in the urine; small quantities are found in the feces. However, antimicrobial activity persists in feces for at least 5 days after therapy is stopped and growth of clindamycin-sensitive microorganisms may be suppressed for 2 weeks.

Clindamycin is inactivated by metabolism to *N*-de-methylclindamycin and clindamycin sulfoxide, which are excreted in the urine and bile. Accumulation of clindamycin can occur in patients with severe hepatic failure, and dosage adjustments may be required.

THERAPEUTIC USES   The oral dose of clindamycin (CLEOCIN) for adults is 150–300 mg every 6 hours; for severe infections, it is 300–600 mg every 6 hours. Children should receive 8–12 mg/kg/day of *clindamycin palmitate hydrochloride* (CLEOCIN PEDIATRIC) in three or four divided doses, or for severe infections, 13–25 mg/kg/day. However, children weighing ≤10 kg should receive half teaspoonful of this preparation (37.5 mg) every 8 hours as a minimal dose.

For serious infections due to aerobic gram-positive cocci and the more sensitive anaerobes, intravenous or intramuscular administration is recommended in dosages of 600–1200 mg/day, divided into three or four equal doses for adults. Clindamycin phosphate *(CLEOCIN PHOSPHATE) is available for intramuscular or intravenous use. For more severe infections, particularly those proven or suspected to be caused by* B. fragilis, Peptococcus, *or* Clostridium *species other than* C. perfringens, *parenteral administration of 1.2–2.4 g/day of clindamycin is suggested. Daily doses as high as 4.8 g have been given intravenously to adults. Children should receive 10–40 mg/kg/day in three or four divided doses; in severe infections, a minimal daily dose of 300 mg is recommended, regardless of body weight.*

Although many infections with gram-positive cocci respond to clindamycin, the high incidence of diarrhea and the occurrence of pseudomembranous colitis limit its use to infections where it is clearly superior to other agents. *Clindamycin is particularly valuable for anaerobic infections, especially those due to* B. fragilis. *Clindamycin is not predictably useful for the treatment of bacterial brain abscesses;* metronidazole, *in combination with penicillin or a third-generation cephalosporin, is preferred.*

Clindamycin is the drug of choice for lung abscess and anaerobic lung and pleural space infections. Clindamycin (600–1200 mg given intravenously every 6 hours) in combination with pyrimethamine (a 200-mg loading dose followed by 75 mg orally each day) and leucovorin is effective for treatment of encephalitis caused by T. gondii *in patients with AIDS. Clindamycin (600 mg intravenously every 8 hours, or 300–450 mg orally every 6 hours for less severe disease) in combination with primaquine (15 mg of base once daily) is useful for mild-to-moderate cases of* P. jiroveci *pneumonia in AIDS patients.*

Clindamycin also is available as a topical solution, gel, or lotion (CLEOCIN T, others) and as a vaginal cream (CLEOCIN). It is effective topically (or orally) for acne vulgaris and bacterial vaginosis.

UNTOWARD EFFECTS   The incidence of diarrhea associated with clindamycin ranges from 2–20%. A number of patients have developed pseudomembranous colitis caused by *C. difficile* toxin, with abdominal pain, fever, and bloody diarrhea. *This syndrome may be lethal.* Drug discontinuation and treatment with metronidazole or vancomycin usually is curative, but relapses can occur. Agents that inhibit peristalsis (*e.g.*,opioids) may worsen the condition.

Rashes occur in ~10% of patients treated with clindamycin and may be more common in HIV-infected patients. Other uncommon reactions include reversible elevation of serum transaminases, granulocytopenia, thrombocytopenia, and anaphylactic reactions. Local thrombophlebitis may follow intravenous administration. Clindamycin may potentiate the effect of a neuromuscular blocking agent administered concurrently.

QUINUPRISTIN/DALFOPRISTIN

Quinupristin/dalfopristin (SYNERCID) combines quinupristin, a streptogramin B, with dalfopristin, a streptogramin A, in a 30:70 ratio. These compounds are more soluble derivatives of pristinamycin and thus are suitable for intravenous administration.

ANTIBACTERIAL ACTIVITY Quinupristin/dalfopristin is active against gram-positive cocci and organisms responsible for atypical pneumonia (*e.g.*, *M. pneumoniae*, *Legionella* spp., and *Chlamydia pneumoniae*), but largely inactive against gram-negative organisms. The combination is bactericidal against streptococci and many strains of staphylococci, but bacteriostatic against *E. faecium*.

MECHANISM OF ACTION Quinupristin and dalfopristin are protein synthesis inhibitors that bind to the 50S ribosomal subunit. Quinupristin binds at the same site as macrolides and also inhibits polypeptide elongation. Dalfopristin binds at an adjacent site, changing the conformation of the 50S ribosome; this synergistically enhances the binding of quinupristin at its target site and also directly interferes with polypeptide-chain formation. The synergistic binding to the ribosome often results in bactericidal activity.

RESISTANCE Resistance to quinupristin is mediated by genes encoding a ribosomal methylase that prevents binding of drug to its target or encoding lactonases that inactivate type B streptogramins. Resistance to dalfopristin is mediated by genes that encode acetyltransferases, which inactivate type A streptogramins, or by staphylococcal genes that encode ATP-binding efflux proteins that pump type A streptogramins out of the cell. Resistance determinants are located on plasmids that may be transferred by conjugation. Resistance to quinupristin/dalfopristin always is associated with a resistance gene for type A streptogramins. Methylase-encoding genes can render the combination bacteriostatic instead of bactericidal, making it ineffective in infections where bactericidal activity is necessary (*e.g.*, endocarditis).

ABSORPTION, DISTRIBUTION, AND EXCRETION Quinupristin/dalfopristin is administered by intravenous infusion over at least 1 hour. The $t_{1/2}$ is 0.85 hour for quinupristin and 0.7 hour for dalfopristin. The volume of distribution is 0.87 L/kg for quinupristin and 0.71 L/kg for dalfopristin. Hepatic metabolism by conjugation is the principal means of clearance, with 80% of an administered dose eliminated by biliary excretion. Renal elimination of active compound accounts for most of the remainder. No dosage adjustment is necessary for renal insufficiency. Pharmacokinetics are not significantly altered by peritoneal dialysis or hemodialysis. Hepatic insufficiency increases the plasma AUC of active component and metabolites by 180% for quinupristin and 50% for dalfopristin.

THERAPEUTIC USES Quinupristin/dalfopristin is approved in the U.S. for treatment of infections caused by vancomycin-resistant strains of *E. faecium* and complicated skin and skin-structure infections caused by methicillin-susceptible strains of *S. aureus* or *S. pyogenes*. In Europe, it also is approved for treatment of nosocomial pneumonia and infections caused by methicillin-resistant strains of *S. aureus*. Cure rates for a variety of infections caused by vancomycin-resistant *E. faecium* were ~70% with quinupristin/dalfopristin at a dose of 7.5 mg/kg every 8–12 hours. Quinupristin/dalfopristin should be reserved for treatment of serious infections caused by multiple-drug-resistant gram-positive organisms such as vancomycin-resistant *E. faecium*.

UNTOWARD EFFECTS The most common side effects are pain and phlebitis at the infusion site, which are minimized by infusion through a central venous catheter. Arthralgias and myalgias are more common in patients with hepatic insufficiency and are managed by reducing the dosing frequency from every 8 to every 12 hours. Quinupristin/dalfopristin inhibits CYP3A4. Coadministration of other CYP3A4 substrates with quinupristin/dalfopristin may cause significant toxicity. Caution and monitoring are recommended for drugs in which the toxic therapeutic window is narrow or for drugs that prolong the QTc interval.

LINEZOLID

Linezolid (ZYVOX) is a synthetic antimicrobial agent of the oxazolidinone class.

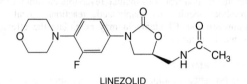

LINEZOLID

ANTIBACTERIAL ACTIVITY Because of its unique mechanism of action, linezolid is active against strains that are resistant to multiple other agents, including penicillin-resistant strains of *S. pneumoniae*; methicillin-resistant, vancomycin-intermediate and vancomycin-resistant strains of staphylococci; and vancomycin-resistant strains of enterococci.

MECHANISM OF ACTION Linezolid inhibits protein synthesis by binding to the P site of the 50S ribosomal subunit and preventing formation of the larger ribosomal-fMet-tRNA complex that initiates protein synthesis. There is no cross-resistance with other drug classes. Resistance in enterococci and staphylococci is due to point mutations of the 23S rRNA. Since bacteria have multiple copies of 23S rRNA genes, resistance generally requires mutations in two or more copies.

ABSORPTION, DISTRIBUTION, AND EXCRETION Linezolid is well absorbed after oral administration and may be taken without regard to food. Dosing for oral and intravenous preparations is the same. The $t_{1/2}$ is ~4–6 hours. Linezolid is 30% protein-bound and distributes widely to well-perfused tissues.

Linezolid is nonenzymatically oxidized to inactive derivatives. Approximately 80% of the drug appears in the urine, 30% as active compound, and 50% as the two primary oxidation products. Ten percent of the administered dose appears as oxidation products in feces. No dose adjustment is needed in renal insufficiency. Linezolid and its breakdown products are eliminated by dialysis; therefore the drug should be administered after hemodialysis.

THERAPEUTIC USES *Linezolid is FDA-approved for treatment of infections caused by vancomycin-resistant E. faecium; nosocomial pneumonia caused by methicillin-susceptible and-resistant strains of S. aureus; community-acquired pneumonia caused by penicillin-susceptible strains of S. pneumoniae; complicated skin and skin-structure infections caused by streptococci and methicillin-susceptible and -resistant strains of S. aureus; and uncomplicated skin and skin-structure infections. Linezolid (600 mg twice daily) has had clinical and microbiological cure rates in the range of 85–90% in treatment of a variety of infections caused by vancomycin-resistant E. faecium. A 400-mg, twice-daily dosage regimen is recommended only for treatment of uncomplicated skin and skin-structure infections.*

Cure rates with linezolid (~60%) were similar to those with vancomycin for nosocomial pneumonia caused by methicillin-resistant or -susceptible S. aureus. Linezolid efficacy also was similar to that of either oxacillin or vancomycin for skin and skin-structure infections, the majority of cases due to by S. aureus. Linezolid appears comparable in efficacy to vancomycin for methicillin-resistant strains. Linezolid may be effective for patients with methicillin-resistant S. aureus infections who are failing vancomycin therapy or whose isolates have reduced susceptibility to vancomycin. Linezolid is bacteriostatic for staphylococci and enterococci and probably should not be used to treat suspected endocarditis.

Linezolid should be reserved as an alternative agent for infections caused by multiple-drug-resistant strains. It should not be used when other agents are likely to be effective. Indiscriminant use and overuse will hasten selection of resistant strains and the eventual loss of this valuable new agent.

UNTOWARD EFFECTS The drug generally has minor side effects (*e.g.*, GI complaints, headache, rash). Myelosuppression, including anemia, leukopenia, pancytopenia, and thrombocytopenia, has been reported. Platelet counts should be monitored in patients with risk of bleeding, preexisting thrombocytopenia, or disorders of platelet function and in patients receiving therapy for >2 weeks. Linezolid is a weak, nonspecific inhibitor of MAO. Patients receiving concomitant therapy with adrenergic or serotonergic agents or consuming more than 100 mg of tyramine daily may have palpitations, headache, or hypertensive crisis. Peripheral and optic neuropathy after prolonged use reverse upon drug discontinuation.

SPECTINOMYCIN

Spectinomycin selectively inhibits protein synthesis in gram-negative bacteria by binding to and affecting the 30S ribosomal subunit. Unlike aminoglycosides, spectinomycin does not cause misreading of messenger RNA and is not bactericidal. Bacterial resistance may be mediated by mutations in the 16S ribosomal RNA or by drug modification by adenylyltransferase.

Spectinomycin is rapidly absorbed after intramuscular injection. The drug is not significantly bound to plasma protein and is renally excreted within 48 hours.

Spectinomycin's only therapeutic use is in the treatment of gonorrhea caused by strains resistant to first-line drugs, or if there are contraindications to the use of these drugs. *For gonococcal infections, spectinomycin is an alternative drug in patients who are intolerant or allergic to β-lactam antibiotics and quinolones. Spectinomycin also is useful in pregnancy for patients are intolerant to β-lactams in whom quinolones are contraindicated. The recommended dose is a single, deep intramuscular injection of 2 g. A disadvantage of this regimen is that spectinomycin has no effect on incubating or established syphilis and is not active against* Chlamydia *spp. It also is less effective for pharyngeal infections; follow-up cultures to document cure should be obtained.*

Spectinomycin produces few significant untoward effects. Local pain, urticaria, chills, fever, dizziness, nausea, and insomnia have been noted.

POLYMYXIN B AND COLISTIN

The polymyxins are a group of closely related antibiotics elaborated by various strains of Bacillus polymyxa. Colistin *is produced by* Bacillus colistinus. *These drugs, which are cationic detergents, are basic peptides of ~1000 Da.*

Colistin (polymyxin E) is available as colistin sulfate for oral use and as colistimethate sodium for parenteral administration (not recommended). The antimicrobial activities of polymyxin B and colistin are restricted to gram-negative bacteria.

Polymyxins are amphipathic agents that interact with phospholipids and disrupt the structure of cell membranes to increase permeability. Polymyxin B sensitivity apparently is related to the phospholipid content of the cell wall–membrane complex, which may prevent access of the drug to the cell membrane.

These drugs are not absorbed when given orally and poorly absorbed from mucous membranes and burn surfaces. They are cleared renally, and dose modification is required with impaired renal function.

Polymyxin B sulfate is available for ophthalmic, otic, and topical use in combination with a variety of other compounds. Colistin is available as otic drops. Parenteral preparations are rarely used, but colistin may be useful as a salvage regimen for infections caused by multiple-drug-resistant organisms.

Infections of the skin, mucous membranes, eye, and ear due to polymyxin B–sensitive microorganisms respond to local application of the antibiotic in solution or ointment. External otitis, frequently due to Pseudomonas, *may be cured by the topical use of the drug.* P. aeruginosa *is a common cause of infection of corneal ulcers; local application or subconjunctival injection of polymyxin B often is curative.*

Because of their extreme nephrotoxicity, these drugs are rarely if ever used except topically. *Polymyxin B applied to intact or denuded skin or mucous membranes produces no systemic reactions because of its almost complete lack of absorption. Hypersensitization is uncommon with topical use. Neurological reactions include muscle weakness and apnea, paresthesias, vertigo, and slurred speech. Polymyxins are nephrotoxic, and coadministration with aminoglycosides should be avoided.*

TEICOPLANIN

Teicoplanin is a glycopeptide antibiotic mixture of related compounds that is approved in the U.S. and Europe. It is like vancomycin in mechanism of action, spectrum of activity, and renal elimination.

MECHANISMS OF ACTION AND RESISTANCE

Teicoplanin inhibits cell-wall synthesis by binding to the D-Ala-D-Ala terminus of cell wall precursor units (Figure 46–4) and is active only against gram-positive bacteria. It is bactericidal against susceptible strains, except for enterococci. It is active against methicillin-susceptible and methicillin-resistant staphylococci, Listeria monocytogenes, Corynebacterium *spp.,* Clostridium *spp., and anaerobic gram-positive cocci. Nonviridans and viridans streptococci,* S. pneumoniae, *and enterococci generally are highly sensitive. Some strains of coagulase-positive and coagulase-negative staphylococci, as well as enterococci and other organisms that are intrinsically resistant to vancomycin, are resistant to teicoplanin.*

Resistance can emerge in susceptible staphylococci during therapy. The Van A phenotype of vancomycin resistance also confers resistance to teicoplanin by altering the cell-wall target so that the glycopeptide does not bind. Strains of enterococci with Van B resistance often remain susceptible to teicoplanin.

ABSORPTION, DISTRIBUTION, AND EXCRETION

Teicoplanin can be given safely by intramuscular injection. It is highly bound by plasma proteins (~90%) and has an extremely long serum elimination $t_{1/2}$ (up to 100 hours) in patients with normal renal function. The dose of teicoplanin in adults is 6–30 mg/kg/day, with higher dosages reserved for serious staphylococcal infections. Once-daily dosing is possible for most infections because of the prolonged serum $t_{1/2}$. Teicoplanin doses must be adjusted in patients with renal insufficiency. For functionally anephric patients, administration once weekly is appropriate, but trough serum drug concentrations should be monitored to determine that the therapeutic range (e.g., 15–20 μg/mL) has been maintained.

THERAPEUTIC USES

Teicoplanin has been used to treat a wide variety of infections, including osteomyelitis and endocarditis, caused by methicillin-resistant and methicillin-susceptible staphylococci, streptococci, and enterococci. Teicoplanin generally is comparable to vancomycin in efficacy, except for treatment failures from low doses used for such serious infections as endocarditis. Teicoplanin is not as efficacious as antistaphylococcal penicillins for treating bacteremia and endocarditis caused by methicillin-susceptible S. aureus (cure rates of 60–70% vs. 85–90% for the penicillins). The efficacy of teicoplanin against S. aureus may be improved by adding an aminoglycoside (e.g., gentamicin) to provide a synergistic effect. Strains of streptococci are uniformly susceptible to teicoplanin. This drug has been very effective in a once-daily regimen for patients with streptococcal osteomyelitis or endocarditis. Teicoplanin is among the most active drugs against enterococci and apparently is effective, although only bacteriostatic, for serious enterococcal infections. It should be combined with gentamicin to achieve a bactericidal effect in the treatment of enterococcal endocarditis.

UNTOWARD EFFECTS

The main side effect reported for teicoplanin is rash, which is dose-related. Hypersensitivity reactions, drug fever, neutropenia, and ototoxicity also have been reported.

DAPTOMYCIN

Daptomycin (CUBICIN) is a cyclic lipopeptide that was resurrected in response to increasing need for bactericidal antibiotics effective against vancomycin-resistant gram-positive bacteria.

ANTIBACTERIAL ACTIVITY

Daptomycin is a bactericidal antibiotic selectively active against aerobic, facultative, and anaerobic gram-positive bacteria. Approximately 90% of strains of staphylococci and streptococci are highly sensitive, as are E. faecalis and E. faecium. Daptomycin may be active against vancomycin-resistant strains.

MECHANISMS OF ACTION AND RESISTANCE

Daptomycin binds to bacterial membranes, resulting in depolarization, loss of membrane potential, and cell death. It has concentration-dependent bactericidal activity. Due to its unique mechanism of action, there are no known resistance mechanisms. Very rarely (~0.2%), clinical resistance to daptomycin has emerged during therapy. Staphylococci with decreased susceptibility to vancomycin have higher daptomycin MICs than fully susceptible strains.

ABSORPTION, FATE, AND EXCRETION

Daptomycin is only administered intravenously. Daptomycin displays linear pharmacokinetics at doses up to 8 mg/kg. Protein binding is 92%. The serum $t_{1/2}$ normally is 8 hours, permitting once-daily dosing. Approximately 80% of the administered dose is recovered in urine; a small amount is excreted in feces. If the creatinine clearance is <30 mL/min, the dose is administered every 48 hours. For hemodialysis patients, the dose should be given immediately after dialysis.

Daptomycin neither inhibits nor induces CYPs and has no important drug–drug interactions. Caution is recommended when daptomycin is coadministered with aminoglycosides or statins because of potential risks of nephrotoxicity and myopathy, respectively.

THERAPEUTIC USES

Daptomycin is indicated for treatment of complicated skin and skin-structure infections caused by methicillin-susceptible and methicillin-resistant strains of S. aureus, *hemolytic streptococci, and vancomycin-susceptible* E. faecalis. *Its efficacy is comparable to that of vancomycin.*

UNTOWARD EFFECTS

Elevations of creatine kinase may occur; this does not require drug discontinuation unless clinical findings suggest an otherwise unexplained myopathy.

BACITRACIN

The bacitracins are a mixed group of polypeptide antibiotics. The major constituent is bacitracin A. Bacitracin inhibits cell wall synthesis. A variety of gram-positive cocci and bacilli, Neisseria, H. influenzae, *and* Treponema pallidum *are sensitive to the drug. A unit of the antibiotic is equivalent to 26 μg of the USP standard.*

Bacitracin is available in ophthalmic and dermatologic ointments; the antibiotic also is available as a powder for the preparation of topical solutions. The ointments are applied directly to the involved surface one or more times daily. A number of topical preparations of bacitracin, to which neomycin *or* polymyxin *or both have been added, are available, and some contain the three antibiotics plus hydrocortisone. For open infections such as infected eczema and infected dermal ulcers, the local application of the antibiotic may be of some help in eradicating sensitive bacteria. Bacitracin rarely produces hypersensitivity. Suppurative conjunctivitis and infected corneal ulcer respond well to the topical use of bacitracin when caused by susceptible bacteria. Bacitracin has been used with limited success for eradication of nasal carriage of staphylococci. Oral bacitracin has been used with some success for the treatment of antibiotic-associated diarrhea caused by* C. difficile. *Serious nephrotoxicity results from the parenteral use of bacitracin. Hypersensitivity reactions rarely result from topical application.*

MUPIROCIN

*Mupirocin (*BACTROBAN*) is active against many gram-positive and selected gram-negative bacteria. It has good activity against* S. pyogenes *and methicillin-susceptible and methicillin-resistant strains of* S. aureus. *It is bactericidal at concentrations achieved with topical application.*

Mupirocin inhibits bacterial protein synthesis by reversible inhibition of Ile tRNA synthase. There is no cross-resistance with other antibiotic classes. Clinically insignificant, low-level resistance results from mutations of the gene encoding Ile tRNA synthase or an extra chromosomal copy of a gene encoding a modified Ile tRNA synthase. High-level resistance is mediated by a plasmid or chromosomal copy of a gene encoding a "bypass" synthetase that binds mupirocin poorly.

Mupirocin is available as a 2% cream or ointment for dermatologic use and as a 2% ointment for intranasal use. The dermatological preparations are indicated for treatment of traumatic skin lesions and impetigo secondarily infected with S. aureus *or* S. pyogenes. *Systemic absorption through intact skin or skin lesions is minimal. Any mupirocin absorbed is rapidly metabolized to inactive monic acid.*

Mupirocin is effective in eradicating S. aureus *carriage. The consensus is that patients who may benefit from mupirocin prophylaxis are those with proven* S. aureus *nasal colonization plus risk factors for distant infection or a history of skin or soft tissue infections.*

Mupirocin may cause irritation and sensitization and contact with the eyes should be avoided. Systemic reactions to mupirocin occur rarely, if at all. Application of the ointment to large surface areas should be avoided in patients with renal failure to avoid accumulation of polyethylene glycol from the ointment.

For a complete Bibliographical listing see Goodman & Gilman's *The Pharmacological Basis of Therapeutics,* **11th ed., or Goodman & Gilman Online at www.accessmedicine.com.**

47

CHEMOTHERAPY OF TUBERCULOSIS, *MYCOBACTERIUM AVIUM* COMPLEX DISEASE, AND LEPROSY

Mycobacteria cause tuberculosis, *Mycobacterium avium* complex (MAC) disease, and leprosy. Tuberculosis remains the leading worldwide cause of death due to infectious disease. "First-line" agents for the chemotherapy of tuberculosis combine the greatest efficacy with an acceptable degree of toxicity (Table 47–1), and the large majority of patients with tuberculosis are treated successfully with these drugs. Occasionally, it may be necessary to resort to "second-line" drugs.

I. DRUGS FOR TUBERCULOSIS

ISONIAZID

Isoniazid (NYDRAZID, others) remains the primary drug for tuberculosis. All patients with disease caused by sensitive strains should receive the drug if they can tolerate it.

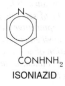

ISONIAZID

ANTIBACTERIAL ACTIVITY AND MECHANISM OF ACTION

Isoniazid is bacteriostatic for "resting" bacilli but bactericidal for dividing microorganisms. Isoniazid is a prodrug that is converted by mycobacterial catalase-peroxidase into an active metabolite. It inhibits biosynthesis of mycolic acids—long, branched lipids that are attached to a unique polysaccharide in the mycobacterial cell wall. Mycolic acids are unique to mycobacteria. The target of the isoniazid derivative is enoyl-ACP reductase of fatty acid synthase II, which converts unsaturated to saturated fatty acids in mycolic acid biosynthesis.

BACTERIAL RESISTANCE

Isoniazid resistance most commonly results from mutations in catalase-peroxidase that decrease its activity, preventing conversion of the prodrug isoniazid to its active metabolite. Mutations in genes involved in mycolic acid biosynthesis also cause resistance.

Isoniazid monotherapy leads to resistance. This resistance typically develops after a few weeks of therapy but can vary. Approximately 1 in 10^6 tubercle bacilli will be genetically resistant to isoniazid; since tuberculous cavities may contain as many as 10^9 microorganisms, it is not surprising that isoniazid selects for resistant bacteria. The incidence of primary resistance to isoniazid in the U.S. is estimated at 8% of isolates but may be much higher in Asian and Hispanic immigrants, large urban areas, and border communities.

ABSORPTION, DISTRIBUTION, AND EXCRETION   Isoniazid is readily absorbed after oral or parenteral administration. Isoniazid diffuses readily into all body fluids and cells. The drug achieves significant quantities in pleural and ascitic fluids; concentrations in the cerebrospinal fluid (CSF) with inflamed meninges are similar to those in the plasma. Isoniazid penetrates well into caseous material and persists in therapeutic concentrations.

From 75 to 95% of a dose of isoniazid is excreted in the urine within 24 hours, mostly as metabolites. The main excretory products in humans result from acetylation (acetylisoniazid) and hydrolysis (isonicotinic acid).

Slow and rapid inactivators (acetylators) of isoniazid differ in the polymorphic arylamine *N*-acetyltransferase type 2 (NAT2); in the U.S., the incidence of "slow acetylators" is ~50%. The serum $t_{1/2}$ in fast acetylators is 1 hour *versus* 2–5 hours in slow acetylators, resulting in serum isoniazid levels in fast acetylators that are 30–50% of those in slow acetylators. Because isoniazid is relatively nontoxic, sufficient drug can be administered to fast acetylators to achieve a therapeutic effect. Hepatic insufficiency also increases drug concentrations, and dosage reduction is recommended for slow acetylators in this setting. Slow acetylators rarely may accumulate toxic concentrations if their renal function is impaired.

Table 47–1

Drugs Used in the Treatment of Tuberculosis, *Mycobacterium avium* Complex, and Leprosy

Mycobacterial Species	First-Line Therapy	Alternative Agents
M. tuberculosis	Isoniazid + rifampin*+ pyrazinamide + ethambutol or streptomycin	Moxifloxacin or gatifloxacin; cycloserine; capreomycin; kanamycin; amikacin; ethionamide; clofazimine; aminosalicylic acid
M. avium complex	Clarithromycin or azithromycin + ethambutol with or without rifabutin	Rifabutin; rifampin; ethionamide; cycloserine; moxifloxacin or gatifloxacin
M. kansasii	Isoniazid + rifampin*+ ethambutol	Trimethoprim-sulfamethoxazole; ethionamide; cycloserine; clarithromycin; amikacin; streptomycin; moxifloxacin or gatifloxacin
M. fortuitum complex	Amikacin + doxycycline	Cefoxitin; rifampin; a sulfonamide; moxifloxacin or gatifloxacin; clarithromycin; trimethoprim-sulfamethoxazole; imipenem
M. marinum	Rifampin + ethambutol	Trimethoprim-sulfamethoxazole; clarithromycin; minocycline; doxycycline
M. leprae	Dapsone + rifampin ± clofazimine	Minocycline; moxifloxacin or gatifloxacin; clarithromycin; ethionamide

*In HIV-infected patients, the substitution of rifabutin for rifampin minimizes drug interactions with the HIV protease inhibitors and nonnucleoside reverse transcriptase inhibitors.

THERAPEUTIC USES Isoniazid is the most important drug for the treatment of tuberculosis. Toxic effects are minimized by prophylactic therapy with *pyridoxine* and careful patient surveillance. For treatment of active infections, the drug is combined with another agent, although it is used alone for prophylaxis.

Isoniazid usually is given orally in a single daily dose of 5 mg/kg, with a maximum of 300 mg. Children should receive 10–20 mg/kg/day (300 mg maximum). After 2 months of daily therapy with isoniazid, rifampin, and pyrazinamide, patients with sensitive strains of M. tuberculosis *may be treated twice-weekly with isoniazid (15 mg/kg orally) plus rifampin (10 mg/kg, up to 600 mg/dose) for 4 months.*

Pyridoxine, vitamin B6, (10–50 mg/day) is coadministered with isoniazid to minimize the risk of peripheral neuropathy and central nervous system (CNS) toxicity in malnourished patients and those predisposed to neuropathy (e.g., *slow acetylators, elderly, pregnant women, human immunodeficiency virus [HIV]-infected subjects, diabetics, alcoholics, and uremics).*

UNTOWARD EFFECTS Adverse reactions to isoniazid occur in ~5%, including rash (2%), fever (1.2%), jaundice (0.6%), and peripheral neuritis (0.2%). Isoniazid hypersensitivity may result in fever, rashes, and hepatitis. Hematological reactions also may occur (*e.g.,* agranulocytosis, eosinophilia, thrombocytopenia, and anemia). Vasculitis associated with antinuclear antibodies may appear but disappears when the drug is stopped.

Peripheral neuritis occurs in ~2% of patients receiving 5 mg/kg of drug daily if pyridoxine is not given concurrently. Prophylactic administration of pyridoxine considerably decreases the risk of peripheral neuritis and other nervous system disorders.

Isoniazid may precipitate convulsions, usually in patients with known seizure disorders. Optic neuritis also has occurred. Muscle twitching, dizziness, ataxia, paresthesias, stupor, and potentially fatal encephalopathy are other manifestations of neurotoxicity. A number of mental abnormalities may appear, including euphoria, transient memory impairment, loss of self-control, and psychosis.

Isoniazid inhibits phenytoin parahydroxylation, and signs and symptoms of toxicity occur in ~25% of patients given both drugs, particularly in slow acetylators. Concentrations of phenytoin in plasma should be monitored, and its dose adjusted if necessary.

Severe hepatic injury leading to death may occur in individuals receiving isoniazid, typically presenting 4–8 weeks after initiation of therapy. Liver biopsy reveals bridging and multilobular *necrosis. Drug continuation after hepatic dysfunction develops may worsen the damage. Alcoholic hepatitis increases the risk, but chronic carriers of the hepatitis B virus tolerate isoniazid. Age is the most important risk factor for isoniazid-induced hepatotoxicity; it is rare in patients <20 years old, occurs in 0.3% of those 20–34 years old, and increases to 1.2% and 2.3% in individuals 35–49 and >50 years of age, respectively. Up to 12% of patients receiving isoniazid may have elevated serum transaminase levels. Patients receiving isoniazid should be evaluated monthly for symptoms of hepatitis and warned to discontinue the drug if symptoms occur. Some clinicians follow serum transaminases at monthly intervals in high-risk individuals (older age, excessive alcohol intake, history of liver disease); an elevation >five times normal is cause for drug discontinuation. Isoniazid should be administered with great care to those with preexisting hepatic disease.*

RIFAMPIN AND OTHER RIFAMYCINS

The rifamycins (rifampin, rifabutin, rifapentine) are related macrocyclic antibiotics produced by *Amycolatopsis mediterrane*; rifampin (RIFADIN; RIMACTANE) is a semisynthetic derivative of rifamycin B.

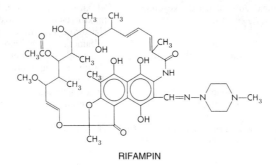

RIFAMPIN

ANTIBACTERIAL ACTIVITY

Rifampin inhibits the growth of most gram-positive and many gram-negative bacteria. Rifampin in concentrations of 0.005–0.2 µg/mL inhibits the growth of M. tuberculosis in vitro. Among nontuberculous mycobacteria, Mycobacterium kansasii is inhibited by 0.25–1 µg/mL. The majority of strains of Mycobacterium scrofulaceum, Mycobacterium intracellulare, and M. avium are suppressed but certain strains may be resistant. Mycobacterium fortuitum is highly resistant to the drug. Rifampin increases the in vitro activity of streptomycin and isoniazid against M. tuberculosis.

MECHANISM OF ACTION AND BACTERIAL RESISTANCE

Rifampin forms a stable complex with DNA dependent RNA polymerase, leading to suppression of initiation of chain formation (but not chain elongation) in RNA synthesis. High concentrations of rifampin can inhibit RNA synthesis in mammalian mitochondria, viral DNA–dependent RNA polymerases, and reverse transcriptases. Rifampin is bactericidal for both intracellular and extracellular microorganisms.

Mycobacteria may rapidly develop rifampin resistance as a one-step process, and 1 of every 10^7–10^8 tubercle bacilli is resistant to the drug; thus, rifampin should not be used alone. Microbial resistance is due to mutations in DNA-dependent RNA polymerase that reduce drug binding to the polymerase.

ABSORPTION, DISTRIBUTION, AND EXCRETION

Following gastrointestinal (GI) absorption, rifampin is eliminated rapidly in the bile, and an enterohepatic circulation ensues. During this time, the drug is progressively deacetylated by hepatic CYPS; after 6 hours, nearly all drug in the bile is in the deacetylated form, which retains antibacterial activity. Intestinal reabsorption is reduced by deacetylation (and by food); thus, metabolism facilitates drug elimination. The rifampin $t_{1/2}$ is progressively shortened (~40%) during the first 14 days of treatment due to induction of hepatic CYPs; $t_{1/2}$ is increased by hepatic dysfunction and may be decreased in slow acetylators concurrently receiving isoniazid. Dosage adjustment is not necessary in patients with renal insufficiency. Rifampin is distributed throughout the body and reaches effective concentrations in the CSF. The drug may impart an orange-red color to bodily fluids.

THERAPEUTIC USES

Rifampin for oral administration is available alone and as a fixed-dose combination with isoniazid (150 mg of isoniazid, 300 mg of rifampin; RIFAMATE) or with isoniazid and pyrazinamide (50 mg of isoniazid, 120 mg of rifampin, and 300 mg pyrazinamide;

RIFATER). A parenteral form of rifampin also is available. *Rifampin and isoniazid are the most effective drugs available for the treatment of tuberculosis.*

The dose of rifampin for tuberculosis treatment in adults is 600 mg daily, given either 1 hour before or 2 hours after a meal. Children should receive 10 mg/kg given in the same way. Rifampin should never be used alone for the treatment of tuberculosis because of the rapidity with which resistance may develop.

Rifampin also is indicated for the prophylaxis of meningococcal disease and Haemophilus influenzae *meningitis. To prevent meningococcal disease, adults may be treated with 600 mg twice daily for 2 days or 600 mg once daily for 4 days; children should receive 10–15 mg/kg, to a maximum of 600 mg. Combined with a β-lactam antibiotic or vancomycin, rifampin is used in selected cases of staphylococcal endocarditis or osteomyelitis. Rifampin may be used to eradicate nasal staphylococci in patients with chronic furunculosis.*

UNTOWARD EFFECTS In usual doses, <4% of patients with tuberculosis have significant adverse reactions to rifampin, most commonly rash (0.8%), fever (0.5%), and nausea and vomiting (1.5%). Rarely, hepatitis and deaths due to liver failure have been observed in patients who received other hepatotoxic agents, or who had preexisting liver disease. Hepatitis from rifampin rarely occurs in patients with normal hepatic function; likewise, the combination of isoniazid and rifampin appears generally safe. Chronic liver disease, alcoholism, and old age increase the risk of severe hepatitis when rifampin is given alone or concurrently with isoniazid.

Rifampin should not be administered less than twice weekly and/or in daily doses of 1.2 g or greater because this is associated with frequent side effects. A flu-like syndrome with fever, chills, and myalgias develops in 20% of patients so treated.

As a potent inducer of hepatic CYPs, rifampin decreases the $t_{1/2}$ of many drugs, including HIV protease and nonnucleoside reverse transcriptase inhibitors, *digoxin, quinidine, disopyramide, mexiletine, tocainide, ketoconazole, propranolol, metoprolol, clofibrate, verapamil, methadone, cyclosporine,* glucocorticoids, oral anticoagulants, *theophylline,* barbiturates, oral contraceptives, *halothane, fluconazole,* and the sulfonylureas. The interaction between rifampin and oral anticoagulants can impair anticoagulation. By enhancing the catabolism of steroids, rifampin can decrease effectiveness of oral contraceptives and induce adrenal insufficiency in patients with marginal adrenal reserve (*see* Chapter 59). The increased metabolism of methadone and other narcotics has led to inadequate pain control or withdrawal symptoms.

GI disturbances produced by rifampin (epigastric distress, nausea, vomiting, abdominal cramps, diarrhea) have occasionally required drug discontinuation. CNS symptoms include fatigue, drowsiness, headache, dizziness, ataxia, confusion, inability to concentrate, generalized numbness, pain in the extremities, and weakness. Hypersensitivity reactions include fever, pruritus, urticaria, various rashes, and eosinophilia. Hemolysis, hemoglobinuria, hematuria, renal insufficiency, and acute renal failure have been observed rarely, likely due to hypersensitivity reactions. Thrombocytopenia, transient leukopenia, and anemia have occurred during therapy. The drug is best avoided during pregnancy.

Rifabutin (MYCOBUTIN) is a rifampin derivative and has the same mechanism of action. Because rifabutin is a less potent inducer of CYPs, it is used in tuberculosis-infected HIV patients treated concurrently with protease inhibitors. Unique side effects of rifabutin include polymyalgia and anterior uveitis. About 25% of rifampin-resistant *M. tuberculosis* isolates are rifabutin-sensitive, so it may have a role in the treatment of multidrug-resistant tuberculosis.

Rifapentine (PRIFTIN) has a longer $t_{1/2}$ than rifampin and rifabutin, which allows once-weekly dosing. It has an intermediate capacity to induce CYPs, between rifabutin and rifampin. In HIV-infected patients, rifapentine may select for rifamycin resistance; rifabutin is therefore preferred in this situation.

ETHAMBUTOL

The structure of ethambutol is:

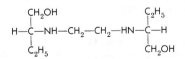

ETHAMBUTOL

ANTIBACTERIAL ACTIVITY, MECHANISM OF ACTION, RESISTANCE

Nearly all strains of M. tuberculosis *and* M. kansasii *and many strains of MAC are sensitive to ethambutol. Sensitivities of other mycobacteria are variable. Ethambutol has no effect on other bacteria. Growth inhibition by ethambutol requires 24 hours and is mediated by inhibition of arabinosyl transferases involved in cell wall biosynthesis. Resistance to ethambutol develops very slowly in* vitro, *but can result from single amino acid mutations when given alone.*

ABSORPTION, DISTRIBUTION, AND EXCRETION

About 80% of an oral dose of ethambutol is absorbed from the GI tract. Concentrations in plasma peak 2–4 hours after the drug is taken and are proportional to the dose. The drug has a $t_{1/2}$ of 3–4 hours. Within 24 hours, 75% of an ingested dose of ethambutol is excreted unchanged in the urine; up to 15% is excreted in the form of aldehyde and dicarboxylic acid derivatives. The drug is renally excreted.

THERAPEUTIC USES Ethambutol (MYAMBUTOL) has been used with notable success in the therapy of tuberculosis when given concurrently with isoniazid and largely has replaced aminosalicylic acid. Ethambutol is available for oral administration in tablets. The usual adult dose is 15 mg/kg given once a day. Some clinicians use 25 mg/kg/day for the first 60 days, followed by 15 mg/kg/day, particularly for those treated previously. Dose adjustment is necessary in patients with impaired renal function. Ethambutol is not recommended for children under 5 years of age because of concern about the ability to test their visual acuity. Children from ages 6–12 years should receive 10–15 mg/kg/day.

UNTOWARD EFFECTS The most important side effect is optic neuritis, resulting in decreased visual acuity and red–green color blindness. The incidence of this reaction is proportional to the dose of ethambutol and is <1% in patients receiving the recommended daily dose of 15 mg/kg. The intensity of the visual difficulty is related to the duration of therapy after visual impairment first becomes apparent and may be unilateral or bilateral. Tests of visual acuity and red–green discrimination prior to the start of therapy and periodically thereafter are recommended. Recovery usually occurs when ethambutol is withdrawn.

Fewer than 2% of patients who received daily doses of 15 mg/kg of ethambutol had adverse reactions, including diminished visual acuity, rash, drug fever, pruritus, joint pain, GI upset, malaise, headache, dizziness, confusion, disorientation, and hallucinations. Numbness and tingling of the fingers owing to peripheral neuritis are infrequent. Anaphylaxis and leukopenia are rare. Therapy with ethambutol increases urate concentration in the blood in ~50% of patients, owing to decreased renal excretion of uric acid.

STREPTOMYCIN

ANTIBACTERIAL ACTIVITY

Streptomycin is bactericidal for the tubercle bacillus in vitro. *The vast majority of strains of* M. tuberculosis *are sensitive.* M. kansasii *is frequently sensitive, but other mycobacteria are only occasionally susceptible. Streptomycin in* vivo *does not eradicate the tubercle bacillus, probably because the drug does not readily enter living cells and thus cannot kill intracellular microbes. The broader pharmacology of streptomycin is covered in chapter 45.*

BACTERIAL RESISTANCE

Primary resistance to streptomycin is found in only 2–3% of isolates of M. tuberculosis. *Selection for resistant tubercle bacilli occurs* in vivo; *the longer therapy, the greater the incidence of resistance.*

THERAPEUTIC USES The use of streptomycin for the treatment of pulmonary tuberculosis has declined sharply. Many clinicians still prefer to give 4 drugs, of which streptomycin may be one, for the most serious forms of tuberculosis, (*e.g.,* disseminated disease or meningitis). Adults should be given 15 mg/kg/day in divided doses given by intramuscular injection every 12 hours, not to exceed 1 g/day. Children should receive 20–40 mg/kg/day in divided doses every 12–24 hours, not to exceed 1 g/day. Therapy usually is discontinued after 2–3 months, or sooner if cultures become negative.

UNTOWARD EFFECTS In tuberculosis patients treated with streptomycin, 8% had adverse reactions; half of which involved the auditory and vestibular functions of the eighth cranial nerve. Other problems included rash and fever.

PYRAZINAMIDE

Pyrazinamide is the synthetic pyrazine analog of nicotinamide and has the following structure:

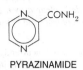

PYRAZINAMIDE

ANTIBACTERIAL ACTIVITY

Pyrazinamide exhibits bactericidal activity in vitro only at a slightly acidic pH; this poses no problem since the drug kills tubercle bacilli residing in acidic phagosomes within the macrophage. The target of pyrazinamide is the mycobacterial fatty acid synthase I gene involved in mycolic acid biosynthesis. Resistance develops rapidly if pyrazinamide is used alone.

ABSORPTION, DISTRIBUTION, AND EXCRETION

Pyrazinamide is well absorbed from the GI tract and widely distributed throughout the body, including the CNS, lungs, and liver. The plasma $t_{1/2}$ is 9–10 hours in patients with normal renal function. The drug is excreted primarily by glomerular filtration. Pyrazinamide is hydrolyzed to pyrazinoic acid and subsequently hydroxylated to 5-hydroxypyrazinoic acid.

THERAPEUTIC USES

Pyrazinamide is an important component of short-term (6-month) multiple-drug therapy of tuberculosis. The daily dose for adults is 15–30 mg/kg in a single oral dose. The maximum dose is 2 g/day, regardless of weight. Children should receive 15–30 mg/kg/day; daily doses also should not exceed 2 g. Pyrazinamide is safe and effective when administered twice or thrice weekly (at increased dosages).

UNTOWARD EFFECTS

Hepatic injury is the most serious side effect of pyrazinamide. Current regimens (15–30 mg/kg/day) are much safer than higher doses used previously. Prior to pyrazinamide administration, all patients should have liver function tests, which should be repeated at frequent intervals. If evidence of significant hepatic damage appears, therapy must be stopped. Pyrazinamide should not be given to individuals with any degree of hepatic dysfunction unless this is absolutely unavoidable.

The drug inhibits urate excretion, rarely precipitating an acute flare of gout. Other adverse effects are arthralgias, nausea and vomiting, dysuria, malaise, and fever.

QUINOLONES

The fluoroquinolones are highly active against *M. tuberculosis* and are important drugs for multidrug-resistant tuberculosis (Table 47–1). Agents such as gatifloxacin (TEQUIN) and moxifloxacin (AVELOX) are most active and least likely to select for quinolone resistance. Mycobacterial resistance to one fluoroquinolone imparts cross-resistance for the entire class.

ETHIONAMIDE

ETHIONAMIDE (TRECATOR-SC) has the following structure:

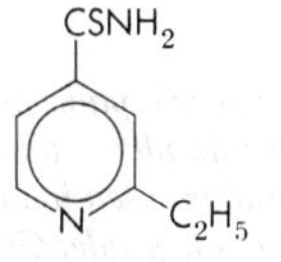

ETHIONAMIDE

MECHANISM OF ACTION AND ANTIBACTERIAL ACTIVITY, RESISTANCE

Ethionamide is a prodrug that is activated by an NADPH-specific monooxygenase to a sulfoxide, and thence to 2-ethyl-4-aminopyridine. Although these products are not toxic, a transient intermediate presumably is the active antibiotic. Like isoniazid, ethionamide inhibits mycobacterial growth by inhibiting the activity of the enoyl-ACP reductase of fatty acid synthase II. Both drugs thus inhibit mycolic acid biosynthesis with consequent impairment of cell-wall synthesis. Resistance can develop rapidly in vivo when ethionamide is used as a single-agent treatment, including low-level cross-resistance to isoniazid.

ABSORPTION, DISTRIBUTION, AND EXCRETION

The $t_{1/2}$ of the drug is 2 hours. Approximately 50% of patients are unable to tolerate a single dose >500 mg because of GI disturbance. Ethionamide is rapidly and widely distributed, with significant concentrations in CSF. Ethionamide is cleared by hepatic metabolism; like aminosalicylic acid, ethionamide inhibits the acetylation of isoniazid in vitro.

THERAPEUTIC USES

Ethionamide is a secondary agent, to be used concurrently with other drugs only when therapy with primary agents is ineffective or contraindicated. The initial dose of ethionamide for adults is 250 mg twice daily given orally; it is increased by 125 mg/day every 5 days until a dose of 15–20 mg/kg/day is achieved. The maximal dose is 1 g daily. The drug is taken with meals in divided doses to minimize gastric irritation. Children should receive 15–20 mg/kg/day in two divided doses, not to exceed 1 g daily.

UNTOWARD EFFECTS

Common reactions to ethionamide are anorexia, nausea and vomiting, gastric irritation, and neurologic symptoms, including depression, drowsiness, and asthenia. Convulsions and peripheral neuropathy are rare. Other neurological manifestations include olfactory disturbances, blurred vision, diplopia, dizziness, paresthesias, headache, restlessness, and tremors. Pyridoxine relieves the neurologic symptoms and its concomitant administration is recommended. Severe allergic skin rashes, purpura, stomatitis, gynecomastia, impotence, menorrhagia, acne, and alopecia also have been observed. Hepatitis has developed in ~5% of cases and reverses when treatment is stopped; hepatic function should be assessed periodically.

AMINOSALICYLIC ACID

ANTIBACTERIAL ACTIVITY

Aminosalicylic acid is bacteriostatic. In vitro, most strains of M. tuberculosis are sensitive to a concentration of 1 μg/mL. Microorganisms other than M. tuberculosis are unaffected.

MECHANISM OF ACTION AND BACTERIAL RESISTANCE

Aminosalicylic acid is a structural analog of para-aminobenzoic acid, and has the same mechanism of action as the sulfonamides (see Chapter 43). Nonetheless, the sulfonamides are ineffective against M. tuberculosis, and aminosalicylic acid is inactive against sulfonamide-susceptible bacteria. Resistant strains of tubercle bacilli emerge slowly in patients treated with aminosalicylic acid.

ABSORPTION, DISTRIBUTION, AND EXCRETION

Aminosalicylic acid is readily absorbed from the GI tract. The drug is distributed throughout total body water; it reaches high concentrations in pleural fluid and caseous tissue, but CSF levels are low. It has a $t_{1/2}$ of 1 hour, and concentrations in plasma are negligible within 4–5 hours after a single dose. Over 80% of the drug is excreted in the urine; >50% as an acetylated derivative; the largest portion of the remainder is the free acid. The drug should not be used in the setting of renal insufficiency.

THERAPEUTIC USES

Aminosalicylic acid (PASER) is a second-line agent in the management of tuberculosis. It is administered orally in a daily dose of 10–12 g. Because of GI irritation, it is administered after meals and divided into 2–4 equal portions. Children should receive 150–300 mg/kg/day in 3–4 divided doses.

UNTOWARD EFFECTS

GI problems (e.g., anorexia, nausea, epigastric pain, and diarrhea) are predominant and often limit patient adherence. Patients with peptic ulcers tolerate the drug especially poorly. Hypersensitivity reactions to aminosalicylic acid are seen in up to 10% of patients. Fever may develop abruptly or may appear gradually and be low-grade. Generalized malaise, arthralgias, and sore throat may be present. Rashes appear as isolated reactions or accompanied by fever. Hematological abnormalities include leukopenia, agranulocytosis, eosinophilia, lymphocytosis, an atypical mononucleosis syndrome, thrombocytopenia, and hemolytic anemia.

CYCLOSERINE

Cycloserine (SEROMYCIN) is a broad-spectrum antibiotic that is used with other drugs in the treatment of tuberculosis when primary agents have failed. Cycloserine is D-4-amino-3-isoxazolidone.

ANTIBACTERIAL ACTIVITY

Cycloserine inhibits M. tuberculosis in concentrations of 5–20 μg/mL in vitro. There is no cross-resistance between cycloserine and other tuberculostatic agents.

MECHANISM OF ACTION

Cycloserine and D-Ala are structural analogs; thus, cycloserine inhibits reactions in which D-Ala is involved in bacterial cell-wall synthesis.

ABSORPTION, DISTRIBUTION, AND EXCRETION

When given orally, 70–90% of cycloserine is rapidly absorbed. Cycloserine is distributed throughout body fluids and tissues. CSF concentrations are comparable to those in plasma. About 50% of a parenteral dose of cycloserine is excreted unchanged in the urine in the first 12 hours; a total of 65% is recoverable in the active form over a period of 72 hours. Very little of the antibiotic is metabolized. The drug may reach toxic concentrations in patients with renal insufficiency; it is removed from the circulation by hemodialysis.

THERAPEUTIC USES

Cycloserine is used only when retreatment is necessary or microorganisms are resistant to other drugs. It must be given together with other effective agents. The usual dose for adults is 250–500 mg twice daily.

UNTOWARD EFFECTS

Side effects typically affect the CNS, appearing within 2 weeks of therapy and disappearing after drug withdrawal. They include: somnolence, headache, tremor, dysarthria, vertigo, confusion, nervousness, irritability, psychotic states, paranoid reactions, catatonic reactions, twitching, ankle clonus, hyperreflexia, visual disturbances, paresis, and seizures. Large doses or concomitant ingestion of alcohol increases the risk of seizures. Cycloserine is contraindicated in individuals with a history of epilepsy and should be used with caution in individuals with a history of depression.

OTHER DRUGS

These agents are all secondary drugs used only for treatment of disease caused by resistant *M. tuberculosis* or by nontuberculous mycobacteria. They all are given parenterally and have similar pharmacokinetics and toxicity. Since these agents are potentially ototoxic and nephrotoxic, no two drugs from this group should be used simultaneously, and they should not be combined with streptomycin.

Amikacin is an aminoglycoside (see Chapter 45) that is extremely active against several mycobacterial species and has a role in the treatment of disease caused by nontuberculous mycobacteria.

Capreomycin (CAPASTAT) is an antimycobacterial cyclic peptide elaborated by Streptococcus capreolus. Bacterial resistance to capreomycin develops when it is given alone; such microorganisms show cross-resistance with kanamycin and neomycin. Capreomycin is used only in conjunction with other appropriate drugs in treatment of pulmonary tuberculosis when bactericidal agents cannot be tolerated or when causative organisms have become resistant.

Capreomycin is given intramuscularly, which may be painful. The daily dose is 15–30 mg/kg/day or up to 1 g for 60–120 days, followed by 1 g two to three times a week. Adverse reactions associated with capreomycin are hearing loss, tinnitus, transient proteinuria, and azotemia. Severe renal failure is rare. Eosinophilia is common, and leukocytosis, leukopenia, rashes, and fever have also been observed.

CHEMOTHERAPY OF TUBERCULOSIS

Most patients are treated in the ambulatory setting, often after diagnosis and initial therapy in a general hospital. Patients must be seen frequently to follow the course of their disease and treatment. The local health department should be notified and contacts should be investigated for the possibility of disease and for the appropriateness of prophylactic therapy.

Most new cases of tuberculosis in the U.S. are caused by microorganisms that are sensitive to isoniazid, rifampin, ethambutol, and pyrazinamide. To prevent the development of resistance to these agents, treatment must include at least 2 drugs to which the bacteria are sensitive. The preferred 6-month treatment program for drug-sensitive tuberculosis in adults and children consists of isoniazid, rifampin, pyrazinamide, and ethambutol for 2 months, followed by isoniazid and rifampin (for sensitive organisms) for 4 additional months. The combination of isoniazid and rifampin for 9 months is equally effective for sensitive tuberculosis. Because of the increasing frequency of drug resistance, the Centers for Disease Control and Prevention (CDC) recommends initial therapy with a 4-drug regimen (isoniazid, rifampin, pyrazinamide, and ethambutol or streptomycin) pending sensitivity results. Directly observed therapy is best and ensures treatment completion rates of ~90%.

Drug interactions are a special concern in patients receiving highly active antiretroviral therapy (HAART). The rifamycins accelerate the metabolism of protease inhibitors and nonnucleoside reverse transcriptase inhibitors. Rifabutin has the least effect on serum levels and is indicated in this setting.

HIV-infected patients may benefit from longer (9–12-month) treatment regimens. Treatment should be initiated with at least a 4-drug regimen consisting of isoniazid, rifabutin, pyrazinamide, and ethambutol or streptomycin. An initial 5- or 6-drug regimen may be appropriate in patients likely infected with multidrug-resistant strains. Treatment should be continued for at least 6 months after three negative cultures have been obtained. If isoniazid or rifampin cannot be used, therapy should be continued for at least 18 months (12 months after cultures become negative). Chemoprophylaxis (*see* below) should be undertaken if a patient with HIV infection has a positive tuberculin test (induration ≥5 mm), a history of a positive tuberculin skin test that was not treated with chemoprophylaxis, or recent close contact with a potentially infectious patient with tuberculosis. Isoniazid does not reduce the incidence of tuberculosis in anergic patients with HIV, so chemoprophylaxis in this setting has been abandoned.

THERAPY OF SPECIFIC TYPES OF TUBERCULOSIS

Therapy for drug-sensitive pulmonary tuberculosis consists of isoniazid (5 mg/kg, up to 300 mg/day), rifampin (10 mg/kg/day, up to 600 mg daily), pyrazinamide (15–30 mg/kg/day or a maximum of 2 g/day), and a fourth agent, typically either ethambutol (usual adult dose of 15 mg/kg once per day) or streptomycin (1 g daily). The streptomycin dose is reduced to 1 g twice weekly after 2 months. Pyridoxine, 15–50 mg/day, also should be included for most adults to minimize adverse reactions to isoniazid. Isoniazid, rifampin, pyrazinamide, and ethambutol or streptomycin are given for 2 months; isoniazid and rifampin are then continued for 4 more months. Doses in children are isoniazid, 10 mg/kg/day (300 mg maximum); rifampin, 10–20 mg/kg/day (600 mg maximum); pyrazinamide, 15–30 mg/kg/day (2 g maximum). Isoniazid, rifampin, and ethambutol are considered safe during pregnancy.

Clinical improvement usually is seen within the first 2 weeks of therapy. Progressive radiological improvement also is evident. Over 90% of patients who receive optimal treatment will have negative cultures within 3–6 months. Cultures that remain positive after 6 months frequently yield resistant microorganisms; the need for an alternative therapeutic program should then be considered.

Chemotherapy failure may be due to (1) irregular or inadequate therapy (resulting in persistent or resistant mycobacteria) caused by poor patient adherence to the protracted therapeutic regimen; (2) the use of a single drug, with interruption necessitated by toxicity or hypersensitivity; (3) an inadequate initial regimen; or (4) primary resistance of the microorganism.

PROBLEMS IN CHEMOTHERAPY

Bacterial Resistance to Drugs

An important problem in the chemotherapy of tuberculosis is bacterial resistance, primarily due to poor patient adherence. To prevent noncompliance and the attendant development of drug-resistant tuberculosis, directly observed therapy is advisable for most patients (i.e., a health care provider observes the patient take the medications 2–5 times weekly).

Where drug resistance is suspected (i.e., in previously treated patients), therapy should be instituted with 5 or 6 drugs, including 2 or 3 that the patient has not previously received. Such a regimen might include isoniazid, rifampin, pyrazinamide, ethambutol, streptomycin, and ethionamide. Some physicians include isoniazid in the therapeutic regimen, even if microorganisms are resistant, on the belief that disease with isoniazid-resistant mycobacteria does not "progress" during such therapy. Others discontinue isoniazid to lessen the possibility of toxicity. Therapy should be continued for at least 24 months.

Nontuberculous (Atypical) Mycobacteria

These microorganisms (not including M. avium *complex) frequently are resistant to many of the commonly used agents; drugs therefore should be selected based on sensitivity in vitro (Table 47–1). Surgical removal of infected tissue followed by long-term treatment with effective drugs may be needed.*
M. kansasii *and* M. tuberculosis *cause similar disease. Therapy of the former with isoniazid, rifampin, and ethambutol has been successful.* Mycobacterium marinum *causes skin lesions. A combination of rifampin and ethambutol is probably effective; minocycline or tetracycline is active in vitro and is used by some physicians.* M. scrofulaceum *is an uncommon cause of cervical lymphadenitis that is treated with surgical excision. Microbes of the* M. fortuitum *complex (including* Mycobacterium chelonae*) may cause chronic lung disease and infections of skin and soft tissues. The microorganisms are highly resistant to most drugs, but amikacin, cefoxitin, and tetracyclines are active* in vitro.

CHEMOPROPHYLAXIS OF TUBERCULOSIS Chemoprophylaxis of tuberculosis involves treating latent infection to prevent progression to active disease. Latent infection may be diagnosed by a positive reaction to a purified protein derivative (PPD) of tuberculosis injected intradermally (the "tuberculin test"). The CDC recommends prophylaxis with isoniazid for 6–9 months or rifampin for 4 months if isoniazid cannot be used. A 2-month regimen of daily rifampin and pyrazinamide has also been used in HIV-infected individuals.

Prophylactic therapy should be considered in patients exposed to tuberculosis who have evidence of infection, including immunosuppressed patients (*e.g.*, HIV-infected) with >5 mm induration on PPD testing; immunocompetent patients with >10 mm induration on PPD testing and risk factors for TB but no apparent disease; and those with a history of tuberculosis in whom the disease is currently "inactive." The main risk of chemoprophylaxis is isoniazid-induced hepatitis. Monitored isoniazid prophylaxis minimizes this risk, even in patients over the age of 35.

Household contacts and other close associates of patients with tuberculosis who have negative tuberculin tests should receive isoniazid for at least 6 months after the contact has been broken, regardless of age. This is especially important for children. If the PPD test becomes positive, therapy should be continued for 12 months.

Patients with "inactive" tuberculosis who have not received adequate therapy should be considered for 1 year of isoniazid treatment. HIV-infected intravenous drug abusers with a positive PPD test have ~8% chance per year of developing active tuberculosis. Isoniazid prophylaxis in HIV-infected persons appears to be as effective as in non-immunocompromised persons. The CDC recommends that isoniazid prophylaxis be continued for 12 months. Persons infected with HIV who are exposed to multidrug-resistant tuberculosis should receive prophylaxis with rifampin and pyrazinamide (with close monitoring for hepatic toxicity) or high-dose ethambutol and pyrazinamide, with or without a fluoroquinolone.

Isoniazid prophylaxis is contraindicated for patients who have active hepatic disease or who have had reactions to the drug. In these individuals, rifampin for 4 months can be given. In pregnant women, prophylaxis usually should be delayed until after delivery. For prophylaxis, isoniazid generally is given to adults in a daily dose of 300 mg. Children should receive 10 mg/kg to a maximal daily dose of 300 mg. Pyridoxine should be coadministered in individuals susceptible to isoniazid-induced neuropathy.

II. DRUGS FOR *MYCOBACTERIUM AVIUM* COMPLEX

Before the advent of HAART and the use of prophylaxis, disseminated MAC infection occurred in 15–40% of patients with HIV infection; MAC infections now are greatly reduced. Patients with MAC infection usually have advanced HIV disease, with CD4 counts <100/mm^3 and symptoms of fever, night sweats, weight loss, and anemia at the time of diagnosis. In non–HIV-infected persons, MAC infection usually is limited to the lungs and presents with a chronic productive cough and radiographic evidence of limited, diffuse, and/or cavitary disease. Although standard antimycobacterial drugs have little activity against MAC, newer agents with activity against MAC are used both to prevent and to treat MAC in AIDS patients.

RIFABUTIN

Rifabutin shares a common mechanism of action with rifampin (inhibition of mycobacterial RNA polymerase) but is more active *in vitro*.

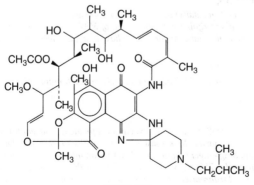

RIFABUTIN

ANTIBACTERIAL ACTIVITY AND BACTERIAL RESISTANCE

Rifabutin has better activity against MAC organisms than rifampin and is active in vitro against MAC bacteria isolated from HIV-infected (typically M. avium*) and non–HIV-infected individuals (~40%* M. intracellulare*). Rifabutin also inhibits the growth of many strains of* M. tuberculosis. *Cross-resistance between rifampin and rifabutin is common in* M. tuberculosis, *although some strains are resistant to rifampin yet sensitive to rifabutin. Most* M. avium *strains resistant to rifampin are still sensitive to rifabutin.*

ABSORPTION, DISTRIBUTION, METABOLISM, AND EXCRETION Rifabutin is given orally, usually at 300 mg/day. Following GI absorption, it is metabolized by hepatic CYPs and eliminated in a biphasic manner with a mean terminal $t_{1/2}$ of ~45 hours, predominantly in urine and bile. Dosage adjustment is not necessary in patients with impaired renal function.

THERAPEUTIC USES Rifabutin is effective for the prevention of MAC infection in HIV-infected individuals and can decrease the frequency of MAC bacteremia. Azithromycin or clarithromycin is more effective and less likely to interact with HAART drugs. Rifabutin also is commonly substituted for rifampin in the treatment of tuberculosis in HIV-infected patients, as it has a less profound CYP-dependent drug interaction. Rifabutin also is used in combination with clarithromycin and ethambutol for the therapy of MAC disease.

UNTOWARD EFFECTS Rifabutin generally is well tolerated in persons with HIV infection; primary reasons for discontinuation of therapy include rash (4%), GI intolerance (3%), and neutropenia (2%). Overall, neutropenia occurred in 25% of patients with severe HIV infection who received rifabutin. Uveitis and arthralgias have occurred in patients receiving rifabutin doses >450 mg daily in combination with clarithromycin or fluconazole. Patients should be cautioned to discontinue the drug if visual symptoms occur. Like rifampin, the drug causes an orange-tan discoloration. Rarely, thrombocytopenia, a flu-like syndrome, hemolysis, myositis, chest pain, and hepatitis have occurred.

Although less potent than rifampin, rifabutin does induce hepatic CYPs and can decrease the $t_{1/2}$ of a number of drugs, including *zidovudine, prednisone,* digitoxin, quinidine, ketoconazole, propranolol, phenytoin, sulfonylureas, and *warfarin.*

MACROLIDES

Clarithromycin and azithromycin are used to treat MAC and other nontuberculous mycobacteria. Clarithromycin alters the metabolism of many other drugs that are metabolized by CYPs, leading to many potential drug interactions. The broader pharmacology of these macrolides is presented in Chapter 46.

ANTIBACTERIAL ACTIVITY AND BACTERIAL RESISTANCE

Clarithromycin is approximately fourfold more active than azithromycin against MAC and is active against most nontuberculous mycobacteria. Azithromycin's lower potency may be compensated for by its greater penetration; tissue levels exceed plasma levels by 100-fold.

Use of clarithromycin or azithromycin alone is associated with the development of resistance, and they therefore should not be used as monotherapy of MAC infection.

THERAPEUTIC USES

Clarithromycin (500 mg twice daily) or azithromycin (500 mg daily) is used in combination with ethambutol, with or without rifabutin, for treatment of MAC infection. Treatment should be lifelong in HIV-infected individuals. Azithromycin has minimal effect on drugs metabolized by CYP3A4.

UNTOWARD EFFECTS

The high doses used to treat MAC infections rarely cause tinnitus, dizziness, and reversible hearing loss.

QUINOLONES

The quinolones (e.g., ciprofloxacin, levofloxacin, moxifloxacin, and gatifloxacin) inhibit MAC bacteria in vitro. M. fortuitum *and* M. kansasii *also are sensitive to these quinolones but* M. chelonae *usually are resistant. Single-agent therapy of* M. fortuitum *infection with ciprofloxacin has led to resistance. Ciprofloxacin, 750 mg twice daily or 500 mg three times daily, has been used in a 4-drug regimen (with clarithromycin, rifabutin, and amikacin) as salvage therapy for MAC infections in HIV-infected patients. Multidrug-resistant tuberculosis has been treated with ofloxacin,*

300 or 800 mg/day, in combination with second-line agents. Moxifloxacin and gatifloxacin are more active than the older fluoroquinolones and would be expected to be useful agents clinically. For more on the quinolones, see Chapter 43.

AMIKACIN

Amikacin (see Chapter 45) may have a role as a third or fourth agent in a multiple-drug regimen for MAC treatment.

CHEMOTHERAPY OF *MYCOBACTERIUM AVIUM* COMPLEX

Clarithromycin and azithromycin both have excellent activity against many strains of MAC, with clinical responses (decrease or elimination of bacteremia, resolution of fever and night sweats) demonstrated even with single-drug therapy. To avoid resistance, most clinicians treat disseminated MAC infections with clarithromycin or azithromycin plus ethambutol. In some situations, rifabutin, clofazimine, and/or a quinolone are added. Drug interactions and adverse drug reactions are common with multiple-drug regimens, necessitating drug discontinuation in ~50% of patients. Clinical improvement is expected in the first 1–2 months of treatment, with sterilization of blood cultures within 3 months of starting therapy. Treatment of MAC infection in HIV-infected individuals typically is lifelong. Isoniazid and pyrazinamide have no role in the treatment of MAC infection.

Prophylaxis of MAC infection with clarithromycin or azithromycin should be strongly considered for HIV-infected persons whose CD4 count is <50/mm³.

III. DRUGS FOR LEPROSY

The worldwide incidence of leprosy (Hansen's disease) has plummeted by nearly 90% to ~534,000. The cornerstone of this global elimination strategy is the provision of effective multidrug chemotherapy, namely dapsone, rifampin, and clofazimine (Table 47–1), to all leprosy patients in the world. The success of the strategy is evident; by the end of 2003, over half of the countries considered endemic for leprosy in 1985 had achieved disease elimination (*i.e.,* a prevalence rate of <1 case per 10,000 inhabitants).

SULFONES

The sulfones are derivatives of 4,4′-diaminodiphenylsulfone (dapsone), all of which share certain pharmacological properties. Only dapsone and sulfoxone are considered here.

ANTIBACTERIAL ACTIVITY, MECHANISM OF ACTION, AND RESISTANCE

Because Mycobacterium leprae does not grow on artificial media, in vivo assays with rat footpads have been used to test potential therapeutic agents. Dapsone is bacteriostatic for M. leprae due to competitive inhibiton of dihydropteroate synthase, which prevents bacterial utilization of para-aminobenzoic acid.

M. leprae may develop drug resistance during therapy, which is termed secondary resistance; this typically occurs in lepromatous (multibacillary) patients treated with a single drug. The incidence is as high as 19%. Partial-to-complete primary resistance in previously untreated patients has been described in 2.5–40% of patients, depending on geographical location.

THERAPEUTIC USES

Dapsone is given orally with a daily dose of 100 mg. Therapy usually is begun with smaller amounts, and doses are increased to those recommended over 1–2 months. Therapy should be continued for at least 3 years and may be necessary for life.

UNTOWARD EFFECTS

Hemolysis is the most common untoward reaction and develops in almost every individual treated with 200–300 mg of dapsone per day. Doses of 100 mg or less in normal healthy persons and 50 mg or less in healthy individuals with glucose-6-phosphate dehydrogenase deficiency do not cause hemolysis. Methemoglobinemia also is common. A genetic deficiency in the NADH-dependent methemoglobin reductase can result in severe methemoglobinemia after dapsone administration. While diminished red-cell survival usually occurs during the use of sulfones—presumably a dose-related effect of their oxidizing activity—hemolytic anemia is unusual unless the patient also has a disorder of either the erythrocytes or the bone marrow. The hemolysis may be so severe that manifestations of hypoxia become striking.

Anorexia, nausea, and vomiting may follow oral administration of sulfones. Isolated instances of headache, nervousness, insomnia, blurred vision, paresthesias, reversible peripheral neuropathy, drug fever, hematuria, pruritus, psychosis, and a variety of rashes have been reported. An infectious mononucleosis-like syndrome occurs occasionally. The sulfones may induce an exacerbation of lepromatous leprosy by a process analogous to the Jarisch-Herxheimer reaction. This "sulfone syndrome" may develop 5–6 weeks after initiation of treatment. Its manifestations include fever, malaise, exfoliative dermatitis, jaundice with hepatic necrosis, lymphadenopathy, methemoglobinemia, and anemia.

Used properly, the sulfones may be given safely for many years in doses adequate for the successful therapy of leprosy. Treatment should be initiated with a small dose and then increased gradually. Patients must be under consistent laboratory and clinical supervision. The reactions induced by the sulfones, especially those related to the "sulfone syndrome," may require the cessation of treatment as well as the institution of specific measures to reduce the threat to life.

ABSORPTION, DISTRIBUTION, AND EXCRETION

Dapsone is absorbed rapidly and nearly completely from the GI tract. Di-substituted sulfones (e.g., sulfoxone) are absorbed incompletely when administered orally and largely excreted in the feces. Peak concentrations of dapsone in plasma are reached within 2–8 hours after administration; the mean $t_{1/2}$ is ~20–30 hours. About 70% of the drug is bound to plasma protein.

The sulfones are distributed throughout total body water and are present in all tissues. They are retained in skin and muscle and especially in liver and kidney. The sulfones persist in the circulation for a long time because of reabsorption from the bile; periodic interruption of treatment is advisable for this reason. Dapsone is acetylated in the liver by the same enzyme that acetylates isoniazid. Daily administration of 50–100 mg results in serum levels exceeding the usual minimal inhibitory concentrations, even in rapid acetylators, in whom the serum $t_{1/2}$ of dapsone is shorter than usual.

Approximately 70–80% of a dose of dapsone is excreted in the urine as an acid-labile mono-N-glucuronide and mono-N-sulfamate.

RIFAMPIN

Rifampin is rapidly bactericidal for M. leprae with a minimal inhibitory concentration of <1 μg/mL. Infectivity of patients is reversed rapidly by therapy that includes rifampin.

CLOFAZIMINE

Clofazimine (LAMPRENE) binds preferentially to GC-rich mycobacterial DNA, increases mycobacterial phospholipase A_2 activity, and inhibits microbial K^+ transport. It is weakly bactericidal against M. intracellulare. The drug also exerts an anti-inflammatory effect and prevents the development of erythema nodosum leprosum. Clofazimine is recommended as a component of multiple-drug therapy for leprosy. It also is useful for treatment of chronic skin ulcers produced by Mycobacterium ulcerans.

Clofazimine is orally absorbed and accumulates in tissues. Human leprosy from which dapsone-resistant bacilli have been recovered has been treated with clofazimine with good results. However, unlike dapsone-sensitive microorganisms, in which killing occurs immediately after dapsone is administered, dapsone-resistant strains do not exhibit an appreciable effect until 50 days after initiation of therapy with clofazimine. The daily dose of clofazimine is usually 100 mg. Patients treated with clofazimine may develop red discoloration of the skin.

CHEMOTHERAPY OF LEPROSY

Leprosy is a continuum between two extremes. At one end of the spectrum is tuberculoid leprosy, *characterized by skin macules with clear centers and well-defined margins. M. leprae is rarely found in smears made from quiescent lesions but may appear during activity. Noncaseating foci are present. The patient's cell-mediated immunity is normal, and a skin test for infection by leprosy is invariably positive. The disease is characterized by prolonged remissions with periodic reactivation.*

The other extreme is the widely disseminated lepromatous form, *characterized by markedly impaired cell-mediated immunity and diffuse infiltration of the skin. M. leprae is demonstrable in smears, and granulomas containing bacteria-laden histiocytes are present. As the disease progresses, large nerve trunks are involved and anesthesia, atrophy of skin and muscle, absorption of small bones, ulceration, and spontaneous amputations may occur.*

Effective therapy heals ulcers and mucosal lesions in months. Cutaneous nodules respond more slowly, and years may be needed to eradicate bacteria from mucous membranes, skin, and nerves. The degree of residual pigmentation or depigmentation, atrophy, and scarring depends upon the extent of the initial involvement. Severe ocular lesions respond poorly to sulfones, but early treatment may prevent progression. Keratoconjunctivitis and corneal ulceration may be secondary to nerve involvement.

The WHO recommends therapy with multiple drugs for all patients with leprosy to reduce the development of resistance, provide adequate therapy when primary resistance already exists, and reduce the duration of therapy. For patients with lepromatous disease, the following regimen is suggested: dapsone, 100 mg/day; plus clofazimine, 50 mg/day (unsupervised); plus rifampin, 600 mg, and clofazimine, 300 mg, once a month under supervision for 1–5 years. Some prefer to treat lepromatous leprosy with daily dapsone (100 mg) and daily rifampin (450–600 mg). All drugs are given orally. The minimal duration of therapy is 2 years, and treatment should continue until acid-fast bacilli are not detected in lesions.

Patients with a small population of bacteria (i.e., with tuberculoid disease) should be treated with dapsone, 100 mg daily, plus rifampin, 600 mg once monthly for a minimum of 6 months. The regimen is repeated if relapse occurs. Single-dose multidrug therapy with rifampin (600 mg), ofloxacin (400 mg), or minocycline (100 mg) also may be as effective.

For a complete Bibliographical listing see Goodman & Gilman's *The Pharmacological Basis of Therapeutics*, 11th ed., or Goodman & Gilman Online at www.accessmedicine.com.

48

ANTIFUNGAL AGENTS

SYSTEMIC ANTIFUNGAL AGENTS

Systemic fungal infections are a major cause of death in patients whose immune system is compromised due to cancer or its chemotherapy, organ transplantation, or HIV-1 infection. Fungi also commonly cause superficial infections of the skin and other soft tissue structures. Many antifungal agents in clinical use are targeted at distinctive components of the fungal cell membrane; others alter cell wall synthesis or nucleic acid synthesis (*see* Figure 48–1).

Amphotericin B

Amphotericin B is the antifungal agent with the broadest spectrum of activity and remains the drug of choice for the vast majority of life-threatening systemic fungal infections. Amphotericin B is a heptaene macrolide; its amphoteric behavior results from a carboxyl group on the main ring and a primary amino group on mycosamine that confer aqueous solubility at pH extremes.

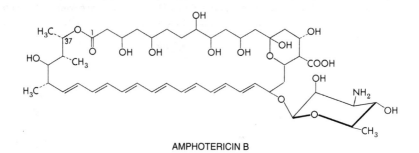

AMPHOTERICIN B

DRUG FORMULATIONS

Amphotericin B is complexed with deoxycholate (C-AMB) and marketed as a lyophilized powder (FUNGIZONE) containing 50 mg of amphotericin B that forms a colloid in water. Three lipid formulations of amphotericin B are marketed in the U.S. Amphotericin B colloidal dispersion (ABCD, AMPHOTEC, AMPHOCIL) contains equimolar amounts of amphotericin B and cholesteryl sulfate. AMBISOME is a small, unilamellar vesicle formulation that combines amphotericin B (50 mg) with 350 mg of lipid (phosphatidylcholine, cholesterol, and distearoylphosphatidylglycerol, in molar ratio of 10:5:4) in an ~10% molar ratio. Amphotericin B lipid complex (ABLC, ABELCET) contains dimyristoylphosphatidylcholine and dimyristoylphosphatidylglycerol in a 7:3 mixture with ~35 mol% of amphotericin B.

The role of lipid formulations of amphotericin B in fungal infections remains to be determined. The risk of adverse effects such as nephrotoxicity is decreased by ~50% with lipid formulations, but they cost 20–50 times more and may be associated with a greater risk of febrile infusion reactions.

ANTIFUNGAL ACTIVITY

Amphotericin B has useful clinical activity against a broad range of pathogenic fungi and against the protozoa, Leishmania braziliensis *and* Naegleria fowleri, *but has no antibacterial activity. The antifungal activity of amphotericin B depends principally on binding the sterol ergosterol in the membrane of sensitive fungi. By virtue of interaction with sterols, amphotericin forms pores that increase membrane permeability and allow leakage of small molecules (Figure 48–1).*

ABSORPTION, DISTRIBUTION, AND EXCRETION   Gastrointestinal (GI) absorption of amphotericin B is negligible and intravenous delivery is used. Amphotericin B in plasma is >90% bound to proteins. Drug elimination apparently is unchanged in anephric patients and those on hemodialysis. Hepatic or biliary disease has no known effect on drug metabolism in humans. The terminal phase of elimination has a $t_{1/2}$ of ~15 days. Concentrations of amphotericin B in fluids from inflamed pleura, peritoneum, synovium, and aqueous humor are approximately two-thirds of plasma trough concentrations. Little amphotericin B penetrates into cerebrospinal fluid (CSF), vitreous humor, or amniotic fluid.

Membrane function
Amphotericin B

Cell wall synthesis
Caspofungin

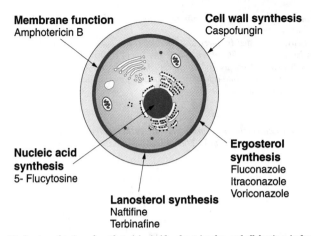

Nucleic acid synthesis
5- Flucytosine

Lanosterol synthesis
Naftifine
Terbinafine

Ergosterol synthesis
Fluconazole
Itraconazole
Voriconazole

FIGURE 48–1 *Mechanism of action of amphotericin, imidazoles, triazoles, and allylamines in fungi.* Amphotericin B and other polyenes, such as nystatin, bind to ergosterol in fungal cell membranes and increase membrane permeability. The imidazoles and triazoles, such as itraconazole and fluconazole, inhibit 14-α-sterol demethylase, prevent ergosterol synthesis, and lead to the accumulation of 14-α-methylsterols. The allylamines, such as naftifine and terbinafine, inhibit squalene epoxidase and prevent ergosterol synthesis. The echinocandins (*e.g.*, caspofungin) inhibit the formation of glucans in the fungal cell wall.

THERAPEUTIC USES
The usual dose of C-AMB is 0.5–0.6 mg/kg, administered in 5% glucose over 4 hours. Candida esophagitis in adults responds to 0.15–0.2 mg/kg daily. Rapidly progressive mucormycosis or invasive aspergillosis is treated with doses of 1–1.2 mg/kg daily until progression is arrested.

Intrathecal infusion of amphotericin B (C-AMB) is used in patients with meningitis caused by Coccidioides. Treatment is initiated with 0.05–0.1 mg and increased on a three-times-weekly schedule to 0.5 mg, as tolerated. Therapy is then continued on a twice-weekly schedule.

Amphotericin B is the treatment of choice for mucormycosis and is used for initial treatment of cryptococcal meningitis, severe or rapidly progressing histoplasmosis, blastomycosis, coccidioidomycosis, penicilliosis marneffei, and in patients not responding to azole therapy of invasive aspergillosis, extracutaneous sporotrichosis, fusariosis, alternariosis, and trichosporonosis. Amphotericin B is given once weekly to prevent relapse in patients with AIDS who have been treated successfully for cryptococcosis or histoplasmosis.

ABCD is approved for patients with invasive aspergillosis who are not responding to or are unable to tolerate C-AMB. Ambisome is approved for empiric therapy of neutopenic patients not responding to appropriate antibacterial agents and for salvage therapy of aspergillosis, cryptococcosis, and candidiasis. ABLC is approved for salvage therapy of deep mycoses.

UNTOWARD EFFECTS
The major acute reaction to intravenous amphotericin B is fever and chills, which typically end spontaneously in ~30 minutes and often abate with subsequent infusions. Tachypnea and modest hypotension may occur, but true bronchospasm or anaphylaxis is rare. Patients with preexisting cardiac or lung disease may become hypotensive or hypoxic. Pretreatment with oral acetaminophen or intravenous glucocorticoids decreases reactions, while meperidine may shorten the duration of established reactions.

Transient azotemia occurs in 80% of patients who receive C-AMB for deep mycoses. Toxicity is dose-dependent and increased by concurrent therapy with other nephrotoxic agents (e.g., aminoglycosides, cyclosporine). Permanent impairment is uncommon in adults with normal renal function unless the cumulative dose is >3–4 g. Renal tubular acidosis and wasting of K^+ and Mg^{2+} also may occur during and for several weeks after therapy, often requiring repletion. Administration of 1 L of normal saline intravenously prior to C-AMB administration is recommended for adults who can tolerate the Na^+ load. Azotemia occurs less frequently with lipid preparations of amphotericin, and saline loading is not needed.

Hypochromic, normocytic anemia is usual with C-AMB and reverses slowly following cessation of therapy. It likely reflects decreased production of erythropoietin and often responds to *erythropoietin. Headache, nausea, vomiting, malaise, weight loss, and phlebitis at peripheral infusion sites are common.*

Arachnoiditis, manifested by fever and headache, can occur with intrathecal injection of C-AMB; it may be decreased by intrathecal administration of 10–15 mg of hydrocortisone. Other serious problems that attend the use of intrathecal injections depend on the injection site. Local injections of amphotericin B into a joint or peritoneal dialysate fluid commonly produce irritation and pain.

Flucytosine

Flucytosine *is an antimetabolite whose spectrum of antigungal activity is considerably more restricted than that of amphotericin B. Flucytosine is a fluorinated pyrimidine:*

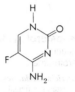

FLUCYTOSINE

ANTIFUNGAL ACTIVITY

Susceptible fungi deaminate flucytosine to 5-fluorouracil, a potent antimetabolite (Figure 48–2). Fluorouracil is metabolized to 5-fluorouracil-ribose monophosphate (5-FUMP) by the enzyme uracil phosphoribosyl transferase (UPRTase). 5-FUMP then is either incorporated into RNA (via synthesis of 5-fluorouridine triphosphate) or metabolized to 5-fluoro-2'-deoxyuridine-5'-monophosphate (5-FdUMP), a potent inhibitor of thymidylate synthetase that thus inhibits DNA synthesis. The selective action of flucytosine is due to the relatively low level of cytosine deaminase in mammalian cells, which prevents metabolism to fluorouracil.

Resistance arising during therapy (secondary resistance) is an important cause of therapeutic failure when flucytosine is used alone for cryptococcosis and candidiasis; it can result from loss of the permease necessary for cytosine transport or decreased activity of UPRTase or cytosine deaminase (Figure 48–2).

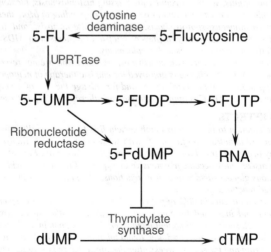

FIGURE 48–2 *Action of flucytosine in fungi.* 5-Flucytosine is transported by cytosine permease into the fungal cell, where it is deaminated to 5-fluorouracil (5-FU). The 5-FU is then converted to 5-fluorouracil-ribose monophosphate (5-FUMP) and then is either converted to 5-fluorouridine triphosphate (5-FUTP) and incorporated into RNA or converted by ribonucleotide reductase to 5-fluoro-2'-deoxyuridine-5'-monophosphate (5-FdUMP), which is a potent inhibitor of thymidylate synthase. 5-FUDP, 5-fluorouridine-5'-diphosphate; dUMP, deoxyuridine-5'-monophosphate; dTMP, deoxyuridine-5'-monophosphate UPRTase, uracil phosphoribosyl transferase.

ABSORPTION, DISTRIBUTION, AND EXCRETION

Flucytosine is absorbed rapidly and well from the GI tract, widely distributed, and minimally bound to plasma proteins. Flucytosine concentration in CSF is 65–90% of that found simultaneously in plasma. Approximately 80% of a dose is excreted unchanged in the urine. The $t_{1/2}$ of the drug normally is 3–6 hours but may reach 200 hours in renal failure. Dose modification is necessary in patients with decreased renal function, and plasma concentrations should be measured periodically to maintain peak concentrations of 50–100 μg/mL. Flucytosine is cleared by hemodialysis, and patients should receive a single dose of 37.5 mg/kg after dialysis; the drug also is removed by peritoneal dialysis.

THERAPEUTIC USES

Flucytosine (ANCOBON) is clinically useful for Cryptococcus neoformans, Candida spp., *and chromoblastomycosis. It is given orally at 100 mg/kg/day, in divided doses at 6-hour intervals and is used predominantly in combination with amphotericin B. An all-oral regimen of flucytosine plus fluconazole has been advocated for therapy of AIDS patients with cryptococcosis, but the combination has substantial GI toxicity without evidence that flucytosine improves the outcome. The combination of flucytosine with C-AMB runs the risk of substantial bone marrow suppression or colitis if the flucytosine dose is not promptly adjusted downward if amphotericin B–induced azotemia occurs. It is common practice in HIV-negative patients with cryptococcal meningitis to begin with C-AMB or AMBISOME plus flucytosine and change to fluconazole after the patient has improved.*

UNTOWARD EFFECTS Flucytosine may cause leukopenia and thrombocytopenia. Rash, nausea, vomiting, diarrhea, and enterocolitis also have been noted. In ~5% of patients, hepatic transaminases are elevated, but this reverses when therapy is stopped. Toxicity is more frequent in patients with AIDS or azotemia or when plasma drug concentrations are >100 μg/mL.

Imidazoles and Triazoles

The azole antifungals include the imidazoles and triazoles. These drugs have the same spectrum of antifungal activity and share a common mechanism by inhibiting fungal CYPs that are essential for ergosterol biosynthesis (Figure 48–1). Of the drugs available in the U.S., *clotrimazole, miconazole, ketoconazole, econazole, butoconazole, oxiconazole, sertaconazole,* and *sulconazole* are imidazoles; *terconazole, itraconazole,* fluconazole, and *voriconazole* are triazoles.

TRIAZOLE

ANTIFUNGAL ACTIVITY Azoles are active against *C. albicans, C. tropicalis, C. parapsilosis, C. glabrata, C. neoformans, Blastomyces dermatitidis, Histoplasma capsulatum, Coccidioides species, Paracoccidioides brasiliensis,* and dermatophytes. *Aspergillus spp., Scedosporium apiospermum (Pseudallescheria boydii), Fusarium,* and *Sporothrix schenckii* are intermediate in susceptibility. *C. krusei* and the agents of mucormycosis are resistant.

Azoles inhibit 14-α-sterol demethylase, a microsomal CYP that is essential for ergosterol biosynthesis (Figure 48–1). This results in the accumulation of 14-α-methylsterols that disrupt the packing of acyl chains of phospholipids and impair the functions of membrane-bound enzymes such as ATPase and those of the electron transport system, resulting in inhibited fungal growth.

Azole resistance has caused clinical failure in patients with far-advanced HIV infection and oropharyngeal or esophageal candidiasis. The primary mechanism of resistance in C. albicans *is accumulation of mutations in the gene encoding 14-α-sterol demethylase; cross-resistance to all azoles results.*

Ketoconazole

Ketoconazole has been replaced by itraconazole for the treatment of all mycoses except when cost is the primary determinant. Itraconazole lacks ketoconazole's corticosteroid suppression, while retaining most of its properties and expanding the antifungal spectrum.

Itraconazole

This synthetic triazole is an equimolar racemic mixture of four diastereoisomers.

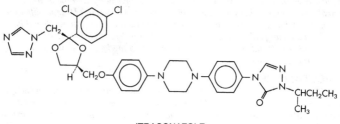

ITRACONAZOLE

ABSORPTION, DISTRIBUTION, AND EXCRETION Itraconazole (SPORONOX) is available as a capsule and solutions for oral or intravenous administration. The capsule is better absorbed with food, but the oral solution is better absorbed in the fasting state and provides peak plasma concentrations that are >150% of those obtained with the capsule. Both the oral solution and intravenous formulations are solubilized in a 40:1 weight ratio of itraconazole:hydroxypropyl-β-cyclodextrin. Itraconazole and its active metabolite hydroxy-itraconazole are >99% bound to plasma proteins and neither appears in urine or CSF. The $t_{1/2}$ of itraconazole is ~30 hours; steady-state levels are not reached for 4 days (7 days for hydroxy-itraconazole); thus, loading doses are used when treating deep mycoses. Severe liver disease increases itraconazole plasma concentrations. Itraconazole should not be used for onychomycosis during pregnancy or in women contemplating pregnancy (category C).

THERAPEUTIC USES

Oral itraconazole is the drug of choice for patients with indolent, nonmeningeal infections due to B. dermatitidis, H. capsulatum, P. brasiliensis, *and* C. immitis *and also is useful for indolent invasive aspergillosis outside the CNS, particularly following initial therapy with amphotericin B. The intravenous formulation is approved for the initial 2 weeks of therapy with blastomycosis, histoplasmosis, and indolent aspergillosis, and for empirical therapy of febrile neutropenic patients not responding to antibiotics and at high risk of fungal infections. The intravenous route is most appropriate for patients unable to tolerate oral drug or unable to absorb itraconazole because of decreased gastric acidity. Approximately half the patients with distal subungual onychomycosis respond to itraconazole. Although not approved, itraconazole is a reasonable choice for pseudallescheriasis, as well as cutaneous and extracutaneous sporotrichosis, tinea corporis, and extensive tinea versicolor. HIV-infected patients with disseminated histoplasmosis or* Penicillium marneffei *infections have a decreased incidence of relapse if given prolonged itraconazole "maintenance" therapy; it is unclear whether patients responding to highly active antiretroviral therapy (HAART) will require less than lifelong therapy. Because of frequent relapses, itraconazole is not recommended for maintenance therapy of cryptococcal meningitis in HIV-infected patients. Long-term therapy has provided clinical improvement in non-HIV–infected patients with allergic bronchopulmonary aspergillosis.*

Itraconazole solution is approved for oropharyngeal and esophageal candidiasis. Because of its GI side effects (see below), itraconazole solution usually is reserved for patients not responding to fluconazole who are not receiving protease inhibitors or other drugs that preclude its use. Itraconazole capsules and oral solution are not bioequivalent and should not be used interchangeably.

UNTOWARD EFFECTS

Itraconazole and other azoles can interact with many drugs by virtue of their effects on CYP3A4 (Table 48–1); these interactions can cause serious toxicity from the companion drug, including fatal cardiac arrhythmias, and may decrease itraconazole concentrations below therapeutic levels.

Itraconazole rarely has led to hepatic failure and death. If symptoms of hepatotoxicity occur, the drug should be discontinued and liver function assessed. Itraconazole can lead to congestive heart failure in patients with impaired ventricular function. In the absence of interacting drugs, itraconazole capsules are well tolerated at 200 mg daily. GI distress occasionally prevents use of 400 mg/day. In patients receiving 50–400 mg/day, nausea and vomiting, hypertriglyceridemia, hypokalemia, elevated serum aminotransferases, and rash occurred in between 2–10% of patients. Occasionally, rash necessitates drug discontinuation, but most other adverse effects

Table 48–1

Interactions of Itraconazole and other Triazoles with Other Drugs

Other Drug Concentration Increased	Itraconazole Concentration Decreased
Alfentanil	Drugs that decrease gastric acidity
Alprazolam	H$_2$-receptor blockers
Amprenavir	Proton pump blockers
Atorvastatin	Simultaneous antacids (includes
Buspirone	didanosine buffer)
Busulfan	Carbamazepine
Cisapride	Isoniazid
Cyclophosphamide	Nevirapine
Cyclosporine	Phenobarbital
Delavirdine	Phenytoin
Diazepam	Rifampin, rifabutin
Digoxin	St. John's wort
Dihydropyridine Ca^{2+} channel blockers	**Itraconazole Concentration Increased**
Docetaxel	Amprenavir
Felodipine	Amprenavir
Haloperidol	Clarithromycin
Indinavir	Grapefruit juice
Loratidine	Indinavir
Lovastatin	Lopinavir
Methylprednisolone	Ritonavir
Midazolam	
Nisoldipine	
Phenytoin	
Pimozide	
Quinidine	
Ritonavir	
Saquinavir	
Sildenafil	
Simvastatin	
Sirolimus	
Sulfonylureas (glyburide, others)	
Tacrolimus	
Triazolam	
Trimetrexate	
Verapamil	
Vinca alkaloids (vincristine, vinblastine)	
Warfarin	

can be handled with dose reduction. Doses of 300 mg twice daily have led to adrenal insufficiency, lower limb edema, hypertension, and rhabdomyolysis; therefore, doses above 400 mg/day are not recommended for long-term use.

Relative to capsules, the oral solution of itraconazole more frequently causes diarrhea, abdominal cramps, anorexia, and nausea. GI side effects are common, but adherence generally is unimpaired. Anaphylaxis and severe rash have rarely occurred.

Intravenous itraconazole has all the adverse effects of capsules but generally is well tolerated. Due to chemical phlebitis, a dedicated catheter port is required, and infusion durations <1 hour are not recommended. The intravenous formulation is contraindicated in patients with a creatinine clearance <30 mL/min.

DOSAGE For deep mycoses, a loading dose of 200 mg of itraconazole is administered three times daily for 3 days. Thereafter, two 100-mg capsules are given twice daily with food. Divided doses allegedly increase the plasma AUC. For maintenance therapy of HIV-infected patients with disseminated histoplasmosis, 200 mg once daily is used. Onychomycosis can be treated with either 200 mg once daily for 12 weeks or with pulse therapy (200 mg twice daily for 1 week out of each month). A loading dose of itraconazole is given as a 200-mg intravenous infusion over 1 hour twice daily for 2 days, followed by 200 mg once daily for 12 days. Itraconazole oral solution should be taken fasting in a dose of 100 mg once daily and swished vigorously in the mouth before swallowing to optimize topical effect. Patients with oropharyngeal or esophageal candidiasis are given 100 mg of the solution twice a day for 2–4 weeks.

Fluconazole

Fluconazole is a fluorinated bistriazole.

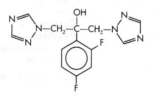

FLUCONAZOLE

ABSORPTION, DISTRIBUTION, AND EXCRETION   Fluconazole is almost completely absorbed from the GI tract irrespective of food or gastric acidity. Only 10% of drug in circulation is protein bound. Renal excretion accounts for >90% of elimination, with a $t_{1/2}$ of ~25 hours. Fluconazole readily diffuses into body fluids, including breast milk, sputum, saliva, and CSF. The dosage interval should be increased from 24–48 hours for a creatinine clearance of 21–40 mL/min and to 72 hours at 10–20 mL/min. In renal failure, a dose of 100–200 mg is given after hemodialysis.

DRUG INTERACTIONS
Fluconazole inhibits CYP3A4 and CYP2C9 and thus significantly increases plasma concentrations of amprenavir, cisapride, cyclosporine, phenytoin, sulfonylureas, tacrolimus, theophylline, telithromycin, and warfarin. Patients receiving >400 mg daily or azotemic patients may experience additional drug interactions. Rifampin decreases the fluconazole AUC by ~25%.

THERAPEUTIC USES
Candidiasis
Fluconazole, 200 mg on the first day and then 100 mg daily for at least 2 weeks, is effective in oropharyngeal candidiasis. Esophageal candidiasis responds to 100–200 mg/day, which also is used to decrease candiduria in high-risk patients. A single dose of 150 mg is effective in uncomplicated vaginal candidiasis. A dose of 400 mg daily decreases the incidence of deep candidiasis in allogeneic bone marrow transplant recipients and is useful in treating candidemia of immunocompetent patients. Fluconazole is not proven to be effective treatment for deep candidiasis in profoundly neutropenic patients.

Cryptococcosis
Fluconazole, 400 mg/day, is used for the initial 8 weeks in the treatment of cryptococcal meningitis in patients with AIDS after the patient has been stabilized with intravenous amphotericin B. Thereafter, the dose is decreased to 200 mg daily and continued indefinitely. If the patient responds to HAART, maintains a CD4 count >200/mm³ for at least 6 months, and has no meningeal symptoms, it is reasonable to discontinue fluconazole as long as the CD4 count is maintained and CSF culture and cryptococcal antigen are negative. For AIDS patients with cryptococcal meningitis and favorable prognostic signs, initial therapy with 400 mg daily may be considered. Fluconazole 400 mg/day has been recommended as continuation therapy in non-AIDS patients with cryptococcal meningitis who have responded to an initial course of C-AMB or AMBISOME and for patients with pulmonary cryptococcosis.

Other Mycoses
Fluconazole is the drug of choice for coccidioidal meningitis and is comparable to itraconazole for other forms of coccidioidomycosis. Fluconazole is less active than itraconazole against

histoplasmosis, blastomycosis, sporotrichosis, and ringworm and neither prevents nor treats aspergillosis or mucormycosis.

UNTOWARD EFFECTS
Nausea and vomiting may occur at doses >200 mg/day; patients receiving 800 mg daily may require parenteral antiemetics. Regardless of dose, side effects in patients receiving >7 days of drug include nausea, headache, skin rash, vomiting, abdominal pain, and diarrhea (all at 1–4%). Reversible alopecia may occur with prolonged therapy at 400 mg daily. Rare deaths due to hepatic failure or Stevens-Johnson syndrome have occurred. Fluconazole is associated with skeletal and cardiac deformities in infants born to women taking high doses during pregnancy and should be avoided during pregnancy (category C).

DOSAGE
Fluconazole (DIFLUCAN, others) is marketed as tablets for oral administration, powder for oral suspension, and intravenous solutions containing 2 mg/mL. Dosage is 50–800 mg once daily for oral or intravenous administration. Children are treated with 3–6 mg/kg once daily.

Voriconazole
Voriconazole (VFEND; UK-109,495) is a triazole that is similar to fluconazole but has increased activity and an expanded spectrum.

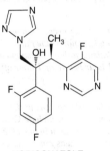

VORICONAZOLE

ABSORPTION, DISTRIBUTION, AND EXCRETION
Oral bioavailability is nearly complete, and gastric acid is not necessary for absorption. The volume of distribution is high (4.6 L/kg), with extensive tissue distribution; metabolism is by hepatic CYPs, especially 2C19. Less than 2% of native drug but most of the inactive metabolites are secreted in the urine. The oral dose is not adjusted for azotemia or hemodialysis.

Plasma elimination $t_{1/2}$ is 6 hours. Voriconazole exhibits nonlinear kinetics, and higher doses disproportionately increase drug exposure. Genetic polymorphisms in CYP2C19 can cause up to a fourfold difference in drug exposure; ~20% of Asians are poor metabolizers compared to 2% of Caucasians and African Americans. Drug exposure is increased considerably in the elderly and in patients with mild or moderate hepatic insufficiency. Patients with hepatic cirrhosis should receive the same loading dose of voriconazole but half the maintenance dose.

The intravenous formulation of voriconazole contains sulfobutyl ether β-cyclodextrin (SBECD), which is excreted by the kidney. Accumulation of SBECD occurs with a creatinine clearance <50 mL/min; in that setting, oral voriconazole is preferred.

DRUG INTERACTIONS
In decreasing rank order, voriconazole is metabolized by, and inhibits, CYP2C19, CYP2C9, and CYP3A4, as does its major metabolite, voriconazole N-oxide. Inhibitors or inducers of these enzymes may increase or decrease voriconazole plasma concentrations, respectively, while voriconazole may increase the plasma concentrations of other drugs metabolized by these enzymes. Coadministration with rifampin, rifabutin, or ritonavir is contraindicated because of accelerated voriconazole metabolism. Efavirenz and perhaps other nonnucleoside reverse transcriptase inhibitors (NNRTIs) significantly increase voriconazole metabolism and slow the metabolism of the NNRTI. When given with phenytoin, the voriconazole dose should be doubled. Drugs that significantly accumulate in patients receiving voriconazole include cyclosporine,

tacrolimus, phenytoin, rifabutin, warfarin, and sirolimus. *Because the sirolimus AUC increases 11-fold when voriconazole is given, coadministration is contraindicated.* Omeprazole *dose should be reduced by half if 40 mg or more per day is given. Until more experience with voriconazole is gained, it is prudent to be observant for drug interactions that occur with other azoles (Table 48–1).*

THERAPEUTIC USES
Voriconazole is superior to C-AMB as primary therapy of invasive aspergillosis. Although not approved, voriconazole has been used for the empirical therapy of neutropenic patients whose fever did not respond to antibacterial therapy. Voriconazole is approved for use in esophageal candidiasis and as salvage therapy in patients with P. boydii *and* Fusarium *infections.*

UNTOWARD EFFECTS
Although the drug is generally well tolerated, hepatotoxicity has been reported and liver function should be monitored. Voriconazole can prolong the QTc interval, which can be significant in patients with other risk factors for torsades de pointes. *Approximately 30% of patients note transient visual changes (e.g., blurred vision, altered color perception, and photophobia) beginning about half an hour after administration and lasting for another half hour. Activities that require keen vision should be avoided, but no sequelae occur. Uncommonly, confusion or transient visual hallucinations occur. Patients receiving their first intravenous infusion have had anaphylactoid reactions requiring drug discontinuation. Rash occurs in 6% of patients. Voriconazole is teratogenic in animals and should not be used in pregnancy (category D).*

DOSAGE
Treatment usually is initiated with 6 mg/kg every 12 hours for two doses, followed by 4 mg/kg every 12 hours, administered at 3 mg/kg/hour. As the patient improves, oral administration is continued at 200 mg every 12 hours. Patients failing to respond may be given 300 mg every 12 hours. Oral drug should be given either 1 hour before or 1 hour after meals.

Echinocandins
Echinocandins *inhibit formation of β(1,3)D-glucans in the cell wall of* Candida *and* caspofungin *is approved for clinical use. Susceptible fungi include* Candida *and* Aspergillus *species. Resistance can be conferred in* C. albicans *by mutation in one of the genes that encodes β(1,3)D-glucan synthase. Azole-resistant isolates of* C. albicans *remain susceptible to echinocandins.*

CASPOFUNGIN
Caspofungin (cancidas, MK-0991) is a water-soluble, lipopeptide synthesized from a fermentation product called pneumocandin Bo. In susceptible yeasts, caspofungin causes lysis.

ABSORPTION, DISTRIBUTION, AND EXCRETION
Caspofungin is not absorbed orally. After intravenous injection, caspofungin is eliminated from the bloodstream with a $t_{1/2}$ of ~10 hours. Catabolism is largely by hydrolysis and N-acetylation, followed by excretion in urine and feces. Mild or moderate hepatic insufficiency increases the AUC by 55% and 76%, respectively. About 97% of serum drug is bound to albumin. Dose adjustment is unnecessary for renal insufficiency or hemodialysis.

THERAPEUTIC USE
Caspofungin is approved for patients with invasive aspergillosis who are failing or intolerant of drugs such as amphotericin B or voriconazole and for esophageal candidiasis. A clinical trial of caspofungin in deeply invasive candidiasis found noninferiority to C-AMB, leading to approval for that indication. Caspofungin also is approved to treat persistently febrile neutropenic patients with suspected fungal infections.

UNTOWARD EFFECTS
Caspofungin is well tolerated, with the exception of phlebitis at the infusion site. Histamine-like effects have occurred with rapid infusions. Other effects are comparable to those in patients receiving fluconazole.

DOSAGE
Caspofungin is administered intravenously once daily over 1 hour. In candidemia and salvage therapy of aspergillosis, the initial dose is 70 mg, followed by 50 mg daily. The dose may be increased to 70 mg daily in patients failing to respond. Esophageal candidiasis is treated with 50 mg daily.

Griseofulvin

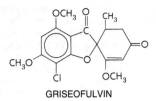

GRISEOFULVIN

ANTIFUNGAL ACTIVITY

Griseofulvin is fungistatic in vitro *for various species of the dermatophytes.*

MECHANISM OF ACTION

Griseofulvin inhibits fungal mitosis, presumably disrupting the mitotic spindle by interacting with polymerized microtubules. Griseofulvin also may bind to a microtubule-associated protein.

ABSORPTION, DISTRIBUTION, AND EXCRETION

Micronized and ultramicronized powders are used to facilitate dissolution (FULVICIN U/F and GRIS-PEG, respectively). Griseofulvin has a $t_{1/2}$ in plasma of ~1 day. The primary metabolite is 6-methylgriseofulvin.

Griseofulvin is deposited in keratin precursor cells and persists in keratin to provide prolonged resistance to fungi. The new growth of hair or nails is the first to become free of disease. As the fungus-containing keratin is shed, it is replaced by normal tissue. Griseofulvin is detectable in the stratum corneum within 4–8 hours of oral administration. Sweat and transepidermal fluid loss play important roles in drug transfer to the stratum corneum. Only a very small fraction of the drug is present in body fluids and tissues.

THERAPEUTIC USES

Readily treatable mycotic infections include those of the hair (tinea capitis) caused by Microsporum canis, M. audouinii, Trichophyton schoenleinii, *and* T. verrucosum; *"ringworm" of the glabrous skin; tinea cruris and tinea corporis caused by* M. canis, T. rubrum, T. verrucosum, *and* Epidermophyton floccosum; *and tinea of the hands (*T. rubrum *and* T. mentagrophytes*) and beard (*Trichophyton *species). Griseofulvin also is effective in "athlete's foot" or epidermophytosis involving the skin and nails, the vesicular form of which is most commonly due to* T. mentagrophytes *and the hyperkeratotic type to* T. rubrum. *Topical therapy is preferred.* T. rubrum *and* T. mentagrophytes *infections may require higher-than-conventional doses. Since very high doses of griseofulvin are carcinogenic and teratogenic in animals, it should not be used systemically to treat trivial infections that respond to topical therapy. Griseofulvin is not effective in treatment of subcutaneous or deep mycoses.*

DOSAGE

The recommended daily dose of griseofulvin is 5–15 mg/kg for children and 0.5–1 g for adults. Doses of 1.5–2 g daily may be used for short periods in severe infections. Best results are obtained when the daily dose is divided and given at 6-hour intervals, although the drug often is given twice per day. Treatment must be continued until infected tissue is replaced by normal hair, skin, or nails, which requires 1 month for scalp and hair ringworm, 6–9 months for fingernails, and at least a year for toenails.

UNTOWARD EFFECTS

Frequent adverse effects include headache (~15% of patients), GI symptoms (e.g., nausea, vomiting, diarrhea, heartburn, flatulence), and rash. More serious reactions include hepatotoxicity, serum sickness reaction, angioedema, and hematologic effects (e.g., leukopenia, neutropenia, punctate basophilia, and monocytosis). Blood studies should be checked weekly during treatment. Estrogen-like effects have been observed in children.

Griseofulvin induces hepatic CYPs and increases metabolism of warfarin, sometimes necessitating dose adjustment; it also may reduce the efficacy of low-estrogen oral contraceptive agents.

Terbinafine

Terbinafine is a synthetic allylamine that is structurally similar to naftifine. *It probably acts by inhibiting fungal squalene epoxidase and blocking ergosterol biosynthesis. Terbinafine is well absorbed, but bioavailability is only 40% because of first-pass hepatic metabolism. Proteins bind*

>99% of the drug in plasma. The drug accumulates in skin, nails, and fat. The initial $t_{1/2}$ of 12 hours extends to 200–400 hours at steady state, and the drug can be found in plasma for weeks after prolonged therapy. Terbinafine is not recommended in patients with marked renal or hepatic failure. Rifampin decreases and cimetidine increases plasma terbinafine concentrations. The drug is well tolerated, with a low incidence of GI distress, headache, or rash. Rarely, hepatotoxicity, severe neutropenia, or toxic epidermal necrolysis may occur. Systemic terbinafine therapy for onychomycosis should be postponed during pregnancy.

Terbinafine (LAMISIL), given as one 250-mg tablet daily, is at least as effective for nail onychomycosis as 200 mg daily of itraconazole, and slightly more effective than pulse itraconazole therapy. Treatment typically is for 3 months. Although not approved for this use, terbinafine (250 mg daily) also is effective in ringworm elsewhere on the body.

TOPICAL ANTIFUNGAL AGENTS

Topical treatment is useful in many superficial fungal infections—*i.e.*, those confined to the stratum corneum, squamous mucosa, or cornea, including dermatophytosis (ringworm), candidiasis, tinea versicolor, piedra, tinea nigra, and fungal keratitis. Topical administration usually is unsuccessful for mycoses of the nails (onychomycosis) and hair (tinea capitis) and has no place in the treatment of subcutaneous mycoses, such as sporotrichosis and chromoblastomycosis. The efficacy of topical agents depends not only on the type of lesion and the mechanism of drug action, but also on the viscosity, hydrophobicity, and acidity of the formulation. Regardless of formulation, penetration of topical drugs into hyperkeratotic lesions often is poor. Removal of thick, infected keratin may be a useful adjunct to therapy.

A plethora of topical agents is available for the treatment of superficial mycoses, the preferred formulations of which usually are creams or solutions. Powders, whether applied by shake containers or aerosols, largely are used for the feet and moist lesions of the groin and other intertriginous areas.

Imidazoles and Triazoles for Topical Use

Indications for topical use include ringworm, tinea versicolor, and mucocutaneous candidiasis. Resistance to imidazoles or triazoles is very rare among the fungi that cause ringworm. Agents for topical use should be selected based on cost and availability.

CUTANEOUS APPLICATION

The preparations for cutaneous use are effective for tinea corporis, tinea pedis, tinea cruris, tinea versicolor, and cutaneous candidiasis. They are applied twice daily for 3–6 weeks.

VAGINAL APPLICATION

Vaginal creams, suppositories, and tablets for vaginal candidiasis are all used once daily for 1–7 days, preferably at bedtime to facilitate retention. None is useful in trichomoniasis. Most vaginal creams are administered in 5-g amounts. Three vaginal formulations—clotrimazole tablets, miconazole suppositories, and terconazole cream—come in both low- and high-dose preparations. A shorter duration of therapy is recommended for the higher doses. These preparations are administered for 3–7 days. Approximately 3–10% of the vaginal dose is absorbed. Although some imidazoles are teratogenic in rodents, no teratogenic effects in humans have been attributed to the vaginal use of imidazoles or triazoles. The most common side effect is vaginal burning or itching. A male sexual partner may experience mild penile irritation. Cross-allergenicity among these compounds is presumed to exist.

ORAL USE

Use of the oral troche of clotrimazole is properly viewed as topical therapy. The only indication for the 10-mg troche is oropharyngeal candidiasis. Antifungal activity is due entirely to local drug action.

Clotrimazole

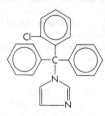

CLOTRIMAZOLE

Absorption of clotrimazole is <0.5% after application to intact skin; from the vagina, it is 3–10%. Fungicidal concentrations remain in the vagina for up to 3 days after drug application. The small amount absorbed is metabolized in the liver and excreted in bile.

Cutaneous clotrimazole occasionally may cause stinging, erythema, edema, vesication, desquamation, pruritus, and urticaria. When it is applied to the vagina, ~1.6% of recipients complain of a mild burning sensation, and rarely of lower abdominal cramps, a slight increase in urinary frequency, or skin rash. The sexual partner may experience penile or urethral irritation. By the oral route, clotrimazole can cause GI irritation. In patients using troches, the incidence of this side effect is ~5%.

THERAPEUTIC USES

Clotrimazole is available as a 1% cream, lotion, and solution (LOTRIMIN, MYCELEX, others), 1% or 2% vaginal cream or vaginal tablets of 100, 200, or 500 mg (GYNE-LOTRIMIN, MYCELEX-G, others), and 10-mg troches (MYCELEX, others). For the vagina, the standard regimens are one 100-mg tablet once a day at bedtime for 7 days, one 200-mg tablet daily for 3 days, one 500-mg tablet inserted only once, or 5 g of cream once a day for 3 days (2% cream) or 7 days (1% cream). For nonpregnant females, one 200-mg tablet may be used once a day for 3 days. Troches are to be dissolved slowly in the mouth five times a day for 14 days.

Clotrimazole cures dermatophyte infections in 60–100% of cases. Cure rates in cutaneous candidiasis are 80–100%. In vulvovaginal candidiasis, the cure rate is usually >80% with the 7-day regimen. A 3-day regimen of 200 mg once a day is similarly effective as is single-dose treatment (500 mg). Recurrences are common after all regimens. The cure rate with oral troches for oral and pharyngeal candidiasis may approach 100% in the immunocompetent host.

Econazole

Econazole is the deschloro derivative of miconazole. Econazole readily penetrates the stratum corneum and achieves effective concentrations down to the mid-dermis. Less than 1% of an applied dose is absorbed into the blood. Approximately 3% of recipients have local erythema, burning, stinging, or itching. Econazole nitrate (SPECTAZOLE, others) is available as a water-miscible cream (1%) to be applied twice a day.

Miconazole

Miconazole is a close chemical congener of econazole with the following structure:

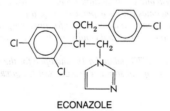

ECONAZOLE

Miconazole readily penetrates the stratum corneum and persists there for >4 days after application. Less than 1% is absorbed into the blood. Systemic absorption from the vagina is <1.3%. Adverse effects from vaginal application include burning, itching, or irritation in ~7% of recipients, and infrequently, pelvic cramps (0.2%), headache, hives, or skin rash. Irritation, burning, and maceration are rare after cutaneous application. Miconazole is considered safe for use during pregnancy.

THERAPEUTIC USES

Miconazole nitrate is available as an ointment, cream, solution, spray, or powder (MICATIN, MONISTAT-DERM, others). To avoid maceration, only the lotion should be applied to intertriginous areas. It is available as a 2% and 4% vaginal cream, and as 100-mg, 200-mg, or 1200-mg vaginal suppositories (MONISTAT 7, MONISTAT 3, others), to be applied at bedtime for 7, 3, or 1 day(s), respectively.

In the treatment of tinea pedis, tinea cruris, and tinea versicolor, the cure rate is >90%. In the treatment of vulvovaginal candidiasis, the cure rate after 1 month is ~80–95%. Pruritus sometimes is relieved after a single application. Some vaginal infections caused by C. glabrata *also respond.*

Terconazole and Butoconazole

Terconazole (TERAZOL, others) is a ketal triazole whose structure is:

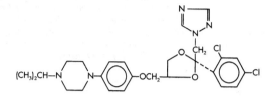

TERCONAZOLE

Its mechanism of action is similar to that of the imidazoles. The 80-mg vaginal suppository is inserted at bedtime for 3 days, while the 0.4% vaginal cream is used for 7 days and the 0.8% cream for 3 days. Clinical efficacy and patient acceptance of both preparations are at least as good as for clotrimazole in patients with vaginal candidiasis.

Butoconazole, an imidazole, is pharmacologically quite comparable to clotrimazole. Butoconazole nitrate (MYCELEX 3, others) is available as a 2% vaginal cream. Because of the slower response during pregnancy, a 6-day course is recommended (during the second and third trimester).

Tioconazole

Tioconazole (VAGISTAT 1, others) is an imidazole that is marketed for treatment of Candida *vulvovaginitis. A single 4.6-g dose of ointment (300 mg) is given at bedtime.*

Oxiconazole, Sulconazole, and Sertaconazole

These imidazole derivatives are used for the topical treatment of infections caused by the common pathogenic dermatophytes. Oxiconazole nitrate (OXISTAT) is available as a cream and lotion; sulconazole nitrate (EXELDERM) as a solution and cream, and sertaconazole (ERTACZO) as a 2% cream.

Ciclopirox Olamine

Ciclopirox olamine *(LOPROX) has broad-spectrum antifungal activity. It is fungicidal to* C. albicans, E. floccosum, M. canis, T. mentagrophytes, *and* T. rubrum. *It also inhibits the growth of* Malassezia furfur. *After application to the skin, it penetrates through the epidermis into the dermis, but even under occlusion, <1.5% is absorbed into the systemic circulation. Because the $t_{1/2}$ is short, 1.7 hours, no systemic accumulation occurs. The drug penetrates into hair follicles and sebaceous glands. It sometimes causes hypersensitivity. It is available as a 0.77% cream and lotion for the treatment of cutaneous candidiasis and for tinea corporis, cruris, pedis, and versicolor. Cure rates in the dermatomycoses and candidal infections range from 81–94%. No topical toxicity has been noted.*

Ciclopirox is also sold as a 0.77% gel and a 1% shampoo for the treatment of seborrheic dermatitis of the scalp, and an 8% topical solution (PENLAC NAIL LACQUER) is sold for the treatment of onychomycosis.

Haloprogin

Haloprogin *is a halogenated phenolic ether. It is fungicidal to* Epidermophyton, Pityrosporum, Microsporum, Trichophyton, *and* Candida. *Irritation, pruritus, burning sensations, vesiculation, increased maceration, and "sensitization" (or exacerbation of the lesion) occasionally occur, especially on the foot if occlusive footgear is worn. Haloprogin is poorly absorbed through the skin, and systemic toxicity from topical application is low.*

Tolnaftate

Tolnaftate is a thiocarbamate. It is effective for most cutaneous mycoses caused by T. rubrum, T. mentagrophytes, T. tonsurans, E. floccosum, M. canis, M. audouinii, M. gypseum, *and* M. furfur *but is ineffective against* Candida. *In tinea pedis, the cure rate is ~80%, compared with ~95% for miconazole. Toxic or allergic reactions to tolnaftate have not been reported.*

Tolnaftate (AFTATE, TINACTIN, others) is available in a 1% concentration as a cream, gel, powder, aerosol powder, and topical solution, or as a topical aerosol liquid. Pruritus is usually relieved in 24–72 hours. Involution of interdigital lesions caused by susceptible fungi is often complete in 7–21 days.

Naftifine

Naftifine is representative of the allylamine drugs that inhibit squalene-2,3-epoxidase and thus inhibit ergosterol biosynthesis. The drug has broad-spectrum fungicidal activity. Naftifine hydrochloride (NAFTIN) is available as a 1% cream or gel. Applied twice daily, it is effective for the topical treatment of tinea cruris and tinea corporis. The drug is well tolerated, although local irritation and contact dermatitis have occurred. Naftifine also may be efficacious off label for cutaneous candidiasis and tinea versicolor.

Terbinafine

Terbinafine 1% cream or spray is applied twice daily and is effective in tinea corporis, tinea cruris, and tinea pedis. Terbinafine is less active against Candida *species and M. furfur, but the cream also can be used in cutaneous candidiasis and tinea versicolor. Oral terbinafine apparently is effective in treatment of ringworm and in some cases of onychomycosis.*

Butenafine

Butenafine hydrochloride *(MENTAX) is a benzylamine derivative with a mechanism of action and spectrum of antifungal activity similar to those of terbinafine, naftifine, and other allylamines.*

Polyene Antifungal Antibiotics

NYSTATIN

Nystatin *is a tetraene macrolide that is structurally similar to amphotericin B and has the same mechanism of action. Nystatin is not absorbed from the GI tract, skin, or vagina.*

Nystatin *(MYCOSTATIN, NILSTAT, others) is used only for candidiasis and is supplied in preparations intended for cutaneous, vaginal, or oral administration for this purpose. Infections of the nails and hyperkeratinized or crusted skin lesions do not respond. Topical preparations include ointments, creams, and powders, each containing 100,000 units per gram. Powders are preferred for moist lesions and are applied two or three times a day. Imadazoles or triazoles are more effective agents than nystatin for vaginal candidiasis.*

An oral suspension that contains 100,000 units per mL of nystatin is given four times a day. Premature and low-birth-weight neonates should receive 1 mL of this preparation, infants 2 mL, and children or adults 4–6 mL per dose. Older children and adults should be instructed to swish the drug around the mouth and then swallow. Nystatin suspension is usually effective for oral candidiasis of the immunocompetent host. Other than the bitter taste and occasional complaints of nausea, adverse effects are uncommon. A 200,000-unit troche (mycostatin pastilles) is available for the treatment of oral candidiasis, and a 500,000-unit oral tablet is sold for the treatment of nonesophageal membrane GI candidiasis.

AMPHOTERICIN B

Topical amphotericin B (FUNGIZONE) also is used for cutaneous candidiasis. A lotion, cream, and ointment are marketed that contain 3% amphotericin B and are applied to the lesion 2–4 times daily.

Miscellaneous Antifungal Agents

UNDECYLENIC ACID

Undecylenic acid *is 10-undecenoic acid. The drug is fungistatic against a variety of fungi, including those that cause ringworm. Undecylenic acid (DESENEX, others) is available in a foam, ointment, cream, powder, spray powder, soap, and liquid.* Zinc undecylenate *is marketed in combination with other ingredients. The zinc provides an astringent action that aids in the suppression of inflammation. Compound undecylenic acid ointment contains both undecylenic acid (~5%) and zinc undecylenate (~20%).* Calcium undecylenate *(CALDESENE, CRUEX) is available as a powder.*

Undecylenic acid preparations are used in the treatment of various dermatomycoses, especially tinea pedis. Concentrations of the acid as high as 10%, as well as those of the acid and salt in the compound ointment, may be applied to the skin. The preparations usually are not irritating to tissue, and sensitization is uncommon. In tinea pedis, the infection frequently persists despite intensive treatment and the clinical "cure" rate is at best ~50%. Other agents therefore are preferred. Undecylenic acid preparations also are approved for use in the treatment of diaper rash, tinea cruris, and other minor dermatological conditions.

For a complete Bibliographical listing see Goodman & Gilman's *The Pharmacological Basis of Therapeutics***, 11th ed., or Goodman & Gilman Online at www.accessmedicine.com.**

49

ANTIVIRAL AGENTS (NONRETROVIRAL)

Viruses are obligate intracellular parasites that contain either double- or single-stranded DNA or RNA enclosed in a protein coat called a *capsid*. Some viruses also possess a lipid envelope that, like the capsid, may contain antigenic glycoproteins. Most viruses contain or encode enzymes essential for viral replication inside a host cell, and they usurp the metabolic machinery of their host cell. Table 49–1 outlines the stages of viral replication and the classes of antiviral agents that act at each stage of replication. Effective antiviral agents inhibit virus-specific replicative events or preferentially inhibit virus-directed rather than host cell–directed nucleic acid or protein synthesis.

Figure 49–1 provides a schematic diagram of the replicative cycle of a DNA virus (*A*) and an RNA virus (*B*). DNA viruses include poxviruses (smallpox), herpesviruses (chickenpox, shingles, oral and genital herpes), adenoviruses (conjunctivitis, sore throat), hepadnaviruses (hepatitis B virus [HBV]), and papillomaviruses (warts). Typically, DNA viruses enter the host cell nucleus, where the viral DNA is transcribed into messenger RNA (mRNA) by host cell polymerase and mRNA is translated into virus-specific proteins.

For RNA viruses, replication in the host cell relies either on enzymes in the virion (the whole infective viral particle) to synthesize its mRNA or on the viral RNA serving as its own mRNA. The mRNA is translated into various viral proteins, including RNA polymerase, which directs the synthesis of more viral mRNA and genomic RNA (Figure 49–1B). Most RNA viruses complete their replication in the cytoplasm, but some, such as influenza, are transcribed in the host cell nucleus. RNA viruses include rubella virus (German measles), rhabdoviruses (rabies), picornaviruses (poliomyelitis, meningitis, colds, hepatitis A), arenaviruses (meningitis, Lassa fever), flaviviruses (West Nile meningoencephalitis, yellow fever, hepatitis C), orthomyxoviruses (influenza), paramyxoviruses (measles, mumps), and coronaviruses (colds, severe acute respiratory syndrome [SARS]).

Retroviruses are RNA viruses that cause diseases such as acquired immunodeficiency syndrome (AIDS) (*see* Chapter 50) and T-cell leukemias (human T-cell lymphotropic virus I [HTLV-I]). They contain a reverse transcriptase that makes a DNA copy of the viral RNA template. The DNA copy integrates into the host genome, at which point it is referred to as a *provirus* and is transcribed into both genomic RNA and mRNA for translation into viral proteins. The polymerase of hepadnaviruses possesses reverse transcriptase activity.

Although many compounds show antiviral activity *in vitro*, most affect some host cell function and are associated with unacceptable toxicity. Effective agents typically have a restricted spectrum of antiviral activity and target a specific viral protein, most often an enzyme involved in viral nucleic acid synthesis (polymerase or transcriptase) or a viral processing protein (protease). Single-nucleotide changes leading to critical amino acid substitutions in a target protein often can cause resistance to antiviral drugs. Most agents inhibit active replication, so viral replication may resume following drug removal, and effective host immune responses are essential for recovery from infection. Clinical failures of antiviral therapy may occur with drug-sensitive virus in immunocompromised patients or following emergence of resistant variants. Most drug-resistant viruses are recovered from immunocompromised patients or those with chronic infections (*e.g.*, HBV) with high viral loads and repeated or prolonged courses of antiviral treatment. Antiviral agents do not eliminate nonreplicating or latent virus, although some drugs are used effectively for chronic suppression of disease reactivation. Clinical efficacy requires inhibitory concentrations at the site of infection, usually within infected cells. For example, nucleoside analogs must be taken up and phosphorylated intracellularly for activity; consequently, concentrations of critical enzymes or competing substrates influence antiviral effects in cells of different types and in different metabolic states. *In vitro* sensitivity tests for antiviral agents generally are not standardized, and results depend on the assay system, cell type, viral inoculum, and laboratory. Therefore, clear relationships among drug concentrations active *in vitro*, those achieved in blood or other body fluids, and clinical response are not established for most agents.

Table 49–2 summarizes currently approved antiviral drugs.

ANTIHERPESVIRUS AGENTS

Herpes simplex virus type 1 (HSV-1) typically causes diseases of the mouth, face, skin, esophagus, or brain. Herpes simplex virus type 2 (HSV-2) usually causes infections of the genitals, rectum, skin, hands, or meninges. Both cause serious infections in neonates.

Table 49–1

Stages of Virus Replication and Possible Targets of Action of Antiviral Agents

Stage of Replication	Classes of Selective Inhibitors
Cell entry	
Attachment	Soluble receptor decoys, antireceptor antibodies,
Penetration	fusion protein inhibitors
Uncoating	Ion channel blockers, capsid stabilizers
Release of viral genome	
*Transcription of viral genome**	Inhibitors of viral DNA polymerase, RNA poly-
Transcription of viral messenger RNA	merase, reverse transcriptase, helicase, primase,
Replication of viral genome	or integrase
Translation of viral proteins	Interferons, antisense oligonucleotides, ribozymes
Regulatory proteins (early)	Inhibitors of regulatory proteins
Structural proteins (late)	
Posttranslational modifications	
Proteolytic cleavage	Protease inhibitors
Myristoylation, glycosylation	
Assembly of virion components	Interferons, assembly protein inhibitors
Release	Neuraminidase inhibitors, antiviral antibodies,
Budding, cell lysis	cytotoxic lymphocytes

*Depends on specific replication strategy of virus, but virus-specified enzyme required for part of process.

Acyclovir is the prototype of antiviral agents that are phosphorylated intracellularly by a viral kinase and subsequently by host cell enzymes to become inhibitors of viral DNA synthesis (Figure 49–2). Related agents include *penciclovir* and *ganciclovir.*

Acyclovir and Valacyclovir

CHEMISTRY AND ANTIVIRAL ACTIVITY Acyclovir is an acyclic guanine nucleoside analog that lacks a 3'-hydroxyl on the side chain. *Valacyclovir* is the L-valyl ester prodrug of acyclovir.

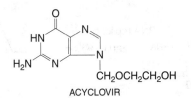

ACYCLOVIR

Acyclovir's clinical use is limited to herpesviruses. Acyclovir is most active against HSV-1, approximately half as active against HSV-2, a tenth as potent against varicella-zoster virus (VZV) and Epstein-Barr virus (EBV), and least active against cytomegalovirus (CMV) and human herpesvirus (HHV-6). Uninfected mammalian cells generally are unaffected by high acyclovir concentrations.

MECHANISMS OF ACTION AND RESISTANCE Acyclovir's selective inhibition of viral DNA synthesis depends on interaction with two distinct viral proteins: HSV thymidine kinase (TK) and DNA polymerase (Figure 49–2). Cellular uptake and initial phosphorylation are facilitated by TK. The affinity of acyclovir for HSV TK is ~200 times greater than for the host enzyme. Cellular enzymes convert the monophosphate to acyclovir triphosphate, which is present in 40- to 100-fold higher concentrations in HSV-infected than in uninfected cells and competes for endogenous deoxyguanosine triphosphate (dGTP). Acyclovir triphosphate competitively inhibits viral DNA polymerases and, to a much smaller extent, cellular DNA polymerases. Acyclovir triphosphate also is incorporated into viral DNA, where it acts as a chain terminator because it lacks a 3 α-hydroxyl group. By *suicide inactivation,* the terminated DNA template containing acyclovir binds the viral DNA polymerase and leads to its irreversible inactivation.

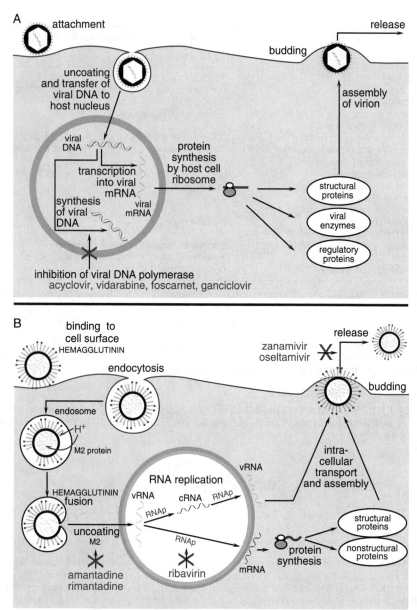

FIGURE 49–1 *Replicative cycles of DNA (A) and RNA (B) viruses.* The replicative cycles of herpesvirus (*A*) and influenza (*B*) are examples of DNA-encoded and RNA-encoded viruses, respectively. Sites of action of antiviral agents also are shown. *Key*: mRNA = messenger RNA; cDNA = complementary DNA; vRNA = viral RNA; DNAp = DNA polymerase; RNAp = RNA polymerase; cRNA = complementary RNA. An X on top of an arrow indicates a block or inhibition. *A.* Replicative cycles of herpes simplex virus, a DNA virus, and the probable sites of action of antiviral agents. Herpes virus replication is a regulated multistep process. After infection, a small number of immediate-early genes are transcribed; these genes encode proteins that regulate their own synthesis and are responsible for synthesis of early genes involved in genome replication, such as thymidine kinases, DNA polymerases, *etc*. After DNA replication, the bulk of the herpes virus genes (called *late genes*) are expressed and encode proteins that either are incorporated into or aid in the assembly of progeny virions. *B.* Replicative cycles of influenza, an RNA virus, and the loci for effects of antiviral agents. The mammalian cell shown is an airway epithelial cell. The M2 protein of influenza virus allows an influx of hydrogen ions into the virion interior, which in turn promotes dissociation of the RNAp segments and release into the cytoplasm (uncoating). Influenza virus mRNA synthesis requires a primer cleared from cellular mRNA and used by the viral RNAp complex. The neuraminidase inhibitors zanamivir and oseltamivir specifically inhibit release of progeny virus. Small capitals indicate virus proteins.

Table 49–2

Nomenclature of Antiviral Agents

Generic Name	Other Names	Trade Names (USA)	Dosage Forms Available
Antiherpesvirus agents			
Acyclovir	ACV, acycloguanosine	ZOVIRAX	IV, O, T, ophth*
Cidofovir	HPMPC, CDV	VISTIDE	IV
Famciclovir	FCV	FAMVIR	O
Foscarnet	PFA, phosphonoformate	FOSCAVIR	IV, O*
Fomivirsen	ISIS 2922	VITRAVENE	Intravitreal
Ganciclovir	GCV, DHPG	CYTOVENE	IV, O, intravitreal
Idoxuridine	IDUR	HERPES, STOXIL, DENDRID	Ophth
Penciclovir	PCV	DENAVIR	T, IV*
Trifluridine	TFT, trifluorothymidine	VIROPTIC	Ophth
Valacyclovir		VALTREX	O
Valganciclovir		VALCYTE	O
Anti-influenza agents			
Amantadine		SYMMETREL	O
Oseltamivir	GS4104	TAMIFLU	O
Rimantadine		FLUMADINE	O
Zanamivir	GG167	RELENZA	Inhaled
Antihepatitis agents			
Adefovir dipivoxil	Bis-pom-PMEA	HEPSERA	O
Interferon-alfa		INTRON A, ROFERON A, INFERGEN, ALFERON N, WELLFERON*	Injected
Lamivudine	3TC	EPIVIR	O
Pegylated interferon alfa		PEGASYS, PEG-INTRON	SC
Other antiviral agents			
Ribavirin		VIRAZOLE, REBETOL, COPEGUS	O, inhaled, IV*
Imiquimod		ALDARA	Topical

*Not currently approved for use in USA.
ABBREVIATIONS: IV, intravenous; O, oral; T, topical; ophth, ophthalmic.

Acyclovir resistance results from three mechanisms: absence or partial production of viral TK, altered TK substrate specificity (*e.g.,* phosphorylation of thymidine but not acyclovir), or altered viral DNA polymerase. Resistant variants are present in native virus populations, and heterogeneous mixtures of viruses occur in isolates from treated patients. The most common resistance mechanism in clinical HSV isolates is absent or deficient viral TK activity; viral DNA polymerase mutants are rare. Resistance typically is defined by inhibitory concentrations of >2–3 μg/mL, which predict failure of therapy in immunocompromised patients.

Similarly, acyclovir resistance in VZV isolates is caused by mutations in its TK or polymerase.

ABSORPTION, DISTRIBUTION, AND ELIMINATION

Oral bioavailability of acyclovir (~10–30%) decreases with increasing dose. Valacyclovir is converted rapidly and virtually completely to acyclovir after oral administration. This conversion reflects first-pass intestinal and hepatic metabolism by enzymatic hydrolysis. Unlike acyclovir, valacyclovir is a substrate for intestinal and renal peptide transporters. The oral bioavailability of acyclovir increases to ~70% following valacyclovir administration. Peak acyclovir concentrations occur ~2 hours after dosing. Peak plasma concentrations of valacyclovir are only 4% of acyclovir levels. Less than 1% of an administered dose of valacyclovir is recovered in the urine, and most is eliminated as acyclovir.

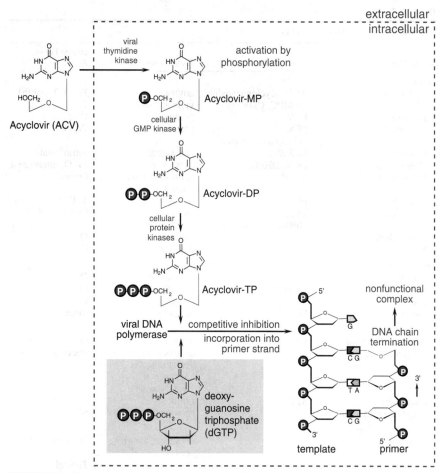

FIGURE 49–2 *Conversion of acyclovir to acyclovir triphosphate leading to DNA chain termination.* Acyclovir is converted to the monophosphate (MP) derivative by a herpes virus thymidine kinase. Acyclovir-MP is then phosphorylated to acyclovir-DP and acyclovir-TP by cellular enzymes. Uninfected cells convert very little or no drug to the phosphorylated derivatives. Thus, acyclovir is selectively activated in cells infected with herpesviruses that code for appropriate thymidine kinases. Incorporation of acyclovir-MP from acyclovir-TP into the primer strand during viral DNA replication leads to chain termination and formation of an inactive complex with the viral DNA polymerase. (Adapted from Elion, 1982, with permission.)

Acyclovir distributes widely in body fluids, including vesicular fluid, aqueous humor, and cerebrospinal fluid (CSF). Compared with plasma, salivary concentrations are low, and vaginal secretion concentrations vary widely. Acyclovir is concentrated in breast milk, amniotic fluid, and placenta. Newborn plasma levels are similar to maternal ones. Percutaneous absorption of acyclovir after topical administration is low.

The plasma elimination half-life of acyclovir is ~2.5 hours in adults with normal renal function, 4 hours in neonates, and 20 hours in anuric patients. Renal excretion of unmetabolized acyclovir by glomerular filtration and tubular secretion is the principal route of elimination.

UNTOWARD EFFECTS

Acyclovir generally is well tolerated. Topical acyclovir may cause mucosal irritation and transient burning when applied to genital lesions.

Oral acyclovir infrequently is associated with nausea, diarrhea, rash, or headache and very rarely with renal insufficiency or neurotoxicity. Valacyclovir also may cause headache, nausea, diarrhea, nephrotoxicity, and CNS symptoms. High doses of valacyclovir have been associated *with confusion and hallucinations, nephrotoxicity, and uncommonly, severe thrombocytopenia, sometimes fatal, in immunocompromised patients. Acyclovir has been associated with neutropenia in neonates. Chronic acyclovir suppression of genital herpes has been used safely for up to 10 years. No excess frequency of congenital abnormalities is recognized in infants born to women exposed to acyclovir during pregnancy.*

The principal dose-limiting toxicities of intravenous acyclovir are renal insufficiency and CNS side effects. Preexisting renal insufficiency, high doses, and acyclovir plasma levels >25 μg/mL are risk factors for both. Reversible renal dysfunction occurs in ~5% of patients, likely related to crystalluria. Manifestations include nausea and vomiting, flank pain, and azotemia. Rapid infusion, dehydration, and inadequate urine flow increase the risk. Infusions should be given at a constant rate over at least an hour. Nephrotoxicity usually resolves with drug cessation and volume expansion. Neurotoxicity occurs in 1–4% of patients and can cause altered sensorium, tremor, myoclonus, delirium, seizures, or extrapyramidal signs. Phlebitis following extravasation, rash, diaphoresis, nausea, hypotension, and interstitial nephritis also may occur. Hemodialysis may be useful in severe cases.

Severe somnolence and lethargy may occur with combinations of zidovudine *and acyclovir.* Concomitant cyclosporine *enhances nephrotoxicity.* Probenecid *decreases acyclovir renal clearance and prolongs the plasma $t_{1/2}$ of elimination. Acyclovir may decrease the renal clearance of other drugs eliminated by active renal secretion (e.g., methotrexate).*

THERAPEUTIC USES In immunocompetent persons, the clinical benefits of acyclovir and valacyclovir are greater in initial HSV infections than in recurrent ones, which typically are milder. These drugs are particularly useful in immunocompromised patients because these individuals experience more frequent and more severe HSV and VZV infections. Since VZV is less susceptible than HSV to acyclovir, higher doses must be used for treating varicella or zoster infections. Oral valacyclovir is as effective as oral acyclovir in HSV infections and more effective for treating herpes zoster.

Herpes Simplex Virus Infections

In initial genital HSV infections, oral acyclovir (200 mg five times daily or 400 mg three times daily for 7–10 days) and valacyclovir (1000 mg twice daily for 7–10 days) significantly reduce virus shedding, symptoms, and time to healing. Intravenous acyclovir (5 mg/kg every 8 hours) has similar effects in patients hospitalized with severe primary genital HSV infections. Topical acyclovir is much less effective. None of these regimens reproducibly reduces the risk of recurrent genital lesions. Patient-initiated acyclovir (200 mg five times daily or 400 mg three times daily for 5 days or 800 mg three times daily for 2 days) or valacyclovir (500 mg twice daily for 3 or 5 days) shortens the manifestations of recurrent genital HSV episodes by 1–2 days. Recurring genital herpes can be suppressed by chronic oral acyclovir (400 mg twice daily or 200 mg three times daily) or valacyclovir (500 mg or, for very frequent recurrences, 1000 mg once daily). The rate of recurrences decreases by ~90% during use, and subclinical shedding is markedly reduced, such that valacyclovir suppression of genital herpes reduces the risk of transmission to a susceptible partner by ~50% over an 8-month period.

Oral acyclovir is effective in primary herpetic gingivostomatitis (600 mg/m² four times daily for 10 days in children) but has only modest benefit in recurrent orolabial herpes. High-dose valacyclovir (2 g twice over one day) shortens the duration of recurrent orolabial herpes by ~1 day. Topical acyclovir is modestly effective in recurrent labial and genital herpes simplex virus infections. Acyclovir prophylaxis (400 mg twice daily for one week) reduces the risk of recurrence by 73% in those with sun-induced recurrences of HSV infections. Acyclovir during the last month of pregnancy reduces the likelihood of viral shedding and frequency of cesarean section in women with primary or recurrent genital herpes.

In immunocompromised patients with mucocutaneous HSV infection, intravenous acyclovir (250 mg/m² every 8 hours for 7 days) shortens healing time, duration of pain, and the period of virus shedding. Oral acyclovir (800 mg five times per day) and valacyclovir (1000 mg twice daily) for 5–10 days are also effective. Recurrences are common after drug cessation and may require long-term suppression. In those with very localized labial or facial HSV infections, topical acyclovir may provide some benefit. Intravenous acyclovir may be beneficial in viscerally disseminating HSV in immunocompromised patients and in patients with HSV-infected burn wounds.

Systemic acyclovir prophylaxis is highly effective in preventing mucocutaneous HSV infections in seropositive patients undergoing immunosuppression. Intravenous acyclovir (250 mg/m² every 8–12 hours) begun prior to transplantation and continuing for several weeks prevents HSV disease in bone marrow transplant recipients. For patients who can tolerate oral medications, oral acyclovir (400 mg five times daily) is effective, and long-term oral acyclovir (200–400 mg three times daily for

6 months) also reduces the risk of VZV infection. In HSV encephalitis, acyclovir (10 mg/kg every 8 hours for at least 10 days) reduces mortality by >50% and improves neurological outcome. Higher doses (15–20 mg/kg every 8 hours) and prolonged treatment (up to 21 days) are recommended by many experts. Intravenous acyclovir (20 mg/kg every 8 hours for 21 days) is more effective than lower doses in viscerally invasive neonatal HSV infections. In neonates and immunosuppressed patients and, rarely, in previously healthy persons, relapses of encephalitis following acyclovir may occur.

An ophthalmic formulation of acyclovir (not available in the U.S.) is effective in herpetic keratoconjunctivitis.

Infection owing to resistant HSV is rare in immunocompetent persons; in immunocompromised hosts, resistant HSV isolates can cause extensive mucocutaneous disease and, rarely, meningoencephalitis, pneumonitis, or visceral disease. Resistant HSV can be recovered from 6% to 17% of immunocompromised patients receiving acyclovir treatment. Recurrences after acyclovir cessation usually are due to sensitive virus but may be due to acyclovir-resistant virus in AIDS patients. In patients with progressive disease, intravenous foscarnet *therapy is effective, but* vidarabine *is not.*

Varicella-Zoster Virus Infections

If begun within 24 hours of rash onset, oral acyclovir is efficacious in varicella of children and adults. In children weighing up to 40 kg, acyclovir (20 mg/kg, up to 800 mg per dose, four times daily for 5 days) reduces fever and new lesion formation by ~1 day. Such use should be considered in those at risk of moderate-to-severe illness (persons >12 years old, secondary household cases, those with chronic cutaneous or pulmonary disorders, or those receiving glucocorticoids or long-term salicylates). *In adults treated within 24 hours, oral acyclovir (800 mg five times daily for 7 days) reduces the time to crusting of lesions by ~2 days, the maximum number of lesions by 50%, and duration of fever. Intravenous acyclovir is effective in varicella pneumonia or encephalitis of previously healthy adults. Oral acyclovir (10 mg/kg four times daily) given between 7 and 14 days after exposure may reduce the risk of varicella.*

In older adults with localized herpes zoster, oral acyclovir (800 mg five times daily for 7 days) reduces pain and healing times if initiated within 72 hours of rash onset. Treatment of zoster ophthalmicus reduces ocular complications. Prolonged acyclovir and concurrent prednisone *for 21 days speed zoster healing and improve quality-of-life compared with either therapy alone. Valacyclovir (1000 mg three times daily for 7 days) provides more rapid relief of zoster-associated pain than acyclovir in adults over 50 with zoster.*

In immunocompromised patients with herpes zoster, intravenous acyclovir (500 mg/m^2 every 8 hours for 7 days) reduces viral shedding, healing time, risks of cutaneous dissemination and visceral complications, and the length of hospitalization. In immunosuppressed children with varicella, intravenous acyclovir decreases healing time and the risk of visceral complications.

Acyclovir-resistant VZV isolates uncommonly have been recovered from HIV-infected children and adults who may manifest chronic hyperkeratotic or verrucous lesions and sometimes meningoradiculitis. Intravenous foscarnet appears to be effective for acyclovir-resistant VZV infections.

Other Viruses

Acyclovir is ineffective in established CMV infections but has been used for CMV prophylaxis in immunocompromised patients. High-dose intravenous acyclovir (500 mg/m^2 every 8 hours for one month) in CMV-seropositive bone marrow transplant recipients is associated with ~50% lower risk of CMV disease and, when combined with prolonged oral acyclovir (800 mg four times daily through 6 months), improves survival. Following engraftment, valacyclovir (2000 mg four times daily to day 100) appears as effective as intravenous ganciclovir prophylaxis. High-dose oral acyclovir or valacyclovir (2000 mg four times daily) suppression for 3 months may reduce the risk of CMV disease and its sequelae in some solid-organ transplant recipients, but oral valganciclovir *is preferred. Compared with acyclovir, high-dose valacyclovir reduces CMV disease in advanced HIV infection but is associated with greater toxicity and possibly shorter survival.*

Cidofovir

CHEMISTRY AND ANTIVIRAL ACTIVITY Cidofovir (1-[(*S*)-3-hydroxy-2-(phosphonomethoxy)-propyl]cytosine dihydrate) is a cytidine nucleotide analog with inhibitory activity against human herpes, papilloma, polyoma, pox, and adenoviruses.

Cidofovir is a phosphonate that is phosphorylated by cellular but not virus enzymes. It inhibits acyclovir-resistant TK-deficient or TK-altered HSV or VZV strains, ganciclovir-resistant CMV strains with UL97 mutations, but not those with DNA polymerase mutations, and some foscarnet-resistant

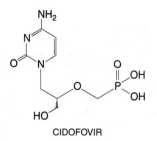

CIDOFOVIR

CMV strains. Cidofovir synergistically inhibits CMV replication in combination with ganciclovir or foscarnet.

MECHANISMS OF ACTION AND RESISTANCE   Cidofovir inhibits viral DNA synthesis by slowing and eventually terminating chain elongation. Cidofovir is metabolized to its active diphosphate form by cellular enzymes; the levels of phosphorylated metabolites are similar in infected and uninfected cells. The diphosphate both acts as a competitive inhibitor with respect to dCTP and an alternative substrate for viral DNA polymerase. The diphosphate has a prolonged intracellular $t_{1/2}$ and competitively inhibits CMV and HSV DNA polymerases at concentrations one-eighth to one six-hundredth of those required to inhibit human DNA polymerases. A phosphocholine metabolite has a prolonged intracellular $t_{1/2}$ (~87 hours) and may serve as an intracellular drug reservoir. The prolonged intracellular $t_{1/2}$ of cidofovir diphosphate allows infrequent dosing regimens.

Cidofovir resistance in CMV is due to mutations in viral DNA polymerase. Low-level resistance to cidofovir develops in up to 30% of retinitis patients by 3 months of therapy. Highly ganciclovir-resistant CMV isolates that possess DNA polymerase and UL97 kinase mutations are resistant to cidofovir, and prior ganciclovir therapy may select for cidofovir resistance. Some foscarnet-resistant CMV isolates show cross-resistance to cidofovir, and triple-drug-resistant variants with DNA polymerase mutations occur.

ABSORPTION, DISTRIBUTION, AND ELIMINATION

Cidofovir has very low oral bioavailability. Plasma levels after intravenous dosing decline biphasically with a terminal $t_{1/2}$ of 2.6 hours. The volume of distribution approximates total-body water. CSF penetration is low. Topical cidofovir gel may result in low plasma concentrations (<0.5 µg/mL) in patients with large mucocutaneous lesions.

Cidofovir is cleared by glomerular filtration and tubular secretion and >90% of the dose is recovered unchanged in the urine. Probenecid (2 g 3 hours before and 1 g 2 and 8 hours after each infusion) blocks tubular transport of cidofovir and reduces renal clearance and associated nephrotoxicity. The $t_{1/2}$ is increased markedly with renal failure. Both peritoneal dialysis and hemodialysis remove >50% of the dose.

UNTOWARD EFFECTS

Nephrotoxicity is the principal dose-limiting side effect of intravenous cidofovir. Proximal tubular dysfunction includes proteinuria, azotemia, glycosuria, and metabolic acidosis. Concomitant oral probenecid and saline prehydration reduce the risk of renal toxicity. On maintenance doses of 5 mg/kg every 2 weeks, up to 50% of patients develop proteinuria, 10–15% show an elevated serum creatinine, and 15–20% develop neutropenia. Anterior uveitis that is responsive to topical glucocorticoids and cycloplegia occur commonly and ocular hypotony occurs infrequently with intravenous cidofovir. Administration with food and pretreatment with antiemetics, antihistamines, and/or acetaminophen may improve tolerance.

Probenecid but not cidofovir alters zidovudine pharmacokinetics such that zidovudine doses should be reduced when probenecid is present, as should the doses of drugs similarly affected by probenecid (e.g., β-lactam antibiotics, nonsteroidal anti-inflammatory drugs [NSAIDs], acyclovir, lorazepam, furosemide, methotrexate, theophylline, and rifampin). Concurrent nephrotoxic agents are contraindicated, and an interval of 1 week before beginning cidofovir treatment is recommended after prior exposure to aminoglycosides, intravenous pentamidine, amphotericin B, foscarnet, NSAIDs, or contrast dye. Cidofovir and oral ganciclovir in combination are poorly tolerated at full doses.

Topical application of cidofovir is associated with local reactions (e.g., burning, pain, and pruritus) in up to one-third of patients and occasionally ulceration.

Cidofovir is considered a potential human carcinogen and is classified as pregnancy category C.

THERAPEUTIC USES

Intravenous cidofovir is approved for the treatment of CMV retinitis in HIV-infected patients. Intravenous cidofovir (5 mg/kg once a week for 2 weeks followed by dosing every 2 weeks) increases the time to progression of CMV retinitis in previously untreated patients and in those failing or intolerant of ganciclovir and foscarnet therapy. CMV viremia may persist during cidofovir administration. Maintenance doses of 5 mg/kg are more effective but less well tolerated than 3 mg/kg doses. Intravenous cidofovir has been used for treating acyclovir-resistant mucocutaneous HSV infection, adenovirus disease in transplant recipients, and progressive multifocal leukoencephalopathy or extensive molluscum contagiosum in HIV patients. Reduced doses (0.25–1 mg/kg every 2–3 weeks) without probenecid may be beneficial in BK virus nephropathy in renal transplant patients.

Topical cidofovir gel eliminates virus shedding and lesions in some HIV-infected patients with acyclovir-resistant mucocutaneous HSV infections and has been used in treating anogenital warts and molluscum contagiosum in immunocompromised patients and cervical intraepithelial neoplasia in women. Intralesional cidofovir induces remissions in adults and children with respiratory papillomatosis.

Docosanol

Docosanol is a long-chain saturated alcohol that is FDA approved as a 10% over-the-counter cream for the treatment of recurrent orolabial herpes. Topical treatment beginning within 12 hours of prodromal symptoms or lesion onset reduces healing time by ~1 day and is well tolerated. Treatment initiation at papular or later stages provides no benefit.

Famciclovir and Penciclovir

CHEMISTRY AND ANTIVIRAL ACTIVITY *Famciclovir* is a diacetyl ester prodrug of 6-deoxy penciclovir. *Penciclovir* (9-[4-hydroxy-3-hydroxymethylbut-1-yl] guanine) is an acyclic guanine nucleoside analog.

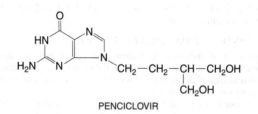

PENCICLOVIR

Penciclovir resembles acyclovir in its spectrum of activity and potency against HSV and VZV. It also inhibits HBV.

MECHANISMS OF ACTION AND RESISTANCE Penciclovir inhibits viral DNA synthesis. In HSV- or VZV-infected cells, penciclovir is phosphorylated initially by viral TK. Penciclovir triphosphate competitively inhibits viral DNA polymerase (Figure 49–2). Although penciclovir triphosphate is approximately one one-hundredth times as potent as acyclovir triphosphate in inhibiting viral DNA polymerase, it is present in infected cells at much higher concentrations and for more prolonged periods. The prolonged intracellular half-life of penciclovir triphosphate, 7–20 hours, provides prolonged antiviral effects. Because penciclovir has a 3'-hydroxyl group, it is not an obligate chain terminator but does inhibit DNA elongation.

Resistance during therapy is low. TK–deficient, acyclovir-resistant herpesviruses are cross resistant to penciclovir.

ABSORPTION, DISTRIBUTION, AND ELIMINATION

Oral penciclovir has low (5%) bioavailability, while famciclovir is well absorbed orally and converted rapidly to penciclovir by side chain deacetylation and purine ring oxidation. The bioavailability of penciclovir is ~70% after oral administration of famciclovir. Food slows absorption without reducing overall bioavailability. A small quantity of the 6-deoxy precursor but no famciclovir is detectable in plasma. The volume of distribution is ~twice the volume of total-body water. The $t_{1/2}$ of elimination of penciclovir is 2 hours, and >90% is excreted unchanged in the urine. Following oral famciclovir administration, nonrenal clearance accounts for ~10% of each dose, *primarily through fecal excretion, but penciclovir (60% of dose) and its 6-deoxy precursor (<10% of dose) mostly are eliminated in the urine. The plasma $t_{1/2}$ is 10 hours when the creatinine clearance is <30 mL/min; hemodialysis effectively removes penciclovir. Lower peak plasma concentrations of penciclovir but equal overall bioavailability occur with compensated hepatic insufficiency.*

UNTOWARD EFFECTS

Oral famciclovir is associated with headache, diarrhea, and nausea. Urticaria, rash, and hallucinations or confusional states (mostly in the elderly) have been reported. Topical penciclovir rarely (~1%) is associated with local reactions. Short-term tolerance of famciclovir is comparable with that of acyclovir.

Penciclovir is mutagenic at high concentrations. Long-term administration (1 year) does not affect spermatogenesis in men. Safety during pregnancy is not established and the drug is pregnancy category B.

THERAPEUTIC USES

Oral famciclovir, topical penciclovir, and intravenous penciclovir are approved for HSV and VZV infections in various countries. Oral famciclovir (250 mg three times a day for 7–10 days) is as effective as acyclovir in treating first-episode genital herpes. In patients with recurrent genital HSV, patient-initiated famciclovir treatment (125 or 250 mg twice a day for 5 days) reduces healing time and symptoms by ~1 day. Famciclovir (250 mg twice a day for up to 1 year) effectively suppresses recurrent genital HSV, but single daily doses are less effective. Higher doses (500 mg twice a day) reduce HSV recurrences in HIV-infected persons. Intravenous penciclovir (5 mg/kg every 8 or 12 hours for 7 days) is comparable with intravenous acyclovir for mucocutaneous HSV infections in immunocompromised hosts. In immunocompetent persons with recurrent orolabial HSV, topical 1% penciclovir cream (applied every 2 hours while awake for 4 days) shortens healing time and symptoms by ~1 day.

In immunocompetent adults with VZV of <3 days duration, famciclovir (500 mg three times a day for 10 days) is at least as effective as acyclovir in reducing healing time and zoster-associated pain, particularly in older individuals. Famciclovir is comparable with valacyclovir in treating zoster and reducing associated pain in older adults. Famciclovir (500 mg three times a day for 7–10 days) also is comparable with high-dose oral acyclovir in treating zoster in immunocompromised patients and in those with ophthalmic zoster.

Famciclovir causes dose-related reductions in HBV DNA and transaminase levels in patients with chronic HBV hepatitis but is less effective than lamivudine. Famciclovir is also ineffective in treating lamivudine-resistant HBV infections owing to emergence of multiply resistant variants.

Fomivirsen

Fomivirsen is a phosphorothioate antisense oligionucleotide complementary to the mRNA sequence for the major immediate-early region of CMV and inhibits CMV replication through sequence-specific and nonspecific mechanisms, including inhibition of virus binding to cells. Fomivirsen is active against CMV strains resistant to ganciclovir, foscarnet, and cidofovir.

Fomivirsen is given by intravitreal injection for patients intolerant of or unresponsive to other therapies for CMV retinitis. Following injection, it is cleared from the vitreous humor with a $t_{1/2}$ of ~55 hours through distribution to the retina and probably local exonuclease digestion. In HIV-infected patients with refractory, sight-threatening CMV retinitis, fomivirsen injections (330 µg weekly for 3 weeks and then every 2 weeks or on days 1 and 15 followed by monthly) significantly delay retinitis progression. Ocular side effects include iritis in up to 25% of patients, which can be managed with topical glucocorticoids, vitritis, cataracts, and increased intraocular pressure in 15–20% of patients. Recent cidofovir use may increase the risk of inflammatory reactions.

Foscarnet

CHEMISTRY AND ANTIVIRAL ACTIVITY Foscarnet (trisodium phosphonoformate) is an inorganic pyrophosphate analog that inhibits herpesviruses and HIV.

High concentrations of 0.5–1 mM reversibly inhibit the proliferation of uninfected cells.

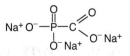

FOSCARNET SODIUM

MECHANISMS OF ACTION AND RESISTANCE Foscarnet inhibits viral nucleic acid synthesis by interacting directly with herpesvirus DNA polymerase or HIV reverse transcriptase (Figure 49–1A). It is taken up slowly by cells and does not undergo significant intracellular metabolism. Foscarnet reversibly and noncompetitively blocks the pyrophosphate binding site of the viral polymerase and inhibits pyrophosphate cleavage from deoxynucleotide triphosphates. Foscarnet has ~100-fold greater inhibitory effects against herpesvirus DNA polymerases than against cellular DNA polymerase α. Herpesviruses resistant to foscarnet have point mutations in the viral DNA polymerase that reduce foscarnet activity.

ABSORPTION, DISTRIBUTION, AND ELIMINATION

Vitreous levels approximate those in plasma, and CSF levels average 66% of those in plasma.

Over 80% of foscarnet is excreted unchanged in the urine. Plasma clearance is proportional to creatinine clearance, and dose adjustments are indicated for small decreases in renal function. Plasma elimination is complex, with an initial $t_{1/2}$ of 4–8 hours and a prolonged terminal $t_{1/2}$ of 4 days. Sequestration in bone with gradual release accounts for a ~10–20% of a given dose. Foscarnet is cleared efficiently by hemodialysis (~50% of a dose).

UNTOWARD EFFECTS

Foscarnet's major dose-limiting toxicities are nephrotoxicity and hypocalcemia. Increases in serum creatinine occur in up to one-half of patients but usually are reversible after drug cessation. High doses, rapid infusion, volume depletion, prior renal insufficiency, and concurrent nephrotoxic drugs are risk factors. Acute tubular necrosis, crystalline glomerulopathy, nephrogenic diabetes insipidus, and interstitial nephritis have been described. Saline loading may reduce the risk of nephrotoxicity.

Foscarnet is highly ionized at physiological pH, and metabolic abnormalities are very common, including increases or decreases in Ca^{2+} and phosphate, hypomagnesemia, and hypokalemia. Concomitant intravenous pentamidine administration increases the risk of hypocalcemia.

CNS side effects include headache, tremor, irritability, and seizures. Other side effects are rash, fever, nausea or vomiting, anemia, leukopenia, abnormal liver function tests, electrocardiographic changes, thrombophlebitis, and painful genital ulcerations. Topical foscarnet may cause local irritation, while oral foscarnet may cause gastrointestinal (GI) disturbance. High foscarnet concentrations in animals are mutagenic and may cause tooth and skeletal abnormalities. Safety in pregnancy or childhood is uncertain.

THERAPEUTIC USES

Intravenous foscarnet is effective for CMV retinitis, including ganciclovir-resistant infections, other types of CMV infection, and acyclovir-resistant HSV and VZV infections. Foscarnet is poorly soluble in aqueous solutions and requires large volumes for administration.

In CMV retinitis in AIDS patients, foscarnet (60 mg/kg every 8 hours or 90 mg/kg every 12 hours for 14–21 days followed by chronic maintenance at 90–120 mg/kg every day in one dose) is associated with clinical stabilization in ~90% of patients. A comparison of foscarnet with ganciclovir in AIDS patients found comparable control of CMV retinitis but improved overall survival in the foscarnet-treated group, possibly related to the drug's intrinsic anti-HIV activity. Patients discontinue foscarnet because of side effects over three times as often as ganciclovir. A combination of foscarnet and ganciclovir is more effective than either drug alone in refractory retinitis; combinations may be useful in treating ganciclovir-resistant CMV infections in solid-organ transplant patients. Foscarnet benefits other CMV syndromes in AIDS or transplant patients but is ineffective as monotherapy in treating CMV pneumonia in bone marrow transplant patients. When used for preemptive therapy of CMV viremia in bone marrow transplant recipients, foscarnet (60 mg/kg every 12 hours for 2 weeks followed by 90 mg/kg daily for 2 weeks) is as effective as intravenous ganciclovir with less neutropenia. Foscarnet may reduce the risk of Kaposi's sarcoma in HIV-infected patients. Intravitreal injections also are used.

In acyclovir-resistant mucocutaneous HSV infections, lower doses of foscarnet (40 mg/kg every 8 hours for 7 days or longer) are associated with cessation of viral shedding and complete healing of lesions in ~75% of patients. Foscarnet also appears to be effective in acyclovir-resistant VZV infections. Topical foscarnet cream may be useful in chronic acyclovir-resistant infections in immunocompromised patients.

Ganciclovir and Valganciclovir

CHEMISTRY AND ANTIVIRAL ACTIVITY Ganciclovir (9-[1,3-dihydroxy-2-propoxymethyl] guanine) is an acyclic guanine nucleoside analog that is similar in structure to

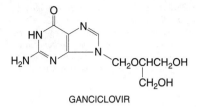

GANCICLOVIR

acyclovir except for an additional hydroxymethyl group on the side chain. Valganciclovir is the L-valyl ester prodrug of ganciclovir.

This agent has inhibitory activity against all herpesviruses but is especially active against CMV. Inhibitory concentrations for human bone marrow progenitors are similar to those inhibitory for CMV replication, a finding consistent with ganciclovir's myelotoxicity in clinical use.

MECHANISMS OF ACTION AND RESISTANCE Ganciclovir inhibits viral DNA synthesis. It is monophosphorylated intracellularly by viral TK during HSV infection and by a viral phosphotransferase encoded by the UL97 gene during CMV infection. Ganciclovir diphosphate and ganciclovir triphosphate are formed by cellular enzymes. At least tenfold higher concentrations of ganciclovir triphosphate are present in CMV-infected than in uninfected cells. The triphosphate competitively inhibits deoxyguanosine triphosphate incorporation into DNA and preferentially inhibits viral rather than host cellular DNA polymerases. Ganciclovir is incorporated into both viral and cellular DNA. Incorporation into viral DNA causes eventual cessation of DNA chain elongation (Figures 49–1A and 49–2).

Intracellular ganciclovir triphosphate concentrations are tenfold higher than those of acyclovir triphosphate and decline much more slowly with an intracellular elimination $t_{1/2}$ >24 hours. These differences may account for ganciclovir's greater anti-CMV activity and provide the rationale for single daily doses in suppressing human CMV infections.

CMV can become resistant to ganciclovir by reduced intracellular ganciclovir phosphorylation owing to mutations in the viral phosphotransferase encoded by the UL97 gene or mutations in viral DNA polymerase. Resistance has been associated primarily with impaired phosphorylation but sometimes only with DNA polymerase mutations. Highly resistant variants with dual UL97 and polymerase mutations are cross-resistant to cidofovir and variably to foscarnet. Ganciclovir also is much less active against acyclovir-resistant TK–deficient HSV strains.

ABSORPTION, DISTRIBUTION, AND ELIMINATION

The oral bioavailability of ganciclovir is ~6–9% following ingestion with food. Oral valganciclovir is well absorbed and hydrolyzed rapidly to ganciclovir; the bioavailability of ganciclovir is ~60% following valganciclovir. Food increases the bioavailability of valganciclovir by ~25%. High oral valganciclovir doses with food provide ganciclovir exposures comparable with intravenous dosing. Following intravenous dosing, vitreous fluid levels equal or exceed those in plasma. Vitreous levels decline with a $t_{1/2}$ of 24 hours.

The plasma $t_{1/2}$ is ~2–4 hours in patients with normal renal function. Over 90% of ganciclovir is eliminated unchanged by renal excretion. Consequently, the plasma $t_{1/2}$ increases almost linearly as creatinine clearance declines and may reach 28–40 hours with severe renal insufficiency.

UNTOWARD EFFECTS

Myelosuppression is the principal dose-limiting toxicity of ganciclovir. Neutropenia occurs in ~15–40% of patients and thrombocytopenia in 5–20%. Neutropenia may be fatal; it appears most commonly during the second week of treatment and usually reverses within 1 week of drug cessation. Recombinant granulocyte colony-stimulating factor (G-CSF, filgrastim, lenograstim) may be useful in treating ganciclovir-induced neutropenia (see Chapter 53). Oral valganciclovir is associated with nausea, pain, and diarrhea in addition to the toxicities associated with intravenous ganciclovir.

CNS side effects occur in 5–15% of patients and range from headache to behavioral changes to convulsions and coma. About one-third of patients will prematurely stop intravenous ganciclovir therapy because of bone marrow or CNS toxicity. Infusion-related phlebitis, azotemia, anemia, rash, fever, liver function test abnormalities, nausea and vomiting, and eosinophilia also have occurred.

Teratogenicity, embryotoxicity, and reproductive toxicity have been observed in ganciclovir-treated animals, and it is classified as pregnancy category C.

Zidovudine and probably other cytotoxic agents increase the risk of myelosuppression, as do nephrotoxic drugs that impair ganciclovir excretion. Probenecid and possibly acyclovir reduce renal clearance of ganciclovir. Zalcitabine increases oral ganciclovir exposure by ~22%. Oral ganciclovir doubles the absorption and peak plasma concentrations of didanosine and increases zidovudine by ~20%.

THERAPEUTIC USES

Ganciclovir is effective for treatment and chronic suppression of CMV retinitis in immunocompromised patients and for prevention of CMV disease in transplant recipients. In CMV retinitis, induction treatment (5 mg/kg intravenously every 12 hours for 10–21 days) is associated with improvement or stabilization in ~85% of patients. Reduced viral excretion is usually evident by 1 week, and funduscopic improvement by 2 weeks. Because of the high risk of relapse, AIDS patients with retinitis require suppressive therapy (a total of 30–35 mg/kg/week, in divided doses). Oral ganciclovir (1000 mg three times daily) is effective for suppression of retinitis after initial intravenous treatment. Oral valganciclovir is comparable with intravenous dosing for initial control (900 mg twice daily for 21 days initial treatment) and sustained suppression (900 mg daily) of CMV retinitis.

Intravitreal ganciclovir injections have been used, and an intraocular sustained-release ganciclovir implant (VITRASERT) is more effective than systemic dosing in suppressing retinitis progression. Ganciclovir therapy (5 mg/kg every 12 hours for 14–21 days) may benefit other CMV syndromes in AIDS patients or solid-organ transplant recipients. Response rates of >67% have been found in combination with a decrease in immunosuppressive therapy. The duration of therapy depends on the clearance of viremia; early switch from intravenous ganciclovir to oral valganciclovir is feasible. Recurrent CMV disease occurs commonly after initial treatment. In bone marrow transplant recipients with CMV pneumonia, ganciclovir alone is ineffective. However, ganciclovir combined with intravenous immunoglobulin or CMV immunoglobulin reduces the mortality of CMV pneumonia by about one-half. Ganciclovir treatment may benefit infants with congenital CMV disease.

Ganciclovir has been used for both prophylaxis and preemptive therapy of CMV infections in transplant recipients. In bone marrow transplant recipients in whom CMV is isolated from bronchoalveolar lavage or other sites, preemptive ganciclovir treatment (5 mg/kg every 12 hours for 7–14 days followed by 5 mg/kg every day to days 100–120 after transplant) is highly effective in preventing CMV pneumonia and appears to reduce mortality. Ganciclovir initiation at the time of engraftment also reduces CMV disease rates but does not improve survival, probably due to infections owing to ganciclovir-related neutropenia.

Intravenous ganciclovir, oral ganciclovir, and oral valganciclovir reduce the risk of CMV disease in solid-organ transplant recipients. Oral ganciclovir (1000 mg three times daily for 3 months) reduces CMV disease risk in liver transplant recipients. Oral valganciclovir prophylaxis generally is more effective than high-dose oral acyclovir. Oral valganciclovir (900 mg once daily) provides somewhat greater antiviral effects and similar reductions in CMV disease as oral ganciclovir in mismatched solid-organ transplant recipients.

In advanced HIV disease, oral ganciclovir (1000 mg three times daily) may reduce the risk of CMV disease in those not receiving didanosine. The addition of oral high-dose ganciclovir (1500 mg three times daily) to the intraocular ganciclovir implant further delays the time to retinitis progression and reduces the risk of new CMV disease and possibly of Kaposi's sarcoma.

Ganciclovir resistance emerges in a minority of transplant patients, especially mismatched solid-organ recipients, and is associated with poor prognosis. The use of antithymocyte globulin and prolonged ganciclovir exposure are risk factors. Recovery of ganciclovir-resistant CMV isolates has been associated with progressive CMV disease in AIDS and other immunocompromised patients. Over one-quarter of retinitis patients have resistant isolates by 9 months of therapy, and resistant CMV has been recovered from CSF, vitreous fluid, and visceral sites.

A ganciclovir ophthalmic gel formulation appears to be effective in treating HSV keratitis. Oral ganciclovir reduces HBV DNA levels and aminotransferase levels in chronic hepatitis B.

Idoxuridine

Idoxuridine (5-iodo-2'-deoxyuridine) is an iodinated thymidine analog that inhibits the in vitro replication of various DNA viruses, including herpesviruses and poxviruses.

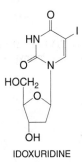

IDOXURIDINE

Inhibitory concentrations of idoxuridine for HSV-1 are at least tenfold higher than those of acyclovir. Idoxuridine lacks selectivity, as low concentrations inhibit the growth of uninfected cells. The triphosphate inhibits viral DNA synthesis and is incorporated into both viral and cellular DNA, increasing their susceptibility to breakage and leading to faulty transcription. Resistance to idoxuridine develops readily.

In the U.S., idoxuridine is approved only for topical treatment of HSV keratitis, although it is available elsewhere for topical treatment of herpes labialis, genitalis, and zoster. In ocular HSV infections, topical idoxuridine is more effective in epithelial than in stromal infections. Adverse reactions include pain, pruritus, inflammation, and edema involving the eye or lids; allergic reactions occur rarely.

Trifluridine

Trifluridine (5-trifluoromethyl-2'-deoxyuridine) is a fluorinated pyrimidine nucleoside with *in vitro* inhibitory activity against HSV types 1 and 2, CMV, vaccinia, and some adenoviruses.

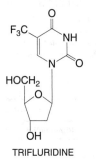

TRIFLURIDINE

Trifluridine inhibits replication of herpesviruses, including acyclovir-resistant strains. Trifluridine also inhibits cellular DNA synthesis at relatively low concentrations.

TRIFLURIDINE INHIBITION OF VIRAL DNA SYNTHESIS   Trifluridine monophosphate irreversibly inhibits thymidylate synthase, and trifluridine triphosphate competitively inhibits thymidine triphosphate incorporation into DNA; trifluridine is incorporated into viral and cellular DNA. Resistance in clinical HSV isolates has been described.

Trifluridine is FDA approved for treatment of primary keratoconjunctivitis and recurrent epithelial keratitis owing to HSV types 1 and 2. Topical trifluridine is more active than idoxuridine and comparable with vidarabine in HSV ocular infections. Adverse reactions include discomfort on instillation and palpebral edema. Hypersensitivity reactions, irritation, and keratopathy are uncommon. Topical trifluridine also is effective in some patients with acyclovir-resistant HSV cutaneous infections.

ANTI-INFLUENZA AGENTS
Amantadine and Rimantadine

CHEMISTRY AND ANTIVIRAL ACTIVITY   *Amantadine* (1-adamantanamine hydrochloride) and its α-methyl derivative *rimantadine* (α-methyl-1-adamantane methylamine hydrochloride) are tricyclic amines.

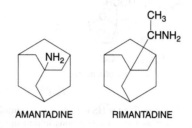

AMANTADINE   RIMANTADINE

Both agents specifically inhibit the replication of influenza A viruses. Rimantadine is 4–10 times more active than amantadine.

MECHANISMS OF ACTION AND RESISTANCE   Amantadine and rimantadine inhibit an early step in viral replication, probably viral uncoating; for some strains, they also have an effect on a late step in viral assembly probably mediated through altering hemagglutinin processing. The primary locus of action is the influenza A virus M2 protein, an integral membrane protein that functions as an ion channel.

Primary drug resistance is uncommon in field isolates but occurs in some avian and swine influenza viruses, including H5N1 human isolates. Resistance is selected readily by virus passage in the presence of drug and is seen in 30% or more of isolates recovered during treatment. Resistance with >100-fold increases in inhibitory concentrations has been associated with single-nucleotide changes leading to amino acid substitutions in the transmembrane region of M2. Amantadine and rimantadine share cross-susceptibility and resistance.

ABSORPTION, DISTRIBUTION, AND ELIMINATION

The pharmacokinetics of amantadine and rimantadine are listed in Table 49–3. The elderly require only one-half the weight-adjusted dose of amantadine to achieve equivalent drug levels. Both drugs have very large volumes of distribution. Nasal secretion and salivary levels of amantadine approximate those found in the serum. Amantadine is excreted in breast milk. Rimantadine

Table 49–3

Pharmacological Characteristics of Antivirals for Influenza

	Amantadine	Rimantadine	Zanamivir	Oseltamivir
Spectrum (types of influenza)	A	A	A, B	A, B
Route/formulations	Oral (tablet/ capsule/syrup)	Oral (tablet/syrup)	Inhaled (powder) Intravenous*	Oral (capsule/ syrup)
Oral bioavailability	>90%	>90%	< 5%[†]	~ 80%[‡]
Effect of meals on AUC	Negligible	Negligible	Not applicable	Negligible
Plasma $t_{1/2, \text{elim}}$, h	12–18	24–36	2.5–5	6–10[‡]
Protein binding, %	67%	40%	<10%	3%[‡]
Metabolism, %	<10%	~ 75%	Negligible	Negligible[‡]
Renal excretion, % (parent drug)	>90%	~ 25%≤	100%	95%[‡]
Dose adjustments	$Cl_{cr} \leq 50$ Age ≥65 yrs	$Cl_{cr} \leq 10$ Age ≥65 years	None	$Cl_{cr} \leq 30$

*Investigational.
[†]Systemic absorption 4–17% after inhalation.
[‡]For antivirally active oseltamivir carboxylate (GS4071).

concentrations in nasal mucus are 50% higher than those in plasma. Amantadine is excreted largely unmetabolized in the urine. Because amantadine's elimination is highly dependent on renal function, the elimination $t_{1/2}$ increases up to twofold in the elderly and even more with renal impairment. Dose adjustment is advised even with mildly decreased renal function. In contrast, rimantadine is metabolized extensively by hydroxylation, conjugation, and glucuronidation; 60–90% is excreted in urine as metabolites.

UNTOWARD EFFECTS

The most common side effects of amantadine and rimantadine are GI and CNS complaints, including nervousness, light-headedness, difficulty concentrating, insomnia, and anorexia or nausea. CNS side effects occur in ~5–33% of patients treated with amantadine at doses of 200 mg/day but are significantly less frequent with rimantadine. Especially in the elderly, the neurotoxic effects of amantadine may be increased by concomitant use of antihistamines and psychotropic or anticholinergic drugs. Amantadine dose reductions are required in older adults (100 mg/day) because of decreased renal function, but 20–40% of infirm elderly experience side effects even at the lower dose. At 100 mg/day, rimantadine is significantly better tolerated in nursing home residents than is amantadine.

High amantadine plasma concentrations (1.0–5.0 µg/mL) have been associated with serious neurotoxic reactions, including delirium, hallucinosis, seizures and coma, and cardiac arrhythmias. Exacerbations of preexisting seizure disorders and psychiatric symptoms may occur with amantadine and possibly with rimantadine. Amantadine is teratogenic in animals and possibly in humans. The safety of these drugs has not been established in pregnancy (category C).

THERAPEUTIC USES

Amantadine and rimantadine are effective for the prevention and treatment of influenza A virus infections. Seasonal prophylaxis with either drug (a total of 200 mg/day in one or two divided doses in young adults) is ~70–90% protective against influenza A illness. Efficacy has been shown during pandemic influenza, in preventing nosocomial influenza, and in curtailing nosocomial outbreaks. Doses of 100 mg/day are better tolerated yet still protective against influenza. Postexposure prophylaxis with either drug provides protection of exposed family contacts if ill young children are not concurrently treated.

Seasonal prophylaxis is an alternative in high-risk patients if the influenza vaccine cannot be administered or may be ineffective due to impaired immunity. Prophylaxis should be started as soon as influenza is identified in a community and continued for the period of risk (usually 4–8 weeks). Alternatively, the drugs can be started in conjunction with immunization and continued for 2 weeks until protective immunity develops.

In uncomplicated influenza A illness of adults, early amantadine or rimantadine treatment (200 mg/day for 5 days) reduces duration of fever and systemic complaints by 1–2 days, speeds functional recovery, and may decrease the duration of virus shedding. In children, rimantadine treatment may be associated with less illness and lower viral titers during the first 2 days of treatment, but treated children have more prolonged virus shedding. The optimal dose and duration of therapy in children are not established.

Resistant variants have been recovered from ~30% of treated outpatient children or adults by the fifth day of therapy. Resistant variants also arise commonly in immunocompromised patients and inpatient children. Illnesses owing to apparent transmission of resistant virus associated with failure of drug prophylaxis have been documented in contacts of drug-treated ill persons in households and in nursing homes. Resistant variants appear to be pathogenic and can cause typically disabling influenza.

Oseltamivir

CHEMISTRY AND ANTIVIRAL ACTIVITY *Oseltamivir carboxylate [(3R, 4R, 5S)-4-acetylamino-5-amino-3(1-ethylpropoxy)-1-cyclohexene-1-carboxylic acid]* is a sialic acid analog that potently inhibits influenza virus neuraminidases.

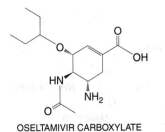

OSELTAMIVIR CARBOXYLATE

Oseltamivir phosphate is an ethyl ester prodrug. Oseltamivir carboxylate has an antiviral spectrum and potency similar to that of *zanamivir*. It inhibits amantadine- and rimantadine-resistant influenza A viruses and some zanamivir-resistant variants.

MECHANISMS OF ACTION AND RESISTANCE   Influenza neuraminidase cleaves terminal sialic acid residues and destroys the receptors recognized by viral hemagglutinin, which are present on the cell surface, in progeny virions, and in respiratory secretions, which is essential for virus release from infected cells. Oseltamivir carboxylate causes a conformational change in neuraminidase's active site and inhibits its activity, leading to viral aggregation at the cell surface and reduced virus spread within the respiratory tract.

Influenza variants selected *in vitro* for resistance to oseltamivir carboxylate contain hemagglutinin and/or neuraminidase mutations. The most commonly recognized resistant variants have reduced infectivity and virulence in animal models. Outpatient oseltamivir therapy has been associated with recovery of resistant variants in ~0.5% of adults and 5.5% of children; a higher frequency (~18%) occurs in hospitalized children.

ABSORPTION, DISTRIBUTION, AND ELIMINATION
Oral oseltamivir phosphate is absorbed rapidly (Table 49–3) and cleaved to the active carboxylate by esterases in the GI tract and liver. The bioavailability of the carboxylate is ~80%; food does not decrease bioavailability but reduces GI symptoms. The carboxylate has a volume of distribution similar to extracellular water. Both prodrug and active metabolite are eliminated primarily unchanged by the kidney.

UNTOWARD EFFECTS
Oral oseltamivir is associated with nausea, abdominal discomfort, and, less often, emesis, probably owing to local irritation. GI complaints usually are relatively mild, resolve in 1–2 days despite continued dosing, and are diminished by administration with food. The frequency of GI complaints is ~10–15% when oseltamivir is used to treat influenza and <5% when used for prophylaxis. An increased frequency of headache in the elderly has been reported.

Oseltamivir phosphate and the carboxylate do not interact with CYPs in vitro. Their protein binding is low. Safety in pregnancy is uncertain (pregnancy category C). Oseltamivir is not approved for children <1 year of age.

THERAPEUTIC USES
Oral oseltamivir is effective in the treatment and prevention of influenza A and B virus infections. Treatment of previously healthy adults (75 mg twice daily for 5 days) or children aged 1–12 years (weight-adjusted dosing) with acute influenza reduces illness duration by ~1–2 days, speeds functional recovery, and reduces the risk of complications requiring antibiotic use by 40–50%. Treatment halves the risk of subsequent hospitalization in adults. When used for prophylaxis during the influenza season, oseltamivir (75 mg once daily) is effective (~70–90%) in reducing the likelihood of influenza illness in both unimmunized working adults and in immunized nursing home residents; short-term use (7–10 days) protects against influenza in household contacts.

Zanamivir

CHEMISTRY AND ANTIVIRAL ACTIVITY   Zanamivir (4-guanidino-2,4-dideoxy-2, 3-dehydro-*N*-acetyl neuraminic acid) is a sialic acid analog that potently and specifically inhibits the neuraminidases of influenza A and B viruses. Depending on the strain, zanamivir competitively inhibits influenza neuraminidase activity but affects neuraminidases from other pathogens and mammalian sources only at much higher concentrations. Zanamivir inhibits *in vitro* replication of influenza A and B viruses, including amantadine- and rimantadine-resistant strains and several oseltamivir-resistant variants.

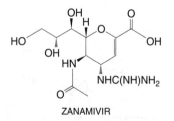

ZANAMIVIR

MECHANISMS OF ACTION AND RESISTANCE Zanamivir inhibits viral neuraminidase and thus causes viral aggregation at the cell surface and reduced spread of virus within the respiratory tract. *In vitro* resistance to zanamivir results from mutations in the viral hemagglutinin and/or neuraminidase. Hemagglutinin variants generally have mutations in or near the receptor binding site that make them less dependent on neuraminidase for release from cells, although they typically retain some drug susceptibility. Hemagglutinin variants are cross-resistant to other neuraminidase inhibitors. Neuraminidase variants contain mutations in the enzyme active site that diminish binding of zanamivir, but the altered enzymes show reduced activity or stability. Zanamivir resistance has not emerged in immunocompetent hosts but has been seen in immunocompromised patients.

ABSORPTION, DISTRIBUTION, AND ELIMINATION

The oral bioavailability of zanamivir is low (<5%) (Table 49–3), and the drug is delivered by oral inhalation. After inhalation, ~15% is deposited in the lower respiratory tract and ~80% in the oropharynx. Overall bioavailability is <20%. The plasma $t_{1/2}$ of zanamivir averages 2.5–5 hours after inhalation but only 1.7 hours following intravenous dosing. Over 90% is eliminated in the urine unmetabolized.

UNTOWARD EFFECTS

Topical zanamivir generally is well tolerated. Wheezing and bronchospasm have been reported in some influenza-infected patients without known airway disease, and acute deteriorations, have occurred in patients with underlying asthma or chronic obstructive airway disease; zanamivir generally is not recommended in these settings.

Preclinical studies of zanamivir revealed no evidence of mutagenic, teratogenic, or oncogenic effects (pregnancy category C).

THERAPEUTIC USES

Inhaled zanamivir is effective for the prevention and treatment of influenza A and B virus infections. Early zanamivir treatment (10 mg twice daily for 5 days) of febrile influenza in ambulatory adults and children >5 years old shortens the duration of illness by 1–3 days and in adults reduces by 40% the risk of lower respiratory tract complications requiring antibiotic use. Once-daily zanamivir is highly protective against community-acquired influenza illness, and when given for 10 days, protects against household transmission.

ANTIHEPATITIS AGENTS
Adefovir

CHEMISTRY AND ANTIVIRAL ACTIVITY *Adefovir dipivoxil (9-[2-[bis[(pivaloyloxy)methoxy]phosphinyl]methoxyl]ethyl]adenine, bis-POM PMEA) is a diester prodrug of adefovir, an acyclic phosphonate nucleotide analog of adenosine monophosphate.*

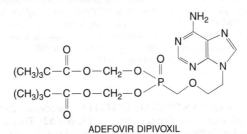

ADEFOVIR DIPIVOXIL

Clinical use is limited to HBV infections, including lamivudine-resistant HBV strains. Oral adefovir dipivoxil shows dose-dependent inhibition of hepadnavirus replication. *In vitro* combinations of adefovir and lamivudine or other anti-HBV nucleosides show enhanced antihepadnavirus activity.

MECHANISMS OF ACTION AND RESISTANCE Adefovir dipivoxil enters cells and is deesterified to adefovir. Cellular enzymes convert adefovir to the diphosphate, which competitively inhibits viral DNA polymerases and reverse transcriptases and also serves as a chain terminator of viral DNA synthesis. Its selectivity relates to a higher affinity for HBV DNA polymerase compared with cellular polymerases. The intracellular $t_{1/2}$ of the diphosphate is prolonged and once-daily dosing is feasible. Adefovir resistance has been detected in ~4% of chronically infected HBV patients during 3 years of treatment, reflecting unique point mutations in the HBV polymerase. The consequences of emerging resistance remain to be determined.

ABSORPTION, DISTRIBUTION, AND ELIMINATION

The parent compound has low oral bioavailability (<12%), whereas the dipivoxil prodrug is absorbed rapidly and hydrolyzed by esterases in the intestine and blood to adefovir. Adefovir bioavailability is ~30–60%. Food does not affect bioavailability. Adefovir has low protein binding (<5%) and has a volume of distribution similar to body water (~0.4 L/kg).

Adefovir is renally excreted. After oral administration of adefovir dipivoxil, ~30–45% of the dose is recovered unchanged in urine within 24 hours; the elimination $t_{1/2}$ is 5–7.5 hours. Dose reductions are indicated for Cl_{Cr} values <50 mL/min. Adefovir is removed by hemodialysis.

UNTOWARD EFFECTS

Adefovir dipivoxil causes dose-related nephrotoxicity, manifested by azotemia and hypophosphatemia, acidosis, glycosuria, and proteinuria, which usually are reversible after discontinuation. The lower dose (10 mg/day) used in chronic HBV infection patients has been associated with few adverse events (e.g., headache, abdominal discomfort, diarrhea, and asthenia) and negligible renal toxicity compared with a threefold higher dose. Adverse events lead to drug discontinuation in ~2% of patients. After 2 years of dosing, the risk of a significant rise in serum creatinine is ~2% but is higher in those with preexisting renal insufficiency. Acute, sometimes severe exacerbations of hepatitis can occur in patients stopping adefovir. Close monitoring is needed, and resumption of antiviral therapy may be required.

No clinically important drug interactions are recognized, although drugs that reduce renal function or compete for active tubular secretion could decrease adefovir clearance. An increased risk of lactic acidosis and hepatic steatosis may exist when adefovir is combined with antiretroviral agents.

High doses in animals cause renal tubular dysfunction, hepatotoxicity, and toxicity to lymphoid tissues. Adefovir dipivoxil is not associated with reproductive toxicity (pregnancy category C).

THERAPEUTIC USES

Adefovir dipivoxil is approved for treatment of chronic HBV infections. In patients with HBV e-antigen (HbeAg)–positive chronic hepatitis B, adefovir dipivoxil (10 mg/day) results in >100-fold reduced serum HBV DNA levels and, in about one-half of patients, improved hepatic histology and normalizes aminotransferase levels by 48 weeks. Continued therapy is associated with increasing frequencies of aminotransferase normalization and HbeAg seroconversion. In patients with HbeAg-negative chronic HBV, adefovir is associated with similar biochemical and histological benefits. Regression of cirrhosis may occur in some patients.

In patients with lamivudine-resistant HBV infections, adefovir dipivoxil results in sustained reductions in serum HBV DNA levels, but lamivudine alone or added to adefovir is not beneficial. In patients with dual HIV and lamivudine-resistant HBV infections, adefovir dipivoxil (10 mg/day) significantly reduces HBV DNA levels and also has been used successfully in patients with lamivudine-resistant HBV infections both before and following liver transplantation. The optimal duration of treatment in different populations, possible long-term effects on HBV complications, and combined use with other anti-HBV agents are under study.

Interferons

CLASSIFICATION AND ANTIVIRAL ACTIVITY   Interferons (IFNs) possess antiviral, immunomodulating, and antiproliferative activities (*see* Chapter 52). They are synthesized by host cells in response to various inducers and stimulate an antiviral state in cells. There are three major classes of human interferons with antiviral activity: α, β, and γ. Clinically used recombinant α IFNs (Table 49–2) are nonglycosylated proteins of ~19,500 Da.

IFN-α and IFN-β are produced by nearly all cells in response to viral infection and a variety of other stimuli, including double-stranded RNA and certain cytokines (*e.g.*, interleukin 1, interleukin 2, and tumor necrosis factor α). IFN-γ production is restricted to T-lymphocytes and natural killer cells responding to antigenic stimuli, mitogens, and specific cytokines. IFN-α and IFN-β have antiviral and antiproliferative actions; stimulate the cytotoxic activity of lymphocytes, natural killer cells, and macrophages; and up-regulate class I major histocompatibility complex (MHC) antigens. IFN-γ has less antiviral activity but more potent immunoregulatory effects. Most animal viruses are inhibited by IFNs, although DNA viruses are relatively insensitive.

MECHANISMS OF ACTION   Following binding to specific cellular receptors, IFNs activate the JAK-STAT pathway and stimulate the transcription of specific genes, leading to synthesis of >20 proteins that contribute to viral resistance at different stages of viral infection (Figure 49–3). For many viruses, the major effect is inhibition of protein synthesis. IFN-induced proteins include $2'$-$5'$-oligoadenylate [2-5(A)] synthetase and a protein kinase, either of which can inhibit protein synthesis in the presence of double-stranded RNA. The protein kinase selectively phosphorylates and inactivates eukaryotic initiation factor 2 (eIF-2). Certain viruses counter IFN effects by blocking production or activity of selected IFN-inducible proteins. For example, IFN resistance in HCV is attributable to inhibition of the IFN-induced protein kinase. IFNs also may modify the immune response; IFN-induced expression of MHC antigens may enhance lytic effects of cytotoxic T-lymphocytes.

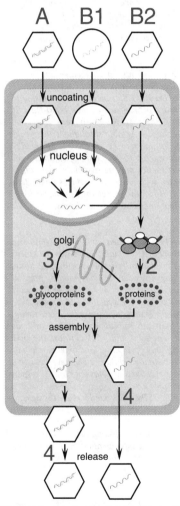

Viruses
A. DNA
B. RNA
1. orthomyxoviruses and retroviruses
2. picornaviruses and most RNA viruses

IFN Effects
1. Transcription inhibition
activates Mx protein
blocks mRNA synthesis

2. Translation inhibition
activates methylase, thereby reducing
mRNA cap methylation

activates 2'5' oligoadenylate synthetase
—> 2'5'A —> inhibits mRNA splicing
and activates RNaseL —> cleaves
viral RNA

activates protein kinase P1 —> blocks
eIF-2α function —> inhibits initiation
of mRNA translation

activates phosphodiesterase —> blocks
tRNA function

3. Protein processing inhibition
inhibits glycosyltransferase, thereby reducing
protein glycosylation

4. Virus maturation inhibition
inhibits glycosyltransferase, thereby reducing
glycoprotein maturation

causes membrane changes —> blocks
budding

FIGURE 49–3 *Interferon-mediated antiviral activity occurs via multiple mechanisms.* The binding of IFN to specific cell surface receptor molecules signals the cell to produce a series of antiviral proteins. The stages of viral replication that are inhibited by various IFN-induced antiviral proteins are shown. Most of these act to inhibit the translation of viral proteins (mechanism 2), but other steps in viral replication also are affected (mechanisms 1, 3, and 4). The roles of these mechanisms in the other actions of IFNs are under study. *Key:* IFN = interferon; mRNA = messenger RNA; Mx = specific cellular protein; tRNA = transfer RNA; RNase L = latent cellular endoribonuclease; $2'5'A = 2'$-$5'$-oligoadenylates; eIF-2α = protein synthesis initiation factor.

Conversely, IFNs may mediate some of the systemic symptoms associated with viral infections and contribute to immunologically mediated tissue damage.

ABSORPTION, DISTRIBUTION, AND ELIMINATION

After intramuscular or subcutaneous injection of IFN-α, absorption is >80%. Plasma levels are dose-related, peaking at 4–8 hours and returning to baseline by 18–36 hours. Levels of 2-5(A) synthetase in peripheral blood mononuclear cells show increases beginning at 6 hours and lasting through 4 days after a single injection. An antiviral state in peripheral blood mononuclear cells peaks at 24 hours and returns to baseline by 6 days after injection. Intramuscular or subcutaneous injections of IFN-β result in negligible plasma levels, although increases in 2-5(A) synthetase levels may occur. After systemic administration, low levels of IFN are detected in respiratory secretions, CSF, eye, and brain.

Because IFNs induce long-lasting cellular effects, their activities are poorly predicted from usual pharmacokinetic measures. After intravenous dosing, clearance of IFN from plasma occurs in a complex manner. With subcutaneous or intramuscular dosing, the plasma elimination $t_{1/2}$ of IFN-α ranges from 3 to 8 hours, largely due to distribution to the tissues, cellular uptake, and catabolism in the kidney and liver. Negligible amounts are excreted in the urine. Clearance of IFN-$α_2$ is reduced by ~70% in dialysis patients.

Attachment of IFN proteins to large, inert polyethylene glycol (PEG) molecules (pegylation) slows absorption, decreases clearance, and provides higher and more prolonged serum concentrations that enable once-weekly dosing. Two pegylated IFNs are available: peginterferon alfa-2a and peginterferon alfa-2b. PegIFN alfa-2b has a 12,000-Da PEG that increases the plasma $t_{1/2}$ from 2 to 3 hours to 30–54 hours. PegIFN alfa-2a contains a branched-chain 40,000-Da PEG bonded to IFN-α2a and has a plasma $t_{1/2}$ of ~80–90 hours. For pegIFN alfa-2a, peak serum concentrations occur up to 120 hours after dosing and remain detectable throughout the weekly dosing interval; steady-state levels occur 5–8 weeks after initiation of weekly dosing. For pegIFN alfa-2a, dose-related maximum plasma concentrations occur at 15–44 hours after dosing and decline by 96–168 hours. These differences in pharmacokinetics may be associated with differences in antiviral effects. Increasing PEG size is associated with longer $t_{1/2}$ and less renal clearance. About 30% of pegIFN alfa-2b is cleared renally; pegIFN alfa-2a is cleared primarily by the liver. Dose reductions in both pegylated IFNs are indicated in end-stage renal disease.

UNTOWARD EFFECTS

Injection of IFN doses of 1–2 million units or greater usually is associated with an acute influenza-like syndrome beginning several hours after injection. Symptoms include fever, chills, headache, myalgia, arthralgia, nausea, vomiting, and diarrhea. Fever usually resolves within 12 hours. Tolerance develops gradually in most patients. Febrile responses can be moderated by pretreatment with antipyretics. Up to one-half of patients receiving intralesional therapy for genital warts experience an initial influenza-like illness, discomfort at the injection site, and leukopenia.

Dose-limiting toxicities of systemic IFN are myelosuppression; neurotoxicity (e.g., somnolence, confusion, depression); autoimmune disorders including thyroiditis; and rarely, cardiovascular effects with hypotension. Elevations in hepatic enzymes and triglycerides, alopecia, proteinuria and azotemia, interstitial nephritis, autoantibody formation, and pneumonia may occur. Alopecia and personality change are common in IFN-treated children. The development of neutralizing antibodies to exogenous IFNs may rarely be associated with loss of clinical responsiveness. Safety during pregnancy is not established (category C).

IFN reduces the metabolism of various drugs by hepatic CYPs. IFNs can increase the hematological toxicity of drugs such as zidovudine and ribavirin, as well as the neuro- and cardiotoxicity of other drugs.

Pegylated IFNs are tolerated about as well as standard IFNs; discontinuation rates range from 2% to 11%, although the frequencies of fever, nausea, local inflammation, and neutropenia may be somewhat higher. Severe neutropenia and the need for dose modifications are higher in HIV-coinfected persons.

THERAPEUTIC USES

Recombinant, natural, and pegylated IFNs are approved in the U.S. for treatment of condyloma acuminatum, chronic HCV infection, chronic HBV infection, Kaposi's sarcoma in HIV-infected patients, other malignancies, and multiple sclerosis.

Hepatitis B Virus

In patients with chronic HBV infection, parenteral administration of IFNs is associated with serological, biochemical, and histological improvement in 25–50% of the patients. Lasting responses *require moderately high IFN doses and prolonged administration (typically 5–10 million units/day in adults and 6 million units/m² in children three times per week for 4–6 months). Plasma HBV DNA and polymerase activity decline promptly in most patients, but complete disappearance is sustained in <33% of patients. Low pretherapy serum HBV DNA levels and high aminotransferase levels predict response. Sustained responses are infrequent in those with vertically acquired infection, anti-HBe positivity, or concurrent immunosuppression owing to HIV. PegIFN alfa-2a is superior to conventional IFN alfa-2a in HbeAg-positive patients, and treatment (180 mg once weekly for 24 weeks) is associated with normalization of aminotransferases in ~60% and sustained viral suppression in ~20% of HBeAg-negative patients. Responses with seroconversion to anti-HBe usually are associated with aminotransferase elevations and often a hepatitis-like illness during the second or third month of therapy, likely related to immune clearance of infected hepatocytes. High-dose IFN can cause myelosuppression and clinical deterioration in those with decompensated liver disease.*

Remissions in chronic hepatitis B induced by IFN are sustained in >80% of patients treated and frequently are followed by loss of HBV surface antigen (HbsAg), histological improvement or stabilization, and reduced risk of liver-related complications and mortality. IFN may benefit some patients with glomerulonephritis owing to chronic HBV infection. Antiviral effects and improvements occur in ~50% of chronic hepatitis D virus (HDV) infections, but relapse is common unless HbsAg disappears. IFN does not appear to be beneficial in acute HBV or HDV infections.

Hepatitis C Virus

In chronic HCV infection, IFN alfa-2b monotherapy (3 million units three times a week) is associated with aminotransferase normalization and loss of plasma viral RNA in ~50–70% of patients; relapse rates are high, and sustained virologic remission is observed in <25% of patients. Sustained viral responses are associated with long-term histological improvement and reduced risk of hepatocellular carcinoma and hepatic failure. Viral genotype and pretreatment RNA level influence treatment response, but early viral clearance is the best predictor of sustained response. Nonresponders generally do not benefit from IFN monotherapy retreatment, but they and patients relapsing after monotherapy may respond to combined pegylated IFN and ribavirin treatment (see below). IFN treatment may benefit HCV-associated cryoglobulinemia and glomerulonephritis. IFN administration during acute HCV infection appears to reduce the risk of chronicity.

Pegylated IFNs are superior to conventional thrice-weekly IFN monotherapy in inducing sustained remissions in treatment-naive patients. Monotherapy with pegIFN alfa-2a (180 μg subcutaneously weekly for 48 weeks) or pegIFN alfa-2b (weight-adjusted doses of 1.5 μg/kg/week) is associated with sustained response in 30–39%, including stable cirrhotic patients, and is a treatment option in patients unable to take ribavirin.

The efficacy of conventional and pegylated IFNs is enhanced by the addition of ribavirin. In previously untreated patients, combined therapy with pegIFN alfa-2a (180 μg once weekly for 48 weeks) and ribavirin (1–1.2 g/day in divided doses) gives higher sustained viral response rates than IFN–ribavirin combinations. The dose and duration of therapy depend on the specific genotype of HCV virus. Approximately 15–20% of those failing to respond to combined IFN–ribavirin will have sustained responses to combined pegIFN–ribavirin. Histological improvement may occur in patients who do not achieve sustained viral responses. In patients with compensated cirrhosis, treatment may reverse cirrhotic changes and possibly reduce the risk of hepatocellular carcinoma.

Papillomavirus

In refractory condylomata acuminata (genital warts), intralesional injection of various IFNs is associated with complete clearance in 36–62% of patients, but other treatments are preferred. Relapse occurs in 20–30% of patients. Verruca vulgaris may respond to intralesional IFN-α. Intramuscular or subcutaneous administration is associated with regression in wart size but greater toxicity. Systemic IFN may provide benefit in recurrent juvenile laryngeal papillomatosis and laryngeal disease in older patients.

Other Viruses

IFNs have effects in various herpesvirus infections including genital HSV infections, localized herpes-zoster infection, and CMV infections of renal transplant patients. IFN generally is associated with more side effects and inferior results relative to conventional antiviral therapies. Topically applied IFN and trifluridine combinations appear active in acyclovir-resistant mucocutaneous HSV infections.

In HIV-infected persons, IFNs have antiretroviral effects, but, the combination of zidovudine and IFN gave only transient benefit and excessive hematological toxicity. IFN-α (3 million units three times weekly) is effective for HIV-related thrombocytopenia resistant to zidovudine therapy.

Except for adenovirus, IFN has broad-spectrum antiviral activity against respiratory viruses. However, prophylactic intranasal IFN-α is protective only against rhinovirus colds, and chronic use is limited by nasal side effects. Intranasal IFN is ineffective in established rhinovirus colds.

Lamivudine

CHEMISTRY AND ANTIVIRAL ACTIVITY Lamivudine, the (–)-enantiomer of 2′,3′-dideoxy-3′-thiacytidine, is a nucleoside analog that inhibits HIV reverse transcriptase and HBV DNA polymerase. Its use in HIV infections is discussed in Chapter 50. It inhibits HBV replication with negligible cellular cytotoxicity. Cellular enzymes convert lamivudine to the triphosphate, which competitively inhibits HBV DNA polymerase and causes chain termination. The intracellular $t_{1/2}$ of the triphosphate is 18 hours in HBV-infected cells, permitting infrequent dosing.

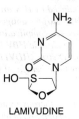

LAMIVUDINE

MECHANISMS OF ACTION AND RESISTANCE Lamivudine triphosphate potently inhibits the DNA polymerase/reverse transcriptase of HBV. Lamivudine has enhanced antiviral activity against hepadnaviruses when combined with adefovir or penciclovir. Point mutations in the HBV DNA polymerase markedly reduce sensitivity. Lamivudine resistance confers cross-resistance to agents such as *emtricitabine* and is often associated with an additional mutation that confers cross-resistance to famciclovir. Lamivudine-resistant HBV retains susceptibility to adefovir and partially to entecavir. Viruses bearing certain mutations are less replication competent than wild-type HBV, but lamivudine resistance is associated with elevated HBV DNA levels, decreased likelihood of HbeAg loss or seroconversion, hepatitis exacerbations, and progressive fibrosis and graft loss in transplant recipients.

ABSORPTION, DISTRIBUTION, AND ELIMINATION

Following oral administration, lamivudine is absorbed rapidly with a bioavailability of ~80% in adults. Lamivudine is distributed widely in a volume comparable with total-body water. The plasma $t_{1/2}$ of elimination averages ~9 hours, and ~70% of the dose is excreted unchanged in the urine. About 5% is metabolized to an inactive trans-sulfoxide *metabolite. In HBV-infected children, doses of 3 mg/kg/day provide drug levels comparable with those in adults receiving 100 mg daily. Dose reductions are indicated for creatinine clearance <50 mL/min.*

UNTOWARD EFFECTS

At doses used for chronic HBV infection, lamivudine generally is well tolerated. Flares in aminotransferase levels occur in ~15% of patients after cessation.

THERAPEUTIC USES

Lamivudine is approved for the treatment of chronic HBV hepatitis in adults and children. In adults, doses of 100 mg/day for 1 year suppress HBV DNA levels, normalize aminotransferase levels in >40% of patients, and reduce hepatic inflammation in >50% of patients. Seroconversion with antibody to HbeAg occurs in <20% of recipients at 1 year. In children aged 2–17 years, lamivudine (3 mg/kg/day to a maximum of 100 mg for 1 year) is associated with normalization of aminotransferase levels in ~50% and seroconversion to anti-Hbe in ~20% of cases. In those without emergence of resistant variants, prolonged therapy is associated with sustained suppression of HBV DNA, histological improvement, and an increased proportion of patients experiencing loss of HbeAg and undetectable HBV DNA. Prolonged therapy halves the risk of clinical progression and development of hepatocellular carcinoma in those with advanced fibrosis or cirrhosis. The frequency of lamivudine-resistant variants increases progressively with continued administration, and frequencies of 38%, 53%, and 67% are found after 2, 3, and 4 years of treatment, respectively. The risk of resistance is higher after transplantation and in HIV/HBV-coinfected patients.

Combined use of IFN or pegIFN alfa-2a with lamivudine has not consistently improved responses in HBeAg-positive patients. The addition of lamivudine to pegINF alfa-2a for 1 year of therapy does not improve posttreatment response rates in HBeAg-negative patients. In HIV and HBV coinfections, higher lamivudine doses are associated with antiviral effects and uncommonly anti-HBe seroconversion. Administration of lamivudine before and after liver transplantation may suppress recurrent HBV infection.

Ribavirin

CHEMISTRY AND ANTIVIRAL ACTIVITY   Ribavirin (1-β-D-ribofuranosyl-1*H*-1,2, 4-triazole-3-carboxamide) is a purine nucleoside analog with a modified base and D-ribose sugar.

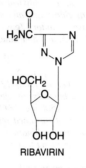

RIBAVIRIN

Ribavirin inhibits the replication of a wide range of RNA and DNA viruses, including orthomyxo-, paramyxo-, arena-, bunya-, and flaviviruses. Therapeutic concentrations reversibly inhibit macromolecular synthesis and proliferation of uninfected cells, suppress lymphocyte responses, and alter cytokine profiles.

MECHANISMS OF ACTION AND RESISTANCE   Ribavirin alters cellular nucleotide pools and inhibits viral mRNA synthesis. Intracellular phosphorylation to the mono-, di-, and triphosphate derivatives is mediated by host cell enzymes. In both uninfected and RSV-infected cells, the predominant derivative is the triphosphate, which has an intracellular $t_{1/2}$ of <2 hours. Ribavirin monophosphate competitively inhibits cellular inosine-5′-phosphate dehydrogenase and interferes with the synthesis of GTP and thus nucleic acid synthesis. Ribavirin triphosphate also competitively inhibits the GTP-dependent 5′ capping of viral messenger RNA and specifically influenza virus transcriptase activity. Ribavirin has multiple sites of action, and some of these (*e.g.,* inhibition of GTP synthesis) may potentiate others (*e.g.,* inhibition of GTP-dependent enzymes). Ribavirin also may enhance viral mutagenesis such that some viruses may be inhibited in effective replication, so-called lethal mutagenesis.

Emergence of viral resistance to ribavirin has been reported in Sindbis and HCV.

ABSORPTION, DISTRIBUTION, AND ELIMINATION

Ribavirin is actively taken up by nucleoside transporters in the proximal small bowel with bioavailability of ~50%. Extensive accumulation occurs in plasma, and steady state is reached by 4 weeks. Food substantially increases plasma levels. With aerosol administration, levels in respiratory secretions are very high.

The volume of distribution for ribavirin is large (~10 L/kg) owing to its cellular uptake. Plasma protein binding is negligible. The plasma $t_{1/2}$ increases to 200–300 hours at steady state, partly because erythrocytes concentrate ribavirin triphosphate and then release it with a $t_{1/2}$ of ~40 days. Hepatic metabolism and renal excretion of ribavirin and its metabolites are the principal routes of elimination. Hepatic metabolism involves deribosylation and hydrolysis to a triazole carboxamide. Ribavirin should be used cautiously in patients with creatinine clearances of <50 mL/min.

UNTOWARD EFFECTS

Aerosolized ribavirin may cause conjunctival irritation, rash, transient wheezing, and occasional reversible deterioration in pulmonary function. When used in conjunction with mechanical ventilation, equipment modifications and frequent monitoring are required to prevent plugging of ventilator valves and tubing. Techniques to reduce environmental exposure of health care workers are recommended.

Systemic ribavirin causes dose-related reversible anemia owing to extravascular hemolysis and bone marrow suppression. Elevations in reticulocyte counts and in serum bilirubin, iron, and uric acid concentrations therefore result. Bolus intravenous infusion may cause rigors. About 20% of chronic HCV infection patients receiving combination IFN–ribavirin therapy discontinue treatment because of side effects. In addition to IFN toxicities, oral ribavirin increases the risk of fatigue, cough, rash, pruritus, nausea, insomnia, dyspnea, depression, and particularly, anemia. Preclinical studies indicate that ribavirin is teratogenic, embryotoxic, oncogenic, and possibly gonadotoxic. To prevent possible teratogenic effects, up to 6 months is required for washout following cessation of long-term treatment.

Pregnant women should not directly care for patients receiving ribavirin aerosol (FDA pregnancy category X).

Ribavirin inhibits the phosphorylation and antiviral activity of pyrimidine nucleoside HIV reverse-transcriptase inhibitors such as zidovudine and stavudine but increases the activity of purine nucleoside reverse-transcriptase inhibitors (e.g., didanosine) in vitro. It appears to increase the risk of mitochondrial toxicity from didanosine (see Chapter 50).

THERAPEUTIC USES

Oral ribavirin in combination with parenteral pegIFN alfa-2a or -2b is standard treatment for chronic HCV infection. Ribavirin monotherapy for 6–12 months reversibly decreases aminotransferases to normal in ~30% of patients but does not affect HCV RNA levels. Combination therapy with pegIFN alfa-2a and oral ribavirin (500 mg, or 600 mg if weight is >75 kg, twice daily for 24–48 weeks) increases the likelihood of sustained responses to ~60%. The combination is superior to IFN or pegIFN monotherapy and combinations of pegIFN alfa-2 and ribavirin in both treatment-naive patients and those not responding to, or relapsing after, IFN monotherapy. Combined ribavirin and pegIFN alfa-2a or -2b is effective in achieving sustained viral responses in a minority of HCV/HIV-coinfected patients. Combined therapy has been used in the management of recurrent HCV infection after liver transplantation.

Ribavirin aerosol is approved in the U.S. for treatment of RSV bronchiolitis and pneumonia in hospitalized children. Aerosolized ribavirin (usual dose of 20 mg/mL as the starting solution in the drug reservoir of the small particle aerosol generator unit for 18 hours' exposure per day for 3–7 days) may reduce some illness measures, but it generally is not recommended. No consistent benefit on duration of hospitalization, ventilatory support, mortality, or long-term pulmonary function has been found. High-dose, reduced-duration therapy (60 mg/mL in the drug reservoir of the small particle aerosol generator unit for 2 hours three times daily) has been used. Aerosol ribavirin combined with intravenous immunoglobulin appears to reduce mortality of RSV infection in bone marrow transplant and other highly immunocompromised patients.

Intravenous and/or aerosol ribavirin has been used occasionally in treating severe influenza virus infection and in the treatment of immunosuppressed patients with adenovirus, vaccinia, parainfluenza, or measles virus infections. Aerosolized ribavirin reduces duration of fever but has no other beneficial effects in influenza infections in hospitalized children. Intravenous ribavirin decreases mortality in Lassa fever and has been used in treating other arenavirus-related hemorrhagic fevers. Intravenous ribavirin is beneficial in hemorrhagic fever with renal syndrome owing to hantavirus infection but ineffective in hantavirus-associated cardiopulmonary syndrome or SARS.

For a complete Bibliographical listing see Goodman & Gilman's *The Pharmacological Basis of Therapeutics*, 11th ed., or Goodman & Gilman Online at www.accessmedicine.com.

50

ANTIRETROVIRAL AGENTS AND TREATMENT OF HIV INFECTION

OVERVIEW OF HIV INFECTION

In 2004, an estimated 42 million people were living with HIV infection worldwide, mostly in resource-poor countries. Of those who would benefit, fewer than 5% were receiving combination antiretroviral therapy, even though such treatment reduces the complications of infection and has the capacity to produce near normal life expectancies for some patients with a previously lethal disease.

Pathogenesis of HIV-Related Disease

Human immunodeficiency viruses (HIVs) are lentiviruses, retroviruses evolved to establish chronic persistent infection with gradual onset of clinical symptoms. Replication is constant following infection; while some infected cells may harbor nonreplicating but infectious virus for years, there generally is no true period of viral latency following infection. Humans and chimpanzees are the only hosts for these viruses.

There are two major families of HIV. Most of the epidemic involves HIV-1; HIV-2 is a close relative whose distribution is concentrated in western Africa. HIV-1 is genetically diverse, with at least five distinct subfamilies or clades. HIV-1 and HIV-2 have similar sensitivities to most antiretroviral drugs, although the nonnucleoside reverse transcriptase inhibitors have no activity against HIV-2.

VIRUS STRUCTURE   HIV has a small RNA genome of 9300 base pairs. Two copies of the genome are contained in a nucleocapsid core surrounded by a lipid bilayer, or envelope, that is derived from the host cell plasma membrane (Figure 50–1). The viral genome includes three major open reading frames: *gag* encodes a polyprotein that is processed to release the major structural proteins; *pol* overlaps gag and encodes three important enzymatic activities—an RNA-dependent DNA polymerase or reverse transcriptase, HIV protease, and the viral integrase; and *env* encodes the large transmembrane envelop protein responsible for cell binding and entry. Several small genes encode regulatory proteins that enhance virus production or combat host defenses, including tat, rev, nef, and vpr.

VIRUS LIFE CYCLE   HIV tropism is controlled by the envelope (env) protein gp160 (Figure 50–1). The major target for env binding is the CD4 receptor present on lymphocytes and macrophages; cell entry also requires binding to a coreceptor, generally the chemokine receptor CCR5 (present on macrophage lineage cells) or CXCR4. Most infected individuals harbor predominantly the CCR5-tropic virus; it is believed that this virus is responsible for sexual transmission of HIV and that the first cells infected in sexual transmission express this coreceptor. A shift from CCR5 to CXCR4 is associated with advancing disease and heralds accelerated loss of CD4 helper T cells and increased risk of immunosuppression. The doligatory role of coreceptors in HIV entry provides a novel target for pharmacotherapy, and the FDA has recently approved a new drug that targets CCR5 to inhibit viral entry.

The gp41 domain of env controls the fusion of the virus lipid bilayer with that of the host cell. Thereafter, full-length viral RNA enters the cytoplasm and is replicated by reverse transcriptase to a short-lived RNA-DNA duplex; the original RNA is degraded by RNase H to allow creation of a full-length double-stranded DNA copy of the virus (Figure 50–1). Because the HIV reverse transcriptase is error-prone and lacks a proofreading function, mutation is quite frequent (~3 bases/9300 base-pair replication). Viral DNA is transported into the nucleus, where it is integrated into a host chromosome by the viral integrase in a random or quasi-random location.

Following integration, the virus may remain quiescent, not producing RNA or protein but replicating as the cell divides. When a cell that harbors the virus is activated, viral RNA and proteins are produced. Structural proteins assemble around full-length genomic RNA to form a nucleocapsid (Figure 50–1). The transmembrane envelope and other structural proteins assemble at the cell surface, concentrated in lipid rafts. The nucleocapsid cores are directed to these sites and bud through the cell membrane, creating a new enveloped HIV particle containing two complete single-stranded RNA genomes. Reverse transcriptase is incorporated into this particle; thus, replication can begin immediately after the virus enters a new cell.

HOW THE VIRUS CAUSES DISEASE   Sexual acquisition of HIV infection is thought to be mediated by one or, at most, a handful of infectious virus particles. Soon after infection, there is a rapid burst of replication peaking at 2–4 weeks, with 10^9 or more cells becoming infected. This peak is associated with a transient dip in the number of peripheral CD4 (helper) T lymphocytes. As

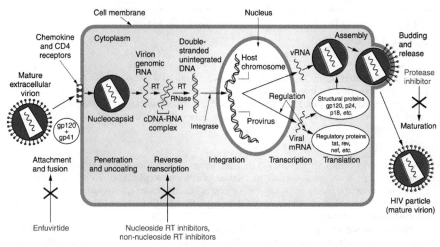

FIGURE 50–1 *Replicative cycle of HIV-1 showing the sites of action of available antiretroviral agents.* Available antiretroviral agents are shown in blue. Key: RT, reverse transcriptase; cDNA, complementary DNA; mRNA, messenger RNA; RNase H, ribonuclease H; gp120 + gp41, extracellular and intracellular domains, respectively, of envelope glycoprotein.

a result of new host immune responses and target cell depletion, the number of infectious virions—as reflected by the plasma HIV RNA concentration (also known as *viral load*)—declines to quasi-steady state. This *set point* of viral activity reflects the interplay between host immunity and the pathogenicity of the infecting virus. In the average infected individual, several billion infectious virus particles are produced every few days.

Eventually, the CD4 lymphocyte count begins a steady decline, accompanied by a rise in the plasma HIV RNA concentration. Once the peripheral CD4 count falls to <200 cell per mm^3, there is an increasing risk of opportunistic infection. Sexual acquisition of CCR5-tropic HIV-1 is associated with a median time to clinical disease—usually an opportunistic infection such as *Pneumocystis carinii* pneumonia—of 8–10 years. Occasional patients can harbor HIV for more than two decades without significant decline in CD4 count or clinical immunosuppression; this may reflect a combination of favorable host immunogenetics and immune responses.

An important question is whether HIV disease is a consequence purely of CD4 lymphocyte depletion or also involves other factors. Most natural history data support the former. Regardless, successful therapy is based on inhibition of HIV replication; treatments designed to boost the host immune system without exerting a direct antiviral effect have had no reliable clinical benefit.

Principles of HIV Chemotherapy

Current treatment assumes that all aspects of the disease derive from direct toxic effects of HIV on host cells, mainly CD4 T lymphocytes. The goal of therapy therefore is to suppress viral replication as much as possible for as long as possible.

Deciding when to initiate therapy has been the subject of some debate. The advent of more effective drugs capable of increasing CD4 cell counts to normal or near normal levels led some to advocate a strategy of early use of combination drug therapy regardless of disease stage or symptoms. It now appears that true eradication of HIV is not possible, at least with current drugs, as there is a reservoir of long-lived, quiescent T cells harboring infectious HIV DNA incorporated into the host chromosome. Natural history studies also point to a low risk of short-term disease progression when the CD4 cell count is >350 cells per mm^3 or plasma HIV RNA concentrations were <50,000 copies per mL. The toxic risks of long-term combination chemotherapy, the need for nearly perfect adherence to prescribed regimens, the inconvenience of some regimens, and the high cost of life-long treatment point to a risk-benefit ratio that favors treating only patients with low CD4 counts and/or very high viral load (Table 50–1).

Drug resistance is also an extensive and serious problem. Because of the high mutation rate of HIV and the tremendous number of infectious virions, there is a high likelihood that any infected individual will harbor viruses with single-amino-acid mutations conferring some degree of resistance

Table 50–1

U.S. Department of Health and Human Services Guidelines for Initiating Therapy in Treatment-Naive HIV-Infected Patients, 2004

A. Patient Characteristics

Clinical Category	CD4 Count	Plasma HIV RNA	Recommendation
AIDS-defining illness* or severe symptoms	Any value	Any value	Treat
Asymptomatic	<200 cells/mm^3	Any value	Treat
Asymptomatic	>200 cells/mm^3, but <350 cells/mm^3	Any value	Offer treatment, following full discussion of pros and cons with each patient
Asymptomatic	>350 cells/mm^3	>100,000 copies/mL	Most physicians recommend deferring therapy, but some will treat
Asymptomatic	>350 cells/mm^3	<100,000 copies/mL	Defer therapy

B. Preferred and Alternative Regimens

Preferred Regimens		Number of Pills per Day
NNRTI-based	EFV + (3TC or FTC) + (AZT or TDF) (not for use in first trimester of pregnancy or in women with high pregnancy potential)	2–3
PI-based	LPV/r + (3TC or FTC) + AZT	8–9

Alternative Regimens		Number of Pills per Day
NNRTI-based	EFV + (3TC or FTC) + (ABC or ddI or d4T**)	2–4
	NVP + (3TC or FTC) + (AZT or d4T or ddI or ABC or TDF)	3–6
PI-based	ATV + (3TC or FTC) + (AZT or d4T or ABC or ddI) or (TDF + RTV 100 mg/d)	3–6
	FosAPV + (3TC or FTC) + (AZT or d4T or ABC or TDF or ddI)	5–8
	FosAPV/RTV† + (3TC or FTC) + (AZT or d4T or ABC or TDF or ddI)	5–8
	IDV/RTV† + (3TC or FTC) + (AZT or d4T or ABC or TDF or ddI)	7–12
	LPV/r + (3TC or FTC) + (d4T or ABC or TDF or ddI)	7–10
	NFV + (3TC or FTC) + (AZT or d4T or ABC or TDF or ddI)	5–8
	SQV/RTV† + (3TC or FTC) + (AZT or d4T or ABC or TDF or ddI)	13–16
3 NRTI-based‡	ABC + AZT + 3TC, only when a preferred or an alternative NNRTI- or a PI-based regimen cannot or should not be used	2

Regimens That Should Not Be Used	Rationale
AZT + d4T	Pharmacologic antagonism between AZT and d4T
ABC + TDF + 3TC once daily as a triple-NRTI regimen	High rate of early virological nonresponse seen in treatment-naive patients
TDF + ddI + 3TC combination once daily as a triple-NRTI regimen	High rate of early virological nonresponse seen in treatment-naive patients

(Continued)

Table 50–1

U.S. Department of Health and Human Services Guidelines for Initiating Therapy in Treatment-Naive HIV-Infected Patients, 2004 *(Continued)*

B. Preferred and Alternative Regimens

Regimens That Should Not Be Used	Rationale
ATV + IDV	Potential additive hyperbilirubinemia
ddI + DDC	Additive peripheral neuropathy
FTC + 3TC	Similar resistance profile with no potential benefit
3TC + DDC	*In vitro* antagonism
SQV hard-gel capsule as single protease inhibitor	Poor oral bioavailability and inferior antiretroviral activity when compared with other protease inhibitors
d4T + DDC	Additive peripheral neuropathy

ABBREVIATIONS: EFV, efavirenz; 3TC, lamivudine; AZT, zidovudine; TDF, tenofovir disoproxil fumarate; d4T, stavudine; LPV/r, lopinavir/ritonavir coformulation; FTC, emtricitabine; NVP, nevirapine; ddI, didanosine; ATV, atazanavir; fosAPV, fosamprenavir; RTV, ritonavir; IDV, indinavir; NFV, nelfinavir; SQV, saquinavir.

*AIDS-defining illness per Centers for Disease Control, 1993. Severe symptoms include unexplained fever or diarrhea >2–4 weeks, oral candidiasis, or >10% unexplained weight loss.
**Higher incidence of lipoatrophy, hyperlipidemia, and mitochondrial toxicities reported with d4T than with other NRTIs.
†Low-dose (100–400 mg) ritonavir per day.
‡The triple-NRTI regimen had reduced efficacy compared with NNRTI-based regimens in one large controlled clinical trial and should be used only when an NNRTI- or PI-based regimen cannot or should not be used as first-line therapy.

to any known antiretroviral drug. A combination of active agents therefore is needed to prevent drug resistance, analogous to strategies employed in the treatment of tuberculosis. Intentional drug holidays (structured treatment interruptions) allow the virus to replicate anew and increase the risk of drug resistance and disease progression; they therefore are not recommended.

The standard of care is to use at least three drugs simultaneously for the entire duration of treatment (Table 50–1). The expected outcome of initial therapy in a previously untreated patient is an undetectable viral load (plasma HIV RNA <50 copies/mL) within 24 weeks of starting treatment. Four or more drugs are often used simultaneously in pretreated patients harboring drug-resistant virus, but the number of agents a patient can take is limited by toxicity and inconvenience. Most clinicians prefer to use drugs that attack at least two different molecular sites (and that thus are from different drug classes). In treatment-naïve patients, a three-drug regimen containing a single drug class is less effective than one that includes drugs from two classes. Regimens containing three or four different classes are reserved for treatment-experienced patients who have failed multiple previous regimens. This acknowledges the benefit of reserving at least one drug class for future treatment in case of failure.

Failure of an antiretroviral regimen involves a persistent increase in plasma HIV RNA in a patient who previously responded or failure to reduce plasma HIV RNA significantly in a patient who has taken the prescribed regimen for more than 12 weeks. This indicates resistance to one or more of the drugs and necessitates a change in treatment. The selection of new drugs is based on the patient's treatment history and viral resistance testing. Treatment failure generally requires a completely new drug combination, as adding a single effective agent to a failing regimen is functionally equivalent to monotherapy. The risk of failing a regimen depends on the percent of prescribed doses taken in any given treatment period. This places an important educational burden on the clinician and requires exceptional patient responsibility.

DRUGS USED TO TREAT HIV INFECTION

Nucleoside and Nucleotide Reverse Transcriptase Inhibitors

The HIV-encoded, RNA-dependent DNA polymerase, also called reverse transcriptase, converts viral RNA into proviral DNA that then is incorporated into a host cell chromosome. Inhibitors of this enzyme are either nucleoside/nucleotide analogs or nonnucleoside inhibitors (Figure 50–2 and Table 50–2). Like all available antiretroviral drugs, nucleoside and nonnucleoside reverse transcriptase inhibitors prevent infection of susceptible cells but have no impact on cells that already

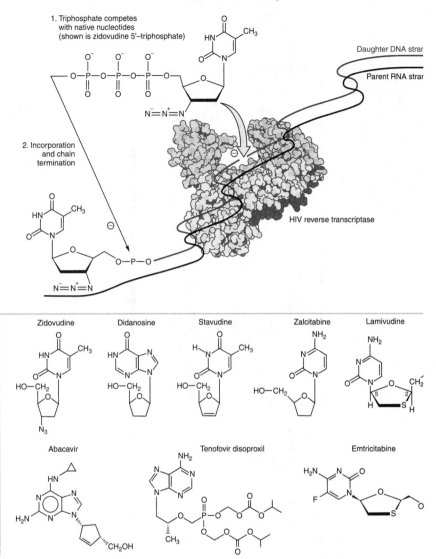

FIGURE 50–2   *Structures and mechanism of nucleoside and nucleotide reverse transcriptase inhibitors.*

harbor HIV. Nucleoside and nucleotide analogs must enter cells and undergo phosphorylation to generate synthetic substrates for the enzyme (Figure 50–3). The fully phosphorylated analogs block replication of the viral genome both by competitively inhibiting incorporation of native nucleotide and by terminating elongation of nascent proviral DNA because they lack a 3'-hydroxyl group.

All but one of the drugs in this class is a nucleoside that must be triphosphorylated at the 5'-hydroxyl to exert activity. The sole exception, tenofovir, is a nucleoside monophosphate analog that requires two phosphates for full activity. These compounds inhibit both HIV-1 and HIV-2 and several have broad-spectrum activity against other retroviruses; some are also active against hepatitis B virus (HBV) or the herpesviruses.

Although many of the drugs in this class induce only a modest decrease in HIV RNA when used as monotherapy, several have favorable safety and tolerability profiles that make them a valuable component of combination regimens.

Table 50–2

Pharmacokinetic Properties of Nucleoside and Nucleotide Reverse Transcriptase Inhibitors*

Parameter	Zidovudine	Lamivudine	Stavudine†	Didanosine‡	Abacavir	Zalcitabine	Tenofovir	Emtricitabine
Oral bioavailability, %	64	86–87	86	42	83	88	25	93
Effect of meals on AUC	↓24% (high fat)	↔	↔	↓55% (acidity)	↔	↓14%	↑40% (high fat)	↔
Plasma $t_{1/2}$ elim, h	1.0	5–7	1.1–1.4	1.5	0.8–1.5	1–2	14–17	10
Intracellular $t_{1/2}$ elim of triphosphate, h	3–4	12–18	3.5	25–40	21	2–3	10–50	39
Plasma protein binding, %	20–38	<35	<5	<5	50	<5	<8	<4
Metabolism, %	60–80 (glucuronidation)	<36	ND	50 (purine metabolism)	>80 (dehydrogenation and glucuronidation)	20	ND	13
Renal excretion of parent drug, %	14	71	39	18–36	<5	60–80	70–80	86

ABBREVIATIONS: *AUC*, area under plasma concentration–time curve; $t_{1/2}$, elim, half-life of elimination; ↑, increase; ↓, decrease; ↔, no effect; ND, not determined.

*Reported mean values in adults with normal renal and hepatic function.
†Parameters reported for the stavudine capsule formulation.
‡Parameters reported for the didanosine chewable tablet formulation.

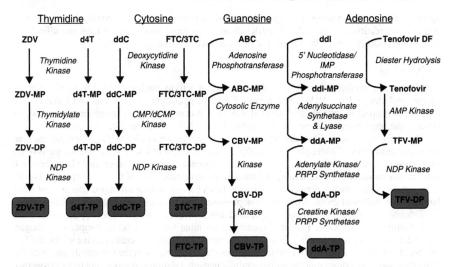

FIGURE 50–3 *Intracellular activation of nucleoside analog reverse transcriptase inhibitors.* Drugs and phosphorylated anabolites are abbreviated; the enzymes responsible for each conversion are spelled out. The active antiretroviral anabolite for each drug is shown in the blue box. Key: ZDV, zidovudine; d4T, stavudine; ddC, dideoxycytidine; FTC, emtricitabine; 3TC, lamivudine; ABC, abacavir; ddI, didanosine; DF, disoproxil fumarate; MP, monophosphate; DP, diphosphate; TP, triphosphate; AMP, adenosine monophosphate; CMP, cytosine monophosphate; dCMP, deoxycytosine monophosphate; IMP, inosine 5′-monophosphate; PRPP, phosphoribosyl pyrophosphate; NDR, nucleoside diphosphate.

Mechanisms of Action and Resistance Resistance to nucleoside reverse transcriptase inhibitors, especially thymidine analogs, occurs slowly relative to the NNRTIs and protease inhibitors. In most cases, high-level resistance requires a minimum of 3–4 codon substitutions, although 1 two-amino-acid insertion is associated with resistance to all drugs in this class. Cross-resistance is common but often confined to drugs having similar chemical structures; for example, zidovudine is a thymidine analog, and a zidovudine-resistant isolate is much more likely to be cross-resistant to the thymidine analog stavudine than to the cytosine analog lamivudine. These mutations are termed *thymidine-analog mutations (TAMs)*. Substitutions at codon 184 are associated with high-level resistance to lamivudine and emtricitabine; these same amino acid substitutions restore sensitivity to zidovudine and reduce the fitness of HIV, perhaps explaining the sustained virologic benefits of combination therapy with lamivudine and zidovudine.

Absorption, Distribution, and Elimination Most nucleoside and nucleotide reverse transcriptase inhibitors are eliminated from the body primarily by renal excretion. The parent compounds are generally eliminated rapidly from plasma with elimination half-lives of 1–10 hours (Table 50–2). Despite rapid clearance from plasma, the critical pharmacological pathway for these agents is production and elimination of the intracellular nucleoside triphosphate or nucleotide diphosphate, which is the active anabolite. These reservoirs allow for less frequent dosing, and all approved nucleoside and nucleotide reverse transcriptase inhibitors are dosed once or twice daily, with the exception of zalcitabine, which is dosed every 8 hours. These drugs are not substrates for hepatic CYPs and thus generally are not involved in clinically significant drug interactions. Specific exceptions to this are described below under the individual drugs.

Adverse Effects The selective toxicity of these drugs depends on their ability to inhibit the HIV reverse transcriptase without inhibiting host cell DNA polymerases. Although these drugs have low affinity for human DNA polymerases α and β, some are capable of inhibiting human DNA polymerase γ, the mitochondrial enzyme. As a result, important toxicities common to this class of drugs result in part from inhibition of mitochondrial DNA synthesis. These toxicities include anemia, granulocytopenia, myopathy, peripheral neuropathy, and pancreatitis. Lactic acidosis with or without hepatomegaly and hepatic steatosis is a rare but potentially fatal complication seen with stavudine, zidovudine, didanosine, and zalcitabine. Risk factors for this lactic acidosis-hepatic steatosis syndrome include female gender, obesity, and prolonged exposure to the causative drugs. Drugs that are subject to mitochondrial toxicities generally should not be coadministered with other agents that can cause neuropathy (*e.g., ethambutol, isoniazid, vincristine, cisplatin, and pentamidine*) or pancreatitis. Phosphorylated emtricitabine, lamivudine, and tenofovir have low affinity for DNA polymerase γ and are largely devoid of mitochondrial toxicity.

Zidovudine

Zidovudine is a synthetic thymidine analog with potent activity against a broad spectrum of retroviruses including HIV-1, HIV-2, and human T-cell lymphotrophic viruses (HTLV) I and II. The drug has no impact in cells already infected with HIV. It is most effective in activated lymphocytes because the phosphorylating enzyme, thymidine kinase, is S-phase specific.

The steps involved in zidovudine phosphorylation are shown in Figure 50–3. Because the conversion of zidovudine 5'-monophosphate to diphosphate is very inefficient, high concentrations of the monophosphate accumulate inside the cell. As a consequence, there is little correlation between extracellular concentrations of parent drug and intracellular concentrations of the active species. The 5'-triphosphate terminates the elongation of proviral DNA because it is incorporated into nascent DNA but lacks a 3'-hydroxyl group, while the monophosphate competitively inhibits thymidylate kinase.

Zidovudine may be taken irrespective of food and undergoes rapid first-pass hepatic metabolism to 5-glucuronyl zidovudine. Patients initiating zidovudine treatment often complain of fatigue, malaise, myalgia, nausea, anorexia, headache, and insomnia, which generally resolve within the first few weeks of therapy. The mitochondrial toxicities shared by this class are commonly encountered. Stavudine and zidovudine compete for intracellular phosphorylation and should not be used together.

Zidovudine is FDA-approved for the treatment of adults and children with HIV infection and for preventing mother-to-child transmission; it also is recommended for postexposure prophylaxis in HIV-exposed healthcare workers, also in combination with other antiretroviral agents. The standard of care for treatment-naïve patients (Table 50–1B) is to combine zidovudine with a potent protease inhibitor and another nucleoside analog or with an NNRTI and another nucleoside analog. The Met-to-Val substitution at reverse transcriptase codon 184 associated with use of lamivudine greatly restores sensitivity to zidovudine, and these drugs are often used in combination.

Didanosine

Didanosine is a purine nucleoside analog active against HIV-1, HIV-2, and HTLV-1. After entering the cell, it is converted by phosphorylation to the active anabolite dideoxyadenosine 5'-triphosphate. Single codon mutations, including TAMs, can contribute to didanosine resistance.

Didanosine is acid labile, and therefore is administered with an antacid buffer. Food decreases bioavailability and all formulations of didanosine must be administered at least 30 minutes before or 2 hours after eating; this complicates dosing of didanosine with other antiretroviral agents that must be administered with food, such as many HIV protease inhibitors. Because of the long intracellular $t_{1/2}$ of the active anabolite, didanosine can be administered once daily.

The most serious toxicities with didanosine are peripheral neuropathy and pancreatitis, both due to mitochondrial toxicity. It should be avoided in patients with a history of pancreatitis or neuropathy and should not be coadministered with other drugs that can cause neuropathy. Diarrhea is reported more frequently with didanosine than with other nucleoside analogs, perhaps related to the antacid in the oral preparations. The buffering agents also can impair the bioavailability of other coadministered drugs.

Stavudine

Stavudine is a synthetic thymidine analog reverse transcriptase inhibitor that is active against HIV-1 and HIV-2. After entering the cell, it is phosphorylated to its active form, stavudine 5'-triphosphate. Unlike zidovudine, the monophosphate does not accumulate within the cell.

Stavudine is well absorbed and its bioavailability is not affected by food. The dose should be adjusted in patients with renal insufficiency. A sustained-release formulation that can be given once daily is FDA-approved.

The most common adverse effect with stavudine is peripheral neuropathy, which occurs in ~12% of patients. Combining stavudine with zidovudine leads to increased risk and severity of peripheral neuropathy and potentially fatal pancreatitis, and these drugs should not be used together under most circumstances. Lactic acidosis and hepatic steatosis also have been seen and are more common with stavudine than with zidovudine or abacavir. Of all the nucleoside analogs, stavudine is most strongly linked to the HIV lipodystrophy syndrome, perhaps due to toxic effects on adipocytes.

Zalcitabine

Zalcitabine is a synthetic cytosine analog reverse transcriptase inhibitor that is active against HIV-1, HIV-2, and hepatitis B virus. After entering the cell, it is phosphorylated to its active anabolite, dideoxycytidine-5'-triphosphate. In addition to DNA polymerase γ, zalcitabine also weakly inhibits DNA polymerase β.

The drug is well absorbed orally and food does not affect bioavailability. The drug is largely excreted unchanged in the urine, and the dose must be reduced in patients with impaired renal function. It is recommended that zalcitabine be administered every 8 hours in patients with normal renal function.

Zalcitabine toxicities are similar to those of the other dideoxynucleotide analogs didanosine and stavudine. Severe peripheral neuropathy has been reported in up to 15% of patients. Pancreatitis occurs rarely with zalcitabine therapy, but coadministration of other drugs that cause pancreatitis should be avoided. One distinctive toxicity of zalcitabine is oral ulceration and stomatitis. An erythematous rash also is common but generally self-limited. The necessity of frequent administration, the risk of toxicities, and the inferior antiviral activity compared to more convenient agents limits the use of zalcitabine in the U.S.

Lamivudine

Lamivudine is a cytosine analog active against HIV-1, HIV-2, and HBV. The molecule is manufactured as the pure cis-(-) enantiomer (Figure 50–2), which is more potent and substantially less toxic. The active species is the intracellular triphosphate derivative, which has low affinity for human DNA polymerases. High-level resistance to lamivudine occurs with single-amino-acid mutations at codon 184 that can reduce in vitro sensitivity to the drug by up to 1000-fold but restore sensitivity to zidovudine. This effect may contribute to the sustained virologic benefits of combination therapy with lamivudine and zidovudine.

The oral bioavailability of lamivudine is >80% and is not affected by food. It is excreted primarily unchanged in the urine, and dose adjustment is recommended for patients with a creatinine clearance of <50 mL/min. Lamivudine is one of the least toxic antiretrovirals and has few significant effects. Neutropenia, headache, and nausea have been reported.

Many trials have confirmed the value of lamivudine in three-drug regimens with other nucleoside analogs, protease inhibitors, and/or NNRTIs. It is a common component of therapy based on its safety, convenience, and efficacy. Since lamivudine and emtricitabine have nearly identical resistance and activity patterns, there is no rationale for their combined use.

Abacavir

Abacavir is a synthetic purine analog that is converted in the cell to carbovir triphosphate, a potent inhibitor of the HIV-1 reverse transcriptase. It is the only approved antiretroviral that is a guanosine analog. Abacavir's oral bioavailability is >80% regardless of food intake. Because of the prolonged $t_{1/2}$ of carbovir triphosphate, the drug can be administered once daily. The most important adverse effect of abacavir is a unique and potentially fatal hypersensitivity reaction that occurs in 2–9% of patients. This reaction typically begins within 6 weeks of drug initiation and is characterized by fever, abdominal pain and other GI complaints, a maculopapular rash, malaise, and fatigue. Less common are respiratory complaints, headache, and paresthesias. The presence of fever, abdominal pain, and rash within 6 weeks of starting abacavir is diagnostic and necessitates immediate drug discontinuation. Patients must be warned about these symptoms, and those who exhibit the hypersensitivity reaction should never be retreated with abacavir. The hypersensitivity syndrome results from an immune reaction that is genetically linked to the HLA-B and the heat shock protein 70 loci, providing one of the most striking pharmacogenetic associations ever described.

Abacavir is widely used in combination with other antiretroviral agents, and is supplied in coformulations with zidovudine or lamivudine for twice-daily administration and with lamivudine for once-daily administration.

Tenofovir

Tenofovir is a derivative of adenosine 5'-monophosphate lacking a complete ribose ring and is the only nucleotide analog currently marketed for the treatment of HIV infection; it is active against HIV-1, HIV-2, and HBV.

Because of poor bioavailability, it is administered as a disoproxil fumarate prodrug. The prodrug is rapidly converted to tenofovir, which then is phosphorylated by cellular kinases to the active metabolite, tenofovir diphosphate (Figure 50–3). It can be dosed once daily. It primarily is excreted unchanged in the urine, and the dose should be decreased in patients with renal insufficiency.

Tenofovir generally is well tolerated, with few adverse events except for flatulence. Rare episodes of acute renal failure and Fanconi's syndrome have been reported, and the drug should be used with caution in patients with preexisting renal disease. It can increase the AUC of didanosine, and the drugs probably should not be used together.

Tenofovir is FDA-approved as a component of combination HIV therapy for adults and has proven value in three-drug regimens with other agents, including other nucleoside analogs, protease inhibitors, and/or NNRTIs.

Emtricitabine

Emtricitabine is a cytosine analog that is chemically related to lamivudine and shares many of its properties. It is active against HIV-1, HIV-2, and HBV.

High-level host resistance to emtricitabine occurs with the same mutation (M184V) that affects lamivudine sensitivity, although the mutation apparently occurs less frequently. This mutation restores sensitivity to zidovudine.

Emtricitabine has excellent oral absorption and can be taken without regard to food. It has a long elimination $t_{1/2}$ and can be administered once daily. It is excreted primarily unchanged in the urine. It is one of the least toxic antiretroviral drugs and has few significant adverse effects. Prolonged exposure has been associated with hyperpigmentation. It is not subject to any known metabolic drug interactions. Emtricitabine is approved in several combination regimens for HIV-1 therapy and has similar efficacy to lamivudine.

Nonnucleoside Reverse Transcriptase Inhibitors

The chemical structures of the three approved NNRTIs are shown in Figure 50–4, and their pharmacokinetic properties are summarized in Table 50–3.

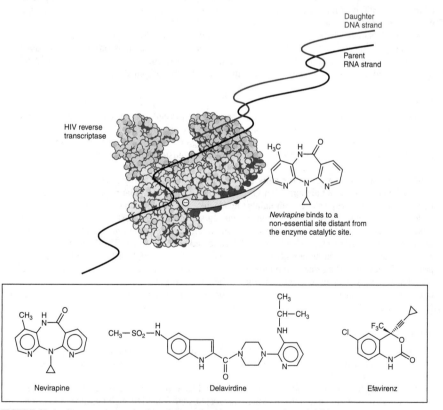

FIGURE 50–4 *Structures an mechanism of nonnucleoside reverse transcriptase inhibitors.*

Table 50–3

Pharmacokinetic Properties of Nonnucleoside Reverse Transcriptase Inhibitors*

Parameter	Nevirapine[†]	Efavirenz[†]	Delavirdine
Oral bioavailability, %	90–93	50	85
Effect of meals on AUC	↔	↑17–28%	↔
Plasma $t_{1/2}$, elim, h	25–30	40–55	2–11
Plasma protein binding, %	60	99	98
Metabolism	CYP3A4 > CYP2B6	CYP2B6 > CYP3A4	CYP3A4
Renal excretion of parent drug, %	<3	<3	<5
Autoinduction of metabolism	Yes	Yes	No
Inhibition of CYP3A	No	Yes	Yes

ABBREVIATIONS: AUC, area under plasma concentration–time curve; $t_{1/2}$, elim, half-life of elimination; ↑, increase; ↓, decrease; ↔, no effect.

*Reported mean values in adults with normal renal and hepatic function.
[†]Values at steady state after multiple oral doses.

MECHANISM OF ACTION AND RESISTANCE These drugs are noncompetitive inhibitors that bind to a peripheral site on HIV-1 reverse transcriptase. The binding site is a hydrophobic pocket in the p66 subunit of reverse transcriptase, distant from the active site and not essential for function. Occupation of the site by an NNRTI induces a conformational change that greatly reduces the enzyme's activity. Because the binding site for NNRTIs is strain-specific, the approved agents are active against HIV-1 but not HIV-2 or other retroviruses. They have no activity against host cell DNA polymerases. NNRTIs do not require intracellular phosphorylation for activity. Resistance can develop rapidly, sometimes within a few days or weeks. Single codon mutations can reduce susceptibility to these drugs by over 100-fold, and cross-resistance to the other NNRTIs is seen with most of these mutations (most often codons 103 or 181 in the hydrophobic binding pocket). Therefore, *any patient who fails treatment with one NNRTI because of a specific resistance mutation should be considered to have failed the entire class.*

Absorption, Distribution, and Elimination These drugs are administered orally and rapidly absorbed. Food generally does not affect their absorption. They are metabolized primarily by hepatic CYPs 3A4 or 2B6. Thus, they are subject to multiple interactions with other drugs that are either substrates or inducers of these enzymes. Efavirenz and nevirapine are moderately potent inducers of CYP3A4, whereas delavirdine is an inhibitor.

Adverse Effects The most frequent adverse effect with these drugs is rash, which typically occurs in 15–25% of patients. The most severe form is life-threatening Stevens-Johnson syndrome. Elevations of hepatic transaminases also are common with all drugs of this class, although the propensity to cause severe hepatitis varies somewhat with the different agents (*see* below).

Nevirapine Nevirapine is FDA-approved for the treatment of HIV-1 infection in adults and children in combination with other antiretroviral agents. Resistance can develop rapidly and the drug should never be used as a single agent or as the sole addition to a failing regimen. Nevirapine readily crosses the placenta and therefore has been used to prevent mother-to-child transmission of HIV-1. In addition to elevated hepatic transaminases, severe and fatal hepatitis has been associated with nevirapine use; this may be more common in women, especially during pregnancy. Although nevirapine is inexpensive and generally well tolerated in intrapartum usage, the high prevalence of nevirapine resistance and the recognition of fatal hepatitis have prompted reexamination of this approach to the prevention of vertical transmission. In particular, the drug should not be initiated in women with CD4 cell counts >250 per mm^3 or men with CD4 counts >400 per mm^3 unless benefits clearly outweigh the risks.

Delavirdine Due to its shorter $t_{1/2}$ and rapid emergence of resistance, delavirdine is the least used of the NNRTIs. Its absorption is best at acid pH and may be decreased by histamine H_2 receptor antagonists or proton pump inhibitors. It is cleared predominantly by CYP3A4 and has an elimination $t_{1/2}$ of 6 hours. It should be avoided with CYP3A4 substrates with a narrow therapeutic index and not combined with potent inducers of CYP3A4 (*e.g.*, carbamazepine, phenobarbital, phenytoin, rifabutin, and rifampin).

Efavirenz Efavirenz (Figure 50–4) is widely used in the developed world because of its convenience, effectiveness, and long-term tolerability. It should only be used in combination with other effective agents and should not be added as the sole new agent to a failing regimen. It is cleared predominantly by CYP2B6 with a prolonged $t_{1/2}$ that permits once-daily dosing. In addition to rash, the predominant adverse effects of efavirenz involve the CNS (*e.g.*, dizziness, impaired concentration, dysphoria, frank psychosis, depression, or hallucinations). Fortunately, these CNS side effects generally lessen or resolve within the first 4 weeks of therapy. Efavirenz is the only antiretroviral drug that is unequivocally teratogenic, causing neural tube defects; thus, women of childbearing potential should use two methods of birth control and avoid pregnancy while taking this drug.

HIV Protease Inhibitors

The HIV protease inhibitors emerged from rational drug design based on the structure of a peptide-enzyme complex. They produce favorable long-term suppression of viremia, elevation of CD4 lymphocyte counts, reduced disease progression, and improved survival when combined with other antiretroviral drugs. These virologic benefits must be balanced against short- and long-term toxicity.

MECHANISM OF ACTION AND RESISTANCE HIV protease inhibitors are peptide-like chemicals that competitively inhibit the action of the virus aspartyl protease. This protease is a homodimer consisting of two 99-amino-acid monomers; each monomer contains an Asp residue that is essential for catalysis. The preferred cleavage site for this enzyme is the N-terminal side of Pro residues, especially between Phe and Pro (Figure 50–5). Human aspartyl proteases contain only one polypeptide chain and are not significantly inhibited by HIV protease inhibitors. These drugs bind reversibly to the active site of the protease and prevent proteolytic cleavage of HIV gag and pol proteins into essential structural and enzymatic components of the virus. This prevents the metamorphosis of HIV virus particles into their mature infectious form. Infected patients treated with HIV protease inhibitors as sole agents experience a 100–1000-fold decrease in plasma HIV RNA concentrations within 12 weeks, an effect similar in magnitude to that produced by NNRTIs.

In patients treated with single protease inhibitors, viral replication in the presence of drug selects for drug resistance. The speed with which HIV develops resistance to protease inhibitors is intermediate between that of nucleoside analogs and NNRTIs, typically with a rebound in HIV RNA levels within 3–4 months. Unlike the NNRTIs, high-level resistance to the protease inhibitors generally requires the accumulation of a minimum of four to five codon substitutions, which may take many months. Primary resistance may result from mutations in the protease-active site that confer resistance only to the specific drug by causing a three- to five-fold decrease in sensitivity. These are followed by secondary mutations, often distant from the active site, that compensate for the reduction in proteolytic efficiency, which often are associated with cross-resistance to multiple HIV protease inhibitors.

Absorption, Distribution, and Elimination The HIV protease inhibitors are all absorbed orally. The absorption of several members is decreased by concomitant use of proton pump inhibitors, suggesting that pH is important. An important shared toxicity for these drugs is the potential for metabolic drug interactions based on their hepatic metabolism (Tables 50–4, 50–5). With the exception of nelfinavir, which is predominantly metabolized by CYP2C19, these drugs are metabolized by and inhibit CYP3A4. The magnitude of this effect varies, with ritonavir by far the most potent. The pharmacokinetic properties of the HIV protease inhibitors also are notable for high interindividual variability, which may reflect differential activity of intestinal and hepatic CYPs. Because of its capacity to inhibit CYP3A4, a low dose of ritonavir is commonly combined with other HIV protease inhibitors to improve their pharmacokinetic profiles by increasing oral bioavailability and prolonging the $t_{1/2}$, often permitting once-daily administration. Following hepatic conversion, these drugs are largely excreted *via* bile in the feces.

Adverse Effects Adverse effects seen commonly with HIV protease inhibitors include nausea and vomiting, anorexia, and diarrhea. Of more consequence, this drug class is frequently associated with the development of lipodystophy, a metabolic syndrome characterized by insulin resistance and dyslipidemia. The long-term impact of the metabolic syndrome on cardiovascular events remains unknown. As a result of their capacity to inhibit CYP3A4 metabolism, protease inhibitors commonly are involved in clinically significant pharmacokinetic drug interactions, and patients and providers must be vigilant for such interactions. These drugs generally should not be coadministered with other CYP3A4 substrates that have a narrow therapeutic index, such as midazolam, triazolam, propafenone, and ergot derivatives.

Specific Drugs

Saquinavir Saquinavir is a peptidomimetic HIV protease inhibitor that inhibits HIV-1 and HIV-2 replication. Of all of the HIV protease inhibitors, saquinavir inhibits CYP3A4 least potently. Typically, saquinavir is administered once or twice daily in combination with ritonavir to improve pharmacokinetics.

Ritonavir Ritonavir is a peptidomimetic HIV protease inhibitor that is active against HIV-1 and HIV-2. Ritonavir is an extremely potent inhibitor of CYP3A4 and is frequently combined with most of the protease inhibitors to enhance their pharmacokinetic profiles and allow a reduction in dose and dosing frequency. Typically, a low dose of ritonavir (100 or 200 mg twice daily) is used, as it is better tolerated and just as effective at inhibiting CYP3A4.

Indinavir Indinavir is a peptidomimetic HIV protease inhibitor that is tenfold more potent against the HIV-1 protease than that of HIV-2. Indinavir is absorbed rapidly after oral administration. Unlike other protease inhibitors, food adversely affects indinavir bioavailability; this can be alleviated by coadministration of ritonavir. Unique adverse effects of indinavir are crystalluria and nephrolithiasis, which stem from its poor solubility; patients should drink at least 2 L of water daily

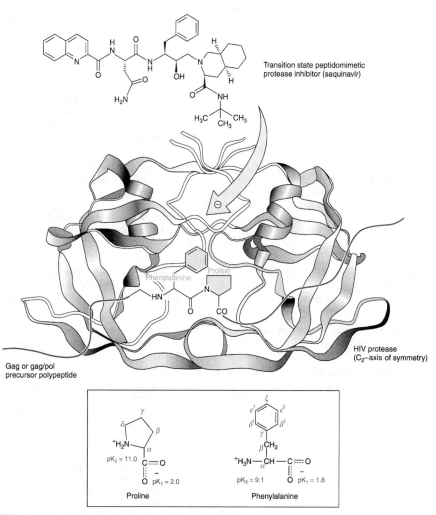

FIGURE 50-5 *Mechanism of action of an HIV protease inhibitor.*

Table 50-4

Drug Interactions Between Nonnucleoside Reverse Transcriptase Inhibitors and HIV Protease Inhibitors*

	Effect of NNRTI on Plasma AUC of PI (% Change)			Effect of PI on Plasma AUC of NNRTI (% Change)		
	Delavirdine	**Nevirapine**	**Efavirenz**	**Delavirdine**	**Nevirapine**	**Efavirenz**
Saquinavir[†]	↑120–400%	↓24–38%	↓62%	↔	↔	↓12%
Indinavir	↑53%	↓31%	↓30–31%	↔	↔	↔
Ritonavir	↑70%	↔	↑18%	↔	↔	↑21%
Nelfinavir	↑107%	↔	↑20%	↓31%	↔	↓12%
Amprenavir	↑130%	NR	↓35%	↓61%	NR	↔
Fosamprenavir	NR	NR	↓13%	NR	NR	NR
Lopinavir[‡]	NR	↓27%	↓19–25%	NR	↑8–9%	↓16
Atazanavir	NR	NR	↓74%	NR	NR	NR

ABBREVIATIONS: NNRTI, nonnucleoside reverse transcriptase inhibitor; PI, HIV protease inhibitor; AUC, area under the plasma concentration–time curve; ↑, increase; ↓, decrease; ↔, no change; NR, not reported.
*Reported mean change in the AUC of the standard dose of the affected drug by the standard dose of the affecting drug; studies using modified dosing regimens were dose-normalized.
†Parameters reported for the saquinavir soft-gel capsule formulation.
‡Lopinavir is only available in a coformulation with ritonavir.

to diminish these complications. Indinavir frequently causes unconjugated hyperbilirubinemia, which is generally asymptomatic and not associated with long-term sequelae. Because indinavir is less soluble at higher pH, antacids or other buffering agents should not be coadministered. Rifampin lowers the indinavir AUC by 90% and is contraindicated, while the dose of rifabutin should be reduced by 50% when coadministered with indinavir.

Nelfinavir Nelfinavir is a nonpeptidic protease inhibitor that is active against HIV-1 and HIV-2. It is absorbed more slowly after oral administration than the other HIV-1 protease inhibitors and is very sensitive to food effects. It undergoes extensive hepatic metabolism, primarily by CYP2C19, to an active metabolite M8. Concomitant use of drugs that induce CYP2C19 may be contraindicated (*e.g.*, rifampin) or may require an increase in the nelfinavir dose (*e.g.*, rifabutin). Although liver disease may prolong the $t_{1/2}$ of the drug, it has been used in HIV-infected patients with significant hepatic dysfunction without evidence of untoward toxicity.

Fosamprenavir Fosamprenavir is a prodrug that is converted to amprenavir, a nonpeptide HIV protease inhibitor; the increased aqueous solubility of the prodrug markedly improves bioavailability. The drug is active against both HIV-1 and HIV-2. Amprenavir is the HIV protease inhibitor that is most likely to produce rash, possibly because it contains a sulfonamide moiety. It generally is combined with ritonavir.

Lopinavir Lopinavir is a peptidomimetic HIV protease inhibitor that is structurally similar to ritonavir and inhibits both HIV-1 and HIV-2. It is only administered in combination with ritonavir, and should be taken with food because oral bioavailability is increased by 50% with a high fat meal.

Atazanavir Atazanavir is a peptide protease inhibitor that is active against both HIV-1 and HIV-2. Absorption is increased by food and it is recommended that the drug be administered with a meal. Absorption may be pH dependent, because proton pump inhibitors substantially reduce drug concentration after oral dosing. Like indinavir, atazanavir frequently causes unconjugated hyperbilirubinemia. The drug may be less likely than other HIV protease inhibitors to cause lipodystrophy.

Tipranavir The FDA recently granted approval for tipranavir, the first member of a new class of nonpeptide inhibitors of the HIV-1 protease, in combination therapy. Although it also binds to the active site of the HIV-1 protease, tipranavir differs in structure from previously available peptidomimetic protease inhibitors and retains activity against HIV-1 isolates that are resistant to other HIV protease inhibitors. Tipranavir, coadministered with ritonavir, is approved for the treatment of HIV-1-infected adults with evidence of viral replication and who have received multiple treatment regimens or have HIV-1 strains resistant to multiple protease inhibitors. As noted in a "black box"

Table 50–5

Drug Interactions Amongst HIV Protease Inhibitors*

Drug Exerting Effect	Drug Affected (Change in Plasma AUC)							
	Saquinavir[†]	Indinavir	Ritonavir	Nelfinavir	Amprenavir	Fosamprenavir	Lopinavir[‡]	Atazanavir
Saquinavir[†]	—	↔	↔	↑18%	↓32%	NR	↔	NR
Indinavir	↑360–620%	—	↔	↑83%	↑33%	NR	↔	NR
Ritonavir	↑1590–1700%	↑320–500%	—	↑150%	↑220–230%	↑110%	↑46%[§]	↑240%
Nelfinavir	↑330–390%	↑51%	↔	—	↔	NR	NR	NR
Amprenavir	↓19%	↓38%	↔	↑15%	—	—	↓15–37%	NR
Fosamprenavir	NR	NR	↔	NR	—	—	↔	NR
Lopinavir[‡]	↑1290–1890%	↑84%	↔	NR	↑180%	↓26%	—	NR
Atazanavir	↑450%	NR	NR	NR	NR	NR	NR	—

ABBREVIATIONS: AUC, area under the plasma concentration–time curve; ↑, increase; ↓, decrease; ↔, no change; NR, not reported.

*Reported mean change in the AUC of the affected drug by the standard dose of the affecting drug; studies using modified dosing regimens were dose-normalized.

[†]Parameters reported for the saquinavir soft-gel capsule formulation.

[‡]Lopinavir is only available in a coformulation with ritonavir.

[§]This represents the impact of additional ritonavir (100 mg bid) on the AUC of lopinavir in the coformulation of 400 mg lopinavir with 100 mg ritonavir bid.

warning, administration of the tipranavir/ritonavir combination has been associated with hepatitis and hepatic decompensation, including fatalities, and special vigilance is indicated in patients with chronic hepatitis B or C coinfection.

Entry Inhibitors

Enfuvirtide is a 36-amino-acid synthetic peptide whose sequence is derived from a part of the transmembrane pg41 region of HIV-1. Enfuvirtide is not active against HIV-2 but has a broad range of potencies against HIV-1 isolates.

MECHANISMS OF ACTION AND RESISTANCE   The peptide blocks the interaction between the N36 and C34 sequences of the gp41 glycoprotein by binding to a hydrophobic groove in the N36 coil. This prevents formation of a six-helix bundle critical for membrane fusion and viral entry into the host cell. Enfuvirtide inhibits infection of CD4 cells by free virus particles, as well as cell-to-cell transmission of HIV-1 in vitro. Because of its unique mechanism of action, enfuvirtide retains activity against viruses that have become resistant to antiretroviral agents of other classes.

HIV-1 can develop resistance to enfuvirtide though specific mutations in the enfuvirtide-binding domain of gp41. Single amino acid substitutions can confer up to 450 times resistance *in vitro*, although high-level clinical resistance is generally associated with two or more amino acid changes.

Absorption, Distribution, and Elimination   Enfuvirtide must be given parentally. Peak concentration after subcutaneous administration occurs on average 4 hours after dosing, with an apparent volume of distribution of 5.5 L. Pharmacokinetics of the subcutaneous drug are not affected by injection site. A deamidated metabolite at the C-terminal Phe is formed in humans, but no other significant metabolites are detected. The mean elimination $t_{1/2}$ is 4 hours, necessitating twice-daily administration. The drug is highly bound by proteins, mainly albumin.

Adverse Effects   The most prominent adverse effects of enfuvirtide are injection site reactions, including pain, erythema, induration, and nodules or cysts. These cause drug discontinuation in ~5% of patients. Use of enfuvirtide has been associated with increased lymphadenopathy and pneumonia. The causal role and underlying mechanism are under investigation.

Therapeutic Use   Enfuvirtide is FDA-approved for use only in treatment-experienced adults who have evidence of HIV-1 replication despite ongoing antiretroviral therapy. Treatment response appears to be much more likely in patients with at least two other active drugs in the regimen, based on history and HIV genotype. Given its cost, inconvenience, and cutaneous toxicity, enfuvirtide is reserved for patients who have failed all other feasible antiretroviral regimens.

CURRENT TREATMENT GUIDELINES

Guidelines for initiating therapy in treatment naïve HIV-infected patients are summarized in Table 50–1. These regulations are based on a consensus assessment of the results of published clinical trials regarding when to initiate treatment, when to change treatment regimens, and which regimens perform best in terms of antiviral efficacy, safety, and tolerability. Practitioners need to be aware that guidelines provide general guidance rather than absolute recommendations for the average uncomplicated patient and may need to be modified based on intercurrent disease, concurrent medications, and other circumstances.

Current treatment guidelines center around two important questions: when to start therapy in treatment-naïve individuals and when to change therapy in individuals who are failing their current regimen. The specific drugs recommended may change as new choices become available. However, *it is likely that future treatment guidelines will continue to be driven by the important principles mentioned earlier; (1) combination therapy in order to prevent the emergence of resistant virus; (2) emphasis on regimen convenience, tolerability, and adherence in order to chronically suppress HIV replication; and (3) the need for life-long treatment under most circumstances.*

For a complete Bibliographical listing see Goodman & Gilman's *The Pharmacological Basis of Therapeutics*, 11th ed., or Goodman & Gilman Online at www.accessmedicine.com.

51

ANTINEOPLASTIC AGENTS

Few categories of medication have a narrower therapeutic index and a greater potential for causing harmful side effects than do the antineoplastic drugs. A thorough understanding of their pharmacology, drug interactions, and clinical pharmacokinetics is essential for safe and effective use. The diversity of agents used to treat neoplastic disease is summarized in Table 51–1. Figure 51–1 shows some of the common targets for chemotherapeutic agents currently used to treat neoplastic disease.

In designing specific regimens for clinical use, many factors must be considered. Drugs are most effective in combination, and may be synergistic because of their biochemical interactions. It is more effective to combine drugs that do not share common mechanisms of resistance and do not overlap in their major toxicities. Cytotoxic drugs should be used as close as possible to their maximum individual doses and should be given as frequently as possible to discourage tumor regrowth and to maximize dose intensity—the dose given per unit time—a key parameter in the success of chemotherapy. Since the tumor cell population in patients with clinically detectable disease exceeds 10^9 cells, and since each cycle of therapy kills <99% of the cells, it is necessary to repeat treatments in multiple cycles to eradicate tumor cells.

THE CELL CYCLE An understanding of cell-cycle kinetics is essential for the proper use of antineoplastic agents (Figure 51–2). Many of the most effective cytotoxic agents damage DNA, and their toxicity is greater during the S, or DNA synthetic, phase of the cell cycle. Others, such as the vinca alkaloids and taxanes, block formation of a functional mitotic spindle in M phase. Human neoplasms that are most susceptible to chemotherapy are those with a high percentage of cells undergoing division. Similarly, normal tissues that proliferate rapidly (*e.g.,* bone marrow, hair follicles, and intestinal epithelium) are most subject to damage by cytotoxic drugs, which often limits their usefulness. Conversely, slowly growing tumors with a small growth fraction (*e.g.,* carcinomas of the colon or non–small cell lung cancer) often are less responsive to cycle-specific drugs. *Understanding of cell-cycle kinetics and the controls of normal and malignant cell growth is crucial to the design of current therapeutic regimens and the search for new drugs.*

ACHIEVING THERAPEUTIC BALANCE AND EFFICACY The treatment of most cancer patients requires a skillful interdigitation of multiple treatment modalities, including surgery and irradiation, with drugs. Each of these forms of treatment carries its own risks and benefits. Not all drug regimens are appropriate for all patients, and factors such as renal and hepatic function, bone marrow reserve, general performance status, and concurrent medical problems must be considered. Beyond those considerations, however, are less quantifiable factors such as the likely natural history of the tumor being treated, the patient's willingness to undergo difficult and potentially dangerous treatments, the patient's physical and emotional tolerance for side effects, and the likely long-term gains and risks involved.

One of the greatest challenges of therapeutics is to adjust dose to achieve a therapeutic, but nontoxic, outcome. While it is customary to base dose on body surface area for individual patients, dose adjustment based on renal function or on pharmacokinetic monitoring can meet specific targets such as desired drug concentration in plasma or area under the concentration–time curve (AUC), a measure of tissue exposure. For example, thrombocytopenia caused by *carboplatin* is a direct function of AUC, which in turn is determined by renal clearance of the parent drug. Basic pharmacokinetic principles can be thus used to achieve a desired AUC for carboplatin based on creatinine clearance. Similarly, therapeutic success during high-dose therapy for pediatric acute lymphoblastic leukemia (ALL) is related to achieving targeted methotrexate concentrations in plasma. Monitoring of steady-state levels of methotrexate allows dose adjustment and improves outcome.

Molecular tests increasingly are used to identify patients likely to benefit from treatment and those at highest risk of toxicity. Pretreatment testing to select patients for response to treatment is standard practice for hormonal therapy of breast cancer and for treatment with antibodies such as

Table 51–1

Chemotherapeutic Agents Useful in Neoplastic Disease

Class/Type of agent	Nonproprietary names (other names)	Disease*
Alkylating agents		
Nitrogen mustards	Mechlorethamine	Hodgkin's disease; non-Hodgkin's lymphoma
	Cyclophosphamide	Acute and chronic lymphocytic leukemia; Hodgkin's disease; non-Hodgkin's lymphoma; multiple myeloma; neuroblastoma; breast, ovary, lung cancer; Wilms' tumor; cervix, testis cancer; soft-tissue sarcoma
	Ifosfamide	
	Melphalan (L-sarcolysin)	Multiple myeloma; breast, ovarian cancer
	Chlorambucil	Chronic lymphocytic leukemia; primary macroglobulinemia; Hodgkin's disease; non-Hodgkin's lymphoma
Ethyleneimines and methylmelamines	Altretamine	Ovarian cancer
	Thiotepa	Bladder, breast, ovarian cancer
Methylhydrazine derivative	Procarbazine (*N*-methylhydrazine, MIH)	Hodgkin's disease
Alkyl sulfonate	Busulfan	Chronic myelogenous leukemia
Nitrosoureas	Carmustine (BCNU)	Hodgkin's disease; non-Hodgkin's lymphoma; primary brain tumor; melanoma
	Streptozocin (streptozotocin)	Malignant pancreatic insulinoma; malignant carcinoid
Triazenes	Dacarbazine (DTIC; dimethyltriazenoimidazole carboxamide), temozolomide	Malignant melanoma; Hodgkin's disease; soft-tissue sarcomas; glioma; melanoma
Platinum coordination complexes	Cisplatin, carboplatin, oxaliplatin	Testicular, ovarian, bladder, esophageal, lung, colon cancer
Antimetabolites		
Folic acid analogs	Methotrexate (amethopterin)	Acute lymphocytic leukemia; choriocarcinoma; breast, head, neck, and lung cancer; osteogenic sarcoma; bladder cancer
	Pemetrexed	Mesothelioma, lung cancer
Pyrimidine analogs	Fluorouracil (5-fluorouracil, 5-FU), capecitabine	Breast, colon, esophageal, stomach, pancreas, head and neck; premalignant skin lesion (topical)
	Cytarabine (cytosine arabinoside)	Acute myelogenous and acute lymphocytic leukemia; non-Hodgkin's lymphoma
	Gemcitabine	Pancreatic, ovarian, lung cancer
Purine analogs and related inhibitors	Mercaptopurine (6-mercaptopurine, 6-MP)	Acute lymphocytic and myelogenous leukemia
	Pentostatin (2'-deoxycoformycin), cladribine, fludarabine	Hairy cell leukemia; chronic lymphocytic leukemia; small cell non-Hodgkin's lymphoma

854

Natural and semi-synthetic products

Vinca alkaloids	Vinblastine, vinorelbine	Hodgkin's disease; non-Hodgkin's lymphoma: breast, lung, and testis cancer
	Vincristine	Acute lymphocytic leukemia; neuroblastoma; Wilms' tumor; rhabdomyosarcoma; Hodgkin's disease; non-Hodgkin's lymphoma
Taxanes	Paclitaxel, docetaxel	Ovarian, breast, lung, bladder, head and neck cancer
Epipodophyllotoxins	Etoposide	Testis, small-cell lung, and other lung cancer; breast cancer; Hodgkin's disease; non-Hodgkin's lymphomas; acute myelogenous leukemia; Kaposi's sarcoma
	Teniposide	Same as etoposide; acute lymphoblastic leukemia in children
Camptothecins	Topotecan, irinotecan	Ovarian cancer; small-cell lung cancer; colon and lung cancer
Antibiotics	Dactinomycin (actinomycin D)	Choriocarcinoma; Wilms' tumor; rhabdomyosarcoma; testis; Kaposi's sarcoma
	Daunorubicin (daunomycin, rubidomycin)	Acute myelogenous and acute lymphocytic leukemia
	Doxorubicin	Soft-tissue, osteogenic, and other sarcoma; Hodgkin's disease; non-Hodgkin's lymphoma; acute leukemia; breast, genitourinary, thyroid, lung, stomach cancer; neuroblastoma and other childhood sarcomas
Anthracenedione	Mitoxantrone	Acute myelogenous leukemia; breast and prostate cancer
	Bleomycin	Testis, and cervical cancer; Hodgkin's disease; non-Hodgkin's lymphoma
	Mitomycin (mitomycin C)	Stomach, anal, and lung cancer
Enzyme	L-Asparaginase	Acute lymphocytic leukemia
Miscellaneous agents		
Substituted urea	Hydroxyurea	Chronic myelogenous leukemia; polycythemia vera; essential thrombocytosis
Differentiating agents	Tretinoin, arsenic trioxide	Acute promyelocytic leukemia
Protein tyrosine kinase inhibitors	Imatinib	Chronic myelocytic leukemia; GI stromal tumors; hypereosinophilia syndrome
	Gefitinib, erlotinib	Non-small-cell lung cancer
	Sunitinib	GI stromal tumors, advanced renal cell carcinoma
Proteasome inhibitor	Bortezomib	Multiple myeloma

(Continued)

855

Table 51–1

Chemotherapeutic Agents Useful in Neoplastic Disease (*Continued*)

Class/Type of agent	Nonproprietary names (other names)	Disease*
Biological response modifiers	Interferon-alfa, interleukin 2	Hairy cell leukemia; Kaposi's sarcoma; melanoma; carcinoid; renal cell; ovary; bladder; non-Hodgkin's lymphoma; mycosis fungoides; multiple myeloma; chronic myelogenous leukemia; malignant melanoma
Antibodies**		
Hormones and antagonists		
Adrenocortical suppressants	Mitotane (*o,p*′-DDD)	Adrenal cortex cancer
	Aminoglutethimide	Breast cancer
Adrenocorticosteroids	Prednisone, others†*	Acute and chronic lymphocytic leukemia; non-Hodgkin's lymphoma; Hodgkin's disease; breast cancer
Progestins	Hydroxyprogesterone caproate, medroxy-progesterone acetate, megestrol acetate	Endometrial, breast cancer
Estrogens	Diethylstilbestrol, ethinyl estradiol†	Breast, prostate cancer
Anti-estrogens	Tamoxifen, toremifene	Breast cancer
Aromatase inhibitors	Anastrozole, letrozole, exemestane	Breast cancer
Androgens	Testosterone propionate, fluoxymesterone, others††	Breast cancer
Anti-androgen	Flutamide, bicalutamide	Prostate cancer
GnRH analog	Leuprolide	Prostate cancer

*Neoplasms are carcinomas unless otherwise indicated. **See Table 51–3 and 51–4. †See Chapter 57. ††See Chapter 58. †*See Chapter 59.

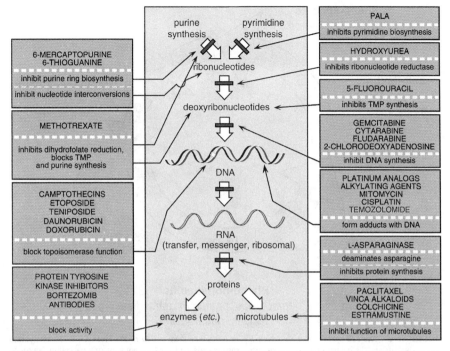

FIGURE 51-1 *Summary of the mechanisms and sites of action of some chemotherapeutic agents useful in neoplastic disease.* PALA = *N*-phosphonoacetyl-L-aspartate; TMP = thymidine monophosphate.

trastuzumab *(her-2/neu receptor)* and rituximab *(CD20). However, in the use of traditional cytotoxic therapy, molecular testing has not been routinely employed. Inherited differences in protein sequence or expression levels (polymorphisms) occur commonly in the population, and affect either toxicity or response. In* 5-fluorouracil *therapy, polymorphisms of drug target genes affect response rates and toxicity. Tandem repeats in the promoter region of the gene encoding thymidylate synthase (TS), the target of 5-fluorouracil, determine the level of expression of the enzyme. Increased numbers of repeats are associated with increased gene expression, a lower incidence of toxicity, and a decreased rate of response in patients with colorectal cancer. Polymorphisms of the dihydropyrimidine dehydrogenase (DPD) gene, which degrades 5-fluorouracil, are associated with decreased enzyme activity and a significant risk of overwhelming drug toxicity, particularly in the rare homozygous individual. Other polymorphisms appear to affect the clearance and therapeutic activity of cancer drugs, including methotrexate, irinotecan, and* 6-mercaptopurine *(see below).*

Specific activating mutations in the epidermal growth factor receptor (EGFR) gene in patients with lung cancer are associated with a high rate of response to the EGFR inhibitor gefitinib. Molecular tests to select patients for specific treatments undoubtedly will shorten the required time for drug testing and approval, improve the outcome of cancer therapy, and realize savings in the cost and toxicity of ineffective drugs.

Despite efforts to anticipate the development of complications, anticancer agents have variable pharmacokinetics and toxicity in individual patients. The causes of this variability are not always clear and often may be related to interindividual differences in drug metabolism, drug interactions, or bone marrow reserves. In dealing with toxicity, the physician must provide vigorous supportive care, including, where indicated, platelet transfusions, antibiotics, and hematopoietic growth factors (*see* Chapter 53). Other delayed toxicities affecting the heart, lungs, or kidneys may lead to permanent organ damage or death. Fortunately, such toxicities can be minimized by adherence to standardized protocols and guidelines for drug use. Clinical practice guidelines for many antineoplastic drugs can be obtained at the National Comprehensive Cancer Network web site (www.nccn.org/ professionals/physician_gls/default.asp).

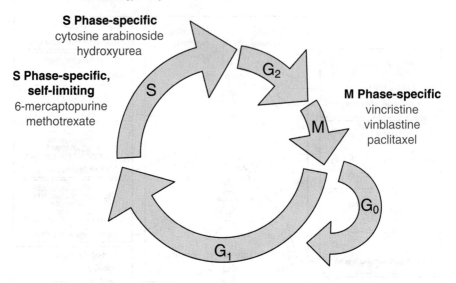

S Phase-specific
cytosine arabinoside
hydroxyurea

S Phase-specific,
self-limiting
6-mercaptopurine
methotrexate

M Phase-specific
vincristine
vinblastine
paclitaxel

Phase-nonspecific
alkylating drugs, nitrosoureas, antitumor antibodies, procarbazine,
cisplatin, dacarbazine

FIGURE 51–2 *The cell cycle and the relationship of antitumor drug action to the cycle.* G_1 is the gap period between mitosis and the beginning of DNA synthesis. Resting cells (cells that are not preparing for cell division) are said to be in a subphase of G_1, G_0. S is the period of DNA synthesis, G_2 the premitotic interval, and M the period of mitosis. Examples of cell cycle–dependent anticancer drugs are listed in *blue* below the phase in which they act. Drugs that are cytotoxic for cells at any point in the cycle are called phase–nonspecific drugs.

I. ALKYLATING AGENTS

In 1942, Goodman, Gilman, and colleagues launched the modern era of cancer chemotherapy with clinical studies of several nitrogen mustards in patients with lymphoma. At present five major types of alkylating agents are used in the chemotherapy of neoplastic diseases: (1) the nitrogen mustards, (2) the ethyleneimines, (3) the alkyl sulfonates, (4) the nitrosoureas, and (5) the triazenes. The methylhydrazine and platinum complexes also are included here, even though they do not formally alkylate DNA and use a different means to form covalent adducts with DNA.

Pharmacological Actions

The most important pharmacological actions of the alkylating agents are those that disturb DNA synthesis and cell division (Figure 51–3). The capacity of these drugs to interfere with DNA integrity and function and to induce cell death in rapidly proliferating tissues provides the basis for their therapeutic and toxic properties. Whereas certain alkylating agents may have damaging effects on tissues with normally low mitotic indices—for example, liver, kidney, and mature lymphocytes—effects in these tissues usually are delayed. Acute effects are manifest primarily against rapidly proliferating tissues. Lethality of DNA alkylation depends on recognition of the adduct, creation of DNA strand breaks by repair enzymes, and an intact apoptotic response.

In normal nondividing cells, DNA damage activates a checkpoint that blocks cell-cycle progression at the G_1/S interface allowing cells to either repair DNA alkylation or undergo apoptosis. Malignant cells with mutant or absent p53 fail to suspend cell-cycle progression, do not undergo apoptosis, and are resistant to these drugs.

While DNA is the ultimate target of all alkylating agents, there is a crucial distinction between the bifunctional agents, in which cytotoxic effects predominate, and the monofunctional methylat-

A   Activation

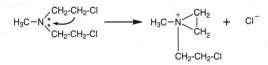

B   Nucleophilic attack
of unstable aziridine ring by electron donor
(–S̈H of protein, –N̈– of protein or DNA base,
=Ö of DNA base or phosphate)

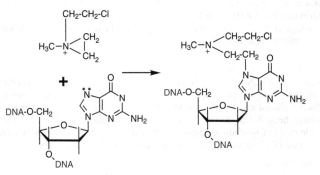

FIGURE 51–3 *Mechanism of action of alkylating agents.*

ing agents (procarbazine, temozolomide), which have greater capacity for mutagenesis and carcinogenesis. This suggests that cross-linking of DNA strands is a much greater threat to cellular survival than effects such as single-base alkylation and the resulting depurination and chain scission. On the other hand, the more frequent methylation may be bypassed by DNA polymerases, leading to mispairing reactions that permanently modify DNA sequence. These new sequences are transmitted to subsequent generations, and may result in mutagenesis or carcinogenesis. Some methylating agents, such as procarbazine, are highly carcinogenic.

Mechanisms of Resistance to Alkylating Agents

Resistance to an alkylating agent develops rapidly when used as a single agent. Specific biochemical changes implicated in the development of resistance include:

1. Decreased permeation of actively transported drugs (mechlorethamine and melphalan);
2. Increased intracellular concentrations of nucleophilic substances, principally thiols such as glutathione, which can conjugate with and detoxify electrophilic intermediates;
3. Increased activity of DNA repair pathways, which may differ for the various alkylating agents. Thus, increased activity of the complex nucleotide excision repair (NER) pathway seems to correlate with resistance to most chloroethyl and platinum adducts. Alkyl guanine transferase (AGT) activity determines response to BCNU and to methylating drugs such as the triazenes, procarbazine, and busulfan;
4. Increased rates of metabolism of the activated forms of cyclophosphamide and ifosfamide to their inactive keto and carboxy metabolites by aldehyde dehydrogenase.

TOXICITIES OF ALKYLATING AGENTS
Bone Marrow Toxicity

The alkylating agents differ in their patterns of antitumor activity and in the sites and severity of their side effects. Most cause dose-limiting toxicity to bone marrow and intestinal mucosa. Most alkylating agents, including nitrogen mustard, melphalan, chlorambucil, cyclophosphamide, and ifosfamide, cause acute myelosuppression, with a nadir of the peripheral blood granulocyte count at 6–10 days and recovery in 14–21 days. Cyclophosphamide has lesser effects on peripheral blood platelet counts than do the other agents. Busulfan suppresses all blood elements, particularly stem cells, and may produce a prolonged and cumulative myelosuppression lasting months or even years. For this reason, it is used in preparation for allogeneic bone marrow transplantation. Carmustine and other chloroethylnitrosoureas cause delayed and prolonged suppression of both platelets and granulocytes, reaching a nadir 4–6 weeks after drug administration and reversing slowly thereafter. Both cellular and humoral immunity are suppressed by alkylating agents, which have been used to treat various autoimmune diseases. Immunosuppression is reversible at doses used in most anticancer protocols.

Mucosal Toxicity

Alkylating agents are highly toxic to dividing mucosal cells, leading to oral mucosal ulceration and intestinal denudation. The mucosal effects are particularly significant in high-dose chemotherapy protocols associated with bone marrow reconstitution, as they predispose to bacterial sepsis arising from the gastrointestinal (GI) tract. In these protocols, cyclophosphamide, melphalan, and thiotepa have the advantage of causing less mucosal damage than the other agents. In high-dose protocols, a number of additional toxicities become limiting (Table 51–2).

Neurotoxicity

Central nervous system (CNS) toxicity is manifest by nausea and vomiting, particularly after intravenous administration of nitrogen mustard or BCNU. Ifosfamide is the most neurotoxic of these agents, producing altered mental status, coma, generalized seizures, and cerebellar ataxia. These side effects have been linked to the release of chloroacetaldehyde from the phosphate-linked chloroethyl side chain of ifosfamide. High-dose busulfan may cause seizures; in addition, it accelerates the clearance of *phenytoin*, an antiseizure medication (*see* Chapter 19).

Other Organ Toxicities

While bone marrow and mucosal toxicities occur predictably and acutely, other organ toxicities may occur after prolonged or high-dose use; these effects can appear after months or years, and may be irreversible and even lethal. All alkylating agents can cause pulmonary fibrosis, usually several months after treatment. In high-dose regimens, particularly those employing busulfan or BCNU, vascular endothelial damage may precipitate veno-occlusive disease (VOD) of the liver, an often-fatal side effect that may be reversed by the investigational drug defibrotide. After multiple cycles of therapy, the nitrosoureas and ifosfamide may lead to renal failure. Cyclophosphamide and ifosfamide release a nephrotoxic and urotoxic metabolite, acrolein, which causes a severe hemorrhagic cystitis; in high-dose regimens, this side effect can be prevented by coadministration of 2-mercaptoethanesulfonate (mesna or MESNEX), which conjugates acrolein. Ifosfamide in high doses for transplant causes a chronic, and often irreversible, renal toxicity. Proximal, and less commonly distal, tubules may be affected, with impaired Ca^{2+} and Mg^{2+} reabsorption, glycosuria, and

Table 51–2

Dose-Limiting Extramedullary Toxicities of Single Alkylating Agents

Drug	MTD,* mg/m²	Fold Increase Over Standard Dose	Major Organ Toxicities
Cyclophosphamide	7000	7	Cardiac, hepatic VOD
Ifosfamide	16,000	2.7	Renal, CNS, hepatic VOD
Thiotepa	1000	18	GI, CNS, hepatic VOD
Melphalan	180	5.6	GI, hepatic VOD
Busulfan	640	9	GI, hepatic VOD
Carmustine (BCNU)	1050	5.3	Lung, hepatic VOD
Cisplatin	200	2	PN, renal
Carboplatin	2000	5	Renal, PN, hepatic VOD

*Maximum tolerated dose (MTD; cumulative) in treatment protocols.

ABBREVIATIONS: GI, gastrointestinal; CNS, central nervous system; PN, peripheral neuropathy; VOD, veno-occlusive disease.

renal tubular acidosis. Nephrotoxicity is correlated with the total dose of drug received and increases in frequency in children <5 years of age. The syndrome has been attributed to chloroacetaldehyde and/or acrolein excreted in the urine. The more unstable alkylating agents (e.g., mechlorethamine and the nitrosoureas) have strong vesicant properties, damage veins with repeated use, and produce ulceration if extravasated. Most alkylating agents cause alopecia. Finally, all alkylating agents have toxic effects on the male and female reproductive systems, causing premature ovarian failure in women and irreversible azoospermia in men.

Leukemogenesis

The alkylating agents are highly leukemogenic. Acute nonlymphocytic leukemia, often associated with partial or total deletions of chromosome 5 or 7, peaks in incidence about 4 years after therapy and may affect 5% of patients treated with regimens containing alkylating drugs. It often is preceded by a period of neutropenia or anemia, and bone marrow morphology consistent with myelodysplasia. Melphalan, the nitrosoureas, and the methylating agent procarbazine have the greatest propensity to cause leukemia, which is less common with cyclophosphamide.

CLINICAL PHARMACOLOGY
Nitrogen Mustards

The unique pharmacological characteristics of the individual agents are considered here.

MECHLORETHAMINE Mechlorethamine was the first clinically used nitrogen mustard and is the most reactive drug in this class.

Severe local reactions of exposed tissues necessitate rapid intravenous injection of mechlorethamine for most uses. In either water or body fluids, at rates affected markedly by pH, mechlorethamine rapidly undergoes chemical degradation as it combines with either water or cellular nucleophiles, and the parent compound disappears within minutes from the bloodstream.

Mechlorethamine HCl (MUSTARGEN) was formerly used primarily in the combination chemotherapy regimen MOPP (mechlorethamine, *vincristine* [ONCOVIN], procarbazine, and *prednisone*) in patients with Hodgkin's disease. It is given by intravenous bolus administration in doses of 6 mg/m^2 on days 1 and 8 of the 28-day cycles of each course of treatment. Mechlorethamine is used topically for treatment of cutaneous T-cell lymphoma as a solution that is rapidly mixed and applied to affected areas of skin. Mechlorethamine has been largely replaced by cyclophosphamide, melphalan, and other more stable alkylating agents.

The major acute toxic manifestations of mechlorethamine are nausea and vomiting, lacrimation, and myelosuppression. Leukopenia and thrombocytopenia limit the amount of drug that can be given in a single course. Like other alkylating agents, mechlorethamine blocks reproductive function and may produce premature ovarian failure in women and oligospermia in men. Since fetal abnormalities can be induced, this drug should not be used in the first trimester of pregnancy and should only be used with caution in later stages of pregnancy. Breast-feeding must be stopped before therapy with mechlorethamine is initiated.

Local reactions to extravasation of mechlorethamine into the subcutaneous tissue result in a severe and persistent induration. If it is obvious that extravasation has occurred, the involved area should be promptly infiltrated with a sterile isotonic solution of sodium thiosulfate (167 mM), which reacts avidly with nitrogen mustard and thereby protects tissue constituents. An ice compress then should be applied intermittently for 6–12 hours.

CYCLOPHOSPHAMIDE The cytotoxic action of this drug is similar to that of other alkylating agents. The drug is not a vesicant, and produces no local irritation. Cyclophosphamide is well absorbed orally and is activated by CYP2B to 4-hydroxycyclophosphamide, which is in a steady state with the acyclic tautomer aldophosphamide. A closely related oxazaphosphorine, ifosfamide, is hydroxylated by CYP3A4. This difference may account for the somewhat slower activation of ifosfamide *in vivo*, and the interpatient variability in toxicity of both molecules. The rate of metabolic activation of cyclophosphamide varies considerably and increases with successive doses in high-dose regimens, but appears to be saturable above infusion rates of 4 g/90 min and concentrations of parent compound >150 μM. 4-Hydroxycyclophosphamide may be oxidized further by aldehyde oxidase, either in liver or in tumor tissue, and perhaps by other enzymes, yielding the inactive metabolites carboxyphosphamide and 4-ketocyclophosphamide; ifosfamide is inactivated in an analogous reaction. The active cyclophosphamide metabolites (e.g., 4-hydroxycyclophosphamide and aldophosphamide) are carried in the circulation to tumor cells, where aldophosphamide cleaves spontaneously, stoichiometrically generating phosphoramide mustard and acrolein. Phosphoramide mustard is responsible for antitumor effects, while acrolein causes hemorrhagic cystitis often seen during therapy with cyclophosphamide.

Ample fluid intake is recommended for routine clinical use, and vigorous intravenous hydration is required during high-dose treatment. Brisk hematuria in a patient receiving daily oral therapy should lead to immediate drug discontinuation. Refractory bladder hemorrhage may require cystectomy for control of bleeding.

The syndrome of inappropriate secretion of antidiuretic hormone has been observed in patients receiving cyclophosphamide, usually at doses >50 mg/kg (see Chapter 29). Since these patients usually are vigorously hydrated to prevent bladder toxicity, water intoxication is a possibility.

Pretreatment with cytochrome (CYP) inducers such as phenobarbital enhances the rate of activation of the azoxyphosphorenes but does not alter total exposure to active metabolites over time and does not affect toxicity or efficacy. Cyclophosphamide is eliminated by hepatic metabolism and can be used at full doses in patients with renal insufficiency. Maximal concentrations in plasma are achieved 1 hour after oral administration; the $t_{1/2}$ of parent drug in plasma is ~7 hours.

Cyclophosphamide (CYTOXAN, NEOSAR, others) is administered orally or intravenously. Recommended doses vary widely; published protocols for the dosage of cyclophosphamide and other chemotherapeutic agents and for the method and sequence of administration should be consulted. As a single agent, a daily oral dose of 100 mg/m² for 14 days has been recommended as adjuvant therapy for breast cancer, and for patients with lymphomas and chronic lymphocytic leukemia (CLL). A higher dosage of 500 mg/m² intravenously every 2–4 weeks in combination with other drugs often is employed in the treatment of breast cancer and lymphomas. The neutrophil nadir of 500–1000 cells/mm³ generally serves as a guide to dosage adjustments in prolonged therapy. In regimens associated with bone marrow or peripheral stem cell rescue, cyclophosphamide may be given in total doses of 5–7 g/m² over a 3–5-day period. GI ulceration, cystitis (counteracted by mesna and diuresis), and less commonly, pulmonary, renal, hepatic, and cardiac toxicities may occur after therapy with total doses >200 mg/kg.

The clinical spectrum of activity for cyclophosphamide is very broad. It is a component of many effective drug combinations for non-Hodgkin's lymphomas, ovarian cancers, and solid tumors in children. Complete remissions and cures have been reported when cyclophosphamide was given as a single agent for Burkitt's lymphoma. It frequently is used in combination with methotrexate (or *doxorubicin*) and fluorouracil as adjuvant therapy after surgery for breast cancer.

Because of its potent immunosuppressive properties, cyclophosphamide has been used to prevent organ rejection after transplantation. It has activity in nonneoplastic disorders, including Wegener's granulomatosis, rheumatoid arthritis, and nephrotic syndrome. Caution is advised when the drug is considered for these conditions, both because of its acute toxic effects and because of its potential for inducing sterility, teratogenic effects, and leukemia.

IFOSFAMIDE Ifosfamide (IFEX), an analog of cyclophosphamide, also is activated by ring hydroxylation in the liver. Severe urinary tract and CNS toxicity initially limited the use of ifosfamide, but adequate hydration and coadministration of mesna have reduced its bladder toxicity. Ifosfamide is approved for use in combination for germ cell testicular cancer and is widely used to treat pediatric and adult sarcomas. It is a common component of high-dose chemotherapy regimens with bone marrow or stem cell rescue; in these regimens, in total doses of 12–14 g/m², it may cause severe neurological toxicity, including hallucinations, coma, and death, with symptoms appearing 12 hours to 7 days after starting the ifosfamide infusion; this toxicity may result from chloroacetaldehyde. Although clinical experience is limited, administration of methylene blue, 50 mg, the day before ifosfamide and 3 times/day during drug infusion, lowers the incidence of neurotoxicity from 30% to near zero. Ifosfamide also causes nausea, vomiting, anorexia, leukopenia, nephrotoxicity, and VOD of the liver.

In nonmyeloablative regimens, ifosfamide is infused intravenously over at least 30 minutes at a dose of up to 1.2 g/m²/day for 5 days. Intravenous mesna is given as bolus injections in a dose equal to 20% of the ifosfamide dose concomitantly and again 4 and 8 hours later, for a total mesna dose of 60% of the ifosfamide dose. Alternatively, mesna may be given concomitantly in a single dose equal to the ifosfamide dose. Patients also should receive at least 2 L of oral or intravenous fluid daily. Treatment cycles usually are repeated every 3–4 weeks.

Ifosfamide has a plasma elimination $t_{1/2}$ of ~15 hours after doses of 3.8–5 g/m² and a somewhat shorter $t_{1/2}$ at lower doses, although its pharmacokinetics are highly variable due to variable rates *of hepatic metabolism. Ifosfamide has virtually the same toxicity profile as cyclophosphamide, although it causes greater platelet suppression, neurotoxicity, nephrotoxicity, and in the absence of mesna, urothelial damage.*

MELPHALAN The pharmacology of melphalan, the Phe derivative of nitrogen mustard, is similar to that of mechlorethamine. The drug is not a vesicant. When given orally, melphalan absorption is incomplete and variable, and 20–50% of the drug is recovered in the stool. The drug has a $t_{1/2}$ in plasma of ~45–90 minutes, and 10–15% of the dose is excreted unchanged in the urine. Patients with decreased renal function may develop unexpectedly severe myelosuppression. Oral *melphalan* (ALKERAN) for multiple myeloma (MM) is used in doses of 6–8 mg daily for a period of 4 days, in combination with other agents. A rest period of up to 4 weeks should then intervene. The usual intravenous dose is 15 mg/m^2 infused over 15–20 minutes. Doses are repeated at 2-week intervals for 4 doses and then at 4–week intervals based on response and tolerance. Dosage adjustments should be considered based on blood cell counts and in patients with renal impairment. Melphalan in a dose of 180–200 mg/m^2 also may be used in myeloablative regimens for bone marrow or peripheral blood stem cell reconstitution. The toxicity of melphalan is mostly hematological and similar to that of other alkylating agents. Nausea and vomiting are less frequent. Alopecia does not occur at standard doses, and changes in renal or hepatic function have not been observed.

CHLORAMBUCIL The cytotoxic effects of chlorambucil on bone marrow, lymphoid organs, and epithelial tissues are similar to those observed with the nitrogen mustards. As an orally administered agent, chlorambucil is well tolerated in small daily doses, and provides flexible titration of blood counts. Nausea and vomiting may result from single oral doses of 20 mg or more. Oral absorption of chlorambucil is adequate and reliable. The drug has a $t_{1/2}$ in plasma of ~1.5 hours; it is almost completely metabolized to phenyl acetic acid mustard and decomposition products. In treating CLL, the standard initial daily dosage of chlorambucil (LEUKERAN) is 0.1–0.2 mg/kg, given once daily and continued for 3–6 weeks. With a fall in the peripheral total leukocyte count or clinical improvement, the dosage is titrated to maintain neutrophils and platelets at acceptable levels. Maintenance therapy (usually 2 mg daily) often is required to maintain clinical remission. It is a standard agent for patients with CLL and Waldenström's macroglobulinemia, and may be used for follicular lymphoma. In CLL, chlorambucil may be given orally for months or years, achieving its effects gradually and often without significant toxicity to a compromised bone marrow. Although it is possible to induce marked hypoplasia of the bone marrow with excessive doses of chlorambucil over long periods, its myelosuppressive action usually is moderate, gradual, and rapidly reversible. GI discomfort, azoospermia, amenorrhea, pulmonary fibrosis, seizures, dermatitis, and hepatotoxicity may rarely be encountered. A marked increase in the incidence of acute myelocytic leukemia (AML) and other tumors was noted in a large controlled study of its use for the treatment of polycythemia vera and in patients with breast cancer receiving chlorambucil as adjuvant chemotherapy.

MISCELLANEOUS ALKYLATING DRUGS

While nitrogen mustards containing chlorethyl groups constitute the most widely used class of alkylating agents, alternative structures with greater chemical stability and defined activity in specific types of cancer continue to have value in clinical practice.

Ethyleneimines and Methylmelamines

ALTRETAMINE Altretamine (HEXALEN), formerly known as hexamethylmelamine, is structurally similar to the alkylating agent triethylenemelamine (*tretamine*), but its precise mechanism of action is unknown. It is used as a palliative treatment for persistent or recurrent ovarian cancer following treatment failure with a cisplatin- or alkylating agent–based combination. The usual dose of altretamine as a single agent in ovarian cancer is 260 mg/m^2 daily in four divided doses, for 14 or 21 consecutive days out of a 28-day cycle, for up to 12 cycles. Following oral administration, altretamine is well absorbed from the GI tract and undergoes rapid demethylation in the liver. Peak plasma levels, which vary widely, are reached between 0.5 and 3 hours. The principal metabolites are pentamethylmelamine and tetramethylmelamine, which are highly bound to plasma proteins (75% and 50%, respectively) and excreted *via* the urine. The elimination $t_{1/2}$ is 4–10 hours.

The main toxicities of altretamine are myelosuppression and neurotoxicity. Altretamine causes both peripheral and central neurotoxicity. CNS symptoms include ataxia, depression, confusion, drowsiness, hallucinations, dizziness, and vertigo. Neurological toxicity appears to be reversible *upon drug discontinuation and may be prevented or decreased by concomitant administration of pyridoxine. Peripheral blood counts and a neurologic examination should be performed before each course of therapy. Therapy should be interrupted for at least 14 days, and subsequently restarted at a lower dose of 200 mg/m² daily, if the white cell count is <2000 cells/mm³ or the platelet count is <75,000 cells/mm³ or if neurotoxic or intolerable GI symptoms occur. If neurologic symptoms fail to stabilize on the reduced dose schedule, altretamine should be discontinued. Nausea and vomiting also are common and may be dose-limiting. Renal toxicity also may be dose-limiting. Rare adverse effects include rashes, alopecia, and hepatic toxicity. Severe, life-threatening orthostatic hypotension developed in patients who received tricylic antidepressants concurrently with altretamine.*

THIOTEPA Thiotepa (THIOPLEX) is composed of three ethyleneimine groups stabilized by attachment to the nucleophilic thiophosphoryl base. Its current use is primarily for high-dose chemotherapy regimens. Both thiotepa and its desulfurated primary metabolite, triethylenephosphoramide (TEPA), to which it is rapidly converted by hepatic CYPs, form DNA cross-links. The aziridine rings open after protonation of the ring-nitrogen, forming a reactive molecule. TEPA becomes the predominant form of the drug in plasma within hours of thiotepa administration. The parent compound has a plasma $t_{1/2}$ of 1.2–2 hours, as compared to a longer $t_{1/2}$ of 3–24 hours for TEPA. Thiotepa pharmacokinetics are essentially the same in children as in adults at conventional doses (up to 80 mg/m²), and drug and metabolite half-lives are unchanged in children receiving high-dose therapy of 300 mg/m²/day for 3 days. Less than 10% of the administered drug appears in urine as the parent drug or the primary metabolite. Multiple secondary metabolites and chemical degradation products account for the remainder of parent.

The toxicities of thiotepa include myelosuppression, and to a lesser extent mucositis. Myelosuppression tends to develop somewhat later than with cyclophosphamide, with leukopenic nadirs at 2 weeks and platelet nadirs at 3 weeks. In high-dose regimens, thiotepa produces neurotoxic symptoms, including coma and seizures.

Alkyl Sulfonates

BUSULFAN Busulfan exerts few pharmacological actions other than myelosuppression at conventional doses and often was used in the chronic phase of chronic myelogenous leukemia (CML) to suppress granulocyte counts. In some patients, a severe and prolonged pancytopenia resulted. In high-dose regimens, pulmonary fibrosis, GI mucosal damage, and VOD of the liver become important. Busulfan is well absorbed after oral administration in doses of 2–6 mg/day, and has a plasma $t_{1/2}$ of 2–3 hours. The drug is conjugated to glutathione by glutathione S-transferase A1A and further degraded by CYP-dependent pathways; its major urinary metabolite is methane sulfonic acid. Children <18 years of age clear the drug 2–4 times faster than adults, and tolerate higher doses. A dose of 40 mg/m² given every 6 hours for 4 days has been suggested for children weighing <20 kg. An intravenous preparation is available for high-dose regimens. There is significant variability in busulfan clearance among patients. VOD is associated with high AUC and peak drug levels (AUC >1500 μM x min) and slow clearance, leading to recommendations for dose adjustment based on drug level monitoring. A target of C_{ss} = 600–900 ng/mL in adults or AUC <1000 μM × min in children appears to achieve an appropriate balance between toxicity and therapeutic benefit.

In treating CML, the initial oral dose of busulfan (MYLERAN, BUSULFEX) varies with the total leukocyte count and the severity of the disease; daily doses from 2 to 8 mg for adults (~60 μg/kg or 1.8 mg/m² for children) are used initially and are adjusted appropriately to subsequent hematological and clinical responses, with the aim of reducing the total leukocyte count to ≤10,000 cells/mm³. A decrease in the leukocyte count is not usually seen during the first 10–15 days of treatment and the leukocyte count may actually increase. Because the leukocyte count may fall for more than a month after discontinuing the drug, it is recommended that busulfan be withdrawn when the total leukocyte count has declined to ~15,000 cells/mm³. A normal leukocyte count usually is achieved within 12–20 weeks. During remission, daily treatment resumes when the total leukocyte count reaches ~50,000 cells/mm³. Daily maintenance doses are 1–3 mg. In high-dose therapy, doses of 1 mg/kg are given every 6 hours for 4 days, with adjustment based on pharmacokinetics.

High doses of busulfan also have been used effectively in combination with high doses of cyclophosphamide to prepare leukemia patients for bone marrow transplantation. In such high-dose regimens, busulfan is given at 0.8 mg/kg every 6 hours for 4 days. Anticonvulsants must be used concomitantly to protect against acute CNS toxicities, including tonic-clonic seizures, which may occur several hours after each dose. Busulfan induces the metabolism of phenytoin. In patients requiring antiseizure medication, drugs such as lorazepam *are recommended as an alternative. When phenytoin is used concurrently, plasma busulfan levels should be monitored and the busulfan dose adjusted.*

The toxic effects of busulfan are related to its myelosuppressive properties; prolonged thrombocytopenia may occur. Occasional patients experience nausea, vomiting, and diarrhea. Long-term use leads to impotence, sterility, amenorrhea, and fetal malformation. Rarely, patients develop asthenia and hypotension. High-dose busulfan causes VOD of the liver in up to 10% of patients, as well as seizures, hemorrhagic cystitis, alopecia, and cataracts. The coincidence of VOD and hepatotoxicity is increased by its coadministration with drugs that inhibit CYPs, including imidazoles and metronidazole, *possibly by inhibition of the clearance of busulfan and/or its toxic metabolites.*

Nitrosoureas

The nitrosoureas are important in the treatment of brain tumors and find occasional use in treating lymphomas and in high-dose regimens with bone marrow reconstitution. They are bifunctional alkylating agents but differ in both pharmacological and toxicological properties from conventional nitrogen mustards. Carmustine (BCNU) and lomustine (CCNU) are highly lipophilic and readily cross the blood–brain barrier, an important property in the treatment of brain tumors. Unfortunately, with the exception of streptozocin, nitrosoureas cause profound and delayed myelosuppression with recovery 4–6 weeks after a single dose. Long-term treatment with the nitrosoureas, especially semustine (methyl-CCNU), has resulted in renal failure. As with other alkylating agents, the nitrosoureas are highly carcinogenic and mutagenic. They generate both alkylating and carbamoylating moieties.

CARMUSTINE (BCNU) Carmustine's major action is its alkylation of DNA at the O^6-guanine position, forming an adduct repaired by AGT. Methylation of the AGT promoter region inhibits its expression in ~30% of primary gliomas and is associated with sensitivity to nitrosoureas. In high doses with bone marrow rescue, carmustine produces hepatic VOD, pulmonary fibrosis, renal failure, and secondary leukemia. It is unstable in aqueous solution and body fluids. After intravenous infusion, it disappears from the plasma with a variable $t_{1/2}$ of 15–90 minutes. Approximately 30–80% of the drug appears in the urine within 24 hours as degradation products. The entry of alkylating metabolites into the cerebrospinal fluid (CSF) is rapid, and their CSF concentrations are 15–30% of concurrent plasma values. When used alone, carmustine (BICNU) usually is administered intravenously at doses of 150–200 mg/m², given by infusion over 1–2 hours and repeated at 6 weeks. Because of its ability to cross the blood–brain barrier, carmustine is used with procarbazine in the treatment of malignant gliomas. An implantable carmustine wafer (GLIADEL) is used as an adjunct to surgery and radiation in newly diagnosed high-grade malignant glioma patients and as an adjunct to surgery for recurrent glioblastoma multiforme.

STREPTOZOCIN This antibiotic has a methylnitrosourea (MNU) moiety attached to C2 of glucose. It has a high affinity for cells of the islets of Langerhans and causes diabetes in experimental animals. After intravenous infusions of 200–1600 mg/m², peak concentrations of streptozocin in the plasma are 30–40 μg/mL; the $t_{1/2}$ of the drug is ~15 minutes. Only 10–20% of a dose is recovered intact in the urine. Streptozocin (ZANOSAR) is useful in the treatment of human pancreatic islet cell carcinoma and malignant carcinoid tumors. It is administered intravenously, 500 mg/m² once daily for 5 days; this course is repeated every 6 weeks. Alternatively, 1000 mg/m² can be given weekly for 2 weeks and the weekly dose then can be increased to a maximum of 1500 mg/m², as tolerated. Nausea is a frequent side effect. Mild, reversible renal or hepatic toxicity occurs in ~two-thirds of cases; in <10% of patients, renal toxicity may be cumulative with each dose and may be fatal. Urinary protein excretion is an early sign of tubular damage and impending renal failure. Streptozocin should not be given with other nephrotoxic drugs. Hematological toxicity—anemia, leukopenia, or thrombocytopenia—occurs in 20% of patients.

Triazenes

DACARBAZINE (DTIC) Dacarbazine functions as a methylating agent after metabolic activation in the liver. The active form is a monomethyl triazeno metabolite, MTIC, which kills cells in all phases of the cell cycle. Resistance has been ascribed to removal of methyl groups from the O^6-guanine bases in DNA by AGT. Dacarbazine is administered intravenously. After an initial rapid phase of disappearance ($t_{1/2}$ ~20 minutes), dacarbazine is removed from plasma with a terminal $t_{1/2}$ of ~5 hours. The $t_{1/2}$ is prolonged in the presence of hepatic or renal disease. Almost 50% of the compound is excreted intact in the urine by tubular secretion. Elevated urinary concentrations of 5-aminoimidazole-4-carboxamide are derived from the catabolism of dacarbazine, rather than by inhibition of *de novo* purine biosynthesis. Dacarbazine (DTIC-DOME, others) for malignant melanoma is given in doses of 3.5 mg/kg/day, intravenously, for a 10-day period, repeated every 28 days. Alternatively, 250 mg/m² can be given daily for 5 days and repeated every 3 weeks. Extravasation of the drug may cause tissue damage and severe pain. At present, dacarbazine is employed in combination regimens for the treatment of Hodgkin's disease. It is less effective against malignant melanoma and adult sarcomas. The toxicity of DTIC includes nausea and vomiting in >90% of patients; vomiting usually develops 1–3 hours after treatment and may last up to 12 hours. Myelosuppression, with both leukopenia and thrombocytopenia, usually is mild to moderate. A flu-like syndrome consisting of chills, fever, malaise, and myalgias may occur during DTIC treatment. Hepatotoxicity, alopecia, facial flushing, neurotoxicity, and dermatologic reactions also have been reported.

TEMOZOLOMIDE Temozolomide (TEMODAR) is a triazene that has significant activity in patients with malignant gliomas, where it is the standard agent in combination with radiation therapy. Temozolomide, like dacarbazine, forms the methylating metabolite MTIC and kills cells in all phases of the cell cycle. Temozolomide is administered orally and its bioavailability approaches 100%. Maximum plasma drug concentration reaches 5 μg/mL, at ~10 μM, 1 hour after administration of a dose of 200 mg, and declines with an elimination $t_{1/2}$ of 1.2 hours. The primary active metabolite MTIC reaches a maximum plasma concentration of 150 ng/mL 90 minutes after a dose and declines with a $t_{1/2}$ of 2 hours. Little intact drug is recovered in the urine, the primary urinary metabolite being the inactive imidazole carboxamide. The pharmacokinetics of temozolomide are linear over the dose range of 100–260 mg/m². The toxicities of temozolomide mirror those of DTIC.

Methylhydrazines

PROCARBAZINE Several methylhydrazine derivatives have anticancer activity, but only procarbazine (*N*-isopropyl-α-(2-methylhydrazino)-*p*-toluamide) is used clinically. The antineoplastic activity of procarbazine results from its conversion by hepatic CYPs to highly reactive alkylating species that methylate DNA. The first step in activation involves oxidation of the hydrazine function, yielding an azo metabolite that exists in equilibrium with its hydrazone tautomer. *N*-Oxidation of azoprocarbazine generates the isomeric benzylazoxy and methylazoxy metabolites, the latter of which liberates an entity resembling diazomethane, a potent methylating reagent. Free-radical intermediates also may be involved. Activated procarbazine can produce chromosomal damage, including chromatid breaks and translocations, consistent with its mutagenic and carcinogenic actions. Exposure to procarbazine leads to inhibition of DNA, RNA, and protein synthesis *in vivo*. Resistance to procarbazine develops rapidly when it is used as a single agent. One mechanism results from the increased ability to repair methylation of guanine *via* AGT.

Procarbazine is efficiently absorbed from the GI tract and rapidly distributes into the CNS. The drug and its metabolites are predominantly eliminated in the urine, with N-isopropyl-terephthalamic acid being the major metabolite, accounting for ~25% of doses given either orally or intravenously. Multiple metabolites of the drug (e.g., azo, methylazoxy, and benzylazoxy derivatives) have been identified in the plasma after oral procarbazine. A marked decrease in the apparent clearance of the drug upon repeated daily oral administration has been observed. Although CYPs have well-defined roles in the activation of procarbazine, the concurrent use of antiseizure drugs that induce hepatic CYPs did not significantly alter the pharmacokinetics of the parent drug in brain cancer patients.

The recommended dose of procarbazine (MATULANE) for adults is 100 mg/m² daily for 10–14 days in combination regimens. The drug rarely is used alone. Procarbazine is used in combination with mechlorethamine, vincristine, and prednisone (the MOPP regimen) for the treatment of Hodgkin's disease. Alternative regimens with less leukemogenic potential have largely replaced MOPP. Of primary importance, procarbazine lacks cross-resistance with other mustard-type alkylating agents. Procarbazine has been used in combination with lomustine and vincristine (the PCV regimen) for treating patients with newly diagnosed or recurrent primary brain tumors.

The most common toxic effects include leukopenia and thrombocytopenia, which begin during the second week of therapy and reverse within 2 weeks following treatment. GI symptoms such as mild nausea and vomiting occur in most patients; neurological and dermatological manifestations have been noted in 5–10% of cases. Behavioral disturbances also have been reported. Because of augmentation of sedative effects, the concomitant use of CNS depressants should be avoided. Since procarbazine is a weak monoamine oxidase inhibitor, hypertensive reactions may result from its use concurrently with sympathomimetic agents, tricyclic antidepressants, or ingestion of foods with high tyramine content. Procarbazine has disulfiram-like actions and the ingestion of alcohol should be avoided. Procarbazine is highly carcinogenic, mutagenic, and teratogenic, and its use in MOPP therapy is associated with a 5–10% risk of acute leukemia; the greatest risk is for patients who also receive radiation therapy. Procarbazine also is a potent immunosuppressive agent, and it causes infertility, particularly in males.

PLATINUM COORDINATION COMPLEXES

Platinum coordination complexes have broad antineoplastic activity and have become the foundation for treatment of testicular cancer, ovarian cancer, and cancers of the head and neck, bladder, esophagus, lung, and colon. Although cisplatin and other platinum complexes do not form carbonium ion intermediates or formally alkylate DNA, they covalently bind to nucleophilic sites on DNA and share many pharmacological attributes with the alkylating agents. Cisplatin, carboplatin, and oxaliplatin enter cells by diffusion and by an active Cu^{2+} transporter. Inside the cell, the chloride atoms of cisplatin are replaced by water, yielding a positively charged molecule that reacts with nucleophilic sites on DNA and proteins. Aquation is favored at the low concentrations of Cl^- inside the cell and in the urine. High concentrations of Cl^- stabilize the drug, explaining the effectiveness of Cl^- diuresis in preventing nephrotoxicity (*see* below). Hydrolysis of carboplatin removes the bidentate cyclobutanedicarboxylato group; this activation reaction occurs slowly. The platinum complexes can react with DNA, forming both intrastrand and interstrand cross-links. DNA adducts formed by cisplatin inhibit DNA replication and transcription and lead to breaks and miscoding, and if recognized by p53 and other checkpoint proteins, induction of apoptosis. The cell cycle specificity of cisplatin appears to differ among cell types, although the effects of cross-linking are most pronounced during S phase. Cisplatin is mutagenic, teratogenic, and carcinogenic. The use of cisplatin- or carboplatin-based chemotherapy for women with ovarian cancer is associated with a fourfold increased risk of developing secondary leukemia.

Resistance to Platinum Analogs

The causes of tumor cell resistance to cisplatin and its analogs are incompletely understood. The various analogs differ in their degree of cross-resistance with cisplatin in experimental tumor systems. Carboplatin shares cross-resistance with cisplatin in most experimental tumors, while oxaliplatin and other tetravalent analogs do not. A number of factors influence cisplatin sensitivity in experimental cells, including intracellular drug accumulation and intracellular levels of glutathione and other sulfhydryls such as metallothionein that bind to and inactivate the drug, and rates of repair of DNA adducts. Repair of cisplatin-DNA adducts occurs through the NER pathway. Inhibition or loss of NER increases sensitivity to cisplatin in ovarian cancer patients, while overexpression of NER components is associated with poor response to cisplatin-based therapy in lung cancer.

Resistance to cisplatin, but not oxaliplatin, is partly mediated by loss of function in mismatch repair (MMR) proteins. By contrast, MMR repair proficiency is not required for oxaliplatin cytotoxicity. In the absence of effective repair of DNA-platinum adducts, sensitive cells cannot replicate or transcribe affected portions of the DNA strand. Some DNA polymerases can bypass adducts, possibly contributing to resistance. Overexpression of Cu^{2+} efflux transporters ATP7A and ATP7B correlates with poor survival after cisplatin-based therapy for ovarian cancer.

Cisplatin

After intravenous administration, cisplatin has an initial plasma elimination $t_{1/2}$ of 25–50 minutes; concentrations of total (bound and unbound) drug fall thereafter, with a $t_{1/2}$ of 24 hours or longer. More than 90% of the platinum in the blood is covalently bound to plasma proteins. The unbound fraction, composed predominantly of parent drug, is cleared within minutes. High concentrations of cisplatin are found in the kidney, liver, intestine, and testes, but CNS penetration is poor. Only a small portion of the drug is excreted by the kidney during the first 6 hours; by 24 hours up to 25% is excreted, and by 5 days up to 43% of the administered dose is recovered in the urine, mostly covalently bound to protein and peptides. Biliary or intestinal excretion of cisplatin is minimal. Cisplatin (PLATINOL-AQ, others) is given only by the intravenous route. The usual dose is 20 mg/m²/day for 5 days, 20–30 mg weekly for 3–4 weeks, or 100 mg/m², given once every 4 weeks. To prevent renal toxicity, it is important to establish a chloride diuresis by the infusion of 1–2 L of normal saline prior to treatment. The appropriate amount of cisplatin then is diluted in a solution of dextrose and saline and administered intravenously over a period of 4–6 hours.

Since aluminum inactivates cisplatin, it is important not to use needles or other infusion equipment that contain aluminum when preparing or administering the drug.

Cisplatin, in combination with *bleomycin*, etoposide, ifosfamide, or *vinblastine*, cures 90% of patients with testicular cancer. Used with paclitaxel, cisplatin induces complete response in most patients with carcinoma of the ovary. Cisplatin produces responses in cancers of the bladder, head and neck, cervix, and endometrium; all forms of carcinoma of the lung; anal and rectal carcinomas; and neoplasms of childhood. The drug sensitizes cells to radiation therapy and enhances control of locally advanced lung, esophageal, and head and neck tumors when given with irradiation.

Cisplatin-induced nephrotoxicity largely has been abrogated by pretreatment hydration and diuresis. Amifostine (ETHYOL) is a thiophosphate cytoprotective agent that is approved for the reduction of renal toxicity associated with repeated administration of cisplatin. Amifostine is dephosphorylated by alkaline phosphatase to a pharmacologically active free thiol metabolite. Faster dephosphorylation and preferential uptake by normal tissues results in a higher concentration of the thiol metabolite available to scavenge reactive cisplatin metabolites in normal tissues. Amifostine also is used to reduce xerostomia in patients undergoing irradiation for head and neck cancer, when the radiation port includes a substantial portion of the parotid glands. Ototoxicity caused by cisplatin is unaffected by diuresis and is manifested by tinnitus and high-frequency hearing loss. The ototoxicity can be unilateral or bilateral, tends to be more frequent and severe with repeated doses, and may be more pronounced in children. Marked nausea and vomiting occur in almost all patients and usually can be controlled with 5-hydroxytryptamine (5-HT$_3$) antagonists, neurokinin-1 (NK1) receptor antagonists, and glucocorticoids (see Chapter 37). At higher doses or after multiple cycles of treatment, cisplatin causes a progressive peripheral motor and sensory neuropathy, which may worsen after drug discontinuation and may be aggravated by subsequent or simultaneous treatment with taxanes or other neurotoxic drugs. Cisplatin causes mild-to-moderate myelosuppression, with transient leukopenia and thrombocytopenia. Anemia may become prominent after multiple cycles of treatment. Electrolyte disturbances, including hypomagnesemia, hypocalcemia, hypokalemia, and hypophosphatemia, are common. Hypocalcemia and hypomagnesemia secondary to renal electrolyte wasting may produce tetany. Routine measurement of Mg^{2+} concentrations in plasma is recommended. Hyperuricemia, hemolytic anemia, and cardiac abnormalities are rare side effects. Anaphylactic-like reactions, characterized by facial edema, bronchoconstriction, tachycardia, and hypotension, may occur within minutes after administration and should be treated by intravenous injection of epinephrine and with glucocorticoids or antihistamines. Cisplatin has been associated with the development of AML, usually 4 years or more after treatment.

Carboplatin

Mechanisms of action and resistance, and the spectrum of clinical activity of carboplatin (CBDCA, JM-8) are similar to those of cisplatin, but the two drugs differ significantly in their chemical, pharmacokinetic, and toxicological properties. Because carboplatin is much less reactive than cisplatin, the majority of drug in plasma remains in its parent form, unbound to proteins. Most eliminatation is via renal excretion, with a t$_{1/2}$ in plasma of ~2 hours. A small fraction of platinum become irreversibly bound to plasma proteins and disappears slowly, with a t$_{1/2}$ >5 days. Carboplatin is relatively well tolerated clinically, with less nausea, neurotoxicity, ototoxicity, and nephrotoxicity than cisplatin. Instead, the dose-limiting toxicity is myelosuppression, primarily evident as thrombocytopenia. Carboplatin and cisplatin appear to be equally effective in the treatment of suboptimally debulked ovarian cancer, non–small cell lung cancer, and extensive small cell lung cancer; however, carboplatin may be less effective than cisplatin in germ cell, head and neck, and esophageal cancers. Carboplatin is an effective alternative for responsive tumors in patients unable to tolerate cisplatin because of impaired renal function, refractory nausea, significant hearing impairment, or neuropathy, but doses must be adjusted for renal function. In addition, it may be used in high-dose therapy with bone marrow or peripheral stem cell rescue. The dose of carboplatin should be adjusted in proportion to the reduction in creatinine clearance for patients with a creatinine clearance <60 mL/min.

Carboplatin (PARAPLATIN) is administered as an intravenous infusion over at least 15 minutes and is given once every 28 days. Carboplatin currently is U.S. Food and Drug Administration (FDA)-approved for use in combination with paclitaxel or cyclophosphamide in patients with advanced ovarian cancer and lung cancer.

Oxaliplatin

Oxaliplatin, like cisplatin, has a very brief plasma t$_{1/2}$, probably due to its rapid uptake by tissues and its reactivity. While the ultrafiltrable component has a slow terminal clearance from plasma (t$_{1/2}$ of 273 hours), most of the low-molecular-weight platinum species represent inactive degradation

*products. These metabolites undergo renal excretion at a rate dependent on the creatinine clear-
ance. However, no dose adjustment is required for patients with creatinine clearances >20 mL/min,
as decreased renal function does not affect the rapid chemical inactivation of the drug and its toxicity at doses of 65–130 mg/m². Oxaliplatin exhibits a wide range of antitumor activity that differs
from other platinum agents, and includes gastric and colorectal cancer; its effectiveness in colorectal cancer is perhaps due to its MMR-independent effects. It also suppresses expression of TS,
the target enzyme of 5-fluorouracil (5-FU) action, which may promote synergy of these two drugs.
In combination with 5-FU, it is approved for treatment of patients with advanced colorectal
cancer.*

*The dose-limiting toxicity of oxaliplatin is peripheral neuropathy. An acute form often is trig-
gered by exposure to cold, and manifests as paresthesias and/or dysesthesias in the upper and
lower extremities, mouth, and throat. A second type of peripheral neuropathy is more closely
related to cumulative dose and similar to that seen with cisplatin; 75% of patients receiving a
cumulative dose of 1560 mg/m² experience some neurotoxicity. Hematologic toxicity is mild to
moderate, and nausea is well controlled with 5-HT₃ receptor antagonists. Oxaliplatin is unstable
in the presence of chloride or alkaline solutions.*

II. ANTIMETABOLITES

FOLIC ACID ANALOGS

Antifolate chemotherapy produced the first cure of a solid tumor, choriocarcinoma. Introduction of
high-dose regimens with "rescue" of host toxicity by the reduced folate, leucovorin (folinic acid,
citrovorum factor, 5-formyl tetrahydrofolate, N^5-formyl FH_4), further extended the effectiveness of
these drugs to both systemic and CNS lymphomas, osteogenic sarcoma, and leukemias. Most
recently, analogs that differ from methotrexate in their transport properties and sites of action have
proven useful in treating other cancers.

*Folic acid is converted by enzymatic reduction to a series of tetrahydrofolate cofactors that pro-
vide carbon groups for the synthesis of precursors of DNA (thymidylate and purines) and RNA
(purines) (see Figure 51–4). The biological functions and therapeutic applications of folic acid
are further described in Chapter 53. To function as a cofactor in one-carbon transfer reactions,
folate must first be reduced by dihydrofolate reductase (DHFR) to tetrahydrofolate (FH_4). Single-
carbon fragments are added enzymatically to FH_4 in various configurations and then may be
transferred in specific synthetic reactions. In a key metabolic event catalyzed by TS, deoxyuridine
monophosphate (dUMP) is converted to thymidine monophosphate (TMP), an essential component of DNA. In this reaction, a one-carbon group is transferred to dUMP from 5,10-methylene
FH_4, and the reduced folate cofactor is oxidized to dihydrofolate (FH_2). To function again as a
cofactor, FH_2 must be reduced to FH_4 by DHFR. Inhibitors such as methotrexate, with a high
affinity for DHFR, prevent the formation of FH_4 and allow a vast accumulation of the toxic
inhibitory substrate, FH_2 polyglutamate, behind the blocked reaction, which inhibits TS and other
enzymes. Methotrexate also undergoes conversion to a series of polyglutamates (MTX-PGs) in
both normal and tumor cells; MTX-PGs constitute an intracellular storage form of folates and
folate analogs, and dramatically increase inhibitory potency of the analog for additional sites,
including TS and two early enzymes in the purine biosynthetic pathway. The one-carbon transfer
reactions crucial for the de novo synthesis of purine nucleotides and thymidylate cease, with the
subsequent interruption of the synthesis of DNA and RNA. Toxic effects of methotrexate can be terminated by administering leucovorin, a fully reduced folate coenzyme that repletes the intracellular pool of tetrahydrofolate cofactors. As with most antimetabolites, methotrexate is only partially
selective for tumor cells and is toxic to all rapidly dividing normal cells, such as those of the intestinal epithelium and bone marrow. Folate antagonists kill cells during the S phase of the cell cycle
and are most effective when cells are proliferating rapidly.*

*Pemetrexed and its polyglutamates have a somewhat different spectrum of biochemical
actions. Like methotrexate, it inhibits DHFR, but as a polyglutamate, even more potently inhibits
glycinamide ribonucleotide formyltransferase (GART) and TS. Unlike methotrexate, it produces
little change in the pool of reduced folates, indicating that the distal sites of inhibition (TS and
GART) predominate. Its pattern of deoxynucleotide depletion also differs, with little effect on
deoxyadenosine triphosphate (dATP), a profile more characteristic of primary TS inhibition.*

*Because folic acid and many of its analogs are hydrophilic, they cross the blood–brain bar-
rier poorly and require specific transport mechanisms to enter mammalian cells. Three inward
folate transport systems are found on mammalian cells: (1) a folate receptor, which has high affinity for folic acid but much reduced ability to transport methotrexate and other analogs; (2) the
reduced folate transporter, the major transit protein for methotrexate, raltitrexed, pemetrexed, and most*

A Thymidylate synthesis

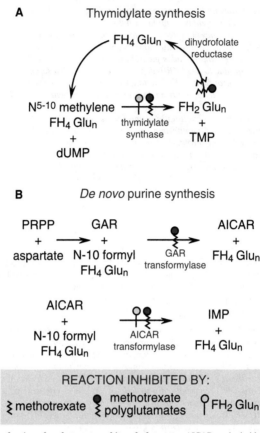

B *De novo* purine synthesis

FIGURE 51–4 *Sites of action of methotrexate and its polyglutamates.* AICAR, aminoimidazole carboxamide; TMP, thymidine monophosphate; dUMP, deoxyuridine monophosphate; FH_2Glu_n, dihydrofolate polyglutamate; FH_4Glu_n, tetrahydrofolate polyglutamate; GAR, glycinamide ribonucleotide; IMP, inosine monophosphate; PRPP, 5-phosphoribosyl-1-pyrophosphate.

analogs; and (3) a poorly characterized transporter that is active at low pH. The reduced folate transporter is highly expressed in the hyperdiploid subtype of ALL, which has extreme sensitivity to methotrexate. Once in the cell, additional glutamyl residues are added to the molecule by the enzyme folylpolyglutamate synthetase. Since these higher polyglutamates are strongly charged and cross cellular membranes poorly, polyglutamation serves as a mechanism of entrapment and may account for the prolonged retention of methotrexate in chorionic epithelium (where it is a potent abortifacient), in tumors derived from this tissue, such as choriocarcinoma cells, and in normal tissues subject to cumulative drug toxicity, such as liver. Polyglutamylated folates and analogs have substantially greater affinity than the monoglutamate form for folate-dependent enzymes required for purine and thymidylate synthesis and have at least equal affinity for DHFR.

New folate antagonists have been identified that are better substrates for the reduced folate carrier and appear to have significant advantages in clinical chemotherapy (see pemetrexed below). In efforts to bypass the obligatory membrane transport system and to facilitate penetration of the blood–brain barrier, lipid-soluble folate antagonists also have been synthesized. Trimetrexate (NEUTREXIN) has modest antitumor activity, primarily in combination with leucovorin rescue. However, it is beneficial in the treatment of Pneumocystis jiroveci pneumonia, where leucovorin provides differential rescue of the host but not the parasite.

The most important new folate analog, MTA or pemetrexed (ALIMTA), is a pyrrole-pyrimidine folate analog. It is avidly transported into cells via the reduced folate carrier, but also may gain entry by a unique folate transport activity found in mesothelioma cell lines. It is readily converted to polyglutamates that inhibit TS and glycine amide ribonucleotide transformylase, as well as DHFR. It has activity against colon cancer, mesothelioma, and non–small cell lung cancer, and is approved for treatment of mesothelioma.

Different biochemical mechanisms of acquired resistance to methotrexate can affect each known step in methotrexate action, including: (1) impaired transport of methotrexate into cells; (2) production of altered forms of DHFR that have decreased affinity for the inhibitor; (3) increased concentrations of intracellular DHFR through gene amplification or altered gene regulation; (4) decreased ability to synthesize methotrexate polyglutamates; and (5) increased expression of a drug efflux transporter, of the MRP (multidrug resistance protein) class.

DHFR levels in leukemic cells increase within 24 hours after treatment of patients with methotrexate; this likely reflects induction of new enzyme synthesis. The unbound DHFR protein may bind to its own mRNA and inhibit its own translation, while the DHFR-MTX complex is ineffective in blocking the DHFR translation. With longer periods of drug exposure, tumor cell populations emerge that contain markedly increased levels of DHFR. These cells contain multiple gene copies of DHFR either in mitotically unstable double-minute chromosomes (extrachromosomal elements) or in stably integrated chromosomal amplicons. Similar gene amplifications of target proteins have been implicated in the resistance to many antitumor agents, including 5-FU and pentostatin (2'-deoxycoformycin). To overcome resistance, high doses of methotrexate may drive entry of drug into transport-defective cells and permit the intracellular accumulation of methotrexate in concentrations that inactivate high levels of DHFR. The understanding of resistance to pemetrexed is incomplete. In various cell lines, resistance to this agent seems to arise either from TS amplification, changes in purine biosynthetic pathways, or both.

The primary toxic effects of methotrexate and other folate antagonists used in cancer chemotherapy are exerted against rapidly dividing cells of the bone marrow and GI epithelium. Mucositis, myelosuppression, and thrombocytopenia reach their maximum in 5–10 days after drug administration, and except in instances of altered drug excretion, reverse rapidly thereafter. In addition to its acute toxicities, methotrexate can cause pneumonitis that regresses upon discontinuation of the drug. In some cases, patients can be rechalleged with drug without toxicity. The etiology is unknown. A second toxicity of particular significance in chronic administration to patients with psoriasis or rheumatoid arthritis is hepatic fibrosis and cirrhosis. Increased hepatic portal fibrosis is detected with higher frequency than in control patients after >6 months of continuous oral methotrexate treatment of psoriasis. Its presence mandates drug discontinuation. Acute, reversible elevation of hepatic enzymes is detected in serum after high-dose administration but rarely is associated with permanent changes. Folic acid antagonists are toxic to developing embryos. Methotrexate is highly effective when used with the prostaglandin analog misoprostol in inducing abortion in first-trimester pregnancy.

Methotrexate is readily absorbed from the GI tract at doses of <25 mg/m^2, but larger doses are absorbed incompletely and are routinely given intravenously. After intravenous administration, the drug disappears from plasma in a triphasic fashion. The rapid distribution phase is followed by a second phase, which reflects renal clearance ($t_{1/2}$ ~2–3 hours). A third phase has a $t_{1/2}$ ~8–10 hours. This terminal phase of disappearance, if unduly prolonged by renal failure, may be responsible for major toxic effects of the drug on the marrow, GI epithelium, and skin. Distribution of methotrexate into body spaces, such as the pleural or peritoneal cavity, occurs slowly. However, if such spaces are expanded (e.g., by ascites or pleural effusion), they may act as a site of storage and slow release of drug, with resultant prolonged elevation of plasma concentrations and more severe toxicity. Approximately 50% of methotrexate is bound to plasma proteins and may be displaced by a number of drugs, including sulfonamides, salicylates, tetracycline, chloramphenicol, and phenytoin; caution should be used if these are given concomitantly. Up to 90% of a given dose is excreted unchanged in the urine within 48 hours, mostly within the first 8–12 hours. A small amount of methotrexate also is excreted in the stool. Metabolism of methotrexate is usually minimal, but with high doses metabolites are readily detectable; these include 7-hydroxymethotrexate, which is potentially nephrotoxic. Renal excretion of methotrexate occurs through a combination of glomerular filtration and active tubular secretion. Therefore, concurrent use of drugs that reduce renal blood flow (e.g., nonsteroidal anti-inflammatory agents), that are nephrotoxic (e.g., cisplatin), or that are weak organic acids (e.g., aspirin or piperacillin) can delay drug excretion and lead to severe myelosuppression. Particular caution must be exercised in treating patients with renal insufficiency, where the dose should be adjusted in proportion to decreases in renal function and high-dose regimens should be avoided if possible. Methotrexate is retained in the form of polyglutamates for long periods—for example, for weeks in the kidneys and for months in the liver. It is important to emphasize that concentrations of methotrexate in CSF are only 3% of those in the systemic circulation at steady state; hence, neoplastic cells in the CNS probably are *not killed by standard regimens. When high doses of methotrexate are given (>1.5 g/m², cytotoxic concentrations of methotrexate may be attained in the CNS.*

Pharmacogenetics may influence the response to antifolates and their toxicity. A mutation in methylenetetrahydrofolate reductase, the enzyme that generates methylenetetrahydrofolate cofactor for TS, reduces its activity and thereby increases methotrexate toxicity. The presence of this polymorphism in leukemic cells confers increased sensitivity to methotrexate, and may also modulate the toxicity and therapeutic effect of pemetrexed, a predominant TS inhibitor. Likewise, polymorphisms in the promoter region of TS affect its expression, and by altering the intracellular levels of TS, modulate the response and toxicity of both antifolates and fluoropyrimidines.

Methotrexate (*amethopterin;* RHEUMATREX, TREXALL, others) has been used in the treatment of severe, disabling psoriasis in doses of 2.5 mg orally for 5 days, followed by a rest period of at least 2 days, or 10–25 mg intravenously weekly. It also is used intermittently at low dosage to induce remission in rheumatoid arthritis.

Methotrexate is a critical drug in the management of ALL in children. Used in high doses, it is of great value in remission induction and consolidation, and in the maintenance of remissions in this highly curable disease. For maintenance therapy, it is administered intermittently at doses of 30 mg/m² intramuscularly weekly in 2 divided doses or in 2-day "pulses" of 175–525 mg/m² at monthly intervals. Outcome of treatment in children correlates inversely with the rate of drug clearance. During methotrexate infusion, high steady-state levels are associated with a lower leukemia relapse rate. Methotrexate is of limited value in adult leukemia, except for treatment and prevention of leukemic meningitis. The intrathecal administration of methotrexate has been employed for treatment or prophylaxis of meningeal leukemia or lymphoma and for treatment of meningeal carcinomatosis. This route of administration achieves high concentrations of methotrexate in the CSF and is also effective in patients whose systemic disease has become resistant to methotrexate. The recommended intrathecal dose in all patients >3 years of age is 12 mg. The dose is repeated every 4 days until malignant cells no longer are evident in the CSF. Leucovorin may be administered to counteract the toxicity of methotrexate that escapes into the systemic circulation, although this generally is not necessary. Since methotrexate administered into the lumbar space distributes poorly over the cerebral convexities, the drug may be more effective when given *via* an intraventricular Ommaya reservoir. Methotrexate is of established value in choriocarcinoma and related trophoblastic tumors of women; cure is achieved in ~75% of advanced cases treated sequentially with methotrexate and *dactinomycin*, and in >90% when early diagnosis is made. In the treatment of choriocarcinoma, 1 mg/kg of methotrexate is administered intramuscularly every other day for 4 doses, alternating with leucovorin (0.1 mg/kg every other day). Courses are repeated at 3-week intervals, toxicity permitting, and urinary β-human chorionic gonadotropin titers are used as a guide for persistence of disease.

Beneficial effects also are observed in the combination therapy of Burkitt's and other non-Hodgkin's lymphomas, and methotrexate is a component of regimens for carcinomas of the breast, head and neck, ovary, and bladder. High-dose methotrexate with leucovorin rescue (HDM-L) is a component of the standard regimen for adjuvant therapy of osteosarcoma, produces a high complete response rate in CNS lymphomas, and is a part of standard curative therapy for childhood ALL. A 6-72-hour infusion of relatively large doses of methotrexate may be employed every 2–4 weeks (from 1 to 7.5 g/m² or more), but only when leucovorin rescue is used. Such regimens produce cytotoxic concentrations of drug in the CSF and protect against leukemic meningitis. A typical regimen includes the infusion of 7.5 g/m² methotrexate for 6 hours followed by leucovorin at a dose of 15 mg/m² every 6 hours for 7 doses, with the goal of rescuing normal cells to prevent toxicity. Other dosage regimens also are used.

The administration of HDM-L has the potential for renal toxicity, probably related to drug precipitation in the acidic tubular fluid. Thus, vigorous hydration and alkalinization of urine are required prior to drug administration. HDM-L should be performed only by experienced clinicians. If methotrexate values measured 48 hours after drug administration are 1 μM or higher, higher doses (100 mg/m²) of leucovorin must be given until the plasma concentration of methotrexate falls below a level of 50 nM. With appropriate hydration and urine alkalinization, and in patients with normal renal function, the incidence of nephrotoxicity following HDM-L approaches 2%. In patients who become oliguric, intermittent hemodialysis is ineffective in reducing methotrexate levels. Continuous-flow hemodialysis can eliminate methotrexate at a rate approximating 50% of the clearance rate in patients with intact renal function. Alternatively, a methotrexate-cleaving enzyme, carboxypeptidase G2, can be obtained from the National Cancer Institute. Methotrexate concentrations in plasma fall by 99% or greater within 5–15 minutes following intravenous enzyme administration, with insignificant rebound. Carboxypeptidase G2 also has received limited evaluation as the sole rescue for high-dose methotrexate, without leucovorin, and was effective. Systemically administered carboxypeptidase G2 has little effect on methotrexate levels in the CSF.

The only FDA-approved indication for pemetrexed is for second-line therapy in mesothelioma; it also is used, however, for refractory non–small cell lung cancer. Promising results have been published in first-line use with cisplatin in both tumors.

The primary toxicities of antifolates affect the bone marrow and the intestinal epithelium. Patients may be at risk for spontaneous hemorrhage or life-threatening infection and may require prophylactic transfusion of platelets and broad-spectrum antibiotics if febrile. Side effects usually reverse completely within 2 weeks, but prolonged myelosuppression may occur in patients with compromised renal function who have delayed drug excretion. The dose of methotrexate (and likely pemetrexed) must be reduced in proportion to any reduction in creatinine clearance. Additional toxicities of methotrexate include alopecia, dermatitis, interstitial pneumonitis, nephrotoxicity, defective oogenesis or spermatogenesis, abortion, and teratogenesis. Elevation of hepatic enzymes is a consistent finding with high-dose methotrexate but usually is reversible. On the other hand, low-dose methotrexate may lead to cirrhosis after long-term continuous treatment, as in patients with psoriasis. Intrathecal administration of methotrexate often causes meningismus and an inflammatory response in the CSF. Seizures, coma, and death may occur rarely. Leucovorin does not reverse neurotoxicity.

Pemetrexed toxicity mirrors that of methotrexate, with the additional feature of a prominent erythematous and pruritic rash in 40% of patients. Dexamethasone, 4 mg twice-daily on days −1, 0, and +1, markedly diminishes this toxicity. Unpredictably severe myelosuppression with pemetrexed, seen especially in patients with preexisting homocystinemia and possibly reflecting folate deficiency, is largely eliminated by concurrent administration of low doses of folic acid, *0.35–1 mg/day, beginning 1–2 weeks prior to pemetrexed and continuing while the drug is administered. Intramuscular vitamin B_{12} (1 mg) is given with the first dose of pemetrexed to correct possible B_{12} deficiency. There is no evidence that these small doses of folate and B_{12} compromise the therapeutic effect.*

PYRIMIDINE ANALOGS

The pyrimidine antimetabolites encompass a diverse group of drugs that inhibit RNA and DNA function in a variety of ways. Some, such as the fluoropyrimidines and the purine base analogs (6-mercaptopurine and *6-thioguanine*) inhibit the synthesis of essential precursors of DNA. Others, particularly the cytidine and adenosine nucleoside analogs, become incorporated into DNA and block its further elongation and its function. Other metabolic effects of these analogs may contribute to their cytotoxicity and even their ability to induce differentiation.

DNA is made up of 2 pyrimidines, thymine and cytosine, and 2 purines, guanine and adenine. RNA differs in that it incorporates uracil instead of thymine. Uracil may serve as a precursor of deoxythymidine monophosphate in the final step of this conversion, TS adds a methyl group to the 5 position of dUMP. Cells can synthesize bases *de novo* and convert them to their active deoxynucleoside triphosphates (dNTPs). The dNTPs then act as substrates for DNA polymerase and become linked in 3′-5′ phosphate ester bonds to form DNA strands. Alternatively, cells can salvage either free bases or their deoxynucleoside from the systemic circulation. Uracil, guanine, and their analogs can be taken up by cells and converted intracellularly to deoxynucleotides by the addition of deoxyribose and phosphate groups. Cytosine, thymine, and adenine cannot be activated by mammalian cells, which lack the ability to add the necessary ribose or deoxy ribose groups to these particular bases. However, preformed deoxynucleosides containing a deoxyribose linked to cytosine or adenine are readily transported into cells and activated by conversion to deoxynucleotides by intracellular kinases.

The limitations of cell uptake and conversion to active triphosphates determine the form in which specific analogs have been synthesized, varying from base analogs such as fluorouracil (5-fluorouracil, or 5-FU) to nucleosides such as cytosine arabinoside, and even to nucleotides such as fludarabine phosphate. Uracil and guanine analogs (such as 5-FU and 6-thioguanine) are efficiently taken up by cells and converted to dNTPs. Because of the inability to activate cytosine or adenine bases, analogs of cytosine and adenine are synthesized as nucleosides (*cytosine arabinoside* [*cytarabine*; Ara-C] and *gemcitabine*, for example), which are readily transported into cells and converted by kinases to the active dNTPs. *Fludarabine phosphate*, a nucleotide, is dephosphorylated rapidly in plasma, releasing the nucleoside that is readily taken up by cells. Analogs may differ from the physiologic bases by alterations in purine or pyrimidine ring or by altering the sugar

attached to the base, as in the arabinoside Ara-C, or by altering both the base and sugar, as in fludarabine phosphate.

*The best-characterized agents in this class are the halogenated pyrimidines, a group that includes
5-FU, floxuridine (5-fluoro-2'-deoxyuridine, or 5-FUdR), and idoxuridine (5-iodo-deoxyuridine)
(see Chapter 49). Iododeoxyuridine behaves as an analog of thymidine, and its primary biological action results from its phosphorylation and ultimate incorporation into DNA in place of
thymidylate. In 5-FU, the smaller fluorine allows the molecule to mimic uracil biochemically.
However, the fluorine–carbon bond is much tighter than that of C—H and prevents the methylation of the 5 position of 5-FU by TS. Instead, in the presence of the physiological cofactor 5,
10-methylene tetrahydrofolate, the fluoropyrimidine locks the enzyme in an inhibited state and
prevents the synthesis of thymidylate, a required DNA precursor.*

*The most clinically important 5-FU analog is capecitabine (N4-pentoxycarbonyl-5'-deoxy-5-
fluorocytidine), a drug active against colon and breast cancers. This orally administered agent is
converted to 5'-deoxy-5-fluorocytidine by carboxylesterase activity in liver and other normal and
malignant tissues, then is converted to 5'-deoxy-fluorodeoxyuridine by the ubiquitous cytidine
deaminase. The final step in its activation occurs when thymidine phosphorylase cleaves the
5'-deoxy sugar, leaving intracellular 5-FU. Tumors with elevated thymidine phosphorylase activity are particularly susceptible to this drug.*

*Cytidine analogs also are potent antitumor agents. The replacement of the ribose of cytidine
with arabinose has yielded a useful chemotherapeutic agent, cytarabine (Ara-C). The arabinose
analog is recognized enzymatically as a 2'-deoxyriboside; it is phosphorylated to a nucleoside
triphosphate that competes with deoxycytidine triphosphate (dCTP) for incorporation into DNA.
When incorporated into DNA, it blocks elongation of the DNA strand and transcription. Other
cytidine analogs include azacitidine (5-azacytidine) and its deoxyanalog, decitabine, which inhibit
DNA methyltransferase. They have antileukemic as well as differentiating actions. The analog
2',2'-difluorodeoxycytidine (gemcitabine) becomes incorporated into DNA and inhibits the elongation of nascent DNA strands. It has useful activity in various human solid tumors, including
pancreatic, lung, and ovarian cancer.*

Fluorouracil and Floxuridine (Fluorodeoxyuridine)

*Fluorouracil (5-FU) requires enzymatic conversion to the nucleotide (ribosylation and phosphory-
lation) in order to exert its cytotoxic activity; these reactions are illustrated in Figure 51–5. The
interaction between FdUMP and TS blocks the synthesis of thymidine triphosphate (TTP), a necessary constituent of DNA. The folate cofactor, 5,10-methylenetetrahydrofolate, and FdUMP form
a covalently bound ternary complex with TS. The transfer of the methylene group and two hydrogen atoms from folate to FdUMP is blocked in the inhibited complex of TS-FdUMP-folate by the
stability of the fluorine carbon bond on FdUMP; sustained inhibition of the enzyme results. In
5-FU–treated cells, both fluorodeoxyuridine triphosphate (FdUTP) and deoxyuridine triphosphate
(dUTP) (the substrate that accumulates behind the blocked TS reaction) incorporate into DNA in
place of the depleted physiological nucleotide, TTP. Presumably, the incorporation of dUTP and/or
FdUTP into DNA activates the excision–repair process. This can lead to DNA strand breakage
because DNA repair requires TTP, which is lacking because of TS inhibition. 5-FU incorporation
into RNA also causes toxicity because of effects on both the processing and functions of RNA.*

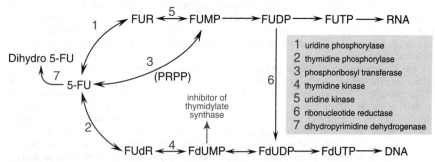

FIGURE 51–5   *Activation pathways for 5-fluorouracil (5-FU) and 5-floxuridine (FUR).* FUDP, floxuridine diphosphate; FUMP, floxuridine monophosphate; FUTP, floxuridine triphosphate; FUdR, fluorodeoxyuridine; FdUDP, fluorodeoxyuridine diphosphate; FdUMP, fluorodeoxyuridine monophosphate; FdUTP, fluorodeoxyuridine triphosphate;
PRPP, 5-phosphoribosyl-1-pyrophosphate.

A number of biochemical mechanisms are associated with resistance to the cytotoxic effects of 5-FU or FUdR. These mechanisms include loss or decreased activity of the enzymes necessary for activation of 5-FU, amplification of TS, and mutation of TS to a form that is not inhibited by FdUMP. The response to 5-FU correlates significantly with low levels of the degradative enzymes dihydrouracil dehydrogenase and thymidine phosphorylase, and a low level of expression of TS. TS levels are finely controlled by an autoregulatory feedback mechanism wherein unbound TS inhibits the translational efficiency of its own mRNA. When TS is bound to FdUMP, inhibition of translation is relieved, and levels of free TS are restored. Thus, TS autoregulation may be an important mechanism by which malignant cells become insensitive to the effects of 5-FU.

Some malignant cells appear to have insufficient concentrations of 5,10-methylene tetrahydrofolate, and thus cannot form maximal levels of the inhibited TS-FdUMP-folate ternary complex. Addition of exogenous folate in the form of leucovorin increases formation of the complex and has enhanced responses to 5-FU.

In addition to leucovorin, a number of other agents have been combined with 5-FU in attempts to enhance the cytotoxic activity through biochemical modulation. Methotrexate, by inhibiting purine synthesis and increasing cellular pools of PRPP, enhances 5-FU activation and increases antitumor activity of 5-FU when given before but not after 5-FU. The combination of cisplatin and 5-FU has yielded impressive responses in tumors of the upper aerodigestive tract, but the molecular basis of their interaction is not well understood. Oxaliplatin is commonly used with 5-FU and leucovorin for treating metastatic colorectal cancer, but the mechanism responsible for the synergistic clinical effect has not been fully elucidated. Oxaliplatin may inhibit catabolism of 5-FU, perhaps by inhibiting DPD, and may inhibit expression of TS. 5-FU with simultaneous irradiation is curative therapy for anal cancer and enhances local tumor control in head and neck, cervical, rectal, gastroesophageal, and pancreatic cancer; the mechanism for this synergism is unclear.

5-FU is administered parenterally, since oral absorption is unpredictable and incomplete. Metabolic degradation occurs in many tissues, particularly the liver. 5-FU is inactivated by reduction of the pyrimidine ring; this reaction is carried out by DPD, which is found in liver, intestinal mucosa, tumor cells, and other tissues. Although rare, inherited deficiency of DPD leads to greatly increased sensitivity to the drug and profound drug toxicity following conventional doses. DPD deficiency can be detected either by enzymatic or molecular assays using peripheral white blood cells, or by determining the plasma ratio of 5-FU to its metabolite, 5-fluoro-5,6-dihydrouracil.

After intravenous administration of 5-FU, plasma clearance is rapid ($t_{1/2}$, 10–20 minutes). Urinary excretion of a single intravenous dose of 5-FU amounts to only 5–10% in 24 hours. Although the liver contains high concentrations of DPD, dosage does not have to be modified in patients with hepatic dysfunction, presumably because of degradation of the drug at extrahepatic sites or by vast excess of this enzyme in the liver. 5-FU enters the CSF in minimal amounts.

Capecitabine is well absorbed orally. It is rapidly de-esterified and deaminated, yielding high plasma concentrations of 5'-deoxy-fluorodeoxyuridine (5'-dFdU), which disappears with a $t_{1/2}$ of ~1 hour. 5-FU levels are <10% of those of 5'-dFdU. The conversion of 5'-dFdU to 5-FU by thymidine phosphorylase occurs in liver, peripheral tissues, and tumors. Liver dysfunction delays the conversion of the parent compound to 5'-dFdU and 5-FU, but there is no consistent effect on toxicity.

5-Fluorouracil   5-Fluorouracil produces partial responses in 10–20% of patients with metastatic colon carcinomas, upper GI carcinomas, and breast carcinomas. The administration of 5-FU in combination with leucovorin in the adjuvant setting is associated with a survival advantage for patients with colorectal cancers and gastric cancers.

For average-risk patients in good nutritional status with adequate hematopoietic function, the weekly dosage regimen is 500-600 mg/m^2 with leucovorin once each week for 6 of 8 weeks. Other regimens use daily doses of 500 mg/m^2 for 5 days, repeated in monthly cycles. When used with leucovorin, doses of daily 5-FU for 5 days must be reduced to 375-425 mg/m^2 because of mucositis and diarrhea. 5-FU is increasingly used as a biweekly loading dose followed by a 48-hour continuous infusion, a schedule that has less overall toxicity as well as superior response rates and progression-free survival for patients with metastatic colon cancer.

Floxuridine (FUdR)

FUdR (fluorodeoxyuridine; FUDR) is used primarily by continuous infusion into the hepatic artery for treatment of metastatic carcinoma of the colon or following resection of hepatic metastases; the response rate to such infusion is 40–50%, or double that observed with intravenous administration. Intrahepatic arterial infusion for 14–21 days may be used with minimal systemic toxicity. However, there is a significant risk of biliary sclerosis if this route is used for multiple cycles of therapy. Treatment should be discontinued at the earliest manifestation of toxicity (usually stomatitis or diarrhea) because the maximal effects of bone marrow suppression and gut toxicity will not be evident until days 7–14.

Capecitabine (XELODA)

Capecitabine is FDA-approved for the treatment of (1) metastatic breast cancer in patients who have not responded to a regimen of paclitaxel and an anthracycline antibiotic; (2) metastatic breast cancer when used in combination with docetaxel *in patients who have had a prior anthracycline-containing regimen; and (3) metastatic colorectal cancer for patients in whom fluoropyrimidine monotherapy is preferred. The recommended dose is 2500 mg/m² daily, given orally in two divided doses with food, for 2 weeks followed by a rest period of 1 week. This cycle is then repeated two more times.*

COMBINATION THERAPY Higher response rates are seen when 5-FU is used in combination with other agents, such as cyclophosphamide and methotrexate (breast cancer), cisplatin (head and neck cancer), and with oxaliplatin or irinotecan in colon cancer. The combination of 5-FU and oxaliplatin or irinotecan has become the standard first-line treatment for patients with metastatic colorectal cancer. The use of 5-FU in combination regimens has improved survival in the adjuvant treatment for breast cancer, and with oxaliplatin and leucovorin, for colorectal cancer. 5-FU also is a potent radiation sensitizer. Beneficial effects also have been reported when combined with irradiation for cancers of the esophagus, stomach, pancreas, cervix, anus, and head and neck. 5-FU is used widely with very favorable results for the topical treatment of premalignant keratoses of the skin and multiple superficial basal cell carcinomas.

The clinical manifestations of toxicity caused by 5-FU and floxuridine are similar and may be difficult to anticipate because of their delayed appearance. The earliest untoward symptoms are anorexia and nausea; these are followed by stomatitis and diarrhea, which are reliable warning signs that a sufficient dose has been administered. Mucosal ulcerations occur throughout the GI tract and may lead to fulminant diarrhea, shock, and death, particularly in patients who are DPD deficient. The major toxic effects of bolus-dose regimens result from the myelosuppressive action of 5-FU. The nadir of leukopenia usually is between days 9 and 14 after the first injection of drug. Thrombocytopenia and anemia also may occur. Loss of hair, occasionally progressing to total alopecia, nail changes, dermatitis, and increased pigmentation and atrophy of the skin may be encountered. Hand-foot syndrome consisting of erythema, desquamation, pain, and sensitivity to touch of the palms and soles also can occur. Neurological manifestations, including an acute cerebellar syndrome, have been reported, and myelopathy has been observed after the intrathecal administration of 5-FU. Cardiac toxicity, particularly acute chest pain with evidence of ischemia in the electrocardiogram, also may occur. In general, myelosuppression, mucositis, and diarrhea occur less often with infusion than bolus regimens, while hand-foot syndrome occurs more often with infusion than bolus regimens. The low therapeutic indices of these agents emphasize the need for very skillful supervision by physicians familiar with the action of the fluorinated pyrimidines and the possible hazards of chemotherapy. Capecitabine causes much the same spectrum of toxicities as 5-FU (diarrhea, myelosuppression), but the hand-foot syndrome occurs more frequently and may require dose reduction or cessation of therapy.

CYTIDINE ANALOGS
Cytarabine (Cytosine Arabinoside; Ara-C)

Cytarabine (1-β-D-arabinofuranosylcytosine; Ara-C) is the single most effective agent for induction of remission in AML. Ara-C is an analog of 2′-deoxycytidine; the 2′-hydroxyl hinders rotation of the pyrimidine base around the nucleosidic bond and interferes with base stacking. Ara-C penetrates cells by a carrier-mediated process shared by physiological nucleosides. In infants and adults with ALL and the t(4;11) MLL translocation, high-dose Ara-C is particularly effective; in these patients, the nucleoside transporter, hENT1, is highly expressed, and its expression correlates with Ara-C sensitivity. At extracellular drug concentrations >10 μM (levels achievable with high-dose Ara-C), the nucleoside transporter no longer limits drug accumulation, and intracellular metabolism to a triphosphate becomes rate limiting.

As with most purine and pyrimidine antimetabolites, Ara-C must be "activated" by conversion to the 5′-monophosphate nucleotide (Ara-CMP), a reaction catalyzed by deoxycytidine kinase. Ara-CMP can then react with appropriate deoxynucleotide kinases to form the diphosphate and triphosphates (Ara-CDP and Ara-CTP). Ara-CTP competes with the physiological substrate deoxycytidine 5′-triphosphate (dCTP) for incorporation into DNA by DNA polymerases. The incorporated Ara-CMP residue potently inhibits DNA polymerase, in both replication and repair. Fragmentation of DNA is observed in Ara-C–treated cells, and there is cytological and biochemical evidence for apoptosis in both tumor and normal tissues.

The optimal interval between bolus doses of Ara-C is ~8–12 hours, a schedule that maintains intracellular concentrations of Ara-CTP at inhibitory levels for at least one cell cycle. Typical schedules for Ara-C administration employ bolus doses every 12 hours for 5–7 days or a continuous infusion for 7 days. Particular subtypes of AML derive benefit from high-dose Ara-C treatment; these include t(8;21), inv(16), t(9;16), and del(16).

Response to Ara-C is strongly influenced by the relative activities of anabolic and catabolic enzymes that determine the proportion of drug converted to Ara-CTP. The rate-limiting enzyme is deoxycytidine kinase, which produces Ara-CMP. An important degradative enzyme is cytidine deaminase, which deaminates Ara-C to a nontoxic metabolite, arauridine. Cytidine deaminase is found in high activity in many tissues, including some human tumors. A second degradative enzyme, dCMP deaminase, converts Ara-CMP to the inactive metabolite, Ara-UMP. Increased synthesis and retention of Ara-CTP in leukemic cells is associated with a longer duration of complete remission in patients with AML. The ability of cells to transport Ara-C also affects the clinical response.

Because drug concentration in plasma rapidly falls below the level needed to saturate transport and activation processes, high-dose regimens (2–3 g/m^2 every 12 hours for 6 doses) to achieve 20–50-times higher serum levels give improved results in remission induction and consolidation for AML. Due to the presence of high concentrations of cytidine deaminase in the GI mucosa and liver, only ~20% of the drug reaches the circulation after oral Ara-C administration; thus, the drug must be given intravenously. Peak plasma concentrations disappear rapidly ($t_{1/2}$ of 10 minutes). Less than 10% of the injected dose is excreted unchanged in the urine within 12–24 hours, while most appears as the inactive deaminated product, arabinosyl uracil. Higher concentrations of Ara-C are found in CSF after continuous infusion than after rapid intravenous injection. After intrathecal administration of the drug at a dose of 50 mg/m^2, relatively little deamination occurs, even after 7 hours, and peak concentrations decline slowly with a half-life of ~3.4 hours. Concentrations above the threshold for cytotoxicity (0.4 µM) are maintained in the CSF for 24 hours or longer. More recently, a formulation of Ara-C (DEPOCYT) has been developed for sustained release into the CSF. After a standard 50-mg dose, cytarabine concentration is maintained at cytotoxic levels for an average of 12 days, thus avoiding the need for repeated lumbar punctures.

Two standard dosage schedules are recommended for administration of cytarabine (CYTOSAR-U, TARABINE PFS, others): (1) rapid intravenous infusion of 100 mg/m^2 every 12 hours for 5–7 days; or (2) continuous intravenous infusion of 100 to 200 mg/m^2 daily for 5–7 days. In general, children tolerate higher doses than do adults. Intrathecal doses of 30 mg/m^2 every 4 days have been used to treat meningeal leukemia. The intrathecal administration of 50–70 mg of the liposomal formulation of cytarabine (DEPOCYT) every 2 weeks seems to be equally effective as the every-4-day regimen. Conventional cytarabine is indicated for induction and maintenance of remission in acute nonlymphocytic leukemia and is useful in the treatment of other leukemias, such as ALL, AML, and CML in the blast phase. Intrathecal cytarabine is indicated for meningeal leukemia. A depot formulation of cytarabine is indicated for the intrathecal treatment of lymphomatous meningitis and may be useful for carcinomatous meningitis. Cytarabine is a potent myelosuppressive agent capable of producing acute, severe leukopenia, thrombocytopenia, and anemia with striking megaloblastic changes. Other toxic manifestations include GI disturbances, stomatitis, conjunctivitis, reversible elevations of hepatic enzymes, noncardiogenic pulmonary edema, and dermatitis. Cerebellar toxicity, manifest as ataxia and slurred speech, and cerebral toxicity, including seizures, dementia, and coma, may follow intrathecal administration or high-dose systemic administration to patients >50 years of age and/or patients with impaired renal function.

Azacitidine (5-Azacytidine)

5-Azacytidine and the closely related investigational drug decitabine (2′-dexoy-5-azacytidine) have antileukemic activity and induce differentiation. 5-Azacytidine is approved for treatment of myelodysplasia; it induces normalization of bone marrow in 15–20% of patients and reduces transfusion requirement in one-third of patients. It becomes incorporated into RNA and DNA and inhibits methylation of DNA, inducing the expression of silenced genes. Thus, it also is used to induce fetal hemoglobin (HbF) synthesis in sickle cell anemia, although it has been largely replaced for this indication by hydroxyurea. It undergoes very rapid deamination by cytidine deaminase, the product hydrolyzing to inactive metabolites. Its major toxicities include myelosuppression, and rather severe nausea and vomiting when given intravenously in large doses (150–200 mg/m^2/day for 5 days). In low-dose daily subcutaneous regimens for myelodysplasia, 30 mg/m^2/day, it is well tolerated.

Gemcitabine

Gemcitabine (2′,2′ difluorodeoxycytidine; dFdC), a difluoro analog of deoxycytidine, is used for patients with metastatic pancreatic cancer, non–small cell lung cancer, ovarian, bladder, esophageal, and head and neck cancer. Gemcitabine enters cells *via* active nucleoside transporters. Intracellularly, deoxycytidine kinase phosphorylates gemcitabine to produce difluorodeoxycytidine monophosphate (dFdCMP), from which point it is converted to difluorodeoxycytidine di- and triphosphate (dFdCDP and dFdCTP). While its anabolism and effects on DNA in general mimic those of cytarabine, there are differences in kinetics of inhibition, additional sites of action, effects of incorporation into DNA, and spectrum of clinical activity. Unlike cytarabine, the cytotoxicity of gemcitabine is not confined to the S phase of the cell cycle. The cytotoxic activity may reflect several actions on DNA synthesis: dFdCTP competes with dCTP as a weak inhibitor of DNA polymerase; dFdCDP is a potent inhibitor of ribonucleotide reductase, resulting in depletion of deoxyribonucleotide pools necessary for DNA synthesis; and incorporation of dFdCTP into DNA leads to DNA strand termination that is apparently resistant to repair. The ability of cells to incorporate dFdCTP into DNA is critical for gemcitabine-induced apoptosis.

Gemcitabine is administered by intravenous infusion. The pharmacokinetics of the parent compound is largely determined by deamination, and the predominant urinary elimination product is the inactive metabolite difluorodeoxyuridine (dFdU). Gemcitabine has a short plasma $t_{1/2}$ (~15 minutes), with women and elderly subjects having slower clearance. Clearance is dose-independent but varies widely among individuals. The standard dosing schedule for gemcitabine (GEMZAR) is a 30-minute intravenous infusion of 1–1.2 g/m² on days 1, 8, and 15 of each 28-day cycle. Similar to that of cytarabine, conversion of gemcitabine to dFdCMP by deoxycytidine kinase is saturated at infusion rates of ~10 mg/m²/min. To increase dFdCTP formation, the duration of infusion at this maximum concentration has been extended to 150 minutes. In contrast to infusion duration of 30 minutes, the 150-minute infusion produces a higher level of dFdCTP within peripheral blood mononuclear cells, increases the degree of myelosuppression, but has uncertain effects on antitumor activity.

The activity of dFdCTP on DNA repair mechanisms may allow for increased cytotoxicity of other chemotherapeutic agents, particularly platinum compounds. Preclinical studies of tumor cell lines show that cisplatin-DNA adducts are enhanced in the presence of gemcitabine, presumably through suppression of nuclear excision repair.

The principal toxicity of gemcitabine is myelosuppression. In general, longer-duration infusions lead to greater myelosuppression. Nonhematologic toxicities including a flu-like syndrome, asthenia, and mild elevation in liver transaminases may occur in 40% or more of patients. Although severe nonhematological toxicities are rare, interstitial pneumonitis may occur and is responsive to glucocorticoids. Rarely, patients on gemcitabine treatment for many months may develop a slowly progressive hemolytic uremic syndrome, necessitating drug discontinuation. Gemcitabine is a very potent radiosensitizer and generally should not be used with radiotherapy.

PURINE ANALOGS

Analogs of naturally occurring purine bases with antileukemic, immunosuppressant, and antiviral properties include mercaptopurine, thioguanine, azathioprine, *acyclovir, ganciclovir, vidarabine,* and *zidovudine.* Other purine analogs important in cancer therapy include pentostatin (2'-deoxycoformycin), *cladribine,* and fludarabine phosphate.

6-Thiopurine Analogs

6-Mercaptopurine (6-MP) and 6-thioguanine (6-TG) are approved for human leukemias and function as analogs of the natural purines, hypoxanthine and guanine. The substitution of sulfur for oxygen on C6 of the purine ring creates compounds that are readily converted to nucleotides in normal and malignant cells. Nucleotides formed from 6-MP and 6-TG inhibit de novo purine synthesis and become incorporated into nucleic acids. Both 6-TG and 6-MP are excellent substrates for hypoxanthine guanine phosphoribosyl transferase (HGPRT) and are converted in a single step to the ribonucleotides 6-thioguanosine-5'-monophosphate (6-thioGMP) and 6-thioinosine-5'-monophosphate (T-IMP), respectively. Because T-IMP is a poor substrate for guanylyl kinase, the enzyme that converts guanosine monophosphate (GMP) to guanosine diphosphate (GDP), T-IMP accumulates intracellularly. T-IMP inhibits the first step in the de novo synthesis of the purine base and thereby inhibits the formation of ribosyl-5-phosphate, as well as conversion of inosine-5'-monophosphate (IMP) to adenine and guanine nucleotides. Of these, the most important point of attack seems to be the reaction of glutamine and 5-phosphoribosyl-1-pyrophosphate (PRPP) to form ribosyl-5-phosphate, the first committed step in the de novo pathway.

The role of incorporation of thiopurines into cellular DNA with regard to therapeutic or toxic effects remains unknown. The incidence of pregnancy-related complications, however, was significantly increased when fathers used mercaptopurine within 3 months of conception. These compounds can cause marked inhibition of the coordinated induction of various enzymes required for DNA synthesis, as well as potentially critical alterations in the synthesis of polyadenylate-containing RNA.

As with other antimetabolites, acquired resistance is a major obstacle. The most common mechanism of 6-MP resistance is deficiency or complete lack of the activating enzyme, HGPRT. Another mechanism of resistance is increased particulate alkaline phosphatase activity. Other potential mechanisms for resistance to 6-MP include: (1) decreased drug transport; (2) alteration in allosteric inhibition of ribosylamine 5-phosphate synthase; (3) altered recognition of DNA breaks and mismatches induced by 6-MP; and (4) increased activity of multidrug resistance protein 5, which exports nucleoside analogs.

Absorption of mercaptopurine is incomplete after oral ingestion and bioavailability is reduced by first-pass metabolism by xanthine oxidase in the liver. Oral bioavailability is only 10–50%, with great interpatient variability and decreased absorption in the presence of food or oral antibiotics. Thus, when used in combination with other drugs, doses should be titrated according to the white blood cell and platelet counts. Bioavailability is increased when mercaptopurine is combined with high-dose methotrexate. After an intravenous dose, the plasma $t_{1/2}$ of the drug is relatively short (~50 minutes in adults), due to rapid metabolic degradation by xanthine oxidase and thiopurine methyltransferase (TPMT). Restricted CNS distribution of mercaptopurine results from an efficient efflux transport system in the blood–brain barrier. In addition to the HGPRT-catalyzed anabolism of mercaptopurine, there are two other pathways for its metabolism. The first involves methylation of the sulfhydryl group and subsequent oxidation of the methylated derivatives. Expression of the TPMT reflects the inheritance of polymorphic alleles; up to 15% of the Caucasian population has decreased enzyme activity which is associated with increased drug toxicity in individual patients and a lower risk of relapse (*see* Chapter 4). High concentrations of 6-methylmercaptopurine nucleotides are formed following 6-MP administration. Substantial amounts of the mono-, di-, and triphosphate nucleotides of 6-methylmercaptopurine ribonucleoside (6-MMPR) are found in cells in the blood and bone marrow of patients treated with 6-MP or azathioprine. They are less potent than 6-MP nucleotides as metabolic inhibitors, and their significance in contributing to the activity of 6-MP is not known. The second major pathway for 6-MP metabolism involves its oxidation by xanthine oxidase to 6-thiouric acid, an inactive metabolite. Oral doses of 6-MP should be reduced by 75% in patients receiving the xanthine oxidase inhibitor allopurinol.

The initial average daily oral dose of mercaptopurine (6-mercaptopurine, 6-MP; PURINETHOL) is 50–100 mg/m², and is adjusted according to white blood cell and platelet counts. The total dose required to produce bone marrow depression in patients with nonhematological malignancies is ~45 mg/kg, ranging from 18 to 100 mg/kg. Hyperuricemia with hyperuricosuria may occur during treatment; the accumulation of uric acid presumably reflects the destruction of cells with release of purines that are oxidized by xanthine oxidase and an inhibition of the conversion of inosinic acid to nucleic acid precursors. This may be an indication for the use of allopurinol. Special caution must be employed if 6-MP or its imidazolyl derivative, azathioprine, is used with allopurinol because the associated delay in catabolism of the purine analog increases the likelihood of severe toxicity. Patients treated simultaneously with both drugs should receive ~25% of the usual dose of mercaptopurine. The combination of methotrexate and 6-MP is synergistic, based on the effects of methotrexate inhibition of the earliest steps in purine synthesis; methotrexate elevates the intracellular concentration of PRPP, which is required for 6-MP activation.

The principal toxicity of 6-MP is bone marrow depression, although this side effect generally develops more gradually than with folic acid antagonists; accordingly, thrombocytopenia, granulocytopenia, or anemia may not be encountered for several weeks. When depression of normal bone marrow elements occurs, dose reduction usually results in prompt recovery. Anorexia, nausea, or vomiting is seen in ~25% of adults, but stomatitis and diarrhea are rare; manifestations of GI effects are less frequent in children than in adults. Jaundice and hepatic enzyme elevations occur in up to one-third of adult patients treated with 6-MP, and usually resolve upon discontinuation of therapy. The long-term complications associated with 6-MP and its derivative azathioprine are opportunistic infection and an increased incidence of squamous cell malignancies of skin. Teratogenic effects during the first trimester are associated with chronic 6-MP, and AML has been reported after prolonged use of 6-MP for Crohn's disease.

Fludarabine Phosphate

A fluorinated deamination-resistant nucleotide analog of the antiviral agent vidarabine (9-β-D-arabinofuranosyl-adenine), this compound is active in CLL and low-grade lymphomas. After rapid extracellular dephosphorylation to the nucleoside fludarabine, it is rephosphorylated intracellularly by deoxycytidine kinase to the active triphosphate derivative. This antimetabolite inhibits DNA polymerase, DNA primase, DNA ligase, and ribonucleotide reductase, and is incorporated into DNA and

RNA. The triphosphate nucleotide is an effective chain terminator when incorporated into DNA, and the incorporation of fludarabine into RNA inhibits RNA function, RNA processing, and mRNA translation. A major effect of this drug may be its activation of apoptosis, which may explain its activity against indolent lymphoproliferative disease, where only a small fraction of cells are in S phase.

Fludarabine phosphate administered intravenously is rapidly converted to fludarabine in the plasma. The terminal $t_{1/2}$ of fludarabine is ~10 hours. The compound is primarily eliminated by renal excretion, and ~23% appears in the urine as fludarabine because of its relative resistance to deamination by adenosine deaminase (ADA).

Fludarabine phosphate (FLUDARA) is available for intravenous use. The recommended dose of fludarabine phosphate is 20–30 mg/m² daily for 5 days. The drug is administered intravenously by infusion during a period of 30 minutes to 2 hours. Dosage may need to be reduced in renal impairment. Treatment may be repeated every 4 weeks, and at these doses gradual improvement usually occurs during a period of 2–3 cycles.

Fludarabine phosphate is used primarily for the treatment of patients with CLL, although experience is accumulating that suggests effectiveness in B-cell lymphomas refractory to standard therapy. In CLL patients previously refractory to a regimen containing a standard alkylating agent, response rates of 32–48% have been reported. Activity also has been seen with indolent non-Hodgkin's lymphoma, promyelocytic leukemia, cutaneous T-cell lymphoma, and Waldenström's macroglobulinemia. In patients with previously untreated low-grade lymphomas, fludarabine phosphate in combination with either cyclophosphamide or with dexamethasone and mitoxantrone has resulted in a high rate of response.

Toxic manifestations include myelosuppression, nausea and vomiting, chills and fever, malaise, anorexia, and weakness. Lymphopenia and thrombocytopenia are dose limiting and possibly cumulative. CD4⁺ T cells are depleted with therapy. Opportunistic infections and tumor lysis syndrome have been reported. Peripheral neuropathy may occur at standard doses. Altered mental status, seizures, optic neuritis, and coma have been observed at higher doses and in older patients. Rarely, CLL patients may develop an acute hemolytic anemia or pure red cell aplasia during fludarabine treatment. Severe pneumonitis responsive to glucocorticoids has been encountered. Because a significant fraction of drug (~25%) is eliminated in the urine, patients with compromised renal function should be treated with caution, and initial doses should be reduced proportionate to serum creatinine levels.

Cladribine

An ADA-resistant purine analog, cladribine (2-chlorodeoxyadenosine; 2-CdA) has demonstrated potent activity in hairy cell leukemia, CLL, and low-grade lymphomas. After intracellular phosphorylation by deoxycytidine kinase and conversion to cladribine triphosphate, it is incorporated into DNA. It produces DNA strand breaks and depletion of NAD and adenosine triphosphate (ATP), as well as apoptosis, and is a potent inhibitor of ribonucleotide reductase. The drug does not require cell division to be cytotoxic. Resistance is associated with loss of the activating enzyme, deoxycytidine kinase, or escape of ribonucleotide reductase from inhibition.

Cladribine is moderately well absorbed orally (55%), but is routinely administered intravenously. The drug is excreted by the kidneys, with a terminal $t_{1/2}$ in plasma of ~7 hours. Cladribine crosses the blood–brain barrier and reaches CSF concentrations of ~25% of those seen in plasma. In patients with meningeal involvement, however, CSF concentrations can approach those in plasma.

Cladribine (LEUSTATIN) is administered as a single course of 0.09 mg/kg/day for 7 days by continuous intravenous infusion. Cladribine is considered the drug of choice in hairy cell leukemia. Eighty percent of patients achieve a complete response after a single course of therapy. The drug also is active in CLL, and is a secondary agent in other leukemias and low-grade lymphomas, Langerhans cell histiocytosis, cutaneous T-cell lymphomas including mycosis fungoides and the Sézary syndrome, and Waldenström's macroglobulinemia.

The major dose-limiting toxicity of cladribine is myelosuppression. Cumulative thrombocytopenia may occur with repeated courses. Opportunistic infections are common and are correlated with decreased CD4⁺ cell counts. Other toxic effects include nausea, infections, high fever, headache, fatigue, skin rashes, and tumor lysis syndrome. Neurological and immunosuppressive adverse effects are less evident than with pentostatin at clinically active doses.

Pentostatin (2′-Deoxycoformycin)

Pentostatin, a transition-state analog of the intermediate in the ADA reaction, is a potent inhibitor of ADA. Its effects mimic the phenotype of genetic ADA deficiency, which is associated with severe immunodeficiency affecting both T- and B-cell functions. Inhibition of ADA by pentostatin leads to accumulation of intracellular adenosine and deoxyadenosine nucleotides, which can block DNA synthesis by inhibiting ribonucleotide reductase. Deoxyadenosine also inactivates S-adenosyl homocysteine hydrolase. The resulting accumulation of S-adenosyl homocysteine is particularly toxic to lymphocytes. Pentostatin also can inhibit RNA synthesis, and its triphosphate derivative is incorporated into DNA, resulting in strand breakage. In combination with 2'-deoxyadenosine, it is capable of inducing apoptosis in human monocytoid leukemia cells. Although the precise mechanism of cytotoxicity is not known, it is probable that the imbalance in purine nucleotide pools accounts for its antineoplastic effect in hairy cell leukemia and T-cell lymphomas.

Pentostatin is administered intravenously, and a single dose of 4 mg/m^2 has a terminal $t_{1/2}$ of 5.7 hours. The drug is eliminated almost entirely by renal excretion, and proportional reduction of dosage is recommended in patients with renal impairment.

Pentostatin (NIPENT) is available for intravenous use. The recommended dosage is 4 mg/m^2 administered every other week. After hydration with 500–1000 mL of 5% dextrose in 0.45% saline, the drug is administered by rapid intravenous injection or by infusion during a period of up to 30 minutes, followed by an additional 500 mL of fluids. Extravasation does not produce tissue necrosis. Pentostatin is extremely effective in producing complete remissions in hairy cell leukemia. Complete responses of 58% and partial responses of 28% have been reported, even in patients who were refractory to interferon-α. Activity also is seen against CLL, CML, promyelocytic leukemia, cutaneous T-cell lymphoma, non-Hodgkin's lymphoma, and Langerhans cell histiocytosis. Pentostatin has no significant activity against solid tumors or MM.

Toxic manifestations include myelosuppression, GI symptoms, rashes, and abnormal liver function studies at standard (4 mg/m^2) doses. Depletion of normal T cells occurs at these doses, and neutropenic fever and opportunistic infections can occur. Immunosuppression may persist for several years after discontinuation of pentostatin therapy. At higher doses (10 mg/m^2), major renal and neurological complications are encountered. The use of pentostatin in combination with fludarabine phosphate may result in severe or even fatal pulmonary toxicity.

III. NATURAL PRODUCTS

ANTIMITOTIC DRUGS
Vinca Alkaloids

Vinblastine and vincristine—alkaloids purified from the periwinkle plant—are used for treatment of leukemias, lymphomas, and testicular cancer. A closely related derivative, *vinorelbine*, has important activity against lung cancer and breast cancer. The vinca alkaloids are cell cycle–specific agents, and in common with other drugs such as *colchicine*, *podophyllotoxin*, and taxanes, block cells in mitosis. The vinca alkaloids bind specifically to β-tubulin and block its ability to polymerize with α-tubulin into microtubules. In the absence of an intact mitotic spindle, duplicated chromosomes cannot align along the division plate and cell division is arrested in metaphase. Cells blocked in mitosis undergo changes characteristic of apoptosis.

In addition to their key role in the formation of mitotic spindles, microtubules are found in high concentration in the brain and are essential to cellular functions such as movement, phagocytosis, and axonal transport. Side effects of the vinca alkaloids, such as their neurotoxicity, may be due to disruption of these functions.

Despite their structural similarity, the vinca alkaloids have unique individual patterns of clinical effectiveness (see below). However, in most experimental systems, they share cross-resistance. Their antitumor effects are blocked by multidrug resistance, in which tumor cells become cross-resistant to a wide range of chemically dissimilar agents after exposure to a single (natural product) drug. Such multidrug-resistant tumor cells display cross-resistance to vinca alkaloids, the epipodophyllotoxins, anthracyclines, and taxanes. Chromosomal abnormalities consistent with gene amplification have been observed in resistant cells in culture, and the cells contain markedly increased levels of the P-glycoprotein, a membrane efflux pump that transports drugs from the cells. Calcium channel blockers such as verapamil can reverse resistance of this type. Other membrane transporters such as the multidrug resistance–associated protein (MRP), and the closely related breast cancer resistance protein, may mediate multidrug resistance. Other forms of resistance to vinca alkaloids stem from mutations in β-tubulin or in the relative expression of its isoforms; both changes prevent the effective binding of the inhibitors to their target.

Vincristine is a standard component of regimens for treating pediatric leukemias, lymphomas, and solid tumors. In large-cell non-Hodgkin's lymphomas, vincristine remains an important drug, particularly when used in the CHOP regimen with cyclophosphamide, doxorubicin, and pred-nisone. As mentioned above, vincristine is more useful for remission induction in lymphocytic leukemia. Vincristine also is a standard component of regimens used to treat pediatric solid tumors such as Wilms' tumor, neuroblastoma, and rhabdomyosarcoma. Vinblastine is employed in bladder cancer, testicular carcinomas, and Hodgkin's disease. Vinorelbine has activity against non–small cell lung cancer and breast cancer. The limited myelosuppressive action of vincristine makes it a valuable component of a number of combination therapy regimens for leukemia and lymphoma, while the lack of neurotoxicity of vinblastine is a decided advantage in lymphomas and in combination with cisplatin against testicular cancer. Vinorelbine, which causes a mild neuro-toxicity as well as myelosuppression, has an intermediate toxicity profile.

The nadir of leukopenia following vinblastine or vinorelbine occurs 7–10 days after drug administration. Vincristine in standard doses, 1.4–2 mg/m², causes little reduction of formed ele-ments in the blood. All three agents cause hair loss and local cellulitis if extravasated. A syndrome of hyponatremia due to inappropriate secretion of vasopressin occurs rarely after vincristine administration (see Chapter 29). While all 3 derivatives may cause neurotoxic symptoms, vin-cristine has predictable cumulative effects. Numbness and tingling of the extremities and loss of deep tendon reflexes are the most common and earliest signs, followed by motor weakness. Sen-sory changes do not usually warrant an immediate reduction in drug dose, but loss of motor func-tion should lead to a reevaluation of the therapeutic plan, and under most circumstances, drug discontinuation. Rarely, patients may experience vocal cord paralysis or loss of extraocular muscle function. High-dose vincristine causes severe constipation. Inadvertent intrathecal vin-cristine administration produces devastating and invariably fatal central neurotoxicity, with seizures and irreversible coma.

The liver extensively metabolizes all three agents, and the conjugates and metabolites are excreted in the bile. Only a small fraction of a dose (<15%) is found in the urine unchanged. In patients with hepatic dysfunction (bilirubin >3 mg/dL), a 75% reduction in dose of any of the vinca alkaloids is advisable. The pharmacokinetics of each of the three drugs are similar, with central and tissue elimination half-lives of 1 and 20 hours for vincristine, 3 and 23 hours for vin-blastine, and 1 and 45 hours for vinorelbine, respectively.

Vinblastine

Vinblastine sulfate (VELBAN, others) is given intravenously; special precautions must be taken against subcutaneous extravasation, since this may cause painful ulceration. The drug should not be injected into an extremity with impaired circulation. After a single dose of 0.3 mg/kg of body weight, myelosuppression reaches its maximum in 7–10 days. If a moderate level of leukopenia (~3000 cells/mm³) is not attained, the weekly dose may be increased gradually by increments of 0.05 mg/kg. In regimens designed to cure testicular cancer, vinblastine is used in doses of 0.3 mg/kg every 3 weeks.

The most important clinical use of vinblastine is with bleomycin and cisplatin (see below) in the curative therapy of metastatic testicular tumors, although it has been supplanted by etoposide or ifosfamide in this disease. It is a component of the standard curative ABVD regimen for Hodgkin's disease (adriamycin, bleomycin, vinblastine, and dacarbazine). It also is active in Kaposi's sar-coma, neuroblastoma, and histiocytosis X, and in carcinoma of the breast and choriocarcinoma.

The nadir of the leukopenia that follows the administration of vinblastine usually occurs within 7–10 days, after which recovery ensues within 7 days. Other toxic effects of include neu-rological manifestations as described above. GI disturbances including nausea, vomiting, anorexia, and diarrhea may be encountered. The syndrome of inappropriate secretion of antidi-uretic hormone has been reported. Loss of hair, stomatitis, and dermatitis occur infrequently. Extravasation during injection may lead to cellulitis and phlebitis. Local injection of hyaluronidase and application of moderate heat to the area may be of help by dispersing the drug.

Vincristine

Vincristine sulfate (ONCOVIN, VINCASAR PFS, others) used together with glucocorticoids is the treat-ment of choice to induce remissions in childhood leukemia; common dosages for these drugs are vincristine, intravenously, 2 mg/m² of body surface area weekly, and prednisone, orally, 40 mg/m² daily. Adult patients with Hodgkin's disease or non-Hodgkin's lymphomas usually receive vin-cristine as part of a complex protocol. When used in the MOPP regimen (see below), the recom-mended dose of vincristine is 1.4 mg/m². Vincristine seems to be better tolerated by children than by adults, who may experience severe, neurological toxicity. Drug administration more frequently than every 7 days or at higher doses seems to increase toxic manifestations without improving the response rate. Maintenance therapy with vincristine is not recommended in children with leukemia.

Precautions also should be used to avoid extravasation during intravenous administration of vincristine.

In large-cell lymphoma, a liposomal formulation of vincristine (ONCO-TCS), given in doses of 2 mg/m², has less neurotoxicity and retains activity in patients who relapse after vincristine therapy. It has the expected advantages of slower elimination and greater tissue distribution as compared to the unmodified drug.

The clinical toxicity of vincristine is mostly neurological. The more severe neurological manifestations may be avoided or reversed either by suspending therapy or reducing the dosage upon occurrence of motor dysfunction. Severe constipation may be prevented by a prophylactic program of laxatives and hydrophilic (bulk-forming) agents and usually is a problem only with doses above 2 mg/m². Alopecia occurs in ~20% of patients given vincristine; however, it is always reversible, frequently without cessation of therapy. Although less common than with vinblastine, leukopenia may occur with vincristine, and thrombocytopenia, anemia, polyuria, dysuria, fever, and GI symptoms have been reported occasionally. The syndrome of inappropriate secretion of antidiuretic hormone occasionally has occurred during vincristine therapy. In view of the rapid action of the vinca alkaloids, it is advisable to prevent hyperuricemia by the administration of allopurinol.

Vinorelbine

Vinorelbine (NAVELBINE, others) is administered in normal saline as an intravenous infusion of 30 mg/m² given over 6–10 minutes. A lower dose (20–25 mg/m²) may be required for patients who have received prior chemotherapy. When used alone, it is initially given every week until progression of disease or dose-limiting toxicity. When used with cisplatin for the treatment of non–small cell lung carcinoma, it is given every 3 weeks. Like the other vinca alkaloids, it is eliminated by hepatic metabolism, and has an elimination $t_{1/2}$ of 24 hours. Its primary toxicity is granulocytopenia, with only modest thrombocytopenia and less neurotoxicity than other vinca alkaloids. It may cause allergic reactions and mild, reversible elevations in liver enzymes. Doses should be reduced in patients with elevated bilirubin or with >75% liver replacement by metastatic disease.

Taxanes

Paclitaxel (TAXOL), a compound first isolated from the bark of the Western yew tree, and its semi-synthetic congener docetaxel (TAXOTERE) exhibit unique pharmacological actions. They differ from the vinca alkaloids and colchicine derivatives in that they bind to a different site on β-tubulin and promote rather than inhibit microtubule formation. The drugs have a central role in the therapy of ovarian, breast, lung, esophageal, bladder, and head and neck cancers. Their optimal dose, schedule, and use in drug combinations still are evolving.

Paclitaxel has very limited solubility and must be administered in a vehicle of 50% ethanol and 50% polyethoxylated castor oil (CREMOPHOR EL), a formation likely responsible for a high rate of hypersensitivity reactions. Patients receiving this formulation are protected by pretreatment with a histamine H_1 receptor antagonist such as diphenhydramine, an H_2 receptor antagonist such as cimetidine (see Chapter 24), and a glucocorticoid such as dexamethasone (see Chapter 59). Docetaxel, which is somewhat more soluble, is administered in polysorbate 80 and causes a lower incidence of hypersensitivity reactions. Pretreatment with dexamethasone is required to prevent progressive, and often disabling, fluid retention.

Paclitaxel binds specifically to β-tubulin and antagonizes the disassembly of microtubules; bundles of microtubules and aberrant structures derived from microtubules appear in the M phase of the cell cycle, causing mitotic arrest. Cell killing is dependent on both drug concentration and duration of cell exposure. Drugs that block cell cycle progression prior to mitosis antagonize the toxic effects of taxanes.

Drug interactions have been noted; the sequence of cisplatin preceding paclitaxel decreases paclitaxel clearance and produces greater toxicity than the opposite schedule. Paclitaxel decreases doxorubicin clearance and enhances cardiotoxicity, while docetaxel has no apparent effect on anthracycline pharmacokinetics.

The basis of clinical drug resistance is not known. Resistance to taxanes in some tumor cells is due to increased expression of the P-glycoprotein; other resistant cells have β-tubulin mutations and may display heightened sensitivity to vinca alkaloids. Cell death occurs by apoptosis.

Paclitaxel is administered as a 3-hour infusion of 135–175 mg/m² every 3 weeks, or as a weekly 1-hour infusion of 80–100 mg/m². Longer infusions (96 hours) have yielded significant response rates in breast cancer patients, but this form of treatment has serious practical limitations. The drug undergoes extensive CYP-mediated hepatic metabolism (primarily CYP2C8), and <10% of *a dose is excreted in the urine intact. The primary metabolite is 6-OH paclitaxel, which is inactive, but multiple additional hydroxylation products are found in plasma.*

Paclitaxel clearance is nonlinear and decreases with increasing dose or dose rate, possibly related to its dissolution in the vehicle of 50% ethanol and 50% polyethoxylated castor oil, and the nonlinearity of concentrations of the diluent. In studies of 96-hour infusion of 35 mg/m²/day, the presence of hepatic metastases >2 cm in diameter decreased clearance and led to high drug concentrations in plasma and greater myelosuppression. Paclitaxel disappears from the plasma compartment with a $t_{1/2}$ of 10–14 hours and a clearance of 15–18 L/hour/m². The critical plasma concentration for inhibiting bone marrow elements depends on duration of exposure, but likely is in the range of 50–100 nM.

Docetaxel pharmacokinetics are similar to those of paclitaxel. Its elimination $t_{1/2}$ is ~12 hours, and its clearance is 22 L/hour/m². Clearance is primarily through CYP3A4- and CYP3A5-mediated hydroxylation, leading to inactive metabolites. Unlike paclitaxel, the pharmacokinetics or docetaxel are linear up to doses of 115 mg/m².

Dose reductions in patients with abnormal hepatic function have been suggested and 50–75% doses of taxanes should be used in the presence of hepatic metastases >2 cm or in patients with abnormal serum bilirubin. Drugs that induce (e.g., phenytoin and phenobarbital) or inhibit (e.g., antifungal imidazoles) CYP2C8 or CYP3A4 significantly alter drug clearance and toxicity. Paclitaxel clearance is markedly delayed by cyclosporine and other drugs that inhibit the P-glycoprotein. This inhibition may be due to a block of CYP-mediated metabolism or effects on biliary excretion of parent drug or metabolites.

Docetaxel and paclitaxel have become central components of regimens for treating metastatic ovarian, breast, lung, and head and neck cancers. Docetaxel has significant activity with estramustine for treatment of hormone-refractory prostate cancer. Either drug is administered once weekly or once every 3 weeks, with comparable response rates and somewhat different patterns of toxicity. Docetaxel produces greater leukopenia and peripheral edema, while paclitaxel causes a higher incidence of hypersensitivity, myalgias, and neuropathy (particularly when used in combination with a platinum analog). The optimal schedule of taxane administration, alone or in combination with other drugs, is still under evaluation.

Paclitaxel exerts its primary toxic effects on the bone marrow. Neutropenia usually occurs 8–11 days after a dose and reverses rapidly by days 15–21. Used with filgrastim (granulocyte-colony stimulating factor; G-CSF), doses as high as 250 mg/m² over 24 hours are well tolerated, and peripheral neuropathy becomes dose limiting. Many patients experience myalgias after receiving paclitaxel. In high-dose schedules, or with prolonged use, a distal sensory neuropathy can be disabling, particularly in patients with underlying diabetic or alcoholic neuropathy or concurrent cisplatin therapy. Mucositis is prominent in 72- or 96-hour infusions and in the weekly schedule.

Hypersensitivity reactions have occurred in patients receiving paclitaxel infusions of short duration (1–6 hours), but largely are averted by pretreatment with dexamethasone, diphenhydramine, and histamine H_2 receptor antagonists. Premedication is not necessary with 96-hour infusions. Many patients experience asymptomatic bradycardia, and occasional episodes of silent ventricular tachycardia also occur and resolve spontaneously during 3- or 24-hour infusions.

Docetaxel tends to cause more severe, but short-lived, neutropenia than does paclitaxel. It causes less severe peripheral neuropathy and asthenia, and less frequent hypersensitivity. Fluid retention is a progressive problem with multiple cycles of therapy, leading to peripheral edema, pleural and peritoneal fluid, and pulmonary edema in extreme cases. Oral dexamethasone, 8 mg/day, begun 1 day prior to drug infusion and continuing for 3 days, greatly ameliorates fluid retention. In rare cases, docetaxel may cause a progressive interstitial pneumonitis, with respiratory failure supervening if the drug is not discontinued.

CAMPTOTHECIN ANALOGS

The camptothecins are potent, cytotoxic antineoplastic agents that target the nuclear enzyme topoisomerase I; the lead compound, *camptothecin*, was isolated from the Chinese tree *Camptotheca acuminata*. The camptothecin analogs, irinotecan and *topotecan*, have activity in colorectal, ovarian, and small cell lung cancer. All camptothecins have a fused five-ring backbone beginning with a weakly basic quinoline moiety and terminating with a lactone ring. Although necessary for the biological activity of the camptothecins, the lactone ring is unstable, undergoing reversible, nonenzymatic, pH-dependent hydrolysis. Consequently, the camptothecins exist as an equilibrium mixture of the intact lactone and opened-ring carboxylate forms in biological fluids. Substituents on the A and B quinoline rings can modulate the equilibrium position between the closed and opened lactone ring forms through effects on their relative affinities for binding to plasma proteins. For instance, the carboxylate form of camptothecin binds to serum albumin with 200 times greater affinity than the intact lactone, and is the predominant form in plasma and whole blood. In contrast, the lactone form of SN-38 (the biologically active metabolite of irinotecan) binds preferentially to serum albumin, shifting the equilibrium in the opposite direction.

The DNA topoisomerases are nuclear enzymes that reduce torsional stress in supercoiled DNA, allowing selected regions of DNA to become sufficiently untangled to permit replication, recombination, repair, and transcription. Two classes of topoisomerase (I and II) mediate DNA strand breakage and resealing, and both have become the target of cancer chemotherapies. Camptothecin analogs inhibit the function of topoisomerase I, while a number of different chemical entities (e.g., *anthracyclines, epipodophyllotoxins, acridines*) *inhibit topoisomerase II. Topoisomerase I binds covalently to double-stranded DNA through a reversible trans-esterification reaction. This reaction yields an intermediate complex and a single-strand DNA break. This "cleavable complex" allows for relaxation of the DNA torsional strain, either by passage of the intact single-strand through the nick, or by free rotation of the DNA about the noncleaved strand. Once the DNA torsional strain has been relieved, the topoisomerase I reseals the cleavage and dissociates from the newly relaxed double helix.*

The camptothecins bind to and stabilize the normally transient DNA-topoisomerase I cleavable complex. Although the initial cleavage action of topoisomerase I is not affected, the religation step is inhibited, leading to the accumulation of single-stranded breaks in DNA. These lesions are not by themselves toxic to the cell. However, the collision of a DNA replication fork with this cleaved strand of DNA causes an irreversible double-strand DNA break, ultimately leading to cell death. Camptothecins are therefore S-phase–specific drugs. This has important clinical implications, because S-phase–specific cytotoxic agents generally require prolonged exposures of tumor cells to drug concentrations above a minimum threshold to optimize therapeutic efficacy. In fact, studies of low-dose, protracted administration of camptothecin analogs has shown less toxicity, and equal or greater antitumor activity than shorter, more intense courses. Since entry into S phase is required to kill tumor cells exposed to camptothecins, drugs that abolish the G_1-S checkpoint enhance camptothecin lethality.

Decreased intracellular drug accumulation has been observed in several cell lines resistant to camptothecin analogs. Topotecan, but not SN-38 or the intact lactone form of irinotecan, is a substrate for P-glycoprotein; however, compared with other substrates, such as etoposide or doxorubicin, it is a relatively poor substrate. Other reports have associated topotecan or irinotecan resistance with the MRP class of transporters. Drug metabolism could have a role in resistance to irinotecan, but the liver and red blood cells may have sufficient carboxylesterase activity to convert irinotecan to the active SN-38. Transient downregulation of topoisomerase I has been demonstrated following prolonged exposure to camptothecins. Moreover, the degree of topoisomerase I downregulation in peripheral blood mononuclear cells is correlated with plasma AUC or neutrophil nadir in ovarian cancer patients treated with a 21-day continuous intravenous infusion of topotecan. Mutations and post-translational modifications leading to reduced topoisomerase I enzyme catalytic activity or DNA binding affinity have been described in association with camptothecin resistance. Finally, exposure of cells to topoisomerase I–targeted agents leads to increased expression of topoisomerase II, providing a rationale for sequential therapy with topoisomerase I and II inhibitors.

Topotecan

Topotecan is only approved for intravenous administration. An oral dosage form for the drug in development has a bioavailability of 30–40% in cancer patients. Topotecan exhibits linear pharmacokinetics and is rapidly eliminated from systemic circulation (biological $t_{1/2}$, 3.5–4.1 hours) compared with other camptothecins. Only 20–35% of the total drug in plasma is found to be in the active lactone form. Elimination of the lactone appears to result mainly from rapid hydrolysis to the carboxylate followed by renal excretion, with 30–40% of the administered dose excreted in the urine within 24 hours. Doses should be reduced in proportion to reductions in creatinine clearance. Although several oxidative metabolites have been identified, hepatic metabolism appears to be a relatively minor route of drug elimination. Plasma protein binding of topotecan is relatively low (7–35%), which may explain its relatively greater CNS penetration.

Topotecan (HYCAMTIN) is indicated for previously treated patients with ovarian and small cell lung cancer. Its significant hematological toxicity has limited its use in combination with other active agents in these diseases (*e.g.*, cisplatin). Promising antitumor activity also has been observed in hematological malignancies, particularly in CML and in myelodysplastic syndromes.

The recommended dosing regimen of topotecan is a 30-minute infusion of 1.5 mg/m²/day for 5 consecutive days every 3 weeks. Since a significant fraction of the topotecan administered is excreted in the urine, severe toxicities have been observed in patients with decreased creatinine clearance. Therefore, the dose of topotecan should be reduced to 0.75 mg/m²/day in patients with moderate renal dysfunction (creatinine clearance 20–40 mL/min), and topotecan should not be administered to patients with creatinine clearance <20 mL/min. Topotecan clearance and toxicity are not significantly altered in patients with hepatic dysfunction, and therefore no dose reduction is necessary in these patients.

The dose-limiting toxicity of topotecan with all schedules is neutropenia, with or without thrombocytopenia. The incidence of severe neutropenia at the recommended phase II dose of 1.5 mg/m² daily for 5 days every 3 weeks may be as high as 81%, with a 26% incidence of febrile neutropenia. In patients with hematological malignancies, GI side effects such as mucositis and diarrhea become dose limiting. Other less common and generally mild topotecan-related toxicities include nausea and vomiting, elevated liver transaminases, fever, fatigue, and rash.

Irinotecan

The conversion of irinotecan to SN-38 is mediated predominantly by carboxylesterases in the liver. Although SN-38 can be measured in plasma shortly after beginning an intravenous infusion of irinotecan, the AUC of SN-38 is only ~4% of the AUC of irinotecan, suggesting that only a relatively small fraction of the dose is ultimately converted to the active form of the drug. Irinotecan exhibits linear pharmacokinetics. In comparison to topotecan, a relatively large fraction of both irinotecan and SN-38 are present in plasma as the biologically active intact lactone form. The biological $t_{1/2}$ of SN-38 is 11.5 hours, which is much longer than topotecan. Oral administration does not appear to be feasible because the bioavailability of irinotecan is only 8%. Plasma protein binding is at least 43% for irinotecan and 92-96% for SN-38.

In contrast to topotecan, hepatic metabolism represents an important route of elimination for both irinotecan and SN-38. Several oxidative metabolites have been identified in plasma, all of which result from CYP3A-mediated reactions directed at the bispiperidine side chain. These metabolites are not significantly converted to SN-38. The total body clearance of irinotecan was found to be two times greater in brain cancer patients who were concurrently taking antiseizure drugs that induce hepatic CYPs, further attesting to the importance of oxidative hepatic metabolism as a route of elimination for this drug.

Conjugation of SN-38 with glucuronic acid through the hydroxyl group at position C10 liberated by cleavage of the bispiperidine promoiety, is the only known metabolite of SN-38. Biliary excretion appears to be the primary elimination route of irinotecan, SN-38, and their metabolites, although urinary excretion also contributes significantly (14–37%). Uridine diphosphate-glucuronosyltransferase (UGT), particularly the UGT1A1 isoform, converts SN-38 to its inactive glucuronidated derivative. The extent of SN-38 glucuronidation is inversely correlated with the risk of severe diarrhea after irinotecan therapy. Polymorphisms of UGT1A1 (which glucuronidates bilirubin) are associated with familial hyperbilirubinemia syndromes such as Crigler-Najjar syndrome and Gilbert syndrome (which occurs in up to 15% of the general population and results in a mild hyperbilirubinemia that may be clinically silent), and may have a major impact on the clinical use of irinotecan. Baseline serum unconjugated bilirubin concentration and both severity of neutropenia and the AUC of irinotecan and SN-38 are positively correlated in patients treated with irinotecan. Severe irinotecan toxicity has been observed in cancer patients with Gilbert syndrome, presumably due to decreased glucuronidation of SN-38.

Approved dosage schedules of irinotecan (CAMPTOSAR) in the U.S. include: 125 mg/m² as a 90-minute infusion administered weekly for 4 out of 6 weeks, 350 mg/m² given every 3 weeks, 100 mg/m² every week, or 150 mg/m² every other week. Irinotecan has significant clinical activity in patients with advanced colorectal cancer. It is the treatment of choice in combination with fluoropyrimidines for advanced colorectal cancer in patients who have not received chemotherapy previously or as a single agent following failure on a 5-FU regimen. Irinotecan may have an increasing role in the treatment of other solid tumors, including small cell and non–small cell lung cancer, cervical cancer, ovarian cancer, gastric cancer, and brain tumors.

The dose-limiting toxicity of irinotecan is delayed diarrhea, with or without neutropenia. In initial studies, up to 35% of patients experienced severe diarrhea. Adoption of an intensive loperamide (see Chapter 38) regimen (4 mg of loperamide starting at the onset of any loose stool beginning more than a few hours after receiving therapy, followed by 2 mg every 2 hours) has effectively reduced this incidence by more than half. However, once severe diarrhea does occur, standard doses of antidiarrheal agents tend to be ineffective, although the diarrhea episode generally resolves within a week and, unless associated with fever and neutropenia, is rarely fatal.

The second most common irinotecan-associated toxicity is myelosuppression. Severe neutropenia occurs in 14–47% of the patients treated with the every-3-week schedule, and is less frequent in patients treated with the weekly schedule. Febrile neutropenia is observed in 3% of patients, and may be fatal, particularly when associated with concomitant diarrhea. A cholinergic syndrome resulting from the inhibition of acetylcholinesterase activity by irinotecan may occur within the first 24 hours after irinotecan administration. Symptoms include acute diarrhea, diaphoresis, hypersalivation, abdominal cramps, visual accommodation disturbances, lacrimation, rhinorrhea, and less often, asymptomatic bradycardia. These effects are short lasting and respond within minutes to atropine. Atropine may be prophylactically administered to patients who have experienced a cholinergic reaction, prior to the administration of additional cycles of irinotecan. Other common and generally manageable toxicities include nausea and vomiting, fatigue, vasodilation or skin flushing, mucositis, elevation in liver transaminases, and alopecia. Finally, there have been case reports of dyspnea and interstitial pneumonitis associated with irinotecan therapy.

ANTIBIOTICS
Dactinomycin (Actinomycin D)

Actinomycin D, first isolated from a species of *Streptomyces*, has beneficial effects in the treatment of solid tumors in children and choriocarcinoma. The actinomycins bind double-helical DNA; the planar phenoxazone ring intercalates between adjacent guanine–cytosine base pairs of DNA and the polypeptide chains extend along the minor groove of the helix, resulting in a dactinomycin-DNA complex with great stability. Binding of dactinomycin blocks transcription of DNA by RNA polymerase. The DNA-dependent RNA polymerases are much more sensitive to the effects of dactinomycin than are the DNA polymerases. In addition, dactinomycin causes single-strand breaks in DNA, possibly through a free-radical intermediate or as a result of the action of topoisomerase II. Dactinomycin inhibits rapidly proliferating cells of normal and neoplastic origin, and is among the most potent antitumor agents known.

Dactinomycin is administered by intravenous injection. The drug is excreted both in bile and in the urine and disappears from plasma with a terminal $t_{1/2}$ of 36 hours. Metabolism of the drug is minimal. Dactinomycin does not cross the blood–brain barrier. The usual daily dose of dactinomycin (actinomycin D; COSMEGEN) is 10–15 µg/kg; this is given intravenously for 5 days. If no manifestations of toxicity are encountered, additional courses may be given at intervals of 2–4 weeks. In other regimens, 3 to 6 µg/kg/day, for a total of 125 µg/kg, and weekly maintenance doses of 7.5 µg/kg have been used.

The most important clinical use of dactinomycin is in the treatment of rhabdomyosarcoma and Wilms' tumor in children, where it is curative in combination with primary surgery, radiotherapy, and other drugs (e.g., vincristine and cyclophosphamide). Antineoplastic activity has been noted in Ewing's tumor, Kaposi's sarcoma, and soft tissue sarcomas. Dactinomycin can be effective in women with advanced cases of choriocarcinoma in combination with methotrexate. Dactinomycin also has been used as an immunosuppressant in renal transplants.

Toxic manifestations include anorexia, nausea, and vomiting, usually beginning a few hours after administration. Hematopoietic suppression with pancytopenia may occur in the first week after completion of therapy. Proctitis, diarrhea, glossitis, cheilitis, and ulcerations of the oral mucosa are common; dermatological manifestations include alopecia, as well as erythema, desquamation, and increased inflammation and pigmentation in areas previously or concomitantly subjected to x-ray radiation. Severe injury may occur as a result of local toxic extravasation.

Daunorubicin, Doxorubicin, Epirubicin, Idarubicin, and Mitoxantrone

These anthracycline antibiotics are among the most important antitumor agents. They are derived from the fungus *Streptococcus peucetius* var. *caesius*. *Idarubicin* and *epirubicin* are analogs of the naturally produced anthracyclines, differing only slightly in chemical structure, but having somewhat distinct patterns of clinical activity. *Daunorubicin and idarubicin have been used primarily in the acute leukemias, whereas doxorubicin and epirubicin display broader activity against human solid tumors.* These agents, which all possess potential for generating free radicals, cause an unusual and often irreversible cardiomyopathy that is related to the total dose of the drug. The structurally similar agent mitoxantrone (an anthracenedione) has useful activity against prostate cancer and AML, is used in high-dose chemotherapy, and has significantly less cardiotoxicity than do the anthracyclines.

The anthracycline antibiotics have a tetracyclic ring structure attached to an unusual sugar, daunosamine. Cytotoxic agents of this class all have quinone and hydroquinone moieties on adjacent rings that permit the gain and loss of electrons. A number of important biochemical effects have been described for the anthracyclines and anthracenediones, all of which could contribute to their therapeutic and toxic effects. These compounds can intercalate with DNA, directly affecting transcription and replication. A more important action is the ability of these drugs to form a *tripartite complex with topoisomerase II and DNA. Formation of the tripartite complex with anthracyclines and with etoposide inhibits the religation of the broken DNA strands, leading to apoptosis. Defects in DNA double-strand break repair sensitize cells to damage by these drugs, while overexpression of transcription-linked DNA repair may contribute to resistance. Anthracyclines can form semiquinone radical intermediates, which in turn can react with oxygen to produce superoxide anion radicals. These can generate both hydrogen peroxide and hydroxyl radicals ($\cdot$OH), which attack DNA and oxidize DNA bases. The production of free radicals is significantly stimulated by the interaction of doxorubicin with iron. Enzymatic defenses such as superoxide dismutase and catalase are believed to have an important role in protecting cells against the toxicity of the anthracyclines, and these defenses can be augmented by exogenous antioxidants such as α tocopherol or by an iron chelator, dexrazoxane (ZINECARD), which protects against cardiac toxicity. Exposure of cells to anthracyclines leads to apoptosis.*

Multidrug resistance is observed in tumor cell populations exposed to anthracyclines. Attempts to reverse or prevent the emergence of resistance through the simultaneous use of inhibitors of P-glycoprotein, such as Ca^{2+} channel blockers, steroidal compounds, and others, have yielded inconclusive results, primarily because of the effects of these inhibitors on anthracycline pharmacokinetics and metabolism. Anthracyclines also are exported from tumor cells by members of the MRP transporter family and by the breast cancer resistance protein. Other biochemical changes in resistant cells include increased glutathione peroxidase activity, decreased activity or mutation of topoisomerase II, and enhanced ability to repair DNA strand breaks.

Daunorubicin, doxorubicin, epirubicin, and idarubicin usually are administered intravenously. Careful infusion over 10–15 minutes is recommended to prevent extravasation, since severe local vesicant action may result. The drugs are cleared by a complex pattern of hepatic metabolism and biliary excretion. The plasma disappearance curve for doxorubicin is multiphasic, with elimination half-lives of 3 hours and ~30 hours. All anthracyclines are converted to an active alcohol intermediate that plays a variable role in their therapeutic activity. Idarubicin has a $t_{1/2}$ of ~15 hours, and its active metabolite, idarubicinol, has a $t_{1/2}$ of ~40 hours. There is rapid uptake of the drugs in the heart, kidneys, lungs, liver, and spleen. They do not cross the blood–brain barrier. Daunorubicin and doxorubicin are eliminated by metabolic conversion to a variety of aglycones and other inactive products. Idarubicin is primarily metabolized to idarubicinol, which accumulates in plasma and likely contributes significantly to its activity. Clearance is delayed in the presence of hepatic dysfunction, and at least a 50% initial reduction in dose should be considered in patients with elevated serum bilirubin levels.

IDARUBICIN AND DAUNORUBICIN

The recommended dosage for idarubicin (IDAMYCIN) is 12 mg/m^2 daily for 3 days by intravenous injection in combination with cytarabine. Daunorubicin (daunomycin, rubidomycin; CERUBIDINE, others) is available for intravenous use. The recommended dosage is 30–60 mg/m^2 daily for 3 days. Total doses of >1000 mg/m^2 are associated with a high risk of cardiotoxicity. A liposomal formulation of daunorubicin citrate (DAUNOXOME) is indicated for the treatment of acquired immunodeficiency syndrome (AIDS)-related Kaposi's sarcoma. It is given in a dose of 40 mg/m^2 infused over 60 minutes and repeated every 2 weeks. Patients should be advised that the drug may impart a red color to the urine. Daunorubicin is primarily used in the treatment of AML in combination with Ara-C and has largely been replaced by idarubicin.

The toxic manifestations of daunorubicin and idarubicin include bone marrow depression, stomatitis, alopecia, GI disturbances, and dermatological manifestations. Cardiac toxicity is a peculiar adverse effect observed with these agents. It is characterized by tachycardia, arrhythmias, dyspnea, hypotension, pericardial effusion, and congestive heart failure that responds poorly to digitalis (see below).

DOXORUBICIN

Doxorubicin (ADRIAMYCIN, others) is available for intravenous use. The recommended dose is 50–75 mg/m^2, administered as a single rapid intravenous infusion that is repeated after 21 days. A doxorubicin liposomal product (DOXIL) is available for treatment of AIDS-related Kaposi's sarcoma and is given intravenously in a dose of 20 mg/m^2 over 30 minutes and repeated every 3 weeks. As for daunorubicin, patients should be advised that the drug may impart a red color to the urine. Doxorubicin is effective in malignant lymphomas but also is active in a number of solid tumors, particularly breast cancer. Used in combination with cyclophosphamide, vinca alkaloids, and other agents, it is an important ingredient for the treatment of lymphomas. It is a valuable component of chemotherapy regimens for adjuvant and metastatic carcinoma of the breast and small cell carcinoma of the lung. The drug also is beneficial in a wide range of pediatric and adult sarcomas, including osteogenic, Ewing's, and soft tissue sarcomas.

The toxic manifestations of doxorubicin are similar to those of daunorubicin. Myelosuppression is a major dose-limiting complication, with leukopenia usually reaching a nadir during the second week of therapy and recovering by the fourth week; thrombocytopenia and anemia follow a similar pattern but usually are less pronounced. Stomatitis, GI disturbances, and alopecia are common but reversible. Erythematous streaking near the site of infusion ("ADRIAMYCIN flare") is a benign local allergic reaction and should not be confused with extravasation. Facial flushing, conjunctivitis, and lacrimation may occur rarely. The drug may produce severe local toxicity in irradiated tissues (e.g., the skin, heart, lung, esophagus, and GI mucosa). Such reactions may occur even when the two therapies are not administered concomitantly.

Cardiomyopathy is the most important long-term toxicity. Two types of cardiomyopathies may occur:

1. An acute form is characterized by abnormal electrocardiographic changes, including ST- and T-wave alterations and arrhythmias. This is brief and rarely a serious problem. An acute reversible reduction in ejection fraction is observed in some patients in the 24 hours after a single dose, and elevation of troponin T is found in a minority of patients in the first few days following drug administration. An exaggerated manifestation of acute myocardial damage, the "pericarditis–myocarditis syndrome," may be characterized by severe disturbances in impulse conduction and frank congestive heart failure, often associated with pericardial effusion.

2. Chronic, cumulative dose-related toxicity (usually at or above total doses of 550 mg/m²) is manifested by congestive heart failure. The mortality rate in patients with congestive failure approaches 50%. Total dosage of doxorubicin as low as 250 mg/m² can cause myocardial changes, including a decrease in the number of myocardial fibrils, mitochondrial changes, and cellular degeneration. Sequential echocardiograms have detected structural abnormalities in 25% of children who received up to 300 mg/m² of doxorubicin, although <10% have clinical manifestations of cardiac disease in long-term follow-up. The frequency of clinically apparent cardiomyopathy is 1–10% at total doses below 450 mg/m², increasing to >20% at total doses higher than 550 mg/m²; this total dosage therefore should be exceeded only under exceptional circumstances or with concomitant use of dexrazoxane, a cardioprotective iron-chelating agent. Cardiac irradiation, administration of high doses of cyclophosphamide or another anthracycline, or concomitant herceptin increases the risk of cardiotoxicity. Late-onset cardiac toxicity, with congestive heart failure years after treatment, may occur in both pediatric and adult populations. In children treated with anthracyclines, there is a three- to tenfold elevated risk of arrhythmias, congestive heart failure, and sudden death in adult life. A total dose limit of 300 mg/m² is advised for pediatric cases; concomitant administration of dexrazoxane may reduce troponin T elevations that predict later cardiotoxicity.

NEWER ANALOGS OF DOXORUBICIN   Valrubicin (VALSTAR) is approved for intravesical therapy of bacille Calmette-Guérin–refractory urinary bladder carcinoma in situ in patients for whom immediate cystectomy would be associated with unacceptable morbidity or mortality. Epirubicin (4'-epidoxorubicin, ELLENCE) is approved as a component of adjuvant therapy following resection of early lymph node–positive breast cancer. A related anthracenedione, mitoxantrone, has been approved for use in AML. Mitoxantrone has limited ability to produce quinone-type free radicals and causes less cardiac toxicity than does doxorubicin. Acute myelosuppression, cardiac toxicity, and mucositis are its major toxicities; the drug causes less nausea and vomiting and alopecia than doxorubicin. It also is used as a component of experimental high-dose chemotherapy regimens, with uncertain efficacy. Mitoxantrone (NOVANTRONE) is supplied for intravenous infusion. To induce remission in acute nonlymphocytic leukemia in adults, the drug is given in a daily dose of 12 mg/m² for 3 days as a component of a regimen that also includes cytosine arabinoside. Mitoxantrone also is used in advanced, hormone-resistant prostate cancer in a dose of 12–14 mg/m² every 21 days. Mitoxantrone is also approved for the treatment of late-stage, secondary progressive multiple sclerosis.

EPIPODOPHYLLOTOXINS

Two of the many semisynthetic derivatives of podophyllotoxins show significant therapeutic activity in several human neoplasms, including pediatric leukemia, small cell carcinomas of the lung, testicular tumors, Hodgkin's disease, and large cell lymphomas. These derivatives, etoposide (VP-16-213) and teniposide (VM-26), have no effect on microtubular structure or function at usual concentrations even though podophyllotoxin binds to tubulin at a site distinct from that for interaction with the vinca alkaloids. Etoposide and teniposide have similar mechanisms of action and activities against different tumors. Unlike podophyllotoxin, but like the anthracyclines, they form a ternary complex with topoisomerase II and DNA and prevent resealing of the break that normally follows topoisomerase binding to DNA. The enzyme remains bound to the free end of the broken DNA strand, leading to an accumulation of DNA breaks and cell death. Cells in the S and G_2 phases of the cell cycle are most sensitive to etoposide and teniposide. Resistant cells demonstrate amplification of the gene that encodes the P-glycoprotein, mutation or decreased expression of topoisomerase II, or mutations of the p53 tumor suppressor gene.

Etoposide

Oral administration of etoposide results in variable absorption that averages ~50%. After intravenous injection, peak plasma concentrations of 30 μg/mL are achieved; there is a biphasic clearance with a terminal $t_{1/2}$ of ~6–8 hours in patients with normal renal function. Approximately 40% of an administered dose is excreted intact in the urine. In patients with compromised renal function, dosage should be reduced in proportion to the reduction in creatinine clearance. In patients with advanced liver disease, low serum albumin and elevated bilirubin (which displaces etoposide from albumin) increase the unbound fraction of drug, increasing the toxicity of any given dose. However, guidelines for dose reduction in this circumstance have not been defined. Drug concentrations in the CSF average 1–10% of those in plasma.

The intravenous dose of etoposide (VEPESID, TOPOSAR, ETOPOPHOS) in combination therapy for testicular cancer is 50–100 mg/m² for 5 days, or 100 mg/m² on alternate days for 3 doses. For small cell carcinoma of the lung, the dose in combination therapy is 50–120 mg/m²/day intravenously for 3 days, or 50 mg/day orally for 21 days. Cycles of therapy usually are repeated every 3–4 weeks. When given intravenously, the drug should be administered slowly during a 30–60-minute infusion to avoid hypotension and bronchospasm, which likely result from the additives used to dissolve etoposide.

A disturbing complication of etoposide therapy is the development of an unusual form of acute nonlymphocytic leukemia with a translocation in chromosome 11 at 11q23. This locus contains the MLL or mixed-lineage leukemia gene that regulates the proliferation of pluripotent stem cells. The leukemic cells have the cytological appearance of acute monocytic or monomyelocytic leukemia. Another distinguishing feature of etoposide-related leukemia is the short time interval between the end of treatment and onset of leukemia (1–3 years), as compared to the 4–5-year interval for secondary leukemias related to alkylating agents, and the absence of a myelodysplastic period preceding leukemia. Patients receiving weekly or twice-weekly doses of etoposide, with cumulative doses above 2000 mg/m², seem to be at higher risk of leukemia.

Etoposide is used primarily for treatment of testicular tumors, in combination with bleomycin and cisplatin, and in combination with cisplatin and ifosfamide for small cell carcinoma of the lung. It also is active against non-Hodgkin's lymphomas, acute nonlymphocytic leukemia, and Kaposi's sarcoma associated with AIDS. Etoposide has a favorable toxicity profile for dose escalation in that its primary acute toxicity is myelosuppression. In combination with ifosfamide and carboplatin, it is frequently used for high-dose chemotherapy in total doses of 1500–2000 mg/m². The dose-limiting toxicity of etoposide is leukopenia, with a nadir at 10–14 days and recovery by 3 weeks. Thrombocytopenia occurs less often and usually is not severe. Nausea, vomiting, stomatitis, and diarrhea occur in ~15% of patients treated intravenously and in ~55% of patients who receive the drug orally. Alopecia is common but reversible. Fever, phlebitis, dermatitis, and allergic reactions including anaphylaxis have been observed. Hepatic toxicity is particularly evident after high-dose treatment. For both etoposide and teniposide, toxicity is increased in patients with decreased serum albumin, an effect related to decreased protein binding of the drug.

Teniposide

Teniposide (VUMON) is administered intravenously. It has a multiphasic pattern of clearance from plasma. After distribution, half-lives of 4 hours and 10–40 hours are observed. Approximately 45% of the drug is excreted in the urine, but in contrast to etoposide, as much as 80% is recovered as metabolites. Anticonvulsants such as phenytoin increase the hepatic metabolism of teniposide and reduce systemic exposure. Dosage need not be reduced for patients with impaired renal function. Less than 1% of the drug crosses the blood–brain barrier. However, teniposide has produced responses in small cell and non–small cell lung cancer metastases in the brain. Teniposide is available for treatment of refractory ALL in children and appears to be synergistic with cytarabine. It is administered by intravenous infusion in doses that range from 50 mg/m²/day for 5 days to 165 mg/m²/day twice weekly. The spectrum of activity includes acute leukemia in children, particularly monocytic leukemia in infants, as well as glioblastoma, neuroblastoma, and brain metastases from small cell carcinomas of the lung. Myelosuppression, nausea, and vomiting are its primary toxic effects.

Bleomycins

The bleomycins are fermentation products of *Streptococcus verticillus*. The drug currently employed clinically is a mixture of bleomycin A_2 and B_2. The bleomycins differ only in their terminal amino acid, which can be altered by the amino acids added to the fermentation medium. Bleomycins have significant antitumor activity against squamous carcinoma of the cervix, and against lymphomas and testicular tumors. They are minimally myelo- and immunosuppressive but cause unusual cutaneous side effects and pulmonary fibrosis. Because their toxicities do not overlap with those of other drugs, and because of their unique mechanism of action, bleomycins maintain an important role in combination chemotherapy.

The core of the bleomycin molecule is a complex metal-binding structure containing a pyrimidine chromophore linked to propionamide, a β-aminoalanine amide side chain, and the sugars L-gulose and 3-O-carbamoyl-D-mannose. Attached to this core are a tripeptide chain and a terminal bithiazole carboxylic acid; this latter segment binds to DNA. The bleomycins form equimolar complexes with metal ions, including Cu^{2+} and Fe^{2+}. Bleomycin's cytotoxic action results from its ability to cause oxidative damage to the deoxyribose of thymidylate and other nucleotides, leading to single- and double-stranded breaks in DNA. Bleomycin causes accumulation of cells in the G_2 phase of the cell cycle, and many of these cells display chromosomal aberrations, including chromatid breaks, gaps, and fragments, as well as translocations. Bleomycin causes scission of DNA by generating reactive oxygen species. In the presence of O_2, Fe^{2+}, and a reducing agent, the metal–drug complex becomes activated and functions mechanistically as a ferrous oxidase, transferring electrons from Fe^{2+} to molecular oxygen to produce activated species of oxygen. Metalloblemycin complexes can be activated by reaction with the flavin enzyme, NADPH-cytochrome P450 reductase. Bleomycin binds to DNA through its amino-terminal peptide, and the activated complex generates free radicals that cleave the deoxyribose backbone of the DNA chain. Bleomycin is degraded by a specific hydrolase found in various normal tissues, including liver. This hydrolase activity is low in skin and lung and bleomycin concentrations in these sites are relatively high, perhaps contributing to skin and pulmonary toxicity. Resistance has been attributed to decreased uptake, cleavage by the hydrolase, repair of strand breaks, or drug inactivation by thiols or thiol-rich proteins.

Bleomycin is administered parenterally, either intravenously or intramuscularly, or instilled into the bladder for local treatment of bladder cancer. Bleomycin crosses the blood–brain barrier poorly. The elimination $t_{1/2}$ is ~3 hours. About two-thirds of the drug normally is excreted in the urine. Concentrations in plasma are greatly elevated if usual doses are given to patients with renal impairment, and such patients are at high risk of developing pulmonary toxicity. Doses of bleomycin should be reduced when the creatinine clearance is <60 mL/min.

The recommended dose of bleomycin (BLENOXANE, others) is 10–30 U/m^2 given weekly by the intravenous or intramuscular route. It also may be administered as a subcutaneous injection or as an intrapleural or intracystic instillation. Total courses exceeding 250 U should be given with great caution because of a marked increase in pulmonary toxicity. However, pulmonary toxicity may occur at lower doses (see below).

Bleomycin is highly effective against germ cell tumors of the testis and ovary. In testicular cancer it is curative when used with cisplatin and vinblastine or cisplatin and etoposide. It is used as a component of the standard ABVD regimen for Hodgkin's disease. Bleomycin also is given intrapleurally (60 U) for malignant pleural effusions.

Because bleomycin causes little myelosuppression, it has significant advantages in combination with other cytotoxic drugs. It does, however, cause significant cutaneous toxicity, including hyperpigmentation, hyperkeratosis, erythema, and even ulceration. These changes begin with tenderness and swelling of the distal digits and progress to erythematous, ulcerating lesions over the elbows, knuckles, and other pressure areas. Skin changes often leave a residual hyperpigmentation at these points and may recur when patients are treated with other antineoplastic drugs.

The most serious adverse reaction to bleomycin is pulmonary toxicity, which begins with a dry cough, fine rales, and diffuse basilar infiltrates on x-ray and may progress to life-threatening pulmonary fibrosis. Approximately 5–10% of patients receiving bleomycin develop clinically apparent pulmonary toxicity, and ~1% die of this complication. Most who recover experience a significant improvement in pulmonary function, but fibrosis may be irreversible. Pulmonary function tests do not predict the early onset of this complication. The risk is related to total dose, with a significant increase above total doses of 250 U, in patients over 70 years of age, and in those with underlying pulmonary disease; single doses of 30 U/m^2 or more also are associated with an increased risk of pulmonary toxicity. High concentrations of inspired oxygen during anesthesia or *respiratory therapy may aggravate or precipitate pulmonary toxicity in patients previously treated with the drug. There is no known therapy for bleomycin pneumonitis except for standard management and pulmonary care.*

Other toxic reactions to bleomycin include hyperthermia, headache, nausea and vomiting, and an acute and sometimes fatal reaction observed in patients with lymphomas that is characterized by profound hyperthermia, hypotension, and sustained cardiorespiratory collapse. This does not appear to be classical anaphylaxis and has occurred in ~1% of patients with lymphomas. Patients should receive a test dose of bleomycin (1 U), followed by a 1-hour period of observation, before the drug is administered on standard dosage schedules. Exacerbations of rheumatoid arthritis also have been reported. Raynaud's phenomenon and coronary artery occlusive events have been reported in patients with testicular tumors treated with bleomycin in combination regimens.

Mitomycin

This antibiotic has limited clinical utility and has been replaced by less toxic and more effective drugs.

ENZYMES

L-ASPARAGINASE   L-*Asparaginase* (L-asp) was introduced into cancer chemotherapy in an effort to exploit a distinct qualitative difference between normal and malignant cells. While most normal tissues can synthesize L-asparagine in amounts sufficient for protein synthesis, some lymphoid malignancies derive the required amino acid from plasma. L-Asp, by catalyzing the hydrolysis of circulating asparagine to Asp and ammonia, deprives these malignant cells of the asparagine necessary for protein synthesis, leading to cell death. L-Asp commonly is used in combination with other agents, including methotrexate, doxorubicin, vincristine, and prednisone, for the treatment of ALL and for high-grade lymphomas. The order of drug administration in these combinations may be critical; synergistic cytotoxicity results when methotrexate precedes the enzyme, but the reverse sequence abrogates methotrexate cytotoxicity. The latter outcome is a consequence of the inhibition of protein synthesis by L-asp, an effect that stops the progression of cells through the cell cycle and negates the effect of methotrexate, a drug that exerts its greatest effect during the DNA synthetic phase of the cell cycle. Resistance arises through induction of asparagine synthetase in tumor cells. For unknown reasons, hyperdiploid ALL cells are particularly sensitive to L-asp.

L-Asparaginase (ELSPAR) is given parenterally. Three preparations of L-asp are used clinically that differ in their pharmacokinetics and immunogenicity. After intravenous administration, Escherichia coli–*derived L-asp has a clearance rate from plasma of 0.035 mL/min/kg, a volume of distribution that approximates the volume of plasma, and a $t_{1/2}$ of 14–24 hours. It is given in doses of 6000–10,000 IU every third day for 3–4 weeks. An* Erwinia *preparation (see below), used in patients hypersensitive to the enzyme from E. coli, has a shorter $t_{1/2}$ (16 hours) and requires administration of higher doses. Pegaspargase (PEG-L-ASPARAGINASE; ONCASPAR) is a preparation in which the enzyme is conjugated to 5 KDa units of polyethylene glycol and is cleared much less rapidly. Its plasma $t_{1/2}$ is 6 days, and it is administered in doses of 2500 IU/m² intramuscularly every week. Pegaspargase has much reduced immunogenicity (<20% of patients develop antibodies).*

Intermittent dosage regimens have an increased risk of anaphylaxis. In hypersensitive patients, circulating antibodies lead to immediate inactivation of the enzyme and L-asp levels rapidly become immeasurable after drug administration. Not all patients with neutralizing antibodies experience hypersensitivity, although enzyme may be inactivated and therapy may be ineffective. In previously untreated ALL, pegaspargase produces more rapid clearance of lymphoblasts from bone marrow than does the E. coli preparation and circumvents the rapid antibody-mediated clearance seen with E. coli enzyme in relapsed patients. Only partial depletion of CSF asparagine is achieved by the various asparaginase preparations in clinical use.

L-Asp has minimal effects on bone marrow and GI mucosa. Its most serious toxicities result from its antigenicity and its inhibition of protein synthesis. Hypersensitivity reactions occur in 5–20% of patients and may be fatal. These reactions are heralded by the appearance of circulating neutralizing antibody in some, but not all, hypersensitive patients. In these patients, pegaspargase is a safe alternative, and the Erwinia *enzyme may be used with caution. Other toxicities result from inhibition of protein synthesis in normal tissues and include hyperglycemia due to insulin deficiency, clotting abnormalities due to deficient clotting factors, and hypoalbuminemia. The clotting problems may take the form of spontaneous thrombosis, or less frequently, hemorrhagic episodes. Brain magnetic resonance imaging (MRI) studies should be considered in patients treated with L-asp who present with seizures, headache, or altered mental status. L-Asp–induced thromboses occur with greater frequency in patients with underlying inherited disorders of coagulation, such as factor V Leiden, elevated serum homocysteine, protein C or S deficiency, antithrombin III deficiency, or the G20210A variant of prothrombin. Intracranial hemorrhage in the first week of L-asp treatment is an infrequent but devastating complication. L-Asp also suppresses immune function. Coma has been attributed to ammonia toxicity resulting from L-asparagine hydrolysis. Pancreatitis also has been observed.*

IV. MISCELLANEOUS AGENTS

HYDROXYUREA

This drug has unique and diverse biological effects that have led to exploration of its clinical utility as an antileukemic drug, radiation sensitizer, and an inducer of HbF in patients with sickle cell disease. Its use has been encouraged because the drug is orally administered and its toxicity in most patients is modest and limited to myelosuppression. Hydroxyurea (HU) inhibits the enzyme ribonucleoside diphosphate reductase, which catalyzes the reductive conversion of ribonucleotides to deoxyribonucleotides and is a crucial rate-limiting step in the biosynthesis of DNA. HU destroys a tyrosyl free radical that binds iron in the catalytic center of the human ribonucleotide reductase subunit hRRM2. The drug is specific for the S phase of the cell cycle, when concentrations of the target reductase are maximal, and causes cells to arrest at or near the G_1–S interface. Since cells are highly sensitive to irradiation in the G_1–S boundary, combinations of HU and irradiation cause synergistic toxicity. Through depletion of deoxynucleotides, HU also may potentiate the antiproliferative effects of DNA-damaging agents such as cisplatin, alkylating agents, or topoisomerase II inhibitors, and facilitates the incorporation of drugs such as Ara-C, gemcitabine, or fludarabine into DNA. HU also induces the expression of a number of genes (*e.g.*, TNF-α, IL-6) and accelerates the loss of extrachromosomally amplified genes present in double-minute chromosomes formed in response to methotrexate therapy.

HU reduces vaso-occlusive events in patients with sickle cell disease. It does so via several mechanisms that ultimately increase synthesis of HbF, which promotes solubility of hemoglobin within red cells. It also reduces adhesion of red cells to vascular endothelium, and by suppressing the production and adhesiveness of neutrophils, decreases their contribution to vascular occlusion. HU reduces the frequency of painful events, acute chest syndrome, and secondary strokes in sickle cell patients.

The oral bioavailability of hydroxyurea is excellent (80–100%), and comparable plasma concentrations are seen after oral or intravenous dosing. Peak plasma concentrations are reached 1–1.5 hours after oral doses of 15–80 mg/kg. Hydroxyurea disappears from plasma with a $t_{1/2}$ of 3.5–4.5 hours. The drug readily crosses the blood–brain barrier, and it appears in significant quantities in breast milk. From 40% to 80% of the drug is recovered in the urine within 12 hours after either intravenous or oral administration. It seems prudent to modify doses for patients with abnormal renal function until individual tolerance can be assessed. In cancer treatment, two dosage schedules for hydroxyurea (HYDREA, DROXIA, others), alone or in combination with other drugs, are most commonly used in a variety of clinical situations: (1) intermittent therapy with 80 mg/kg administered orally as a single dose every third day; or (2) continuous therapy with 20–30 mg/kg administered as a single daily dose. In patients with essential thrombocythemia and in sickle cell disease, HU is given in daily dose of 15–30 mg/kg, depending on tolerance and myelosuppression. Dosage should be adjusted according to the number of leukocytes in the peripheral blood. Treatment is typically continued for a period of 6 weeks to determine its effectiveness; if satisfactory results are obtained, therapy can be continued indefinitely, although leukocyte counts at weekly intervals are advised.

The principal use of HU has been as a myelosuppressive agent in myeloproliferative syndromes, particularly in essential thrombocythemia with platelet counts >1.5 million cells/mm³ or history of arterial or venous thrombosis. It dramatically lowers the risk of thrombosis by lowering the platelet count, through its effect on neutrophil and red cell counts, and by reducing L-selectin expression and increasing NO production of neutrophils.

In CML, HU largely has been replaced by imatinib. HU has produced anecdotal, temporary remissions in patients with advanced cancers (e.g., head and neck or genitourinary carcinomas, melanoma). HU has been incorporated into several schedules with concurrent irradiation, as it can synchronize cells into a radiation-sensitive phase of the cell cycle.

HU (DROXIA) is FDA-approved for the treatment of adult patients with sickle cell disease, and appears to be effective in children and in patients with sickle cell–α-thalassemia and sickle cell–hemoglobin C disease.

Hematopoietic depression—involving leukopenia, megaloblastic anemia, and occasionally thrombocytopenia—is the major toxic effect; bone marrow recovery usually is prompt if the drug is discontinued for a few days. Other adverse reactions include a desquamative interstitial pneumonitis, GI disturbances, and mild dermatological reactions. More rarely, stomatitis, alopecia, and neurological manifestations have occurred. Increased skin and fingernail pigmentation and painful leg ulcers may occur. Hydroxyurea has uncertain effect on the risk of secondary leukemia in patients with myeloproliferative disorders and should be used with caution in nonmalignant diseases. Hydroxyurea is a potent teratogen in animals and should not be used in women who may become pregnant.

DIFFERENTIATING AGENTS

A hallmark of malignant transformation is a block in differentiation. A number of chemical entities, including vitamin D and its analogs, retinoids, benzamides and other inhibitors of histone deacetylase, various cytotoxics and biological agents, and inhibitors of DNA methylation, can induce differentiation in tumor cell lines.

Retinoids

TRETINOIN   The biology and pharmacology of retinoids are discussed in detail in Chapter 62. The most important of these for cancer treatment is *tretinoin* (all-trans retinoic acid; ATRA), which induces a high rate of complete remission in acute promyelocytic leukemia (APL) as a single agent, and in combination with anthracyclines, has become part of a curative regimen for this disease. Under physiologic conditions, the RAR-α receptor dimerizes with the retinoid X receptor (RXR) to form a complex that binds ATRA tightly, displacing a repressor of differentiation. In APL cells, there is a t(15;17) translocation that results in a fusion protein (PML-RAR-α) that binds retinoids with much decreased affinity, lacks PML transcription factor function (*i.e.*, inhibition of proliferation and promotion of myeloid differentiation), and blocks the function of transcription factors such as C/EBP, which promote myeloid differentiation. Physiologic concentrations of retinoid are inadequate but pharmacologic concentrations displace the repressor from the fusion protein, activating the differentiation program and promoting degradation of the PML-RAR-α fusion protein. Resistance to ATRA arises by further mutation of the fusion gene that abolishes ATRA binding or by loss of expression of the fusion gene.

The usual dosing regimen of orally administered ATRA is 45 mg/m²/day until remission is achieved. ATRA as a single agent reverses the hemorrhagic diathesis associated with APL and induces a high rate of temporary remission. In combination with an anthracycline, ATRA achieves >70% relapse-free, long-term survival. ATRA reaches a plasma concentration of 400 ng/ml and is cleared by CYP-mediated elimination with a $t_{1/2}$ of <1 hour. Treatment with CYP inducers increases drug metabolism and may result in resistance to ATRA. Remission rate and time to remission induction improve with the inclusion of other chemotherapy. When used as a single agent, especially in patients with >5000 leukemic cells per mm³ in the peripheral blood, ATRA induces an outpouring of cytokines and mature appearing neutrophils of leukemic origin. These cells can clog small vessels in the pulmonary circulation and elsewhere, resulting in the "retinoic acid syndrome" characterized by fever, respiratory distress, pulmonary infiltrates, pleural or pericardial effusions, and mental status changes. Glucocorticoids and chemotherapy decrease the occurrence of the retinoic acid syndrome. Retinoids as a class, including ATRA, cause dry skin, cheilitis, reversible hepatic enzyme abnormalities, bone tenderness, and hyperlipidemia.

Arsenic Trioxide (ATO)

ATO is administered as a 2-hour intravenous infusion in doses of 0.15 mg/kg/day for up to 60 days, until remission is documented. Further consolidation therapy resumes after a 3-week break. The primary mechanism of elimination is by enzymatic methylation to metabolites that have uncertain biological effects. Peak concentrations of ATO in plasma reach 5–7 µM with rapid conversion to metabolites. Little drug appears in the urine. No dose reductions are indicated for hepatic or renal dysfunction.

Pharmacological doses of ATO are well tolerated. Patients may experience reversible side effects including hyperglycemia, hepatic enzyme elevations, fatigue, dysesthesias, and lightheadedness. Ten percent or fewer of patients will experience a leukocyte maturation syndrome similar to that seen with ATRA. O_2, glucocorticoids, and temporary discontinuation of ATO lead to full reversal of this syndrome. Another important and potentially dangerous side effect is lengthening of the QT interval on the electrocardiogram in 40% of patients. The basis for this conduction defect appears to be enhanced Ca^{2+} flux and an inhibition of K^+ channels in myocardial tissue by

As_2O_3, which leads to atrial or ventricular arrhythmias in a small minority of patients. Daily monitoring of the ECG and repletion of serum K^+ in patients with hypokalemia are standard measures in ATO therapy.

PROTEIN TYROSINE KINASE INHIBITORS

Abnormal activation of specific protein tyrosine kinases has been demonstrated in many human neoplasms, making them attractive molecular targets for cancer therapy. There currently are 3 small-molecular-weight protein tyrosine kinase inhibitors that are FDA-approved and many others in clinical trials.

Imatinib

IMATINIB MESYLATE

Imatinib mesylate (GLEEVEC, GLIVEC; 4-[(4-methyl-1-piperazinyl) methyl]-N-[4-methyl-3-[[4-(3-pyridinyl)-2-pyrimidinyl] amino]-phenyl]benzamidemethanesulfonate) was developed through combined use of high throughput screening and medicinal chemistry. Imatinib inhibits protein tyrosine kinase activities of ABL and its activated derivatives v-ABL, BCR-ABL, and EVT6-ABL, the platelet-derived growth factor receptor (PDGFR), and KIT receptor tyrosine kinases. Imatinib binds in the ATP-binding site of the kinase domain and exhibits a high level of selectivity towards these three kinases. Complete inhibition of proliferation with cell death through apoptosis occurs in cells dependent on activated ABL, KIT, or PDGFR for proliferation. This includes cells expressing BCR-ABL in CML, mutant KIT isoforms associated with gastrointestinal stromal tumors (GISTs), the ETV6-PDGFR fusion associated with a subset of chronic myelomonocytic leukemia (CMML), and the FIP1L1-PDGFRA fusion associated with hypereosinophilic syndrome (HES).

Resistance to imatinib can be manifested by a failure to achieve a specific desired response (i.e., primary) or by the loss of a desired response (i.e., secondary). Secondary resistance predominantly results from mutations in the kinase domain that render it less sensitive to imatinib, although some patients have amplification of the kinase target.

Imatinib is nearly completely absorbed after oral administration with peak plasma concentrations achieved within 2–4 hours. Following oral administration in healthy volunteers, the elimination $t_{1/2}$ of imatinib and its major active metabolite, the N-desmethyl derivative, are ~18 and 40 hours, respectively. There is no significant change in the pharmacokinetics of imatinib on repeated dosing or with administration of food. Doses >300 mg/day achieve trough levels of 1 μM, which corresponds to in vitro levels required to kill BCR-ABL–expressing cells. Improved responses may be observed with doses of 600 or 800 mg/day compared to 400 mg/day, consistent with dose-dependent inhibition of the kinase.

CYP3A4 is the major enzyme responsible for metabolism of imatinib. Other CYPs play a minor role in imatinib's metabolism. Imatinib increased the peak plasma concentration and AUC of simvastatin by 2 and 3.5 times, respectively, and coadministration with rifampin, an inducer of CYP3A4, reduces plasma imatinib AUC by ~70%. Elimination of imatinib occurs predominantly in the feces, mostly as metabolites.

Imatinib has efficacy in diseases in which the ABL, KIT, or PDGFR have dominant roles in driving the proliferation of the tumor because of mutations that result in constitutive activation of the kinase, either by fusion with another protein or point mutations. Thus, imatinib shows remarkable therapeutic benefits in patients with CML (BCR-ABL), GIST (KIT mutation positive), CMML (EVT6-PDGFR), HES (FIP1L1-PDGFR), and dermatofibrosarcoma protuberans (constitutive production of the ligand for PDGFR). The situation in GIST is particularly instructive, as patients with an exon 11 mutation of KIT have a significantly higher partial response rate (72%) than those with no detectable KIT mutations (9%). Thus, KIT mutational status predicts response. The currently recommended dose of imatinib is 400–600 mg/day.

The most frequently reported drug-related adverse events are nausea, vomiting, edema, and muscle cramps. Most events are mild to moderate, and only 2–5% of patients permanently discontinue therapy, most commonly because of rashes and elevations of transaminases (each in <1% of patients). Edema can manifest at any site, most commonly in the ankles and periorbital tissues. Severe fluid retention (pleural effusion, pericardial effusion, pulmonary edema, and ascites) is reported in 1–2% of patients taking imatinib. The probability of edema increases with higher imatinib doses and in persons >65 years old. Neutropenia and thrombocytopenia are consistent findings in all studies in leukemia patients, with a higher frequency at doses ≥750 mg. The occurrence of cytopenias also is dependent on the stage of CML, with a frequency of severe neutropenia and thrombocytopenia between two- and threefold higher in blast crisis and accelerated phase compared to chronic phase. In solid tumor patients, severe neutropenia has been reported in <5% of patients. Thrombocytopenia is much less common.

Gefitinib

The EGFR belongs to the ERB family of receptor tyrosine kinases. The EGFR type 1 (ErbB1 or HER1) is overexpressed in many common malignancies, and may be activated by autocrine loops in many others. A truncated version of the EGFR (EGFRvIII) that has lost a portion of the extracellular ligand-binding domain and is constitutively activated is found in a subset of patients with glioblastoma.

Gefitinib (IRESSA; 4-(3-chloro-4-fluoroanilino)-7-methoxy-6-(3-morpholinopropoxy) quinazoline) was discovered by screening a library for compounds that inhibited EGFR tyrosine kinase activity. Gefitinib is a specific inhibitor of the EGFR tyrosine kinase that competitively inhibits ATP binding. Gefitinib is 100 times less potent against highly related tyrosine kinases such as HER2 (ErbB2/neu) and does not inhibit a variety of serine/threonine kinases. The predominant problem with the clinical use of gefitinib has been relatively low response rates. Levels of EGFR expression do not correlate with clinical responses; however, patients whose non–small cell lung tumors have point mutations in the EGFR respond dramatically to gefitinib, similar to imatinib response in GIST with KIT mutations (see above). Thus, primary resistance could result from tumors that are not uniquely dependent on EGFR activity for survival. Although target inhibition by gefitinib has been demonstrated in normal skin, it is possible that poor tumor penetration of the drug could lead to incomplete EGFR inhibition. Alternatively, drug efflux, unappreciated mutations that affect drug sensitivity, or a variety of other factors may mediate lack of responsiveness.

Following oral administration of gefitinib, peak plasma concentrations are achieved within 3–7 hours. Mean absolute bioavailability of the oral formulation is 59%. Exposure to gefitinib is not significantly altered by food; however, coadministration of drugs that cause sustained elevations in gastric pH to ≥5 reduce mean gefitinib AUC by 47%. Administration of gefitinib once daily results in two- to eightfold accumulation with steady-state achieved after 7–10 doses. At steady state, circulating plasma concentrations typically are maintained within a two- to threefold range over the 24-hour dosing interval. The mean terminal $t_{1/2}$ is 41 hours.

Metabolism of gefitinib is predominantly via CYP3A4. The major metabolite in plasma is O-desmethyl gefitinib; it is 14 times less potent than gefitinib. Inducers of CYP3A4 activity may increase metabolism and decrease gefitinib plasma concentrations. Coadministration with rifampin (a CYP3A4 inducer) reduced mean gefitinib AUC by 83%. Coadministration with itraconazole (a CYP3A4 inhibitor) resulted in an 80% increase in the mean AUC of gefitinib. Elimination of gefitinib is primarily by metabolism and excretion in feces.

Gefitinib is approved for the treatment of patients with non–small cell lung cancer who have failed standard chemotherapy. Single-agent responses in these heavily pretreated patients are in the 12–18% range. However, there is a subset of patients who respond dramatically to gefitinib and these are predominantly nonsmoking women with bronchoalveolar tumors. This subset of patients has EGFR mutations that render the EGFR hypersensitive to ligand and to gefitinib. Many of the same EGFR mutations are found in tumors from patients that respond to another small molecule EGFR inhibitor, erlotinib (TARCEVA). The recommended dose of gefitinib is one 250-mg tablet daily, taken with or without food.

The most common adverse drug reactions are diarrhea, rash, acne, pruritus, dry skin, nausea, vomiting, and anorexia. A higher rate of most of these adverse events is observed in patients treated with 500 mg/day of gefitinib as compared to treatment with 250 mg/day. Most adverse events are of mild-to-moderate grade. Less than 2% of patients have permanently discontinued therapy. Adverse drug reactions usually occur within the first month of therapy and generally are reversible. Asymptomatic increases in liver transaminases have been observed and periodic liver function testing should be performed. Interstitial lung disease, which may be acute in onset, has been observed uncommonly in patients receiving gefitinib, and some cases have been fatal. The overall frequency of interstitial lung disease is ~0.3% outside of Japan and ~2% in Japan.

Erlotinib

Erlotinib (TARCEVA; [N-(3-ethynylphenyl)-6,7-bis(2-methoxyethoxy)-4-quinazolinamine]) is a human HER1/EGFR tyrosine kinase inhibitor. It is indicated for treatment of patients with locally advanced or metastatic non–small cell lung cancer. Erlotinib is ~60% absorbed after oral administration and its bioavailability is increased to almost 100% by food. Peak plasma levels occur 4 hours after an oral dose. Following absorption, erlotinib is ~93% protein-bound to albumin and α_1-acid glycoprotein. Its $t_{1/2}$ is ~36 hours. Erlotinib is metabolized primarily by CYP3A4 and to a lesser extent by CYP1A2 and CYP1A1. The most common adverse reactions in patients receiving erlotinib were diarrhea and rash. Serious interstitial lung disease also has been reported. Other adverse effects include elevated liver enzymes and bleeding, especially in patients receiving warfarin. Coadministration of CYP3A4 inhibitors is expected to increase toxicity to erlotinib.

THALIDOMIDE AND LENALIDOMIDE

Thalidomide has been reintroduced to clinical practice as an oral agent for the management of erythema nodosum leprosum (ENL) and in other disease settings, most notably MM. *Lenalidomide* is a thalidomide derivative with improved potency and safety profile compared to thalidomide. Thalidomide is a nonpolar racemic mixture of cell permeable and rapidly interconverting S(–) and R(+) isomers. The precise mechanisms responsible for thalidomide's clinical activity remain to be elucidated. Multiple distinct, but potentially complementary, mechanisms have been proposed to explain the antitumor activity of thalidomide and its derivatives, including stimulation of T cells and NK cells, inhibition of angiogenesis and tumor cell proliferation, and modulation of hematopoietic stem cell differentiation (Figure 51–6).

Thalidomide absorption from the GI tract is slow and highly variable (4 hours to reach peak concentration, with a range of 1–7 hours). It is widely distributed throughout most tissues and organs, with a large apparent volume of distribution. Thalidomide metabolism via hepatic CYPs is limited, and no induction of its own metabolism is noted with prolonged use. Elimination of thalidomide is mainly by spontaneous nonenzymatic hydrolysis, which occurs in all body fluids, with an apparent mean clearance of 10 L/h for the (R)-enantiomer and 21 L/h for the (S)-enantiomer in adults. Thalidomide and over 50 metabolites are rapidly excreted in the urine, while the nonabsorbed portion of the drug is excreted unchanged in feces. Both single and multiple dosing of thalidomide in elderly prostate cancer patients shows significantly longer $t_{1/2}$ at higher doses (1200 mg daily) versus lower doses (200 mg daily). Conversely, no effect of increased age on elimination $t_{1/2}$ was identified in the age range of 55–80 years. The impact of renal or hepatic dysfunction on thalidomide clearance remains to be defined.

Lenalidomide is rapidly absorbed following oral administration, with peak plasma levels occurring 0.6–1.5 hours postdose. The AUC values increase proportionately with increasing dose, both over a single-dose range of 5–400 mg and after multiple dosing with 100 mg daily. The $t_{1/2}$ increases with dose, from ~3 hours at the 5-mg dose, to ~9 hours at the 400-mg dose (the higher dose is believed to provide a better estimate of the $t_{1/2}$ due to the prolonged elimination phase). Approximately 70% of the orally administered dose of lenalidomide is excreted by the kidney.

Thalidomide (THALOMID) is used to treat patients with relapsed and refractory MM, as well as early stage disease. The National Comprehensive Cancer Network (NCCN; www.nccn.org) Clinical Practice Guidelines for Multiple Myeloma includes thalidomide as an option for salvage therapy in patients with relapsed or refractory MM, or as initial therapy in combination with dexamethasone for patients with advanced myeloma. Thalidomide is also in clinical trials for use in treating a variety of solid tumors and myelodysplasias.

Lenalidomide (REVLIMID) is approved for treatment of transfusion-dependent anemia due to low- or intermediate-risk myelodysplastic syndromes associated with the 5q cytogenetic deletion, with or without additional cytogenetic abnormalities. It is being examined for use in combination with dexamethasone in newly diagnosed patients with MM, and in combination with agents such as bortezomib in relapsed and refractory MM. It is also being evaluated for use in treating many of the same neoplasias for which thalidomide might be useful, including myelodysplastic syndromes and certain solid tumors.

Thalidomide generally is well tolerated at doses <200 mg daily, the typical doses used to treat MM and ENL. The most common adverse effects reported in cancer patients are sedation and constipation, while the most serious one is treatment-emergent peripheral neuropathy, which occurs in 10–30% of patients with MM or other malignancies in a dose- and time-dependent manner. Thalidomide-related neuropathy is an asymmetric, painful, peripheral paresthesia with sensory loss, commonly presenting with numbness of toes and feet, muscle cramps, weakness, signs of pyramidal tract involvement, and carpal tunnel syndrome. The incidence of peripheral neuropathy increases with higher cumulative doses of thalidomide, especially in elderly patients. Although clinical improvement typically occurs upon drug discontinuation, long-standing residual sensory loss can occur. Particular caution should be applied in cancer patients with preexisting neuropathy (e.g., related to diabetes) or prior exposure to drugs that can cause peripheral neuropathy (e.g., vinca alkaloids or bortezomib). An increasing incidence of thromboembolic events in

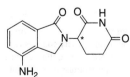

LENALIDOMIDE   THALIDOMIDE

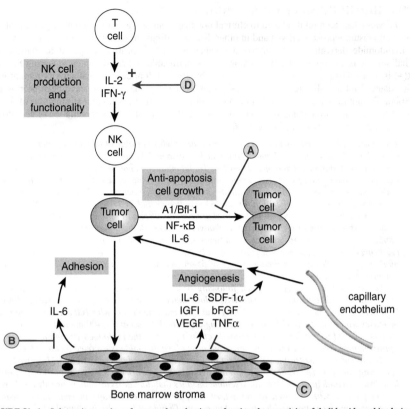

FIGURE 51–6 *Schematic overview of proposed mechanisms of antimyeloma activity of thalidomide and its derivatives.* Some biological hallmarks of the malignant phenotype are indicated in light gray boxes. The proposed sites of action for thalidomide (dark blue letters within circles) are hypothesized to be operative for thalidomide derivatives also. *A.* Direct anti-MM effect on tumor cells including G1 growth arrest and/or apoptosis, even against MM cells resistant to conventional therapy. This is due to the disruption of the anti-apoptotic effect of Bcl-2 family members, blocking NF-κB signaling, and inhibition of the production of IL-6. *B.* Inhibition of MM cell adhesion to bone marrow stromal cells due partially to the reduction in IL-6 release. *C.* Decreased angiogenesis due to the inhibition of cytokine and growth factor production and release. *D.* Enhanced T-cell production of cytokines, such as IL-2 and IFN-g, that increase the number and cytotoxic functionality of natural killer (NK) cells.

thalidomide-treated patients has been reported. This appears to be very rare in patients treated with thalidomide as a single agent and generally occurs when thalidomide is combined with glucocorticoids or particularly anthracycline-based chemotherapy. The 2006 NCCN Practice Guidelines for Multiple Myeloma (www.nccn.org) include the possible prophylactic use of anticoagulants in patients receiving thalidomide therapy.

Ongoing studies are characterizing the adverse-effect profile of lenalidomide and addressing its potential for interactions with other drugs. More clinical experience is required to determine whether lenalidomide is completely devoid of some of thalidomide's side effects. Because of the risk of teratogenic effects, thalidomide and lenalidomide are regulated by the FDA to prevent fetal drug exposure (see System for Thalidomide Education and Prescribing Safety (STEPS) Program [www.thalomid.com/steps_program.aspx] and RevAssist [www.revlimid.com/default.aspx]).

ESTRAMUSTINE

Estramustine (EMCYT), a combination of *estradiol* coupled to *normustine* (nornitrogen mustard) by a carbamate link, has weaker estrogenic and antineoplastic activity than estradiol and other alkylating agents, respectively. While the combination was intended to enhance the uptake of the alkylating agent into estradiol-sensitive prostate cancer cells, estramustine does not appear to function as an alkylating agent. Rather, estramustine binds to β-tubulin and microtubule-associated proteins, causing microtubule disassembly and antimitotic actions. Estramustine is used for the treatment of metastatic or progressive prostate cancer at a usual initial dose of 10–16 mg/kg daily in 3 or 4 divided doses. Following oral administration, at least 75% of a dose of estramustine is absorbed from the GI tract and rapidly dephosphorylated. Estramustine is found in the body mainly as its oxidized 17-keto analog isomer, estromustine; both forms accumulate in the prostate. Some hydrolysis of the carbamate linkage occurs in the liver, releasing estradiol, estrone, and the normustine group. Estramustine and estromustine have plasma $t_{1/2}$ of 10–20 hours, respectively, and are excreted with their metabolites, mainly in the feces. In addition to myelosuppression, estramustine also possesses estrogenic side effects (gynecomastia, impotence, and elevated risk of thrombosis, and fluid retention) and is associated with hypercalcemia, acute attacks of porphyria, impaired glucose tolerance, and hypersensitivity reactions including angioedema.

Bortezomib

Bortezomib (VELCADE); (1R)-3-methyl-1-[[(2S)-1-oxo-3-phenyl-2-[pyrazinylcarbonyl)amino] propyl]butyl]boronic acid binds to the 20S core of the 26S proteasome and reversibly inhibits its chymotrypsin-like activity. Inhibition of the proteasome disrupts multiple signaling cascades within the cell, often leading to cell death. The most important consequences of proteasome inhibition are believed to result from downregulation of NF-κB, a key transcription factor that promotes cell survival. In a similar manner, bortezomib disrupts ubiquitin-proteasome regulation of p21, p27, and p53, which are key regulatory proteins in the cell cycle and initiators of apoptosis. The antineoplastic activity of bortezomib in tumors is likely due to a greater dependence on cell proliferating pathways in cancer relative to normal tissues.*

After intravenous administration of 1–1.3 mg/m² of bortezomib in patients without renal or hepatic impairment, there is a rapid distribution phase (<10 minutes), followed by a longer elimination phase of 5–15 hours. Plasma protein binding averaged 83%. The mean terminal elimination in preclinical studies was 5.4 hours, with an average clearance of 66 L/h. Peak pharmacodynamic activity (proteasome inhibition) occurred at 1 hour with a mean of 61% inhibition and a $t_{1/2}$ of ~24 hours. Inhibition of the 20S subunit was 10–30% at 96 hours. Proteasome inhibition is highly concentration dependent.

Bortezomib is primarily metabolized to an inactive metabolite by hepatic CYPs. Deboronation accounts for >90% of total metabolism, with CYP3A4 being more active than CYP2D6. Ongoing studies in patients with hepatic or renal impairment should define pathways of elimination that will help guide dose reduction in such patients. Bortezomib is a poor inhibitor of hepatic CYPs.

Bortezomib is available for intravenous injection only. Each vial contains 3.5 mg of bortezomib as a sterile lyophilized powder and 35 mg of mannitol. Prior to use, the contents of each vial are reconstituted with 3.5 mL of normal (0.9%) saline. The reconstituted product should be clear and colorless and should be administered to patients within 8 hours. The recommended starting dose of bortezomib is 1.3 mg/m² given as an intravenous bolus, and this should be given on days 1, 4, 8, and 11 of every 21-day cycle (10-day rest period per cycle). At least 72 hours should elapse between doses. For severe nonhematologic and hematologic toxicities, the drug should be held until resolution and subsequent doses should be reduced by 25%. In clinical trials, some patients have received 2 mg/m² without severe toxicity.

Bortezomib is FDA-approved for patients with MM who have received 2 prior therapies and are progressing on their current therapy. The drug is being studied in combination with other drugs in MM as well as other hematologic neoplasms and solid tumors. Escalating doses of bortezomib have resulted in dose-limiting GI, hematopoietic, lymphatic, and renal toxicities. At the standard dose and schedule, serious toxicities encountered in >5% of patients included thrombocytopenia, fatigue, peripheral neuropathy, neutropenia, anemia, nausea and vomiting, diarrhea, limb pain, dehydration, and weakness. Peripheral neuropathy was encountered more frequently in patients with a prior history of neuropathy or preexisting numbness, pain, or burning, where dose reductions of bortezomib are recommended. Usually, the neuropathy improves or resolves completely after several months off treatment. Hypotension associated with the injection of bortezomib has been rarely encountered, and caution should be taken with patients who are volume-depleted, have a history of syncope, or who are on antihypertensive medications.

Zoledronic Acid

Zoledronic acid (ZOMETA) is a bisphosphonate (*see* Chapter 61) indicated for the treatment of patients with bony metastases and for patients with MM. A direct antitumor effect on myeloma cells has been proposed; some data suggest that inhibition of bone matrix–degrading proteinases may inhibit tumor cell invasion in breast and prostate cancers.

Mitotane

The principal application of *mitotane* (*o,p'*-DDD) is in the treatment of neoplasms derived from the adrenal cortex. The drug causes a rapid reduction in the levels of corticosteroids and their metabolites in blood and urine, a response that is useful both in guiding dosage and in following the course of hypercorticism resulting from an adrenal tumor or adrenal hyperplasia.

Mitotane (LYSODREN) is administered in initial daily oral doses of 2–6 g, usually given in 3 or 4 divided portions, but the maximal tolerated dose may vary from 2 to 16 g/day. Treatment should be continued for at least 3 months; if beneficial effects are observed, therapy should be maintained indefinitely. Spironolactone should not be administered concomitantly, since it interferes with the adrenal suppression produced by mitotane. Treatment with mitotane is indicated for the palliation of inoperable adrenocortical carcinoma, producing symptomatic benefit in 30–50% of such patients. Although the administration of mitotane produces anorexia and nausea in ~80% of patients, somnolence and lethargy in 34%, and dermatitis in 15–20%, these effects do not contraindicate the use of the drug at lower doses. Since this drug damages the adrenal cortex, administration of corticosteroids is indicated, particularly in patients with evidence of adrenal insufficiency, shock, or severe trauma.

BIOLOGICAL RESPONSE MODIFIERS

In contrast to small molecules, biological response modifiers include biological agents that beneficially affect the patient's biological response to a neoplasm. Included are agents that mediate their antitumor effects indirectly (*e.g.*, by enhancing the immunologic response to neoplastic cells) or directly on the tumor cells (*e.g.*, differentiating agents). Recombinant proteins with potent effects on the function and growth of both normal and neoplastic cells that currently are in clinical trials include the interferons (*see* Chapters 49 and 52), interleukins (*see* Chapter 52), hematopoietic growth factors (*see* Chapter 53) such as *erythropoietin*, filgrastim (granulocyte colony-stimulating factor [G-CSF]), and *sargramostim* (granulocyte-macrophage colony-stimulating factor [GM-CSF]), *tumor necrosis factor* (TNF), and monoclonal antibodies such as trastuzumab, *cetuximab*, and rituximab. Among the agents now approved for clinical use in specific neoplastic diseases are *interferon-α* for use in hairy cell leukemia, condylomata acuminata, CML, and Kaposi's sarcoma associated with AIDS; *interleukin-2* (IL-2) for kidney cancer; trastuzumab for breast cancer; and rituximab for B-cell lymphomas.

Interleukin-2 (IL-2, ALDESLEUKIN, PROLEUKIN)

IL-2 is not directly cytotoxic to cancer cells; rather, it induces and expands a T-cell response that is cytolytic for tumor cells. Clinical trials have studied the antitumor activity of IL-2 both as a single agent and with adoptive cellular therapy using IL-2–stimulated autologous lymphocytes obtained by leukopheresis, termed *lymphokine-activated killer* (LAK) *cells*; addition of LAK cells to the treatment regimen has not improved overall response rates.

Because the $t_{1/2}$ of IL-2 in humans is short (13 minutes for α and 85 minutes for β), most clinical schedules have explored either continuous infusion or multiple intermittent dosing. The most significant antitumor activity has been demonstrated with the most intense dosing schedules: continuous intravenous infusion for 5 days every other week for 2 cycles, or intravenous bolus dosing every 8 hours daily for 5 days every other week.

The toxicities of IL-2 likely are related to the activation and expansion of cytotoxic lymphocytes in organs and within vessels, resulting in inflammation and vascular leak, and to the secondary release by activated cells of other cytokines, such as TNF-α and interferon. When given at maximally tolerated doses of 600,000 units/kg every 8 hours for up to 5 days, IL-2 causes hypotension, arrhythmias, peripheral edema, prerenal azotemia, elevated liver transaminases, anemia, thrombocytopenia, nausea, vomiting, diarrhea, confusion, and fever.

Reproducible antitumor activity has been reported in advanced MM and renal cell cancer, where response rates (partial and complete) are seen in 20–30% of patients. Complete responses, seen in ~5–10% of patients, appear to be durable, with some patients free of disease beyond 5 years. IL-2 is being studied in the treatment of AML, where it is capable of inducing remission in relapsed patients. Given following bone marrow transplantation, it appears that IL-2 can lengthen the remission duration compared to historical controls.

Monoclonal Antibodies

Cancer cells express a variety of antigens that are attractive targets for monoclonal antibody–based therapy (Table 51–3). Several monoclonal antibodies are FDA-approved for treating lymphoid and solid tumor malignancies, including rituximab and *alemtuzumab* for lymphoid malignancies, and trastuzumab for breast cancer. Because murine monoclonal antibodies have a short $t_{1/2}$ and induce a human anti-mouse antibody immune response, they usually are chimerized or humanized when used as therapeutic agents. The nomenclature adopted for therapeutic monoclonal antibodies is to terminate the name in *-ximab* for chimeric antibodies and *-umab* for humanized antibodies. A variety of mechanism(s) of cell killing have been described for naked monoclonal antibodies, including antibody-dependent cellular cytotoxicity (ADCC), complement-dependent cytotoxicity (CDC) and direct induction of apoptosis, but the clinically relevant mechanisms remain uncertain. Monoclonal antibodies also may be engineered to combine the antibody with a toxin (immunotoxins), such as *gemtuzumab ozogamicin* (MYLOTARG) or *denileukin diftitox* (ONTAK), or combined with a radioactive isotope, as in the case of 90Y-*ibritumomab tiuxetan* (ZEVALIN) (Table 51–3). More recently, antibodies have been engineered to contain a second specificity, known as bi-specific antibodies.

Naked Monoclonal Antibodies

RITUXIMAB Rituximab (RITUXAN) is a chimeric monoclonal antibody that targets the CD20 B-cell antigen (Tables 51–3 and 51–4), which is found on cells from the pre–B-cell stage through terminal differentiation to plasma cells and is expressed on 90% of B-cell neoplasms. Monoclonal antibody binding to CD20 generates transmembrane signals in B-cells, but it is not known how ligation of the CD20 receptor produces cell death independent of ADCC or complement-mediated pathways. Rituximab initially was approved for relapsed indolent lymphomas and has shown activity in a wide variety of clinical settings. Recent studies have demonstrated significant activity of rituximab in mantle cell lymphoma, relapsed aggressive B-cell lymphomas, and CLL. The use of maintenance rituximab has gained increased acceptance, based on demonstration of delayed time to progression, but effects on survival have not been demonstrated. Rituximab and chemotherapy are synergistic, suggesting it sensitizes lymphoma cells to the apoptotic effects of chemotherapy by directly acting on tumor cells; rituximab is being clinically combined with agents such as fludarabine and combinations such as CHOP. The addition of rituximab to CHOP chemotherapy significantly improves the event-free survival of diffuse large B-cell lymphoma.

Rituximab demonstrates dose-dependent pharmacokinetics. At a dose of 375 mg/m², the mean serum $t_{1/2}$ was 76 hours after one dose and 206 hours after the last dose, with considerable interindividual variation. The wide range of $t_{1/2}$ likely reflects differences in patient tumor burden and normal B-cell populations. Rituximab toxicities are mostly related to infusion reactions, although there are increasing reports of late-onset neutropenia and rare reports of severe skin toxicity (Table 51–4).

ALEMTUZUMAB Alemtuzumab (CAMPATH) targets the CD52 antigen present on normal neutrophils and lymphocytes as well as most B- and T-cell lymphomas (Tables 51–3 and 51–4). CD52 is expressed at reasonable levels and does not modulate with antibody binding, making it a good target for unconjugated monoclonal antibodies. Alemtuzumab induces tumor cell death through ADCC and CDC (Table 51–4). Clinical activity has been demonstrated in low-grade lymphomas and CLL, including patients with disease refractory to purine analogs.

Alemtuzumab demonstrates dose-dependent pharmacokinetics. Alemtuzumab has a mean $t_{1/2}$ of 12 days and steady-state levels are reached ~week 6 of treatment, although there is significant variability. The most concerning side effects are acute infusion reactions and the depletion of hematopoietic cells and T cells (Table 51–4). Opportunistic infections are a serious and sometimes fatal side effect, particularly in patients who have received purine analogs. The broad expression of CD52 in T cells has led to the testing of alemtuzumab in T-cell lymphomas. Studies have shown a high response rate in mycosis fungoides, and combination chemotherapy trials are being conducted in aggressive T-cell lymphomas.

TRASTUZUMAB Trastuzumab (HERCEPTIN) targets the HER2/neu (ErbB-2) member of the EGF family of protein tyrosine kinase receptors. Activation of HER2/neu enhances metastatic potential and inhibits apoptosis. HER2/neu is overexpressed in up to 30% of breast cancers and is associated with clinical resistance to cytotoxic and hormone therapy. Trastuzumab can initiate Fcγ-receptor–mediated ADCC and directly induce apoptosis.

Trastuzumab is approved for HER2/neu overexpressing metastatic breast cancer in combination with paclitaxel as initial treatment or as monotherapy following chemotherapy relapse. Trastuzumab also is synergistic with other cytotoxic agents, but only in HER2/neu–overexpressing cancers. HER2/neu expression also is found in other solid tumors and responses have been reported in colorectal and non–small cell lung cancer. Other tumors that express HER2/neu at relatively high frequency include pancreas and stomach.

Table 51–3

Monoclonal Antibodies Approved for Hematopoietic and Solid Tumors

Antigen and tumor cell targets	Antigen function	Naked antibodies	Radioisotope-based antibodies	Toxin-based antibodies
Antigen: CD20 Tumor type: B-cell lymphoma and CLL	Proliferation/differentiation	Rituximab (chimeric)	^{131}I-tositumomab; ^{90}Y-ibritumomab tiuxetan	None
Antigen: CD52 Tumor type: B-cell CLL and T-cell lymphoma	Unknown	Alemtuzumab (humanized)	None	None
Antigen: CD25 α subunit	Activation antigen	Daclizumab (humanized)	None	Denileukin diftitox (diphtheria toxin)
Antigen: CD33 Tumor type: T-cell mycosis fungoides	Unknown	Gemtuzumab (humanized)	None	Gemtuzumab ozogamicin
Antigen: HER2/neu (ErbB-2) Tumor type: acute myeloid leukemia	Tyrosine kinase	Trastuzumab (humanized)	None	None
Antigen: EGFR (ErbB-1) Tumor type: breast cancer	Tyrosine kinase	Cetuximab (chimeric)	None	None
Antigen: VEGF Tumor type: colorectal; NSCLC; pancreatic, breast	Angiogenesis	Bevacizumab (humanized)	None	None
Tumor type: colorectal cancer				

ABBREVIATIONS: CLL, chronic lymphocytic leukemia; EGFR, epidermal growth factor receptor; NSCLC, non-small cell lung cancer; VEGF, vascular endothelial growth factor.

Table 51–4

Dose and Toxicity of Monoclonal Antibody–Based Drugs

Drug	Mechanism	Dose and Schedule	Major Toxicity
Rituximab	ADCC; CDC; apoptosis	375 mg/m^2 IV infusion weekly for 4 weeks	Infusion-related toxicity with fever, rash, and dyspnea; B-cell depletion; late-onset neutropenia
Alemtuzumab	ADCC; CDC; apoptosis	Escalation 3, 10, 30 mg/m^2 IV 3 times per week followed by 30 mg/m^2 3 times per week for 4 to 12 weeks	Infusion-related toxicity, T-cell depletion with increased infection; hematopoietic suppression; pancytopenia
Trastuzumab	ADCC; apoptosis; inhibition of HER2 signaling with G$_1$ arrest	Loading dose of 4 mg/kg infusion followed by 2 mg/kg weekly	Cardiomyopathy; infusion-related toxicity
Cetuximab	Inhibition of EGFR signaling; apoptosis; ADCC	Loading dose of 400 mg/kg infusion followed by 250 mg/kg weekly	Infusion-related toxicity; skin rash in 75%
Bevacizumab	Inhibition of angiogenesis/ neovascularization	5 mg/kg IV every 14 days until disease progression	Hypertension; pulmonary hemorrhage; gastrointestinal perforation; proteinuria; congestive heart failure
Denileukin diftitox	Targeted diphtheria toxin with inhibition of protein synthesis	9–18 μg/kg per day IV for the first 5 days every 3 weeks	Fever; arthralgia; asthenia; hypotension
Gemtuzumab ozogamicin	Double DNA strand breaks and apoptosis	2 doses of 9 mg/m^2 IV separated by 14 days	Infusion-related toxicity; hematopoietic suppression; mucosal hepatic (VOD); and skin toxicity
^{90}Y-ibritumomab tiuxetan	Targeted radiotherapy	0.4 mCi/kg IV	Hematologic toxicity; myelodysplasia
^{131}I-tositumomab	Targeted radiotherapy	Patient-specific dosimetry	Hematologic toxicity; myelodysplasia

ABBREVIATIONS: ADCC, antibody-dependent cellular cytotoxicity; CDC, complement-dependent cytotoxicity; EGFR, epidermal growth factor receptor; VOD, veno-occlusive disease.

Trastuzumab has dose-dependent pharmacokinetics with a mean $t_{1/2}$ of 5.8 days at the 2-mg/kg maintenance dose. Steady-state levels were achieved between the 16th and the 32nd weeks. The infusion effects of trastuzumab are typical of other monoclonal antibodies and include fever, chills, nausea, dyspnea, and rashes. Allergic reactions also may be observed. Cardiac dysfunction is an unexpected and potentially serious side effect that was observed in the pivotal trial of trastuzumab chemotherapy. Left ventricular dysfunction was seen most commonly in those patients who received doxorubicin and cyclophosphamide.

CETUXIMAB Cetuximab (ERBITUX) recognizes the EGF receptor (EGFR; also termed ErbB1 or HER1). Activation of EGFR tyrosine kinase activity is associated with proliferation, survival, and angiogenesis. EGFR expression is found in 60–75% of colorectal cancers, where it has been linked to tumor progression and a poor prognosis. Multiple epithelial cancers, such as breast, lung, kidney, prostate, brain, pancreas, bladder, and head and neck malignancies, also express EGFR and are potential therapeutic targets of cetuximab. Although the mechanism of tumor cell killing by cetuximab is uncertain, it is likely to involve inhibition of EGF binding and signaling. The role of more classical immune mechanisms, such as ADCC, is unclear. Cetuximab is FDA-approved for the treatment of EGFR-positive metastatic colorectal cancer as a single agent in patients who were unable to tolerate irinotecan-based therapy, or in combination with irinotecan for refractory patients. Studies in head and neck cancer in combination with radiation therapy suggest that cetuximab improves local control.

Cetuximab displays nonlinear pharmacokinetics. Following the recommended dose regimen, steady-state levels are achieved by the third weekly infusion. The mean $t_{1/2}$ is 114 hours (range, 75–188 hours). Toxic side effects observed with cetuximab include infusion reactions. The incidence of rash is significantly greater than that observed with other monoclonal antibodies; it may occur in 75% of patients, and may be severe in 16%. Interestingly, there is a correlation between development and intensity of rash and duration of benefit from cetuximab.

BEVACIZUMAB *Bevacizumab* (AVASTIN) targets the vascular-endothelial growth factor (VEGF) and inhibits its interaction with the VEGFR1 and VEGFR2 receptors. VEGF is an angiogenic growth factor that regulates vascular proliferation and permeability and inhibits apoptosis of new blood vessels. VEGF expression is increased in several tumor types, including breast, ovarian, non–small cell lung, and colorectal cancer, and its expression correlates with neovascularization within tumors. In colorectal cancer, microvessel density is associated with progression of adenomas to carcinomas and with metastatic potential and poor prognosis. Bevacizumab is FDA-approved for metastatic colorectal cancer in combination with 5-FU. There also is evidence of bevacizumab efficacy in clear-cell renal cancer as a single agent and in non–small cell lung cancer and breast cancer in combination with chemotherapy.

The pharmacokinetics of bevacizumab varies by sex, body weight, and tumor burden. Clearance is higher in patients with greater tumor burden, but the relationship with clinical outcome has not been explored. Bevacizumab has an estimated $t_{1/2}$ of 20 days (range, 11–50 days) and a predicted time to reach steady state of 100 days at the therapeutic dose. Infusion-related toxicities are relatively uncommon. However, this agent has a number of unique and potentially serious toxicities, including severe hypertension, proteinuria, congestive heart failure, hemorrhage, and GI perforation.

Monoclonal Antibody-Cytotoxic Conjugates

GEMTUZUMAB OZOGAMICIN Gemtuzumab ozogamicin (MYLOTARG) comprises a monoclonal antibody against CD33 covalently linked to a semisynthetic derivative of *calicheamicin*, a potent enediyne antitumor antibiotic. The CD33 antigen is found on most hematopoietic cells, on >80% of AML, and in most myelodysplasias. Following binding to CD33, gemtuzumab ozogamicin undergoes endocytosis with cleavage of calicheamicin within the lysosome, which ultimately causes double-strand DNA breaks and cell death. Gemtuzumab ozogamicin is FDA-approved for the treatment of CD33-positive AML in first relapse in patients >60 years old who are not candidates for conventional cytotoxic therapy. Studies exploring new roles for gemtuzumab ozogamicin are being conducted, including treatment of refractory and previously untreated AML.

Pharmacokinetics of gemtuzumab ozogamicin at the standard 9 mg/m² dose showed half-lives of total and unconjugated calicheamicin of 41 and 143 hours, respectively. Following a second dose, the $t_{1/2}$ increased to 64 hours and the AUC was twice that of the initial dose. Serious toxicities may occur with gemtuzumab ozogamicin. Like other monoclonal antibodies, infusion-related toxicities occur with the first infusion but are ameliorated by glucocorticoids. The primary toxicities are *bone marrow suppression and hepatic toxicity. Hepatic toxicity can be serious and may lead to fatal VOD. In the phase 2 study, significant hyperbilirubinemia was observed in 23% of patients; this may represent subclinical VOD in some cases.*

Radioimmuno-Conjugates

Radioimmuno-conjugates use monoclonal antibody to target radioactive particles to tumor cells (Tables 51–3 and 51–4). [131]Iodine (^{131}I) is a commonly used radioisotope; the γ emission of ^{131}I can be used for both imaging and therapy, but releasing free ^{131}I and ^{131}I-tyrosine into the blood presents a potential health hazard to caregivers. The β emitter, [90]Yttrium (^{90}Y), is an attractive alternative to ^{131}I, based on its higher energy and longer path length, which may be more effective in tumors with larger diameters. It also has a short $t_{1/2}$ and remains conjugated, even after endocytosis, providing a safer profile for outpatient use. However, disadvantages include its inability to image, limited availability, and expense.

Radioimmuno-conjugates have been developed with monoclonal antibodies against CD20 conjugated with [131]I (^{131}I-tositumomab or BEXXAR) and ^{90}Y-ibritumomab tiuxetan (ZEVALIN) that have response rates in relapsed lymphoma of 65–80%. These agents are well tolerated with most toxicity attributable to bone marrow suppression. However, there are reports of secondary leukemias (Table 51–4). Pretargeting has been used to increase the therapeutic index of radioimmuno-conjugates by initially treating with avidin-labeled monoclonal antibody, followed 1–2 days later by ^{90}Y-conjugated biotin. This technique may improve the specificity of radioisotope delivery to tumor cells and increase the therapeutic index.

Immunotoxin

DENILEUKIN DIFTITOX Denileukin diftitox (ONTAK) is an immunotoxin made from the genetic recombination of IL-2 and the catalytically active fragment of diphtheria toxin. The human IL-2 receptor (IL-2R) is not expressed on resting T cells, but is constitutively expressed on malignant lymphocytes of both T-cell and B-cell origin. Denileukin diftitox is FDA-approved for the treatment of recurrent/refractory cutaneous T-cell lymphomas. Denileukin diftitox is being evaluated in patients with CD25-negative tumors and modulators of CD25 expression are being combined in an attempt to increase response rates. *Bexarotene* increases the level of CD25 expression on malignant T cells and provides a rationale for combining these agents.

Systemic exposure to denileukin diftitox is variable but proportional to dose. It has a distribution $t_{1/2}$ of 2–5 minutes with a terminal $t_{1/2}$ of ~70 minutes. Immunologic reactivity to denileukin diftitox can be detected in virtually all patients after treatment but does not preclude clinical benefit with continued treatment. Denileukin diftitox clearance in later cycles of treatment is accelerated by two- to threefold as a result of development of antibodies, but serum levels are greater than required to produce cell death in IL-2R–expressing cell lines (1–10 ng/mL for more than 90 minutes). Patients with a history of hypersensitivity reactions to diphtheria toxin or IL-2 should not be treated. Significant toxicities associated with denileukin diftitox are acute hypersensitivity reactions, a vascular leak syndrome, and constitutional toxicities; glucocorticoid premedication significantly decreases toxicity.

Colony-Stimulating Factors

Many agents used for cancer chemotherapy suppress bone marrow production of hematopoietic cells, often limiting the delivery of chemotherapy on schedule and at prescribed doses. The availability of recombinant growth factors for erythrocytes (*i.e.,* erythropoietin), granulocytes (*i.e.,* granulocyte colony-stimulating factor), and granulocytes and macrophages (*i.e.,* granulocyte-macrophage colony-stimulating factor) have enormously advanced the ability to use combination therapy or high-dose therapy with diminished complications such as febrile neutropenia. Whether this will result in improved survival rates for specific cancers remains to be determined. The individual growth factors and specifics of therapy are described in detail in Chapter 53.

V. HORMONES AND RELATED AGENTS

GLUCOCORTICOIDS

The glucocorticoids are discussed in detail in Chapter 59. Because of their lympholytic effects and their ability to suppress mitosis in lymphocytes, the greatest value of glucocorticoids as cytotoxic agents is in the treatment of acute leukemia in children and malignant lymphoma in children and adults. In acute lymphoblastic or undifferentiated leukemia of childhood, glucocorticoids may produce prompt clinical improvement and objective hematological remissions in up to 30% of children. Although these responses frequently are characterized by complete disappearance of all detectable leukemic cells from the peripheral blood and bone marrow, the remission is brief. Remissions occur more rapidly with glucocorticoids than with antimetabolites, and there is no evidence of cross-resistance to unrelated agents. For these reasons, therapy is initiated with prednisone and vincristine, often followed by an anthracycline or methotrexate, and L-asparaginase. Glucocorticoids are a valuable component of curative regimens for Hodgkin's disease and non-Hodgkin's lymphoma, as well as for treatment of MM and CLL. Glucocorticoids are extremely helpful in controlling autoimmune hemolytic anemia and thrombocytopenia associated with CLL.

Dexamethasone is used in conjunction with radiotherapy to reduce edema related to tumors in critical areas such as the superior mediastinum, brain, and spinal cord. Doses of 4–6 mg every 6 hours have dramatic effects in restoring neurological function in patients with cerebral metastases, but these effects are temporary. Because acute changes in dosage can lead to a rapid recrudescence of symptoms, dexamethasone should not be discontinued abruptly in patients receiving radiotherapy or chemotherapy for brain metastases. Gradual tapering of the dosage may be undertaken if a clinical response to definitive antitumor therapy has been achieved.

Several glucocorticoids are available and at equivalent dosages exert similar effects (see Chapter 59). Prednisone, for example, usually is administered orally in doses as high as 60–100 mg, or even higher, for the first few days and gradually reduced to levels of 20–40 mg/day.

PROGESTINS
Progestational agents (*see* Chapter 57) have been used as second-line hormonal therapy for metastatic hormone-dependent breast cancer and in the management of endometrial carcinoma previously treated by surgery and radiotherapy. In addition, progestins stimulate appetite and restore a sense of well-being in cachectic patients with advanced stages of cancer and AIDS.

ESTROGENS AND ANDROGENS
Carcinomas arising from the prostate and mammary gland often retain some of the hormonal responsiveness of their normal counterparts for varying periods of time. By changing the hormonal environment of such tumors, it is possible to alter the course of the neoplastic process.

ANTIANDROGEN THERAPY IN PROSTATE CANCER
Although the antiandrogenic treatment of metastatic prostate carcinoma is palliative, life expectancy is increased and thousands of patients have benefited. When distant metastases already are present, hormonal therapy becomes the primary treatment for prostate cancer. Pharmacological approaches to reduce the concentrations of endogenous androgens or inhibit their action include antiandrogens, or more commonly, the administration of gonadotropin-releasing hormone (GnRH) agonists or antagonists with or without antiandrogens (*see* below).

Among men with metastatic prostate cancer, >90% have an initial favorable response to primary hormonal therapy with androgen deprivation therapy (ADT). This is manifest as disease regression or stabilization and relief of cancer-related symptoms. The average time to progression is 18–36 months, making ADT one of the longest-lasting beneficial treatments in any advanced solid tumor. There is a survival benefit to ADT. Disease progression after ADT signifies an androgen-independent state, with subsequent median survival of only 12 months. However, many men will respond to secondary hormonal therapy even after failure of ADT. Secondary hormonal treatments include androgen receptor (AR) blockers, adrenal androgen synthesis inhibitors, and estrogenic agents. Responses are more variable than to primary hormonal therapy, but a substantial portion of men benefit from these well-tolerated forms of treatment. When patients become refractory to any form of hormonal therapy, their management usually involves chemotherapeutic agents.

Common side effects of all forms of antiandrogen hormonal therapy include vasomotor flushing, loss of libido, gynecomastia, increased weight, decreased bone mineral density (BMD), and loss of muscle mass. There is variability to these side effects. For example, AR blockers cause more gynecomastia compared with GnRH agonists but less vasomotor flushing and loss of BMD. Importantly, the increased cardiovascular toxicity observed with high doses of estrogen is not observed with other forms of ADT.

Gonadotropin-Releasing Hormone Agonists and Antagonists

The most common form of ADT involves suppression of the pituitary with GnRH agonists. GnRH agonists cause an initial surge in levels of luteinizing hormone (LH) and follicle-stimulating hormone (FSH), followed by inhibition of gonadotropin release (*see* Chapter 55). One important side effect, a transient flare of disease due to the initial gonadotropin surge, can be avoided by temporary (2–4 weeks) administration of AR blockers or by the use of GnRH antagonists (*see* below).

Complete androgen blockade (CAB) refers to combination therapy with androgen-receptor blockers and GnRH agonists. However, the advantages of long-term CAB over GnRH agonists alone are questionable.

Treatment with GnRH antagonists rapidly reduces serum testosterone levels, without the transient initial increase observed after GnRH agonists. *Abarelix* (PLENAXIS) effectively reduces serum testosterone to castrate levels within a week in most men. Other than avoidance of the initial flare, GnRH antagonist therapy offers no advantage compared with GnRH agonists, and GnRH antagonists for prostate cancer are available only in the 1-month depot formulation.

Androgen Receptor Blockers

Compounds that competitively inhibit natural ligands of the AR are called AR blockers or antiandrogens (*see* Chapter 58). AR blockers as monotherapy are not indicated as routine treatment for patients with advanced prostate cancer, although some evidence points to reduced adverse effects of AR blockers relative to GnRH agonists on BMD and body composition. The AR blockers are often given in combination with GnRH agonists, where they act to block potential deleterious effects resulting from transient increases in gonadotropins and testosterone. The most commonly used drugs are members of the nonsteroidal class of AR blockers, including flutamide (EULEXIN, others), *nilutamide* (NILANDRON), and *bicalutamide* (CASODEX).

ESTROGENS AND ANDROGENS IN THE TREATMENT OF BREAST CANCER

Antagonizing the effects of estrogen in breast cancer frequently is effective, and the use of antiestrogens such as *tamoxifen* is now a standard part of hormonal therapy of breast cancer. Immunohistochemical detection of estrogen receptors (ER) and progesterone receptors (PR) has improved selection of patients for hormone therapies. Most patients with ER- or PR-positive tumors will respond to hormonal therapy; these patients also have a better overall prognosis independent of the type of therapy. In contrast, ER- and PR-negative carcinomas rarely respond to hormonal therapy. Clinically detectable responses to hormone therapy usually take 8–12 weeks to detect. If the disease responds or remains stable on a given treatment, the medication typically is continued indefinitely until the disease progresses or unwanted toxicities develop. The duration of an induced remission averages 6–12 months but sometimes can last for many years.

Antiestrogen Therapy

Antiestrogen approaches for the therapy of hormone-receptor positive breast cancer include the use of selective estrogen-receptor modulators (SERMs), selective estrogen receptor downregulators (SERDs), and aromatase inhibitors (AIs).

SELECTIVE ESTROGEN RECEPTOR MODULATORS SERMs bind to the ER and exert either estrogenic or antiestrogenic effects depending on the specific organ. The recent decline in breast cancer mortality is believed to be in part due to the widespread utilization of tamoxifen. In addition to its estrogen antagonist effects on breast cancer, tamoxifen also exerts undesirable estrogenic agonist effects in nonbreast tissues. Several novel antiestrogen compounds have been developed that offer the potential for enhanced efficacy and reduced toxicity compared with tamoxifen, which can be divided into tamoxifen analogs (*e.g., toremifene, droloxifene,* and *idoxifene*), "fixed ring" compounds (*e.g., raloxifene, lasofoxifene, arzoxifene, miproxifene, levormeloxifene,* and EM652), and the SERDs (*e.g., fulvestrant*), the latter also termed "pure antiestrogens").

TAMOXIFEN Tamoxifen's broad use is related to its anticancer activity and good tolerability profile allowing chronic daily dosing. Tamoxifen is prescribed for the prevention of breast cancer in high-risk patients, for the adjuvant therapy of early-stage breast cancer, and for the therapy of advanced breast cancer. Other organs affected by tamoxifen include the uterine endometrium (endometrial hypertrophy, vaginal bleeding, and endometrial cancer), the coagulation system (thromboembolism), bone metabolism (increase in BMD), and liver function (alterations of blood lipid profile).

The use of tamoxifen in the hormonal therapy of breast cancer is described in detail in Chapter 57. Alternative or additional antiestrogen strategies in premenopausal women include oophorectomy or GnRH analogs (see Chapter 55). Tamoxifen also has shown effectiveness in initial trials for preventing breast cancer in women at increased risk. A similar decrease in the incidence of breast cancer also was observed with raloxifene.

TOREMIFENE Toremifene (FARESTON) is a triphenylethylene derivative of tamoxifen and has a similar pharmacological profile. Toremifene is indicated for the treatment of breast cancer in women with tumors that are ER-positive or of unknown receptor status. Toremifene has ~40 times lower estrogen agonist effect than tamoxifen *in vitro*, which may make toremifene more effective in combination with an aromatase inhibitor than tamoxifen.

Selective Estrogen Receptor Downregulators

SERDs, also termed "pure antiestrogens," include compounds such as fulvestrant, RU 58668, SR 16234, ZD 164384, and ZK 191703. SERDs, unlike SERMs, are devoid of any estrogen agonist activity and function as pure antagonists.

FULVESTRANT Fulvestrant (FASLODEX) is the first FDA-approved agent in the new class of ER downregulators. Fulvestrant is approved for postmenopausal women with ER-positive metastatic breast cancer that has progressed despite antiestrogen therapy. Fulvestrant binds to the ER with an affinity >100 times that of tamoxifen; its long, bulky side-chain at the 7α position sterically hinders receptor dimerization, leading to increased ER turnover and disruption of nuclear localization. Unlike tamoxifen, which stabilizes or even increases ER expression, fulvestrant reduces the number of ER molecules in cells.

This ER "downregulation," can completely suppress the expression of estrogen-dependent genes, which likely explains why fulvestrant demonstrates efficacy against tamoxifen-resistant breast cancer. Maximum plasma concentrations are reached about 7 days after intramuscular administration of fulvestrant and are maintained over a period of 1 month. The plasma $t_{1/2}$ is approximately 40 days. Steady-state concentrations are reached after 3–6 monthly injections.

Fulvestrant generally is well tolerated with the most common adverse events being nausea, asthenia, pain, vasodilation (hot flushes), and headache. Injection site reactions, seen in ~7% of patients, are reduced by giving the injection slowly. In the study comparing anastrozole and fulvestrant, quality-of-life outcome measures were maintained over time with no significant difference between the drugs.

AROMATASE INHIBITORS

AIs are drugs that inhibit aromatase, the enzyme that carries out the final step in the conversion of androgens to estrogen. These drugs have achieved wide use and considerable success in the treatment of early and advanced breast cancer, as described in Chapter 57.

For a complete Bibliographical listing see Goodman & Gilman's *The Pharmacological Basis of Therapeutics*, 11th ed., or Goodman & Gilman Online at www.accessmedicine.com.

52

IMMUNOSUPPRESSANTS, TOLEROGENS, AND IMMUNOSTIMULANTS

THE IMMUNE RESPONSE

The immune system evolved to discriminate self from nonself. Innate, or natural, immunity is broadly reactive, does not require priming, and is of relatively low affinity. Adaptive, or learned, immunity is antigen-specific, depends upon antigen exposure or priming, and can be of very high affinity. The two arms of immunity work closely together, with the innate immune system being more active early in an immune response and adaptive immunity becoming progressively dominant over time. The major effectors of innate immunity are complement, granulocytes, monocytes/macrophages, natural killer cells, mast cells, and basophils. The major effectors of adaptive immunity are B and T lymphocytes. B lymphocytes make antibodies; T lymphocytes function as helper, cytolytic, and regulatory (suppressor) cells. These cells are important in the normal immune response to infection and tumors but also mediate transplant rejection and autoimmunity.

Immunoglobulins (antibodies) on the B lymphocyte surface are receptors for a large variety of specific structural conformations. In contrast, T lymphocytes recognize antigens as peptide fragments in the context of self major histocompatibility complex (MHC) antigens [called human leukocyte antigens (HLA)] on the surface of antigen-presenting cells (APCs), such as dendritic cells, macrophages, and other cell types expressing MHC class I and class II antigens. Once activated by specific antigen recognition *via* their respective clonally restricted cell-surface receptors, both B and T lymphocytes are triggered to differentiate and divide, leading to release of soluble mediators (cytokines, lymphokines) that are effectors and regulators of the immune response.

The impact of the immune system in human disease is enormous. Immunological diseases (*e.g.*, rheumatoid arthritis, type 1 diabetes mellitus, and asthma; solid tumors and hematologic malignancies) are growing at epidemic proportions that require aggressive and innovative approaches to develop new treatments. Immune system–mediated graft rejection remains a formidable obstacle to widespread use of organ transplantation.

IMMUNOSUPPRESSION

In transplantation, the major classes of immunosuppressive drugs are: (1) *glucocorticoids*, (2) *calcineurin inhibitors*, (3) *antiproliferative/antimetabolic agents*, and (4) *biologics (antibodies)*. These drugs have achieved a high degree of clinical success in treating conditions such as acute immune rejection of organ transplants and severe autoimmune diseases. However, such therapies require lifelong use and nonspecifically suppress the entire immune system, exposing patients to considerably higher risks of infection and cancer. The calcineurin inhibitors and glucocorticoids are nephrotoxic and diabetogenic, respectively, thus restricting their usefulness in a variety of clinical settings.

Monoclonal and polyclonal antibodies directed at reactive T cells are important adjunct therapies and provide a unique opportunity to target specifically immune-reactive cells. Finally, newer small molecules and antibodies have expanded the arsenal of immunosuppressives. In particular, mTOR (*m*ammalian *t*arget *o*f *r*apamycin) inhibitors (*sirolimus, everolimus*) and anti-CD25 (interleukin [IL]-2 receptor) antibodies (*basiliximab, daclizumab*) target growth factor pathways, substantially limiting clonal expansion and potentially promoting tolerance.

General Approach to Organ Transplantation Therapy

A multitiered approach, similar to that in cancer chemotherapy, is employed in immunosuppressive drug therapy for organ transplants. Several agents are used simultaneously, each of which is directed at a different molecular target within the allograft response (Table 52–1). Synergistic effects permit use of the various agents at relatively low doses, thereby limiting specific toxicities while maximizing the immunosuppressive effect. Greater immunosuppression is required to gain early engraftment and/or to treat established rejection than to maintain long-term immunosuppression. Therefore, intensive induction and lower-dose maintenance protocols are employed.

Table 52–1

Sites of Action of Selected Immunosuppressive Agents on T-Cell Activation

Drug	Site of Action
Glucocorticoids	Glucocorticoid response elements in DNA (regulate gene transcription)
Muromonab-CD3	T-cell receptor complex (blocks antigen recognition)
Cyclosporine	Calcineurin (inhibits phosphatase activity)
Tacrolimus	Calcineurin (inhibits phosphatase activity)
Azathioprine	Deoxyribonucleic acid (false nucleotide incorporation)
Mycophenolate Mofetil	Inosine monophosphate dehydrogenase (inhibits activity)
Daclizumab, Basiliximab	IL-2 receptor (block IL-2–mediated T-cell activation)
Sirolimus	Protein kinase involved in cell-cycle progression (mTOR) (inhibits activity)

BIOLOGIC INDUCTION THERAPY

In many transplant centers, induction therapy with biologic agents is used to delay the use of the nephrotoxic calcineurin inhibitors or to intensify the initial immunosuppressive therapy in patients at high risk of rejection (i.e., repeat transplants, broadly presensitized patients, African American patients, or pediatric patients). Most of the limitations of murine-based mAbs generally were overcome by the introduction of chimeric or humanized mAbs that lack antigenicity and have prolonged serum half-lives. The anti–interleukin-2 receptor (IL-2R) mAbs—frequently termed anti-CD25—were the first biologics proven to be effective as induction agents.

Biologic agents for induction therapy in the prophylaxis of rejection currently are used in ~70% of de novo transplant patients. Biologics for induction can be divided into two groups: depleting agents and immune modulators. Depleting agents consist of lymphocyte immune globulin, antithymocyte globulin, and muromonab-CD3 mAb (the latter also produces immune modulation); their efficacy derives from their ability to deplete the recipient's CD3-positive cells at the time of transplantation and antigen presentation. The second group, the anti–IL-2R mAbs, does not deplete T lymphocytes, but rather block IL-2–mediated T-cell activation by binding to the α chain of IL-2R.

For patients with high levels of anti-HLA antibodies, humoral rejection mediated by B cells can be modified by plasmapheresis, usually given every other day for 4–5 treatments followed by intravenous immunoglobulin to suppress antibody production.

MAINTENANCE IMMUNOTHERAPY

Therapy typically involves a calcineurin inhibitor (e.g., cyclosporine or tacrolimus), glucocorticoids, and mycophenolate mofetil (a purine metabolism inhibitor; see below), each directed at a discrete site in T-cell activation. Alternatively, sirolimus can be used to limit exposure to the nephrotoxic calcineurin inhibitors. Glucocorticoids, azathioprine, cyclosporine, tacrolimus, mycophenolate mofetil, sirolimus, and various monoclonal and polyclonal antibodies are all approved for use in transplantation.

THERAPY FOR ESTABLISHED REJECTION

Although low doses of prednisone, calcineurin inhibitors, purine metabolism inhibitors, or sirolimus are effective in preventing acute cellular rejection, they are less effective in blocking activated T lymphocytes and thus are not very effective against established, acute rejection or for the total prevention of chronic rejection. Therefore, treatment of established rejection requires the use of agents directed against activated T cells. These include glucocorticoids in high doses (pulse therapy), polyclonal antilymphocyte antibodies, or muromonab-CD3 mAb.

Glucocorticoids

Glucocorticoid chemistry, pharmacokinetics, and drug interactions are described in Chapter 59. Prednisone, prednisolone, and other glucocorticoids are used alone and in combination with other immunosuppressive agents for treatment of transplant rejection and autoimmune disorders.

MECHANISM OF ACTION

Glucocorticoids have broad anti-inflammatory effects on multiple components of cellular immunity. The mechanisms of glucocorticoid action (i.e., gene regulation, suppression of proinflammatory cytokines, etc.) are detailed in Chapter 59.

THERAPEUTIC USES   Glucocorticoids commonly are combined with other immunosuppressive agents to prevent and treat transplant rejection. High dose pulses of intravenous *methylprednisolone sodium succinate* (SOLU-MEDROL, A-METHAPRED) are used to reverse acute transplant rejection and acute exacerbations of selected autoimmune disorders. Glucocorticoids also are efficacious for treatment of graft-*versus*-host disease in bone marrow transplantation. Glucocorticoids are used routinely to treat autoimmune disorders (*see* Chapter 59) and acute exacerbations of multiple sclerosis (*see* below). In addition, glucocorticoids limit allergic reactions that occur with other immunosuppressive agents and are used in transplant recipients to block first-dose cytokine storm caused by treatment with muromonad-CD3 and to a lesser extent thymoglobulin (*see* below).

TOXICITY   Unfortunately, chronic use of steroids often results in disabling and life-threatening adverse effects, as described in Chapter 59. The advent of combined glucocorticoid/cyclosporine regimens has allowed reduced doses of steroids, but steroid-induced morbidity remains a major problem in many transplant patients.

Calcineurin Inhibitors

Perhaps the most effective immunosuppressive drugs in routine use are the calcineurin inhibitors, *cyclosporine* and *tacrolimus*, which target intracellular signaling pathways induced as a consequence of T-cell–receptor activation. Although they are structurally unrelated and bind to distinct molecular targets, they inhibit normal T-cell signal transduction essentially by the same mechanism (*see* Figure 52–1).

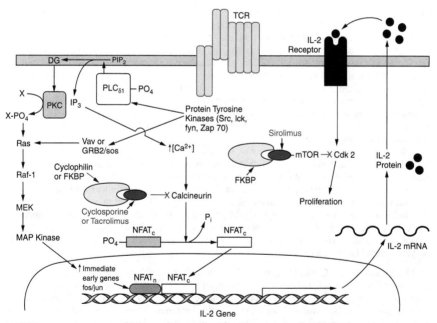

FIGURE 52–1   *Mechanisms of action of cyclosporine, tacrolimus, and sirolimus on T cells.* Both cyclosporine and tacrolimus bind to immunophilins (cyclophilin and FK506-binding protein [FKBP], respectively), forming a complex that binds the phosphatase calcineurin and inhibits the calcineurin-catalyzed dephosphorylation essential to permit nuclear movement of the nuclear factor of activated T cells (NFAT) into the nucleus. In the nucleus, NFAT interacts with transcription factor AP-I (fos/jun), an interaction required for transcription of interleukin-2 (IL-2) and other growth and differentiation–associated cytokines (lymphokines). Sirolimus (rapamycin) works at a later stage in T-cell activation, downstream of the IL-2 receptor. Sirolimus also binds FKBP, but the FKBP-sirolimus complex binds to and inhibits the mammalian target of rapamycin (mTOR), a kinase involved in cell-cycle progression (proliferation). TCR, T-cell receptor.

CYCLOSPORINE

Chemistry

Cyclosporine (cyclosporin A), a cyclic undecapeptide, is produced by the fungus Beauveria nivea. *Cyclosporine is lipophilic and highly hydrophobic, and is formulated for clinical administration using castor oil or other strategies to ensure solubilization.*

Mechanism of Action

Cyclosporine suppresses humoral immunity but is much more effective against T-cell–dependent immune mechanisms that underlie transplant rejection and some forms of autoimmunity. It preferentially inhibits antigen-triggered signal transduction in T lymphocytes, blunting expression of many lymphokines, including IL-2, and the expression of antiapoptotic proteins (Figure 52–1). Cyclosporine also increases expression of transforming growth factor-β, a potent inhibitor of IL-2–stimulated T-cell proliferation and generation of cytotoxic T lymphocytes (CTL).

Disposition and Pharmacokinetics Cyclosporine is administered intravenously or orally. The intravenous preparation (SANDIMMUNE Injection) is dissolved in an ethanol-polyoxyethylated castor oil vehicle that must be further diluted in 0.9% NaCl or 5% dextrose solution before injection. The oral dosage forms include soft gelatin capsules and oral solutions. Cyclosporine supplied in the original soft gelatin capsule (SANDIMMUNE) is absorbed slowly with 20–50% bioavailability. A modified microemulsion formulation (NEORAL) has more uniform and slightly increased bioavailability compared to SANDIMMUNE and is provided as 25-mg and 100-mg soft gelatin capsules and a 100-mg/mL oral solution. SANDIMMUNE and its generics are not the same as NEORAL and its generics, such that one preparation cannot be substituted for another without risk of inadequate immunosuppression or increased toxicity.

Drug monitoring is essential to optimize therapy. Because both radioimmunoassays and high-performance liquid chromatography assays are used, the clinician should ensure that the methods are consistent when monitoring an individual patient. Blood is most conveniently sampled at 2 hours after a dose administration (*i.e.*, C_2 levels) rather than prior to dosing. In complex patients with delayed absorption, such as diabetics with gastoparesis, the C_2 level may underestimate the peak cyclosporine level obtained; in rapid absorbers, the C_2 level may have peaked before the blood sample is drawn. If a patient has clinical signs or symptoms of toxicity or there is unexplained rejection or renal dysfunction, a pharmacokinetic profile (*see* Chapter 1) can be used to estimate exposure to the drug.

Cyclosporine absorption is incomplete following oral administration and varies with the individual patient and the formulation used. The elimination of cyclosporine from the blood is generally biphasic, with a terminal $t_{1/2}$ of 5–18 hours. After intravenous infusion, clearance is ~5–7 mL/min/kg in adult recipients of renal transplants, but results differ by age and patient populations (*e.g.*, slower in cardiac transplant patients, faster in children). Thus, the intersubject variability is so large that individual monitoring is required.

After oral administration of cyclosporine (as NEORAL), the time to peak blood concentrations is 1.5–2 hours. Administration with food delays and decreases absorption. High- and low-fat meals consumed within 30 minutes of administration decrease the AUC by ~13% and the maximum concentration by 33%. This makes it imperative to individualize dosage regimens for outpatients.

Cyclosporine is extensively metabolized in the liver by CYP3A and to a lesser degree by the gastrointestinal (GI) tract and kidneys. Cyclosporine and its metabolites are excreted principally through the bile into the feces. Cyclosporine also is excreted in human milk. In the presence of hepatic dysfunction, dosage adjustments are required. No adjustments generally are necessary for dialysis or renal failure patients.

Therapeutic Uses Clinical indications for cyclosporine are kidney, liver, heart, and other organ transplantation; rheumatoid arthritis; and psoriasis. Its use in dermatology is discussed in Chapter 62. Cyclosporine usually is combined with other agents, especially glucocorticoids and either azathioprine or mycophenolate mofetil, and most recently, sirolimus. The dose of cyclosporine varies, depending on the organ transplanted and the other drugs used in the specific treatment protocol(s). The initial dose generally is not given before the transplant because of the concern about nephrotoxicity. Especially for renal transplant patients, algorithms have been developed to delay cyclosporine introduction until a threshold renal function has been attained. Dosage is guided by signs of rejection (too low a dose), renal or other toxicity (too high a dose), and close monitoring of blood levels. Great care must be taken to differentiate renal toxicity from rejection in kidney transplant patients. Ultrasound-guided allograft biopsy is the best way to assess the reason for renal dysfunction. Because adverse reactions have been ascribed more frequently to the intravenous formulation, this route of administration is discontinued as soon as the patient is able to take the drug orally.

In rheumatoid arthritis, cyclosporine is used in severe cases that have not responded to *methotrexate.* Cyclosporine can be combined with methotrexate, but the levels of both drugs must be monitored closely. In psoriasis, cyclosporine is indicated for treatment of adult immunocompetent patients with severe and disabling disease for whom other systemic therapies have failed. Because of its mechanism of action, cyclosporine also has been used successfully in inflammatory bowel disease (*see* Chapter 38).

Toxicity The principal adverse reactions to cyclosporine therapy are renal dysfunction, tremor, hirsutism, hypertension, hyperlipidemia, and gum hyperplasia. Hyperuricemia may lead to worsening of gout, increased P-glycoprotein activity, and hypercholesterolemia. Nephrotoxicity occurs in the majority of patients treated and is the major indication for cessation or modification of therapy. Hypertension occurs in ~50% of renal transplant and almost all cardiac transplant patients. Combined use of calcineurin inhibitors and glucocorticoids is particularly diabetogenic, although this apparently is more problematic in patients treated with tacrolimus (*see* below). Especially at risk are obese patients, African American or Hispanic recipients, or those with family history of type 2 diabetes or obesity. Cyclosporine, as opposed to tacrolimus, is more likely to produce elevations in low-density lipoprotein (LDL) cholesterol.

Drug Interactions Cyclosporine interacts with a wide variety of commonly used drugs, and close attention must be paid to drug interactions. Any drug that affects microsomal enzymes, especially the CYP3A system, may impact cyclosporine blood concentrations. Substances that inhibit this enzyme can decrease cyclosporine metabolism and increase blood concentrations. These include Ca^{2+} channel blockers (*e.g., verapamil, nicardipine*), antifungal agents (*e.g., fluconazole, ketoconazole*), antibiotics (*e.g., erythromycin*), glucocorticoids (*e.g., methylprednisolone*), and HIV-protease inhibitors (*e.g., indinavir*). Grapefruit and grapefruit juice block CYP3A and the multidrug efflux pump and should be avoided by patients taking cyclosporine because these effects can increase cyclosporine blood concentrations. In contrast, drugs that induce CYP3A activity can increase cyclosporine metabolism and decrease blood concentrations. Such drugs include antibiotics (*e.g., nafcillin, rifampin*), anticonvulsants (*e.g., phenobarbital, phenytoin*), and others (*e.g., octreotide, ticlopidine*). In general, close monitoring of cyclosporine blood levels and the levels of other drugs is required when such combinations are used.

Interactions between cyclosporine and sirolimus (*see* below) have led to the recommendation that administration of the two drugs be separated by time. Sirolimus aggravates cyclosporine-induced renal dysfunction, while cyclosporine increases sirolimus-induced hyperlipidemia and myelosuppression. Other drug interactions of concern include additive nephrotoxicity when cyclosporine is coadministered with nonsteroidal anti-inflammatory drugs and other drugs that cause renal dysfunction; elevation of methotrexate levels when the two drugs are coadministered; and reduced clearance of *prednisolone, digoxin,* and statins.

TACROLIMUS Tacrolimus (PROGRAF, FK506) is a macrolide antibiotic produced by *Streptomyces tsukubaensis.*

Like cyclosporine, tacrolimus inhibits T-cell activation by inhibiting calcineurin. Tacrolimus binds to an intracellular protein, FK506-binding protein-12 (FKBP-12), an immunophilin structurally related to cyclophilin. A complex of tacrolimus-FKBP-12, Ca^{2+}, calmodulin, and calcineurin then forms, and calcineurin phosphatase activity is inhibited. As described for cyclosporine and depicted in Figure 52–1, the inhibition of phosphatase activity prevents dephosphorylation and nuclear translocation of NFAT and inhibits T-cell activation. Thus, although the intracellular receptors differ, cyclosporine and tacrolimus target the same pathway for immunosuppression.

Disposition and Pharmacokinetics

Tacrolimus is available for oral administration as capsules (0.5, 1, and 5 mg) and as a sterile solution for injection (5 mg/mL). Immunosuppressive activity resides primarily in the parent drug. Because of intersubject variability in pharmacokinetics, individualized dosing is required for optimal therapy. Whole blood, rather than plasma, is the most appropriate sampling compartment to describe tacrolimus pharmacokinetics. For tacrolimus, the trough level seems to correlate better with clinical events than it does for cyclosporine. Target concentrations in many centers are 200–400 ng/mL in the early preoperative period and 100–200 ng/mL 3 months after transplantation. GI absorption is incomplete and variable. Food decreases the rate and extent of absorption. Plasma protein binding of tacrolimus is 75–99%, involving primarily albumin and α_1-acid glycoprotein. Tacrolimus is extensively metabolized in the liver by CYP3A, with a $t_{1/2}$ of ~12 hours; at least some of the metabolites are active. The bulk of excretion of the parent drug and metabolites is in the feces.

Therapeutic Uses

Tacrolimus is indicated for the prophylaxis of solid-organ allograft rejection in a manner akin to cyclosporine and as rescue therapy in patients with rejection despite "therapeutic" levels of cyclosporine. Dosages are intended to achieve blood trough levels of 5–15-ng/mL. Pediatric patients generally require higher doses than do adults.

Toxicity

Nephrotoxicity, neurotoxicity (tremor, headache, motor disturbances, seizures), GI complaints, hypertension, hyperkalemia, hyperglycemia, and diabetes are all associated with tacrolimus use. As with cyclosporine, nephrotoxicity is limiting. Tacrolimus has a negative effect on pancreatic β cells, and glucose intolerance and diabetes mellitus are well-recognized complications of tacrolimus-based immunosuppression. As with other immunosuppressive agents, there is an increased risk of secondary tumors and opportunistic infections. Notably, tacrolimus does not adversely affect uric acid or LDL cholesterol.

Drug Interactions

Because of its potential for nephrotoxicity, tacrolimus blood levels and renal function should be monitored closely, especially when tacrolimus is used with other potentially nephrotoxic drugs. Coadministration with cyclosporine results in additive or synergistic nephrotoxicity; therefore, a delay of at least 24 hours is required when switching a patient from cyclosporine to tacrolimus. Since tacrolimus is metabolized mainly by CYP3A, the potential interactions described above for cyclosporine also apply for tacrolimus.

Antiproliferative and Antimetabolic Drugs

SIROLIMUS Sirolimus (*rapamycin*; RAPAMUNE) is a macrocyclic lactone produced by *Streptomyces hygroscopicus.*

Mechanism of Action

Sirolimus inhibits T-lymphocyte activation and proliferation downstream of the IL-2 and other T-cell growth factor receptors (Figure 52–1). Like cyclosporine and tacrolimus, therapeutic action of sirolimus requires formation of a complex with an immunophilin, in this case FKBP-12. The sirolimus–FKBP-12 complex does not affect calcineurin activity but rather inhibits a protein kinase that is a key enzyme in cell-cycle progression, designated mTOR. Inhibition of mTOR blocks cell-cycle progression at the $G_1 \rightarrow S$ phase transition.

Disposition and Pharmacokinetics After oral administration, sirolimus is absorbed rapidly and reaches a peak blood concentration within ~1 hour after a single dose in healthy subjects and within ~2 hours after multiple oral doses in renal transplant patients. Systemic availability is ~15%, and blood concentrations are proportional to doses between 3 and 12 mg/m². A high-fat meal decreases peak blood concentration by 34%; sirolimus therefore should be taken consistently either with or without food, and blood levels should be monitored closely. About 40% of sirolimus in plasma is protein bound, especially to albumin. The drug partitions into formed elements of blood, with a blood:plasma ratio of 38 in renal transplant patients. Sirolimus is extensively metabolized by CYP3A4 and is transported by P-glycoprotein. Although some of its metabolites are active, sirolimus itself is the major active component in whole blood and contributes >90% of the immunosuppressive effect. The blood $t_{1/2}$ after multiple doses in stable renal transplant patients is 62 hours. A loading dose of three times the maintenance dose usually provides nearly steady-state concentrations within 1 day.

Therapeutic Uses Sirolimus is indicated for prophylaxis of organ transplant rejection in combination with a calcineurin inhibitor and glucocorticoids. In patients experiencing or at high risk for calcineurin inhibitor–associated nephrotoxicity, sirolimus has been used with glucocorticoids and mycophenolate mofetil to avoid permanent renal damage. The initial dosage in patients 13 years or older who weigh <40 kg should be adjusted based on body surface area (1 mg/m²/day) with a loading dose of 3 mg/m². Data regarding doses for pediatric and geriatric patients are lacking. It is recommended that the maintenance dose be reduced by approximately one-third in patients with hepatic impairment. Sirolimus also has been incorporated into stents to inhibit local cell proliferation and blood vessel occlusion.

Toxicity The use of sirolimus in renal transplant patients is associated with a dose-dependent increase in serum cholesterol and triglycerides. While immunotherapy with sirolimus *per se* is not nephrotoxic, patients treated with cyclosporine plus sirolimus have impaired renal function compared to patients treated with cyclosporine alone. Sirolimus also may prolong delayed graft function in deceased donor kidney transplants, presumably because of its antiproliferative action. Renal function must be monitored closely in such patients. Lymphocele, a surgical complication associated with renal transplantation, is increased in a dose-dependent fashion by sirolimus, requiring close postoperative follow-up. Other adverse effects include anemia, leukopenia, thrombocytopenia, hypo- or hyperkalemia, fever, and GI effects. Delayed wound healing may occur. As with other immunosuppressive agents, there is an increased risk of neoplasms, especially lymphomas, and infections. Prophylaxis for *Pneumocystis jiroveci* pneumonia and cytomegalovirus is recommended.

Drug Interactions Since sirolimus is a substrate for CYP3A4 and is transported by P-glycoprotein, close attention to interactions with other drugs that are metabolized or transported by these proteins is required. As noted above, cyclosporine and sirolimus interact, and their administration should be separated by time. Dose adjustment may be required when sirolimus is coadministered with *diltiazem* or rifampin.

EVEROLIMUS Everolimus (40-*O*-[2-hydroxy] ethyl-rapamycin) is closely related chemically and clinically to sirolimus but has distinct pharmacokinetics. The main difference is a shorter $t_{1/2}$ and thus a shorter time to achieve steady-state concentrations of the drug. Dosage on a milligram per kilogram basis is similar to sirolimus. Aside from the shorter $t_{1/2}$, no studies have compared everolimus with sirolimus in standard immunosuppressive regimens. As with sirolimus, the combination of a calcineurin inhibitor and an mTOR inhibitor produces worse renal function at 1 year than does calcineurin inhibitor therapy alone, suggesting a drug interaction between the mTOR inhibitors and the calcineurin inhibitors to enhance toxicity and to reduce rejection. The toxicity of everolimus and the drug interactions seem to be the same as with sirolimus.

AZATHIOPRINE Azathioprine (IMURAN) is a purine antimetabolite. It is an imidazolyl derivative of 6-mercaptopurine.

Mechanism of Action

Following exposure to nucleophiles such as glutathione, azathioprine is cleaved to 6-mercaptopurine, which in turn is converted to additional metabolites that inhibit de novo *purine synthesis (see Chapter 51). 6-Thio-IMP, a fraudulent nucleotide, is converted to 6-thio-GMP and finally to 6-thio-GTP, which is incorporated into DNA. Cell proliferation is thereby inhibited, impairing a variety of lymphocyte functions. Azathioprine appears to be a more potent immunosuppressive agent than 6-mercaptopurine.*

Disposition and Pharmacokinetics Azathioprine is well absorbed orally and reaches maximum blood levels within 1–2 hours after administration. The $t_{1/2}$ of azathioprine is ~10 minutes, while that of its metabolite 6-mercaptopurine is about an hour. Blood levels have limited predictive value because of extensive metabolism, significant activity of many different metabolites, and high tissue levels attained. Azathioprine and *mercaptopurine* are moderately bound to plasma proteins and are partially dialyzable. Both are rapidly removed from the blood by oxidation or methylation in the liver and/or erythrocytes. Renal clearance has little impact on biological effectiveness or toxicity, but the dose should be reduced in patients with renal failure.

Therapeutic Uses Azathioprine is indicated as an adjunct for prevention of organ transplant rejection and in severe rheumatoid arthritis. Although the dose of azathioprine required to prevent organ rejection and minimize toxicity varies, 3–5 mg/kg/day is the usual starting dose. Lower initial doses (1 mg/kg/day) are used for rheumatoid arthritis. Complete blood count and liver function tests should be monitored.

Toxicity The major side effect of azathioprine is bone marrow suppression, including leukopenia (common), thrombocytopenia (less common), and/or anemia (uncommon). Other important adverse effects include increased susceptibility to infections (especially varicella and herpes simplex viruses), hepatotoxicity, alopecia, GI toxicity, pancreatitis, and increased risk of neoplasia.

Drug Interactions Xanthine oxidase, a key enzyme in the catabolism of azathioprine metabolites, is blocked by allopurinol. If azathioprine and allopurinol are used concurrently, the azathioprine dose must be decreased to 25–33% of the usual dose; it is best not to use these two drugs together. Adverse effects resulting from coadministration of azathioprine with other myelosuppressive agents or angiotensin-converting enzyme inhibitors include leukopenia, thrombocytopenia, and anemia as a result of myelosuppression.

MYCOPHENOLATE MOFETIL *Mycophenolate mofetil* (CELLCEPT) is the 2-morpholinoethyl ester of mycophenolic acid (MPA).

Mechanism of Action

Mycophenolate mofetil is a prodrug that is rapidly hydrolyzed to MPA, a selective, noncompetitive, and reversible inhibitor of inosine monophosphate dehydrogenase (IMPDH), an important enzyme in the de novo *pathway of guanine nucleotide synthesis. B and T lymphocytes are highly dependent on this pathway for cell proliferation, while other cell types can use salvage pathways; MPA therefore selectively inhibits lymphocyte proliferation and functions, including antibody formation, cellular adhesion, and migration.*

Disposition and Pharmacokinetics Mycophenolate mofetil is rapidly and completely metabolized to MPA after oral or intravenous administration. MPA, in turn, is metabolized to the inactive glucuronide MPAG. The parent drug is cleared from the blood within a few minutes. The $t_{1/2}$ of MPA is ~16 hours. Negligible (<1%) amounts of MPA are excreted in the urine. Most (87%) is excreted in the urine as MPAG. Plasma concentrations of MPA and MPAG are increased in patients with renal insufficiency. In early renal transplant patients (<40 days post-transplant), plasma concentrations of MPA after a single dose of mycophenolate mofetil are approximately half of those found in healthy volunteers or stable renal transplant patients.

Therapeutic Uses Mycophenolate mofetil is indicated for prophylaxis of transplant rejection, and it typically is used in combination with glucocorticoids and a calcineurin inhibitor, but not with azathioprine. Combined treatment with sirolimus is possible, although potential drug interactions necessitate careful monitoring of drug levels. For renal transplants, 1 g is administered orally or intravenously (over 2 hours) twice daily (2 g/day). A higher dose, 1.5 g twice daily (3 g/day), is recommended for African American renal transplant patients and all cardiac transplant patients.

Toxicity The principal toxicities of mycophenolate mofetil are leukopenia, diarrhea, and vomiting. There also is an increased incidence of some infections, especially sepsis associated with cytomegalovirus. Tacrolimus in combination with mycophenolate mofetil has been associated with devastating viral infections including polyoma nephritis.

Drug Interactions There appear to be no untoward effects produced by combination therapy of mycophenolate mofetil with cyclosporine, trimethoprim-sulfamethoxazole, or oral contraceptives. Unlike cyclosporine, tacrolimus delays elimination of mycophenolate mofetil by impairing the conversion of MPA to MPAG. This may enhance GI toxicity. Mycophenolate mofetil has not been tested with azathioprine. Coadministration with antacids containing aluminum or magnesium hydroxide decreases absorption of mycophenolate mofetil; thus, these drugs should not be administered simultaneously. Mycophenolate mofetil should not be administered with *cholestyramine* or other drugs that affect enterohepatic circulation. Such agents decrease plasma MPA concentrations, probably by binding free MPA in the intestines. Acyclovir and *ganciclovir* may compete with MPAG for tubular secretion, possibly resulting in increased concentrations of both MPAG and the antiviral agents in the blood, an effect that may be compounded in patients with renal insufficiency.

OTHER ANTIPROLIFERATIVE AND CYTOTOXIC AGENTS Many of the cytotoxic and antimetabolic agents used in cancer chemotherapy (*see* Chapter 51) are immunosuppressive due to their action on lymphocytes and other cells of the immune system. Other cytotoxic drugs that have been used as immunosuppressive agents include methotrexate, *cyclophosphamide* (CYTOXAN), *thalidomide*, and *chlorambucil* (LEUKERAN). Methotrexate is used for treatment of graft-*versus*-host disease, rheumatoid arthritis, and psoriasis, as well as in cancer therapy (*see* Chapter 51). Cyclophosphamide and chlorambucil are used in treating childhood nephrotic syndrome and a variety of malignancies (*see* Chapter 51). Cyclophosphamide also is used widely for treatment of severe systemic lupus erythematosus and other vasculitides such as Wegener's granulomatosis. *Leflunomide* (ARAVA) is a pyrimidine-synthesis inhibitor indicated for the treatment of adults with rheumatoid arthritis; it increasingly is used in the treatment of polyomavirus nephropathy seen in immunosuppressed renal transplant recipients. There are no studies showing efficacy compared with control patients treated with withdrawal or reduction of immunosuppression alone in BK virus nephropathy. It is hepatotoxic and can cause fetal injury when administered to pregnant women.

FTY720

FTY720 is the first agent in a new class of small molecules, sphingosine 1-phosphate receptor (S1P-R) agonists. It is a prodrug that reduces recirculation of lymphocytes from the lymphatic system to the blood and peripheral tissues, including inflammatory lesions and organ grafts.

Antibodies

Both polyclonal and monoclonal antibodies against lymphocyte cell-surface antigens are widely used for prevention and treatment of organ transplant rejection. Monoclonal reagents have overcome the problems of variability in efficacy and toxicity seen with the polyclonal products, but they are more limited in their target specificity. First-generation murine monoclonal antibodies generally have been replaced by newer chimeric or humanized monoclonal antibodies that lack antigenicity, have prolonged half-lives, and can be mutagenized to alter their affinity to Fc receptors. Both polyclonal and monoclonal products have a place in immunosuppressive therapy (Figure 52–2).

ANTITHYMOCYTE GLOBULIN Antithymocyte globulin is a purified gamma globulin from the serum of rabbits immunized with human thymocytes.

Mechanism of Action

Antithymocyte globulin contains cytotoxic antibodies that bind to CD2, CD3, CD4, CD8, CD11a, CD18, CD25, CD44, CD45, and HLA class I and II molecules on the surface of human T lymphocytes. The antibodies deplete circulating lymphocytes by direct cytotoxicity (both complement and cell-mediated) and block lymphocyte function by binding to cell surface molecules involved in the regulation of cell function.

Therapeutic Uses Antithymocyte globulin is used for induction immunosuppression, although the only approved indication is in the treatment of acute renal transplant rejection in combination with other immunosuppressive agents. Antilymphocyte-depleting agents (THYMOGLOBULIN, ATGAM) are thought to improve graft survival. A course of antithymocyte-globulin treatment often is given to

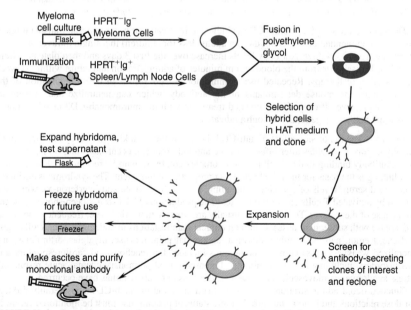

FIGURE 52–2 *Generation of monoclonal antibodies.* Mice are immunized with the selected antigen, and spleen or lymph node is harvested and B cells separated. These B cells are fused to a suitable B-cell myeloma that has been selected for its inability to grow in medium supplemented with hypoxanthine, aminopterin, and thymidine (HAT). Only myelomas that fuse with B cells can survive in HAT-supplemented medium. The hybridomas expand in culture. Those of interest based upon a specific screening technique are then selected and cloned by limiting dilution. Monoclonal antibodies can be used directly as supernatants or ascites fluid experimentally but are purified for clinical use. HPRT, hypoxanthine-guanine phosphoribosyl transferase.

renal transplant patients with delayed graft function to avoid early treatment with the nephrotoxic calcineurin inhibitors and thereby aid in recovery from ischemic reperfusion injury. The recommended dose for acute rejection of renal grafts is 1.5 mg/kg/day (given intravenously over 4–6 hours) for 7–14 days. Mean T-cell counts fall by day 2 of therapy. Antithymocyte globulin also is used for acute rejection of other types of organ transplants and for prophylaxis of rejection.

Toxicity Polyclonal antibodies are xenogeneic proteins that can elicit major side effects, including fever and chills with the potential for hypotension. Premedication with glucocorticoids, *acetaminophen*, and/or an antihistamine and administration of the antiserum by slow infusion (over 4–6 hours) into a large-diameter vein minimize such reactions. Serum sickness and glomerulonephritis can occur; anaphylaxis is rare. Hematologic complications include leukopenia and thrombocytopenia. As with other immunosuppressive agents, there is an increased risk of infection and malignancy, especially when multiple immunosuppressive agents are combined. No drug interactions have been described; anti-ATG antibodies develop but do not limit repeated use.

MONOCLONAL ANTIBODIES

Anti-CD3 Monoclonal Antibodies Antibodies directed at the ε chain of CD3, a trimeric molecule adjacent to the T-cell receptor on the surface of human T lymphocytes, have been used with considerable efficacy in human transplantation. The original mouse IgG_{2a} antihuman CD3 monoclonal antibody, muromonab-CD3 (OKT3, ORTHOCLONE OKT3), still is used to reverse glucocorticoid-resistant rejection episodes.

Mechanism of Action

Muromonab-CD3 binds to the ε chain of CD3, a component of the T-cell receptor complex involved in antigen recognition, cell signaling, and proliferation. Antibody treatment induces rapid internalization of the T-cell receptor, thereby preventing subsequent antigen recognition. Administration of the antibody is followed rapidly by depletion and extravasation of a majority of T cells from the bloodstream and peripheral lymphoid organs such as lymph nodes and spleen following, margination of T cells onto vascular endothelial walls, and redistribution of T cells to nonlymphoid organs such as the lungs. Muromonab-CD3 also reduces function of the remaining T cells, as defined by lack of IL-2 production and great reduction in the production of multiple cytokines.

Therapeutic Uses Muromonab-CD3 is indicated for treatment of acute organ transplant rejection. The recommended dose is 5 mg/day (in adults; less for children) in a single intravenous bolus (<1 minute) for 10–14 days. Antibody levels increase over the first 3 days and then plateau. Circulating T cells disappear from the blood within minutes of administration and return within ~1 week after cessation of therapy. Repeated use of muromonab-CD3 results in the immunization of the patient against the mouse determinants of the antibody, which can neutralize and prevent its immunosuppressive efficacy. Thus, repeated treatment with the muromonab-CD3 or other mouse monoclonal antibodies generally is contraindicated.

Toxicity The major side effect of anti-CD3 therapy is the "cytokine release syndrome," which typically begins 30 minutes after infusion of the antibody (but can occur later) and may persist for hours. Antibody binding to the T-cell receptor complex combined with Fc receptor (FcR)–mediated cross-linking is the basis for the initial activating properties of this agent. The syndrome is attributed to increased serum levels of cytokines (including TNF-α, IL-2, IL-6, and interferon-γ), which are released by activated T cells and/or monocytes. The production of TNF-α has been shown to be the major cause of the toxicity. The symptoms usually are worst with the first dose; frequency and severity decrease with subsequent doses. Common clinical manifestations include high fever, chills/rigor, headache, tremor, nausea/vomiting, diarrhea, abdominal pain, malaise, myalgias, arthralgias, and generalized weakness. Less common complaints include skin reactions and cardiorespiratory and CNS disorders, including aseptic meningitis. Potentially fatal pulmonary edema, acute respiratory distress syndrome, cardiovascular collapse, cardiac arrest, and arrhythmias have occurred.

Glucocorticoid administration before the injection of muromonab-CD3 considerably reduces first-dose reactions and is now standard. Volume status of patients also must be monitored carefully before therapy; steroids and other premedications should be given, and a fully competent resuscitation facility must be immediately available for patients receiving their first several doses.

Other toxicities associated with anti-CD3 therapy include anaphylaxis and the usual infections and neoplasms associated with immunosuppressive therapy. "Rebound" rejection has been observed when muromonab-CD3 treatment is stopped. Anti-CD3 therapies may be limited by anti-idiotypic or anti-murine antibodies in the recipient.

Anti-IL-2 Receptor (Anti-CD25) Antibodies Daclizumab (ZENAPAX), a humanized murine complementarity-determining region (CDR)/human IgG_1 chimeric monoclonal antibody, and basiliximab (SIMULECT), a murine-human chimeric monoclonal antibody, are produced by recombinant DNA technology. Daclizumab consists of human (90%) constant domains of IgG_1 and variable framework regions of the Eu myeloma antibody and murine (10%) CDR of the anti-Tac antibody.

Mechanism of Action

The exact mechanism of action of the anti-CD25 mAbs is not completely understood but likely results from the binding of the anti-CD25 mAbs to the IL-2 receptor on the surface of activated, but not resting, T cells. Significant depletion of T cells does not appear to play a major role in the mechanism of action of these mAbs. Therapy with the anti-IL-2R mAbs is thought to result in a relative decrease of the expression of the α chain, either from depletion of coated lymphocytes or modulation of the α chain secondary to decreased expression or increased shedding.

Therapeutic Uses Daclizumab and basiliximab are used for prophylaxis of acute organ rejection in adult patients. In Phase III trials, daclizumab was administered in five doses (1 mg/kg given intravenously over 15 minutes in 50–100 mL of normal saline) starting immediately preoperatively, and subsequently at biweekly intervals. The $t_{1/2}$ of daclizumab was 20 days, resulting in saturation of the IL-2Rα on circulating lymphocytes for up to 120 days after transplantation. Daclizumab has been used with maintenance immunosuppression regimens (cyclosporine, azathioprine, and glucocorticoids; cyclosporine and glucocorticoids) and with maintenance triple-therapy regimen—either with cyclosporine or tacrolimus, glucocorticoids, and mycophenolate mofetil (MMF) substituting for azathioprine. Basiliximab, administered in a fixed dose of 20 mg preoperatively and on days 0 and 4 after transplantation, resulted in a concentration sufficient to saturate IL-2R on circulating lymphocytes for 25–35 days after transplantation. The $t_{1/2}$ of basiliximab was 7 days. Basiliximab has been used with a maintenance regimen consisting of cyclosporine and prednisone.

There is no marker or test to monitor the effectiveness of anti–IL-2R therapy, as saturation of α chain on circulating lymphocytes during anti–IL-2R mAb therapy does not predict rejection. The duration of IL-2R blockade by basiliximab was similar in patients with or without acute rejection episodes.

Toxicity No cytokine-release syndrome has been observed with these antibodies, but anaphylaxis can occur. Although lymphoproliferative disorders and opportunistic infections may occur, the incidence ascribed to anti-CD25 treatment is remarkably low. No significant drug interactions with anti–IL-2-receptor antibodies have been described.

Campath-1H *Campath-1H* (ALEMTUZUMAB) is a humanized mAb that is approved for use in chronic lymphocytic leukemia. The antibody targets CD52, a glycoprotein expressed on lymphocytes, monocytes, macrophages, and natural killer cells; thus, the drug causes extensive lympholysis by inducing apoptosis of targeted cells. It has achieved some use in renal transplantation because it produces prolonged T- and B-cell depletion and allows drug minimization. Although short-term results are promising, further clinical experience is needed.

Anti-TNF Reagents

Infliximab *Infliximab* (REMICADE) is a chimeric anti–TNF-α monoclonal antibody containing a human constant region and a murine variable region. It binds with high affinity to TNF-α and prevents the cytokine from binding to its receptors.

TNF-α is implicated in the pathogenesis of a number of autoimmune diseases, including rheumatoid arthritis and Crohn's disease. Infliximab plus methotrexate improves the signs and symptoms of rheumatoid arthritis more than methotrexate alone. Patients with active Crohn's disease who had not responded to other therapies, including those with fistulae, also improved when treated with infliximab. Infliximab is approved in the U.S. for treating the symptoms of rheumatoid arthritis and is used in combination with methotrexate in patients who do not respond to methotrexate alone. Infliximab also is approved for treatment of symptoms of moderate-to-severe Crohn's disease in patients who have failed to respond to conventional therapy and in treatment to reduce the number of draining fistulae in Crohn's disease patients (*see* Chapter 38).

About one of six patients receiving infliximab experience an infusion reaction, characterized by fever, urticaria, hypotension, and dyspnea, within 1–2 hours after antibody administration. Serious infections also have occurred in infliximab-treated patients, most frequently in the upper respiratory and urinary tracts. The development of antinuclear antibodies, and rarely a lupus-like syndrome, has been reported after treatment with infliximab.

Although not a monoclonal antibody, *etanercept* (ENBREL) also targets TNF-α. Etanercept contains the ligand-binding portion of a human TNF-α receptor fused to the Fc portion of human IgG$_1$, and binds to TNF-α and prevents it from interacting with its receptors. It is approved in the U.S. for treatment of rheumatoid arthritis in patients who have not responded to other treatments. Etanercept can be used in combination with methotrexate in patients who have not responded adequately to methotrexate alone. As with infliximab, serious infections have occurred. Injection-site reactions (erythema, itching, pain, or swelling) have occurred in more than one-thirds of etanercept-treated patients.

Adalimimab (HUMIRA) is recombinant human IgG$_1$ monoclonal anti-TNF for intravenous use in rheumatoid arthritis.

LFA-1 Inhibition *Efalizumab* (RAPTIVA) is a humanized IgG$_1$ mAb targeting the CD11a chain of LFA-1 (lymphocyte function associated antigen). Efalizumab binds to LFA-1 and prevents the LFA-1–ICAM (intercellular adhesion molecule) interaction to block T-cell adhesion, trafficking, and activation. Efalizumab is approved for use in patients with psoriasis. Efalizumab is given as weekly subcutaneous injections. The first dose is 0.7 mg/kg of body weight. Thereafter, each weekly dose is 1 mg/kg (up to a maximum single dose of 200 mg). Pharmacokinetic and pharmacodynamic studies showed that efalizumab produced saturation and 80% modulation of CD11a within 24 hours of therapy. In a subset of 10 patients who received higher dose efalizumab (2 mg/kg) with full-dose cyclosporine, mycophenolate mofetil, and glucocorticoids, 3 patients developed post-transplant lymphoproliferative diseases. While efalizumab appears to be an effective immunosuppressive agent, for transplant rejection, it may be best used in a lower dose and with an immunosuppressive regimen that avoids calcineurin inhibitors.

TOLERANCE

Immunosuppression has concomitant risks of opportunistic infections and secondary tumors. Therefore, the ultimate goal of research on organ transplantation and autoimmune diseases is to induce and maintain immunologic tolerance, the active state of antigen-specific nonresponsiveness. If attainable, tolerance would represent a true cure for conditions discussed above without the side effects of the various immunosuppressive therapies. The calcineurin inhibitors prevent tolerance induction in some, but not all, preclinical models. In these same model systems, sirolimus does not prevent tolerance and may even promote tolerance induction.

IMMUNOSTIMULATION

General Principles

In contrast to immunosuppressive agents that inhibit the immune response in transplant rejection and autoimmunity, a few immunostimulatory drugs have applicability to infection, immunodeficiency, and cancer.

LEVAMISOLE

Levamisole *(ERGAMISOL) was synthesized originally as an anthelmintic but appears to "restore" depressed immune function of B lymphocytes, T lymphocytes, monocytes, and macrophages. Its only clinical indication is as adjuvant therapy with 5-fluorouracil after surgical resection in patients with Dukes' stage C colon cancer. It occasionally has been associated with fatal agranulocytosis.*

THALIDOMIDE

Thalidomide *(THALOMID) is best known for the severe birth defects it caused when administered to pregnant women. For this reason, it is available only under a restricted distribution program and can be prescribed only by specially licensed physicians who understand that thalidomide should never be taken by women who are pregnant or who could become pregnant while taking the drug. Nevertheless, it is indicated for the treatment of patients with erythema nodosum leprosum (see Chapter 47) and also is used in conditions such as multiple myeloma. Its mechanism of action is unclear.*

BACILLUS CALMETTE-GUÉRIN (BCG)

Live bacillus Calmette-Guérin *(BCG; TICE BCG, THERACYS) is an attenuated culture of the bacillus of Calmette and Guérin strain of* Mycobacterium bovis, *which induces a granulomatous reaction at the site of administration. By unclear mechanisms, this preparation is active against tumors and is indicated for treatment and prophylaxis of carcinoma* in situ *of the urinary bladder and for prophylaxis of primary and recurrent stage Ta and/or T1 papillary tumors after transurethral resection. Adverse effects include hypersensitivity, shock, chills, fever, malaise, and immune complex disease.*

RECOMBINANT CYTOKINES

Interferons Although interferons (α, β, and γ) initially were identified by their antiviral activity, these agents also have important immunomodulatory activities. The interferons bind to specific cell-surface receptors that initiate a series of intracellular events: induction of certain enzymes, inhibition of cell proliferation, and enhancement of immune activities, including increased phagocytosis by macrophages and augmentation of specific cytotoxicity by T lymphocytes. Recombinant *interferon alfa-2b* (IFN-alpha 2, INTRON A) is obtained by recombinant expression in *E. coli*. It is a member of a family of naturally occurring small proteins with molecular weights of 15–27.6 KDa, produced and secreted by cells in response to viral infections and other inducers. Interferon alfa-2b is indicated in the treatment of a variety of tumors, including hairy cell leukemia, malignant melanoma, follicular lymphoma, and AIDS-related Kaposi's sarcoma. It also is indicated for chronic hepatitis B infection and condylomata acuminata. It is supplied in combination with *ribavirin* (REBETRON) for treatment of chronic hepatitis C in patients with compensated liver function not treated previously with interferon alfa-2b or who have relapsed after interferon alfa-2b therapy.

Flu-like symptoms, including fever, chills, and headache, are the most common adverse effects after interferon alfa-2b administration. Adverse effects involving the cardiovascular system (hypotension, arrhythmias, and rarely cardiomyopathy and myocardial infarction) and CNS (depression, confusion) are less frequent.

Interferon gamma-1b (ACTIMMUNE) is a recombinant polypeptide that activates phagocytes and induces their generation of oxygen metabolites that are toxic to a number of microorganisms. It is indicated to reduce the frequency and severity of serious infections associated with chronic granulomatous disease. Adverse reactions include fever, headache, rash, fatigue, GI distress, anorexia, weight loss, myalgia, and depression.

Interferon beta-1a (AVONEX, REBIF), a 166–amino acid recombinant glycoprotein, and *interferon beta-1b* (BETASERON), a 165–amino acid recombinant protein, have antiviral and immunomodulatory properties. They are FDA-approved for the treatment of relapsing and relapsing-remitting multiple sclerosis to reduce the frequency of clinical exacerbations (*see* below). The mechanism of their action in multiple sclerosis is unclear. Flu-like symptoms (fever, chills, myalgia) and injection-site reactions are common adverse effects. The use of these and other interferons in the treatment of viral diseases is discussed in Chapter 49.

Interleukin-2 Human recombinant IL-2 (*aldesleukin,* PROLEUKIN; des-alanyl-1, serine-125 human IL-2) differs from native IL-2 in that it is not glycosylated, has no amino terminal Ala, and has an Ser substituted for the Cys at amino acid 125. The potency of the preparation is represented in International Units in a lymphocyte proliferation assay such that 1.1 mg of recombinant IL-2 protein equals 18 million International Units. Aldesleukin has the following *in vitro* biologic activities of native IL-2: enhancement of lymphocyte proliferation and growth of IL-2–dependent cell lines; enhancement of lymphocyte-mediated cytotoxicity and killer cell activity; and induction of interferon-γ activity. *In vivo* administration of aldesleukin in animals produces multiple immunologic effects in a dose-dependent manner. Cellular immunity is profoundly activated with lymphocytosis, eosinophilia, thrombocytopenia, and release of multiple cytokines (*e.g.*, TNF-α, IL-1, interferon-γ). Aldesleukin is indicated for the treatment of adults with metastatic renal cell carcinoma and melanoma. Administration of aldesleukin has been associated with serious cardiovascular toxicity resulting from capillary leak syndrome, which involves loss of vascular tone and leak of plasma proteins and fluid into the extravascular space. Hypotension, reduced organ perfusion, and death may occur. An increased risk of disseminated infection due to impaired neutrophil function also has been associated with aldesleukin treatment.

Immunization

Active immunization involves stimulation with an antigen to develop immunologic defenses against a future exposure, while passive immunization involves administration of preformed antibodies to an individual who is already exposed or is about to be exposed to an antigen.

VACCINES Active immunization, or vaccination, involves administration of an antigen as a whole, killed organism, attenuated (live) organism, or a specific protein or peptide constituent of an organism. Booster doses often are required, especially when killed (inactivated) organisms are used as the immunogen. In the U.S., vaccination has sharply curtailed or practically eliminated a variety of major infections, including polio, smallpox, diphtheria, measles, mumps, pertussis, rubella, tetanus, *Haemophilus influenzae* type b, and pneumococcus.

Although most vaccines have targeted infectious diseases, a new generation of vaccines may provide complete or limited protection from specific cancers or autoimmune diseases. Because T cells optimally are activated by peptides and costimulatory ligands that both are present on antigen-presenting cells, one approach for vaccination has consisted of immunizing patients with APCs expressing a tumor antigen.

Multiple studies have demonstrated the efficacy of DNA vaccines in models of infectious diseases and cancer. The advantage of DNA vaccination over peptide immunization is that it permits generation of entire proteins, enabling determinant selection to occur in the host without having to restrict immunization to patients bearing specific HLA alleles. However, a safety concern about this technique is the potential for integration of the plasmid DNA into the host genome, possibly disrupting important genes and thereby leading to phenotypic mutations or carcinogenicity. A final approach to generate or enhance immune responses against specific antigens consists of infecting cells with recombinant viruses that encode the protein antigen of interest.

IMMUNE GLOBULIN   Passive immunization is indicated when an individual is deficient in antibodies because of a congenital or acquired immunodeficiency, when an individual with a high degree of risk is exposed to an agent and there is inadequate time for active immunization (*e.g.*, measles, rabies, hepatitis B), or when a disease is already present but can be ameliorated by passive antibodies (*e.g.*, botulism, diphtheria, tetanus). Passive immunization may be provided by several different products (Table 52–2). Nonspecific immunoglobulins or highly specific immunoglobulins may be provided based upon the indication. The protection provided usually lasts from 1 to 3 months. Immune globulin is derived from pooled plasma of adults by an alcohol-fractionation procedure. It contains largely IgG (95%) and is indicated for antibody-deficiency disorders, exposure to infections such as hepatitis A and measles, and specific immunologic diseases such as immune thrombocytopenic purpura and Guillain-Barré syndrome. In contrast, specific immune globulins (hyperimmune) differ from other immune globulin preparations in that donors are selected for high titers of the desired antibodies. Specific immune globulin preparations are available for hepatitis B, rabies, tetanus, varicella-zoster, cytomegalovirus, and respiratory syncytial virus. Rho(D) immune globulin is a specific hyperimmune globulin for prophylaxis against hemolytic disease of the newborn due to Rh incompatibility between mother and fetus. All such plasma-derived products carry the theoretical risk of transmission of infectious disease.

Table 52–2

Selected Immune Globulin Preparations

Immune globulin intravenous	BAYGAM
	GAMMAGARD S/D
	GAMMAR-P.I.V
	IVEEGAM
	SANDOGLOBULIN I.V.
	others
Cytomegalovirus immune globulin	CYTOGAM
Respiratory syncytial virus immune globulin	RESPIGAM
Hepatitis B immune globulin	BAYHEP B
	HYPERHEP
	H-BIG
Rabies immune globulin	BAYRAB
	IMOGAM RABIS-HT
	HYPER-AB
Rho(D) immune globulin	BAY-RHO-D
	WINRHO SDF
	MICRHOGAM
	RHOGAM
	others
Tetanus immune globulin	BAYTET
	HYPERTET

RHO(D) IMMUNE GLOBULIN   The commercial forms of Rho(D) immune globulin (Table 52–2) consist of IgG containing a high titer of antibodies against the Rho(D) antigen on the surface of red blood cells. All donors are carefully screened to reduce the risk of transmitting infectious diseases. Fractionation of the plasma is performed by precipitation with cold alcohol followed by passage through a viral clearance system.

Mechanism of Action

Rho(D) immune globulin binds Rho antigens, thereby preventing sensitization. Rh-negative women may be sensitized to the "foreign" Rh antigen on red blood cells via the fetus at the time of birth, miscarriage, ectopic pregnancy, or any transplacental hemorrhage. If the women go on to have a primary immune response, they will make antibodies to Rh antigen that can cross the placenta and damage subsequent fetuses by lysing red blood cells. This syndrome, called hemolytic disease of the newborn, is life-threatening. The form due to Rh incompatibility is largely preventable by Rho(D) immune globulin.

Therapeutic Use   Rho(D) immune globulin is indicated whenever fetal red blood cells are known or suspected to have entered the circulation of an Rh-negative mother unless the fetus is known also to be Rh-negative. The drug is given intramuscularly. The $t_{1/2}$ of circulating immunoglobulin is ~21–29 days.

Toxicity   Injection site discomfort and low-grade fever have been reported. Systemic reactions are extremely rare, but myalgia, lethargy, and anaphylactic shock have been reported. As with all plasma-derived products, there is a theoretical risk of transmission of infectious diseases.

INTRAVENOUS IMMUNOGLOBULIN   Indications for the use of intravenous immunoglobulin (IVIG) have expanded beyond replacement therapy for agammaglobulinemia and other immunodeficiencies to include a variety of bacterial and viral infections and an array of autoimmune and inflammatory diseases as diverse as thrombocytopenic purpura, Kawasaki's disease, and autoimmune skin, neuromuscular, and neurologic diseases. The mechanism of action of IVIG in immune modulation is unknown. Although IVIG is effective in many autoimmune diseases, its spectrum of efficacy and appropriate dosing (especially duration of therapy) are unknown. Additional controlled studies of IVIG are needed to identify proper dosing, cost-benefit, and quality-of-life parameters.

A CASE STUDY: IMMUNOTHERAPY FOR MULTIPLE SCLEROSIS

CLINICAL FEATURES AND PATHOLOGY   Multiple sclerosis (MS) is a demyelinating inflammatory disease of the CNS white matter that displays a triad of pathogenic features: mononuclear cell infiltration, demyelination, and scarring (gliosis). The peripheral nervous system is spared. The disease, which may be episodic or progressive, occurs in early to middle adulthood with prevalence increasing from late adolescence to 35 years and then declining. MS is roughly twice as common in females as in males and occurs mainly in higher latitudes of the temperate climates. Epidemiologic studies suggest a role for environmental factors in the pathogenesis of MS; despite many suggestions, associations with infectious agents have proven inconclusive, even though several viruses can cause similar demyelinating diseases in laboratory animals and humans. A stronger linkage is genetic: people of Northern European origin have a higher susceptibility to MS, and studies in twins and siblings suggest a genetic component. One genetic determinant of MS may be the class II (or HLA-DR) domain of the MHC on chromosome 6 that encodes the histocompatibility antigens. There is also substantial evidence of an autoimmune component to MS: in MS patients, there are activated T cells and antibodies that are reactive to different myelin antigens including myelin basic protein (MBP). These antibodies may act with pathogenic T cells to produce some of the cellular pathology of MS. The neurophysiological result is altered conduction (both positive and negative) in myelinated fibers within the CNS (cerebral white matter, brain stem, cerebellar tracts, optic nerves, spinal cord); some alterations appear to result from exposure of voltage-dependent K^+ channels that are normally covered by myelin.

Attacks are classified by type and severity. Thus, physicians refer to acute MS (an acute attack), relapsing-remitting MS (the form in 85% of younger patients), secondary progressive MS (progressive neurologic deterioration following a long period of relapsing-remitting disease), and primary progressive MS (~15% of patients, wherein deterioration with relatively little inflammation is apparent at onset).

PHARMACOTHERAPY FOR MS   Specific therapies are aimed at resolving acute attacks, reducing recurrences and exacerbations, and slowing the progression of disability (Table 52–3).

Table 52–3

Pharmacotherapy of Multiple Sclerosis

Therapeutic Agent	TRADE NAME (dose, regimen)	Indications	Results	Mechanism of Action
IFNβ-1a	AVONEX (30 µg, IM, weekly) REBIF (22 or 44 µg, SC, 3 times weekly)	Treatment of RRMS	Reduction of relapses by one-third Reduction of new MRI T2 lesions and the volume of enlarging T2 lesions Reduction in the number and volume of Gd-enhancing lesions Slowing of brain atrophy	Acts on blood–brain barrier by interfering with T-cell adhesion to the endothelium by binding VLA-4 on T cells or by inhibiting the T cell expression of MMP Reduction in T cell activation by interfering with HLA class II and costimulatory molecules B7/CD28 and CD40:CD40L Immune deviation of Th2 over Th1 cytokine profile
IFNβ-1b	BETASERON (0.3 µg, SC, every other day)	Treatment of RRMS	Same as IFNβ-1a	Same as IFNβ-1a
Glatiramer acetate	COPAXONE (20 µg, SC, daily)	Treatment of RRMS	Reduction of relapses by one-third Reduction in the number and volume of Gd-enhancing lesions	Induces T-helper type 2 cells that enter the CNS; mediates bystander suppression at sites of inflammation
Mitoxantrone	NOVANTRONE (12 mg/m², as short [5–15 min] IV infusion every 3 months)	Worsening forms of RRMS SPMS	Reduction in relapses by 67% Slowed progression on EDSS, ambulation index, and MRI disease activity	Intercalates DNA (*see* Chapter 51) Suppresses cellular and humoral immune response

IFN, interferon; IM, intramuscularly; RRMS, relapsing-remitting MS; SC, subcutaneously; SPMS, secondary progressive MS; IV, intravenously. Gd, gadolinium, used in Gd-enhanced MRI to assess number and size of inflammatory brain lesions; EDSS, Expanded Disability Status Scale, a neurologic assessment scale for MS pathology; MMP, matrix metalloprotease.

Nonspecific therapies focus on maintaining function and quality of life. For acute attacks, pulse glucocorticoids are often employed (typically, 1 g/day of methylprednisolone administered intravenously for 3–5 days). There is no evidence that tapered doses of oral prednisone are useful.

For relapsing-remitting attacks, immunomodulatory therapies are approved: beta-1 interferons (interferon beta-1a, interferon beta-1b, and *glatiramer acetate* [COPAXONE]). The interferons suppress the proliferation of T lymphocytes, inhibit their movement into the CNS from the periphery, and shift the cytokine profile from pro- to anti-inflammatory types.

Random polymers that contain amino acids commonly used as MHC anchors and T-cell receptor contact residues have been proposed as possible "universal altered peptide ligands." Glatiramer acetate (GA) is a random sequence polypeptide consisting of four amino acids (alanine [A], lysine [K], glutamate [E], and tyrosine [Y] at a molar ratio of A:K:E:Y of 4.5:3.6:1.5:1) with an average length of 40–100 amino acids. Directly labeled GA binds efficiently to different murine H2 I-A molecules, as well as to their human counterparts, the MHC class II DR molecules, but does not bind MHC class II DQ or MHC class I molecules *in vitro*. In clinical trials,

GA, administered subcutaneously to patients with relapsing-remitting MS, decreased the rate of exacerbations by ~30%. *In vivo* administration of GA induces highly cross-reactive CD4$^+$ T cells that are immune-deviated to secrete Th2 cytokines and prevents the appearance of new lesions detectable by MRI. This represents one of the first successful uses of an agent that ameliorates autoimmune disease by altering signals through the T-cell receptor complex.

For relapsing-remitting attacks and for secondary progressive MS, cyclophosphamide and the anthracenedionene-derivative *mitoxantrone* (NOVATRONE) are used in patients refractory to other immunomodulators. These agents, used primarily for cancer chemotherapy, have significant toxicities (*see* Chapter 51). While cyclophosphamide in patients with MS may not be limited by an accumulated dose exposure, mitoxantrone can be tolerated only up to an accumulated dose of 100–140 mg/m^2. The utility of interferon therapy in patients with secondary progressive MS is unclear. In primary progressive MS, with no discrete attacks and less observed inflammation, suppression of inflammation seems to be less helpful. A minority of patients at this stage will respond to high doses of glucocorticoids. Table 52–3 summarizes immunomodulatory therapies for MS.

Each agent has adverse effects and contraindications that may be limiting: infections (for glucocorticoids); hypersensitivity and pregnancy (for immunomodulators); and prior anthracycline/ anthracenedione use, mediastinal irradiation, or cardiac disease (mitoxantrone). With all of these agents, it is clear that the earlier they are used, the more effective they are in preventing disease relapses. What is not clear is whether any of these agents will prevent or diminish the later onset of secondary progressive disease, which causes the more severe form of disability.

For a complete Bibliographical listing see Goodman & Gilman's *The Pharmacological Basis of Therapeutics*, 11th ed., or Goodman & Gilman Online at www.accessmedicine.com.

DRUGS ACTING ON THE BLOOD AND THE BLOOD-FORMING ORGANS

53

HEMATOPOIETIC AGENTS
Growth Factors, Minerals, and Vitamins

The finite life span of most mature blood cells requires their continuous replacement, a process termed hematopoiesis. New cell production must respond to basal needs and states of increased demand. Red blood cell production can increase >20-fold in response to anemia or hypoxemia, white blood cell production increases dramatically in response to a systemic infection, and platelet production can increase 10–20-fold when platelet consumption results in thrombocytopenia.

The regulation of blood cell production is complex. Hematopoietic stem cells are rare marrow cells that manifest self-renewal and lineage commitment, resulting in cells destined to differentiate into the nine distinct blood-cell lineages. For the most part, this process occurs in the marrow cavities of the skull, vertebral bodies, pelvis, and proximal long bones; it involves interactions among hematopoietic stem and progenitor cells and the cells and complex macromolecules of the marrow stroma, and is influenced by a number of soluble and membrane-bound hematopoietic growth factors. A number of these hormones and cytokines have been identified and cloned, permitting their production in quantities sufficient for therapeutic use. Clinical applications range from the treatment of primary hematological diseases to use as adjuncts in the treatment of severe infections and in the management of patients who are undergoing cancer chemotherapy or marrow transplantation.

Hematopoiesis also requires an adequate supply of minerals (*e.g.*, iron, cobalt, and copper) and vitamins (*e.g.*, folic acid, vitamin B_{12}, pyridoxine, ascorbic acid, and riboflavin), and deficiencies generally result in characteristic anemias, or, less frequently, a general failure of hematopoiesis. Therapeutic correction of a specific deficiency state depends on the accurate diagnosis of the anemic state and knowledge about the correct dose, the use of these agents in various combinations, and the expected response.

I. HEMATOPOIETIC GROWTH FACTORS

GROWTH FACTOR PHYSIOLOGY   Steady-state hematopoiesis encompasses the production of more than 400 billion blood cells each day. This production is tightly regulated and can be increased severalfold with increased demand. The hematopoietic organ also is unique in adult physiology in that several mature cell types are derived from a much smaller number of multipotent progenitors, which develop from a more limited number of pluripotent hematopoietic stem cells. Such cells are capable of maintaining their own number and differentiating under the influence of cellular and humoral factors to produce the large and diverse number of mature blood cells (*see* Figure 53–1).

Stem cell differentiation involves a series of steps that produce so-called burst-forming units (BFU) and colony-forming units (CFU) for each of the major cell lines. Colonies of morphologically distinct cells form under the control of an overlapping set of additional growth factors (G-CSF, M-CSF, erythropoietin, and thrombopoietin). Proliferation and maturation of the CFU for each cell line can amplify the resulting mature cell product by another 30-fold or more, generating >1000 mature cells from each committed stem cell.

Hematopoietic and lymphopoietic growth factors are active at very low concentrations and typically affect more than one committed cell lineage. Most interact synergistically with other factors and also stimulate production of additional growth factors, a process called *networking*. Growth factors generally exert actions at several points in the processes of cell proliferation and differentiation and in mature cell function. However, the network of growth factors that contributes to any given cell lineage depends absolutely on a nonredundant, lineage-specific factor, such that absence of factors that stimulate developmentally early progenitors is compensated for by redundant cytokines, but loss of the lineage-specific factor leads to a specific cytopenia.

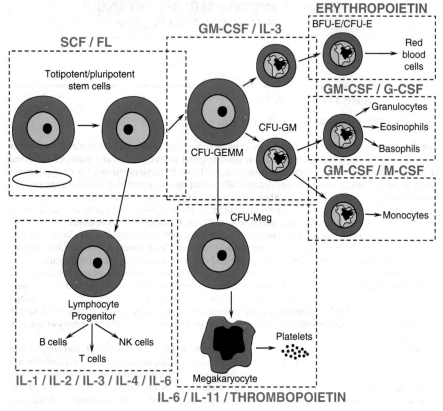

FIGURE 53–1 *Sites of action of hematopoietic growth factors in the differentiation and maturation of marrow cell lines.* A self-sustaining pool of marrow stem cells differentiates under the influence of specific hematopoietic growth factors to form a variety of hematopoietic and lymphopoietic cells. Stem cell factor (SCF), ligand (FL), interleukin-3 (IL-3), and granulocyte-macrophage colony-stimulating factor (GM-CSF), together with cell–cell interactions in the marrow, stimulate stem cells to form a series of burst-forming units (BFU) and colony-forming units (CFU): CFU-GEMM (granulocyte, erythrocyte, monocyte and megakaryocyte), CFU-GM (granulocyte and macrophage), CFU-Meg (megakaryocyte), BFU-E (erythrocyte), and CFU-E (erythrocyte). After considerable proliferation, further differentiation is stimulated by synergistic interactions with growth factors for each of the major cell lines—granulocyte colony–stimulating factor (G-CSF), monocyte/macrophage-stimulating factor (M-CSF), thrombopoietin, and erythropoietin. Each of these factors also influences the proliferation, maturation, and in some cases the function of the derivative cell line.

ERYTHROPOIETIN

While not the sole growth factor responsible for erythropoiesis, erythropoietin is the most important regulator of the proliferation of committed progenitors (CFU-E) and their immediate progeny. In its absence, severe anemia invariably results. Erythropoiesis is controlled by a highly responsive feedback system in which a sensor in the kidney detects changes in O_2 delivery to modulate the erythropoietin secretion. The sensor mechanism is now understood at the molecular level. Hypoxia-inducible factor (HIF-1) is a heterodimeric (*HIF-1α and HIF-1β*) transcription factor that enhances expression of multiple hypoxia-inducible genes, such as vascular endothelial growth factor and erythropoietin. *HIF-1α is labile due to its prolyl hydroxylation and subsequent polyubiquitination and degradation, aided by the von Hippel-Lindau (VHL) protein. During states of hypoxia, the prolyl hydroxylase is inactive, allowing the accumulation of HIF-1α* and activating erythropoietin expression, which in turn stimulates a rapid expansion of erythroid progenitors. Specific alteration of VHL leads to an O_2-sensing defect, characterized by constitutively elevated levels of HIF-1α and erythropoietin, with a resultant polycythemia. Erythropoietin is expressed primarily in peritubular interstitial cells of the kidney. Erythropoietin contains 193 amino acids, the first 27 of which are cleaved during secretion. The final hormone is heavily glycosylated and has a molecular mass of ~30,000 Da. After secretion, erythropoietin binds to a membrane receptor on committed erythroid progenitors in the marrow and is internalized. With anemia or hypoxemia, synthesis rapidly increases by 100-fold or more, serum erythropoietin levels rise, and marrow progenitor cell survival, proliferation, and maturation are dramatically stimulated. This feedback loop can be disrupted by kidney disease, marrow damage, or a deficiency in iron or an essential vitamin. With an infection or inflammation, erythropoietin secretion, iron delivery, and progenitor proliferation all are suppressed by inflammatory cytokines, but this accounts for only part of the resultant anemia; interference with iron metabolism also is an effect of inflammatory mediator effects on the hepatic protein hepcidin.

Recombinant human erythropoietin (*epoetin alfa*) is nearly identical to the endogenous hormone. The carbohydrate modification pattern of the recombinant form differs slightly from that of the native protein, but this difference apparently does not alter kinetics, potency, or immunoreactivity of the drug. However, modern assays can detect these differences, which is of significance for detecting athletes who use the recombinant product for "blood doping."

Available preparations of epoetin alfa include EPOGEN, PROCRIT, and EXPREX, supplied in single-use vials of from 2000 to 40000 U/mL for intravenous or subcutaneous administration. When injected intravenously, epoetin alfa is cleared from plasma with a $t_{1/2}$ of 4–8 hours. However, the effect on marrow progenitors is sufficiently sustained that it need only be given three times a week to achieve an adequate response. Combination of the weekly dose into a single injection also can achieve virtually identical results. No significant allergic reactions have been associated with the intravenous or subcutaneous administration of epoetin alfa, and—except as noted below—antibodies have not been detected even after prolonged administration.

More recently, novel erythropoiesis-stimulating protein (NESP) or darbepoetin alfa (ARANESP) also has been approved for clinical use in patients with indications similar to those for epoetin alfa. It is a genetically modified form of erythropoietin in which four amino acids have been mutated such that additional carbohydrate side chains are added during its synthesis, prolonging the circulatory survival of the drug to ~24 hours.

THERAPEUTIC USES, MONITORING, AND ADVERSE EFFECTS

Recombinant erythropoietin therapy, in conjunction with adequate iron intake, can be highly effective in a number of anemias, especially those associated with a poor erythropoietic response. There is a clear dose-response relationship between the epoetin alfa dose and the rise in hematocrit in anephric patients. Epoetin alfa is effective in the treatment of anemias associated with surgery, AIDS, cancer chemotherapy, prematurity, and certain chronic inflammatory conditions. Darbepoetin alfa also is approved for use in patients with anemia associated with chronic kidney disease and is under review for several other indications.

During erythropoietin therapy, absolute or functional iron deficiency may develop. Functional iron deficiency (i.e., normal ferritin levels but low transferrin saturation) presumably results from the inability to mobilize iron stores rapidly enough to support the increased erythropoiesis. Virtually all patients eventually will require supplemental iron to increase or maintain transferrin saturation to levels that will adequately support stimulated erythropoiesis. Supplemental iron therapy is recommended for all patients whose serum ferritin is <100 μg/L or whose serum transferrin saturation is <20% (see below).

During initial therapy and after any dosage adjustment, the hematocrit is determined once a week (HIV-infected and cancer patients) or twice a week (renal failure patients) until it has stabilized in the target range (establishing the maintenance dose); the hematocrit then is monitored at regular intervals. If the hematocrit increases by more than 4 points in any 2-week period, the dose should be decreased. Due to the time required for erythropoiesis and the erythrocyte $t_{1/2}$, hematocrit changes lag behind dosage adjustments by 2–6 weeks. The dose of darbepoetin should be decreased if the hemoglobin (Hb) increase exceeds 1 g/dL in any 2-week period because of the association of excessive rate of rise of Hb with adverse cardiovascular events.

During hemodialysis, patients receiving epoetin alfa or darbepoetin may require increased anticoagulation. Serious thromboembolic events have been reported, including migratory thrombophlebitis, microvascular thrombosis, pulmonary embolism, and thrombosis of the retinal artery and temporal and renal veins. Because the higher risk of cardiovascular events from erythropoietic therapies may be associated with higher Hb, the dose should be adjusted to avoid exceeding an Hb level of 12 g/dL. Although epoetin alfa is not associated with direct pressor effects, blood pressure may rise during the early phases of therapy. Erythropoietins should be withheld in patients with preexisting uncontrolled hypertension. Patients may require initiation of, or increases in, antihypertensive therapy. Hypertensive encephalopathy and seizures have occurred *in chronic renal failure patients treated with epoetin alfa. The incidence of seizures appears to be higher during the first 90 days of therapy with epoetin alfa in patients on dialysis (occurring in ~2.5% of patients) when compared with subsequent 90-day periods. Headache, tachycardia, edema, shortness of breath, nausea, vomiting, diarrhea, injection site stinging, arthralgias, and myalgias also have been reported in conjunction with epoetin alfa therapy. Pure red cell aplasia in association with neutralizing antibodies to native erythropoietin has been observed in patients treated with recombinant erythropoietins. Other causes of failure to respond to erythropoietin include underlying infectious, inflammatory, or malignant processes; occult blood loss; underlying hematologic diseases (e.g., thalassemia, refractory anemia, or other myelodysplastic disorders); folic acid or vitamin B_{12} deficiency; hemolysis; aluminum intoxication; bone marrow fibrosis; and osteitis fibrosa cystica.*

Anemia of Chronic Renal Failure

Patients with anemia secondary to chronic kidney disease are ideal candidates for epoetin alfa therapy. The response in predialysis, peritoneal dialysis, and hemodialysis patients depends on the severity of renal failure, the erythropoietin dose and route of administration, and iron availability. Subcutaneous administration is preferred because absorption is slower and the amount of drug required is reduced by 20–40%.

The dose of epoetin alfa should be adjusted to obtain a gradual rise in the hematocrit over a 2–4-month period to a final Hb of 11–12 g/dL. Treatment to a Hb level >13 g/dL showed a higher incidence of myocardial infarction and death. The drug should not be used to replace emergency transfusion in patients who need immediate correction of a life-threatening anemia.

Patients are started on doses of 80–120 U/kg of epoetin alfa, given subcutaneously, 3 times/week. It can be given on a once-a-week schedule, but somewhat more drug is required for an equivalent effect. If the response is poor, the dose should be progressively increased. The final maintenance dose of epoetin alfa can vary from as little as 10 units/kg to more than 300 units/kg, with an average dose of 75 units/kg, 3 times/week. Children younger than 5 years generally require a higher dose. Resistance to therapy is common in patients who develop an inflammatory illness or become iron deficient, so close monitoring of general health and iron status is essential. Less common causes of resistance include occult blood loss, folic acid deficiency, carnitine deficiency, inadequate dialysis, aluminum toxicity, and osteitis fibrosa cystica secondary to hyperparathyroidism.

The most common side effect of epoetin alfa therapy is aggravation of hypertension, which occurs in 20–30% of patients and most often is associated with a rapid rise in hematocrit. Blood pressure usually can be controlled either by increasing antihypertensive therapy or ultrafiltration in dialysis patients or by reducing the epoetin alfa dose to slow the hematocrit response.

Darbepoetin alfa also is approved for use in patients who are anemic secondary to chronic kidney disease. The recommended starting dose is 0.45 µg/kg administered intravenously or subcutaneously once weekly, with dose adjustments depending on the response. Like epoetin alfa, side effects tend to occur when patients experience a rapid rise in Hb concentration; a rise of less than 1 g/dL every 2 weeks generally is considered safe.

Anemia in AIDS Patients

Epoetin alfa therapy is approved for the treatment of HIV-infected patients, especially those on zidovudine therapy. Excellent responses to doses of 100–300 U/kg, given subcutaneously three times a week, generally are seen in patients with zidovudine-induced anemia.

Cancer-Related Anemias

Epoetin alfa therapy, 150 U/kg 3 times/week or 450–600 U/kg once a week, can reduce the transfusion requirement in cancer patients undergoing chemotherapy when Hb levels fall below 10 g/dL. For anemia associated with hematologic malignancies, recombinant erythropoietin is useful in patients with low-grade myelodysplastic syndrome. A baseline serum erythropoietin level may help to predict the response; most patients with blood levels of more than 500 U/L are unlikely to respond to any dose of the drug. Most patients treated with epoetin alfa experienced an improvement in their anemia, sense of well being, and quality of life. This improved sense of well being, particularly in cancer patients, may not be solely due to the rise in the hematocrit.

Case reports have suggested a direct effect of both epoetin alfa and darbepoetin alfa in stimulation of tumor cells, a possibility that is being evaluated by the U.S. Food and Drug Administration (FDA) and warrants serious attention.

Surgery

Epoetin alfa has been used perioperatively to treat anemia and reduce the need for transfusion. Patients undergoing elective orthopedic and cardiac procedures have been treated with 150–300

U/kg of epoetin alfa once daily for the 10 days preceding surgery, on the day of surgery, and for 4 days after surgery. This can correct a moderately severe preoperative anemia (i.e., hematocrit 30–36%) and reduce the need for transfusion.

MYELOID GROWTH FACTORS

The myeloid growth factors are produced naturally by a number of different cells, including fibroblasts, endothelial cells, macrophages, and T cells (Figure 53–1). They are active at extremely low concentrations and act *via* membrane receptors of the cytokine receptor superfamily to activate the JAK/STAT signal transduction pathway.

GRANULOCYTE-MACROPHAGE COLONY-STIMULATING FACTOR (GM-CSF)

Recombinant human GM-CSF (*sargramostim*) is a 127–amino acid glycoprotein produced in yeast. Except for the substitution of a Leu in position 23 and variable levels of glycosylation, sargramostim is identical to endogenous human GM-CSF. Sargramostim's primary therapeutic effect is to stimulate myelopoiesis. The initial clinical application of sargramostim was in patients undergoing autologous bone marrow transplantation. By shortening the duration of neutropenia, transplant morbidity was significantly reduced without a change in long-term survival or risk of inducing an early relapse of the malignant process.

The role of GM-CSF therapy in allogeneic transplantation is less clear. Its effect on neutrophil recovery is less pronounced in patients receiving prophylactic treatment for graft-versus-host disease (GVHD), and studies have failed to show a significant effect on transplant mortality, long-term survival, the appearance of GVHD, or disease relapse. However, it may improve survival in transplant patients who exhibit early graft failure. It also has been used to mobilize CD34[+] progenitor cells for peripheral blood stem cell (PBSC) collection for transplantation after myeloablative chemotherapy. Sargramostim has been used to shorten the period of neutropenia and reduce morbidity in patients receiving intensive cancer chemotherapy. It also stimulates myelopoiesis in some patients with cyclic neutropenia, myelodysplasia, aplastic anemia, or AIDS-associated neutropenia.

Sargramostim (LEUKINE) is administered by subcutaneous injection or slow intravenous infusion at doses of 125–500 µg/m²/day. Plasma levels of GM-CSF rise rapidly after subcutaneous injection and then decline with a $t_{1/2}$ of 2–3 hours. With the initiation of therapy, there is a transient decrease in the absolute leukocyte count secondary to margination and sequestration in the lungs. This is followed by a dose-dependent, biphasic increase in leukocyte counts over the next 7–10 days. Once the drug is discontinued, the leukocyte count returns to baseline within 2–10 days. When GM-CSF is given in lower doses, the response is primarily neutrophilic, while monocytosis and eosinophilia are observed at larger doses. After hematopoietic stem cell transplantation or intensive chemotherapy, sargramostim is given daily during the period of maximum neutropenia until a sustained rise in the granulocyte count is observed. Frequent blood counts are essential to avoid an excessive rise in the granulocyte count. Higher doses are associated with more pronounced side effects, including bone pain, malaise, flu-like symptoms, fever, diarrhea, dyspnea, and rash. Sensitive patients exhibit an acute reaction to the first dose, characterized by flushing, hypotension, nausea, vomiting, and dyspnea, with a fall in arterial O_2 saturation due to granulocyte sequestration in the pulmonary circulation. With prolonged administration, a few patients may develop a capillary leak syndrome, with peripheral edema and pleural and pericardial effusions. Other serious side effects include transient supraventricular arrhythmias, dyspnea, and elevation of serum creatinine, bilirubin, and hepatic enzymes.

GRANULOCYTE COLONY-STIMULATING FACTOR (G-CSF)
Recombinant human G-CSF *filgrastim* (NEUPOGEN) is a 175–amino acid glycoprotein produced in *Escherichia coli*. Unlike natural G-CSF, it is not glycosylated and carries an extra N-terminal Met. The principal action of filgrastim is the stimulation of CFU-G to increase neutrophil production (Figure 53–2). It also enhances the phagocytic and cytotoxic functions of neutrophils.

Filgrastim is effective in the treatment of severe neutropenia after autologous hematopoietic stem cell transplantation and high-dose cancer chemotherapy. Like GM-CSF, filgrastim shortens the period of severe neutropenia and reduces morbidity secondary to bacterial and fungal infections. When used as a part of an intensive chemotherapy regimen, it can decrease the frequency of hospitalization for febrile neutropenia and interruptions in the chemotherapy protocol; a positive impact on survival has not been demonstrated. G-CSF also is effective in the treatment of severe congenital neutropenias. In patients with cyclic neutropenia, G-CSF therapy will increase the level of neutrophils and shorten the length of the cycle sufficiently to prevent recurrent bacterial infections. Filgrastim therapy can improve neutrophil counts in some patients with myelodysplasia or

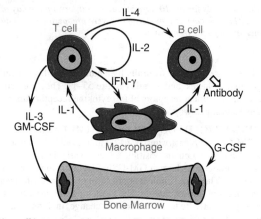

FIGURE 53–2 *Cytokine–cell interactions.* Macrophages, T cells, B cells, and marrow stem cells interact *via* several cytokines (IL-1, IL-2, IL-3, IL-4, IFN [interferon]-γ, GM-CSF, and G-CSF) in response to a bacterial or a foreign antigen challenge.

marrow damage (*e.g.*, moderately severe aplastic anemia or tumor infiltration of the marrow). The neutropenia of AIDS patients receiving zidovudine also can be partially or completely reversed. Filgrastim is routinely used in patients undergoing PBSC collection for stem cell transplantation. It promotes the release of CD34$^+$ progenitor cells from the marrow, reducing the number of collections necessary for transplant. Moreover, filgrastim-mobilized PBSCs appear more capable of rapid engraftment. PBSC-transplanted patients require fewer days of platelet and red blood cell transfusions and a shorter duration of hospitalization than do patients receiving autologous bone marrow transplants.

Filgrastim is administered by subcutaneous injection or intravenous infusion over at least 30 minutes at doses of 1–20 μg/kg/day. The usual starting dose in a patient receiving myelosuppressive chemotherapy is 5 μg/kg/day. The distribution and clearance rate from plasma ($t_{1/2}$ ~3.5 hours) are similar for both routes of administration. As with GM-CSF therapy, filgrastim given daily after hematopoietic stem cell transplantation or intensive cancer chemotherapy increases granulocyte production and shortens the period of severe neutropenia. Frequent blood counts should be obtained to determine the effectiveness of the treatment and guide dosage adjustment. In patients who received intensive myelosuppressive cancer chemotherapy, daily administration of G-CSF for 14–21 days or longer may be necessary to correct the neutropenia. With less intensive chemotherapy, fewer than 7 days of treatment may suffice. In AIDS patients on zidovudine or patients with cyclic neutropenia, chronic G-CSF therapy often is required.

Adverse reactions to filgrastim include mild-to-moderate bone pain in patients receiving high doses over a protracted period, local skin reactions following subcutaneous injection, and rare cutaneous necrotizing vasculitis. Patients with a history of hypersensitivity to proteins produced by E. coli *should not receive the drug. Marked granulocytosis, with counts >100,000/μL, can occur in patients receiving filgrastim over a prolonged period of time. Mild-to-moderate splenomegaly has been observed in patients on long-term therapy.*

Pegylated recombinant human G-CSF *pegfilgrastim* (NEULASTA) is generated by conjugation of a polyethylene glycol moiety (20 kDa) to the *N*-terminal Met residue of the G-CSF glycoprotein produced in *E. coli*. The clearance of pegfilgrastim by glomerular filtration is minimized, thus making neutrophil-mediated clearance the primary route of elimination. Consequently the circulating $t_{1/2}$ of pegfilgrastim is longer than that of filgrastim, allowing for more sustained duration of action and less frequent dosing. The recommended dose for pegfilgrastim is 6 mg administered subcutaneously.

THROMBOPOIETIC GROWTH FACTORS

INTERLEUKIN-11 Interleukin-11 is a 23 kDa cytokine that stimulates hematopoiesis, intestinal epithelial cell growth, and osteoclastogenesis and inhibits adipogenesis. IL-11 enhances megakaryocyte maturation.

Recombinant human interleukin-11 *oprelvekin* (NEUMEGA) is a bacterially derived, 19 kDa polypeptide that lacks the amino terminal Pro residue and is not glycosylated. The recombinant protein has a 7-hour $t_{1/2}$ after subcutaneous injection. In normal subjects, daily administration of oprelvekin leads to a thrombopoietic response in 5–9 days.

The drug is administered at 25–50 μg/kg/day subcutaneously. Oprelvekin is approved for use in patients undergoing chemotherapy for nonmyeloid malignancies who display severe thrombocytopenia (platelet count <20,000/μL) on a prior cycle of the same chemotherapy and is administered until the platelet count is >100,000/μL. The major complications of therapy are fluid retention and associated cardiac symptoms, such as tachycardia, palpitation, edema, and shortness of breath; this is a significant concern in elderly patients and often requires concomitant therapy with diuretics. Fluid retention reverses upon drug discontinuation, but volume status should be carefully monitored in elderly patients, those with a history of heart failure, or those with preexisting pleural or pericardial effusions or ascites. Also reported are blurred vision, injection-site rash or erythema, and paresthesias.

THROMBOPOIETIN Thrombopoietin is a glycoprotein (45–75 kDa, 332 amino acids) produced by the liver, marrow stromal cells, and many other organs and is the primary regulator of platelet production. Two forms of recombinant thrombopoietin have been developed. One is a truncated version of the native polypeptide, termed recombinant *human megakaryocyte growth and development factor* (rHuMGDF), covalently modified with polyethylene glycol to increase the circulatory $t_{1/2}$. The second is the full-length polypeptide termed *recombinant human thrombopoietin* (rHuTPO).

Results with these agents have been mixed. In cancer patients, recombinant human thrombopoietin therapy has reduced the duration of severe thrombocytopenia and the need for platelet transfusions. On the other hand, in patients treated for 7 days with standard therapy for acute leukemia, the addition of recombinant thrombopoietin failed to accelerate platelet recovery.

II. DRUGS EFFECTIVE IN IRON DEFICIENCY AND OTHER HYPOCHROMIC ANEMIAS

IRON AND IRON SALTS

Iron deficiency is the most common nutritional cause of anemia in humans. It can result from inadequate iron intake, malabsorption, blood loss, or an increased requirement, as with pregnancy. When severe, it results in a characteristic microcytic, hypochromic anemia. Iron is an essential component of myoglobin; heme enzymes such as the cytochromes, catalase, and peroxidase; and the metalloflavoprotein enzymes, including xanthine oxidase and the mitochondrial enzyme α-glycerophosphate oxidase. Iron deficiency can affect metabolism in muscle independent of the effect of anemia on O_2 delivery, possibly due to a reduction in the activity of iron-dependent mitochondrial enzymes. Iron deficiency also has been associated with behavioral and learning problems in children, abnormalities in catecholamine metabolism, and impaired heat production.

METABOLISM OF IRON The body store of iron (Table 53–1) is divided between essential iron-containing compounds and excess iron, which is held in storage. Hb (molecular weight, 64,500), contains 4 atoms of iron/molecule, amounting to 1.1 mg of iron/milliliter of red blood cells. Other forms of essential iron include myoglobin and a variety of heme and nonheme iron-dependent enzymes. Ferritin is a protein-iron storage complex that exists as individual molecules or as aggregates. Apoferritin has a molecular weight of ~450 and is composed of 24 polypeptide subunits that

Table 53–1

The Body Content of Iron

	mg/kg of body weight	
	Male	Female
Essential iron		
Hemoglobin	31	28
Myoglobin and enzymes	6	5
Storage iron	13	4
Total	50	37

form an outer shell that surrounds a storage cavity for polynuclear hydrous ferric oxide phosphate. More than 30% of the weight of ferritin may be iron (4000 atoms of iron per ferritin molecule). Ferritin aggregates, referred to as *hemosiderin* and visible by light microscopy, constitute about one-third of normal stores.

The two predominant sites of iron storage are the reticuloendothelial system and the hepatocytes.

Internal exchange of iron is accomplished by the plasma protein transferrin. This 76 kDa β_1-glycoprotein has 2 binding sites for ferric iron. Iron is delivered from transferrin to intracellular sites by means of specific transferrin receptors in the plasma membrane. The iron–transferrin complex binds to the receptor, and the ternary complex is taken up by receptor-mediated endocytosis. Iron subsequently dissociates in the acidic, intracellular vesicular compartment (the endosomes), and the receptor returns the apotransferrin to the cell surface, where it is released into the extracellular environment. Cells regulate their expression of transferrin receptors and intracellular ferritin in response to the iron supply. Apoferritin synthesis is regulated post-transcriptionally by 2 cytoplasmic binding proteins (IRP-1 and IRP-2) and an iron-regulating element on its mRNA (IRE).

The flow of iron through the plasma is 30–40 mg/day in the adult (about 0.46 mg/kg of body weight). The major internal circulation of iron involves the erythron and reticuloendothelial cells (Figure 53–3). About 80% of the iron in plasma goes to the erythroid marrow to be packaged into new erythrocytes; these normally circulate for ~120 days before being catabolized by the reticuloendothelial system. At that time, a portion of the iron is immediately returned to the plasma bound to transferrin, while another portion is incorporated into the ferritin stores of reticuloendothelial cells and returned to the circulation more gradually. With abnormalities in erythrocyte maturation, the predominant portion of iron assimilated by the erythroid marrow may be rapidly localized in the reticuloendothelial cells as defective red cell precursors are broken down; this is termed *ineffective erythropoiesis*. The rate of iron turnover in plasma may be reduced by one-half or more with red cell aplasia, with all the iron directed to the hepatocytes for storage.

A remarkable feature of iron metabolism is the degree to which body stores are conserved. Only 10% of the total is lost per year by normal men, *i.e.*, ~1 mg/day. Two-thirds of this iron is excreted from the GI tract as extravasated red cells, iron in bile, and iron in exfoliated mucosal

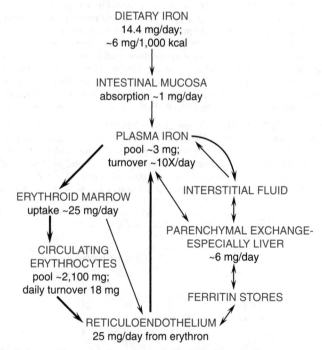

FIGURE 53–3 *Pathways of iron metabolism in human beings (excretion omitted).*

Table 53–2

Iron Requirements for Pregnancy

	Average, mg	Range, mg
External iron loss	170	150–200
Expansion of red cell mass	450	200–600
Fetal iron	270	200–370
Iron in placenta and cord	90	30–170
Blood loss at delivery	150	90–310
Total requirement*	980	580–1340
Cost of pregnancy†	680	440–1050

*Blood loss at delivery not included.
†Iron lost by the mother; expansion of red cell mass not included.

cells. The other third includes small amounts of iron in desquamated skin and in the urine. Additional losses of iron occur in women due to menstruation; pregnancy and lactation impose even greater requirements (Table 53–2). Other causes of iron loss include blood donation, the use of anti-inflammatory drugs that cause bleeding from the gastric mucosa, and GI disease with associated bleeding.

IRON REQUIREMENTS AND THE AVAILABILITY OF DIETARY IRON Iron requirements are determined by obligatory physiological losses and the needs imposed by growth. Thus, adult men require only 13 μg/kg/day (~1 mg of iron), whereas menstruating women require ~21 μg/kg/day (~1.4 mg). In the last two trimesters of pregnancy, requirements increase to ~80 μg/kg/day (5–6 mg), and infants have similar requirements due to their rapid growth. These requirements (Table 53–3) must be considered in the context of the amount of dietary iron available for absorption.

In developed countries, the normal adult diet contains about 6 mg of iron per 1000 calories, providing an average daily intake for adult men of between 12 and 20 mg and for adult women of between 8 and 15 mg. Foods high in iron (>5 mg/100 g) include organ meats such as liver and heart, brewer's yeast, wheat germ, egg yolks, oysters, and certain dried beans and fruits; foods low in iron (<1 mg/100 g) include milk and milk products and most nongreen vegetables. Iron also may be added when food is cooked in iron pots.

Although the iron content of the diet is important, of greater nutritional significance is the bioavailability of iron in food. Heme iron, which constitutes only 6% of dietary iron, is far more available and is absorbed independent of the diet composition; it represents 30% of iron absorbed.

The nonheme fraction represents by far the largest amount of dietary iron ingested by the economically underprivileged. In a vegetarian diet, nonheme iron is absorbed very poorly because of the inhibitory action of a variety of dietary components, particularly phosphates. Ascorbic acid and meat facilitate the absorption of nonheme iron. Ascorbate forms complexes with and/or reduces ferric to ferrous iron. Meat facilitates the absorption of iron by stimulating production of gastric

Table 53–3

Daily Iron Intake and Absorption

Subject	Iron Requirement, mg/kg	Available Iron in Poor Diet–Good Diet, mg/kg	Safety Factor, available iron/requirement
Infant	67	33–66	0.5–1
Child	22	48–96	2–4
Adolescent (male)	21	30–60	1.5–3
Adolescent (female)	20	30–60	1.5–3
Adult (male)	13	26–52	2–4
Adult (female)	21	18–36	1–2
Mid-to-late pregnancy	80	18–36	0.22–0.45

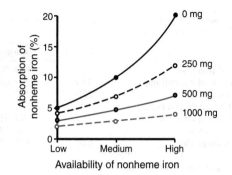

FIGURE 53–4 *Effect of iron status on the absorption of nonheme iron in food.* The percentages of iron absorbed from diets of low, medium, and high bioavailability in individuals with iron stores of 0, 250, 500, and 1000 mg are portrayed.

acid; other effects also may be involved. Thus, assessment of available dietary iron should include both the amount of iron ingested and an estimate of its availability (Figure 53–4).

IRON DEFICIENCY   Iron deficiency is the most common nutritional disorder, and leads to progressive changes in erythropoiesis that are outlined in Figure 53–5. The prevalence of iron-deficiency anemia in the U.S. is 1–4%, depending on the economic status of the population. In developing countries, up to 20–40% of infants and pregnant women may be affected. Better iron balance has resulted from the practice of fortifying flour, the use of iron-fortified formulas for infants, and the prescription of medicinal iron supplements during pregnancy.

Iron-deficiency anemia results from dietary intake of iron that is inadequate to meet normal requirements (nutritional iron deficiency), blood loss, or interference with iron absorption. Most nutritional iron deficiency in the U.S. is mild. More severe iron deficiency is usually the result of blood loss, either from the GI tract, or in women, from the uterus. Impaired absorption of iron from food results most often from partial gastrectomy or malabsorption in the small intestine. Finally, erythropoietin therapy can result in a functional iron deficiency.

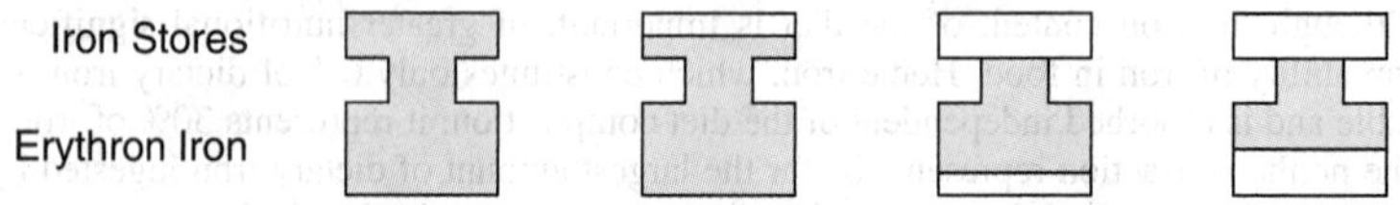

	Normal	Iron Depletion	Iron-Deficient Erythropoiesis	Iron-Deficiency Anemia
Iron Stores				
Erythron Iron				
RE marrow Fe	2–3+	0–1+	0	0
Transferrin	330 ± 30	360	390	410
µg/100 mL (µM)	(59 ± 5)	(64)	(70)	(73)
Plasma ferritin, µg/L	100 ± 60	20	10	<10
Iron absorption, %	5–10	10–15	10–20	10–20
Plasma iron	115 ± 50	115	<60	<40
µg/100 mL (µM)	(21 ± 9)	(21)	(<11)	(<7)
Transferrin saturation, %	35 ± 15	30	<15	<10
Sideroblasts, %	40–60	40–60	<10	<10
RBC protoporphyrin				
µg/100 mL RBC	30	30	100	200
(µmol/L RBC)	(0.53)	(0.53)	(1.8)	(3.5)
Erythrocytes	Normal	Normal	Normal	Microcytic/ hypochromic

FIGURE 53–5 *Sequential changes (from left to right) in the development of iron deficiency in the adult.* Rectangles enclose abnormal test results that identify the stage of Fe-deficiency. RE marrow Fe, reticuloendothelial hemosiderin; RBC, red blood cells.

Iron deficiency in infants and young children can lead to behavioral disturbances and can impair development, effects that may not be fully reversible. Iron deficiency in children also can lead to an increased risk of lead toxicity secondary to pica and an increased absorption of heavy metals. Premature and low-birth-weight infants are at greatest risk for developing iron deficiency, especially if they are not breast-fed and/or do not receive iron-fortified formula. After age 2–3, the requirement for iron declines until adolescence, when rapid growth combined with irregular dietary habits again increase the risk of iron deficiency. Adolescent girls are at greatest risk; the dietary iron intake of most girls ages 11–18 is insufficient to meet their requirements.

Treatment of Iron Deficiency

GENERAL THERAPEUTIC PRINCIPLES The response of iron-deficiency anemia to iron therapy is influenced by several factors, including the severity of anemia, the ability of the patient to tolerate and absorb medicinal iron, and the presence of other complicating illnesses. Therapeutic effectiveness is best measured by the resulting increase in the rate of production of red cells. The magnitude of the marrow response to iron therapy is proportional to the severity of the anemia (level of erythropoietin stimulation) and the amount of iron delivered to marrow precursors.

The patient's ability to tolerate and absorb medicinal iron is a key factor in determining the rate of response to therapy. The small intestine regulates absorption, and with increasing doses of oral iron, limits iron uptake. This provides a natural ceiling on how much iron can be supplied by oral therapy. In the patient with a moderately severe iron-deficiency anemia, tolerable doses of oral iron will deliver, at most, 40–60 mg of iron/day to the erythroid marrow. This is an amount sufficient for production rates of two to three times normal.

Complicating illness also can interfere with the response of an iron-deficiency anemia to iron therapy. By decreasing the number of red cell precursors, intrinsic disease of the marrow can blunt the response. Inflammatory illnesses suppress the rate of red cell production, both by reducing iron absorption and reticuloendothelial release and by direct inhibition of erythropoietin and erythroid precursors. Continued blood loss can mask the response as measured by recovery of the Hb or hematocrit.

Clinically, the effectiveness of iron therapy is best evaluated by tracking the reticulocyte response and the rise in the Hb or the hematocrit. An increase in the reticulocyte count is not observed for at least 4–7 days after beginning therapy. An increase in the Hb level takes even longer. A decision as to the effectiveness of treatment should not be made until 3–4 weeks after the start of treatment, when an increase in the Hb concentration (2 g/dL is considered a positive response, assuming that no other change in the patient's clinical status can account for the improvement and that the patient has not been transfused.

If the response to oral iron is inadequate, the diagnosis must be reconsidered. A full laboratory evaluation should be conducted, and poor compliance by the patient or the presence of a concurrent inflammatory disease must be explored. A source of continued bleeding obviously should be sought. If no other explanation can be found, an evaluation of the patient's ability to absorb oral iron should be considered. There is no justification for merely continuing oral iron therapy beyond 3–4 weeks if a favorable response has not occurred.

THERAPY WITH ORAL IRON Orally administered *ferrous sulfate* is the treatment of choice for iron deficiency. Ferrous salts are absorbed about three times as well as ferric salts, and the discrepancy increases at high dosages. Variations in the particular ferrous salt have relatively little effect on bioavailability.

Ferrous sulfate (FEOSOL, others) is the hydrated salt, $FeSO_4 \cdot 7H_2O$, which contains 20% iron. Ferrous fumarate (FEOSTAT, others) contains 33% iron and is moderately soluble in water, stable, and almost tasteless. Ferrous gluconate (FERGON, others), which contains 12% iron, also is used in the therapy of iron-deficiency anemia. Polysaccharide–iron complex (NIFEREX, others), a compound of ferrihydrite and carbohydrate, has comparable absorption. The effective dose of these preparations is based on iron content.

The average dose for the treatment of iron-deficiency anemia is about 200 mg of iron/day (2–3 mg/kg/day), given in three equal doses of 65 mg. Children weighing 15–30 kg can take half the average adult dose, while small children and infants can tolerate relatively large doses of iron (e.g., 5 mg/kg). The dose used is a compromise between the desired therapeutic action and the adverse effects. Prophylaxis and mild nutritional iron deficiency may be managed with modest doses. When the object is the prevention of iron deficiency in pregnant women, for example, doses of 15–30 mg of iron/day are adequate to meet the 3–6 mg daily requirement of the last 2 trimesters.

Table 53–4

Average Response to Oral Iron

Total Dose (mg Fe/day)	Estimated Absorption		Increase in Hemoglobin (g/L of blood/day)
	%	mg	
35	40	14	0.7
105	24	25	1.4
195	18	35	1.9
390	12	45	2.2

When the purpose is to treat iron-deficiency anemia, but the circumstances do not demand haste, a total dose of about 100 mg (35 mg three times daily) may suffice.

The responses expected for different dosage regimens of oral iron are given in Table 53–4. These effects are modified by the severity of the iron-deficiency anemia and by the time of ingestion of iron relative to meals. Bioavailability of iron ingested with food is probably 33–50% of that seen in the fasting subject. Antacids also reduce iron absorption if given concurrently. It is always preferable to administer iron in the fasting state, even if the dose must be reduced because of GI side effects. For patients who require maximal therapy to encourage a rapid response or to counteract continued bleeding, as much as 120 mg of iron may be administered four times a day. Sustained high rates of red cell production require an uninterrupted supply of iron, and oral doses should be spaced equally to maintain a continuous high concentration of iron in plasma.

The duration of treatment is governed by the rate of recovery of Hb and the desire to create iron stores. The former depends on the severity of the anemia. With a daily rate of repair of 0.2 g of Hb/dL of whole blood, the red cell mass usually is reconstituted within 1–2 months. Thus, an individual with an Hb of 5 g/dL may achieve a normal complement of 15 g/dL in about 50 days, whereas an individual with an Hb of 10 g/dL may take only half that time. The creation of stores of iron requires many months of oral iron administration. The rate of absorption decreases rapidly after recovery from anemia, and after 3–4 months of treatment, stores may increase at a rate of not much more than 100 mg/month. Much of the strategy of continued therapy depends on the estimated future iron balance. Patients with an inadequate diet may require continued therapy with low doses of iron. If the bleeding has stopped, no further therapy is required after the Hb has returned to normal. With continued bleeding, long-term therapy clearly is indicated.

UNTOWARD EFFECTS OF ORAL PREPARATIONS OF IRON Intolerance to oral preparations of iron primarily is a function of the amount of soluble iron in the upper GI tract and of psychological factors. Side effects include heartburn, nausea, upper gastric discomfort, and diarrhea or constipation. A good policy is to initiate therapy at a small dosage, to demonstrate freedom from symptoms at that level, and then gradually to increase the dosage to that desired. With a dose of 200 mg of iron per day divided into three equal portions, symptoms occur in ~25% of treated individuals *versus* 13% among those receiving placebo; this increases to ~40% when the dosage of iron is doubled. Nausea and upper abdominal pain are increasingly common at high dosage. Constipation and diarrhea, perhaps related to iron-induced changes in the intestinal bacterial flora, are not more prevalent at higher dosage, nor is heartburn. If a liquid is given, one can place the iron solution on the back of the tongue with a dropper to prevent transient staining of teeth.

Normal individuals apparently control absorption of iron despite high intake, and only individuals with underlying disorders that augment the absorption of iron run the hazard of developing iron overload (hemochromatosis). However, hemochromatosis is a relatively common genetic disorder, present in 0.5% of the population.

IRON POISONING

Large amounts of ferrous salts are toxic, but fatalities in adults are rare. Most deaths occur in children, particularly between the ages of 12 and 24 months. As little as 1–2 g of iron may cause death, but 2–10 g usually is ingested in fatal cases. The frequency of iron poisoning relates to its availability in the household, particularly the supply that remains after a pregnancy. The colored sugar coating of many of the commercially available tablets gives them the appearance of candy. All iron preparations should be kept in childproof bottles.

Signs and symptoms of severe poisoning may occur within 30 minutes after ingestion or may be delayed for several hours. They include abdominal pain, diarrhea, or vomiting of brown or bloody stomach contents containing pills. Of particular concern are pallor or cyanosis, lassitude, *drowsiness, hyperventilation due to acidosis, and cardiovascular collapse. The corrosive injury to the stomach may result in pyloric stenosis or gastric scarring. Hemorrhagic gastroenteritis and hepatic damage are prominent findings at autopsy. In the evaluation of a child thought to have ingested iron, a color test for iron in the gastric contents and an emergency determination of the concentration of iron in plasma can be performed. If the latter is <63 μm (3.5 mg/L), the child is not in immediate danger. However, vomiting should be induced when there is iron in the stomach, and an x-ray should be taken to evaluate the number of radio-opaque pills remaining in the small bowel. When the plasma concentration of iron exceeds the total iron-binding capacity (63 μm; 3.5 mg/L), deferoxamine should be administered (see Chapter 65). Shock, dehydration, and acid-base abnormalities should be treated in the conventional manner. Most important is the speed of diagnosis and therapy. With early effective treatment, the mortality from iron poisoning can be reduced from as high as 45% to ~1%.*

THERAPY WITH PARENTERAL IRON When oral iron therapy fails, parenteral iron administration may be an effective alternative. Common indications are iron malabsorption (*e.g.*, sprue, short bowel syndrome), severe intolerance of oral iron, as a routine supplement to total parenteral nutrition, and in patients who are receiving erythropoietin. Parenteral iron also has been given to iron-deficient patients and pregnant women to create iron stores, something that would take months to achieve by the oral route. *Parenteral iron therapy should be used only when clearly indicated, since acute hypersensitivity, including anaphylactic reactions, can occur.* The belief that the response to parenteral iron, especially *iron dextran*, is faster than oral iron is open to debate. In otherwise healthy individuals, the rate of Hb response is determined by the balance between the severity of the anemia (the level of erythropoietin stimulus) and the delivery of iron to the marrow from iron absorption and iron stores. When a large intravenous dose of iron dextran is given to a severely anemic patient, the hematologic response can exceed that seen with oral iron for 1–3 weeks. Subsequently, the response is no better than that seen with oral iron.

FDA-approved preparations for parenteral therapy include sodium ferric gluconate complex in sucrose (FERRLECIT), iron sucrose (VENOFER), and iron dextran (INFED, DEXFERRUM). Unlike iron dextran, which requires macrophage processing that may require several weeks, ~80% of sodium ferric gluconate is delivered to transferrin with 24 hours. Sodium ferric gluconate has a much lower risk of serious anaphylactic reactions than iron dextran.

Iron dextran injection (INFED, DEXFERRUM) is a colloidal solution of ferric oxyhydroxide complexed with polymerized dextran (molecular weight ~180 kDa) that contains 50 mg/mL of elemental iron. It can be administered by either intravenous (preferred) or intramuscular injection. When given by deep intramuscular injection, it is gradually mobilized via the lymphatics and transported to reticuloendothelial cells; the iron then is released from the dextran complex. Intravenous administration gives a more reliable response. Given intravenously in a dose of less than 500 mg, the iron dextran complex is cleared with a plasma $t_{1/2}$ of 6 hours. When 1 g or more is administered intravenously as total dose therapy, reticuloendothelial cell clearance is constant at 10–20 mg/h. This slow rate of clearance results in a brownish discoloration of the plasma for several days and an elevation of the serum iron for 1–2 weeks.

Intramuscular injection of iron dextran should only be initiated after a test dose of 0.5 mL (25 mg of iron). If no adverse reactions are observed, the injections can proceed. The daily dose ordinarily should not exceed 0.5 mL (25 mg of iron) for infants weighing less than 4.5 kg (10 lb), 1 mL (50 mg of iron) for children weighing less than 9 kg (20 lb), and 2 mL (100 mg of iron) for other patients. Iron dextran should be injected only into the muscle mass of the upper outer quadrant of the buttock using a z-track technique (displacement of the skin laterally before injection).

A test injection of 0.5 mL of undiluted iron dextran or an equivalent amount (25 mg of iron) diluted in saline also should precede intravenous administration of a therapeutic dose of iron dextran. The patient should be observed for signs of immediate anaphylaxis, and for an hour after injection for any signs of vascular instability or hypersensitivity, including respiratory distress, hypotension, tachycardia, or back or chest pain. When widely spaced, total-dose infusion therapy is given, a test dose injection should be given before each infusion because hypersensitivity can appear at any time. The patient should be monitored closely throughout the infusion for signs of cardiovascular instability. Delayed hypersensitivity reactions also are observed, especially in patients with rheumatoid arthritis or a history of allergies. Fever, malaise, lymphadenopathy, arthralgias, and urticaria can develop days or weeks following injection and last for prolonged periods of time. Therefore, iron dextran should be used with extreme caution in patients with rheumatoid arthritis or other connective tissue diseases, and during the acute phase of an inflammatory illness. Once hypersensitivity is documented, iron dextran therapy must be abandoned.

When hemodialysis patients are started on erythropoietin, oral iron therapy alone generally is insufficient to guarantee an optimal Hb response. It therefore is recommended that sufficient parenteral iron be given to maintain a plasma ferritin level between 100 and 800 µg/L and a transferrin saturation of 20–50%. One approach is to administer an initial intravenous dose of 200–500 mg, followed by weekly or every-other-week injections of 25–100 mg of iron dextran to replace ongoing blood loss. With repeated doses of iron dextran—especially multiple, total-dose infusions such as those sometimes used in the treatment of chronic GI blood loss—accumulations of slowly metabolized iron dextran stores in reticuloendothelial cells can be impressive. The plasma ferritin level also can rise to levels associated with iron overload. While disease-related hemochromatosis has been associated with an increased risk of infections and cardiovascular disease, this has not been shown to be true in hemodialysis patients treated with iron dextran. It seems prudent, however, to withhold the drug if the plasma ferritin exceeds 800 µg/L.

Reactions to intravenous iron include headache, malaise, fever, generalized lymphadenopathy, arthralgias, urticaria, and in some patients with rheumatoid arthritis, exacerbation of the disease. Phlebitis may occur with prolonged infusions of a concentrated solution or when an intramuscular preparation containing 0.5% phenol is used in error. Of greatest concern is the rare anaphylactic reaction, which may be fatal despite treatment.

COPPER

Copper deficiency is extremely rare, and there is no evidence that copper ever need be added to a normal diet. Even in clinical states associated with hypocupremia (sprue, celiac disease, and nephrotic syndrome), effects of copper deficiency usually are not demonstrable. Anemia due to copper deficiency has been described in individuals who have undergone intestinal bypass surgery, in those who are receiving parenteral nutrition, in malnourished infants, and in patients ingesting excessive amounts of zinc. While an inherited disorder affecting copper transport (Menkes' disease) is associated with reduced activity of several copper-dependent enzymes, this disease is not associated with hematological abnormalities.

The outstanding findings in copper deficiency are leukopenia, particularly granulocytopenia, and anemia; the anemia is not always microcytic. When a low plasma copper concentration is determined in the presence of leukopenia and anemia, a therapeutic trial with copper is appropriate. Daily doses up to 0.1 mg/kg of *cupric sulfate* have been given by mouth, or 1–2 mg/day may be added to the solution of nutrients for parenteral administration.

PYRIDOXINE

Patients with sideroblastic anemia characteristically have impaired Hb synthesis and accumulate iron in the perinuclear mitochondria of erythroid precursors, so-called ringed sideroblasts. Oral therapy with pyridoxine is of proven benefit in correcting the sideroblastic anemias associated with the antituberculosis drugs *isoniazid* and *pyrazinamide,* which act as vitamin B_6 antagonists. A daily dose of 50 mg of pyridoxine completely corrects the defect without interfering with treatment, and routine pyridoxine supplementation is recommended (*see* Chapter 47). In contrast, if pyridoxine is given to counteract the sideroblastic abnormality associated with administration of levodopa, the effectiveness of levodopa in controlling Parkinson's disease is decreased. Pyridoxine therapy does not correct the sideroblastic abnormalities produced by chloramphenicol or lead. Patients with idiopathic-acquired sideroblastic anemia generally fail to respond to oral pyridoxine; those few individuals who appear to have a pyridoxine-responsive anemia require prolonged therapy with large doses of the vitamin, 50–500 mg/day.

III. VITAMIN B_{12}, FOLIC ACID, AND THE TREATMENT OF MEGALOBLASTIC ANEMIAS

Vitamin B_{12} and *folic acid* are essential vitamins; the deficiency of either impairs DNA synthesis in any cell in which chromosomal replication and division are taking place. Since tissues with the greatest rate of cell turnover show the most dramatic changes, the hematopoietic system is especially sensitive to deficiencies of these vitamins.

RELATIONSHIPS BETWEEN VITAMIN B_{12} AND FOLIC ACID   The major roles of vitamin B_{12} and folic acid in intracellular metabolism are summarized in Figure 53–6. Intracellular vitamin B_{12} is maintained as two active coenzymes: methylcobalamin and deoxyadenosylcobalamin. Deoxyadenosylcobalamin (deoxyadenosyl B_{12}) is a cofactor for the mitochondrial mutase enzyme that catalyzes the isomerization of L-methylmalonyl CoA to succinyl CoA, an important

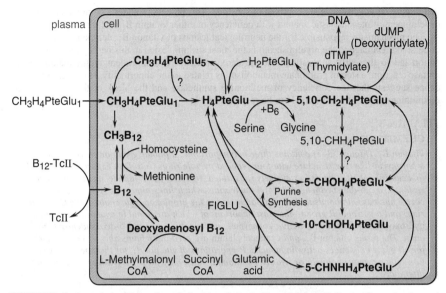

FIGURE 53–6 *Interrelationships and metabolic roles of vitamin B_{12} and folic acid.* See text for explanation and Figure 53–9 for structures of the various folate coenzymes. FIGLU, formiminoglutamic acid, which arises from the catabolism of histidine; TcII, transcobalamin II; $CH_3H_4PteGlu_1$, methyltetrahydrofolate.

reaction in carbohydrate and lipid metabolism. This reaction has no direct relationship to the metabolic pathways that involve folate. In contrast, methylcobalamin (CH_3B_{12}) supports the methionine synthetase reaction, which is essential for normal metabolism of folate. Methyl groups contributed by methyltetrahydrofolate ($CH_3H_4PteGlu_1$) are used to form methylcobalamin, which then acts as a methyl group donor for the conversion of homocysteine to methionine. This folate–cobalamin interaction is pivotal for normal synthesis of purines and pyrimidines, and therefore of DNA. The methionine synthetase reaction is largely responsible for the control of the recycling of folate cofactors; the maintenance of intracellular concentrations of folylpolyglutamates; and, through the synthesis of methionine and its product, *S*-adenosylmethionine (SAM), the maintenance of a number of methylation reactions.

Since methyltetrahydrofolate is the principal folate congener supplied to cells, the transfer of the methyl group to cobalamin is essential for the adequate supply of tetrahydrofolate ($H_4PteGlu_1$), the substrate for a number of metabolic steps. Tetrahydrofolate is a precursor for the formation of intracellular folylpolyglutamates; it also acts as the acceptor of a one-carbon unit in the conversion of Ser to Gly, with the resultant formation of 5,10-methylenetetrahydrofolate ($5,10-CH_2H_4PteGlu$). The latter derivative donates the methylene group to deoxyuridylate (dUMP) for the synthesis of thymidylate (dTMP)—an extremely important reaction in DNA synthesis. In the process, the $5,10-CH_2H_4PteGlu$ is converted to dihydrofolate ($H_2PteGlu$). The cycle then is completed by the reduction of the $H_2PteGlu$ to $H_4PteGlu$ by dihydrofolate reductase, the step that is blocked by folate antagonists such as methotrexate (*see* Chapter 51). As shown in Figure 53–6, other pathways also lead to the synthesis of 5,10-methylenetetrahydrofolate. These pathways are important in the metabolism of formiminoglutamic acid (FIGLU) and purines and pyrimidines.

Deficiency of either vitamin B_{12} or folate decreases the synthesis of methionine and *SAM*, thereby interfering with protein biosynthesis, a number of methylation reactions, and the synthesis of polyamines. In addition, the cell responds to the deficiency by redirecting folate metabolic pathways to supply increasing amounts of methyltetrahydrofolate; this tends to preserve essential methylation reactions at the expense of nucleic acid synthesis. With vitamin B_{12} deficiency, methylenetetrahydrofolate reductase activity increases, directing available intracellular folates into the methyltetrahydrofolate pool (not shown in Figure 53–6). The methyltetrahydrofolate then is trapped by the lack of sufficient vitamin B_{12} to accept and transfer methyl groups, and subsequent steps in folate metabolism that require tetrahydrofolate are deprived of substrate. This process provides a common basis for the development of megaloblastic anemia with deficiency of either vitamin B_{12} or folic acid.

The mechanisms responsible for the neurological lesions of vitamin B_{12} deficiency are less well understood. Damage to the myelin sheath is the most striking lesion in this neuropathy; this observation led to the early suggestion that the deoxyadenosyl B_{12}–dependent methylmalonyl CoA mutase reaction, a step in propionate metabolism, is related to the abnormality. However, other evidence suggests that the deficiency of methionine synthetase and the block of the conversion of methionine to *SAM* are more likely to be responsible.

VITAMIN B_{12}

CHEMISTRY

Vitamin B_{12} (Figure 53–7) contains three major portions: a planar group or corrin nucleus— a porphyrin-like ring structure with four reduced pyrrole rings (A to D in Figure 53–7) linked to a central cobalt atom and extensively substituted with methyl, acetamide, and propionamide residues; a 5,6-dimethylbenzimidazolyl nucleotide, which links almost at right angles to the corrin nucleus with bonds to the cobalt atom and to the propionate side chain of the C pyrrole ring; and a variable R group—the most important of which are found in cyanocobalamin and hydroxocobalamin *and the active coenzymes methylcobalamin and 5-deoxyadenosylcobalamin. The terms vitamin B_{12} and cyanocobalamin are used interchangeably as generic terms for all of the cobamides active in humans. Preparations of vitamin B_{12} for therapeutic use contain either cyanocobalamin or hydroxocobalamin, since only these derivatives remain active after storage.*

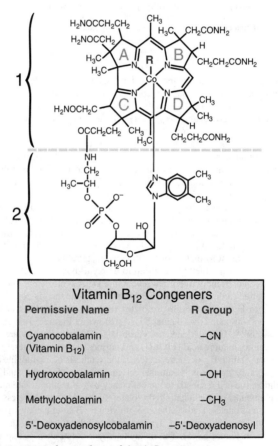

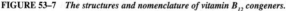

Vitamin B_{12} Congeners

Permissive Name	R Group
Cyanocobalamin (Vitamin B_{12})	–CN
Hydroxocobalamin	–OH
Methylcobalamin	–CH_3
5'-Deoxyadenosylcobalamin	–5'-Deoxyadenosyl

FIGURE 53–7 *The structures and nomenclature of vitamin B_{12} congeners.*

METABOLIC FUNCTIONS The active coenzymes methylcobalamin and 5-deoxyadeno-sylcobalamin are essential for cell growth and replication. Methylcobalamin is required for the conversion of homocysteine to methionine and its derivative, *SAM*. In addition, when concentrations of vitamin B_{12} are inadequate, folate becomes "trapped" as methyltetrahydrofolate, causing a functional deficiency of other required intracellular forms of folic acid (*see* Figures 53–6 and 53–7 and discussion above). The hematological abnormalities in vitamin B_{12}–deficient patients result from this process. 5-Deoxyadenosylcobalamin is required for the isomerization of L-methylmalonyl CoA to succinyl CoA (Figure 53–6).

SOURCES IN NATURE Humans depend on exogenous sources of vitamin B_{12}. Vegetables are free of vitamin B_{12} unless they are contaminated with microorganisms, so that we depend on synthesis in our own alimentary tract or the ingestion of animal products containing vitamin B_{12}. The daily nutritional requirement of 3–5 μg must be obtained from animal by-products in the diet. Despite this, strict vegetarians rarely develop vitamin B_{12} deficiency, probably because some vitamin B_{12} is available from legumes and because they often fortify their diets with vitamins and minerals.

ABSORPTION, DISTRIBUTION, ELIMINATION, AND DAILY REQUIREMENTS In the presence of gastric acid and pancreatic proteases, dietary vitamin B_{12} is released from food and bound to gastric intrinsic factor. When the vitamin B_{12}–intrinsic factor complex reaches the ileum, it interacts with a receptor on the mucosal cell surface and is actively transported into circulation. Adequate intrinsic factor, bile, and sodium bicarbonate (to provide a suitable pH) all are required for ileal transport of vitamin B_{12}. Vitamin B_{12} deficiency in adults rarely results from a deficient diet *per se;* rather, it usually reflects a defect in one or another aspect of this sequence of absorption (Figure 53–8). Achlorhydria and decreased secretion of intrinsic factor by parietal cells secondary to gastric atrophy or gastric surgery is a common cause of vitamin B_{12} deficiency in adults. Antibodies to parietal cells or intrinsic factor complex also can play a prominent role. A number of intestinal diseases can interfere with absorption, including pancreatic disorders (loss of pancreatic protease secretion), bacterial overgrowth, intestinal parasites, sprue, and localized damage to ileal mucosal cells by disease or as a result of surgery.

Once absorbed, vitamin B_{12} binds to transcobalamin II, a plasma β-globulin, for transport to tissues. Two other transcobalamins (I and III) also are present in plasma; their concentrations are related to the rate of turnover of granulocytes. They may represent intracellular storage proteins that

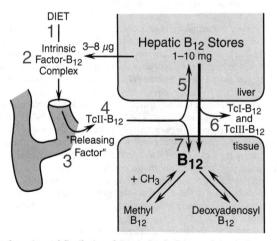

FIGURE 53–8 *The absorption and distribution of vitamin B_{12}.* Deficiency of vitamin B_{12} can result from a congenital or acquired defect in any one of the following: (1) inadequate dietary supply; (2) inadequate secretion of intrinsic factor (classical pernicious anemia); (3) ileal disease; (4) congenital absence of transcobalamin II (TcII); or (5) rapid depletion of hepatic stores by interference with reabsorption of vitamin B_{12} excreted in bile. The utility of measurements of the concentration of vitamin B_{12} in plasma to estimate supply available to tissues can be compromised by liver disease and (6) the appearance of abnormal amounts of transcobalamins I and III (TcI and III) in plasma. Finally, the formation of methylcobalamin requires (7) normal transport into cells and an adequate supply of folic acid as $CH_3H_4PteGlu_1$.

are released with cell death. Vitamin B_{12} bound to transcobalamin II is rapidly cleared from plasma and preferentially distributed to hepatic parenchymal cells, which comprise a storage depot for other tissues. In normal adults, as much as 90% of the body's stores of vitamin B_{12}, from 1 to 10 mg, is in the liver. Vitamin B_{12} is stored as the active coenzyme with a turnover rate of 0.5–8 μg/day, depending on the size of the body stores. The recommended daily intake of the vitamin in adults is 2.4 μg.

Approximately 3 μg of cobalamins is secreted into bile each day, 50–60% of which is not destined for reabsorption. This enterohepatic cycle is important because interference with reabsorption by intestinal disease can progressively deplete hepatic stores of the vitamin. This process may help explain why patients can develop vitamin B_{12} deficiency within 3–4 years of major gastric surgery, even though a daily requirement of 1–2 μg would not be expected to deplete hepatic stores of more than 2–3 mg during this time.

The supply of vitamin B_{12} available for tissues is directly related to the size of the hepatic storage pool and the amount of vitamin B_{12} bound to transcobalamin II (Figure 53–8). The plasma concentration of vitamin B_{12} normally ranges from 150 to 660 pmol (about 200–900 pg/mL), and deficiency should be suspected whenever the concentration is <150 pmol. The correlation is excellent except when the plasma concentrations of transcobalamin I and III are increased, as occurs with hepatic disease or myeloproliferative disorders. Because the vitamin B_{12} bound to these transport proteins is relatively unavailable to cells, tissues can become deficient when the concentration of vitamin B_{12} in plasma is normal or even high. In subjects with congenital absence of transcobalamin II, megaloblastic anemia occurs despite relatively normal plasma concentrations of vitamin B_{12}; the anemia will respond to parenteral doses of vitamin B_{12} that exceed the renal clearance.

Defects in intracellular metabolism of vitamin B_{12} have been reported in children with methylmalonic aciduria and homocystinuria. Potential mechanisms include an inability of cells to transport vitamin B_{12} or accumulate the vitamin because of a failure to synthesize an intracellular acceptor, a defect in the formation of deoxyadenosylcobalamin, or a congenital lack of methylmalonyl CoA isomerase.

VITAMIN B_{12} DEFICIENCY Vitamin B_{12} deficiency is recognized by its impact on the hematopoietic and nervous systems. The sensitivity of the hematopoietic system relates to its high rate of cell turnover. Other tissues with high rates of cell turnover (*e.g.,* mucosa and cervical epithelium) also have high requirements for the vitamin.

As a result of an inadequate supply of vitamin B_{12}, DNA replication becomes highly abnormal. Once a hematopoietic stem cell is committed to enter a programmed series of cell divisions, the defect in chromosomal replication results in an inability of maturing cells to complete nuclear divisions while cytoplasmic maturation continues at a relatively normal rate. This results in the production of morphologically abnormal cells and death of cells during maturation, a phenomenon known as *ineffective hematopoiesis.* Maturation of red cell precursors is highly abnormal (megaloblastic erythropoiesis). Those cells that do leave the marrow also are abnormal, and many cell fragments, poikilocytes, and macrocytes appear in the peripheral blood. The mean red cell volume increases to values greater than 110 fL. Severe deficiency affects all cell lines, and a pronounced pancytopenia results.

The diagnosis of a vitamin B_{12} deficiency usually can be made using measurements of the serum vitamin B_{12} and/or serum methylmalonic acid. The latter is somewhat more sensitive and has been used to identify metabolic deficiency in patients with normal serum vitamin B_{12} levels. As part of the clinical management of a patient with severe megaloblastic anemia, a therapeutic trial using very small doses of the vitamin can be used to confirm the diagnosis. Serial measurements of the reticulocyte count, serum iron, and hematocrit are performed to define the characteristic recovery of normal red cell production. The Schilling test can be used to quantitate the absorption of the vitamin and delineate the mechanism of the deficiency. By performing the Schilling test with and without added intrinsic factor, it is possible to discriminate between intrinsic factor deficiency by itself and primary ileal disease.

Vitamin B_{12} deficiency can irreversibly damage the nervous system. Progressive swelling of myelinated neurons, demyelination, and neuronal cell death are seen in the spinal column and cerebral cortex. This causes a wide range of neurological manifestations, including paresthesias, decreased vibration and position senses with resultant unsteadiness, decreased deep tendon reflexes, and in the later stages, confusion, moodiness, loss of memory, and even a loss of central vision. The patient may exhibit delusions, hallucinations, or even overt psychosis. Since the neurological damage can be dissociated from the changes in the hematopoietic system, vitamin B_{12} deficiency must be considered in elderly patients with dementia or psychiatric disorders, even if they are not anemic.

VITAMIN B$_{12}$ THERAPY Vitamin B$_{12}$ is available for injection or oral administration; combinations with other vitamins and minerals also can be given orally or parenterally. The choice of a preparation always depends on the cause of the deficiency. Although oral preparations may be used to supplement deficient diets, they are of limited value in the treatment of patients with deficiency of intrinsic factor or ileal disease. Even though small amounts of vitamin B$_{12}$ may be absorbed by simple diffusion, the oral route of administration cannot be relied upon for effective therapy in the patient with a marked deficiency of vitamin B$_{12}$ and abnormal hematopoiesis or neurological deficits. Therefore, the treatment of choice for vitamin B$_{12}$–deficiency is cyanocobalamin administered by intramuscular or subcutaneous injection.

Effective use of vitamin B$_{12}$ depends on accurate diagnosis and an understanding of the following principles:

1. Vitamin B$_{12}$ should be given prophylactically only when there is a reasonable probability that a deficiency exists or will exist. Dietary deficiency in the strict vegetarian, the predictable malabsorption of vitamin B$_{12}$ in patients who have had a gastrectomy, and certain diseases of the small intestine constitute such indications. When GI function is normal, an oral prophylactic supplement of vitamins and minerals, including vitamin B$_{12}$, may be indicated. Otherwise, the patient should receive monthly injections of cyanocobalamin.
2. The relative ease of treatment with vitamin B$_{12}$ should not prevent a full investigation of the etiology of the deficiency. The initial diagnosis usually is suggested by a macrocytic anemia or an unexplained neuropsychiatric disorder. Full understanding of the etiology of vitamin B$_{12}$ deficiency involves studies of dietary supply, GI absorption, and transport.
3. Therapy always should be as specific as possible. While a large number of multivitamin preparations are available, the use of "shotgun" vitamin therapy in the treatment of vitamin B$_{12}$ deficiency can be dangerous. With such therapy, there is the danger that sufficient folic acid will be given to result in a hematological recovery, which can mask continued vitamin B$_{12}$ deficiency and permit neurological damage to develop or progress.
4. Although a therapeutic trial with small amounts of vitamin B$_{12}$ can help confirm the diagnosis, acutely ill, elderly patients may not be able to tolerate the delay in the correction of a severe anemia. Such patients require supplemental blood transfusions and immediate therapy with folic acid and vitamin B$_{12}$ to guarantee rapid recovery.
5. Long-term therapy with vitamin B$_{12}$ must be evaluated at intervals of 6–12 months in patients who are otherwise well. If there is an additional illness or a condition that may increase the requirement for the vitamin (*e.g.*, pregnancy), reassessment should be performed more frequently.

FOLIC ACID

CHEMISTRY AND METABOLIC FUNCTIONS

Pteroylglutamic acid (PteGlu) (Figure 53–9) contains a pteridine ring linked by a methylene bridge to para-aminobenzoic acid, which is joined by an amide linkage to glutamic acid. While pteroylglutamic acid is the common pharmaceutical form of folic acid, it is neither the principal folate congener in food nor the active coenzyme for intracellular metabolism. After absorption, PteGlu is rapidly reduced at the 5, 6, 7, and 8 positions to tetrahydrofolic acid (H$_4$PteGlu), which then acts as an acceptor of a number of one-carbon units. These are attached at either the 5 or the 10 position of the pteridine ring or may bridge these atoms to form a new five-membered ring. The most important forms of the coenzyme that are synthesized by these reactions are listed in Figure 53–9. Each plays a specific role in intracellular metabolism (see "Relationships Between Vitamin B$_{12}$ and Folic Acid," above, as well as Figure 53–6)

Conversion of homocysteine to methionine. This reaction requires CH$_3$H$_4$PteGlu as a methyl donor and utilizes vitamin B$_{12}$ as a cofactor.

Conversion of serine to glycine. This reaction requires tetrahydrofolate as an acceptor of a methylene group from Ser and utilizes pyridoxal phosphate as a cofactor. It results in the formation of 5,10-CH$_2$H$_4$PteGlu, an essential coenzyme for the synthesis of thymidylate.

Synthesis of thymidylate. 5,10-CH$_2$H$_4$PteGlu donates a methylene group and reducing equivalents to deoxyuridylate for the synthesis of thymidylate—a rate-limiting step in DNA synthesis.

Histidine metabolism. H$_4$PteGlu also acts as an acceptor of a formimino group in the conversion of formiminoglutamic acid to glutamic acid.

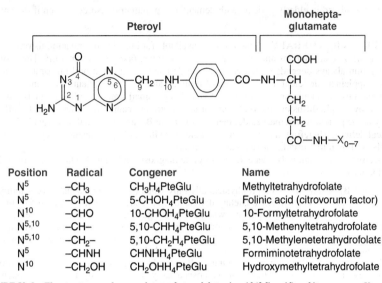

Position	Radical	Congener	Name
N^5	$-CH_3$	$CH_3H_4PteGlu$	Methyltetrahydrofolate
N^5	$-CHO$	$5\text{-}CHOH_4PteGlu$	Folinic acid (citrovorum factor)
N^{10}	$-CHO$	$10\text{-}CHOH_4PteGlu$	10-Formyltetrahydrofolate
$N^{5,10}$	$-CH-$	$5,10\text{-}CHH_4PteGlu$	5,10-Methenyltetrahydrofolate
$N^{5,10}$	$-CH_2-$	$5,10\text{-}CH_2H_4PteGlu$	5,10-Methylenetetrahydrofolate
N^5	$-CHNH$	$CHNHH_4PteGlu$	Formiminotetrahydrofolate
N^{10}	$-CH_2OH$	$CH_2OHH_4PteGlu$	Hydroxymethyltetrahydrofolate

FIGURE 53–9 *The structures and nomenclature of pteroylglutamic acid (folic acid) and its congeners.* X represents additional residues of glutamate; polyglutamates are the storage and active forms of the vitamin. The subscript that designates the number of residues of glutamate is frequently omitted because this number is variable.

Synthesis of purines. Two steps in the synthesis of purine nucleotides require the participation of derivatives of folic acid. Glycinamide ribonucleotide is formylated by 5,10-CHH$_4$PteGlu; 5-aminoimidazole-4-carboxamide ribonucleotide is formylated by 10-CHOH$_4$PteGlu. By these reactions, carbon atoms at positions 8 and 2, respectively, are incorporated into the growing purine ring.

Utilization or generation of formate. *This reversible reaction utilizes H$_4$PteGlu and 10-CHOH$_4$PteGlu.*

DAILY REQUIREMENTS Many food sources are rich in folates, especially green vegetables, liver, yeast, and some fruits, but lengthy cooking can destroy up to 90% of the folate content. Generally, a standard U.S. diet provides 50–500 μg of folate/day, although individuals with high intakes of fresh vegetables and meats may ingest as much as 2 mg/day. In the normal adult, the recommended daily intake is 400 μg, while pregnant or lactating women and patients with high rates of cell turnover (*e.g.*, patients with hemolytic anemia) may require 500–600 μg/day or more. For prevention of neural tube defects, a daily intake of at least 400 μg of folate in food or in supplements, beginning a month before pregnancy and continued for at least the first trimester, is recommended. Folate supplementation also is being considered in patients with elevated levels of plasma homocysteine (*see* below).

ABSORPTION, DISTRIBUTION, AND ELIMINATION As with vitamin B$_{12}$, the diagnosis and management of folic acid deficiency depend on an understanding of the transport pathways and intracellular metabolism of the vitamin (Figure 53–10). Folates present in food are largely in the form of reduced polyglutamates, and absorption requires transport and the action of a pteroylglutamyl carboxypeptidase associated with mucosal cell membranes. The mucosae of the duodenum and upper part of the jejunum are rich in dihydrofolate reductase and can methylate most or all of the reduced folate that is absorbed. Since most absorption occurs in the proximal small intestine, it is not unusual for folate deficiency to occur with jejunal disease. Both nontropical and tropical sprues are common causes of folate deficiency.

Once absorbed, folate is transported rapidly to tissues as CH$_3$H$_4$PteGlu. While certain plasma proteins do bind folate derivatives, they have a greater affinity for nonmethylated analogs; their role in folate homeostasis is not well understood. An increase in binding capacity is detected in folate deficiency and in certain disease states (*e.g.*, uremia, cancer, and alcoholism).

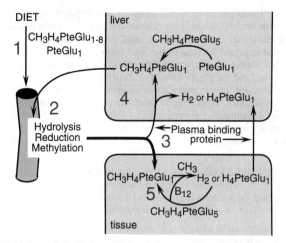

FIGURE 53–10 *Absorption and distribution of folate derivatives.* Dietary sources of folate polyglutamates are hydrolyzed to the monoglutamate, reduced, and methylated to $CH_3H_4PteGlu_1$ during GI transport. Folate deficiency commonly results from (1) inadequate dietary supply and (2) small intestinal disease. In patients with uremia, alcoholism, or hepatic disease there may be defects in (3) the concentration of folate binding proteins in plasma and (4) the flow of $CH_3H_4PteGlu_1$ into bile for reabsorption and transport to tissue (the folate enterohepatic cycle). Finally, vitamin B_{12} deficiency will (5) "trap" folate as $CH_3H_4PteGlu_1$ thereby, reducing the availability of $H_4PteGlu_1$ for its essential roles in purine and pyrimidine synthesis.

A constant supply of $CH_3H_4PteGlu$ is maintained by food and by an enterohepatic cycle of the vitamin. The liver actively reduces and methylates PteGlu (and H_2 or $H_4PteGlu$) and then transports the $CH_3H_4PteGlu$ into bile for reabsorption by the gut and subsequent delivery to tissues. This pathway may provide 200 μg or more of folate each day for recirculation to tissues. The importance of the enterohepatic cycle is suggested by animal studies that show a rapid reduction of the plasma folate concentration after either drainage of bile or ingestion of alcohol, which apparently blocks the release of $CH_3H_4PteGlu$ from hepatic parenchymal cells.

Following uptake into cells, $CH_3H_4PteGlu$ acts as a methyl donor for the formation of methylcobalamin and as a source of $H_4PteGlu$ and other folate congeners. Folate is stored within cells as polyglutamates.

FOLATE DEFICIENCY Folate deficiency is a common complication of diseases of the small intestine, which interfere with the absorption of dietary folate and the recirculation of folate through the enterohepatic cycle. In acute or chronic alcoholism, daily intake of dietary folate may be severely restricted, and the enterohepatic cycle of the vitamin may be impaired by toxic effects of alcohol on hepatic parenchymal cells; this is the most common cause of folate-deficient megaloblastic erythropoiesis. However, it also is the most amenable to therapy, inasmuch as the reinstitution of a normal diet is sufficient to overcome the effect of alcohol. Disease states characterized by a high rate of cell turnover, such as hemolytic anemias, also may be complicated by folate deficiency. Additionally, drugs that inhibit dihydrofolate reductase (*e.g.,* methotrexate and trimethoprim) or that interfere with the absorption and storage of folate in tissues (*e.g.,* certain anticonvulsants and oral contraceptives) can lower the concentration of folate in plasma and may cause a megaloblastic anemia.

Folate deficiency has been implicated in neural tube defects, including spina bifida, encephaloceles, and anencephaly. This is true even in the absence of folate-deficient anemia or alcoholism. An inadequate intake of folate also can result in elevations in plasma homocysteine. Since even moderate hyperhomocysteinemia is considered an independent risk factor for coronary artery and peripheral vascular disease and for venous thrombosis, the role of folate as a methyl donor in the homocysteine-to-methionine conversion is getting increased attention. Patients who are heterozygous for one or another enzymatic defect and have high normal to moderate elevations of plasma homocysteine may improve with folic acid therapy.

Folate deficiency is recognized by its impact on the hematopoietic system, again reflecting the increased requirement associated with high rates of cell turnover. The megaloblastic anemia that results from folate deficiency cannot be distinguished from that caused by vitamin B_{12} deficiency. This finding is to be expected because of the final common pathway of the major intracellular metabolic roles of the 2 vitamins. In contrast, folate deficiency is rarely if ever associated with neurological abnormalities, and the observation of characteristic abnormalities in vibratory and position sense and in motor and sensory pathways is incompatible with isolated folate deficiency.

After deprivation of folate, megaloblastic anemia develops much more rapidly than it does following interruption of vitamin B_{12} absorption (*e.g.*, gastric surgery). This observation reflects the fact that body stores of folate are limited. Although the rate of induction of megaloblastic erythropoiesis may vary, a folate-deficiency state may appear in 1–4 weeks, depending on the individual's dietary habits and stores of the vitamin.

GENERAL PRINCIPLES OF THERAPY   The therapeutic use of folic acid is limited to the prevention and treatment of deficiencies of the vitamin. As with vitamin B_{12} therapy, effective use of the vitamin depends on accurate diagnosis and an understanding of the mechanisms that are operative in a specific disease state. The following general principles of therapy apply:

1. Prophylactic administration of folic acid should be undertaken for clear indications. Dietary supplementation is necessary when there is a requirement that may not be met by a "normal" diet. The daily ingestion of a multivitamin preparation containing 400–500 μg of folic acid has become standard practice before and during pregnancy to reduce the incidence of neural tube defects and for as long as a woman is breastfeeding. In women with a history of a pregnancy complicated by a neural tube defect, an even larger dose of 4 mg/day has been recommended. Patients on total parenteral nutrition should receive folic acid supplements because liver folate stores are limited. Adult patients with a disease state characterized by high cell turnover (*e.g.*, hemolytic anemia) generally require larger doses, 1 mg of folic acid given once or twice a day. The 1-mg dose also has been used in the treatment of patients with elevated levels of homocysteine.
2. As with vitamin B_{12} deficiency, any patient with folate deficiency and a megaloblastic anemia should be evaluated carefully to determine the underlying cause of the deficiency state. This should include evaluation of the effects of medications, the amount of alcohol intake, the patient's history of travel, and the function of the GI tract.
3. Therapy always should be as specific as possible. Multivitamin preparations should be avoided unless there is good reason to suspect deficiency of several vitamins.
4. *The potential danger of mistreating a patient who has vitamin B_{12} deficiency with folic acid must be kept in mind.* The administration of large doses of folic acid can result in an apparent improvement of the megaloblastic anemia, inasmuch as PteGlu is converted by dihydrofolate reductase to H_4PteGlu; this circumvents the methylfolate "trap." However, folate therapy does not prevent or alleviate the neurological defects of vitamin B_{12} deficiency, and these may progress and become irreversible.

For a complete Bibliographical listing see Goodman & Gilman's *The Pharmacological Basis of Therapeutics*, 11th ed., or Goodman & Gilman Online at www.accessmedicine.com.

54

BLOOD COAGULATION AND ANTICOAGULANT, THROMBOLYTIC, AND ANTIPLATELET DRUGS

OVERVIEW OF HEMOSTASIS: PLATELET FUNCTION, BLOOD COAGULATION, AND FIBRINOLYSIS

Hemostasis is the cessation of blood loss from a damaged vessel. Platelets first adhere to macromolecules in the subendothelial regions of the injured blood vessel and then aggregate to form the primary hemostatic plug. Platelets stimulate local activation of plasma coagulation factors, leading to generation of a fibrin clot that reinforces the platelet aggregate. Later, as wound healing occurs, the platelet aggregate and fibrin clot are degraded. The processes of platelet aggregation and blood coagulation are summarized in Figures 54–1 and 54–2. The pathway of clot removal, fibrinolysis, is shown in Figure 54–3, along with sites of action of fibrinolytic agents.

Coagulation involves a series of zymogen activation reactions (Figure 54–2). At each stage, a precursor protein, or *zymogen,* is converted to an active protease by cleavage of one or more peptide bonds in the precursor molecule. The components at each stage include a protease from the preceding stage, a zymogen, a nonenzymatic protein cofactor, Ca^{2+}, and an organizing surface provided by a phospholipid emulsion *in vitro* or by platelets *in vivo*. The final protease generated is thrombin (factor IIa).

INITIATION OF COAGULATION   Coagulation is initiated *in vivo* by the extrinsic pathway. Small amounts of factor VIIa in the plasma bind to subendothelial tissue factor following vascular injury. Tissue factor accelerates activation of factor X by VIIa, phospholipids, and Ca^{2+} by ~30,000-fold. VIIa also can activate IX in the presence of tissue factor, providing a convergence between the extrinsic and intrinsic pathways.

Clotting by the intrinsic pathway is initiated *in vitro* when XII, prekallikrein, and high-molecular-weight kininogen interact with kaolin, glass, or another surface to generate small amounts of XIIa. Activation of XI to XIa and IX to IXa follows. IXa then activates X in a reaction that is accelerated by VIIIa, phospholipids, and Ca^{2+}. Activation of factor X by IXa appears to occur by a mechanism similar to that for activation of prothrombin and may also be accelerated by platelets *in vivo*. Activation of factor XII is not required for hemostasis, since patients with deficiency of XII, prekallikrein, or high-molecular-weight kininogen do not bleed abnormally, even though their aPTT values (see below) are prolonged. Factor XI deficiency is associated with a variable and usually mild bleeding disorder. The mechanism for activation of factor XI *in vivo* is not known, although thrombin activates factor XI *in vitro*.

Fibrinolysis and Thrombolysis

The fibrinolytic system dissolves intravascular clots as a result of the action of plasmin, an enzyme that digests fibrin. Plasminogen, an inactive precursor, is converted to plasmin by cleavage of a single peptide bond. Plasmin is a relatively nonspecific protease; it digests fibrin clots and other plasma proteins, including several coagulation factors. Therapy with thrombolytic drugs can dissolve both pathological thrombi and fibrin deposits at sites of vascular injury; thus, such drugs also may promote also hemorrhage.

The fibrinolytic system is regulated such that unwanted fibrin thrombi are removed, while fibrin in wounds persists to maintain hemostasis. *Tissue plasminogen activator (t-PA)* is released from endothelial cells in response to various signals, including stasis produced by vascular occlusion. It is rapidly cleared from blood or inhibited by circulating inhibitors, plasminogen activator inhibitor-1 and plasminogen activator inhibitor-2, and thus exerts little effect on circulating plasminogen. t-PA binds to fibrin and converts plasminogen, which also binds to fibrin, to plasmin. Plasminogen and plasmin bind to fibrin at binding sites located near their amino termini that are rich in Lys residues (*see* below). These sites also are required for plasmin binding to the inhibitor α_2-antiplasmin. Therefore, fibrin-bound plasmin is protected from inhibition. Any plasmin that escapes this local milieu is rapidly inhibited. Some α_2-antiplasmin is bound covalently to fibrin and thereby protects fibrin from premature lysis. When plasminogen activators are administered for thrombolytic therapy, massive fibrinolysis is initiated, and the inhibitory controls are overwhelmed. The pathway of fibrinolysis and sites of drug action are summarized by Figure 54–3.

COAGULATION IN VITRO   The time in which recalcified plasma will clot after addition of kaolin is termed the *activated partial thromboplastin time* (aPTT); normal values are from

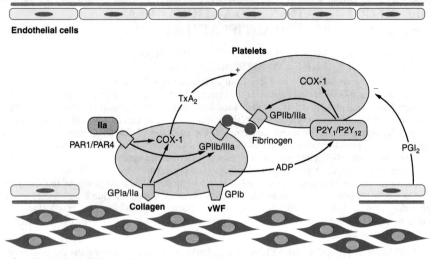

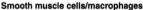

FIGURE 54–1 *Platelet adhesion and aggregation.* GPIa/IIa and GPIb are platelet membrane proteins that bind to collagen and von Willebrand factor (vWF), causing platelets to adhere to the subendothelium of a damaged blood vessel. PAR1 and PAR4 are protease-activated receptors that respond to thrombin (IIa); $P2Y_1$ and $P2Y_{12}$ are receptors for ADP (adenosine diphosphate); when stimulated by agonists, these receptors activate the fibrinogen-binding protein GPIIb/IIIa and COX-1 to promote platelet aggregation and secretion. Thromboxane A_2 (TxA_2) is the major product of COX-1 involved in platelet activation. Prostacyclin (PGI_2) synthesized by endothelial cells inhibits platelet activation.

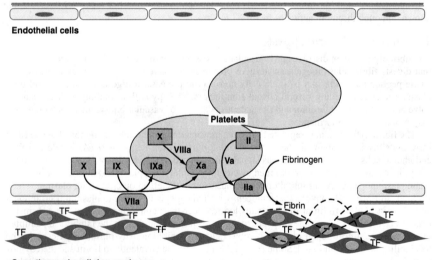

FIGURE 54–2 *Major reactions of blood coagulation.* Shown are interactions among proteins of the "extrinsic" (tissue factor and factor VII), "intrinsic" (factors IX and VIII), and "common" (factors X, V, and II) coagulation pathways that are important *in vivo*. Boxes enclose the coagulation factor zymogens (indicated by Roman numerals) and the rounded boxes represent the active proteases. TF, tissue factor; activated coagulation factors are followed by the letter "a." II, prothrombin; IIa, thrombin.

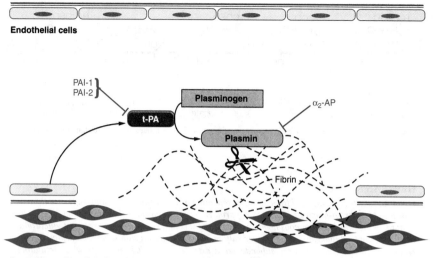

Smooth muscle cells/macrophages

FIGURE 54–3 *Fibrinolysis.* Endothelial cells secrete tissue plasminogen activator (t-PA) at sites of injury. t-PA binds to fibrin and cleaves plasminogen to plasmin, resulting in fibrin digestion. Plasminogen activator inhibitors-1 and -2 (PAI-1, PAI-2) inactivate t-PA; α_2-antiplasmin (α_2-AP) inactivates plasmin.

26 to 33 seconds. Alternatively, the time required for recalcified plasma to clot after the addition of "thromboplastin" (a mixture of tissue factor and phospholipids is termed the *prothrombin time* (PT); a normal value is from 12 to 14 seconds. Because of considerable variation in the performance of the PT, results typically are normalized to an international standard and reported as the "International Normalized Time", or INR. Typically, the aPTT is used to follow anticoagulation with heparin, while the INR is used to monitor anticoagulation with oral anticoagulants (*see* below).

NATURAL ANTICOAGULANT MECHANISMS Platelet activation and coagulation normally do not occur within an intact blood vessel. Thrombosis is prevented by several regulatory mechanisms that require a normal vascular endothelium. Prostacyclin (prostaglandin I_2; PGI_2) is synthesized by endothelial cells and inhibits platelet aggregation and secretion (*see* Chapter 25). Antithrombin is a plasma protein that inhibits coagulation factors of the intrinsic and common pathways (*see* below). Heparan sulfate proteoglycans synthesized by endothelial cells stimulate the activity of antithrombin. Protein C is a plasma zymogen that is homologous to factors II, VII, IX, and X; its activity depends on the binding of Ca^{2+} to γ-carboxyglutamate (Gla) residues within its amino-terminal domain. Activated protein C, in combination with its nonenzymatic Gla-containing cofactor (protein S), degrades cofactors Va and VIIIa and thereby greatly diminishes the activation of prothrombin and factor X. Protein C is activated by thrombin only in the presence of thrombomodulin, an integral membrane protein of endothelial cells. Like antithrombin, protein C exerts an anticoagulant effect in the vicinity of intact endothelial cells. Tissue factor pathway inhibitor (TFPI) is found in the lipoprotein fraction of plasma. When bound to factor Xa, TFPI inhibits factor Xa and the factor VIIa–tissue factor complex. By this mechanism, factor Xa may regulate its own production.

PARENTERAL ANTICOAGULANTS
Heparin

BIOCHEMISTRY Heparin is a glycosaminoglycan found in the secretory granules of mast cells. It is synthesized from UDP-sugar precursors as a polymer of alternating D-glucuronic acid and *N*-acetyl-D-glucosamine residues (Figure 54–4). About 10–15 glycosaminoglycan chains, each containing 200–300 monosaccharide units, are attached to a core protein and yield a proteoglycan of 750–1000 kDa. The glycosaminoglycan is modified to yield a variety of oligosaccharide structures. After the heparin proteoglycan has been transported to the mast cell granule, an endo-β-D-glucuronidase degrades the glycosaminoglycan chains to fragments of ~12,000 Da (~40 monosaccharide units) over a period of hours.

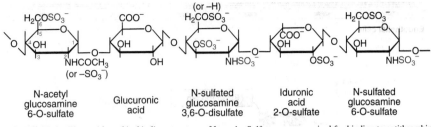

N-acetyl glucosamine 6-O-sulfate	Glucuronic acid	N-sulfated glucosamine 3,6-O-disulfate	Iduronic acid 2-O-sulfate	N-sulfated glucosamine 6-O-sulfate

FIGURE 54–4 *The antithrombin-binding structure of heparin.* Sulfate groups required for binding to antithrombin are indicated in blue.

HEPARAN SULFATE

Heparan sulfate is synthesized from the same repeating disaccharide precursor (D-glucuronic acid linked to N-acetyl-D-glucosamine) as is heparin. However, heparan sulfate undergoes less modification of the polymer than does heparin and therefore contains higher proportions of glucuronic acid and N-acetylglucosamine and fewer sulfate groups. Heparan sulfate on the surface of vascular endothelial cells or in the subendothelial extracellular matrix interacts with circulating antithrombin (see below) to provide a natural antithrombotic mechanism.

SOURCE

Heparin is commonly extracted from porcine intestinal mucosa or bovine lung. Despite the heterogeneity in composition among different commercial preparations of heparin, their biological activities are similar (~150 USP units/mg). The USP unit is the quantity of heparin that prevents 1 mL of citrated sheep plasma from clotting for 1 hour after the addition of 0.2 mL of 1% CaCl₂.

Low-molecular-weight heparins (~ 4500 Da, or 15 monosaccharide units) are isolated from standard heparin by gel filtration chromatography, precipitation with ethanol, or partial depolymerization with nitrous acid and other chemical or enzymatic reagents. Low-molecular-weight heparins differ from standard heparin and from each other in their pharmacokinetic properties and mechanism of action (see below). The biological activity of low-molecular-weight heparin is generally measured with a factor Xa inhibition assay, which is mediated by antithrombin.

MECHANISM OF ACTION Heparin catalyzes the inhibition of several coagulation proteases by antithrombin, a glycosylated, single-chain polypeptide (432 amino acids). Antithrombin is synthesized in the liver and circulates in plasma at an approximate concentration of 2.6 μM. It inhibits activated coagulation factors of the intrinsic and common pathways, including thrombin, Xa, and IXa; however, it has relatively little activity against factor VIIa. Antithrombin is a "suicide substrate" for these proteases; inhibition occurs when the protease attacks a specific Arg-Ser peptide bond in the reactive site of antithrombin and becomes trapped as a stable 1:1 complex.

Heparin increases the rate of the thrombin-antithrombin reaction at least 1000-fold by serving as a catalytic template to which both the inhibitor and the protease bind. Binding of heparin also induces a conformational change in antithrombin that makes the reactive site more accessible to the protease. Once thrombin has become bound to antithrombin, the heparin molecule is released from the complex. The binding site for antithrombin on heparin is a specific pentasaccharide sequence that contains a 3-O-sulfated glucosamine residue (Figure 54–4). This structure occurs in ~30% of heparin molecules and less abundantly in heparan sulfate. Heparin molecules containing fewer than 18 monosaccharide units (<5400 Da) do not catalyze inhibition of thrombin by antithrombin, since they cannot bind thrombin and antithrombin simultaneously. In contrast, the pentasaccharide shown in Figure 54–4 catalyzes inhibition of factor Xa by antithrombin. In this case, catalysis may occur solely by induction of a conformational change in antithrombin that facilitates reaction with the protease. Low-molecular-weight heparin preparations produce an anticoagulant effect mainly through inhibition of Xa by antithrombin, because the majority of molecules are of insufficient length to catalyze inhibition of thrombin.

Miscellaneous Pharmacological Effects

High doses of heparin can interfere with platelet aggregation and thereby prolong bleeding time. It is unclear to what extent the antiplatelet effect of heparin contributes to the hemorrhagic complications of treatment with the drug. Heparin "clears" lipemic plasma in vivo by causing the release of lipoprotein lipase into the circulation. Lipoprotein lipase hydrolyzes triglycerides to glycerol and free fatty acids. The clearing of lipemic plasma may occur at concentrations of heparin below those necessary to produce an anticoagulant effect.

CLINICAL USE   Heparin is used to initiate treatment of venous thrombosis and pulmonary embolism because of its rapid onset of action. An oral anticoagulant usually is started concurrently, and heparin is continued for at least 4–5 days to allow the oral anticoagulant to achieve its full therapeutic effect. Patients who experience recurrent thromboembolism despite adequate oral anticoagulation (*e.g.,* patients with Trousseau's syndrome) may benefit from long-term heparin administration. Heparin is used in the initial management of patients with unstable angina or acute myocardial infarction, during and after coronary angioplasty or stent placement, and during surgery requiring cardiopulmonary bypass. Heparin also is used to treat selected patients with disseminated intravascular coagulation. Low-dose heparin regimens are effective in preventing venous thromboembolism in certain high-risk patients.

Low-molecular-weight heparin preparations were first approved for prevention of venous thromboembolism. They are also effective in the treatment of venous thrombosis, pulmonary embolism, and unstable angina. Their principal advantage of over standard heparin is a more predictable pharmacokinetic profile, which allows weight-adjusted subcutaneous administration without laboratory monitoring. Thus, therapy of many patients with acute venous thromboembolism can be provided in the outpatient setting. Other advantages of low-molecular-weight heparin include a lower incidence of heparin-induced thrombocytopenia and possibly lower risks of bleeding and osteopenia.

In contrast to warfarin, heparin does not cross the placenta and is not associated with fetal malformations; therefore it is the drug of choice for anticoagulation during pregnancy. Heparin does not appear to increase the incidence of fetal mortality or prematurity. If possible, the drug should be discontinued 24 hours before delivery to minimize the risk of postpartum bleeding. Safety and efficacy of low-molecular-weight heparin use during pregnancy have not been adequately evaluated.

ABSORPTION AND PHARMACOKINETICS   Heparin is not absorbed through the gastrointestinal (GI) mucosa and must be given by continuous intravenous infusion or subcutaneous injection. Heparin has an immediate onset of action when given intravenously; there is considerable variation in the bioavailability of heparin given subcutaneously, and the onset of action is delayed 1–2 hours. Low-molecular-weight heparins are absorbed more uniformly.

The $t_{1/2}$ of heparin in plasma depends on the dose administered. When doses of 100, 400, or 800 units/kg of heparin are injected intravenously, the half-lives of the anticoagulant activities are ~1, 2.5, and 5 hours. Heparin appears to be cleared and degraded primarily by the reticuloendothelial system; a small amount of undegraded heparin appears in the urine. The $t_{1/2}$ of heparin may be shortened in patients with pulmonary embolism and prolonged in patients with hepatic cirrhosis or end-stage renal disease. Low-molecular-weight heparins have longer biological half-lives than do standard preparations of the drug.

ADMINISTRATION AND MONITORING   Full-dose heparin therapy usually is administered by continuous intravenous infusion. Treatment of venous thromboembolism is initiated with a bolus injection of 5000 units, followed by 1200–1600 units/h delivered by an infusion pump. Therapy routinely is monitored by the aPTT; the target is an elevation to 1.8–2.5 times the normal value. The risk of recurrence of thromboembolism is greater in patients who do not achieve a therapeutic level of anticoagulation within the first 24 hours. Initially, the aPTT should be measured and the infusion rate adjusted every 6 hours; dose adjustments may be aided by use of a nomogram. Once a steady dosage schedule has been established, daily monitoring is sufficient.

Subcutaneous administration of heparin can be used for the long-term management of patients in whom warfarin is contraindicated (*e.g.,* during pregnancy). A total daily dose of ~35,000 units administered as divided doses every 8–12 hours usually is sufficient to achieve an aPTT of 1.5 times the control value (measured midway between doses). Monitoring generally is unnecessary once a steady dosage schedule is established.

Low-dose heparin therapy is used prophylactically to prevent deep venous thrombosis and thromboembolism in susceptible patients, to whom it should be administered every 8 hours in a hospital setting; laboratory monitoring is unnecessary in this setting.

LOW-MOLECULAR-WEIGHT HEPARIN PREPARATIONS   *Enoxaparin* (LOVENOX), *dalteparin* (FRAGMIN), *tinzaparin* (INNOHEP, others), *ardeparin* (NORMIFLO), *nadroparin* (FRAXIPARINE,* others), and *reviparin* (CLIVARINE) differ considerably in composition, and it cannot be assumed that two preparations with similar anti–factor Xa activity will produce equivalent antithrombotic effects. The more predictable pharmacokinetic properties of low-molecular-weight heparins permit subcutaneous administration in a fixed or weight-adjusted dosage regimen 1–2 times daily. Since they have a minimal effect on tests of clotting *in vitro,* monitoring is not done routinely. Patients with end-stage renal failure may require monitoring with an anti–factor Xa assay because this condition may prolong the $t_{1/2}$ of low-molecular-weight heparin. Specific dosage recommendations for various low-molecular-weight heparins may be obtained from the manufacturers' literature. Nadroparin and reviparin are not available in the U.S.

SYNTHETIC HEPARIN DERIVATIVES *Fondaparinux* (ARIXTRA) is a synthetic pentasaccharide based on the structure of the antithrombin binding region of heparin. It mediates inhibition of factor Xa by antithrombin but does not cause thrombin inhibition due to its short polymer length. Fondaparinux is administered by subcutaneous injection, reaches peak plasma levels in 2 hours, and is excreted in the urine with a $t_{1/2}$ of 17–21 hours. It should not be used in patients with renal failure. Because it does not interact significantly with blood cells or plasma proteins other than antithrombin, fondaparinux can be given once a day at a fixed dose without coagulation monitoring. Fondaparinux appears to be much less likely than heparin or low-molecular-weight heparin to trigger the syndrome of heparin-induced thrombocytopenia (*see* below). Fondaparinux is approved for thromboprophylaxis of patients undergoing hip or knee surgery and for the therapy of pulmonary embolism and deep venous thrombosis.

TOXICITIES

Bleeding Bleeding is the primary untoward effect of heparin. Major bleeding occurs in 1–5% of patients treated with intravenous heparin for venous thromboembolism, somewhat less in patients treated with low-molecular-weight heparin for this indication. Often an underlying cause for bleeding is present, such as recent surgery, trauma, peptic ulcer disease, or platelet dysfunction.

The anticoagulant effect of heparin disappears within hours of drug discontinuation. Mild bleeding due to heparin usually can be controlled without the administration of an antagonist. If life-threatening hemorrhage occurs, the effect of heparin can be reversed quickly by the slow intravenous infusion of *protamine sulfate,* a mixture of basic polypeptides that bind tightly to heparin and thereby neutralize its anticoagulant effect. Use the minimal amount of protamine required to neutralize the heparin present in the plasma, ~1 mg of protamine for every 100 units of heparin remaining in the patient, giving it intravenously at a slow rate (up to 50 mg over 10 minutes).

Anaphylactic reactions occur in ~1% of patients with diabetes mellitus who have received protamine-containing insulin (*NPH insulin* or *protamine zinc insulin*) but are not limited to this group. A less common reaction consisting of pulmonary vasoconstriction, right ventricular dysfunction, systemic hypotension, and transient neutropenia also may occur after protamine administration.

Heparin-Induced Thrombocytopenia Heparin-induced thrombocytopenia (platelet count <150,000/μL or a 50% decrease from pretreatment value) occurs in ~0.5% of medical patients, typically 5–10 days after initiation of therapy with standard heparin. The incidence of thrombocytopenia is lower with low-molecular-weight heparin. Thrombotic complications that can be life-threatening or lead to amputation occur in about one-half of the affected heparin-treated patients and may precede the onset of thrombocytopenia. The incidence of heparin-induced thrombocytopenia and thrombosis is higher in surgical patients. Venous thromboembolism occurs most commonly, but arterial thromboses causing limb ischemia, myocardial infarction, and stroke also occur. Bilateral adrenal hemorrhage, skin lesions at the site of subcutaneous heparin injection, and a variety of systemic reactions may accompany heparin-induced thrombocytopenia. The development of IgG antibodies against complexes of heparin with platelet factor 4 (or, rarely, other chemokines) appears to cause all of these reactions. These complexes activate platelets by binding to FcγIIa receptors, which results in platelet aggregation, release of more platelet factor 4, and thrombin generation. The antibodies also may trigger vascular injury by binding to platelet factor 4 attached to heparan sulfate on the endothelium.

Heparin should be discontinued immediately if unexplained thrombocytopenia or any of the clinical manifestations mentioned above occur 5 or more days after beginning heparin therapy, regardless of the dose or route of administration. The onset of heparin-induced thrombocytopenia may occur earlier in patients who have received heparin within the previous 3–4 months and have residual circulating antibodies. The diagnosis of heparin-induced thrombocytopenia can be confirmed by a heparin-dependent platelet activation assay or an assay for antibodies that react with heparin/platelet factor 4 complexes. Since thrombotic complications may occur after cessation of therapy, an alternative anticoagulant such as *lepirudin, argatroban,* or *danaparoid* (*see* below) should be administered to patients with heparin-induced thrombocytopenia. Low-molecular-weight heparins should be avoided, because these drugs often cross-react with standard heparin in heparin-dependent antibody assays. Warfarin may precipitate venous limb gangrene or multicentric skin necrosis in patients with heparin-induced thrombocytopenia and should not be used until the thrombocytopenia has resolved and the patient is adequately anticoagulated with another agent.

Other Parenteral Anticoagulants

LEPIRUDIN Lepirudin (REFLUDAN) is a recombinant derivative (Leu^1-Thr^2-63-desulfohirudin) of hirudin, a direct thrombin inhibitor present in the salivary glands of the medicinal leech. It is a 65-amino-acid protein that binds tightly to both the catalytic site and the extended substrate recognition site of thrombin. Lepirudin is approved in the U.S. for treatment of patients with heparin-induced thrombocytopenia. It is administered intravenously at a dose adjusted to maintain the aPTT at 1.5–2.5 times the median of the laboratory's normal range. The drug is excreted by the kidneys with a t$_{1/2}$ of ~1.3 hours. Lepirudin should be used cautiously in patients with renal failure, since it can accumulate and cause bleeding. Occasionally, patients may develop antihirudin antibodies that paradoxically increase the aPTT; therefore, daily monitoring of the aPTT is recommended. There is no antidote for lepirudin.

BIVALIRUDIN Bivalirudin (ANGIOMAX) is a synthetic, 20-amino-acid polypeptide that directly inhibits thrombin. Bivalirudin contains the sequence Phe^1-Pro^2-Arg^3-Pro^4, which occupies the catalytic site of thrombin, followed by a polyGly linker and a hirudin-like sequence that binds to exosite I. Thrombin slowly cleaves the Arg^3-Pro^4 peptide bond and thus regains activity. Bivalirudin is administered intravenously and is used as an alternative to heparin in patients undergoing coronary angioplasty. The t$_{1/2}$ of bivalirudin in patients with normal renal function is 25 minutes; dosage reductions are recommended for patients with moderate or severe renal impairment.

ARGATROBAN Argatroban, a synthetic compound based on the structure of L-Arg, binds reversibly to the catalytic site of thrombin. Administered intravenously, it has an immediate onset of action and a t$_{1/2}$ of 40–50 minutes. Argatroban is metabolized by hepatic CYPs and is excreted in the bile; therefore dosage reduction is required for patients with hepatic insufficiency. The dosage is adjusted to maintain an aPTT of 1.5–3 times the baseline value. Argatroban can be used as an alternative to lepirudin for prophylaxis or treatment of patients with or at risk of developing heparin-induced thrombocytopenia.

DANAPAROID Danaparoid (ORGARAN) is a mixture of nonheparin glycosaminoglycans isolated from porcine intestinal mucosa (84% heparan sulfate, 12% dermatan sulfate, 4% chondroitin sulfate) with a mean mass of 5500 Da. Danaparoid is used for prophylaxis of deep venous thrombosis. It also is an effective anticoagulant for patients with heparin-induced thrombocytopenia and has a low rate of cross-reactivity with heparin in platelet-activation assays. Danaparoid mainly promotes inhibition of factor Xa by antithrombin, but it does not prolong the PT or aPTT at the recommended dosage. Danaparoid is administered subcutaneously at a fixed dose for prophylactic use and intravenously at a higher, weight-adjusted dose for full anticoagulation. Its t$_{1/2}$ is ~24 hours. Patients with renal failure may require monitoring with an anti–factor Xa assay because of a prolonged t$_{1/2}$ of the drug. No antidote is available. Danaparoid is no longer available in the U.S.

DROTRECOGIN ALFA Drotrecogin alfa (XIGRIS) is a recombinant form of human activated protein C that inhibits coagulation by proteolytic inactivation of factors Va and VIIIa. It also has anti-inflammatory effects. A 96-hour continuous infusion of drotrecogin alfa decreases mortality in adult patients at high risk for death from severe sepsis if given within 48 hours of the onset of organ dysfunction (*e.g.,* shock, hypoxemia, oliguria). The major adverse effect is bleeding.

ORAL ANTICOAGULANTS
Warfarin
CHEMISTRY

Numerous anticoagulants have been synthesized as derivatives of 4-hydroxycoumarin and of the related compound, indan-1,3-dione (Figure 54–5). Only the coumarin derivatives are widely used; the 4-hydroxycoumarin residue, with a nonpolar carbon substituent at the 3 position, is the

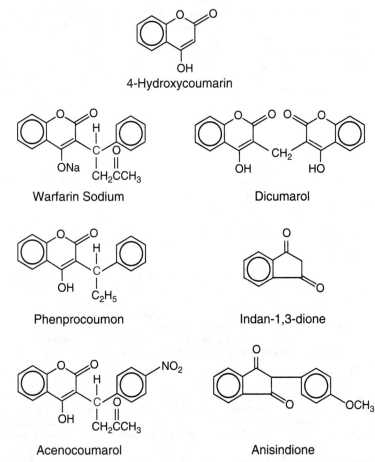

4-Hydroxycoumarin

Warfarin Sodium

Dicumarol

Phenprocoumon

Indan-1,3-dione

Acenocoumarol

Anisindione

FIGURE 54–5 *Structural formulas of the oral anticoagulants.* 4-Hydroxycoumarin and indan-1,3-dione are the parent molecules from which the oral anticoagulants are derived. The asymmetrical carbon atoms in the coumarins are shown in blue.

minimal structural requirement for activity. This carbon is asymmetrical in warfarin (and in phenprocoumon *and* acenocoumarol). *The enantiomers differ in anticoagulant potency, metabolism, elimination, and interactions with other drugs. Commercial preparations of these anticoagulants are racemic mixtures. No advantage of administering a single enantiomer has been established.*

MECHANISM OF ACTION The oral anticoagulants are antagonists of vitamin K (*see* below). Coagulation factors II, VII, IX, and X and the anticoagulant proteins C and S are synthesized mainly in the liver and are biologically inactive unless 9–13 of the amino-terminal glutamate residues are carboxylated to form the Ca^{2+}-binding γ-carboxyglutamate (Gla) residues. This reaction of the descarboxy precursor protein requires CO_2, O_2, and reduced vitamin K, and is catalyzed by γ-glutamyl carboxylase in the rough endoplasmic reticulum (Figure 54–6). Carboxylation is directly coupled to the oxidation of vitamin K to its corresponding epoxide.

Therapeutic doses of warfarin decrease by 30–50% the total amount of each vitamin K–dependent coagulation factor made by the liver; in addition, the secreted molecules are undercarboxylated, resulting in diminished biological activity (10–40% of normal). Congenital deficiencies of the procoagulant proteins to these levels cause mild bleeding disorders. Oral anticoagulants have no effect on the activity of fully carboxylated molecules in the circulation. Thus, the time required for the activity of each factor in plasma to reach a new steady state after therapy is initiated or adjusted depends on its individual rate of clearance. The approximate half-lives (in hours) are: factor VII, 6;

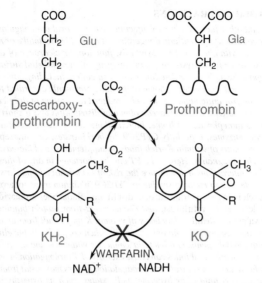

FIGURE 54–6 *The vitamin K cycle: γ-glutamyl carboxylation of vitamin K–dependent proteins.* The enzyme γ-glutamyl carboxylase couples the oxidation of the reduced hydroquinone form (KH_2) of vitamin K_1 or K_2, to γ-carboxylation of Glu residues on vitamin K–dependent proteins, generating the epoxide of vitamin K (KO) and γ-carboxyglutamate (Gla) residues in vitamin K–dependent precursor proteins in the endoplasmic reticulum. A 2,3-epoxide reductase regenerates vitamin KH_2 and is the warfarin-sensitive step. The R on the vitamin K molecule represents a 20-carbon phytyl side chain in vitamin K_1 and a 5- to 65-carbon prenyl side chain in vitamin K_2.

factor IX, 24; factor X, 36; factor II, 50; protein C, 8; and protein S, 30. Because of the long half-lives of some of the coagulation factors, in particular factor II, the full antithrombotic effect of warfarin is not achieved for several days, even though the PT may be prolonged soon after administration due to the more rapid reduction of factors with a shorter $t_{1/2}$, in particular factor VII.

DOSAGE The usual adult dose of warfarin (COUMADIN) is 5 mg/day for 2–4 days, followed by 2–10 mg/day as indicated by measurements of the INR. A lower initial dose should be given to patients with an increased risk of bleeding, including the elderly; age correlates with increased sensitivity to oral anticoagulants. Warfarin usually is administered orally but also can be given intravenously without dose modification. Intramuscular injection is not recommended because of the risk of hematoma formation.

ABSORPTION

The bioavailability of warfarin is nearly complete when the drug is administered orally, intravenously, or rectally. Different commercial preparations of warfarin tablets vary in their rate of dissolution, and this causes some variation in the rate and extent of absorption. Food in the GI tract also can decrease the rate of absorption. Warfarin usually is detectable in plasma within 1 hour of its oral administration, and concentrations peak in 2–8 hours.

DISTRIBUTION

Warfarin is almost completely (99%) bound to plasma proteins, principally albumin, and the drug distributes rapidly into a volume equivalent to the albumin space (0.14 L/kg). Concentrations in fetal plasma approach the maternal values, but active warfarin is not found in milk (unlike other coumarins and indandiones).

BIOTRANSFORMATION AND ELIMINATION

Warfarin is a racemic mixture of R (weak) and S (potent) anticoagulant enantiomers. S-warfarin is transformed into inactive metabolites by CYP2C9 and R-warfarin is transformed by CYP1A2, CYP2C19 (minor pathway), and CYP3A4 (minor pathway). The inactive metabolites of warfarin are excreted in urine and stool. The $t_{1/2}$ ranges from 25 to 60 hours (mean ~40 hours); the duration of action of warfarin is 2–5 days.

DRUG AND OTHER INTERACTIONS

The list of drugs and other factors that may affect the action of oral anticoagulants is prodigious. Any substance or condition is potentially dangerous if it alters (1) the uptake or metabolism of the oral anticoagulant or vitamin K; (2) the synthesis, function, or clearance of any factor or cell involved in hemostasis or fibrinolysis; or (3) the integrity of any epithelial surface. Patients must be educated to report the addition or deletion of any medication, including nonprescription drugs, herbal remedies and food supplements. Some of the more commonly described factors that cause a decreased effect of oral anticoagulants include: reduced absorption of drug caused by binding to cholestyramine *in the GI tract; increased volume of distribution and a short $t_{1/2}$ secondary to hypoproteinemia, as in nephrotic syndrome; increased metabolic clearance of drug secondary to induction of hepatic enzymes, especially CYP2C9, by barbiturates,* carbamazepine, *or* rifampin; *ingestion of large amounts of vitamin K–rich foods or supplements; and increased levels of coagulation factors during pregnancy. Hence, the PT can be shortened in any of these cases.*

Frequently cited interactions that enhance the risk of hemorrhage in patients taking oral anticoagulants include decreased metabolism due to CYP2C9 inhibition by amiodarone, *azole antifungals,* cimetidine, clopidogrel, cotrimoxazole, disulfiram, fluoxetine, isoniazid, metronidazole, sulfinpyrazone, tolcapone, *or* zafirlukast, *and displacement from protein binding sites caused by loop diuretics or* valproate. *Relative deficiency of vitamin K may result from inadequate diet* (e.g., *postoperative patients on parenteral fluids), especially when coupled with the elimination of intestinal flora by antimicrobial agents. Gut bacteria synthesize vitamin K and are an important source of this vitamin. Consequently, antibiotics can cause excessive PT prolongation in patients adequately controlled on warfarin. Low concentrations of coagulation factors may result from impaired hepatic function, congestive heart failure, or hypermetabolic states, such as hyperthyroidism; generally, these conditions increase the prolongation of the PT. Serious interactions that do not alter the PT include inhibition of platelet function by agents such as* aspirin *and gastritis or frank ulceration induced by anti-inflammatory drugs. Agents may have more than one effect; for example,* clofibrate *increases the rate of turnover of coagulation factors and inhibits platelet function.*

SENSITIVITY TO WARFARIN

Approximately 10% of patients require <1.5 mg/day of warfarin to achieve an INR of 2–3. These patients are more likely to possess one or two polymorphic alleles of CYP2C9, the major enzyme responsible for converting the S-enantiomer warfarin to its inactive metabolites. In comparison with the wild-type CYP2C9*1 allele, the variant alleles CYP2C9*2 and CYP2C9*3 have been shown to inactivate S-warfarin much less efficiently in vitro. The variant alleles are present in 10–20% of Caucasians, but in <5% of African Americans or Asians. Polymorphic variations in VKORC1, which encodes a component of the Vitamin K reductase complex (see Figure 54–6), also determine warfarin sensitivity.

TOXICITIES

Bleeding Bleeding is the major toxicity of oral anticoagulant drugs. The risk of bleeding increases with the intensity and duration of anticoagulant therapy, the use of other medications that interfere with hemostasis, and the presence of a potential anatomical source of bleeding. The incidence of major bleeding episodes is generally <5% per year in patients treated with a target INR of 2–3. The risk of intracranial hemorrhage increases dramatically with an INR >4, especially in older patients. In a large outpatient anticoagulation clinic, the most common factors associated with a transient elevation of the INR (>6) were use of a new medication known to potentiate warfarin (*e.g.*, acetaminophen), advanced malignancy, recent diarrheal illness, decreased oral intake, and taking more warfarin than prescribed. Patients must be informed of the signs and symptoms of bleeding, and laboratory monitoring should be done at frequent intervals during intercurrent illnesses or any changes of medication or diet.

If the INR is above the therapeutic range but <5 and the patient is not bleeding or in need of a surgical procedure, warfarin can be discontinued temporarily and restarted at a lower dose once the INR is within the therapeutic range. If the INR is ≥5, vitamin K_1 (*phytonadione,* MEPHYTON, AQUAMEPHYTON) can be given orally at a dose of 1–2.5 mg (for an INR of 5–9) or 3–5 mg (for an INR >9). These doses of oral vitamin K_1 generally cause the INR to fall substantially within 24–48 hours without rendering the patient resistant to further warfarin therapy. Higher doses may be required if more rapid correction of the INR is necessary. The effect of vitamin K_1 is delayed for at least several hours, because reversal of anticoagulation requires synthesis of fully carboxylated coagulation factors. If immediate hemostatic competence is necessary because of serious bleeding or profound warfarin overdosage (INR >20), adequate concentrations of vitamin K–dependent coagulation factors can be restored by transfusion of fresh frozen plasma (10–20 mL/kg), supplemented with 10 mg of vitamin K_1, given by slow intravenous infusion. Transfusion of plasma may need to be repeated, since the transfused factors (particularly factor VII) are cleared from the circulation more rapidly than the residual oral anticoagulant. Vitamin K_1 administered intravenously carries the risk of anaphylactoid reactions, and therefore should be used cautiously. Patients who receive high doses of vitamin K_1 may become unresponsive to warfarin for several days, but heparin can be used if continued anticoagulation is required.

Birth Defects

Administration of warfarin during pregnancy causes birth defects and abortion. Central nervous system (CNS) abnormalities have been reported following exposure during the second and third trimesters. Fetal or neonatal hemorrhage and intrauterine death may occur, even when maternal PT values are in the therapeutic range. Oral anticoagulants should not be used during pregnancy; heparin can be used safely in this circumstance.

Toxicities

A reversible, sometimes painful, bluish discoloration of the plantar surfaces and sides of the toes that blanches with pressure and fades with elevation (purple toe syndrome) may develop 3–8 weeks after initiation of therapy with warfarin; cholesterol emboli released from atheromatous plaques have been implicated as the cause. Infrequent reactions include alopecia, urticaria, dermatitis, fever, nausea, diarrhea, abdominal cramps, and anorexia.

Clinical Use

Oral anticoagulants are used to prevent the progression or recurrence of acute deep vein thrombosis or pulmonary embolism following an initial course of heparin. They also are effective in preventing venous thromboembolism in patients undergoing orthopedic or gynecological surgery and in preventing systemic embolization in patients with acute myocardial infarction, prosthetic heart valves, or chronic atrial fibrillation.

Prior to initiation of therapy, laboratory tests are used in conjunction with the patient's history and physical examination to uncover hemostatic defects that might make the use of oral anticoagulant drugs more dangerous (congenital coagulation factor deficiency, thrombocytopenia, hepatic or renal insufficiency, vascular abnormalities, *etc.*). Thereafter, the INR calculated from the patient's PT is used to monitor efficacy and compliance. Therapeutic ranges for various clinical indications have been established empirically and reflect dosages that reduce the morbidity from thromboembolic disease while minimally increasing the risk of serious hemorrhage. For most indications the target INR is 2–3. A higher target INR (*e.g.*, 2.5–3.5) generally is recommended for patients with mechanical prosthetic heart valves.

For treatment of acute venous thromboembolism, heparin usually is continued for at least 4–5 days after oral anticoagulation is begun and until the INR is in the therapeutic range on 2 consecutive days. This overlap allows for adequate depletion of the vitamin K–dependent coagulation factors with long half-lives, especially factor II. Daily INR measurements are indicated at the onset of therapy to guard against excessive anticoagulation in the unusually sensitive patient. The testing interval can be lengthened gradually to weekly and then to monthly for patients on long-term therapy in whom test results have been stable.

Other Oral Anticoagulants

PHENPROCOUMON AND ACENOCOUMAROL These agents are not available in the U.S. but are prescribed in Europe and elsewhere. Phenprocoumon (MARCUMAR) has a longer plasma $t_{1/2}$ (5 days) than warfarin, as well as a somewhat slower onset of action and a longer duration of action (7–14 days). It is administered in daily maintenance doses of 0.75–6 mg. Acenocoumarol (SINTHROME) has a shorter $t_{1/2}$ (10–24 hours), a more rapid effect on the PT, and a shorter duration of action (2 days). The maintenance dose is 1–8 mg daily.

XIMELAGATRAN *Ximelagatran* is a novel drug that is readily absorbed after oral administration and is rapidly metabolized to *melagatran*, a direct thrombin inhibitor. The drug has not yet been approved for use in the U.S.

FIBRINOLYTIC DRUGS

The fibrinolytic pathway is summarized by Figure 54–3. The action of fibrinolytic agents is best understood in conjunction with an understanding of the characteristics of the physiologic components.

PLASMINOGEN

Plasminogen is a single-chain glycoprotein of 791 amino acids; it is converted to an active protease by cleavage at Arg 560. High-affinity binding sites mediate the binding of plasminogen (or plasmin) to carboxyl-terminal Lys residues in partially degraded fibrin; this enhances fibrinolysis. A plasma carboxypeptidase termed thrombin-activatable fibrinolysis inhibitor *(TAFI) can remove these Lys residues and thereby attenuate fibrinolysis. The Lys binding sites are in the amino-terminal "kringle" domain of plasminogen, and they also promote formation of complexes of plasmin with* α_2-antiplasmin, *the major physiological plasmin inhibitor. A degraded form of plasminogen termed* Lys-plasminogen *binds to fibrin more rapidly than does intact plasminogen.*

α_2-ANTIPLASMIN

α_2-Antiplasmin *is a 452 amino acid glycoprotein that forms a stable complex with plasmin, thereby inactivating it. Plasma concentrations of* α_2-antiplasmin *(1 μM) are sufficient to inhibit ~50% of potential plasmin. When massive activation of plasminogen occurs, the inhibitor is depleted, and free plasmin causes a "systemic lytic state," in which hemostasis is impaired. In this state, fibrinogen is destroyed and fibrinogen degradation products impair formation of fibrin and therefore increase bleeding from wounds.* α_2-Antiplasmin *inactivates plasmin nearly instantaneously, as long as the Lys binding sites on plasmin are unoccupied by fibrin or other antagonists, such as* aminocaproic acid *(see below).*

STREPTOKINASE *Streptokinase* (STREPTASE) is a 47,000 Da protein produced by β-hemolytic streptococci. It forms a stable, noncovalent 1:1 complex with plasminogen, producing a conformational change that exposes the active site on plasminogen that cleaves Arg 560 on free plasminogen to form free plasmin. Streptokinase is rarely used clinically for fibrinolysis since the advent of newer agents.

TISSUE PLASMINOGEN ACTIVATOR (t-PA) t-PA is a serine protease that is a poor plasminogen activator in the absence of fibrin. t-PA binds to fibrin *via* Lys binding sites at its amino terminus and activates bound plasminogen several hundredfold more rapidly than it activates plasminogen in the circulation. The Lys binding sites on t-PA are in a "finger" domain that is homologous to similar sites on fibronectin. Under physiological conditions (t-PA concentrations of 5–10 ng/mL), the specificity of t-PA for fibrin limits systemic formation of plasmin and induction of a systemic lytic state. During therapeutic infusions of t-PA, however, concentrations rise to 300–3000 ng/mL. Clearance of t-PA primarily occurs by hepatic metabolism, with a $t_{1/2}$ of 5–10 minutes. t-PA is effective in lysing thrombi during treatment of acute myocardial infarction. t-PA (*alteplase,* ACTIVASE) is produced by recombinant DNA technology. The currently recommended ("accelerated") regimen for coronary thrombolysis is a 15 mg intravenous bolus, followed by 0.75 mg/kg of body weight over 30 minutes (not to exceed 50 mg) and 0.5 mg/kg (up to 35 mg accumulated dose) over the following hour. Recombinant mutant variants of t-PA are available (*reteplase,* RETAVASE and *tenecteplase,* TNKASE). They differ from native t-PA by having increased plasma half-lives that allow convenient bolus dosing (2 doses of 15 milliunits given 30 minutes apart). They also are relatively resistant to inhibition by plasma activator inhibitor-1. Despite these apparent advantages, these agents are similar to t-PA in efficacy and toxicity.

HEMORRHAGIC TOXICITY OF THROMBOLYTIC THERAPY The major toxicity of all thrombolytic agents is hemorrhage, which results from two factors: (1) the lysis of fibrin in "physiological thrombi" at sites of vascular injury; and (2) a systemic lytic state that results from systemic formation of plasmin, which produces fibrinogenolysis and destruction of other coagulation factors (especially factors V and VIII). The actual toxicities of streptokinase and t-PA are difficult to assess. In early clinical trials, many bleeding episodes resulted from the extensive invasive monitoring of therapy that was required by the protocol. Many studies to evaluate thrombolysis involved concurrent systemic heparinization, which also contributes to bleeding complications. Analysis of more recent clinical trials suggests that heparin confers no benefit in patients receiving fibrinolytic therapy plus aspirin.

The contraindications to fibrinolytic therapy are listed in Table 54–1. Patients with these conditions should not receive such treatment, and invasive procedures (*e.g.,* cardiac catheterization and arterial blood gases) should be avoided. If heparin is used concurrently with either streptokinase or t-PA, serious hemorrhage will occur in 2–4% of patients. Intracranial hemorrhage is by far the most serious problem. Hemorrhagic stroke occurs with all regimens and is more common when heparin is used. The efficacies of t-PA and streptokinase in treating myocardial infarction are essentially identical, with ~30% reductions in death and reinfarction in regimens containing aspirin.

Table 54–1

Contraindications to Thrombolytic Therapy

1. Surgery within 10 days, including organ biopsy, puncture of noncompressible vessels, serious trauma, cardiopulmonary resuscitation
2. Serious gastrointestinal bleeding within 3 months
3. History of hypertension (diastolic pressure >110 mm Hg)
4. Active bleeding or hemorrhagic disorder
5. Previous cerebrovascular accident or active intracranial process
6. Aortic dissection
7. Acute pericarditis

Inhibition of Fibrinolysis

AMINOCAPROIC ACID

Aminocaproic acid (AMICAR) is a Lys analog that competes for Lys binding sites on plasminogen and plasmin, thus blocking the interaction of plasmin with fibrin. Aminocaproic acid is thereby a potent inhibitor of fibrinolysis and can reverse states that are associated with excessive fibrinolysis. The main problem with its use is that thrombi that form during treatment with the drug are not lysed. For example, in patients with hematuria, ureteral obstruction by clots may lead to renal failure after treatment with aminocaproic acid. Aminocaproic acid has been used to reduce bleeding after prostatic surgery or after tooth extractions in hemophiliacs. Aminocaproic acid is absorbed rapidly after oral administration, and 50% is excreted unchanged in the urine within 12 hours. For intravenous use, a loading dose of 4–5 g is given over 1 hour, followed by an infusion of 1 g/h until bleeding is controlled. No more than 30 g should be given in a 24-hour period. Rarely, the drug causes myopathy and muscle necrosis.

ANTIPLATELET DRUGS

Platelets provide the initial hemostatic plug at sites of vascular injury. They also participate in pathological thromboses that lead to myocardial infarction, stroke, and peripheral vascular thromboses. Potent inhibitors of platelet function have been developed. These drugs act by discrete mechanisms, and thus in combination their effects are additive or even synergistic. Their availability has led to a revolution in cardiovascular medicine, whereby angioplasty and vascular stenting of lesions now is feasible with low rates of restenosis and thrombosis when effective platelet inhibition is employed.

ASPIRIN

In platelets, the major cyclooxygenase product is thromboxane A_2, a labile inducer of platelet aggregation and a potent vasoconstrictor. Aspirin blocks production of thromboxane A_2 by acetylating a Ser residue near the active site of platelet cyclooxygenase (COX-1). Since platelets do not synthesize new proteins, the action of aspirin on platelet cyclooxygenase is permanent, lasting for the life of the platelet (7–10 days). Thus, repeated doses of aspirin produce a cumulative effect on platelet function. Complete inactivation of platelet COX-1 is achieved when 160 mg of aspirin is taken daily. Therefore, aspirin is maximally effective as an antithrombotic agent at doses much lower than those required for other actions of the drug. Numerous trials indicate that aspirin, used as an antithrombotic drug, is maximally effective at doses of 50–320 mg/day. Higher doses do not improve efficacy and potentially are less efficacious because of inhibition of prostacyclin production, which can be largely spared by using lower doses of aspirin. Higher doses also increase toxicity, especially bleeding.

Other nonsteroidal anti-inflammatory drugs (NSAIDs) that are reversible inhibitors of COX-1 have not been shown to have antithrombotic efficacy and in fact may even interfere with low-dose aspirin regimens.

DIPYRIDAMOLE

Dipyridamole *(PERSANTINE) is a vasodilator that, in combination with warfarin, inhibits embolization from prosthetic heart valves. A single study suggests that dipyridamole plus aspirin reduces strokes in patients with prior strokes or transient ischemic attack. A formulation containing 200 mg of dipyridamole, in an extended-release form, and 25 mg of aspirin (AGGRENOX) is available.*

Dipyridamole interferes with platelet function by increasing the cellular concentration of cyclic AMP. This effect is mediated by inhibition of cyclic nucleotide PDEs and/or by blockade of uptake of adenosine, which acts at adenosine A_2 receptors to stimulate platelet adenylyl cyclase. The only recommended use of dipyridamole is in combination with warfarin for postoperative primary prophylaxis of thromboemboli in patients with prosthetic heart valves.

TICLOPIDINE The agonists of purinergic receptors are extracellular nucleotides. Platelets contain two purinergic receptors, $P2Y_1$ and $P2Y_{12}$; both are GPCRs for ADP. The ADP-activated platelet $P2Y_1$ receptor couples to the G_q-PLC-IP_3-Ca^{2+} pathway and induces a shape change and aggregation. Activation of the $P2Y_{12}$ receptor by ADP couples *via* G_i to inhibit adenylyl cyclase, resulting in lower levels of cyclic AMP and thereby less cyclic AMP–dependent inhibition of platelet activation. Apparently, both receptors must be stimulated for platelet activation, and inhibition of either receptor is sufficient to block platelet activation. *Ticlopidine* (TICLID) is a thienopyridine that inhibits the $P2Y_{12}$ receptor. Ticlopidine is a prodrug that requires conversion to the active thiol metabolite by a hepatic CYP. It is rapidly absorbed and highly bioavailable. It permanently inhibits the $P2Y_{12}$ receptor by forming a disulfide bridge between the thiol on the drug and a free Cys residue in the extracellular region of the receptor; thus, the effect is prolonged, even though the free drug has a short $t_{1/2}$. Maximal inhibition of platelet aggregation is not seen until 8–11 days after starting therapy; loading doses of 500 mg sometimes are given to achieve a more rapid onset of action. The usual dose is 250 mg twice/day. Inhibition of platelet aggregation persists for a few days after the drug is stopped.

Adverse Effects

The most common side effects are nausea, vomiting, and diarrhea. The most serious is severe neutropenia (absolute neutrophil count <1500/μL), which occurred in 2.4% of stroke patients given the drug during premarketing clinical trials. Fatal agranulocytosis with thrombopenia can occur within the first 3 months of therapy; therefore, frequent blood counts should be obtained during the first few months of therapy, with immediate discontinuation of therapy if cell counts decline. Platelet counts also should be monitored. Rare cases of thrombotic thrombocytopenic purpura (TTP)-hemolytic uremic syndrome have been associated with ticlopidine, with a reported incidence of 1 in 1600–4800 patients when the drug is used after cardiac stenting; the mortality associated with these cases is reported to be as high as 18–57%. Remission of TTP has been reported when the drug is stopped.

Therapeutic Uses

Ticlopidine has been shown to prevent cerebrovascular events in secondary prevention of stroke and is at least as good as aspirin in this regard. Ticlopidine also reduces cardiac events in patients with unstable angina; however, its only FDA-approved indication is to reduce the risk of thrombotic stroke in patients who have experienced stroke precursors and in patients who have had a completed thrombotic stroke. Since ticlopidine has a mechanism of action distinct from that of aspirin, combining the drugs should produce additive or even synergistic effects. This appears to be the case, and the combination has been used in patients undergoing angioplasty and stenting for coronary artery disease, with a very low (<1%) frequency of stent thrombosis occurring over a short, 30-day follow-up . As ticlopidine is associated with life-threatening blood dyscrasias and a relatively high rate of TTP, it is generally reserved for patients who are intolerant or allergic to aspirin or who have failed aspirin therapy.

CLOPIDOGREL The thienopyridine clopidogrel (PLAVIX) is closely related to ticlopidine and appears to have a slightly more favorable toxicity profile with less frequent thrombocytopenia and leukopenia, although TTP has been reported. Clopidogrel is a prodrug with a slow onset of action. The usual dose is 75 mg/day with or without an initial loading dose of 300 mg. The drug is equivalent to aspirin in the secondary prevention of stroke, and in combination with aspirin it appears to be as effective as ticlopidine and aspirin. It is used with aspirin after angioplasty and should be continued for at least 1 year. In one study, the combination of clopidogrel and aspirin clearly was superior to aspirin alone; this finding suggests that the actions of the two drugs are synergistic. FDA-approved indications for clopidogrel are to reduce the rate of stroke, myocardial infarction (MI), and death in patients with recent MI or stroke, established peripheral arterial disease, or acute coronary syndrome.

GLYCOPROTEIN IIb/IIIa INHIBITORS Glycoprotein IIb/IIIa is a platelet-surface integrin designated $\alpha_{IIb}\beta_3$. This dimeric glycoprotein is a receptor for fibrinogen and von Willebrand factor, which anchor platelets to foreign surfaces and to each other, thereby mediating aggregation.

The integrin heterodimer/receptor is activated by platelet agonists such as thrombin, collagen, or thromboxane A_2 to develop binding sites for its ligands, which do not bind to resting platelets. Inhibition of binding to this receptor blocks platelet aggregation induced by any agonist. Thus, inhibitors of this receptor are potent antiplatelet agents that act by a mechanism distinct from that of aspirin or the thienopyridine platelet inhibitors. Three agents are approved for use at present, with others under development.

ABCIXIMAB *Abciximab* (REOPRO) is the Fab fragment of a humanized monoclonal antibody directed against the $\alpha_{IIb}\beta_3$ receptor. It also binds to the vitronectin receptor on platelets, vascular endothelial cells, and smooth muscle cells. The antibody is used in conjunction with percutaneous angioplasty for coronary thromboses, and when used in conjunction with aspirin and heparin, has been shown to be quite effective in preventing restenosis, recurrent myocardial infarction, and death. The reduction in total events is ~50% in various large trials. The unbound antibody is cleared from the circulation with a $t_{1/2}$ of ~30 minutes, but antibody remains bound to the $\alpha_{IIb}\beta_3$ receptor and inhibits platelet aggregation as measured *in vitro* for 18–24 hours after infusion is stopped. It is given as a 0.25-mg/kg bolus followed by 0.125 μg/kg/min for 12 hours or longer.

Adverse Effects

The major side effect of abciximab is bleeding, and contraindications are similar to those for fibrinolytic agents. The frequency of major hemorrhage in clinical trials varies from 1% to 10%, depending on the intensity of anticoagulation with heparin. Thrombocytopenia of <50,000 platelets/μL is seen in ~2% of patients and may be due to development of neo-epitopes induced by bound antibody. Since the duration of action is long, if major bleeding or emergent surgery occurs, platelet transfusions can reverse the aggregation defect, because free antibody concentrations fall rapidly after cessation of infusion. Readministration of antibody has been performed in a small number of patients without evidence of decreased efficacy or allergic reactions.

Eptifibatide *Eptifibatide* (INTEGRILIN) is a cyclic peptide inhibitor of the fibrinogen binding site on $\alpha_{IIb}\beta_3$. The drug blocks platelet aggregation *in vitro* after intravenous infusion. Eptifibatide is given as a bolus of 180 μg/kg followed by 2 μg/kg/min for up to 96 hours. It is used to treat acute coronary syndrome and for angioplastic coronary interventions. In the latter case, myocardial infarction and death have been reduced by ~20%. Although direct comparisons are lacking, the benefit from eptifibatide seems to be somewhat less than that obtained with abciximab, perhaps because eptifibatide is specific for $\alpha_{IIb}\beta_3$ and does not react with the vitronectin receptor. The duration of action of the drug is relatively short and platelet aggregation is restored within 6–12 hours after cessation of infusion. Eptifibatide generally is administered in conjunction with aspirin and heparin.

Adverse Effects

The major side effect is bleeding. The frequency of major bleeding in trials was ~10%, compared with ~9% in a placebo group, which included heparin. Thrombocytopenia has been seen in 0.5–1% of patients.

Tirofiban *Tirofiban* (AGGRASTAT) is a nonpeptide, small-molecule inhibitor of $\alpha_{IIb}\beta_3$ that appears to have a similar mechanism of action as eptifibatide. Tirofiban has a short duration of action and has efficacy in non-Q-wave myocardial infarction and unstable angina. Reductions in death and myocardial infarction have been ~20% compared to placebo, results similar to those with eptifibatide. Side effects also are similar to those of eptifibatide. The agent is specific to $\alpha_{IIb}\beta_3$ and does not react with the vitronectin receptor. Meta-analysis of trials using $\alpha_{IIb}\beta_3$ inhibitors suggests that their value in antiplatelet therapy after acute myocardial infarction is limited. Tirofiban is administered intravenously at an initial rate of 0.4 μg/kg/min for 30 minutes, and then continued at 0.1 mg/kg/min for 12–24 hours after angioplasty or atherectomy. It is used in conjunction with heparin.

THE ROLE OF VITAMIN K

Green plants are a nutritional source of vitamin K, an essential cofactor in the γ-carboxylation of multiple Glu residues of several clotting factors and anticoagulant proteins. The vitamin K–dependent formation of γ-carboxy-glutamate (Gla) residues permits the appropriate interactions of clotting factors, Ca^{2+}, and membrane phospholipids and modulator proteins (Figures 54–1, 54–2, and 54–3). Oral anticoagulant drugs (*e.g.,* coumadin, Figure 54–5) block Gla formation and thereby inhibit clotting; excess vitamin K_1 can reverse these effects.

CHEMISTRY AND OCCURRENCE

Vitamin K activity is associated with at least two distinct natural substances, designated as vitamin K_1 and vitamin K_2. Vitamin K_1, or phylloquinone (phytonadione), *is 2-methyl-3-phytyl-1, 4-naphthoquinone; it is found in plants and is the only natural vitamin K available for therapeutic use. Vitamin K_2 is actually a series of compounds (the menaquinones) in which the phytyl side chain of phylloquinone has been replaced by a side chain built up of 2–13 prenyl units. Considerable synthesis of menaquinones occurs in gram-positive bacteria; indeed, intestinal flora synthesize the large amounts of vitamin K contained in human and animal feces. In animals, menaquinone-4 can be synthesized from the vitamin precursor menadione (2-methyl-1,4-naphthoquinone), or vitamin K_3. Depending on the bioassay system used, menadione is at least as active on a molar basis as phylloquinone.*

PHYSIOLOGICAL FUNCTIONS AND PHARMACOLOGICAL ACTIONS

Phylloquinone and menaquinones are virtually devoid of pharmacodynamic activity. However, in subjects deficient in vitamin K, the vitamin performs its normal physiological function: to promote the biosynthesis of the γ-carboxy-glutamate (Gla) forms of factors II (prothrombin), VII, IX, and X, anticoagulant proteins C and S, protein Z (a cofactor to the inhibitor of Xa), the bone Gla protein osteocalcin, matrix Gla protein, and growth arrest–specific protein 6 (Gas6). Figure 54–6 summarizes the coupling of the vitamin K cycle with glutamate carboxylation. Vitamin K, as KH_2, the reduced hydroquinone, is an essential cofactor for γ-glutamyl carboxylase. Using KH_2, O_2, CO_2, and the glutamate-containing substrate, the enzyme forms a γ-carboxy-glutamatyl protein (Gla protein) and concomitantly, the 2,3-epoxide of vitamin K. A coumarin-sensitive 2,3-epoxide reductase regenerates KH_2. The γ-glutamyl carboxylase and epoxide reductase are integral membrane proteins of the endoplasmic reticulum and function as a multicomponent complex. Two natural mutations in γ-glutamyl carboxylase lead to bleeding disorders. With respect to proteins affecting blood coagulation, these reactions occur in the liver, but γ-carboxylation of Glu also occurs in lung, bone, and other cell types.

HUMAN REQUIREMENTS

In patients made vitamin K–deficient by a starvation diet and antibiotic therapy for 3–4 weeks, the minimum daily requirement is estimated to be 0.03 μg/kg of body weight and possibly as high as 1 μg/kg, which is approximately the recommended intake for adults (70 μg/day).

SYMPTOMS OF DEFICIENCY

*The chief manifestation of vitamin K deficiency is an increased bleeding tendency (*see discussion of hypoprothrombinemia in section on oral anticoagulants, above*). Ecchymoses, epistaxis, hematuria, GI bleeding, and postoperative hemorrhage are common; intracranial hemorrhage may occur. Hemoptysis is uncommon. The discovery of a vitamin K–dependent protein in bone suggests that the fetal bone abnormalities associated with the administration of oral anticoagulants during the first trimester of pregnancy ("fetal warfarin syndrome") may be related to a deficiency of the vitamin.*

Evidence indicates a role for vitamin K in adult skeletal maintenance and osteoporosis. Low concentrations of the vitamin are associated with deficits in bone mineral density and fractures; vitamin K supplementation increases the carboxylation state of osteocalcin and also improves bone mineral density, but the relationship of these two effects is unclear. Bone mineral density in adults is not changed by therapeutic use of oral anticoagulants, but new bone formation may be impaired.

ABSORPTION, FATE, AND EXCRETION

The mechanism of intestinal absorption of compounds with vitamin K activity varies with their solubility. In the presence of bile salts, phylloquinone and the menaquinones are adequately absorbed from the intestine, almost entirely by way of the lymph. Phylloquinone is absorbed by an energy-dependent, saturable process in proximal portions of the small intestine; menaquinones are absorbed by diffusion in the distal portions of the small intestine and in the colon. Following absorption, phylloquinone is incorporated into chylomicrons in close association with triglycerides and lipoproteins. The extremely low phylloquinone levels in newborns may be partly related to very low plasma lipoprotein concentrations at birth and may lead to an underestimation of vitamin K tissue stores. Absorbed phylloquinone and menaquinones are concentrated in the liver, but the concentration of phylloquinone declines rapidly. Menaquinones, produced in the lower bowel, are less biologically active than phylloquinone due to their long side chain. Very little vitamin K accumulates in other tissues.

Apparently, there is only modest storage of vitamin K in the body. Under circumstances in which lack of bile interferes with absorption of vitamin K, hypoprothrombinemia develops slowly over a period of several weeks.

THERAPEUTIC USES

Vitamin K is used therapeutically to correct the bleeding tendency or hemorrhage associated with its deficiency. Vitamin K deficiency can result from inadequate intake, absorption, or utilization of the vitamin, or as a consequence of the action of a vitamin K antagonist.

Phylloquinone (AQUAMEPHYTON, KONAKION, MEPHYTON) is available as tablets and in a dispersion with buffered polysorbate and propylene glycol (KONAKION) or polyoxyethylated fatty acid derivatives and dextrose (AQUAMEPHYTON). KONAKION is administered only intramuscularly. AQUAMEPHYTON should be given by subcutaneous or intramuscular injection because severe reactions resembling anaphylaxis have followed its intravenous administration.

Inadequate Intake

After infancy, coagulopathy due to dietary deficiency of vitamin K is extremely rare: Vitamin K is present in many foods and also is synthesized by intestinal bacteria. Occasionally, the use of a broad-spectrum antibiotic may produce a hypoprothrombinemia that responds readily to small doses of vitamin K and reestablishment of normal bowel flora. Hypoprothrombinemia can occur in patients receiving prolonged intravenous alimentation. Patients on total parenteral nutrition should receive phylloquinone (1 mg/week, the equivalent of ~150 µg/day).

Hypoprothrombinemia of the Newborn

Healthy newborn infants show decreased plasma concentrations of vitamin K–dependent clotting factors for a few days after birth, the time required to obtain an adequate dietary intake of the vitamin and to establish a normal intestinal flora. In premature infants and in infants with hemorrhagic disease of the newborn, the concentrations of clotting factors are particularly depressed, possibly reflecting vitamin K deficiency. Measurements of non-γ-carboxylated prothrombin suggest that true vitamin K deficiency occurs in ~3% of live births.

Hemorrhagic disease of the newborn has been associated with breast-feeding; human milk has low concentrations of vitamin K. In addition, the intestinal flora of breast-fed infants may lack microorganisms that synthesize the vitamin. Commercial infant formulas are supplemented with vitamin K.

In the neonate with hemorrhagic disease of the newborn, the administration of vitamin K raises the concentration of these clotting factors to the level normal for the newborn infant and controls the bleeding tendency within ~6 hours. The routine administration of 1 mg phylloquinone intramuscularly at birth is required by law in the U.S.. This dose may have to be increased or repeated if the mother has received anticoagulant or anticonvulsant drug therapy or if the infant develops bleeding tendencies. Alternatively, some clinicians treat mothers who are receiving anticonvulsants with oral vitamin K prior to delivery (10–20 mg/day for 2 weeks).

Inadequate Absorption

Vitamin K is poorly absorbed in the absence of bile. Thus, hypoprothrombinemia may be associated with either intrahepatic or extrahepatic biliary obstruction or a severe defect in the intestinal absorption of fat from other causes.

Biliary Obstruction or Fistula

Bleeding that accompanies obstructive jaundice or biliary fistula responds promptly to the administration of vitamin K. Oral phylloquinone administered with bile salts is both safe and effective and should be used in the care of the jaundiced patient, both preoperatively and postoperatively. In the absence of significant hepatocellular disease, the prothrombin activity of the blood rapidly returns to normal. If oral administration is not feasible, a parenteral preparation of vitamin K should be used; the usual dose is 10 mg/day.

Malabsorption Syndromes

Among the disorders that result in inadequate absorption of vitamin K from the GI tract are: cystic fibrosis, sprue, inflammatory bowel disease, dysentery, and extensive bowel resection. Since drugs that greatly reduce the bacterial population of the bowel are used frequently in these disorders, the availability of the vitamin may be further reduced. Moreover, dietary restrictions also may limit the availability of the vitamin. For immediate correction of the deficiency, parenteral therapy should be used.

Drug-Induced Hypoprothrombinemia

Anticoagulant drugs such as warfarin act as competitive antagonists of vitamin K and interfere with the hepatic biosynthesis of Gla-containing clotting factors. The treatment of bleeding caused by oral anticoagulants is discussed above. Vitamin K may be of help in combating the bleeding and hypoprothrombinemia that follow the bite of the tropical American pit viper or other species whose venom destroys or inactivates prothrombin.

For a complete Bibliographical listing see Goodman & Gilman's *The Pharmacological Basis of Therapeutics*, 11th ed., or Goodman & Gilman Online at www.accessmedicine.com.

55

PITUITARY HORMONES AND THEIR HYPOTHALAMIC RELEASING HORMONES

Anterior pituitary hormones are classified into three different groups based on their structural features. *Growth hormone* (GH) and *prolactin* (PRL) belong to the somatotropic family, which in humans also includes *placental lactogen*. The glycoprotein hormones—*thyroid-stimulating hormone* (TSH, also called thyrotropin), *luteinizing hormone* (LH), and *follicle-stimulating hormone* (FSH)—share a common α-subunit but have different β-subunits that determine their distinct biological activities. Placenta-derived *human chorionic gonadotropin* (hCG) also is a member of the glycoprotein hormone family. *Corticotropin* (adrenocorticotropic hormone; ACTH) and α-*melanocyte-stimulating hormone* (α-MSH) are part of a family of peptides derived from *pro-opiomelanocortin* (POMC) by proteolytic processing (*see* Chapter 21). *Hypothalamic releasing hormones*, peptides released by hypothalamic neurons in the median eminence, positively regulate the secretion of anterior pituitary hormones. These releasing factors include *growth hormone-releasing hormone* (GHRH), *gonadotropin-releasing hormone* (GnRH), *thyroid-releasing hormone* (TRH), and *corticotropin-releasing hormone* (CRH). The hypothalamic peptide *somatostatin* (SST) negatively regulates pituitary secretion of GH and TSH.

The posterior pituitary gland, also known as the neurohypophysis, contains the endings of nerve axons arising from distinct populations of neurons in the supraoptic and paraventricular nuclei that synthesize either *arginine vasopressin* or *oxytocin*. Arginine vasopressin plays an important role in water homeostasis (*see* Chapter 29); oxytocin plays important roles in labor and parturition and in milk letdown, as discussed below.

GROWTH HORMONE

Growth hormone, the most abundant anterior pituitary hormone, is synthesized and secreted by somatotropes, which account for about 40% of hormone-secreting cells of the anterior pituitary. Due to alternative splicing of the GH gene, the anterior pituitary secretes a heterogeneous mixture of GH peptides; an appreciable fraction of which circulates bound to a protein corresponding to the extracellular domain of the GH receptor. Bound GH has a biological $t_{1/2}$ ten times that of unbound GH, suggesting that the binding protein may provide a reservoir that dampens acute fluctuations in GH levels associated with its pulsatile secretion. Obesity and estrogen treatment increase circulating levels of GH binding proteins and thus may affect the clinical response to exogenous GH.

Regulation of Growth Hormone Secretion

Daily GH secretion varies throughout life; secretion is high in children, reaches maximal levels at puberty, and then declines in an age-related manner in adulthood. GH is secreted in discrete but irregular pulses. The amplitude of secretory pulses is maximal at night; the most consistent period of GH secretion is shortly after the onset of deep sleep.

The regulation of GH secretion (Figure 55–1) incorporates many of the features of the classic negative feedback systems seen in other endocrine axes. GH and its predominant peripheral effector, insulin-like growth factor-1 (IGF-1), act in negative feedback loops to suppress GH secretion. IGF-1 predominantly inhibits GH secretion through direct effects on the anterior pituitary gland. Somatostatin (SST) and ghrelin also contribute to the negative regulation of GH.

Ghrelin is a 28-amino-acid peptide, octanoylated at Ser³, that is synthesized by endocrine cells in the fundus of the stomach and stimulates appetite and food intake through central mechanisms.

SST is synthesized by widely distributed neurons, as well as by neuroendocrine cells in the gastrointestinal (GI) tract and pancreas. SST is synthesized as a prohormone precursor and processed by proteolytic cleavage to generate two predominant forms: SST-14 and SST-28. The somatostatins exert their effects by binding to and activating a family of five related GPCRs that signal through G_i to inhibit cyclic AMP accumulation and to activate K^+ channels and phosphotyrosine phosphatases.

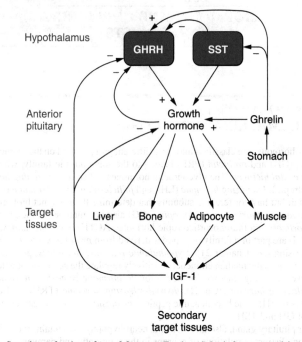

FIGURE 55–1 *Secretion and actions of growth hormone.* Two hypothalamic factors, growth hormone-releasing hormone (GHRH) and somatostatin (SST), act on the somatotropes in the anterior pituitary to regulate growth hormone secretion. SST also inhibits GHRH release. Growth hormone exerts direct effects on target tissues and indirect effects mediated by stimulating the release of insulin-like growth factor-1 (IGF-1). The gastric peptide ghrelin enhances growth hormone release, directly by actions at the anterior pituitary and indirectly by multiple actions on the hypothalamus. IGF-1 feeds back at the anterior pituitary to inhibit growth hormone secretion and at the hypothalamus to inhibit further GHRH release.

Each of the SST receptor subtypes (abbreviated SSTR or sstr) binds SST with nanomolar affinity; whereas receptor types 1–4 (SSTR1–4) bind the two SSTs with approximately equal affinity, type 5 (SSTR5) has a 10–15-fold greater selectivity for SST-28. SSTR2 and SSTR5 are the most important for regulation of GH secretion. SST exerts direct effects on somatotropes in the pituitary and indirect effects mediated *via* GHRH neurons in the arcuate nucleus. As discussed below, SST analogs play a key role in the therapy of syndromes of GH excess.

Several neurotransmitters, drugs, metabolites, and other stimuli modulate the release of GHRH and/or SST and thereby affect GH secretion. Dopamine, 5-hydroxytryptamine, and α_2 adrenergic receptor agonists stimulate GH release, as do hypoglycemia, exercise, stress, emotional excitement, and ingestion of protein-rich meals. In contrast, β adrenergic receptor agonists, free fatty acids, IGF-1, and GH itself inhibit release, as does the administration of glucose to normal subjects in an oral glucose tolerance test.

These observations form the basis for provocative tests to assess the ability of the pituitary to secrete GH. Provocative stimuli include Arg, glucagon, insulin-induced hypoglycemia, clonidine, and the dopamine precursor levodopa; each can increase circulating GH levels in normal subjects within 45–90 minutes.

Molecular and Cellular Bases of Growth Hormone Action

All effects of GH result from its interactions with the GH receptor, as evidenced by the severe phenotype of rare patients with homozygous mutations of the GH receptor gene (the Laron syndrome of GH-resistant dwarfism). The GH receptor is a widely distributed cell-surface receptor that belongs to the cytokine receptor superfamily. Like other members of the cytokine receptor family, the GH receptor contains an extracellular domain that binds GH, a single membrane-spanning

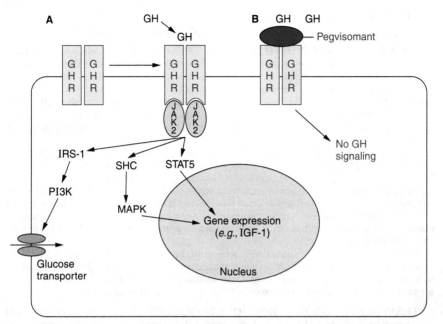

FIGURE 55–2 *Mechanisms of growth hormone and prolactin action and of GH receptor antagonism.* **A.** The binding of GH to two molecules of the growth hormone receptor (GHR) induces autophosphorylation of JAK2. JAK2 then phosphorylates cytoplasmic proteins that activate downstream signaling pathways, including STAT5 and mediators upstream of mitogen-activated protein kinase (MAPK), which ultimately modulate gene expression. The structurally related prolactin receptor also is a ligand-activated homodimer that recruits the JAK-STAT signaling pathway (*see* text for further details). The GHR also activates the IRS-1, which may mediate the increased expression of glucose transporters on the plasma membrane. The diagram does not reflect the localization of the intracellular molecules, which presumably exist in multicomponent signaling complexes. **B.** Pegvisomant, a recombinant pegylated variant of human GH, contains mutations that increase the affinity for the GHR but do not activate downstream signaling by the GHR. It thus interferes with GH signaling in target tissues. JAK2, Janus kinase 2; IRS-1, insulin receptor substrate-1; PI3K, phosphatidyl inositol-3 kinase; STAT, signal transducer and activator of transcription; MAPK, mitogen-activated protein kinase; SHC, Src homology containing.

region, and an intracellular domain that mediates signal transduction. Receptor activation results from the binding of a single GH molecule to two identical receptor molecules, forming a ligand-occupied receptor dimer that presumably brings the intracellular domains of the receptors into close proximity to activate cytosolic components critical for cell signaling.

The ligand-occupied receptor dimer does not have inherent tyrosine kinase activity but, rather, provides docking sites for 2 molecules of JAK2, a cytoplasmic tyrosine kinase of the Janus kinase family. The juxtaposition of 2 JAK2 molecules leads to *trans*-phosphorylation and autoactivation of JAK2, with consequent tyrosine phosphorylation of cytoplasmic proteins that mediate downstream signaling events (Figure 55–2).

Physiological Effects of Growth Hormone

The most striking physiological effect of GH is the stimulation of the longitudinal growth of bones. GH also increases bone mineral density after longitudinal growth ceases and epiphyses have closed. GH stimulates myoblast differentiation (in experimental animals), increases muscle mass (in human subjects with GH deficiency), increases glomerular filtration rate, and stimulates preadipocyte differentiation into adipocytes.

GH acts directly on adipocytes to increase lipolysis and on hepatocytes to stimulate gluconeogenesis, but its anabolic and growth-promoting effects are mediated indirectly through the induction of IGF-1 (Figure 55–2). The U.S. Food and Drug Administration (FDA) has approved a new drug application for recombinant human IGF-1 to treat short stature in patients resistant to GH (*see* below).

Clinical Disorders of Growth Hormone

Both GH deficiency and excess are associated with defined diseases in human beings.

INDICATIONS FOR GROWTH HORMONE TREATMENT   GH deficiency in children is a well-accepted cause of short stature; replacement therapy is used to treat children with severe GH deficiency. GH therapy has been extended to children with other conditions associated with short stature despite adequate GH production, including Turner's syndrome, Prader-Willi syndrome (in the absence of morbid obesity or obstructive sleep apnea), chronic renal insufficiency, children born small for gestational age, and children with idiopathic short stature (*i.e.,* more than 2.25 standard deviations below mean height for age and sex but normal laboratory indices of GH levels).

In adults, GH deficiency is associated with a defined endocrinopathy that includes increased mortality from cardiovascular causes, probably secondary to deleterious changes in fat distribution, increases in circulating lipids, and increased inflammation; decreased muscle mass and exercise capacity; decreased bone density; and impaired psychosocial function. In GH-deficient adults, the consensus is that the most severely affected GH-deficient adults may benefit the most from GH replacement therapy. The FDA also has approved GH therapy for AIDS-associated wasting and for malabsorption associated with the short bowel syndrome. In this latter setting, GH is administered once daily for 4 weeks.

GH increases mortality in patients with acute critical illness due to complications after open heart or abdominal surgery, multiple accidental trauma, or acute respiratory failure and should not be used in these settings. GH also should not be used in patients who have any evidence of neoplasia, and antitumor therapy should be completed before initiation of GH therapy.

TREATMENT OF GROWTH HORMONE DEFICIENCY   Humans do not respond to GH from nonprimate species. GH for clinical use corresponds in sequence to the human hormone and is produced by recombinant DNA technology.

GH is used for replacement therapy in GH-deficient children, whether the deficiency is congenital or acquired. By convention, *somatropin* refers to the many GH preparations whose sequences match that of native GH (GENOTROPIN, HUMATROPE, NORDITROPIN, NUTROPIN, OMNITROPE, SEROSTIM, TEV-TROPIN, ZORBTIVE), while *somatrem* refers to a derivative of GH with an additional methionine at the amino terminus (PROTROPIN). To mimic the normal pattern of secretion, these preparations typically are administered to GH-deficient children in a dose of 40 μg/kg/day subcutaneously in the evening; although the circulating $t_{1/2}$ of GH is only 20 minutes, its biological $t_{1/2}$ is in the range of 9–17 hours, and once-daily administration is sufficient. Higher daily doses (*e.g.,* 50 μg/kg) are employed for patients with Turner's syndrome, who have partial GH resistance. In children with overt GH deficiency, measurements of serum IGF-1 levels are used to monitor initial response and compliance; long-term response is monitored by close evaluation of height, sometimes in conjunction with measurements of serum IGF-1 levels. Although the most pronounced increase in growth velocity occurs within the first 2 years of therapy, GH is continued until the epiphyses are fused, and also may be extended into the transition period from childhood to adulthood. The response to GH can be variable. In part, this variability has been attributed to the differential expression of two splice variants of the GH receptor in the human population that differ in their GH responsiveness.

In view of the increased appreciation of the effects of GH on bone density and the manifestations of GH deficiency in adults, some experts continue therapy into adulthood for children with GH deficiency; it is essential to confirm GH deficiency in adulthood so as to identify those patients who will benefit from continuing GH treatment. Clinical response is monitored by serum IGF-1 levels, which should be restored to the mid-normal range adjusted for age and sex. Because estrogen increases the levels of GH binding proteins, women taking oral—but not transdermal—estrogen often require larger GH doses to achieve the target IGF-1 level.

Growth impairment also may be associated with elevated GH levels and GH resistance, most frequently secondary to mutations in the GH receptor (Laron dwarfism). These patients can be treated effectively with subcutaneous administration of recombinant human IGF-1 (INCRELEX, IPLEX). Although this therapy clearly is beneficial in promoting growth, the optimal regimen remains to be established.

In addition to GH, *sermorelin acetate* (GEREF), a synthetic form of human GHRH containing residues 1-29, is FDA-approved for diagnostic purposes. Sermorelin used therapeutically (30 μg/kg/day given subcutaneously) was less effective than GH in clinical trials. This agent will not work in patients whose GH deficiency results from defects in the anterior pituitary.

Side Effects of GH Therapy In children, GH therapy is associated with remarkably few side effects. Rarely, patients develop intracranial hypertension, with papilledema, visual changes, headache, nausea, and/or vomiting. This generally occurs within the first 8 weeks of therapy, and funduscopic examination is recommended at the initiation of therapy and periodically thereafter. Leukemia has been reported in some children receiving GH therapy; conditions associated with GH deficiency (*e.g.,* Down's syndrome, cranial irradiation for central nervous system [CNS] tumors) probably explain the apparent association. Despite this, the consensus is that GH should not be administered in the first year after treatment of pediatric tumors, including leukemia, or during the first 2 years after therapy for medulloblastomas or ependymomas. An increased incidence of type 2 diabetes mellitus has been reported. Finally, too-rapid growth may be associated with slipped epiphyses or scoliosis.

In adults, side effects associated with the initiation of GH therapy include peripheral edema, carpal tunnel syndrome, arthralgias, and myalgias. These symptoms, which occur most frequently in patients who are older or more obese, generally respond to a decrease in dose.

Syndromes of GH Excess

If the epiphyses are unfused, GH excess causes increased longitudinal growth, resulting in gigantism. In adults, GH excess causes acromegaly. Life expectancy is shortened in these patients due to increased incidences of cardiovascular disease, upper airway obstruction, and GI malignancies (possibly). Because the traditional treatment options, transsphenoidal surgery and radiation, have attendant complications, more attention has been given to pharmacological management of acromegaly.

SOMATOSTATIN ANALOGS The development of analogs of SST (Figure 55-3) revolutionized the medical treatment of acromegaly. Active SST analogs retain the amino acids in positions 7-10 [FWKT] as a core segment constrained in a cyclic structure. The most widely used somatostatin analog is octreotide (SANDOSTATIN), an 8-amino-acid synthetic derivative of somatostatin that has a longer $t_{1/2}$ and binds preferentially to SSTR2 and SSTR5 receptors. Typically, octreotide (100 μg) is administered subcutaneously 3 times daily; bioactivity is virtually 100%, peak effects are seen within 30 minutes, serum $t_{1/2}$ is approximately 90 minutes, and duration of action is ~12 hours. The goal of treatment is to decrease GH levels to <2 ng/mL after an oral glucose tolerance test and to bring IGF-1 levels to within the normal range for age and sex.

In addition to its effect on GH secretion, octreotide can decrease tumor size, although tumor growth generally resumes after octreotide treatment is stopped. Octreotide also has a significant inhibitory effect on thyrotropin secretion, and is the treatment of choice for patients who have thyrotrope adenomas that oversecrete TSH and are not good candidates for surgery. The use of octreotide in GI disorders is discussed in Chapter 37.

GI side effects—including diarrhea, nausea, and abdominal pain—occur in up to 50% of patients receiving octreotide. In most patients, these symptoms diminish over time and do not require cessation of therapy. Approximately 25% of patients receiving octreotide develop gallstones, presumably due to decreased gallbladder contraction and GI transit time. In the absence of symptoms, gallstones are not a contraindication to continued use of octreotide. Compared to somatostatin, octreotide reduces insulin secretion to a lesser extent and only infrequently affects glycemic control.

A long-acting, depot form of octreotide (SANDOSTATIN LAR) can be administered intramuscularly once every 4 weeks; the recommended dose is 20 or 30 mg.

Somatostatin-28 (Prosomatostatin):

Ser-Ala-Asn-Ser-Asn-Pro-Ala-Met-Ala-Pro-Arg-Glu-Arg-Lys-Ala-Gly-Cys-Lys-Asn-Phe-Phe-Trp-Lys-Thr-Phe-Thr-Ser-Cys

Somatostatin-14:   Ala-Gly-Cys-Lys-Asn-Phe-Phe-Trp-Lys-Thr-Phe-Thr-Ser-Cys

Octreotide: D-Phe-Cys-Phe-D-Trp-Lys-Thr-Cys-Thr-ol

Lanreotide: D-Nal-Cys-Tyr-D-Trp-Lys-Val-Cys-Thr-NH$_2$

FIGURE 55-3 *Structures of the somatostatins and clinically available analogs.* The amino acid sequences of the synthetic somatostatin analogs, octreotide and lanreotide are shown. D-Nal, 3-(2-naphthyl)-D-alanyl.

Lanreotide (SOMATULINE LA) is another long-acting octapeptide analog of somatostatin that causes prolonged suppression of GH secretion when administered in a 30-mg dose intramuscularly. Although its efficacy appears comparable to that of the long-acting formulation of octreotide, its duration of action is shorter; thus, it must be administered either at 10- or 14-day intervals. A 60-mg formulation of lanreotide (SOMATULINE AUTOGEL) reduces the required dosing frequency to once every 4 weeks. Lanreotide has not been approved by the FDA for use in the U.S.

GROWTH HORMONE ANTAGONISTS

Pegvisomant (SOMAVERT) is a GH receptor antagonist that is FDA-approved for the treatment of acromegaly. Pegvisomant binds to the GH receptor but does not activate JAK-STAT signaling or stimulate IGF-1 secretion (Figure 55–2). It is administered subcutaneously as a 40-mg loading dose under medical supervision, followed by self-administration of 10 mg/day. Based on serum IGF-1 levels, the dose is titrated at 4- to 6-week intervals to a maximum of 40 mg/day. Liver function should be monitored in all patients, and pegvisomant should not be used in patients with elevated levels of liver transaminases. Because there are concerns that loss of negative feedback by GH and IGF-1 may increase the growth of GH-secreting adenomas, careful follow-up of the pituitary by MRI is mandatory.

PROLACTIN
Secretion

Prolactin is related structurally to GH. Whereas serum prolactin levels remain low throughout life in normal males, they are elevated somewhat in normal cycling females. Prolactin levels rise markedly during pregnancy, reach a maximum at term, and decline thereafter unless the mother breast-feeds the infant. Suckling or breast manipulation in nursing mothers stimulates circulating prolactin levels, which can rise 10–100-fold within 30 minutes of stimulation. This response is neurally transmitted from the breast to the hypothalamus and is distinct from milk letdown, which is mediated by oxytocin release from the posterior pituitary gland. The precise mechanism for suckling-induced prolactin secretion is not known but involves both decreased secretion of dopamine by tuberoinfundibular neurons and possibly increased release of factors that stimulate prolactin secretion (*see* below). The suckling response becomes less pronounced after several months of breast-feeding, and prolactin concentrations eventually decline to prepregnancy levels.

Prolactin detected in maternal and fetal blood originates from maternal and fetal pituitaries, respectively. Prolactin also is synthesized by decidual cells near the end of the luteal phase of the menstrual cycle and early in pregnancy; the latter source is responsible for the very high levels of prolactin in amniotic fluid during the first trimester.

Many of the factors that influence prolactin secretion are similar to those that affect GH secretion. Thus, sleep, stress, hypoglycemia, exercise, and estrogen increase the secretion of both hormones.

Like other anterior pituitary hormones, prolactin is secreted in a pulsatile manner. Prolactin is unique among the anterior pituitary hormones in that hypothalamic regulation of its secretion is predominantly inhibitory. The major regulator of prolactin secretion is dopamine, which is released by tuberoinfundibular neurons and interacts with the D_2 receptor on lactotropes to inhibit prolactin secretion. A number of putative prolactin-releasing factors have been described, but their physiological roles are unclear. Under certain pathophysiological conditions, such as severe primary hypothyroidism, persistently elevated levels of TRH can induce hyperprolactinemia and consequent galactorrhea.

Molecular and Cellular Bases of Prolactin Action

The effects of prolactin result from interactions with specific receptors that are widely distributed among a variety of cell types within many tissues. The prolactin receptor is encoded by a single gene, alternative splicing of which gives rise to multiple forms of the receptor, including soluble forms found in the circulation that correspond to the extracellular domain of the receptor. The membrane-bound prolactin receptor is related structurally to receptors for GH and several cytokines and uses similar signaling mechanisms. Like the GH receptor, the prolactin receptor lacks intrinsic tyrosine kinase activity; prolactin induces a conformational change leading to recruitment and activation of JAK kinases (Figure 55–2). The activated JAK2 kinase, in turn, induces phosphorylation, dimerization, and nuclear translocation of the transcription factor STAT5. Unlike human GH and placental lactogen, which bind to the prolactin receptor and are lactogenic, prolactin binds specifically to the prolactin receptor and has no somatotropic (GH-like) activity.

Physiological Effects of Prolactin

Prolactin plays an important role in inducing growth and differentiation of the ductal and lobuloalveolar epithelium, which is essential for lactation. Prolactin receptors are present in many other sites; however, the physiological effects of prolactin at these sites remain poorly characterized.

Agents Used to Treat Syndromes of Prolactin Excess

Prolactin has no therapeutic uses. Hyperprolactinemia is a relatively common endocrine abnormality that most often is caused by prolactin-secreting pituitary adenomas. Hyperprolactinemia also can result from: hypothalamic or pituitary diseases that interfere with the delivery of inhibitory dopaminergic signals; primary hypothyroidism associated with increased TRH levels; renal failure; treatment with dopamine receptor antagonists. Manifestations of prolactin excess in women include galactorrhea, amenorrhea, and infertility. In men, hyperprolactinemia causes loss of libido, impotence, and infertility.

The therapeutic options for patients with prolactinomas include transsphenoidal surgery, radiation, and treatment with dopamine-receptor agonists that suppress prolactin production *via* activation of D_2 dopamine receptors. Inasmuch as initial surgical cure rates are only 50–70% with microadenomas and 30% with macroadenomas, most patients with prolactinomas ultimately require drug therapy. Thus, dopamine-receptor agonists have become the initial treatment of choice for many patients. These agents generally decrease both prolactin secretion and the size of the adenoma, thereby improving the endocrine abnormalities, as well as the neurological symptoms caused directly by the adenoma (including visual field deficits). It is worth noting, however, that they typically are not curative.

BROMOCRIPTINE

Bromocriptine *(PARLODEL) is the dopamine-receptor agonist against which newer agents are compared. Bromocriptine is a semisynthetic ergot alkaloid that interacts with D_2 dopamine receptors to inhibit spontaneous and TRH-induced release of prolactin; to a lesser extent, it also activates D_1 receptors. Bromocriptine normalizes serum prolactin levels in 70–80% of patients with prolactinomas and decreases tumor size in more than 50% of patients, including those with macroadenomas.*

Frequent side effects of bromocriptine include nausea and vomiting, headache, and postural hypotension—particularly on initial use. Less-frequent side effects include nasal congestion, digital vasospasm, and CNS effects such as psychosis, hallucinations, nightmares, or insomnia. Starting at a low dose (1.25 mg), administered at bedtime, can diminish these side effects. If clinical symptoms persist or serum prolactin levels remain elevated, the dose can be increased gradually, every 3–7 days, to 5 mg twice daily or 2.5 mg three times a day as tolerated. Patients often develop tolerance to the side effects of bromocriptine. Those who do not respond to bromocriptine or who have intractable side effects may respond to a different dopamine agonist. Although a high fraction of the oral dose of bromocriptine is absorbed, only 7% of the dose reaches the systemic circulation because of extensive first-pass hepatic metabolism. Bromocriptine has a relatively short elimination $t_{1/2}$ (2–8 hours). Longer acting forms of bromocriptine have been developed but are not available for use in the U.S. At higher concentrations, bromocriptine is used in the management of acromegaly and at still higher concentrations is used in the management of Parkinson's disease.

Patients with prolactinomas who wish to become pregnant comprise a special subset of hyperprolactinemic patients. Because experience with bromocriptine is more extensive than that with any other D_2 receptor agonist, bromocriptine is recommended as the first-line treatment in this setting. Bromocriptine relieves the inhibitory effect of prolactin on ovulation and permits most patients with prolactinomas to become pregnant without apparent detrimental effects on pregnancy or fetal development.

PERGOLIDE

Pergolide *(PERMAX), an ergot derivative approved by the FDA for treatment of Parkinson's disease, also is used "off label" to treat hyperprolactinemia. It induces many of the same side effects as does bromocriptine, but it can be given once a day, starting at 0.025 mg at bedtime and increased gradually to a maximum daily dose of 0.5 mg.*

CABERGOLINE

Cabergoline *(DOSTINEX) is an ergot derivative with a longer $t_{1/2}$ (~65 hours), higher affinity, and greater selectivity for the D_2 receptor (~4 times more potent) than bromocriptine. It is FDA-approved for the treatment of hyperprolactinemia and likely will play an increasing role in the* *treatment of this syndrome. Compared to bromocriptine, cabergoline has a much lower tendency to induce nausea, although it still may cause hypotension and dizziness. In some clinical trials, cabergoline has been more effective than bromocriptine in decreasing serum prolactin in patients with hyperprolactinemia, although this may reflect improved adherence to therapy due to decreased side effects. Therapy is initiated at a dose of 0.25 mg twice a week or 0.5 mg once a week. If the serum prolactin remains elevated, the dose can be increased to a maximum of 1.5–2 mg two or three times a week as tolerated; however, the dose should not be increased more often than once every 4 weeks.*

QUINAGOLIDE

Quinagolide *(NORPROLAC) is a nonergot* D_2 *dopamine agonist with a half-life of 22 hours. Quinagolide is administered once daily at doses of 0.1–0.5 mg/day. It is not approved by the FDA but has been used extensively in Europe.*

GONADOTROPIN-RELEASING HORMONE AND GONADOTROPINS

LH and FSH were named initially based on their actions on the ovary. These pituitary hormones, together with the related placental hormone hCG, are collectively referred to as the gonadotropins because of their actions on the gonads. The regulation of gonadotropin secretion is described in detail in Chapters 57 and 58. LH and FSH are synthesized and secreted by gonadotropes; hCG is synthesized the syncytiotrophoblast of the placenta. Pituitary gonadotropin production is stimulated by GnRH and is further regulated by feedback effects of the gonadal hormones (Figure 55–4; *see also* Figure 57–2).

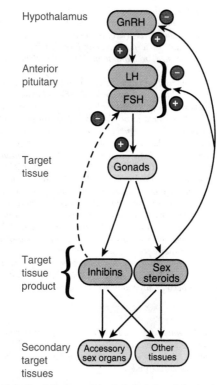

FIGURE 55–4 *The hypothalamic-pituitary-gonadal axis.* A single hypothalamic releasing factor, GnRH, controls the synthesis and release of both gonadotropins (LH and FSH) in males and females. Gonadal steroid hormones (androgens, estrogens, and progesterone) cause feedback inhibition at the level of the pituitary and the hypothalamus. The preovulatory surge of estrogen also can exert a stimulatory effect at the level of the pituitary and the hypothalamus. Inhibins, polypeptide hormones produced by the gonads, specifically inhibit FSH secretion by the pituitary.

Table 55–1

Gnrh and Gnrh Analogs

Analog (TRADE NAME)	Dosage Form
Agonists	
Gnrh (FACTREL)	IV, SC
Leuprolide (LUPRON, ELIGARD, VIADUR)	IM, SC depot
Buserelin (SUPREFACT)	SC, IN
Nafarelin (SYNAREL)	IN
Deslorelin (SOMAGARD)	SC, IM, depot
Histrelin (SUPPRELIN)	SC
Triptorelin (TRELSTAR DEPOT, LA)	IM
Goserelin (ZOLADEX)	SC implant
Antagonists	
Cetrorelix (CETROTIDE)	SC
Ganirelix (ANTAGON)	SC
Abarelix (PLENAXIS)	SC depot

ABBREVIATIONS: IM, intramuscular; IN, intranasal; IV, intravenous; SC, subcutaneous.

REGULATION OF RELEASE OF Gnrh   Gnrh is a decapeptide with blocked amino and carboxyl termini (Table 55–1) that is derived by proteolytic cleavage of a 92-amino-acid precursor peptide. Gnrh release is intermittent and is governed by a hypothalamic neural pulse generator, primarily in the arcuate nucleus, that controls the frequency and amplitude of Gnrh release. The intermittent release of Gnrh is crucial for the proper synthesis and release of the gonadotropins; the continuous administration of Gnrh leads to desensitization and down-regulation of Gnrh receptors on pituitary gonadotropes. This downregulation forms the basis for the clinical use of long-acting Gnrh analogs to suppress gonadotropin secretion (*see* below).

MOLECULAR AND CELLULAR BASES OF GNRH ACTION   Gnrh signals through a specific GPCR on gonadotropes that activates $G_{q/11}$ and stimulates the PLC-IP_3-Ca^{2+} pathway (*see* Chapter 1), resulting in increased synthesis and secretion of LH and FSH.

OTHER REGULATORS OF GONADOTROPIN PRODUCTION   Gonadal steroids regulate gonadotropin production at the level of the pituitary and the hypothalamus, but effects on the hypothalamus predominate. The feedback effects of gonadal steroids are sex-, dosage-, and time-dependent. In women, low levels of estradiol and progesterone inhibit gonadotropin production, largely through opioid action on the neural pulse generator that controls Gnrh secretion. Higher and more sustained levels of estradiol have positive feedback effects that ultimately result in the gonadotropin surge that precedes ovulation. In men, testosterone inhibits gonadotropin secretion, both directly and after its conversion to estradiol.

Gonadotropin secretion also is regulated by the *inhibins*, which are members of the bone morphogenetic protein family of secreted signaling proteins. Inhibins are made by granulosa cells in the ovary and Sertoli cells in the testis in response to the gonadotropins and local growth factors. They act directly in the pituitary to selectively inhibit FSH secretion without affecting that of LH.

Molecular and Cellular Bases of Gonadotropin Action

The gonadotropins (LH, FSH, and hCG) are glycosylated heterodimers, each containing a common α-subunit and a distinct β-subunit that confers specificity of action. The longer $t_{1/2}$ of hCG has some clinical relevance for its use in assisted reproduction technologies (*see* below).

The actions of LH and hCG are mediated by the LH receptor, while those of FSH are mediated by the FSH receptor. These receptors couple to G_s to activate the adenylyl cyclase–cyclic AMP pathway and most, if not all, of the actions of the gonadotropins can be mimicked by cyclic AMP analogs.

Physiological Effects of Gonadotropins

In men, LH acts on testicular Leydig cells to stimulate *de novo* synthesis of testosterone from cholesterol. Testosterone is required for gametogenesis within the seminiferous tubules and for maintenance of libido and male secondary sexual characteristics (*see* Chapter 58). FSH acts on the

Sertoli cells to stimulate the production of proteins and nutrients required for sperm maturation, thereby indirectly supporting germ cell maturation.

In women, the actions of FSH and LH are more complicated. FSH stimulates the growth of developing ovarian follicles and induces the expression of LH receptors on theca and granulosa cells. FSH also regulates the activity of aromatase in granulosa cells, thereby stimulating the production of estradiol. LH acts on the theca cells to stimulate the *de novo* synthesis of androstenedione, the major precursor of ovarian estradiol in premenopausal women (*see* Figure 57–1). LH also is required for the rupture of the dominant follicle during ovulation and for the synthesis of progesterone by the corpus luteum.

CLINICAL USES OF GnRH

Synthetic GnRH (*gonadorelin hydrochloride*) and GnRH analogs are used clinically (Table 55–1). The analogs exhibit enhanced potency and a prolonged duration of action compared to GnRH, which has a $t_{1/2}$ of 2–4 minutes. The prolonged actions of the analogs serve to desensitize the GnRH receptor to GnRH, thereby downregulating gonadotropin secretion.

Pure GnRH antagonists also have been developed; these do not cause the initial increase in gonadotropin secretion seen when long-acting GnRH agonists are used.

Therapeutic Uses of GnRH Analogs

SUPPRESSION OF GONADOTROPIN SECRETION Long-acting GnRH agonists markedly inhibit gonadotropin secretion and decrease the production of gonadal steroids by desensitizing GnRH signaling pathways. This pharmacological castration is useful in disorders that respond to reductions in gonadal steroids. A clear indication for this therapy is in children with GnRH-dependent precocious puberty, whose premature sexual maturation can be arrested with minimal side effects by chronic administration of a GnRH agonist.

Long-acting GnRH agonists are used for palliative therapy of hormonally responsive tumors (*e.g.*, prostate or breast cancer), generally in conjunction with agents that block steroid biosynthesis or action to avoid effects of transient increases in hormone levels (*see* Chapter 51). Because it does not transiently increase sex steroid production, an extended-release form of the GnRH antagonist *abarelix* (PLENAXIS) is marketed for use in prostate cancer patients in whom serious adverse consequences might accompany any stimulus to tumor growth (*e.g.*, in patients with spinal cord metastases where increased tumor growth could lead to paralysis).

The GnRH agonists also are used to suppress steroid-responsive conditions such as endometriosis, uterine leiomyomas, and acute intermittent porphyria. *Nafarelin* (SYNAREL) is administered by nasal spray for endometriosis. Depot preparations of *goserelin* (ZOLADEX), *leuprolide* (LUPRON DEPOT, ELEGARD) or *triptorelin* (TRELSTAR LA), which can be administered subcutaneously or intramuscularly monthly or every 3 months, can be used in these settings and may be particularly useful for pharmacological castration in disorders such as paraphilia, for which strict patient compliance is problematic.

The long-acting agonists generally are well tolerated, and side effects are those that would be predicted to occur when gonadal steroidogenesis is inhibited (*e.g.*, hot flashes, vaginal dryness and atrophy, decreased bone density). Because of these effects, therapy in non–life-threatening diseases such as endometriosis or uterine leiomyomas generally is limited to 6 months unless add-back therapy with estrogens and/or progestins is incorporated into the regimen. In addition to these predicted effects, *abarelix* has been associated with a significant incidence of hypersensitivity reactions, and its therapeutic role remains to be defined. For safety reasons, abarelix distribution is limited to physicians who are enrolled in the manufacturer's prescribing program.

MANAGEMENT OF INFERTILITY Two GnRH antagonists, *ganirelix* (ANTAGON) and *cetrorelix* (CETROTIDE) (Table 55–1), have been used to suppress the LH surge and thus prevent premature follicular luteinization in ovarian-stimulation protocols that are part of assisted reproduction techniques.

Therapeutic Uses of Gonadotropins

Gonadotropins are purified from human urine or prepared using recombinant DNA technology. *Chorionic gonadotropin* (PREGNYL, NOVAREL, PROFASI, others), which mimics the action of LH, is obtained from the urine of pregnant women. Urine from postmenopausal women also is the source of *menotropins* (PERGONAL, REPRONEX), which contain roughly equal amounts of FSH and LH, as well as a number of other urinary proteins. Because of their relatively low purity, menotropins are administered intramuscularly to decrease the incidence of hypersensitivity reactions. *Urofollitropin* (UFSH; BRAVELLE) is a highly purified FSH prepared by immunoconcentration with monoclonal antibodies and pure enough to be administered subcutaneously, as is a purified preparation of FSH and LH derived from urine (MENOPURE).

Recombinant preparations of gonadotropins increasingly are used in clinical practice. The two rFSH preparations that are available (*follitropin α* [GONAL-F] and *follitropin β* [PUREGON, FOLLISTIM]) both exhibit less interbatch variability than do preparations purified from urine and can be administered subcutaneously, since they are considerably purer. The relative advantages of the recombinant preparations (*i.e.*, efficacy, lower frequency of side effects such as ovarian hyperstimulation) have not been definitively established despite much debate in the published literature.

Recombinant forms of hCG (choriogonadotropin alfa; OVIDREL) and LH (LUVERIS, LHADI) also are available.

CRYPTORCHIDISM   Cryptorchidism, the failure of one or both testes to descend into the scrotum, affects up to 3% of full-term male infants, becoming less prevalent with advancing postnatal age. Cryptorchid testes have defective spermatogenesis and are at increased risk for developing germ cell tumors. Hence, the current approach is to reposition the testes as early as possible, typically at 1 year of age but definitely before 2 years of age. The local actions of androgens stimulate descent of the testes; thus, hCG can be used to induce testicular descent if the cryptorchidism is not secondary to anatomical blockage. Therapy usually consists of injections of hCG (3000 IU/m^2 body surface area) intramuscularly every other day for 6 doses.

OXYTOCIN
Biosynthesis of Oxytocin

Oxytocin is a cyclic nonapeptide that differs from vasopressin by only 2 amino acids (*see* Chapter 29). It is synthesized as a larger precursor molecule in cell bodies of the paraventricular nucleus, and to a lesser extent, the supraoptic nucleus in the hypothalamus. The precursor is rapidly converted by proteolysis to the active hormone and its neurophysin, packaged into secretory granules as an oxytocin-neurophysin complex, and secreted from nerve endings that terminate primarily in the posterior pituitary gland. In addition, oxytocinergic neurons that regulate the autonomic nervous system project to regions of the hypothalamus, brainstem, and spinal cord. Other sites of oxytocin synthesis include the luteal cells of the ovary, the endometrium, and the placenta.

Stimuli for oxytocin secretion include sensory stimuli arising from dilation of the cervix and vagina and from suckling at the breast. Estradiol stimulates oxytocin secretion, whereas the ovarian polypeptide relaxin inhibits release. Other factors that primarily affect vasopressin secretion also have some impact on oxytocin release (e.g., ethanol inhibits release, while pain, dehydration, hemorrhage, and hypovolemia stimulate release).

Physiological Roles of Oxytocin

UTERUS   Because loss of pituitary oxytocin apparently does not compromise labor and delivery, the physiological role of oxytocin in pregnancy has been highly debated; however, the finding that the oxytocin antagonist *atosiban* (TRACTOCILE) is effective in suppressing preterm labor (*see* below) supports the physiological importance of oxytocin in this setting. Exogenous oxytocin stimulates the frequency and force of uterine contractions. The responsiveness to oxytocin roughly parallels the increase in spontaneous activity that constitutes the initiation of labor and is highly dependent on estrogen, which increases the expression of the oxytocin receptors. Thus, the uterus is more responsive to oxytocin in late pregnancy than in early pregnancy. Progesterone antagonizes the stimulant effect of oxytocin *in vitro,* and a decline in progesterone receptor signaling in late pregnancy may contribute to the normal initiation of human parturition.

BREAST   Oxytocin plays an important physiological role in milk ejection. Stimulation of the breast through suckling or mechanical manipulation induces oxytocin secretion, causing contraction of the myoepithelium that surrounds alveolar channels in the mammary gland. This action forces milk from the alveolar channels into large collecting sinuses, where it is available to the suckling infant.

Mechanism of Action

In the human myometrium, oxytocin acts *via* specific GPCRs, coupled to G_q and G_{11}, to activate the PLCβ-IP$_3$-Ca^{2+} pathway and enhance activation of voltage-sensitive Ca^{2+} channels. Oxytocin also increases local prostaglandin production, which further stimulates uterine contractions.

Clinical Use of Oxytocin

INDUCTION OF LABOR Oxytocin (PITOCIN, SYNTOCINON) is the drug of choice for labor induction. Indications for induction of labor include situations in which the risk of continued pregnancy to the mother or fetus is considered to be greater than the risks of delivery or of pharmacological induction. Such circumstances include premature rupture of the membranes, isoimmunization, fetal growth restriction, and uteroplacental insufficiency (as in diabetes, preeclampsia, or eclampsia). Before labor is induced, it is essential to verify that the fetal lungs are sufficiently mature and to exclude potential contraindications (*e.g.*, abnormal fetal position, evidence of fetal distress, placental abnormalities, or previous uterine surgery that predisposes to uterine rupture).

Oxytocin is administered by intravenous infusion of a diluted solution (typically 10 mIU/mL), preferably by means of an infusion pump. If uterine hyperstimulation occurs, as evidenced by too-frequent contractions or the development of uterine tetany, the oxytocin should be discontinued immediately. The $t_{1/2}$ of intravenous oxytocin is short (~3 minutes); thus, the hyperstimulatory effects of oxytocin should dissipate over several minutes after the infusion is stopped. Because of its structural similarity to vasopressin, oxytocin at higher doses activates the vasopressin V_2 receptor causing antidiuretic effects. Particularly if hypotonic fluids (*e.g.*, dextrose in water) are infused too liberally, water intoxication may result causing convulsions, coma, and even death. Vasodilating actions of oxytocin also have been noted, particularly at high doses, which may provoke hypotension and reflex tachycardia. Deep anesthesia may exaggerate the hypotensive effect of oxytocin by preventing the reflex tachycardia.

AUGMENTATION OF DYSFUNCTIONAL LABOR To augment hypotonic contractions in dysfunctional labor, it rarely is necessary to exceed an infusion rate of 10 mIU/min, and doses of >20 mIU/min rarely are effective when lower concentrations fail. Potential complications of overstimulation include trauma of the mother or fetus due to forced passage through an incompletely dilated cervix, uterine rupture, and compromised fetal oxygenation due to decreased uterine perfusion. Oxytocin usually is effective when there is a prolonged latent phase of cervical dilation and when, in the absence of cephalopelvic disproportion, there is an arrest of dilation or descent.

THIRD STAGE OF LABOR AND PUERPERIUM Postpartum hemorrhage is a significant problem in developed nations and is of even greater importance in underdeveloped countries. After delivery of the fetus or after therapeutic abortion, a firm, contracted uterus greatly reduces the incidence and extent of hemorrhage. Oxytocin (10 IU intramuscularly) often is given immediately after delivery to help maintain uterine contractions and tone. Alternatively, 20 IU of oxytocin is diluted in 1 L of intravenous solution and infused at a rate of 10 mL/min until the uterus is contracted. Then the infusion rate is reduced to 1–2 mL/min until the mother is ready for transfer to the postpartum unit. If this is ineffective, ergot alkaloids such as *ergonovine maleate* (ERGOTRATE) or its methyl analog *methylergonovine maleate* (METHERGINE) or the prostaglandin analog *misoprostol* may be used in normotensive patients. The ergot alkaloids are discussed in more detail in Chapter 11; prostaglandins are discussed in Chapter 25.

Oxytocin-Receptor Antagonists

A peptide analog that competitively inhibits the interaction of oxytocin with its membrane receptor, atosiban *(TRACTOCILE), has been introduced in a number of countries for the treatment of preterm labor.* Atosiban *decreases the frequency of uterine contractions and increases the number of women who remained undelivered. Its efficacy is comparable to β adrenergic agonists but the incidence of side effects is lower. It should be noted, however, that studies to date have failed to demonstrate a significant improvement in infant outcome when preterm labor is delayed.*

56

THYROID AND ANTITHYROID DRUGS

The thyroid gland is the source of two fundamentally different types of hormones, iodothyronines and calcitonin. The iodothyronine hormones—thyroxine (T_4) and triiodothyronine (T_3)—are essential for normal growth and development and play an important role in energy metabolism. Calcitonin is discussed in Chapter 61.

The principal hormones of the thyroid gland are iodine-containing amino acid derivatives of thyronine: T_4 and T_3 (see Figure 56–1). T_4 is a prohormone that is converted to the biologically active form, T_3. The 3′-monosubstituted compounds are more active than the 3′,5′-disubstituted molecules. The affinity of iodothyronines for thyroid hormone receptors (TRs) generally parallels their biological potency.

BIOSYNTHESIS OF THYROID HORMONES The thyroid hormones are synthesized and stored as amino acid residues of thyroglobulin, a complex glycoprotein that forms the bulk of thyroid follicular colloid. The thyroid gland uniquely stores great quantities of potential hormone in this way, and extracellular thyroglobulin can represent a large portion of the thyroid mass.

The major steps in the synthesis, storage, release, and interconversion of thyroid hormones are summarized in Figure 56–2: (1) uptake of iodide ion (I^-) by the gland; (2) oxidation of iodide and the iodination of tyrosyl groups of thyroglobulin; (3) coupling of iodotyrosine residues by ether linkage to generate the iodothyronines; (4) resorption of the thyroglobulin colloid from the lumen into the cell; (5) proteolysis of thyroglobulin and the release of T_4 and T_3 into the blood; (6) recycling of the iodine within the thyroid cell via de-iodination of the mono- and diiodotyrosines and reuse of the I^-; and (7) conversion of T_4 to T_3 in peripheral tissues and in the thyroid.

1. *Uptake of Iodide.* Dietary iodine reaches the circulation as iodide. Normally, its concentration in the blood is very low (0.2–0.4 $\mu g/dL$; about 15–30 nM), but the thyroid actively transports the ion via a specific, membrane-bound protein termed the sodium-iodide symporter (NIS). The ratio of thyroid to plasma iodide concentration is usually between 20 and 50 and can far exceed 100 when the gland is stimulated. The NIS is inhibited by a number of ions such as thiocyanate and perchlorate (Figure 56–3). Thyrotropin (see below) stimulates the NIS, which is controlled by an autoregulatory mechanism. Thus, decreased stores of thyroid iodine enhance iodide uptake, and the administration of iodide can reverse this situation by decreasing NIS protein expression.

2. *Oxidation and Iodination.* The oxidation of iodide to its active form and the iodination of tyrosine are catalyzed by thyroid peroxidase, a heme-containing enzyme that utilizes hydrogen peroxide (H_2O_2) as the oxidant. The peroxidase is membrane-bound and concentrated at the apical surface of the thyroid cells. The reaction forms mono- and diiodotyrosyl residues in thyroglobulin just prior to its extracellular storage in the lumen of the thyroid follicle. H_2O_2 is formed near its site of utilization and is stimulated by a rise in cytosolic Ca^{2+}.

3. *Formation of Thyroxine and Triiodothyronine from Iodotyrosines.* The remaining synthetic step is the coupling of two diiodotyrosyl residues to form T_4 or of one monoiodotyrosyl and one diiodotyrosyl residues to form T_3. The same peroxidase catalyzes these oxidative reactions. The conformation of thyroglobulin apparently renders it uniquely efficient for the coupling reaction. T_4 predominantly is formed at the amino terminus of thyroglobulin, while T_3 is preferentially localized to the carboxy terminus.

The relative rates of synthetic activity at the various sites depend on the concentration of thyroid-stimulating hormone (TSH) and the availability of iodide, possibly accounting for the varying proportions of T_4 and T_3 depending on iodine supply. Limited iodine is utilized more efficiently in the synthesis of T_3, the transcriptionally active form, which contains three-fourths as much iodine as T_4. Eventually, iodine deficiency impairs synthesis of both T_4 and T_3 and hypothyroidism results. In addition to the coupling reaction, intrathyroidal and secreted T_3 is generated by the 5′-deiodination of T_4.

4. *Resorption; 5. Proteolysis of Colloid; 6. Secretion of Thyroid Hormones.* Since T_4 and T_3 are synthesized and stored within thyroglobulin, proteolysis is an important part of the secretory process. This process is initiated by endocytosis of colloid from the follicular lumen at the apical surface, with the participation of a thyroglobulin receptor, megalin. This "ingested" thyroglobulin appears as intracellular colloid droplets, which apparently fuse with lysosomes containing the requisite proteolytic enzymes. TSH enhances the degradation of thyroglobulin by increasing the activity of several lysosomal thiol endopeptidases, which selectively cleave

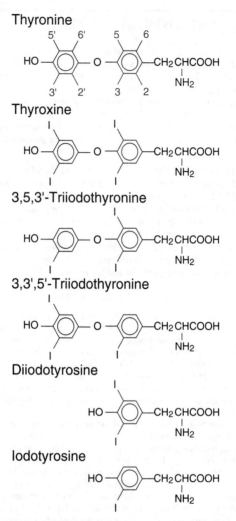

FIGURE 56–1 *Thyronine, thyroid hormones, and precursors.*

thyroglobulin to hormone-containing intermediates that subsequently are processed by exopeptidases. The liberated hormones then exit the cell.

7. ***Peripheral Conversion of Thyroxine to Triiodothyronine.*** The normal daily production of T_4 is 70–90 μg, while that of T_3 is 15–30 μg. Although the thyroid does secrete some T_3, monodeiodination of T_4 in peripheral tissues accounts for about 80% of circulating T_3 (Figure 56–3). Removal of the 5′-, or outer ring, iodine leads to the formation of T_3 in the "activating" metabolic pathway. The major nonthyroidal site of conversion of T_4 to T_3 is the liver. Thus, when T_4 is given to hypothyroid patients in doses that normalize its plasma concentration, the plasma concentration of T_3 also normalizes. Most peripheral tissues utilize T_3 derived from the circulating hormone. Notable exceptions are the brain and pituitary, where local generation of T_3 is the major source of intracellular hormone. Removal of the iodine on position 5 of the inner ring produces the metabolically inactive 3,3′,5′-triiodothyronine (reverse T_3; Figure 56–1). Normally, about 40% of T_4 is converted to T_3, about 40% is converted to reverse T_3, and about 20% is metabolized *via* other pathways, such as conjugation in the liver and excretion in the bile. Normal plasma concentrations of T_4 range from 4.5 to 11 μg/dL, while those of T_3 are 60–180 ng/dL.

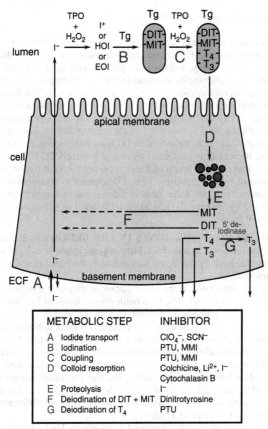

FIGURE 56–2 *Major pathways of thyroid hormone biosynthesis and release.*

ABBREVIATIONS: Tg, thyroglobulin; DIT, diiodotyrosine; MIT, monoiodotyrosine; TPO, thyroid peroxidase; HOI, hypoiodous acid; EOI, enzyme-linked species; PTU, propylthiouracil; MMI, methimazole; ECF, extracellular fluid.

METABOLIC STEP		INHIBITOR
A	Iodide transport	ClO$_4^-$, SCN$^-$
B	Iodination	PTU, MMI
C	Coupling	PTU, MMI
D	Colloid resorption	Colchicine, Li^{2+}, I$^-$
		Cytochalasin B
E	Proteolysis	I$^-$
F	Deiodination of DIT + MIT	Dinitrotyrosine
G	Deiodination of T$_4$	PTU

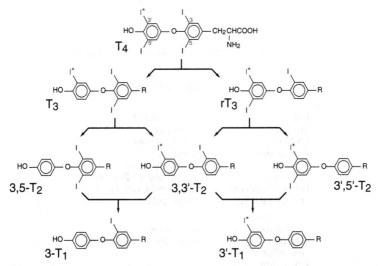

FIGURE 56–3 *Pathways of iodothyronine deiodination.*

Two distinct 5'-deiodinase enzymes convert T_4 to T_3; they are selenoproteins that are encoded by distinct genes and are differentially expressed and regulated. The type I 5'-deiodinase (D1)—which is expressed in the liver, kidney, and thyroid—generates circulating T_3 that is used by most peripheral target tissues. D1 is inhibited by a number of drugs, including the antithyroid drug *propylthiouracil* (*see* below), *propranolol, amiodarone*, and *glucocorticoids*. The decreased plasma T_3 levels observed in a variety of nonthyroidal illnesses result from inhibition of D1 and decreased entrance of T_4 into cells. D1 is upregulated in hyperthyroidism and downregulated in hypothyroidism. Type II 5'-deiodinase (D2) is expressed in the brain, pituitary, and skeletal and cardiac muscle and supplies intracellular T_3 to these tissues. D2 has a much lower Km for T_4 than does D1 (nM *vs.* uM values) and its activity is unaffected by propylthiouracil. D2 is dynamically regulated by its substrate T_4, such that elevated levels of the enzyme are found in hypothyroidism and suppressed levels are found in hyperthyroidism. Thus, D2 appears to autoregulate the intracellular supply of T_3 in the brain and pituitary. Inner ring- or 5-deiodination, a major inactivating pathway for T_4 and T_3, is catalyzed by the type III deiodinase (D3), another selenoprotein that is found in placenta, skin, uterus, and brain.

TRANSPORT OF THYROID HORMONES IN THE BLOOD Iodine circulates as both organic iodine (95%) and inorganic iodide (5%). Most organic iodine is in T_4 (90–95%), while T_3 contains approximately 5%. Both T_4 and T_3 are transported in the blood in strong but noncovalent association with plasma proteins.

Thyroxine-binding globulin (TBG) is the major carrier of thyroid hormones. An acidic glycoprotein with a molecular weight of ~63,000, TBG binds one molecule of T_4 with very high affinity ($K_a \sim 10^{10}$ M^{-1}). T_3 is bound less avidly. T_4, but not T_3, also is bound by transthyretin (thyroxine-binding prealbumin), a retinol-binding protein. This protein is present in higher concentration than TBG but has a lower affinity ($K_a \sim 10^7$ M^{-1}). Albumin can also bind T_4 when the more avid carriers are saturated, but the physiological significance of this binding generally is unclear.

Binding of thyroid hormones to plasma proteins protects the hormones from metabolism and excretion and prolongs their half-lives in circulation. The free (unbound) hormone is a small percentage (about 0.03% of T_4 and 0.3% of T_3) of the total hormone in plasma. The differential binding affinities for plasma proteins also are reflected in the 10–100-fold differences in circulating hormone concentrations and half-lives of T_4 and T_3.

Because of the high degree of binding of thyroid hormones to TBG, changes in TBG concentration can have major effects on total serum hormone levels. Certain drugs and a variety of pathological and physiological conditions (*e.g.*, changes in estrogen levels during pregnancy or with administration of oral estrogens) can alter both the amount of TBG and its binding of thyroid hormones (Table 56–1). The increase in TBG induced by estrogen is due to an increase in its sialic acid content that decreases TBG clearance. Since the pituitary responds to and regulates circulating free

Table 56–1

Factors That Alter Binding of Thyroxine to Thyroxine-Binding Globulin

Increase Binding	Decrease Binding
Drugs	
Estrogens	Glucocorticoids
Methadone	Androgens
Clofibrate	L-Asparaginase
5-Fluorouracil	Salicylates
Heroin	Mefenamic Acid
Tamoxifen	Antiseizure medications
Selective estrogen	(phenytoin, carbamazepine)
receptor modulators	Furosemide
Systemic Factors	
Liver disease	Inheritance
Porphyria	Acute and chronic illness
HIV infection	
Inheritance	

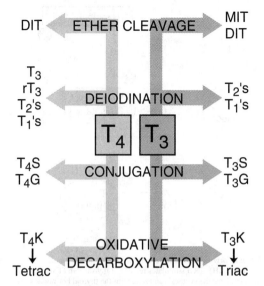

FIGURE 56–4 *Pathways of metabolism of thyroxine (T_4) and triiodothyronine (T_3).*

ABBREVIATIONS: DIT, diiodotyrosine; MIT, monoiodotyrosine; T_4S, T_4 sulfate; T_4G, T_4 glucuronide; T_3S, T_3 sulfate; T_3G, T_3 glucuronide; T_4K, T_4 pyruvic acid; T_3K, T_3 pyruvic acid; Tetrac, tetraiodothyroacetic acid; Triac, triiodothyroacetic acid.

hormone levels, which are the metabolically active species, minimal changes in free hormone concentrations are seen when the pituitary-thyroid axis is intact; however, laboratory tests that measure only total hormone levels can be misleading in these settings.

DEGRADATION AND EXCRETION T_4 is eliminated from the body with a $t_{1/2}$ of 6–8 days. In hyperthyroidism, the $t_{1/2}$ is shortened to 3 or 4 days; in hypothyroidism, it may be 9–10 days. These differing half-lives presumably reflect altered rates of hormone metabolism. In conditions associated with increased binding to TBG, such as pregnancy, clearance is retarded. The opposite effect is observed when there is reduced TBG or when certain drugs inhibit thyroid hormone binding (Table 56–1). T_3, which is less avidly bound to protein, has a $t_{1/2}$ of ~1 day.

The liver is the major site of nondeiodinative degradation of thyroid hormones; T_4 and T_3 are conjugated with glucuronic and sulfuric acids through the phenolic hydroxyl group and excreted in the bile. Some thyroid hormone is liberated by hydrolysis of the conjugates in the intestine and reabsorbed. A portion of the conjugated material reaches the colon unchanged, where it is hydrolyzed and eliminated in the feces. Steps in breakdown *via* deiodination to inactive metabolites are summarized in Figure 56–4.

REGULATION OF THYROID FUNCTION Thyroid hormone levels are tightly regulated by complex, reciprocal interactions among the hypothalamus, anterior pituitary, and thyroid (Figure 56–5). Thyrotropin-releasing hormone (TRH), which is made and secreted by the TRH neurons in the hypothalamus, stimulates the synthesis and secretion of TSH. TSH, made and secreted by pituitary thyrotropes, stimulates the biosynthesis and release of thyroid hormone. Superimposed on this positive regulatory loop is a negative feedback loop wherein circulating thyroid hormone acts in the hypothalamus and pituitary to decrease TSH stimulation of thyroid hormone release.

Thyrotropin-Releasing Hormone TRH is a tripeptide (L-pyroglutamyl-L-histidyl-L-proline amide) that is synthesized in the hypothalamus and released into the hypophyseal-portal circulation. TRH binds to its receptor, a GPCR, stimulates the G_q-PLC-IP$_3$-Ca^{2+} pathway, and activates PKC, ultimately stimulating the synthesis and release of TSH by the thyrotropes. Although TRH is the dominant regulator of TSH secretion, somatostatin, dopamine, and pharmacological doses of glucocorticoids inhibit TRH-stimulated TSH secretion.

Actions of TSH on the Thyroid TSH is a glycoprotein hormone with α and β subunits analogous to those of the gonadotropins (*see* Chapter 55). It is secreted in a pulsatile manner

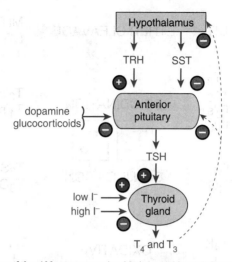

FIGURE 56–5 *Regulation of thyroid hormone secretion.* Myriad neural inputs influence hypothalamic secretion of thyrotropin-releasing hormone (TRH). TRH stimulates release of thyrotropin (TSH, thyroid-stimulating hormone) from the anterior pituitary; TSH stimulates the synthesis and release of the thyroid hormones T_3 and T_4. T_3 and T_4 feed back to inhibit the synthesis and release of TRH and TSH. Somatostatin (SST) can inhibit TRH action, as can dopamine and high concentrations of glucocorticoids. Low levels of I^- are required for thyroxine synthesis, but high levels inhibit thyroxine synthesis and release.

and circadian pattern, its levels in circulation being highest during sleep. Its secretion is precisely controlled by the levels of TRH and by the concentration of free thyroid hormones in the circulation. It is the key direct stimulator of thyroid hormone synthesis and release.

The first measurable effect of TSH on thyroid hormone metabolism is increased secretion, which is detectable within minutes. All phases of hormone synthesis and secretion are eventually stimulated: iodide uptake and organification, endocytosis, and proteolysis of thyroglobulin. There also is increased vascularity of the gland and hypertrophy and hyperplasia of thyroid cells.

The TSH receptor is a GPCR that is structurally similar to the receptors for luteinizing hormone and follicle-stimulating hormone (*see* Chapter 55). These receptors all have large extracellular domains that are involved in hormone binding. TSH binding to its receptor stimulates the G_s-adenylyl cyclase-cyclic AMP pathway. Higher concentrations of TSH activate the G_q-PLC pathway. Both signaling pathways apparently mediate effects of TSH on thyroid function in human beings.

Mutations of the TSH receptor result in clinical thyroid dysfunction. Germline mutations can present as autosomal dominant toxic thyroid hyperplasia (gain-of-function mutations) or as gestational hyperthyroidism due to receptor hypersensitivity to hCG. Somatic mutations that result in constitutive activation of the receptor are associated with hyperfunctioning thyroid adenomas.

RELATION OF IODINE TO THYROID FUNCTION Normal thyroid function requires an adequate intake of iodine; without this, thyroid hormone cannot be made, TSH is secreted in excess, and the thyroid becomes hyperplastic and hypertrophic. The enlarged and stimulated thyroid becomes remarkably efficient at extracting the residual traces of iodide from the blood, developing an iodide gradient that may be 10 times normal. In mild-to-moderate iodine deficiency, the thyroid usually succeeds in producing sufficient hormone, in part by preferentially secreting T_3. In more severe deficiency, as is common in some parts of the world, adult hypothyroidism or cretinism may occur.

The daily requirement for iodine in adults is 1–2 μg/kg body weight. In the U.S., recommended daily allowances for iodine range from 40 to 120 μg for children, 150 μg for adults, 220 μg for pregnancy, and 270 μg for lactation. Dairy products and fish have relatively high iodine contents. Because of concerns of iodine insufficiency, iodine supplementation has been widely used for prophylaxis and therapy. The most practical form of this supplementation has been addition of iodide or iodate (now preferred) to table salt. In the U.S., such supplementation is optional and iodized salt provides 100 μg of iodine/g.

ACTIONS OF THYROID HORMONES Most actions of thyroid hormones are mediated by nuclear TRs that are members of the nuclear receptor superfamily. T_3 binds to high-affinity TRs, which then bind to specific DNA sequences (thyroid hormone response elements, TREs) in the promoter/regulatory regions of target genes to modulate gene transcription, and ultimately, protein synthesis. The unliganded TR is bound to the TREs in the basal state, typically repressing gene transcription. Binding by T_3 may activate gene transcription by relieving this repression; the T_3-TR complex may also have direct activation or repression functions. Like many nuclear receptors, TR typically activates transcription as a heterodimer with the retinoid X receptor. These transcriptional effects are mediated by interactions with a complex group of coactivator and corepressor proteins. Despite its capacity to bind to TRs, T_4 has not been shown to alter gene transcription and probably serves as a prohormone whose actions are manifested following conversion to T_3.

Two distinct genes encode 2 families of TRs, TRα and TRβ, and both genes encode multiple receptor isoforms. Certain isoforms (*e.g.*, TRα$_1$ and TRβ$_1$) are found in virtually all thyroid hormone-responsive tissues, whereas TRβ$_2$ is expressed only in the anterior pituitary. Resistance to thyroid hormone has been described in patients with mutations in the TRβ gene. In addition to nuclear receptor-mediated actions, there are several well-characterized, nongenomic actions of thyroid hormones, including those occurring at the plasma membrane and on the cellular cytoarchitecture.

Growth and Development Thyroid hormone plays a critical role in brain development. The absence of thyroid hormone during the period of active neurogenesis (up to 6 months postpartum) leads to irreversible mental retardation (cretinism) and is accompanied by multiple morphological alterations in the brain that reflect disturbed neuronal migration, deranged axonal projections, and decreased synaptogenesis. Thyroid hormone supplementation during the first 2 weeks of life prevents the development of these abnormalities.

Perhaps the most striking illustration of the pervasive developmental effects of thyroid hormones is provided by children with severe thyroid hormone deficiency from early childhood, a condition termed *cretinism*. This may either be endemic in regions of severe iodine deficiency or sporadic due to failure of the thyroid to develop normally or defects in the synthesis of thyroid hormone. Affected children are dwarfed with short extremities, have mental retardation, and are inactive and listless. Other manifestations include facial puffiness, enlarged tongue, dry and doughy skin, slow heart rate, and decreased body temperature. For full recovery, treatment of patients with cretinism must be initiated before these florid features are apparent. Thus, pregnant women in areas of endemic cretinism due to iodine deficiency are supplemented with iodine and all newborns are screened for thyroid hormone deficiency in many developed nations.

Calorigenic Effects In homeothermic animals, a characteristic response to thyroid hormone is increased O_2 consumption. Most peripheral tissues contribute to this response; heart, skeletal muscle, liver, and kidney are stimulated markedly by thyroid hormone. Indeed, 30–40% of the thyroid hormone-dependent increase in O_2 consumption can be attributed to stimulation of cardiac contractility. The mechanism of the calorigenic effect of thyroid hormone appears to reflect an integrated program by which thyroid hormone regulates the set-point of energy expenditure and maintains the metabolic machinery necessary to sustain it. Even small changes in L-thyroxine replacement dose may significantly alter the set-point for resting energy expenditure in the hypothyroid patient.

Cardiovascular Effects Thyroid hormones directly and indirectly influence cardiac function, and cardiovascular manifestations are prominent clinical consequences of thyroid disease. In hyperthyroidism, there is tachycardia, increased stroke volume, increased cardiac index, cardiac hypertrophy, decreased peripheral vascular resistance, and increased pulse pressure. In hypothyroidism, there is bradycardia, decreased cardiac index, pericardial effusion, increased peripheral vascular resistance, decreased pulse pressure, and elevation of mean arterial pressure.

Metabolic Effects

Thyroid hormones stimulate metabolism of cholesterol to bile acids and increase the concentration of receptors for low-density lipoprotein on hepatocytes, perhaps explaining the hypercholesterolemia that is characteristic in hypothyroid states.

Thyroid hormones enhance the lipolytic responses of fat cells to other hormones (e.g., catecholamines) and elevated plasma free fatty acid levels are seen in hyperthyroidism. Hyperthyroidism is an insulin resistant state, as manifested by depleted glycogen stores and enhanced gluconeogenesis; this may precipitate diabetes mellitus or worsen glycemic control in diabetics on treatment. Conversely, insulin requirements are reduced in diabetics who become hypothyroid.

Clinical Aspects of Thyroid Dysfunction

Clinical disorders of the thyroid can result from excessive or deficient production of thyroid hormone or from disorders of thyroid growth.

Assays of thyroid function Advances in thyroid function tests (TFTs), including the development of sensitive assays for TSH and the use of analog assays that provide a reasonable estimate of the free T_4 level, have markedly improved the diagnosis and treatment of thyroid disorders. These assays nonetheless can be misleading, as the TSH level can remain low for weeks to months after a hyperthyroid patient is restored to a euthyroid state and the analog assays of free T_4 can provide misleading results in certain settings such as critical illness.

A considerable advance in the management of thyroid cancer has resulted from the introduction of recombinant human TSH (THYROGEN). A dose of 0.9 mg is administered intramuscularly, followed by an identical dose 24 hours later. The serum thyroglobulin is then measured 48–72 hours after the second TSH injection; this has become the preferred diagnostic test for following patients with differentiated thyroid cancer who have had thyroidectomy and ablation of any remnant tissue with radioactive iodine. This regimen can also be used to stimulate iodine uptake by malignant cells in a total body scan (*see* below).

The percent uptake of a tracer dose of radioactive iodine (the radioactive iodine uptake, or RAIU) can provide important information about the pathogenesis of thyrotoxic states (*see* below).

Thyroid Hyperfunction Thyrotoxicosis is the term applied to any condition caused by elevated levels of circulating free thyroid hormones, while hyperthyroidism is restricted to those conditions in which thyroid hormone production and release are caused by gland hyperfunction.

Graves' disease, a frequent cause of hyperthyroidism, is an autoimmune disorder caused by IgG antibodies that bind to and activate the TSH receptor. Because of the persistent activation of the TSH receptor, the RAIU is increased. Other manifestations of Graves' disease include infiltrative ophthalmopathy and skin involvement (pretibial myxedema). Toxic multinodular goiter or hyperfunctioning adenomas account for 10–40 % of cases of hyperthyroidism and are more common in older patients. Destructive processes involving the thyroid (e.g., thyroiditis) can cause thyrotoxicosis due to leakage of preformed thyroid hormone from the gland. In this case, as with patients taking excessive doses of exogenous thyroid hormone, the RAIU will be suppressed.

Most of the signs and symptoms of thyrotoxicosis stem from excessive heat production, increased motor activity, and increased activity of the sympathetic nervous system. Eventually, the increased energy expenditure is often associated with weight loss. Cardiac manifestations include tachycardia and bounding pulses; older patients or those with underlying heart disease may exhibit angina, arrhythmias (especially atrial fibrillation), and high-output heart failure.

The most severe form of hyperthyroidism is thyroid storm, a rare but life-threatening disease that usually is precipitated by an intercurrent medical problem. Precipitating factors include infections, stress, trauma, thyroidal or nonthyroidal surgery, diabetic ketoacidosis, labor, heart disease, and rarely, radioactive iodine ablation. Clinical features are similar to those of thyrotoxicosis, but are more severe. Cardinal features include fever and tachycardia out of proportion to the fever. Nausea, vomiting, diarrhea, agitation, and confusion are frequent presentations. The abnormalities in TFTs are not necessarily worse than those in uncomplicated thyrotoxicosis and thyroid storm is a clinical diagnosis.

Thyroid Hypofunction Hypothyroidism is the most common disorder of thyroid function. It can be divided into patients who have a failure of the thyroid gland to produce sufficient thyroid hormone (primary hypothyroidism) and patients in which pituitary or hypothalamic disease is associated with impaired TSH stimulation (central or secondary hypothyroidism). Worldwide, primary hypothyroidism is caused most often by iodine deficiency. In areas where iodine is sufficient, chronic autoimmune thyroiditis (Hashimoto's thyroiditis) accounts for most cases. Other causes include postpartum thyroiditis, surgical removal, or radioactive iodine ablation of the gland. Hypothyroidism present at birth (cretinism) is the most common preventable cause of mental retardation in the world.

Hypothyroidism, when mild, can be subtle in its presentation. When severe, the signs are overt and the presentation is pathognomonic. The face is puffy and pallid, the skin is cold and dry, and the hair is coarse. The voice is husky, mentation is impaired, and depression may be present. The appetite is poor and constipation is common. The pulse is slow and a pericardial effusion may be present. Patients are lethargic and often complain of cold intolerance and weight gain.

The most severe expression of severe, long-standing hypothyroidism is myxedema coma. This medical emergency occurs most commonly in the elderly, particularly during winter months. Common precipitating factors include pneumonia, cerebrovascular accidents, and congestive heart failure. The clinical course—lethargy proceeding to stupor and then coma—is often hastened by drugs, especially sedatives, narcotics, antidepressants, and tranquilizers. Cardinal features of myxedema coma are (1) hypothermia, which may be profound; (2) respiratory depression; and (3) unconsciousness. Other clinical features include bradycardia, macroglossia, delayed reflexes, and dry skin. Hyponatremia is common and may be severe. Although the diagnosis is confirmed by measuring TFTs, myxedema coma is a clinical diagnosis.

Disorders of Thyroid Growth   Disorders of thyroid growth include diffuse enlargement of the thyroid gland, or goiter, nodular thyroid disease, and thyroid cancer. Goiter may be associated with hypothyroidism and the resultant TSH-induced hypertrophy and hyperplasia of thyroid cells.

Nodular thyroid disease is the most common endocrinopathy; when sensitive techniques such as ultrasound are used, the prevalence of thyroid nodules approaches 50% by age 60. Although these nodules can cause hyperthyroidism due to autonomous function, TFTs often are in the normal range. In this setting, it is important to distinguish benign nodules (solitary or multinodular) from the 5% to 10% that are malignant. Fine needle aspiration for cytopathology is the preferred diagnostic test.

Most thyroid cancers retain many functional aspects of normal thyroid cells. Although the treatment of choice for these tumors—as for all thyroid cancers—is surgical removal, the fact that these differentiated thyroid cancers retain some features of normal thyroid cells has important implications for both diagnosis and therapy (see below).

THERAPEUTIC USES OF THYROID HORMONE   The major indications for the therapeutic use of thyroid hormone are for hormone replacement therapy in patients with hypothyroidism or cretinism and for TSH suppression therapy in patients with thyroid cancer and occasionally those with nontoxic goiter.

The synthetic preparations used are the sodium salts of the natural isomers of the thyroid hormones. Levothyroxine *sodium (L-T_4, SYNTHROID, LEVOXYL, LEVOTHROID, UNITHROID, others) is available in tablets in a variety of doses and as a lyophilized powder for injection. L-T_4 has a narrow therapeutic index, and the FDA has mandated demonstration of bioequivalence for brand and generic preparations by the various producers.* Liothyronine *sodium (L-T_3) is available in tablets (CYTOMEL) and in an injectable form (TRIOSTAT). A mixture of L-T_4 and L-T_3 is marketed as* liotrix *(THYROLAR). Desiccated thyroid preparations, derived from whole animal thyroids and containing both T_4 and T_3, have highly variable biologic activity and are much less desirable.*

Thyroid Hormone Replacement Therapy

L-T_4 is preferred for thyroid hormone replacement because of its consistent potency and prolonged duration of action. Absorption of L-T_4 in the small intestine is variable and incomplete (50–80% of the dose absorbed, slightly increased when taken on an empty stomach). Certain drugs may interfere with L-T_4 absorption, including cholestyramine, iron and calcium supplements, aluminum hydroxide, *and soy products. Enhanced biliary excretion of L-T_4 occurs during the co-administration of drugs that induce hepatic CYPs, such as* phenytoin, carbamazepine, *and* rifampin, *often necessitating an increase in the dose. L-T_3 may be used occasionally when a quicker onset of action is desired, as in patients with myxedema coma, or when a shorter duration of action is desired, as when preparing a patient for ^{131}I therapy for thyroid cancer. It is less desirable for chronic therapy because it is more expensive, must be dosed more frequently, and causes transient elevations of serum T_3 above the normal range.*

The average daily adult replacement dose of L-T_4 in a 70-kg person is 112 μg given as a single dose, while that for L-T_3 is 50–75 μg in divided doses. In healthy younger individuals, therapy can be initiated at the full replacement dose. Because of the prolonged $t_{1/2}$ of T_4 (1 week), steady state levels will not be achieved until 5 weeks after a change in dose; thus, reevaluation of TFTs should not be performed at intervals of less than 6–8 weeks. The goal is to achieve a TSH value in the normal range, since suppression of TSH by overreplacement may be associated with osteoporosis and cardiac dysfunction. In patients with markedly elevated TSH (>50 mIU /mL), it may take more than 8 weeks for the TSH to reach a steady state. In patients with central hypothyroidism, the dose should be adjusted based on the free T_4 and patient well-being. In noncompliant young patients, the total weekly dose of L-T_4 can safely be administered as a single dose once weekly. In individuals over age 60, initiation of therapy at lower doses of L-T_4 (25–50 μg/day) *minimizes the risk of exacerbating undiagnosed heart disease. For individuals with preexisting cardiac disease, L-T$_4$ is initiated at 12.5 μg/day, with increases of 12.5–25 μg/day every 6–8 weeks. Because of its long t$_{1/2}$, a lapse of several days of L-T$_4$ therapy is unlikely to have significant consequences; if more prolonged interruption is necessary, L-T$_4$ can be given parenterally at a dose 25–50% less than the daily oral requirement.*

Thyroid Hormone Replacement during Pregnancy Due to estrogen-induced increases in TBG and transplacental passage of L-T$_4$ from mother to fetus, a higher dose of L-T$_4$ often is required in hypothyroid patients who become pregnant (typically 25–40% over basal). Because even mild hypothyroidism may be associated with impaired psychomotor development, any woman whose TSH is elevated should be treated during pregnancy. Serum TSH should be determined during the first trimester in all patients with preexisting hypothyroidism and in those at risk for developing the disorder. Some screen all pregnant women in the first trimester. Therapy with L-T$_4$ should be administered to keep the TSH in the normal range and adjusted based on the serum TSH throughout the pregnancy.

Treatment of Myxedema Coma

Myxedema coma is the extreme expression of severe, long-standing hypothyroidism. In addition to supportive care and treatment of the precipitating cause, treatment with thyroid hormone is essential. Based on uncertain oral absorption, thyroid hormone generally is given parenterally (e.g., a loading dose of 200–300 μg of L-T$_4$ intravenously followed by a second dose of 100 μg 24 hours later). A daily maintenance dose is then continued intravenously until the patient has improved sufficiently for oral therapy. Because of its more rapid onset of action, some clinicians add L-T$_3$ (10 μg intravenously every 8 hours) until the patient is stable. Overly aggressive treatment with either L-T$_4$ or L-T$_3$ may be associated with increased mortality.

Treatment of Cretinism

An initial daily dose of L-T$_4$ of 10–15 μg/kg is recommended to rapidly normalize the serum T$_4$ concentration, which will increase the serum T$_4$ concentration to the upper half of the normal range within 1–2 weeks. Individual L-T$_4$ doses are then adjusted at 4–6-week intervals during the first 6 months, at 2-month intervals during the 6–18-month period, and then at 3–6-month intervals to maintain serum free T$_4$ levels in the upper half of the normal range, or even slightly above the normal range, with a normal TSH. Clinical guides for assessing response include growth, motor development, bone maturation, and developmental progress.

Treatment of Thyroid Nodules

Thyroid hormone is sometimes used to suppress growth in patients with a benign solitary thyroid nodule and a normal TSH, but such therapy generally is not recommended. Suppression therapy is of no value if the nodule is autonomous, as indicated by a subnormal TSH. Once TSH is suppressed, a radioisotope scan should be performed; if significant uptake persists, the gland is non-suppressible and L-T$_4$ therapy should be discontinued. Suppression therapy should not be used in patients with known coronary artery disease, since the risks of precipitating cardiac arrhythmias or angina are considerable.

Thyroid Cancer

L-T$_4$ therapy to suppress TSH stimulation to growth of differentiated thyroid cancers is the cornerstone of therapy following surgical removal and radioactive ablation with ^{131}I (see below). In tumors with more worrisome prognostic features, the goal is to suppress the TSH to undetectable levels. For tumors judged to be of lower risk, the L-T$_4$ dose is typically adjusted so that the TSH is below the normal range but still detectable.

ANTITHYROID DRUGS AND OTHER THYROID INHIBITORS

A large number of compounds interfere either directly or indirectly with the synthesis, release, or action of thyroid hormones (Table 56–2). Inhibitors are classified into four categories: (1) antithyroid drugs, which interfere directly with the synthesis of thyroid hormones; (2) ionic inhibitors, which block the iodide transport mechanism; (3) high concentrations of iodine itself, which decrease release of thyroid hormones and may also decrease hormone synthesis; and (4) radioactive iodine, which damages the gland with ionizing radiation. Adjuvant therapy with drugs that have no specific effects on thyroid hormone synthesis is useful in controlling the peripheral manifestations of thyrotoxicosis, including inhibitors of the peripheral deiodination of T$_4$ to T$_3$, β adrenergic receptor antagonists, and Ca^{2+} channel blockers.

Table 56–2

Antithyroid Compounds

Process Affected	Examples of Inhibitors
Active transport of iodide	Complex anions: perchlorate, fluoborate, pertechnetate, thiocyanate
Iodination of thyroglobulin	Thionamides: propylthiouracil, methimazole, carbimazole
	Thiocyanate; iodide
	Aniline derivatives; sulfonamides
Coupling reaction	Thionamides; sulfonamides
Hormone release	Lithium salts; iodide
Iodotyrosine deiodination	Nitrotyrosines
Peripheral iodothyronine deiodination	Thiouracil derivatives; amiodarone
	Oral cholecystographic agents
Hormone excretion/ inactivation	Inducers of hepatic drug-metabolizing enzymes: phenobarbital, rifampin, carbamazepine, phenytoin
Hormone action	Thyroxine analogs; amiodarone
Binding in gut	Cholestyramine

Antithyroid Drugs

The antithyroid drugs that have greatest clinical utility are the thioureylenes, which belong to the family of thionamides (Figure 56–6).

MECHANISM OF ACTION Antithyroid drugs inhibit the formation of thyroid hormones by interfering with the incorporation of iodine into tyrosyl residues of thyroglobulin; they also inhibit the coupling of these iodotyrosyl residues to form iodothyronines. The inhibition of hormone synthesis eventually results in depletion of stores of iodinated thyroglobulin as the protein is hydrolyzed and the hormones are released into the circulation. Clinical effects only become apparent when the preformed hormone is reduced and the concentrations of circulating thyroid hormones begin to decline.

In addition to blocking hormone synthesis, propylthiouracil also inhibits the peripheral deiodination of T_4 to T_3; this added effect provides a rationale for the choice of propylthiouracil over methimazole in the treatment of severe hyperthyroid states such as thyroid storm.

ABSORPTION, METABOLISM, AND EXCRETION The antithyroid drugs used in the U.S. are propylthiouracil (6-*n*-propylthiouracil) and methimazole (1-methyl-2-mercaptoimidazole; TAPAZOLE). In Europe, carbimazole (NEO-MERCAZOLE), a carbethoxy derivative that is converted to methimazole, also is used. Some pharmacological properties of propylthiouracil and methimazole are shown in Table 56–3. Because of its shorter $t_{1/2}$, propylthiouracil must be dosed more frequently than methimazole. In severe hyperthyroid states, even a 500-mg dose of propylthiouracil must be dosed every 6-8 hours to yield complete thyroid inhibition, while doses of 20-40 mg of methimazole may be given once-daily. The drugs are concentrated in the thyroid and drugs and metabolites largely are excreted in the urine. Propylthiouracil and methimazole cross the placenta equally and also can be found in milk. Their use in pregnancy is discussed below.

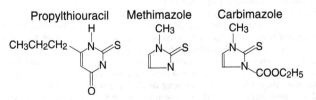

FIGURE 56–6 *Antithyroid drugs of the thionamide type.*

Table 56–3

Selected Pharmacokinetic Features of Antithyroid Drugs

	Propylthiouracil	Methimazole
Plasma protein binding	~75%	Nil
Plasma $t_{1/2}$	75 minutes	~4–6 hours
Volume of distribution	~20 L	~40 L
Concentrated in thyroid	Yes	Yes
Metabolism of drug during illness		
Severe liver disease	Normal	Decreased
Severe kidney disease	Normal	Normal
Dosing frequency	1–4 times daily	Once or twice daily
Transplacental passage	Low	Low
Levels in breast milk	Low	Low

UNTOWARD REACTIONS The most serious adverse effect of the antithyroid drugs is agranulocytosis, which can occur in up to 0.2% of patients. The development of agranulocytosis apparently is dose related with methimazole but not with propylthiouracil. Agranulocytosis usually occurs during the first few weeks of therapy but may occur later. Surveillance white blood cell counts are of limited value, and patients should be warned to report immediately sore throat or fever that may herald the onset of this reaction. Agranulocytosis is reversible upon discontinuation of the offending drug. Mild granulocytopenia, if noted, may be due to thyrotoxicosis or may be the first sign of this dangerous drug reaction; frequent leukocyte counts are then required.

The most common adverse reaction is an urticarial rash that often subsides spontaneously without drug discontinuation and may be relieved by antihistamines or glucocorticoids or by changing antithyroid drugs (cross-sensitivity to propylthiouracil and methimazole is uncommon). Other less common manifestations include arthralgias, paresthesias, headache, nausea, skin pigmentation, and hair loss. Drug fever, hepatitis, and nephritis are rare, although abnormal liver function tests are not infrequent with higher does of propylthiouracil.

THERAPEUTIC USES

The antithyroid drugs are used as definitive treatment of hyperthyroidism, to control the disorder in anticipation of a spontaneous remission in Graves' disease, while awaiting the effects of radiation, and in preparation for thyroid surgery.

A typical starting dose of propylthiouracil is 100 mg every 8 hours or 150 mg every 12 hours. When doses >300 mg/day are needed in severely hyperthyroid patients, the drug should be administered at least every 8 hours. In thyroid storm, propylthiouracil is preferred due to its inhibition of peripheral conversion of T_4 to T_3; doses of 200–400 mg every 4 hours are typically employed. In less severely hyperthyroid patients, methimazole often is effective when given once daily (10–30 mg), which may improve patient adherence. Response to therapy is followed by TFTs, remembering that the TSH may remain suppressed even after the patient has become euthyroid. Once euthyroidism is achieved, usually within 12 weeks, the dose can be reduced but should not be stopped lest the hyperthyroid state recur. Continued overtreatment with antithyroid drugs can induce hypothyroidism, often heralded by increased gland size.

Although remission of Graves' disease does occur, experience in the U.S. suggests that this happens in less than 50% of patients. Thus, many endocrinologists in the U.S. prefer radioactive iodine ablation for definitive therapy (see below).

Pregnant women with thyrotoxicosis comprise a special subset of patients. In this setting, radioactive iodine is clearly contraindicated. Propylthiouracil and methimazole cross the placenta equally and either can be used in pregnancy. The dose of antithyroid drug should be minimized to avoid possible hypothyroidism in the fetus; the goal is to keep the free T_4 in the upper half of the normal range or even slightly elevated. Because Graves' disease often improves during pregnancy, TFTs should be followed at 4–6-week intervals, with dose decreases as indicated. In nursing mothers, propylthiouracil is the drug of choice, since very small amounts of drug are found in breast milk and impaired thyroid function has not been demonstrated in suckling babies whose mothers were taking this drug; methimazole also appears to be safe in this setting.

Ionic Inhibitors

The ionic inhibitors interfere with iodide concentration by the thyroid gland. Effective agents are monovalent hydrated anions of a size similar to that of iodide. The best studied, thiocyanate, is unique among these agents because it is not concentrated by the thyroid gland. Perchlorate (ClO_4^-) blocks the entrance of iodide into the thyroid by competitively inhibiting the NIS. Perchlorate at higher doses (2–3 g daily) has caused fatal aplastic anemia; lower doses (750 mg/day) have been used to treat patients with hyperthyroidism due to the administration of pharmacological doses of iodide (see below). Although concern has been raised about potential effects of perchlorate contamination of the water supply, there is no definitive evidence of deleterious effects on thyroid function.

Iodide

High concentrations of iodide inhibit iodide uptake, organification and coupling, and the release of thyroid hormone. In hyperthyroid patients, the response to iodide therapy can be striking. Over time, however, the beneficial effects disappear, even with ongoing therapy. Thus, iodide is often used for the preoperative treatment of hyperthyroidism in anticipation of thyroid surgery, where it causes a salutary decrease in gland vascularity. Iodide also can be administered prophylactically to protect the thyroid from radioactive iodine following a nuclear accident. In euthyroid individuals, the administration of doses of iodide from 1.5 to 150 mg daily does not significantly impair thyroid hormone synthesis. However, euthyroid patients with a wide variety of underlying thyroid disorders (*e.g.*, treated Graves' disease, Hashimoto's thyroiditis, postpartum thyroiditis) may develop iodine-induced hypothyroidism when exposed to large amounts of iodine present in many commonly prescribed drugs, most often certain expectorants, topical antiseptics, amiodarone, and radiological contrast agents.

Occasional individuals show marked hypersensitivity to intravenous administration of iodide or organic preparations of iodine. Angioedema is the cardinal manifestation, and laryngeal edema may lead to suffocation. Later, a serum sickness-like reaction may develop. These reactions to radiographic contrast agents are not due to the iodine *per se.*

Radioactive Iodine

^{131}I has a t$_{1/2}$ of 8 days and emits both γ rays and β particles. Radioactive ablation with ^{131}I is used for the treatment of hyperthyroidism and for adjuvant therapy of differentiated thyroid cancer. The only absolute contraindication to the use of ^{131}I therapy is pregnancy, as the fetal thyroid after the first trimester can concentrate the isotope and thus will be damaged. There is no evidence for increased total cancer mortality or increased incidence of leukemia in treated patients. One study found an increased incidence of colorectal cancer following ^{131}I therapy, leading to the recommendation that laxatives be given prophylactically to all patients receiving ^{131}I. The short-lived ^{123}I is primarily a γ-emitter that is used for diagnostic purposes in thyroid uptake and scans.

Hyperthyroidism

^{131}I is highly useful in the treatment of hyperthyroidism and is viewed by many as the treatment of choice for this condition. There is little benefit from individualized dosing based on thyroid weight and RAIU, and a total dose of approximately 15 mCi is typically employed. Patients who have been pretreated with propylthiouracil to control their hyperthyroidism may need a higher dose; no such effect is seen with methimazole. The course of a patient who has received an effective dose of ^{131}I is characterized by progressive recovery, beginning within a few weeks after treatment and continuing for a period of 2–4 months thereafter. If therapy has been inadequate, the need for further treatment should be apparent within 6–12 months. Adjuvant therapy with β adrenergic antagonists, antithyroid drugs, or both can be used while awaiting the full effects of therapy. The antithyroid drug should be withheld for a few days before and after the ^{131}I to avoid inhibiting iodine uptake and organification.

Radioactive iodine ablation therapy for hyperthyroidism is relatively inexpensive, does not require hospitalization, and is relatively free of adverse effects. It is associated with a high incidence of permanent hypothyroidism, and all patients must be warned of this and followed thereafter for the onset of hypothyroidism. Because thyroid hormone replacement therapy is generally well accepted by the patient, many specialists prefer to treat with relatively higher ^{131}I doses to rapidly and predictably induce hypothyroidism. Another adverse effect of ^{131}I ablation therapy for Graves' disease is the possible worsening of the Graves' ophthalmopathy, particularly if the patient is allowed to become hypothyroid. Although rare, thyroid storm has occurred after therapy with ^{131}I.

Thyroid Carcinoma

Following surgical removal, the most important intervention in the treatment of differentiated thyroid cancer is L-T_4 suppression of serum TSH (see above). Radioactive iodine ablation with ^{131}I also plays an important therapeutic role. While most well-differentiated thyroid carcinomas accumulate iodine inefficiently, stimulation of iodine uptake with TSH often is used efficiently to treat residual cervical disease or metastases. Following near total thyroidectomy—the preferred surgical approach—the patient is allowed to become hypothyroid until the TSH is over 30 mIU/L. Thereafter, the patient is given 30–150 mCi of ^{131}I and a total body scan is obtained at one week. Alternatively, recombinant human TSH can be administered to stimulate the uptake of radioactive iodine. The ^{131}I dose is repeated if a rising serum thyroglobulin level or persistent iodine uptake on a total body scan suggests that there is tumor recurrence. Particularly at higher doses, salivary gland dysfunction may occur after radioactive iodine therapy.

For a complete Bibliographical listing see Goodman & Gilman's *The Pharmacological Basis of Therapeutics*, 11th ed., or Goodman & Gilman Online at www.accessmedicine.com.

57

ESTROGENS AND PROGESTINS

Estrogens and *progestins* are steroid hormones with numerous physiological actions. In women, these include developmental effects, control of ovulation, cyclical preparation of the reproductive tract for fertilization and implantation, and metabolic actions. Estrogens also have important actions in males, including effects on bone, spermatogenesis, and behavior. Estrogens and progestins are used in menopausal hormone therapy (MHT) and contraception in women. Estrogen- and progesterone-receptor antagonists also are available. Antiestrogens are employed in treating hormone-responsive breast cancer and infertility. The main use of antiprogestins has been for medical abortion. Selective estrogen receptor modulators (SERMs) with tissue-selective agonist or antagonist activities are increasingly available.

ESTROGENS

CHEMISTRY AND BIOSYNTHESIS

Many steroidal and nonsteroidal compounds possess estrogenic activity (Table 57–1 and Figure 57–1). The most potent endogenous estrogen is 17β-estradiol, followed by estrone and estriol. The phenolic A ring is the principal structural feature responsible for selective, high-affinity binding to the estrogen receptors (ERs). Ethinyl substitutions at C17 increase oral potency by inhibiting first-pass hepatic metabolism.

Nonsteroidal compounds with estrogenic or antiestrogenic activity—including flavones, isoflavones (e.g., genistein), and coumestan derivatives—occur in plants and fungi. Synthetic agents—including pesticides (e.g., p,p'-DDT), plasticizers (e.g., bisphenol A), and other industrial chemicals (e.g., polychlorinated biphenyls)—also have hormonal or antihormonal activity. While their affinity is relatively weak, their large number, bioaccumulation, and persistence in the environment raise concerns about their potential toxicity in humans and wildlife.

Steroidal estrogens arise from androstenedione or testosterone (Figure 57–1) by aromatization of the A ring, a reaction catalyzed by aromatase (CYP19), an enzyme found in ovarian granulosa cells, testicular Sertoli and Leydig cells, adipose stroma, placental syncytiotrophoblast, preimplantation blastocysts, bone, various brain regions, and other tissues. Ovaries are the principal source of circulating estrogen in premenopausal women. Gonadotropins, acting via receptors that couple to the G_s-adenylyl cyclase–cyclic AMP pathway, increase the activities of aromatase and the cholesterol side-chain cleavage enzyme. The ovary contains the type I isoform of 17β-hydroxysteroid dehydrogenase, which favors the production of testosterone and estradiol from androstenedione and estrone, respectively. In the liver, the type II isoform oxidizes circulating estradiol to estrone, which then is converted to estriol (Figure 57–1). These estrogens are excreted in the urine along with their glucuronide and sulfate conjugates. In postmenopausal women, the principal source of circulating estrogen is adipose tissue stroma, where estrone is synthesized from dehydroepiandrosterone (DHEA) secreted by the adrenals. In men, the testes produce estrogens but extragonadal aromatization of circulating androstenedione and DHEA accounts for most circulating estrogens.

Local production of estrogens by the aromatization of androgens may play a causal role in the development or progression of diseases such as breast cancer. Estrogens also may be produced from androgens by CYP19 in the central nervous system (CNS) and other tissues and exert local effects near their production site (e.g., in bone they increase bone mineral density).

Physiological and Pharmacological Actions

DEVELOPMENTAL ACTIONS Estrogens in girls cause growth and development of the vagina, uterus, and fallopian tubes, and contribute to breast enlargement, molding the body contours, shaping the skeleton, and causing the pubertal growth spurt of the long bones and epiphyseal closure. Growth of axillary and pubic hair, pigmentation of the genital region, and the regional pigmentation of the nipples and areolae that occur after the first trimester of pregnancy are also estrogenic actions.

Estrogens also play developmental roles in males. In boys, estrogen deficiency diminishes the pubertal growth spurt and delays skeletal maturation and epiphyseal closure so that linear growth continues into adulthood. Estrogen deficiency in men leads to elevated gonadotropins, macroorchidism, and increased testosterone levels and also may affect carbohydrate and lipid metabolism and fertility.

Table 57–1

Structural Formulas of Selected Estrogens

Steroidal Estrogens			Nonsteroidal Compounds with Estrogenic Activity

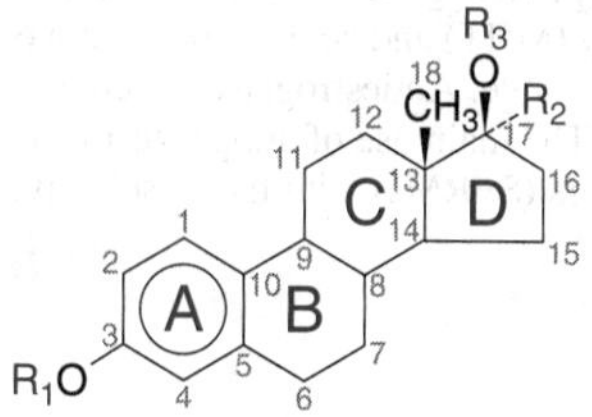

Diethylstilbestrol

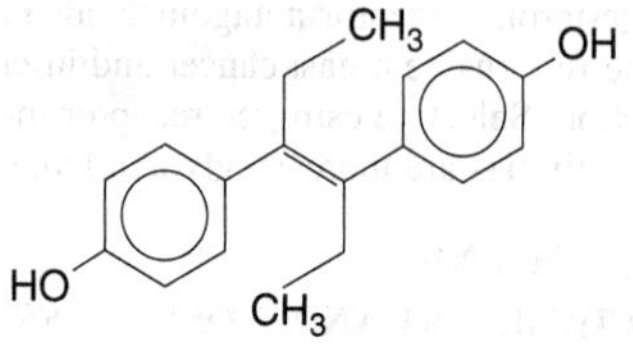

Derivative	R_1	R_2	R_3
Estradiol	—H	—H	—H
Estradiol valerate	—H	—H	$-\overset{\displaystyle O}{\overset{\displaystyle \|}{C}}(CH_2)_3CH_3$
Ethinyl estradiol	—H	—C≡CH	—H
Mestranol	—CH$_3$	—C≡CH	—H
Estrone sulfate	—SO$_3$H	—*	=O*
Equilin†	—H	—*	=O*

Bisphenol A

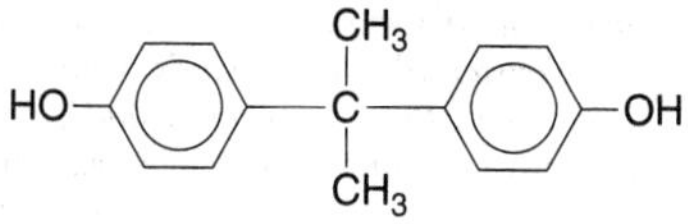

Genistein

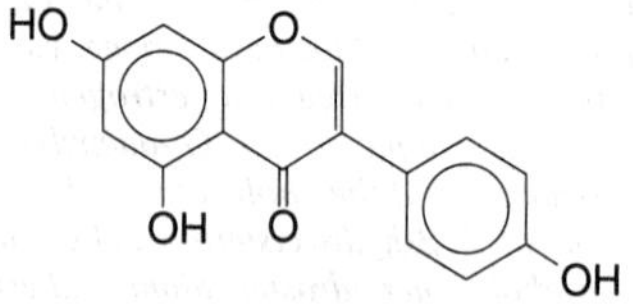

*Designates C17 ketone.
†Also contains 7, 8 double bond.

NEUROENDOCRINE CONTROL OF THE MENSTRUAL CYCLE A neuroendocrine cascade involving the hypothalamus, pituitary, and ovaries controls the menstrual cycle (Figure 57–2). A neuronal oscillator or "clock" in the hypothalamus fires at intervals that coincide with bursts of gonadotropin-releasing hormone (GnRH) release into the hypothalamic-pituitary portal vasculature (*see* Chapter 55). GnRH interacts with its receptor on pituitary gonadotropes to cause release of luteinizing hormone (LH) and follicle-stimulating hormone (FSH). The frequency of the GnRH pulses, which varies in the different phases of the menstrual cycle (*see* below), controls the relative secretion of FSH and LH.

The gonadotropins (LH and FSH) regulate the growth and maturation of follicles in the ovary and ovarian production of estrogen and progesterone, which then exert feedback regulation on the pituitary and hypothalamus.

Because GnRH release is intermittent, LH and FSH secretion is pulsatile. The pulse *frequency* is determined by the *hypothalamic GnRH pulse generator* (Figure 57–2), but the amount of gonadotropin released in each pulse (*i.e.,* the pulse *amplitude*) is largely controlled by the actions of estrogens and progesterone on the pituitary. The intermittent, *pulsatile* nature of hormone release is essential for the maintenance of normal ovulatory menstrual cycles; constant infusion of GnRH inhibits gonadotropin release and ovarian steroid production (*see* Chapter 55).Ovarian steroids, primarily progesterone, regulate the frequency of GnRH release by direct and indirect effects on GnRH neurons.

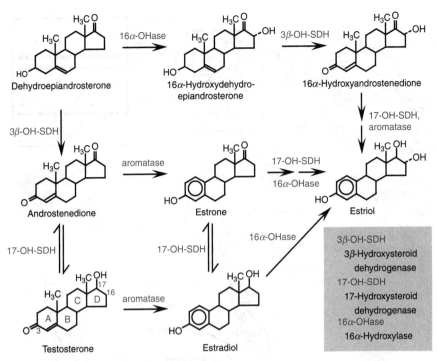

FIGURE 57-1 *The biosynthetic pathway for the estrogens.*

Figure 57-3 summarizes the profiles of gonadotropin and gonadal steroid levels in the menstrual cycle. In the early follicular phase, GnRH is secreted in pulses with a frequency of ~1/h. These pulses cause a corresponding pulsatile release of LH and FSH from pituitary gonadotropes; FSH in particular causes the graafian follicle to mature and secrete estrogen. Effects of estrogens at this time decrease LH and FSH release, so gonadotropin levels gradually fall. The ovarian peptide inhibin also exerts a negative feedback to selectively decrease serum FSH. At midcycle, serum estradiol rises above a threshold level of 150–200 pg/mL for approximately 36 hours, exerting a brief positive feedback at the pituitary to trigger the preovulatory surge of LH and FSH. The midcycle surge in gonadotropins stimulates follicular rupture and ovulation within 1–2 days. The ruptured follicle then develops into the corpus luteum, which produces large amounts of progesterone under the influence of LH during the second half of the cycle. In the absence of pregnancy, the corpus luteum ceases to function, steroid levels drop, and menstruation occurs. When steroid levels drop, the pulse generator reverts to the follicular phase pattern, the entire system then resets, and a new cycle occurs.

Progesterone decreases the frequency of GnRH pulses and also exerts a direct pituitary effect to oppose the inhibitory actions of estrogens and thus enhance the amount of LH released. These steroid feedback effects, coupled with the intrinsic activity of the GnRH neurons, lead to relatively frequent LH pulses of small amplitude in the follicular phase, and less frequent pulses of larger amplitude in the luteal phase.

In males, testosterone regulates the hypothalamic-pituitary-gonadal axis at both the hypothalamic and pituitary levels, and its negative feedback effect is mediated to a substantial degree by estrogen formed via aromatization.

EFFECTS OF CYCLICAL GONADAL STEROIDS ON THE REPRODUCTIVE TRACT

The cyclical changes in estrogen and progesterone production by the ovaries regulate corresponding events in the fallopian tubes, uterus, cervix, and vagina. Physiologically, these changes prepare the uterus for implantation and pregnancy. If pregnancy does not occur, the uterine endometrium is shed as the menstrual discharge (Figure 57–3).

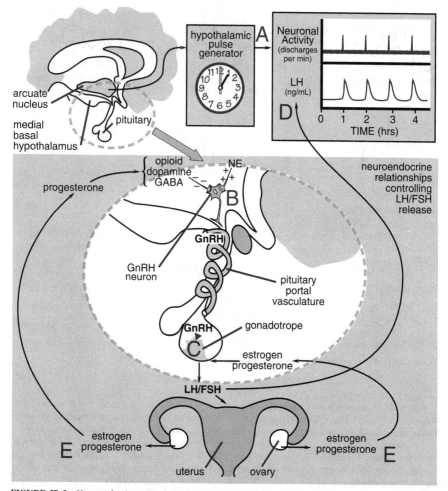

FIGURE 57–2 *Neuroendocrine control of gonadotropin secretion in females.* The hypothalamic pulse generator functions as a neuronal "clock" that fires at regular hourly intervals (**A**), resulting in the periodic release of gonadotropin-releasing hormone (GnRH) from GnRH neurons into the hypothalamic-pituitary portal vasculature (**B**). GnRH neurons (**B**) receive inhibitory input from opioid, dopamine, and GABA neurons and stimulatory input from noradrenergic neurons (NE, norepinephrine). The pulses of GnRH trigger the intermittent release of luteinizing hormone (LH) and folli-cle-stimulating hormone (FSH) from pituitary gonadotropes (**C**), resulting in the pulsatile plasma profile (**D**). FSH and LH regulate ovarian production of estrogen and progesterone, which exert feedback controls (**E**). (See text and Figure 57–3 for additional details.)

    Menstruation marks the start of the menstrual cycle. During the follicular (or proliferative) phase, estrogen stimulates proliferation and differentiation. One important effect of estrogen in the endometrium and other tissues is induction of the progesterone receptor (PR), which enables cells to respond to this hormone during the second half of the cycle.

    In the luteal (or secretory) phase of the cycle, elevated progesterone limits the proliferative effect of estrogens on the endometrium by stimulating differentiation. Progesterone is thus important in preparation for implantation and for the decidual reaction that takes place in the uterus at the implantation site. There is a narrow "window of implantation," spanning days 19–24 of the cycle, when the epithelial cells of the endometrium are receptive to blastocyst implantation.

    If implantation occurs, human chorionic gonadotropin, produced initially by the trophoblast and later by the placenta, maintains steroid hormone synthesis by the corpus luteum during the early stages of pregnancy. Thereafter, the placenta itself becomes the major site of estrogen and progesterone synthesis.

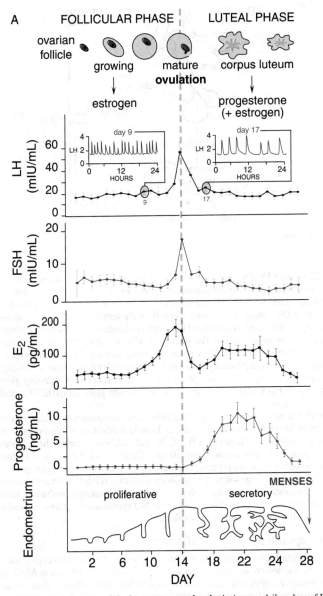

FIGURE 57–3 *Hormonal relationships of the human menstrual cycle.* **A**. Average daily values of LH, FSH, estradiol (E_2), and progesterone in plasma samples from women exhibiting normal 28-day menstrual cycles. Changes in the ovarian follicle (*top*) and endometrium (*bottom*) also are illustrated schematically.

Frequent plasma sampling reveals pulsatile patterns of gonadotropin release. Characteristic profiles are illustrated schematically for the follicular phase (day 9, inset on left) and luteal phase (day 17, inset on right). Both the frequency (number of pulses per hour) and amplitude (extent of change of hormone release) of pulses vary throughout the cycle. *(Redrawn with permission from Thorneycroft et al., 1971).*

B. Major regulatory effects of ovarian steroids on hypothalamic-pituitary function. Estrogen decreases the amount of follicle-stimulating hormone (FSH) and luteinizing hormone (LH) released (*i.e.*, gonadotropin pulse amplitude) during most of the cycle and triggers a surge of LH release only at mid-cycle. Progesterone decreases the frequency of GnRH release from the hypothalamus and thus decreases the frequency of plasma gonadotropin pulses. Progesterone also increases the amount of LH released (*i.e.*, the pulse amplitude) during the luteal phase of the cycle.

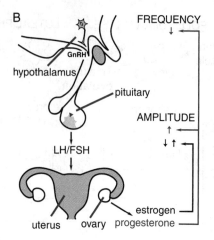

FIGURE 57–3 (*Continued*)

METABOLIC EFFECTS   *Estrogens increase bone mass, largely by decreasing the number and activity of osteoclasts, thereby decreasing bone resorption* (*see* Chapter 61). Estrogens increase high-density lipoprotein (HDL) levels and decrease the levels of low-density lipoprotein (LDL) and Lp(a) (*see* Chapter 35). Estrogens also increase biliary cholesterol secretion and decrease bile acid secretion, leading to increased saturation of bile with cholesterol that results in gallstone formation in some women receiving estrogens. The decline in bile acid biosynthesis may contribute to the decreased incidence of colon cancer in women receiving combined estrogen-progestin treatment. Estrogens affect many serum proteins, particularly those involved in hormone binding and clotting cascades. In general, estrogens increase plasma levels of corticosteroid-binding globulin (CBG), thyroxine-binding globulin (TBG), and sex hormone–binding globulin (SHBG), which binds both androgens and estrogens.

Estrogens alter a number of pathways that affect the cardiovascular system. Systemic effects include changes in lipoprotein metabolism and in hepatic production of plasma proteins. Estrogens slightly increase coagulation factors II, VII, IX, X, and XII, and decrease the anticoagulation factors protein C, protein S, and antithrombin III (*see* Chapter 54). Fibrinolytic pathways also are affected; several studies of women treated with estrogen or estrogen with a progestin demonstrate decreased levels of plasminogen-activator inhibitor protein-1 (PAI-1) with a concomitant increase in fibrinolysis. Thus, estrogens increase both coagulation and fibrinolytic pathways. Estrogen actions on the vascular wall include induction of inducible NO synthase and increased production of NO and prostacyclin, all of which promote vasodilation.

Estrogen Receptors; Mechanism of Action

Estrogens exert their effects *via* receptors that are members of the nuclear receptor superfamily. The two ER genes are located on separate chromosomes: *ESR1* encodes ERα, and *ESR2* encodes ERβ. Both ERs are estrogen-dependent transcription factors that have different tissue distributions and transcriptional regulatory effects on a wide number of target genes. Both genes encode multiple isoforms due to differential promoter use and alternative splicing. There are significant differences between the two receptors in their ligand-binding and transactivation domains, and they appear to have different biological functions and respond differently to various estrogenic compounds. However, the high homology in their DNA-binding domains suggests that both receptors recognize similar DNA sequences and hence regulate many of the same target genes.

ERα is expressed most abundantly in the female reproductive tract—especially the uterus, vagina, and ovaries—as well as in the mammary gland, hypothalamus, endothelial cells, and vascular smooth muscle. ERβ is expressed most highly in the prostate and ovaries, with lower expression in lung, brain, bone, and vasculature. Many cells express both ERα and ERβ.

Both ERs are ligand-activated transcription factors that increase or decrease the transcription of target genes. After entering the cell, the hormone binds to an ER in the nucleus. Upon bind-

ing estrogen, a change in ER conformation dissociates heat-shock proteins and causes receptor dimerization, which increases receptor binding to DNA. The ER dimer binds to estrogen response elements (EREs), typically located in the promoter region of target genes. The ER/DNA complex recruits a cascade of coactivators and other proteins to the promoter region of target genes. Interaction of ERs with antagonists also promotes dimerization and DNA binding but antagonists produce a conformation of ER that facilitates binding of corepressors, which inhibit target gene expression. In addition, both MAP kinase and PI-3-kinase–activated Akt can directly phosphorylate ERα to induce ligand-independent activation of estrogen-target genes. This cross-talk between membrane-bound receptor pathways (i.e., EGF/IGF-1) and the nuclear ER may have implications for diseases such as breast cancer.

Rapid, non-genomic actions of estrogen are mediated by membrane-localized ERs encoded by ESR1.

Absorption, Fate, and Elimination

Various estrogens are available for oral, parenteral, transdermal, or topical administration. For many uses, preparations are available as an estrogen alone or in combination with a progestin. Oral administration may utilize estradiol, conjugated estrogens, esters of estrone and other estrogens, and *ethinyl estradiol*. A micronized preparation of estradiol (ESTRACE, others) can be given orally, but high doses must be used due to first-pass metabolism. Ethinyl estradiol is used orally, as the ethinyl substitution at C17 inhibits first-pass hepatic metabolism. Other common oral preparations contain conjugated equine estrogens (PREMARIN); *esterified esters*; or mixtures of conjugated estrogens prepared from plant-derived sources (CENESTIN).

Transdermal administration of estradiol (ESTRADERM, VIVELLE, ALORA, CLIMARA, others) provides slow, sustained release of the hormone, systemic distribution, and more constant blood levels than oral dosing. Estradiol is also available as a topical cream (ESTRASORB) or as a gel (ESTROGEL). The transdermal route does not lead to the high level of the drug that enters the liver via the portal circulation after oral administration and is thus may decrease estrogen effects on hepatic protein synthesis, lipoprotein profiles, and triglyceride levels. Estradiol and conjugated estrogen creams also are available for topical administration to the vagina. These are effective locally, but systemic effects also are possible due to significant absorption. A 3-month vaginal ring (ESTRING, FEMRING) may be used for slow release of estradiol, and tablets are also available for vaginal use (VAGIFEM). Other preparations are available for intramuscular injection. The esters of estradiol become less polar as the size of the substituents increases; thus, the rate of absorption of oily preparations is progressively slowed, and the duration of action can be prolonged. A single intramuscular injection of compounds such as estradiol valerate (DELESTROGEN) or estradiol cypionate (DEPO-ESTRADIOL) in oil may be absorbed over several weeks.

Estrogens are extensively bound to plasma proteins. Estradiol and other naturally occurring estrogens are bound mainly to SHBG; ethinyl estradiol is bound extensively to serum albumin but not SHBG. Due to their size and lipophilic nature, unbound estrogens distribute rapidly and extensively.

Estrogens undergo rapid hepatic biotransformation, with a plasma $t_{1/2}$ measured in minutes. Estradiol is converted primarily by 17β-hydroxysteroid dehydrogenase to estrone, which undergoes conversion by 16α-hydroxylation and 17-keto reduction to estriol, the major urinary metabolite. A variety of sulfate and glucuronide conjugates also are excreted in the urine. Estrogen conjugates also undergo enterohepatic recirculation.

Ethinyl estradiol is cleared more slowly than is estradiol due to decreased hepatic metabolism, with an elimination $t_{1/2}$ of 13–27 hours. Its primary route of biotransformation is via 2-hydroxylation and subsequent formation of the corresponding 2- and 3-methyl ethers.

Untoward Responses

The amount of estrogens (and progestins) in oral contraceptives has been markedly decreased, significantly diminishing the risks associated with their use.

CONCERN ABOUT CARCINOGENIC ACTIONS

Early studies established that estrogens can induce tumors of the breast, uterus, testis, bone, kidney, and other tissues in various animal species. Thereafter, an increased incidence of vaginal and cervical adenocarcinoma was noted in female offspring of mothers who had taken diethylstilbestrol during the first trimester of pregnancy. Estrogen use during pregnancy also can increase the incidence of nonmalignant genital abnormalities in both male and female offspring; pregnant women should not be given estrogens.

The use of unopposed estrogen in postmenopausal women increases the risk of endometrial carcinoma by 5–15-fold, an increase that can be prevented if a progestin is coadministered with the estrogen. Randomized, clinical trials of estrogen-progestin and estrogen-only use in post-menopausal women have established a small but significant increase in the risk of breast cancer, apparently due to the medroxyprogesterone. In women without a uterus who received estrogen alone, the relative risk of breast cancer was insignificantly decreased. Thus, the data suggest that the progestin component in hormone-replacement therapy plays a major role in this increased risk of breast cancer. Importantly, the excess risk of breast cancer associated with menopausal hormone use apparently abates within 5 years after discontinuing therapy.

METABOLIC AND CARDIOVASCULAR EFFECTS

Although they may slightly elevate plasma triglycerides, estrogens generally have favorable over-all effects on plasma lipoprotein profiles. However, concurrent administration of progestins may reduce these favorable actions. Currently prescribed doses of estrogens do not increase the risk of hypertension.

Observational studies, clinical trials using surrogate markers of cardiovascular disease, and animal studies suggested that estrogen therapy in postmenopausal women would reduce the risk of cardiovascular disease. In randomized clinical trials, however, conjugated equine estrogens alone or in combination with medroxyprogesterone acetate (MPA) did not protect against coronary heart disease (CHD). It is unclear whether these results (single dose; relatively older population) apply to other preparations, doses, and patient populations (e.g., women closer to age 50 who typically initiate hormone therapy for relief of vasomotor symptoms). Clearly, oral estrogens significantly increase the risk of thromboembolic disease in healthy women and in women with preexisting cardiovascular disease.

EFFECTS ON COGNITION

Retrospective studies suggested that estrogens had beneficial effects on cognition and delayed the onset of Alzheimer's disease. However, in randomized trials, no protective effect was observed, and the incidence of dementia in the treated group was actually increased.

OTHER POTENTIAL UNTOWARD EFFECTS

Nausea and vomiting occur in some women but often disappear with time and may be minimized by taking estrogens with food or just prior to sleeping. Breast fullness and tenderness and edema may occur, which may be diminished by lowering the dose. A more serious concern is that estrogens may cause severe migraine in some women. Estrogens also may reactivate or exacerbate endometriosis.

Therapeutic Uses

The two major uses of estrogens are as components of combination oral contraceptives (*see* below) and for MHT. Historically, conjugated estrogens have been the most common agents for post-menopausal use (typically 0.625 mg/day). In contrast, most combination oral contraceptives in current use employ 20–35 μg/day of ethinyl estradiol. The "effective" dose of estrogen used for MHT is less than that in oral contraceptives when one considers potency. The doses of estrogens employed in both settings have decreased substantially in recent years and untoward effects have a lower incidence and severity than those reported in older studies.

MENOPAUSAL HORMONE THERAPY Established benefits of estrogen therapy in post-menopausal women include amelioration of vasomotor symptoms and the prevention of bone fractures and urogenital atrophy.

Vasomotor Symptoms

The decline in ovarian function at menopause is associated with vasomotor symptoms, typically hot flashes. Treatment of vasomotor symptoms with estrogen is specific and is the most efficacious pharmacotherapy.

Osteoporosis

Osteoporosis is associated with the loss of bone mass and an increased incidence of fractures. Estrogen therapy clearly is efficacious in decreasing the incidence of fractures, although bone loss resumes when treatment is discontinued. However, because of potential risks associated with estrogen use, first-line use of other drugs should be carefully considered (see Chapter 61). Estrogens are more effective at preventing than restoring bone loss and are most effective if initiated before significant bone loss occurs.

Vaginal Dryness and Urogenital Atrophy

Loss of tissue lining the vagina or bladder in postmenopausal women leads to a variety of symptoms, including dryness and itching of the vagina, dyspareunia, swelling of tissues in the genital region, pain during urination, a need to urinate urgently or often, and sudden or unexpected urinary incontinence. When estrogens are being used solely for relief of vulvar and vaginal atrophy, local administration as a vaginal cream, ring device, or tablets may be considered.

Cardiovascular Disease

Prospective studies unexpectedly indicated that the incidence of heart disease and stroke in older postmenopausal women treated with conjugated estrogens and a progestin was initially increased, although the trend reversed with time. While it is not clear if similar results would occur with different drugs/doses or in different patient populations, estrogens (alone or in combination with a progestin) should not be used for the treatment or prevention of cardiovascular disease.

MENOPAUSAL HORMONE REGIMENS *Estrogen-replacement therapy*, or ERT (i.e., estrogens alone), in postmenopausal women was associated with an increased incidence of endometrial carcinoma; this led to the use of *hormone-replacement therapy*, or HRT, which includes a progestin to limit estrogen-related endometrial hyperplasia. "Hormone-replacement" therapy (now generally referred to as "menopausal hormone" therapy) with both an estrogen and progestin now is recommended for postmenopausal women with a uterus. For women who have undergone a hysterectomy, estrogen alone avoids the possible deleterious effects of progestins. Regardless of the specific agent or regimen, MHT with estrogens should use the lowest dose and shortest duration necessary to achieve an appropriate therapeutic goal.

Conjugated estrogens and MPA have been used most commonly in menopausal hormone regimens, although estradiol, estrone, and estriol have been used as estrogens, and norethindrone, norgestimate, levonorgestrel, norethisterone, and progesterone also have been widely used (especially in Europe). Various "continuous" or "cyclic" regimens that include drug-free days have been used. An example of a cyclic regimen is: (1) administration of an estrogen for 25 days, (2) the addition of MPA for the last 12–14 days of estrogen treatment, and (3) 5–6 days with no hormone treatment, during which withdrawal bleeding normally occurs due to breakdown and shedding of the endometrium. Continuous administration of combined estrogen plus progestin does not lead to regular, recurrent endometrial shedding, but may cause intermittent spotting or bleeding. Other regimens include a progestin intermittently (e.g., every third month), but the long-term endometrial safety of these regimens remains to be firmly established. PREMPRO (conjugated estrogens plus MPA given as a fixed dose daily) and PREMPHASE (conjugated estrogens given for 28 days plus MPA given for 14 out of 28 days) are widely used combinations. Other combination products available in the U.S. are FEMHRT (ethinyl estradiol plus norethindrone acetate), ACTIVELLA (estradiol plus norethindrone), and PREFEST (estradiol and norgestimate).

Another pharmacological consideration is the route of administration. Oral administration exposes the liver to higher concentrations of estrogens than transdermal administration and may increase SHBG, other binding globulins, angiotensinogen; and the cholesterol content of bile. Transdermal estrogen appears to cause smaller beneficial changes in LDL and HDL profiles but may be preferred in women with hypertriglyceridemia.

Tibolone (LIVIAL) is widely used in Europe for treatment of vasomotor symptoms and prevention of osteoporosis but is not approved in the U.S. The parent compound is metabolized in a tissue-selective manner to metabolites that have predominantly estrogenic, progestogenic, and androgenic activities. The drug increases bone mineral density and decreases vasomotor symptoms without stimulating the endometrium, but its effects on fractures, breast cancer, and long-term outcomes remain to be established.

ESTROGEN TREATMENT IN THE FAILURE OF OVARIAN DEVELOPMENT

In several conditions (e.g., Turner's syndrome), the ovaries do not develop and puberty does not occur. Estrogen therapy at the appropriate time replicates the events of puberty; androgens (see Chapter 58) and/or growth hormone (see Chapter 55) may be used concomitantly to promote normal growth. While estrogens and androgens promote bone growth, they also accelerate epiphyseal fusion, and their premature use can thus shorten ultimate height.

SELECTIVE ESTROGEN RECEPTOR MODULATORS AND ANTIESTROGENS

SERMs: TAMOXIFEN, RALOXIFENE, AND TOREMIFENE Selective ER modulators, or SERMs, exert tissue-selective actions. Their pharmacological goal is to produce beneficial estrogenic actions in certain tissues (*e.g.*, bone, brain, and liver) but antagonist activity in others (*e.g.*, breast and endometrium). Currently approved SERMs in the U.S. are *tamoxifen* (NOLVADEX, OTHERS), *raloxifene* (EVISTA), and *toremifene* (FARESTON).

ANTIESTROGENS: CLOMIPHENE AND FULVESTRANT These compounds are pure antagonists in all tissues. Clomiphene (CLOMID, SEROPHENE, others) is approved for the treatment of infertility in anovulatory women; *fulvestrant* (FASLODEX, ICI 182,780) is used to treat breast cancer in women with disease progression after tamoxifen.

CHEMISTRY

Structures of the trans-*isomer of tamoxifen, raloxifene,* trans-*clomiphene (enclomiphene), and fulvestrant are:*

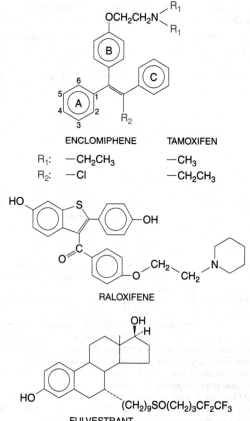

	ENCLOMIPHENE	TAMOXIFEN
R_1:	$-CH_2CH_3$	$-CH_3$
R_2:	$-Cl$	$-CH_2CH_3$

RALOXIFENE

FULVESTRANT

Hepatic metabolism of tamoxifen produces N-desmethyltamoxifen, which has affinity for ER comparable to that of tamoxifen, and lesser amounts of the highly active metabolites 4-hydroxytamoxifen and endoxifen, which have 25–50 times higher affinity for both ERα and ERβ. Raloxifene is a nonsteroidal, polyhydroxylated compound. Clomiphene has two isomers: zuclomiphene (cis-clomiphene), a weak estrogen agonist, and enclomiphene (trans-clomiphene), a potent antagonist. Fulvestrant is a 7α-alkylamide derivative of estradiol.

Pharmacological Effects

All of these agents bind to the ligand-binding pockets of both ERα and ERβ and competitively block estradiol binding. However, the conformation of the ligand-bound ERs differs with different ligands. The distinct ER-ligand conformations recruit different coactivators and corepressors onto the promoter of a target gene. While 17β-estradiol induces a conformation that recruits coactivators to the receptor, tamoxifen induces a conformation that recruits co-repressors to both

ERα and ERβ. The agonist activity of tamoxifen in tissues such as the endometrium is mediated by ERα.

Tamoxifen exhibits antiestrogenic, estrogenic, or mixed activity depending on the target gene measured. Tamoxifen inhibits the proliferation of cultured human breast cancer cells and reduces tumor size and number in women, yet it stimulates proliferation of endometrial cells. The drug has an antiresorptive effect on bone and decreases total cholesterol, LDL, and Lp(a) but does not increase HDL and triglycerides. Tamoxifen approximately doubles the relative risk of deep vein thrombosis and pulmonary embolism and endometrial carcinoma. Tamoxifen produces hot flashes and other adverse effects, including cataracts, nausea, and hepatic steatosis. Due to its agonist activity in bone, it does not increase the incidence of fractures.

Raloxifene is an estrogen agonist in bone and reduces the number of vertebral fractures by up to 50% in a dose-dependent manner. The drug also acts as an estrogen agonist in reducing total cholesterol and LDL but does not increase HDL or normalize plasminogen-activator inhibitor 1 in postmenopausal women. Raloxifene does not cause proliferation of the endometrium. Raloxifene has an antiproliferative effect on ER-positive breast tumors and on proliferation of ER-positive breast cancer cell lines and significantly reduces the risk of ER-positive but not ER-negative breast cancer. Raloxifene does not alleviate the vasomotor symptoms associated with menopause. Adverse effects include hot flashes and leg cramps and a threefold increase in deep vein thrombosis and pulmonary embolism.

In women with a functional hypothalamic-hypophyseal-ovarian system and adequate endogenous estrogen production, clomiphene is used to induce ovulation in conditions such as polycystic ovarian syndrome and dysfunctional bleeding with anovulatory cycles.

Fulvestrant binds to ERα and ERβ with an affinity comparable to estradiol but represses transactivation. Fulvestrant also stimulates the proteolytic degradation of ERα, which may explain its efficacy in tamoxifen-resistant breast cancer.

Absorption, Fate, and Excretion

Tamoxifen given orally reaches peak plasma levels after 4–7 hours; it has two elimination phases (half-lives of 7–14 hours and 4–11 days; thus, 3–4 weeks of treatment are required to reach steady-state plasma levels). Tamoxifen is metabolized by hepatic CYPs, some of which it also induces. In humans, the potent antiestrogens 4-hydroxytamoxifen and endoxifen are produced in the liver. The major route of elimination involves N-demethylation and deamination. The drug undergoes enterohepatic circulation, and excretion is primarily in the feces as conjugates of the deaminated metabolite.

Raloxifene has an oral bioavailability of about 2%. The drug has a $t_{1/2}$ of about 28 hours and is eliminated primarily in the feces after hepatic glucuronidation.

Clomiphene is well absorbed following oral administration, and the drug and its metabolites are eliminated primarily in the feces. The long plasma $t_{1/2}$ (5–7 days) is due largely to plasma-protein binding, enterohepatic circulation, and accumulation in fatty tissues.

Fulvestrant is administered monthly by intramuscular depot injections. Plasma concentrations peak in 7 days and then are maintained for a month. The drug is eliminated primarily via the feces.

Therapeutic Uses

BREAST CANCER Tamoxifen is highly efficacious in the palliation of advanced breast cancer in women with ER-positive tumors and for hormonal treatment of both early and advanced breast cancer in women of all ages. Response rates are ~50% in women with ER-positive tumors and 70% for ER-positive, PR-positive tumors. Tamoxifen increases disease-free and overall survival; a 5-year treatment period is more efficacious than shorter treatments. Tamoxifen reduces by 50% the risk of developing contralateral breast cancer in women at high risk and is approved for primary prevention in this setting. Prophylactic treatment should be limited to 5 years. The most frequent side effect is hot flashes. Tamoxifen increases the risk of endometrial cancer and thromboembolic disease by two- to threefold.

Toremifene has therapeutic actions similar to tamoxifen. Fulvestrant may be efficacious in women who become resistant to tamoxifen, perhaps by downregulating ERα. Untoward effects of fulvestrant include hot flashes, GI symptoms, headache, back pain, and pharyngitis.

OSTEOPOROSIS Raloxifene reduces the rate of bone loss and may increase bone mass at certain sites. Raloxifene increased lumbar bone mineral density by more than 2% and reduced the rate of vertebral fractures by 30–50%, but did not significantly reduce nonvertebral fractures. Raloxifene does not appear to increase the risk of endometrial cancer. The drug has beneficial actions on lipoprotein metabolism, reducing both total cholesterol and LDL; HDL is not increased. Adverse effects include hot flashes, deep vein thrombosis, and leg cramps.

INFERTILITY Clomiphene is used primarily for treatment of female infertility due to anovulation. By increasing FSH levels, clomiphene enhances follicular recruitment. The drug is relatively inexpensive, orally active, and requires less extensive monitoring than do other fertility protocols. Untoward effects include ovarian hyperstimulation, increased incidence of multiple births, ovarian cysts, hot flashes, and blurred vision. Prolonged use (*e.g.*, 12 or more cycles) may increase the risk of ovarian cancer. Clomiphene should not be administered to pregnant women due to reports of teratogenicity in animals, although there is no evidence of this in humans.

Estrogen-Synthesis Inhibitors

Continual administration of GnRH agonists prevents ovarian synthesis of estrogens but not their synthesis from adrenal androgens (*see* Chapter 55). The recognition that locally produced estrogens may play a significant role in breast cancer has greatly stimulated interest in the use of aromatase inhibitors to selectively block estrogen production. Both steroidal (*e.g., formestane* and *exemestane* [AROMASIN]) and nonsteroidal agents (*e.g., anastrozole* [ARIMIDEX], *letrozole* [FEMARA], and *vorozole*) are available. Steroidal (type 1) agents are substrate analogs that act as suicide inhibitors to irreversibly inactivate aromatase, while the nonsteroidal (type 2) agents interact reversibly with the heme groups of CYPs. Exemestane, letrozole, and anastrozole are approved in the U.S. for the treatment of breast cancer. The structures of exemestane and anastrozole are shown in the 11th edition of the parent text:

These agents may be used as first-line treatment of breast cancer or as second-line drugs after tamoxifen. They are highly efficacious and actually superior to tamoxifen in some adjuvant settings; unlike tamoxifen, they do not increase the risk of uterine cancer or venous thromboembolism. Because they dramatically reduce circulating and local levels of estrogens, they produce hot flashes. The marked decreases in estrogen levels are likely to be associated with significant bone loss, but long-term studies are needed.

PROGESTINS

The progestins (Figure 57–4) are widely used with estrogens for MHT and other situations in which a selective progestational effect is desired; a depot form of MPA is used as a long-acting injectable contraceptive. The 19-nortestosterone derivatives were developed for use as progestins in oral contraceptives; their predominant activity is progestational, but they also exhibit androgenic activity. The gonanes are "19-nor" compounds that have diminished androgenic activity.

CHEMISTRY

Unlike the ER, which requires a phenolic A ring for high-affinity binding, the PR favors a Δ^4-3-one A-ring structure in an inverted 1β, 2α-conformation. Some synthetic progestins (especially the 19-nor compounds) display limited binding to glucocorticoid, androgen, and mineralocorticoid receptors.

One class of agents is similar to progesterone and its metabolite 17α-hydroxyprogesterone (Figure 57–4). Compounds such as hydroxyprogesterone caproate have progestational activity but must be used parenterally due to first-pass hepatic metabolism. Further substitutions at the 6-position of the B ring yield orally active compounds with selective progestational activity, such as MPA and megestrol acetate.

A second class of agents includes 19-nor testosterone derivatives. Lacking the C19 methyl group, these testosterone derivatives display primarily progestational rather than androgenic activity. An ethinyl substituent at C17 decreases hepatic metabolism and yields orally active 19-nortestosterone analogs such as norethindrone, norethynodrel, and ethynodiol diacetate. The activity of the latter two compounds is due primarily to their rapid conversion to norethindrone. These compounds have varying degrees of androgenic activity, and to a lesser extent, estrogenic and antiestrogenic activities.

Replacement of the 13-methyl group of norethindrone with a 13-ethyl substituent yields the gonane norgestrel, which is a more potent progestin than the parent compound but has less androgenic activity. Other gonanes—including norgestimate, desogestrel, and gestodene (not available in the U.S.)—reportedly have little if any androgenic activity at therapeutic doses.

Newer steroidal progestins include the gonane dienogest; 19-nor-progestin derivatives (e.g., nomegestrol, nestorone, and trimegestone), which have increased selectivity for the PR and less androgenic activity than estranes; and the spironolactone derivative drospirenone, which is used in a combination oral contraceptive. Like spironolactone, drospirenone is also a mineralocorticoid receptor antagonist.

Agents Similar to Progesterone (Pregnanes)

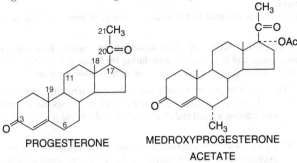

PROGESTERONE

MEDROXYPROGESTERONE
ACETATE

Agents Similar to 19-Nortestosterone (Estranes)

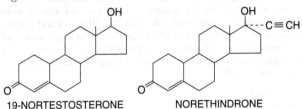

19-NORTESTOSTERONE

NORETHINDRONE

Agents Similar to Norgestrel (Gonanes)

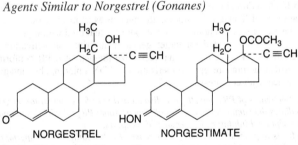

NORGESTREL

NORGESTIMATE

FIGURE 57–4 *Structural features of various progestins.*

BIOSYNTHESIS AND SECRETION

Progesterone is secreted by the corpus luteum during the second half of the menstrual cycle under the stimulus of LH (Figure 57–3). After fertilization, the trophoblast secretes hCG into the maternal circulation, which also acts through the LH receptor to sustain the corpus luteum. During the second or third month of pregnancy, the developing placenta begins to secrete estrogen and progesterone in collaboration with the fetal adrenal glands, and thereafter the corpus luteum is not essential. Estrogen and progesterone then continue to be secreted in large amounts by the placenta throughout gestation.

Physiological and Pharmacological Actions

NEUROENDOCRINE ACTIONS Progesterone produced in the luteal phase of the cycle decreases the frequency of GnRH pulses, which is one mechanism of action of progestin-containing contraceptives.

REPRODUCTIVE TRACT Progesterone decreases estrogen-driven endometrial proliferation and induces a secretory endometrium (Figure 57–3); the abrupt decline in progesterone at the end of the cycle is the main determinant of the onset of menstruation. Progesterone also influences the endocervical glands, changing the abundant watery secretion of the estrogen-stimulated structures to a scant, viscid material. These and other effects of progestins decrease penetration of the cervix by sperm.

Finally, progesterone is essential to maintain pregnancy, at least partly by suppressing uterine contractility.

MAMMARY GLAND Mammary gland development requires both estrogen and progesterone. During pregnancy, and to a minor degree during the luteal phase of the cycle, progesterone acts with estrogen to induce proliferation of the acini of the mammary gland.

CNS EFFECTS Progesterone increases basal body temperature by about 0.6°C at midcycle when ovulation occurs. Progesterone also increases the ventilatory response of the respiratory centers to CO_2 and leads to reduced arterial and alveolar P_{CO_2} in the luteal phase of the menstrual cycle and during pregnancy.

METABOLIC EFFECTS Progesterone increases basal insulin and postprandial insulin levels but does not normally alter glucose tolerance. However, long-term administration of more potent progestins, such as norgestrel, may decrease glucose tolerance. Progesterone and analogs (*e.g.*, MPA) increase LDL and cause either no effect or modest reduction in serum HDL levels. Because of their androgenic activity, the 19-norprogestins may have more pronounced effects on plasma lipids. In one study, MPA decreased the favorable HDL increase caused by conjugated estrogens during postmenopausal hormone replacement, but did not significantly affect the beneficial effect of estrogens to lower LDL. In contrast, micronized progesterone does not significantly affect beneficial estrogen effects on either HDL or LDL. Progesterone also may diminish the effects of aldosterone in the renal tubule.

Mechanism of Action

A single gene encodes two isoforms of the PR, PR_A and PR_B, by differential use of two distinct estrogen-dependent promoters; the ratios of the individual isoforms vary in reproductive tissues. Since the ligand-binding domains of the PR isoforms are identical, there is no difference in ligand binding. In the absence of ligand, PR resides in the nucleus as an inactive monomer. Upon progesterone binding, the receptors form homo- and heterodimers that bind with high selectivity to progesterone response elements located on target genes. Transcriptional activation by PR occurs primarily by recruitment of co-activators that recognize the activated PR conformation. Progesterone antagonists also facilitate receptor dimerization and DNA binding, but antagonist-bound PR preferentially interacts with corepressors.

The biological activities of PR_A and PR_B are distinct and vary for different target genes. In most cells, PR_B mediates the stimulatory activities of progesterone; PR_A inhibits this action of PR_B and is also a transcriptional inhibitor of other steroid receptors.

Certain effects of progesterone, such as increased Ca^{2+} mobilization in sperm, occur within minutes and reflect nongenomic mechanisms involving membrane-bound PRs that are not derived from the gene encoding PR_A/PR_B.

Absorption, Fate, and Excretion

Progesterone undergoes rapid first-pass metabolism, but high-doses (e.g., 100–200 mg) of micronized progesterone (PROMETRIUM) are orally effective. Progesterone also is available in oil solution for injection, as a vaginal gel (CRINONE, PROCHIEVE), and as a slow-release intrauterine device (PROGESTASERT) for contraception.

Esters [e.g., hydroxyprogesterone caproate (HYALUTIN) and MPA (DEPO-PROVERA)] are available for intramuscular administration, and MPA (PROVERA, others) and megestrol acetate (MEGACE) may be used orally due to decreased hepatic metabolism. The 19-nor-steroids have good oral activity because the ethinyl substituent at C17 slows hepatic metabolism. Implants and depot preparations for prolonged release of synthetic progestins are widely available.

Progesterone in circulation is bound by albumin and CBG but not by SHBG. 19-Nor compounds, such as norethindrone, norgestrel, and desogestrel, bind to SHBG and albumin, and esters such as MPA bind primarily to albumin. Total binding of these synthetic compounds to plasma proteins exceeds 90%.

The elimination $t_{1/2}$ of progesterone is ~5 minutes; the hormone is metabolized primarily in the liver to hydroxylated metabolites and their sulfate and glucuronide conjugates, which are eliminated in the urine. The synthetic progestins have much longer half-lives (~7 hours for norethindrone, 16 hours for norgestrel, 12 hours for gestodene, and 24 hours for MPA). Metabolism of synthetic progestins is primarily hepatic, and elimination is generally in the urine as conjugates and various polar metabolites.

Therapeutic Uses

The two most frequent uses of progestins are for contraception, either alone or with an estrogen, and in combination with estrogen for hormone therapy of postmenopausal women. Progestins also are used for secondary amenorrhea, abnormal uterine bleeding in patients without underlying fibroids or cancer, luteal-phase support to treat infertility, and premature labor.

Progestins are used diagnostically to test for estrogen secretion and for responsiveness of the endometrium: after progesterone administration to amenorrheic women for 5–7 days, withdrawal bleeding will occur if the endometrium has been stimulated by endogenous estrogens.

Progestins are highly efficacious in decreasing the occurrence of endometrial hyperplasia and carcinoma caused by unopposed estrogens; in this setting, there appears to be less irregular uterine bleeding with sequential rather than continuous administration. Progestins are also used palliatively for metastatic endometrial carcinoma. Megestrol acetate is used as a second-line treatment for breast cancer and also is used off-label for AIDS-related wasting.

ANTIPROGESTINS AND PROGESTERONE-RECEPTOR MODULATORS

The antiprogestin, RU 38486 (often referred to as RU-486) or *mifepristone*, is available for the termination of pregnancy. Antiprogestins have several other potential applications, including uses as contraceptives, to induce labor, and to treat uterine leiomyomas, endometriosis, meningiomas, and breast cancer.

Mifepristone

Mifepristone effectively competes with both progesterone and glucocorticoids for binding to their respective receptors. Mifepristone is considered a PR modulator (PRM) due to its context-dependent antagonist/agonist activity. Another antiprogestin is onapristone, which contains a methyl substituent in the 13α rather than 13β orientation. The structures of mifepristone and onapristone are shown in the 11th edition of the parent text.

PHARMACOLOGICAL ACTIONS   In the presence of progestins, mifepristone is a competitive antagonist of both PRs and, in certain contexts, may also be an agonist. In contrast, onapristone appears to be a pure progesterone antagonist. Mifepristone also exerts antiglucocorticoid and antiandrogenic actions. Onapristone has less antiglucocorticoid activity than does mifepristone.

Absorption, Fate, and Excretion

Mifepristone has good oral bioavailability. Plasma levels peak within several hours, and the drug is cleared with a plasma $t_{1/2}$ of 20–40 hours, in part because it is bound by α_1-acid glycoprotein. Metabolites are primarily mono- and di-demethylated products (which may have pharmacological activity) formed via CYP3A4, and to a lesser extent, hydroxylated compounds. The drug undergoes hepatic metabolism and enterohepatic circulation; metabolic products are found predominantly in the feces.

THERAPEUTIC USES

Mifepristone (MIFEPREX) is used to terminate early pregnancy. A prostaglandin (e.g., intramuscular sulprostone, intravaginal gemeprost, or oral misoprostol) is given 48 hours after the mifepristone to ensure expulsion of the detached blastocyst. The success rate with such regimens is >90% among women with pregnancies of <7 weeks' duration. The most severe untoward effect is vaginal bleeding, which typically lasts from 1 to 2 weeks but is rarely severe enough to require blood transfusions (0.1% of patients). High percentages of women also experience abdominal pain and uterine cramps, nausea, vomiting, and diarrhea due to the prostaglandin. A "black box" warning added to product labeling details the risk of serious, and sometimes fatal, infections and bleeding following mifepristone use for medical abortion. Women should be informed of these risks and cautioned to seek immediate medical attention if symptoms of these conditions occur. Women receiving chronic glucocorticoid therapy should not be given mifepristone because of its antiglucocorticoid activity. The drug should be used very cautiously in women who are anemic or receiving anticoagulants. Women over 35 years old with cardiovascular risk factors should not be given sulprostone because of possible heart failure.

HORMONAL CONTRACEPTIVES

Oral contraceptives are widely used worldwide and have had a revolutionary impact by providing a convenient, affordable, and reliable means of contraception. Myriad agents with substantially different components, doses, and side effects provide real therapeutic options. In addition to contraceptive actions, these agents have substantial health benefits.

Types of Hormonal Contraceptives

COMBINATION ORAL CONTRACEPTIVES The most frequently used agents in the U.S. are combination oral contraceptives containing both an estrogen and a progestin. Their theoretical efficacy is considered to be 99.9%. Ethinyl estradiol and mestranol are the two estrogens used (with ethinyl estradiol being much more frequently used). The progestins are 19-nor compounds in the estrane or gonane series that have varying degrees of androgenic, estrogenic, and antiestrogenic activities that may be responsible for some side effects. Compounds such as desogestrel and norgestimate have less androgenic activity than other 19-nor compounds. Combination oral contraceptives are generally provided in 21-day packs with an additional 7 pills containing no active hormone. For monophasic agents, fixed amounts of the estrogen and progestin are present in each pill, which is taken daily for 21 days, followed by a 7-day "drug-free" period. The biphasic and triphasic preparations provide two or three different pills containing varying amounts of active ingredients, for different days in the 21-day cycle. This reduces the total amount of steroids administered and more closely approximates the estrogen-to-progestin ratios that occur during the menstrual cycle. Predictable menstrual bleeding generally occurs during the 7-day "off" period each month. The FDA recently approved a levonorgestrel–ethinyl estradiol combination (LYBREL) that is taken continuously for the full 90 days, eliminating any menstrual periods. Additional options include a once-monthly medroxyprogesterone–estradiol cypionate injectable (LUNELLE), an ethinyl estradiol– *norelgestromin* (the active metabolite of norgestimate) patch (ORTHO EVRA) applied weekly, and an ethinyl estradiol–*etonogestrel* (the active metabolite of desogestrel) flexible vaginal ring (NUVARING) used for 3 weeks (followed by a removal for 1 week that leads to menstrual bleeding).

The estrogen content ranges from 20 to 50 μg; most contain 30–35 μg. Preparations containing ≤35 μg of an estrogen are termed "low-dose" pills. The progestin dose is more variable because of different potencies of the compounds. Monophasic pills available in the U.S. contain 0.4–1 mg of norethindrone, 0.1–0.15 mg of levonorgestrel, 0.3–0.5 mg of norgestrel, 1 mg of ethynodiol diacetate, 0.25 mg of norgestimate, and 0.15 mg of desogestrel, with slightly different dose ranges in biphasic and triphasic preparations.

PROGESTIN-ONLY CONTRACEPTIVES Progestin-only contraceptives are only slightly less efficacious than combination oral contraceptives, with theoretical efficacy of 99%. Specific preparations include the "minipill"; low doses of progestins (*e.g.*, 350 μg of norethindrone [NOR-QD, MICRONOR] or 75 μg of norgestrel [OVRETTE]) taken daily without interruption; subdermal implants of 216 mg of norgestrel (NORPLANT II, JADELLE) for slow release and resultant long-term contraceptive action (*e.g.*, up to 5 years); and crystalline suspensions of MPA (DEPO-PROVERA) for intramuscular injection of 150 mg of drug, which provides effective contraception for 3 months.

An intrauterine device (PROGESTASERT) that releases low amounts of progesterone locally is available for insertion on a yearly basis. Its effectiveness is considered to be 97–98%; contraceptive action probably is due to local effects on the endometrium. Another intrauterine device (MIRENA) releases levonorgestrel for up to 5 years. It again is thought to act primarily by local effects.

POSTCOITAL OR EMERGENCY CONTRACEPTIVES The FDA has approved two preparations for postcoital contraception. PLAN-B is two doses of the "minipill" (0.75 mg levonorgestrel per pill) separated by 12 hours; PLAN-B will soon be available without a prescription for women 18 years old and older. PREVEN is two 2-pill doses of a high-dose oral contraceptive (0.25 mg of levonorgestrel and 0.05 mg of ethinyl estradiol per pill) separated by 12 hours. The FDA also has declared other products with the same or very similar composition safe and effective for use as emergency contraceptive pills.

The first dose of such preparations should be taken within 72 hours after intercourse, and this should be followed 12 hours later by a second dose. These treatments reduce the risk of pregnancy following unprotected intercourse by approximately 60–80%. With either preparation, effectiveness appears to increase the sooner after intercourse the pills are taken.

Mechanism of Action

COMBINATION ORAL CONTRACEPTIVES Combination oral contraceptives act by preventing ovulation. Plasma LH and FSH levels are suppressed, the midcycle surge of LH is absent, endogenous steroid levels are diminished, and ovulation does not occur. While either component alone can exert these effects, the combination synergistically decreases plasma gonadotropin levels and suppresses ovulation more consistently than either alone.

Oral contraceptives exert hypothalamic and pituitary effects. Progesterone diminishes the frequency of GnRH pulses, and oral contraceptives also decrease pituitary responsiveness to GnRH. Estrogens also suppress FSH release from the pituitary during the follicular phase of the menstrual cycle, which likely contributes to the lack of follicular development in oral contraceptive users. The progestin may also inhibit the estrogen-induced LH surge at midcycle. Other effects may contribute to a minor extent to the efficacy of oral contraceptives, including impaired oocyte transport in the fallopian tubes. Progestin also leads to a thick, viscous mucus that reduces sperm penetration and induces an endometrium that is not receptive to implantation.

PROGESTIN-ONLY CONTRACEPTIVES Progestin-only pills and levonorgestrel implants are highly efficacious for contraception. The pills block ovulation in only 60–80% of cycles; effectiveness is thought to be due largely to local effects in the cervix and uterus; such effects also account for the efficacy of intrauterine devices that release progestins. Depot injections of MPA yield plasma levels of drug high enough to prevent ovulation in virtually all patients, presumably by decreasing the frequency of GnRH pulses.

Untoward Effects

COMBINATION ORAL CONTRACEPTIVES The consensus is that low-dose oral contraceptives pose minimal health risks in women who have no predisposing risk factors and also provide many beneficial health effects.

Cardiovascular Effects

There is no significant increase in the risk of myocardial infarction or stroke in nonsmokers without other risk factors such as hypertension or diabetes. There is a 28% increase in relative risk for venous thromboembolism, but the estimated absolute increase is very small because these events are rare in women without other predisposing factors. Nevertheless, the risk is significantly increased in women who smoke or have other factors that predispose to thrombosis. The incidence of hypertension is much lower with low-dose preparations, and most reported changes in blood pressure are not significant. The cardiovascular risk associated with oral contraceptive use apparently does not persist after drug cessation. Studies of low-dose oral contraceptives have not found significant changes in total serum cholesterol or lipoprotein profiles.

Cancer

There is not a widespread association between oral contraceptives and cancer. Combined oral contraceptives may increase the risk of cervical cancer by about twofold, but only in long-term users with human papilloma virus infection. There are reported increases in the incidence of hepatic adenoma and hepatocellular carcinoma in oral contraceptive users (perhaps a doubling in the risk of liver cancer after 4–8 years of use) but these are rare cancers and the absolute increases are small.

The risk of breast cancer in women of childbearing age is very low, and current oral contraceptive users in this group have only a very small increased relative risk of 1.1–1.2 that is not substantially affected by duration of use, dose or type of component, age at first use, or parity. Importantly, 10 years after discontinuation of oral contraceptives, breast cancer incidence is comparable in past users and never users. In addition, breast cancers diagnosed in women who have used oral contraceptives are more likely to be localized to the breast and thus easier to treat. Thus, overall there is no significant difference in the cumulative risk of breast cancer between those who have ever used oral contraceptives and those who have never used them.

Combination oral contraceptives actually cause a 50% decrease in the incidence of endometrial cancer that lasts 15 years after the pills are stopped. This is thought to be due to the inclusion of a progestin, which opposes estrogen-induced proliferation, throughout the entire 21 days. These agents also decrease the incidence of ovarian cancer and may decrease the risk of colorectal cancer.

Metabolic and Endocrine Effects

Current low-dose combination contraceptives do not impair and may even improve insulin sensitivity and lipid profiles. In women who smoke, the ethinyl estradiol in oral contraceptives appears to cause a dose-dependent increase in several serum factors that may shift the hemostatic profile toward a hypercoagulable condition.

The estrogenic component of oral contraceptives may increase hepatic synthesis of a number of serum proteins, including CBG, TBG, and SHBG. While physiological feedback mechanisms generally adjust hormone synthesis to maintain normal "free" hormone levels, these changes can affect endocrine function tests that measure total plasma hormone levels and may necessitate dose adjustment in patients receiving thyroid-hormone replacement.

Miscellaneous Effects

Nausea, edema, and mild headache occur in some individuals; migraine headaches may be precipitated by oral contraceptives in a smaller fraction of women. Some patients may experience breakthrough bleeding during the 21-day cycle when the active pills are being taken. Withdrawal bleeding may fail to occur in a small fraction of women during the 7-day "off" period, thus causing confusion about a possible pregnancy. Acne and hirsutism are thought to be mediated by the androgenic activity of the 19-nor progestins.

PROGESTIN-ONLY CONTRACEPTIVES   Episodes of irregular, unpredictable spotting and breakthrough bleeding are the most frequent untoward effect and the major reason women discontinue use of progestin-only contraceptives. With time, the incidence of these bleeding episodes decreases; amenorrhea becomes common after a year or more of use.

Progestin-only minipill preparations do not increase thromboembolic events or blood pressure or cause nausea and breast tenderness. Acne may result from the androgenic activity of norethindrone-containing preparations. These preparations may be attractive for nursing mothers because they do not decrease lactation as do products containing estrogens.

Aside from bleeding irregularities, headache is the most commonly reported untoward effect of depot MPA. Mood changes and weight gain also have been reported. Of more concern, many studies have found decreases in HDL levels and increases in LDL levels and decreased bone density. The labeling information for depot MPA for contraceptive injection contains a "black box" warning about increased risk of osteoporosis. There are no increases in breast, endometrial, cervical, or ovarian cancer in women receiving MPA.

Norethindrone implants may be associated with infection, local irritation, pain at the insertion site, and rarely, expulsion of the inserts. Headache, weight gain, mood changes, and acne occur in some patients.

EMERGENCY CONTRACEPTIVE PILLS

Nausea and vomiting are the main untoward effects and may be severe. Emergency contraceptive pills are contraindicated in cases of confirmed pregnancy.

Contraindications

Modern oral contraceptives can contribute to the incidence and severity of certain diseases if other risk factors are present. *The following conditions are considered absolute contraindications for combination oral contraceptives: the presence or history of thromboembolic disease, cerebrovascular disease, myocardial infarction, coronary artery disease, or congenital hyperlipidemia; known or suspected carcinoma of the breast, carcinoma of the female reproductive tract, or other hormone-dependent/responsive neoplasias; abnormal undiagnosed vaginal bleeding; known or suspected pregnancy; and past or present liver tumors or impaired liver function.* The risk of serious cardiovascular side effects is particularly marked in women over 35 years of age who smoke heavily (e.g., *>15 cigarettes/day); even low-dose oral contraceptives are contraindicated in such patients.*

Other relative contraindications should be considered on an individual basis, including migraine headaches, hypertension, diabetes mellitus, obstructive jaundice of pregnancy or prior oral contraceptive use, and gallbladder disease. If elective surgery is planned, many physicians discontinue oral contraceptives for several weeks to minimize the possibility of thromboembolism. These agents should be used with care in women with prior gestational diabetes or uterine fibroids; low-dose pills are preferred in such cases.

Progestin-only contraceptives are contraindicated in the presence of undiagnosed vaginal bleeding, benign or malignant liver disease, and known or suspected breast cancer. Depot MPA and levonorgestrel inserts are contraindicated in women with a history or predisposition to thrombophlebitis or thromboembolic disorders.

Choice of Contraceptive Preparations

Treatment should generally begin with preparations containing the minimum dose of steroids that provides effective contraceptive coverage. This is typically a pill with 30–35 μg of estrogen, but preparations with 20 μg may be adequate for lighter women or those over 40 with perimenopausal symptoms, while a preparation containing 50 μg of estrogen may be required for heavier women. Breakthrough bleeding may occur if the estrogen-to-progestin ratio is too low to produce a stable endometrium, and this may be prevented by switching to a pill with a higher ratio.

In women for whom estrogens are contraindicated or undesirable, progestin-only contraceptives are an option. The progestin-only minipill may have enhanced effectiveness in nursing mothers and women over 40 in whom fertility may be decreased.

Concomitant administration of medications that may increase metabolism of estrogens (e.g., rifampin, barbiturates, and phenytoin*) or reduce their enterohepatic recycling (e.g., tetracyclines and* ampicillin*) may decrease the effectiveness of oral contraceptives.*

The choice of preparation also may be influenced by the specific 19-nor progestin component, since this component may have varying degrees of androgenic and other activities. The androgenic activity of this component may contribute to untoward effects such as weight gain, acne, and un-favorable lipoprotein profiles. These side effects are greatly reduced in low-dose contraceptives, but any patients exhibiting such side effects may benefit by switching to pills that contain a progestin with less androgenic activity. Of the progestins commonly found in oral contraceptives, norgestrel has the most androgenic activity and desogestrel, norgestimate, and drospirenone have the least androgenic activity.

The FDA has approved a triphasic, low-dose combination oral contraceptive (ORTHO TRI-CYCLEN) containing ethinyl estradiol and norgestimate for the treatment of moderate acne vulgaris. Similar preparations (DEMULEN 1/35, DESOGEN, others) also are effective. The mechanism appears to be a decrease in free plasma testosterone due to an increase in plasma SHBG.

Noncontraceptive Health Benefits

Combination oral contraceptives have substantial health benefits unrelated to their contraceptive use. They significantly reduce the incidence of ovarian and endometrial cancer within 6 months of use, a protective effect that persists for up to 15 years after oral contraceptives are discontinued. Depot MPA injections also reduce substantially the incidence of uterine cancer. These agents also decrease the incidence of ovarian cysts and benign fibrocystic breast disease.

Oral contraceptives have major benefits related to menstruation, including more regular menstruation, reduced menstrual blood loss and less iron-deficiency anemia, and decreased frequency of dysmenorrhea. There also is a decreased incidence of pelvic inflammatory disease and ectopic pregnancies, and endometriosis may be ameliorated.

Combination oral contraceptives prevent thousands of deaths, episodes of various diseases, and cases of hospitalization each year in the U.S. alone. Fertility regulation by oral contraceptives is substantially safer than pregnancy or childbirth for most women, even without considering these additional health benefits.

For a complete Bibliographical listing see Goodman & Gilman's *The Pharmacological Basis of Therapeutics*, 11th ed., or Goodman & Gilman Online at www.accessmedicine.com.

58

ANDROGENS

TESTOSTERONE AND OTHER ANDROGENS

SYNTHESIS, SECRETION, AND TRANSPORT OF TESTOSTERONE Leydig cells in the testes synthesize testosterone by the pathways shown in Figure 58–1. In women, testosterone primarily serves as a precursor to estrogens but also is the predominant circulating androgen. Testosterone secretion is greater in men than in women at almost all stages of life, a difference that explains almost all other differences between men and women. In the first trimester *in utero,* placental human chorionic gonadotropin (hCG) induces testosterone secretion by the fetal testes (Figure 58–2); this testosterone is essential for virilization of the male internal genitalia. By the beginning of the second trimester, the circulating testosterone level (~250 ng/dL) is close to that of midpuberty. Testosterone production then falls by the end of the second trimester, but by birth the value is again about 250 ng/dL, possibly due to stimulation of the fetal Leydig cells by luteinizing hormone (LH) from the fetal pituitary gland. The testosterone value falls again in the first few days after birth, rises and peaks again at about 250 ng/dL at 2–3 months, and falls to <50 ng/dL by 6 months, where it remains until puberty. During puberty, the serum testosterone concentration in males increases to a much greater degree than in females, so that by early adulthood the serum testosterone concentration is 500–700 ng/dL in men, compared to 30–50 ng/dL in women. This greater testosterone concentration induces the pubertal changes that further differentiate men from women. As men age, their serum testosterone concentrations gradually decrease, which may contribute to some effects of aging.

LH, secreted by the pituitary gonadotropes (*see* Chapter 55), is the principal stimulus of testosterone secretion in men, perhaps potentiated by follicle-stimulating hormone (FSH), also secreted by gonadotropes. LH secretion is stimulated by hypothalamic gonadotropin-releasing hormone (GnRH), while testosterone directly inhibits LH secretion in a negative feedback loop (*see* Chapter 55). GnRH and LH are released in pulses that occur approximately every 2 hours and are greater in magnitude in the morning. Pulsatile administration of GnRH to men who are hypogonadal due to hypothalamic disease restores normal LH pulses and testosterone secretion, but continuous administration does not. Testosterone secretion is likewise pulsatile and diurnal, with the highest plasma concentrations occurring at about 8 AM and the lowest at about 8 PM. The morning peaks diminish as men age.

Sex hormone–binding globulin (SHBG) binds about 40% of circulating testosterone with high affinity, such that testosterone bound to SHBG is unavailable for biological effects. Albumin binds almost 60% of circulating testosterone with low affinity, leaving approximately 2% unbound or free. In some testosterone assays, the latter two components are considered as "bioavailable" testosterone.

METABOLISM OF TESTOSTERONE TO ACTIVE AND INACTIVE COMPOUNDS Testosterone has many different effects in tissues, both directly and after its metabolism to two other active steroids, dihydrotestosterone and estradiol (Figure 58–3). The enzyme 5α-reductase catalyzes the conversion of testosterone to dihydrotestosterone. Although testosterone and dihydrotestosterone both act *via* the androgen receptor (AR), dihydrotestosterone binds with higher affinity and activates gene expression more efficiently. Two forms of 5α-reductase have been identified: type I, found predominantly in nongenital skin, liver, and bone, and type II, found predominantly in urogenital tissue in men and genital skin in men and women. The enzyme complex aromatase (CYP19), which is present in many tissues, converts testosterone to estradiol. This conversion results in approximately 85% of circulating estradiol in men; the remainder is secreted directly by the testes.

Testosterone is metabolized in the liver to androsterone and etiocholanolone (Figure 58–3), which are biologically inactive. Dihydrotestosterone is metabolized to androsterone, androstanedione, and androstanediol.

Physiological and Pharmacological Effects of Androgens

The biological effects of testosterone can be considered by the receptor it activates and by the tissues in which its effects occur at various stages of life. Testosterone can act as an androgen either directly, by binding to the AR, or indirectly by conversion to dihydrotestosterone, Testosterone also can converted to estradiol, which activates the estrogen receptor (Figure 58–4).

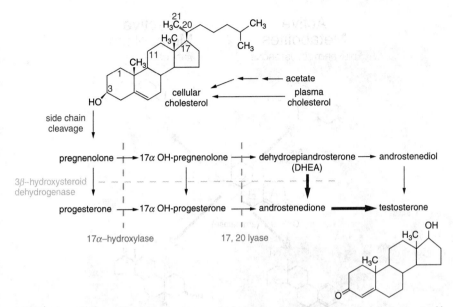

FIGURE 58–1 *Pathway of synthesis of testosterone in the Leydig cells of the testes.* Leydig cells express steroid 17α-hydroxylase (CYP17), which carries out sequential 17-hydroxylation and C17-20 lyase reactions in the biosynthetic pathway to produce androgens. Bold arrows indicate favored pathways.

EFFECTS THAT OCCUR VIA THE ANDROGEN RECEPTOR Testosterone and dihydrotestosterone act as androgens *via* the AR. The AR is a member of the nuclear receptor superfamily that contains amino-terminal, DNA-binding, and ligand-binding domains. After testosterone and dihydrotestosterone bind to the ligand-binding domain, they cause a conformational change that allows the ligand-AR complex to translocate to the nucleus, bind *via* the DNA-binding domain to androgen response elements on certain responsive genes, and regulate their transcription. One

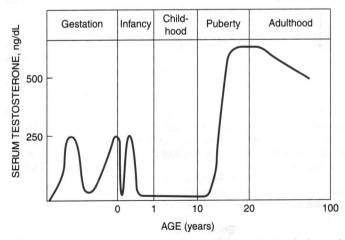

FIGURE 58–2 *Schematic representation of the serum testosterone concentration in males from early gestation to old age.*

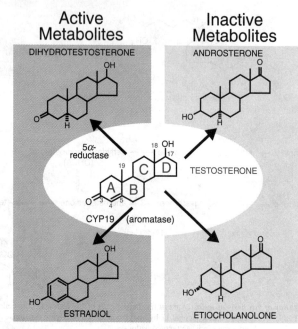

FIGURE 58–3   *Metabolism of testosterone to its major active and inactive metabolites.*

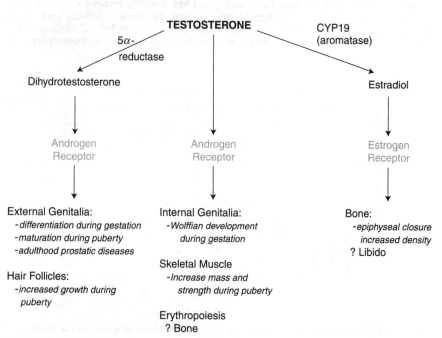

FIGURE 58–4   *Direct effects of testosterone and indirect effects mediated by dihydrotestosterone or estradiol.*

mechanism by which androgens have different actions in diverse tissues is the higher affinity with which dihydrotestosterone binds to and activates the AR compared to testosterone. Another mechanism involves tissue-specific coactivators and corepressors.

Mutations in the AR cause resistance to the actions of testosterone and dihydrotestosterone. Male sexual differentiation and pubertal development therefore are incomplete. Other AR mutations occur in patients who have spinal and bulbar muscular atrophy, known as Kennedy's disease. These patients have an expansion of the CAG repeat, which codes for glutamine, at the amino terminus of the AR; they exhibit very mild androgen resistance—manifest principally by gynecomastia—but progressively severe motor neuron atrophy, the basis of which is poorly understood.

Metastatic prostate cancer often regresses initially in response to androgen-deprivation treatment but then becomes unresponsive to continued deprivation. The AR not only continues to be expressed in androgen-independent prostate cancer, but its signaling remains active in the absence of testosterone. This ligand-independent signaling may result from mutations in the AR gene or from changes in AR coregulatory proteins.

EFFECTS THAT OCCUR VIA THE ESTROGEN RECEPTOR   Certain effects of testosterone are mediated after its conversion to estradiol by CYP19 (Figures 58–3 and 58–4). In the rare males deficient in CYP19 or the estrogen receptor, the epiphyses do not fuse, long-bone growth continues indefinitely, and the bones are osteoporotic. Estradiol administration corrects the bone abnormalities in patients with CYP19 deficiency, but not if there is an estrogen-receptor defect. Because men have larger bones than women, and bone cells express the AR, testosterone also may have a direct effect on bone *via* the AR. Administration of estradiol to a man with CYP19 deficiency increased his libido, suggesting that the effect of testosterone on male libido may be mediated by conversion to estradiol.

EFFECTS OF ANDROGENS AT DIFFERENT STAGES OF LIFE

In Utero

The fetal testes, stimulated by hCG, begin to secrete testosterone at about the eighth week of gestation, and the high local concentration of testosterone around the testes induces the nearby wolffian ducts to differentiate into the male internal genitalia: the epididymis, vas deferens, and seminal vesicles. Farther away, in the anlage of the external genitalia, testosterone is converted to dihydrotestosterone, which causes the development of the male external genitalia—the penis and scrotum—and the prostate. The increase in testosterone at the end of gestation (Figure 58–2) may result in further phallic growth.

Puberty

Puberty in boys begins at a mean age of 12 years when pulsatile GnRH stimulates the secretion of FSH and LH from the gonadotropes. The first sign of puberty is a gonadotropin-induced increase in testes size. The increase in testosterone production by Leydig cells, along with the effects of FSH on the Sertoli cells, stimulates the development of the seminiferous tubules, eventually producing mature sperm. Increased secretion of testosterone into the systemic circulation affects many tissues simultaneously; most changes occur gradually over the course of several years. The phallus enlarges in length and width, the scrotum becomes rugated, and the prostate begins secreting the fluid it contributes to the semen. The skin becomes coarser and oilier due to increased sebum production, which contributes to the development of acne. Sexual hair begins to grow, initially pubic and axillary hair (driven also by adrenal androgens), and then other body hair and facial hair. Muscle mass and strength increase, and subcutaneous fat decreases. Epiphyseal bone growth accelerates, resulting in the pubertal growth spurt, but epiphyseal maturation leads eventually to a slowing and then cessation of growth. Bones also become thicker. The increase in the mass of muscle and bone results in a pronounced increase in body weight. Erythropoiesis increases, resulting in higher hematocrit in men than boys or women. The larynx thickens, resulting in a lower voice. Libido develops.

Adulthood

The serum testosterone concentration and the characteristics of the adult male are largely maintained during early adulthood and midlife. One change during this time is the gradual development of male pattern baldness. Two conditions that can develop are of much greater medical significance: benign prostatic hyperplasia and prostate cancer. Prostatic hyperplasia occurs to a variable degree in almost all men, sometimes obstructing urine outflow by compressing the urethra as it passes through the prostate, and is mediated by the conversion of testosterone to dihydrotestosterone by 5α-reductase II within prostatic cells. Although there is no proven causal role, prostate cancer is dependent on testosterone, at least to some degree and at some time in its course. This dependency is the basis for treating metastatic prostate cancer by lowering the serum testosterone concentration or by blocking its action.

Senescence

As men age, the serum testosterone concentration gradually declines, and the SHBG concentration gradually increases; by age 80, the total testosterone concentration is approximately 80% and the free testosterone is approximately 40% of that present at age 20. This decline in serum testosterone may contribute to several other changes that occur with increasing age in men, including decreased energy, libido, muscle mass and strength, and bone mineral density. A causal role is suggested by the occurrence of similar changes in men who develop hypogonadism at a younger age.

Consequences of Androgen Deficiency

During Fetal Development Testosterone deficiency in a male fetus during the first trimester causes incomplete sexual differentiation. Complete deficiency of testosterone secretion results in entirely female external genitalia; less severe testosterone deficiency impairs virilization of the external genitalia proportionate to the degree of deficiency. Testosterone deficiency at this stage of development also leads to failure of the wolffian ducts to differentiate into the vas deferens and seminal vesicles, but the Müllerian ducts do not form the female internal genitalia as long as the testes secrete Müllerian-inhibiting substance. Similar changes occur if the action of testosterone is diminished because of an abnormality of the AR or of 5α-reductase. Abnormalities of the AR can have quite varied effects. The most severe form results in complete absence of androgen action and a female phenotype; moderately severe forms result in partial virilization of the external genitalia; and the mildest forms permit normal virilization *in utero* and result only in impaired spermatogenesis in adulthood. Abnormal 5α-reductase results in incomplete virilization of the external genitalia *in utero* but normal development of the male internal genitalia, which requires only testosterone.

Testosterone deficiency during the third trimester impairs phallus growth, a condition called microphallus, and causes cryptorchidism—the failure of the testes to descend into the scrotum. These conditions occur commonly in boys whose LH secretion is impaired (*see* Chapter 55).

Before Completion of Puberty Postnatal defects in testosterone synthesis acquired before the anticipated age of puberty result in failure to initiate or complete puberty. All of the pubertal changes described above, including those of the external genitalia, sexual hair, muscle mass, voice, and behavior, are impaired to a degree proportionate to the abnormality of testosterone secretion. If growth hormone secretion remains intact when testosterone secretion is subnormal, the epiphyses do not close, and the long bones continue to lengthen. The result is longer arms and legs relative to the trunk. Another consequence of subnormal testosterone secretion during the age of expected puberty is enlargement of glandular breast tissue (gynecomastia).

After Completion of Puberty Regression of the pubertal effects of testosterone depends on both the degree and the duration of testosterone deficiency. When the deficiency is severe, libido and energy decrease within a week or two, but other testosterone-dependent characteristics decline more slowly. A clinically detectable decrease in muscle mass does not occur for several years. A pronounced decrease in hematocrit and hemoglobin will occur within several months. A decrease in bone mineral density probably is detectable within 2 years by dual-energy x-ray absorptiometry, but an increase in fracture incidence would not be likely to occur for many years. A loss of sexual hair takes many years.

In Women Loss of androgen secretion in women results in a decrease in sexual hair, but not for many years. Some experts have proposed that the loss of androgens, especially the severe loss of both ovarian and adrenal androgens that occurs in panhypopituitarism, is associated with decreased libido, energy, muscle mass and strength, and bone mineral density. Testosterone preparations that yield physiological serum testosterone concentrations in women currently are being developed and tested in clinical trials.

Therapeutic Androgen Preparations

Androgen therapy is complicated by the fact that orally ingested testosterone undergoes rapid hepatic metabolism, and hypogonadal men generally cannot ingest testosterone in sufficient amounts

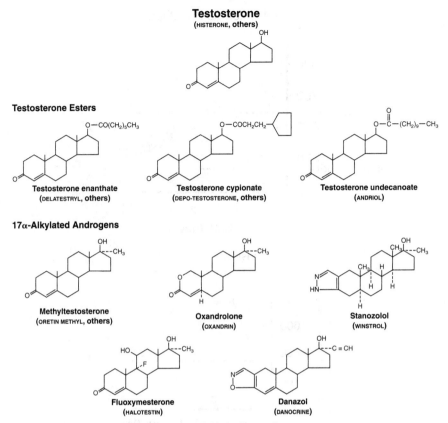

FIGURE 58–5 *Structures of some androgens available for therapeutic use.*

and with sufficient frequency to maintain a normal serum concentration. Therefore, most pharmaceutical preparations of androgens are designed to bypass the liver.

TESTOSTERONE ESTERS Esterifying a fatty acid to the 17α-hydroxyl group of testosterone makes it even more lipophilic than testosterone. When esters such as *testosterone enanthate (heptanoate)* (Figure 58–5) or *cypionate (cyclopentylpropionate)* are dissolved in oil and administered intramuscularly every 2 weeks to hypogonadal men, the ester hydrolyzes *in vivo* and results in serum testosterone concentrations that range from higher-than-normal in the first few days after the injection to low-normal just before the next injection (Figure 58–6). Attempts to decrease the frequency of injections by increasing the amount of each injection result in wider fluctuations and poorer therapeutic outcomes. The undecanoate ester of testosterone (Figure 58–5), when dissolved in oil and ingested orally, is absorbed into the lymphatic circulation, thus bypassing first-pass hepatic metabolism. *Testosterone undecanoate* in oil also can be injected and produces stable serum testosterone concentrations for a month. The undecanoate ester of testosterone is not currently marketed in the U.S.

ALKYLATED ANDROGENS Adding an alkyl group to the 17α position of testosterone (Figure 58–5) retards its hepatic metabolism. Consequently, 17α-alkylated androgens are androgenic when administered orally; however, they are less androgenic than testosterone itself and cause hepatotoxicity, whereas native testosterone does not.

TRANSDERMAL DELIVERY SYSTEMS Attempts to avoid hepatic first-pass inactivation of testosterone have used chemicals called excipients to facilitate the cutaneous absorption of native

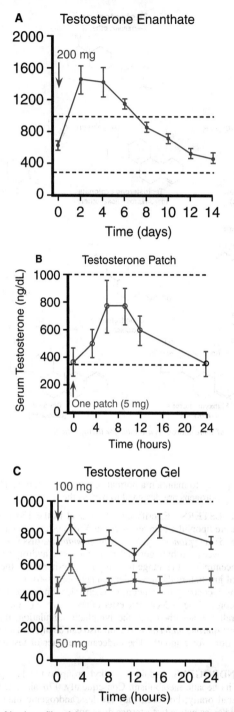

FIGURE 58–6 *Pharmacokinetic profiles of three testosterone preparations during their chronic administration to hypogonadal men.* Doses of each were given at time 0. Dashed lines indicate range of normal levels.

testosterone in a controlled fashion. These transdermal preparations provide more stable serum testosterone concentrations than do injections of testosterone esters. The first such preparations were patches, one of which (ANDRODERM) is still available. Newer preparations include gels (ANDROGEL, TESTIM) and a buccal tablet (STRIANT). These preparations produce mean serum testosterone concentrations within the normal range in hypogonadal men (Figure 58–6).

Attempts to Design Selective Androgens

ALKYLATED ANDROGENS Decades ago, investigators attempted to synthesize analogs of testosterone that possessed greater anabolic effects than androgenic effects compared to native testosterone. These compounds, most are 17α-alkylated androgens, were called anabolic steroids. None has been convincingly demonstrated to have such a differential effect in human beings. Nonetheless, they have enjoyed considerable popularity among athletes who seek to enhance their performance, as described below.

Therapeutic Uses of Androgens

MALE HYPOGONADISM The best-established indication for androgen administration is to treat male hypogonadism (testosterone deficiency in men). Any of the transdermal testosterone preparations or testosterone esters described above can be used with good efficacy.

Monitoring for Efficacy

The goal of testosterone therapy in hypogonadal men is to mimic as closely as possible the normal serum concentration; therefore, serum testosterone concentration must be monitored. With transdermal patches, the serum testosterone concentration fluctuates during the 24-hour period, with a peak value 6–9 hours after application and a nadir (about 50% of the peak) just before the next patch is applied (Figure 58–6). With testosterone gels, the mean serum testosterone concentration is relatively constant from one application to the next. Occasional random fluctuations can occur, so measurements should be repeated for any dose. When the enanthate or cypionate esters of testosterone are administered once every 2 weeks (typically in a dose of 200 mg), the serum testosterone concentration measured midway between doses should be normal; if not, the dose should be adjusted accordingly.

Normalization of the serum testosterone concentration induces virilization in prepubertal boys and restores virilization in men who became hypogonadal as adults. Within a few months, and often sooner, libido, energy, and hematocrit return to normal. Within 6 months, muscle mass increases and fat mass decreases. Bone density, however, continues to increase for 2 years.

Monitoring for Adverse Effects

As long as the dose is not excessive, testosterone has no "side effects" (i.e., no effects that endogenously secreted testosterone does not have). Modified testosterone compounds, such as the 17α-alkylated androgens, may have undesirable effects even when dosages are targeted at physiologic replacement. Raising the serum testosterone concentration from prepubertal or midpubertal levels to that of an adult male at any age can result in undesirable effects similar to those that occur during puberty, including acne, gynecomastia, and more aggressive sexual behavior. Replacement of physiological levels of testosterone may occasionally have undesirable effects in the presence of concomitant illnesses. For example, in patients with chronic pulmonary disease, stimulation of erythropoiesis may raise the hematocrit above normal and cause polycythemia. Similarly, the mild degree of sodium and water retention seen with testosterone replacement may exacerbate preexisting congestive heart failure. If the testosterone dose is excessive, erythrocytosis, and uncommonly, salt and water retention and peripheral edema can occur, even in men who have no predisposition to these conditions. Men over 40 whose serum testosterone concentrations have been in the normal adult male range for many years are subject to testosterone-dependent diseases such as benign prostatic hyperplasia and prostate cancer.

The principal side effects of the 17α-alkylated androgens are hepatic, including cholestasis, and uncommonly, peliosis hepatis (blood-filled hepatic cysts). Hepatocellular cancer has rarely been reported. When administered at high doses, these androgens are more likely than others to affect serum lipid concentrations, specifically to decrease high-density lipoprotein cholesterol and increase low-density lipoprotein cholesterol.

All androgens suppress gonadotropin secretion when taken in high doses and thereby suppress endogenous testicular function. This decreases endogenous testosterone and sperm production, resulting in diminished fertility. If administration continues for many years, testicular size may diminish. Testosterone and sperm production usually return to normal within a few months of discontinuation but may take longer. High doses of androgens also cause erythrocytosis.

When administered in high doses, androgens that can be converted to estrogens, such as testosterone, cause gynecomastia. Androgens with A ring modifications that prevent aromatization, such as dihydrotestosterone, do not cause gynecomastia, even in high doses.

Monitoring at the Anticipated Time of Puberty Administration of testosterone to testosterone-deficient boys at the anticipated time of puberty must be guided by the fact that testosterone accelerates epiphyseal maturation, leading initially to a growth spurt but then to epiphyseal closure and permanent cessation of linear growth. Thus, boys who are short because of growth-hormone deficiency should be treated with growth hormone before their hypogonadism is treated with testosterone.

MALE SENESCENCE Increasing the serum testosterone concentration of men whose serum levels are subnormal for no reason other than their age will increase their bone mineral density and lean mass and decrease their fat mass. It is uncertain at this time if such treatment will worsen benign prostatic hyperplasia or increase the incidence of clinically significant prostate cancer.

ENHANCEMENT OF ATHLETIC PERFORMANCE
Athletes seeking to enhance their performance have taken virtually all androgens produced for human or veterinary purposes. Belated support for this use came from randomized, controlled trials, which showed that normal young men who received testosterone experienced an increase in muscle strength compared to those who received placebo. When this abuse began more than three decades ago, the favored compounds were 17α-alkylated androgens and other compounds that were thought to have greater anabolic effects than androgen effects relative to testosterone (so-called "anabolic steroids"). Because these compounds are readily detected, preparations that increase the serum concentration of testosterone itself, such as the testosterone esters or hCG, have increased in popularity. Testosterone precursors, such as androstenedione and dehydroepiandrosterone (DHEA), also have been used because they have been considered "nutritional supplements."

Certain side effects of anabolic steroid abuse occur specifically in women and children. Both experience virilization, including facial and body hirsutism, temporal hair recession in a male pattern, and acne. Boys experience phallic enlargement, and women experience clitoral enlargement. Boys and girls whose epiphyses have not yet closed experience premature closure and stunting of linear growth.

MALE CONTRACEPTION
Scientists long have sought to use androgens—either alone or in combination with other drugs—as a male contraceptive. Because the high concentration of testosterone within the testes, approximately one hundred times that in the peripheral circulation, is necessary for spermatogenesis, suppression of endogenous testosterone production greatly diminishes spermatogenesis. Initial use of testosterone alone required supraphysiologic doses, while addition of GnRH agonists required daily injections. An alternative approach is to combine a progestin with a physiological dose of testosterone to attempt to suppress LH secretion and spermatogenesis but provide a normal serum testosterone concentration; clinical trials are ongoing.

CATABOLIC AND WASTING STATES
Because of its anabolic effects, testosterone has been used to ameliorate catabolic and muscle-wasting states, generally without benefit. One exception is in the treatment of muscle wasting associated with acquired immunodeficiency syndrome (AIDS), which often is accompanied by hypogonadism. Treatment of men with AIDS-related muscle wasting and subnormal serum testosterone concentrations increases their muscle mass and strength.

ANGIOEDEMA
Angioedema is caused by hereditary impairment of C1-esterase inhibitor or acquired development of antibodies against it. The 17α-alkylated androgens, such as stanozolol and danazol, stimulate hepatic synthesis of the esterase inhibitor and thereby decrease the frequency of acute attacks. In women, virilization is a potential side effect. In children, virilization and premature epiphyseal

closure prevent chronic prophylactic use of androgens, although they are used occasionally to treat acute episodes.

ANTIANDROGENS

Because some effects of androgens are undesirable, agents have been developed to inhibit androgen synthesis or action.

INHIBITORS OF TESTOSTERONE SECRETION Analogs of GnRH effectively inhibit testosterone production by inhibiting LH secretion. They are used to suppress precocious puberty, in assisted reproductive technologies, and to treat prostate cancer (*see* Chapter 55).

Some antifungal drugs such as ketoconazole (*see* Chapter 48) inhibit CYPs and thereby block the synthesis of steroid hormones, including testosterone and cortisol. Because they may induce adrenal insufficiency and are associated with hepatotoxicity, these drugs generally are not used to inhibit androgen synthesis, but sometimes are employed in cases of glucocorticoid excess.

Inhibitors of Androgen Action

These drugs inhibit the binding of androgens to the AR or inhibit 5α-reductase.

ANDROGEN RECEPTOR ANTAGONISTS

Flutamide, Bicalutamide, and Nilutamide These relatively potent AR antagonists have limited efficacy when used alone because the increased LH secretion elevates serum testosterone concentrations. They primarily are used in conjunction with a GnRH analog in the treatment of metastatic prostate cancer, where they block the action of adrenal androgens that are not inhibited by GnRH analogs. AR antagonists used in this fashion include *flutamide* (EULEXIN), *bicalutamide* (CASODEX), or *nilutamide* (NILANDRON). Bicalutamide is replacing flutamide for this purpose because it has less hepatotoxicity and is taken once daily. Nilutamide apparently has worse side effects than flutamide and bicalutamide. Flutamide also has been used effectively to treat hirsutism in women, but the association with hepatotoxicity argues against its routine use for this cosmetic purpose.

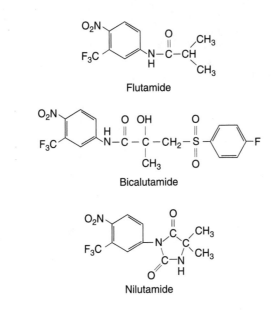

Flutamide

Bicalutamide

Nilutamide

Spironolactone

Spironolactone *(ALDACTONE) (see Chapter 28) is an aldosterone antagonist that also is a weak AR antagonist and a weak inhibitor of testosterone synthesis, apparently inhibiting CYP17. When used to treat fluid retention or hypertension in men, gynecomastia is a common side effect.*

5α-REDUCTASE INHIBITORS *Finasteride* (PROSCAR) is an inhibitor of 5α-reductase, especially the type II isozyme; *dutasteride* (AVODART) is a dual inhibitor of types I and II; both drugs block the conversion of testosterone to dihydrotestosterone, especially in the male external genitalia. These agents are approved for benign prostatic hyperplasia in the U.S. and many other countries. When administered to men with moderately severe symptoms due to obstruction of urinary tract outflow, serum and prostatic concentrations of dihydrotestosterone decrease, prostatic volume decreases, and urine flow rate increases. Impotence is a well-documented, albeit infrequent, side effect of this use. Finasteride (PROPECIA) also is approved for use in the treatment of male pattern baldness and appears to be as effective as flutamide or the combination of estrogen and *cyproterone* in the treatment of hirsutism.

Finasteride

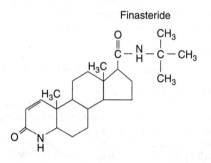

For a complete Bibliographical listing see Goodman & Gilman's *The Pharmacological Basis of Therapeutics,* **11th ed., or Goodman & Gilman Online at www.accessmedicine.com.**

59

ADRENOCORTICOTROPIC HORMONE; ADRENOCORTICAL STEROIDS AND THEIR SYNTHETIC ANALOGS; INHIBITORS OF THE SYNTHESIS AND ACTIONS OF ADRENOCORTICAL HORMONES

Corticosteroids and their biologically active synthetic derivatives are classified according to their metabolic (glucocorticoid) and electrolyte-regulating (mineralocorticoid) activities. These agents are employed at physiological doses for replacement therapy when endogenous production is impaired. In addition, glucocorticoids potently suppress inflammation, and their usefulness in a variety of inflammatory and autoimmune diseases making them among the most frequently prescribed classes of drugs. Because they exert effects on almost every organ system, the clinical use of and withdrawal from corticosteroids are complicated by a number of serious side effects, some of which are life-threatening. Therefore, the decision to institute therapy with corticosteroids always requires careful consideration of the relative risks and benefits in each patient.

ADRENOCORTICOTROPIC HORMONE (ACTH; CORTICOTROPIN)

Adrenocorticotropic hormone (ACTH) a peptide of 39 amino acids, is synthesized as part of a larger precursor protein, pro-opiomelanocortin (POMC), and is liberated along with α, β, and γ melanocyte-stimulating hormone (MSH) and other physiologically important peptides from the precursor through proteolytic cleavage at dibasic residues by prohormone convertases (*see* Chapter 21). The actions of ACTH and MSH are mediated by their specific interactions with five melanocortin receptor (MCR) subtypes comprising a distinct subfamily of G protein-coupled receptors (GPCRs). The well-known effects of MSH on pigmentation result from interactions with the MC1R on melanocytes. MC1Rs also are found on cells of the immune system and are thought to mediate the anti-inflammatory effects of α-MSH in experimental models of inflammation. ACTH, which is identical to α-MSH in its first 13 amino acids, exerts its effects on the adrenal cortex through the MC2R. ACTH has a much higher affinity for the MC2R than for the MC1R; however, under pathological conditions in which ACTH levels are markedly elevated, such as primary adrenal insufficiency, ACTH can signal through the MC1R and cause hyperpigmentation. The α-MSH-responsive MC3R and MC4R receptors in the hypothalamus play key roles in the regulation of appetite and body weight, and they therefore are the subject of considerable investigation as possible targets for drugs that affect appetite. The role of MC5R is less well-defined.

ACTIONS ON THE ADRENAL CORTEX Acting *via* MC2R, ACTH stimulates the adrenal cortex to secrete glucocorticoids, mineralocorticoids, and the androgen precursor dehydroepiandrosterone (DHEA), which can be converted peripherally into more potent androgens. The adrenal cortex is comprised of three zones that produce different steroid products under different regulatory influences. The outer zona glomerulosa secretes the mineralocorticoid aldosterone, the middle zona fasciculata secretes the glucocorticoid cortisol, and the inner zona reticularis secretes DHEA and its sulfated derivative (Figure 59–1).

Cells of the outer zone have receptors for angiotensin II (AngII) and express aldosterone synthase (CYP11B2), an enzyme that catalyzes the terminal reactions in mineralocorticoid biosynthesis. Although ACTH acutely stimulates mineralocorticoid production by the zona glomerulosa, this zone is regulated predominantly by AngII (*see* Chapter 30) and extracellular K^+ and does not undergo atrophy in the absence of ongoing stimulation by the pituitary gland. In the setting of persistently elevated ACTH, mineralocorticoid levels initially increase and then return to normal (a phenomenon termed *ACTH escape*).

Cells of the zona fasciculata have fewer receptors for AngII and express two enzymes, steroid 17α-hydroxylase (CYP17) and 11β-hydroxylase (CYP11B1), which catalyze the production of glucocorticoids. In the zona reticularis, CYP17 carries out a second C17-20 lyase reaction that converts C21 corticosteroids to C19 androgen precursors.

In the absence of the anterior pituitary and ACTH stimulation, the inner zones of the cortex atrophy, and the production of glucocorticoids and adrenal androgens is markedly impaired. Persistently elevated levels of ACTH, due either to repeated administration of large doses of ACTH or to excessive endogenous production, induce hyperplasia and hypertrophy of the inner cortical zones, with overproduction of cortisol and adrenal androgens. Adrenal hyperplasia is most marked

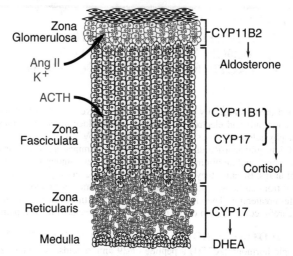

FIGURE 59–1 *The adrenal cortex contains three anatomically and functionally distinct compartments.* The major functional compartments of the adrenal cortex are shown, along with the steroidogenic enzymes that determine the unique profiles of corticosteroid products. Also shown are the predominant physiologic regulators of steroid production: AngII and K+ for the zona glomerulosa and ACTH for the zona fasciculata. The physiologic regulator(s) of dehydroepiandrosterone (DHEA) production by the zona reticularis are not known, although ACTH acutely increases DHEA biosynthesis.

in congenital disorders of steroidogenesis, in which ACTH levels are continuously elevated as a secondary response to impaired cortisol biosynthesis.

MECHANISM OF ACTION ACTH stimulates the production of adrenocortical steroids by increasing *de novo* biosynthesis. ACTH, binding to MC2R, activates the G_s-adenylyl cyclase-cyclic AMP-PKA pathway. Cyclic AMP is an obligatory second messenger for most, if not all, effects of ACTH on steroidogenesis. Temporally, the response of adrenocortical cells to ACTH has two phases. The acute phase, which occurs within seconds to minutes, largely reflects increased delivery of cholesterol substrate to the steroidogenic enzymes. The chronic phase, which occurs over hours to days, results largely from increased transcription of the steroidogenic enzymes. Pathways of adrenal steroid biosynthesis and structures of the major steroid intermediates and products of the human adrenal cortex are shown in Figure 59–2. The rate-limiting step in steroid hormone production is the conversion of cholesterol to pregnenolone, a reaction catalyzed by CYP11A1, the cholesterol side-chain cleavage enzyme. Most of the enzymes required for steroid hormone biosynthesis, including CYP11A1, are members of the cytochrome P450 superfamily (*see* Chapter 3). The rate-limiting components in this reaction regulate the mobilization of substrate cholesterol and its delivery to CYP11A1 in the inner mitochondrial matrix.

REGULATION OF ACTH SECRETION
Hypothalamic-Pituitary-Adrenal Axis The rate of glucocorticoid secretion is determined by fluctuations in the release of ACTH by pituitary corticotropes. These corticotropes, in turn, are regulated by corticotropin-releasing hormone (CRH), a peptide hormone released by CRH neurons of the endocrine hypothalamus. These three organs collectively are referred to as the hypothalamic-pituitary-adrenal (HPA) axis, an integrated system that maintains appropriate levels of glucocorticoids (*see* Figure 59–3). There are 3 characteristic modes of regulation of the HPA axis: diurnal rhythm in basal steroidogenesis, negative feedback regulation by glucocorticoids, and marked increases in steroidogenesis in response to stress. The diurnal rhythm is entrained by higher neuronal centers in response to sleep-wake cycles, such that levels of ACTH peak in the early morning hours, causing the circulating glucocorticoid levels to peak at approximately 8 AM. As discussed below, negative feedback regulation occurs at multiple levels of the HPA axis and is the major mechanism that maintains circulating glucocorticoid levels in the appropriate range. Stress can override the normal negative feedback control mechanisms, leading to marked increases in plasma concentrations of glucocorticoids.

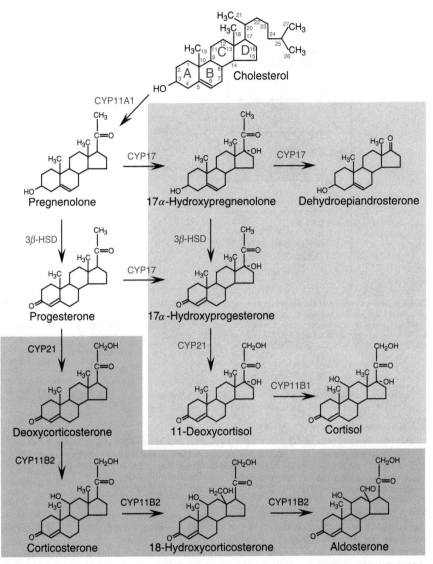

FIGURE 59–2 *Pathways of corticosteroid biosynthesis.* The steroidogenic pathways used in the biosynthesis of the corticosteroids are shown, along with the structures of the intermediates and products. The pathways that are unique to the zona glomerulosa are shown in blue, whereas those that occur in the inner zona fasciculata and zona reticularis are shown in gray. The zona reticularis does not express 3β-HSD, and thus preferentially synthesizes DHEA. CYP11A1, cholesterol side-chain cleavage enzyme; 3β-HSD, 3β-hydroxysteroid dehydrogenase; CYP17, steroid 17α-hydroxylase; CYP21, steroid 21-hydroxylase; CYP11B2, aldosterone synthase; CYP11B1, steroid 11β-hydroxylase.

DIAGNOSTIC APPLICATIONS OF ACTH

Because all known therapeutic effects of ACTH can be achieved with corticosteroids, synthetic steroid hormones generally are used therapeutically instead of ACTH. A synthetic derivative of ACTH comprised of the first 24 amino acids of the natural hormone, cosyntropin (CORTROSYN, SYN-ACTHEN), is used principally in the diagnostic assessment of the HPA axis. In the standard cosyntropin test, cosyntropin is used at the considerably supraphysiological dose of 250 μg to maximally stimulate adrenocortical steroidogenesis. Cosyntropin is readily absorbed from

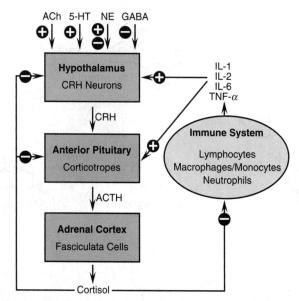

FIGURE 59–3 *Overview of the hypothalamic-pituitary-adrenal (HPA) axis and the immune inflammatory network.* Also shown are inputs from higher neuronal centers that regulate CRH secretion. + indicates a positive regulator, – indicates a negative regulator, +/– indicates a mixed effect. IL-1, interleukin-1; IL-2, interleukin-2; IL-6, interleukin-6; TNF-α, tumor necrosis factor-α; CRH, corticotropin-releasing hormone; ACh, acetylcholine; 5-HT, 5-hydroxytryptamine (serotonin); NE, norepinephrine; GABA, γ-aminobutyric acid.

parenteral sites and rapidly disappears from the circulation after intravenous administration; the plasma $t_{1/2}$ *is ~15 minutes, primarily due to rapid enzymatic hydrolysis.*

CRH Stimulation Test

Synthetic forms of ovine CRH (corticorelin [ACTHREL]) and human CRH are available for diagnostic testing of the HPA axis, with the former used in the U.S. and the latter preferred in Europe. In patients with documented ACTH-dependent hypercorticism, CRH testing in conjunction with petrosal sinus sampling can differentiate between a pituitary source (i.e., Cushing's disease) and an ectopic source of ACTH.

ADRENOCORTICAL STEROIDS

The adrenal cortex synthesizes two classes of steroids: the *corticosteroids*, which have 21 carbon atoms, and the *androgens*, which have 19 (Figure 59–2). The actions of corticosteroids are classified as glucocorticoid (carbohydrate metabolism–regulating) and mineralocorticoid (electrolyte balance–regulating), reflecting their preferential activities. In humans, *cortisol (hydrocortisone)* is the main glucocorticoid and aldosterone is the main mineralocorticoid. Typically cortisol is secreted at a rate of 10 mg/day whereas aldosterone is secreted at a rate of 0.125 mg/day. The concentrations of cortisol in peripheral plasma are considerably higher in the morning (16 μg/dL at 8 AM) than in the late afternoon (4 μg/dL at 4 PM) reflecting diurnal regulation, whereas the plasma concentrations of aldosterone are lower and more constant (0.01 μg/dL) throughout the day. The daily production of cortisol can rise at least tenfold in the setting of severe stress.

Although adrenal DHEA is an important precursor of testosterone and estradiol synthesis in women, patients with adrenal insufficiency can be restored to normal life expectancy by replacement therapy with glucocorticoids and mineralocorticoids. Nevertheless, some studies suggest that addition of DHEA to the standard replacement regimen in women with adrenal insufficiency improves subjective well-being and sexuality. The finding that the levels of DHEA and its sulfated derivative DHEA-S fall progressively after the third decade of life has prompted speculation that DHEA may at least partly reverse the adverse consequences of aging. This has led to the wide use of DHEA as a nutritional supplement despite the absence of definitive data.

Physiological Functions and Pharmacological Effects

PHYSIOLOGICAL ACTIONS   The effects of corticosteroids are numerous and widespread, and include alterations in carbohydrate, protein, and lipid metabolism; maintenance of fluid and electrolyte balance; and preservation of normal function of the cardiovascular system, the immune system, the kidney, skeletal muscle, the endocrine system, and the nervous system. In addition, corticosteroids endow the organism with the capacity to resist such stressful circumstances as noxious stimuli and environmental changes. In the absence of the adrenal cortex, survival is made possible only by maintaining an optimal environment, including adequate and regular feedings, ingestion of relatively large amounts of sodium chloride, and maintenance of an appropriate environmental temperature; stresses such as infection and trauma can be life-threatening when adrenal function is impaired.

The actions of corticosteroids are interrelated to those of other hormones. In the absence of glucocorticoids, epinephrine and norepinephrine have only minor effects on lipolysis. Administration of a small dose of glucocorticoid, however, markedly potentiates their lipolytic action. Those effects of corticosteroids that involve concerted actions with other hormonal regulators are termed *permissive* and most likely reflect steroid-induced changes in protein synthesis that, in turn, modify tissue responsiveness to other hormones.

Corticosteroids traditionally are divided into mineralocorticoids and glucocorticoids according to their relative potencies in Na^+ retention and effects on carbohydrate metabolism (*i.e.*, hepatic deposition of glycogen and gluconeogenesis) In general, potencies of steroids to sustain life in adrenalectomized animals closely parallel their mineralocorticoid activity, while potencies as anti-inflammatory agents closely parallel their effects on glucose metabolism. The effects on Na^+ retention and the carbohydrate/anti-inflammatory actions are not closely related and reflect selective actions at distinct receptors.

Estimates of potencies of representative steroids in these actions are listed in Table 59–1. Some steroids that are classified predominantly as glucocorticoids (*e.g.*, cortisol) also possess modest but significant mineralocorticoid activity and thus may affect fluid and electrolyte handling in the clinical setting. At doses used for replacement therapy in patients with primary adrenal insufficiency (*see* below), the mineralocorticoid effects of these "glucocorticoids" are insufficient to replace that of aldosterone, and concurrent therapy with a more potent mineralocorticoid generally is needed. In contrast, aldosterone is exceedingly potent with respect to Na^+ retention, but has only modest potency for effects on carbohydrate metabolism. At normal rates of secretion by the adrenal cortex or in doses that maximally affect electrolyte balance, aldosterone has no significant glucocorticoid activity and thus acts as a pure mineralocorticoid.

GENERAL MECHANISMS FOR CORTICOSTEROID EFFECTS   Corticosteroids interact with specific receptor proteins in target tissues to regulate the expression of corticosteroid-responsive

Table 59–1

Relative Potencies and Equivalent Doses of Representative Corticosteroids

Compound	Anti-inflammatory Potency	Na^+-Retaining Potency	Duration of Action*	Equivalent Dose,[†] mg
Cortisol	1	1	S	20
Cortisone	0.8	0.8	S	25
Fludrocortisone	10	125	I	‡
Prednisone	4	0.8	I	5
Prednisolone	4	0.8	I	5
6α-Methylprednisolone	5	0.5	I	4
Triamcinolone	5	0	I	4
Betamethasone	25	0	L	0.75
Dexamethasone	25	0	L	0.75

*S, short (*i.e.*, $t_{1/2} \approx$ 8–12 h; I, intermediate (*i.e.*, $t_{1/2} \approx$ 12–36 h); L, long (*i.e.*, $t_{1/2} \approx$ 36–72 h).
[†]These dose relationships apply only to oral or intravenous administration, as glucocorticoid potencies may differ greatly following intramuscular or intraarticular administration.
[‡]This agent is not used for glucocorticoid effects.

genes, thereby changing the levels and array of proteins synthesized by the various target tissues. As a consequence of the time required to effect these changes, most effects of corticosteroids are not immediate but become apparent after several hours. This fact is of clinical significance, because a delay generally is seen before beneficial effects of corticosteroid therapy become manifest. Although corticosteroids predominantly act to increase expression of target genes, there are well-documented examples in which glucocorticoids decrease transcription. In addition to these genomic effects, some immediate actions of corticosteroids may be mediated by membrane-bound receptors.

Regulation of Gene Expression by Glucocorticoids

The GR resides predominantly in the cytoplasm in an inactive form until it binds glucocorticoids. The inactive GR is complexed with other proteins, including heat-shock proteins and an immunophilin. After ligand binding, the GR dissociates from its associated proteins and translocates to the nucleus. There, it interacts with specific DNA sequences called glucocorticoid responsive elements *(GREs) within the regulatory regions of affected genes. These GREs thus provide specificity to the regulation of gene transcription by glucocorticoids.*

Regulation of Gene Expression by Mineralocorticoids

Like the GR, the MR also is a ligand-activated transcription factor and binds to a very similar, if not identical, hormone responsive element. The selective actions of GR and MR are thought to result from interactions with other transcription factors that also are recruited to the promoter regions of target genes as well as from the restricted pattern of expression of the MR. Unlike the GR, which has a more ubiquitous distribution, the MR is expressed principally in the kidney (distal cortical tubule and cortical collecting duct), colon, salivary glands, sweat glands, and hippocampus.

Receptor-Independent Mechanism for Corticosteroid Specificity

Biochemical studies of the GR and MR led to the surprising finding that aldosterone (a classic mineralocorticoid) and cortisol (predominantly a glucocorticoid) bind the MR with equal affinity. This raised the question of how the apparent specificity of the MR for aldosterone was maintained in the face of much higher circulating levels of cortisol. We now know that the type 2 isozyme of 11β-hydroxysteroid dehydrogenase (11\betaHSD2) plays a key role in corticosteroid specificity, particularly in the kidney, colon, and salivary glands. This enzyme metabolizes glucocorticoids such as cortisol to receptor-inactive 11-keto derivatives such as cortisone (Figure 59–4) and thus forms an enzymatic barrier that prevents cortisol from reaching the MR. Because its predominant form in physiological settings is the hemiacetal derivative (Figure 59–4), aldosterone is resistant to this inactivation and maintains mineralocorticoid activity.

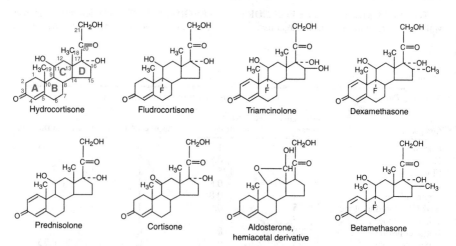

FIGURE 59–4 *Structure and nomenclature of corticosteroid products and selected synthetic derivatives.* The structure of hydrocortisone is represented in two dimensions. The steroid ring system is not completely planar and the orientation of the groups attached to the steroid rings is an important determinant of the biological activity. The methyl groups at C18 and C19 and the hydroxyl group at C11 project upward (forward in the two-dimensional representation and shown by a solid line connecting the atoms) and are designated β. The hydroxyl at C17 projects below the plane (behind in the two-dimensional representation, and represented by the dashed line connecting the atoms) and is designated α.

CARBOHYDRATE AND PROTEIN METABOLISM Corticosteroids profoundly affect carbohydrate and protein metabolism. Teleologically, these effects of glucocorticoids on intermediary metabolism can be viewed as protecting glucose-dependent tissues (*e.g.*, the brain and heart) from starvation. They stimulate the liver to form glucose from amino acids and glycerol and to store glucose as liver glycogen. In the periphery, glucocorticoids diminish glucose utilization, increase protein breakdown and the synthesis of glutamine, and activate lipolysis, thereby providing amino acids and glycerol for gluconeogenesis. The net result is to increase blood glucose levels. Because of their effects on glucose metabolism, glucocorticoids can worsen glycemic control in patients with overt diabetes and can precipitate the onset of diabetes in patients who are otherwise predisposed.

LIPID METABOLISM Two effects of corticosteroids on lipid metabolism are firmly established. The first is the dramatic redistribution of body fat that occurs in settings of endogenous or pharmacologically induced hypercorticism, such as Cushing's syndrome. The other is the permissive facilitation of the lipolytic effect of other agents, such as growth hormone and β adrenergic receptor agonists, resulting in an increase in free fatty acids after glucocorticoid administration. With respect to fat distribution, there is increased fat in the back of the neck ("buffalo hump"), face ("moon facies"), and supraclavicular area, coupled with a loss of fat in the extremities.

ELECTROLYTE AND WATER BALANCE Aldosterone is by far the most potent endogenous corticosteroid with respect to fluid and electrolyte balance. Thus, electrolyte balance is relatively normal in patients with adrenal insufficiency due to pituitary disease, despite the loss of glucocorticoid production by the inner cortical zones. Mineralocorticoids act on the distal tubules and collecting ducts of the kidney to enhance reabsorption of Na^+ from the tubular fluid; they also increase the urinary excretion of K^+ and H^+.

These actions on electrolyte transport, in the kidney and in other tissues (*e.g.*, colon, salivary glands, and sweat glands), appear to account for the physiological and pharmacological activities that are characteristic of mineralocorticoids. Thus, the primary features of hyperaldosteronism are positive Na^+ balance with consequent expansion of extracellular fluid volume, normal or slight increases in plasma Na^+ concentration, hypokalemia, and alkalosis. Mineralocorticoid deficiency, in contrast, leads to Na^+ wasting and contraction of the extracellular fluid volume, hyponatremia, hyperkalemia, and acidosis. Chronically, hyperaldosteronism can cause hypertension, whereas aldosterone deficiency can lead to hypotension and vascular collapse.

Glucocorticoids also exert effects on fluid and electrolyte balance, largely due to permissive effects on tubular function and actions that maintain glomerular filtration rate. In part, the inability of patients with glucocorticoid deficiency to excrete free water results from the increased secretion of vasopressin, which stimulates water reabsorption in the kidney.

In addition to their effects on monovalent cations and water, glucocorticoids also exert multiple effects on Ca^{2+} metabolism. Steroids interfere with Ca^{2+} uptake in the gut and increase Ca^{2+} excretion by the kidney. These effects collectively lead to decreased total body Ca^{2+} stores.

CARDIOVASCULAR SYSTEM The most striking cardiovascular effects of corticosteroids result from mineralocorticoid-induced changes in renal Na^+ excretion, as is evident in primary aldosteronism. The resultant hypertension can lead to a diverse group of adverse effects on the cardiovascular system (*see* Chapter 32). Consistent with the known actions of mineralocorticoids in the kidney, restriction of dietary Na^+ can lower the blood pressure considerably in mineralocorticoid excess.

Studies also have shown direct effects of aldosterone on the heart and vascular lining; aldosterone induces hypertension and interstitial cardiac fibrosis in animal models. The increased cardiac fibrosis is proposed to result from direct mineralocorticoid actions in the heart rather than from the effect of hypertension, because treatment with spironolactone, a MR antagonist, blocks the fibrosis without altering blood pressure. Similar effects of mineralocorticoids on cardiac fibrosis in human beings may explain, at least in part, the beneficial effects of spironolactone in patients with congestive heart failure (*see* Chapter 33).

The second major action of corticosteroids on the cardiovascular system is to enhance vascular reactivity to other vasoactive substances. Hypoadrenalism is associated with reduced response to vasoconstrictors such as norepinephrine and AngII, perhaps due to decreased expression of adrenergic receptors in the vascular wall. Conversely, hypertension is seen in patients with excessive glucocorticoid secretion, occurring in most patients with Cushing's syndrome and in a subset of patients treated with synthetic glucocorticoids (even those lacking any significant mineralocorticoid action).

SKELETAL MUSCLE Permissive concentrations of corticosteroids are required for the normal function of skeletal muscle, and diminished work capacity is a prominent sign of adrenocortical insufficiency. In patients with Addison's disease, weakness and fatigue are frequent symptoms. Excessive amounts of either glucocorticoids or mineralocorticoids also impair muscle function. In primary aldosteronism, muscle weakness results primarily from hypokalemia rather than from direct effects of mineralocorticoids on skeletal muscle. In contrast, glucocorticoid excess over prolonged periods, either secondary to glucocorticoid therapy or endogenous hypercorticism, causes skeletal muscle wasting. This effect, termed *steroid myopathy*, accounts in part for weakness and fatigue in patients with glucocorticoid excess.

CENTRAL NERVOUS SYSTEM Corticosteroids exert a number of indirect effects on the CNS, through maintenance of blood pressure, plasma glucose concentrations, and electrolyte concentrations. Increasingly, direct effects of corticosteroids on the CNS have been recognized, including effects on mood, behavior, and brain excitability. Patients with adrenal insufficiency exhibit a diverse array of psychiatric manifestations, including apathy, depression, and irritability; some patients are frankly psychotic. Appropriate replacement therapy corrects these abnormalities. Conversely, most patients receiving glucocorticoids respond with mood elevation, which may impart a sense of well-being despite the persistence of underlying disease. Some patients exhibit more pronounced behavioral changes, such as euphoria, insomnia, restlessness, and increased motor activity. A smaller but significant percentage of patients treated with glucocorticoids become anxious, depressed, or overtly psychotic.

FORMED ELEMENTS OF BLOOD Glucocorticoids exert minor effects on hemoglobin and erythrocyte content of blood, as evidenced by the occurrence of polycythemia in Cushing's syndrome and of normochromic, normocytic anemia in adrenal insufficiency. More profound effects are seen in the setting of autoimmune hemolytic anemia, in which the immunosuppressive effects of glucocorticoids can diminish erythrocyte destruction.

Corticosteroids also affect circulating white blood cells. Addison's disease is associated with an increased mass of lymphoid tissue and lymphocytosis. In contrast, Cushing's syndrome is characterized by lymphocytopenia and decreased mass of lymphoid tissue. The administration of glucocorticoids leads to a decreased number of circulating lymphocytes, eosinophils, monocytes, and basophils. A single dose of hydrocortisone decreases these circulating cells within 4–6 hours; this effect persists for 24 hours and results from the redistribution of cells away from the periphery rather than from increased destruction. In contrast, glucocorticoids increase circulating polymorphonuclear leukocytes as a result of increased release from the marrow, diminished rate of removal from the circulation, and increased demargination from vascular walls. Finally, certain lymphoid malignancies are destroyed by glucocorticoid treatment, an effect that may relate to the ability of glucocorticoids to activate programmed cell death.

ANTI-INFLAMMATORY AND IMMUNOSUPPRESSIVE ACTIONS In addition to their effects on lymphocyte number, corticosteroids profoundly alter immune response. These effects are important facets of the anti-inflammatory and immunosuppressive actions of the glucocorticoids. Glucocorticoids can prevent or suppress inflammation in response to multiple inciting events, including radiant, mechanical, chemical, infectious, and immunological stimuli. Although the use of glucocorticoids as anti-inflammatory agents does not address the underlying cause of the disease, the suppression of inflammation is of enormous clinical utility and has made these drugs among the most frequently prescribed agents. Similarly, glucocorticoids are of immense value in treating diseases that result from undesirable immune reactions. These diseases range from conditions that predominantly result from humoral immunity, such as urticaria (*see* Chapter 62), to those that are mediated by cellular immune mechanisms, such as transplant rejection (*see* Chapter 52). The immunosuppressive and anti-inflammatory actions of glucocorticoids are inextricably linked, perhaps because they both involve inhibition of leukocyte functions.

Multiple mechanisms are involved in the suppression of inflammation by glucocorticoids. There is decreased release of vasoactive and chemoattractive factors, diminished secretion of lipolytic and proteolytic enzymes, decreased extravasation of leukocytes to areas of injury, and ultimately, decreased fibrosis. Glucocorticoids can also reduce expression of proinflammatory enzymes, such as COX-2 and NOS.

Absorption, Transport, Metabolism, and Excretion

ABSORPTION Hydrocortisone and numerous congeners, including the synthetic analogs, are orally effective. Certain water-soluble esters of hydrocortisone and its synthetic congeners are administered intravenously to rapidly achieve high concentrations of drug in body fluids. More prolonged effects are obtained by intramuscular injection of suspensions of hydrocortisone, its esters, and congeners. Minor changes in chemical structure may markedly alter the rate of absorption, time of onset of effect, and duration of action.

Glucocorticoids also are absorbed systemically from sites of local administration, such as synovial spaces, the conjunctival sac, skin, and respiratory tract. When administration is prolonged, when the site of application is covered with an occlusive dressing, or when large areas of skin are involved, the absorption may be sufficient to cause systemic effects, including suppression of the HPA axis.

TRANSPORT, METABOLISM, AND EXCRETION After absorption, >90% of cortisol in plasma is reversibly bound to protein under normal circumstances. Only the fraction of corticosteroid that is unbound can enter cells to mediate corticosteroid effects. Two plasma proteins account for almost all of the steroid-binding capacity: corticosteroid-binding globulin (CBG; also called transcortin), and albumin. CBG is an α-globulin secreted by the liver that has high affinity (association constant of ~7.6 $\times$ 10^7 M^{-1}) for steroids but relatively low total binding capacity, whereas albumin has low affinity (association constant of 1 $\times$ 10^3 M^{-1}) but relatively large binding capacity. CBG has relatively high affinity for cortisol and most of its synthetic congeners and low affinity for aldosterone and glucuronide-conjugated steroid metabolites; thus, greater percentages of these latter steroids are found in the free form.

A special state of physiological hypercorticism occurs during pregnancy. The elevated circulating estrogen levels induce CBG production, and CBG and total plasma cortisol increase severalfold. The physiological significance of these changes remains to be established.

All of the biologically active adrenocortical steroids and their synthetic congeners have a double bond in the 4,5 position and a ketone group at C3 (Figure 59–4). The metabolism of steroid hormones generally involves sequential additions of oxygen or hydrogen atoms, followed by conjugation to form water-soluble derivatives. Reduction of the 4,5 double bond occurs at both hepatic and extrahepatic sites, yielding inactive compounds. Subsequent reduction of the 3-ketone substituent to the 3-hydroxyl derivative, forming tetrahydrocortisol, occurs only in the liver. Most of these A ring–reduced steroids are conjugated through the 3-hydroxyl group with sulfate or glucuronide by enzymatic reactions that take place in the liver, and to a lesser extent in the kidney. The resultant sulfate esters and glucuronides are water-soluble and are the predominant forms excreted in urine. Neither biliary nor fecal excretion is of quantitative importance in humans. The role of 11βHSD2 in the conversion of cortisol to its inactive 11-keto derivative, cortisone, is discussed above. The type 1 isozyme (11βHSD1), expressed predominantly in the liver but also in adipocytes, skin, bone and the eye, metabolizes cortisone to cortisol.

Structure–Activity Relationships

The structures of hydrocortisone (cortisol) and some of its major derivatives are shown in Figure 59–4. Chemical modifications to the cortisol molecule have generated derivatives with greater separations of glucocorticoid and mineralocorticoid activity; for a number of synthetic glucocorticoids, the effects on electrolytes are minimal even at the highest doses used (Table 59–1). In addition, these modifications have led to derivatives with greater potencies and longer durations of action. A vast array of steroid preparations is available for oral, parenteral, and topical use. None of the available derivatives effectively separates anti-inflammatory effects from effects on carbohydrate, protein, and fat metabolism, or from suppressive effects on the HPA axis. Note that synthetic steroids with an 11-keto substituent, such as cortisone and prednisone, *must be metabolized to their corresponding 11β-hydroxy derivatives before they are biologically active.*

Toxicity of Adrenocortical Steroids

Two categories of toxic effects result from the therapeutic use of corticosteroids: those resulting from withdrawal of steroid therapy and those resulting from continued use at supraphysiological doses. The side effects from both categories are potentially life-threatening and mandate a careful assessment of the risks and benefits in each patient.

WITHDRAWAL OF THERAPY The most frequent problem in steroid withdrawal is flareup of the underlying disease for which steroids were prescribed. There are several other complications associated with steroid withdrawal. The most severe complication of steroid cessation, acute adrenal insufficiency, results from overly rapid withdrawal of corticosteroids after prolonged therapy has suppressed the HPA axis. Treatment with supraphysiological doses of glucocorticoids for 2–4 weeks may cause some degree of HPA impairment. The therapeutic approach to acute adrenal insufficiency is detailed below. There is significant variation among patients with respect to the degree and duration of adrenal suppression after glucocorticoid therapy, making it difficult to establish the relative risk in any given patient. Many patients recover from glucocorticoid-induced HPA suppression within several weeks to months; however, in some individuals the time to recovery can be one year or longer.

CONTINUED USE OF SUPRAPHYSIOLOGICAL GLUCOCORTICOID DOSES
Since the pharmacological and physiological actions of corticosteroids are mediated by the same receptors, supraphysiological doses of the various glucocorticoid derivatives generally cause side effects that are exaggerated manifestations of their physiological effects. Besides the consequences that result from HPA suppression, other complications of prolonged therapy include fluid and electrolyte abnormalities, hypertension, hyperglycemia, increased susceptibility to infection, osteoporosis, myopathy, behavioral disturbances, cataracts, growth arrest, and the characteristic habitus of steroid overdose, including fat redistribution, striae, and ecchymoses.

Therapeutic Uses

With the exception of replacement therapy in deficiency states, the use of glucocorticoids largely is empirical. Based on extensive clinical experience, a number of therapeutic principles can be proposed. Given the number and severity of potential side effects, the decision to institute therapy with glucocorticoids always requires a careful consideration of the relative risks and benefits in each patient. For any disease and in any patient, the appropriate dose to achieve a given therapeutic effect must be determined by trial and error and must be reevaluated periodically as the activity of the underlying disease changes or as complications of therapy arise. A single dose of glucocorticoid, even a large one, is virtually without harmful effects, and a short course of therapy (up to one week), in the absence of specific contraindications, is unlikely to be harmful. As the duration of glucocorticoid therapy is increased beyond one week, there are time- and dose-related increases in the incidence of disabling and potentially lethal effects. Except in patients receiving replacement therapy, glucocorticoids are neither specific nor curative; rather, they are palliative by virtue of their anti-inflammatory and immunosuppressive actions. Finally, abrupt cessation of glucocorticoids after prolonged therapy is associated with the risk of adrenal insufficiency, which may be fatal.

These principles have several implications for clinical practice. When glucocorticoids are to be given over long periods, the dose must be determined by trial and error and must be the smallest one that will achieve the desired effect. When the therapeutic goal is relief of painful or distressing symptoms not associated with an immediately life-threatening disease, complete relief is not sought, and the steroid dose is reduced gradually until worsening symptoms indicate that the minimal acceptable dose has been found. Where possible, the substitution of other medications, such as nonsteroidal anti-inflammatory drugs, may facilitate the tapering process once the initial benefit of glucocorticoid therapy has been achieved. When therapy is directed at a life-threatening disease (*e.g.*, pemphigus or lupus cerebritis), the initial dose should be a large one aimed at achieving rapid control of the crisis. If some benefit is not observed quickly, then the dose should be doubled or tripled. After initial control in a potentially lethal disease, dose reduction should be carried out under conditions that permit frequent, accurate observations of the patient. It is always essential to weigh carefully the relative dangers of therapy and of the disease being treated.

REPLACEMENT THERAPY   Adrenal insufficiency can result from structural or functional lesions of the adrenal cortex (primary adrenal insufficiency or Addison's disease) or from structural or functional lesions of the anterior pituitary or hypothalamus (secondary adrenal insufficiency). In developed countries, primary adrenal insufficiency most frequently is secondary to autoimmune adrenal disease, whereas tuberculous adrenalitis is the most frequent etiology in underdeveloped countries. Other causes include adrenalectomy, bilateral adrenal hemorrhage, neoplastic infiltration of the adrenal glands, acquired immunodeficiency syndrome, inherited disorders of the steroidogenic enzymes, and X-linked adrenoleukodystrophy. Secondary adrenal insufficiency resulting from pituitary or hypothalamic dysfunction generally presents in a more insidious manner than does the primary disorder, probably because mineralocorticoid biosynthesis is preserved.

Acute Adrenal Insufficiency   This life-threatening disease is characterized by GI symptoms (nausea, vomiting, and abdominal pain), dehydration, hyponatremia, hyperkalemia, weakness, lethargy, and hypotension. It usually is associated with disorders of the adrenal rather than the pituitary or hypothalamus, but sometimes follows abrupt withdrawal of glucocorticoids used at high doses or for prolonged periods.

The immediate management of patients with acute adrenal insufficiency includes intravenous therapy with isotonic sodium chloride solution supplemented with 5% glucose and corticosteroids and appropriate therapy for precipitating causes such as infection, trauma, or hemorrhage. Because cardiovascular function often is reduced in the setting of adrenocortical insufficiency, the patient should be monitored for evidence of volume overload such as pulmonary edema. After an initial intravenous bolus of 100 mg, hydrocortisone (cortisol) should be given by continuous infusion at a rate of 50–100 mg every 8 hours. At this dose, which approximates the maximum daily rate of cortisol secretion in response to stress, hydrocortisone overwhelms the 11βHSD2 barrier in mineralocorticoid-responsive tissues and has sufficient mineralocorticoid activity to meet all requirements. As the patient stabilizes, the hydrocortisone dose may be decreased to 25 mg every 6–8 hours. Thereafter, patients are treated in the same fashion as those with chronic adrenal insufficiency (*see* below).

For the treatment of suspected but unconfirmed acute adrenal insufficiency, 4 mg of *dexamethasone sodium phosphate* can be substituted for hydrocortisone, since dexamethasone does not cross-react in the cortisol assay and will not interfere with the measurement of cortisol (either basally or in response to the cosyntropin stimulation test). A failure to respond to cosyntropin in this setting is diagnostic of adrenal insufficiency. Often, plasma ACTH also is measured to provide information about the underlying etiology if the diagnosis of adrenocortical insufficiency is established.

Chronic Adrenal Insufficiency   Patients with chronic adrenal insufficiency present with many of the same manifestations seen in adrenal crisis, but with lesser severity. These patients require daily treatment with corticosteroids. Traditional replacement regimens have used hydrocortisone in doses of 20–30 mg/day. *Cortisone acetate*, which is inactive until converted to cortisol by 11βHSD1, also has been used in doses ranging from 25 to 37.5 mg/day. In an effort to mimic the normal diurnal rhythm of cortisol secretion, these glucocorticoids generally are given in divided doses, with two-thirds of the dose given in the morning and one-third given in the afternoon. Based on revised estimates of daily cortisol production and clinical studies showing that subtle degrees of glucocorticoid excess can decrease bone density in patients on traditional replacement regimens, many authorities advocate a lower daily hydrocortisone dose of 15–20 mg/day divided into either two doses (*e.g.,* 10–15 mg on awakening and 5 mg in late afternoon) or three doses (*e.g.,* 10 mg on awakening, 5 mg at lunch, and 5 mg in late afternoon). Others prefer to use intermediate-acting (*e.g.,* prednisone) or long-acting (*e.g.,* dexamethasone) glucocorticoids, since no regimen employing shorter-acting steroids can reproduce the peak serum glucocorticoid levels that normally occur before awakening in the morning. The superiority of any one of these regimens has not been rigorously demonstrated. Although some patients with primary adrenal insufficiency can be maintained on hydrocortisone and liberal salt intake, most of these patients also require mineralocorticoid replacement; *fludrocortisone* generally is used in doses of 0.05–0.2 mg/day. For patients with secondary adrenal insufficiency, the administration of a glucocorticoid alone is generally adequate, as the zona glomerulosa, which makes mineralocorticoids, is intact. When initiating treatment in patients with panhypopituitarism, it is important to administer glucocorticoids before initiating treatment with thyroid hormone, because the administration of thyroid hormone may precipitate acute adrenal insufficiency by increasing cortisol metabolism.

The adequacy of corticosteroid replacement therapy is judged by clinical criteria and biochemical measurements. The subjective well-being of the patient is an important clinical parameter in primary and secondary disease. In primary adrenal insufficiency, the disappearance of hyperpigmentation and the resolution of electrolyte abnormalities are valuable indicators of adequate replacement. Overtreatment may cause manifestations of Cushing's syndrome; in children, linear growth may be decreased. Plasma ACTH levels may be used to monitor therapy in patients with primary adrenal insufficiency; the early-morning ACTH level should not be suppressed, but should be less than 100 pg/mL (20 pmol/L).

Standard doses of glucocorticoids often must be adjusted upward in patients who also are taking drugs that increase their metabolic clearance (*e.g., phenytoin*, barbiturates, or *rifampin*). Dosage adjustments also are needed to compensate for the stress of intercurrent illness, and proper patient education is essential for the execution of these adjustments. All patients with adrenal insufficiency should wear a medical alert bracelet or tag that lists their diagnosis and carries information about their steroid regimen. During minor illness, the glucocorticoid dose should be doubled. Patients should be instructed to contact their physician if nausea and vomiting preclude the retention of oral medications. The patient and family members should also be trained to administer parenteral dexamethasone (4 mg subcutaneously or intramuscularly) in the event that severe nausea or vomiting precludes the oral administration of medications; they then should seek medical attention immediately. Based largely on empirical data, glucocorticoid doses also are adjusted when patients with adrenal insufficiency undergo either elective or emergency surgery. In this setting, the doses are designed to approximate or exceed the maximal cortisol secretory rate of 200 mg/day; a standard regimen is hydrocortisone, 80–100 mg parenterally every 8 hours. Following surgery, the dose is halved each day until it is reduced to routine maintenance levels. Although some data suggest that increases in dose to this degree are not essential for survival even in major surgery, this approach remains the standard clinical practice.

Congenital Adrenal Hyperplasia (CAH) This term denotes a group of genetic disorders in which the activity of one of the several enzymes required for the biosynthesis of cortisol is deficient. The impaired production of cortisol and the consequent lack of negative feedback inhibition lead to increased release of ACTH. As a result, other hormonally active steroids that are proximal to the enzymatic block in the steroidogenic pathway are produced in excess. CAH includes a spectrum of disorders whose precise clinical presentation, laboratory findings, and treatment depend on which of the steroidogenic enzymes is deficient. In approximately 90% of patients, CAH results from mutations in CYP21, the enzyme that carries out the 21-hydroxylation reaction (Figure 59–3).

All patients with classical CAH require replacement therapy with hydrocortisone or a suitable congener, and those with salt wasting also require mineralocorticoid replacement. The goals of therapy are to restore levels of physiological steroid hormones to the normal range and to suppress ACTH, thereby abrogating the effects that result from overproduction of other steroids such as the adrenal androgens. The typical oral dose of hydrocortisone is approximately 0.6 mg/kg daily in 2 or 3 divided doses. The mineralocorticoid used is fludrocortisone acetate (0.05–0.2 mg/day). Many experts also administer table salt to infants (one-fifth of a teaspoon dissolved in formula daily) until the child is eating solid food. Therapy is guided by gain in weight and height, by plasma levels of 17-hydroxyprogesterone, and by blood pressure. Elevated plasma renin activity suggests that the patient is receiving an inadequate dose of mineralocorticoid. Sudden spurts in linear growth often indicate inadequate pituitary suppression and excessive androgen secretion, whereas growth failure suggests overtreatment with glucocorticoid.

THERAPEUTIC USES IN NONENDOCRINE DISEASES Outlined below are important uses of glucocorticoids in diseases that do not directly involve the HPA axis. The disorders discussed are not inclusive; rather, they illustrate the principles governing glucocorticoid use in selected diseases for which these drugs are more frequently employed. The dosage of glucocorticoids varies considerably depending on the nature and severity of the underlying disorder. For convenience, approximate doses of a representative glucocorticoid (generally prednisone) are provided. This choice is not an endorsement of one particular glucocorticoid preparation over other congeners and is made for illustrative purposes only.

Rheumatic Disorders

Glucocorticoids are used widely in the treatment of a variety of rheumatic disorders and are a mainstay in the treatment of the more serious inflammatory rheumatic diseases, such as systemic lupus erythematosus, and a variety of vasculitic disorders, such as polyarteritis nodosa, Wegener's granulomatosis, Churg-Strauss syndrome, and giant cell arteritis.

Glucocorticoids are often used in conjunction with other immunosuppressive agents such as cyclophosphamide and methotrexate, which offer better long-term control than steroids alone. The exception is giant cell arteritis, for which glucocorticoids remain superior to other agents. Caution should be exercised in the use of glucocorticoids in some forms of vasculitis (e.g., polyarteritis nodosa), for which underlying infections with hepatitis viruses may play a pathogenetic role. Intermediate-acting glucocorticoids such as prednisone and methylprednisolone are generally preferred over longer-acting steroids such as dexamethasone.

In rheumatoid arthritis, glucocorticoids are used as temporizing agents for progressive disease and provide relief until other, slower-acting anti-rheumatic drugs, such as methotrexate or newer agents targeted at tumor necrosis factor take effect. A typical starting dose is 5–10 mg/day of prednisone. In the setting of an acute exacerbation, higher doses of glucocorticoids may be employed (typically 20–40 mg/day of prednisone or equivalent), with rapid taper thereafter. Alternatively, patients with major symptomatology confined to one or a few joints may be treated with intra-articular steroid injections. Depending on joint size, typical doses are 5–20 mg of triamcinolone acetonide *or its equivalent.*

In noninflammatory degenerative joint diseases (e.g., osteoarthritis) or in a variety of regional pain syndromes (e.g., tendinitis or bursitis), glucocorticoids may be administered by local injection for the treatment of episodic disease flares. Intra-articular injections should be performed with intervals of at least 3 months to minimize painless joint destruction, a potential side effect of this treatment.

Renal Diseases

Patients with nephrotic syndrome secondary to minimal change disease generally respond to steroid therapy, and glucocorticoids clearly are the first-line treatment in both adults and children. Initial daily doses of prednisone are 1–2 mg/kg for 6 weeks, followed by a gradual tapering of the dose over 6–8 weeks, although some nephrologists advocate alternate-day therapy. Objective evidence of response, such as diminished proteinuria, is seen within 2–3 weeks in 85% of patients, and more than 95% of patients will have remission within 3 months. Patients with renal disease secondary to systemic lupus erythematosus also are generally given a therapeutic trial of glucocorticoids.

Allergic Disease

The onset of action of glucocorticoids in allergic diseases is delayed, and patients with severe allergic reactions such as anaphylaxis require immediate therapy with epinephrine. The manifestations of allergic diseases of limited duration—such as hay fever, urticaria, drug reactions, bee stings, and angioedema—can be suppressed by adequate doses of glucocorticoids given as supplements to the primary therapy. In severe disease, intravenous glucocorticoids (methylprednisolone 125 mg intravenously every 6 hours, or equivalent) are appropriate. In allergic rhinitis, intranasal steroids are now viewed by many experts as the drug of choice.

Bronchial Asthma

The use of glucocorticoids in bronchial asthma is discussed in Chapter 27.

Preterm Infants

Glucocorticoids such as betamethasone (12 mg intramuscularly every 24 hours for two doses) or dexamethasone (6 mg intramuscularly every 12 hours for four doses) are used frequently in the setting of premature labor to decrease the incidence of respiratory distress syndrome, intraventricular hemorrhage, and death in babies delivered prematurely.

Ocular Diseases

Ocular pharmacology, including consideration of the use of glucocorticoids, is discussed in Chapter 63.

GI Diseases

Glucocorticoid therapy is indicated in selected patients with inflammatory bowel disease (chronic ulcerative colitis and Crohn's disease; see Chapter 38).

Malignancies

Glucocorticoids are used in the chemotherapy of acute lymphocytic leukemia and lymphomas because of their antilymphocytic effects (see Chapter 51).

Organ Transplantation

In organ transplantation, most patients are kept on a regimen that includes glucocorticoids in conjunction with other immunosuppressive agents (see Chapter 52).

Spinal Cord Injury

Multicenter trials have shown significant decreases in neurological defects in patients with acute spinal cord injury treated within 8 hours of injury with large doses of methylprednisolone (30 mg/kg initially followed by an infusion of 5.4 mg/kg/h for 23 hours).

Diagnostic Applications of Adrenocortical Steroids

In addition to their therapeutic uses, glucocorticoids also are used for diagnostic purposes. The overnight dexamethasone suppression test is used to determine if patients with clinical manifestations suggestive of hypercortisolism have biochemical evidence of increased cortisol biosynthesis.

INHIBITORS OF THE BIOSYNTHESIS AND ACTION OF ADRENOCORTICAL STEROIDS

Four pharmacologic agents are useful inhibitors of adrenocortical secretion. *Mitotane* (o,p′-DDD), an adrenocorticolytic agent, is discussed in Chapter 51. The other inhibitors of steroid hormone biosynthesis are *aminoglutethimide, ketoconazole,* and *trilostane.* Aminoglutethimide and ketoconazole are discussed below. Trilostane is a competitive inhibitor of the conversion of pregnenolone to progesterone, a reaction catalyzed by 3β-hydroxysteroid dehydrogenase. All of these agents pose the common risk of precipitating acute adrenal insufficiency; thus, they must be used in appropriate doses, and the status of the patient's HPA axis must be carefully monitored.

AMINOGLUTETHIMIDE Aminoglutethimide (α-ethyl-*p*-aminophenyl-glutarimide; CYTADREN) primarily inhibits CYP11A1, which catalyzes the initial step in the biosynthesis of all physiological steroids. As a result, the production of all classes of steroid hormones is impaired. Aminoglutethimide also inhibits CYP11B1 and CYP19 (aromatase), which converts androgens to estrogens. Aminoglutethimide has been used primarily to decrease hypersecretion of cortisol in patients with Cushing's syndrome secondary to autonomous adrenal tumors or ectopic production of ACTH. Dose-dependent GI and neurological side effects are relatively common, as is a transient, maculopapular rash. The usual dose is 250 mg every 6 hours, with gradual increases of 250 mg/day at 1–2-week intervals until the desired biochemical effect is achieved, side effects prohibit further increases, or a daily dose of 2 g is reached. Because aminoglutethimide can cause frank adrenal insufficiency, glucocorticoid replacement therapy is necessary, and mineralocorticoid supplements also may be indicated. Aminoglutethimide accelerates the metabolism of dexamethasone, and this steroid therefore should not be used for glucocorticoid replacement in this setting.

KETOCONAZOLE Ketoconazole (NIZORAL) is used primarily as an antifungal agent (*see* Chapter 48). In doses higher than those employed in antifungal therapy, it inhibits adrenal and gonadal steroidogenesis, primarily by inhibiting the activity of CYP17 (17α-hydroxylase). At even higher doses, ketoconazole also inhibits CYP11A1, effectively blocking steroidogenesis in all primary steroidogenic tissues. Ketoconazole is the most effective inhibitor of steroid hormone biosynthesis in patients with Cushing's disease, though this use of the drug is not FDA-approved. In most cases, a dosage regimen of 600–800 mg/day (in two divided doses) is required, and some patients may require up to 1200 mg/day given in 2–3 doses. Side effects include hepatic dysfunction, which ranges from asymptomatic elevations of transaminase levels to severe hepatic injury. The potential of ketoconazole to interact with a number of CYP enzymes can lead to drug interactions of serious consequence (*see* Chapter 3).

ANTIGLUCOCORTICOIDS

The progesterone receptor antagonist *mifepristone* [RU-486; (11β-4-dimethylaminophenyl)-17β-hydroxy-7α-(propyl-1-ynyl)estra-4,9-dien-3-one] is used as an antiprogestin to terminate early pregnancy (*see* Chapter 57). At higher doses, mifepristone also inhibits the GR and thus has been studied as a potential therapeutic agent in patients with hypercorticism. Currently, it can be recommended only for patients with inoperable causes of cortisol excess that have not responded to other agents.

For a complete Bibliographical listing see Goodman & Gilman's *The Pharmacological Basis of Therapeutics,* 11th ed., or Goodman & Gilman Online at www.accessmedicine.com.

60

INSULIN, ORAL HYPOGLYCEMIC AGENTS, AND THE PHARMACOLOGY OF THE ENDOCRINE PANCREAS

Developed nations are witnessing a striking increase in the prevalence of diabetes mellitus (DM), predominantly related to lifestyle changes and the resulting surge in obesity. The metabolic consequences of prolonged hyperglycemia and dyslipidemia, including accelerated atherosclerosis, chronic kidney disease, and blindness, pose an enormous burden on patients with DM and on society. Improvements in our understanding of the pathogenesis of diabetes and its complications and in the prevention and therapy of diabetes are critical to meeting this challenge.

INSULIN

CHEMISTRY

Insulin is a peptide hormone (MW = 5734); it contains an A peptide of 21 amino acids and a B subunit of 30 amino acids, linked by one intrasubunit and two intersubunit disulfide bonds (Figure 60–1). The two chains of insulin form a highly ordered structure with α-helical regions in each of the chains. In solution, insulin can exist as a monomer, dimer, or hexamer. Two molecules of Zn^{2+} are coordinated in the hexamer, and this form of insulin presumably is stored in the β cell granules. Insulin hexamers also comprise most of the highly concentrated preparations used for therapy. As the concentration falls to physiological levels (nM), the hormone dissociates into monomers, which likely are the biologically active form.

Insulin is a member of the insulin-like growth factor (IGF) family. *IGF-1 and IGF-2 have structures that are homologous to that of proinsulin, but their short equivalents of the proinsulin C peptide are not removed in the mature proteins. In contrast to insulin, the IGFs are produced in many tissues and likely play a more important function in the regulation of growth than in the regulation of metabolism.*

Synthesis, Secretion, Distribution, and Degradation of Insulin

INSULIN PRODUCTION   The islet of Langerhans contains four major cell types, each of which synthesizes and secretes a distinct polypeptide hormone: insulin in the β (B) cell, *glucagon* in the α (A) cell, *somatostatin* in the δ (D) cell, and pancreatic polypeptide in the PP or F cell. The β cells make up 60–80% of the islet and form its central core with the α, δ and F cells in a discontinuous mantle around this core. The geographical organization of islet cells facilitates coordinated control of groups of cells. Blood in the islet flows from the β cells to α and δ cells. Thus, the β cell is the primary glucose sensor for the islet, and the other cell types presumably are exposed to particularly high concentrations of insulin.

The β cells synthesize insulin from a single-chain precursor of 110 amino acids termed preproinsulin. *The 24-amino-acid N-terminal signal peptide of preproinsulin is rapidly cleaved in the endoplasmic reticulum to form proinsulin (Figure 60–1). Subsequent processing of proinsulin in the secretory granule removes the connector C peptide, giving rise to mature insulin.*

The prohormone convertases, PC2 and PC3, convert proinsulin to insulin by proteolytic cleavage of four basic amino acids and removal of the C peptide (Figure 60–1). These Ca^{2+}-dependent endopeptidases are found in the islet cell granules and in other neuroendocrine cells. The conversion of proinsulin to insulin is nearly complete at the time of secretion. Thus, equimolar amounts of inactive C peptide and insulin are released into the circulation, and C peptide serves as a useful index of insulin secretion in assessing β cell mass and in identifying patients with factitious insulin injection or insulin-producing tumors. Since the $t_{1/2}$ of proinsulin in the circulation is much longer than that of insulin, up to 20% of immunoreactive insulin in plasma may reflect proinsulin and intermediates.

Regulation of Insulin Secretion

Insulin secretion is tightly regulated to maintain stable concentrations of glucose in blood during both fasting and feeding. This regulation is achieved by the coordinated interplay of various nutrients, gastrointestinal (GI) hormones, pancreatic hormones, and autonomic neurotransmitters. Glucose, amino acids, fatty acids, and ketone bodies stimulate insulin secretion. In general, any condition that activates the sympathetic nervous system (e.g., hypoxia, hypoglycemia, exercise, hypothermia, surgery, or severe burns) suppresses the secretion of insulin by stimulation of α_2 adrenergic receptors. Predictably, α_2 adrenergic receptor antagonists increase basal concentrations of insulin in plasma, while β_2 adrenergic receptor antagonists decrease them.

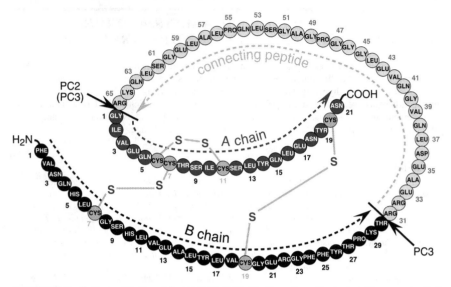

FIGURE 60–1 *Human proinsulin and its conversion to insulin.* The amino acid sequence of human proinsulin is shown. By proteolytic cleavage, four basic amino acids (residues 31, 32, 64, and 65) and the connecting peptide are removed, converting proinsulin to insulin. The sites of action of the endopeptidases PC2 and PC3 are shown.

Glucose, the principal stimulus to insulin secretion, is permissive for the action of many other secretagogues. Glucose provokes insulin secretion more effectively when taken orally than when administered intravenously because the oral route induces the release of GI hormones and stimulates vagal activity. Several GI hormones promote insulin secretion, the most potent of which are glucose-dependent insulinotropic peptide (GIP, also known as gastrointestinal inhibitory peptide) and glucagon-like peptide-1 (GLP-1).

Glucose-induced insulin secretion is biphasic: The first phase reaches a peak after 1–2 minutes and is short-lived; the second phase has a delayed onset but longer duration.

The resting β cell is hyperpolarized, and its glucose-induced depolarization leads to insulin secretion. Glucose enters the β cell by facilitated transport mediated by GLUT2, a specific subtype of glucose transporter. The sugar then is phosphorylated by glucokinase to yield glucose-6-phosphate (G-6-P). Its relatively high K_m (10–20 mM) allows glucokinase to play an important regulatory role at physiological glucose concentrations. Glucokinase's role as a glucose sensor was validated by its association with type 2 maturity-onset diabetes of the young (MODY), a rare monogenic form of diabetes. These glucokinase mutations, which compromise its ability to phosphorylate glucose, raise the threshold for glucose-stimulated insulin release and eventually result in DM.

The increase in oxidizable substrates (e.g., glucose and G-6-P) enhances ATP production, thereby inhibiting an ATP-sensitive K^+ channel. This decrease in K^+ conductance causes E_m to rise, opening a voltage-sensitive Ca^{2+} channel; Ca^{2+} then acts as the insulin secretagogue. The ATP-sensitive K^+ channel in β cells is an octamer composed of four Kir 6.2 and four SUR1 subunits. Both subunits contain nucleotide-binding domains; Kir 6.2 appears to mediate the inhibitory response to ATP; SUR1 binds ADP, the channel activator diazoxide, and the channel inhibitors (and promoters of insulin secretion) sulfonylureas and meglitinide.

DISTRIBUTION AND DEGRADATION OF INSULIN   Insulin circulates in blood as a monomer, and its volume of distribution approximates the volume of extracellular fluid. Under fasting conditions, the pancreas secretes about 40 μg (1 unit) of insulin/h into the portal vein to achieve a concentration of insulin in portal blood of 2–4 ng/mL (50–100 μunits/mL) and in the peripheral circulation of 0.5 ng/mL (12 μunits/mL) or ~0.1 nM. After ingestion of a meal, there is a rapid rise in the concentration of insulin in portal blood, followed by a parallel but smaller rise in the peripheral circulation.

The plasma $t_{1/2}$ of insulin normally is ~5–6 minutes but may be increased in diabetics who develop anti-insulin antibodies. The $t_{1/2}$ of proinsulin is longer than that of insulin, and proinsulin accounts for ~10% of the immunoreactive insulin in plasma. Since proinsulin is only 2% as potent as insulin, the biologically effective concentration of insulin is lower than estimated by immunoassay. C peptide is secreted in equimolar amounts with insulin, but its molar concentration in plasma is higher because of its considerably longer $t_{1/2}$ (~30 minutes).

Degradation of insulin occurs primarily in liver, kidney, and muscle. About 50% of the insulin that reaches the liver *via* the portal vein is destroyed and never reaches the general circulation. Insulin is filtered by the renal glomeruli and is reabsorbed by the tubules, which also degrade it. Severe impairment of renal function affects insulin clearance to a greater extent than does hepatic disease. Hepatic degradation of insulin operates near its maximal capacity and cannot compensate for diminished renal breakdown.

CELLULAR ACTIONS OF INSULIN   Key insulin target tissues for regulation of glucose homeostasis are liver, muscle, and fat, but insulin also exerts potent regulatory effects on other cell types. Insulin stimulates intracellular use and storage of glucose, amino acids, and fatty acids and inhibits catabolic processes such as the breakdown of glycogen, fat, and protein. It does this by stimulating the transport of substrates and ions into cells, promoting the translocation of proteins between cellular compartments, activating and inactivating specific enzymes, and changing the amounts of proteins by altering the rates of transcription and mRNA translation (Figure 60–2).

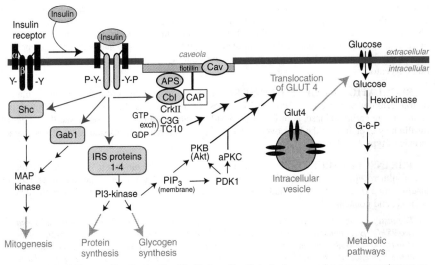

FIGURE 60–2   *Pathways of insulin signaling.* The binding of insulin to its plasma membrane receptor activates a cascade of downstream signaling events. Insulin binding activates the intrinsic tyrosine kinase activity of the receptor dimer, resulting in the tyrosine phosphorylation (Y-P) of the receptor's β subunits and a small number of specific substrates (light blue shapes): the insulin receptor substrate (IRS) proteins, Gab-1 and Shc; within the membrane, a caveolar pool of insulin receptor phosphorylates caveolin (Cav), APS, and Cbl. These tyrosine-phosphorylated proteins interact with signaling cascades *via* SH2 and SH3 domains to mediate the effects of insulin, with specific effects of insulin resulting from each pathway. In target tissues such as skeletal muscle and adipocytes, a key event is the translocation of the GLUT4 glucose transporter from intracellular vesicles to the plasma membrane; this translocation is stimulated by both the caveolar and noncaveolar pathways. In the noncaveolar pathway, the activation of PI3K is crucial, and PKB/Akt (anchored at the membrane by PIP_3) and/or an atypical form of PKC is involved. In the caveolar pathway, the caveolar protein flotillin localizes the signaling complex to the caveola; the signaling pathway involves series of SH2 domain interactions that add the adaptor protein CrkII, the guanine nucleotide exchange protein C3G, and small GTP-binding protein, TC10. The pathways are inactivated by specific phosphoprotein phosphatases (*e.g.*, PTB1B) and possibly by actions of Ser/Thr protein kinases. In addition to the actions shown, insulin also stimulates the plasma membrane Na^+,K^+-ATPase by a mechanism that is still being elucidated; the result is an increase in pump activity and a net accumulation of K^+ in the cell.

ABBREVIATIONS: APS, adaptor protein with PH and SH2 domains; CAP, Cbl associated protein; CrkII, chicken tumor virus regulator of kinase II; GLUT4, glucose transporter 4; Gab-1, Grb-2 associated binder; MAP kinase, mitogen-activated protein kinase; PDK, phosphoinositide-dependent kinase; PI3 kinase, phosphatidylinositol-3-kinase; PIP3, phosphatidylinositol trisphosphate; PKB, protein kinase B (also called Akt); aPKC, atypical isoform of protein kinase C; Y, tyrosine residue; Y-P, phosphorylated tyrosine residue.

Some effects of insulin occur within seconds or minutes, including the activation of glucose and ion transport systems, the covalent modification of enzymes (*i.e.,* phosphorylation or dephosphorylation), and some effects on gene transcription (*i.e.,* inhibition of the phosphoenolpyruvate carboxykinase gene). Effects on protein synthesis and gene transcription require hours, while those on cell proliferation and differentiation may take days.

REGULATION OF GLUCOSE TRANSPORT Stimulation of glucose transport into muscle and adipose tissue is a key response to insulin. Glucose enters cells by facilitated diffusion through one of a family of five glucose transporters, GLUTs 1–5, that mediate Na^+-independent facilitated diffusion of glucose into cells. Insulin stimulates glucose transport by promoting translocation of intracellular vesicles that contain the GLUT4 and GLUT1 glucose transporters to the plasma membrane (Figure 60–2). The transporters return to the intracellular pool on removal of insulin.

REGULATION OF GLUCOSE METABOLISM The facilitated diffusion of glucose into cells down a concentration gradient is ensured by glucose phosphorylation. The conversion of glucose to glucose-6-phosphate (G-6-P) is accomplished by one of a family of hexokinases. Hexokinase IV, or *glucokinase,* is coexpressed with GLUT2 in liver and pancreatic β cells and is regulated by insulin. Hexokinase II is found in association with GLUT4 in skeletal and cardiac muscle and in adipose tissue, and also is regulated transcriptionally by insulin.

G-6-P is a branch-point substrate that can enter several pathways. Following isomerization to G-1-P, G-6-P can be stored as glycogen (insulin enhances the activity of glycogen synthase); G-6-P can enter the glycolytic pathway (leading to ATP production); and G-6-P can also enter the pentose phosphate pathway (providing NADPH). Effects of insulin on cellular metabolic enzymes are myriad and generally are mediated by modulating activities of protein kinases and phosphoprotein phosphatases. Figure 60–2 depicts the signaling events following the binding of insulin to its membrane receptor.

REGULATION OF GENE TRANSCRIPTION A major action of insulin is the regulation of transcription of more than 100 specific genes. Insulin inhibits the transcription of phosphoenolpyruvate carboxykinase, contributing to insulin's inhibition of gluconeogenesis; this effect of insulin may explain why the liver overproduces glucose in the insulin-resistant state that is characteristic of type 2 DM.

THE INSULIN RECEPTOR Insulin initiates its actions by binding to its cell-surface receptor. Insulin receptors are present in virtually all cells, including not only the classic targets for insulin action (*i.e.,* liver, muscle, and fat) but also nonclassic targets such as circulating blood cells, neurons, and gonadal cells.

The insulin receptor is a transmembrane glycoprotein composed of two 135 kDa α subunits and two 95 kDa β subunits; the subunits are linked by disulfide bonds to form a β-α-α-β heterotetramer (Figure 60–2). Both subunits are derived from a single-chain precursor molecule that contains the entire sequence of the α and β subunits separated by a processing site consisting of four basic amino acid residues. The α subunits are entirely extracellular and contain the insulin-binding domain, whereas the β subunits are transmembrane proteins that possess tyrosine protein kinase activity. After insulin is bound, receptors aggregate and are internalized rapidly. Since bivalent (but not monovalent) anti-insulin receptor antibodies cross-link adjacent receptors and mimic the actions of insulin, it has been suggested that receptor dimerization is essential for signal transduction. After internalization, the receptor may be degraded or recycled back to the cell surface.

TYROSINE PHOSPHORYLATION AND THE INSULIN ACTION CASCADE
Receptors for insulin and IGF-1 belong to the family of receptor tyrosine kinases, and tyrosine kinase activity is essential for insulin signaling (Figure 60–2). The activated receptors undergo autophosphorylation, which activates their tyrosine kinase activity toward other substrates, principally the four insulin receptor substrates IRS-1, 2, 3, and 4 and Shc Tyrosine phosphorylated IRS proteins recruit signaling cascades via the interaction of SH2 domains with phosphotyrosines, recruiting such proteins as SHP2, Grb2, and SOS and resulting in the activation of MAP kinases and PI3K, which transduce many of insulin's cellular effects. The IGF-1 receptor resembles the insulin receptor and uses similar signaling pathways; furthermore, the two receptors bind each other's ligand, albeit with lower affinity. In addition, IGF-1 and insulin-receptor heterodimers can combine to form hybrid heterotetramers.

Diabetes Mellitus and the Physiological Effects of Insulin

DM consists of a group of disorders characterized by hyperglycemia; altered metabolism of lipids, carbohydrates, and proteins; and an increased risk of complications from vascular disease. Most patients can be classified clinically as having either type 1 or type 2 DM. The American Diabetes Association (ADA) criteria for the diagnosis of DM include symptoms (*e.g.*, polyuria, polydipsia, and unexplained weight loss) and a random plasma glucose concentration of greater than 200 mg/dL (11.1 mM), a fasting plasma glucose concentration of greater than 126 mL/dL (7 mM), or a plasma glucose concentration of greater than 200 mg/dL (11 mM) 2 hours after the ingestion of an oral glucose load.

The incidence of diabetes varies widely throughout the world. In the U.S., 5–10% of all diabetic patients have type 1 DM, with an incidence of 18/100,000 inhabitants/year. The vast majority of diabetic patients (~90% in the U.S.) have type 2 DM. Incidence rates of type 2 DM increase with age, with a mean rate of about 440/100,000/year by the sixth decade in males in the U.S.

Both environmental and genetic components affect the risk of developing DM. These factors are more clearly defined for type 2 DM. Obesity is a major risk factor, and 80–90% of type 2 DM subjects in the U.S. are obese. Studies also support a strong genetic basis for type 2 DM. In a small subset of patients, the genetic basis for type 2 DM is clearly established. Mutations in glucokinase cause the autosomal dominant disorder MODY2; these patients have an increased glycemic threshold for insulin release that results in persistent mild hyperglycemia. Other single-gene mutations cause the other types of MODY, including those affecting pancreatic transcription factors.

For type 1 DM, the concordance rate for identical twins is only 25–50% and environmental influences must have an important role. Type 1 DM involves an autoimmune attack on the pancreatic β cells. Antibodies to islet cell antigens are detected in up to 80% of patients with type 1 DM shortly after diagnosis or even prior to the onset of clinical disease. Type 1 DM is associated with specific human leukocyte antigen (HLA) alleles, especially at the B and DR loci, and the HLA complex is known to play critical roles in the immune response. However, the trigger for the immune response remains unknown. In about 10% of new cases of type 1 DM, there is no evidence of autoimmune insulitis. The ADA and the World Health Organization (WHO) therefore subdivide this disease into autoimmune (1A) and idiopathic (1B) subtypes.

Whatever the causes, the final result in type 1 DM is an extensive and selective loss of pancreatic β cells and a state of absolute insulin deficiency. In type 2 DM, β-cell mass is generally reduced by ~50%. At diagnosis, virtually all persons with type 2 DM have a profound defect in first-phase insulin secretion in response to an intravenous glucose challenge, although some of these β-cell abnormalities may be secondary to desensitization by chronic hyperglycemia.

Virtually all forms of DM result from a decrease in the circulating concentration of insulin (insulin deficiency) and a decrease in the response of peripheral tissues to insulin (insulin resistance). These abnormalities lead to alterations in the metabolism of carbohydrates, lipids, ketones, and amino acids; the central feature of the syndrome is hyperglycemia.

Insulin lowers the concentration of glucose in blood by inhibiting hepatic glucose production and by stimulating the uptake and metabolism of glucose by muscle and adipose tissue (Table 60–1). These two important effects occur at different concentrations of insulin. Glucose production is inhibited half maximally by an insulin concentration of about 20 μunits/mL, whereas glucose utilization is stimulated half maximally at about 50 μunits/mL.

Table 60–1

Hypoglycemic Actions of Insulin

Liver	Muscle	Adipose Tissue
Inhibits hepatic glucose production (decreases gluconeogenesis and glycogenolysis)	Stimulates glucose uptake	Stimulates glucose uptake (amount is small compared to muscle)
Stimulates hepatic glucose uptake	Inhibits flow of gluconeogenic precursors to the liver (*e.g.*, alanine, lactate, and pyruvate)	Inhibits flow of gluconeogenic precursor to liver (glycerol) and reduces energy substrate for hepatic gluconeogenesis (nonesterfied fatty acids)

In both types of diabetes, glucagon (elevated in untreated patients) opposes the hepatic effects of insulin by stimulating glycogenolysis and gluconeogenesis but has relatively little effect on peripheral glucose utilization. Thus, in the diabetic patient (depressed insulin signaling and hyperglucagonemia) there is increased hepatic glucose production, decreased peripheral glucose uptake, and decreased conversion of glucose to glycogen in the liver.

Alterations in insulin and glucagon secretion also profoundly affect lipid, ketone, and protein metabolism. At concentrations below those needed to stimulate glucose uptake, insulin inhibits hormone-sensitive lipase in adipocytes and inhibits the hydrolysis of triglyceride stores. This counteracts the lipolytic action of catecholamines, cortisol, and growth hormone and reduces the concentrations of glycerol (a substrate for gluconeogenesis) and free fatty acids (a substrate for production of ketone bodies and a necessary fuel for gluconeogenesis). These actions of insulin are deficient in DM, leading to increased gluconeogenesis and ketogenesis.

The liver produces ketone bodies by oxidizing free fatty acids to acetyl CoA, which then is converted to acetoacetate and β-hydroxybutyrate. The initial step in fatty acid oxidation is transport of the fatty acids into the mitochondria. The essential enzyme in this process, acylcarnitine transferase, is inhibited by intramitochondrial malonyl CoA, one of the products of fatty acid synthesis. Normally, insulin inhibits lipolysis, stimulates fatty acid synthesis (thereby increasing the concentration of malonyl CoA), and decreases the hepatic concentration of carnitine; these factors all decrease the production of ketone bodies. Conversely, glucagon stimulates ketone body production by increasing fatty acid oxidation and decreasing concentrations of malonyl CoA. In patients with type 1 DM, insulin deficiency and glucagon in excess provide a hormonal milieu that favors ketogenesis and may lead to ketoacidosis.

Insulin also enhances the transcription of lipoprotein lipase in the capillary endothelium. Thus, hypertriglyceridemia and hypercholesterolemia often occur in untreated or undertreated diabetics. In addition, insulin deficiency may be associated with increased production of VLDL.

The key role of insulin in protein metabolism usually is evident only in diabetic patients with persistently poor glycemic control. Insulin stimulates amino acid uptake and protein synthesis and inhibits protein degradation in muscle and other tissues. The increased conversion of amino acids to glucose also results in increased production and excretion of urea and ammonia. In addition, there are increased circulating concentrations of branched-chain amino acids as a result of increased proteolysis, decreased protein synthesis, and increased release of branched-chain amino acids from the liver.

A nearly pathognomonic feature of diabetes mellitus is thickening of the capillary basement membrane. The progressive narrowing of the vessel lumina causes inadequate perfusion of certain organs, contributing to the major complications of diabetes, including premature atherosclerosis, intercapillary glomerulosclerosis, retinopathy, neuropathy, and ulceration and gangrene of the extremities.

It was hypothesized that the factor responsible for the development of most complications of DM is the prolonged exposure of tissues to elevated concentrations of glucose. The results from the Diabetes Control and Complications Trial (DCCT) definitively demonstrated that most diabetic complications arise from prolonged exposure of tissue to elevated glucose concentrations. The DCCT demonstrated unequivocally that improving day-to-day glycemic control in type 1 DM patients can dramatically decrease diabetic complications. A follow-up study showed that intensive therapy reduced cardiovascular adverse events and that the reduction in the risk of progressive retinopathy and nephropathy persists for at least 4 years, even if tight glycemic control is not maintained. Rigorous control of blood glucose provides similar benefits to patients with type 2 diabetes.

The toxic effects of hyperglycemia may relate to the formation and accumulation of products such as glycosylated proteins and lipids. Advanced glycosylation end-products (AGEs) signal through receptors for AGEs (RAGEs) to alter oxidative stress, inflammatory injury, and a variety of other responses that may contribute to the sequelae of diabetes. In the face of elevated blood glucose, hemoglobin (Hb) becomes glycosylated on its amino terminal valine, forming Hb A_{1c}, the concentration of which reflects the severity and duration of the hyperglycemic state and may be assessed clinically.

A serious complication of intensive therapy is an increased incidence of severe hypoglycemia. Therefore, ADA guidelines for treatment include a contraindication for implementing tight metabolic control in infants younger than 2 years old and an extreme caution in children of 2–7 years of age in whom hypoglycemia may impair brain development. Older patients with significant arteriosclerosis also may be vulnerable to permanent injury from hypoglycemia. Current therapies for type 1 and type 2 DM therefore aim for tight metabolic control, always keeping in mind the risks of severe hypoglycemia in individual patients.

Insulin Therapy

Insulin is the mainstay for treatment of virtually all type 1 DM and many type 2 DM patients. When necessary, insulin may be administered intravenously or intramuscularly; however, long-term treatment relies predominantly on subcutaneous injections of the hormone. Subcutaneous administration of insulin differs from physiological secretion of insulin in at least two major ways: The kinetics do not reproduce the normal rapid rise and decline of insulin secretion in response to ingestion of nutrients, and the insulin diffuses into the peripheral circulation instead of being released into the portal circulation; the direct effect of secreted insulin on hepatic metabolic processes thus is eliminated. Nonetheless, when such treatment is performed carefully, considerable success is achieved.

Insulin preparations are classified according to their duration of action into rapid, short, intermediate, and long acting and by their species of origin—human or porcine. Human insulin (HUMULIN, NOVOLIN) is widely available, as is porcine insulin, which differs from human insulin by one amino acid (alanine instead of threonine in position B30. Human insulin, produced using recombinant DNA technology, is more water soluble than porcine insulin owing to the presence of an extra hydroxyl group. The vast majority of preparations now are supplied at neutral pH, which improves stability and permits storage for several days at room temperature.

UNITAGE

Insulin doses are expressed in units. One unit of insulin equals the amount required to reduce the concentration of blood glucose in a fasting rabbit to 45 mg/dL. The current international standard is a mixture of bovine and porcine insulins and contains 24 units/mg. Homogeneous preparations of human insulin contain between 25 and 30 units/mg. Almost all commercial preparations of insulin are supplied at a concentration of 100 units/mL, which is about 3.6 mg insulin per milliliter (0.6 mM). Insulin also is available in a more concentrated solution (500 units/mL) for patients who are resistant to the hormone.

CLASSIFICATION OF INSULINS

Short- and Rapid-Acting Insulins

Traditionally, the short-acting insulins were solutions of regular, crystalline zinc insulin (insulin injection) dissolved in a buffer at neutral pH. These preparations have a rapid onset of action but short duration (Table 60–2). More recently, modified recombinant insulins have been introduced with even more rapid onset and shorter duration of action; they therefore are termed "rapid-acting" insulins.

Table 60–2

Properties of Currently Available Insulin Preparations

Type	Appearance	Added Protein	Zinc Content, mg/100 units	Buffer*	Action, Hours† Onset	Peak	Duration
Rapid/Short							
Regular soluble (crystalline)	Clear	None	0.01–0.04	None	0.5–0.7	1.5–4	5–8
Lispro	Clear	None	0.02	Phosphate	0.25	0.5–1.5	2–5
Aspart	Clear	None	0.0196	Phosphate	0.25	0.6–0.8	3–5
Glulisine	Clear	None	None	None	—	0.5–1.5	1–2.5
Intermediate							
NPH (isophane)	Cloudy	Protamine	0.016–0.04	Phosphate	1–2	6–12	18–24
Lente	Cloudy	None	0.2–0.25	Acetate	1–2	6–12	18–24
Slow							
Ultralente	Cloudy	None	0.2–0.25	Acetate	4–6	16–18	20–36
Protamine zinc	Cloudy	Protamine	0.2–0.25	Phosphate	4–6	14–20	24–36
Glargine	Clear	None	0.03	None	2–5	5–24	18–24
Detemir	Clear	None	0.065	Phosphate	1–2	4–14	6–24

*Most insulin preparations are supplied at pH 7.2–7.4. Glargine and Detemir are supplied at a pH of 4.0.
†These are approximate figures. There is considerable variation from patient to patient and from time to time in a given patient.

Short-acting (i.e., regular) insulin usually is injected subcutaneously 30–45 minutes before meal, and also may be given intravenously or intramuscularly. After intravenous injection, the blood glucose concentration diminishes swiftly, usually reaching a nadir in 20–30 minutes. In the absence of a sustained infusion of insulin, the hormone is cleared rapidly, and counter-regulatory hormones (e.g., glucagon, epinephrine, cortisol, and growth hormone) restore plasma glucose to baseline in 2–3 hours. In the absence of a normal counter-regulatory response (e.g., in diabetic patients with autonomic neuropathy), plasma glucose will remain suppressed for many hours following an insulin bolus of 0.15 units/kg because the cellular actions of insulin are prolonged far beyond its clearance from plasma.

Regular insulin typically is given subcutaneously, often in combination with an intermediate- or long-acting preparation. Special buffered formulations of regular insulin are available for use in subcutaneous infusion pumps that are less likely to crystallize in the tubing during the slow infusion associated with this type of therapy.

Native insulin in regular insulin forms hexamers that slow absorption and reduce postprandial peaks of subcutaneously injected insulin. These pharmacokinetics stimulated the development of rapid-acting insulin analogs that retain a monomeric or dimeric configuration. Several such compounds are now available for clinical use. These analogs are absorbed three times more rapidly from subcutaneous sites than is human insulin. Consequently, there is a more rapid increase in plasma insulin concentrations and an earlier hypoglycemic response. Injection of the analogs 15 minutes before a meal affords glycemic control similar to that from an injection of human insulin given 30 minutes before the meal.

Owing to their fast onset, the rapid-acting insulin analogs all may be injected immediately before or after a meal. Factors such as gastroparesis or anorexia may cause many diabetic patients to eat fewer calories than anticipated. Due to their pharmacokinetics, the rapid-acting analogs may be administered postprandially based on the amount of food actually consumed, possibly providing smoother glycemic control and decreasing the risk of hypoglycemia.

Insulin lispro (HUMALOG) differs from human insulin only at positions B28 and B29, which are reversed to match the sequence in IGF-1, which does not self-associate. Relative to regular insulin, the prevalence of hypoglycemia is reduced by 20–30% with insulin lispro, and glucose control, as assessed by Hb A$_{1c}$, is modestly but significantly improved (0.3–0.5%).

Insulin aspart (NOVOLOG) is formed by the replacement of proline at B28 with aspartic acid. Comparison of single subcutaneous doses of insulin aspart and insulin lispro in patients with type 1 DM revealed similar plasma insulin profiles. In clinical trials, insulin aspart and insulin lispro have had similar effects, with lower rates of nocturnal hypoglycemia as compared with regular insulin.

A third rapid-acting insulin analog, insulin glulisine (APIDRA), is available for use in the U.S. In this compound, glutamic acid replaces lysine at B29, and lysine replaces asparagine at B23, again reducing self-association and permitting rapid dissociation into active monomers with kinetics similar to insulin aspart and lispro. Insulin glulisine also is FDA-approved for continuous subcutaneous insulin infusion (CSII) pump use.

The FDA recently approved inhaled insulin for use in patients with type 1 or type 2 DM. This powdered formulation of recombinant human insulin (EXUBERA) is inhaled through the mouth before eating using a special inhalation device. Although the efficacy of inhaled insulin is more clearly documented for patients with type 2 DM, approval also was given for use in subjects with type 1 DM. Some concerns have been expressed about the use of the inhaled formulation in patients with chronic obstructive pulmonary disease and asthma, and additional studies are ongoing in these settings. The inhaled insulin preparation was associated with high titers of anti-insulin antibodies, but this has not been shown to affect the pharmacokinetics of the drug or to impair its glucose-lowering activity.

Intermediate-Acting Insulins

These insulins are formulated to dissolve more gradually when administered subcutaneously; thus, their durations of action are longer. The two preparations used most frequently are neutral protamine Hagedorn (NPH) insulin (isophane insulin suspension) *and* lente insulin (insulin zinc suspension). *NPH insulin is a suspension of insulin in a complex with zinc and protamine in a phosphate buffer. Lente insulin is a mixture of crystallized (ultralente) and amorphous (semilente) insulins in an acetate buffer, which minimizes the solubility of insulin. The pharmacokinetic properties of human intermediate-acting insulins are slightly different from those of porcine preparations. Human insulin has a more rapid onset and shorter duration of action than does porcine insulin. This difference may create a problem with optimal timing for evening therapy; human insulin preparations taken before dinner may not have a sufficient duration of action to prevent hyperglycemia by morning. There is no evidence that lente or NPH insulin has different pharmacodynamic effects when used in combination with regular (soluble) insulin in a twice-daily regimen. Intermediate-acting insulins usually are given either once a day before breakfast or twice a day.*

In patients with type 2 DM, intermediate-acting insulin given at bedtime may help normalize fasting blood glucose. When lente insulin is mixed with regular insulin, some of the regular insulin may form a complex with the protamine or Zn^{2+} after several hours, which may slow absorption of the short-acting insulin. NPH insulin does not retard the action of regular insulin when the two are mixed vigorously by the patient or when they are supplied as a mixture.

Long-Acting Insulins

Ultralente insulin (extended insulin zinc suspension) is a long-acting insulin that has a slower onset and a prolonged peak of action. This insulin has been advocated to provide a low basal concentration of insulin throughout the day. Doses given once or twice daily are adjusted according to the fasting blood glucose concentration. The long $t_{1/2}$ of ultralente insulin makes it difficult to determine the optimal dosage because several days of treatment are required before a steady-state concentration of circulating insulin is achieved. Protamine zinc insulin is no longer available in the U.S. Preparations of insulin that are available for clinical use in the U.S. are shown in Table 60–3.

The pharmacokinetic limitations of ultralente insulin have prompted efforts to develop insulin analogs that do not have significant peaks in their action. Insulin glargine (LANTUS) is a long-acting analog of human insulin that has two arginine residues added to the C terminus of the B chain, and glycine replaces an asparagine molecule in position A21 on the A chain. Glargine is a clear solution with a pH of 4.0 that stabilizes the insulin hexamer and results in a prolonged and predictable absorption from subcutaneous tissues. Owing to its acidic pH, insulin glargine cannot be mixed with currently available short-acting or rapid-acting insulin preparations that are formulated at neutral pH. In clinical studies, insulin glargine results in less hypoglycemia, has a sustained "peakless" absorption profile, and provides a better once-daily 24-hour insulin coverage than ultralente or NPH insulin. Glargine may be administered at any time during the day with equivalent efficacy and no difference in the frequency of hypoglycemic episodes. Glargine does not accumulate after several injections.

Insulin glargine can be used in combination with various oral antihyperglycemic agents (see below) to effectively lower plasma glucose levels. Combination of insulin glargine with sulfonylureas and/or metformin can reduce both fasting (basal) and postprandial glucose levels. The use of a long-acting basal insulin alone will not control postprandial glucose elevations in insulin-deficient type 1 or type 2 DM. Glargine has been shown in clinical studies to normalize fasting glucose levels following once-daily administration in patients with type 2 DM. Rarely, the glargine dose may need to be divided in very lean, insulin-sensitive type 1 DM patients to achieve good fasting glucose levels. Unlike traditional insulin preparations, the site of administration does not influence the time–action profile of glargine. Similarly, exercise does not influence glargine's unique absorption kinetics, even when the insulin is injected into a working limb.

Table 60–3

Insulin Preparations Available in the United States

Type	Human	Porcine
Rapid/Short		
Insulin injection (regular)	R, C	P, S
Lispro	R	—
Aspart	R	—
Glulisine	R	—
Intermediate		
Isophane insulin suspension (NPH)	R	P
Insulin zinc suspension (lente)	R	P
Slow		
Extended insulin zinc suspension (ultralente)	R	—
Insulin glargine	R	—
Insulin detemir	R	—
Mixtures		
70% NPH/30% Regular	R	—
50% NPH/50% Regular	R	—
75% Lispro Protamine/25% Lispro	R	—
70% Aspart Protamine/30% Aspart	R	—

ABBREVIATIONS: S, standard insulins; P, purified insulins; C, concentrated insulin; R, recombinant or semisynthetic human insulins.

Another approach to prolong the action of soluble insulin analogs is to add a saturated fatty acid to the ε amino group of LysB29, yielding a myristoylated insulin called insulin detemir. *When insulin detemir is injected subcutaneously, it binds to albumin via its fatty acid chain. When administered twice a day, insulin detemir has a smoother time–action profile and a reduced prevalence of hypoglycemia as compared with NPH insulin. Insulin determir (LEVEMIR) is FDA-approved for use in adult patients with type 1 or type 2 DM who require long-acting insulin. It should not be mixed with any other insulin preparations.*

INDICATIONS AND GOALS FOR THERAPY Subcutaneous administration of insulin is the primary treatment for all patients with type 1 DM, for patients with type 2 DM that is not controlled adequately by diet and/or oral hypoglycemic agents, and for patients with postpancrea-tectomy diabetes or gestational diabetes. In addition, insulin is critical for the management of diabetic ketoacidosis, and it has an important role in the treatment of hyperglycemic, nonketotic coma and in the perioperative management of both type 1 and type 2 DM. In all cases, the goal is to normalize not only blood glucose but also all aspects of metabolism; the latter is difficult to achieve. Optimal treatment requires a coordinated approach to diet, exercise, and insulin administration.

In many patients, near-normoglycemia can be attained with multiple daily doses of insulin or with infusion pump therapy. The goal is a fasting blood glucose concentration of between 90 and 120 mg/dL (5–6.7 mM) and a 2-hour postprandial value below 150 mg/dL (8.3 mM). Goal Hb A_{1c} values should be below 7% (below 6.5% for some experts). In patients with defective counter-regulatory responses, it may be necessary to accept higher fasting [e.g., 140 mg/dL (7.8 mM)] and 2-hour postprandial [e.g., 200–250 mg/dL (11.1–13.9 mM)] blood glucose concentrations.

DAILY REQUIREMENTS

Insulin production by a normal, thin, healthy person is between 18 and 40 units/day (~0.2–0.5 units/kg/day). About half this amount is secreted in the basal state and about half in response to meals. Thus, basal secretion is about 0.5–1 units/h; after an oral glucose load, insulin secretion may increase to 6 units/h. In obese and insulin-resistant individuals, insulin secretion may be increased fourfold or more.

In type 1 DM patients, the average dose of insulin is usually 0.6–0.7 units/kg/day, with a range of 0.2–1 units/kg/day. Obese patients generally require more (about 2 units/kg/day) because of resistance of peripheral tissues to insulin. As in nondiabetics, the daily requirement for insulin can be divided into basal and postprandial needs. The basal dose (usually 40–60% of the total daily dose) suppresses lipolysis, proteolysis, and hepatic glucose production. The dose necessary for disposition of nutrients after meals usually is given before meals. Insulin often has been adminis-tered as a single daily dose of intermediate-acting insulin, alone or in combination with regular insulin. This rarely achieves true euglycemia; since hyperglycemia is the major determinant of long-term diabetic complications, more complex regimens that include combinations of intermediate- or long-acting insulins with regular insulin are used to reach this goal.

Several commonly used dosage regimens that include mixtures of insulin given in two or three daily injections are depicted in Figure 60–3. The most frequently used is the so-called split-mixed regimen involving prebreakfast and presupper injections of a mixture of regular and intermediate-acting insulins (Figure 60–3A). When the presupper NPH or lente insulin is not sufficient to con-trol hyperglycemia throughout the night, the evening dose may be divided into a presupper dose of regular insulin followed by NPH or lente insulin at bedtime (Figure 60–3B). Both normal and diabetic individuals have an increased requirement for insulin in the early morning; this dawn phenomenon *makes the kinetics and timing of the evening insulin dose extremely important.*

A regimen that is gaining widespread use involves multiple daily injections consisting of basal administration of long-acting insulin (e.g., insulin glargine or detemir) either before breakfast or at bedtime and prandial injections of a short- or rapid-acting insulin (Figure 60–3C). This method, called basal/bolus, *is very similar to the pattern of insulin administration achieved with a subcutaneous infusion pump (Figure 60–3E). Following the successful demonstration that inten-sive glycemic control can reduce the risk of complications in patients with type 2 DM, there has been increased interest in using insulin earlier in the treatment of these patients. Data indicate that 50% of relative β-cell insulin secretory capacity is lost for every 6 years of type 2 DM. This pro-gressive insulin deficiency as type 2 DM progresses makes it increasingly difficult to achieve glycemic control with oral antihyperglycemic agents. An option in this setting is to introduce basal-acting insulin in combination with oral hypoglycemic agents. The exact combination of therapies should be guided by the β-cell secretory reserve in each patient. Thus, in an individual with some exogenous insulin secretory capacity (i.e., a measurable circulating C peptide), combining an oral insulin secretagogue (see below) with basal insulin may provide smooth and efficient glycemic*

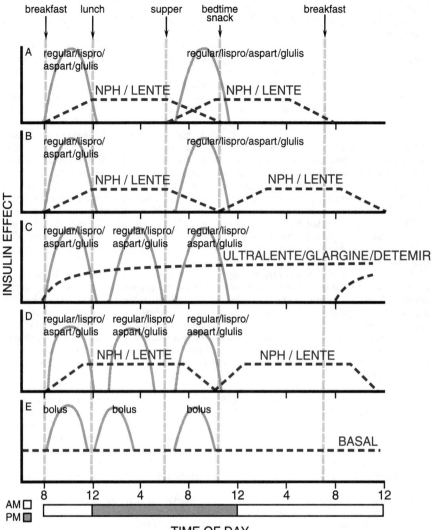

FIGURE 60–3 *Common multidose insulin regimens.* **A.** Typical split-mixed regimen consisting of twice-daily injections of a mixture of regular (regular/lispro/aspart/glulis) and intermediate-acting (NPH or lente) insulin. **B.** A variation in which the evening dose of intermediate-acting insulin is delayed until bedtime to increase the amount of insulin available the next morning. **C.** A regimen that incorporates ultralente or glargine insulin. **D.** A variation that includes premeal short-acting insulin with intermediate-acting insulin at breakfast and bedtime. **E.** Patterns of insulin administration with a regimen of continuous subcutaneous insulin infusion.

control. The addition of a second oral agent, such as an insulin sensitizer (see below), either alone or in combination with an oral insulin secretagogue, also may provide good therapeutic results. This combination allows the oral agents to provide postprandial glycemic control while the basal insulin provides the foundation for normalizing fasting or "basal" glucose levels. In all patients, careful monitoring of therapeutic end points directs the insulin dose used. This approach is facilitated by the use of home glucose monitors and measurements of Hb A_{1c}.

FACTORS THAT AFFECT INSULIN ABSORPTION The degree of control of plasma glucose may be modified by changes in insulin absorption, factors that alter insulin action, diet, exercise, and other factors. Factors that determine the rate of absorption of insulin after subcutaneous administration include the site of injection, the type of insulin, subcutaneous blood flow, smoking, regional muscular activity at the site of the injection, and the volume and concentration of the injected insulin.

Insulin usually is injected subcutaneously in the abdomen, buttock, anterior thigh, or dorsal arm. Rotation of insulin injection sites traditionally has been advocated to avoid lipohypertrophy or lipoatrophy. The abdomen is the preferred site of injection in the morning because insulin is absorbed more rapidly from that site than from the arm. If the patient refuses to inject into the abdomen, it is preferable to select a consistent injection site for each component of insulin treatment (*e.g.,* prebreakfast dose into the thigh, evening dose into the arm).

Increased subcutaneous blood flow (brought about by hot baths or exercise) increases the rate of insulin absorption. In the upright posture, subcutaneous blood flow diminishes considerably in the legs and to a lesser extent in the abdominal wall. An altered volume or concentration of injected insulin affects the rate of absorption and the duration of action. When regular insulin is mixed with lente or ultralente insulin, some of the regular insulin becomes modified, causing a partial loss of the short-acting component. Injections of mixtures of insulin preparations thus should be made without delay. There is less delay in absorption of regular insulin when it is mixed with NPH insulin. Stable, mixed combinations of NPH and regular insulin in proportions of 50:50, 60:40, 70:30, and 80:20, respectively, are available commercially; only the 70:30 and 50:50 combinations are available in the U.S. Combinations of lispro protamine-Lispro (75/25, HUMALOG MIX), aspart protamine-aspart (70/30, NOVOLOG MIX), and glusine are also available in the U.S. (Table 60–3).

Subcutaneous insulin administration may result in anti-insulin IgG antibody formation. In most patients, circulating anti-insulin antibodies do not alter the pharmacokinetics of the injected hormone. Rarely, the pharmacokinetics of the insulin preparations can be altered, potentially leading to increased postprandial hyperglycemia (owing to decreased action of regular insulin) but nighttime hypoglycemia (owing to the prolonged action of intermediate insulin). Because of concerns that IgG anti-insulin antibodies could cross the placenta and cause fetal hyperglycemia by neutralizing fetal insulin or cause fetal or neonatal hypoglycemia due to unpredictable release of insulin from antigen-antibody complexes, it is recommended that only human insulin be used during pregnancy.

CONTINUOUS SUBCUTANEOUS INSULIN INFUSION A number of pumps are available for continuous *subcutaneous* insulin *infusion* (CSII) therapy. CSII, or "pump," therapy is not suitable for all patients because it demands considerable attention, especially during the initial phases of treatment. For patients interested in intensive insulin therapy, a pump may be an attractive alternative to several daily injections. Most pumps provide a constant basal infusion of insulin and have the option of different infusion rates during the day and night to help avoid the dawn phenomenon and bolus injections that are programmed according to the size and nature of a meal.

Pump therapy presents some unique problems. Since all the insulin used is short-acting or rapid-acting and there is a minimal amount of insulin in the subcutaneous pool at any given time, insulin deficiency and ketoacidosis may develop rapidly if therapy is interrupted accidentally. Although pumps have warning devices that detect changes in line pressure, mechanical problems may occur. There also is a possibility of subcutaneous abscesses and cellulitis. Patient selection is extremely important for success with pump therapy. Offsetting these potential problems, pump therapy can produce a more physiological profile of insulin replacement that apparently decreases the risk of hypoglycemia.

ADVERSE REACTIONS

Hypoglycemia Hypoglycemia is the most common adverse reaction to insulin and may result from an inappropriately large dose, from a mismatch between the time of peak delivery of insulin and food intake, or from additional factors that increase insulin sensitivity (*e.g.,* adrenal or pituitary insufficiency) or that increase insulin-independent glucose uptake (*e.g.,* exercise). More vigorous efforts to achieve euglycemia are accompanied by more frequent episodes of hypoglycemia. In the DCCT, the incidence of severe hypoglycemic reactions was tripled in the intensive therapy group. Hypoglycemia is the major risk that always must be weighed against benefits of intensive therapy.

There is a hierarchy of physiological responses to hypoglycemia. Endogenous insulin secretion is reduced at a plasma glucose of about 70 mg/dL (3.9 mM); thereafter, counter-regulatory hormones—epinephrine, glucagon, growth hormone, cortisol, and norepinephrine—are released. Autonomic symptoms of hypoglycemia are first discerned at a plasma glucose level of 60–80 mg/dL (3.3–4.4 mM) and include sweating, hunger, paresthesias, palpitations, tremor, and anxiety. Difficulty in concentrating, confusion, weakness, drowsiness, a feeling of warmth, dizziness, blurred vision, and loss of consciousness (*i.e., the neuroglycopenic symptoms*) usually occur at lower plasma glucose levels than do autonomic symptoms.

Glucagon and epinephrine are the predominant counter-regulatory hormones in acute hypoglycemia in normal subjects and in newly diagnosed type 1 DM patient. In patients with type 1 DM of longer duration, the glucagon response to hypoglycemia becomes deficient, but epinephrine maintains effective glucose counter-regulation. If this epinephrine response becomes deficient, as in diabetics of long duration who have autonomic neuropathy, the incidence of severe hypoglycemia increases. The absence of both glucagon and epinephrine can lead to prolonged hypoglycemia, particularly during the night, and can cause convulsions and coma.

In addition to autonomic neuropathy, several related syndromes of defective counter-regulation in intensively treated type 1 DM patients contribute to their increased incidence of severe hypoglycemia. These include hypoglycemic unawareness, altered thresholds for release of counter-regulatory hormones, and deficient secretion of counter-regulatory hormones.

With the ready availability of home glucose monitoring, hypoglycemia can be documented in most patients with suggestive symptoms. Nocturnal hypoglycemia is suggested by a history of morning headaches, night sweats, or symptoms of hypothermia; if confirmed, the predinner or bedtime insulin dose should be decreased.

All diabetic patients who receive insulin should be aware of the symptoms of hypoglycemia, carry some form of easily ingested glucose, and carry an identification card or bracelet containing pertinent medical information. When possible, patients who suspect that they are experiencing hypoglycemia should document the glucose concentration with a measurement. Mild-to-moderate hypoglycemia may be treated simply by ingestion of glucose. When hypoglycemia is severe, it should be treated with intravenous glucose or injection of glucagon (see below).

Insulin Allergy and Resistance

The most frequent allergic manifestations are IgE-mediated local cutaneous reactions, although patients rarely may develop life-threatening systemic responses or insulin resistance owing to IgG antibodies. Attempts should be made to identify the underlying cause of the hypersensitivity response by measuring insulin-specific IgG and IgE antibodies. Skin testing also is useful, although false-positive results are not uncommon. If patients have allergic reactions to porcine insulin, human insulin should be used. If allergy persists, desensitization may be successful in about 50% of cases. Antihistamines may provide relief in patients with cutaneous reactions, whereas glucocorticoids have been used in patients with resistance to insulin or more severe systemic reactions.

Lipoatrophy and Lipohypertrophy

Atrophy of subcutaneous fat at the site of insulin injection (lipoatrophy) is probably an immune response to insulin, whereas lipohypertrophy (enlargement of subcutaneous fat depots) is ascribed to the lipogenic action of high local concentrations of insulin. Both problems are rare with more purified preparations. However, hypertrophy may occur with human insulin if patients inject themselves repeatedly in the same site. The recommended treatment is to avoid the hypertrophic areas by using other injection sites and to inject insulin into the periphery of the atrophic sites in an attempt to restore the subcutaneous adipose tissue.

Insulin Edema

Edema, abdominal bloating, and blurred vision develop in many diabetic patients with severe hyperglycemia or ketoacidosis that is brought under control with insulin. The edema usually disappears spontaneously within several days to a week and is attributed primarily to renal retention of Na^+.

INSULIN TREATMENT OF KETOACIDOSIS AND OTHER SPECIAL SITUATIONS

Intravenous administration of insulin is used in patients with diabetic ketoacidosis. In this setting, infusion of a relatively low dose of insulin (0.1 units/kg/h) will produce plasma concentrations of insulin of ~100 μunits/mL, level sufficient to inhibit lipolysis and gluconeogenesis completely and to stimulate near-maximal glucose uptake. In most patients with diabetic ketoacidosis, blood glucose concentrations will fall by about 10% per hour; the acidosis corrects more slowly. As treatment proceeds, it often is necessary to administer glucose along with the insulin to prevent hypoglycemia but to allow clearance of all ketones. Patients with nonketotic hyperglycemic coma typically are more sensitive to insulin than are those with ketoacidosis. Appropriate replacement of fluid and electrolytes is an integral part of the therapy in both situations because there is always a major deficit. The key to effective therapy is careful and frequent monitoring of the patient's clinical status, glucose, and electrolytes. A frequent error in the management of such patients is the failure to administer subcutaneous insulin at least 30 minutes before intravenous therapy is discontinued.

Intravenous administration of insulin also is well suited to the treatment of diabetic patients during the perioperative period and during childbirth. Two widely used protocols for intravenous insulin administration are the variable-rate regimen and the glucose–insulin–potassium (GIK) infusion method. Both protocols provide stable plasma glucose, fluid, and electrolyte levels during the operative and postoperative period. Other physicians give patients half their normal daily dose of insulin subcutaneously before the procedure and then maintain glucose concentration by administering 5% dextrose in water. Protocols that rely on intermediate-acting insulin subcutaneously on the morning of an operation with 5% dextrose infusions during surgery to maintain glucose concentrations provide less minute-to-minute control than is possible with intravenous regimens and also may increase the likelihood of hypoglycemia.

DRUG INTERACTIONS AND GLUCOSE METABOLISM

Many drugs can cause hypoglycemia or hyperglycemia or alter the response of diabetic patients to their existing therapeutic regimens. Aside from insulin and oral hypoglycemic drugs, drug-induced hypoglycemia is most often caused by ethanol, β adrenergic receptor antagonists, and salicylates. The primary action of ethanol is to inhibit gluconeogenesis. In diabetics, β adrenergic receptor antagonists pose a risk of hypoglycemia because of their capacity to inhibit catecholamine effects on gluconeogenesis and glycogenolysis. These agents also may mask the autonomic symptoms associated with hypoglycemia (e.g., tremor and palpitations). Salicylates enhance β-cell sensitivity to glucose and potentiate insulin secretion and also have a weak insulin-like action in the periphery. A number of drugs have no direct hypoglycemic action but may potentiate the actions of sulfonylureas (see below).*

An equally large number of drugs may cause hyperglycemia in normal individuals or impair metabolic control in diabetic patients. Many of these agents have direct effects on peripheral tissues that counter the actions of insulin; examples include epinephrine, glucocorticoids, atypical antipsychotic drugs such as clozapine and olanzapine, and drugs used in HIV-1 infection (especially the protease inhibitors). Other drugs cause hyperglycemia by inhibiting insulin secretion directly (e.g., phenytoin, clonidine, and Ca^{2+}-channel blockers) or indirectly via depletion of K$^+$ (diuretics). It is important to be aware of such interactions and to modify treatment regimens for diabetic patients accordingly.*

ORAL HYPOGLYCEMIC AGENTS
Sulfonylureas
CHEMISTRY
The sulfonylureas are divided into two generations whose structural relationships are shown in Table 60–4. All are substituted arylsulfonylureas that differ by substitutions at the para position on the benzene ring (R_1) and at one nitrogen residue of the urea moiety (R_2). The first generation of sulfonylureas includes tolbutamide, acetohexamide, tolazamide, *and* chlorpropamide. *Second generation sulfonylureas include* glyburide (glibenclamide), glipizide, gliclazide, *and* glimepiride.

MECHANISM OF ACTION Sulfonylureas stimulate insulin release from pancreatic β cells. The acute administration of sulfonylureas to type 2 DM patients increases insulin release from the pancreas. In the initial months of sulfonylurea treatment, fasting plasma insulin levels and insulin responses to oral glucose challenge are increased. With chronic administration, circulating insulin levels decline to those that existed before treatment; despite this, reduced plasma glucose levels are maintained, possibly because reduced plasma glucose increases insulin sensitivity of its target tissues and improves the impaired insulin secretion caused by chronic hyperglycemia.

Sulfonylureas bind to the SUR1 subunits and block the ATP-sensitive K$^+$ channel. The drugs thus resemble physiological secretagogues (*e.g.*, glucose, leucine).

Table 60–4

Structural Formulas of the Sulfonylureas

General Formula:

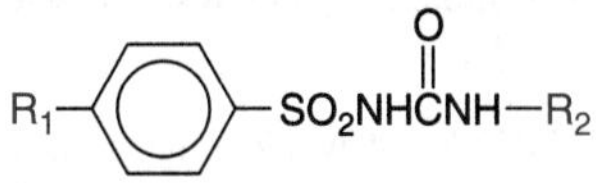

$$R_1 - \bigcirc - SO_2NHCNH - R_2$$

with a carbonyl O above the C

First-Generation Agents	R_1	R_2
Tolbutamide (ORINASE, others)	H_3C-	$-C_4H_9$
Chlorpropamide (DIABINESE, others)	$Cl-$	$-C_3H_7$
Tolazamide (TOLINASE, others)	H_3C-	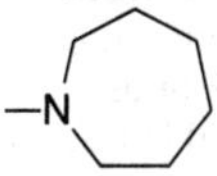 —N (seven-membered ring)
Acetohexamide (DYMELOR, others)	H_3CCO-	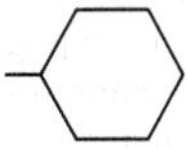 (cyclohexyl ring)

Second-Generation Agents	R_1	R_2
Glyburide (Glibenclamide, MICRONASE, DIABETA, others)	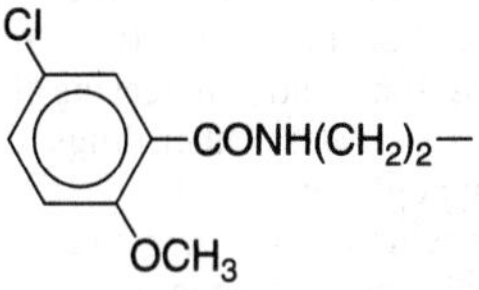 (chlorinated methoxy-benzene with $-CONH(CH_2)_2-$); Cl and OCH_3 substituents	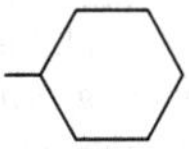 (cyclohexyl ring)
Glipizide (GLUCOTROL, others)	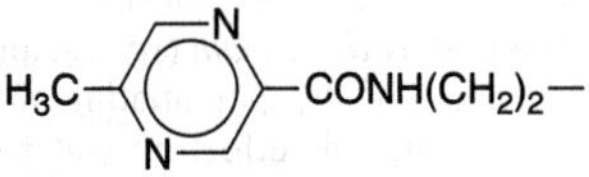 H_3C- (pyrazine ring with two N) $-CONH(CH_2)_2-$	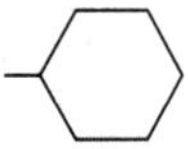 (cyclohexyl ring)
Gliclazide (DIAMICRON, others; unavailable in the U.S.)	H_3C-	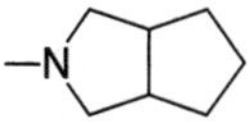 —N (fused bicyclic ring)
Glimepiride (AMARYL)	pyrrolinedione ring: H_3C, H_5C_2 substituents, $N-C$ with carbonyl, $NH-CH_2-CH_2-$	(cyclohexyl)$-CH_3$

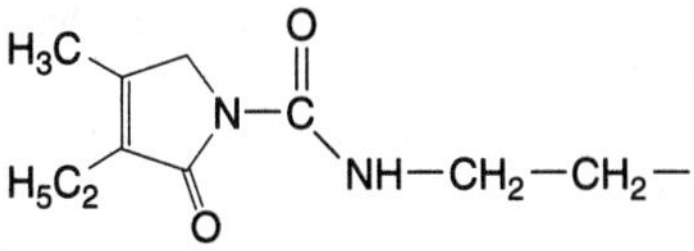

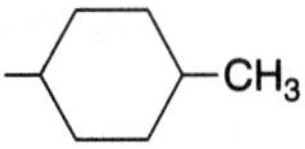

ABSORPTION, FATE, AND EXCRETION The sulfonylureas have similar spectra of activities; thus, their pharmacokinetics are their most distinctive characteristics. All are effectively absorbed from the gastrointestinal tract, although food and hyperglycemia can reduce the absorption. In view of the time required for absorption, sulfonylureas with short half-lives may be more effective when given 30 minutes before eating. Sulfonylureas in plasma are largely (90–99%) bound to protein, especially albumin. The volumes of distribution of most of the sulfonylureas are about 0.2 L/kg.

The first-generation sulfonylureas vary considerably in their half-lives and extents of metabolism. The $t_{1/2}$ of acetohexamide is short, but it is reduced to an active compound whose $t_{1/2}$ is similar to those of tolbutamide and tolazamide (4–7 hours). These drugs may require divided daily doses. Chlorpropamide has a long $t_{1/2}$ (24–48 hours). The second-generation agents are approximately

100 times more potent than are those in the first generation. Although their half-lives are short (3–5 hours), their hypoglycemic effects persist for 12–24 hours, and they often can be administered once daily. All sulfonylureas are metabolized by the liver, and the metabolites are excreted in the urine. Thus, sulfonylureas should be administered with caution to patients with either renal or hepatic insufficiency.

ADVERSE REACTIONS Adverse effects of the sulfonylureas occur in about 4% of patients taking first-generation drugs and perhaps slightly less often with the second-generation agents. Not unexpectedly, sulfonylureas may cause hypoglycemic reactions, including coma, particularly in elderly patients with impaired hepatic or renal function who are taking longer-acting sulfonylureas. Sulfonylureas can be ranked in order of decreasing risk of causing hypoglycemia. With first-generation agents, longer-acting sulfonylureas result in a greater risk of hypoglycemia (*i.e.,* chlorpropamide > tolbutamide). Second-generation sulfonylureas have very differing risks of hypoglycemia despite similar half-lives. Thus, glyburide (glibenclamide) reportedly results in hypoglycemia in up to 20–30% of users, whereas glimepiride results in hypoglycemia in only 2–4% of users. A long-acting version of glipizide also results in a lower hypoglycemia frequency than gliburide, apparently because glucose-dependent inhibition of insulin secretion during hypoglycemia occurs with glimepiride but not with glyburide.

Severe hypoglycemia in the elderly can present as an acute neurological emergency that may mimic a cerebrovascular accident. Thus, it is important to check the plasma glucose level of any elderly patient presenting with acute neurological symptoms. Because of the long $t_{1/2}$ of some sulfonylureas, it may be necessary to treat elderly hypoglycemic patients for 24–48 hours with an intravenous glucose infusion.

Many other drugs may potentiate the effects of the sulfonylureas, particularly the first-generation agents, by inhibiting their metabolism or excretion. Some drugs also displace the sulfonylureas from binding proteins, thereby transiently increasing the free concentration. These include other sulfonamides, *clofibrate,* and salicylates. Other drugs, especially ethanol, may enhance the action of sulfonylureas by causing hypoglycemia.

Other side effects of sulfonylureas include nausea and vomiting, cholestatic jaundice, agranulocytosis, aplastic and hemolytic anemias, generalized hypersensitivity reactions, and rashes. About 10–15% of patients who receive these drugs, particularly chlorpropamide, develop an alcohol-induced flush similar to that caused by *disulfiram* (*see* Chapter 23). Sulfonylureas, especially chlorpropamide, may induce hyponatremia by potentiating the effects of vasopressin on the renal collecting duct (*see* Chapter 29), and this effect on water retention has been used to therapeutic advantage in patients with mild forms of central diabetes insipidus.

THERAPEUTIC USES Sulfonylureas are used to control hyperglycemia in type 2 DM patients who cannot achieve appropriate control with diet alone. In all patients, continued dietary restrictions are essential to maximize the efficacy of the sulfonylureas. Contraindications to the use of these drugs include type 1 DM, pregnancy, lactation, and for the first-generation agents, significant hepatic or renal insufficiency.

Between 50% and 80% of properly selected patients will respond initially to oral hypoglycemic agents. Concentrations of glucose often are lowered sufficiently to relieve symptoms of hyperglycemia but may not reach normal levels. About 5–10% of patients per year who respond initially to sulfonylureas become secondary failures, as defined by unacceptable levels of hyperglycemia. This may occur as a result of a change in drug metabolism, progression of β-cell failure, change in dietary compliance, or misdiagnosis of a patient with slow-onset type 1 DM. Additional oral agent(s) can produce a satisfactory response, but most of these patients eventually will require insulin. Treatment with the sulfonylureas must be guided by the patient's response, which must be monitored frequently.

The usual initial daily dose and maximum effective dose are as follows (initial/maximum): tolbutamide 500 mg/3000 mg; tolazamide 100 mg/1000 mg; chlorpropamide 250 mg/750 mg; glyburide 2.5–5 mg/20 mg; glipizide 5 mg/40 mg (divided when the daily dose >15 mg); gliclazide 40–80 mg/320 mg; glimepiride 0.5 mg/8 mg.

Combinations of insulin and sulfonylureas have been used in some patients with type 1 and type 2 DM. In type 1 DM patients, there is no evidence that glucose control is improved by combination therapy, while some type 2 DM patients have shown significant improvements in metabolic control. A prerequisite for a beneficial effect of combination therapy is residual β-cell activity; a short duration of diabetes also may predict a good response.

Repaglinide

Repaglinide (PRANDIN) is an oral insulin secretagogue of the meglitinide class.

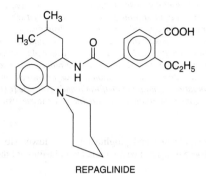

REPAGLINIDE

Like sulfonylureas, repaglinide stimulates insulin release by closing ATP-dependent K⁺ channels in pancreatic β cells. The drug is absorbed rapidly from the GI tract, and peak blood levels are obtained within 1 hour with a $t_{1/2}$ of ~1 hour. These features permit multiple preprandial use as compared with the classical once- or twice-daily dosing of sulfonylureas. Repaglinide is metabolized primarily by the liver to inactive derivatives and should be used cautiously in patients with hepatic insufficiency. Caution is also indicated in patients with renal insufficiency. The major adverse effect of repaglinide is hypoglycemia.

Nateglinide

Nateglinide (STARLIX) is derivative of D-phenylalanine that stimulates insulin secretion by blocking ATP-sensitive K⁺ channels in pancreatic β cells. Nateglinide promotes a more rapid but less sustained secretion of insulin than do other available oral antidiabetic agents. The drug's major therapeutic effect is reducing postprandial glycemic elevations in type 2 DM patients. Nateglinide is FDA-approved for use in type 2 DM and is most effective if administered in a dose of 120 mg, 1–10 minutes before a meal. Nateglinide is metabolized primarily by the liver and should be used cautiously in patients with hepatic insufficiency. Dosage adjustment is unnecessary in renal failure. Nateglinide may produce fewer episodes of hypoglycemia than most other oral insulin secretagogues, including repaglinide.

Metformin

Metformin is antihyperglycemic, not hypoglycemic. It does not stimulate insulin release from the pancreas and generally does not cause hypoglycemia, even in large doses. Metformin reduces glucose levels primarily by decreasing hepatic glucose production and by increasing insulin action in muscle and fat. These actions are mediated at least partly by activation of AMP-activated protein kinase (AMP kinase). The mechanism by which metformin reduces hepatic glucose production is controversial, but most data support an effect on reducing gluconeogenesis.

ABSORPTION, EXCRETION, AND DOSING

Metformin is absorbed mainly from the small intestine. The drug is stable, does not bind to plasma proteins, and is excreted unchanged in the urine. It has a $t_{1/2}$ of ~2 hours. The maximum recommended daily dose of metformin is 2.5 g divided into three doses with meals.

PRECAUTIONS AND ADVERSE EFFECTS
Patients with renal impairment should not receive metformin. Other contraindications include hepatic disease, a history of lactic acidosis, cardiac failure requiring drug therapy, or chronic hypoxic lung disease. These conditions all predispose to the potentially fatal complication of lactic acidosis. Metformin should be discontinued temporarily prior to the administration of intravenous *contrast media* and prior to any surgical procedure. The drug should not be readministered any sooner than 48 hours after such procedures and should be withheld until renal function is determined to be normal.

Acute side effects of metformin occur in up to 20% of patients and include diarrhea, abdominal discomfort, nausea, metallic taste, and anorexia. These usually can be minimized by increasing the dosage of the drug slowly and taking it with meals. Intestinal absorption of vitamin B_{12} *and* folate *may be decreased during chronic metformin therapy.*

Consideration should be given to stopping treatment with metformin if the plasma lactate level exceeds 3 mM or in the setting of decreased renal or hepatic function. It also is prudent to stop metformin if a patient is undergoing a prolonged fast or is treated with a very low calorie diet. Myocardial infarction or septicemia mandates immediate drug discontinuation.

Metformin lowers Hb A_{1c} values by about 2%, an effect comparable with that of the sulfonylureas. Metformin does not promote weight gain and can reduce plasma triglycerides by 15–20%. Metformin is the only drug that has been demonstrated to reduce macrovascular events in type 2 DM. Metformin can be administered in combination with sulfonylureas, thiazolizinediones, and/or insulin. Fixed-dose combinations containing metformin and glyburide (GLUCOVANCE, others), glipizide (METAGLIP), rosiglitazone (AVANDAMET), and pioglitazone (ACTOPLUSMET) are available.

Thiazolidinediones

The thiazolidinediones, rosiglitazone and pioglitazone, can lower Hb A_{1c} levels by 1–1.5% in patients with type 2 DM. These drugs can be combined with insulin or other classes of oral glucose-lowering agents.

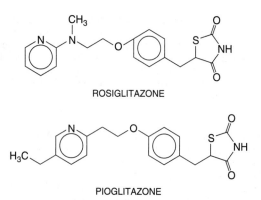

ROSIGLITAZONE

PIOGLITAZONE

MECHANISM OF ACTION Thiazolidinediones are agonists for the peroxisome proliferator–activated receptor γ (PPARγ). PPARγ, activates insulin-responsive genes that regulate carbohydrate and lipid metabolism. Thiazolidinediones principally act by increasing insulin sensitivity in peripheral tissues—and thus are effective only when insulin is present—but also may lower hepatic glucose production. Thiazolidinediones increase glucose transport into muscle and adipose tissue by enhancing the synthesis and translocation of specific forms of the glucose transporters. The thiazolidinediones also activate genes that regulate fatty acid metabolism in peripheral tissue. Some peripheral actions may be secondary to the stimulation of adiponectin release by adipocytes. Adiponectin increases insulin sensitivity, reportedly by elevating AMP kinase, which stimulates glucose transport into muscle and increases fatty acid oxidation.

ABSORPTION, EXCRETION, AND DOSING Rosiglitazone (AVANDIA) and pioglitazone (ACTOS) are taken once a day. Both agents are absorbed within about 2 hours; maximum clinical effect requires 6–12 weeks. The thiazolidinediones are metabolized by the liver and should not be used if there is active hepatic disease or significant elevations of hepatic transaminases.

Rosiglitazone is metabolized by hepatic CYP2C8, whereas pioglitazone is metabolized by CYP3A4 and CYP2C. Other drugs that induce or inhibit these enzymes can cause drug interactions. Clinically significant interactions between the available thiazolidinediones and other drugs have not been described.

PRECAUTIONS AND ADVERSE EFFECTS Pioglitazone and rosiglitazone rarely have been associated with hepatotoxicity, and liver function should be monitored in patients receiving these drugs. Hepatotoxicity can occur several months after drug initiation. Any patient who has suffered any hepatotoxicity (even abnormal liver function tests) while on a thiazolidinediones should not receive any drugs in this class. Thiazolidinediones also reportedly cause anemia, weight gain, edema, and plasma volume expansion. Edema is more likely when these drugs are combined with insulin; they should not be used in patients with New York Heart Association class 3 or 4 heart failure. Fluid retention and even overt heart failure can occur, usually within 6 months of initiating thiazolidinedione therapy. In most cases, the subjects had no past history of heart failure, but all had underlying abnormal cardiac function. Obese hypertensive individuals and those with cardiac diastolic dysfunction are at greatest risk for fluid retention with thiazolidinediones. Thiazolidinediones also can induce peripheral edema independent of heart failure. Exacerbations of fluid retention and/or heart failure should be treated, and the thiazolidinedione should be discontinued. A recent meta-analysis of results from clinical trials also raised the possibility that rosiglitazone is associated with an increased risk of adverse cardiovascular events, including myocardial infarction.

α-Glucosidase Inhibitors

α-Glucosidase inhibitors reduce intestinal absorption of starch, dextrin, and disaccharides by inhibiting the action of α-glucosidase in the intestinal brush border. Consequent to this delayed carbohydrate absorption, the postprandial rise in plasma glucose is blunted in both normal and diabetic subjects.

α-Glucosidase inhibitors may be used as monotherapy in elderly patients or in patients with predominantly postprandial hyperglycemia. α-Glucosidase inhibitors typically are used in combination with other oral antidiabetic agents and/or insulin. The drugs should be administered at the start of a meal.

Acarbose (PRECOSE), an oligosaccharide, and *miglitol* (GLYSET), a desoxynojirimycin derivative, also competitively inhibit glucoamylase and sucrase but have weak effects on pancreatic α-amylase. They reduce postprandial plasma glucose levels in type 1 and type 2 DM subjects. α-Glucosidase inhibitors can significantly improve Hb A$_{1c}$ levels in severely hyperglycemic type 2 DM patients. However, in patients with mild-to-moderate hyperglycemia, the glucose-lowering potential of α-glucosidase inhibitors is about 30–50% of that of other oral antidiabetic agents.

α-Glucosidase inhibitors do not result in hypoglycemia but do cause dose-related malabsorption, flatulence, diarrhea, and abdominal bloating. Titrating the drug dose over weeks to months reduces GI side effects. Smaller doses are given with snacks. Acarbose is most effective when given with a starchy, high-fiber diet with restricted amounts of glucose and sucrose. If hypoglycemia occurs when α-glucosidase inhibitors are used with insulin or an insulin secretagogue, glucose rather than sucrose, starch, or maltose should be administered.

Reduction in the Incidence of Type 2 DM

Type 2 DM is a worldwide health problem and the number of individuals who have impaired glucose tolerance (often termed *prediabetes*) may equal or even exceed the number of people with diabetes. In the U.S., nearly 20 million individuals are diagnosed with diabetes; perhaps twice that number have *impaired glucose tolerance* (IGT), defined as a fasting plasma glucose concentration of 100–126 mg/dL (5.6–7 mM) or 2-hour value in the oral glucose tolerance test of 140–199 mg/dL (7.8–11 mM). The rate of progression of IGT to overt diabetes ranges from 9 to 15%. Particularly troubling is the rapid increase in the incidence of type 2 DM in children, which has increased by tenfold over the last generation. Several clinical trials have investigated the effects of lifestyle modification and/or drugs on reducing the incidence of type 2 DM; lifestyle modification (*e.g.*, exercise and weight loss), metformin, troglitazone (a thiazolidinedione that is no longer available), acarbose, and *Orlistat* (a GI lipase inhibitor used for weight loss) all have shown some protection in various high-risk populations.

Glucagon-like Peptide 1

Oral, as compared with intravenous, delivery of glucose produces a greater release of insulin. Two hormones—*glucose-dependent insulinotropic polypeptide* (GIP) and *glucagon-like peptide-1* (GLP-1)—are released from the upper and lower bowel and augment glucose-dependent insulin secretion. These hormones are termed *incretins*. GLP-1 significantly augments glucose-dependent insulin secretion and consequently has become an attractive target for therapeutic development in type 2 DM. GLP-1 also reduces glucagon secretion, slows gastric emptying, and decreases appetite. Thus, the compound reduces postprandial glucose excursions (*i.e.,* increase in insulin, reduction of glucagon, slowing of gastric emptying) and also induces weight loss. Offsetting these advantages, circulating GLP-1 is rapidly (1–2 minutes) inactivated by the dipeptidyl peptidase IV enzyme (DPP-IV). Thus, GLP-1 must be infused continuously to have therapeutic benefits.

Two synthetic GLP-1 analogs have entered clinical trials. Exendin-4, derived from the salivary gland of the Gila monster, has 53% homology with human GLP-1. Exendin-4 is resistant to DPP-IV *and has full agonist activity at GLP-1 receptors. Exendin-4 (exenatide, BYETTA) is effective in lowering Hb A$_{1c}$ (~1–1.3%) and also promotes weight loss in type 2 DM. The compound is administered subcutaneously twice-daily; studies are planned to test longer-acting formulations. The FDA has approved exenatide for twice-daily injection in combination therapy with other agents in subjects with type 2 DM. Side effects include a self-limiting nausea in 15–30% of patients; hypoglycemia can occur when GLP-1 agonists are used in conjunction with oral insulin secretagogues. A second long-acting analog of GLP-1, NN2211, contains a hexadeconyl fatty acid covalently linked to GLP-1. NN2211 resists the action of DPP-IV but also must be injected. Studies suggest that NN2211 is effective in lowering Hb A$_{1c}$ but may not induce as much weight loss as exendin-4. Nausea and hypoglycemia also occur with NN2211 when used with oral hypoglycemic agents.*

An alternative approach to GLP-1 therapy is to inactivate the DPP-IV protease, thereby increasing endogenous GLP-1 levels. A number of orally effective DPP-IV inhibitors are in clinical trials, and sitagliptin (JANLLVIA) is now available for therapy of type 2 DM in th U.S. One study in type 2 DM reported similar reductions in Hb A$_{1c}$ as compared with the GLP-1 receptor analogs. These agents are well tolerated and appear to result in less nausea than the GLP-1 analogs. However, since DPP-IV can metabolize a wide range of peptides, there is some concern about their long-term safety. Furthermore, the potency of the DPP-IV inhibitors may be limited by endogenous production of GLP-1. In contrast, pharmacological amounts of injectable GLP-1 analogs can be given with possibly increased therapeutic effect.

Amylin

Amylin is a 37-amino-acid peptide that is produced in pancreatic β cells and cosecreted with insulin. It is structurally related to calcitonin, calcitonin gene–related peptide, and adrenomedullin, and interacts with GPCRs to inhibit glucagon secretion, delay gastric emptying, and suppress appetite. Pramlintide is a modified amylin peptide in which Pro residues are substituted at positions 25, 28, and 29, thereby decreasing the tendency to self-aggregate into amyloid-like plaques. Pramlintide (SYMLIN) is FDA-approved for the treatment of patients with type 1 and type 2 DM who are inadequately controlled with insulin therapy.

Several clinical trials have shown beneficial effects of pramlintide on HbA$_{1c}$ levels without concomitant weight gain. For patients with type 1 DM, the starting dose is 15 μg subcutaneously before major meals, and the dose can be titrated to a maximum of 60 μg/injection. For patients with type 2 DM, the starting dose is 60 μg before major meals, with a maximum dose of 120 μg/ injection. Adverse effects include nausea and vomiting, anorexia, and headache. In conjunction with insulin, pramlintide can cause hypoglycemia within 3 hours of the pramlintide injection, particularly in patients with type 1 DM. To minimize the likelihood of this serious adverse effect, the patient should be instructed about the signs and symptoms of hypoglycemia and the preprandial dose of short-acting or rapid-acting insulin should be decreased by 50% when pramlintide therapy is initiated, with upward titration thereafter as needed.

GLUCAGON

CHEMISTRY

Glucagon is a single-chain polypeptide of 29 amino acids. It has significant homology with several other polypeptide hormones, including secretin, vasoactive intestinal peptide (VIP), and GIP. Glucagon is synthesized from preproglucagon, a 180-amino-acid precursor. An amino-terminal signal peptide is followed by glicentin-related pancreatic peptide, glucagon, GLP-1, and glucagon-like peptide-2. Processing of the protein occurs in a tissue-specific fashion; this results in different secretory peptides in pancreatic α cells and intestinal α-like cells (L cells).

In the pancreatic α cell, the granule consists of a central core of glucagon surrounded by a halo of glicentin. Intestinal L cells contain only glicentin and presumably lack the enzyme required to process this precursor to glucagon. Enteroglucagon binds to hepatic glucagon receptors and stimulates adenylyl cyclase with 10–20% of the potency of glucagon. GLP-1 is an extremely potent potentiator of insulin secretion (see above), although it apparently lacks significant hepatic actions.

REGULATION OF SECRETION

Glucagon secretion is regulated by dietary glucose, insulin, amino acids, and fatty acids. The effect of glucose is lost in untreated or undertreated type 1 DM patients and in isolated pancreatic α cells, indicating that at least part of the effect is secondary to stimulation of insulin secretion. Somatostatin also inhibits glucagon secretion, as do free fatty acids and ketones.

Most amino acids stimulate the release of both glucagon and insulin. This coordinated response to amino acids may prevent insulin-induced hypoglycemia in individuals who ingest a meal of pure protein. Secretion of glucagon also is regulated by the autonomic innervation of the islets. Stimulation of sympathetic nerves or administration of sympathomimetic amines increases glucagon secretion.

GLUCAGON IN DIABETES MELLITUS

Plasma glucagon concentrations are elevated in poorly controlled diabetic patients. Because it enhances gluconeogenesis and glycogenolysis, glucagon exacerbates the hyperglycemia of diabetes. However, this abnormality of glucagon secretion appears to be secondary to the diabetic state and is corrected with improved control of the disease. Although somatostatin-mediated inhibition of glucagons secretion does not restore glucose metabolism to normal, it significantly slows the rate of development of hyperglycemia and ketonemia in insulin-deficient subjects with type 1 DM. In normal individuals, glucagon secretion increases in response to hypoglycemia, but this important defense mechanism against insulin-induced hypoglycemia is lost in type 1 DM.

DEGRADATION

Glucagon is degraded in liver, kidney, plasma, and other sites. Its $t_{1/2}$ in plasma is approximately 3–6 minutes. Proteolytic removal of the amino-terminal histidine residue leads to loss of biological activity.

CELLULAR AND PHYSIOLOGICAL ACTIONS

Glucagon interacts with a GPCR that signals through the G_s-cyclic AMP-PKA pathway to activate phosphorylase and inactivate glycogen synthase, enhancing glycogenolysis and inhibiting glycogen synthesis. In the liver, cyclic AMP also stimulates phosphorylation of the bifunctional enzyme 6-phosphofructo-2-kinase/fructose-2,6-bisphosphatase (PFK2/FBP2), which determines the cellular concentration of fructose-2,6-bisphosphate, a regulator of gluconeogenesis and glycogenolysis. When [glucagon] is high relative to insulin (i.e., when glucose is scarce), PFK2/FBP2 is phosphorylated and acts as a phosphatase, reducing hepatic [fructose-2, 6-bisphosphate], which reduces the rate of phosphofructokinase-1 (PFK-1, which is rate limiting in glycolysis), and thence the rate of glycolysis. Under these conditions, glucagon inhibits glycolysis, stimulates gluconeogenesis, and stimulates fatty acid oxidation and ketone body production. Conversely, when insulin predominates (the "fed" state, when glucose is abundant), PFK2/FBP2 is dephosphorylated, favoring its PFK2 activity and raising the level of fructose-2,6-bisphosphate, which stimulates PFK-1 and hepatic glycolysis.

Glucagon also affects tissues other than liver, especially at higher concentrations. It increases lipolysis in adipocytes and the force of cardiac contraction. Glucagon has relaxant effects on the GI tract.

THERAPEUTIC USE

Glucagon extracted from bovine and porcine pancreas has a sequence identical to that of the human hormone. For hypoglycemic reactions, 1 mg is administered intravenously, intramuscularly, or subcutaneously. The first two routes are preferred. The hyperglycemic action of glucagon is transient and may be inadequate if glycogen hepatic stores are depleted. After the initial response to glucagon, patients should be given glucose or urged to eat to prevent recurrent hypoglycemia. Nausea and vomiting are the most frequent adverse effects.

Glucagon also is used to facilitate radiographic examination of the upper and lower GI tract in various procedures. The hormone also has been used as a cardiac inotropic agent for the treatment of shock, particularly when prior administration of a β adrenergic receptor antagonist has rendered β adrenergic receptor agonists ineffective.

SOMATOSTATIN (SST)

In the gut, SST influences the functions of adjacent cells—a paracrine effect—and also acts in an autocrine manner to inhibit its own pancreatic release. The δ cell is the last islet cell to receive blood flow; thus, SST likely regulates insulin and glucagons secretion by β and α cells only via the systemic circulation.

SST is released in response to many of the nutrients and hormones that stimulate insulin secretion, including glucose, arginine, leucine, glucagon, VIP, and cholecystokinin. SST in pharmacological doses inhibits virtually all endocrine and exocrine secretions of the pancreas, gut, and gallbladder. SST also inhibits nutrient absorption from the intestine, decreases intestinal motility, and reduces splanchnic blood flow.

The major therapeutic use of SST is to block hormone release in endocrine-secreting tumors, Available SST analogs and their clinical uses are described in Chapter 55. Since the analog octreotide also can decrease blood flow to the GI tract, it has been used to treat bleeding esophageal varices, peptic ulcers, and postprandial orthostatic hypotension.

DIAZOXIDE

Diazoxide is an antihypertensive benzothiadiazine with potent hyperglycemic *actions when given orally. Diazoxide interacts with the ATP-sensitive K⁺ channel on the β-cell membrane and either prevents its closing or prolongs the open time to inhibit insulin secretion; this effect is opposite to that of the sulfonylureas. Diazoxide (PROGLYCEM) is used to treat patients with various forms of hypoglycemia. The usual oral dose is 3–8 mg/kg/day in adults and 8–15 mg/kg/day in infants and neonates. The drug can cause nausea and vomiting and thus usually is given in divided doses with meals. Diazoxide has a $t_{1/2}$ of ~48 hours. Thus, the patient should be maintained at any dosage for several days before evaluating the therapeutic result.*

Adverse effects, including Na⁺ retention, edema, hyperuricemia, hypertrichosis (especially in children), thrombocytopenia, and leucopenia, sometimes limit its use, but the drug may be quite useful in patients with inoperable insulinomas and in children with hyperinsulinism due to nesidioblastosis.

For a complete Bibliographical listing see Goodman & Gilman's *The Pharmacological Basis of Therapeutics*, 11th ed., or Goodman & Gilman Online at www.accessmedicine.com.

61

AGENTS AFFECTING MINERAL ION HOMEOSTASIS AND BONE TURNOVER

PHYSIOLOGY OF MINERAL HOMEOSTASIS AND BONE METABOLISM

Calcium

Adult men and women possess about 1300 g and 1000 g of calcium respectively, more than 99% of which is in bone and teeth. Although the absolute amount of calcium in the extracellular fluid is small, this fraction is stringently regulated. Normal serum calcium ranges from 8.5 to 10.4 mg/dL (4.25–5.2 mEq/L, 2.1–2.6 mM) and includes three components: *ionized* (~50%), *protein-bound* (~40%, predominantly to albumin; a decrease in albumin of 1.0 g/dL from the normal value of 4.0 g/dL typically decreases total serum calcium by ~0.8 mg/dL), and *complexed to anions* such as phosphate and citrate (~10%) (Figure 61–1).

It is the ionized Ca^{2+} (~1.2 mM) that exerts biological effects (*see* Figure 33–2) and this fraction is tightly regulated. Hormones regulate plasma Ca^{2+} by controlling Ca^{2+} entry from the intestine and Ca^{2+} excretion by the kidney. When needed, these same hormones regulate Ca^{2+} withdrawal from the large skeletal reservoir.

CALCIUM STORES   Skeletal calcium largely is in a crystalline form that resembles the mineral hydroxyapatite with other ions in the crystal lattice. The steady-state content of calcium in bone reflects the net effect of bone resorption and bone formation (*see* below).

CALCIUM ABSORPTION AND EXCRETION   In the U.S., ~75% of dietary calcium is obtained from milk and dairy products. The recommended adequate daily intake value for calcium is 1300 mg in adolescents, 1000 mg in adults, and 1250–1500 mg in postmenopausal women; typical intake is only ~50% of these values.

Figure 61–2 illustrates the components of calcium turnover. Calcium enters the body only through the intestine (~300 mg/day), both by facilitated diffusion throughout the small intestine and by active transport in the proximal duodenum. The former accounts for the majority of total calcium uptake, whereas active transport is the process that is regulated by vitamin D. The efficiency of intestinal calcium absorption is inversely related to total calcium intake. Certain drugs such as *glucocorticoids* or *phenytoin* depress intestinal calcium transport. Opposed to uptake is an obligatory calcium loss of 150 mg/d due to mucosal and biliary secretions and sloughing of intestinal cells; diseases associated with chronic diarrhea or malabsorption promote fecal calcium loss.

Calcium excretion in the kidney also is highly regulated. About 9 g of Ca^{2+} is filtered in the glomeruli, of which >98% is reabsorbed in the tubules. The efficiency of tubular reabsorption is tightly regulated by parathyroid hormone (PTH) but also is influenced by filtered Na^+, the presence of non–reabsorbed anions, and diuretics.

Phosphate

Phosphate is present in plasma, extracellular fluid, cell membrane phospholipids, intracellular fluid, collagen, and bone. More than 80% of total body phosphate is found in bone and ~15% in soft tissues. Phosphorus (P) in the body exists in both organic and inorganic forms. Organic forms include phospholipids and various organic esters. In extracellular fluid, the bulk of phosphorus exists as inorganic phosphate (P_i) in the form of NaH_2PO_4 and Na_2HPO_4. The aggregate level of P_i modifies tissue concentrations of Ca^{2+} and plays a major role in renal acid excretion. Within bone, phosphate is complexed with calcium as hydroxyapatite and calcium phosphate.

ABSORPTION, DISTRIBUTION, AND EXCRETION   Phosphate is a component of many foods; thus, dietary insufficiency rarely causes phosphate depletion. Intestinal uptake of phosphate primarily is passive, although an active component is stimulated by several factors, including vitamin D. In adults, about two-thirds of ingested phosphate is absorbed, almost all of which is excreted into the urine. In children, phosphate balance is positive and the plasma concentration of phosphate is higher than in adults.

Phosphate excretion by the kidney also is highly regulated. More than 90% of plasma phosphate is filtered at the glomeruli, >80% of which is reabsorbed in the tubules. Renal phosphate reabsorption is regulated by a variety of factors, including PTH and dietary phosphate. Vitamin D has minimal effects on renal phosphate excretion.

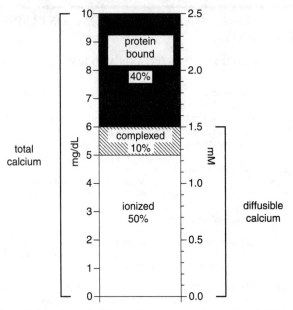

FIGURE 61–1 *Pools of calcium in serum.* Concentrations are expressed as mg/dL on the left-hand axis and as mM on the right. The total serum calcium concentration is 10 mg/dL or 2.5 mM, divided into three pools: protein-bound (40%), complexed with small anions (10%), and ionized calcium (50%). The complexed and ionized pools represent the diffusible forms of calcium.

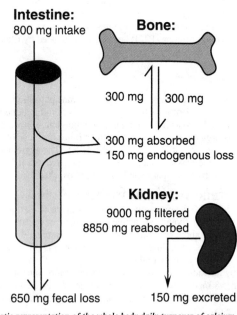

FIGURE 61–2 *Schematic representation of the whole body daily turnover of calcium.*

PHYSIOLOGY OF CALCIUM AND PHOSPHATE REGULATION

A number of hormones interact to regulate the Ca^{2+} and phosphate concentrations. The most important are PTH and 1,25-dihydroxyvitamin D (1,25-$(OH)_2$D; calcitriol), which regulate mineral homeostasis by effects on the kidney, intestine, and bone (Figure 61–3).

Parathyroid Hormone

PTH is a polypeptide hormone that regulates plasma Ca^{2+} by affecting bone formation/resorption, renal Ca^{2+} excretion/reabsorption, and calcitriol synthesis (thereby indirectly regulating GI calcium absorption).

CHEMISTRY

Human PTH consists of a single polypeptide chain of 84 amino acids (molecular weight ~9500). Biological activity is associated with the N-terminal portion and residues 1-27 are required for optimal binding and activation of the PTH receptor. PTH (1-84) has a $t_{1/2}$ in plasma of 2–5 minutes and is predominantly (~90%) cleared by the liver and kidney.

PHYSIOLOGICAL FUNCTIONS The primary function of PTH is to maintain a constant concentration of Ca^{2+} in the extracellular fluid. The principal processes regulated are renal Ca^{2+} reabsorption and mobilization of bone Ca^{2+} (Figure 61–3). The actions of PTH on tissues are mediated by at least two GPCRs that couple to G_s and G_q in cell-specific manners.

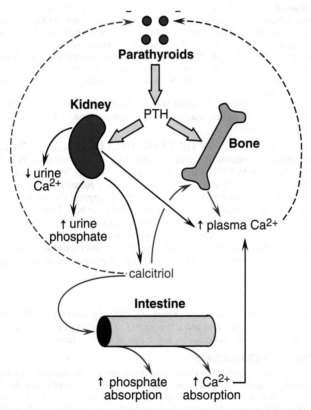

FIGURE 61–3 *Calcium homeostasis and its regulation by parathyroid hormone (PTH) and 1,25-dihydroxyvitamin D.* PTH has stimulatory effects on bone and kidney, including the stimulation of 1α-hydroxylase activity in kidney mitochondria leading to the increased production of the biologically active hormone 1,25-dihydroxyvitamin D (calcitriol) from 25-hydroxyvitamin D (*see* Figure 61–5). Solid lines indicate a positive effect; dashed lines refer to negative feedback.

Regulation of Secretion   Plasma Ca^{2+} is the major regulator of PTH secretion; hypocalcemia stimulates and hypercalcemia inhibits PTH secretion. Sustained hypocalcemia also induces parathyroid hypertrophy and hyperplasia. Changes in Ca^{2+} modulate PTH secretion by parathyroid cells *via* the calcium-sensing receptor (CaSR), a GPCR that couples with G_q-PLC and G_i. Occupancy of the CaSR by Ca^{2+} inhibits PTH secretion; thus, the extracellular concentration of Ca^{2+} is controlled by an endocrine negative-feedback system, the afferent limb of which senses the ambient activity of Ca^{2+} and the efferent limb of which releases PTH that then acts to increase Ca^{2+}. The active vitamin D metabolite calcitriol directly suppresses PTH gene expression.

Effects on Bone   PTH increases bone resorption and thereby increases Ca^{2+} delivery to the extracellular fluid. The apparent cellular target for PTH is the osteoblast. PTH also recruits osteoclast precursors to form new bone remodeling units (*see* below).

Effects on Kidney   In the kidney, PTH enhances the efficiency of Ca^{2+} reabsorption, inhibits tubular reabsorption of phosphate, and stimulates conversion of 25-OHD to calcitriol (Figure 61–3, *see* below). As a result, filtered Ca^{2+} is avidly retained and its plasma concentration increases, whereas phosphate is excreted and its plasma concentration falls. Newly synthesized calcitriol interacts with specific high-affinity vitamin D receptors (VDRs) in the intestine to increase the efficiency of calcium absorption, thereby also increasing the plasma Ca^{2+} concentration.

PTH increases tubular reabsorption of Ca^{2+}, primarily in the distal nephron, with concomitant decreases in urinary Ca^{2+} excretion. Many of these effects are mediated by G_s-induced increases in intracellular cyclic AMP, and subsequent stimulation of the epithelial Ca^{2+} channel TRPV5. As the plasma Ca^{2+} concentration increases, the filtered load of Ca^{2+} also increases; the tubular capacity to reabsorb Ca^{2+} is exceeded and hypercalciuria results. Conversely, reduction of serum PTH depresses tubular reabsorption of Ca^{2+} and thereby increases urinary Ca^{2+} excretion. When the plasma Ca^{2+} concentration falls below 7 mg/dL, the filtered load of Ca^{2+} declines to the point that Ca^{2+} is almost completely reabsorbed despite reduced tubular capacity.

PTH increases renal excretion of P_i by decreasing its reabsorption, an effect mediated by retrieval of the Na-P_i cotransporter from the luminal membrane rather than a decrease in the number of cotransporters. Fibroblast growth factor 23 also plays important roles in regulating phosphate reabsorption.

The final step in the activation of vitamin D to calcitriol occurs in the kidney proximal tubular cells. The key enzyme in this process, 1α-hydroxylase, is a mitochondrial CYP that is regulated by PTH, P_i, and Ca^{2+} (see below).

INTEGRATED REGULATION OF EXTRACELLULAR Ca^{2+} CONCENTRATION BY PTH   Even modest reductions of serum Ca^{2+} stimulate PTH secretion. Acutely, the regulation of tubular Ca^{2+} reabsorption by PTH suffices to maintain plasma Ca^{2+} homeostasis. With more prolonged hypocalcemia, renal 1α-hydroxylase is stimulated; this enhances the synthesis and release of calcitriol, which directly stimulates intestinal calcium absorption (Figure 61–3). Finally, PTH and the resulting increase in calcitriol also stimulate Ca^{2+} release from bone.

When plasma Ca^{2+} rises, PTH secretion is suppressed and tubular Ca^{2+} reabsorption decreases. The reduced PTH promotes renal phosphate conservation, and both the decreased PTH and the increased phosphate reduce calcitriol production and thereby decrease intestinal Ca^{2+} absorption. Finally, bone remodeling is suppressed. These physiological events provide an integrated response to positive or negative excursions of plasma Ca^{2+} concentration.

Vitamin D

Vitamin D traditionally was viewed as a permissive factor in calcium metabolism, facilitating efficient absorption of dietary calcium and allowing full expression of PTH action. Vitamin D is a hormone, rather than a vitamin, and plays an active role in calcium homeostasis.

CHEMISTRY AND OCCURRENCE

Ultraviolet irradiation of several animal and plant sterols converts them to compounds possessing vitamin D activity. In animals, the principal precursor sterol is 7-dehydrocholesterol, which is synthesized in the skin; exposure to ultraviolet light in sunlight converts 7-dehydrocholesterol to cholecalciferol (vitamin D_3; Figure 61–4). Ergosterol, which is present only in plants, is the precursor to vitamin D_2 (ergocalciferol) and its derivatives. Derivatives of vitamin D_2 and vitamin D_3 are both biologically active—although some data suggest that the D_3 hormones may be more potent in certain settings—and are widely available in a variety of commercial vitamin preparations.

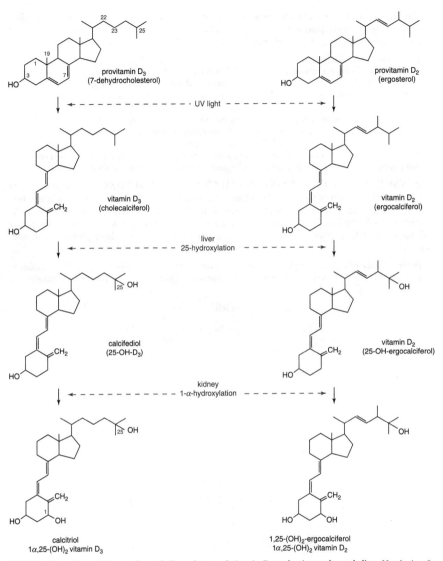

FIGURE 61–4 *Photobiology and metabolic pathways of vitamin D production and metabolism.* Numbering for select positions discussed in the text is shown.

HUMAN REQUIREMENTS AND UNITS The recommended daily dose of vitamin D is 400 IU, or 10 μg. Vitamin D intake in many individuals (*e.g.,* premature infants, the elderly, and African Americans) may be inadequate; contributory factors include decreased intake of dairy products, decreased sun exposure and increased use of sunscreen, and increased prevalence and duration of exclusive breast-feeding.

ABSORPTION, FATE, AND EXCRETION Both vitamins D_2 and D_3 are absorbed from the small intestine and transported as chylomicrons in the lymphatics. Bile salts are essential for adequate absorption. The primary route of vitamin D excretion also is the bile. Severe shortening or inflammation of the small bowel or hepatic or biliary dysfunction may cause overt vitamin D deficiency.

In the blood, vitamin D circulates bound to vitamin D-binding protein. Its plasma $t_{1/2}$ is ~24 hours, but it is stored in fat for prolonged periods.

METABOLIC ACTIVATION Whether endogenously synthesized or acquired from diet, vitamin D requires modification to become biologically active. The primary active metabolite of vitamin D is calcitriol, which is formed by two successive hydroxylations (Figure 61–4).

The initial 25-hydroxylation occurs in the liver to form 25-OH-cholecalciferol or 25-OH-ergocalciferol (collectively termed 25-OHD). 25-OHD has a circulating $t_{1/2}$ of 19 days, and normal levels are 30–80 ng/mL. Because of its prolonged $t_{1/2}$ and precursor role in the production of calcitriol, measurement of serum 25-OHD is the preferred test to evaluate sufficiency of body stores of vitamin D.

After production in the liver, 25-OHD enters the circulation, largely bound by vitamin D-binding protein. Final activation occurs predominantly in the kidney, where 1α-hydroxylase in the proximal tubule converts 25-OHD to calcitriol. This process is highly regulated (Figure 61–5). Calcitriol and 25-OHD also can be hydroxylated by another renal enzyme, 24-hydroxylase, to make compounds that have considerably lower biological activity and presumably are destined for excretion.

PHYSIOLOGICAL FUNCTIONS AND MECHANISM OF ACTION Calcitriol augments absorption and retention of Ca^{2+} and phosphate. The action of calcitriol is mediated by interaction with the VDR, a member of the nuclear receptor family. After binding to calcitriol, the VDR translocates to the nucleus and regulates the transcription of its target genes, likely as a heterodimer with the retinoid X receptor. Calcitriol also exerts nongenomic effects whose physiological relevance is unclear.

In the absence of calcitriol, calcium absorption throughout the small intestine is inefficient and involves passive diffusion via *the paracellular pathway. Calcitriol in the proximal duodenum*

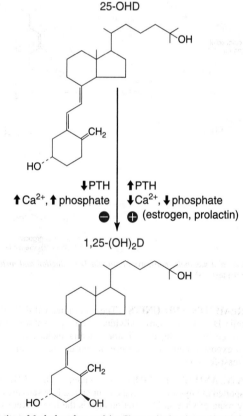

FIGURE 61–5 *Regulation of 1a-hydroxylase activity.* Changes in the plasma levels of PTH, Ca^{2+}, and phosphate modulate the hydroxylation of 25-OH vitamin D to the active form, 1,25-dihydroxyvitamin D.

ABBREVIATIONS: 25-OHD, 25-hydroxycholecalciferol; 1,25-(OH)₂D, calcitriol; PTH, parathyroid hormone.

stimulates the TRPV6 Ca^{2+} channels and also induces the synthesis of calbindin D$_{9K}$, calbindin D$_{28K}$ and the serosal membrane Ca^{2+}-ATPase. The net effect of these actions is to stimulate active calcium uptake.

Calcitriol's effects on bone are predominantly mediated by its actions to stimulate intestinal calcium uptake, although large doses can directly stimulate bone resorption. Similarly, there are direct effects of calcitriol to stimulate Ca^{2+} reabsorption in the distal tubule. The physiological impact of these effects is unknown.

The VDR is distributed widely throughout the body, and calcitriol actions extend well beyond calcium homeostasis. For example, calcitriol and synthetic analogs have been evaluated as antiproliferative agents for therapy of skin diseases (e.g., psoriasis) and cancer.

Calcitonin

Calcitonin is produced by the C cells of the thyroid gland; its actions generally oppose those of PTH. Calcitonin is a single-chain polypeptide hormone of 32 amino acids with an intrachain disulfide bridge. Salmon calcitonin, which differs from the human sequence at approximately half of the residues, is used therapeutically because it is more potent and is cleared more slowly from the circulation.

REGULATION OF SECRETION   Calcitonin secretion increases with hypercalcemia and decreases when plasma Ca^{2+} is low; the hormone in circulation has a t$_{1/2}$ of 10 minutes. Circulating concentrations are normally low (<15 pg/mL in males and 10 pg/mL in females) but can be markedly elevated with C cell hyperplasia or medullary thyroid cancer.

MECHANISM OF ACTION   Calcitonin actions are mediated by the calcitonin receptor, a GPCR that couples through multiple G proteins to diverse signal transduction pathways. The hypocalcemic and hypophosphatemic effects of calcitonin result primarily from direct inhibition of osteoclast bone resorption.

BONE PHYSIOLOGY

The skeleton is the primary structural support for the body and also provides a protected environment for hematopoiesis. It contains both a large mineralized matrix and a highly active cellular component.

A process called modeling drives the growth and development of endochondral bone. Once new bone is laid down, it is subject to a continuous process of breakdown and renewal, called remodeling, by which bone mass is adjusted throughout adult life. This remodeling is carried out by multiple independent bone remodeling units throughout the skeleton (Figure 61–6). In response to physical

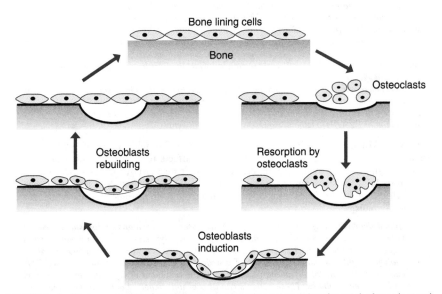

FIGURE 61–6   *The bone remodeling cycle.* Osteoclast precursors fuse and are activated to resorb a lacuna in a previously quiescent surface. These cells are replaced by osteoblasts that deposit new bone to restore the integrity of the tissue.

or biochemical signals, mononuclear precursors are recruited to the bone surface, where they fuse to form the characteristic multinucleated osteoclasts that excavate a cavity into the bone called the resorption lacuna.

Osteoclast production is regulated by osteoblast-derived cytokines. One particularly important factor is RANK ligand (previously called osteoclast differentiation factor), which induces osteoclast formation by activating its RANK receptor. Osteoblasts also produce osteoprotegerin, a decoy ligand that inhibits osteoclast differentiation by blocking the RANK receptor. Estrogen induces osteoprotegerin, which may be one mechanism by which estrogens inhibit osteoclast function and bone resorption in postmenopausal women.

The resorption phase is followed by ingress of preosteoblasts into the base of the resorption cavity. These cells become osteoblasts and elaborate new bone matrix constituents that help form the osteoid. Once the osteoid reaches a thickness of ~15–20 μm, mineralization begins. A complete remodeling cycle normally requires about 3–6 months.

The remodeling process is imperfect and small bone deficits persist on completion of each cycle. Lifelong accumulation of these remodeling deficits underlies the age-related bone loss that begins shortly after growth ceases. Alterations in remodeling activity represent the final pathway through which diverse stimuli—such as dietary insufficiency, hormones, and drugs—affect bone balance.

DISORDERS OF MINERAL HOMEOSTASIS AND BONE
Abnormal Calcium Metabolism

HYPERCALCEMIA The degree and rapidity of onset of hypercalcemia largely dictate the extent of symptoms. Chronic elevation of serum Ca^{2+} to 12–14 mg/dL (3–3.5 mM) generally causes few manifestations, whereas an acute rise to the same level may cause marked neuromuscular manifestations by increasing the threshold for nerve and muscle excitation. Symptoms include fatigue, weakness, anorexia, depression, diffuse abdominal pain, and constipation.

The most common cause of hypercalcemia in outpatients is primary hyperparathyroidism, due either to a single adenoma or diffuse hyperplasia. Primary hyperparathyroidism is often associated with significant hypophosphatemia due to PTH effects on renal phosphate reabsorption. The diagnosis is generally apparent from the elevated serum Ca^{2+} associated with an inappropriately high PTH level. In contrast, secondary hyperparathyroidism is a disorder in which PTH levels are elevated in response to persistent threats to normal calcium homeostasis such as hyperphosphatemia from chronic renal disease.

Hypercalcemia in hospitalized patients is caused most often by a malignancy, either with or without bone metastases. The degree of hypercalcemia here often exceeds considerably that seen with primary hyperparathyroidism (often >13 mg/dL) and lethargy, weakness, and volume depletion may be profound. PTH-related peptide, which is produced by squamous cell and other tumors, can interact with the PTH receptor to cause humoral hypercalcemia. An assay for PTH-related peptide is often diagnostic in these patients, while the PTH level is suppressed due to feedback by the elevated serum Ca^{2+}.

Pharmacologic overdoses of vitamin D may cause hypercalcemia if sufficient 25-OHD is present to stimulate intestinal calcium absorption. Measurement of the serum 25-OHD level is diagnostic. More often, granulomatous disorders such as sarcoidosis are associated with increased production of $1,25(OH)_2D$ due to expression of 1α-hydroxylase.

HYPOCALCEMIA Mild hypocalcemia (*i.e.*, serum Ca^{2+} in the range of 8–8.5 mg/dL) is usually asymptomatic. Again, the rapidity of onset affects the clinical manifestations. The signs and symptoms of hypocalcemia include tetany, paresthesias, increased neuromuscular excitability, laryngospasm, muscle cramps, and tonic-clonic seizures. Nail and tooth changes and calcification of the basal ganglia are encountered with chronic hypocalcemia due to hypoparathyroidism.

Combined deprivation of Ca^{2+} and vitamin D, as observed in malabsorption states, readily promotes hypocalcemia. Serum phosphate also will be low. Hypoparathyroidism is most often a consequence of thyroid or neck surgery, but also may be due to genetic or autoimmune disorders. Pseudohypoparathyroidism, a rare group of genetic disorders associated with decreased PTH action, results from mutations in the gene encoding the α subunit of G_s, which mediates PTH action in the renal tubules. These patients can also exhibit impaired action of multiple other hormones that couple to G_s, but the impaired response to PTH is most severe.

Disturbed Phosphate Metabolism

Dietary inadequacy rarely causes phosphate depletion. Sustained use of aluminum-containing antacids can severely limit phosphate absorption and cause clinically significant phosphate depletion. If severe, hypophosphatemia can cause malaise, muscle weakness, and a bone disorder termed *osteomalacia* that is characterized by undermineralized bone osteoid.

Hyperphosphatemia occurs commonly in chronic renal failure. The increased phosphate level directly stimulates PTH secretion and also has secondary effects due to the reduction in serum Ca^{2+}. Because renal function is impaired, the increased PTH is unable to increase phosphate excretion sufficiently to avoid ongoing phosphate retention. The chronic secondary hyperparathyroidism may result in a bone disease called renal osteodystrophy.

Disorders of Vitamin D

HYPERVITAMINOSIS D The acute or chronic administration of excessive amounts of vitamin D can cause hypervitaminosis D and hypercalcemia. The amount of vitamin D necessary to induce this condition varies widely. As an approximation, prolonged daily ingestion of 50,000 U or more can cause poisoning. The signs and symptoms are those associated with hypercalcemia.

VITAMIN D DEFICIENCY Vitamin D deficiency is associated with inadequate absorption of calcium and phosphate. The resulting decrease in Ca^{2+} stimulates PTH secretion, which acts to restore plasma Ca^{2+} at the expense of bone. Plasma phosphate concentration will remain low due to the phosphaturic effect of PTH. In children, the failure to mineralize newly formed bone results in rickets, a growth disorder in which the long bones may be bowed due to inadequate calcification.

In adults, vitamin D deficiency results in osteomalacia, a disease characterized by generalized accumulation of undermineralized bone matrix. Severe osteomalacia may be associated with extreme bone pain and tenderness and proximal muscle weakness. A low serum level of 25-OHD is diagnostic.

Conditions associated with abnormalities in calcitriol synthesis or response can cause rickets in children and osteomalacia in adults. Specific disorders include X-linked hypophosphatemic rickets due to mutations in the PHEX endoprotease, Vitamin D-dependent rickets due to mutations in 1α-hydroxylase, and hereditary 1,25-(OH)$_2$D resistance due to mutations in the VDR.

SPECIFIC DISORDERS OF BONE

Osteoporosis

Osteoporosis is a condition of low bone mass and microarchitectural disruption that results in fractures with minimal trauma. Characteristic sites of fracture include vertebral bodies, the distal radius, and the proximal femur, but osteoporotic individuals have generalized skeletal fragility, and fractures at sites such as ribs and long bones also occur. Fracture risk increases exponentially with age, related both to decreased bone density and to factors such as decreased muscle strength and increased risk of falls.

Osteoporosis can be categorized as primary (idiopathic) or secondary to a systemic illness or medication such as glucocorticoids or phenytoin. A major factor in the former category is the decline in estrogen levels, and the resulting sharp decrease in bone mass that accompanies menopause in women.

PAGET'S DISEASE

Paget's disease affects up to 3% of the population over age 60. It is characterized by single or multiple foci of disordered bone remodeling. The primary pathologic abnormality is increased bone resorption followed by exuberant formation of disorganized bone of poor quality. The altered bone structure can lead to bowing and stress fractures and also is associated with secondary problems such as deafness, spinal cord compression, high-output cardiac failure, and pain. Malignant degeneration to osteogenic sarcoma is a rare but potentially lethal complication.

Renal Osteodystrophy

Bone disease is a frequent consequence of chronic renal failure and dialysis. Pathologically, the lesions are typical of hyperparathyroidism, adynamic bone disease, deficiency of vitamin D (osteomalacia), or a combination of the above. The underlying defect reflects increased phosphate and decreased calcium, leading to secondary events that strive to preserve circulating levels of Ca^{2+} at the expense of bone.

PHARMACOLOGICAL TREATMENT OF DISORDERS OF MINERAL ION HOMEOSTASIS AND BONE METABOLISM

HYPERCALCEMIA Hypercalcemia can be life-threatening. Because hypercalcemia compromises renal concentrating mechanisms, such patients frequently are severely volume depleted. Thus, fluid resuscitation with large volumes of isotonic saline is essential. Loop diuretics that augment renal Ca^{2+} excretion may help to counteract the effect of plasma volume expansion with saline but should not be used until volume is replete.

Calcitonin (CALCIMAR, MIACALCIN) can rapidly reduce Ca^{2+}, but the response is generally transient and the magnitude of response is less than with other agents. The recommended stating dose is 4 U/kg administered subcutaneously every 12 hours; if there is no response within 1 or 2 days, the dose may be increased to 8 U/kg every 12 hours, or then to a maximum of 8 U/kg every 6 hours.

Intravenous bisphosphonates (*pamidronate, zoledronate*) have proven very helpful in the management of hypercalcemia (*see* below for further discussion of biphosphonates). Typically, a 60–90-mg dose of pamidronate (AREDIA) is given by intravenous infusion over 4 hours. Alternatively, zoledronate (ZOMETA) can be given in a dose of 4 mg over 15 minutes. Resolution of the hypercalcemia generally occurs within several days and persists for several weeks.

Once the hypercalcemic crisis has resolved, or in patients with milder calcium elevations, long-term therapy can be initiated. Parathyroidectomy remains the definitive therapy for primary hyperparathyroidism. As described below, a Ca^{2+} mimetic that stimulates the CaSR is a promising therapy for hyperparathyroidism. If the hypercalcemia results from malignancy, therapy ideally is directed at the underlying cancer. When this is not possible, intermittent dosing of parenteral bisphosphonates has been used to keep serum Ca^{2+} within an acceptable range.

HYPOCALCEMIA AND OTHER THERAPEUTIC USES OF CALCIUM

Hypoparathyroidism is treated primarily with vitamin D and calcium supplementation. In severe hypocalcemia, symptoms are best treated intravenously. Calcium chloride, calcium gluceptate, and calcium gluconate all can be administered intravenously; the latter two are preferred because they are less irritating. The gluceptate salt also can be administered intramuscularly when the intravenous route is unavailable.

For milder hypocalcemic symptoms, oral calcium suffices, frequently in combination with vitamin D or one of its active metabolites. A number of calcium salts are available. Calcium carbonate is prescribed most frequently, whereas calcium citrate may be absorbed most efficiently. Cost and palatability often outweigh modest differences in efficacy.

THERAPEUTIC USES OF VITAMIN D

SPECIFIC FORMS OF VITAMIN D Calcitriol (1,25-dihydroxycholecalciferol; CALCIJEX, ROCALTROL) is available for oral and parenteral use. A number of derivatives are also used therapeutically (Figure 61–7). Doxercalciferol (1α-hydroxyvitamin D_2, HECTORAL), a prodrug that must be activated by hepatic 25-hydroxylation, is approved for treating secondary hyperparathyroidism. Dihydrotachysterol (DHT, ROXANE) is a reduced form of vitamin D_2 that is converted in the liver to its active form, 25-hydroxydihydrotachysterol. It is active at high doses in mobilizing bone Ca^{2+} and therefore can be used to maintain plasma Ca^{2+} in hypoparathyroidism. 1α-hydroxycholecalciferol (1-OHD$_3$, alphacalcidol; ONE-ALPHA) is a synthetic vitamin D_3 analog that is already hydroxylated in the 1α position and is rapidly converted by 25-hydroxylase to 1,25-(OH)$_2D_3$. Because it does not require renal activation, it has been used to treat renal osteodystrophy. Ergocalciferol (CALCIFEROL, DRISDOL) is vitamin D_2; it is available for oral, intramuscular, or intravenous administration. It is indicated for the prevention and treatment of vitamin D deficiency and for the treatment of hypoparathyroidism and the genetic disorders of vitamin D synthesis or action described above.

Calcitriol Analogs Several vitamin D analogs suppress PTH secretion by the parathyroid glands but have less or negligible hypercalcemic activity (Figure 61–7). They therefore have advantages in treating secondary hyperparathyroidism. Calcipotriol (calcipotriene) is a synthetic derivative of calcitriol with a modified side chain that is used topically for psoriasis (*see* Chapter 62). Paricalcitol (1,25-dihydrox-19-norvitamin D_2, ZEMPLAR) is a synthetic D_2 derivative that is FDA-approved for intravenous treatment of secondary hyperparathyroidism in patients with chronic renal failure. 22-oxacalcitriol (1,25-dihydroxy-22-oxavitamin D_3, OCT, maxacalcitol, OXAROL) has a low affinity for vitamin D-binding protein and thus has a shorter $t_{1/2}$. It is used in patients with secondary hyperparathyroidism due to renal failure.

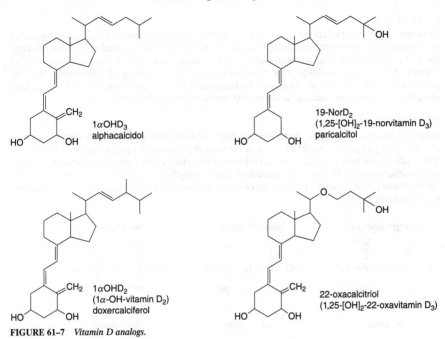

FIGURE 61–7 *Vitamin D analogs.*

Indications for Therapy with Vitamin D

NUTRITIONAL RICKETS

Nutritional rickets results from inadequate exposure to sunlight or deficiency of dietary vitamin D. Its incidence in the U.S. apparently is increasing. Breast-fed infants should receive 400 U of vitamin D daily as a supplement. Since the fetus acquires more than 85% of its calcium stores during the third trimester, premature infants are especially susceptible to rickets and may also require supplemental vitamin D. Treatment of fully developed rickets requires a larger dose of vitamin D. Although 1000 U/day probably is sufficient, daily doses of 3000–4000 U/day are frequently used to promote more rapid healing. Vitamin D may be given prophylactically in conditions that impair its absorption (e.g., diarrhea, steatorrhea, and biliary obstruction), sometimes by the parenteral route.

OSTEOMALACIA AND RENAL OSTEODYSTROPHY

Osteomalacia, distinguished by undermineralization of the bone matrix, occurs commonly during sustained phosphate depletion. Patients with chronic renal disease are at risk for developing osteomalacia, but also may develop the complex bone disease called renal osteodystrophy. In this setting, bone metabolism is stimulated by an increase in PTH and by a delay in bone mineralization due to decreased renal synthesis of calcitriol. Either a high turnover state reminiscent of primary hyperparathyroidism or a state of adynamic bone may result. The former is treated with dietary phosphate restriction and phosphate binders such as sevelamer (RENAGEL) and lanthanum carbonate (FOSRENOL). Renal osteodystrophy associated with adynamic bone disease may be due to overly aggressive suppression of PTH with calcitriol or other vitamin D analogs. Vitamin D therapy should be discontinued if the 25-OHD and serum calcium levels are elevated.

HYPOPARATHYROIDISM

Vitamin D and its analogs are the mainstay of the therapy of hypoparathyroidism. Dihydrotachysterol has a faster onset, shorter duration of action than 25-OHD, and traditionally has been the preferred agent. Calcitriol also is effective and often is used acutely while awaiting effects of slower-acting forms of vitamin D.

CALCITONIN

Measurement of serum calcitonin is used diagnostically to detect medullary thyroid cancer, especially in the setting of multiple endocrine neoplasia, type 2. Therapeutically, it is used in the acute management of hypercalcemia. It also is approved for Paget's disease, generally by subcutaneous injection because of limited bioavailability of the intranasal form, and for the therapy of osteoporosis. After initial therapy at 100 units/day, the dose typically is reduced to 50 units three times a week. Side effects include allergic reactions, nausea, hand swelling, urticaria, and rarely intestinal cramping.

BISPHOSPHONATES

Bisphosphonates are pyrophosphate analogs (Figure 61–8); they contain 2 phosphonate groups attached to a germinal (central) carbon that replaces the oxygen in pyrophosphate. They have a strong affinity for bone, especially areas undergoing remodeling. They are used extensively in conditions characterized by osteoclast-mediated bone resorption, including osteoporosis, steroid-induced osteoporosis, Paget's disease, tumor-associated osteolysis, breast and prostate cancer, and hypercalcemia.

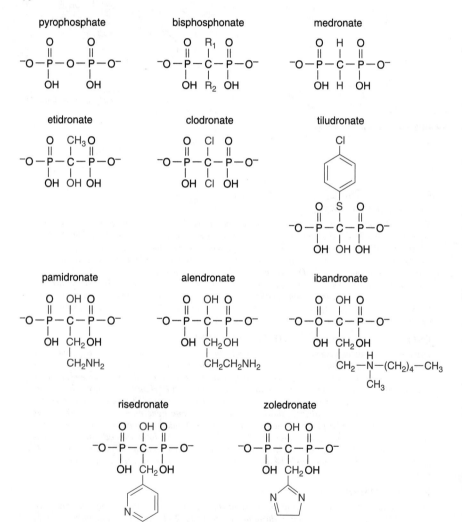

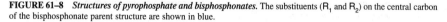

FIGURE 61–8 *Structures of pyrophosphate and bisphosphonates.* The substituents (R_1 and R_2) on the central carbon of the bisphosphonate parent structure are shown in blue.

Based on their side chains, the bisphosphonates are grouped into first-, second-, and third-generation drugs. First-generation drugs (*e.g.*, medronate, clodronate, and etidronate) contain minimally modified side-chains or a chlorophenyl group (*e.g.*, tiludronate) and are the least potent agents. Second-generation aminobisphosphonates (*e.g.*, pamidronate, alendronate, and ibandronate) contain an *N*-atom in the side chain and are 10–100 times more potent than the first-generation drugs. Third-generation drugs (*e.g.*, risedronate and zoledronate) contain an *N*-atom within a heterocyclic ring and are up to 10,000 times more potent than first-generation drugs.

Bisphosphonates concentrate at sites of active remodeling and are incorporated into the bone matrix. When the bone is remodeled, they are released in the acid environment of the resorption lacunae and induce apoptosis in the osteoclasts.

Available Bisphosphonates

Several bisphosphonates are available in the U.S. (Figure 61–8). Etidronate (DIDRONEL) is used for the treatment of Paget's disease but largely has been supplanted by pamidronate and zoledronate for hypercalcemia. Pamidronate (AREDIA) is approved in the U.S. for parenteral treatment of hypercalcemia (60–90 mg infused over 4 hours), and also is used for Paget's disease.

Several bisphosphonates are approved for the treatment of Paget's disease, including tiludronate (SKELID), alendronate (FOSAMAX), and risedronate (ACTONEL), typically at higher doses than those employed in osteoporosis. Zoledronate (ZOMETA) also appears to be quite effective as a single infusion of 4 mg.

ABSORPTION, FATE, AND EXCRETION

All oral bisphosphonates have very limited bioavailability. They should be administered with a full glass of water following an overnight fast and at least 30 minutes before breakfast. They are excreted primarily by the kidneys and are not recommended for patients with a creatinine clearance of less than 30 mL/min.

ADVERSE EFFECTS

Although oral bisphosphonates are generally well tolerated, some patients will experience symptoms of esophagitis. Symptoms often abate with fastidious adherence to recommendations for taking these drugs. If symptoms persist, a proton pump inhibitor at bedtime may be helpful. The oral drugs may be better tolerated when taken once weekly or monthly, with no reduction in efficacy. Patients with active upper GI disease should not be given oral bisphosphonates. Mild fever and aches may accompany the first infusion of pamidronate. These symptoms are short-lived and generally do not recur. Zoledronate has been associated with deterioration of renal function. Thus, zoledronate should be given over at least 15 minutes at a maximum dose of 4 mg. and renal function should be assessed periodically.

Therapeutic Uses

HYPERCALCEMIA Pamidronate is used parenterally in the management of malignancy-associated hypercalcemia. Zoledronate is also FDA-approved for this indication and appears to be more effective than pamidronate, at least as safe, and can be infused over 15 minutes rather than 4 hours.

POSTMENOPAUSAL OSTEOPOROSIS The use of bisphosphonates in the prevention and therapy of osteoporosis is described below.

CANCER Second- and third-generation bisphosphonates also may act as anticancer drugs by inhibiting the activation of cancer-associated proteins, such as Ras, through suppression of geranylgeranylation and farnesylation.

PARATHYROID HORMONE

Continuous administration of PTH or high circulating PTH levels achieved in primary hyperthyroidism causes bone demineralization and osteopenia. Paradoxically, intermittent PTH administration promotes bone growth. The FDA has approved human recombinant PTH (1-34) for treating severe osteoporosis, and full-length PTH is also undergoing clinical trials.

ABSORPTION, FATE, AND EXCRETION

Pharmacokinetics and systemic actions of PTH (1-34) (teriparatide, FORTEO) are identical to those for endogenous PTH. Teriparatide is administered by once-daily subcutaneous injection of 20 μg into the thigh or abdomen. With this regimen, serum PTH levels peak at 30 minutes after the injection and decline to undetectable levels within 3 hours. Teriparatide is eliminated by non-specific enzymatic mechanisms in the liver and kidney.

CLINICAL EFFECTS

In postmenopausal women with osteoporosis, teriparatide increases bone mineral density and reduces the risk of vertebral and nonvertebral fractures. The precise role of this agent relative to other agents used for osteoporosis, alone or in combination, remains to be determined. Candidates for teriparatide therapy at this time are women with a history of an osteoporotic fracture who have multiple risk factors for fracture and who are intolerant or have failed other therapies. The drug is also approved to increase bone mass in men with idiopathic or hypogonadal osteoporosis who are at high risk for fracture.

ADVERSE EFFECTS

In rats, teriparatide increased the incidence of bone tumors, including osteogenic sarcoma. The clinical relevance of this is unclear, especially since higher PTH levels in patients with primary hyperparathyroidism are not associated with an increased tumor risk. Nevertheless, teriparatide use should be limited to 24 months, and the drug should not be used in patients at increased risk for osteosarcoma (e.g., those with Paget's disease, unexplained elevations of alkaline phosphatase, open epiphyses, or prior radiation therapy involving the skeleton).

CALCIUM SENSOR MIMETICS: CINACALCET

Calcimimetics mimic the action of calcium via the CaSR to inhibit PTH secretion by the parathyroid glands. Because of this enhanced sensitivity, they decrease PTH secretion for any given level of Ca^{2+}. The calcimimetic cinacalcet (SENSIPAR) is FDA-approved for the treatment of secondary hyperparathyroidism due to chronic renal disease and for patients with hypercalcemia associated with parathyroid carcinoma (Figure 61–9). In clinical trials, cinacalcet also effectively reduced PTH levels in patients with primary hyperparathyroidism and normalized serum calcium without altering bone mineral density for up to 2 years.

Cinacalcet given orally achieves peak serum levels at 2–6 hours, with maximum biological action (suppression of PTH) at 2–4 hours after administration. After absorption, the drug is eliminated, primarily by the kidney, with a $t_{1/2}$ of 30–40 hours. The drug is also metabolized by multiple hepatic CYPs.

The recommended starting dose of cinacalcet for secondary hyperparathyroidism is 30 mg once daily, with a maximum of 180 mg/day. For the treatment of parathyroid carcinoma, a starting dose of 30 mg twice daily is recommended, with a maximum dose of 90 mg four times daily. The dose is titrated upward every 2–4 weeks to maintain the serum PTH level between 150 and 300 pg/mL (secondary hyperparathyroidism) or to normalize the serum calcium (parathyroid carcinoma). Cinacalcet likely will interact with other drugs that are metabolized by hepatic CYPs.

The principal adverse effect of cinacalcet is hypocalcemia. The drug should not be used if the initial serum calcium is <8.4 mg/dL; serum calcium and phosphate concentrations should be measured within one week and PTH should be measured within 4 weeks of therapy initiation. Adynamic bone disease may develop in patients with secondary hyperparathyroidism, so the drug should be discontinued or the dose decreased if the PTH level falls below 150 pg/mL.

INTEGRATED APPROACH TO OSTEOPOROSIS PREVENTION AND TREATMENT

Osteoporosis is a growing problem in developed nations, causing fractures in 30–50% of older women and 15–30% of older men. Drugs used to manage osteoporosis act by decreasing the rate of bone resorption, thereby slowing the rate of bone loss (antiresorptive therapy), or by promoting bone formation (anabolic therapy). Since bone remodeling is a coupled process, antiresorptive

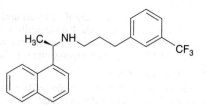

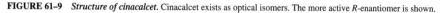

FIGURE 61–9 *Structure of cinacalcet.* Cinacalcet exists as optical isomers. The more active *R*-enantiomer is shown.

drugs ultimately decrease the rate of bone formation and therefore do not promote substantial gains in bone mineral density. Pharmacotherapy of osteoporosis is aimed at restoring bone strength and preventing fractures. The linchpin of this approach has long been antiresorptive drugs such as the bisphosphonates, estrogen, or more recently, the selective estrogen receptor modulator (SERM) raloxifene. These drugs inhibit osteoclast-mediated bone loss, thereby reducing bone turnover. The increases in bone density that they produce are variable and depend on the site and the specific drug (Figure 61–10).

Therapeutic options for osteoporosis were expanded in 2002 when the FDA approved teriparatide for use in treating postmenopausal women with osteoporosis and to increase bone mass in men with osteoporosis. Pharmacotherapy likely will evolve as newer treatment strategies are developed and combinations of antiresorptive and anabolic agents are introduced.

ANTIRESORPTIVE AGENTS

Bisphosphonates Bisphosphonates have emerged as the most effective drugs for treatment and prevention of osteoporosis. Second- and third-generation oral agents (*e.g.,* alendronate, risedronate, ibandronate) have sufficient potency to suppress bone resorption at doses that generally do not inhibit mineralization. They generally are well tolerated (especially when given weekly or monthly). For patients in whom the oral drugs cause severe esophageal distress despite countermeasures, ibandronate (BONIVA, 3 mg every 3 months) can be given intravenously for skeletal protection. A formulation of alendronate in combination with vitamin D (FOSAMAX PLUS D) is approved for treatment of osteoporosis.

Calcium The utility of supplemental calcium to protect bone has been the subject of considerable debate. While the impact of supplementation in adolescents, young adults, or early postmenopausal women is argued, some studies do suggest that supplemental calcium in the elderly, typically in combination with vitamin D, suppresses bone turnover, improves bone mineral density, and decreases the incidence of fractures. Typical dosing has been in the range of 1000 mg/day in adolescents and young adults and 1500 mg/day in the elderly. Calcium supplements are most often taken with meals to improve absorption.

Vitamin D and Its Analogs The role for oral supplementation with vitamin D also has been controversial; at least one prospective trial found that neither vitamin D nor calcium had a major impact on prevention of osteoporotic fractures in women. Nonetheless, supplemental vitamin D may be of value in patients whose intake appears inadequate based on dietary assessment.

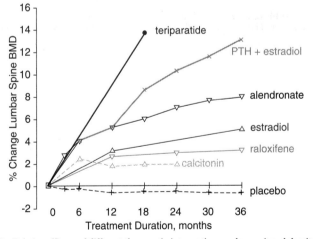

FIGURE 61–10 *Relative efficacy of different therapeutic interventions on bone mineral density of the lumbar spine.* Teriparatide (40 μg), PTH (25 μg) + estradiol, alendronate (10 mg), estradiol (0.625 mg/day), raloxifene (120 mg), calcitonin (200 IU). Typical results with placebo treatment underscore the inexorable bone loss without intervention. Some of the indicated treatment interventions involved combination therapy, and absolute comparisons should not be made.

Estrogen   Postmenopausal status or estrogen deficiency at any age significantly increases the risk for osteoporosis. Likewise, overwhelming evidence supports the positive impact of post-menopausal estrogen replacement on bone conservation and protection against osteoporotic frac-tures. The apparently increased risk of adverse cardiovascular events in prospective studies has led to the recommendation that hormone replacement therapy should not be first-line therapy for pre-vention or treatment of osteoporosis.

Selective Estrogen Receptor Modulators   Raloxifene (EVISTA) acts as an estrogen agonist on bone and liver, is inactive on the uterus, and acts as an estrogen antagonist on the breast. In post-menopausal women, raloxifene modestly increases bone mineral density and has been shown to reduce the risk of vertebral compression fractures; in this setting, it is approved for both the pre-vention and treatment of osteoporosis. The major adverse effect is worsened vasomotor symptoms; the drug also increases the incidence of deep venous thrombosis.

Calcitonin   Calcitonin modestly increases bone mass in patients with osteoporosis, particu-larly those with high bone turnover and is approved for the treatment of established osteoporosis in postmenopausal women.

Combination Therapies

Simultaneous use of PTH and bisphosphonates may inhibit the increase in bone mineral density typically caused by the anabolic agent. A rational strategy is to use anabolic agents (*e.g.*, teri-paratide) to increase bone formation, followed by antiresorptive therapy with agents such as bis-phosphonates to maintain bone density. The efficacy of such combination therapy in preventing fractures remains to be established in clinical trials.

Paget's Disease

Indications for pharmacotherapy in Paget's disease include severe pain, nerve compression, progressive deformity, hypercalcemia, high-output congestive heart failure, and high fracture risk (i.e., involvement of weight-bearing bones). Bisphosphonates and calcitonin decrease the high rate of bone turnover, often with a salutary decrease in symptoms and alkaline phosphatase level. Either oral or intravenous administration can be used; in patients in whom oral administration is ineffective or poorly tolerated, pamidronate or zoledronate infusions every few months are often effective, with repeat dosing guided by symptoms and alkaline phosphatase levels. Calcitonin generally is viewed as second-line therapy.

For a complete Bibliographical listing see Goodman & Gilman's *The Pharmacological Basis of Therapeutics*, 11th ed., or Goodman & Gilman Online at www.accessmedicine.com.

62

DERMATOLOGICAL PHARMACOLOGY

THE STRUCTURE AND FUNCTION OF SKIN

A unique aspect of dermatological pharmacology is the direct accessibility of the skin as a target organ for diagnosis and treatment (Figure 62–1). The skin acts as a two-way barrier to prevent absorption or loss of water and electrolytes. The barrier resides in the outermost layer of the epidermis, the stratum corneum, as evidenced by approximately equal rates of penetration of chemicals through isolated stratum corneum or whole skin. Having lost their nuclei and cytoplasmic organelles, the corneocytes of the stratum corneum are nonviable. The cells are flattened, and the fibrous keratins are aligned into disulfide cross-linked macrofibers in association with filaggrin, the major protein component of the keratohyalin granule. Each cell develops a cornified envelope resulting from cross-linking of involucrin and keratohyalin, forming an insoluble exoskeleton that acts as a rigid scaffold for the internal keratin filaments. The intercellular spaces are filled with hydrophobic lamellar lipids derived from membrane-coating granules. The combination of hydrophilic cornified cells in hydrophobic intercellular material provides a barrier to both hydrophilic and hydrophobic substances. In dermatological diseases, the thickened epidermis may further diminish the penetration of pharmacological agents into the dermis.

DRUG DELIVERY IN DERMATOLOGICAL DISEASES

Topical Preparations

Appropriate use of topical agents requires an appreciation of the factors that influence percutaneous absorption (*see* Chapter 1). Molecules can penetrate the skin by three routes: through intact stratum corneum, through sweat ducts, or through the sebaceous follicle. The surface of the stratum corneum presents more than 99% of the total skin surface available for percutaneous drug absorption. Passage through this outermost layer is the rate-limiting step for percutaneous absorption. The major steps involved in percutaneous absorption include the establishment of a concentration gradient, which provides the driving force for drug movement across the skin; release of drug from the vehicle (partition coefficient); and drug diffusion across the layers of the skin (diffusion coefficient). Preferable characteristics of topical drugs include low molecular mass (600 Da), adequate solubility in oil and water, and a high partition coefficient. Except for very small particles, water-soluble ions and polar molecules do not penetrate intact stratum corneum.

Metabolism

The viable epidermis contains a variety of enzyme systems capable of metabolizing drugs that reach this compartment, including CYPs, epoxide hydrolase, transferases such as *N*-acetyl-transferases, and diverse enzymes including glucuronyl transferases and sulfatases. Transporter proteins that influence influx (OATP) or efflux (MDR and LRD) of certain xenobiotics are present in human keratinocytes. While substrate turnover is considerably less than that for hepatic CYPs, these enzymes influence concentrations of xenobiotics in the skin.

General Guidelines for Topical Therapy

ALTERED BARRIER FUNCTION   In many dermatological diseases, such as psoriasis, the stratum corneum is abnormal, and barrier function is compromised. In these settings, percutaneous absorption may be increased to the point that standard drug doses can result in systemic toxicity (*e.g.*, hypothalamic–pituitary–adrenal axis suppression can result from systemic absorption of potent topical glucocorticoids).

HYDRATION   Drug absorption is increased with *hydration*. Methods of hydration include occlusion with an impermeable film, application of lipophilic occlusive vehicles such as ointments, and soaking dry skin before occlusion.

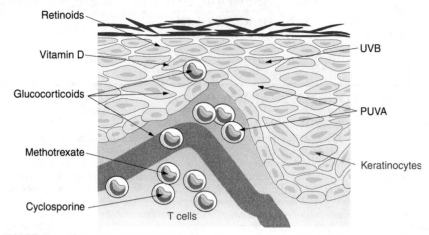

FIGURE 62–1 *Skin as a pharmacological target.* The skin is a multicellular organ containing numerous indigenous cells and structures as well as circulating cells that are potential targets for pharmacological intervention (*black arrows*). UVB, ultraviolet radiation (290–320 nm); PUVA, psoralen activated by UVA radiation (320–400 nm).

VEHICLE Most topical medications are incorporated into bases or vehicles that are applied directly to the skin. The chosen vehicle can influence drug absorption and provide therapeutic efficacy; for example, an ointment is more occlusive and has superior emollient properties than a cream or a lotion base.

Newer vehicles include liposomes and microgel formulations. Liposomes are concentric spherical shells of phospholipids in an aqueous medium that may enhance percutaneous absorption. Variations in size, charge, and lipid content can influence liposome function substantially. Liposomes penetrate compromised epidermal barriers more efficiently. Microgels are polymers that may enhance solubilization of certain drugs, thereby enhancing penetration and diminishing irritancy.

Transfersomes are a drug-delivery technology based on highly deformable, ultraflexible lipid vesicles that penetrate the skin when applied nonocclusively. Finally, pressure waves generated by intense laser radiation can permeabilize the stratum corneum and may provide a novel system for transdermal drug delivery.

Age

Children have a greater ratio of surface area to mass than adults, so a given amount of topical drug results in a greater systemic dose. Based on transepidermal water loss and percutaneous absorption studies, term infants seem to possess a stratum corneum with barrier properties comparable with adults.

Application Frequency

For certain drugs, once-daily application of a larger dose may be as effective as more frequent applications of smaller doses. The stratum corneum may act as a drug reservoir that allows gradual penetration into the viable skin layers over a prolonged period. Intermittent pulse therapy— treatment for several days or weeks alternating with treatment-free periods—may prevent development of tachyphylaxis associated with drugs such as topical glucocorticoids.

Intralesional Administration

Intralesional drug administration is used mainly for inflammatory lesions but also can be used for treatment of warts and selected neoplasms. Medications injected intralesionally have the advantages of direct contact with the underlying pathologic process, no first-pass metabolism, and the formation of a slowly absorbed depot of drug. In considering the use of intralesional medications, it is important to be cognizant of the possibility of systemic absorption of the medication.

GLUCOCORTICOIDS

Glucocorticoids are prescribed frequently for their immunosuppressive and anti-inflammatory properties. They are administered locally, through topical and intralesional routes, and systemically, through intramuscular, intravenous, and oral routes.

Mechanisms of glucocorticoid action are numerous, as discussed in Chapter 59. These include apoptosis of lymphocytes, inhibitory effects on the arachidonic acid cascade, depression of production of many cytokines, and myriad effects on inflammatory cells.

Topical glucocorticoids (*see* Chapter 59, Table 59–4) can be grouped based on potency and many of the more potent drugs have a fluorinated hydrocortisone backbone.

THERAPEUTIC USES Many inflammatory skin diseases respond to topical or intralesional administration of glucocorticoids. Absorption varies among body areas; the steroid is selected on the basis of its potency, the site of involvement, and the severity of the skin disease. Often, a more potent steroid is used initially, followed by a less potent agent. Twice-daily application is sufficient, and more frequent application does not improve response. In general, only nonfluorinated glucocorticoids should be used on the face or in occluded areas such as the axillae or groin.

Intralesional preparations of glucocorticoids include insoluble preparations of *triamcinolone acetonide* (KENALOG-10, others) and *triamcinolone hexacetonide* (KENOLOG-40 and ARISTOSPAN), which solubilize gradually and therefore have a prolonged duration of action.

TOXICITY AND MONITORING Chronic use of potent topical glucocorticoids (*e.g.,* diflorasone diacetate 0.05%, betamethasone dipropionate 0.05%) can cause skin atrophy, striae, telangiectasias, purpura, and acneiform eruptions. Because perioral dermatitis and rosacea can develop after the use of fluorinated compounds on the face, they should not be used in this site.

Systemic Glucocorticoids

THERAPEUTIC USES Systemic glucocorticoid therapy is used for severe dermatological illnesses. In general, it is best to reserve this method for allergic contact dermatitis to plants (*e.g.,* poison ivy) and for life-threatening vesiculobullous dermatoses such as pemphigus vulgaris and bullous pemphigoid. Chronic administration of oral glucocorticoids is problematic, given the side effects associated with their long-term use (*see* Chapter 59).

Daily morning dosing with *prednisone* generally is preferred, although divided doses are used occasionally to enhance efficacy. Fewer side effects are seen with alternate-day dosing, and if required for chronic therapy, prednisone is tapered to every other day as soon as it is practical. Pulse therapy using large intravenous doses of *methylprednisolone sodium succinate* (SOLU-MEDROL) is an option for severe resistant pyoderma gangrenosum, pemphigus vulgaris, systemic lupus erythematosus with multisystem disease, and dermatomyositis. The dose usually is 0.5–1 g given over 2–3 hours. More rapid infusion has been associated with increased rates of hypotension, electrolyte shifts, and cardiac arrhythmias.

TOXICITY AND MONITORING Most side effects are dose-dependent. Long-term use is associated with a number of complications, including psychiatric problems, cataracts, myopathy, osteoporosis, avascular bone necrosis, glucose intolerance or overt diabetes mellitus, and hypertension. In addition, psoriatic patients treated with parenteral or topical glucocorticoids may have a pustular flare, particularly if the steroid is tapered rapidly.

RETINOIDS

Retinoids include natural compounds and synthetic derivatives of retinol that exhibit vitamin A activity. First-generation retinoids include *retinol, tretinoin* (all-*trans*-retinoic acid), *isotretinoin* (13-*cis*-retinoic acid), and *alitretinoin* (9-*cis*-retinoic acid). Second-generation retinoids, also known as *aromatic retinoids*, were created by alteration of the cyclic end group and include *acitretin*. Third-generation retinoids contain further modifications and are called *arotinoids*. Members of this generation include *tazarotene* and *bexarotene*. *Adapalene*, a derivative of naphthoic acid with retinoid-like properties, does not fit precisely into any of the three generations.

Retinoic acid (RA) exerts its effects on gene expression by activating two families of receptors—*retinoic acid receptors* (RARs) and the *retinoid X receptors* (RXRs)—that are members of the nuclear receptor superfamily. Retinoids (ligands) bind transcription factors (nuclear receptors), and the ligand–receptor complex then binds to the promoter regions of target genes to regulate their expression. The gene products formed contribute to the desirable pharmacological effects of these drugs and their unwanted side effects. Additional complexity arises because each receptor has three isoforms (α, β, and γ) that form homo- and heterodimers. Retinoid-responsive tissues express one or more RAR and RXR subtypes in various combinations that determine activity locally. Human skin contains mainly RARα and RARβ.

First- and second-generation retinoids can bind to several retinoid receptors because of the flexibility imparted by their alternating single and double bonds. This relative lack of receptor specificity may lead to greater side effects. The structures of third-generation retinoids are much less flexible than those of earlier-generation retinoids and therefore are more selective.

Acute retinoid toxicity is similar to vitamin A intoxication. Side effects of retinoids include dry skin, nosebleeds from dry mucous membranes, conjunctivitis, and hair loss. Less frequently, musculoskeletal pain, pseudotumor cerebri, and mood alterations occur. Oral retinoids are potent teratogens and cause severe fetal malformations. Because of this, *systemic retinoids should be used with great caution in females of childbearing potential.*

Retinoids are used in the treatment of diverse diseases and are effective in the treatment of inflammatory skin disorders, skin malignancies, hyperproliferative disorders, photoaging, and many other disorders. Topical retinoids can normalize disordered keratinization in sebaceous follicles and reduce inflammation, and they may enhance the penetration of other topical medications.

Tretinoin

Tretinoin (RETIN-A, others) is used to reduce the hyperkeratinization that leads to microcomedone formation, the initial lesion in acne. Follicular corneocytes become less cohesive as a result of shedding of desmosomes, decreasing tonofilaments, and increasing keratinocyte autolysis and intracellular deposition of glycogen.

In addition to treating acne, tretinoin improves photodamaged human skin. Ultraviolet radiation activates growth factor and cytokine receptors on epidermal keratinocytes and dermal cells. These receptors stimulate MAP kinases, which, in turn, induce c-Jun expression. This transcription factor heterodimerizes with c-Fos to form activated AP-1 complexes that induce the transcription of metalloproteinases that degrade dermal collagens and other proteins. Epidermal effects of tretinoin include increased epidermal and granular layer thickness, decreased melanocytic activity, and increased secretion of a glycosaminoglycan-like substance into the intercellular space. In the dermis, blood vessel vasodilation and angiogenesis and increased papillary dermal collagen synthesis have been documented. Clinically, this translates to modest attenuation of fine and coarse wrinkling, smoother texture, increased pinkness, and diminished hyperpigmentation.

Tretinoin is approved for the treatment of acne vulgaris and as an adjunctive agent for treating photoaging. Topical preparations contain from 0.01% to 0.1% tretinoin in cream, gel, and solution formulations. Initiation of therapy with lower-strength preparations and progression to higher strengths may be useful because individual sensitivity is unpredictable. Tretinoin formulations with a cream base are indicated for dry skin, whereas gel-based formulations are indicated for oily skin. The medication is applied once daily before bedtime to minimize photodegradation. Maximum clinical response in acne may require several months, and maintenance therapy is necessary. A formulation of tretinoin with active drug incorporated into microsponges (RETIN-A MICRO) decreases irritation by slowing the release of the medication and enhances efficacy by targeting delivery to the sebaceous follicle.

A 0.5% emollient cream formulation of tretinoin (RENOVA) is approved for treatment of photoaged skin. Nightly application produces maximum response within 1 year, and application 1–3 times weekly is said to maintain improvement. Treatment must be combined with a rigorous program of photoprotection, including sunscreens, sun avoidance, and photoprotective clothing.

Adapalene

Adapalene (DIFFERIN), a derivative of naphthoic acid, is a synthetic retinoid-like compound that is available in solution, cream, and gel formulations for topical use. In addition to displaying typical retinoid effects, it also has anti-inflammatory properties. Adapalene has similar efficacy to tretinoin, but unlike tretinoin, it is stable in sunlight and tends to be less irritating.

Tazarotene

Tazarotene (TAZORAC) is a third-generation retinoid approved for the treatment of psoriasis and acne vulgaris. This retinoid binds to all three RARs.

Tazarotene gel, applied once daily to dry skin, may be used as monotherapy or in combination with other medications, such as topical corticosteroids, for the treatment of localized plaque psoriasis. This is the first topical retinoid approved by the FDA for the treatment of psoriasis. Side effects of burning, itching, and skin irritation are relatively common, and patients should avoid sun exposure.

Alitretinoin

Alitretinoin (PANRETIN) is a retinoid that binds all types of retinoid receptors and is approved only for treatment of the skin manifestations of Kaposi's sarcoma. Approximately 50% of patients in an open-label trial responded positively to topical application of this drug.

TOXICITY AND MONITORING   Adverse effects of all topical retinoids include erythema, desquamation, burning, and stinging. These effects often decrease spontaneously with time and are lessened by concomitant use of emollients. Photosensitivity can occur as a result of epidermal thinning, with a resulting greater potential for phototoxic reactions such as sunburn. Although there is little systemic absorption of tretinoin and no alteration in plasma vitamin A levels with its use as a topical agent, most physicians do not prescribe tretinoin during pregnancy and it is category X for pregnant women.

Isotretinoin

Oral isotretinoin (ACCUTANE) is approved for the treatment of severe nodulocystic acne vulgaris. The drug has remarkable efficacy in severe acne and may induce prolonged remissions after a single course of therapy. It normalizes keratinization in the sebaceous follicle, reduces sebocyte number with decreased sebum synthesis, and reduces *Propionibacterium acnes,* the organism that produces inflammation in acne.

THERAPEUTIC USES   Isotretinoin is administered orally. The recommended dose is 0.5–2 mg/kg/day for 15–20 weeks. Lower doses are effective but are associated with shorter remissions. The cumulative dose also is important, so smaller doses for longer periods can be used to achieve a total dose in the range of 120 mg/kg. Approximately 40% of patients will relapse, usually within 3 years of therapy, and may require retreatment. Preteens and patients with acne conglobata or androgen excess are at increased risk of relapse. However, mild relapses may respond to conventional management with topical and systemic antiacne agents.

Isotretinoin is prescribed for severe, recalcitrant nodular acne, moderate acne unresponsive to oral antibiotics, and acne that produces scarring. It also is used commonly for other related disorders, such as gram-negative folliculitis, acne rosacea, and hidradenitis suppurativa.

TOXICITY AND MONITORING   Dose-dependent adverse effects on the skin and mucous membranes are observed most commonly, including cheilitis, mucous membrane dryness, epistaxis, dry eyes, blepharoconjunctivitis, erythematous eruptions, and xerosis. Alteration of epidermal surfaces may facilitate *Staphylococcus aureus* colonization and, rarely, subsequent infection. Hair loss, exuberant granulation tissue formation, photosensitivity, and decreased night vision are rarer occurrences.

Systemic side effects generally are less significant with short-term therapy. Transitory elevations in serum transaminases occur rarely. Hyperlipidemia is frequent, with 25% of patients developing increased triglyceride levels and, less frequently, increased cholesterol and low-density lipoproteins, and decreased high-density lipoproteins. Myalgias and arthralgias are common complaints. Headaches occur and rarely are a symptom of pseudotumor cerebri. Use of isotretinoin concomitantly with *tetracycline* antibiotics may increase the risk of pseudotumor cerebri.

Some physicians have proposed a causal relationship with mood changes and depression in a limited number of patients. These uncontrolled clinical observations have not been examined in a rigorous, prospective manner. In addition, there is a paucity of data on the effect of retinoids on adult brain function. Long-term therapy may produce skeletal side effects, including diffuse idiopathic skeletal hyperostoses, extraskeletal ossification (particularly at tendinous insertions), and premature epiphyseal closure in children.

Teratogenicity is a major problem; it occurs if the drug is given within the first 3 weeks of gestation and is not dose-related. Teratogenic effects include CNS, cardiac, thymus, and craniofacial abnormalities. Spontaneous abortion occurs in one-third of patients. *Pregnancy is an absolute contraindication to the use of isotretinoin.* Two forms of birth control (one of which must be surgical or hormonal) must be practiced during therapy and for 1 month both before beginning therapy and after completion of therapy; pregnancy tests should be repeated monthly. Patients should not donate blood for transfusion during treatment and for 1 month after treatment.

Other laboratory evaluations should include a complete blood count, liver function tests, and fasting lipid determination before initiating therapy. Testing should be repeated after 1 month of therapy and thereafter only as abnormalities indicate.

Acitretin

Acitretin (SORIATANE) is the major metabolite of *etretinate*, an aromatic retinoid that formerly was approved for psoriasis but withdrawn from the market because of its undesirable pharmacokinetics. Acitretin has an elimination $t_{1/2}$ of 2–3 days.

Acitretin is readily esterified *in vivo* to produce etretinate, especially in the presence of *ethanol*. The optimal dosing range for acitretin in adults is 25–50 mg/day, providing efficacy with an acceptable level of side effects. Improvement of plaque psoriasis requires up to 3–6 months for optimal results. As monotherapy, acitretin has an overall rate of complete remission of <50%; response rates are higher when the drug is combined with other modalities. At doses of 10–25 mg/day, both pustular and erythrodermic psoriasis usually respond more rapidly than common plaque psoriasis. Excellent control of these conditions usually can be achieved with acitretin. Common side effects include dry skin and mucous membranes, xerophthalmia, and hair thinning. Less frequently, arthralgias and decreased night vision have been noted. Serious side effects (*e.g.,* hepatotoxicity or pseudotumor cerebri) are rare. *Acitretin is a potent teratogen and should not be used by females who intend to become pregnant during therapy or at any time for at least 3 years following discontinuation of therapy.* The same precautions regarding blood donation described earlier for isotretinoin should be followed. Laboratory monitoring should include a baseline pregnancy test in all female patients and a complete blood count, lipid profile, and hepatic profile in all patients. Serial follow-up of laboratory tests should be conducted every 1–2 weeks until stable and thereafter as clinically indicated.

Bexarotene

Bexarotene (TARGRETIN) is a retinoid that selectively binds RXRs. Bexarotene has been used in patients with cutaneous T-cell lymphoma with a suggested dose of 300 mg/m^2/day. Inhibitors of CYP3A4 (*e.g., imidazole antifungals* and *macrolide antibiotics*) will increase and inducers of the CYP3A4 system will decrease plasma levels of bexarotene. Side effects include lipid abnormalities, hypothyroidism secondary to a reversible RXR-mediated suppression of *TSH* gene expression, pancreatitis, leukopenia, and GI symptoms. Blood lipids and thyroid function should be measured before initiating therapy and periodically thereafter.

CANCER CHEMOPREVENTION WITH RETINOIDS   Systemic and topical retinoids have been used successfully to treat premalignant skin conditions and may have a role in chemoprevention of skin malignancies. High-dose isotretinoin (2 mg/kg/day) has suppressed skin cancers in patients with increased risk of skin malignancy from congenital disorders such as xeroderma pigmentosa and nevoid basal cell carcinoma syndrome. To achieve an anticancer effect, toxic doses of retinoids generally are required. Acitretin at a dose of 25 mg/day or more appears to reduce the risk of skin cancer by ~25% among patients with psoriasis who are at high risk for squamous cell carcinoma. Isotretinoin also is effective for oral leukoplakia. Topical tazarotene has shown efficacy in some basal cell carcinomas. Cutaneous T-cell lymphoma has been shown to respond to several types of topical and systemic retinoids, including bexarotene. The benefits of long-term retinoid use in malignant lymphomas such as cutaneous T-cell lymphoma are balanced by appreciation of retinoid toxicity and the chronicity of the disease.

PHOTOCHEMOTHERAPY

Electromagnetic radiation is defined by its wavelength and frequency; for convenience, it can be classified into different regions based on its photon energy. For therapeutic purposes, dermatologists are most concerned with the ultraviolet (UV) B (290–320 nm), A-I (320–340 nm), and A-II (340–400 nm) and visible (400–800 nm) spectrum. UVB is the most erythrogenic and melanogenic. It is the major action spectrum for sunburn, tanning, skin cancer, and photoaging. The longer wavelengths of UVA are a thousand times less erythrogenic than UVB; however, they penetrate more deeply into the skin and contribute substantially to photoaging and photosensitivity diseases. They also enhance UVB-induced erythema and increase the risk of skin carcinogenesis. Visible radiation may augment the severity of some photosensitive eruptions.

Electromagnetic radiation has proven to be highly efficacious in the treatment of numerous dermatologic diseases. Phototherapy and photochemotherapy are treatment methods in which ultraviolet or visible radiation is used to induce a therapeutic response either alone or in the presence of a photosensitizing drug. Phototherapy using UVB or high-dose UVA-I is efficacious in selected dermatological diseases. To be effective, the incident radiation must be absorbed by a target or chromophore in the skin—which in phototherapy is endogenous and in photochemotherapy must be administered exogenously. Patients treated with these modalities should be monitored for concomitant use of other potential photosensitizing medications before initiation of therapy. Such drugs include phenothiazines, thiazides, sulfonamides, nonsteroidal anti-inflammatory agents, sulfonylureas, *tetracyclines, and* benzodiazepines.

PUVA: Psoralens and UVA

Orally administered 8-methoxypsoralen *followed by UVA (PUVA) is FDA-approved for the treatment of vitiligo, psoriasis, and cutaneous T-cell lymphoma.*

CHEMISTRY

Psoralens belong to the furocoumarin class of compounds. They occur naturally in many plants, including limes, lemons, figs, and parsnips. Two psoralens, 8-methoxypsoralen (methoxsalen) *and 4, 5, 8-trimethylpsoralen* (trioxsalen, TRISORALEN) *are available in the U.S. Methoxsalen is used primarily because of its superior GI absorption.*

PHARMACOKINETICS The psoralens are absorbed rapidly after oral administration. Photosensitivity typically is maximal 1–2 hours after ingestion of methoxsalen. There is significant but saturable first-pass elimination in the liver, which may account for variations in plasma levels among individuals after a standard dose. Methoxsalen has a serum $t_{1/2}$ of approximately 1 hour, but the skin remains sensitive to light for 8–12 hours. Despite widespread drug distribution throughout the body, it is photoactivated only in the skin where the UVA penetrates.

MECHANISM OF ACTION The action spectrum for oral PUVA is between 320 and 400 nm. Two distinct photoreactions take place. Type I reactions involve the oxygen-independent formation of mono- and bifunctional adducts in DNA. Type II reactions are oxygen-dependent and involve sensitized transfer of energy to molecular O_2. The therapeutic effects of PUVA in psoriasis may result from a decrease in DNA-dependent proliferation after adduct formation. Perhaps more important, PUVA can alter cytokine profiles and cause immunocyte apoptosis, thereby interrupting immunopathologic processes.

THERAPEUTIC USES Methoxsalen is supplied in soft gelatin capsules (OXSORALEN-ULTRA) and hard gelatin capsules (8-MOP). The dose is 0.4 mg/kg for the soft capsule and 0.6 mg/kg for the hard capsule taken 1.5–2 hours before UVA exposure. A lotion containing 1% methoxsalen (OXSORALEN) also is available for topical application. It can be diluted for use in bath water to minimize systemic absorption. The risk of phototoxicity is increased with topical PUVA therapy. In studies of PUVA for the treatment of psoriasis, initial clearance rates approaching 90% were achieved. Relapse occurs within 6 months of cessation of treatment in many patients, which has prompted efforts to design maintenance protocols.

PUVA also is used to repigment the leukoderma of vitiligo. Success rates are highest in young individuals with recent onset of disease involving nonacral areas. Localized vitiligo can be treated with topical PUVA and more extensive disease with systemic administration. PUVA also is employed in the treatment of cutaneous T-cell lymphoma, atopic dermatitis, alopecia areata, lichen planus, urticaria pigmentosa, and as a preventive modality in some forms of photosensitivity.

TOXICITY AND MONITORING The major acute side effects of PUVA include nausea, blistering, and painful erythema. PUVA-induced redness and blistering generally peak within 48–72 hours.

Chronic PUVA therapy accelerates photoaging and the development of actinic keratoses, nonmelanoma skin cancer, and melanoma. Squamous cell carcinomas occur at 10 times the expected frequency. In patients receiving 250 or more treatments, there is an increased risk of melanoma. Careful monitoring of patients for cutaneous carcinoma therefore is essential.

PHOTOPHERESIS Extracorporeal photopheresis (ECP) has proven effective in the treatment of cutaneous T-cell lymphoma. After oral administration of methoxsalen, leukocytes are separated from whole blood and then exposed to UVA radiation. The irradiated cells then are returned to the patient. Multiple mechanisms probably contribute to the effectiveness of this procedure. ECP simultaneously and efficiently induces apoptosis of disease-causing T cells and conversion of monocytes to functional dendritic cells. By processing and presenting the unique antigenic determinants of pathogenic T-cell clones, the dendritic cells can either initiate a clinically relevant anti–cutaneous T-cell lymphoma cytotoxic response or suppress the activity of autoreactive T-cell clones.

PHOTODYNAMIC THERAPY (PDT)   This modality combines the use of photosensitizing drugs and visible light for the treatment of various dermatological disorders, particularly nonmelanoma skin cancer and precancerous actinic keratoses. The concept is predicated on the insight that tumor tissue selectively absorbs greater amounts of porphyrins than surrounding nontumor tissue. The agents most widely employed in photodynamic therapy (PDT) are *porphyrins,* their precursors, or derivatives. The photosensitized chemical reaction is oxygen-dependent. Light delivered to the skin is absorbed by porphyrin molecules. These molecules transfer their energy to oxygen, forming reactive oxygen species that result in injury or destruction of lipid-rich membranes and subsequent tissue damage.

Early studies with PDT employed complex mixtures of poorly defined porphyrins known as hematoporphyrin derivative *(PHOTOFRIN I) or a partially purified mixture known as* porfimer sodium *(PHOTOFRIN II) that was administered parenterally with subsequent irradiation using polychromatic light sources. The major problem with this approach was the prolonged period (4–6 weeks) of photosensitivity caused by skin retention of the porphyrin formulations. This led to a search for compounds that could be administered topically and that were eliminated more readily from the skin. The porphyrin precursor δ-aminolevulinic acid (ALA) is converted to various porphyrins, particularly* protoporphyrin *(PROTO), in tissues including the skin (see below). Protoporphyrin subsequently is eliminated rapidly from the body, thereby minimizing the period of skin photosensitivity to a few hours. Topically applied ALA HCl (20% w/v) and, more recently, the methyl ester of ALA have been used successfully for the PDT of various types of nonmelanoma skin cancers and premalignant lesions.*
Incoherent (nonlaser) and laser light sources have been used for PDT. The wavelengths chosen must include those within the action spectrum of protoporphyrin and ideally those that permit maximum skin penetration. Light sources in use emit energy predominantly in the blue portion (maximum porphyrin absorption) or the red portion (better tissue penetration) of the visible spectrum. Nonhypertrophic actinic keratoses and superficial basal cell carcinomas and Bowen's disease seem to respond best to PDT. Topical ALA products for PDT approved by the FDA include LEVULAN KERASTICK, BLU-U *blue light, and* METVIX.

ANTIHISTAMINES

Histamine is a potent vasodilator, bronchial smooth muscle constrictor, and stimulant of nociceptive itch nerves. In addition to histamine, multiple chemical itch mediators can act as pruritogens on C-fibers, including *neuropeptides, prostaglandins, serotonin, acetylcholine,* and *bradykinin.*

Human skin mast cells express H_1, H_2, and H_4 receptors but not H_3 receptors. H_1 and H_2 receptors are involved in wheal formation and erythema, whereas only H_1 receptor agonists cause pruritus. Complete blockade of H_1 receptors does not totally relieve itching, and combinations of H_1 and H_2 blockers may be superior to H_1 blockers alone.

Oral *antihistamines,* particularly H_1-receptor antagonists, have some anticholinergic activity and are sedating (*see* Chapter 24), making them useful for the control of pruritus. First-generation sedating H_1 receptor antagonists include *hydroxyzine hydrochloride* (ATARAX), which is given in a dose of 0.5 mg/kg every 6 hours; *diphenhydramine* (BENADRYL; others); *promethazine* (PHENERGAN); and *cyproheptadine* (PERIACTIN). *Doxepin* (ADAPIN, SINEQUAN), which has tricyclic antidepressant and sedative antihistamine effects (*see* Chapter 17), is a good alternative for severe pruritus. A topical formulation of doxepin also is available as a 5% cream (ZONALON), which can be used in conjunction with low-to-moderate potency topical glucocorticoids. The systemic effect from topical doxepin is comparable with that of low-dose oral therapy.

Second-generation H_1-receptor antagonists lack anticholinergic side effects and are described as nonsedating largely because they do not cross the blood–brain barrier. They include *cetirizine* (ZYRTEC), *loratadine* (CLARITIN), *desloratadine* (CLARINEX), and *fexofenadine hydrochloride* (ALLEGRA). While second-generation nonsedating H_1-receptor blockers are as effective as the first-generation H_1 blockers, they are metabolized by CYP3A4 and, to a lesser extent, by CYP2D6 and should not be coadministered with medications that inhibit these enzymes (*e.g.,* imidazole antifungals and macrolide antibiotics).

H_2-receptor blockers include *cimetidine* (TAGAMET), *ranitidine* (ZANTAC), *famotidine* (PEPCID), and *nizatidine* (AXID). Besides their use in combination with H_1-receptor blockers for pruritus, the H_2-receptor blockers have immunomodulating effects, and this property has been exploited in children to treat warts.

ANTIMICROBIAL AGENTS
Antibiotics

These drugs are used commonly to treat superficial cutaneous infections (pyoderma) and noninfectious diseases. Topical agents are very effective for the treatment of superficial bacterial infections and acne vulgaris. Systemic antibiotics also are prescribed commonly for acne and for deeper bacterial infections. The pharmacology of individual antibacterial agents is discussed in Section VIII, Chemotherapy of Microbial Diseases. Only the topical and systemic antibacterial agents principally used in dermatology are discussed here.

Acne vulgaris is the most common dermatologic disorder treated with either topical or systemic antibiotics. The anaerobe *P. acnes* is a component of normal skin flora that proliferates in the obstructed, lipid-rich lumen of the pilosebaceous unit, where O_2 tension is low. *P. acnes* generates free fatty acids that are irritants and may lead to microcomedo formation and result in the inflammatory lesions of acne. Suppression of cutaneous *P. acnes* with antibiotic therapy is correlated with clinical improvement.

Resistant strains of *P. acnes* are emerging that may respond to judicious use of retinoids in combination with antibiotics. Commonly used topical antimicrobials in acne include *erythromycin, clindamycin* (CLEOCIN-T), and *benzoyl peroxide* and antibiotic–benzoyl peroxide combinations (BENZAMYCIN, BENZACLIN, others). Other antimicrobials used in treating acne include *sulfacetamide* (KLARON), *sulfacetamide/sulfur combinations* (SULFACET-R), *metronidazole* (METROCREAM, METROGEL, NORITATE), and *azelaic acid* (AZELEX). *Systemic therapy* is prescribed for patients with more extensive disease and acne that is resistant to topical therapy. Effective agents include tetracycline (SUMYCIN, others), *minocycline* (MINOCIN, others), erythromycin (ERYC, others), clindamycin (CLEOCIN), and *trimethoprim–sulfamethoxazole* (BACTRIM, others). Antibiotics usually are administered twice daily, and doses are tapered after control is achieved. Tetracycline is the most commonly employed antibiotic because it is inexpensive, safe, and effective. The initial daily dose is usually 1 g in divided doses. Although tetracycline is an antimicrobial agent, its efficacy in acne may be more dependent on its anti-inflammatory activity.

Minocycline has better GI absorption than tetracycline and may be less photosensitizing than either tetracycline or doxycycline. Side effects of minocycline include dizziness and hyperpigmentation of the skin and mucosa, serum-sickness-like reactions, and drug-induced lupus erythematosus. With all the tetracyclines, vaginal candidiasis is a common complication that is readily treated with local administration of antifungal drugs.

In healthy individuals taking oral antibiotics for acne, laboratory monitoring is not necessary. Orally administered antibiotics also may be indicated in other noninfectious conditions, including acne rosacea, perioral dermatitis, hidradenitis suppurativa, autoimmune blistering diseases, sarcoidosis, and pyoderma gangrenosum.

Cutaneous Infections

Gram-positive organisms, including S. aureus *and* Streptococcus pyogenes, *are the most common cause of pyoderma. Skin infections with gram-negative bacilli are rare, although they can occur in diabetics and patients who are immunosuppressed; appropriate parenteral antibiotic therapy is required for their treatment.*

Topical therapy frequently is adequate for impetigo, the most superficial bacterial infection of the skin caused by S. aureus *and* S. pyogenes. *Pseudomonic acid (MUPIROCIN, BACTROBAN), produced by* Pseudomonas fluorescens, *is effective for such localized infections. It inhibits protein synthesis by binding to bacterial isoleucyl-tRNA synthetase. Mupirocin is highly active against staphylococci and all streptococci except those of group D. It is less active against gram-negative organisms, but it has* in vitro *activity against* Haemophilus influenzae, *Neisseria gonorrhoeae,* Pasteurella multocida, Moraxella catarrhalis, *and* Bordetella pertussis. *Its antibacterial activity is enhanced by the acid pH of the skin surface. Mupirocin is available as a 2% ointment or cream (BACTODERM, BACTROBAN, BACTROBAN NASAL, EISMYCIN) and is applied three times daily.*

Topical therapy often is employed for prophylaxis of superficial infections caused by wounds and injuries. Neomycin *is active against staphylococci and most gram-negative bacilli. It may cause allergic contact dermatitis, especially on disrupted skin.* Bacitracin *inhibits staphylococci, streptococci, and gram-positive bacilli.* Polymyxin B *is active against aerobic gram-negative bacilli. Bacitracin and polymyxin B are combined in a number of over-the-counter preparations.*

Deeper bacterial infections of the skin include folliculitis, erysipelas, cellulitis, and necrotizing fasciitis. Since streptococcal and staphylococcal species also are the most common causes of deep cutaneous infections, penicillins *(especially β-lactamase-resistant β-lactams), and* cephalosporins *are the systemic antibiotics used most frequently in their treatment (see Chapter 44). A growing concern is the increased incidence of skin and soft tissue infections with hospital- and community-acquired methicillin-resistant* S. aureus *(MRSA) and drug-resistant pneumococci. Infection with community-acquired MRSA often is susceptible to trimethoprim–sulfamethoxazole.*

Antifungal Agents

Fungal infections are among the most common causes of skin disease in the U.S., and numerous effective topical and oral antifungal agents have been developed. *Griseofulvin,* topical and oral *imidazoles, triazoles,* and *allylamines* are the most effective agents available. The pharmacology, uses, and toxicities of antifungal drugs are discussed in Chapter 48. Recommendations for cutaneous antifungal therapy are summarized in Table 62–1.

The azoles miconazole *(MICATIN, others)* and econazole *(SPECTRAZOLE, others) and the allylamines* naftifine *(NAFTIN)* and terbinafine *(LAMISIL, others) are effective topical agents for the treatment of localized tinea corporis and uncomplicated tinea pedis. Topical therapy with the azoles is preferred for localized cutaneous candidiasis and tinea versicolor.*

Systemic therapy is necessary for the treatment of tinea capitis. Oral griseofulvin (FULVICIN V/F, P/G, others) has been the traditional medication for treatment of tinea capitis. Oral terbinafine is a safe and effective alternative to griseofulvin in treating tinea capitis in children.

TINEA PEDIS Topical therapy with the azoles and allylamines is effective for tinea pedis. Macerated toe web disease may require the addition of antibacterial therapy. *Econazole nitrate,* which has a limited antibacterial spectrum, can be useful in this situation. Systemic therapy with griseofulvin, terbinafine, or *itraconazole* (SPORANOX, others) is used for more extensive tinea pedis. It should be recognized that long-term topical therapy may be necessary in some patients after courses of systemic antifungal therapy.

ONYCHOMYCOSIS Fungal infection of the nails is caused most frequently by dermatophytes and *Candida.* Mixed infections are common. The nail must be cultured or clipped for histological examination before initiating therapy because up to a third of dystrophic nails that appear clinically to be onychomycosis are actually due to psoriasis or other conditions.

Despite the availability of topical treatments, systemic therapy is necessary for effective management of onychomycosis. Treatment of toenails with griseofulvin for 12–18 months produces a cure rate of 50% and a relapse rate of 50% after 1 year. Terbinafine and itraconazole quickly produce high drug levels in the nail, which persist after therapy is discontinued. Additional advantages include a broader spectrum of coverage with itraconazole and few drug interactions with terbinafine. Treatment of toenail onychomycosis requires 3 months with terbinafine (250 mg/day) or itraconazole (pulsed dosing 1 week per month for 3 months). Cure rates of 75% or greater have been achieved with both drugs.

Antiviral Agents

Viral infections of the skin are very common and include verrucae (human papillomavirus [HPV]), herpes simplex (HSV), condyloma acuminatum (HPV), molluscum contagiosum (poxvirus), and chicken pox (varicella-zoster virus [VZV]). *Acyclovir* (ZOVIRAX), *famciclovir* (FAMVIR), and *valacyclovir* (VALTREX) frequently are used systemically to treat herpes simplex and varicella infections

Table 62–1

Recommended Cutaneous Antifungal Therapy

Condition	Topical Therapy	Oral Therapy
Tinea corporis, localized	Azoles, allylamines	—
Tinea corporis, widespread	—	Griseofulvin, terbinafine, itraconazole, fluconazole
Tinea pedis	Azoles, allylamines	Griseofulvin, terbinafine, itraconazole, fluconazole
Onychomycosis	—	Griseofulvin, terbinafine, itraconazole, fluconazole
Candidiasis, localized	Azoles	—
Candidiasis, widespread and mucocutaneous	—	Ketaconazole, itraconazole, fluconazole
Tinea versicolor, localized	Azoles, allylamines	
Tinea versicolor, widespread	—	Ketaconazole, itraconazole, fluconazole

(*see* Chapter 49). *Cidofovir* (VISTIDE) may be useful in treating acyclovir-resistant HSV or VZV and other cutaneous viral infections. Topically, acyclovir, *docosanol* (ABREVA), and *penciclovir* (DENAVIR) are available for treating mucocutaneous HSV. *Podophyllin* (25% solution) and *podofilox* (CONDYLOX; 0.5% solution) are used to treat condylomata. The immune response modifier *imiquimod* (ALDARA) is discussed below. Interferons α-2b (INTRONA), α-n1 (not commercially available in the U.S.), and α-n3 (ALFERON N) may be useful for treating refractory or recurrent warts.

Agents Used to Treat Infestations

Infestations with ectoparasites such as body lice and scabies are common throughout the world. These conditions have a significant impact on public health in the form of disabling pruritus, secondary infection, and in the case of the body louse, transmission of life-threatening illnesses such as typhus. Topical and oral medications are available to treat these infestations.

Perhaps the best known antiectoparasitic medication is 1% *γ-benzene hexachloride* lotion, also known as *lindane*.

Lindane has been used as a commercial insecticide as well as a topical medication. It is highly effective in the treatment of ectoparasites. Neurotoxicity, although a concern with the use of lindane, is a rare side effect when the medication is used correctly. However, the FDA has defined lindane as a second-line drug in treating pediculosis and scabies and has highlighted the potential for neurotoxicity in children and adults weighing <110 lb. The lotion is applied in a thin layer from the neck down, left in place for 8–12 hours or overnight, and removed by thorough washing at the end of the 8–12-hour period. The treatment may be repeated in 1 week. To avoid problems with neurotoxicity, the lotion should be applied only in a thin coat to dry skin, should not be applied immediately after bathing, and should be kept away from the eyes, mouth, and open cuts or sores. A 1% lindane shampoo also is available for head and body lice.

A second topical agent that is very useful in the treatment of ectoparasites is *permethrin*, a synthetic derivative of the insecticide pyrethrum, which was obtained originally from *Chrysanthemum cinerariifolium*. Neurotoxicity associated with this compound is rare. A 5% cream (ACTICIN, ELIMITE, others) is available for the treatment of scabies. This is used as an 8–12-hour or overnight application. A 1% permethrin cream rinse (NIX) also is available for the treatment of head lice.

Ivermectin (STROMECTOL), an anthelmintic drug (*see* Chapter 41) used traditionally to treat onchocerciasis, also is effective in the off-label treatment of scabies.

Because ivermectin does not cross the blood–brain barrier, there is no major CNS toxicity. Ivermectin, available as a 6-mg tablet, is given at a dose of 250–400 μg/kg, which is repeated in a week. Cure rates of 70% after one dose and 95% after two doses given 2 weeks apart have been achieved. For treatment of scabies outbreaks in large groups, this drug has obvious advantages as compared with topical therapy.

ANTIMALARIAL AGENTS

The major antimalarials used commonly in dermatology include *chloroquine* (ARALEN), *hydroxychloroquine* (PLAQUENIL), and to a lesser extent, *quinacrine* (no longer available in the U.S.); all three drugs are useful because of their anti-inflammatory effects, especially in connective tissue disorders and photosensitivity diseases (*see* Chapter 39).

The mechanism of action of the immunological and anti-inflammatory effects of antimalarials include inhibition of phospholipase A$_2$, inhibition of platelet aggregation, a range of lysosomal effects (e.g., an increase in pH, membrane stabilization, and inhibition of release and activity of lysosomal enzymes), inhibition of phagocytosis, an increase in intracellular pH in cytoplasmic vacuoles leading to decreased stimulation of autoimmune CD4$^+$ T cells, decreased cytokine release from lymphocytes and stimulated monocytes, inhibition of immune complex formation, and antioxidant activity. In patients with porphyria cutanea tarda, chloroquine and hydroxychloroquine bind to porphyrins and/or iron to facilitate their hepatic clearance. The ability to bind to melanin and other pigments may contribute to the retinal toxicity seen occasionally when antimalarial agents are used.

THERAPEUTIC USES   FDA-approved dermatological uses of hydroxychloroquine include treatment of discoid and systemic lupus erythematosus. Unapproved but first-line uses include treatment of dermatomyositis, porphyria cutanea tarda, polymorphous light eruption, sarcoidosis, eosinophilic fasciitis, lymphocytic infiltrate of Jessner, lymphocytoma cutis, solar urticaria, granuloma annulare, and some forms of panniculitis.

Usual doses of antimalarials are hydroxychloroquine, 200 mg twice a day; chloroquine, 250–500 mg/day; and quinacrine, 100–200 mg/day. Usually, hydroxychloroquine is started first, and if no improvement is noted in 3 months, quinacrine is added. Alternatively, chloroquine is used as a single agent. Dosing should be adjusted for low-weight individuals so that chloroquine dosing is 2.5 mg/kg/day and hydroxychloroquine is 6.5 mg/kg/day. Antimalarial agents are the treatment of choice for widespread forms of cutaneous lupus that do not respond to topical glucocorticoids and sunscreens. Clinical improvement may be delayed for several months.

Porphyria cutanea tarda, characterized by fluid-filled vesicles and bullae on sun-exposed areas, can be either genetic or associated with alcohol abuse or hepatitis C. Although the associated iron overload is treated with phlebotomy, the dermatologic manifestations sometimes are treated with antimalarial agents. These patients require reduced doses because of the potential for hepatotoxicity, as manifested by elevated transaminase levels, and the rapid excretion of large amounts of uroporphyrins in the urine that can occur with usual doses. Low-dose twice-weekly administration is effective and avoids these side effects.

TOXICITY AND MONITORING The toxic effects of antimalarial agents are described in Chapter 39. The incidence of retinopathy from chloroquine and hydroxychloroquine is low, as long as the doses are as described above and the medication is used for less than 10 years in patients with normal renal function.

Quinacrine does not cause retinopathy. Eye examinations every 6 months or even yearly after a baseline examination probably are sufficient, provided dosing guidelines are followed. Although caution is required, there is evidence that antimalarial agents probably are safe in pregnancy and in children. Rare hematological side effects include agranulocytosis, aplastic anemia, and hemolysis in patients with glucose-6-phosphatase deficiency. Liver function tests and complete blood counts should be performed monthly at the start of therapy and at least every 4–6 months throughout treatment.

CYTOTOXIC AND IMMUNOSUPPRESSANT DRUGS

Cytotoxic and immunosuppressive drugs are used in dermatology for immunologically mediated diseases such as psoriasis, the autoimmune blistering diseases, and leukocytoclastic vasculitis. These agents are discussed in detail in Chapters 51 and 52.

Antimetabolites

METHOTREXATE The antimetabolite methotrexate suppresses immunocompetent cells in the skin, and it also decreases the expression of cutaneous lymphocyte-associated antigen (CLA)–positive T cells and endothelial cell E-selectin, which may account for its efficacy in psoriasis. It is useful in treating a number of other dermatological conditions, including pityriasis lichenoides et varioliformis, lymphomatoid papulosis, sarcoidosis, pemphigus vulgaris, pityriasis rubra pilaris, lupus erythematosus, dermatomyositis, and cutaneous T-cell lymphoma.

Methotrexate (RHEUMATREX, others) is equally effective as orally administered *cyclosporine* for the treatment of moderate-to-severe chronic plaque psoriasis. Methotrexate is used often in combination with phototherapy and photochemotherapy or other systemic agents, and it also may be useful in combination with the biologics. A usual starting dose for methotrexate therapy is 5–7.5 mg/week (maximum of 15 mg/week). This dose may be increased gradually to 20–30 mg/week if needed. Widely used regimens include three oral doses given at 12-hour intervals once weekly or weekly intramuscular injections. Doses must be decreased for patients with impaired renal clearance. *Methotrexate should never be coadministered with trimethoprim–sulfamethoxazole, probenecid, salicylates, or other drugs that can compete with it for protein binding and thereby raise plasma concentrations to levels that may result in bone marrow suppression.* Fatalities have occurred because of concurrent treatment with methotrexate and nonsteroidal anti-inflammatory agents.

Methotrexate exerts significant antiproliferative effects on the bone marrow; therefore, complete blood counts should be monitored. *Folinic acid (leucovorin)* can be used to rescue patients with hematologic crises caused by methotrexate-induced bone marrow suppression. Careful monitoring of liver function tests is necessary but may not be adequate to identify early hepatic fibrosis in patients receiving chronic methotrexate therapy. Liver biopsy is recommended when the cumulative dose reaches 1–1.5 g. A baseline liver biopsy also is recommended for patients with increased potential risk for hepatic fibrosis, such as a history of alcohol abuse or infection with hepatitis B or C. Patients with significantly abnormal liver function tests, symptomatic liver disease, or evidence of hepatic fibrosis should not use this drug. Pregnancy and lactation are absolute contraindications to methotrexate use.

Azathioprine (IMURAN) is discussed in detail in Chapters 38 and 52. In dermatologic practice, the drug is used as a steroid-sparing agent for autoimmune and inflammatory dermatoses, including pemphigus vulgaris, bullous pemphigoid, dermatomyositis, atopic dermatitis, chronic actinic dermatitis, lupus erythematosus, psoriasis, pyoderma gangrenosum, and Behçet's disease. The usual starting dose is 1–2 mg/kg/day. Since it often takes 6–8 weeks to achieve therapeutic effect, azathioprine often is started early in the course of disease management. Careful laboratory monitoring is important. Thiopurine *S*-methyltransferase is critical for the metabolism of azathioprine to nontoxic metabolites. Homozygous deficiency of this enzyme may raise plasma levels of the drug and cause myelosuppression, and some experts advocate measuring this enzyme before initiating azathioprine therapy (*see* Chapter 38).

Fluorouracil (5-FU) interferes with DNA synthesis by blocking the methylation of deoxyuridylic acid to thymidylic acid. Topical formulations (CARAC, EFUDEX, FLUOROPLEX) are used in multiple actinic keratoses, actinic cheilitis, Bowen's disease, and superficial basal cell carcinomas not amenable to other treatments.

Fluorouracil is applied twice daily for 2–4 weeks. The treated areas may become severely inflamed during treatment, but the inflammation subsides after the drug is stopped. Intralesional injection of 5-FU has been used for keratoacanthomas, warts, and porokeratoses.

ALKYLATING AGENTS *Cyclophosphamide* (CYTOXAN, NEOSAR) is an effective cytotoxic and immunosuppressive agent.

Both oral and intravenous preparations of cyclophosphamide are used in dermatology. Cyclophosphamide is FDA-approved for treatment of advanced cutaneous T-cell lymphoma. Other uses include treatment of pemphigus vulgaris, bullous pemphigoid, cicatricial pemphigoid, paraneoplastic pemphigus, pyoderma gangrenosum, toxic epidermal necrolysis, Wegener's granulomatosis, polyarteritis nodosa, Churg-Strauss angiitis, Behçet's disease, scleromyxedema, and cytophagic histiocytic panniculitis. The usual oral dose is 2–3 mg/kg/day in divided doses, and there is often a 4–6-week delay in onset of action. Alternatively, intravenous pulse administration of cyclophosphamide may offer advantages, including lower cumulative dose and a decreased risk of bladder cancer.

Cyclophosphamide has many adverse effects, including the risk of secondary malignancy and myelosuppression, and thus is used only in the most severe, recalcitrant dermatological diseases. The secondary malignancies have included bladder, myeloproliferative, and lymphoproliferative malignancies and have been seen with the use of cyclophosphamide alone or in combination with other antineoplastic drugs.

Mechlorethamine hydrochloride (MUSTARGEN) and *carmustine* (*bischloronitrosourea*, BCNU, BICNU) are used topically to treat cutaneous T-cell lymphoma. Both can be applied as a solution or in ointment form. It is important to monitor complete blood counts and liver function tests because systemic absorption can cause bone marrow suppression and hepatitis. Other side effects include allergic contact dermatitis, irritant dermatitis, secondary cutaneous malignancies, and pigmentary changes. Carmustine also can cause erythema and posttreatment telangiectasias.

CALCINEURIN INHIBITORS Cyclosporine (SANDIMMUNE, NEORAL, SANGCYA) is a potent immunosuppressant isolated from the fungus *Tolypocladium inflatum*. Its mechanism of action is discussed in Chapter 52. The presence of calcineurin in Langerhans' cells, mast cells, and keratinocytes may explain the therapeutic efficacy of cyclosporine and the other calcineurin inhibitors (*e.g.,* tacrolimus and pimecrolimus; *see* below). Cyclosporine is FDA-approved for the treatment of psoriasis. Other cutaneous disorders that typically respond well to cyclosporine are atopic dermatitis, alopecia areata, epidermolysis bullosa acquisita, pemphigus vulgaris, bullous pemphigoid, lichen planus, and pyoderma gangrenosum. The usual initial oral dose is 3–5 mg/kg/day given in divided doses.

Hypertension and renal dysfunction are the major adverse effects associated with the use of cyclosporine. These risks can be minimized by monitoring serum creatinine (which should not rise more than 30% above baseline), calculating creatinine clearance or glomerular filtration rate in patients on long-term therapy or with a rising creatinine, maintaining a daily dose of less than 5 mg/kg, and regular monitoring of blood pressure. Alternation with other therapeutic modalities may diminish cyclosporine toxicity. *Laboratory monitoring during therapy is essential.* Cyclosporine is not mutagenic. However, as with other immunosuppressive agents, patients with psoriasis treated with cyclosporine are at increased risk of cutaneous, solid organ, and lymphoproliferative malignancies. The risk of cutaneous malignancies is compounded if patients have received phototherapy with PUVA.

Tacrolimus (FK506, PROGRAF), a metabolite of *Streptomyces tsukubaensis*, is a potent macrolide immunosuppressant traditionally used to prevent kidney, liver, and heart allograft rejection (*see* Chapter 52). Like cyclosporine, tacrolimus works mainly by inhibiting early activation of T lymphocytes, thereby inhibiting the release of IL-2, suppressing humoral and cell-mediated immune responses, and suppressing mediator release from mast cells and basophils. In contrast to cyclosporine, this effect is mediated by binding to intracellular FK506-binding protein 12, generating a complex that inhibits the phosphatase activity of calcineurin.

Tacrolimus is available in oral and topical forms for the treatment of skin disease. Systemic tacrolimus has shown some efficacy in the treatment of inflammatory skin diseases such as psoriasis, pyoderma gangrenosum, and Behçet's disease. When administered systemically, the most common side effects are hypertension, nephrotoxicity, neurotoxicity, GI symptoms, hyperglycemia, and hyperlipidemia. Topical formulations of tacrolimus penetrate into the epidermis.

In commercially available topical formulations (0.03% and 0.1%), tacrolimus ointment (PROTOPTIC) is effective in and approved for the treatment of atopic dermatitis in adults (0.03% and 0.1%) and children (0.03%). Other uses in dermatology include intertriginous psoriasis, vitiligo, mucosal lichen planus, graft-versus-host disease, allergic contact dermatitis, and rosacea. It is applied to the affected area twice a day and generally is well tolerated.

A major benefit of topical tacrolimus compared with topical glucocorticoids is that tacrolimus does not cause skin atrophy and therefore can be used safely in locations such as the face and intertriginous areas. Common side effects at the site of application are transient erythema, burning, and pruritus, which tend to improve with continued treatment. Systemic absorption generally is very low and decreases with resolution of the dermatitis. However, topical tacrolimus should be used with extreme caution in patients with Netherton's syndrome because these patients have been shown to develop elevated blood levels of the drug after topical application. It is recommended that patients using tacrolimus use sunscreen and avoid excessive UV exposure.

Pimecrolimus 1% cream (ELIDEL), a macrolide derived from azomycin, is FDA-approved for the treatment of atopic dermatitis in patients >2 years of age. Its mechanism of action and side effect profile are similar to those of tacrolimus. Burning, while occurring in some patients, appears to be less common with pimecrolimus than with tacrolimus. In addition, pimecrolimus has less systemic absorption. Similar precautions with regard to UV exposure should be taken during treatment with pimecrolimus.

MISCELLANEOUS IMMUNOSUPPRESSANT AND ANTI-INFLAMMATORY AGENTS

Mycophenolate mofetil (CELLCEPT) is an immunosuppressant approved for prophylaxis of organ rejection in patients with renal, cardiac, and hepatic transplants (*see* Chapter 52). Mycophenolic acid depletes guanosine nucleotides essential for DNA and RNA synthesis, and functions as a specific inhibitor of T- and B-lymphocyte activation and proliferation. The drug also may enhance apoptosis.

Mycophenolate mofetil is used increasingly to treat inflammatory and autoimmune diseases in dermatology in doses ranging from 1 to 2 g/day orally. Mycophenolate mofetil is particularly useful as a corticosteroid-sparing agent in the treatment of autoimmune blistering disorders, including pemphigus vulgaris, bullous pemphigoid, cicatricial pemphigoid, and pemphigus foliaceus. It also has been used effectively in the treatment of inflammatory diseases such as psoriasis, atopic dermatitis, and pyoderma gangrenosum.

Imiquimod (ALDARA) is a synthetic imidazoquinoline amine believed to exert immunomodulatory effects by acting as a ligand at toll-like receptors in the innate immune system and inducing the cytokines interferon-α (IFN-α), tumor necrosis factor-α (TNF-α), and IL-1, IL-6, IL-8, IL-10, and IL-12.

Approved for the treatment of genital warts imiquimod is applied to genital or perianal lesions three times a week usually for a 16-week period that may be repeated as necessary. Imiquimod is also approved for the treatment of actinic keratoses. In this capacity, imiquimod is applied three times a week for 16 weeks to the face, scalp, and arms. Phase 2 trials evaluating imiquimod for the treatment of nodular and superficial basal cell carcinomas suggest that imiquimod may prove useful when applied daily over 6–12 weeks, and the drug is FDA-approved for this indication. Off-label applications include the treatment of nongenital warts, molluscum contagiosum, extramammary Paget's disease, and Bowen's disease. Irritant reactions occur in virtually all patients, and some develop edema, vesicles, erosions, or ulcers. It appears that the degree of inflammation parallels therapeutic efficacy. No systemic effects have been reported.

Systemic *vinblastine* (VELBAN, others) is approved for use in Kaposi's sarcoma and advanced cutaneous T-cell lymphoma. Intralesional vinblastine also is used to treat Kaposi's sarcoma. Intralesional *bleomycin* (BLENOXANE, others) is used for recalcitrant warts and has cytotoxic and proinflammatory effects. Intralesional injection of bleomycin into the digits has been associated with a vasospastic response that mimics Raynaud's phenomenon, local skin necrosis, and flagellate hyperpigmentation. Intralesional bleomycin has been used for palliative treatment of squamous cell carcinoma. Systemic bleomycin has been used for Kaposi's sarcoma (*see* Chapter 51 for a more complete discussion of these agents). Liposomal anthracyclines [specifically *doxorubicin* (DOXIL, CAELYX)] may provide first-line monotherapy for advanced Kaposi's sarcoma.

Dapsone (4,4′-diaminodiphenylsulfone) is used in dermatology for its anti-inflammatory properties, particularly in sterile (noninfectious) pustular diseases of the skin. Dapsone prevents the respiratory burst from myeloperoxidase, suppresses neutrophil migration by blocking integrin-mediated adherence, inhibits adherence of antibodies to neutrophils, and decreases the release of eicosanoids and blocks their inflammatory effects; all these actions are likely to be important in autoimmune skin diseases.

Dapsone is approved for use in dermatitis herpetiformis and leprosy. It is particularly useful in the treatment of linear immunoglobulin A (IgA) dermatosis, bullous systemic lupus erythematosus, erythema elevatum diutinum, and subcorneal pustular dermatosis.

An initial dose of 50 mg/day is prescribed, followed by increases of 25 mg/day at weekly intervals, always with appropriate laboratory testing. Potential side effects of dapsone include methemoglobinemia and hemolysis. The glucose-6-phosphate dehydrogenase (G6PD) level should be checked in all patients before initiating dapsone therapy because dapsone hydroxylamine, the toxic metabolite of dapsone formed by hydroxylation, depletes glutathione within G6PD-deficient cells. The nitroso derivative then causes peroxidation reactions, leading to rapid hemolysis. A maximum dose of 150–300 mg/day should be given in divided doses to minimize the risks of methemoglobinemia. The H_2 blocker cimetidine, at a dose of 400 mg 3 times daily, alters the degree of methemoglobinemia by competing with dapsone for CYPs. Toxicities include agranulocytosis, peripheral neuropathy, and psychosis.

Thalidomide (THALOMID) is an anti-inflammatory, immunomodulating, antiangiogenic agent (*see* Figure 51–6) that also can increase keratinocyte migration and proliferation.

Thalidomide is FDA-approved for the treatment of erythema nodosum leprosum. There are reports suggesting its efficacy in actinic prurigo, aphthous stomatitis, Behçet's disease, Kaposi's sarcoma, and the cutaneous manifestations of lupus erythematosus, as well as prurigo nodularis and uremic prurigo. Thalidomide has been associated with increased mortality when used to treat toxic epidermal necrolysis. It also may cause an irreversible neuropathy. *Because of its teratogenic effects, thalidomide use is restricted to specially licensed physicians who fully understand the risks. Thalidomide should never be taken by women who are pregnant or who could become pregnant while taking the drug.*

BIOLOGICAL AGENTS

Biological agents (*see* Chapters 38 and 52) are highly specialized systemic therapies that target specific mediators of the immunologic/inflammatory reactions that are, at least in part, responsible for the clinical manifestations of a disease. The rapidly advancing knowledge of cutaneous immunology has brought with it equally impressive innovations in the therapy of malignant disorders such as cutaneous T-cell lymphoma and of immunologic diseases such as psoriasis and psoriatic arthritis. Investigational studies are evaluating a variety of biological agents for the treatment of malignancy and autoimmune diseases. This section will focus on agents that have been well studied or applied widely to the treatment of dermatological disease.

Once thought to be primarily a disorder of keratinocyte hyperproliferation, psoriasis now is known to be an autoimmune process mediated by T lymphocytes that can react with epidermal keratinocytes (Figure 62–2). The mechanism of biological therapies in psoriasis can be illustrated

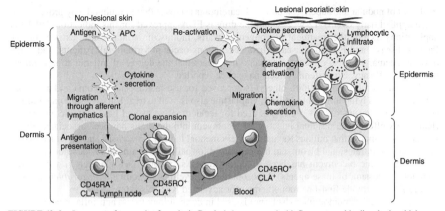

FIGURE 62–2 *Immunopathogenesis of psoriasis.* Psoriasis is a prototypical inflammatory skin disorder in which specific T-cell populations are stimulated by as yet undefined antigen(s) presented by antigen-presenting cells. The T cells release proinflammatory cytokines such as TNF-α and IFN-γ that induce keratinocyte and endothelial cell proliferation.

by a conceptual model that outlines four strategies in the treatment of psoriasis: (1) reduction of pathogenic T cells; (2) inhibition of T-cell activation; (3) immune deviation (from a T_H1 to a T_H2 immune response); and (4) blockade of the activity of inflammatory cytokines.

Although there are limited long-term data regarding the efficacy and safety of biological agents solely for the treatment of psoriasis, similar, if not identical, therapies have been used extensively in the treatment of rheumatoid arthritis and Crohn's disease. The major advantage of biological agents in the treatment of psoriasis appears to be that they specifically target the activity of T lymphocytes and cytokines that mediate inflammation with fewer side effects than traditional systemic immunosuppressive/cytotoxic agents.

Alefacept (AMEVIVE) was the first immunobiological agent approved for the treatment of moderate-to-severe psoriasis in patients who are candidates for systemic therapy. Alefacept consists of a recombinant fully human fusion protein composed of the binding site of the leukocyte function–associated antigen 3 (LFA-3) protein and a human IgG1 Fc domain. The LFA-3 portion of the alefacept molecule binds to CD2 on the surface of T cells, thus blocking a necessary costimulation step in T-cell activation (Figure 62–3). Importantly, since CD2 is expressed preferentially on memory-effector T cells, naive T cells largely are unaffected by alefacept. A second important action of alefacept is its ability to induce apoptosis of memory-effector T cells through simultaneous binding of its IgG1 portion to immunoglobulin receptors on cytotoxic cells and its LFA-3 portion to CD2 on T cells, thus inducing granzyme-mediated apoptosis of memory-effector T cells.

Alefacept is administered by intramuscular injection at a dose of 15 mg/week for 12 weeks. An additional 12-week course can be initiated if required, and a continuous 24-week regimen is under investigation. Significant reductions in psoriatic lesions have been shown for significant numbers of patients. Alefacept may induce longer remissions than do other biological agents. Adverse effects include a reduction in CD4$^+$ lymphocyte counts, requiring a baseline T-lymphocyte count before initiating alefacept and weekly monitoring of T cells during therapy.

Efalizumab (RAPTIVA) is a humanized monoclonal antibody against the CD11a molecule of LFA-1. By binding to CD11a on T cells, efalizumab prevents binding of LFA-1 to intercellular adhesion molecule 1 (ICAM-1) on the surface of antigen-presenting cells, vascular endothelial cells, and cells in the dermis and epidermis (*see* Figure 62–3), thereby interfering with T-cell activation and migration and cytotoxic T-cell function. Efalizumab is FDA-approved for the treatment of moderate-severe psoriasis in patients who are candidates for systemic therapy.

The drug is administered by subcutaneous injection once a week at a dose of 1 mg/kg, usually for 12 or 24 weeks. Significant reductions in psoriatic lesions have been shown for significant numbers of patients. After discontinuation of therapy, patients may experience rebound of disease. It is recommended that periodic evaluation of platelet levels be performed during therapy. Side effects

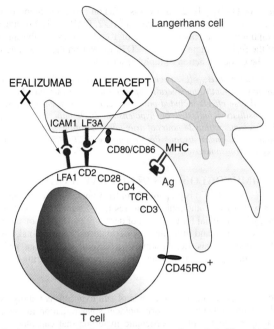

FIGURE 62-3 *Mechanisms of action of selected biological agents in psoriasis.* Newer biological agents can interfere with one or more steps in the pathogenesis of psoriasis, resulting in clinical improvement. *See* text for details.

generally are mild, and there is no evidence to date of increased risk of malignancy, infection, or end-organ toxicity.

Etanercept (ENBREL) is FDA-approved for the treatment of psoriasis, psoriatic arthritis, rheumatoid arthritis, juvenile rheumatoid arthritis, and ankylosing spondylitis. Etanercept is a soluble, recombinant, fully human TNF receptor fusion protein consisting of two molecules of the ligand-binding portion of the TNF receptor fused to the Fc portion of IgG1. As a dimeric molecule, it can bind two molecules of TNF-α. Etanercept binds soluble and membrane-bound TNF-α, thereby inhibiting the action of TNF-α.

Etanercept is administered by subcutaneous injection at doses of either 25 or 50 mg twice a week. As with alefacept and efalizumab, significant reductions in psoriatic lesions have been shown for significant numbers of patients. Except for injection-site reactions, the drug is well tolerated. Monthly complete blood counts with a differential should be monitored for the first 3 months of treatment. Potential side effects include aplastic anemia, increased risk of infection, and exacerbation of congestive heart failure and demyelinating disorders. The risk of malignancy is unknown but may be increased with the use of etanercept.

Infliximab (REMICADE) is a mouse–human chimeric monoclonal antibody that binds to soluble and membrane-bound TNF-α and inhibits binding with its receptors. Infliximab is a complement-fixing antibody that induces complement-dependent and cell-mediated lysis when bound to cell-surface-bound TNF-α. It also induces proinflammatory cytokines, such as IL-1 and IL-6, and enhances leukocyte migration. Infliximab is FDA-approved for the treatment of Crohn's disease and rheumatoid arthritis, but it is also in phase 3 trials for the treatment of psoriasis.

Infliximab is administered by intravenous infusion over 2 hours at doses of 3 or 5 mg/kg, usually at weeks 0, 2, and 6. As with the other biological agents discussed above, significant reductions in psoriatic lesions have been shown for significant numbers of patients. Complications of therapy include infusion reactions, reactivation of latent tuberculosis infection, exacerbation of congestive heart failure, and multiple sclerosis–like syndromes. Purified protein derivative (PPD) testing is required before initiating therapy. Neutralizing antibodies to infliximab may develop, and concomitant administration of methotrexate or glucocorticoids may suppress antibody formation.

Denileukin diftitox or DAB$_{389}$–IL-2, (ONTAK) is a fusion protein composed of diphtheria toxin fragments A and B and the receptor-binding portion of IL-2. DAB$_{389}$–IL-2 is indicated for advanced cutaneous T-cell lymphoma in patients with >20% of T cells expressing the surface marker CD25. The IL-2 portion of the fusion protein binds the CD25 marker on the T cell and promotes destruction of the T cell by the cytocidal action of diphtheria toxin.

When 9 or 18 µg/kg/day of DAB$_{389}$–IL-2 is given as an intravenous infusion for 5 consecutive days every 3 weeks for up to 6 months, the overall response rate was 36% with 18 µg/kg/day and 23% with 9 µg/kg/day. Adverse effects included pain, fevers, chills, nausea, vomiting, and diarrhea. Immediate hypersensitivity manifested by hypotension, back pain, dyspnea, and chest pain occurred in 60% of patients within 24 hours of drug administration; other serious side effects are edema, hypoalbuminemia, and/or hypotension, occurring in 20–30% of patients, and elevated blood levels of hepatic transaminases.

INTRAVENOUS IMMUNOGLOBULIN IN DERMATOLOGY

Intravenous immunoglobulin (IVIG) is prepared from fractionated pooled human sera derived from thousands of donors with various antigenic exposures (*see* Chapter 52). At the present time it is unclear if IVIG therapy is beneficial for treatment of dermatoses. Reports of successful use of IVIG in the treatment of autoimmune and inflammatory dermatoses are anecdotal. IVIG has been used to treat toxic epidermal necrolysis, dermatomyositis, chronic recalcitrant urticaria/angioedema, atopic dermatitis, systemic lupus erythematosus, and autoimmune blistering disorders.

SUNSCREENS

Photoprotection from the acute and chronic effects of sun exposure is readily available with sunscreens that include chemical agents to absorb incident solar radiation in the UVB and/or UVA ranges and physical agents that contain particulate materials that can block or reflect incident energy and reduce its transmission to the skin. Many of the sunscreens available are mixtures of organic chemical absorbers and particulate physical substances. Ideal sunscreens provide a broad spectrum of protection and are formulations that are photostable and remain intact for sustained periods on the skin. They also should be nonirritating, invisible, and nonstaining to clothing. No single sunscreen ingredient possesses all these desirable properties, but many are quite effective nonetheless.

UVA Sunscreen Agents

Currently available UVA filters in the U.S. include (1) avobenzone, also known as Parsol 1789; (2) oxybenzone (2-hydroxy-4-methoxy-benzophenone); (3) titanium dioxide; and (4) zinc oxide. Additional UVA sunscreens, including ecamsule (MEXORYL SX and XL), bisethylhexyloxyphenol methoxyphenyl triazine (TINOSORB S), and methylene bisbenzotriazolyl tetramethylbutylphenol (TINSORB M), are available in Europe and elsewhere but not in the U.S.

UVB Sunscreen Agents

There are numerous UVB filters, including (1) PABA esters (e.g., padimate O); (2) cinnamates (octinoxate); (3) octocrylene (2-ethylhexyl-2-cyano-3,3 diphenylacrylate); and (4) salicylates (octisalate).

The major measurement of sunscreen photoprotection is the sun protection factor *(SPF), which defines a ratio of the minimal dose of incident sunlight that will produce erythema or redness (sunburn) on skin with the sunscreen in place (protected) and the dose that evokes the same reaction on skin without the sunscreen (unprotected). The SPF provides valuable information regarding UVB protection but is useless in documenting UVA efficacy because no standard systems have been developed to measure UVA protection. Such protocols are needed because more than 85% of solar ultraviolet radiation reaching earth's surface is UVA, which penetrates more deeply into human skin than does UVB and appears to play an important role in photoaging and photocarcinogenesis.*

There is evidence that the regular use of sunscreens can reduce the risk of actinic keratoses and squamous cell carcinomas of the skin.

THE TREATMENT OF PRURITUS

The term *pruritus* is derived from the Latin *prurire*, which means "to itch." Pruritus is a symptom unique to skin that occurs in a multitude of dermatologic disorders, including dry skin or xerosis, atopic eczema, urticaria, and infestations. Itching also may be a sign of internal disorders, including malignant neoplasms, chronic renal failure, and hepatobiliary disease. The treatment of pruritus varies greatly depending on the underlying disorder.

General measures employing copious application of emollients usually are sufficient for xerosis. Inflammatory disorders such as atopic dermatitis, contact dermatitis, and lichen simplex chronicus may respond better to potent topical glucocorticoids and oral doses of sedating antihistamines. Antihistamines are useful in histamine-induced pruritus and in other pruritic disorders in which the sedating effects of these drugs facilitate sleep and reduce scratching at night, when most pruritic disorders are more symptomatic.

Cholestasis-associated pruritus may respond to *cholestyramine* (QUESTRAN, others; *see* Chapter 35), *ursodeoxycholic acid* (ACTIGALL, others; *see* Chapter 37), *ondansetron* (ZOFRAN; *see* Chapter 37), or *rifampin* (*see* Chapter 47). Recently, *nalmefene* (REVEX) (20 mg twice per day) has been shown to be effective in cholestatic pruritus.

The pruritus of uremia is treated most effectively with UVB radiation. Prurigo, a ubiquitous disorder associated with itchy nodules of the skin, is notoriously difficult to treat. In addition to topical and intralesional steroids, prurigo may respond to the opioid antagonist *naltrexone* (*see* Chapter 21) at a dose of 50 mg/day or to the proton pump inhibitor *omeprazole* (*see* Chapter 36).

Gold will ameliorate the itching palm (*see* Chapter 26) but the relief is generally only temporary.

DRUGS FOR HYPERKERATOTIC DISORDERS

Keratolytic agents—including *lactic acid, glycolic acid, salicylic acid, urea,* and *sulfur*—are employed to treat various forms of hyperkeratosis ranging from calluses and verrucae to severe xerosis. Lactic and glycolic acid are α-hydroxy acids that are thought to disrupt ionic bonds and thus diminish corneocyte cohesion.

Salicylic acid is a β-hydroxy acid that is thought to function through solubilization of intercellular cement, again reducing corneocyte adhesion. It appears to eliminate the stratum corneum layer by layer from the outermost level downward. This contrasts with the α-hydroxy acids, which preferentially diminish cellular cohesion between the corneocytes at the lowest levels of the stratum corneum.

Urea is an antimicrobial agent that denatures and dissolves proteins and increases skin absorption and retention of water. Sulfur is antiseptic, antiparasitic, antiseborrheic, and keratolytic, accounting for its myriad uses in dermatology.

Keratolytics are available in numerous formulations for treating skin diseases. Prolonged use of salicylic acid preparations over large areas, especially in children and patients with renal and hepatic impairment, can result in salicylism (*see* Chapter 26). Irritation is a common side effect with higher concentrations. Lactic acid (LAC-HYDRIN, others) is an emollient that contains 12% lactic acid that is an effective moisturizer indicated for the treatment of xerosis and ichthyosis vulgaris.

Glycolic acid is marketed in multiple cosmetic preparations (4–10%) and is used for the treatment of xerosis, ichthyosis, and photoaging.

Destructive Agents

Podophyllin (podophyllum resin) is a mixture of chemicals from the plant Podophyllum peltatum *(mandrake or May apple). The major constituent of the resin is podophyllotoxin (podofilox). It binds to microtubules and causes mitotic arrest in metaphase. Podophyllum resin (10–40%) is applied and left in place for 2–6 hours weekly for the treatment of anogenital warts. Irritation and ulcerative local reactions are the major side effects. It should not be used in the mouth or during pregnancy. Podofilox (*CONDYLOX, *others) is available as a 0.5% solution for application twice daily for 3 consecutive days. Weekly cycles may be repeated.*

DRUGS FOR ANDROGENETIC ALOPECIA

Androgenetic alopecia, commonly known as male and female pattern baldness, is the most common cause of hair loss in adults older than age 40. Up to 50% of men and women are affected. Androgenetic alopecia is a genetically inherited trait with variable expression. In susceptible hair follicles, dihydrotestosterone binds to the androgen receptor, and the hormone–receptor complex activates the genes responsible for the gradual transformation of large terminal follicles into miniaturized vellus follicles. Treatment of androgenetic areata is aimed at reducing hair loss and maintaining existing hair. The capacity to stimulate substantial regrowth of human hair remains a formidable pharmacological challenge.

*Minoxidil (*ROGAINE*) was first developed as an antihypertensive agent (see Chapter 32) and was noted to be associated with hypertrichosis in some patients. A topical formulation of minoxidil* *then was developed to exploit this side effect. Topical minoxidil is available as a 2% solution (ROGAINE) and a 5% solution (ROGAINE EXTRA STRENGTH FOR MEN). Minoxidil enhances follicular size, resulting in thicker hair shafts, and stimulates and prolongs the anagen phase of the hair cycle, resulting in longer and increased numbers of hairs. Treatment must be continued, or any drug-induced hair growth will be lost. Allergic and irritant contact dermatitis can occur, and care should be taken in applying the drug because hair growth may emerge in undesirable locations. This is reversible on stopping the drug. Patients should be instructed to wash their hands after applying minoxidil.*

Finasteride (PROPECIA) inhibits the type II isozyme of 5α-reductase, the enzyme that converts testosterone to dihydrotestosterone (see Chapter 58). The type II 5α-reductase is found in hair follicles. Balding areas of the scalp are associated with increased dihydrotesterone levels and smaller hair follicles than nonbalding areas. Orally administered finasteride (1 mg/day) has been shown to variably increase hair growth in men over a 2-year period, increasing hair counts in the vertex and the frontal scalp. Finasteride is approved for use only in men. Pregnant women should not be exposed to the drug because of the potential for inducing genital abnormalities in male fetuses. Adverse effects of finasteride include decreased libido, erectile dysfunction, ejaculation disorder, and decreased ejaculate volume. Each of these occurs in <2% of patients. Like minoxidil, treatment with finasteride must be continued, or any new hair growth will be lost.

TREATMENT OF HYPERPIGMENTATION

Hyperpigmentation is treated with products containing *hydroquinone* that produce reversible depigmentation of the skin by inhibiting the enzymatic oxidation of tyrosine to 3,4-dihydroxyphenylalanine and also inhibiting other melanocyte metabolic processes. It is indicated for the gradual bleaching of hyperpigmented skin in conditions such as melasma, freckles, and solar lentigines. Concomitant application of SPF 15–30 sunscreens and meticulous photoprotection are essential to minimize sun-induced exacerbation of hyperpigmentation. Numerous preparations are available (SOLAQUIN FORTE, others).

MISCELLANEOUS AGENTS

Capsaicin is a naturally occurring substance derived from hot chili peppers of the genus *Capsicum*. Capsaicin interacts with the vanilloid receptor (VR1) on sensory afferents. VR1 is a gated cation channel of the TRP family, modulated by a variety of noxious stimuli. Chronic exposure to capsaicin stimulates and desensitizes this channel. Capsaicin also causes local depletion of substance P, an endogenous neuropeptide involved in sensory perception and pain transmission. Capsaicin is available as a 0.025% cream (ZOSTRIX, others) and a 0.075% cream (ZOSTRIX HP, others) to be applied 3–4 times daily. Capsaicin is FDA-approved for the treatment of postherpetic neuralgia and painful diabetic neuropathy, although its efficacy in relieving pain is debatable.

Masoprocol, a dicatechol compound with an aliphatic spacer, is derived from the plant *Larrea divaricata;* it is a potent 5-lipoxygenase inhibitor with antitumor activity. It is effective for the topical therapy of actinic keratoses. Masoprocol is available as a cream (ACTINEX) and is applied twice daily for approximately 1 month. Common side effects include redness, scaling, and pruritus.

For a complete Bibliographical listing see Goodman & Gilman's *The Pharmacological Basis of Therapeutics,* **11th ed., or Goodman & Gilman Online at www.accessmedicine.com.**

63

OCULAR PHARMACOLOGY

OVERVIEW OF OCULAR ANATOMY, PHYSIOLOGY, AND BIOCHEMISTRY

The eye is a specialized sensory organ that is relatively secluded from systemic access by the blood–retinal, blood–aqueous, and blood–vitreous barriers; as a consequence, the eye exhibits some unusual pharmacodynamic and pharmacokinetic properties. No organ in the body is more accessible or visible for observation; however, the eye also presents some unique opportunities as well as challenges for drug delivery.

PHARMACOKINETICS AND TOXICOLOGY OF OCULAR THERAPEUTIC AGENTS

Drug Delivery Strategies

Properties of varying ocular routes of administration are outlined in Table 63–1. Several formulations prolong the time a drug remains on the surface of the eye. These include gels, ointments, solid inserts, soft contact lenses, and collagen shields. Prolonging the time in the cul-de-sac facilitates drug absorption. Ophthalmic gels (*e.g., pilocarpine* gel) release drugs by diffusion following erosion of soluble polymers. The polymers used include cellulosic ethers, polyvinyl alcohol, carbopol, polyacrylamide, polymethylvinyl ether–maleic anhydride, poloxamer 407, and puronic acid. Ointments usually contain mineral oil and a petrolatum base and are helpful in delivering antibiotics, cycloplegic drugs, or miotic agents. Solid inserts, such as the *ganciclovir* intravitreal implant, provide a zero-order rate of delivery over several months to treat cytomegalovirus retinitis in patients with AIDS.

Pharmacokinetics

Classical pharmacokinetic models of systemically administered drugs (*see* Chapter 1) do not fully apply to many ophthalmic drugs. Most ophthalmic medications are formulated to be applied topically or may be injected by subconjunctival, sub-Tenon's, and retrobulbar routes (Figure 63–1 and Table 63–1). Although similar principles of absorption, distribution, metabolism, and excretion determine drug disposition in the eye, these alternative routes of drug administration introduce other variables in compartmental analysis.

ABSORPTION

After topical instillation of a drug, the rate and extent of absorption are determined by the time the drug remains in the cul-de-sac and precorneal tear film, elimination by nasolacrimal drainage, drug binding to tear proteins, drug metabolism by tear and tissue proteins, and diffusion across the cornea and conjunctiva. A drug's residence time may be prolonged by changing its formulation. Residence time also may be extended by blocking the egress of tears from the eye by closing the tear drainage ducts with plugs or cautery. (Figure 63–2.) Nasolacrimal drainage contributes to systemic absorption of topically administered ophthalmic medications. Absorption from the nasal mucosa avoids so-called first-pass metabolism by the liver, and consequently significant systemic side effects may be caused by topical medications, especially when used chronically. Possible absorption pathways of an ophthalmic drug following topical application to the eye are shown schematically in Figure 63–3.

Transcorneal and transconjunctival/scleral absorption are the desired routes for localized ocular drug effects. The time period between drug instillation and its appearance in the aqueous humor is defined as the lag *time. The drug concentration gradient between the tear film and the cornea and conjunctival epithelium provides the driving force for passive diffusion across these tissues. Other factors that affect a drug's diffusion capacity are the size of the molecule, chemical structure, and steric configuration. Transcorneal drug penetration is a differential solubility process due to the cornea's trilamellar "fat-water-fat" composition. The epithelium and endothelium represent barriers for hydrophilic substances, while the stroma is a barrier for hydrophobic compounds. Hence, a drug with both hydrophilic and lipophilic properties is best suited for transcorneal absorption.*

Table 63–1

Some Characteristics of Ocular Routes of Drug Administration*

Route	Absorption Pattern	Special Utility	Limitations and Precautions
Topical	Prompt, depending on formulation	Convenient, economical, relatively safe	Compliance, corneal and conjunctival toxicity, nasal mucosal toxicity, systemic side effects from nasolacrimal absorption
Subconjunctival, sub-Tenon's, and retrobulbar injections	Prompt or sustained, depending on formulation	Anterior segment infections, posterior uveitis, cystoid macular edema	Local toxicity, tissue injury, globe perforation, optic nerve trauma, central retinal artery and/or vein occlusion, direct retinal drug toxicity with inadvertent globe perforation, ocular muscle trauma, prolonged drug effect
Intraocular (intracameral) injections	Prompt	Anterior segment surgery, infections	Corneal toxicity, intraocular toxicity, relatively short duration of action
Intravitreal injection or device	Absorption circumvented, immediate local effect, potential sustained effect	Endophthalmitis, retinitis	Retinal toxicity

*See text for more complete discussion of individual routes.

Drug penetration into the eye is approximately linearly related to its concentration in the tear film. Certain disease states, such as corneal ulcers and other corneal epithelial defects, may increase drug penetration when anatomic barriers are compromised or removed. Experimentally, drugs may be screened for their potential clinical utility by assessing their corneal permeability coefficients. These pharmacokinetic data combined with the drug's octanol/water partition coefficient (for lipophilic drugs) or distribution coefficient (for ionizable drugs) yield a parabolic

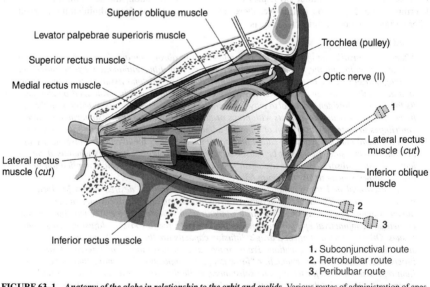

1. Subconjunctival route
2. Retrobulbar route
3. Peribulbar route

FIGURE 63–1 *Anatomy of the globe in relationship to the orbit and eyelids.* Various routes of administration of anesthesia are demonstrated by the needle pathways numbered in blue.

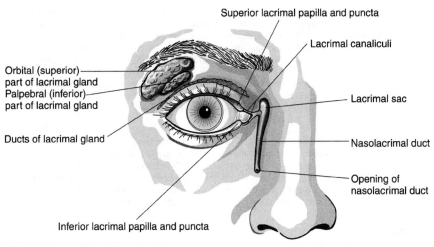

FIGURE 63–2 *Anatomy of the lacrimal system.*

relationship that is a useful parameter for predicting ocular absorption. Of course, other factors also affect corneal absorption in vivo, *such as epithelial integrity, blink rate, dilution by tear flow, nasolacrimal drainage, drug binding to proteins and tissue, and transconjunctival absorption.*

DISTRIBUTION

Topically administered drugs may undergo systemic distribution primarily by nasal mucosal absorption and possibly by local ocular distribution by transcorneal/transconjunctival absorption.

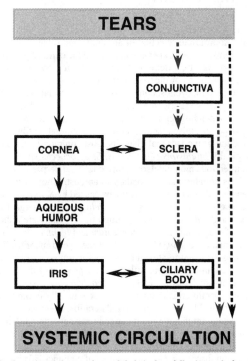

FIGURE 63–3 *Possible absorption pathways of an ophthalmic drug following topical application to the eye.* Solid black arrows represent the corneal route; *dashed blue arrows* represent the conjunctival/scleral route; the *black dashed line* represents the nasolacrimal absorption pathway.

Following transcorneal absorption, the aqueous humor accumulates the drug, which then is distributed to intraocular structures and potentially to the systemic circulation via the trabecular meshwork pathway (Figure 63–4). Melanin binding of certain drugs is an important factor in some ocular compartments. For example, the mydriatic effect of α adrenergic receptor agonists is slower in onset in humans with darkly pigmented irides compared to those with lightly pigmented irides; drug–melanin binding is also a potential reservoir for sustained drug release. Another clinically important consideration for drug–melanin binding involves the retinal pigment epithelium: accumulation of chloroquine (see *Chapter 39) causes a toxic retinal lesion that is associated with decreased visual acuity.*

METABOLISM

Local enzymatic biotransformation of ocular drugs may be significant since a variety of enzymes, including esterases, oxidoreductases, lysosomal enzymes, peptidases, glucuronide and sulfate transferases, glutathione-conjugating enzymes, catechol-O-methyl-transferase, monoamine oxidase, and 11β-hydroxysteroid dehydrogenase are found in the eye. The esterases have been of particular interest because of the development of prodrugs for enhanced corneal permeability; in the treatment of glaucoma, for example, dipivefrin hydrochloride *is a prodrug for* epinephrine, *and* latanoprost *is a prodrug for* PGF$_{2\alpha}$.

TOXICOLOGY

All ophthalmic medications are potentially absorbed into the systemic circulation (Figure 63–3), so undesirable systemic side effects may occur, as well as potential local toxic effects due to hypersensitivity reactions or to direct toxic effects on the cornea, conjunctiva, periocular skin, and nasal mucosa. Eyedrops and contact lens solutions commonly contain preservatives such as benzalkonium chloride, chlorobutanol, and chelating agents for their antimicrobial effectiveness. In particular, benzalkonium chloride may cause a punctate keratopathy or toxic ulcerative keratopathy.

THERAPEUTIC AND DIAGNOSTIC APPLICATIONS OF DRUGS IN OPHTHALMOLOGY

Chemotherapy of Microbial Diseases in the Eye

ANTIBACTERIAL AGENTS   A number of antibiotics have been formulated for topical ocular use (Table 63–2). Appropriate selection of antibiotic and route of administration is dependent on the patient's symptoms, the clinical examination, and the culture/sensitivity results. Specially formulated antibiotics also may be extemporaneously prepared by pharmacists for serious eye infections such as corneal infiltrates or ulcers and endophthalmitis.

Infectious diseases of the skin, eyelids, conjunctivae, and lacrimal excretory system are encountered regularly in clinical practice. Periocular skin infections are divided into preseptal and postseptal or orbital cellulitis. Depending on the clinical setting (*i.e.,* preceding trauma, sinusitis, age of patient, relative immunocompromised state), oral or parenteral antibiotics are administered. *Dacryoadenitis,* an infection of the lacrimal gland, is most common in children and young adults. It may be bacterial (typically *Staphylococcus aureus, Streptococcus* species) or viral (most commonly seen in mumps, infectious mononucleosis, influenza, and herpes zoster). In infants and children, the disease usually is unilateral and secondary to an obstruction of the nasolacrimal duct. In adults, dacryocystitis and canalicular infections may be caused by *S. aureus, Streptococcus* species, *Diphtheroids, Candida* species, and *Actinomyces israelii.* Any discharge from the lacrimal sac should be sent for smears and cultures. Systemic antibiotics typically are indicated.

Infectious processes of the eyelids include *hordeolum* and *blepharitis.* A hordeolum, or stye, is an infection of the meibomian, Zeis, or Moll glands at the eyelid margins. The typical offending bacterium is *S. aureus,* and the usual treatment consists of warm compresses and topical antibiotic ointment. Blepharitis is a common bilateral inflammatory process of the eyelids characterized by irritation and burning, and is usually associated with a *Staphylococcus* species. Local hygiene is the mainstay of therapy; topical antibiotics frequently are used, usually in ointment form, particularly when the disease is accompanied by conjunctivitis and keratitis. Systemic *tetracycline, doxycycline, minocycline,* and *erythromycin* often are effective in reducing severe eyelid inflammation, but must be used for weeks to months.

Conjunctivitis is an inflammatory process of the conjunctiva that varies in severity from mild hyperemia to severe purulent discharge. Common causes of conjunctivitis include viruses, allergies, environmental irritants, contact lenses, and chemicals. Less common causes include other infectious pathogens, immune-mediated reactions, associated systemic diseases, and tumors of the conjunctiva

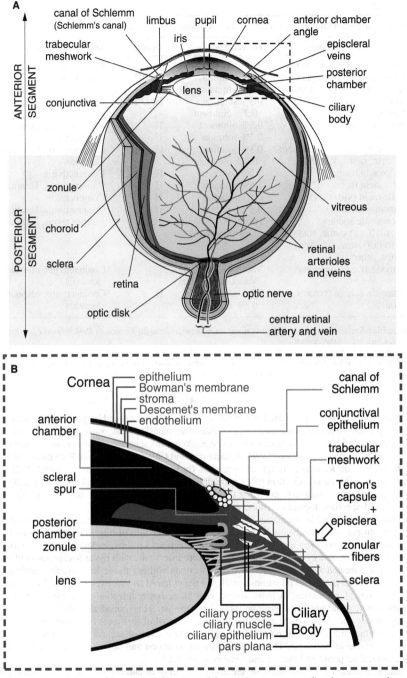

FIGURE 63–4 *A. Anatomy of the eye. B. Enlargement of the anterior segment revealing the cornea, angle structures, lens, and ciliary body.*

Table 63–2

Topical Antibacterial Agents Commercially Available for Ophthalmic Use[*]

Generic Name (TRADE NAME)	Formulation[†]	Toxicity[†]	Indications for Use
Bacitracin zinc (AK-TRACIN)	500 units/g ointment	H	Conjunctivitis, blepharitis
Chloramphenicol (AK-CHLOR, CHLOROMYCETIN, CHLOROPTIC)	0.5% solution, 1% ointment	H, BD	Conjunctivitis, keratitis
Ciprofloxacin hydrochloride (CILOXAN)	0.3% solution, 0.3% ointment	H, D-RCD	Conjunctivitis, keratitis
Erythromycin (ILOTYCIN)	0.5% ointment	H	Blepharitis, conjunctivitis
Gatifloxacin (ZYMAR)	0.3% solution	H	Conjunctivitis
Gentamicin sulfate (GARAMYCIN, GENOPTIC, GENT-AK, GENTACIDIN)	0.3% solution, 0.3% ointment	H	Conjunctivitis, blepharitis, keratitis
Levofloxacin (QUIXIN)	0.5% solution	H	Conjunctivitis
Levofloxacin (IQUIX)	1.5% solution	H	Conjunctivitis, keratitis
Moxifloxacin (VIGAMOX)	0.5% solution	H	Conjunctivitis
Ofloxacin (OCUFLOX)	0.3% solution	H	Conjunctivitis, keratitis
Sulfacetamide sodium (BLEPH-10, CETAMIDE, SULF-10, ISOPTO CETAMIDE, SULAMYD SODIUM, others)	10, 15, 30% solution, 10% ointment	H, BD	Conjunctivitis, keratitis
Polymyxin B combinations[‡]	Various solutions Various ointments		Conjunctivitis, blepharitis, keratitis
Tobramycin sulfate (TOBREX, AKTOB)	0.3% solution, 0.3% ointment	H	Conjunctivitis, blepharitis, keratitis

[*]For specific information on dosing, formulation, and trade names, refer to the *Physician's Desk Reference for Ophthalmology*, which is published annually.
[†]ABBREVIATIONS: H, hypersensitivity; BD, blood dyscrasia; D-RCD, drug-related corneal deposits.
[‡]Polymyxin B is formulated for delivery in combination with bacitracin, neomycin, gramicidin, oxytetracycline, or trimethoprim. *See* Chapters 43 through 46 for further discussion of these antibacterial agents.

or eyelid. More commonly reported infectious agents are adenovirus and herpes simplex virus, followed by other viral (*e.g.,* enterovirus, coxsackievirus, measles virus, varicella zoster virus, and vaccinia-variola virus) and bacterial sources (*e.g., Neisseria* species, *Streptococcus pneumoniae, Haemophilus* species, *S. aureus, Moraxella lacunata,* and *Chlamydial* species). Rare causes of conjunctivitis include *Rickettsia,* fungi, and parasites (in both cyst and trophozoite form). Effective management is based on selection of an appropriate antibiotic for suspected bacterial pathogens. Unless an unusual causative organism is suspected, bacterial conjunctivitis is treated empirically with a broad-spectrum topical antibiotic without obtaining a culture.

Keratitis, or corneal inflammation, can occur at any level of the cornea (*e.g.,* epithelium, subepithelium, stroma, and endothelium). It can be due to noninfectious or infectious causes. Numerous microbial agents have been identified as causes of infectious keratitis, including bacteria, viruses, fungi, spirochetes, and cysts and trophozoites. Severe infections, with tissue loss (corneal ulcers), generally are treated more aggressively than infections without tissue loss (corneal infiltrates). Mild, small, more peripheral infections usually are not cultured and the eyes are treated with broad-spectrum topical antibiotics. In more severe, central, or larger infections, corneal scrapings for smears, cultures, and sensitivities are performed and the patient is immediately started on intensive hourly, around-the-clock topical antibiotic therapy. The goal of treatment is to eradicate the infection and reduce the amount of corneal scarring and the chance of corneal perforation and severe decreased vision or blindness. The initial medication selection and dosage are adjusted according to the clinical response and culture and sensitivity results.

Endophthalmitis is a potentially severe and devastating inflammatory, and usually infectious, process involving the intraocular tissues. When the inflammatory process encompasses the entire globe, it is called *panophthalmitis.* Endophthalmitis is usually caused by bacteria or fungi, or rarely by spirochetes. The typical case occurs during the early postoperative course (*e.g.,* after cataract, glaucoma, cornea, or retinal surgery), following trauma, or by endogenous seeding in the immunocompromised host or intravenous drug user. Acute postoperative endophthalmitis requires a prompt vitreous tap for smears and cultures and empirical injection of intravitreal antibiotics. Immediate vitrectomy (*i.e.,* surgical removal of the vitreous) is beneficial for patients who have light perception–only vision. Vitrectomy for other causes of endophthalmitis (*e.g.,* glaucoma bleb–related, posttraumatic, or endogenous) may be beneficial. In cases of endogenous seeding, parenteral antibiotics have a role in eliminating the infectious source, but the efficacy of systemic antibiotics with trauma is not well established.

ANTIVIRAL AGENTS The antiviral drugs used in ophthalmology are summarized in Table 63–3 (*see* Chapter 49 for more details about these agents). The primary indications for antiviral drugs in ophthalmology are viral keratitis, herpes zoster ophthalmicus, and retinitis. There currently are no antiviral agents for the treatment of viral conjunctivitis caused by adenoviruses, which usually has a self-limited course and is treated by symptomatic relief of irritation.

Viral keratitis, an infection of the cornea that may involve either the epithelium or stroma, is most commonly caused by herpes simplex type I and varicella zoster viruses. Less common viral etiologies include herpes simplex type II, Epstein-Barr virus, and cytomegalovirus. Topical antiviral agents are indicated for the treatment of epithelial disease due to herpes simplex infection. *When treating viral keratitis topically, there is a very narrow margin between the therapeutic topical antiviral activity and the toxic effect on the cornea*; hence, patients must be followed very closely. Topical glucocorticoids are contraindicated in herpetic epithelial keratitis due to active viral replication. In contrast, for herpetic disciform keratitis, which is presumed to predominantly involve a cell-mediated immune reaction, topical glucocorticoids accelerate recovery. For recurrent herpetic stromal keratitis, there is clear benefit from treatment with oral *acyclovir* in reducing the risk of recurrence.

Herpes zoster ophthalmicus is a latent reactivation of a varicella zoster infection in the first division of the trigeminal cranial nerve. Systemic acyclovir, *valacyclovir,* and *famciclovir* are effective in reducing the severity and complications of herpes zoster ophthalmicus. Currently, there are no ophthalmic preparations of acyclovir approved by the FDA, although an ophthalmic ointment is available for investigational use.

Viral retinitis may be caused by herpes simplex virus, cytomegalovirus (CMV), adenovirus, and varicella zoster virus. With the highly active antiretroviral therapy (*see* Chapter 50), CMV retinitis does not appear to progress when specific anti-CMV therapy is discontinued, but some patients develop an immune recovery uveitis. Treatment usually involves long-term parenteral administration of antiviral drugs. Intravitreal administration of ganciclovir has been found to be an effective

Table 63–3

Antiviral Agents for Ophthalmic Use[*]

Generic Name (TRADE NAME)	Route of Administration	Ocular Toxicity[†]	Indication for Use
Trifluridine (VIROPTIC)	Topical (1% solution)	PK, H	Herpes simplex keratitis and conjunctivitis
Vidarabine (VIRA-A)	Topical (3% ointment)	PK, H	Herpes simplex keratitis and conjunctivitis
Acyclovir (ZOVIRAX)	Oral, intravenous (200-mg capsules, 400- and 800-mg tablets)		Herpes zoster ophthalmicus Herpes simplex iridocyclitis
Valacyclovir (VALTREX)	Oral (500-mg, 1000-mg tablets)		Herpes simplex keratitis Herpes zoster ophthalmicus
Famciclovir (FAMVIR)	Oral (125-mg, 250-mg, 500-mg tablets)		Herpes simplex keratitis Herpes zoster ophthalmicus
Foscarnet (FOSCAVIR)	Intravenous, Intravitreal		Cytomegalovirus retinitis
Ganciclovir (CYTOVENE) (VITRASERT)	Intravenous, oral, Intravitreal implant		Cytomegalovirus retinitis
Formivirsen (VITRAVENE)	Intravitreal injection		Cytomegalovirus retinitis
Cidofovir (VISTIDE)	Intravenous		Cytomegalovirus retinitis

[*]For additional details, *see* Chapter 49.
[†]ABBREVIATIONS: PK, punctate keratopathy; H, hypersensitivity.

alternative to the systemic route. Acute retinal necrosis and progressive outer retinal necrosis, most often caused by varicella zoster virus, can be treated by various combinations of oral, intravenous, intravitreal injection, and intravitreal implantation of antiviral medications.

ANTIFUNGAL AGENTS The only currently available topical ophthalmic antifungal preparation is a polyene, *natamycin* (NATACYN). Other antifungal agents may be extemporaneously compounded for topical, subconjunctival, or intravitreal routes of administration (Table 63–4; *see* Chapter 48 for details). As with systemic fungal infections, the incidence of ophthalmic fungal infections has risen with the growing number of immunocompromised hosts. Ophthalmic indications for antifungal medications include fungal keratitis, scleritis, endophthalmitis, mucormycosis, and canaliculitis. Risk factors for fungal keratitis include trauma, chronic ocular surface disease, and immunosuppression (including topical steroid use). When fungal infection is suspected, samples of the affected tissues are obtained for smears, cultures, and sensitivities to guide drug selection.

ANTIPROTOZOAL AGENTS Parasitic infections involving the eye usually manifest themselves as a form of *uveitis,* an inflammatory process of either the anterior or posterior segments, and less commonly as conjunctivitis, keratitis, and retinitis. In the U.S., the most commonly encountered protozoal infections include *Acanthamoeba* and *Toxoplasma gondii.* In contact-lens wearers who develop keratitis, clinicians should be highly suspicious of the presence of *Acanthamoeba.* Additional risk factors for *Acanthamoeba* keratitis include poor contact lens hygiene, wearing contact lenses in a pool or hot tub, and ocular trauma. Treatment usually consists of a combination topical antibiotic, such as *polymyxin B sulfate, bacitracin zinc,* and *neomycin sulfate* (NEOSPORIN), and sometimes an imidazole (*e.g., clotrimazole, miconazole,* or *ketoconazole*). In the UK, the aromatic diamidines (*i.e., propamidine isethionate* in both topical aqueous and ointment forms, BROLENE) have been used successfully to treat this relatively resistant infectious keratitis. The cationic antiseptic agent *polyhexamethylene biguanide* (PHMB) also is typically used in drop form for acanthamoeba keratitis, although it is not an FDA-approved antiprotozoal agent. Topical *chlorhexidine* is an alternative to PHMB. Oral itraconazole or ketoconazole often are used in addition to the topical medications. Resolution of *Acanthamoeba* keratitis may require many months of treatment.

Toxoplasmosis may present as a posterior (*e.g.,* focal retinochoroiditis, papillitis, vitritis, or retinitis) or occasionally as an anterior uveitis. Treatment is indicated when inflammatory lesions encroach upon the macula and threaten central visual acuity. Several regimens have been recommended with concurrent use of systemic steroids: (1) *pyrimethamine, sulfadiazine,* and *folinic acid (leucovorin);* (2) pyrimethamine, sulfadiazine, *clindamycin,* and folinic acid; (3) sulfadiazine and

Table 63–4

Antifungal Agents for Ophthalmic Use*

Drug Class/Agent	Method of Administration	Indications for Use
Polyenes		
Amphotericin B	0.1–0.5% (typically 0.15%) topical solution	Yeast and fungal keratitis and endophthalmitis
	0.8–1 mg subconjunctival	Yeast and fungal endophthalmitis
	5 µg intravitreal injection	Yeast and fungal endophthalmitis
	Intravenous	Yeast and fungal endophthalmitis
Natamycin	5% topical suspension	Yeast and fungal blepharitis, conjunctivitis, keratitis
Imidazoles		
Fluconazole	Oral, intravenous	Yeast keratitis and endophthalmitis
Itraconazole	Oral	Yeast and fungal keratitis and endophthalmitis
Ketoconazole	Oral	Yeast keratitis and endophthalmitis
Miconazole	1% topical solution	Yeast and fungal keratitis
	5–10 mg subconjunctival	Yeast and fungal endophthalmitis
	10 µg intravitreal injection	Yeast and fungal endophthalmitis

*Only natamycin (NATACYN) is commercially available for ophthalmic use. The other antifungal drugs must be formulated for the given method of administration. For further dosing information, refer to the *Physicians' Desk Reference for Ophthalmology.* For additional discussion of these antifungal agents, *see* Chapter 48.

clindamycin; (4) clindamycin; and (5) *trimethoprim-sulfamethoxazole* with or without clindamycin.

Other protozoal infections (*e.g.,* giardiasis, leishmaniasis, and malaria) and helminths are less common eye pathogens in the U.S. Systemic pharmacological management as well as vitrectomy may be indicated.

Use of Autonomic Agents in the Eye

Autonomic drugs are used extensively for diagnostic and surgical purposes and for the treatment of glaucoma, uveitis, and strabismus. The autonomic agents used in ophthalmology as well as the responses (*i.e.,* mydriasis and cycloplegia) to muscarinic cholinergic antagonists are summarized in Table 63–5 (also see Chapters 6 through 10).

Glaucoma Characterized by progressive optic nerve cupping and visual field loss, glaucoma is responsible for the bilateral blindness of 90,000 Americans (half of whom are African American or Hispanic), and about 2.2 million have the disease (1.9% of the population over age 40). Risk factors associated with glaucomatous nerve damage include increased intraocular pressure (IOP), positive family history of glaucoma, African American heritage, and possibly myopia and hypertension. Elevated IOP is a risk factor for glaucoma. Several clinical trials have determined that reducing IOP can delay glaucomatous nerve damage. Although markedly elevated IOPs (*e.g.,* greater than 30 mm Hg) usually will lead to optic nerve damage, the optic nerves in certain patients apparently can tolerate IOPs in the mid-to-high twenties. These patients are referred to as *ocular hypertensives.* A recent prospective trial found that prophylactic medical reduction of IOP reduced the risk of progression to glaucoma from 10% to 5%. Other patients have progressive glaucomatous optic nerve damage despite having IOPs in the normal range, and this form of the disease sometimes is called *normal-* or *low-tension* glaucoma. A reduction of IOP by 30% reduces disease progression from ~35% to ~10%, even for normal-tension glaucoma patients. Despite overwhelming evidence that IOP reduction is a helpful treatment, the pathophysiological processes involved in glaucomatous optic nerve damage and the relationship to aqueous humor dynamics are not understood.

Current pharmacotherapies are targeted to decrease the production of aqueous humor at the ciliary body and to increase outflow through the trabecular meshwork and uveoscleral pathways. There is no consensus on the best IOP–lowering technique for glaucoma therapy. General principles of patient management based on the patient's health, age, and ocular status include: (1) asthma and chronic obstructive pulmonary disease with a bronchospastic component are relative contraindications to the use of topical β adrenergic receptor antagonists because of the risk of significant side effects from systemic absorption via the nasolacrimal system; (2) some cardiac dysrhythmias (i.e., bradycardia and heart block) also are relative contraindications to β adrenergic antagonists for similar reasons; (3) history of nephrolithiasis can be a contraindication for carbonic anhydrase inhibitors (CAIs); (4) young patients usually are intolerant of miotic therapy secondary to visual blurring from induced myopia; (5) direct miotic agents are preferred over cholinesterase inhibitors in "phakic" patients (i.e., those patients who have their own crystalline lens), since the latter drugs can promote cataract formation; and (6) in patients who have an increased risk of retinal detachment, miotics should be used with caution since retinal tears could occur due to altered forces at the vitreous base produced by drug-induced ciliary body contraction.

The goal of glaucoma therapy is to prevent progressive glaucomatous optic-nerve damage with minimum risk and side effects. A stepped medical approach may begin with a topical prostaglandin analog. Due to their once-daily dosing, low incidence of systemic side effects, and potent IOP lowering effect, prostaglandin analogs have largely replaced β adrenergic receptor antagonists as first-line medical therapy for glaucoma. The $PGF_{2\alpha}$ analogs consist of latanoprost (XALATAN), travoprost (TRAVATAN), bimatoprost (LUMIGAN), and unoprostone (RESCULA). $PGF_{2\alpha}$ analogs appear to lower IOP by facilitating aqueous outflow through the accessory uveoscleral outflow pathway. The mechanism by which this occurs is unclear.

The β receptor antagonists are the next most common topical medical treatment. There are two classes of topical β blockers. The nonselective ones bind to both β_1 and β_2 receptors and include timolol, levobunolol, metipranolol, and carteolol. There is one β_1-selective antagonist, betaxolol, available for ophthalmic use. It is less likely to cause breathing difficulty than nonselective β blockers, but it is less efficacious than the nonselective β blockers since the β receptors of the ciliary body epithelium and ocular blood vessels are 75–90% β_2 subtype. The molecular basis of β blockade leading to decreased aqueous production and reduced IOP is uncertain.

Table 63-5

Autonomic Drugs for Ophthalmic Use*

Drug Class (TRADE NAME)	Formulation	Indications for Use	Ocular Side Effects
Cholinergic agonists			
Acetylcholine (MIOCHOL-E)	1% solution	Intraocular use for miosis in surgery	Corneal edema
Carbachol (MIOSTAT, ISOPTO CARBACHOL, others)	0.01–3% solution	Intraocular use for miosis in surgery, glaucoma	Corneal edema, miosis, induced myopia, decreased vision, brow ache, retinal detachment
Pilocarpine (AKARPINE, ISOPTO CARPINE, PILOCAR, PILAGAN, PILOPINE-HS, PILOPTIC, PILOSTAT, others)	0.25–10% solution, 4% gel	Glaucoma	Same as for carbachol
Anticholinesterase agents			
Physostigmine (ESERINE)	0.25% ointment	Glaucoma, accommodative esotropia, louse and mite infestation of lashes	Retinal detachment, miosis, cataract, pupillary block glaucoma, iris cysts, brow ache, punctal stenosis of the nasolacrimal system
Echothiophate (PHOSPHOLINE IODIDE)	0.125% solution	Glaucoma, accommodative esotropia	Same as for physostigmine
Muscarinic antagonists			
Atropine (ATROPISOL, ATROPINE-CARE, ISOPTO ATROPINE)	0.5–2% solution, 1% ointment	Cycloplegic retinoscopy, dilated funduscopic exam, cycloplegia†	Photosensitivity, blurred vision
Scopolamine (ISOPTO HYOSCINE)	0.25% solution	Same as for atropine	Same as for atropine
Homatropine (ISOPTO HOMATROPINE)	2 & 5% solution	Same as for atropine	Same as for atropine
Cyclopentolate (AK-PENTOLATE, CYCLOGYL, PENTOLAIR)	0.5, 1, & 2% solution	Same as for atropine	Same as for atropine
Tropicamide (MYDRIACYL, TROPICACYL, OPTICYL)	0.5 & 1% solution	Same as for atropine	Same as for atropine
Sympathomimetic agents			
Dipivefrin (PROPINE, AKPRO)	0.1% solution	Glaucoma	Photosensitivity, conjunctival hyperemia, hypersensitivity
Epinephrine (EPINAL, EPIFRIN, GLAUCON)	0.1, 0.5, 1, & 2% solution	Glaucoma	Same as for dipivefrin
Phenylephrine (AK-DILATE, MYDFRIN, NEO-SYNEPHRINE, others)	0.12, 2.5, & 10% solution	Mydriasis	Same as for dipivefrin
Apraclonidine (IOPIDINE)	0.5 & 1% solution	Glaucoma, pre- & postlaser prophylaxis of intraocular pressure spike	Same as for dipivefrin

Sympathomimetic agents (Continued)			
Brimonidine (ALPHAGAN)	0.15 and 0.2% solution	Glaucoma	Same as for dipivefrin
Cocaine	1–4% solution	Topical anesthesia, evaluate anisocoria	
		Evaluate anisocoria	
Hydroxyamphetamine (PAREDRINE)	1% solution		
Naphazoline (AK-CON, ALBALON, CLEAR EYES, NAPHCON, VASOCLEAR, VASOCON REGULAR, others)	0.012–0.1% solution	Decongestant	Same as for dipivefrin
Tetrahydrozoline (COLLYRIUM FRESH, MURINE PLUS, VISINE MOISTURIZING, others)	0.05% solution	Decongestant	Same as for dipivefrin
α & β Adrenergic antagonists			
Dapiprazole (α) (REV-EYES)	0.5% solution	Reverse mydriasis	Conjunctival hyperemia
Betaxolol (β_1-selective) (BETOPTIC, BETOPTIC-S)	0.25 and 0.5% suspension	Glaucoma	
Carteolol (β) (OCUPRESS)	1% solution	Glaucoma	
Levobunolol (β) (BETAGAN, AKBETA)	0.25 & 0.5% solution	Glaucoma	
Metipranolol (β) (OPTIPRANOLOL)	0.3% solution	Glaucoma	
Timolol (β) (TIMOPTIC, TIMOPTIC XE, BETIMOL)	0.25 & 0.5% solution & gel	Glaucoma	

*Refer to *Physicians' Desk Reference for Ophthalmology* for specific indications and dosing information.

†Mydriasis and cycloplegia, or paralysis of accommodation, of the human eye occurs after one drop of atropine 1%, scopolamine 0.5%, homatropine 1%, cyclopentolate 0.5% or 1%, and tropicamide 0.5% or 1%. Recovery of mydriasis is defined by return to baseline pupil size to within 1 mm. Recovery of cycloplegia is defined by return to within two diopters of baseline accommodative power. The maximal mydriatic effect of homatropine is achieved with a 5% solution, but cycloplegia may be incomplete. Maximal cycloplegia with tropicamide may be achieved with a 1% solution.

Times to development of maximal mydriasis and to recovery, respectively, are: for *atropine*, 30–40 minutes and 7–10 days; for *scopolamine*, 20–130 minutes and 3–7 days; for homatropine, 40–60 minutes and 1–3 days; for *cyclopentolate*, 30–60 minutes and 1 day; for *tropicamide*, 20–40 minutes and 6 hours.

Times to development of maximal cycloplegia and to recovery, respectively, are: for *atropine*, 60–180 minutes and 6–12 days; for *scopolamine*, 30–60 minutes and 3–7 days; for *homatropine*, 30–60 minutes and 1–3 days; for *cyclopentolate*, 25–75 minutes and 6 hours to 1 day; for *tropicamide*, 30 minutes and 6 hours.

When there are medical contraindications to the use of prostaglandin analogs or β-receptor antagonists, other agents, such as an α_2 adrenergic receptor agonist or topical carbonic anhydrase inhibitor may be first-line therapy. The α_2 adrenergic agonists improve the pharmacologic profile of the nonselective sympathomimetic agent epinephrine and its prodrug derivative, dipivefrin (PROPINE). Epinephrine stimulates both α and β adrenergic receptors. The drug appears to decrease IOP by enhancing both conventional (via a β_2 receptor mechanism) and uveoscleral outflow (perhaps via prostaglandin production) from the eye. Although effective, epinephrine is poorly tolerated, principally due to localized irritation and hyperemia. Dipivefrin is an epinephrine prodrug that is converted into epinephrine by esterases in the cornea. It is much better tolerated but still is prone to cause epinephrine-like side effects. The α_2 adrenergic agonist apraclonidine (IOPIDINE) is highly ionized at physiologic pH and therefore does not cross the blood–brain barrier to cause sedation. Brimonidine (ALPHAGAN, others) is also a selective α_2 adrenergic agonist, but is lipophilic, enabling easy corneal penetration. Both apraclonidine and brimonidine reduce aqueous production and may enhance some uveoscleral outflow. Both appear to bind to pre- and postsynaptic α_2 receptors. By binding to the presynaptic receptors, the drugs reduce the amount of neurotransmitter release from sympathetic nerve stimulation and thereby lower IOP (Figure 63–3). By activating postsynaptic α_2 receptors, these drugs stimulate the G_i pathway, reducing cyclic AMP production and thereby reducing aqueous humor production.

The development of a topical carbonic anhydrase inhibitor was prompted by the poor side-effect profile of oral CAIs. Dorzolamide (TRUSOPT) and brinzolamide (AZOPT) both work by inhibiting carbonic anhydrase (isoenzyme II), which is found in the ciliary body epithelium. This reduces the formation of bicarbonate ions, which reduces fluid transport and thus IOP.

Any of these four drug classes can be used as additive second- or third-line therapy. The β receptor antagonist timolol has been combined with the carbonic anhydrase inhibitor dorzolamide in a single medication (COSOPT) that may improve compliance.

Topical miotic agents are less commonly used today because of their numerous side effects and inconvenient dosing. Miotics lower IOP by causing muscarinic-induced contraction of the ciliary muscle, which facilitates aqueous outflow. They do not affect aqueous production. Pilocarpine and carbachol are cholinomimetics that stimulate muscarinic receptors. Echothiophate (PHOSPHOLINE IODIDE) is an organophosphate inhibitor of acetylcholinesterase; it is relatively stable in aqueous solution, and by virtue of its quaternary ammonium structure, is positively charged and poorly absorbed.

If combined topical therapy fails to achieve the target IOP or fails to halt glaucomatous optic nerve damage, then systemic therapy with CAIs is a final medication option before resorting to laser or incisional surgical treatment. The best-tolerated oral preparation is acetazolamide in sustained-release capsules (see Chapter 28), followed by methazolamide. The least well-tolerated are acetazolamide tablets.

Toxicity of Agents in Treatment of Glaucoma

Ciliary body spasm is a muscarinic cholinergic effect that can lead to induced myopia and changing refraction due to iris and ciliary body contraction as the drug effect waxes and wanes between doses. Headaches can occur from the iris and ciliary body contraction. Epinephrine-related compounds, effective in IOP reduction, can cause a vasoconstriction-vasodilation rebound phenomenon leading to a red eye. Ocular and skin allergies from topical epinephrine, related prodrug formulations, apraclonidine, and brimonidine are common. Brimonidine is less likely to cause ocular allergy and is therefore more commonly used. These agents can cause CNS depression and apnea in neonates and are contraindicated in children under the age of 2.

Systemic absorption of epinephrine-related drugs and β adrenergic antagonists can induce all the side effects found with direct systemic administration. The systemic use of CAIs may give some patients significant problems with malaise, fatigue, depression, paresthesias, and nephrolithiasis; the topical CAIs may minimize these relatively common side effects.

Uveitis   Inflammation of the uvea, or uveitis, has both infectious and noninfectious causes, and medical treatment of the underlying cause (if known) is essential in addition to the use of topical therapy. *Cyclopentolate,* or sometimes even longer-acting antimuscarinic agents such as atropine, *scopolamine,* and *homatropine,* frequently are used to prevent posterior synechia formation between the lens and iris margin and to relieve ciliary muscle spasm causes much of the pain associated with anterior uveitis. If posterior synechiae already have formed, an α adrenergic agonist may be used to break the synechiae by enhancing pupillary dilation. A solution containing scopolamine 0.3% in combination with 10% *phenylephrine* is available for this purpose. Topical glucocorticoids usually are adequate to decrease inflammation, but sometimes must be supplemented by systemic glucocorticoids.

Strabismus   Strabismus, or ocular misalignment, has numerous causes and may occur at any age. Besides causing *diplopia* (double vision), strabismus in children may lead to *amblyopia* (reduced vision). Nonsurgical efforts to treat amblyopia include occlusion therapy, orthoptics, optical devices, and drugs. An eye with *hyperopia*, or farsightedness, must accommodate to focus distant images. In some hyperopic children, the synkinetic accommodative-convergence response leads to excessive convergence and a manifest *esotropia* (turned-in eye). The brain rejects diplopia and suppresses the image from the deviated eye. If proper vision is not restored by about the age of 7, the brain never learns to process visual information from that eye. The result is that the eye appears structurally normal but does not develop normal visual acuity and is therefore amblyopic. Unfortunately this is a fairly common cause of visual disability. In this setting, atropine (1%) instilled in the preferred seeing eye produces cycloplegia and the inability of this eye to accommodate, thus forcing the child to use the amblyopic eye. Echothiophate iodide also has been used in the setting of accommodative strabismus. Accommodation drives the near reflex, the triad of miosis, accommodation, and convergence. An irreversible cholinesterase inhibitor such as echothiophate causes miosis and an accommodative change in the shape of the lens; hence, the accommodative drive to initiate the near reflex is reduced, and less convergence will occur.

Surgery and Diagnostic Purposes   For certain surgical procedures and for clinical funduscopic examination, it is desirable to maximize the view of the retina and lens. Muscarinic cholinergic antagonists and α_2 adrenergic agonists frequently are used singly or in combination for this purpose (Table 63–5). Intraoperatively, there are circumstances when miosis is preferred, and two cholinergic agonists are available for intraocular use, *acetylcholine* and carbachol. Patients with myasthenia gravis may first present to an ophthalmologist with complaints of double vision (diplopia) or eyelid droop (ptosis); the *edrophonium test* is helpful in diagnosing these patients (*see* Chapter 8).

Use of Immunomodulatory Drugs for Ophthalmic Therapy

GLUCOCORTICOIDS   Glucocorticoids have an important role in managing ocular inflammatory diseases; their chemistry and pharmacology are described in Chapter 59. Currently the glucocorticoids formulated for topical administration to the eye are *dexamethasone* (DECADRON, others), *prednisolone* (PRED FORTE, others), *fluorometholone* (FML, others), *loteprednol* (ALREX, LOTEMAX), *medrysone* (HMS), and *rimexolone* (VEXOL). Because of their anti-inflammatory effects, topical glucocorticoids are used in managing significant ocular allergy, anterior uveitis, external eye inflammatory diseases associated with some infections and ocular cicatricial pemphigoid, and postoperative inflammation following refractive, corneal, and intraocular surgery. After glaucoma filtering surgery, topical glucocorticoids can delay the wound-healing process by decreasing fibroblast infiltration, thereby reducing potential scarring of the surgical site. Glucocorticoids are commonly given systemically and by sub-Tenon's capsule injection to manage posterior uveitis. Intravitreal injection of glucocorticoids is used to treat a variety of retinal conditions including age-related macular degeneration, diabetic retinopathy, and cystoid macular edema. Parenteral glucocorticoids followed by tapering oral doses are the preferred treatment for optic neuritis.

Toxicity of Glucocorticoids   Glucocorticoid drops, pills, and creams are associated with ocular problems, as are intravitreal and intravenous steroids. Ocular complications include the development of posterior subcapsular cataracts, secondary infections (*see* Chapter 59), and secondary open-angle glaucoma. There is a significant increase in risk for developing secondary glaucoma when there is a positive family history of glaucoma. In the absence of a family history of open-angle glaucoma, only about 5% of normal individuals respond to topical or long-term systemic steroids with a marked increase in IOP. With a positive family history, moderate-to-marked glucocorticoid-induced IOP elevations may occur in up to 90% of patients. Typically, glucocorticoid-induced IOP elevation is reversible once drug administration ceases. However, intraocular or sub-Tenon's steroid-related pressure elevation may persist for months and may require treatment with glaucoma medication or even filtering surgery. Newer topical glucocorticoids, so called "soft steroids" (*e.g.*, loteprednol), reduce but do not eliminate the risk of elevated IOP.

NONSTEROIDAL ANTI-INFLAMMATORY AGENTS (NSAIDs)   There are five topical NSAIDs approved for ocular use: *diclofenac* (VOLTAREN), *flurbiprofen* (OCUFEN), *ketorolac* (ACULAR), *bromfenac* (XIBROM), and *nepafenac* (NEVANAC). Diclofenac and flurbiprofen are discussed in Chapter 26. Flurbiprofen is used to counter unwanted intraoperative miosis during cataract surgery. Ketorolac is given for seasonal allergic conjunctivitis. Diclofenac, bromfenac, and nepafenac are used for postoperative inflammation; nepafenac may be used to relieve pain following cataract surgery. Ketorolac and diclofenac are effective in treating cystoid macular edema occurring after cataract surgery. In patients treated with prostaglandin analogs (*e.g.*, latanoprost or bimatoprost), ketorolac and diclofenac may decrease postoperative inflammation. They also are useful in decreasing pain after corneal refractive surgery. Topical NSAIDs occasionally have been associated with sterile corneal melts and perforations, especially in older patients with ocular surface disease, such as dry eye syndrome.

ANTIHISTAMINES AND MAST-CELL STABILIZERS   *Pheniramine* (*see* Chapter 24) and *antazoline*, both H_1 receptor antagonists, are formulated in combination with *naphazoline*, a vasoconstrictor, for relief of allergic conjunctivitis. Topical antihistamines include *emedastine difumarate* (EMADINE) and *levocabastine hydrochloride* (LIVOSTIN). *Cromolyn sodium* (CROLOM), which prevents the release of histamine and other autacoids from mast cells (*see* Chapter 27), has found limited use in treating conjunctivitis that is thought to be allergen-mediated, such as vernal conjunctivitis. *Lodoxamide tromethamine* (ALOMIDE) and *pemirolast* (ALAMAST), mast-cell stabilizers, also are available for ophthalmic use. *Nedocromil* (ALOCRIL) also is primarily a mast-cell stabilizer with some antihistamine properties. *Olopatadine hydrochloride* (PATANOL), *ketotifen fumarate* (ZADITOR), and *azelastine* (OPTIVAR) are H_1 antagonists with mast cell–stabilizing properties. *Epinastine* (ELESTAT) antagonizes H_1 and H_2 receptors and exhibits mast cell–stabilizing activity.

IMMUNOSUPPRESSIVE AND ANTIMITOTIC AGENTS   The principal application of immunosuppressive and antimitotic agents to ophthalmology relates to the use of 5-fluorouracil and mitomycin C in corneal and glaucoma surgeries. Interferon α-2b also has occasionally been used. Certain systemic diseases with serious vision-threatening ocular manifestations—such as Behçet's disease, Wegener's granulomatosis, rheumatoid arthritis, and Reiter's syndrome—require systemic immunosuppression (*see* Chapter 52). In glaucoma surgery, both fluorouracil and mitomycin (MUTAMYCIN), which also are antineoplastic agents (*see* Chapter 51), improve the success of filtration surgery by limiting the postoperative wound-healing process. Mitomycin is used intraoperatively as a single subconjunctival application at the trabeculectomy site. Meticulous care is used to avoid intraocular penetration, since mitomycin is extremely toxic to intraocular structures. Fluorouracil may be used intraoperatively at the trabeculectomy site and/or subconjunctivally during the postoperative course. Although both agents work by limiting the healing process, sometimes this can result in thin, ischemic, avascular tissue that is prone to breakdown. The resultant leaks can cause hypotony (low IOP) and increase the risk of infection. In cornea surgery, mitomycin has been used topically after excision of pterygium, a fibrovascular membrane that can grow onto the cornea. Mitomycin can be used to reduce the risk of scarring after certain procedures to remove corneal opacities and also prophylactically to prevent corneal scarring after excimer laser surface ablation (photorefractive and phototherapeutic keratectomy). Mitomycin also is used to treat certain conjunctival and corneal tumors. Interferon α-2b has been used in the treatment of conjunctival papilloma and certain conjunctival tumors. Although the use of mitomycin for both corneal surgery and glaucoma filtration surgeries augments the success of these surgical procedures, caution is advocated in light of potentially serious delayed ocular complications.

IMMUNOMODULATORY AGENT   Topical *cyclosporine* (RESTASIS) is approved for the treatment of chronic dry eye associated with inflammation. Cyclosporine is an immunomodulatory agent that inhibits T-cell activation. Use of cyclosporine is associated with decreased inflammatory markers in the lacrimal gland, increased tear production, and improved vision and comfort.

Drugs and Biological Agents Used in Ophthalmic Surgery

ADJUNCTS IN ANTERIOR SEGMENT SURGERY   *Viscoelastic* substances assist in ocular surgery by maintaining spaces, moving tissue, and protecting surfaces. These substances are prepared from hyaluronate, chondroitin sulfate, or hydroxypropylmethylcellulose, share the following important physical characteristics: viscosity, shear flow, elasticity, cohesiveness, and coatability, and are broadly characterized as dispersive or cohesive. They are used almost exclusively in anterior segment surgery. Complications associated with viscoelastic substances are related to transient elevation of IOP after the procedure.

OPHTHALMIC GLUE   Cyanoacrylate tissue adhesive (ISODENT, DERMABOND, HISTOACRYL), while not FDA-approved for the eye, is widely used in the management of corneal ulcerations and perforations. It is applied in liquid form and polymerized into a solid plug. Fibrinogen glue (TISSEEL) is increasingly being used on the ocular surface to secure tissue such as conjunctiva, amniotic membrane, and lamellar corneal grafts.

CORNEAL BAND KERATOPATHY *Edetate disodium* (disodium EDTA; ENDRATE) is a chelating agent that can be used to treat band keratopathy (*i.e.,* a calcium deposit at the level of Bowman's membrane on the cornea). After the overlying corneal epithelium is removed, it is applied topically to chelate the calcium deposits from the cornea.

ANTERIOR SEGMENT GASES Sulfur hexafluoride (SF_6) and perfluoropropane gases have long been used as vitreous substitutes during retinal surgery. In the anterior segment, they are used in nonexpansile concentrations to treat Descemet's detachments, typically after cataract surgery. These detachments can cause mild-to-severe corneal edema. The gas is injected into the anterior chamber to push Descemet's membrane up against the stroma, where ideally it reattaches and clears the corneal edema.

VITREOUS SUBSTITUTES The primary use of vitreous substitutes is reattachment of the retina following vitrectomy and membrane-peeling procedures for complicated proliferative vitreoretinopathy and traction retinal detachments. Several compounds are available, including gases, perfluorocarbon liquids, and silicone oil (Table 63–6). With the exception of air, the gases expand because of interaction with systemic oxygen, carbon dioxide, and nitrogen, and this property makes them desirable to temporarily tamponade areas of the retina. However, use of these expansile gases carries the risk of complications from elevated IOP, subretinal gas, corneal edema, and cataract formation. The gases are absorbed over a time period of days (for air) to 2 months (for perfluoropropane).

The liquid perfluorocarbons, with specific gravities between 1.76 and 1.94, are denser than vitreous and are helpful in flattening the retina when vitreous is present. If a lens becomes dislocated into the vitreous, a perfluorocarbon liquid injection posteriorly will float the lens anteriorly, facilitating surgical retrieval. This liquid can be an important tool for flattening and unrolling severely detached and contorted retinas such as those found in giant retinal tears and proliferative vitreoretinopathy but are potentially toxic if it remains in chronic contact with the retina.

Silicone oil has had extensive use for long-term tamponade of the retina. Complications from silicone oil use include glaucoma, cataract formation, corneal edema, corneal band keratopathy, and retinal toxicity.

SURGICAL HEMOSTASIS AND THROMBOLYTIC AGENTS Hemostasis has an important role in most surgical procedures and usually is achieved by temperature-mediated coagulation. In some intraocular surgeries, thrombin has a valuable role in hemostasis. Intravitreal administration of thrombin can assist in controlling intraocular hemorrhage during vitrectomy. When used intraocularly, a potentially significant inflammatory response may occur, but this reaction can be minimized by thorough irrigation after hemostasis is achieved. This coagulation factor also may be applied topically *via* soaked sponges to exposed conjunctiva and sclera, where hemostasis may be a challenge due to the rich vascular supply. Topical *aminocaproic acid* (CAPROGEL) has been advocated to prevent rebleeding after traumatic *hyphema* (blood in the anterior chamber), but recent clinical trials report mixed success. Depending on the intraocular location of a clot, there may be significant problems relating to IOP, retinal degeneration, and persistent poor vision. *Tissue plasminogen activator* (t-PA) (*see* Chapter 54) has been used during intraocular surgeries to assist evacuation of a hyphema, subretinal clot, or nonclearing vitreous hemorrhage. t-PA also has been administered subconjunctivally and intracamerally (*i.e.,* controlled intraocular administration into the anterior segment) to lyse blood clots obstructing a glaucoma filtration site. The main complication related to the use of t-PA is bleeding.

BOTULINUM TOXIN TYPE A IN THE TREATMENT OF STRABISMUS, BLEPHAROSPASM, AND RELATED DISORDERS *Botulinum toxin type A* (BOTOX) is used to treat strabismus, blepharospasm, Meige's syndrome, spasmodic torticollis hemifacial spasm, facial wrinkles, and certain migraine headaches (*see also* Chapter 9). By preventing acetylcholine release at the neuromuscular junction, botulinum toxin A usually causes a temporary paralysis of the locally injected muscles. The variability in duration of paralysis may be related to the rate of developing antibodies to the toxin, upregulation of nicotinic cholinergic postsynaptic receptors, and aberrant regeneration of motor nerve fibers at the neuromuscular junction. Complications related to this toxin include double vision (diplopia) and lid droop (ptosis).

Table 63–6

Vitreous Substitutes

Vitreous Substitute	Chemical Structure	Characteristics (Duration of Viscosity)
Nonexpansile gases		
Air, Ar, CO_2, He, Kr, N_2, O_2, Xe		Duration of 5–7 days
Expansile gases		
Sulfur hexafluoride		Duration of 1 day
Octafluorocyclobutane		Duration of 10–14 days
Perfluoromethane		Duration of 10–14 days
Perfluoroethane	$F_3C—CF_3$	Duration of 30–35 days
Perfluoropropane	$F_3C—CF_2—CF_3$	Duration of 55–65 days
Perfluoro-*n*-butane	$F_3C—(CF_2)_2—CF_3$	
Perfluoropentane	$F_3C—(CF_2)_3—CF_3$	
Silicone oils		
Nonfluorinated silicone oils	$(CH_3)_3SiO[(CH_3)_2SiO]_nSi(CH_3)_3$	Viscosity range from 1000 to 30,000 cs*
Fluorosilicone	$(CH_3)_3SiO[(C_3H_4F_3)(CH_3)SiO]_n Si(CH_3)_3$	Viscosity range from 1000 to 10,000 cs*
"High-tech" silicone oils	$(CH_3)_3SiO[(C_6H_5)(CH_3)SiO]_n Si(CH_3)_3$	May terminate as trimethylsiloxy (shown) or polyphenylmethylsiloxane, viscosity not reported

*cs, centistoke (unit of viscosity).

BLIND AND PAINFUL EYE   Retrobulbar injection of either absolute or 95% ethanol may provide relief from chronic pain associated with a blind and painful eye. Retrobulbar chlorpromazine also has been used. This treatment is preceded by administration of local anesthesia. Local infiltration of the ciliary nerves provides symptomatic relief from pain, but other nerve fibers may be damaged, causing paralysis of the extraocular muscles, including those in the eyelids, or neuroparalytic keratitis. The sensory fibers of the ciliary nerves may regenerate, and repeated injections sometimes are needed.

SYSTEMIC AGENTS WITH OCULAR SIDE EFFECTS   Just as certain systemic diseases have ocular manifestations, certain systemic drugs have ocular side effects. These can range from mild and inconsequential to severe and vision threatening.

Retina Numerous drugs have toxic side effects on the retina. The antiarthritis and antimalarial medicines *hydroxychloroquine* (PLAQUENIL) and chloroquine can cause a central retinal toxicity. With normal dosages, toxicity does not appear until about 6 years after the drug is started. Stopping the drug will not reverse the damage but will prevent further toxicity. *Sildenafil* (VIAGRA) inhibits PDE5 in the corpus cavernosum for the purpose of helping to achieve and maintain penile erection. The drug also mildly inhibits PDE6, which controls the levels of cyclic GMP in the retina. Visually, this can result in seeing a bluish haze or experiencing light sensitivity. Although no retinal damage has been reported, no long-term studies have been reported. Two newer PDE5 inhibitors, *vardenafil* (LEVITRA) and *tadalafil* (CIALIS), are associated with similar visual disturbances.

Optic Nerve Multiple medications can cause a toxic optic neuropathy characterized by gradually progressive bilateral central scotomas and vision loss. There can be accompanying optic nerve pallor. These medicines include *ethambutol, chloramphenicol,* and *rifampin.* Systemic or ocular glucocorticoids can cause elevated IOP and glaucoma. If the glucocorticoids cannot be stopped, glaucoma medications, and even filtering surgery, often are required.

Anterior Segment Glucocorticoids also have been implicated in cataract formation. If vision is reduced, cataract surgery may be necessary. *Rifabutin,* if used in conjunction with *clarithromycin* or *fluconazole* for treatment of *Mycobacterium avium complex* (MAC) opportunistic infections in AIDS, is associated with an iridocyclitis and even hypopyon. This will resolve with glucocorticoids or by stopping the medication.

Ocular Surface *Isotretinoin* (ACCUTANE) has a drying effect on mucous membranes and is associated with dry eye.

CORNEAL SIDE EFFECTS OF SYSTEMIC MEDICATIONS The cornea, conjunctiva, and even eyelids can be affected by systemic medications. One common drug deposit found in the cornea is from the cardiac medication *amiodarone.* It deposits in the inferior and central cornea in a whorl-like pattern termed *cornea verticillata.* It appears as fine tan or brown pigment in the epithelium that seldom affects vision and rarely causes discontinuation. The deposits disappear slowly if the medication is stopped. Other medications can cause a similar pattern, including *indomethacin, atovaquone,* chloroquine, and hydroxychloroquine.

The phenothiazines, including *chlorpromazine* and *thioridazine,* can cause brown pigmentary deposits in the cornea, conjunctiva, and eyelids. The deposits generally are found in Descemet's membrane and the posterior cornea and typically do not affect vision. The ocular deposits generally persist after discontinuation of the medication and can even worsen, perhaps because the medication deposits in the skin are slowly released and accumulate in the eye. Tetracyclines can cause a yellow discoloration of the light-exposed conjunctiva. Systemic minocycline can induce a blue-gray scleral pigmentation that is most prominent in the interpalpebral zone.

Agents Used to Assist in Ocular Diagnosis

A number of agents are used in an ocular examination (*e.g.,* mydriatic agents and topical anesthetics, and dyes to evaluate corneal surface integrity) to facilitate intraocular surgery (*e.g.,* mydriatic and miotic agents, topical and local anesthetics) and to help in making a diagnosis in cases of anisocoria and retinal abnormalities (*e.g.,* intravenous contrast agents). The autonomic agents have been discussed earlier. The diagnostic and therapeutic uses of topical and intravenous dyes and of topical anesthetics are discussed below.

ANTERIOR SEGMENT AND EXTERNAL DIAGNOSTIC USES Epiphora (excessive tearing) and surface problems of the cornea and conjunctiva are common external ocular disorders. The dyes *fluorescein, rose bengal,* and *lissamine green* are used in evaluating these problems. Available both as a 2% alkaline solution and as an impregnated paper strip, fluorescein reveals epithelial defects of the cornea and conjunctiva and aqueous humor leakage that may occur after trauma or ocular surgery. In the setting of epiphora, fluorescein is used to help determine the patency of the nasolacrimal system. In addition, this dye is used as part of the procedure of *applanation tonometry* (IOP measurement) and to assist in determining the proper fit of rigid and semirigid contact lenses. Fluorescein in combination with *proparacaine* or *benoxinate* is available for procedures in which a disclosing agent is needed in conjunction with a topical anesthetic. *Fluorexon* (FLUORESOFT), a high-molecular-weight fluorescent solution, is used when fluorescein is contraindicated (as when soft contact lenses are in place). Rose bengal and lissamine green, which also are available as a 1% solution and as saturated paper strips, stain devitalized tissue on the cornea and conjunctiva.

POSTERIOR SEGMENT DIAGNOSTIC AND THERAPEUTIC USES The integrity of the blood–retinal and retinal pigment epithelial barriers may be examined directly by retinal angiography using intravenous administration of either *fluorescein sodium* or *indocyanine green*. These agents commonly cause nausea and may precipitate serious allergic reactions in susceptible individuals.

Verteporfin (VISUDYNE) is a photosensitizing agent approved for photodynamic therapy of the exudative form of age-related macular degeneration with predominantly classic choroidal neovascular membranes. Verteporfin also is used in the treatment of predominantly classic choroidal neovascularization caused by conditions such as pathological myopia and presumed ocular histoplasmosis syndrome. Verteporfin is administered intravenously, and once it reaches the choroidal circulation, the drug is light-activated by a nonthermal red laser source. Depending on the size of the neovascular membrane and concerns of occult membranes and recurrence, multiple photodynamic treatments may be necessary. Activation of the drug in the presence of oxygen generates free radicals, which cause vessel damage and subsequent platelet activation, thrombosis, and occlusion of choroidal neovascularization. The $t_{1/2}$ of the drug is 5–6 hours. It is eliminated predominantly in the feces. Potential side effects include headache, injection site reactions, and visual disturbances. The drug causes temporary photosensitization, and patients must avoid exposure of skin or eyes to direct sunlight or bright indoor lights for 5 days after treatment.

Use of Anesthetics in Ophthalmic Procedures

Topical anesthetic agents used clinically in ophthalmology include *cocaine,* proparacaine, and *tetracaine* drops and *lidocaine* gel (*see* Chapter 14). Proparacaine and tetracaine are used topically to perform tonometry, to remove foreign bodies on the conjunctiva and cornea, to perform superficial corneal surgery, and to manipulate the nasolacrimal canalicular system. They also are used topically to anesthetize the ocular surface for refractive surgery using either the excimer laser or placement of intrastromal corneal rings. Cocaine may be used intranasally in combination with topical anesthesia for cannulating the nasolacrimal system. Lidocaine and *bupivacaine* are used for infiltration and retrobulbar block anesthesia for surgery. Potential complications and risks relate to allergic reactions, globe perforation, hemorrhage, and vascular and subdural injections. Both preservative-free lidocaine (1%), which is introduced into the anterior chamber, and lidocaine jelly (2%), which is placed on the ocular surface during preoperative patient preparation, are used for cataract surgery performed under topical anesthesia. This form of anesthesia eliminates the risks of the anesthetic injection and allows for more rapid visual recovery after surgery. General anesthetics and sedation are important adjuncts for patient care for surgery and examination of the eye, especially in children and uncooperative adults. Most inhalational agents and central nervous system depressants are associated with a reduction in IOP. An exception is *ketamine,* which has been associated with an elevation in IOP. In the setting of a patient with a ruptured globe, the anesthesia should be selected carefully to avoid agents that depolarize the extraocular muscles, which may result in expulsion of intraocular contents.

Other Agents for Ophthalmic Therapy
VITAMINS AND TRACE ELEMENTS

Table 63–7 summarizes the vitamin deficiencies related to eye function and disease, especially vitamin A. Vitamin A plays an essential role in retinal function; the active vitamin is retinal (vitamin A aldehyde). Vitamin A deficiency interferes with vision in dim light, a condition known as night blindness (nyctalopia). Photoreception is accomplished by two types of specialized retinal cells, termed rods and cones. Rods are especially sensitive to light of low intensity; cones act as receptors of high-intensity light and are responsible for color vision. The initial step is the absorption of light by a chromophore attached to the receptor protein. 11-cis-retinal is the chromophore of both rods and cones. The holoreceptor in rods is termed rhodopsin—a combination of the protein opsin and 11-cis-retinal attached as a prosthetic group. In the synthesis of rhodopsin, 11-cis-retinol is converted to 11-cis-retinal, which then combines with the ε-amino group of a specific Lys residue in opsin to form rhodopsin. Most rhodopsin is located in the membranes of the discs situated in the outer segments of the rods. The polypeptide chain of rhodopsin spans the membrane seven times, a characteristic shared by all GPCRs. The visual cycle is initiated by the absorption of a photon of light, followed by the photodecomposition, or bleaching, of rhodopsin, leading ultimately to the isomerization of 11-cis-retinal to the all-trans form and dissociation of the opsin moiety. Activated rhodopsin interacts rapidly with a G protein termed transducin or G_t. Transducin stimulates a cyclic GMP–specific phosphodiesterase (PDE6). The resultant decline in cyclic GMP concentration

Table 63–7

Ophthalmic Effects of Selected Vitamin Deficiencies and Zinc Deficiency

Deficiency	Effects in Anterior Segment	Effects in Posterior Segment
Vitamin		
A (retinol)	Conjunctiva (Bitot's spots, xerosis) Cornea (keratomalacia, punctate keratopathy)	Retina (nyctalopia, impaired rhodopsin synthesis); retinal pigment epithelium (hypopigmentation)
B_1 (thiamine)		Optic nerve (temporal atrophy with corresponding visual field defects)
B_6 (pyridoxine)	Cornea (neovascularization)	Retina (gyrate atrophy)
B_{12} (cyanocobalamin)		Optic nerve (temporal atrophy with corresponding visual field defects)
C (ascorbic acid)	Lens (?cataract formation)	
E (tocopherol)		Retina and retinal pigment epithelium (?macular degeneration)
Folic acid		Vein occlusion
K	Conjunctiva (hemorrhage) Anterior chamber (hyphema)	Retina (hemorrhage)
Zinc		Retina and retinal pigment epithelium (?macular degeneration)

causes a decreased conductance of cyclic GMP–gated Na^+ channels in the plasma membrane and an increased transmembrane potential; this primary receptor potential leads to the generation of action potentials that travel to the brain via the optic nerve. All-trans-retinal can isomerize to 11-cis-retinal, or alternatively, all-trans-retinal can cycle through all-trans-retinol and 11-cis-retinol to 11-cis-retinal, which combines with opsin to regenerate rhodopsin.

Humans deficient in vitamin A lose their ability for dark adaptation. Rod vision is affected more than cone vision. Upon depletion of retinol from liver and blood, the concentrations of retinol and rhodopsin in the retina fall. Unless the deficiency is overcome, opsin, lacking the stabilizing effect of retinal, decays and anatomical deterioration of the rods' outer segments occurs. In rats maintained on a vitamin A–deficient diet, irreversible ultrastructural changes leading to blindness then supervene, a process that takes ~10 months. Following short-term deprivation of vitamin A, dark adaptation can be restored to normal by the addition of retinol to the diet, but this restoration takes several weeks. The reason for this delay is unknown.

The functional and structural integrity of epithelial cells throughout the body requires an adequate supply of vitamin A, which plays a major role in the induction and control of epithelial differentiation in mucus-secreting or keratinizing tissues. In the presence of retinol or retinoic acid, basal epithelial cells are stimulated to produce mucus. Excessive concentrations of the retinoids lead to the production of a thick layer of mucin, the inhibition of keratinization, and the display of goblet cells. In the absence of vitamin A, goblet mucous cells disappear and are replaced by basal cells that have been stimulated to proliferate. These undermine and replace the original epithelium with a stratified, keratinizing epithelium. The suppression of normal secretions leads to irritation and infection. When this process happens in the cornea, severe hyperkeratinization (xerophthalmia) may lead to permanent blindness, one of the most common causes of blindness worldwide.

Nutritional vitamin A deficiency causes xerophthalmia, a progressive disease characterized by night blindness, xerosis (dryness), and keratomalacia (corneal thinning), which may lead to perforation; xerophthalmia may be reversed with vitamin A therapy. However, rapid, irreversible blindness ensues once the cornea perforates. Vitamin A also is involved in epithelial differentiation and may have some role in corneal epithelial wound healing. There is no evidence to support using topical vitamin A for keratoconjunctivitis sicca in the absence of a nutritional deficiency.

The current recommendation for retinitis pigmentosa is to administer 15,000 IU of vitamin A palmitate daily under the supervision of an ophthalmologist and to avoid high-dose vitamin E.

One recent clinical trial found a reduction in the risk of progression of some types of age-related macular degeneration in subjects who received high doses of vitamins C (500 mg), E (400 IU), β-carotene (15 mg), cupric oxide (2 mg), and zinc (80 mg), and other studies are ongoing.

WETTING AGENTS AND TEAR SUBSTITUTES

The management of dry eyes usually includes instilling artificial tears and ophthalmic lubricants. Tear substitutes generally are hypotonic or isotonic solutions composed of electrolytes, surfactants, preservatives, and some viscosity-increasing agent that prolongs the residence time in the cul-de-sac and precorneal tear film. Common viscosity agents include cellulose polymers (e.g., carboxymethylcellulose, hydroxyethyl cellulose, hydroxypropyl cellulose, hydroxypropyl methylcellulose, and methylcellulose), polyvinyl alcohol, polyethylene glycol, polysorbate, mineral oil, glycerin, and dextran. The tear substitutes are available as preservative-containing or preservative-free preparations. The viscosity of the tear substitute depends on its exact formulation and can range from watery to gel-like. Some tear formulations also are combined with a vasoconstrictor, such as naphazoline, phenylephrine, or tetrahydrozoline. In other countries, (but not the U.S.), hyaluronic acid sometimes is used as a viscous agent.

The lubricating ointments are composed of a mixture of white petrolatum, mineral oil, liquid or alcohol lanolin, and sometimes a preservative. These highly viscous formulations cause considerable blurring of vision, and consequently they are used primarily at bedtime, in critically ill patients, or in very severe dry eye conditions.

Such aqueous and ointment formulations are only fair substitutes for the precorneal tear film, a poorly understood lipid, aqueous, and mucin trilaminar barrier (see above). Many local eye conditions and systemic diseases may affect the precorneal tear film. Local eye disease, such as blepharitis, ocular rosacea, ocular pemphigoid, chemical burns, or corneal dystrophies, may alter the ocular surface and change the tear composition. Appropriate treatment of the symptomatic dry eye includes treating the accompanying disease and possibly the addition of tear substitutes. There also are a number of systemic conditions that may manifest themselves with symptomatic dry eyes, including Sjögren's syndrome, rheumatoid arthritis, vitamin A deficiency, Stevens-Johnson syndrome, and trachoma. Treating the systemic disease may not eliminate the symptomatic dry eye complaints; chronic therapy with tear substitutes or surgical occlusion of the lacrimal drainage system may be indicated.

OSMOTIC AGENTS AND DRUGS AFFECTING CARBONIC ANHYDRASE

The main osmotic drugs for ocular use include glycerin, mannitol (see *Chapter 28), and hypertonic saline. Ophthalmologists occasionally use glycerin and mannitol for short-term management of acute rises in IOP. Sporadically, these agents are used intraoperatively to dehydrate the vitreous prior to anterior segment surgical procedures. Many patients with acute glaucoma do not tolerate oral medications because of nausea; therefore, intravenous administration of mannitol and/or acetazolamide may be preferred. These agents should be used with caution in patients with congestive heart failure or renal failure.*

Corneal edema is a clinical sign of corneal endothelial dysfunction, and topical osmotic agents may effectively dehydrate the cornea. Identifying the cause of corneal edema will guide therapy, and topical osmotic agents, such as hypertonic saline, may temporize the need for surgical intervention in the form of a corneal transplant. Sodium chloride is available in either aqueous or ointment formulations. Topical glycerin also is available; however, because it causes pain upon contact with the cornea and conjunctiva, its use is limited to urgent evaluation of filtration-angle structures. In general, when corneal edema occurs secondary to acute glaucoma, the use of an oral osmotic agent to help reduce IOP is preferred to topical glycerin, which simply clears the cornea temporarily. Reducing IOP will help clear the cornea more permanently to allow both a view of the filtration angle by gonioscopy and a clear view of the iris as required to perform laser iridotomy.

For a complete Bibliographical listing see Goodman & Gilman's *The Pharmacological Basis of Therapeutics*, 11th ed., or Goodman & Gilman Online at www.accessmedicine.com.

64

PRINCIPLES OF TOXICOLOGY
AND TREATMENT OF POISONING

The clinician must evaluate the possibility that a patient's signs and symptoms may be caused by toxic chemicals present in the environment or administered as therapeutic agents. Many adverse effects of drugs mimic symptoms of disease. Appreciation of the principles of toxicology is necessary for the recognition and management of such clinical problems.

DOSE–RESPONSE RELATIONSHIPS; RISK ASSESSMENT

There is a graded dose–response relationship in an *individual* and a quantal dose–response relationship in the *population* (*see* Chapters 1 and 5). Graded doses of a drug given to an individual usually result in a greater magnitude of response as the dose is increased. In a quantal dose–response relationship, the percentage of the population affected increases as the dose is raised; the relationship is quantal in that the effect is specified to be either present or absent in a given individual (*see* Figure 5–4). This quantal dose–response phenomenon is used to determine the *median lethal dose* (LD_{50}) of drugs and other chemicals.

There are marked differences in the LD_{50} values of various chemicals. Some result in death at extremely low doses (LD_{50} for botulinum toxin = 10 pg/kg); others may be relatively harmless in doses of several grams or more (*e.g.*, penicillin). Even a single chemical may be safe at low doses and quite toxic at higher doses, or safe acutely but harmful over time. Thus, it is not possible to categorize all chemicals as either safe or toxic. The real concern is the *risk* associated with use of the chemical. Depending on the use and disposition of a chemical, a very toxic compound ultimately may be less harmful than a relatively nontoxic one.

There is much concern about the risk from exposure to chemicals that produce cancer in laboratory animals. Whether these chemicals are human carcinogens is generally unknown. Regulatory agencies take one of three approaches to potential chemical carcinogens. For food additives, the U.S. Food and Drug Administration (FDA) is very cautious because large numbers of people are likely to be exposed to the chemicals, and they are not likely to have beneficial effects to individuals. For drugs, the FDA weighs the relative risks and benefits of the drugs for patients. Thus, it is unlikely that the FDA will approve the use of a drug that produces tumors in laboratory animals for a mild ailment, but it may approve its use for a serious disease. In fact, most cancer chemotherapeutic drugs also are chemical carcinogens.

In the regulation of environmental carcinogens, agencies such as the Environmental Protection Agency (EPA) attempt to limit lifetime exposure such that the incidence of cancer due to the chemical is no more than one in a million people. To determine the daily allowable exposure for humans, mathematical models are used to extrapolate doses of chemicals that produce a particular incidence of tumors in laboratory animals (often in the range of 10–20%) to those that should produce cancer in no more than one person in a million in a lifetime. The models used are conservative and are thought to provide adequate protection from undue risks from exposure to potential carcinogens. As discussed in Chapter 3, variations in drug metabolism often result in substantial differences between the biological responses of humans and rodents (the common laboratory test animals).

ACUTE *VERSUS* CHRONIC EXPOSURE   Effects of acute exposure to a chemical often differ from those of chronic exposure. Evaluation of *cumulative* toxic effects is receiving increased attention because of chronic exposure to low concentrations of various natural and synthetic chemical substances in the environment.

CHEMICAL FORMS OF DRUGS THAT PRODUCE TOXICITY

Both therapeutic and toxic effects of drugs can be due to the administered agent or metabolites of the drug produced by enzymes, light, or reactive oxygen species. In considering the toxicity of drugs and chemicals, it is important to understand their metabolism, activation, or decomposition. For instance, most organophosphate insecticides are biotransformed by CYPs (cytochromes P450)

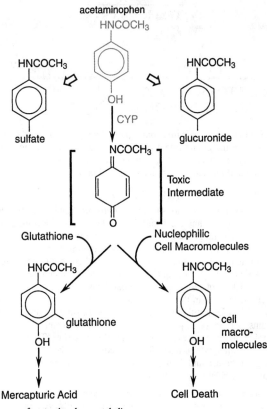

FIGURE 64–1 *Pathways of acetaminophen metabolism.*

to produce the active toxin: parathion is biotransformed to paraoxon, a stable metabolite that binds to and inactivates cholinesterase (see *Chapter 8*). *Some drug metabolites are not chemically stable and are referred to as* reactive intermediates; *consider the metabolite of* acetaminophen *(Figure 64–1), which binds to nucleophiles such as glutathione; when cellular glutathione is depleted, the metabolite binds to cellular macromolecules, the mechanism by which acetaminophen kills liver cells* (see *Chapters 3 and 26*). *Both parathion and acetaminophen are more toxic under conditions in which CYPs are increased, such as following* ethanol *or* phenobarbital *exposure, because CYPs produce the toxic metabolites.*

Some chemicals can be activated in the skin by ultraviolet (UV) and/or visible radiation. In photoallergy, radiation absorbed by a drug, such as a sulfonamide, results in its conversion to a more potent allergen than the parent compound. Phototoxic reactions to drugs, in contrast to photoallergic ones, do not have an immunological component. Drugs that are either absorbed locally into the skin or have reached the systemic circulation may be the object of photochemical reactions within the skin; this can lead directly either to chemically induced photosensitivity reactions or to enhancement of the usual effects of sunlight. Tetracyclines, sulfonamides, chlorpromazine, and nalidixic acid are examples of phototoxic chemicals; generally, they are innocuous to skin if not exposed to light.

SPECTRUM OF UNDESIRED EFFECTS

In therapeutics, a drug typically produces numerous effects, but usually only one is sought as the primary goal of treatment; most of the other effects are referred to as *undesirable effects* of that drug for that therapeutic indication. *Side effects* of drugs usually are nondeleterious; they include effects such as dry mouth occurring with tricyclic antidepressant therapy. Some side effects may be *adverse* or *toxic*. Mechanistic categorization of *toxic* effects is a necessary prelude to their avoidance or, if they occur, to effect their rational and successful management.

TYPES OF TOXIC REACTIONS   Toxic effects of drugs may be classified as pharmacological, pathological, or genotoxic (alterations of DNA), and their incidence and seriousness are related, at least over some range, to the concentration of the toxic chemical in the body. An example of a pharmacological toxicity is excessive depression of the central nervous system (CNS) by barbiturates; of a pathological effect, hepatic injury produced by acetaminophen; of a genotoxic effect, a neoplasm produced by a *nitrogen mustard*. If the concentration of chemical in the tissues does not exceed a critical level, the effects usually will be reversible. The pharmacological effects usually disappear when the concentration of drug or chemical in the tissues is decreased by biotransformation or excretion from the body. Pathological and genotoxic effects may be repaired. If these effects are severe, death may ensue within a short time; if more subtle damage to DNA is not repaired, cancer may appear in a few months or years in laboratory animals or in a decade or more in humans.

Local *versus* Systemic Toxicity

Local toxicity occurs at the site of first contact between the biological system and the toxicant. Systemic toxicity requires absorption and distribution of the toxicant; most substances, with the exception of highly reactive chemical species, produce systemic toxic effects. The two categories are not mutually exclusive. Tetraethyl lead, for example, injures skin at the site of contact and deleteriously affects the CNS after it is absorbed into the circulation (see Chapter 65).

Most systemic toxicants predominantly affect one or a few organs. The target organ of toxicity is not necessarily the site of accumulation of the chemical. For example, lead is concentrated in bone, but its primary toxic action is on soft tissues; DDT (chlorophenothane) is concentrated in adipose tissue but produces no known toxic effects there.

The CNS is involved in systemic toxicity most frequently because many compounds with prominent effects elsewhere also affect the brain. Next in order of frequency of involvement in systemic toxicity are the heart and circulatory system; the blood and hematopoietic system; visceral organs such as liver, kidney, and lung; and the skin. Muscle and bone are least often affected. With substances that have a predominantly local effect, the frequency of tissue reaction depends largely on the portal of entry (skin, GI tract, or respiratory tract).

Reversible and Irreversible Toxic Effects

The effects of drugs on humans, whenever possible, must be reversible; otherwise, the drugs would be prohibitively toxic. If a chemical produces injury to a tissue, the capacity of the tissue to regenerate or recover largely will determine the reversibility of the effect. Injuries to a tissue such as liver, which has a high capacity to regenerate, usually are reversible; injury to the CNS is largely irreversible because the highly differentiated neurons of the brain have a more limited capacity to divide and regenerate.

Delayed Toxicity

Most toxic effects of drugs occur at a predictable (usually short) time after administration. However, such is not always the case. For example, aplastic anemia caused by chloramphenicol *may appear weeks after the drug has been discontinued. Carcinogenic effects of chemicals usually have a long latency period: 20–30 years may pass before tumors are observed. Because such delayed effects cannot be assessed during any reasonable period of initial evaluation of a chemical, there is an urgent need for reliably predictive short-term tests for such toxicity, as well as for systematic surveillance of the long-term effects of marketed drugs and other chemicals (see Chapter 5).*

CHEMICAL CARCINOGENS   Chemical carcinogens are classified as *genotoxic* or *nongenotoxic*. Genotoxic carcinogens interact with DNA; nongenotoxic carcinogens do not. Chemical carcinogenesis is a multistep process. Most genotoxic carcinogens are themselves unreactive (*procarcinogens* or *proximate carcinogens*) but are converted to *primary* or *ultimate carcinogens* in the body. The drug-metabolizing enzymes often convert the proximate carcinogens to reactive electrophilic intermediates (*see* Chapter 3). These reactive intermediates can interact with nucleophilic centers in DNA to produce a mutation. Such interaction of the ultimate carcinogen with DNA in a cell is thought to be the initial step in chemical carcinogenesis. The DNA may revert to normal if DNA repair mechanisms operate successfully; if not, the transformed cell may grow into a tumor that becomes apparent clinically.

Nongenotoxic carcinogens, or *promoters*, do not produce tumors alone but do potentiate the effects of genotoxic carcinogens. The time from initiation to the development of a tumor probably depends on the presence of such promoters; for many human tumors, the latent period is 15–45 years.

Two main types of laboratory tests are used to screen for potential carcinogenicity. One is performed to determine whether the chemical is mutagenic, since many carcinogens are also mutagens. Such studies often use assays such as the Ames test. This reverse mutation test uses a strain of Salmonella typhimurium that has a mutant gene for the enzyme phosphoribosyl adenosine triphosphate (ATP) synthetase. This enzyme is required for histidine synthesis, and the bacterial strain is unable to grow in a histidine-deficient medium unless a reverse mutation is induced. Because many chemicals are not mutagenic or carcinogenic unless activated by enzymes on the endoplasmic reticulum, rat hepatic microsomes usually are added to the medium containing the mutant bacteria and the drug. The Ames test is rapid and sensitive; its usefulness for the prediction of genotoxic carcinogens is widely accepted; it does not, however, detect nongenotoxic carcinogens (promoters). The second type consists of feeding laboratory rodents the chemical at high dosages for their entire life span, after which autopsies and histopathological examinations are performed on each animal. This latter study can detect both promoters and genotoxic carcinogens.

ALLERGIC REACTIONS Chemical allergy is an adverse reaction that results from previous sensitization to a particular chemical or to one that is structurally similar. Such reactions are mediated by the immune system. The terms *hypersensitivity* and *drug allergy* often are used to describe the allergic state.

For a low-molecular-weight chemical to cause an allergic reaction, it or its metabolic product usually acts as a hapten, combining with an endogenous protein to form an antigenic complex. Such antigens induce the synthesis of antibodies, usually after a latent period of at least 1–2 weeks. Subsequent exposure of the organism to the chemical results in an antigen–antibody interaction that provokes the typical manifestations of allergy. Dose–response relationships usually are not apparent for the provocation of allergic reactions.

Allergic responses have been divided into four general categories based on the mechanism of immunological involvement. Type I, or anaphylactic, reactions are mediated by immunoglobulin (IgE) antibodies. The Fc portion of IgE can bind to receptors on mast cells and basophils (see Chapter 27). If the Fab portion of the antibody molecule then binds antigen, various mediators (e.g., histamine, leukotrienes, and prostaglandins) are released and cause vasodilation, edema, and an inflammatory response. The main targets of this type of reaction are the GI tract (food allergies), the skin (urticaria and atopic dermatitis), the respiratory system (rhinitis and asthma), and the vasculature (anaphylactic shock). These responses tend to occur quickly after challenge with an antigen to which the individual has been sensitized and are termed immediate hypersensitivity reactions.

Type II, or cytolytic, reactions are mediated by both IgG and IgM antibodies and usually are attributed to their ability to activate the complement system. The major target tissues for cytolytic reactions are the cells in the circulatory system. Examples of type II allergic responses include penicillin-*induced hemolytic anemia,* methyldopa-*induced autoimmune hemolytic anemia,* quinidine-*induced thrombocytopenic purpura, and* sulfonamide-*induced granulocytopenia. These autoimmune reactions to drugs usually subside within several months after removal of the offending agent.*

Type III, or Arthus, reactions are mediated predominantly by IgG; the mechanism involves the generation of antigen–antibody complexes that subsequently fix complement. The complexes are deposited in the vascular endothelium, where a destructive inflammatory response called serum sickness occurs. This phenomenon contrasts with the type II reaction, in which the inflammatory response is induced by antibodies directed against tissue antigens. The signs and symptoms of serum sickness include urticarial skin eruptions, arthralgia or arthritis, lymphadenopathy, and fever. These reactions usually last for 6–12 days and then subside after the offending agent is eliminated. Several drugs (e.g., sulfonamides, penicillins, certain anticonvulsants, and iodides) can induce serum sickness. Stevens-Johnson syndrome, such as that caused by sulfonamides, is a more severe form of immune vasculitis; manifestations include erythema multiforme, arthritis, nephritis, CNS abnormalities, and myocarditis.

Type IV, or delayed-hypersensitivity, reactions are mediated by sensitized T-lymphocytes and macrophages. When sensitized cells come in contact with antigen, an inflammatory reaction is generated by the production of lymphokines and the subsequent influx of neutrophils and macrophages. An example of type IV or delayed hypersensitivity is the contact dermatitis caused by poison ivy.

IDIOSYNCRATIC REACTIONS

Idiosyncrasy is an abnormal reactivity to a chemical that is peculiar to a given individual. The idiosyncratic response may take the form of extreme sensitivity to low doses or extreme insensitivity to high doses of chemicals. Certain idiosyncratic reactions can result from genetic polymorphisms that cause individual differences in drug pharmacokinetics; for example, an increased incidence of peripheral neuropathy is seen in patients with inherited deficiencies in acetylation when isoniazid *is used to treat tuberculosis. The polymorphisms also can be due to pharmacodynamic factors such as drug-receptor interactions (e.g., ~10% of black males develop a serious hemolytic anemia when they receive* primaquine *as an antimalarial therapy; such individuals have a deficiency of erythrocyte glucose-6-phosphate dehydrogenase [see Chapter 39]). Genetically determined resistance to the anticoagulant action of* warfarin *is due to an alteration in the vitamin K epoxide reductase, whereas inherent sensitivity to warfarin is due to polymorphisms in CYP2C9* (see *Chapter 54).*

INTERACTIONS BETWEEN CHEMICALS

Concurrent exposures may alter the pharmacokinetics of drugs by changing rates of absorption, the degree of protein binding, or the rates of biotransformation or excretion of one or both interacting compounds. The pharmacodynamics of chemicals can be altered by competition at the receptor; for example, atropine *is used to treat organophosphate insecticide toxicity because it blocks muscarinic cholinergic receptors and prevents their stimulation by the excess acetylcholine accruing from inhibition of acetylcholinesterase by the insecticide. Nonreceptor pharmacodynamic drug interactions also can occur when two drugs have different mechanisms of action:* Aspirin *and* heparin *given together can cause unexpected bleeding. The response to combined toxicants thus may be equal to, greater than, or less than the sum of the effects of the individual agents.*

Numerous terms describe pharmacological and toxicological interactions. An additive *effect describes the combined effect of two chemicals that equals the sum of the effect of each agent given alone; the additive effect is the most common. A* synergistic *effect is one in which the combined effect of two chemicals exceeds the sum of the effects of each agent given alone. For example, both carbon tetrachloride and ethanol are hepatotoxins, but together they produce much more injury to the liver than expected from the sum of their individual effects.* Potentiation *is the increased effect of a toxic agent acting simultaneously with a nontoxic one. Isopropanol alone, for example, is not hepatotoxic; however, it greatly increases the hepatotoxicity of carbon tetrachloride.* Antagonism *is the interference of one chemical with the action of another. An antagonistic agent is often desirable as an antidote. Functional* or *physiological antagonism occurs when two chemicals produce opposite effects on the same physiological function. For example, this principle is applied to the use of intravenous infusion of dopamine to maintain perfusion of vital organs during certain severe intoxications characterized by marked hypotension.* Chemical antagonism *or inactivation is a reaction between two chemicals to neutralize their effects. For example,* dimercaprol *chelates various metals to decrease their toxicity (see Chapter 65).* Dispositional antagonism *is the alteration of the disposition of a substance (its absorption, biotransformation, distribution, or excretion) so that less of the agent reaches the target organ or its persistence there is reduced.* Antagonism at the receptor *for the chemical entails the blockade of the effect of an agonist with an appropriate antagonist that competes for the same site. For example, the antagonist* naloxone *is used to treat respiratory depression produced by opioids* (see *Chapter 21).*

INCIDENCE OF ACUTE POISONING

The true incidence of poisoning in the U.S. is not known, but in 2003, nearly 2.4 million cases were voluntarily reported to the American Association of Poison Control Centers. The number of actual poisonings almost certainly exceeds by far the number reported. Deaths in the U.S. owing to poisoning number more than 1100 per year. The incidence of poisoning in children younger than 5 years of age has decreased dramatically over the past four decades (e.g., there were no reported childhood deaths from aspirin in 2003, compared with ~140 deaths/year in the early 1960s). This favorable trend probably is due to safety packaging of drugs, drain cleaners, turpentine, and other household chemicals; improved medical training and care; and increased public awareness of potential poisons.

The substances involved most frequently in human poison exposures are shown in Table 64–1. Analgesic drugs lead the list, followed by two nondrug entries, cleaning agents and cosmetics. However, the top five categories of substances that produce deaths are drugs (Table 64–2). The categories most commonly associated with fatalities are analgesics (e.g., acetaminophen and salicylates), sedative-hypnotics/antipsychotics, antidepressants, stimulants and street drugs (including opiates *and* cocaine*), and cardiovascular drugs (including* digoxin *and* Ca^{2+} *channel blockers). The most common categories of nonpharmaceutical poisons were alcohols (particularly methanol) and fumes (principally carbon monoxide). Most of the people who die from poisoning are adults, and the deaths often result from intentional rather than accidental exposure. Children younger than 6 years of age account for 52% of the poisoning incidents reported but only 3% of the deaths. Children between 1 and 2 years of age have the highest incidence of accidental poisoning. Fortunately, most of the substances available to these young children are not highly toxic. Iron and pesticides are the leading cause of pediatric accidental poisoning fatalities.*

Table 64–1

Substances Most Frequently Involved in Human Poison Exposures in the U.S.

Substance	Number	%*
Analgesics	256,843	10.8
Cleaning substances	225,578	9.5
Cosmetics and personal care products	219,877	9.2
Foreign bodies	110,000	5.0
Sedative-hypnotics/antipsychotics	111,001	4.7
Topicals	105,815	4.4
Cough and cold preparations	100,612	4.2
Antidepressants	99,800	4.2
Bites/envenomations	98,585	4.1
Pesticides	96,112	4.0
Plants	84,578	3.6
Food products, food poisoning	75,813	3.2
Alcohols	69,215	2.9
Antihistamines	69,107	2.9
Antimicrobials	63,372	2.7
Cardiovascular drugs	61,056	2.6
Hydrocarbons	59,132	2.5
Chemicals	54,623	2.3

NOTE: Despite a high frequency of involvement, these substances are not necessarily the most toxic, but rather may only be the most readily accessible.

*Percentages are based on total number of known ingested substances in the U.S. rather than the total number of human exposure cases.

From Watson *et al.*, 2004.

Table 64–2

Categories with Largest Numbers of Deaths*

Category	Number	% of All Exposures
Analgesics	659	0.257
Sedative-hypnotics/antipsychotics	364	0.328
Antidepressants	318	0.316
Stimulants and street drugs	242	0.528
Cardiovascular drugs	181	0.295
Alcohols	139	0.200
Chemicals	50	0.091
Anticonvulsants	65	0.181
Gases and fumes	44	0.106
Antihistamines	71	0.103
Muscle relaxants	52	0.260
Hormones and hormone antagonists	33	0.062
Cleaning substances	33	0.013
Automotive products	30	0.213
Cough and cold preparations	22	0.022
Pesticides	18	0.019

*This list is for deaths in the U.S. From Watson *et al.*, 2004.

The incidence of serious and fatal adverse drug reactions (ADRs) in U.S. hospitals is high. An estimated 2 million hospitalized patients have serious ADRs each year, and about 100,000 suffer fatal ADRs. If this estimate is correct, then more people die annually from medication errors than from highway accidents, breast cancer, or AIDS.

MAJOR SOURCES OF INFORMATION ON POISONING

The web site of the American Association of Poison Control Centers (*http://www.aapcc.org/*) lists 78 members, including 11 regional centers. Valuable information can be obtained from these centers by telephone (800-222-1222). The National Library of Medicine maintains a very informative Web site on toxicology and environmental health (*http://sis.nlm.nih.gov/Tox/ToxMain.html*), including a link to ToxNet (*http://toxnet.nlm.nih.gov/*), a cluster of databases on toxicology, hazardous chemicals, and related areas. Pharmacology textbooks are a good source of information on the treatment of poisoning by drugs.

PREVENTION AND TREATMENT OF POISONING

For clinical purposes, toxic agents can be divided into two classes: those for which a specific treatment or antidote exists and those for which there is no specific treatment. For the vast majority of drugs and other chemicals, there is no specific treatment; symptomatic medical care that supports vital functions is the only strategy.

Supportive therapy is the mainstay of the treatment of drug poisoning. The adage, "Treat the patient, not the poison," remains the most basic and important principle of clinical toxicology. Maintenance of respiration and circulation takes precedence. Serial measurement and charting of vital signs and important reflexes help to judge the progress of intoxication, response to therapy, and need for additional treatment. This monitoring usually requires hospitalization. The classification in Table 64–3 helps to define the severity of CNS intoxication. Treatment with large doses of stimulants and sedatives often causes more harm than the poison. Chemical antidotes should be used judiciously; heroic measures seldom are necessary.

Treatment of acute poisoning must be prompt. The first goal is to maintain the vital functions if their impairment is imminent. The second goal is to keep the concentration of poison in the crucial tissues as low as possible by preventing absorption and enhancing elimination. The third goal is to combat the pharmacological and toxicological effects at the effector sites.

Prevention of Further Absorption of Poison

EMESIS   The routine induction of emesis in emergency rooms is declining. Although emesis still may be indicated for immediate intervention after poisoning by oral ingestion of chemicals, it is

Table 64–3

Signs and Symptoms of CNS Intoxication

Degree of Severity	Characteristics
Depressants	
0	Asleep, but can be aroused and can answer questions
I	Semicomatose, withdraws from painful stimuli, reflexes intact
II	Comatose, does not withdraw from painful stimuli, no respiratory or circulatory depression, most reflexes intact
III	Comatose, most or all reflexes absent, but without depression of respiration or of circulation
IV	Comatose, reflexes absent, respiratory depression with cyanosis or circulatory failure and shock, or both
Stimulants	
I	Restlessness, irritability, insomnia, tremor, hyperreflexia, sweating, mydriasis, flushing
II	Confusion, hyperactivity, hypertension, tachypnea, tachycardia, extrasystoles, sweating, mydriasis, flushing, mild hyperpyrexia
III	Delirium, mania, self-injury, marked hypertension, tachycardia, arrhythmias, hyperpyrexia
IV	As in III, plus convulsions, coma, and circulatory collapse

contraindicated in certain situations: (1) if the patient has ingested a corrosive poison, such as a strong acid or alkali (*e.g.*, drain cleaners), emesis increases the likelihood of gastric perforation and further necrosis of the esophagus; (2) if the patient is comatose or in a state of stupor or delirium, emesis may cause aspiration of the gastric contents; (3) if the patient has ingested a CNS stimulant, further stimulation associated with vomiting may precipitate convulsions; and (4) if the patient has ingested a petroleum distillate (*e.g.*, kerosene, gasoline, or petroleum-based liquid furniture polish), regurgitated hydrocarbons can be aspirated readily and cause chemical pneumonitis. In contrast, emesis *should* be considered if the ingested solution contains potentially dangerous compounds, such as pesticides.

The ability of various hydrocarbons to produce pneumonitis is generally inversely proportional to their viscosity: If the viscosity is high, as with oils and greases, the risk is limited; if the viscosity is low, as with mineral seal oil found in liquid furniture polishes, the risk of aspiration is high.

Vomiting can be induced mechanically by stroking the posterior pharynx. However, this technique is not as effective as the administration of ipecac *or* apomorphine.

IPECAC   The most common household emetic is syrup of ipecac (not ipecac fluid extract, which is 14 times more potent and may cause fatalities). Syrup of ipecac is available OTC in 15 and 30 mL containers. The drug can be given orally, but it takes 15–30 minutes to produce emesis (comparable to the time required for adequate gastric lavage). The oral dose is 15 mL in children from 6 months to 12 years of age and 30 mL in older children and adults. Because emesis may not occur when the stomach is empty, administration of ipecac should be followed by a drink of water.

The current consensus is *that syrup of ipecac should not be administered routinely in the management of poisoned patients.* In studies with various marker substances, the beneficial effects of ipecac-induced emesis were highly variable and diminished rapidly with time. In addition, initial use of ipecac in fact may be counterproductive by reducing the efficacy of other, later, and presumably more effective treatments such as use of activated charcoal, oral antidotes, and whole bowel irrigation (WBI). Ipecac may be indicated when it can be administered to conscious, alert patients within 60 minutes of poisoning.

Ipecac acts as an emetic because of its local irritant effect on the enteric tract and its effect on the chemoreceptor trigger zone (CTZ) in the area postrema of the medulla. Ipecac is not benign; it can produce toxic effects on the heart (due to emetine); this usually is not a problem with the dose used for emesis. If emesis does not occur, ipecac should be removed by gastric lavage. Chronic abuse of ipecac for weight reduction can result in cardiomyopathy, ventricular fibrillation, and death.

Apomorphine

Apomorphine stimulates the CTZ and causes emesis. The drug is unstable in solution and must be prepared just prior to use. Apomorphine is not effective orally and must be given parenterally, usually subcutaneously, 6 mg for adults and 0.06 mg/kg for children. Vomiting ensues in 3–5 minutes. Subcutaneous administration can be an advantage with an uncooperative patient. Because apomorphine is a respiratory depressant, it should not be used if the patient has been poisoned by a CNS depressant or if the patient's respiration is slow and labored. At present, apomorphine is used rarely as an emetic.

GASTRIC LAVAGE   Gastric lavage is accomplished by inserting a tube into the stomach and washing the stomach with water, normal saline, or one-half normal saline to remove the unabsorbed poison. The procedure should be performed as soon as possible, but only if vital functions are adequate or supportive procedures have been implemented. The contraindications to this procedure generally are the same as for emesis, and there is the additional potential complication of mechanical injury to the throat, esophagus, and stomach. The current consensus amongst clinical toxicologists is that *gastric lavage should not be used routinely in the management of the poisoned patient but should be reserved for patients who have ingested a potentially life-threatening amount of poison and when the procedure can be undertaken within 60 minutes of ingestion.*

CHEMICAL ADSORPTION   Activated charcoal avidly adsorbs many drugs and chemicals on the surfaces of the charcoal particles, thereby preventing absorption and toxicity. Charcoal does not absorb all chemicals (*e.g.*, alcohols, hydrocarbons, metals, and corrosives). The effectiveness of charcoal also depends on the time since the ingestion and on the dose of charcoal; one should attempt to achieve a charcoal–drug ratio of at least 10:1. Activated charcoal also can interrupt the enterohepatic circulation of drugs and enhance the net rate of diffusion of the chemical from the body into the GI tract. For example, serial doses of activated charcoal have been shown to enhance the elimination of *theophylline* and phenobarbital.

During the last two decades, there has been an increase in the use of activated charcoal and a corresponding decrease in the use of ipecac-induced emesis and gastric lavage in the treatment of poisoning. Studies in patients with drug overdoses and in normal subjects fail to show a benefit of treatment with ipecac or lavage plus activated charcoal as compared with charcoal alone. Based on these findings, American and European clinical toxicologists issued a position paper in 1999 on the use of multidose-activated charcoal in treatment of acute poisoning. They concluded that while experimental and clinical trials demonstrate that elimination of some drugs can be enhanced by treatment with activated charcoal, rarely has charcoal been demonstrated to reduce morbidity or mortality in a controlled study. The position paper recommends consideration of activated charcoal treatment only if a patient has ingested a life-threatening amount of *carbamazepine, dapsone*, phenobarbital, *quinine*, or theophylline.

Activated charcoal usually is prepared as a mixture of at least 50 g (about 10 heaping tablespoons) in a glass of water. The mixture is then administered either orally or via a gastric tube. Because most poisons do not appear to desorb from the charcoal if charcoal is present in excess, the adsorbed poison need not be removed from the GI tract. Charcoal also may adsorb and decrease the effectiveness of specific antidotes.

Activated charcoal must be distinguished from the so-called universal antidote, which consists of two parts burned toast (not activated charcoal), one part tannic acid (strong tea), and one part magnesium oxide. In practice, the universal antidote is ineffective.

CHEMICAL INACTIVATION

Antidotes can change the chemical nature of a poison by rendering it less toxic or preventing its absorption. Formaldehyde poisoning can be treated with ammonia to promote formation of hexamethylenetetramine; sodium formaldehyde sulfoxylate can convert mercuric ion to the less soluble metallic mercury; and sodium bicarbonate converts ferrous iron to ferrous carbonate, which is poorly absorbed. Chemical inactivation techniques seldom are used today, however, because valuable time may be lost, whereas emetics, activated charcoal, and gastric lavage are rapid and effective. The treatment of choice for ingestion of either acids or alkalis is dilution with water or milk. Similarly, burns produced by acid or alkali on the skin should be treated with copious amounts of water.

PURGATION

The rationale for using an osmotic cathartic is to minimize absorption by hastening the passage of the toxicant through the GI tract. Few, if any, controlled clinical data are available on the effectiveness of cathartics in the treatment of poisoning. Cathartics generally are considered harmless unless the poison has injured the GI tract. Cathartics are indicated after the ingestion of enteric-coated tablets, when the time after ingestion is >1 hour, and for poisoning by volatile hydrocarbons. Sorbitol is the most effective, but sodium sulfate and magnesium sulfate also are used; all act promptly and usually have minimal toxicity. However, $MgSO_4$ should be used cautiously in patients with renal failure or in those likely to develop renal dysfunction, and Na^+-containing cathartics should be avoided in patients with congestive heart failure.

Whole-bowel irrigation (WBI) promotes defecation and eliminates the entire contents of the intestines. This technique uses a high-molecular-weight polyethylene glycol and isomolar electrolyte solution (PEG-E S) that does not alter serum electrolytes. It is available commercially as GOLYTELY and COLYTE. The current consensus amongst clinical toxicologists is that WBI should not be used routinely in the management of the poisoned patient. WBI may be considered in cases of acute poisoning by sustained-release or enteric-coated drugs and possibly toxic ingestions of iron, lead, zinc, or packets of illicit drugs.

INHALATION AND DERMAL EXPOSURE TO POISONS

When a poison has been inhaled, the first priority is to remove the patient from the source of exposure. Similarly, if the skin has had contact with a poison, it should be washed thoroughly with water. Contaminated clothing should be removed. Initial treatment of all types of chemical injuries to the eye must be rapid; thorough irrigation of the eye with water for 15 minutes should be performed immediately.

Enhanced Elimination of the Poison

BIOTRANSFORMATION

Many chemicals are biotransformed into toxic forms. Thus, inhibition of biotransformation should decrease the toxicity. For example, ethanol is used to inhibit the conversion of methanol to its highly toxic metabolite, formic acid, by alcohol dehydrogenase (see Chapter 22). Acetaminophen is converted by the CYP system to an electrophilic metabolite that is detoxified by glutathione, a cellular nucleophile (Figure 64–1). Acetaminophen does not cause hepatotoxicity until glutathione is depleted, whereupon the reactive metabolite binds to essential macromolecular constituents of the hepatocyte, resulting in cell death. The liver can be protected by maintenance of the concentration of glutathione, which can be accomplished by the administration of N-acetylcysteine (see Chapter 26).

Some drugs are detoxified by conjugation with glucuronic acid or sulfate before elimination from the body, and the availability of the endogenous cosubstrates for conjugation may limit the rate of elimination; such is the case in the detoxication of acetaminophen. Repletion of these compounds will provide an additional mechanism to treat poisoning. For instance, detoxication of cyanide by conversion to thiocyanate can be accelerated by the administration of thiosulfate.

BILIARY EXCRETION

The liver excretes many drugs and other foreign chemicals into bile, but little is known about efficient ways to enhance biliary excretion of xenobiotics for the treatment of acute poisoning. Inducers of microsomal enzyme activity enhance biliary excretion of some xenobiotics, but the effect is slow in onset.

URINARY EXCRETION

Drugs and poisons are excreted into the urine by glomerular filtration and active tubular secretion (see Chapter 28); they can be reabsorbed into the blood if they are in a lipid-soluble form that will penetrate the tubule or if there is an active mechanism for their transport.

There are no methods known to accelerate the active transport of poisons into urine, and enhancement of glomerular filtration is not a practical means to facilitate elimination of toxicants. However, passive reabsorption from the tubular lumen can be altered. Diuretics inhibit reabsorption by decreasing the concentration gradient of the drug from the lumen to the tubular cell and by increasing flow through the tubule. Furosemide is used most often, but osmotic diuretics also are employed (see Chapter 28). Forced diuresis should be used with caution, especially in patients with renal, cardiac, or pulmonary complications.

Nonionized compounds are reabsorbed far more rapidly than ionized polar molecules; therefore, a shift from the nonionized to the ionized species of the toxicant by alteration of the pH of the tubular fluid may hasten elimination (*see* Chapter 1). Acidic compounds such as phenobarbital and salicylates are cleared much more rapidly in alkaline than in acidic urine. Clinical toxicologists have issued a position paper on the use of urine alkalinization in treatment of acute poisoning. Urine alkalinization increases the urine elimination of *chlorpropamide, 2,4-dichlorophenoxyacetic acid, diflunisal, fluoride, mecoprop, methotrexate,* phenobarbital, and salicylate. However, urine alkalinization is recommended as first-line treatment only for patients with moderately severe salicylate poisoning who do not meet the criteria for hemodialysis. Urine alkalinization and high urine flow (approximately 600 mL/h) should also be considered in patients with severe 2,4-dichlorophenoxyacetic acid and mecoprop poisoning. Urine alkalinization is not recommended as first-line treatment in cases of phenobarbital poisoning because multiple-dose activated charcoal has been shown to be superior. Urine alkalinization is contraindicated in the case of compromised renal function or failure. Hypokalemia is the most common complication but can be corrected by giving potassium supplements. Intravenous sodium bicarbonate is used to alkalinize the urine.

Renal excretion of basic drugs such as *amphetamine* theoretically can be enhanced by acidification of the urine. Acidification can be accomplished by the administration of ammonium chloride or ascorbic acid. Urinary excretion of an acidic compound is particularly sensitive to changes in urinary pH if its pK_a is within the range of 3.0–7.5; for bases, the corresponding pH range is 7.5–10.5.

DIALYSIS

Hemodialysis or hemoperfusion usually has limited use in the treatment of intoxication with chemicals. However, under certain circumstances, such procedures can be lifesaving. The utility of dialysis depends on the amount of poison in the blood relative to the total-body burden. Thus, if a poison has a large volume of distribution, as is the case for the tricyclic antidepressants, the plasma will contain too little of the compound for effective removal by dialysis. Extensive binding of the compound to plasma proteins impairs dialysis greatly. The elimination of a toxicant by dialysis also depends on dissociation of the compound from binding sites in tissues; for some chemicals, this rate may be slow and limiting.

Although peritoneal dialysis requires a minimum of personnel and can be started as soon as the patient is admitted to the hospital, it is too inefficient to be of value for the treatment of acute intoxications. Hemodialysis (extracorporeal dialysis) is much more effective than peritoneal dialysis and may be essential in a few life-threatening intoxications, such as with methanol, ethylene glycol, and salicylates.

Passage of blood through a column of charcoal or adsorbent resin (hemoperfusion) is a technique for the extracorporeal removal of a poison. Because of the high adsorptive capacity and affinity of the material in the column, some chemicals that are bound to plasma proteins can be removed. The principal side effect of hemoperfusion is depletion of platelets.

ANTAGONISM OR CHEMICAL INACTIVATION OF AN ABSORBED POISON

If a patient is poisoned with a compound that acts as an agonist at a receptor for which a specific blocking agent is available, administration of the receptor antagonist may be highly effective. Functional antagonism also can be valuable for support of the patient's vital functions. For example, anticonvulsant drugs are used to treat chemically induced convulsions. However, drugs that stimulate antagonistic physiological mechanisms are not always of clinical value and may even decrease survival because it often is difficult to titrate the effect of one drug against another when the two act on opposing systems. An example of such a complication is the use of CNS stimulants to attempt to reverse respiratory depression. Convulsions are a typical complication of such therapy; mechanical support of respiration is preferred. In addition, the duration of action of the poison and the antidote may differ, sometimes leading to poisoning with the antidote.

Specific chemical antagonists of a toxicant, such as opioid antagonists (see Chapter 21) and atropine as an antagonist of pesticide-induced acetylcholine excess (see Chapter 7), are rare. A recently approved antagonist is fomepizole, an inhibitor of alcohol dehydrogenase, approved for treatment for poisoning by ethylene glycol and methanol. Chelating agents with high selectivity for certain metal ions are used more commonly (see Chapter 65). Antibodies offer the potential for the production of specific antidotes; a notable example is the use of purified digoxin-specific Fab fragments of antibodies in the treatment of potentially fatal cases of poisoning with digoxin (see Chapter 33). The development of human monoclonal antibodies directed against specific toxins has significant potential.

For a complete Bibliographical listing see Goodman & Gilman's *The Pharmacological Basis of Therapeutics,* **11th ed., or Goodman & Gilman Online at www.accessmedicine.com.**

65

HEAVY METALS AND HEAVY-METAL ANTAGONISTS

Heavy metals exert their toxic effects by combining with one or more reactive groups (ligands) essential for normal physiological functions. Heavy-metal antagonists (*chelating agents*) are designed specifically to compete with these groups for the metals and thereby prevent or reverse toxic effects and enhance the excretion of metals.

HEAVY-METAL ANTAGONISTS

A *chelate* is a complex formed between a metal and a compound that contains two or more potential ligands. The product of such a reaction is a heterocyclic ring. Five- and six-membered chelate rings are the most stable, and polydentate (multiligand) chelators typically form more stable chelates than chelators with only one ligand atom.

The stability of chelates varies with the metal and the ligand atoms. For example, lead and mercury have greater affinities for sulfur and nitrogen than for oxygen ligands; calcium, however, has a greater affinity for oxygen than for sulfur and nitrogen. These differences in affinity serve as the basis for selectivity of action of a chelating agent in the body.

The effectiveness of a chelating agent for the treatment of poisoning by a heavy metal depends on numerous factors: the relative affinity of the chelator for the heavy metal as compared with essential body metals, the distribution of the chelator in the body as compared with the distribution of the metal, and the capacity of the chelator to remove the metal from the body once chelated. Consider the properties of an ideal chelating agent: high solubility in water, resistance to biotransformation, ability to reach sites of metal storage, capacity to form nontoxic complexes with toxic metals, ability to retain chelating activity at the pH of body fluids, and ready excretion of the chelate. A low affinity for Ca^{2+} also is desirable because Ca^{2+} in plasma is readily available for chelation, and a drug might produce hypocalcemia despite high affinity for heavy metals. A therapeutic chelating agent must bind the metal more avidly than endogenous ligands bind the metal. The large number of endogenous ligands is a formidable barrier to the effectiveness of a chelating agent. Observations *in vitro* on chelator–metal interactions provide only a rough guide to the treatment of heavy-metal poisoning. Empirical observations *in vivo* are necessary to determine the clinical utility of a chelator.

Edetate Calcium Disodium

Ethylenediaminetetraacetic acid (EDTA) is a polycarboxylic acid chelator; its sodium salt (*edetate disodium*, Na_2EDTA), and a number of closely related compounds chelate many divalent and trivalent metals. The cation used to make a water-soluble salt of EDTA has an important role in the toxicity of the chelator. Na_2EDTA causes hypocalcemic tetany. However, *edetate calcium disodium* ($CaNa_2EDTA$) can be used for treatment of poisoning by metals that have higher affinity for the chelating agent than does Ca^{2+}.

MECHANISM OF ACTION

The pharmacological effects of $CaNa_2EDTA$ result from formation of chelates with divalent and trivalent metals in the body. Accessible metal ions (both exogenous and endogenous) with an affinity for $CaNa_2EDTA$ that is higher than that of Ca^{2+} will be chelated, mobilized, and usually excreted. Because EDTA is charged at physiological pH, it does not significantly penetrate cells; its volume of distribution approximates extracellular fluid space. Experimental studies in mice have shown that administration of $CaNa_2EDTA$ mobilizes several endogenous metallic cations, including those of zinc, manganese, and iron. The main therapeutic use of $CaNa_2EDTA$ is in the treatment of metal intoxications, especially lead intoxication (see below).

$CaNa_2EDTA$ is available as edetate calcium disodium (CALCIUM DISODIUM VERSENATE). Intramuscular administration of $CaNa_2EDTA$ results in good absorption, but pain occurs at the injection site; consequently, the chelator injection often is mixed with a local anesthetic or administered intravenously. For intravenous use, $CaNa_2EDTA$ is diluted in either 5% dextrose or 0.9% saline and is administered slowly by intravenous drip. A dilute solution is necessary to avoid thrombophlebitis. To minimize nephrotoxicity, adequate urine production should be established prior to and during treatment with $CaNa_2EDTA$. However, in patients with lead encephalopathy and increased intracranial pressure, excess fluids must be avoided. In such cases, conservative replacement of fluid is advised, and intramuscular administration of $CaNa_2EDTA$ is recommended.

Indications: Lead Poisoning

The successful use of CaNa$_2$EDTA in the treatment of lead poisoning is due, in part, to the capacity of lead to displace calcium from the chelate. Enhanced mobilization and excretion of lead indicate that the metal is accessible to EDTA. Bone provides the primary source of lead that is chelated by CaNa$_2$EDTA. After such chelation, lead is redistributed from soft tissues to the skeleton.

Mercury poisoning, by contrast, does not respond to the drug despite the fact that mercury displaces calcium from CaNa$_2$EDTA in vitro. Mercury is unavailable to the chelate, perhaps because it is too tightly bound by –SH groups or sequestered in body compartments that are not penetrated by CaNa$_2$EDTA.

Although the lay press has reported that chelation therapy with CaNa$_2$EDTA could minimize development of atherosclerotic plaques (which can accumulate calcium deposits), such use of CaNa$_2$EDTA is without therapeutic rationale and not efficacious.

ABSORPTION, DISTRIBUTION, AND EXCRETION

Less than 5% of CaNa$_2$EDTA is absorbed from the GI tract. After intravenous administration, CaNa$_2$EDTA disappears from the circulation with a $t_{1/2}$ of 20–60 minutes. In blood, all of the drug is found in plasma. About 50% is excreted in urine in 1 hour and >95% in 24 hours. For this reason, adequate renal function is necessary for successful therapy. Renal clearance of the compound in dogs equals that of inulin, and glomerular filtration accounts entirely for urinary excretion. Altering either the pH or the rate of flow of urine has no effect on the rate of excretion. There is very little metabolic degradation of EDTA. The drug is distributed mainly in the extracellular fluids, but very little gains access to the spinal fluid (5% of the plasma concentration).

TOXICITY

Rapid intravenous administration of Na$_2$EDTA causes hypocalcemic tetany. However, a slow infusion (<15 mg/min) administered to a normal individual elicits no symptoms of hypocalcemia because of the ready availability of extracirculatory stores of Ca^{2+}. In contrast, CaNa$_2$EDTA can be administered intravenously in relatively large quantities with no untoward effects because the change in the concentration of Ca^{2+} in the plasma and total body is negligible.

Renal Toxicity

The principal toxic effect of CaNa$_2$EDTA is on the kidney. Repeated large doses of the drug cause hydropic vacuolization of the proximal tubule, loss of the brush border, and eventually, degeneration of proximal tubular cells. Changes in distal tubules and glomeruli are less conspicuous. The early renal effects usually are reversible, and urinary abnormalities disappear rapidly on cessation of treatment. Renal toxicity may be related to the large amounts of chelated metals that transit the renal tubule in a relatively short period during drug therapy. Some dissociation of chelates may occur because of competition for the metal by physiological ligands or because of pH changes in the cell or the lumen of the tubule. However, a more likely mechanism of toxicity may be interaction between the chelator and endogenous metals in proximal tubular cells.

Other Side Effects

Other less serious side effects have been reported with use of CaNa$_2$EDTA, including malaise, fatigue, and excessive thirst, followed by the sudden appearance of chills and fever. This, in turn, may be followed by severe myalgia, frontal headache, anorexia, occasional nausea and vomiting, and rarely, increased urinary frequency and urgency. Other possible undesirable effects include sneezing, nasal congestion, and lacrimation; glycosuria; anemia; dermatitis with lesions strikingly similar to those of vitamin B$_6$ deficiency; transitory hypotension; prolonged prothrombin time; and T-wave inversion on the electrocardiogram.

Pentetic Acid (DTPA)

Diethylenetriaminepentaacetic acid (DTPA) is a polycarboxylic acid chelator with a somewhat greater affinity for most heavy metals than EDTA and with a spectrum of clinical effectiveness similar to that of EDTA. Because of its relatively greater affinity for metals, DTPA has been tried in cases of heavy-metal poisoning that do not respond to EDTA, particularly poisoning by radioactive metals. Unfortunately, success has been limited probably because DTPA also has limited access to intracellular sites of metal storage. Because DTPA rapidly binds Ca^{2+}, CaNa$_3$DTPA is employed. The use of DTPA is investigational.

Dimercaprol

Dimercaprol (2,3-dimercaptopropanol) was developed during World War II as an antidote to lewisite, a vesicant arsenical war gas, hence its alternative name, *British antilewisite* (BAL).

Arsenicals and other heavy metals form a very stable and relatively nontoxic chelate ring with the dimercaprol. It is an oily fluid with a pungent, disagreeable odor typical of mercaptans. Because of its instability in aqueous solutions, peanut oil is the solvent employed in pharmaceutical preparations. Dimercaprol and related thiols are readily oxidized.

MECHANISM OF ACTION   The pharmacological actions of dimercaprol result from formation of chelation complexes between its -SH groups and metals. The molecular properties of the dimercaprol–metal chelate have considerable practical significance. With metals such as mercury, gold, and arsenic, the strategy is to attain a stable complex to promote elimination of the metal. Dissociation of the complex and oxidation of dimercaprol can occur *in vivo*. Furthermore, the sulfur–metal bond may be labile in the acidic tubular urine, which may increase delivery of metal to renal tissue and increase toxicity. The dosage regimen therefore is designed to maintain a concentration of dimercaprol in plasma adequate to favor the continuous formation of the more stable 2:1 (BAL–metal) complex and its rapid excretion. However, because of pronounced and dose-related side effects, excessive plasma concentrations must be avoided. The concentration in plasma therefore must be maintained by repeated fractional dosage until the heavy metal can be excreted.

Dimercaprol is much more effective when given as soon as possible after exposure to the metal because it is more effective in preventing inhibition of sulfhydryl enzymes than in reactivating them. Dimercaprol antagonizes the biological actions of metals that form mercaptides with essential cellular -SH groups, principally arsenic, gold, and mercury. It also is used in combination with CaNa$_2$EDTA to treat lead poisoning, especially when evidence of lead encephalopathy exists. Intoxication by selenites, which also oxidize sulfhydryl enzymes, is not influenced by dimercaprol.

ABSORPTION, DISTRIBUTION, AND EXCRETION   Dimercaprol cannot be administered orally; it is given by deep intramuscular injection as a 100 mg/mL solution in peanut oil; thus it should not be used in patients who are allergic to peanuts or peanut products. Peak concentrations in blood are attained in 30–60 minutes. The $t_{1/2}$ is short, and metabolic degradation and excretion are essentially complete within 4 hours.

TOXICITY   The administration of dimercaprol produces a number of side effects that usually are more alarming than serious. Reactions to dimercaprol occur in ~50% of subjects receiving 5 mg/kg intramuscularly. The effects of repeated administration of this dose are not cumulative if an interval of at least 4 hours elapses between injections. One of the most consistent responses to dimercaprol is a rise in blood pressure, accompanied by tachycardia. The rise in pressure may be as great as 50 mm Hg in response to the second of 2 doses (5 mg/kg) given 2 hours apart. The pressure rises immediately, but returns to normal within 2 hours.

Other signs and symptoms of dimercaprol toxicity, many of which tend to parallel the change in blood pressure in time and intensity, are, in approximate order of frequency: nausea and vomiting; headache; a burning sensation in the lips, mouth, and throat; and a feeling of constriction, sometimes pain, in the throat, chest, or hands; conjunctivitis, blepharospasm, lacrimation, rhinorrhea, and salivation; tingling of the hands; a burning sensation in the penis; sweating of the forehead, hands, and other areas; abdominal pain; and the occasional appearance of painful sterile abscesses at the injection site. Symptoms often are accompanied by a feeling of anxiety and unrest. Because the dimercaprol–metal complex breaks down easily in an acidic medium, production of alkaline urine protects the kidney during therapy. Children react as do adults, although ~30% also may experience a fever that disappears on withdrawal of the drug. A transient reduction in the percentage of polymorphonuclear leukocytes may be observed. Dimercaprol also may cause hemolytic anemia in patients deficient in glucose-6-phosphate dehydrogenase. Dimercaprol is contraindicated in patients with hepatic insufficiency, except when this is a result of arsenic poisoning.

Succimer

Succimer (2,3-dimercaptosuccinic acid, CHEMET) is an orally effective chelator that is chemically similar to dimercaprol but contains two carboxylic acids that modify both the distribution and chelating spectrum of the drug. After its absorption in humans, succimer is biotransformed to a mixed disulfide with cysteine.

Succimer produces a lead diuresis with a subsequent lowering of blood lead levels and attenuation of the untoward biochemical effects of lead, manifested by normalization of δ-aminolevulinate (δ-ALA) dehydrase activity. The succimer–lead chelate also is eliminated in bile and enters enterohepatic circulation.

A desirable feature of succimer is that it does not significantly mobilize essential metals such as zinc, copper, or iron. Animal studies suggest that succimer is effective as a chelator of arsenic, cadmium, mercury, and other metals. Succimer has been approved in the U.S. for treatment of children with blood lead levels >45 µg/dL.

Toxicity with succimer is less than that with dimercaprol, perhaps because its relatively lower lipid solubility minimizes its uptake into cells. Nonetheless, transient elevations in hepatic transaminases are observed following treatment with succimer. The most commonly reported adverse effects of succimer treatment are nausea, vomiting, diarrhea, and loss of appetite. Rashes also have been reported that may necessitate discontinuation of therapy.

Penicillamine

The D-isomer of penicillamine, D-β,β-dimethylcysteine, is used clinically, although the L-isomer also forms chelation complexes. Penicillamine is an effective chelator of copper, mercury, zinc, and lead and promotes the excretion of these metals in the urine.

ABSORPTION, DISTRIBUTION, AND EXCRETION

Penicillamine is well absorbed (40–70%) from the GI tract and therefore has a decided advantage over many other chelating agents. Food, antacids, and iron reduce its absorption. Peak concentrations in blood are obtained 1–3 hours after administration. Unlike cysteine, its nonmethylated parent compound, penicillamine, is somewhat resistant to attack by cysteine desulfhydrase or L-amino acid oxidase and is relatively stable in vivo. Hepatic biotransformation is responsible for most of the degradation of penicillamine, and very little is excreted unchanged. Metabolites are found in both urine and feces.

THERAPEUTIC USES

Penicillamine (CUPRIMINE, DEPEN) is available for oral administration. For chelation therapy, the usual adult dose is 11.5 g/day in 4 divided doses (see sections under individual metals). The drug should be given on an empty stomach to avoid interference by metals in food.

In addition to its use as a chelating agent for the treatment of copper, mercury, and lead poisoning, penicillamine is used in Wilson's disease (hepatolenticular degeneration owing to an excess of copper), cystinuria, and rheumatoid arthritis (rarely). For the treatment of Wilson's disease, 1–2 g/day usually is administered in 4 doses. The urinary excretion of copper should be monitored to determine whether the dosage of penicillamine is adequate. N-Acetylpenicillamine is more effective than penicillamine in protecting against the toxic effects of mercury presumably because it is even more resistant to metabolism.

The rationale for the use of penicillamine in cystinuria is that penicillamine reacts with the poorly soluble cysteine in a thiol–disulfide exchange reaction and forms a relatively water-soluble cysteine–penicillamine mixed disulfide. In cystinuria, the urinary excretion of cystine is used to adjust dosage, although 2 g/day in 4 divided doses usually is employed.

The mechanism of action of penicillamine in rheumatoid arthritis remains uncertain, although suppression of the disease may result from marked reduction in concentrations of immunoglobulin (IgM) rheumatoid factor. A single daily dose of 125–250 mg usually is used to initiate therapy, with dosage increases at intervals of 1–3 months as necessary to a typical range of 500–750 mg/day. Because of toxicity, the drug is used rarely today in this setting.

Other experimental uses of penicillamine include the treatment of primary biliary cirrhosis and scleroderma. The mechanism of action of penicillamine in these diseases also may involve effects on immunoglobulins and immune complexes.

TOXICITY

With long-term use, penicillamine induces several cutaneous lesions, including urticaria, macular or papular reactions, pemphigoid lesions, lupus erythematosus, dermatomyositis, adverse effects on collagen, and other less serious reactions, such as dryness and scaling. Cross-reactivity with penicillin may be responsible for some episodes of urticarial or maculopapular reactions with generalized edema, pruritus, and fever that occur in as many as one-third of patients taking penicillamine. The hematological system also may be affected severely; reactions include leukopenia, aplastic anemia, and agranulocytosis. These may occur at any time during therapy, and they may be fatal. Patients obviously must be monitored carefully. Renal toxicity induced by penicillamine usually is manifested as reversible proteinuria and hematuria, but it may progress to the nephrotic syndrome with membranous glomerulopathy. More rarely, fatalities have been reported from Goodpasture's syndrome. Toxicity to the pulmonary system is uncommon, but severe dyspnea has been reported from penicillamine-induced bronchoalveolitis. Myasthenia gravis also has been induced by long-term therapy with penicillamine. Less serious side effects include nausea, vomiting, diarrhea, dyspepsia, anorexia, and a transient loss of taste for sweet and salt, which is relieved by supplementation of the diet with copper. Contraindications to penicillamine therapy include pregnancy, a previous history of penicillamine-induced agranulocytosis or aplastic anemia, or the presence of renal insufficiency.

Trientine

Penicillamine is the drug of choice for treatment for Wilson's disease. However, the drug produces undesirable effects (*see* above) and some patients become intolerant. For these individuals, *trientine* (triethylenetetramine dihydrochloride) is an acceptable alternative. Trientine is an effective cupruretic agent (although possibly less potent than penicillamine) that is effective orally. Maximal daily doses of 2 g for adults or 1.5 g for children are taken in 2–4 divided portions on an empty stomach. Trientine may cause iron deficiency; this can be overcome with short courses of iron therapy, but iron and trientine should not be ingested within 2 hours of each other.

Deferoxamine

Deferoxamine is isolated as the iron chelate from *Streptomyces pilosus* and is treated chemically to obtain the metal-free ligand. Deferoxamine has the desirable properties of a remarkably high affinity for ferric iron ($K_a = 10^{31}$ M^{-1}) coupled with a very low affinity for calcium ($K_a = 10^{2}$ M^{-1}). Studies *in vitro* have shown that it removes iron from hemosiderin and ferritin and, to a lesser extent, from transferrin. Iron in hemoglobin or cytochromes is not removed by deferoxamine.

Deferoxamine (*deferoxamine mesylate*, DESFERAL MESYLATE) is poorly absorbed after oral administration, and parenteral administration is required in most cases. For severe iron toxicity (serum iron levels >500 μg/dL), the intravenous route is preferred. The drug is administered at 10–15 mg/kg/h by constant infusion. Faster rates of infusion (45 mg/kg/h) have been used in a few cases; rapid boluses usually are associated with hypotension. Deferoxamine may be given intramuscularly in moderately toxic cases (serum iron 350–500 μg/dL) at a dose of 50 mg/kg with a maximum dose of 1 g. Hypotension also can occur with the intramuscular route.

For chronic iron intoxication (*e.g.*, thalassemia), an intramuscular dose of 0.5–1.0 g/day is recommended, although continuous subcutaneous administration (1–2 g/day) is almost as effective as intravenous administration. When blood is being transfused to patients with thalassemia, 2 g deferoxamine (per unit of blood) should be given by slow intravenous infusion (rate not to exceed 15 mg/kg/h) during the transfusion but not by the same intravenous line. Deferoxamine is not recommended in primary hemochromatosis; phlebotomy is the treatment of choice. Deferoxamine also has been used for the chelation of aluminum in dialysis patients. Deferoxamine is metabolized principally by plasma enzymes, but the pathways have not been defined. The drug also is excreted readily in the urine.

Deferoxamine causes a number of allergic reactions, including pruritus, wheals, rash, and anaphylaxis. Other adverse effects include dysuria, abdominal discomfort, diarrhea, fever, leg cramps, and tachycardia. Occasional cases of cataract formation have been reported. Deferoxamine may cause neurotoxicity during long-term, high-dose therapy for transfusion-dependent thalassemia major; both visual and auditory changes have been described. A "pulmonary syndrome" has been associated with high-dose (10–25 mg/kg/h) deferoxamine therapy; tachypnea, hypoxemia, fever, and eosinophilia are prominent manifestations. Contraindications to the use of deferoxamine include renal insufficiency and anuria; during pregnancy, the drug should be used only if clearly indicated.

An orally effective iron chelator now under clinical investigation, *deferiprone* (1,2-dimethyl-3-hydroxypyridin-4-one), may be of value in patients with thalassemia major who are unable or unwilling to receive deferoxamine. Combination therapy with deferoxamine also is under investigation.

HEAVY METAL TOXICITY
Lead Poisoning

Through natural occurrence and its industrial use, lead is ubiquitous in the environment. The removal of tetraethyl lead from gasoline has resulted in a decline in blood levels from 13 µg/dL in the 1980s to <5 µg/dL in the general U.S. population. However, many children living in central portions of large cities still have blood lead concentrations >10 µg/dL. The primary sources of environmental exposure to lead are leaded paint and drinking water; most of the overt toxicity from lead results from environmental and industrial exposures.

ACUTE LEAD POISONING

Acute lead poisoning is relatively infrequent and follows ingestion of acid-soluble lead compounds or inhalation of lead vapors. Local actions in the mouth produce marked astringency, thirst, and a metallic taste. Nausea, abdominal pain, and vomiting ensue. The vomitus may be milky from the presence of lead chloride. Although the abdominal pain is severe, it is unlike that of chronic poisoning. Stools may be black from lead sulfide, and there may be diarrhea or constipation. If large amounts of lead are absorbed rapidly, a shock syndrome may develop as the result of massive GI loss of fluid. Acute CNS symptoms include paresthesias, pain, and muscle weakness. An acute hemolytic crisis sometimes causes severe anemia and hemoglobinuria. The kidneys are damaged, and oliguria and urinary changes are evident. Death may occur in 1–2 days. If the patient survives the acute episode, characteristic signs and symptoms of chronic lead poisoning are likely to appear.

CHRONIC LEAD POISONING

Signs and symptoms of plumbism (lead poisoning) include GI, neuromuscular, CNS, hematological, renal, and other disturbances, occurring separately or in combination. The neuromuscular and CNS syndromes usually result from intense exposure, whereas the GI syndrome more commonly reflects a very slowly and insidiously developing intoxication. The CNS syndrome, or lead encephalopathy, is more common among children; the GI syndrome is more prevalent in adults. The CNS syndrome is the most serious manifestation of lead poisoning; early signs include clumsiness, vertigo, ataxia, falling, headache, insomnia, restlessness, and irritability. As the encephalopathy develops, the patient may first become excited and confused; delirium with repetitive tonic-clonic convulsions or lethargy and coma follow. Vomiting, a common sign, usually is projectile. Visual disturbances also are present. The mortality rate among patients who develop cerebral involvement is ~25%. When chelation therapy is begun after the symptoms of acute encephalopathy appear, ~40% of survivors have neurological sequelae (e.g., mental retardation, electroencephalographic abnormalities or frank seizures, cerebral palsy, optic atrophy, or dystonia musculorum deformans).

Exposure to lead occasionally produces clear-cut progressive mental deterioration in children, with normal development during the first 12–18 months of life or longer, followed by a steady loss of motor skills and speech; they may have severe hyperkinetic and aggressive behavior disorders and a poorly controllable convulsive disorder. The lack of sensory perception severely impairs learning. Elevated blood lead levels in infancy and early childhood later may be manifested as decreased attention span, reading disabilities, and failure to graduate from high school. Most studies report a 2–4-point IQ deficit for each µg/dL increase in blood lead within the range of 5–35 µg/dL. Blood lead concentrations ≥10 µg/dL indicate excessive absorption of lead in children and constitute grounds for environmental assessment, cleanup, and/or intervention. Chelation therapy should be considered when blood lead concentrations exceed 25 µg/dL. The CDC recommends universal screening of children beginning at 6 months of age.

In the absence of a positive history of abnormal exposure to lead, the diagnosis of lead poisoning is missed easily because the signs and symptoms of lead poisoning are shared by other diseases. For example, the signs of encephalopathy may resemble those of various degenerative conditions. Physical examination does not easily distinguish lead colic from other abdominal disorders. Clinical suspicion should be confirmed by determinations of the concentration of lead in blood and protoporphyrin in erythrocytes. A common hematological manifestation of chronic lead intoxication is a hypochromic microcytic anemia, which is observed more frequently in children and is morphologically similar to that resulting from iron deficiency. The anemia is thought to result from two factors: a decreased life span of the erythrocytes and an inhibition of heme synthesis. Lead at low concentrations decreases heme synthesis at several enzymatic steps (Figure 65–1). This leads to buildup of the diagnostically important substrates δ-ALA, coproporphyrin (both measured in urine), and zinc protoporphyrin (measured in the red cell as erythrocyte protoporphyrin). For children, the erythrocyte protoporphyrin level is insufficiently sensitive to identify children with elevated blood lead levels <25 µg/dL, and the screening test of choice is blood lead measurement.

The concentration of lead in blood is an indication of recent absorption of the metal. Clinical manifestations associated with increasing concentrations of lead in blood are shown in Figure 65–2. Children with concentrations of lead in blood >10 µg/dL are at risk of developmental disabilities. Adults with concentrations <30 µg/dL exhibit no known functional injury or symptoms; however, they will have a definite decrease in δ-ALA dehydratase activity, a slight increase in urinary excretion of δ-ALA, and an increase in erythrocyte protoporphyrin. Patients with a blood lead concentration of 30–75 µg/dL have all the preceding laboratory abnormalities and, usually, nonspecific, mild symptoms of lead poisoning. Clear symptoms of lead poisoning are associated

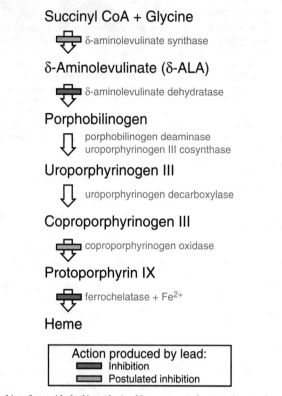

Succinyl CoA + Glycine

δ-aminolevulinate synthase

δ-Aminolevulinate (δ-ALA)

δ-aminolevulinate dehydratase

Porphobilinogen

porphobilinogen deaminase
uroporphyrinogen III cosynthase

Uroporphyrinogen III

uroporphyrinogen decarboxylase

Coproporphyrinogen III

coproporphyrinogen oxidase

Protoporphyrin IX

ferrochelatase + Fe^{2+}

Heme

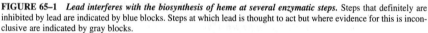

Action produced by lead:
Inhibition
Postulated inhibition

FIGURE 65–1 *Lead interferes with the biosynthesis of heme at several enzymatic steps.* Steps that definitely are inhibited by lead are indicated by blue blocks. Steps at which lead is thought to act but where evidence for this is inconclusive are indicated by gray blocks.

with concentrations of >75 μg/dL of whole blood, and lead encephalopathy usually is apparent when lead concentrations exceed 100 μg/dL.

The urinary concentration of lead in normal adults generally is <80 μg/L (0.4 μM). Most patients with lead poisoning show concentrations of lead in urine of 150–300 μg/L (0.7–1.4 μM). However, in persons with chronic lead nephropathy or other forms of renal insufficiency, urinary excretion of lead may be within the normal range, even though blood lead concentrations are significantly elevated.

Because the onset of lead poisoning usually is insidious, it often is desirable to estimate the body burden of lead in individuals who are exposed to an environment that is contaminated with the metal. In the past, the edetate calcium disodium ($CaNa_2EDTA$) provocation test was used to determine whether there is an increased body burden of lead in those for whom exposure occurred much earlier. The provocation test is performed by intravenous administration of a single dose of $CaNa_2EDTA$ (50 mg/kg) followed by collection of urine for 8 hours. The test is positive for children when the lead excretion ratio (μg of lead excreted in the urine per mg of $CaNa_2EDTA$ administered) is >0.6; it also may be useful for therapeutic chelation in children with blood levels of 25–45 μg/dL. This test is not used in symptomatic patients or in those whose concentration of lead in blood is >45 μg/dL because these patients require the proper therapeutic regimen with chelating agents (see below).

ORGANIC LEAD POISONING

Tetraethyl lead and tetramethyl lead are lipid-soluble compounds that are absorbed readily from the skin, GI tract, and lungs. The toxicity of tetraethyl lead is believed to be due to its metabolic conversion to triethyl lead and inorganic lead. The major symptoms of intoxication with tetraethyl lead are referable to the CNS: insomnia, nightmares, anorexia, nausea and vomiting, diarrhea, headache, muscular weakness, and emotional instability. Subjective CNS symptoms such as

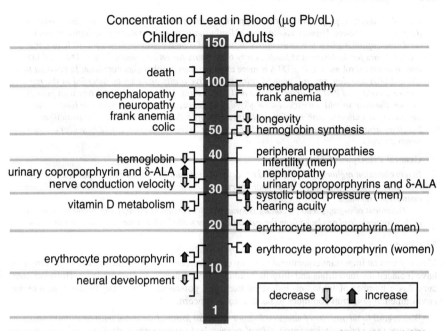

FIGURE 65–2 *Manifestations of lead toxicity associated with varying concentrations of lead in blood of children and adults.* δ-ALA = δ-aminolevulinate.

irritability, restlessness, and anxiety are next evident, usually accompanied by hypothermia, bradycardia, and hypotension. With continued exposure, or in the case of intense short-term exposure, CNS manifestations progress to delusions, ataxia, exaggerated muscular movements, and finally, a maniacal state.

The diagnosis of poisoning by tetraethyl lead is established by relating these signs and symptoms to a history of exposure. The urinary excretion of lead may increase markedly, but the concentration of lead in blood remains nearly normal. Anemia and basophilic stippling of erythrocytes are uncommon in organic lead poisoning. There is little effect on the metabolism of porphyrins, and erythrocyte protoporphyrin concentrations are inconsistently elevated. In the case of severe exposure, death may occur within a few hours or may be delayed for several weeks. If the patient survives the acute phase of organic lead poisoning, recovery usually is complete; however, instances of residual CNS damage have been reported.

TREATMENT OF LEAD POISONING

Initial treatment of the acute phase of lead intoxication involves supportive measures. Prevention of further exposure is important. Seizures are treated with diazepam *or* phenytoin *(see Chapter 19), fluid and electrolyte balances must be maintained, and cerebral edema is treated with* mannitol *and* dexamethasone *or controlled hyperventilation. The concentration of lead in blood should be determined or at least a blood sample obtained for analysis prior to initiation of chelation therapy. Chelation therapy is indicated in symptomatic patients or in patients with a blood lead concentration in excess of 50–60 μg/dL (about 2.5 μM). Four chelators are employed: edetate calcium disodium (CaNa₂EDTA), dimercaprol, D-penicillamine, and succimer (2,3–dimercaptosuccinic acid [DMSA], CHEMET). CaNa₂EDTA and dimercaprol usually are used in combination for lead encephalopathy.*

CaNa₂EDTA is initiated at a dose of 30–50 mg/kg/day in 2 divided doses either by deep intramuscular injection or slow intravenous infusion for up to 5 consecutive days. The first dose of CaNa₂EDTA should be delayed until 4 hours after the first dose of dimercaprol. An additional course of CaNa₂EDTA may be given after an interruption of 2 days. Each course of therapy with CaNa₂EDTA should not exceed a total dose of 500 mg/kg. Urine output must be monitored because the chelator–lead complex is believed to be nephrotoxic. Treatment with CaNa₂EDTA can alleviate symptoms quickly. Colic may disappear within 2 hours; paresthesia and tremor cease after 4–5 days; coproporphyrinuria, stippled erythrocytes, and gingival lead lines tend to decrease in 4–9 days. Urinary elimination of lead usually is greatest during the initial infusion.

Dimercaprol is given intramuscularly at a dose of 4 mg/kg every 4 hours for 48 hours, then every 6 hours for 48 hours, and finally, every 6–12 hours for an additional 7 days. The combination of dimercaprol and CaNa₂EDTA is more effective than is either chelator alone. In contrast to CaNa₂EDTA and dimercaprol, penicillamine is effective orally and may be included in the regimen at a dosage of 250 mg given 4 times daily for 5 days. During chronic therapy with penicillamine, the dose should not exceed 40 mg/kg/day. Succimer is the first orally active lead chelator available for children, with a safety and efficacy profile that surpasses that of D-penicillamine. Succimer usually is given every 8 hours (10 mg/kg) for 5 days and then every 12 hours for an additional 2 weeks.

General Principles of Therapy

In any chelation regimen, the blood lead concentration should be reassessed 2 weeks after the regimen has been completed; an additional course of therapy may be indicated if blood lead concentrations rebound.

Treatment of organic lead poisoning is symptomatic. Chelation therapy will promote excretion of the inorganic lead produced from the metabolism of organic lead, but the increase is not dramatic.

Mercury

Mercury was an important constituent of many drugs for centuries, but other modes of therapy now have replaced the mercurials and drug-induced mercury poisoning has become rare. However, mercury has a number of important industrial uses, and poisoning from occupational exposure and environmental pollution continues to be an area of concern.

With regard to the toxicity of mercury, 3 major chemical forms of the metal must be distinguished: mercury vapor (elemental mercury), salts of mercury, and organic mercurials. Elemental mercury is the most volatile of the metal's inorganic forms. Human exposure to mercury vapor is mainly occupational. Extraction of gold with mercury and then heating the amalgam to drive off the mercury is a technique that still is used today in some developing countries. Chronic exposure to mercury in ambient air after inadvertent mercury spills in poorly ventilated rooms can produce toxic effects. Mercury vapor also can be released from silver–amalgam dental restorations (the main source of mercury exposure to the general population), but the amount of mercury released does not appear to be of significance for human health except for allergic contact eczema seen in a few individuals.

Salts of mercury exist in 2 states of oxidation—as monovalent mercurous salts or as divalent mercuric salts. Mercurous chloride (Hg_2Cl_2), or calomel, was used in some skin creams as an antiseptic and as a diuretic and cathartic. Mercuric salts are the more irritating and acutely toxic form of the metal. Mercuric nitrate was commonly used in the felt-hat industry; the neurological and behavioral changes depicted by the Mad Hatter in Lewis Carroll's Alice's Adventures in Wonderland illustrate the toxic effects of mercuric salts. Mercuric salts still are employed widely in industry, and industrial discharge into rivers has introduced mercury into the environment. The main uses of inorganic mercury today are in chloralkali production, the manufacture of electronics, plastics, fungicides, and germicides, and the formulation of amalgams in dentistry.

The organomercurials in use today contain mercury with one covalent bond to a carbon atom. The alkylmercury salts are by far the most dangerous of these compounds; methylmercury is the most common. Alkylmercury salts have been used widely as fungicides. Major incidents of human poisoning from the inadvertent consumption of mercury-treated seed grain have occurred in Iraq, Pakistan, Ghana, and Guatemala. The most catastrophic incident occurred in Iraq in 1972, when treated grain was ground into flour and made into bread, hospitalizing 6530 and killing 500. Minamata disease results from methylmercury poisoning; residents of Minamata, Japan, were poisoned after eating fish contaminated by mercury from a chemical plant that emptied its effluent directly into Minamata Bay. Eventually, 121 persons were poisoned and 46 died. Because of concerns about methylmercury accumulation in fish, the U.S. Food and Drug Administration (FDA) recommends that pregnant or nursing women, women of childbearing age, and young children avoid eating large fish (e.g., shark, swordfish, king mackerel, and tilefish) and limit their intake of albacore tuna to 6 oz/week.

The possible health risks of thimerosal (CH_3CH_2—Hg—S—C_6H_4—$COOH$), an antibacterial preservative used in vaccines, have been debated. The FDA has determined that that there is a significant safety margin incorporated into all the acceptable mercury exposure limits, and there are no data or evidence of any harm caused by the level of exposure that some children may have encountered in following the existing immunization schedule. Nevertheless, the availability of vaccines with alternate preservatives led to the removal of all vaccines containing thimerosal.

CHEMISTRY AND MECHANISM OF ACTION

Mercury readily forms covalent bonds with sulfur, and it is this property that accounts for most of the biological properties of the metal. When the sulfur is in the form of sulfhydryl groups, divalent mercury replaces the hydrogen atom to form mercaptides, X—Hg—SR and Hg(SR)$_2$, where X is an electronegative radical and R is protein. Organic mercurials form mercaptides of the type R—Hg—SR'. Even in low concentrations, mercurials are capable of inactivating -SH groups of enzymes, thus interfering with cellular metabolism and function. The affinity of mercury for thiols provides the basis for treatment of mercury poisoning with such agents as dimercaprol and penicillamine. Mercury also combines with phosphoryl, carboxyl, amide, and amine groups.

TOXICITY

Elemental Mercury

Elemental mercury is not particularly toxic when ingested because of very low absorption from the GI tract; this is due to the formation of droplets and because the metal in this form cannot react with biologically important molecules. However, inhaled mercury vapor is completely absorbed by the lung and then is oxidized to the divalent mercuric cation by catalase in erythrocytes. Short-term exposure to the vapor of elemental mercury may produce symptoms within several hours, including weakness, chills, metallic taste, nausea, vomiting, diarrhea, dyspnea, cough, and a feeling of tightness in the chest. Pulmonary toxicity may progress to an interstitial pneumonitis with severe compromise of respiratory function. Recovery, although usually complete, may be complicated by residual interstitial fibrosis. Chronic exposure to mercury vapor produces a more insidious form of toxicity that is dominated by neurological effects. The concentrations of mercury vapor in the air and mercury in urine that are associated with the various effects are shown in Figure 65–3.

Inorganic Salts of Mercury

Inorganic ionic mercury (e.g., mercuric chloride) *can produce severe acute toxicity. Precipitation of mucous membrane proteins by mercuric salts results in an ashen-gray appearance of the mucosa of the mouth, pharynx, and intestine and also causes intense pain, which may be*

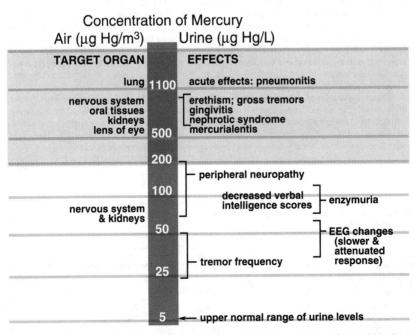

Concentration of Mercury
Air (µg Hg/m³)   Urine (µg Hg/L)

TARGET ORGAN		EFFECTS
lung	1100	acute effects: pneumonitis
nervous system oral tissues kidneys lens of eye	500	⎡erethism; gross tremors gingivitis nephrotic syndrome ⎣mercurialentis
	200	
	100	⎤ peripheral neuropathy
nervous system & kidneys	50	decreased verbal intelligence scores ⎤ enzymuria
	25	⎤ EEG changes (slower & attenuated tremor frequency ⎦ response)
	5	← upper normal range of urine levels

FIGURE 65–3 *The concentration of mercury vapor in the air and related concentrations of mercury in urine associated with a variety of toxic effects.*

accompanied by vomiting. The vomiting is perceived to be protective because it removes unabsorbed mercury from the stomach; if the patient is awake and alert, vomiting should not be inhibited. The local corrosive effect of ionic inorganic mercury on the GI mucosa results in severe hematochezia with evidence of mucosal sloughing in the stool. Hypovolemic shock and death can occur in the absence of proper treatment, which can overcome the local effects of inorganic mercury.

Systemic toxicity may begin within a few hours of exposure to mercury and last for days. A strong metallic taste is followed by stomatitis with gingival irritation, foul breath, and loosening of the teeth. The most serious and frequent systemic effect of inorganic mercury is renal toxicity. Acute tubular necrosis occurs after short-term exposure, leading to oliguria or anuria. Renal injury also follows long-term exposure to inorganic mercury, where glomerular injury predominates.

Organic Mercurials

Most human toxicological data about organic mercury concern methylmercury. More than 90% of methylmercury is absorbed from the human GI tract. The organic mercurials distribute more uniformly to the various tissues than do the inorganic salts; they also cross the blood–brain barrier and the placenta and thus produce more neurological and teratogenic effects. A significant portion of the body burden of organic mercurials is in the red blood cells; for methylmercury, the red cell-plasma ratio is ~20:1. Symptoms of exposure to methylmercury are mainly neurological; Table 65–1 lists frequency of symptoms and corresponding blood levels of methylmercury. Effects of methylmercury on the fetus can occur even when the mother is asymptomatic; mental retardation and neuromuscular deficits have been observed.

DIAGNOSIS OF MERCURY POISONING

A history of exposure to mercury, either industrial or environmental, is obviously valuable in making the diagnosis of mercury poisoning. Otherwise, clinical suspicions can be confirmed by laboratory analysis. The upper limit of a nontoxic concentration of mercury in blood generally is considered to be 3–4 μg/dL (0.15–0.20 μM). A concentration of mercury in blood >4 μg/dL (0.20 μM) is unexpected in normal, healthy adults and suggests the need for environmental evaluation and medical examination to assess the possibility of adverse health effects. Because methylmercury is concentrated in erythrocytes and inorganic mercury is not, the distribution of total mercury between red blood cells and plasma may indicate whether the patient has been poisoned with inorganic or organic mercury. Measurement of total mercury in red blood cells gives a better estimate of the body burden of methylmercury than it does for inorganic mercury. Concentrations of mercury in plasma provide a better index of the body burden of inorganic mercury, but the relationship between body burden and the concentration of inorganic mercury in plasma is not well documented. This may relate to the importance of timing of measurement of the blood sample relative to the last exposure to mercury. The relationship between the concentration of inorganic mercury in blood and toxicity also depends on the form of exposure. For example, exposure to vapor results in concentrations in brain approximately 10 times higher than those that follow an equivalent dose of inorganic mercuric salts.

The concentration of mercury in the urine also has been used as a measure of the body burden of the metal. The normal upper limit for excretion of mercury in urine is 5 μg/L. There is a linear relationship between plasma concentration and urinary excretion of mercury after exposure to vapor; in contrast, the excretion of mercury in urine is a poor indicator of the amount of methylmercury in the blood because methylmercury is eliminated mainly in feces.

Table 65–1

Frequency of Symptoms of Methylmercury Poisoning in Relation to Concentration of Mercury in Blood

Mercury in Blood, μg/mL (μM)	Cases with Symptoms (%)					
	Paresthesias	Ataxia	Visual Defects	Dysarthria	Hearing Defects	Death
0.1–0.5 (0.5–2.5)	5	0	0	5	0	0
0.5–1 (2.5–5)	42	11	21	5	5	0
1–2 (5–10)	60	47	53	24	5	0
2–3 (10–15)	79	60	56	25	13	0
3–4 (15–20)	82	100	58	75	36	17
4–5 (20–25)	100	100	83	85	66	28

Hair is rich in -SH groups, and the concentration of mercury in hair is about 300 times that in blood. Human hair grows about 20 cm/year, and a history of exposure may be obtained by analysis of different segments of hair.

CHELATION THERAPY FOR MERCURY POISONING

Inorganic or Elemental Mercury

Chelation therapy with dimercaprol (for high-level exposures or symptomatic patients) or penicillamine (for low-level exposures or asymptomatic patients) is used routinely to treat poisoning with either inorganic or elemental mercury. Recommended treatment includes dimercaprol 5 mg/kg intramuscularly initially, followed by 2.5 mg/kg intramuscularly every 12–24 hours for 10 days. Penicillamine (250 mg orally every 6 hours) may be used alone or following treatment with dimercaprol. The duration of chelation therapy will vary, and progress can be monitored by following concentrations of mercury in urine and blood. The orally effective chelator succimer appears to be an effective chelator for mercury, although not FDA-approved for this purpose.

The dimercaprol–mercury chelate is excreted into both bile and urine, whereas the penicillamine–mercury chelate is excreted only into urine. Thus, penicillamine should be used with extreme caution when renal function is impaired. In fact, hemodialysis may be necessary in the poisoned patient whose renal function declines. Chelators still may be used because the dimercaprol–mercury complex is removed by dialysis.

Organic Mercury

The short-chain organic mercurials, especially methylmercury, are the most difficult forms of mercury to mobilize from the body, presumably because of their poor reactivity with chelating agents. Dimercaprol is contraindicated in methylmercury poisoning because it increases brain concentrations of methylmercury in experimental animals. Although penicillamine facilitates the removal of methylmercury from the body, it is not clinically efficacious, and large doses (2 g/day) are needed. During the initial 1–3 days of administration of penicillamine, the concentration of mercury in the blood increases before it decreases, probably reflecting the mobilization of metal from tissues to blood at a rate more rapid than that for excretion of mercury into urine and feces.

Methylmercury compounds undergo extensive enterohepatic recirculation; therefore, introduction of a nonabsorbable mercury-binding substance into the intestinal tract should facilitate their removal from the body. A polythiol resin has been used for this purpose in humans and appears to be effective. The resin has certain advantages over penicillamine. It does not cause redistribution of mercury in the body with a subsequent increase in the concentration of mercury in blood, and it has fewer adverse effects than do sulfhydryl agents that are absorbed. Clinical experience with various treatments for methylmercury poisoning in Iraq indicates that penicillamine, N-acetylpenicillamine, and an oral nonabsorbable thiol resin all can reduce blood concentrations of mercury; however, clinical improvement was not clearly related to reduction of the body burden of methylmercury.

Conventional hemodialysis is of little value in the treatment of methylmercury poisoning because methylmercury concentrates in erythrocytes, and little is contained in the plasma. However, it has been shown that L-cysteine can be infused into the arterial blood entering the dialyzer to convert methylmercury into a diffusible form. Both free cysteine and the methylmercury–cysteine complex form in the blood and then diffuse across the membrane into the dialysate. This method has been shown to be effective in humans. Studies in animals indicate that succimer may be more effective than cysteine in this regard.

Arsenic

Arsenic is found in soil, water, and air as a common environmental toxicant. The average daily human intake of arsenic is about 10 µg, largely ingested with food and water. The major source of occupational exposure to arsenic-containing compounds is from the manufacture of arsenical herbicides and pesticides. Arsenic is used as arsine and as arsenic trioxide in the manufacture of most computer chips using silicon-based technology. Gallium arsenide is used in the production of compound (types III–V) semiconductors that are used for making light-emitting diodes (LEDs), as well as laser and solar devices. Chromated copper arsenate (CCA) was used as a common treatment for outdoor lumber until 2004; this should not pose a health risk unless treated wood is burned in fireplaces or woodstoves. Federal restrictions on the allowable content of arsenic in food and in the occupational environment not only have improved safety procedures and decreased the number of intoxications but also have decreased the amount of arsenic in use; only the annual production of arsenic-containing herbicides is increasing. The incidence of accidental, homicidal, and suicidal arsenic poisoning has diminished greatly in recent decades.

CHEMISTRY AND MECHANISM OF ACTION

The toxicity of a given arsenical is related to the rate of its clearance from the body and therefore to its degree of accumulation in tissues. In general, toxicity increases in the sequence of organic arsenicals $<As^{5+} <As^{3+} <$ arsine (AsH_3). The organic arsenicals contain arsenic covalently linked to a carbon atom, where arsenic exists in the trivalent or pentavalent state. Arsphenamine contains trivalent arsenic; sodium arsanilate contains arsenic in the pentavalent form. The organic arsenicals usually are excreted more rapidly than are the inorganic forms.

Arsenate (pentavalent) uncouples mitochondrial oxidative phosphorylation by a mechanism whereby arsenate substitutes for inorganic phosphate in the formation of ATP, with subsequent formation of an unstable arsenate ester that is hydrolyzed rapidly. This process is termed arsenolysis.

Trivalent arsenicals, including inorganic arsenite, are regarded primarily as -SH reagents. As such, trivalent arsenicals inhibit many enzymes by reacting with biological ligands containing available -SH groups. The pyruvate dehydrogenase system is especially sensitive to trivalent arsenicals because of their interaction with two -SH groups of lipoic acid to form a stable 6-membered ring.

ACUTE ARSENIC POISONING

GI discomfort usually is experienced within an hour after intake of an arsenical, although it may be delayed as much as 12 hours after oral ingestion if food is in the stomach. Burning lips, constriction of the throat, and difficulty in swallowing may be the first symptoms, followed by excruciating gastric pain, projectile vomiting, and severe diarrhea. Oliguria with proteinuria and hematuria usually is present; eventually, anuria may occur. The patient often complains of marked skeletal muscle cramps and severe thirst. As the loss of fluid proceeds, symptoms of shock appear. Hypoxic convulsions may occur terminally; coma and death ensue. In severe poisoning, death can occur within an hour, but the usual interval is 24 hours. With prompt application of corrective therapy, patients may survive the acute phase of the toxicity only to develop neuropathies and other disorders. The motor system appears to be spared only in the mildest cases; severe crippling is common.

CHRONIC ARSENIC POISONING

The most common early signs of chronic arsenic poisoning are muscle weakness and aching, skin pigmentation (especially of the neck, eyelids, nipples, and axillae), hyperkeratosis, and edema. GI involvement is less prominent in long-term exposures. Other signs and symptoms that should arouse suspicion of arsenic poisoning include garlic odor of the breath and perspiration, excessive salivation and sweating, stomatitis, generalized itching, sore throat, coryza, lacrimation, numbness, burning or tingling of the extremities, dermatitis, vitiligo, and alopecia. Poisoning may begin insidiously with symptoms of weakness, languor, anorexia, occasional nausea and vomiting, and diarrhea or constipation. Subsequent symptoms may simulate acute coryza. Dermatitis and keratosis of the palms and soles are common features. Mee's lines are found characteristically in the fingernails (white transverse lines of deposited arsenic that usually appear 6 weeks after exposure). Desquamation and scaling of the skin may initiate an exfoliative process involving many epithelial structures of the body. The liver may enlarge, and obstruction of the bile ducts may result in jaundice. Eventually, cirrhosis may occur from the hepatotoxic action. Renal dysfunction also may be encountered. As intoxication advances, encephalopathy may develop. Peripheral neuritis results in motor and sensory paralysis of the extremities; in contrast to lead palsy, the legs usually are more severely affected than the arms. The bone marrow is seriously damaged by arsenic, and all hematological elements may be affected with severe exposure.

CHELATION THERAPY FOR ARSENIC POISONING

Chelation therapy often is begun with dimercaprol (3–4 mg/kg intramuscularly every 4–12 hours) until abdominal symptoms subside and charcoal (if given initially) is passed in the feces. Oral treatment with penicillamine then may be substituted for dimercaprol and continued for 4 days. Penicillamine is given in 4 divided doses to a maximum of 2 g/day. If symptoms recur after cessation of chelation therapy, a second course of penicillamine may be instituted. Succimer (2,3-dimercaptosuccinic acid), a derivative of dimercaprol, is efficacious in the treatment of arsenic poisoning but is FDA-approved only for lead chelation in children.

After long-term exposure to arsenic, treatment with dimercaprol and penicillamine also may be used, but oral penicillamine alone usually is sufficient. The duration of therapy is determined by the clinical condition of the patient, and the decision is aided by periodic determinations of urinary arsenic concentrations. Adverse effects of the chelating agents may limit the usefulness of therapy. Dialysis may become necessary with severe arsenic-induced nephropathy; successful removal of arsenic by dialysis has been reported.

ARSINE

Arsine gas, generated by electrolytic or metallic reduction of arsenic in nonferrous metal products, is a rare cause of industrial intoxication. Rapid and often fatal hemolysis is a unique characteristic of arsine poisoning and probably results from arsine combining with hemoglobin and then reacting with oxygen to cause hemolysis. The classic arsine triad of hemolysis, abdominal pain, and hematuria is noteworthy. If the patient survives the severe hemolysis, death may result from renal failure. Because the hemoglobin–arsine complex cannot be dialyzed, exchange transfusion is recommended in severe cases; forced alkaline diuresis also may be employed (see Chapter 64). Dimercaprol has no effect on the hemolysis, and beneficial effects on renal function have not been established; it therefore is not recommended.

Cadmium

Cadmium ranks close to lead and mercury as a metal of current toxicological concern. Cadmium is used in electroplating and galvanization, and in plastics, paint pigments (cadmium yellow), and nickel–cadmium batteries. Because <5% of the metal is recycled, environmental pollution is an important consideration. Coal and other fossil fuels contain cadmium, and their combustion releases the element into the environment. Extraction and processing of zinc and lead also lead to environmental contamination with cadmium. Workers in smelters and other metal-processing plants may be exposed to high concentrations of cadmium in the air; however, for most of the population, food is the major source of cadmium.

Cadmium occurs only in one valency state (2$^+$) and does not form stable alkyl compounds or other organometallic compounds of known toxicological significance. Cadmium initially is distributed to the liver and then redistributes slowly to the kidney as cadmium–metallothionein (Cd–MT), with ~50% of the total-body burden in the liver and kidney after distribution. Cadmium and several other metals induce the expression of metallothionein, a cysteine-rich protein with high affinity for metals such as cadmium and zinc. Metallothionein protects cells against cadmium toxicity by preventing the interaction of cadmium with other proteins.

ACUTE CADMIUM POISONING

Acute poisoning usually results from inhalation of cadmium dusts and fumes (usually cadmium oxide) or from the ingestion of cadmium salts. The early toxic effects are due to local irritation. In the case of oral intake, these include nausea, vomiting, salivation, diarrhea, and abdominal cramps; the vomitus and diarrhea often are bloody. In the short term, inhaled cadmium is more toxic. Signs and symptoms, which appear within a few hours, include irritation of the respiratory tract with severe, early pneumonitis, chest pains, nausea, dizziness, and diarrhea. Toxicity may progress to fatal pulmonary edema or residual emphysema with peribronchial and perivascular fibrosis.

CHRONIC CADMIUM POISONING

The toxic effects of long-term exposure to cadmium differ somewhat with the route of exposure. The kidney is affected following either pulmonary or GI exposure; marked effects are observed in the lungs only after exposure by inhalation. Excretion of β_2-microglobulin in urine is a sensitive but not specific index of cadmium-induced nephrotoxicity. Measurement of urine β_2-microglobulin is part of the Occupational Safety and Health Administration (OSHA) standard for monitoring cadmium poisoning. Retinol-binding protein may be a better marker, but its measurement generally is not available. Cadmium is classified as a human carcinogen based mainly on epidemiological studies from workers exposed occupationally to cadmium. These investigations primarily have identified tumors of the lungs and, to a lesser extent, prostate, kidney, and stomach.

TREATMENT OF CADMIUM POISONING BY CHELATION THERAPY

Effective therapy for cadmium poisoning is difficult to achieve. Although there is no proven benefit, some clinicians recommend chelation therapy with CaNa$_2$EDTA. The dose of CaNa$_2$EDTA is 75 mg/kg/day in 3–6 divided doses for 5 days. After a minimum of 2 days without treatment, a second 5-day course is given. The total dose of CaNa$_2$EDTA per 5-day course should not exceed 500 mg/kg. Animal studies suggest that chelation therapy should be instituted as soon as possible after cadmium exposure because a rapid decrease in effectiveness of chelation therapy occurs in parallel with distribution to sites inaccessible to the chelators. The use of dimercaprol and substituted dithiocarbamates appears promising for individuals chronically exposed to cadmium.

Iron

Although iron is not an environmental poison, accidental intoxication with ferrous salts used to treat iron deficiency is a frequently encountered source of poisoning in young children. Iron is discussed further in Chapter 53.

Radioactive Heavy Metals

The widespread production and use of radioactive heavy metals for nuclear generation of electricity, nuclear weapons, laboratory research, manufacturing, and medical diagnosis have generated unique problems in dealing with accidental poisoning by such metals. Because the toxicity of radioactive metals is almost entirely a consequence of ionizing radiation, the therapeutic objective following exposure is chelation of the metals and their removal from the body as rapidly and completely as possible. Treatment of the acute radiation syndrome is largely symptomatic. Attempts have been made to investigate the effectiveness of organic reducing agents, such as mercaptamine (cysteamine), administered to prevent the formation of free radicals; success has been limited.

Major products of a nuclear accident or the use of nuclear weapons include ^{239}Pu, ^{137}Cs, ^{144}Ce, and ^{90}Sr. Isotopes of Sr and Ra are extremely difficult to remove from the body with chelating agents. Several factors are involved in the relative resistance of radioactive metals to chelation therapy; these include the affinity of these particular metals for individual chelators and the observation that radiation from Sr and Ra in bone destroys nearby capillaries, thereby decreasing blood flow and isolating the radioisotopes. Many chelating agents have been used experimentally, including $CaNa_3DTPA$ (pentetic acid), which has been shown to be effective against ^{239}Pu. One gram of $CaNa_3DTPA$, administered by slow intravenous drip on alternate days three times per week has enhanced excretion 50-100-fold in animals and in human subjects exposed in accidents. As is seen commonly with heavy-metal poisoning, effectiveness of treatment diminishes very rapidly with an increasing delay between exposure and the initiation of therapy.

For a complete Bibliographical listing see Goodman & Gilman's *The Pharmacological Basis of Therapeutics*, 11th ed., or Goodman & Gilman Online at www.accessmedicine.com.

PRINCIPLES OF PRESCRIPTION ORDER WRITING AND PATIENT COMPLIANCE

THE MECHANICS OF WRITING PRESCRIPTION ORDERS

The written prescription consists of the superscription, the inscription, the subscription, the signa, and the name and signature of the prescriber, all contained on a single form (Figure A–1). The *superscription* includes the date the prescription order is written; the name, address, weight, and age of the patient; and the Rx (or *recipe*). The body of the prescription, or *inscription*, contains the name and amount or strength of the drug to be dispensed, or the name and strength of each ingredient to be compounded. The *subscription* is the instruction to the pharmacist, usually consisting of a short sentence such as: "make a solution," "mix and place into 30 capsules," or "dispense 30 tablets." The *signa* or *Sig* is the instruction for the patient as to how to take the prescription, interpreted and transposed onto the prescription label by the pharmacist. In the U.S., these generally are written in English. Many physicians continue to use Latin abbreviations; for example, "1 cap tid pc," will be interpreted by the pharmacist as "take one capsule three times daily after meals." However, the use of Latin abbreviations only mystifies the prescription, which can hinder proper patient-physician communication and may lead to errors. Since the pharmacist always writes the label in English (or as appropriate in the language of the patient), the use of such abbreviations or symbols is unnecessary and discouraged.

The instruction "take as directed" should be avoided; Such directions can only be seen as inadequate by the pharmacist, who must determine the intent of the physician before dispensing the medication, and who shares the responsibility for safe and proper use of the medication by the patient. The best directions to the patient include a reminder of the intended purpose of the medication by including such phrases as "for relief of pain," or "to relieve itching." The correct route of administration is reinforced by the choice of the first word of the directions. For an oral dosage form, the directions would begin with "take" or "give"; for externally applied products, the word "apply"; for suppositories, "insert"; and for eye, ear, or nose drops, "place" is preferable to "instill."

Prescriptive Authority

In many states in the U.S., health care practitioners other than M.D. and D.O. physicians (*e.g.,* physician's assistants, nurse practitioners, and pharmacists) can write prescriptions in certain circumstances.

Avoiding Confusion

Units of measure can lead to confusion and medication errors. Older systems of measure such as minims for volume (15 minims = 1 mL) and grains for weight (1 grain = 60 mg) are obscure and should not be used. Doses always should be listed by metric weight of active ingredient; doses for liquid medications should include the volume. Writing "μg" for micrograms can very easily be misinterpreted as milligrams (mg). Thus, if abbreviated, micrograms should be written "mcg" and milligrams as "mg"; a zero should be used before a decimal (0.X mg, rather than .X mg) but not after (use X mg rather than X.0 mg). The metric system should be used in place of common household measurements such as "dropperful" and "teaspoon" in the patient directions, and both the doctor and the pharmacist should be sure that the patient understands the measurement prescribed. For medical purposes, a "teaspoon" or "teaspoonful" dose is considered to be equivalent to 5 mL and a "tablespoon" to 15 mL, but the actual volumes held by ordinary household teaspoons and tablespoons vary too widely to be used reliably for measurement of medications. Prescribing oral medications in "drops" likewise can cause problems when accuracy of dose is important unless the patient understands that only the calibrated dropper provided by the manufacturer or pharmacist should be used to dispense the medication. Thus, one possible dosage for a pediatric iron product would be more accurately written "15 mg (0.6 mL) three times daily" instead of "one dropperful three times daily."

Abbreviations can cause dispensing errors. A prescription intending every-other-day dosing (qod) may be miswritten as "od" by the physician for "other-day dosing"; the pharmacist will interpret "od" as the abbreviation of the Latin for "right eye." Once-daily dosing at bedtime (qhs) may be misinterpreted as "qhr" for every hour. The use of slash marks (/) to separate names and doses

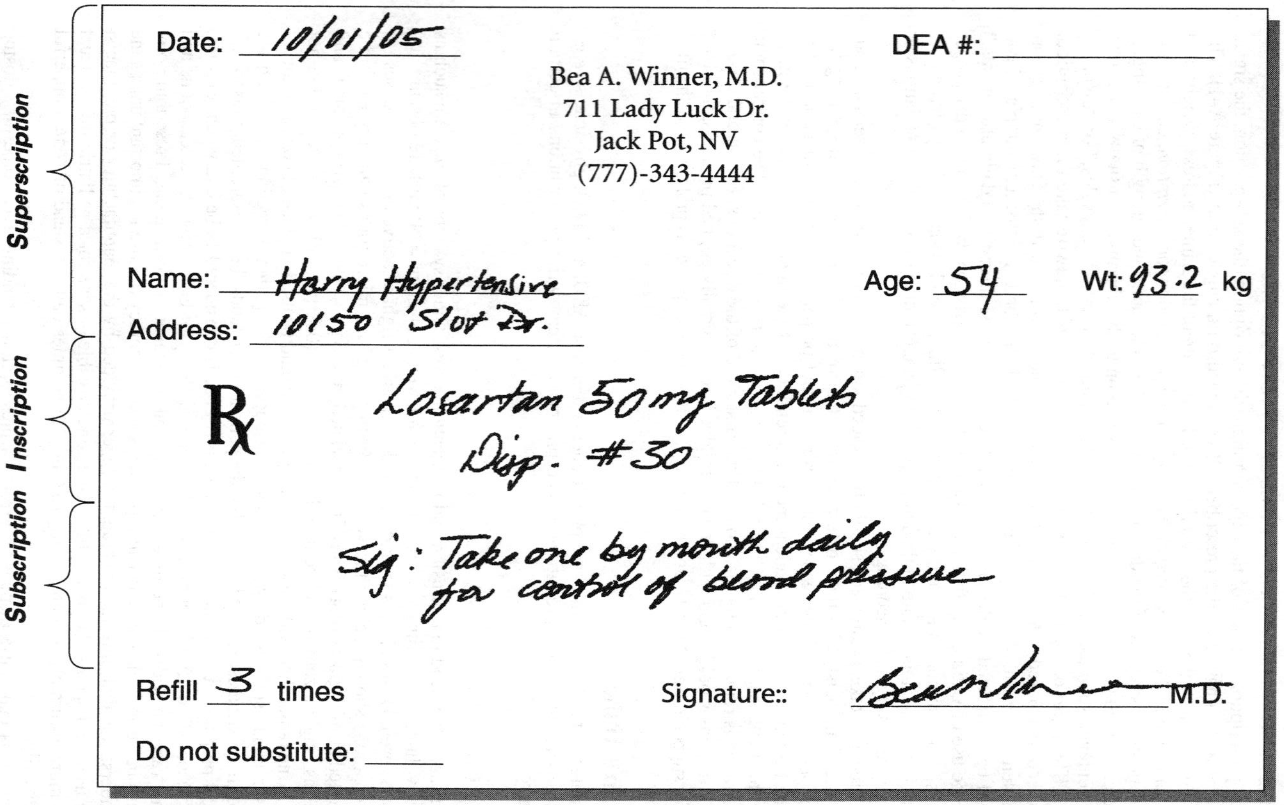

Date: _10/01/05_

Bea A. Winner, M.D.
711 Lady Luck Dr.
Jack Pot, NV
(777)-343-4444

DEA #: _____

Age: _54_ **Wt** _93.2_ kg

Name: _Harry Hypertensive_

Address: _10150 Slot Dr._

R _Losartan 50 mg Tablets_
        Disp. #30

      Sig: Take one by mouth daily
          for control of blood pressure

Signature:: _Bea Winner_ M.D.

Refill _3_ times

Do not substitute: _____

Superscription

Inscription | Subscription

FIGURE A-1 *The prescription.* The prescription must be carefully prepared to identify the patient and the medication to be dispensed, as well as the manner in which the drug is to be administered. Accuracy and legibility are essential. Use of abbreviations, particularly Latin, is discouraged, as it leads to dispensing errors. Inclusion of the purpose of the medication in the *subscription* (e.g., *"for control of blood pressure"*) can prevent errors in dispensing. For example, the use of losartan for the treatment of hypertension may require 100 mg/day (1.4 mg/kg per day), whereas treatment of congestive heart failure with this angiotensin II–receptor antagonist should not generally exceed 50 mg/day. Including the purpose of the prescription can also assist patients in organizing and understanding their medications. Including the patient's weight on the prescription can be useful in avoiding dosing errors, particularly when drugs are administered to children.

can result in the incorrect drug or dose being dispensed; the slash mark may be interpreted as a letter or number. When medications are measured in units or international units, the abbreviation "U" or "IU" must NOT be used; this can lead to errors such as misinterpretation of "U" as zero or four, or "IU" as 10 or 14. The word "unit" should be written as such. Drug products available in the U.S. that are dosed in units (*e.g., corticotropin*) or international units (*e.g.,* heparin) are "harmonized" by those responsible for drug standardization to avoid errors in dosing (*see* Drug Standards and Classification, below). *The critical message is that practitioners in the U.S. must write out the Rx fully in English if errors are to be avoided.*

Proper Patient Information

The patient's name and address are needed on the order to assure that the correct medication goes to the correct patient and also for identification and recordkeeping purposes. For medications whose dosage involves a calculation, pertinent factors such as the patient's weight, age, or body surface area also should be listed on the prescription.

Prescribers often commit errors in dosage calculations that can be prevented. When prescribing a drug whose dosage involves a calculation based on body weight or surface area, it is good practice to include both the calculated dose and the dosage formula used, such as "240 mg every 8 hours (40 mg/kg per day)" to allow another health care professional to double-check the prescribed dosage. Pharmacists always should recalculate dosage equations when filling these prescriptions. In hospitals and some clinic settings, medication orders for antibiotics or antiseizure medications that are sometimes difficult to adequately dose (*e.g., phenytoin*) can specify the patient diagnosis and desired drug and request dosing by the clinical pharmacist.

All prescriptions should be written in ink; this practice is compulsory for schedule II prescriptions under the Controlled Substances Act of 1970, as erasures on a prescription easily can lead to dispensing errors or diversion of controlled substances.

Prescription pad blanks normally are imprinted with a heading that gives the name of the physician and the address and phone number of the practice site (Figure A–1). When using institutional blanks that do not bear the physician's information, the physician always should print his or her name and phone number on the face of the prescription to clearly identify the prescriber and facilitate communication with other health care professionals if questions arise. U.S. law requires that prescriptions for controlled substances include the name, address, and Drug Enforcement Agency (DEA) registration number of the physician.

The date of the prescription is an important part of the patient's medical record, and it can assist the pharmacist in recognizing potential problems. Compliance behavior also can be estimated using the dates when a prescription is filled and refilled. The U.S. Controlled Substances Act requires that all orders for controlled substances (Table A–1) be dated and signed on the day issued and prohibits filling or refilling orders for schedule III or IV substances more than 6 months after their date of issuance. When writing the original prescription, the physician should designate the number of refills the patient may have. For maintenance medications without abuse potential, it is reasonable to write for a 1-month supply and to mark the prescription form for refills to be dispensed over a period sufficient to supply the patient until the next scheduled visit to the physician. A statement such as "refill prn" (refill as needed) is inappropriate, as it could allow the patient to misuse the medicine or neglect medical appointments. If no refills are desired, "zero" (rather than "0") should be written in the refill space to prevent alteration of the doctor's intent. Refills for controlled substances are discussed below.

Concern about the rising cost of health care has favored the dispensing of so-called "generic" drugs. A drug can be called by its generic name (in the U.S., this is the U.S. Adopted Name or USAN) or the manufacturer's proprietary name, called the trademark, trade name, or brand name. In most states in the U.S., pharmacists have the authority to dispense generic drugs rather than brand-name medications. The physician can request that the pharmacist not substitute a generic for a branded medication by indicating this on the prescription ("do not substitute"), although this is generally unnecessary since the FDA requires that generic medications meet the same bioequivalence standards as their brand-named counterparts. In some jurisdictions, prescriptions may not be filled with a generic substitution unless specifically permitted as stated on the prescription. Substituting generic medications is discouraged for drugs with specialized release systems and narrow therapeutic indices, or when substantial patient confusion and potential noncompliance may occur.

Table A–1

Controlled Substance Schedules

Schedule I (examples: heroin, methylene dioxymethamphetamine, lysergic acid diethylamide, mescaline, and all salts and isomers thereof):
1. High potential for abuse.
2. No accepted medical use in the U.S. or lacks accepted safety for use in treatment in the U.S. May be used for research purposes by properly registered individuals.

Schedule II (examples: morphine, oxycodone, fentanyl, meperidine, dextroamphetamine, cocaine, amobarbital):
1. High potential for abuse.
2. Has a currently accepted medical use in the U.S.
3. Abuse of substance may lead to severe psychological or physical dependence.

Schedule III (examples: anabolic steroids, nalorphine, ketamine, certain schedule II substances in suppositories, mixtures, or limited amounts per dosage unit):
1. Abuse potential less than substances in schedule I or schedule II.
2. Has a currently accepted medical use in the U.S.
3. Abuse of substance may lead to moderate or low physical dependence or high psychological dependence.

Schedule IV (examples: alprazolam, phenobarbital, meprobamate, modafinil):
1. Abuse potential less than substances in schedule III.
2. Has a currently accepted medical use in the U.S.
3. Abuse of substance may lead to limited physical or psychological dependence relative to substances in schedule III.

Schedule V (examples: buprenorphine, products containing a low dose of an opioid plus a non-narcotic ingredient such as codeine + guaifenesin cough syrup or diphenoxylate + atropine tablets):
1. Low potential for abuse relative to schedule IV.
2. Has a currently accepted medical use in the U.S.
3. Some schedule V products may be sold in limited amounts without a prescription at the discretion of the pharmacist; however, if a physician wishes a patient to receive one of these products, it is preferable to provide a prescription.

Choice of Drug Product

It cannot be assumed that a drug's therapeutic promise or popularity is proof of its overall efficacy or safety. Prescribers must rely on unbiased sources when seeking drug information (*see* Chapter 5).

Electronic Prescription Writing

Both government and healthcare businesses have called for the widespread use of electronic medical records by 2014 to help lower costs, reduce medical errors, improve quality of care, and provide better information for patients and providers. Electronic prescriptions are a central part of this strategy; while no national standard for either the technology or format of this record exists, electronic prescriptions are being used in many parts of the country. The advantages of electronic prescription writing include convenience for the prescriber (*e.g.,* use of hand-held devices permits prescribing at the time of therapeutic decision making); convenience for the patient, and electronic screening for appropriate drug choices, interactions with existing therapy, *etc.* The high probability that electronic prescription writing will reduce medication errors is, in and of itself, justification to make the change from current practice. Whatever the specific format of the electronic prescription, the essential features of writing the prescription described here are unchanged.

THE PRESCRIPTION AS A COMMODITY

Prescribers must be aware that patients may visit their doctor to "get a prescription." Indeed, in an era when the time spent between physician and patient is ever shorter, patients may view a trip to the doctor that does not result in a new prescription as a failed visit or a lost opportunity. Similarly, physicians may feel that they have fulfilled their role if the patient leaves with a prescription. Physicians must be careful to educate their patients about the importance of viewing medicines as only to be used when really needed and that remaining on a particular medicine when their condition is stable may be preferable to seeking the newest medications available.

PRESCRIPTION DRUG ADVERTISING

The benefits of direct-to-consumer (DTC) advertising of drugs, including internet advertising, are controversial. DTC advertising has alerted consumers to the existence of new drugs and the conditions they treat but has also increased consumer demand for drugs. This demand has increased the number of prescriptions being dispensed (raising sales revenues), which has led to higher pharmaceutical costs borne by health insurers, government, and consumers. In the face of a growing demand for particular brand name drugs driven by advertising, physicians and pharmacists must be able to counsel patients effectively and provide evidence-based drug information to their patients.

ERRORS IN DRUG ORDERS

The Institute of Medicine (IOM) estimates that between 44,000 and 98,000 deaths annually in the U.S. result from medical errors. While there is some debate about this estimate, it is clear that medication errors are common and result in significant adverse effects, including death. Databases of anonymously reported errors are maintained jointly by the Institute for Safe Medication Practices (ISMP), the U.S. Pharmacopeia Medication Errors Reporting Program (USP MERP), and the FDA's MedWatch program. Adverse drug events occur in ~3% of hospitalizations, and this number is larger for special populations such as those in pediatric and neonatal intensive care units.

By examining aspects of prescription writing that can cause errors and by modifying prescribing habits accordingly, the physician can improve the chance that the patient will receive the correct prescription, whether in a hospital or an outpatient setting. Vigilance for common problems that can occur with medication orders and improved communication among physicians, pharmacists, and other healthcare professionals can reduce medication errors. Areas of particular concern in the preparation of medication orders in both the institutional and outpatient settings are summarized below:

- All orders should be written using metric measurements of weight and volume.
- Arabic (decimal) numerals are preferable to Roman numerals; in some instances, it is preferable for numbers to be spelled out.
- Use leading zeros (0.125 mg, not .125 mg); never use trailing zeros (5 mg, not 5.0 mg).
- Avoid abbreviating drug names since this leads to numerous errors due to sound-alike names. For instance, NEUMEGA, an interleukin-11 product abbreviated IL-11, can be dispensed as PRO-LEUKIN, an interleukin-2 derivative, if Roman rather than Arabic numerals are used.
- Avoid abbreviating directions for drug administration; write directions out clearly in English.
- Some drug names sound alike when spoken and may look alike when spelled out. The USP MERP maintains a current list of drug names that can be confused (http://www.usp.org), including over 750 pairs of potentially confusing names that could lead to prescribing or dispensing errors harmful to patients. The alliterative drug names can be particularly problematic when giving verbal orders to pharmacists or other healthcare providers.
- The single most important measure to prevent dispensing errors based on sound-alike or look-alike drug names is for the physician to provide the patient's diagnosis on the prescription order. For instance, an order for administration of *magnesium sulfate* must not be abbreviated "MS," as this may result in administration of morphine sulfate. Including the therapeutic purpose and/or the patient's diagnosis can prevent this error.
- Poor handwriting is a well-known and preventable cause of dispensing errors. Both physician and pharmacist share in the responsibility to prevent adverse drug events by writing prescriptions clearly and questioning intent whenever an order is ambiguous or potentially ambiguous.

Controlled Substances

DEA regulates each step of the handling of controlled substances from manufacture to dispensing. State agencies may impose additional regulations such as requiring that prescriptions for controlled substances be printed on triplicate or state-issued prescription pads or restricting the use of a particular class of drugs for specific indications. The most stringent law always takes precedence, whether it is federal, state, or local. Substances that come under the jurisdiction of the Federal Controlled

Substances Act (CSA) are divided into five schedules (Table A–1); individual states may have additional schedules. Criminal offenses and penalties for misuse generally depend on the schedule of a substance as well as the amount of drug in question.

Physicians must be authorized to prescribe controlled substances by the jurisdiction in which they are licensed and they must be registered with the DEA or exempted from registration as defined under the CSA. The number on the certificate of registration must be indicated on all prescription orders for controlled substances.

PRESCRIPTION ORDERS FOR CONTROLLED SUBSTANCES

To be valid, a prescription for a controlled substance must be issued for a *legitimate medical purpose* by an *individual practitioner* acting in the *usual course of his or her professional practice*. An order that does not meet these criteria, such as a prescription issued as a means to obtain controlled substances for the doctor's office use or to maintain addicted individuals, is not considered a legitimate prescription and thus does not protect either the issuing physician or the dispensing pharmacist. Most states prohibit physicians from prescribing controlled substances for themselves; it is prudent to comply with this guideline even when not mandated by local law.

Execution of the Order

Prescriptions for controlled substances should be dated and signed on the day of their issuance and must bear the full name and address of the patient and the printed name, address, and DEA number of the practitioner; they should be signed as one would sign a legal document. Preprinted orders are not allowed in most states, and presigned blanks are prohibited by federal law. When oral orders are not permitted (schedule II), the prescription must be written with ink or typewritten. The order may be prepared by a member of the physician's staff, but the prescriber is responsible for the signature and any errors that the order may contain.

Oral Order

Prescriptions for schedule III, IV, and V medications may be telephoned to a pharmacy by a physician or by trusted staff in the same manner as a prescription for a noncontrolled substance, although it is in the physician's best interest to keep his or her DEA number as private as reasonably possible (*see* Preventing Diversion, below). Schedule II prescriptions may be telephoned to a pharmacy only in *emergency* situations. To be an emergency: (1) immediate administration is necessary; (2) no appropriate alternative treatment is available; and (3) it is not reasonably possible for the physician to provide a written prescription prior to the dispensing.

For an emergency prescription, the quantity must be limited to the amount adequate to treat the patient during the emergency period, and the physician must have a written prescription delivered to the pharmacy for that emergency within 72 hours. If mailed, the prescription must be postmarked within 72 hours. The pharmacist must notify the DEA if this prescription is not received.

Refills

No prescription order for a schedule II drug may be refilled under any circumstance. For schedule III and IV drugs, refills may be issued either orally or in writing, not to exceed five refills or 6 months after the issue date, whichever comes first. Beyond this time, a new prescription must be ordered. For schedule V drugs, there are no restrictions on the number of refills allowed, but if no refills are noted at the time of issuance, a new prescription must be made for additional drug to be dispensed.

Preventing Diversion

Prescription blanks often are stolen and used to sustain abuse of controlled substances and to divert legitimate drug products to the illicit market. To prevent such diversion, prescription pads should be protected in the same manner as one would protect a personal checkbook. A prescription blank should never be pre-signed for a staff member to fill in at a later time. Also, a minimum number of pads should be stocked, and they should be kept in a locked, secure location except when in use. If a pad or prescription is missing, it should be reported immediately to local authorities and pharmacies; some areas have systems in place to allow the rapid dissemination of such information.

Ideally, the physician's full DEA number should not be preprinted on the prescription pad; most prescriptions will not be for controlled substances and will not require the registration number, and anyone in possession of a valid DEA number may find it easier to commit prescription fraud. Some physicians may intentionally omit part or all of their DEA number on a prescription and instead write "pharmacist call to verify" or "call for registration number." This practice works only when the pharmacist may independently verify the authenticity of the prescription, and patients must be advised to fill the prescription during the prescriber's office hours. Pharmacists can ascertain the likely authenticity of a physician's DEA number using an algorithm.

Another method employed by the drug-seeker is to alter the face of a valid prescription to increase the number of units or refills. By spelling out the number of units and refills authorized instead of giving numerals, the prescriber essentially removes this option for diversion. Controlled substances should not be prescribed excessively or for prolonged periods, as the continuance of a patient's addiction is not a legitimate medical purpose.

DRUG STANDARDS AND CLASSIFICATION

The U.S. Pharmacopeial Convention, Inc. is a nongovernmental organization that promotes the public health and benefits practitioners and patients by disseminating authoritative standards and information on medicines and other health care technologies. This organization is home to the U.S. Pharmacopeia (USP), which together with the FDA, the pharmaceutical industry, and health professions, establishes authoritative drug standards. Drug monographs are published in the USP/National Formulary (USP-NF), the official drug standards compendium that organizes drugs into categories based on pharmacological actions and therapeutic uses.

The USP is also home to the USAN (The USP Dictionary of *U.S. Adopted Names* and International Drug Names). This compendium is recognized throughout the healthcare industry as the authoritative dictionary of drugs. The USP maintains an electronic Web site that can be accessed for useful drug naming, classification, and standards information (http://www.usp.org).

In the U.S., drug products are also coded under the National Drug Code. Each drug product listed under the Federal Food, Drug, and Cosmetic Act is assigned a unique 10-digit, 3-segment number. This number, known as the National Drug Code (NDC) number, identifies the labeler/vendor, product, and package size. The labeler code is assigned by the FDA. The second segment, the product code, identifies a specific strength, dosage form, and formulation for a particular drug company. The third segment, the package code, identifies package sizes. Both the product and package codes are assigned by the manufacturer.

Drugs are also grouped by their potential for misuse under British and United Nations legal classifications as class A, B, or C. The classes are linked to maximum legal penalties in a descending order of severity, from A to C. A separate FDA classification scheme is used to rate the risk to the fetus of drugs taken during pregnancy in five categories from Category A (safest) through Categories B, C, D, and Category X (contraindicated in pregnancy). The possible risk increases in categories B, C, and D. In Category D, for example, there is positive evidence of human fetal risk, but the benefits from use in pregnant women may be acceptable despite the risk (*e.g.,* if the drug is needed in a life-threatening situation or for a serious disease for which safer drugs cannot be used or are ineffective).

COMPLIANCE

Compliance may be defined as the extent to which the patient follows a prescribed regimen. The assumption that the patient follows directions on the prescription is unrealistic. The patient is the final and most important determinant of how successful a therapeutic regimen will be and should be engaged as an active participant with a vested interest in its success. The prescriber must promote a collaborative interaction with the patient in which each helps to determine the course of therapy. The patient's quality-of-life beliefs may differ from the clinician's therapeutic goals, and the patient will have the last word when there is an unresolved conflict. Suggestions for improving patient compliance are listed in Table A–2.

Even the most carefully prepared prescription for the ideal therapy will be useless if the patient's level of compliance is inadequate. Noncompliance, thought to occur 50% of the time, may be manifest in drug therapy as intentional or accidental errors in dosage or schedule, overuse, underuse, early termination of therapy, or not having a prescription filled. Noncompliance always should be considered in evaluating therapeutic failures.

Table A–2

Suggestions for Improving Patient Compliance

Provide respectful communication; ask patient how he takes medicine.
Develop satisfactory, collaborative relationship between doctor and patient; encourage pharmacist involvement.
Provide and encourage use of medication counseling.
Give precise, clear instructions, with most important information given first.
Support oral instructions with easy-to-read written information.
Simplify whenever possible.
Use mechanical compliance aids as needed (sectioned pill boxes or trays, compliance packaging, color-coding).
Use optimal dosage form and schedule for the individual patient.
Assess patient's literacy and comprehension and modify educational counseling as needed. Don't rely on patient knowledge about his or her disease, alone, to improve compliance.
Find solutions when physical or sensory disabilities are present (use nonsafety caps on bottles, use large type on labels and written material, place tape marks on syringes).
Enlist support and assistance from family or caregivers.
Use behavioral techniques such as goal setting, self-monitoring, cognitive restructuring, skills training, contracts, and positive reinforcement.

THE PATIENT–PROVIDER RELATIONSHIP

Patient satisfaction with the physician has a significant impact on compliance behavior and is one of the few factors that the physician can directly influence. When deciding upon a course of therapy, it can be useful to discuss a patient's habits and daily routine as well as the therapeutic options with the patient. This information can help suggest cues for remembrance, such as storing a once-daily medicine atop the books on the bedside table for a patient who reads nightly, or in the cabinet with the coffee cups if it is to be taken in the morning (noting that the bathroom can be the worst place to store a medication in terms of its physical and chemical preservation). The information also can help tailor the regimen to the patient's lifestyle. A lack of information about a patient's lifestyle can lead to situations such as prescribing a medication to be taken with meals three times daily for a patient who only eats twice a day or who works a night shift and sleeps during the day. Rarely is there only one treatment option for a given problem, and it may be better to prescribe an adequate regimen that the patient will follow instead of an ideal regimen that the patient will not. Involving patients in the control of any appropriate aspects of their therapy may improve compliance, by aiding memory, making the dosage form or schedule more agreeable or convenient, giving patients a feeling of empowerment, and emphasizing their responsibility for the treatment outcome.

Behavioral models suggest that patients are more likely to be compliant when they *perceive* that they are susceptible to the disease, that the disease may have serious negative impact, that the therapy will be effective, that the benefits outweigh the costs, and when they believe in their own efficacy to execute the therapy. Education of the patient about his or her condition alone will not improve compliance.

Pharmacists have a legal and professional responsibility to offer medication counseling in many situations—even though practice environments are not always conducive to its provision—and can educate and support patients by discussing prescribed medications and their use. Because they often see the patient more frequently than does the physician, pharmacists who take the time to inquire about a patient's therapy can help identify compliance and other problems and notify the physician as appropriate.

Elderly patients often face a number of barriers to compliance related to their age. Such barriers include increased forgetfulness and confusion; altered drug disposition and higher sensitivity to some drug effects; decreased social and financial support; decreased dexterity, mobility, or sensory abilities; and an increased number of concurrent medicines used (both prescription and over-the-counter), whose attendant toxicities and interactions may cause decreased mental alertness or intolerable side effects.

Credits

FIGURE 4-1 Reproduced from Vesell ES: Genetic and environmental factors causing variation in drug response. *Mutat Res* 247:241–257, 1991. Copyright 1991 with permission from Elsevier.

FIGURE 4-6 Reproduced, with permission, from Murphy GM Jr *et al.*: Pharmacogenomics of antidepressant medication intolerance. *Am J Psychiatry* 160:1830–1835, 2003. Copyright 2003 American Psychiatric Association.

FIGURE 4-7 Reproduced from Herrington DM *et al.*: Estrogen-receptor polymorphisms and effects of estrogen replacement on high-density lipoprotein cholesterol in women with coronary disease. *N Engl J Med.* 346:967–974, 2002. Copyright 2002 Massachusetts Medical Society. All rights reserved.

FIGURE 10-2 Modified from Allwood MJ *et al.*: Peripheral vascular effects of noradrenaline, isopropylnoradrenaline, and dopamine. *Br Med Bull* 19:132–136, 1963. By permission of Oxford University Press.

FIGURE 10-4 Reproduced from Toda N: Vasodilating β-adrenoceptor blockers as cardiovascular therapeutics. *Pharmacol Ther* 100:215–234, 2003. Copyright 2003 with permission from Elsevier.

FIGURE 13-2 Reproduced from Reves JG *et al.*: Intravenous nonopioid anesthetics. In: *Anesthesia*, 6th ed. RD Miller (ed). Philadelphia, Elsevier, 2005. Copyright 2005 with permission from Elsevier.

FIGURE 13-4 Reproduced from Eger EI II: Uptake and distribution. In: *Anesthesia*, 6th ed. RD Miller (ed). Philadelphia, Elsevier, 2005. Copyright 2005 with permission from Elsevier.

FIGURE 14-2 Adapted from Catterall WA: From ionic currents to molecular mechanisms: the structure and function of voltage-gated sodium channels. *Neuron* 26:13–25, 2000. Copyright with permission from Elsevier.

TABLE 14-1 Adapted, with permission, from Carpenter RL, Mackey DC: Local anesthetics. In: *Clinical Anesthesia*, 3rd ed. PG Barash *et al.* (eds). Philadelphia, Lippincott Williams & Wilkins, 1997.

FIGURE 20-2 Adapted, with permission, from Cooper JR, Bloom FE, Roth RH: *The Biochemical Basis of Neuropharmacology*, 7th ed. Oxford University Press, 1996.

TABLE 21-5 Modified from Agency for Health Care Policy and Research. *Acute Pain Management in Infants, Children, and Adolescents: Operative and Medical Procedures.* No. 92-0020. U.S. Dept. of Health and Human Services, Rockville, MD, 1992.

FIGURE 23-2A Reprinted by permission of Macmillan Publishers Ltd: Benowitz NL *et al.*: Nicotine absorption and cardiovascular effects with smokeless tobacco use: comparison with cigarettes and nicotine gum. *Clin Pharmacol* 44:23–28, 1988. Copyright 1988.

FIGURE 23-2B Reproduced from Srivastava ED *et al.*: Sensitivity and tolerance to nicotine in smokers and nonsmokers. *Psychopharmacology* 105:63–68, 1991. With kind permission from Springer Science and Business Media.

TABLE 23-2 Reproduced from Anthony JC *et al.*: Comparative epidemiology of dependence on tobacco, alcohol, controlled substances and inhalants: basic findings from the national comorbidity survey. *Exp Clin Psychopharmacol* 2:244–268, 1994.

FIGURE 30-5 Modified from Jackson EK *et al.*: Physiological functions of the renal prostaglandin, renin, and kallikrein systems. In: *The Kidney: Physiology and Pathophysiology.* DW Seldin and G Giebisch (eds). New York, Raven, 1985.

FIGURE 35-2 Adapted, with permission, from Thompson GR, Barter PJ: Clinical lipidology at the end of the millennium. *Curr Opin Lipidol* 10:521–526, 1999.

FIGURE 36-4 Adapted from Wolfe MM, Sachs G: Acid suppression: optimizing therapy for gastroesophageal ulcer healing, gastroesopageal reflux disease, and stress-related syndrome. *Gastroenterology.* 118:S9–S31, 2000. Copyright 2000 with permission from Elsevier.

FIGURE 37-1 Reprinted, with permission, from Kunze WA, Furness JB: The enteric nervous system and regulation of intestinal motility. *Annu Rev Physiol* 61:117–142, 1999. Copyright 1999 by Annual Reviews www. annualreviews.org

TABLE 37-2 Modified, with permission, from Kreck MJ: Constipation syndromes. In: *A Pharmacologic Approach to Gastrointestinal Disorders.* JH Lewis (ed). Philadelphia, Lippincott Williams & Wilkins, 1994.

TABLE 37-7 Adapted, with permission, from Grunberg SM, Hesketh PJ: Control of chemotherapy-induced emesis. *N Eng J Med* 329:1790–1796, 1993. Copyright 1993 Massachusetts Medical Society. All rights reserved.

TABLE 38-1 Reproduced from Sands BE: Therapy of inflammatory bowel disease. *Gastroenterology* 118:S68–S82, 2000. Copyright 2000 with permission from Elsevier.

FIGURE 42-1 Courtesy of Hiroshi Nikaido

FIGURE 43-3 From Cozzarelli NR: DNA gyrase and the supercoiling of DNA. *Science* 207:953–960, 1980. Reprinted with permission from AAAS.

FIGURE 44-3 Fig. 4.11, p. 83 from MICROBIOLOGY: An Introduction, 3rd ed. by Gerard J. Tortora, Berdell R. Funke and Christine L. Case. Copyright 1989, 1986, 1982 by The Benjamin/Cummings Publishing Company, Inc. Reprinted by permission of Pearson Education, Inc.

FIGURE 45-1 From Moellering RC: Microbiological considerations in the use of tobramycin and related aminoglycosidic aminocyclitol antibiotics. *MJA* 1977; 2S: 4–8. Copyright 1977. The Medical Journal of Australia – reproduced with permission.

FIGURE 49-3 Modified, with permission, from Baron S *et al.*: Introduction to the interferon system. In: *Interferons: Principles and Medical Applications.* S Baron *et al.* (eds). Galveston, University of Texas, 1992.

FIGURE 49-2 Adapted from Elion GB: Mechanism of action and selectivity of acyclovir. *Am J Med* 73:7–13, 1982. Copyright 1982 with permission from Elsevier.

FIGURE 52-1 Reproduced, with permission, from Clayberger C, Krensky AM: Mechanisms of allograft refection. In: *Immunologic Renal Diseases*, 2nd ed. EG Neilson, WG Couser (eds). Philadelphia, Lippincott Williams & Wilkins, 2001.

FIGURE 52-2 Reproduced, with permission, from Krensky AM, Clayberger C: Transplantation immunobiology. In: *Pediatric Nephrology*, 5th ed. ED Avner *et al.* (eds). Philadelphia, Lippincott Williams & Wilkins, 2004.

FIGURE 53-4 Reproduced from Monsen ER *et al.*: Estimation of available dietary iron. *Amer J Clin Nutr* 31:134–141, 1978. With permission from the American Society for Nutrition.

FIGURE 53-5 From Hillman RS, Finch CA: *Red Cell Manual*, 7th ed. Philadelphia. FA Davis, 1996, p 72, with permission.

TABLE 53-2 From Council on Foods and Nutrition: Iron deficiency in the United States. *JAMA* 203:407–412, 1968. Copyright 1968 American Medical Association. All rights reserved.

FIGURE 56-2 Adapted, with permission, from Taurog A: Hormone synthesis: thyroid iodine metabolism. In: *Werner and Ingbar's The Thyroid*, 7ᵗʰ ed. LE Braverman, RD Utiger (eds). Philadelphia, Lippincott Williams & Wilkins, 1996.

FIGURE 57-3A Reproduced from Thorneycroft IH *et al.*: The relation of serum 17-hydroxyprogesterone and estradiol-17β levels during the human menstrual cycle. *Am J Obstet Gynecol* 111:947–951, 1971. Copyright 1971 with permission from Elsevier.

FIGURE 61-2 Adapted, with permission, from Yanagawa N, Lee DBN: Renal handling of calcium and phosphorus. In: *Disorders of Bone and Mineral Metabolism.* FL Coe, MJ Favus (eds). Philadelphia, Lippincott Williams & Wilkins, 1992.

FIGURE 63-3 Modified from Chien DS *et al.*: Corneal and conjuctival/scleral penetration of *p*-aminoclonidine, AGN 190342, and clonidine in rabbit eyes. *Curr Eye Res* 9:1051–1059, 1990. Copyright 1990 by Informa Healthcare – Journals. Reproduced with permission of Informa Healthcare via Copyright Clearance Center.

FIGURE 63-4B Adapted with permission from Riordan-Eva P, Tabbara KF: Anatomy and embryology of the eye. In: *General Ophthalmology*, 13th ed. D Vaughan, T Asbury, P Riordan-Eva (eds). Appleton & Lange, Stamford, CT, 1992.

TABLE 64-1 and TABLE 64-2 Reproduced from Watson WA *et al.*: 2003 annual report of the American Association of Poison Control Centers Toxic Exposure Surveillance System. *Am J Emerg Med* 22:335–404, 2004. Copyright 2004 with permission from Elsevier.

INDEX

Page numbers followed by *f* refer to illustrations; page numbers followed by *t* refer to tables.

A

Abacavir (ABC), 839*t*, 841*f*, 842*t*, 843*f*, 845
Abarelix, 907, 975*t*, 976
ABCD (amphotericin B), 798
Abciximab, 963
ABC transporters. *See* ATP-binding cassette (ABC) transporters
ABILIFY (aripiprazole), 308*t*
ABLC (amphotericin B), 798
Abortifacients, 423, 871
ABREVA (docosanol), 1085
Absence seizures, 320*t*, 322
pharmacotherapy, 328, 334
Absorption, 1–4, 2*f*, 10–11. *See also specific agents*
Abuse, substance, 385. *See also* Dependence; *specific agents*
Acamprosate, 384, 390
Acanthamoeba, 1102
ACARBOSE, 1055
ACCOLATE (zafirlukast), 467
ACCUPRIL (quinapril), 521
ACCUTANE (isotretinoin), 1079
ACE. *See* Angiotensin-converting enzyme
Acebutolol, 175*t*, 179
ACE inhibitors. *See* Angiotensin-converting enzyme (ACE) inhibitors
Acenocoumarol, 956*f*, 959
ACEON (perindopril), 521–522
Acetaminophen (paracetamol), 430*t*, 445–446, 1116*f*
toxicity of/poisoning with, 446, 1123–1124
Acetazolamide, 477, 479*f*, 480–481, 480*t*, 1106
Acetic acid derivatives, 430*t*, 446–449. *See also specific agents*
Acetohexamide, 1051, 1051*t*
Acetylation. *See* N-acetylation
Acetylcholine (ACh), 96–97, 114–118, 116*t*, 117, 1104*t*, 1107
as neurotransmitter, 210*t*, 215
receptors. *See* Muscarinic receptor(s); Nicotinic acetylcholine receptor(s)
vasopressin secretion and, 501

Acetylcholinesterase (AChE)
in cholinergic transmission, 97–98
inhibition. *See* Anticholinesterase agents
Acetylsalicylic acid. *See* Aspirin
Acid–base balance, salicylates and, 441, 444
Acid-peptic disease. *See* Gastroesophageal reflux disease; Peptic ulcer disease
ACIPHEX (rabeprazole), 621
Acitretin, 1080
Acne rosacea, therapy for, 1079, 1088
Acne vulgaris, therapy for, 1011, 1078, 1079, 1083
Acrivastine, 409*t*
Acromegaly, 971, 972
ACTH. *See* Adrenocorticotropic hormone
ACTHREL (corticorelin), 1026
ACTICIN (permethrin), 1085
ACTIGALL (ursodeoxycholic acid), 652
ACTIMMUNE (IFN-γ-1b), 921
ACTINEX (masoprocol), 1094
Actinic cheilitis, 5-fluorouracil for, 1087
Actinic dermatitis, azathioprine for, 1087
Actinic keratosis
therapy for, 1082, 1087, 1088, 1094
Actinomycin D. *See* Dactinomycin
Actinomycosis, treatment for, 736, 765
Action potentials, cardiac, 578, 581*f*, 582
ACTIVASE (alteplase), 960
Activated charcoal, for poisoning, 445, 1122–1123
Activated partial thromboplastin time (aPTT), 949
ACTIVELLA (estradiol/norethindrone), 1001
Active transport, 29
ACTONEL (risedronate), 1071
ACTOS (pioglitazone), 1054
ACULAR (ketorolac), 1107
Acute coronary syndrome, 531–532

drug-eluting endovascular stents for, 543
heparin therapy in, 532, 953
Acute lymphocytic leukemia (ALL)
therapy for, 872, 877, 890, 892
Acute myelogenous leukemia (AML)
chlorambucil and, 863
cisplatin and, 868
etoposide and, 890
mercaptopurine and, 879
pharmacogenetics, 68
therapy for, 877, 879, 887, 888, 889, 900, 904
Acute myocardial infarction. *See* Myocardial infarction
Acute promyelocytic leukemia (APL), tretinoin for, 894
Acute radiation syndrome, 1140
Acute tubular necrosis, mannitol for, 482
Acyclovir, 813, 815–819, 815*t*, 816*f*
for herpes simplex virus infections, 817–818, 1084
interactions
with ganciclovir, 824
with mycophenolate mofetil, 916
for varicella-zoster virus infections, 818, 1084, 1101, 1101*t*
ADALAT (nifedipine), 535*t*
Adalimumab, 920
Adapalene, 1078
ADAPIN (doxepin), 279*t*
ADBR1, ADBR2, 66*t*
ADDERAL XR (amphetamine), 169
Addiction, 385. *See also* Dependence; *specific agents*
Addison's disease, 1032
Adducin, 66*t*
Adefovir dipivoxil, 815*t*, 829–830
ADENOCARD (adenosine), 592
Adenosine, 587, 587*t*, 592, 593*t*
receptors, 212*t*
as neurotransmitter, 217–218
Adenovirus infection
cidofovir for, 820
ribavirin for, 836
ADH (antidiuretic hormone). *See* Vasopressin

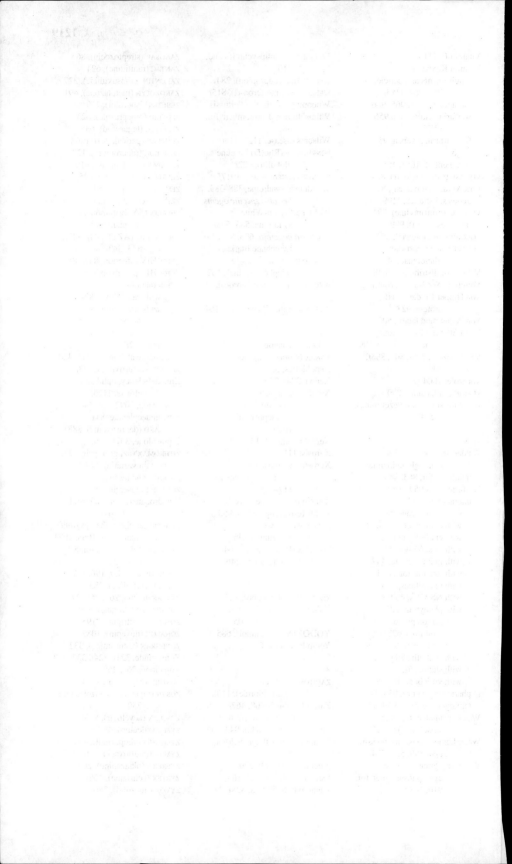